W. B. SAUNDERS COMPANY
Harcourt Brace Jovanovich, Inc.

The Curtis Center
Independence Square West
Philadelphia, PA 19106

Library of Congress Cataloging-in-Publication Data

Clinical management of poisoning and drug overdose / [edited by] Lester M. Haddad, James F. Winchester.—2nd ed.

p. cm.

Includes bibliographical references.

ISBN 0–7216–2342–5

1. Poisoning. 2. Medical abuse. 3. Toxicology. 4. Drugs-Overdosage. I. Haddad, Lester M. II. Winchester, James F. [DNLM: 1. Poisoning—therapy. QV 600 C639]

RA1211.C584 1983

615.9′08—dc20

DNLM/DLC 89–10799

esigner: W. B. Saunders Staff
oduction Manager: Ken Neimeister
nuscript Editor: Wynette Kommer
stration Coordinator: Peg Shaw
exer: Ellen Murray
r Designer: Ellen Bodner

al Management of Poisoning and Drug Overdose, Second Edition ISBN 0–7216–2342–5

n the United States of America

is the print number: 9 8 7 6 5 4 3 2

Clinical Management of

POISONING AND DRUG OVERDOSE

Second Edition

LESTER M. HADDAD, M.D., FACEP
Director, Emergency Department
Beaufort Memorial Hospital
Beaufort, South Carolina
Attending Physician
Emergency Medicine Residency Program
Richland Memorial Hospital/USC School of Medicine
Consultant and Adjunct Professor
USC Palmetto State Poison Center
Columbia, South Carolina

JAMES F. WINCHESTER, M.D., FRCP
Professor of Medicine and Acting Director
Division of Nephrology
Department of Medicine
Consultant, National Capital Poison Center
Georgetown University Medical Center
Washington, D.C.

1990
W.B. SAUNDERS COMPANY
Harcourt Brace Jovanovich, Inc.
Philadelphia ■ London ■ Montreal ■ Toronto ■ Sydne

TO OUR LOVING PARENTS,

Sara Mary Marshall Haddad
and in memory of Lester M. Haddad, Sr.

Alexander G. Clegg Winchester
and in memory of Elizabeth Mary McKillop Winchester

CONTRIBUTORS

John Adriani, M.D. *(deceased)*
Late Professor of Pharmacology, Anesthesiology, and Clinical Surgery, Louisiana State School of Medicine; Late Director Emeritus, Department of Anesthesiology, Charity Hospital, New Orleans, Louisiana
General Anesthetics

John J. Ambre, M.D., Ph.D.
Associate Professor, Department of Medicine, Northwestern University Medical School; Attending Physician, Northwestern Memorial Hospital, Chicago, Illinois
Principles of Pharmacology for the Clinician

Kathryn D. Anderson, M.D.
Professor of Surgery and Pediatrics, George Washington University; Senior Attending Surgeon, Children's National Medical Center, Washington, D.C.
Alkali Injury and Esophageal Burns

John S. Andrews, Jr., M.D.
Assistant Director for Science, Agency for Toxic Substances and Disease Registry, Centers for Disease Control, Atlanta, Georgia
Environmental Toxicology: Polychlorinated Dibenzo-P-Dioxins

Jay M. Arena, M.D.
Professor (Emeritus) of Pediatrics and Director (Emeritus), Poison Control Center, Duke University School of Medicine and Medical Center, Durham, North Carolina
Phosphorus

Regine Aronow, M.D.
Associate Professor, Department of Pediatrics, Wayne State University School of Medicine; Director, Poison Control Center, Children's Hospital of Michigan, Detroit, Michigan
Mercury; Bromides and Bromates; Iodine

W. Lynn Augenstein, M.D.
Assistant Professor, Division of Emergency Medicine, University Medical Center, Jacksonville, Florida
Acetaminophen

Lydia L. Baltarowich, M.D.
Senior Staff Physician, Department of Emergency Medicine, Henry Ford Hospital, Detroit, Michigan
Bromides and Bromates

Patrice A. Barish, M.D.
Clinical Instructor, Department of Surgery, University of Michigan, Ann Arbor, Michigan; Attending Staff, Department of Emergency Medicine, William Beaumont Hospital, Royal Oak, Michigan
Designer Drugs

Robert R. Bass, M.D., FACEP
Assistant Professor of Emergency Medicine, Eastern Virginia Graduate School of Medicine; Director, Emergency Department, Obici Hospital, Suffolk, Virginia
The Antipsychotic Drugs

Charles E. Becker, M.D.
Professor of Medicine, University of California, San Francisco; Head, Division of Occupational Medicine and Toxicology, San Francisco General Hospital; Director, Northern California Occupational Health Center, San Francisco, California
Toxicology of Dependency: The Alcoholic Patient

Neal L. Benowitz, M.D.
Professor of Medicine and Chief, Division of Clinical Pharmacology and Experimental Therapeutics, University of California, San Francisco; Attending Physician, Department of Medicine, San Francisco General Hospital Medical Center; Medical Advisor, San Francisco Bay Area Poison Center, San Francisco, California
Cardiac Disturbances; Beta-Adrenoceptor Blocker Poisoning; Calcium Entry Blocker Poisoning; Quinidine, Procainamide, and Disopyramide; Lidocaine, Mexiletine, and Tocainide

Jeffrey L. Blumer, Ph.D., M.D.
Professor of Pediatrics, University of Virginia; Chief, Division of Pediatric Pharmacology and Critical Care, University of Virginia Hospital, Charlottesville, Virginia
Developmental Toxicology; Drug-Drug Interactions; Antimicrobial Agents

John C. Bradford, D.O., FACEP
Assistant Professor of Emergency Medicine, Northeastern Ohio Universities College of Medicine, Rootstown; Program Director, Department of Emergency Medicine, Akron General Medical Center, Akron, Ohio
Methyl Bromide and Related Compounds

Joseph M. Brandwein, M.D., FRCPC
Leukemia Research Fund Fellow, Division of Hematology-Oncology, Department of Medicine, Toronto General Hospital, Toronto, Ontario, Canada
Hematologic Consequences of Poisoning

Terry Branson, M.D., FACEP
Private Practice, North Park Hospital, Hixson, Tennessee
Anthelminthics

Jeffrey Brent, M.D., Ph.D.
Assistant Professor of Pediatrics and Surgery, University of Colorado Health Sciences Center; Assistant Medical Director, Rocky Mountain Poison Center; Attending Physician, Department of Medicine, Division of Clinical Toxicology, Denver General Hospital, Denver, Colorado
Mushrooms

Clyde M. Burnett
Director of Toxicology, Clairol, Inc., Research Division, Stamford, Connecticut
Cosmetics and Toilet Articles

Peter A. Campochiaro, M.D.
Associate Professor of Ophthalmology, University of Virginia School of Medicine, Charlottesville, Virginia
Chemical and Drug Injury to the Eye

Louis A. Cannon, M.D.
Clinical Research Fellow, Department of Cardiovascular Diseases; Instructor, Department of Emergency/Trauma Medicine, University of Cincinnati and University Hospital; Research Review Board, University Hospital, Cincinnati, Ohio
Benzene and the Aromatic Hydrocarbons; Ammonia, Nitrogen, Nitrous Oxides, and Related Compounds

Thomas R. Caraccio, Pharm.D.
Visiting Assistant Professor of Pharmacology and Toxicology, New York College of Osteopathic Medicine, Old Westbury; Adjunct Assistant Professor of Clinical Pharmacy, St. John's University College of Pharmacy, Jamaica; Clinical Coordinator, Long Island Regional Poison Control Center, and Clinical Pharmacist, Nassau County Medical Center, East Meadow, New York
Sodium and Sodium Chloride; Fluorine and Fluoride

Stanley L. Cohan, M.D., Ph.D.
Associate Professor, Department of Neurology, Georgetown University School of Medicine; Attending Neurologist, Georgetown University Hospital, Washington, D.C.
Central Nervous System Disturbances and Brain Death

Dale G. Deutsch, Ph.D.
Associate Professor, Department of Biochemistry, State University of New York at Stony Brook, Stony Brook, New York
Laboratory Diagnosis and Drug Testing

J. Ward Donovan, M.D., FACEP
Assistant Professor of Medicine, Emergency Medicine Division, The Pennsylvania State University School of Medicine; Medical Director, Capital Area Poison Center, The Milton S. Hershey Medical Center, Hershey, Pennsylvania
Nitrates, Nitrites, and Other Sources of Methemoglobinemia

James M. Dougherty, M.D., FACEP
Assistant Professor of Emergency Medicine, Northeastern Ohio Universities School of Medicine, Rootstown; Research Director and Senior Staff Physician, Department of Emergency Medicine, Akron General Medical Center, Akron, Ohio
Freon and Other Inhalants

Constance J. Doyle, M.D., FACEP
Clinical Instructor, Department of Surgery, Section of Emergency Services, University of Michigan School of Medicine; Emergency Physician, University of Michigan Hospitals, Ann Arbor, and Foote Memorial Hospital, Jackson, Michigan
Disaster Management of Massive Toxic Exposure

David N. Dunbar, M.D.
Assistant Professor of Medicine, University of Minnesota; Department of Medicine, Division of Cardiology, Hennepin County Medical Center, Minneapolis, Minnesota
New Cardiac Antiarrhythmic Agents

Philip A. Edelman, M.D.
Assistant Clinical Professor, Departments of Medicine, Pathology, and Occupational Medicine, University of California, Irvine; Chief, Toxicology Service and Regional Poison Center, University of California, Irvine, Medical Center, Irvine, California
Industrial Toxicology: The Microelectronics Industry

Sally M. Ehlers, M.D.
Assistant Professor of Medicine, University of Minnesota Medical School; Director of Dialysis and Acting Chief of Nephrology, Department of Medicine, St. Paul–Ramsey Medical Center, St. Paul, Minnesota
Theophylline

Mark A. Eilers, M.D., FACEP
Assistant Professor, Department of Emergency Medicine, and Education Coordinator, Wright State University School of Medicine; Active Staff, Kettering Medical Center and Good Samaritan Hospital; Academic Staff, Miami Valley Hospital; Courtesy Staff, St. Elizabeth's Medical Center, Dayton, Ohio
Smoke Inhalation

Teddi F. Eisen, M.D.
Clinical Fellow, Pediatrics, Harvard Medical School; Fellow, Division of Clinical Pharmacology and Toxicology, The Children's Hospital, Boston, Massachusetts
Iron

Michael E. Ervin, M.D.
Associate Clinical Professor, Wright State University School of Medicine; Director, Emergency and Trauma Center, Miami Valley Hospital, Dayton, Ohio
Petroleum Distillates and Turpentine

Richard Feldman, M.D., FACEP
Assistant Professor of Clinical Emergency Medicine, Department of Surgery, University of Illinois College of Medicine at Chicago; Chairman, Department of Emergency Medicine, Illinois Masonic Medical Center, Chicago, Illinois
The Volatile Oils

Jerry A. Fogle, M.D.
Assistant Clinical Professor, University of Virginia, Charlottesville, Virginia, and West Virginia University, Morgantown, West Virginia; Staff Ophthalmologist, City Hospital Inc., Martinsburg, West Virginia
Chemical and Drug Injury to the Eye

Susanne Freeman, M.D.
Lecturer, St. Vincent's Hospital, University of New South Wales; Visiting Dermatologist at St. Vincent's Hospital; Head, Contact and Occupational Dermatitis Clinic, Skin and Cancer Foundation, Sydney, New South Wales, Australia
Dermatologic Toxicity

Lorne K. Garrettson, M.D.
Associate Professor of Pediatrics, Emory University School of Medicine; Director, Georgia Poison Control Center; Attending Physician, Grady Memorial Hospital and Henrietta Egleston Hospital for Children, Atlanta, Georgia
Lead

Shawn Gazaleh, M.D., FACEP
Clinical Instructor, Medicine, University of Tennessee College of Medicine, Chattanooga Unit, Chattanooga, Tennessee; Medical Director, Emergency Care Department, Hamilton Medical Center, Dalton, Georgia
Anthelminthics; Cyanoacrylate (Super Glue)

Johanna Goldfarb, M.D.
Assistant Professor of Pediatrics, Department of Pediatrics, Case Western Reserve University School of Medicine; Attending Pediatrician, Division of Pediatric Infectious Diseases, Rainbow Babies and Childrens Hospital, Cleveland, Ohio
Antimicrobial Agents

Nora Goldschlager, M.D.
Professor of Clinical Medicine, University of California, San Francisco; Director, Coronary Care Unit, and Director, Electrocardiographic Laboratory, San Francisco General Hospital, San Francisco, California
Cardiac Disturbances

Lloyd S. Goodman, M.D., FACC
Associate Clinical Professor, Department of Medicine, School of Medicine, Medical College of Georgia; Associate Professor of Internal Medicine, School of Medicine, Mercer University; Medical Director, Department of Cardiology, Memorial Medical Center, Savannah, Georgia
Digitalis

Richard E. Gradisek, M.D., FACEP
Assistant Professor of Emergency Medicine, Northeastern Ohio Universities College of Medicine, Rootstown; Senior Staff Physician, Department of Emergency Medicine, Akron General Medical Center, Akron, Ohio
Freon and Other Inhalants

David R. Graham, M.D.
Senior Registrar, Mersey Regional Health Authority and Fazakeney Hospital, Liverpool, England
Tear Gas and Riot Control Agents; Solvent Abuse

Philip S. Guzelian, M.D.
Professor and Chairman, Division of Clinical Toxicology and Environmental Medicine, Medical College of Virginia, Richmond, Virginia
Environmental Toxicology: Overview

Lester M. Haddad, M.D., FACEP
Director, Emergency Department, Beaufort Memorial Hospital, Beaufort; Attending Physician, Emergency Medicine Residency Program, Richland Memorial Hospital/University of South Carolina School of Medicine; Consultant and Adjunct Professor, USC Palmetto State Poison Center, Columbia, South Carolina

A General Approach to the Emergency Management of Poisoning; Poisonous Snakebite; Toxic Marine Life; Tricyclic and Newer Antidepressants; Cocaine; Organophosphates and Other Insecticides; Phenol and Related Agents; Miscellany

Alan H. Hall, M.D.
Assistant Professor of Pediatrics, University of Colorado Health Sciences Center; Senior Consultant, Rocky Mountain Poison and Drug Center, Denver General Hospital, Denver, Colorado
Arsenic and Other Heavy Metals; Cyanide

Lorraine Hartnett, M.D., FAAP
Staff Physician, Emergency Services, Department of Surgery, North Shore University Hospital, Manhasset, New York; Consultant, New York City Poison Control Center, New York, New York
Toxic Emergencies in the Neonate

Darell E. Heiselman, D.O., FACP, FACC, FCCP
Associate Professor, Internal Medicine, Northeastern Ohio Universities College of Medicine, Rootstown; Chief, Critical Care Medicine, and Co-Director, Intensive Care Unit, Akron General Medical Center, Akron, Ohio
Benzene and the Aromatic Hydrocarbons

Thomas S. Herman, Ph.D., DABCC
Technical Director, National Health Laboratories, Tampa Division, Tampa, Florida
Appendix: Chemical Conversions of Toxicologic Laboratory Values

Thomas J. Hetrick, M.D., FACEP
Assistant Professor of Emergency Medicine, Northeastern Ohio Universities College of Medicine, Rootstown; Senior Attending Staff Physician, Akron General Medical Center, Akron, Ohio
Ammonia, Nitrogen, Nitrous Oxides, and Related Compounds; Freon and Other Inhalants

David J. Holbrook, Ph.D.
Associate Professor, Department of Biochemistry, and Director of Graduate Studies, Curriculum in Toxicology, School of Medicine, University of North Carolina, Chapel Hill, North Carolina
Environmental Toxicology: Carcinogenesis

Kathleen C. Hubbell, M.D. FACEP
Assistant Professor, Department of Medicine, Louisiana State University School of Medicine in New Orleans, and Director, Louisiana State University Emergency Medicine Residency Program; Acting Director, Accident Room, Charity Hospital of Louisiana in New Orleans, New Orleans, Louisiana
Opiates and Narcotics

Kenneth V. Iserson, M.D., M.B.A., FACEP
Associate Professor and Residency Director in Emergency Medicine, University of Arizona College of Medicine; Attending Physician, University Medical Center, Tucson, Arizona
Caffeine and Nicotine

Lt. Andy S. Jagoda, M.D., M.C., USNR
Lieutenant, Naval Medical Command, Medical Department, ASU Bahrain, FPO New York, New York
Phencyclidine and the Hallucinogens

David S. Jallo, R.Ph.
Instructor, Environmental Science, University of Phoenix; Lead Environmental Scientist, Arizona Public Service Company, Phoenix, Arizona
Ergot

Jeffrey S. Jones, M.D.
Assistant Professor, Division of Emergency Medicine, Michigan State University College of Human Medicine, East Lansing; Research Director and Staff Physician, Department of Emergency Medicine,

Butterworth Hospital, Grand Rapids, Michigan
Industrial Toxicology: General Concepts

Richard L. Jones, M.D.
Associate Clinical Professor of Pediatrics, Georgetown University Hospital, Washington, D.C.
Evaluation of Drug Use in the Adolescent

Armand Keating, M.D., FRCP(C)
Director, University of Toronto Autologous Bone Marrow Transplant Program; Director of Research, Division of Hematology-Oncology, Department of Medicine, Toronto General Hospital, Toronto, Ontario, Canada
Hematologic Consequences of Poisoning

Brian F. Keaton, M.D., FACEP
Assistant Professor in Emergency Medicine, Northeastern Ohio Universities College of Medicine, Rootstown; Attending Physician, Department of Emergency Medicine, St. Thomas Medical Center, Akron, Ohio
Chlorinated Hydrocarbons

Michael T. Kelley, M.D., FACEP
Assistant Professor of Preventive Medicine, Division of Emergency Medicine, Ohio State University; Pediatrics/Pharmacology/Toxicology, Ohio State University Hospital; Department of Pharmacology/Toxicology, Columbus Children's Hospital, Columbus, Ohio
Sympathomimetics

Daniel E. Keyler, Pharm.D.
Clinical Assistant Professor, College of Pharmacy, University of Minnesota; Clinical Assistant Professor, Division of Clinical Toxicology and Pharmacology, Department of Medicine, Hennepin County Medical Center, Minneapolis, Minnesota
Tricyclic and Newer Antidepressants

Robert P. Kimberly, M.D.
Associate Professor of Medicine, Cornell University Medical College; Associate Attending Physician, The New York Hospital and The Hospital for Special Surgery, New York, New York
Nonsteroidal Anti-Inflammatory Drugs and Colchicine

Mark Kirk, M.D.
Clinical Toxicology Fellow, University of Colorado Health Sciences Center, Rocky Mountain Poison and Drug Center; Attending Physician, Denver General Hospital, Denver, Colorado
Anticholinergics

Robert C. Kopelman, M.D.
Clinical Assistant Professor of Medicine, University of California, Los Angeles; Active Staff, Mercy, San Joaquin, Memorial, and Bakersfield Community Hospitals and Kern Medical Center, Bakersfield, California
Camphor

Ken Kulig, M.D., FACEP
Assistant Professor, Department of Surgery, Trauma and Emergency Medicine Section, University of Colorado Medical School; Medical Director, Rocky Mountain Poison Center, University of Colorado Health Services Center; Clinical Attending Staff, Denver General Hospital, University Hospital, and Porter Memorial Hospital, Denver, Colorado
Mushrooms; Anticholinergics; Other Herbicides and Fungicides; Strychnine

Donald B. Kunkel, M.D.
Associate in Pharmacology and Toxicology, College of Pharmacy, The University of Arizona, Tucson; Medical Director, Department of Medical Toxicology and Samaritan Regional Poison Center, Good Samaritan Regional Medical Center, Phoenix, Arizona
Poisonous Arthropods: Spiders and Scorpions; Poisonous Plants; Ergot

Peter G. Lacouture, Ph.D.
Instructor, Pediatrics, Harvard Medical School; Research

Coordinator, Massachusetts Poison Control System, The Children's Hospital, Boston, Massachusetts
Iron

Paul W. Ladenson, M.D.
Associate Professor of Medicine, Johns Hopkins University School of Medicine; Director, Division of Endocrinology and Metabolism, Johns Hopkins Hospital, Baltimore, Maryland
Thyroid

Joseph LaDou, M.D.
Clinical Professor and Chief, Division of Occupational and Environmental Medicine, University of California, San Francisco; Attending Physician, O'Connor Hospital, San Jose, California
Industrial Toxicology: The Microelectronics Industry

Richard F. Lee, Ph.D.
Professor of Oceanography, Skidaway Institute of Oceanography, University of Georgia System, Savannah, Georgia
Toxic Marine Life

Toby Litovitz, M.D., FACEP
Associate Professor, Emergency Medicine, Georgetown University School of Medicine; Director, National Capital Poison Center, Georgetown University Hospital, Washington, D.C.
Alkali Injury: The Miniature Battery Hazard

Neal E. Little, M.D., FACEP
Clinical Instructor, University of Michigan Medical School; Emergency Physician, St. Joseph Mercy Hospital, Ann Arbor, Michigan
Disaster Management of Massive Toxic Exposure

Frederick H. Lovejoy, M.D.
Professor of Pediatrics, Harvard Medical School; Associate Physician-in-Chief, The Children's Hospital, Boston, Massachusetts
Prevention of Childhood Poisonings; Isoniazid; Iron

Timothy J. Mader, M.D.
Senior Resident, Department of Emergency Medicine, Richland Memorial Hospital/University of South Carolina School of Medicine, Columbia, South Carolina
Geriatric Toxicology

John F. Maher, M.D.
Professor of Medicine, Uniformed Services University of the Health Sciences, Bethesda, Maryland; Attending Staff, Walter Reed Army Medical Center, Washington, D.C., and Naval Hospital, Bethesda, Maryland
Renal Considerations: Acute Renal Failure

C. Patrick Mahoney, M.D.
Clinical Professor of Pediatrics, University of Washington School of Medicine; Attending Physician, Children's Hospital and Medical Center and Virginia Mason Medical Center, Seattle, Washington
Vitamins A and D and Their Analogues

Howard I. Maibach, M.D.
Professor, University of California Medical School and Hospital, San Francisco, California
Dermatologic Toxicity

Anthony S. Manoguerra, Pharm.D., DABAT
Professor of Clinical Pharmacy, School of Pharmacy, University of California, San Francisco; Director, San Diego Regional Poison Center, University of California, San Diego, Medical Center, San Diego, California; Immediate Past-President, American Association of Poison Control Centers
The Poison Information Telephone Call

Michael G. Manske, M.D.
Clinical Instructor, Wright State University School of Medicine, Dayton, Ohio; Attending Physician, St. Mary's Hospital, Racine, Wisconsin
Petroleum Distillates and Turpentine

Celeste Martin Marx, Pharm.D.
Assistant Professor of Pediatrics, Case Western Reserve University School of Medicine; Pediatric Clinical Pharmacist, Rainbow Babies and Childrens Hospital, Cleveland, Ohio
Developmental Toxicology

James F. McAnally, M.D., FACC, FACP
Clinical Associate Professor of Medicine, Seton Hall University Graduate School of Medicine; Chief of Nephrology, St. Elizabeth's Hospital; Director of Nephrology, Alexian Brothers Hospital, Elizabeth, New Jersey
Acid-Base Balance

Michael McGuigan, M.D.
Assistant Professor of Pediatrics and Pharmacology, Faculty of Medicine, University of Toronto; Medical Director, Poison Information Centre, Hospital for Sick Children, Toronto, Ontario, Canada
Hydrofluoric Acid

Terrance P. McHugh, M.D., FACEP
Attending Physician, Emergency Medicine Residency Program, Richland Memorial Hospital/ University of South Carolina School of Medicine, Columbia, South Carolina
Borates

Thomas W. McKee, M.D.
Director, Pediatric Intensive Care Unit, Memorial Medical Center, Savannah, Georgia
Fluids and Electrolytes II: The Pediatric Patient

M. Jo McMullen, M.D., FACEP
Assistant Professor of Emergency Medicine, Northeastern Ohio Universities College of Medicine, Rootstown; Senior Attending Staff Physician, Akron General Medical Center, Akron, Ohio
Industrial Toxicology: General Concepts; Ammonia, Nitrogen, Nitrous Oxides, and Related Compounds

Brooks C. Metts, Jr., Pharm.D.
Associate Professor of Clinical Pharmacy, University of South Carolina; Director, Palmetto Poison Center, University of South Carolina and Richland Memorial Hospital, Columbia, South Carolina
Other Rodenticides

Edith P. Mitchell, M.D.
Assistant Professor of Medicine, University of Missouri–Columbia, Columbia, Missouri
Chemotherapeutic Agents

Howard C. Mofenson, M.D.
Professor of Clinical Pediatrics, State University of New York at Stony Brook; Visiting Professor of Pharmacology and Toxicology, New York College of Osteopathy; Professor of Clinical Pharmacy, St. John's University College of Pharmacy, Jamaica; Attending in Pediatrics, Director of Long Island Regional Poison Control Center, and Director of Clinic for Children with Diabetes Mellitus, Nassau County Medical Center, East Meadow, New York
Sodium and Sodium Chloride; Fluorine and Fluoride

Roy A. M. Myers, M.D., FRCS (Edin.)
Clinical Assistant Professor of Surgery, University of Maryland, Baltimore, and Georgetown University, Washington, D.C.; Clinical Assistant Professor of Medicine, Pennsylvania State University, Hershey, Pennsylvania; Director of Hyperbaric Medicine, Maryland Institute for Emergency Medical Services Systems; University of Maryland Hospital, Montebello Rehabilitation Hospital, and Maryland General Hospital, Baltimore, Maryland
Carbon Monoxide Poisoning

Larry L. Needham, Ph.D.
Chief, Toxicology Branch, Centers for Disease Control, Atlanta, Georgia
Environmental Toxicology: Polychlorinated Dibenzo-P-Dioxins

Donald G. Patterson, Jr., Ph.D.
Chief, Dioxin and Related Compounds Laboratory, Centers for Disease Control, Atlanta, Georgia
Environmental Toxicology: Polychlorinated Dibenzo-P-Dioxins

Paul R. Pentel, M.D.
Associate Professor of Medicine, University of Minnesota Medical School; Department of Medicine, Hennepin County Medical Center, Division of Clinical Pharmacology and Toxicology, Minneapolis, Minnesota
Tricyclic and Newer Antidepressants; New Cardiac Antiarrhythmic Agents

George Podgorny, M.D., FICS
Associate Professor of Clinical Surgery, Bowman Gray School of Medicine, Wake Forest University; Visiting Professor of Emergency Medicine, East Carolina University School of Medicine; Attending Physician, Department of Emergency Medicine, Moses H. Cone Memorial Hospital, Winston-Salem, North Carolina
Poisonous Snakebite; Poisonous Arthropods: Spiders and Scorpions

John F. Pope, M.D.
Fellow in Pediatric Pharmacology, University of Virgina; Fellow, Division of Pediatric Pharmacology and Critical Care, University of Virginia Hospital, Charlottesville, Virginia
Developmental Toxicology

Daniel Carl Postellon, M.D.
Assistant Professor of Pediatrics, Wayne State University; Attending Physician, Children's Hospital of Michigan, Detroit, Michigan
Iodine

A. T. Proudfoot, B.Sc., FRCPE
Director, Regional Poison Treatment Centre, Edinburgh Royal Infirmary, Edinburgh, Scotland
Salicylates and Salicylamide

James I. Raymond, M.D., FACEP
Director of Education and Professional Services, Department of Emergency Medicine and Program Director, Emergency Medicine Residency Training Program, Richland Memorial Hospital/ University of South Carolina School of Medicine; Medical Director, South Carolina State Emergency Medical Service, Department of Health and Environmental Control, Columbia, South Carolina
Geriatric Toxicology

Michael D. Reed, Pharm.D.
Associate Professor of Pediatrics, Division of Pediatric Pharmacology and Critical Care, Department of Pediatrics, University of Virginia Children's Medical Center, University of Virginia Health Sciences Center, Charlottesville, Virginia
Drug-Drug Interactions

Betty S. Riggs, M.D.
Associate Director, Clinical Research and Development, Wyeth-Ayerst Research, Philadelphia, Pennsylvania
Other Herbicides and Fungicides; Strychnine

Timothy J. Rittenberry, M.D., FACEP
Assistant Professor of Clinical Emergency Medicine, Department of Surgery, University of Illinois College of Medicine at Chicago; Director of Emergency Medicine Education, Illinois Masonic Medical Center, Chicago, Illinois
The Volatile Oils

James R. Roberts, M.D., FACEP
Associate Professor, Emergency Medicine, Medical College of Pennsylvania; Director, Emergency Medicine, Misericordia Hospital, Philadelphia, Pennsylvania
A General Approach to the Emergency Management of Poisoning; Benzodiazepines; Clonidine

William O. Robertson, M.D.
Professor of Pediatrics, Department of Pediatrics, University of

Washington School of Medicine; Medical Director, Seattle Poison Center, Children's Hospital and Medical Center; Medical Director, Washington Poison Network, Seattle, Washington; President, American Association of Poison Control Centers
Arsenic and Other Heavy Metals

Marilyn Rogers, M.D., FACEP
Emergency Physician, Erlanger Medical Center, Chattanooga, Tennessee
Cyanoacrylate (Super Glue)

Carlos Rotellar, M.D.
Assistant Professor of Medicine, Georgetown University School of Medicine, Washington, D.C.
Renal Considerations: Chronic Drug Nephropathy

Barry H. Rumack, M.D.
Professor of Pediatrics, University of Colorado School of Medicine; Director, Rocky Mountain Poison and Drug Center; Attending Physician, University of Colorado Health Sciences Center, Denver General Hospital, and The Children's Hospital, Denver, Colorado
Mushrooms; Anticholinergics; Acetaminophen; Cyanide

Philip S. Schein, M.D.
Adjunct Professor of Medicine and Pharmacology, University of Pennsylvania School of Medicine, Philadelphia; Clinical Professor of Medicine and Pharmacology, Georgetown University School of Medicine, Washington, D.C.; President and Chief Executive Officer, U.S. Bioscience, Blue Bell, Pennsylvania
Chemotherapeutic Agents

Daniel T. Schelble, M.D., FACEP
Associate Professor, Department of Emergency Medicine, Northeastern Ohio Universities College of Medicine, Rootstown; Chairman, Department of Emergency Medicine, Akron General Medical Center, Akron, Ohio
Phosphine and Phosgene

George E. Schreiner, M.D., FACP, FRCPS(GLAS)
Distinguished Professor of Medicine, Georgetown University School of Medicine, Washington, D.C.
Renal Considerations: Chronic Drug Nephropathy

Andre Schuh, M.D., FRCP(C)
Postdoctoral Fellow, Mt. Sinai Hospital Research Institute, Department of Medical Genetics, Faculty of Medicine, University of Toronto, Toronto, Ontario, Canada
Anticoagulants

Janice B. Schwartz, M.D.
Assistant Professor of Medicine and Pharmacy, University of California at San Francisco; Attending Physician, Moffitt-Long Hospital, San Francisco, California
Calcium Entry Blocker Poisoning

Donna Seger, M.D., FACEP, ABMT
Assistant Professor of Surgery and Medicine, Section of Emergency Medicine, Vanderbilt University Medical Center; Acting Director, Vanderbilt Poison Control Center, Nashville, Tennessee
Phenytoin and Other Anticonvulsants

Brad S. Selden, M.D.
Fellow, Department of Medical Toxicology, Good Samaritan Regional Medical Center, Phoenix, Arizona
Poisonous Arthropods: Spiders and Scorpions

Günter Seyffart, M.D.
Dialysis Center, Bad Homburg, Germany
Antihistamines and Other Sedatives

Michael W. Shannon, M.D., M.P.H.
Clinical Instructor in Pediatrics, Harvard Medical School; Assistant in Medicine, The Children's Hospital; Medical Consultant, The

Massachusetts Poison Control System, Boston, Massachusetts
Isoniazid

Suzanne M. Shepherd, M.D., FACEP
Assistant Professor of Emergency Medicine, Georgetown University Medical Center; Attending Physician, Department of Emergency Medicine, Georgetown University Hospital, Washington, D.C.
Phencyclidine and the Hallucinogens

Richard O. Shields, Jr., M.D., FACEP
Chairman, Department of Emergency Medicine and Medical Director of the Emergency Department, Memorial Medical Center, Savannah, Georgia
Amphetamines

L. Reed Shirley, M.D.
Assistant Professor of Pediatrics and Immunology and Microbiology, Medical University of South Carolina; Attending Physician, Medical University of South Carolina, Charleston Memorial Hospital, and Roper Hospital, Charleston, South Carolina
Poisonous Arthropods: Stinging Insects

Corey M. Slovis, M.D., FACP, FACEP
Associate Professor of Emergency Medicine and Medicine and Director, Emergency Medicine, University of Rochester School of Medicine and Dentistry; Director, Department of Emergency Medicine, Strong Memorial Hospital, Rochester, New York
Food Poisoning

Wayne R. Snodgrass, M.D., Ph.D.
Head, Clinical Pharmacology-Toxicology Unit; Medical Director, Texas Poison Center; Associate Professor of Pediatrics and Pharmacology-Toxicology, University of Texas Medical Branch; Attending Physician, Pediatic Intensive Care Unit, Child Health Center; John Sealy Hospital; and University of Texas Medical Branch, Galveston, Texas
Air Pollution: Air Quality Index and Ozone

Daniel A. Spyker, Ph.D., M.D.
Director of Clinical Services, Pharmaceutical Research Associates, Inc., Charlottesville, Virginia
Chemical and Drug Injury to the Eye

Thomas Stair, M.D.
Associate Professor of Emergency Medicine and Acting Director, Department of Emergency Medicine, Georgetown University School of Medicine, Washington, D.C.
Chlorine; Baby Powder

Alice D. Stark, Dr.P.H., M.P.H.
Associate Professor, Department of Epidemiology/Department of Anthropology, State University of New York–Albany, Albany, New York
Environmental Toxicology: Hormonal, Growth, and Other Effects; Formaldehyde

N. John Stewart, M.D., FACEP
Attending Physician, Department of Emergency Medicine, Richland Memorial Hospital; Medical Director, Palmetto Poison Center, Columbia, South Carolina
Borates

Williamson B. Strum, M.D.
Clinical Member, Scripps Clinic and Research Foundation; Attending Physician, Green Hospital of Scripps Clinic, La Jolla, California
Gastrointestinal Effects of Poisoning

John B. Sullivan, Jr., M.D.
Associate Professor, Emergency Medicine; Medical Director, Arizona Poison Center; Attending Physician, University of Arizona Health Sciences Center and University Medical Center, Tucson, Arizona
Immunologic Consequences of Poisoning

Stephen Szara, M.D., D.Sc.
Chief, Biomedical Branch, National

Institute on Drug Abuse, Rockville, Maryland
Marijuana

John A. Tafuri, M.D.
Clinical Instructor, Emergency Medicine, Northeastern Ohio Universities College of Medicine, Rootstown; Staff Physician, Department of Emergency Medicine, Western Reserve Care System, Cleveland, Ohio
Benzodiazepines

Angelo M. Taveira Da Silva, M.D., Ph.D.
Associate Professor of Medicine and Pharmacology, Georgetown University School of Medicine; Director, Medical Intensive Care Unit, Georgetown University Hospital, Washington, D.C.
Management of Respiratory Complications

Anthony R. Temple, M.D.
Adjunct Associate Professor, University of Pennsylvania, Philadelphia; Director, Regulatory and Medical Affairs, McNeil Consumer Products Company, Fort Washington, Pennsylvania
Bleach, Soaps, and Detergents

W. J. Tilstone, Ph.D.
Director, State Forensic Science, Adelaide, South Australia
Laboratory Diagnosis and Drug Testing

Judith E. Tintinalli, M.D.
Clinical Assistant Professor of Emergency Medicine, University of Michigan, Ann Arbor; Associate Chief, Emergency Medicine, William Beaumont Hospital, Royal Oak, Michigan
Designer Drugs

Mark J. Upfal, M.D., M.P.H.
Clinical Instructor, Wayne State University, School of Medicine, Division of Occupational Health; Attending Physician, Grace Hospital Division, Detroit, Michigan
Disaster Management of Massive Toxic Exposure

Jonathan Vargas, M.D., FACEP
Residency Director and Assistant Professor of Emergency Medicine, Eastern Virginia Graduate School of Medicine; Attending Physician, Norfolk General Hospital, Norfolk, Virginia
The Antipsychotic Drugs

Ingrid M. O. Vicas, M.D., C.M.
Clinical Associate Professor, Pharmacology, and Clinical Assistant Professor, Internal Medicine, University of Calgary; Director, Poison and Drug Information Service, Division of Emergency Medicine, Foothills Hospital; Department of Emergency Medicine, Alberta Children's Hospital, Alberta, Canada
Hydrogen Sulfide and Carbon Disulfide

Richard B. Warner, M.D.
Director, Emergency Psychiatric Service, The Kansas Institute, Overland Park, Kansas
Psychiatric Evaluation of the Suicidal Patient

Michael S. Weinstock, M.D., FAAP, FACEP
Assistant Clinical Professor, Emergency Medicine, Georgetown University School of Medicine, Washington, D.C.; Director, Emergency Medical Services, North Shore University Hospital, Manhasset, New York
Toxic Emergencies in the Neonate

Daniel D. Whitcraft, III, M.D., FACEP
Director, Emergency Department, Memorial Medical Center of Long Beach, Long Beach, California
Hydrogen Sulfide and Carbon Disulfide

J. Douglas White, M.D.
Associate Professor of Emergency Medicine and Internal Medicine,

Georgetown University School of Medicine; Clinical Director, Emergency Department, Georgetown University Medical Center, Washington, D.C.
Thyroid

James F. Winchester, M.D., FRCP
Professor of Medicine and Acting Director, Division of Nephrology, Department of Medicine, Georgetown University School of Medicine; Co-Director, Hemodialysis, Hemoperfusion, and Transplantation Services; Associate Director, Clinical Nephrology Service; Director, Self-Care Dialysis Program; Consultant to National Capital Poison Center, Georgetown University Hospital, Washington, D.C.
Fluids and Electrolytes I: General Principles; Active Methods for Detoxification; Lithium; Methanol, Isopropyl Alcohol, Higher Alcohols, Ethylene Glycol, Cellosolves, Acetone, and Oxalate; Barbiturates, Methaqualone, and Primidone; Acids and Antacids; Paraquat and the Bipyridyl Herbicides; Nitroprusside and Selected Antihypertensives

Alan Woolf, M.D., M.P.H.
Assistant Professor of Pediatrics, Harvard Medical School; Assistant in Medicine, The Children's Hospital, Boston, Massachusetts
Prevention of Childhood Poisonings

Richard B. Yow, M.D.
Chief of Radiology Department, Beaufort Memorial Hospital and Beaufort Naval Hospital, Beaufort, South Carolina
Radiation Poisoning

Hyman J. Zimmerman, M.D.
Distinguished Scientist, Armed Forces Institute of Pathology; Professor of Medicine, Emeritus, George Washington University School of Medicine; Clinical Professor of Medicine, Uniformed Services University of Health Sciences; Consultant, Veterans Administration Medical Center, George Washington University Medical Center, Clinical Center, NIH, U.S. Naval Medical Center, Bethesda, Maryland and Walter Reed Medical Center, Washington, D.C.
Chemical Hepatic Injury

Brian J. Zink, M.D.
Assistant Professor, Emergency Medicine, Albany Medical College, Albany, New York
Clonidine

PREFACE

The Second Edition of this textbook finds toxicology established in the public eye. This past decade has made toxicology a world concern, with such catastrophic events as Bhopal, Chernobyl, the "crack" and "ice" epidemics, and the development of the ozone "hole" over the South Pole. New expressions such as "acid rain" and "greenhouse effect" have been coined to describe new phenomena, pointing up world concern over environmental contamination from industrial and atmospheric pollution. Trafficking in illegal drugs has multiplied, and a world initiative in the "war against drugs" has begun. International cooperation has begun to tackle these problems that threaten the life of our planet and its inhabitants.

Since the First Edition was published, patient management and toxicology research have advanced. We have, however, continued to stress the most important aspect of toxicology, namely, care of the poisoned patient. Our text also highlights the renewed interest in poisoning by specialists in academic emergency medicine, toxicology, internal medicine, pediatrics, and others; presents a lively discourse on new aspects of patient management; and enters into some controversy—for example, the approach to gastric decontamination.

As in the First Edition, we strove to maintain uniformity of opinion in patient management, although this has not always been possible; the controversial viewpoints expressed in this book, however, lend credence to the ever-changing and exciting nature of the discipline of clinical toxicology.

The text has been completely updated, with the addition of 19 new chapters: examples are Developmental, Neonatal, and Geriatric Toxicology, and an expanded section on Environmental Toxicology. We feel the addition of these topics offers the reader a more complete treatise on the global importance of poisoning.

We are especially grateful to our contributors, those outstanding, knowledgeable, and experienced individuals in their fields of expertise, without whom this text would not have been possible. We appreciate the tireless efforts of the staff at W. B. Saunders, particularly Wynette Kommer, William Lamsback, Bonnie Karfeld, Carolyn Naylor, and Kenneth Neimeister. We appreciate the helpful suggestions and comments of our medical colleagues.

We wish to thank our families, especially our children Craig and Jane Winchester and Matthew, Joseph, Jeanne, Charlene, Daniel, Elizabeth Anne, and Madeleine Haddad for their enthusiastic support, and we hope the knowledge herein will make them aware of the threat of illegal drugs to themselves, their friends, and the world at large.

We extend to our readers the hope that this text will benefit them in their pursuit of knowledge and in their clinical knowledge of medicine.

LESTER M. HADDAD
JAMES F. WINCHESTER

CONTENTS

PART I

GENERAL INTRODUCTORY CHAPTERS

PART II

SPECIFIC POISONS

SECTION A

SECTION B

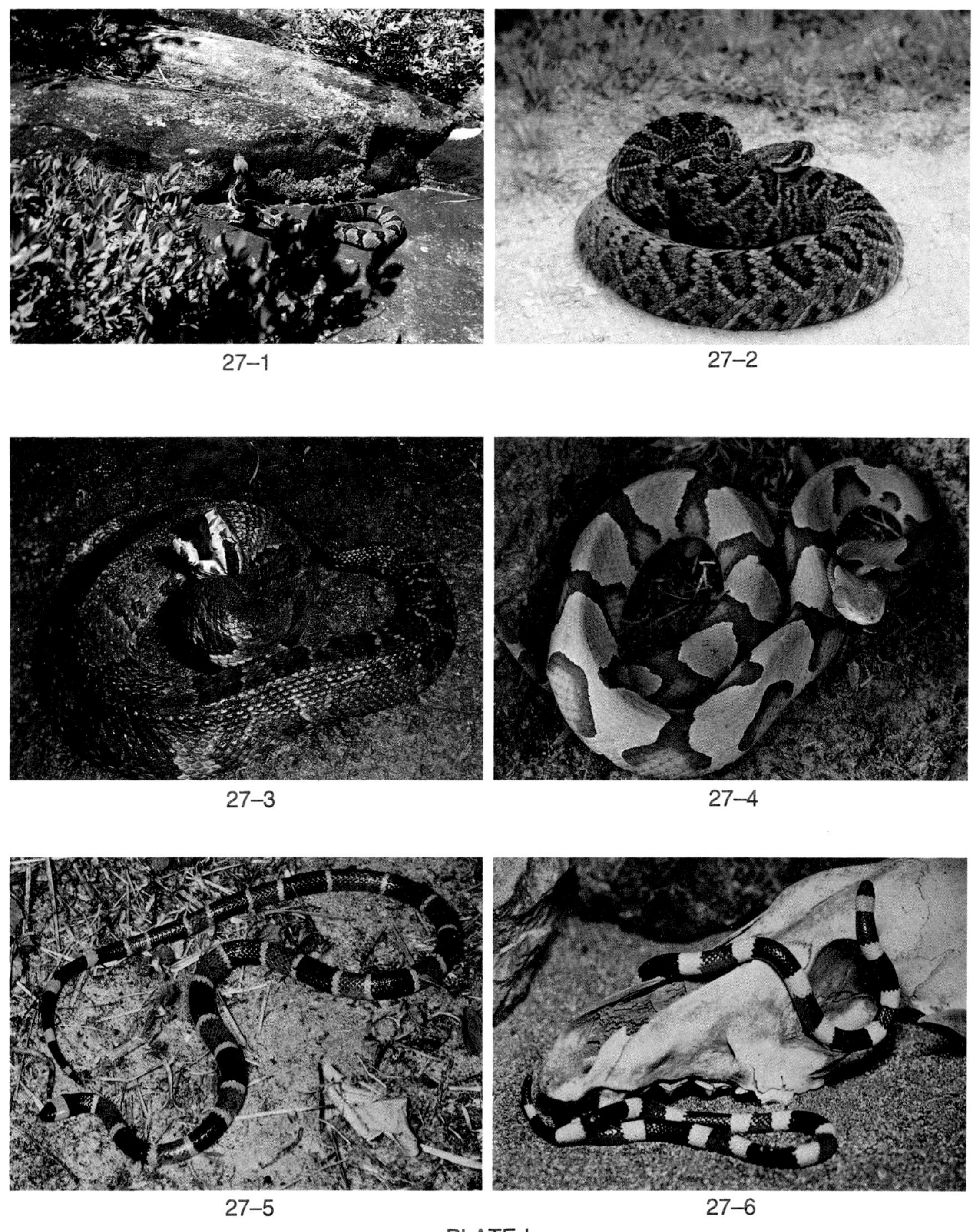

PLATE I

Figure 27–1. The timber rattlesnake *Crotalus horridus.* (Courtesy of the Savannah Science Museum, Savannah, Georgia.)
Figure 27–2. The eastern diamondback rattlesnake *Crotalus adamanteus.* (Courtesy of the Savannah Science Museum, Savannah, Georgia.)
Figure 27–3. The water moccasin, or cottonmouth, *Agkistrodon piscivorus,* named for the cotton-white interior of its mouth. Fond of swamps, rivers, and ditches, this snake does not retreat when confronted, unlike the harmless water snakes. (Courtesy of Winchester Seyle, herpetologist, and the Savannah Science Museum, Savannah, Georgia.)
Figure 27–4. The copperhead *Agkistrodon contortrix.* (Courtesy of the Savannah Science Museum, Savannah, Georgia.)
Figure 27–5. The eastern coral snake *Micrurus fulvius* "Red next to yellow, kill a fellow." (Courtesy of Murray E. Fowler, D.V.M.)
Figure 27–6. The Arizona coral snake *Micruroides euryxanthus.* (Courtesy of Murray E. Fowler, D.V.M.)

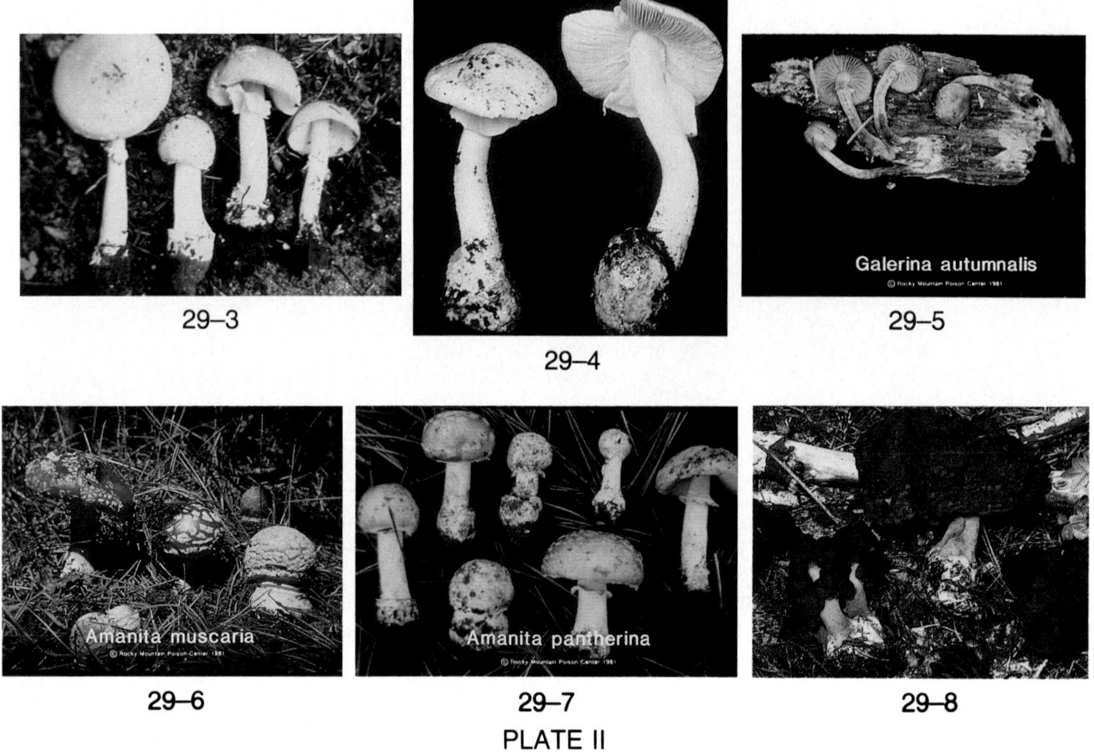

PLATE II

Figure 29–3. Amanita verna (cyclopeptide). Courtesy of Linea Gilman, Denver.

Figure 29–4. Amanita virosa (cyclopeptide). Courtesy of Linea Gilman, Denver.

Figure 29–5. Galerina autumnalis (cyclopeptide). Courtesy of Linea Gilman and the Rocky Mountain Poison Center, Denver.

Figure 29–6. Amanita muscaria (muscimol, ibotenic acid). Courtesy of Linea Gilman and the Rocky Mountain Poison Center, Denver.

Figure 29–7. Amanita pantherina (muscimol, ibotenic acid). Courtesy of Linea Gilman and the Rocky Mountain Poison Center, Denver.

Figure 29–8. Gyromitra esculenta (monomethylhydrazine). (From Arora D: Mushrooms Demystified. © 1979, 1986 by David Arora. Berkeley, CA, Ten Speed Press, 1986.)

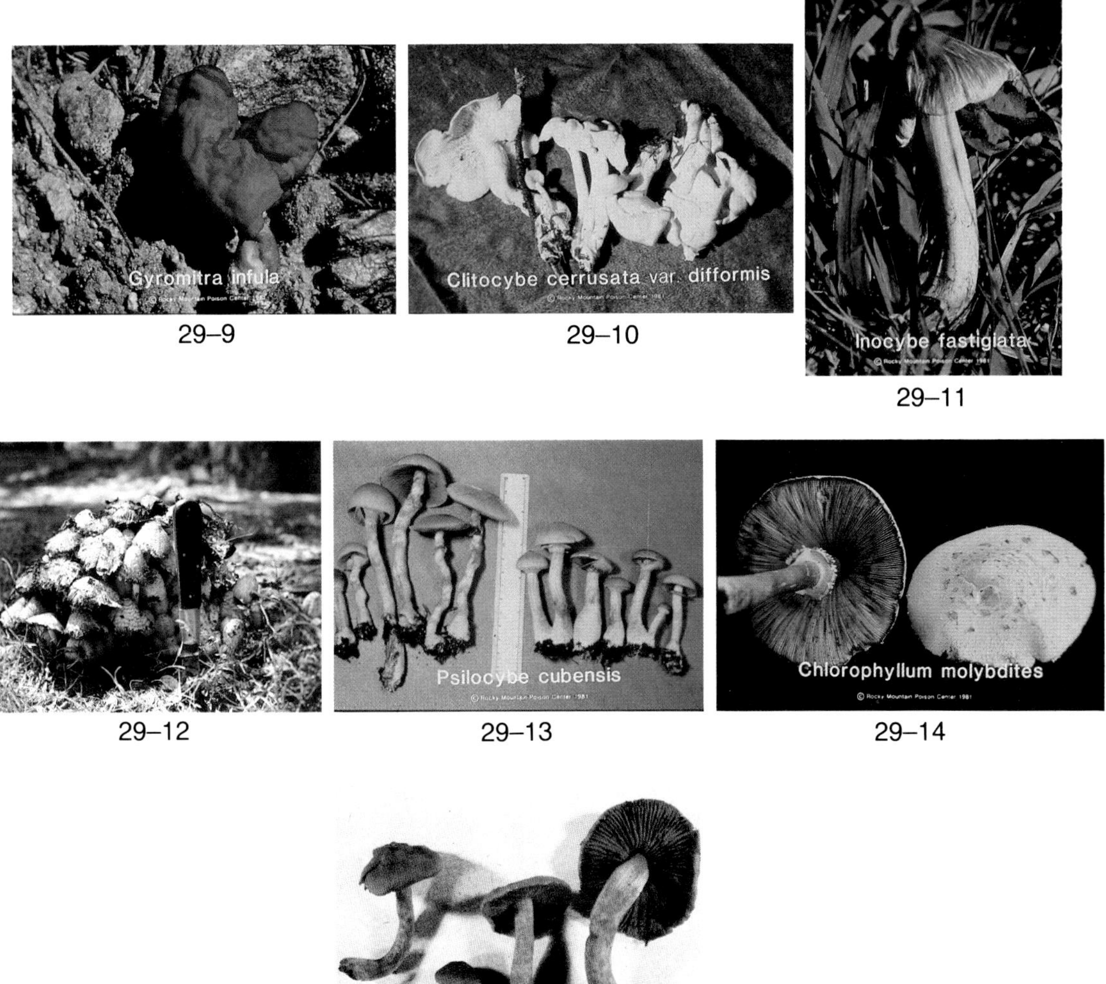

PLATE III

Figure 29–9. Gyromitra infula (monomethylhydrazine). Courtesy of George Grimes and the Rocky Mountain Poison Center, Denver.

Figure 29–10. Clitocybe cerrusata (muscarine). Courtesy of Linea Gilman and the Rocky Mountain Poison Center, Denver.

Figure 29–11. Inocybe fastigiata (muscarine). Courtesy of George Grimes and the Rocky Mountain Poison Center, Denver.

Figure 29–12. Coprinus atramentarius (coprine). Courtesy of Joe H. Restivo, Department of Biology, Armstrong College, Savannah.

Figure 29–13. Psilocybe cubensis (indole). Courtesy of the Rocky Mountain Poison Center, Denver.

Figure 29–14. Chlorophyllum molybdites. Courtesy of George Grimes and the Rocky Mountain Poison Center, Denver.

Figure 29–15. Cortinarius speciosissinus (orelline, orellanine). (From Lampe KF (ed): AMA Handbook of Poisonous and Injurious Plants. Chicago, American Medical Association, 1985. Reprinted with permission.)

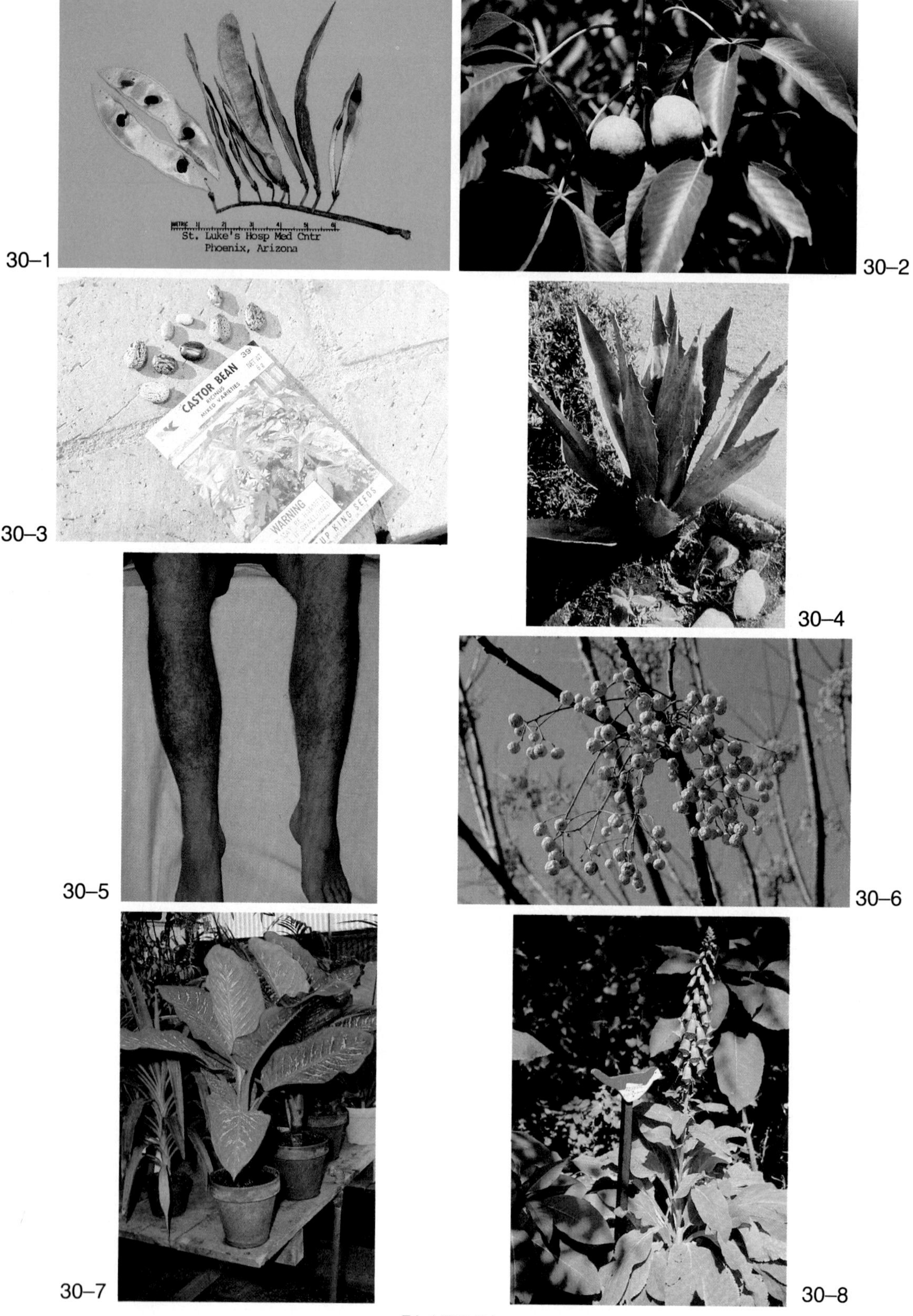
30–1
St. Luke's Hosp Med Cntr
Phoenix, Arizona
30–2
30–3
CASTOR BEAN
RICINUS
MIXED VARIETIES
WARNING
30–4
30–5
30–6
30–7
30–8

PLATE IV

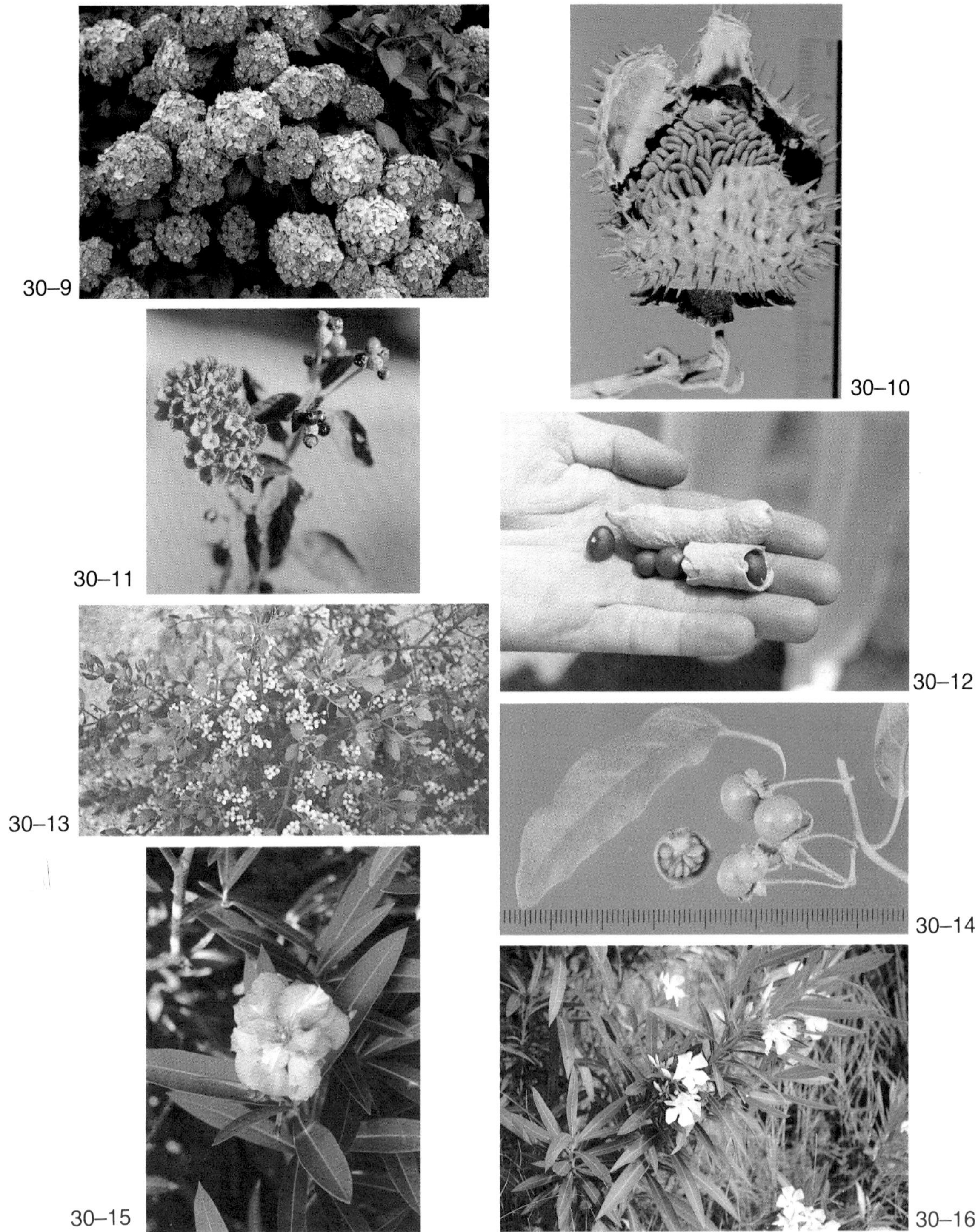

PLATE V

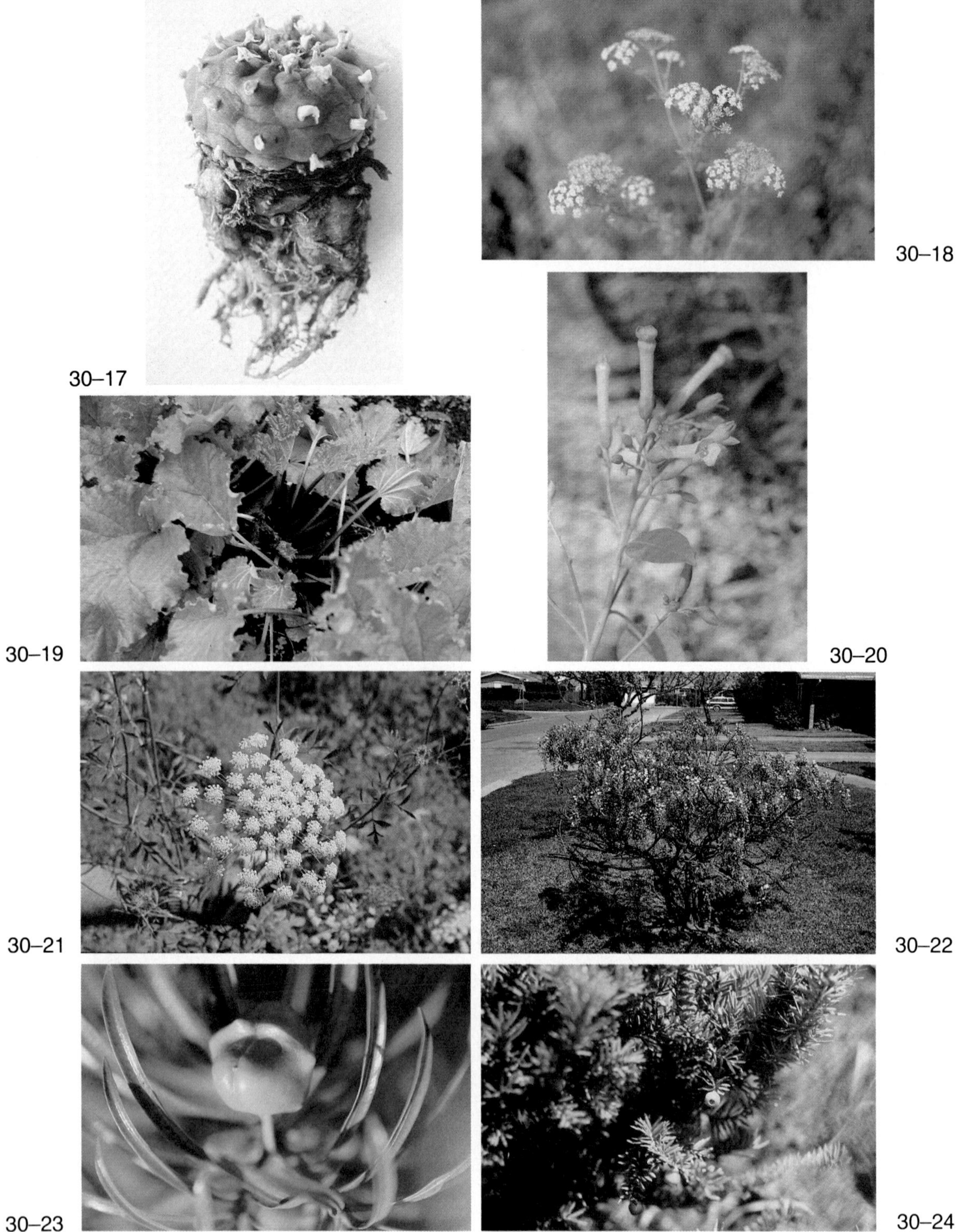

PLATE VI

Figure 30–1. Black locust pods and seeds.

Figure 30–2. Tainted buckeye.

Figure 30–3. Castor bean. Note warning label on package.

Figure 30–4. Century plant.

Figure 30–5. Hemorrhagic rash from century plant sap contact.

Figure 30–6. Chinaberry (drying fruit).

Figure 30–7. Dieffenbachia.

Figure 30–8. Digitalis, foxglove. (From Ellis MD: Dangerous Plants, Snakes, Arthropods and Marine Life—Toxicity and Treatment. Drug Intelligence Publications, Inc., Hamilton, IL, 1975. With permission.)

Figure 30–9. Hydrangea. (From Ellis MD: Dangerous Plants, Snakes, Arthropods and Marine Life—Toxicity and Treatment. Drug Intelligence Publications, Inc., Hamilton, IL, 1975. With permission.)

Figure 30–10. Jimson weed pod and seeds.

Figure 30–11. Lantana.

Figure 30–12. Mescal bean or Texas mountain laurel.

Figure 30–13. American mistletoe. (From Ellis MD: Dangerous Plants, Snakes, Arthropods and Marine Life—Toxicity and Treatment. Drug Intelligence Publications, Inc., Hamilton, IL, 1975. With permission.)

Figure 30–14. Silverleaf nightshade.

Figure 30–15. Pink oleander.

Figure 30–16. White oleander. (From Ellis MD: Dangerous Plants, Snakes, Arthropods and Marine Life—Toxicity and Treatment. Drug Intelligence Publications, Inc., Hamilton, IL, 1975. With permission.)

Figure 30–17. Peyote.

Figure 30–18. Poison hemlock.

Figure 30–19. Rhubarb.

Figure 30–20. Tree tobacco.

Figure 30–21. Water hemlock. (From Ellis MD: Dangerous Plants, Snakes, Arthropods and Marine Life—Toxicity and Treatment. Drug Intelligence Publications, Inc., Hamilton, IL, 1975. With permission.)

Figure 30–22. Wisteria. (From Ellis MD: Dangerous Plants, Snakes, Arthropods and Marine Life—Toxicity and Treatment. Drug Intelligence Publications, Inc., Hamilton, IL, 1975. With permission.)

Figure 30–23. Yellow oleander ("lucky nut").

Figure 30–24. Yew.

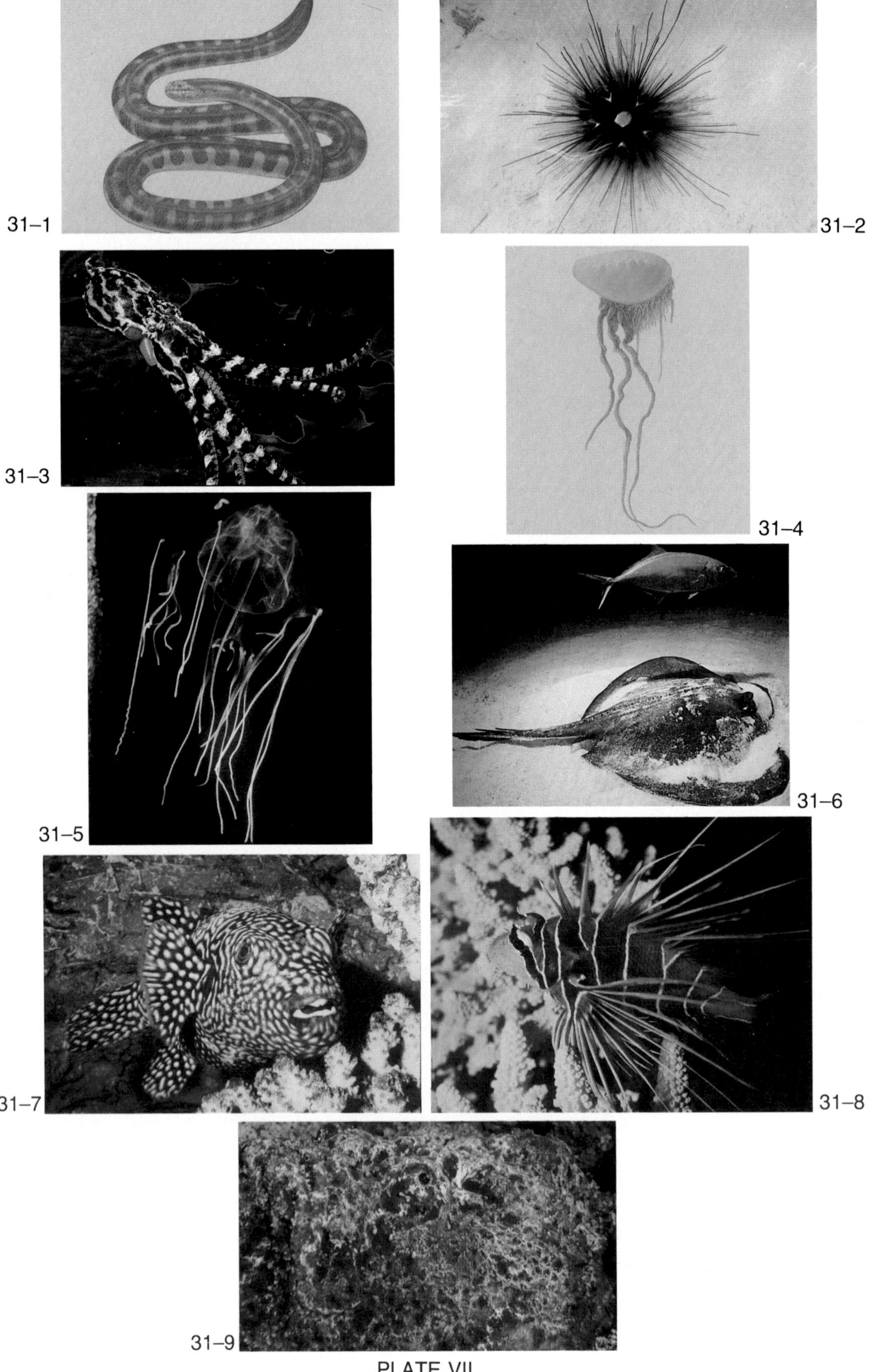

PLATE VII

Figure 31–1. The sea snake, *Enhydrina schistosa* daudin. (Courtesy of Bruce W. Halstead and the World Life Research Institute, California.)

Figure 31–2. The sea urchin, *Diadema setosum*. (Courtesy of Bruce W. Halstead and The World Life Research Institute, California.)

Figure 31–3. The Australian blue-ringed octopus, *Octopus maculosa*. (Courtesy of David Parer, *In* John VanDenbeld: Nature of Australia; A Portrait of the Island Continent. Facts on File, New York, in cooperation with the Australian Broadcasting Corporation, 1988; © D. Parer and E. Parer Cook, Auscape International.)

Figure 31–4. Portuguese man-of-war, *Physalia physalis*. (Courtesy of Bruce W. Halstead and the World Life Research Institute, California.

Figure 31–5. The sea wasp, *Chironex fleckeri*. (Courtesy of Bruce W. Halstead and the World Life Research Institute, California.)

Figure 31–6. Blunt-nosed stingray, or raia (Brazil), *Dasyatis sayi*. (Courtesy of Bruce W. Halstead and the World Life Research Institute, California.)

Figure 31–7. The puffer fish, *Arophron meleagris*. (Courtesy of Sea World, Florida.)

Figure 31–8. The zebra, or lionfish, or turkeyfish, *Dendrochirus zebra*. (Courtesy of Sea World, Florida.)

Figure 31–9. The stonefish, *Synanjeca verrucosa*. (Courtesy of Sea World, Florida.)

PART 1

GENERAL INTRODUCTORY CHAPTERS

CHAPTER 1

A GENERAL APPROACH TO THE EMERGENCY MANAGEMENT OF POISONING

Lester M. Haddad, M. D., FACEP
James R. Roberts, M. D., FACEP

The emergency management of poisoning is currently undergoing critical reappraisal.[1] For example, an entire spectrum of opinion can presently be found in the medical literature with regard to gastric decontamination. The role of specific antidotes is continually evolving, and promising new antidotes are on the horizon. In order to provide the reader with an understanding of basic concepts, we herein present a traditional outline of the general approach to the emergency management of poisoning.

The final mortality statistics for poisoning and drug overdose, as published by the National Center for Health Statistics[2] (primarily a review of death certificates), attributes 9976 deaths in 1986 to poisoning: 4187 were accidental; 2796, intentional; 1449 caused by drug dependence; 553 from nondependent use of drugs; 30, homicidal; 5 from drug psychoses; and 956 from undetermined causes. Carbon monoxide remains the number one cause of toxic death, with 3664 fatalities. In contrast, the total number of poisoning deaths reported by the National Center for Health Statistics in 1978 was 12,171.

The National Institute of Drug Abuse also publishes morbidity and mortality statistics relating specifically to drugs of abuse, primarily through DAWN (Drug Abuse Warning Network), which surveys emergency department visits. In 1986, DAWN reported 119,163 drug-related emergency department visits and 4138 deaths related to drug abuse. In 1986, the DAWN survey revealed that cocaine was the drug most frequently involved in emergency department visits and was the third leading cause of drug-related death (outranked only by heroin/morphine and alcohol/drug combinations).[3]

The American Association of Poison Control Centers also publishes morbidity and mortality figures derived from information phone calls to the nation's poison control centers. The 1987 Annual Report of the AAPCC National Data Collection System collected 1,166,940 human exposure cases reported by 63 poison centers: 88.9 per cent were accidental, 77.5 per cent were by ingestion, and 74.5 per cent were managed at home or as outpatients.[4] Fatalities numbered 397, with the largest group being victims of tricyclic and other antidepressants (105), followed by analgesics (93), then stimulants and street drugs (54). The three leading causes of death reported by the AAPCC were carbon monoxide (28), cocaine (27), and amitriptyline (25).

Data from all three sources, however, cannot accurately measure the scope of human illness and injury from poisoning. For example, the data do not include the deaths by trauma, drowning, or fire of intoxicated patients; carbon monoxide deaths from fires; or medical complications from therapy, anesthesia, or adverse drug reactions. Morbidity (examples: heart disease specifically from nicotine and cocaine, cirrhosis from alcohol) or long-term effects of environmental hazards are not included and probably are impossible to quantify. Unintentional poisoning is currently the fifth leading cause of unintentional injury in the United States,[3] and the alarming increase in drug abuse and overdose in the United States reflects a worldwide trend.

Definition of Terms

Poisoning, as defined by Webster's Dictionary (1984), is "to injure or kill with 'poison,' a substance that through its chemical action usually kills, injures, or impairs an organism." Thus, *poisoning connotes clinical symptomatology.* Poisoning also implies that the toxic exposure was accidental (example: an elderly patient who misreads a label), unintentional (an inquisitive toddler or a child who gives drugs to a sibling when playing "doctor"), or unknown to the patient (the victim of an intended homicide).

In contrast, the term *overdose* implies an intentional toxic exposure, although this may occur either in the form of a suicide attempt or as an inadvertent overdose secondary to intentional drug abuse.

The age of the patient may or may not be helpful in identifying whether or not a toxic exposure was intentional. Poisoning occurs most commonly in the 1 to 5 year old age group and in elderly people. Overdose, motivated by suicidal intent or secondary gain or for purposes of abuse, is recognized from age 12 years through adulthood but should also be suspected in poisonings of children. The cause of toxic exposure from age 6 to 12 years, generally an unusual age for intentional poisoning or overdose, is often difficult to determine, and each case must be assessed individually. A critical decision to make is whether or not the toxic ingestion was intentional, in order to provide appropriate psychotherapy in follow-up care.

History

The history of poisons dates to antiquity; their usage originally was the province of ancient magicians and priests. It was once believed that poisons were mystical substances that would prove lethal to a guilty person while remaining harmless to someone innocent.

Perhaps the first documented recognition of the existence of poisons comes from Egypt. The Smith Papyrus (1600 BC) cites "the use of charms against snake poison."[5] The Hearst Medical Papyrus and the Ebers Papyrus refer to both poisonous and therapeutic agents and are considered to have been written about 1500 BC.

The recognition of poisonous fishes in biblical times is clearly depicted when in the Bible Moses admonishes the Israelites: "These you shall eat of all that are in the waters which have fins and scales; and whatsoever hath not fins and scales you may not eat, for it is unclean" (Deuteronomy 14:9–10).

Mithridates, King of Pontus, in the first century before Christ, in his quest for the universal antidote was the first person to develop antidotes.

The earliest recognized poisons were plant and animal poisons, used for murder or official executions. Plato reported the death of Socrates by hemlock (*Conium maculatum*). A 9 year old student wrote about his death succinctly: "Socrates was a Greek. He was a wise man. He went about the country telling people what they should be doing . . . they poisoned him."

In his work *De Venenis* in the thirteenth century, Peter of Abanos reviewed collections of Arabic thought and divided all poisons into the three Arabic categories of animal, vegetable, and mineral.

Paracelsus in the sixteenth century was the first to relate poisoning to dosage of the toxic substance. He is the author of the historic comment "Dosage alone determines poisoning."

Modern Era

Modern clinical approaches to the field of toxicology were initiated primarily in the specialty of pediatrics. In 1952, the American Academy of Pediatrics established an Accident Prevention Committee. The Committee's first task was to survey the Academy's then 3000 members for information on the most common household factors associated with children's accidents. This survey unearthed an unexpected finding, which surprised the Academy's members: 50 per cent of the reported accidents involved some type of poisoning.[6]

Analysis of the poisoning cases showed that most were nonfatal and were caused by common household agents and over-the-counter and prescription drugs. Flavored children's aspirin, which had been introduced in the mid-1940s at a dosage of 2.5 grains (150 mg) in bottle holding 100 or more tablets, was responsible for 25 per cent of the poisoning in children under 5 years of age, with an annual mortality of approximately 400 patients. Dr. Jay M. Arena, a pediatrician at Duke University, worked with the Plough Company, makers of St. Joseph's Aspirin, to develop the safety closure cap.[7] Use of the safety closure cap, which was introduced in 1959, was finally made mandatory by Federal law in 1972, the same year Dr. Arena served as president of the American Academy of Pediatrics. This cap over the years has eliminated aspirin as a major factor in childhood poisoning, as well as helped reduce the overall incidence of death from childhood poisoning. In 1977, for example, only 2 deaths from aspirin in children under 5 years of age were reported, and the overall incidence of poisoning deaths in 1980 fell to under 100 in children under 5 years of age.

On October 21, 1958, the first meeting of the American Association of Poison Control Centers was held in Chicago. The AAPCC has been a leader in the poison control movement and has done an outstanding job in developing standards. Recently it has been especially active in developing standards for the proper rendering of poison information by regional poison centers.[8]

Death by drug overdose became almost commonplace in the late 1950s and early 1960s, typified by the tragic death of Marilyn Monroe at age 36 years on August 4, 1962 from an overdose of barbiturates. The use of dialysis for removal of drugs was introduced and became accepted as a therapeutic regimen primarily through the work of the nephrologist George Schreiner at Georgetown University.[9]

The nationwide growth of hospital emergency departments and the proliferation of LSD, Quaaludes, and other street drugs in the late 1960s necessitated rapid involvement in toxicology by emergency physicians. In fact, 99 per cent of all significant poisonings present first to an emergency department.[10] Microfiche systems such as POISINDEX[11] did much to disseminate poison information to hospitals throughout the United States. In 1978, the American College of Emergency Physicians established its Committee on Toxicology and has been active in improving standards of care in poison treatment.

There has been considerable improvement in the management of the toxicologic patient in the past 10 years, primarily as a result of the development of regional poison centers and emergency medical service systems, the burgeoning specialty of emergency medicine and improved emergency department care, and greater access to laboratory diagnostic studies. A recent review of 90 inpatients at the Boston Children's Hospital in 1981 and 1982 revealed that 85 per cent of the patients had gastric lavage or emesis, and 69 per cent had a positive drug screen.[12] The use of ipecac or gastric lavage/charcoal/cathartic has become established as a cornerstone of emergency department management of the toxicologic patient.[12]

The American Board of Medical Toxicology has developed a certification examination in toxicology. Clinical fellowships in toxicology are now coming into vogue.

Emergency Medicine was established as the 22nd primary medical specialty by the American Board of Medical Specialties on September 21, 1989, and the American College of Emergency Physicians created a section on toxicology that same month.

The future should bring further development and recognition of the subspecialty of toxicology, as emergency physicians, pediatricians, internists, and others refine this exciting and dynamic new field.

DIAGNOSIS AND GENERAL APPROACH

GENERAL APPROACH

The diagnosis of poisoning may be completely straightforward, or it may be most difficult to ascertain. The diagnosis is obvious in the child who ingests mother's iron tablets in her presence. It is not rare for the diagnosis to be made in the hospital when a drug screen has been ordered as an afterthought, after a patient has been admitted to a psychiatric hospital, or even after death. Patients or family who are embarrassed about drug addiction or fear legal reprisal may purposefully withhold information from the physician.

Any patient who presents with multisystem involvement of unknown etiology should be suspected of poisoning until proved otherwise. In addition, poisoning or overdose should always be considered in the following: any adult or child with an unexplained change in mental status; patients with head injury; a psychiatric patient with sudden decompensation; a trauma victim (especially a young individual or when other circumstances do not offer a plausible cause for a motor vehicle accident or fall); a young patient with chest pain or life-threatening arrhythmia or any patient with an arrhythmia of unknown etiology; and patients rescued from a fire or found symptomatic in a work environment where chemicals or other toxins are present. Patients who have a metabolic acidosis of unknown etiology likewise should be evaluated for poisoning. Children with unexplained lethargy, neurologic symptoms, bizarre behavior, and other puzzling presentations must be evaluated with respect to poisoning. *In summary, the clinician must main-*

tain a high index of suspicion to be able to arrive at the often difficult diagnosis of poisoning.

Patients often present with exposure to commonly available household products that are nontoxic, such as those listed in Table 1–1. The poison information center is usually the best resource to aid the physician in determining toxicity of household products. If ingestion produces no symptomatology, aggressive therapy is unnecessary, and the patient may be reassured and sent home for observation.

The general approach to the poisoning patient may be divided into seven phases:

- 1. Emergency management
- 2. Clinical evaluation
- 3. Elimination of poison from the gastrointestinal tract, skin, eyes, or the site of exposure in inhalation poisoning
- 4. Administration of a specific antidote (if available)
- 5. Elimination of the absorbed substance
- 6. Supportive therapy
- 7. Observation and disposition

1. EMERGENCY MANAGEMENT

Adequate ventilation and perfusion must be established in the critical patient before specific evaluation or therapy for overdose is begun. Patients presenting with a history or signs and symptoms of overdose should be given priority evaluation and placed in an area of the emergency room that allows continuous monitoring and observation. Since the clinical course of poisoning is unpredictable and decompensation is often precipitous, in all but the most clearly benign overdoses an intravenous infusion of normal saline should be begun. The patient should be placed on a cardiac monitor, and oxygen should be administered following blood gas determination (if possible). A patient may present in cardiac arrest, and not until the patient is resuscitated and evaluation is completed is the cause of the arrest identified as poisoning.

All patients in coma should be given naloxone hydrochloride (2 mg in an adult, up to 0.1 mg per kg in a child) intravenously. Since hypoglycemia is often a cause of coma or altered mental status, all patients presenting in such manner should be given an intravenous bolus of 1 ml per kg of 50 per cent glucose. Infants and children should be given glucose in only 10 to 20 per cent concentrations. Blood for glucose determination and appropriate blood and toxicologic studies should be obtained before glucose or other medications are administered. Many authorities also routinely administer thiamine, 100 mg intramuscularly, especially if supplemental glucose has been given or the patient has

Table 1–1. NONTOXIC INGESTIONS

abrasives	deodorizers, spray and refrigerator	perfumes
adhesives	Elmer's glue	petroleum jelly (Vaseline)
antacids	Etch-A-Sketch	Play-Doh
antibiotics	fabric softeners	Polaroid picture coating fluid
baby product cosmetics	fish bowl additives	porous tip marking pens
ballpoint pen inks	glues and pastes	Prussian blue (ferricyanide)
bathtub floating toys	hand lotions and creams	putty (less than 2 oz)
bath oil (castor oil and perfume)	3% hydrogen peroxide, medicinal	rubber cement
birth control pills	incense	sachets (essential oils, powder)
bleach (less than 5% sodium hypochlorite)	indelible markers	shampoos (liquid)
body conditioners	ink (black, blue)	shaving creams and lotions
bubble bath soaps (detergents)	iodophil disinfectant	soap and soap products
calamine lotion	laxatives	spackles
candles (beeswax or paraffin)	lipstick	suntan preparations
chalk (calcium carbonate)	lubricant	sweetening agents (saccharin)
cigarettes or cigars (nicotine)	Magic Markers	teething rings (water sterility)
colognes	makeup (eye, liquid, facial)	thermometers (mercury)
cosmetics	matches	toothpaste with or without fluoride
crayons marked AP, CP	mineral oil	toy pistol caps (potassium chlorate)
dehumidifying packets (silica or charcoal)	modeling clay	vitamins with or without fluoride
deodorants	newspaper	watercolors
	pencil (graphite lead, coloring)	zinc oxide
		zirconium oxide

(Adapted from Mofenson HC, Greensher J: The non-toxic ingestion. Pediatr Clin North Am *17*:583, 1970.)

a history of alcoholism. In hospitals that do not routinely record methemoglobin levels as a routine part of arterial blood gases, this is a convenient time to perform the methemoglobinemia filter paper test in patients who appear cyanotic. A methemoglobin level of 15 mg per dl or greater is present if a drop of the patient's blood turns chocolate brown when placed on filter paper. Physostigmine or central nervous stimulants are *not* used as a general antidote in the comatose patient.

2. CLINICAL EVALUATION

A thorough history and physical examination are critical to the diagnosis of the toxicologic patient, and laboratory tests are helpful in rounding out the assessment of the patient. While the initial manifestations of poisoning and overdose are legion, *a patient with significant poisoning often presents with coma, cardiac arrhythmia, metabolic acidosis, seizures, and/or gastrointestinal disturbance, either together as symptom complexes or as isolated events.* For example, mercury or iron ingestion initially results in gastrointestinal symptoms alone, whereas patients with tricyclic antidepressant overdose may present with coma, cardiac arrhythmia, and seizures. Symptom complexes, or *toxidromes,* may give clues to an unknown poisoning[13] (Table 1–2). *Hepatic, renal, respiratory, and hematologic disturbances are generally delayed manifestations of poisoning.*

The clinical evaluation, in addition to the history, physical examination, and laboratory studies, includes an assessment of the five major modes of presentation, in order to properly diagnose and manage poisoning.

History

The primary goal is to identify the toxic agent when one suspects poisoning or drug overdose. Prior medical and psychiatric history, current medications, and allergies should be obtained from family or friends if the patient is unable to relate the information. Often the old records or previous emergency department charts offer valuable information. A prior history of drug overdose should always be sought. An occupational or vocational history may suggest a toxic exposure.

The EMS Paramedics can be a most valuable source of information in obtaining the history of the event. Paramedics should be questioned about the specific circumstances they encountered when arriving on the scene, whether the noncomatose patient offered any history, whether empty bottles were found nearby, or whether there was evidence of trauma or inhalation exposure. It should be determined whether any home remedies were administered—the cure may have been worse than the disease. Is the patient on a special diet, using vitamins or health foods or over-the-counter medications? The history from the patient is often inaccurate, however, owing to such factors as fear, confusion, or disorientation. A patient who has ingested a street drug may be totally unaware of what actually has been taken.

Does the patient have two simultaneous disorders? For example, an accident victim may have had the accident because of an overdose. Often an intoxicated patient will have underlying trauma, such as a fall down the stairs. Or a patient with an overdose may develop an acute episode of diabetic ketoacidosis.

Accurate statistics are lacking, but one review reported that a careful history and physical examination and routine laboratory analyses were sufficient to identify the *principal* drug involved in self-poisoning in 86 per cent of cases.[14] Often, however, drugs or toxins are not identified by the clinical history alone, and clinicians can be misled if they rely only on the history. In an analysis of 140 drug overdoses, one investigator reported that drugs often are not taken, or cannot be detected by routine screening; or unsuspected drugs frequently are the culprit; or the history of drug ingestion may be totally incorrect and not the cause of the current condition. Patients both exaggerate and underestimate the variety and amount of drug ingested.[15]

Physical Examination

The physical examination can help determine the extent of poisoning and may reveal the presence of a toxic syndrome, of any underlying disease, and of concomitant trauma.

Vital Signs. As part of the initial evaluation, all patients must have a complete record

Table 1–2. EXAMPLES OF SYMPTOM COMPLEXES, OR TOXIDROMES

TOXIDROME OR COMPLEX	CONSCIOUSNESS	RESPIRATIONS	PUPILS	OTHER	POSSIBLE TOXIC AGENT
Cholinergic	Coma	⇅	Pinpoint	Fasciculations Incontinence Salivation, wheezing Lacrimation Bradycardia	Organophosphate insecticides, carbamates, nicotine
Anticholinergic	Agitated, hallucinating	↑	Dilated	Fever, flushing Dry skin and mucous membranes Urinary retention	Anticholinergics (Atropine, Jimson weed) (Antihistamines)
Opioid	Coma	↓	Pinpoint	Tracks Hypothermia Hypotension	Opiates, Lomotil, Pentazocine, Darvon
Structural	Coma	Apneustic	Pinpoint	Decerebrate Babinski sign	Pontine (brain stem) structural lesions
Extrapyramidal	Awake	↑	—	Torsion head/neck	Phenothiazines, haloperidol
Phenothiazine	Coma	↓	Pinpoint	Cardiac arrhythmia Orthostatic hypotension, anticholinergic findings	Phenothiazines
Tricyclic antidepressant	Coma (initially agitated)	↓	Dilated	Cardiac arrhythmia Convulsions Hypotension QT interval prolongation Cardiac conduction defect Myoclonus, hyperreflexia	Tricyclic antidepressants
Uremia	Coma	↑	—	Uremic frost Detectable shunt Hyperkalemia Acidosis	(Uremia)
Sedative/hypnotic	Coma	↓	Dilated	Hypothermia Decreases reflexes Hypotension	Sedatives, barbiturates
Salicylates	Semicoma, agitation	↑	—	Diaphoresis Tinnitus Agitation Alkalosis (early) Acidosis (late) Fever	Salicylates Oil of wintergreen
Sympathomimetic	Agitated, hallucinations	↑	Dilated	Seizures Tachycardia Hypertension Diaphoresis Metabolic acidosis Tremor Hyperreflexic	Cocaine Theophylline Amphetamines Caffeine

of initial vital signs and these must be repeated and recorded frequently throughout the hospital stay. An extremely important vital sign in toxicology is the *temperature*, and obtaining a core temperature is often necessary. An elevated temperature can occur with a number of ingestions and systemic disorders, but it is the hallmark of poisoning with salicylates, cocaine, anticholinergics, dinitrophenols, and monoamine oxidase inhibitors. Occasionally life-threatening malignant hyperthermia is the result of drug overdose. Hypothermia can be present because of exposure or hypoglycemia, or it can result from overdose from a number of agents, especially barbiturates, narcotics, sedative-hypnotics, and phenothiazines. Bradycardia can be seen with digitalis, cholinergics, beta-blockers, and calcium-entry blockers, but also it can be found with spinal cord or head trauma or hypothermia. Hypertension is characteristic of cocaine, phencyclidine, amphetamines, and sympathomimetics. An overdose of almost any drug may result in hypotension or tachycardia.

Skin. The skin should be examined for needle tracks, burns, bruises, or lacerations. Needle tracks may be confined to the groin or other areas not readily visible. A "boiled lobster" appearance suggests borate poisoning, particularly in a child who may have ingested roach powder insecticide. Flushing suggests an allergic reaction, niacin, anticholinergic poisoning, fever, the toxic shock syndrome, or an alcohol-disulfiram reaction.

Diaphoresis points to hypoglycemia, organophosphate or salicylate poisoning, a severe extrapyramidal reaction, acetaminophen ingestion, cocaine toxicity, hyperthyroidism, or drug or alcohol withdrawal. Jaundice and hepatic coma suggest causes other than poisoning, but if the patient has been transferred from an outlying hospital, delayed hepatic failure could result from poisoning, such as acetaminophen, carbon tetrachloride, or arsenic. Petechiae and ecchymoses suggest a coagulopathy, a coumadin or aspirin overdose, or meningococcemia. Myxedema or hypocalcemia should be suspected in a patient with a thyroidectomy scar. Bullous lesions are secondary to skin hypoxia or prolonged pressure and are seen with most sedative-hypnotics (especially barbiturates), carbon monoxide poisoning, and thermal burns. Bullous lesions or soft tissue swelling demands an evaluation for rhabdomyolysis, a common finding in patients with malignant hyperthermia or prolonged coma.

Breath. It is important to smell the patient's breath. Alcohol is probably the most common odor detected on the breath of an overdose patient. The accurate identification of other odors varies greatly among physicians. A fruity odor may be detectable with diabetic ketoacidosis, but ketosis is also seen with isopropyl alcohol ingestion. If the breath smells like silver polish, consider cyanide poisoning. A cleaning fluid smell suggests carbon tetrachloride. Phenol, camphor, paraldehyde, hydrogen sulfide, disulfiram, methyl salicylate, ether, turpentine, gasoline, and organophosphate insecticides all have a characteristic odor. Arsenic smells like garlic.

ENT. An ear, nose, and throat examination may disclose hidden needle marks (ears), or a nasal examination may suggest chronic snorting of cocaine. An edematous, often elongated uvula is highly suggestive of marijuana abuse.[16]

Lungs. Lung auscultation may offer diagnostic clues. In tricyclic antidepressant or narcotic overdose, pulmonary edema may be a complication, and in all overdose patients, aspiration pneumonitis is a possibility. Wheezing, in addition to being heard in asthma and allergic response, is noted in organophosphate poisoning, inhalation of toxic gases, and cardiogenic pulmonary edema from myocardial depressants. Auscultation may reveal a pneumothorax secondary to trauma. Mediastinal emphysema from marijuana or crack cocaine smoking also may be detected by auscultation.

Heart. The heart is examined in the usual manner. An arrhythmia in a young patient can suggest overdose, especially cocaine, or an electrolyte disturbance. Sinus tachycardia is an indirect tip to fever, hypoxia, or hypotension but also is seen in overdose with sympathomimetics or anticholinergics. Atrial fibrillation may be noted during an ethanol binge ("holiday heart" syndrome).[17] A murmur may signify endocarditis in an intravenous drug abuser.

Abdomen. An examination of the abdomen may reveal an adynamic ileus, common in many serious overdoses. A boardlike abdomen with the history of spider bite indicates black widow envenomation. Evidence of trauma over the upper abdomen can suggest a ruptured spleen or liver laceration. A distended abdomen may signal perforation from acid ingestion or ischemic bowel. In patients with abdominal pain, a surgical abdomen must be ruled out. Hepatomegaly suggests an etiology for coma other than poisoning, such as Reye's syndrome.

Neurologic. All patients should be evaluated with a careful neurologic examination. Issues of major concern are concomitant head and spinal cord trauma. Reflexes should be examined carefully for focality. The neurologic examination is discussed under assessment of coma.

Extremities. Evaluate the extremities to detect thrombophlebitis, fracture or dislocation, or vascular insufficiency. Rhabdomyolysis and the compartment syndrome are concerns in overdose patients, especially those with prolonged coma or underlying trauma.

Assessment of Major Toxic Signs

The acute toxicologic patient may present in one of five major modes: coma, cardiac arrhythmia, metabolic acidosis, gastrointestinal disturbances, and seizures.

Coma

One of the most common manifestations of acute poisoning is coma. The principles of managing coma are relatively straightforward. Patients in coma must be stabilized initially by establishment of an airway, insertion of an intravenous line with normal saline, and resuscitation if necessary. In general, comatose patients should be intubated. Draw blood and order appropriate studies to rule out other causes of coma. Save urine and the initial gastric aspirate. Oxygen, dextrose, and naloxone (Narcan) should be administered as discussed.

The clinical evaluation of the comatose patient[17] is invaluable not only in providing diagnostic clues but also in providing a baseline for repeated clinical assessment.

Level of consciousness. Consciousness is defined as an awareness of self and environment. Coma is defined as unarousable unresponsiveness.[17] Wakefulness is having the ability to be aroused. These functions are mediated by the ascending reticular activating system, a tract that courses through the diencephalon, midbrain, and pons (the brain stem).[17] Diseases produce coma either by diffusely affecting the brain or by directly encroaching upon the brain stem. This may be effected by (1) a supratentorial mass lesion, such as a subdural hematoma; (2) a brain stem lesion (uncommon); or (3) metabolic disorders that widely depress or interrupt brain function.[17]

Other causes of coma, such as head trauma, cardiovascular accident, anoxia, meningitis, Reye's syndrome, hypothermia, and diabetes must be ruled out or, if present, must be treated.

Supratentorial structural lesions are suggested by a rapid progression of signs, such as changes in respiratory pattern, disconjugate gaze, lateralizing signs, loss of doll's eyes movements, and other signs of trauma in the patient.

A metabolic cause of coma is indicated by the persistence of the pupillary light reflex; a depression of respiration and consciousness more pronounced than other neurologic signs; coma preceded by altered mental states; asterixis, fasciculations, or both; presence of a ciliospinal reflex; and extracranial signs such as jaundice or uremic frost.[17]

Repeated assessment of the comatose patient is critical to proper management of the poisoned patient.

Pupils. Evaluation of the patient's pupils is most helpful. Midpoint fixed pupils or unilateral dilated pupils suggest a structural lesion. Pinpoint pupils are significant in that they suggest overdose by opiates, clonidine, organophosphate insecticides, chloral hydrate, phenothiazines, or nicotine; the use of pilocarpine eye drops; or a structural pontine lesion. Dilated pupils are nonspecific.

Respirations. Review the pattern of breathing in your patient. Posthyperventilation apnea, Cheyne-Stokes respirations, apneustic breathing, and ataxic breathing strongly suggest a structural lesion as the etiology of the patient's coma. Whereas central neurogenic hyperventilation is a classic presentation of brain stem injury, the differential diagnosis of rapid, deep breathing is a challenge in itself. Salicylate poisoning, dinitrophenol insecticide poisoning, Kussmaul's breathing in the diabetic, pulmonary embolus, carbon monoxide poisoning, or hypoxia from any cause may produce a similar pattern. Compensatory hyperventilation may accompany methanol, ethylene glycol, or other toxin-producing metabolic acidosis. Respiratory arrest is a common means of presentation in the overdose patient.

Ocular Movements. A disturbance of ocular movements (for example: loss of doll's eyes movements) suggests a structural lesion.

Motor Function. Decorticate and decerebrate posturing may suggest a structural lesion, but these may also be seen in a patient with a metabolic cause of coma (see Chapter 11).

It is important to realize that patients with drug overdose initially may appear brain dead, with fixed, dilated pupils; unresponsive coma; and absent cold caloric response, yet recover fully when the offending substance is metabolized.

Cardiac Arrhythmia

Obtain an electrocardiogram for any patient with significant poisoning and place the person on a cardiac monitor. A patient may not have arrhythmia, but the electrocardiogram can provide important diagnostic clues, such as a prolonged QT interval in phenothiazine overdose or a widened QRS interval in tricyclic antidepressant, quinine, or quinidine poisoning. Whereas many drugs cause a sinus tachycardia, sinus bradycardia is significant, as discussed. Table 1–3 lists some toxic causes of cardiac arrhythmia.

The patient with life-threatening ventricular arrhythmia or cardiac arrest should be managed using the basic principles of advanced cardiac life support. If cyclic antidepressant overdose is suspected, sodium bicarbonate is indicated for ventricular arrhythmia or for conduction disturbances. In a referral patient with ventricular arrhythmia or cardiac arrest, the etiology of arrhythmia may be hyperkalemia, as renal failure may have already ensued, and intravenous sodium bicarbonate or glucose/insulin or calcium chloride may be warranted. In all toxic patients, correction of hypoxia, metabolic acidosis, and fluid or electrolyte disturbance will serve to reduce the incidence of cardiac arrhythmias (see Chapter 4).

Metabolic Acidosis

Causes of a high anion gap metabolic acidosis are listed in Table 1–4. Chronic toluene sniffing may produce a hyperchloremic metabolic acidosis. Metabolic acidosis should be considered to be of toxicologic origin and dealt with appropriately. The assessment of metabolic acidosis must include not only arterial blood gas analysis but also determinations of serum sodium, potassium, chloride, carbon dioxide, BUN, glucose, acetone, serum osmolality, and urine pH. Determining the anion gap[18] in the differential diagnosis of poisoning is essential.

Table 1–3. COMMON TOXIC CAUSES OF CARDIAC ARRHYTHMIA

tricyclic antidepressants	quinine
phenothiazines	chloroquine
carbon monoxide	chloral hydrate
cyanide	phenol
cocaine	arsenic
digitalis	dinitrophenols
calcium channel blockers	fluoroacetate
beta-blockers	succinylcholine chloride
physostigmine	ethanol
clonidine	

Table 1–4. CAUSES OF A HIGH ANION GAP METABOLIC ACIDOSIS

Uremia
Diabetic ketoacidosis
Lactic acidosis
Salicylate toxicity
Methanol poisoning
Ethylene glycol poisoning
Nondiabetic alcoholic ketoacidosis
Paraldehyde toxicity
Cyanide poisoning
Isoniazid overdose
Iron overdose

The serum osmolality can be measured either directly by determining the freezing point, or by calculation. The formula for calculating osmolality is

$$\text{Serum osmolality} = 2 \times \text{Na (mEq/L)} + \frac{\text{BUN (mg/dl)}}{2.8} + \frac{\text{glucose (mg/dl)}}{18}$$

The normal serum osmolality is 280 to 295 milliosmols (mOsm). An osmometer measurement indicating a serum osmolality that is more than 10 mOsm greater than the calculated osmolality is termed an osmolal gap, and this suggests the presence of osmotically active substances that are not accounted for by the calculated osmolality. Substances such as ethyl alcohol, methanol, isopropyl alcohol, ethylene glycol, glycerol, or mannitol produce an increase in the measured osmolality over the calculated osmolality. Clinically, alcohols are the most common cause of an elevated osmolal gap. A substance contributes to osmolality only if it achieves relatively high blood levels and has a low molecular weight. Most drugs or intoxicants cannot be detected by using the osmolal gap (see Chapters 6 and 7).

Gastrointestinal Disturbance

Iron, mercury, lithium, phosphorus, arsenic, mushrooms, theophylline, colchicine, fluoride, and organophosphate poisoning are some common toxic causes of vomiting or diarrhea or both. The patient with iron poisoning will have severe, repeated episodes of vomiting and may develop gastrointestinal hemorrhage. Arsenic poisoning characteristically causes massive diarrhea, and patients with theophylline poisoning typically have persistent emesis. A patient with mercury poisoning usually has marked salivation and mucous-type diarrhea, with later development of hemorrhagic colitis. One of the most striking presentations is caused by phosphorus poisoning, which produces luminescent vomitus and flatus.

The management of gastrointestinal disturbances is specific to each agent. Hypovolemia should be treated by fluid replacement with normal saline. Blood should be transfused when there is hemorrhage. It is important to control persistent vomiting with the judicious use of parenteral antiemetics to avoid a Mallory-Weiss tear, and to limit fluid and electrolyte depletion.

Seizures

Common agents causing seizures are listed in Table 1–5. Almost any drug or toxin in massive overdose is capable of producing a seizure. Delayed seizures occurring during a recovery period may be a sign of drug or alcohol withdrawal.

Seizures should be managed first by establishing an airway and oxygenation. Simple isolated seizures may require only observation and supportive care, whereas repetitive seizures or status epilepticus can be life-threatening and should be treated aggressively. Some seizures are particularly difficult to control, such as those seen with theophylline or amoxapine overdose. Other drug-induced seizures require specific maneuvers, such as pyridoxine for isoniazid-induced seizures, or naloxone for propoxyphene-induced seizures (Table 1–6). Head trauma, eclampsia, meningitis, malignant hypertension, hypoxia, or hypoglycemia should always be considered in any patient experiencing a seizure.

Table 1–5. COMMON TOXIC CAUSES OF SEIZURES

amoxapine	LSD
anticholinergics	oral hypoglycemics
camphor	parathion
carbon monoxide	phencyclidine
cocaine	phenothiazines
ergotamine	propoxyphene hydrochloride
insulin	propranolol
isoniazid	strychnine
lead	theophylline
lindane	tricyclic antidepressants
lithium	

The standard regimen for seizure control in an unknown overdose is to use full therapeutic doses of benzodiazepines, such as diazepam or lorazepam, followed by phenytoin or phenobarbital or both. For resistant life-threatening status epilepticus unresponsive to the usual measures, paralysis with EEG monitoring and pentobarbital-induced coma and/or the addition of pancuronium bromide may be necessary (Table 1–7).

Laboratory Evaluation

In every significant poisoning or overdose, routine studies include a complete blood count (CBC), levels of serum electrolytes, BUN, glucose, arterial blood gases, prothrombin time, and a 12-lead electrocardiogram. Arterial blood gas analysis is necessary to evaluate respiratory status and acid/base abnormalities, especially in the comatose patient or one with seizures. A baseline prothrombin time is helpful in assessing delayed hepatic effects, because the prothrombin time is often the earliest indication of hepatotoxicity. In selected cases, specific studies are of diagnostic and therapeutic significance, such as the use of hepatic enzymes to evaluate acetaminophen toxicity and serum calcium levels in serious hydrofluoric acid burns.

It is important to maintain a proper perspective in the use of the toxicology drug screen and not to overemphasize its value in treating the routine overdose. In a recent study of 209 cases, unexpected toxicology findings on the drug screen led to changes in therapy in only 3 cases, and *none* of these changes appeared to have a major impact on outcome.[19] A far greater yield than the drug screen is obtained by determining acetaminophen, salicylate, and ethanol levels, as these are common principal and co-ingested drugs.

Furthermore, no drug screen is ever complete: Table 1–8 lists common substances not routinely identified in many so-called complete drug screens. The old adage, "Treat the patient, not the lab" is still true today. In

Table 1–6. SPECIFIC INTERVENTIONS FOR TOXIC-RELATED SEIZURES

DRUG/TOXIN-RELATED CONDITION	TREATMENT
Insulin/oral hypoglycemics	Glucose
Carbon monoxide* Hypoxia	Oxygen
Hydrofluoric acid Ethylene glycol–induced hypocalcemia† Phosphate–induced hypocalcemia† Hypoparathyroidism	Calcium chloride
Lead	BAL/EDTA
Isoniazid	Pyridoxine
Propoxyphene (Darvon)	Naloxone
Seizure caused by drug-induced ventricular fibrillation	Defibrillation
Severe hyponatremia	Hypertonic saline
Increased intracranial pressure‡	Lidocaine
Severe or malignant hypertension§	Nitroprusside/phentolamine

The drugs in this table are not generally considered anticonvulsants and are not meant to replace the standard therapy for seizures. However, these may be effective when standard therapy fails or as an adjunct to the treatment outlined in Table 1–7.

*May require hyperbaric oxygen.
†Extremely rare.
‡Secondary to tumor or trauma.
§Secondary to amphetamines/cocaine, MAO inhibitor.

Table 1–7. MANAGEMENT OF STATUS EPILEPTICUS*

DRUG OF CHOICE	INITIAL IV DOSE	COMMENTS
1. Lorazepam OR	adults: 2 mg children: 0.05 mg/kg	Lorazepam may have less respiratory depression than diazepam. Assisted ventilation may be necessary Second drug necessary, such as phenytoin or barbiturate, to control EEG seizure activity
Diazepam	adults: 5–10 mg children: 0.25–0.5 mg/kg	IV infusion rate in adults of 0.1 mg/kg/hr: diazepam, 100 mg, diluted in 500 ml D5W, infused at 40 ml/hr Second drug necessary to control EEG seizure activity.
2. Phenytoin AND/OR	15 mg/kg	Administer under EKG monitoring Rapid infusion may produce hypotension or bradycardia or ventricular arrhythmia: infusion not to exceed 40 mg/min
Phenobarbital	15 mg/kg	Infusion rate not to exceed 30 mg/min in children, 50 mg/min in adults
3. FOR REFRACTORY STATUS EPILEPTICUS:		
Pentobarbital AND AS NEEDED	5 mg/kg IV, then 25–50 mg IV q 5 min	Titration end-point of EEG evidence of burst suppression every 15 sec Maintenance infusion of 5 mg/kg/hr
Pancuronium bromide	0.1 mg/kg	Successful in controlling motor activity only; EEG control of electrical seizure activity with another agent mandatory, such as phenytoin and/or barbiturate; ventilatory support required.

*Dosages listed may require modification according to specific clinical conditions.

Table 1–8. A PARTIAL LIST OF DRUGS AND TOXINS NOT COMMONLY DETECTED WITH ROUTINE DRUG SCREENING

ethylene glycol
digitalis
lithium
carbon monoxide
hydrocarbons
most antiarrhythmics
most antihypertensive medications
venom
LSD
newer benzodiazepines (e.g., lorazepam)
organophosphates/carbamates
isoniazid
cyanide
heavy metals (arsenic, mercury, thallium, and so on)
iron
paraquat
poisonous mushrooms
hypoglycemics

proper perspective, however, the laboratory can help in the diagnosis and management of the poisoning victim, such as determining whether drug ingestion is truly the cause of coma.

Any significant emergency department should have access to the following quantitative toxicologic studies on a 24-hour basis: acetaminophen, barbiturate, phenytoin, salicylate, iron, theophylline, ethanol, methemoglobin, serum cholinesterase, carboxyhemoglobin, methanol, ethylene glycol, and lithium. A blood ammonia level may be indicated to rule out Reye's syndrome or confirm hepatic coma from other causes. A serum pregnancy test is usually indicated in women of child-bearing age.

Whereas a specific blood level can direct therapy, treatment regimens are rarely dictated by serum levels alone, and in many instances qualitative rather than quantitative analysis is all that is required. For instance, one probably would not dialyze or institute aggressive therapy in a patient with a toxic lithium or theophylline level who is minimally symptomatic, nor alter therapy based on the cyclic antidepressant or benzodiazepine level.

However, when drugs form concretions or bezoars (examples: salicylates, iron, meprobamate, carbromal, barbiturates, glutethimide) in the stomach and produce prolonged or confusing symptoms, serial quantitative blood levels may be of diagnostic or therapeutic significance. Serial blood levels are also helpful in guiding hemodialysis therapy.

The intravenous drug abuser requires special blood testing, such as evaluation for the human immunodeficiency virus, a hepatitis profile, blood cultures for septicemia, and evaluation for rhabdomyolysis and myoglobinuria.

The urine is the best specimen to use for "screening" purposes. In patients with poisoning of unknown etiology, save all urine for the first 24 hours for diagnostic studies. Many agents, such as ethylene glycol, mercury, and carbon tetrachloride, can cause delayed renal failure. Urine pH monitoring is helpful in the management of salicylate overdose. A urine dipstick positive for blood in the absence of erythrocytes on the microscopic analysis usually means rhabdomyolysis.

The chest film is an aid for diagnosing aspiration pneumonia or pulmonary edema. A plain abdominal radiograph is seldom useful: potassium chloride, ferrous sulfate, and calcium carbonate are strongly radiopaque.[20] A computed tomography scan may be necessary if a structural central nervous system lesion is suspected. Finally, lumbar puncture may be indicated to rule out meningitis in a patient with fever and coma.

3. ELIMINATION OF POISON FROM THE EYES, SKIN, AND GASTROINTESTINAL TRACT

Aggressive removal of substances from the eyes, skin, and gastrointestinal tract may be necessary to limit toxic effects. In the event of inhalation poisoning, such as from carbon monoxide, hydrogen sulfide, or chlorine gas, removal of the patient from the exposure site and administration of 100 per cent oxygen is indicated.

Eyes. Caustic alkalis and acids should be removed from the eyes with copious irrigation for no less than 30 minutes with normal saline. Measuring the pH of the tears may direct further irrigation. All patients with eye exposures should be examined with a slit lamp and have visual acuity tested. In the event of significant caustic alkali exposure, ophthalmologic consultation is necessary.

Skin. Irritants, acids, and chemicals should be removed from the skin by copious irrigation for 15 to 30 minutes; caustic alkalis warrant irrigation for at least 30 minutes. A patient exposed to insecticide poisoning should immediately remove all clothing and shower for 30 minutes, as residual insecticide spray on the clothes will be continuously absorbed.

Gastrointestinal Tract. The majority of poisonings occur via the gastrointestinal tract. Perhaps the most controversial area of research in emergency medicine today is the approach to gastric decontamination. This area of management is presently undergoing critical reappraisal. Both the role of ipecac[21] and the routine use of gastric lavage[22, 23] have been questioned. Activated charcoal now has an undisputed role in the emergency management of poisoning,[1, 24] and serial administration of oral activated charcoal is now advocated in significant poisoning with agents such as cyclic antidepressants,[25] digitoxin,[26] phenobarbital,[27] and theophylline.[28]

Traditionally, it was recommended to induce emesis in the alert patient with syrup of ipecac; gastric lavage followed by activated charcoal was indicated for the comatose or lethargic patient.[29] Curtis and associates showed that activated charcoal/magnesium sulfate alone was superior to ipecac alone and ipecac/activated charcoal in inhibiting the absorption of multiple aspirin tablets.[21] Kulig and colleagues, in a prospective study of 592 drug overdose patients, compared gastric emptying with no gastric emptying—without relation to the specific drug ingested—and suggested that gastric emptying is generally not of benefit unless gastric lavage is performed within 1 hour of ingestion.[22] This study, inconclusive as it may be with respect to any particular agent, certainly challenged the concept of performing gastric lavage on all comatose or lethargic patients with drug overdose. In a well-designed study by Tandberg and colleagues, gastric lavage appeared to be superior overall to ipecac-induced emesis, based on the per cent removal of an ingested marker drug (mean of 45 per cent for lavage versus 28 per cent for emesis).[30] However, the amount removed by each procedure varied greatly (19 to 68 per cent for lavage and 6 to 70 per cent for emesis), and in a few patients, emesis was more efficacious. Numerous studies on the efficacy of ipecac versus lavage have been published; each procedure has its advocates and data are conflicting. The selection of a gastric emptying procedure at present should be individualized and should be based on patient cooperation, the specific ingestion, and the patient's clinical state.

A toxin can be neutralized or eliminated from the gastrointestinal tract by the use of milk, syrup of ipecac, activated charcoal, gastric lavage, demulcents, neutralizers, and cathartics when appropriate.

Milk. Milk is an immediate first aid remedy that is readily available in the home. It is indicated promptly following ingestion of a caustic.

In fact, when a caller to the poison center reports that he or she has no syrup of ipecac, we advise the person to give milk to all awake patients who have ingested any toxic substance except phosphorus. Milk provides dilution, it is a demulcent, and its high protein content can provide a substrate for agents such as caustics. Milk does not affect the time of ipecac-induced emesis.[31] In addition, giving milk provides the caller, often a mother, with something to do, a tremendous psychologic support at a critical moment.

Water is an alternative to milk.

Syrup of Ipecac. Ever since Robertson showed in 1962 that 88 per cent of children had emesis within 30 minutes following use of ipecac,[32] syrup of ipecac has become the agent of choice for gastric emptying in the awake patient and remains so for the pediatric age group. Spontaneous emesis, frequently seen following the ingestion of many substances (iron, theophylline, salicylates), is ineffective in removing sufficient quantities of toxic material from the stomach.[33] Production of emesis by gagging or means of insertion of a blunt object in the throat is also ineffective.[34] Administration of copper sulfate[35, 36] or sodium chloride[37, 38] has been abandoned owing to the significant toxicity of these agents. Although apomorphine produces emesis the quickest, it has never been accepted because it produces central nervous depression and occasionally protracted vomiting.[39]

Ipecac is the dried root or rhizome of *Cephaelis ipecacuanha* and *acuminata,* plants indigenous to Brazil and Central America. The principal alkaloids are emetine, which is cardiotoxic, and cephaeline. Fluid extract of ipecac, 14 times as concentrated as syrup of ipecac, has been replaced because of its cardiotoxicity.

Syrup of ipecac has been a nonprescription drug since 1966, because of an excellent safety record. Syrup of ipecac has little acute toxicity when used in recommended dosages, but the chronic use of ipecac by patients with eating disorders has proved lethal.[40] Syrup of ipecac is sold over-the-counter in 15- and 30-ml containers; syrup of ipecac with an expired date also has been shown to be effective.[41]

Syrup of ipecac produces vomiting through stimulation of the chemoreceptor trigger zone of the central nervous system. The following dosages of syrup of ipecac are recommended: age 6 to 12 months, 10 ml;[42] age 1 to 12 years, 15 ml; and age 12 years to adulthood, 30 ml. A recent study indicated that the amount of fluid voume did not influence the number of patients having emesis following ipecac.[43] Syrup of ipecac is effective even following ingestion of antiemetic medications[44] and may be followed by activated charcoal without reducing its effectiveness.[45, 46]

A review of 23,790 calls to the Massachusetts Poison Control System showed that syrup of ipecac is safe for home use;[47] there was little use of ipecac without medical consultation (less than 1 per cent), with no complications.

Contraindications to the use of syrup of ipecac include caustic or petroleum distillate ingestion, impending or frank coma, or seizures.

Gastric Lavage. Ever since Matthew and associates showed in 1966 that gastric lavage and aspiration could remove over 200 mg of barbiturate within 4 hours of ingestion, and up to 20 gm of salicylate up to 9 hours after ingestion, gastric lavage followed by administration of activated charcoal and a cathartic has been a traditional cornerstone of therapy.[48] There is an increasing trend to administer charcoal prior to lavage in order to halt further absorption immediately, remove the drug-charcoal complex via gastric lavage and aspiration, and again administer charcoal, followed by a cathartic. We prefer to use charcoal/gastric lavage/charcoal over ipecac-induced emesis in cases of life-threatening overdoses, such as cyclic antidepressants, theophylline, salicylates, barbiturates, and lithium, and in symptomatic patients with an unknown overdose of drug(s). Lavage is preferred because patient compliance is not an issue, the 20 to 30 minute delay for ipecac to work may allow significant absorption, and charcoal can be administered easily via the lavage tube.

Major points about gastric lavage include:

1. Use the largest-bore tube possible. In adults, pass a premeasured No. 36 French Ewald tube and confirm the position before lavage.
2. Protect the airway. Endotracheal intubation is necessary in the comatose patient but not required in the awake patient (remove the lavage tube immediately in the awake patient who vomits during lavage, to allow the patient to protect the airway).
3. Tap water is sufficient for lavage in adults. Saline theoretically should be used in children since they are more susceptible to fluid and electrolyte imbalance. Warmed lavage fluid may have some benefit.
4. Place the patient in the head down, left lateral decubitus position.
5. Manually agitate the stomach during the lavage.
6. Use the oral route to avoid nasal trauma, but be gentle to avoid esophageal or pharyngeal injury.
7. Lavage until clear and instill charcoal before removing the tube.
8. Replace the lavage tube with a nasogastric tube if repeated doses of activated charcoal are to be used.

Although gastric lavage is considered most effective within 1 hour of ingestion,[22] because of delayed gastric emptying time with certain agents such as salicylates, cyclic antidepressants, and anticholinergics, gastric lavage may remove drugs hours after ingestion.

Endoscopy may be necessary for the management of concretions in the stomach if warm saline lavage with abdominal massage is ineffective.[49]

The decision whether or not to intubate in the lethargic or comatose but responsive patient or the patient with altered mental status is often difficult. Clinical judgment should decide whether nasotracheal intubation prior to lavage, with or without succinylcholine, *or* gastric lavage in the left lateral decubitus position with the medical staff in constant attendance is indicated. In one study, succinylcholine was determined safe[50] and may be useful in experienced hands.

In the awake asymptomatic or mildly symptomatic adult with a reliable history of either insignificant ingestion, or ingestion of a known substance that may be only mildly toxic, activated charcoal without gastric lavage is indicated.[22]

Contraindications to gastric lavage include caustic alkali ingestion.

Activated Charcoal. Activated charcoal has

an undisputed role in the management of the overdose patient.[24] There are no absolute contraindications to charcoal, but repeated doses in patients with ileus may predispose to vomiting. Charcoal alone will cause vomiting in about 10 to 15 per cent of patients. Charcoal will make gastroscopy impossible. Aspirated charcoal produces no direct pulmonary damage, but it is often mixed with oral bacteria and stomach acid. Aspirated charcoal may cause respiratory distress because of physical obstruction. Large amounts of vomited charcoal can impair vision enough to make tracheal intubation difficult.

Charcoal is the residue from the destructive distillation of various organic materials by burning such substances as wood, pulp, bone, starch, lactose, sucrose, and coconut shells.[24] The adsorptive capacity of charcoal is increased, or "activated," by treatment with substances such as steam or air at high temperatures (600 to 900° C). This process fragments carbon granules and creates a greater surface area for binding. The surface area of the standard activated charcoal now available is 950 m^2/gm. The new product Super-Char, or super-activated charcoal, has a surface area of up to 2500 to 3000 m^2/gm.

Maximum prevention of drug absorption occurs the sooner activated charcoal follows administration of the drug. One should also attempt to achieve an activated charcoal:drug ratio of at least 10:1.

An adult should be given 50 to 100 gm of activated charcoal mixed in 8 ounces of water. The pediatric dose is 1 gm per kg, or 25 to 50 gm in 4 ounces of water. Charcoal is traditionally mixed with a cathartic to hasten transit. Most drugs will be absorbed on the surface of activated charcoal. Substances with minimal adsorption are listed in Table 1–9.

Examples of commercially available activated charcoal preparations are (1) *Norit* USP (Activated Charcoal Powder USP), from American Norit Company of Jacksonville; (2) *Actidose* (premixed activated charcoal suspension with 70 per cent sorbitol; each 4-ounce bottle contains 25 gm of activated charcoal in 48 gm of sorbitol; each milliliter of the solution contains 208 mg of activated charcoal in 400 mg of sorbitol), from Paddock of Minneapolis; and (3) *Super Char Liquid* (premixed 30 gm of super-activated charcoal in sorbitol or aqueous solution), from Gulf Bio-Systems of Dallas.

Table 1–9. DRUGS OR TOXINS NOT EFFECTIVELY ADSORBED BY ACTIVATED CHARCOAL

alcohols	hydrocarbons
ethylene glycol	organophosphates/carbamates
lithium	cyanide
heavy metals	acids
iron	alkali caustics

N-Acetylcysteine (NAC) given concomitantly for acute acetaminophen overdose will be adsorbed by activated charcoal, but only minimally. Often it happens that one gives activated charcoal to overdose patients and finds later that they have co-ingested toxic doses of acetaminophen. Two approaches for this situation are to perform gastric lavage to remove the activated charcoal prior to NAC administration, or to increase the loading dose of NAC by 40 per cent to compensate for activated charcoal adsorption or repeat the NAC loading dose in 4 hours.[51]

Serial administration of oral activated charcoal has had a role in the inpatient management of overdoses of drugs that enter the enterohepatic circulation, such as cyclic antidepressants,[25] digitoxin,[26] and glutethimide.[52] Serial administration of activated charcoal can also recover drugs such as phenobarbital[27] and theophylline[28] that diffuse from the plasma into the gastrointestinal lumen. Serial charcoal (1 gm per kg q 4 hr) also may be indicated for digoxin,[53] cyclosporin,[54] and dapsone; [55] further indications no doubt will be forthcoming.

Neutralizers. There are specific instances in which a neutralizing agent instead of activated charcoal has empirically been clinically indicated:

Mercury Poisoning. Sodium formaldehyde sulfoxylate (20-gm ampule) is an effective neutralizing agent because it reduces mercuric chloride and other mercury salts to metallic mercury, which is considerably less soluble and thus nonabsorbable.

Iron Poisoning. Sodium bicarbonate lavage is indicated in iron poisoning because sodium bicarbonate converts the ferrous ion to ferrous carbonate, which is poorly absorbed. After lavage, 200 to 300 ml of the bicarbonate solution sould be left in the stomach.

Iodine Poisoning. A solution of 75 gm of starch in 1 liter of water provides an effective lavage solution for neutralization following iodine ingestion. Lavage should be continued until the gastric aspirate is no longer blue.

Strychnine, Nicotine, and Quinine Poisoning.

Potassium permanganate is an effective neutralizing agent. A 1:10,000 solution is prepared by dissolving a 100-mg tablet in 1 liter of water.

Demulcents. The most common demulcent is milk. An example of a demulcent used in the management of poisoning includes Mylanta or other antacids to provide symptomatic relief for the patient with acute gastritis from salicylate overdose.

Cathartics. Cathartics are given as a means of eliminating poisons from the gastrointestinal tract and to augment the passage of activated charcoal. An actual benefit of cathartics in decreasing morbidity and mortality has not been convincingly demonstrated. The most rapid and potent catharsis is achieved with the osmotic agent sorbitol (1 to 2 ml per kg of a 70 per cent solution).[56] Magnesium sulfate (Epsom salt) and magnesium citrate are also acceptable, but their onset of action is slower, and magnesium levels should be monitored in patients with renal failure. Cathartics, especially repeated or large doses of sorbitol, should be used with great caution in infants and in adults with cardiovascular instability. The osmosis-mediated fluid loss with sorbitol may cause hypotension or hypovolemic shock in these patients.[57] Recently a new form of catharsis, termed *whole bowel irrigation,* has been recommended as an efficient and rapid way to cleanse the bowel.[58] Its role in treating acute overdose is not yet defined. This procedure uses a nonabsorbable, osmotically active compound (such as polyethylene glycol, Golytely), and it may be especially useful in patients who have ingested large quantities of pills or substances that cannot be removed with emesis or lavage (such as sustained-release capsules, iron tablets, cocaine packets, "crack" vials, or lead pellets). This procedure produces voluminous diarrhea, and the large volume of fluid required for whole bowel irrigation (4 to 6 liters over 1 to 2 hours) usually necessitates instillation via a nasogastric tube.

4. ANTIDOTE ADMINISTRATION

Unfortunately, specific antidotes to drugs and poisons are uncommon. Table 1–10 lists some generally accepted antidotes. True antidotes are divided into physiologic and specific. Many "general" or "supportive" antidotes are also available—for example, activated charcoal or sodium bicarbonate. They are not antidotes in the true sense but are helpful in treating symptoms of overdose. Atropine and 2-PAM chloride, used in organophosphate poisoning, are examples of physiologic and specific antidotes, respectively. Organophosphates inhibit the enzyme cholinesterase, probably by phosphorylation. Toxic signs are considered to be an indirect consequence of this enzyme inactivation, for there is a local accumulation of acetylcholine. The clinical effects of organophosphate poisoning are thus, in effect, due to acetylcholine rather than the organophosphate directly. Atropine physiologically blocks acetylcholine, whereas 2-PAM chloride is a specific antidote for the organophosphates since it cleaves the alkyl phosphate parathion-cholinesterase bond and thus liberates (regenerates) cholinesterase and allows cholinesterase to metabolize acetylcholine.

An example of a general or nonspecific "antidote" is sodium bicarbonate. This drug will aid in the therapy for acidosis or for the treatment of hypotension or ventricular arrhythmias seen with tricyclic antidepressant overdose. Although bicarbonate may be considered an antidote, it does not have a specific physiologic effect on tricyclic antidepressants, nor does it in any way antagonize them in the true pharmacologic sense.

A new approach to antidote therapy is through the use of drug-binding antibodies. Antibodies capable of binding and neutralizing digitalis (Digibind) have dramatically altered the course of this once fatal poisoning.[59, 60] Some experimental antidotes that may significantly benefit selected overdoses are on the horizon. Flumazenil is currently being investigated as a benzodiazepine antagonist. Hydroxycobalamin and the chelating agent DMSA may soon be available in this country for the treatment of cyanide and heavy metal poisoning, respectively.

5. ELIMINATION OF ABSORBED SUBSTANCE

Methods available for the elimination of the absorbed substance when an antidote is not available include forced diuresis; acidification or alkalinization of the urine; dialysis and hemoperfusion; and a modality finding

Table 1–10. COMMON EMERGENCY ANTIDOTES

POISON	ANTIDOTE	ADULT DOSAGE*	COMMENTS
acetaminophen	*N*-Acetylcysteine	140 mg/kg initial dose, followed by 70 mg/kg q 4 hr × 17 doses	Most effective within 16 hr
arsenic	See mercury		
atropine	Physostigmine	Initial dose 0.5–2 mg (IV)	Can produce convulsions, bradycardia
beta-blockers	Glucagon	1 mg/ml ampule; 5–10 mg (IV) initially	Stimulates cyclic AMP synthesis, increasing myocardial contractility
calcium channel blockers	Calcium	Calcium chloride 10% up to 1 gm (10 ml) (IV) as initial dose	Each syringe contains 1 gm or 10 ml of 10% calcium chloride. Each ml contains 100 mg of calcium chloride, or 1.4 mEq of Ca^{++}
carbon monoxide	Oxygen		
cyanide	Amyl nitrate; *then*	Pearls every 2 min	Methemoglobin cyanide complex
	Sodium nitrite	10 ml of 3% solution over 3 min (IV) 0.33 ml (10 mg 3% sol)/kg initially for children	Causes hypotension. Dosage assumes normal hemoglobin
	Sodium thiosulfate	25% solution—50 ml (IV) over 10 min; 1.65 ml/kg for children	Forms harmless sodium thiocyanate
ethylene glycol	See methyl alcohol		
gold	See mercury		
iron	Deferoxamine	Initial dose: 40–90 mg/kg (IM) not to exceed 1 gm; 15 mg/kg/hr (IV)	Deferoxamine mesylate—forms excretable ferrioxamine complex
lead	Calcium disodium edetate	1 ampule/250 ml D5W over 1 hr	5-ml ampule (IV) 20% solution. Dilute to less than 3% solution—Calcium displaced by lead
mercury (arsenic, gold)	BAL (British antilewisite)	5 mg/kg (IM) as soon as possible	Each ml BAL in oil has dimercaprol, 100 mg, in 210 mg (21%) benzyl benzoate and 680 mg peanut oil—Forms stable, nontoxic, excretable cyclic compound
methyl alcohol (ethylene glycol)	Ethyl alcohol in conjunction with dialysis	1 ml/kg of 100% ethanol initially in glucose solution; dilute ethanol to 10%; maintain blood level of 100 mg/dl	Competes for alcohol dehydrogenase; prevents formation of formic acid, oxalates
nitrites	Methylene blue	0.2 ml/kg of 1% solution (IV) over 5 min	Often exchange transfusion is needed for severe methemoglobinemia
opiates, Darvon, Lomotil	Naloxone	0.4–2.0 mg (IV) 0.01 mg/kg (IV)—children	Naloxone—no respiratory depression (0.4 mg/1 ml ampule)
organophosphates	Atropine	Initial dose: 0.5–2 mg (IV) 0.05 mg/kg (IV) initially for children	Physiologic: Blocks acetylcholine. Up to 5 mg (IV) every 15 min may be necessary in the critical adult patient
	Pralidoxime (2-PAM chloride) (Protopam)	Initial dose: 1 gm (IV) Children: 25–50 mg/kg (IV)	Specific: Breaks alkyl phosphate-cholinesterase bond. Up to 500 mg every hour may be necessary in the critical adult patient

*Dosages listed may require modification according to specific clinical conditions; see each specific chapter for details.

(Updated and adapted from the American College of Emergency Physicians poster on poisoning, Dallas, Texas, 1980.)

its place in modern medicine, hyperbaric oxygen.

Forced Diuresis

Several years ago, when barbiturates were one of the most common causes of overdose, fluid loading and forced diuresis were accepted means of management for barbiturate poisoning. Unfortunately, these means were extrapolated to all forms of poisoning. The clinical course of the majority of drug and toxin poisonings is unaffected by diuresis, and an excessive fluid load may produce volume overload or electrolyte disturbances.

Forced diuresis is used infrequently, since most overdose agents are metabolized in the liver. In addition, the tricyclic antidepressants and many sedative-hypnotics cause a susceptibility to drug-induced interstitial pulmonary edema, and fluid loading is contraindicated. When drugs are markedly protein-bound, forced diuresis has no place in treatment. Thus, forced diuresis should be used only when specifically indicated, such as in poisoning by phenobarbital, bromides, lithium, salicylate, and amphetamines. The urine flow for forced diuresis is 3 to 5 ml per kg per hr, and this may require a diuretic. Furosemide is usually the agent of choice, although osmotic diuresis with mannitol can be more useful in some instances.

Acidification

Acidification of the urine is of theoretic value in overdose with phencyclidine and amphetamines, but it is rarely used. Many patients with these overdoses already have a metabolic acidosis. In addition, an acid urine may predispose to renal damage in the presence of myoglobinuria. Acidification may impair the excretions of other drugs, such as salicylates and phenobarbital.

Alkalinization

Alkalinization of the blood is helpful in reducing arrhythmias secondary to tricyclic antidepressants. Alkalinization of the urine ionizes weak acids, such as salicylates and barbiturates, and prevents reabsorption by the renal tubule, thus increasing excretion. Systemic alkalinization may produce severe hypokalemia.

Charcoal Hemoperfusion and Dialysis

Charcoal hemoperfusion and hemodialysis can be valuable adjuncts to treatment, but many drugs are not significantly removed with these invasive and complicated procedures. Both specific and general indications for dialysis or hemoperfusion are discussed in Chapter 8.

A patient who requires only removal of a drug that is adsorbed by charcoal (theophylline, barbiturates) benefits most from charcoal hemoperfusion. Hemodialysis is indicated in the patient who in addition has severe metabolic acidosis, electrolyte abnormality, or renal failure, as in salicylate and methanol poisoning. Peritoneal dialysis is generally not effective in altering the clinical course of poisoned patients and is inferior to hemodialysis.

Specific indications for dialysis include significant poisoning with methyl alcohol, ethylene glycol, and lithium and severe salicylate poisoning.[61]

Dialysis is not indicated in a patient who has ingested a substance that is markedly protein-bound, such as tricyclic antidepressant; in a drug ingestion in which the agent is rarely, if ever, lethal, such as benzodiazepine; when the plasma concentration of the drug is not significant enough to ensure drug removal, as with digitalis; when the action of the agent is irreversible, as with cyanide; when the patient is in shock; or when the dangers of hemodialysis outweigh the benefits.

Hyperbaric Oxygen

Hyperbaric oxygenation can provide oxygen at pressures greater than normal atmospheric pressure, which is given as 1 ATA (atmosphere absolute) or 760 mm Hg. Three ATA is the maximal pressure humans can tolerate over a reasonable period of time, although hyperbaric medicine units generally do not exceed 2.5 to 2.8 ATA.

The use of hyperbaric oxygen is becoming standard therapy for patients with critical carbon monoxide poisoning[62–64] *when available.* Chapter 74 provides a discussion of the indications for hyperbaric oxygen in the treatment of carbon monoxide poisoning. The use of hyperbaric oxygen in cyanide (Chapter 70) and hydrogen sulfide (Chapter 83) is presently being evaluated. No doubt new applications for hyperbaric medicine will be found in toxicology in this rapidly expanding field of expertise.

6. SUPPORTIVE THERAPY

Supportive therapy is the mainstay of treatment for the poisoned patient and is all that is required in many cases. Overaggressive therapy and the indiscriminate use of unproved antidotes often produce more complications than the overdose itself. All too often the agent is unknown, multiple drugs have been taken, or the patient is too unstable to withstand invasive therapy. The following are axioms of supportive care for the overdose patient:

- Frequent vital sign assessment, including temperature, is mandatory.
- Hypothermia or hyperthermia must be assessed and treated.
- Multiple system monitoring is indicated, and upon indication of any particular system failure, appropriate subspecialty consultation is indicated.
- Intensive nursing care is essential to detect acute or subtle changes in the patient's condition and to avoid complications such as aspiration or decubiti.
- Intravenous fluids are indicated to provide *maintenance* needs and replace losses, or to provide forced diuresis when indicated.
- Frequent arterial blood gas analysis should be obtained when using alkaline therapy or if the patient is on a ventilator.
- Indiscriminate use of drugs or antidotes should be avoided if not indicated or necessary.
- The management of hypotension may be difficult and must be individualized and based on the ingested poison.

7. OBSERVATION AND DISPOSITION

Inhospital observation of the patient following management of drug overdose may be necessary for numerous reasons. First, some drugs, such as iron, mercury, acetaminophen, paraquat, carbon tetrachloride, and *Amanita phalloides* toxin, have a latent phase, in which the patient appears to recover from the initial insult only to decompensate 24 to 72 hours postingestion. Rarely, the cyclic antidepressants have been known to cause fatal arrhythmia up to 6 days following ingestion.[65–67]

Some effects are not seen until later, such as hypertension following phencyclidine ingestion, hemorrhagic colitis following mercury ingestion, and disseminated intravascular coagulation (DIC) following snakebite. The delayed manifestations of poisoning, such as renal (Chapter 9), pulmonary (Chapter 10), hepatic (Chapter 13), and hematologic (Chapter 14), must be watched for.

Second, the patient may need observation because of an underlying disease that may be exacerbated because of the overdose; for example, the onset of diabetic ketoacidosis.

Third, observation may be necessary to evaluate and treat complications. For example, a skull fracture or other signs of trauma may not be evident until the overdose has been managed. Aspiration pneumonia or interstitial pulmonary edema may develop during the course of therapy.

The intravenous use of drugs brings multiple complications with their use, and observation is especially indicated for entities such as bacterial endocarditis, rhabdomyolysis, and neurologic and other sequelae.

The disposition of the toxicologic patient may involve medical and psychiatric as well as social service follow-up. It is suggested that all patients admitted to the hospital with intentional overdose warrant close observation and suicide precautions and be appropriately restrained to prevent further injury or additional overdose attempts. Overt or subtle attempts or gestures indicate the need for psychiatric consultation. Some ingestions in the pediatric age group will require outpatient follow-up the next day—for example, a kerosene ingestion in a patient with a negative chest radiograph and no respiratory distress. In addition, the question of child abuse or neglect always should be considered when treating a pediatric poisoning or overdose. Long-term follow-up may be indicated, such as testing for hepatitis and AIDS in the intravenous drug abuser.

References

1. Haddad LM: The emergency management of poisoning. Pediatr Ann *16*:900, 1987.
2. National Center for Health Statistics: Vital Statistics of the United States, 1986. Vol II: Mortality; Part B. Washington, DC, Government Printing Office, 1988.
3. Morbidity and Mortality Weekly Report 38:153, Mar 17, 1989.
4. Litovitz TL, Schmitz BF, Matyunas N, Martin TG: 1987 Annual Report of the American Association of Poison Control Centers National Data Collection System. Am J Emerg Med *6*:479, 1988.
5. Halstead BW: Poisonous and Venomous Marine Animals of the World. Rev ed. Princeton, NJ, Darwin Science Press, 1978.
6. Arena JM: Foreword—A brief history of the poison

control movement. *In* Haddad LM, Winchester JF: Clinical Management of Poisoning and Drug Overdose. Philadelpia, WB Saunders, 1983.
7. Arena JM: Safety closure caps. JAMA *169*:1187, 1959.
8. Lovejoy FH Jr, Caplan DL, Rowland T, Fazen L: A statewide plan for care of the poisoned patient: the Massachusetts Poison Control System. N Engl J Med *300*:363, 1979.
9. Schreiner GE: The role of hemodialysis (artificial kidney) in acute poisoning. Arch Intern Med *102*:896, 1958.
10. Haddad LM: Emergency physicians and poison treatment. N Engl J Med *300*:1223, 1979.
11. Rumack BH: POISINDEX. Denver, 1st ed. Micromedex, June 1, 1974.
12. Fazen LE, Lovejoy FH, Crone RK: Acute poisoning in a children's hospital: A 2 year experience. Pediatrics *77*:144, 1986.
13. Mofenson HC, Greensher J: The unknown poison. Pediatrics *54*:336, 1974.
14. Rygnestad T: Evaluation of benefits of drug analysis in the routine clinical management of acute self-poisoning. Clin Toxicol *22*:51, 1984.
15. Wright N: An assessment of the unreliability of the history given by self-poisoned patients. Clin Toxicol *16*:381, 1980.
16. Haddad LM: Marijuana uvula (letter). Am J Emerg Med *8*:4, 1990.
17. Plum P, Posner JB: Diagnosis of Stupor and Coma. 3rd ed. Philadelphia, FA Davis, 1980.
18. Oh MS, Carroll HJ: The anion gap. N Engl J Med *295*:814, 1977.
19. Brett AS: Implications of discordance between clinical impression and toxicology analysis in drug overdose. Arch Intern Med *148*:437, 1988.
20. Savitt DL, Hawkins HH, Roberts JR: The radiopacity of ingested medications. Ann Emerg Med *16*:331, 1987.
21. Curtis RA, Barone J, Giacona N: Efficacy of ipecac and activated charcoal/cathartic. Arch Intern Med *144*:48, 1984.
22. Kulig K, Bar-Or D, Cantrill SV, Rosen P, Rumack BH: Management of acutely poisoned patients without gastric emptying. Ann Emerg Med *14*:562, 1985.
23. Blake DR, Bramble MG, Evans JG: Is there excessive use of gastric lavage in the treatment of self-poisoning? Lancet 2:1362, 1978.
24. Park GD, Spector R, Goldberg MJ, Johnson GF: Expanded role of charcoal therapy in the poison and drug overdose patient. Arch Intern Med *146*:969, 1986.
25. Crome P, Dawling S, Braithwaite RA, Masters J, Walker R: Effect of activated charcoal on absorption of nortriptyline. Lancet 2:1203, 1977.
26. Pond S, Jacobs M, Marks J, Garner J, Goldschlager N, Hansen D: Treatment of digitoxin overdose with oral activated charcoal. Lancet 2:1177, 1981.
27. Berg MJ, Berlinger WG, Goldberg MJ, Spector R, Johnson GF: Acceleration of the body clearance of phenobarbital by oral activated charcoal. N Engl J Med *307*:642, 1982.
28. Berlinger WG, Spector R, Goldberg MJ, Johnson GF, Quee CK, Berg MJ: Theophylline clearance by oral activated charcoal. Clin Pharmacol Ther *33*:351, 1983.
29. American College of Emergency Physicians poster on poisoning. Dallas, ACEP, 1980.
30. Tandberg D, Diven BG, McLeod JW: Ipecac-induced emesis versus gastric lavage: A controlled study in normal adults. Am J Emerg Med *4*:205, 1986.
31. Grbcich PA, Lacouture PG, Lewander WJ, Lovejoy FH Jr: Effect of milk on ipecac-induced emesis. J Pediatr *110*:973, 1987.
32. Robertson WO: Syrup of ipecac—a fast or slow emetic? Am J Dis Child *103*:136, 1962.
33. Easom JM, Lovejoy FH: Efficacy and safety of gastrointestinal decontamination in the treatment of oral poisoning. Pediatr Clin North Am *26*:827, 1979.
34. Dabbous IA, Bergman AB, Robertson WO: The ineffectiveness of mechanically-induced vomiting. J Pediatr *66*:952, 1965.
35. Stein RS, Jenkins D, Korns ME: Death after use of cupric sulfate as emetic. JAMA *235*:801, 1976.
36. Chuttani HK, Gupta PS, Gulati S, Gupta DN: Acute copper sulfate poisoning. Am J Med *39*:849, 1965.
37. Calvin ME, Knepper R, Robertson WO: Salt poisoning. N Engl J Med *270*:625, 1964.
38. DeGenaro F, Nyhan WL: Salt—a dangerous antidote. J Pediatr *78*:1048, 1971.
39. MacLean WC: A comparison of ipecac syrup and apomorphine in the immediate treatment of ingestion of poisons. J Pediatr *82*:121, 1973.
40. Adler AG, Walinsky P, Krall RA, Cho SY: Death resulting from ipecac syrup poisoning. JAMA *243*:1927, 1980.
41. Grbcich PA, Lacouture PG, Kresel JJ, Russell MT, Lovejoy FH: Expired ipecac syrup efficacy. Pediatrics *78*:1085, 1986.
42. Litovitz TL, Klein-Schwartz W, Oderda GM, Matyunas NJ, Wiley S, Gorman RL: Ipecac administration in children younger than 1 year of age. Pediatrics *76*:761, 1985.
43. Grbcich PA, Lacouture PG, Lovejoy FH: Effect of fluid volume on ipecac-induced emesis. J Pediatr *110*:970, 1987.
44. Thoman ME, Verhulst HL: Ipecac syrup in antiemetic ingestion. JAMA *196*:433, 1966.
45. Krenzelok EP, Freedman GE, Pasternak S: Preserving the emetic effect of syrup of ipecac with concurrent activated charcoal administration: A preliminary study. J Toxicol Clin Toxicol *24*:159, 1986.
46. Freedman GE, Pasternak S, Krenzelok EP: A clinical trial using syrup of ipecac and activated charcoal concurrently. Ann Emerg Med *16*:164, 1987.
47. Chafee-Bahamon C, Lacouture PG, Lovejoy FH Jr: Risk assessment of ipecac in the home. Pediatrics *75*:1105, 1985.
48. Matthew H, Mackintosh TF, Tompsett SL, Cameron JC: Gastric aspiration and lavage in acute poisoning. Br Med J *1*:1333, 1966.
49. Marstellar H, Gugler R: Endoscopic management of toxic masses in the stomach. N Engl J Med *196*:1003, 1977.
50. Dronen SC, Merigian KS, Hedges JR, Hoekstra JW, Borron SW: A comparison of blind nasotracheal and succinylcholine-assisted intubation in the poisoned patient. Ann Emerg Med *16*:650, 1987.
51. Ekins BR, Ford DC, Thompson MIB, Bridges RR, Rollins DE, Jenkins RD: The effect of activated charcoal on *N*-acetylcysteine absorption in normal subjects. Am J Emerg Med *5*:483, 1987.
52. Fiser RH, Maetz HM, Treuting JJ, Decker WJ: Activated charcoal in barbiturate and glutethimide poisoning. J Pediatr *78*:1045, 1971.
53. Lake KD, Brown DC, Peterson CD: Digoxin toxicity: Enhanced systemic elimination during oral activated charcoal therapy. Pharmacotherapy *4*:161, 1984.
54. Honcharik N, Anthone S: Activated charcoal in acute cyclosporin overdose. Lancet 2:1051, 1985.
55. Neuvonen PJ, Elonen E, Mattila MJ: Oral activated

charcoal and dapsone elimination. Clin Pharmacol Ther *27*:823, 1980.
56. Krenzelok EP: Gastrointestinal times of cathartics used with activated charcoal. Clin Pharm 4:446, 1985.
57. Farley TA: Severe hypernatremic dehydration after use of an activated charcoal-sorbitol suspension. J Pediatr *109*:719, 1986.
58. Tenenbein M: Whole bowel irrigation as a gastrointestinal decontamination procedure after acute poisoning. Med Toxicol *3*:77, 1988.
59. Smith TW, Haber E, Yeatman L, Butler VP Jr: Reversal of advanced digoxin intoxication with Fab fragments of digoxin-specific antibodies. N Engl J Med *294*:797, 1976.
60. Smith TW, Butler VP, Haber E, Fozzar H, Marcus FI, Bremner WR, Schulman IC, Phillips A: Treatment of life-threatening digitalis intoxication with digoxin-specific Fab antibody fragments. Experience in 26 cases. N Engl J Med *307*:1357, 1982.
61. Winchester JF: Active methods for detoxification: Oral sorbents, forced diuresis, hemoperfusion, and hemodialysis. *In* Haddad LM, Winchester JF (eds): Clinical Management of Poisoning and Drug Overdose. Philadelphia, WB Saunders, 1983, pp 154–169.
62. Myers RAM, Snyder SK, Linberg S, Cowley RA: Value of hyperbaric oxygen in suspected carbon monoxide poisoning. JAMA *246*:2478, 1981.
63. Myers RAM, Snyder SK, Emhoff TA: Subacute sequelae of carbon monoxide poisoning. Ann Emerg Med *14*:1163, 1985.
64. Norkool DM, Kirkpatrick JN: Treatment of acute carbon monoxide poisoning: A review of 115 cases. Ann Emerg Med *14*:1168, 1985.
65. Freeman JW, Mundy GR, Beattie RR, Ryan C: Cardiac abnormalities in poisoning with tricyclic antidepressants. Br Med J *2*:610, 1969.
66. Sedal L, Korman MG, Williams PO, Mushin G: Overdosage of tricyclic antidepressants: A report of 2 deaths and a prospective study of 24 patients. Med J Aust 2:74, 1972.
67. McAlpine SB, Calabro JJ, Robinson MD, Burkle FM: Late death in tricyclic antidepressant overdose revisited. Ann Emerg Med *15*:1349, 1986.

CHAPTER 2

PRINCIPLES OF PHARMACOLOGY FOR THE CLINICIAN

John Ambre, M.D., Ph.D.

Certain basic knowledge is necessary for a rational approach to clinical problems. This chapter discusses general principles of pharmacology, illustrated by specific examples, in an attempt to relate the principles to the diagnosis and treatment of drug overdose and poisoning. Throughout this chapter the term *drug* refers not only to therapeutic agents but also to other exogenous chemicals or toxic agents.

DRUG AND TOXIN DISPOSITION

Toxin exposure results from environmental contamination or accidental or intentional administration of a toxin. Intoxication is the result of the presence of a drug or toxin in a critical concentration at the site of toxic action in the body. The factors determining the concentration, in addition to the dose, are the rates of absorption, distribution, metabolism, and excretion.

All these disposition processes involve passage across cell and capillary membranes. Drugs pass cell membranes by diffusing through aqueous pores in the membrane, or they pass directly through the lipoprotein membrane structure by dissolving in it and diffusing out the other side. These are passive processes (not requiring chemical energy), and they occur in response to and in the direction of a concentration difference (gradient). Dissolution in the lipoprotein membrane structure requires that the drug have some degree of lipid solubility. Lipophilicity is usually expressed as an in vitro oil-water partition ratio. Movement across the membrane occurs until the concentration of diffusible substance on each side is the same. Filtration through cell membrane pores involves the flow of water in response to a hydrostatic or osmotic gradient. Water-soluble substances are transported if they are sufficiently small in molecular size to move through the pore.

Drugs may pass capillary membranes by crossing capillary endothelial cell membranes. The capillary endothelial cell has relatively large membrane pores. However, the primary mode of passage across capillaries, with the exception of those capillaries in the central nervous system, is by flow through intercellular spaces. This is the process involved, for example, in filtration across glomerular capillaries. The absence of such spaces between endothelial cells in capillaries of the central nervous system constitutes the anatomic basis for the blood-brain barrier.

Specialized transport mechanisms are available for some drugs. Active transport refers to a process having characteristic ability to move substances against a concentration gradient, relative selectivity for certain chemical structures, saturability, requirement for metabolic energy, and susceptibility to inhibition. Facilitated diffusion processes have the characteristics related to carrier mediation (selectivity, saturability, and susceptibility to inhibition) but do not require energy or work against a gradient.

ABSORPTION

Absorption basically means movement from a drug deposit site into the blood. Of the various sites for drug deposit, the gastrointestinal tract is by far the most important, since a majority of acute poisoning problems involve drug ingestion. It is worthwhile to consider briefly the factors that influence absorption from the stomach and intestines. Gastrointestinal absorption involves diffusion across lipid cell membranes of the lining epithelium, since movement between lining cells is limited by tight intercellular junctions.

Absorption, therefore, takes place most readily with nonionized, lipid-soluble chemical species. Lipid-soluble nonelectrolytes such as methanol and ethanol are rapidly absorbed, limited only by factors that reduce their contact with the membrane, such as the presence of food.

For drugs that are weak electrolytes, the pH at the absorption site may influence the degree of ionization and thereby influence absorption, since membrane passage is easiest for the nonionized form. The extent of ionization at a particular pH depends upon the ionization constant (pK) of the weak acid or base. The pK is the pH at which the electrolyte exists half in the ionized and half in the nonionized form (Fig. 2–1). Absorption will be best from the medium in which the drug is least ionized. As shown in Figure 2–2, the nonionized form moves in response to its concentration gradient until concentrations are equal on each side of the membrane. Since the degree of ionization changes as the drug moves to the plasma compartment, total concentration of the acidic drug becomes greater in the plasma. Likewise for a basic drug, concentration in the plasma will be favored by an alkaline-absorbing medium. Obviously, the pH of the gastrointestinal tract can be influenced by disease (e.g., achlorhydria) or by administration of antacids, and this, in turn, can influence absorption from these sites.

Strong electrolytes are absorbed to a limited extent. They are not influenced by pH, since they are essentially completely ionized at any pH in the physiologic range. They diffuse slowly or depend on specialized mechanisms for absorption.

A few substances can be absorbed by specialized active transport processes, apparently because their chemical structure closely resembles those of natural substances that are normally transported by the system. The

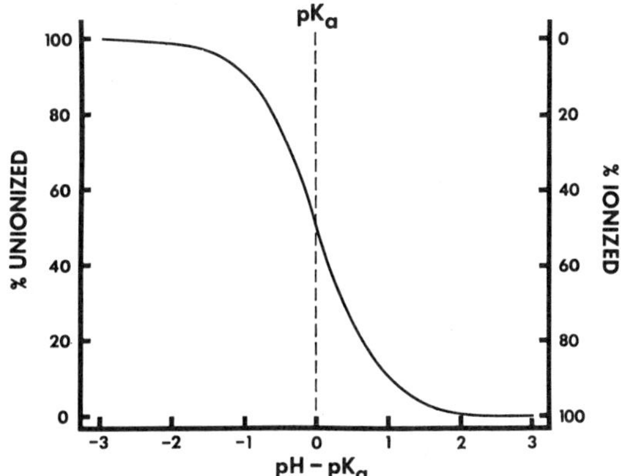

Figure 2–1. The effect of pH on the ionization of a weak acid. The acid is 50 per cent ionized at a pH = pK_a. At higher pH values, it becomes increasingly more ionized; at lower pH values, it becomes increasingly more nonionized. The rate of change of ionization is greatest at pH values near the pK_a. (From LaDu BN, Mandel HG, Way EL: Fundamentals of Drug Metabolism and Disposition. Baltimore, Williams & Wilkins, © 1971, p 5.)

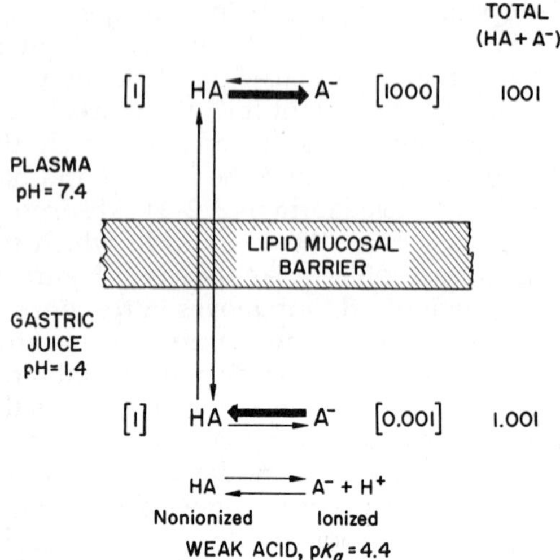

Figure 2–2. Influence of pH on the distribution of a weak acid between plasma and gastric juice, separated by a lipid barrier. (From Mayer SE, Melmon KL, Gilman AG: Introduction: The dynamics of drug absorption, distribution, and elimination. In Gilman AG, Goodman, LS, Gilman A (eds): The Pharmacological Basis of Therapeutics. New York, Macmillan, 1980, p 4.)

antitumor drug 5-fluorouracil is actively carried across intestinal mucosa by a process that transports the natural pyrimidine bases uracil and thymine.[1]

In general, drugs in solution are better absorbed than those in solid form. Since dissolution in the aqueous contents of the gut is required for presentation to the lipid gut membrane, a certain degree of aqueous solubility is also required for efficient absorption. Some highly lipid-soluble drugs are poorly absorbed for that reason. Finely divided, small particulate substances are better absorbed than larger particles.

Other factors modifying absorption that apply to gastrointestinal and other absorption sites are the concentration of the drug at the absorption site, the presence of food or binding agents, the total area of the absorbing surface, the rate of gastric emptying, blood flow to the site, and intestinal motility.

A high concentration of drug at the absorption site maximizes the concentration gradient into blood. The presence of food or other binding substances essentially reduces the concentration of absorbable drug. The large absorbing surface of the small intestine makes it the primary site of gastrointestinal absorption for most substances, the area being so great that other factors such as pH may become relatively insignificant. The effect of rate of gastric emptying on absorption is probably the result of hastening or retarding delivery of gastric contents to the large absorptive surface of the intestine. Blood flow to the stomach and intestines via the splanchnic vessels ordinarily is not rate limiting for absorption but presumably could be in the shock state. An increase in intestinal motility might reduce absorption by shortening intestinal transit time and reducing contact time with the absorbing surface. In the intoxicated patient, decreased motility might reduce absorption by allowing formation of tablet masses or might increase absorption by prolonging transit time.

The value of thinking about these various influences on absorption is in knowing that the therapist can alter some of them. The drug or poison may affect these factors in such a way that intoxication is more severe or prolonged than need be. The physician can aid recovery by recognizing and reversing drug effects that are detrimental or by influencing these factors in the patient's favor. For example, in a patient with tricyclic antidepressant or glutethimide overdose, the anticholinergic effects on the gastrointestinal tract might include delayed gastric emptying and decreased intestinal motility. Retention of some drug in the stomach may allow removal by lavage. Decreased intestinal motility may reduce absorption from a tablet mass but may also prevent expulsion of unabsorbed tablets. Administration of activated charcoal may bind a drug and reduce the absorbable drug concentration, but the charcoal may also form a stagnant mass in the intestine that eventually takes on the consistency of concrete. Administration of a cathartic should aid in rectal passage of undissolved tablets and charcoal-bound drug.

Skin Absorption

The skin, to a great extent, is an effective barrier to toxic chemical absorption. The intact skin behaves qualitatively like cellular membranes. Thus, drugs penetrate the skin at rates determined by their lipid solubility. Lipid-soluble organophosphate insecticides are readily absorbed from skin and thereby present a hazard to medical personnel who handle the patient. Organic solvents, such as carbon tetrachloride, methanol, and others that are present as vehicles for some industrial toxins, may enhance skin absorption. Dimethyl sulfoxide, a common commercial solvent, is particularly efficient as a carrier in skin absorption. Inflammation, rubbing, and other causes of increased skin blood flow may increase absorption, while application of tourniquets or local application of ice may retard absorption.

Absorption from the Respiratory Tract

Certain toxic fumes, particulates, and noxious gases may be absorbed via the lungs. Particle size is an important factor in lung retention of a particulate substance, since only particles less than 1 micron (1μ) in diameter can penetrate to the lower airways. Generally, the only means of reducing lung absorption is by removing the patient from the toxic atmosphere.

DISTRIBUTION

After absorption, which involves movement into blood, and mechanical displacement with the blood into the various body organs by the action of the heart, the drug or toxin moves into organ tissues. This is the process of distribution.

Concept of Volume of Distribution

As a rule, the amount of drug or poison at the specific site of its toxic action is a very small part of the total amount of drug in the body. Each drug distributes to the tissues of the body in a definite pattern. This pattern is established when drug concentrations in the various tissues are in equilibrium. Equilibrium does not mean that all tissue concentrations are equal; it means there is no net transfer of drug from one tissue to another. Usually, it is not possible or practical to measure drug concentrations in each tissue or at the drug's site of action. Actually, even in the target tissue, most of the drug present will be associated with tissue membranes or molecules having nothing to do with the drug's action; that is, only a fraction of the drug is bound to specific receptors. Since plasma is the tissue in which drug concentration is most easily measured and since plasma is the medium of distribution, drug distribution is usually related to plasma concentrations.

The volume of distribution is the *apparent* volume in which the drug is distributed. It is the volume the drug would occupy if it were present elsewhere at the same concentration found in plasma. The volume of distribution is clinically useful because it tends to be characteristic of the drug and is constant over a wide range of doses. It allows prediction of the plasma concentrations that will be produced by a given dose of the drug.

Factors Influencing Distribution

The rate at and extent to which a drug reaches the tissues of each organ is determined by the blood flow through the organ, the drug's ability to cross capillary and cell membranes, and the drug's relative partitioning between blood and tissue.

Blood Flow. The early phase of drug distribution is primarily a reflection of the rate of blood flow to various organs. Distribution of drug into highly perfused tissues, such as the brain, liver, and kidney, is faster than distribution into adipose tissue and muscle. This feature is dramatically illustrated by the time course of blood and tissue concentrations after an intravenous dose of thiopental (Fig. 2–3).

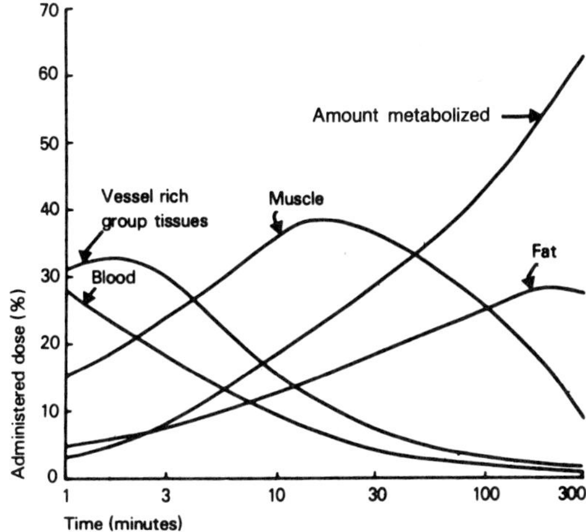

Figure 2–3. Distribution of thiopental after an intravenous injection. The time course of distribution is a reflection of tissue blood flow. The drug moves quickly into highly perfused tissues, such as brain, liver, and kidney, and more slowly to muscle and fat tissue. (From Ghoneim MM, Korttila K: Pharmacokinetics of intravenous anaesthetics: Implications for clinical use. Clin Pharmacokinet 2:344, 1977. Used with permission.)

Capillary Membrane Passage. Movement from blood into the extracellular or interstitial space of tissues (except for brain) occurs readily, since most drugs are considerably smaller than albumin and are able to pass the intercellular channels of the capillary endothelial membrane. Lipid-soluble drugs may also move directly across capillary endothelial cells to reach interstitial space. Lipid-insoluble drugs are not able to pass cell membranes, as explained in a following section, and may be therefore limited to the extracellular tissue spaces.

The term *blood-brain barrier* refers to the brain capillary membranes' lack of intercellular channels, or pores; movement directly across cell membranes is the only means of access to brain extracellular fluid. The blood-brain barrier is therefore essentially a lipid barrier, and, in general, lipid-insoluble substances have limited access to and therefore little effect on the central nervous system.

Cell Membrane Passage. The ability to cross cell membranes is a function of the lipid solubility of the drug and the degree of protein binding. The same factors influencing membrane passage that were considered under the section on absorption will apply here. Lipid-soluble nonelectrolytes pass readily, while strong electrolytes pass poorly into cells. Passage by weak electrolytes depends upon their ionization state and the relative lipid solubility of their unionized form.

EFFECT OF pH

It is generally assumed that only the nonionized forms of organic acids and bases are lipid soluble enough to pass cell membranes. The ionized form is too polar to penetrate the membrane. Since many drugs are weak organic acids or bases, the relative pH of blood and tissue fluids will influence the proportion of ionized to nonionized species in these fluids and therefore the amount in the form capable of penetrating cell membranes. Normal pH differences between bodily fluids and tissues, therefore, influence the normal distribution pattern of these drugs. Influence of changes in pH on distribution is seen only with drugs whose pK is in a range such that their ionization state changes substantially with pH changes within the physiologic range. The pK of a weak acid or base is the pH at which it exists half in the ionized and half in the nonionized form; as pH decreases, weak bases become more ionized, while weak acids become more ionized with a pH increase. The distribution of these substances is altered if they move into a tissue fluid in which the pH, and consequently their ionization state, are different.

The practical application of this phenomenon can be seen in the effect systemic pH changes have on the anesthesia produced by the weak acid phenobarbital. When phenobarbital is administered and blood pH is lowered, there is a drop in plasma drug level, an increase in brain levels, and a deepening of anesthesia. Blood alkalosis produces the opposite effects.[2] This phenomenon must be considered when the physician is deciding on which method will be used to alkalinize the urine to hasten phenobarbital excretion (discussed in a following section).

PROTEIN BINDING

Many drugs and poisons are bound to some extent to plasma proteins, particularly albumin. The binding usually involves reversible, weak electrostatic, hydrophobic, or Van der Waals' forces but, in some cases, may involve formation of covalent bonds. The extent of binding varies greatly. Some lipophilic organic acids are more than 90 per cent bound, whereas small, neutral hydrophilic organic bases may also bind to plasma proteins, but albumin tends to bind acids more strongly and extensively than bases. Some basic drugs are bound to other plasma components, such as the acute phase reactant α_1-acid glycoprotein.

Binding in the plasma limits movement of drug through capillaries and into the tissues. Only the unbound drug crosses cell membranes because the large molecular size of drug-protein complexes limits such movement. Equilibrium is established between the unbound drug in plasma and the tissue water. Since a drug ordinarily must pass some membranes to reach its site of action, only the unbound portion represents active drug. Drug binding may influence the processes of liver uptake and renal excretion, as will be discussed later.

In the case of drug overdose, drug distribution may be altered by increasing drug concentrations if plasma protein binding sites become saturated. Then, as the concentration rises, the fraction unbound also rises, and the volume of distribution increases. More drug would move into tissues and penetrate to the site of toxic action. This concentration-dependent decrease in protein binding could be responsible for poor correlation between total (free plus bound) plasma concentrations and the clinical status of the patient.

An interesting converse of the above process may be the basis for an exciting new approach to therapy of drug intoxication. New hybridoma techniques may allow production of large quantities of drug-specific antibodies. The high affinity-specific antibodies (or their Fab fragments) might be administered to bind the drug in an inactive complex while awaiting excretion. The process is illustrated by the administration of digoxin-specific Fab fragments (Fig. 2–4).[3] Free digoxin in the serum is bound immediately, and digoxin in the tissues is redistributed back to the vascular system, where in turn it is also bound. Signs of toxicity dissipate. Total serum digoxin consisting almost entirely of bound inactive drug rises 10-fold, reflecting the influx of digoxin from tissue, and then begins to decline at a rate determined by the excretion of the Fab-drug complex.

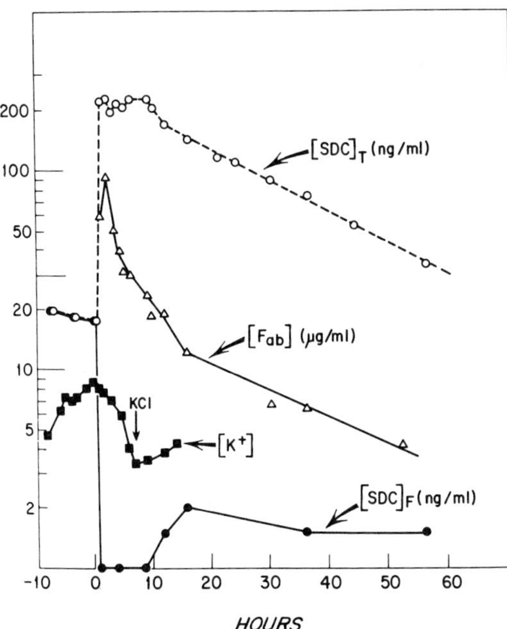

Figure 2–4. Fab therapy of digoxin toxicity. (From Smith TW, et al: Reversal of advanced digoxin toxicity with Fab fragments of digoxin-specific antibodies. N Engl J Med 294:797–800, 1976.)

REDISTRIBUTION

Movement of drug into more slowly penetrated tissues may be responsible in some cases for termination of drug effect rather than metabolism and excretion of the drug. The best example is the redistribution of lipid-soluble thiopental from its site of action in the brain to the more slowly perfused muscle and fat tissues. After single intravenous doses, redistribution to these tissues is primarily responsible for terminating its anesthetic effect, as initially high levels in rapidly perfused brain tissue continue to equilibrate with falling blood levels (see Fig. 2–3). In circumstances in which repeated administration or continuous infusion is used, these more slowly perfused muscle and fat tissues equilibrate and accumulate the lipophilic drug. When infusion is stopped, the anesthetic effect disappears at the slower rate, dependent on metabolism rather than redistribution.

TISSUE RESERVOIRS

For lipophilic drugs like thiopental, slowly perfused muscle and fat tissues may serve as a reservoir to store the drug. For other drugs, slowly mobilized intracellular drug present in many tissues may function as a reservoir. In toxicology, the reservoir effect is most evident in situations in which drug removal from plasma is augmented by artificial means, such as hemodialysis or hemoperfusion. Plasma concentrations of the drug may be seen to rise again when dialysis is stopped as tissue-bound drug re-enters the plasma from the reservoir.

Glutethimide is a lipophilic drug that will move into fat tissues during the course of a large overdose. As shown in Figure 2–5, plasma concentrations may rise at termination of dialysis because of redistribution of drug from tissue stores.

The drug lithium, after a single dose, is initially distributed to extracellular fluid and then more slowly moves inside cells. With repeated dosing, it eventually has a distribution volume similar to that of total body water and has fairly uniform concentration in all body tissues.[4] Plasma concentrations are lowered very efficiently by hemodialysis. When dialysis is discontinued, however, plasma levels may rise again, owing to

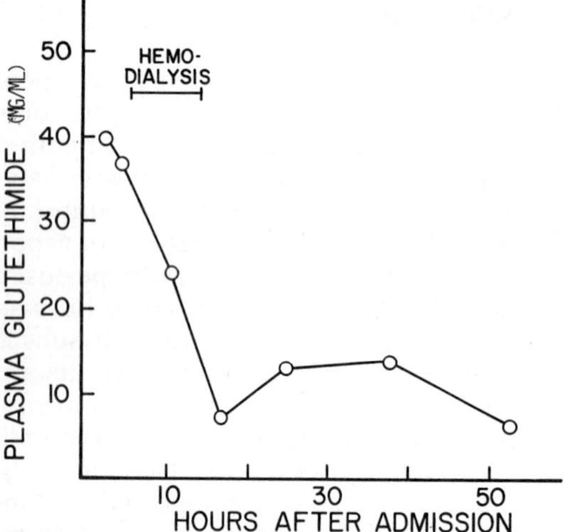

Figure 2–5. Plasma glutethimide levels in a comatose patient who had ingested 20 gm of glutethimide several hours before hospital admission. Glutethimide clearance is augmented by dialysis over a 10-hour period. Plasma glutethimide levels rise after dialysis is discontinued, owing to redistribution of drug from tissue stores.

movement of lithium out of cellular stores (Fig. 2–6).

BIOTRANSFORMATION PATHWAYS

Most foreign chemicals introduced into the body undergo a chemical transformation before excretion. This process has been called *metabolism* to draw a parallel between it and the chemical transformations undergone by normal or endogenous bodily chemicals. The term *biotransformation* is now more widely used to describe the process, but the products are generally called *metabolites*.

When the study of drug and foreign chemical biotransformation was relatively new, transformation was considered a process of detoxification. The title of the first textbook dealing with the subject, published in 1947 by R. T. Williams, was *Detoxication Mechanisms*.[5] Now, it is appreciated that transformation of drugs and chemicals can be the source of substances more active or toxic than the original chemical. In general, biotransformations can be characterized as processes that produce more water-soluble or polar compounds. Metabolites are, therefore, chemical forms that are less able to move through biomembranes; more restricted in their distribution to tissues; less readily reabsorbed from renal tubules, bile duct, or intestine; and ultimately more easily excreted.

Biotransformation may occur in any tissue, including the blood. However, it is generally most active or quantitatively most important in the liver. The metabolizing enzymes are present in various parts of the liver cell. Their location is conventionally indicated by the in vitro fraction of the homogenized liver tissue in which the enzymatic activity is present, rather than the subcellular structure with which the enzyme is associated in vivo. Drug-metabolizing enzymes are therefore referred to as *soluble, mitochondrial*, or *microsomal* enzymes. The microsomes are spherical fragments of the hepatocyte endoplasmic reticulum, which are formed by the process of liver homogenization. The mitochondria, microsomes, and other cellular components are sedimented out of liver tissue homogenates by ultracentrifugation under well-defined conditions. The supernatant solution contains the cytosol and is called the *soluble* fraction.

Drugs and other foreign chemicals may undergo three general types of biotransformation: oxidation/reduction, hydrolysis, and conjugation. Drug-metabolizing enzymes

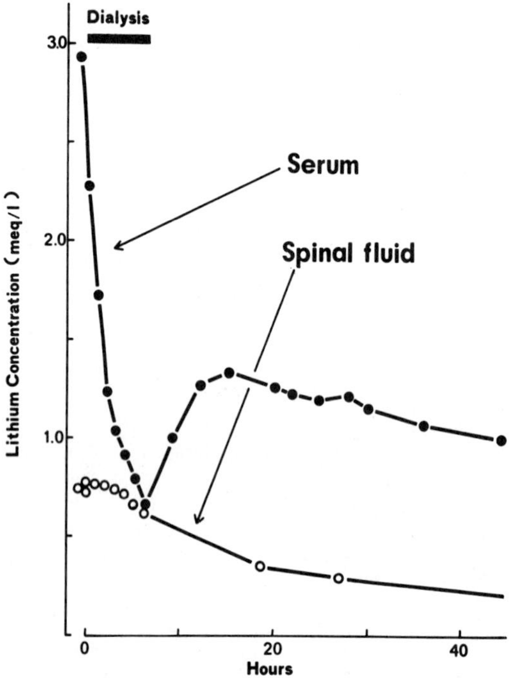

Figure 2–6. Serum and spinal fluid lithium levels in a 48 year old lithium-intoxicated man who was anuric. Serum levels decline rapidly with dialysis and rise again as lithium redistributes from tissues. Spinal fluid levels respond slowly to changes in serum level. (From Amdisen A, Skjoldborg H: Haemodialysis for lithium poisoning. Lancet 2:213, 1969.)

subserving oxidation reactions are primarily found in the microsomes (Table 2–1), whereas hydrolytic and conjugating enzymes may be found in the cytosol or may be found extracellularly in the plasma. Drugs that chemically resemble endogenous substances may be metabolized by the same enzymes as these normal body constituents.

Most of the reactions involved in drug metabolism may be considered chemical oxidations. A hemoprotein involved in many of the microsomal reactions as an electron transport function is cytochrome P-450. An outline of the electron transport chain involving P-450 and the oxidation of drugs by the hepatic endoplasmic reticulum is shown in Figure 2–7. NADPH is oxidized by the flavoprotein cytochrome P-450 reductase, and an electron is transferred to the oxidized form of cytochrome P-450, which has formed a complex with the drug. The reduced form of the P-450 drug complex binds oxygen, and another electron is introduced to generate oxidized drug, oxidized P-450, and water.

The cytochrome P-450 system was originally thought to consist of a few hemoproteins with broad substrate activity. It is now known that there are several classes or families of P-450 isozymes with varying substrate specificity. Different inducers of drug metabolism, such as phenobarbital and other chemicals (mentioned in a following section), may promote the formation of specific isozymes. Different P-450 isozymes may also be preferentially involved in production of different metabolites from a particular drug.

Table 2–1. SITES OF DRUG METABOLISM

METABOLIC PATHWAYS	LOCATION OF ENZYMES*
Oxidations	
Hydroxylation	M
Dealkylation	M
Epoxidation	M
S- and N-Oxidation	M
Desulfuration	M
Dehalogenation	M
Deamination	M, mitochondria
Alcohol oxidation	M, S
Aldehyde oxidation	S
Reductions	
Aldehyde reduction	S
Azoreduction	M
Nitroreduction	M, S
Hydrolyses	
De-esterification	M, S, plasma
Deamidation	M, S
Conjugations	
Glucuronidation	M
Sulfation	S
Glutathione conjugation	S
Methylation	S
Acylation	S

*M, microsomes (endoplasmic reticulum); S, soluble fraction (cytosol).

Other routes of chemical metabolism involve chemical reduction, hydrolysis, and glucuronide conjugation. Figure 2–8 illustrates specific examples of the major pathways of drug metabolism.

Many drugs undergo sequential reactions; a common example is hydroxylation followed by conjugation with glucuronic acid or activated sulfate on the hydroxyl group, or both. This process is so common that drug metabolism is often described as taking place in two phases.[6] The first phase is an oxidation, reduction, or hydrolysis step that introduces or unmasks a functionality such as hydroxyl (-OH), sulfhydryl (-SH), amine (-NH_2), or carboxyl (-COOH) group on the drug structure. These are primarily microsomal (endoplasmic reticulum) enzymatic reactions. The second phase consists of a synthetic or conjugation reaction in which the drug or a phase-one metabolite is linked through the functional group to an endogenous compound such as glucuronic acid or sulfate to form a conjugate. These are primarily cytosol or soluble-phase enzymes. The conjugate is not only more water soluble and ionizable but may also be handled by the acid transport mechanism of the excretory systems.

The sedative drug glutethimide (Doriden) provides an example of this metabolic pattern (Fig. 2–9). Hydroxylation takes place at several sites on the drug molecule, and these oxidized compounds are subsequently conjugated. The various glutethimide metabolites illustrate the variety of compounds that can be produced by a single general pathway of metabolism (i.e., hydroxylation). This, together with the fact that a variety of general pathways are available, indicates the potential complexity of drug metabolism.

As indicated previously, important conjugation reactions and some oxidative, reductive, and hydrolytic enzyme systems are available for drug metabolism at nonmicrosomal sites in liver, in other tissues, and in plasma (see Table 2–1).

Microsomal drug-metabolizing enzymes are subject to induction. Some common

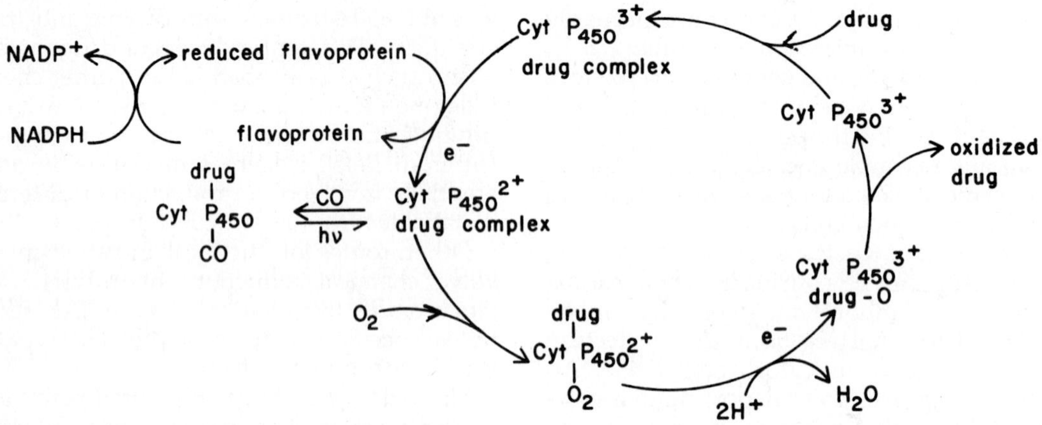

NADP$^+$ reduced flavoprotein Cyt $P_{450}{}^{3+}$ drug complex drug
NADPH flavoprotein Cyt $P_{450}{}^{3+}$ oxidized drug
drug | Cyt P_{450} | CO   CO   hν e^- Cyt $P_{450}{}^{2+}$ drug complex
Cyt $P_{450}{}^{3+}$ drug-O
O_2 drug | Cyt $P_{450}{}^{2+}$ | O_2 e^- $2H^+$ H_2O

Figure 2–7. Electron flow pathway in microsomal drug metabolizing system. NADPH is oxidized by the flavoprotein cytochrome P-450 reductase (cyt P-450), and an electron is transferred to the oxidized form of cytochrome P-450 that has formed a complex with the drug. The reduced form of cytochrome P-450 drug complex binds oxygen and another electron and is introduced to generate oxidized drug, oxidized P-450, and water. The oxidized cytochrome P-450 is then available to bind another drug molecule and continue the cycle. (Adapted from Goldstein A, Aronow L, Kalman S: Principles of Drug Action. 2nd ed. New York, John Wiley & Sons, 1974, p 243. Used with permission.)

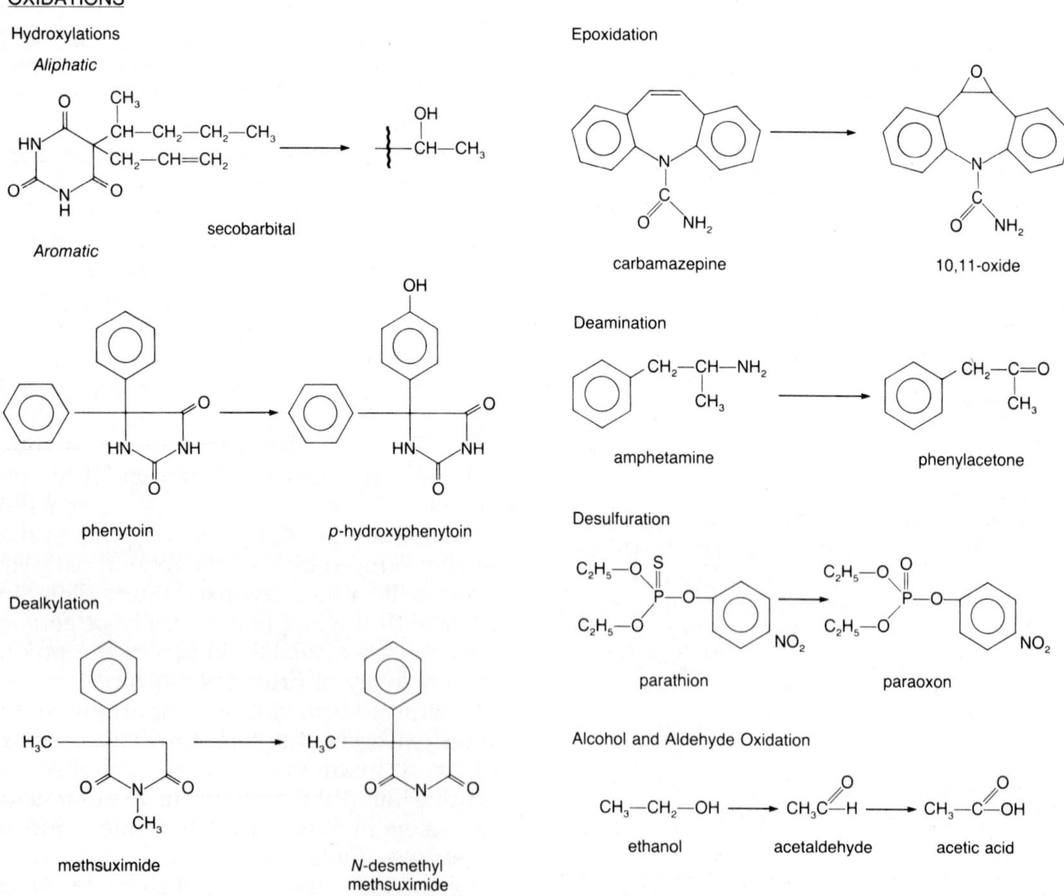

Figure 2–8. Typical metabolic reactions.

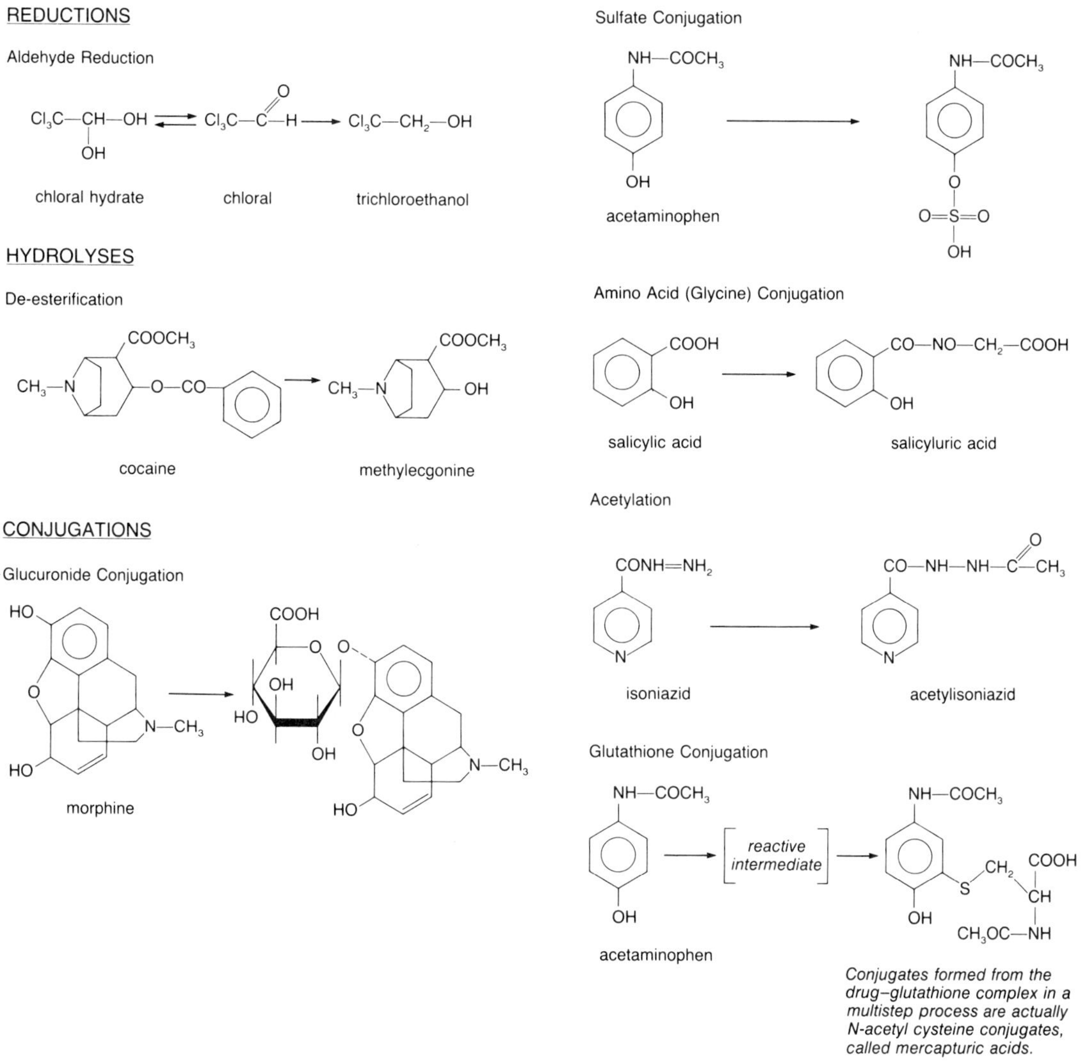

REDUCTIONS

Aldehyde Reduction

chloral hydrate   chloral   trichloroethanol

HYDROLYSES

De-esterification

cocaine   methylecgonine

CONJUGATIONS

Glucuronide Conjugation

morphine

Sulfate Conjugation

acetaminophen

Amino Acid (Glycine) Conjugation

salicylic acid   salicyluric acid

Acetylation

isoniazid   acetylisoniazid

Glutathione Conjugation

acetaminophen

Conjugates formed from the drug–glutathione complex in a multistep process are actually N-acetyl cysteine conjugates, called mercapturic acids.

Figure 2–8 *Continued*

drugs, such as phenobarbital and various environmental chemicals, are capable of inducing the rate of metabolism of many other drugs processed by microsomal enzymes. Phenobarbital and glutethimide, which induce the metabolism of other drugs, also induce their own rate of metabolism with repeated administration. Unfortunately, induction of the rate of drug metabolism is not useful in the treatment of acute intoxication because the process requires synthesis of new enzyme and takes place over a period of days. A compound that "activates" enzyme already present in the liver might be useful in this manner, but such a compound is not available.

Metabolizing enzymes are also subject to inhibition of their activity on one drug (substrate) by *competition* from alternate drugs (substrates). Inhibition may also be *noncompetitive,* resulting from inactivation of metabolizing enzymes by highly reactive substances. Inhibition is a phenomenon that can take place acutely. Significant competitive inhibition is likely only when the drug has saturated its metabolizing enzyme system. Few drugs or toxins saturate the system even in overdose. Exceptions are salicylates, methanol, ethanol, theophylline, acetaminophen, and phenytoin. Ethyl alcohol can induce microsomal drug metabolism chronically and inhibit it acutely. For example, when sober, alcoholic subjects have a faster than normal rate of pentobarbital metabolism, which slows when alcohol is also present in their blood. Inhibition of metabolism has a definite

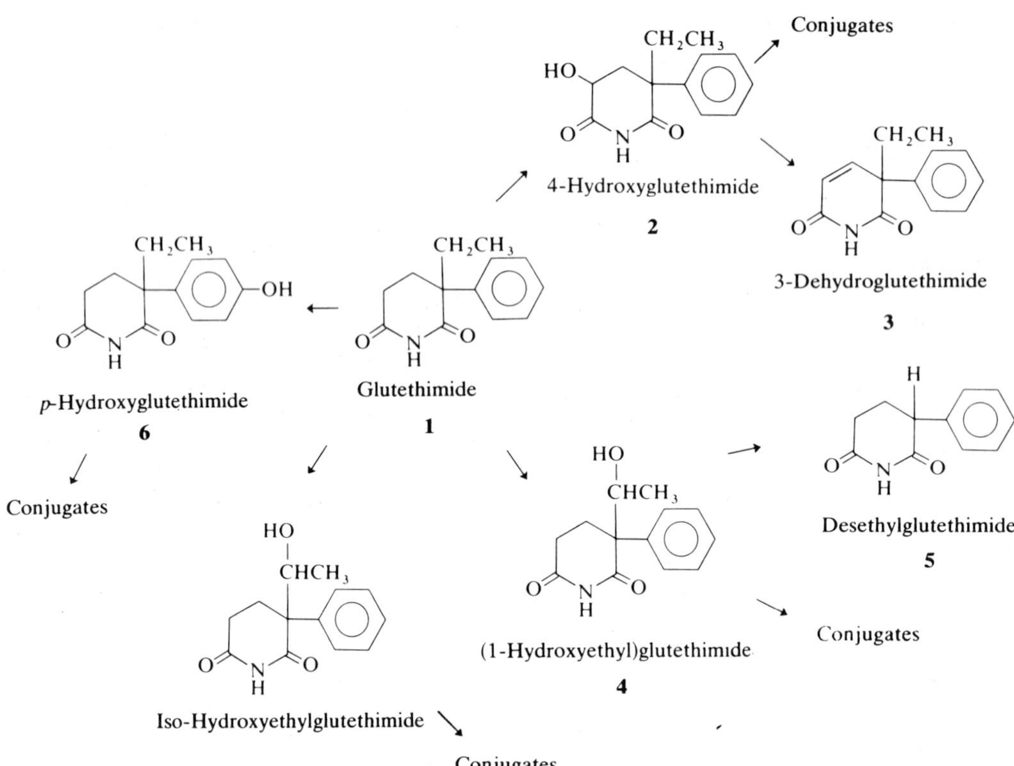

Figure 2–9. The sedative-hypnotic drug glutethimide (Doriden) is metabolized by hydroxylation at several positions on the parent structure. These hydroxylated metabolites are conjugated with glucuronic acid prior to excretion in the urine. (From Kennedy KA, Ambre JJ, Fischer LJ: A selected ion monitoring method for glutethimide and six metabolites: Application to blood and urine from humans intoxicated with glutethimide. Biomed Mass Spec 5:679, 1978.)

but limited place in the treatment of acute intoxication. The best example involving inhibition of metabolism in the treatment of acute intoxication is inhibition of methanol metabolism to formate by administration of ethanol, and more recently, by 4-methylpyrazole.[7]

The phenomenon of induction and inhibition of microsomal drug metabolism is superimposed on a normal interindividual variation in rates of metabolism of approximately 3- to 20-fold.[8]

It is widely believed, as a result of Vesell's[8] studies in identical and fraternal twins, that the major cause of the large interindividual differences in rates of drug metabolism is genetic. Using drugs such as antipyrine, bishydroxycoumarin, and phenylbutazone, for which the plasma half-lives are related to their rate of metabolism, it was found that the plasma half-lives of these drugs were virtually the same in identical twins, whereas fraternal twins given the same drugs exhibited interindividual differences in plasma half-lives similar to those of the general population. Environmental factors seemed to play a minor role. Individuals with the slowest rates of metabolism were subject to the greatest degree of induction when treated with phenobarbital, an inducer of microsomal drug metabolism. The extent to which variation in rates of drug metabolism makes different individuals more or less susceptible to drug toxicity has not been fully explored.[9]

Nonmicrosomal enzyme systems exhibit similar interindividual variation in rates, and some, such as the cholinesterase system in plasma, exhibit genetic polymorphism. However, they are generally not subject to enzyme induction.

Some drugs may be metabolized nonenzymatically (chemical decomposition) within the body. Benzoylecgonine, a major metabolite of cocaine, probably arises from cocaine by spontaneous hydrolysis.[10]

ACTIVE METABOLITES (Tables 2–2 and 2–3)

Toxicity in some cases is directly related to the products of drug metabolism.[11] These

Table 2–2. ACTIVE METABOLITES OF THERAPEUTIC AGENTS

AGENT	METABOLITE
acetohexamide	hydroxyhexamide
acetylmethadol	noracetylmethadol dinoracetylmethadol
allopurinol	oxypurinol
amitriptyline	nortriptyline 10-hydroxynortriptyline
carbamazepine	carbamazepine epoxide
chlordiazepoxide	*N*-desmethylchlordiazepoxide demoxepam
diazepam	*N*-desmethyldiazepam oxazepam
disopyramide	*N*-desalkyldisopyramide
flurazepam	*N*-desalkylflurazepam
glutethimide	4-hydroxyglutethimide
imipramine	desipramine
lidocaine	MEGX, GX
meperidine	normeperidine
phenylbutazone	oxyphenbutazone
procainamide	*N*-acetylprocainamide
propranolol	4-hydroxypropranolol
sulindac	sulfide metabolite
tolbutamide	hydroxytolbutamide
verapamil	norverapamil

(Adapted from Wilkinson GR, Rawlins MD (eds): Drug Metabolism and Disposition: Considerations in Clinical Pharmacology. Boston, MTP Press, 1985.)

products may be major metabolites that accumulate in the systemic circulation, or they may be quantitatively minor, acting locally in the cell where they are formed.

Toxicity due to accumulation of an active metabolite characteristically exhibits a latency that is due to the time required for accumulation. Clinically, the patient exhibits increasing toxic effect rather than improvement in the hours after hospital admission.

When taken in an overdose the sedative-hypnotic drug glutethimide produces a coma similar to that produced by barbiturates. The only distinguishing clinical signs are the result of glutethimide's anticholinergic effects on the pupils and gastrointestinal tract. The clinical course of the coma is unusually long, and many patients seem to have a recurrence of deep coma after having shown signs of awakening. Several reports have indicated a poor correlation between the concentrations of unchanged glutethimide in plasma and the clinical course of the intoxicated patients in that the patients remained in a coma when glutethimide concentration had fallen to low levels. These features can be explained by the accumulation of an active metabolite, 4-hydroxyglutethimide, in patients who have taken a large overdose of glutethimide. Hansen and associates showed that a combined plot of glutethimide and 4-hydroxyglutethimide concentrations correlated with the clinical status of a glutethimide-intoxicated patient (Fig. 2–10).[12] The hydroxy metabolite, tested in mice, has twice the potency of glutethimide as a sedative and toxic agent.[13]

Methanol is another example of a substance whose toxicity is enhanced by metab-

Table 2–3. TOXIC AGENTS WITH ACTIVE METABOLIC INTERMEDIATES

AGENT	ACTIVE PRODUCT
acetaminophen	*N*-hydroxylated intermediate
acetylhydrazine	*N*-hydroxylated intermediate and rearrangement
aflatoxin B_1	epoxide
benzene	epoxide
benzo[*a*]pyrene	epoxide
carbon tetrachloride	free radical form
chloroform	phosgene
cyclophosphamide	hydroxylation and rearrangement
halothane	free radical form
parathion	paraoxon
vinyl chloride	epoxide

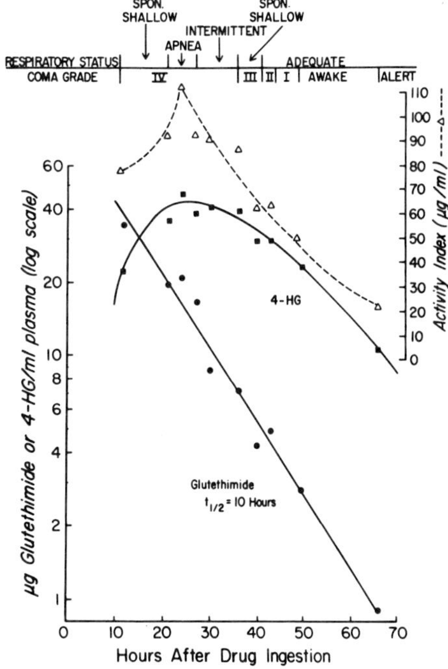

Figure 2–10. Semi-log plot of concentrations of glutethimide (●) and 4-HG (■) in the plasma of a patient poisoned with glutethimide. The activity index (–△–) is a measure of total drug activity in plasma. Also shown are the respiratory status of the patient and the grade of coma. (From Hansen AR, Kennedy KA, Ambre JJ, Fischer LJ: Glutethimide poisoning; A metabolite contributes to morbidity and mortality. N Engl J Med *292*:250, 1975.)

olism. The active metabolite in this case is formic acid. Formate is responsible for the ocular toxicity of methanol and may account for the metabolic acidosis in human beings.[14] The time required for metabolite accumulation is responsible for the usual 10- to 20-hour latent period between methanol ingestion and development of clinical signs and symptoms. As already mentioned, it is possible to inhibit the metabolism of methanol to formate by administration of ethanol, which has much greater affinity for the alcohol-oxidizing enzyme system. Most recently, 4-methylpyrazole, a potent inhibitor of alcohol dehydrogenase has been proposed as an antidote to methanol and ethylene glycol intoxication.[7]

The clinical course following ingestion of a single large overdose of the anticonvulsant drug methsuximide (Celontin) is strikingly biphasic. The initially stuporous patient appears to recover and then lapses into deep coma several hours later. The prolonged second phase of coma is apparently due to accumulation of the active metabolite *N*-desmethylmethsuximide.[15]

Other active, toxic metabolites are not quantitatively prominent and do not accumulate systemically but act locally as the proximate toxin. These metabolites are reactive intermediates that are ordinarily inactivated by protective mechanisms in the cell. Two examples of reactive metabolites formed by microsomal oxidations are epoxides and quinones (Fig. 2–11). The sulfhydryl compound glutathione appears to function in the cell as a "scavenger" of reactive chemical species. Combination with glutathione results in formation of an inactive conjugate. When a large overdose of acetaminophen is taken, the limited glutathione stores of the cell are depleted by excessive formation of the reactive metabolites, and the conjugation process is overwhelmed. The intermediate then reacts with vital cell components, and cell damage occurs. Induction of the microsomal oxidation pathway producing the reactive product may lead to glutathione depletion and tissue damage in circumstances in which excessive therapeutic amounts of the drug are taken.

The finding that the availability of glutathione in liver cells correlated inversely with the extent of liver necrosis induced by acetaminophen was an important step in understanding this mechanism of drug toxicity.[16] Since exogenous glutathione cannot enter the liver cell, the search for an acetaminophen antidote involved trials of various other sulfhydryl compounds that might substitute for glutathione. *N*-Acetylcysteine was found to be effective and well tolerated.

Polycyclic aromatic hydrocarbons, naphthalene, monohalogenated benzene, aflatoxins, and presumably benzene are metabolized to epoxides. Halogenated benzenes are hepatotoxins that produce liver damage in a manner analogous to that of acetaminophen. Polycyclic aromatic hydrocarbons and aflatoxins are carcinogenic substances that apparently interact with DNA by means of the reactive epoxide intermediates to initiate the neoplastic transformation of cells. Possibly, individual susceptibility to the carcinogenic effects of these chemicals is related to the level of activity of the cellular oxidative enzyme producing the toxic metabolite.[17, 18]

EXCRETION

Excretion processes are of primary importance in toxicology. Often, the therapeutic effort is directed to supporting the patient long enough for excretion processes to remove the intoxicant. At other times, the main goal is to protect and to enhance excretion of the drug and thereby shorten the course of intoxication. The kidneys play the most important role in the excretion of drugs and poisons, some in unchanged form and some as metabolites. With few exceptions, excretion into bile is of little quantitative or practical importance. To a great extent, this may be due to the process of enterohepatic recirculation of the excreted drug or to the fact that the excreted material has already been inactivated by metabolism.

Biliary and/or Enteric Excretion

Drugs and other chemicals excreted into the bile enter the intestine and are subsequently either reabsorbed into the blood or eliminated in the feces. The same factors, mentioned previously, that influence absorption will determine the extent of gastrointestinal reabsorption. Drugs excreted in the form of more water-soluble glucuronide conjugates may be hydrolyzed by intestinal bacteria, resulting in reformation of the lipid-

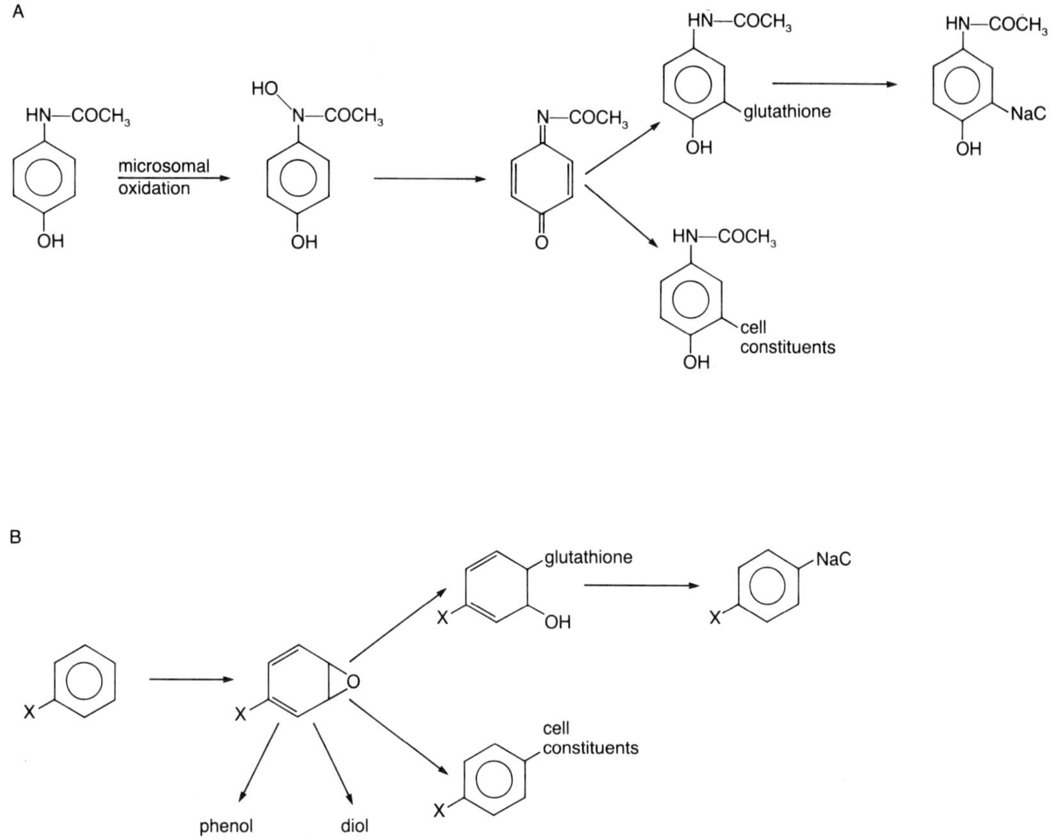

Figure 2–11. *A*, Acetaminophen may react with tissue components by formation of a quinone intermediate. Normally, the quinone form reacts with liver cell glutathione and is excreted as the mercapturic conjugate. *B*, An aromatic compound such as monohalogenated benzene may be metabolized to an epoxide. This reactive intermediate is converted spontaneously to the phenol or by further oxidation to the dihydroxy compound (diol). It may also react with glutathione and eventually be excreted as a mercapturic conjugate. If glutathione is not available, the epoxide may react with tissue components.

soluble parent drug or primary metabolite, which is readily absorbed. The resultant excretion-reabsorption cycle is referred to as enterohepatic recirculation. Morphine is an example of a common drug that undergoes this cycle. The major part of administered morphine is conjugated as morphine 3-glucuronide. Most of this metabolite is excreted into bile and then enters the intestine. A portion is lost in the feces, but most is recycled. Eventually, about 75 per cent of the morphine in the glucuronide form escapes the cycle and is eliminated in the urine.

Attempts have been made to hasten elimination of drugs by interrupting an enterohepatic cycle. Cholestyramine, which can bind digitalis glycosides and other substances in the gut, has been used to interrupt the recycling of digitoxin.[19]

For the vast majority of drugs and toxic chemicals, insufficient information exists on the biliary excretion of the drug in humans to make any estimate of the usefulness of therapy based on biliary excretion. Animal studies are not reliable indicators of the quantitative aspects of biliary excretion in humans. There is marked species variation in the extent of biliary excretion of chemicals. Rats tend to be more extensive biliary excretors of most drugs. Plaa has compiled data on the excretion of various drugs into bile and on interspecies differences in biliary excretion.[20]

The metabolism of glutethimide, a sedative, has been studied extensively. It has been speculated that the recurrence of coma in glutethimide-intoxicated patients is due to enterohepatic recirculation of active drug. In rats with biliary fistulas, 70 per cent of radiolabeled glutethimide was excreted into bile.[21] The only information on the quantitative importance of biliary excretion of glutethimide in humans consists of a single experiment on a single subject, and only 15 per cent of a sedative dose of radioactive drug and/or metabolites was collected from bile.[22] Furthermore, only a small fraction of the material in human bile is unchanged glutethimide.[23] No data exist on how much of the active metabolite is excreted in bile or how much is recycled.

Because of the scarcity of information on biliary excretion of drugs in humans, there appear to be no definite indications for biliary diversion procedures in any acute intoxication syndrome. An interesting future possibility would be direct drainage of bile from a catheter placed endoscopically in the common duct.

The usefulness of cholestyramine as a binding agent may not be confined to treatment of toxicity due to substances excreted in bile. Adsorbents in the gut may also interrupt any enteroenteric recirculation.[24] This pathway of enteric or intestinal excretion was suspected, for example, when data in rats and humans suggested that the pesticide chlordecone (Kepone) entered the gastrointestinal tract from a second source in addition to the bile, possibly by transport directly across the intestinal mucosa.[25] Entry of chlordecone into the intestine by this nonbiliary pathway and excretion in the feces was enhanced by cholestyramine.[26] Workers exposed to chlordecone excreted more chlordecone in bile than in feces, indicating that it might undergo enterohepatic recirculation. A single human subject, requiring biliary surgery for other reasons, was studied in detail (Table 2–4). Chlordecone and its alcoholic metabolite were excreted in bile at a rate four times as high as in feces when the biliary system was intact. When bile was diverted from the intestine through a T tube, fecal excretion of chlordecone alcohol was abolished, presumably because of interruption of its passage in bile to the intestine. However, the amount of chlordecone in feces increased rather than disappeared, indicating that chlordecone entered the intestine from a nonbiliary source. With the biliary system intact, cholestyramine also increased the fecal excretion of chlordecone and its metabolite severalfold.[27]

Subsequently, it was shown that clearance of several other drugs or chemicals could be enhanced by a program of repeated oral doses of activated charcoal (and laxative to ensure passage of the charcoal load through the gut), including drugs with no appreciable biliary excretion or enterohepatic circulation.[28] The serum half-life of intravenous phenobarbital was significantly shortened by a six-hourly charcoal-sorbitol dosing program.[29]

The drugs diffuse into the gastrointestinal tract from the general circulation along a concentration gradient, which is analogous to the process operating in the other direction discussed under sections on absorption mechanisms. The activated charcoal or other binding agent maintains or enhances the gradient by adsorbing the drug from intestinal fluids, thereby continually reducing active drug concentrations on the enteric side of the intestinal membrane. Bound drug is eliminated with the charcoal as it passes in the feces, and additional charcoal is provided to continue the process.

This method of increasing clearance of drug via the gastrointestinal tract has been termed *gastrointestinal dialysis*.[30] In some cases, it may be an additional or alternative measure useful in treating an intoxicated patient. It is important to understand, however, that only a few drugs have been shown to be amenable to this method of removal. The degree of lipid solubility of the drug molecule seems to be an important determinant.[24] Even when the method has been shown to be effective, its effectiveness relative to traditional methods of hemodialysis and hemoperfusion may not be entirely clear.[30]

Table 2–4. CHLORDECONE (KEPONE) EXCRETION IN A HUMAN SUBJECT

	BILE		FECES	
	Chlordecone μ*g/24 hr*	*Metabolite* μ*g/24 hr*	*Chlordecone* μ*g/24 hr*	*Metabolite* μ*g/24 hr*
Intact biliary system	365	469	40	160
Intact biliary system and cholestyramine	235	312	185	162
Diversion of bile (T tube)	180	263	314	—

Data of Boylan JJ, Cohn WJ, Egle JL, et al: Excretion of chlordecone by the gastrointestinal tract. Evidence for a nonbiliary mechanism. Clin Pharmacol Ther *25*:579, 1979.

Urinary Excretion

Drugs and other chemicals are handled by the same renal processes as are endogenous substances, namely glomerular filtration, tubular reabsorption, and secretion. Physicians are generally acquainted with these concepts and the mechanisms involved. Only a very brief discussion is appropriate here.

Most drugs are of small molecular size and therefore are filtered at the glomerulus. The degree of protein binding in blood limits filtration. Once in the tubule, the substance may remain there and eventually be excreted, or it may be passively reabsorbed across the tubule wall into the blood stream. The chemical principles governing this diffusion process are the same as those considered in discussing drug distribution and the passage of lipid membranes. Relatively lipophilic substances will diffuse back to some extent, whereas polar substances and ions will remain in the tubule. The tubular reabsorption and therefore excretion of drugs or poisons that are weak acids or bases is influenced by the pH of urine. The pK of a weak acid or base is the pH at which it is half ionized. As pH decreases, weak bases become more ionized, as do weak acids when pH increases. These substances are able to pass membranes such as the kidney tubule only in the nonionized form. The phenomenon of "ion trapping" refers to the movement of a weak acidic or basic drug across a membrane into a compartment or into bodily fluid having a pH in which it becomes more ionized. It thereby becomes trapped in the compartment in which ionization occurs because the ionic form cannot diffuse out again. By this mechanism, when tubular filtrate (urine) is made more basic relative to plasma, weak acidic drugs are retained in the tubular fluid after filtration and thereby are excreted more rapidly. On the other hand, when urine is more acid relative to plasma, weak basic drugs are excreted more rapidly. The classic practical application of this principle is the hastening of salicylate or phenobarbital excretion by alkalinization and of amphetamine excretion by acidification of urine.

Alkalinization of the urine may be accomplished by administration of bicarbonate, and acidification may be accomplished by administration of ammonium chloride or hydrochloric acid with careful monitoring. It is prudent to avoid the use of carbonic-anhydrase–inhibiting drugs such as acetazolamide to alkalinize the urine unless bicarbonate is administered concurrently. These drugs alkalinize urine by blocking net endogenous bicarbonate reabsorption, and they produce systemic metabolic acidosis. This has the effect, as noted earlier, of favoring distribution of the weak acids salicylate and phenobarbital out of blood into tissues by the ion-trapping mechanism.[31]

Drugs may also appear in the tubule fluid as a result of active secretion by the tubule cells. In contrast to filtration, both free and protein-bound drug are available for secretion. There are at least two active secretion processes; both are located in the proximal tubule. One process handles acids while the other transports bases. Like other active processes, they require a chemical energy source and are subject to substrate competition and saturation.

DIURESIS

Oliguria due to inadequate fluid therapy is obviously not consistent with efficient renal excretion of poisons. The effect of increased urine flow in enhancing drug or poison excretion varies among different substances. A drug that is handled only by glomerular filtration may be excreted in amounts proportional to urine volume. There are few such substances, however, and whether increased urine flow significantly enhances excretion is not known for most substances. Unless specific information of this type is available for a particular drug or poison, the best approach might be to administer sufficient fluid to produce a reasonable urine flow of approximately 2 ml per minute while avoiding circulatory overload. In those instances when forced diuresis is useful, urine pH alteration is usually required.

It is also important, in considering forced diuresis, to be sure that a major portion of the active agents (either parent drug or parent drug and active metabolites) is normally excreted in the urine. This rather obvious point is often forgotten. If, for example, only 10 per cent of the drug is removed by forced diuresis, the potential benefit may not balance the hazards of such therapy.

PHARMACOKINETICS

Clinical pharmacokinetics is the study of the time course of human drug or toxin concentrations that results from drug administration or toxin exposure by whatever route. The study of kinetics is a complex of mathematics and biology aimed at interpretation of concentration data and development of models that allow prediction of drug disposition as a function of administration or exposure variables. Pharmacodynamics describes the relationship between concentrations and effects.

An understanding of kinetic fundamentals is useful in relating drug or toxin concentration data to the status of the intoxicated patient, in selecting appropriate therapy, and in evaluating effectiveness of therapy.

Most drugs are absorbed, eliminated, and moved between compartments in the body by first-order processes. *First order* is a term borrowed from chemical reaction kinetics, indicating an exponential or logarithmic process. A constant fraction of the drug present is handled per unit time. *A characteristic of first-order disappearance of a drug from plasma* is that the time required for the plasma level to fall to half a given value (the half-life) is the same regardless of where on the disappearance curve the measurement is made. A plot of the plasma concentrations versus time is linear on a semilogarithmic graph.

Under certain conditions, some drugs are handled by zero-order, constant, or linear processes. In such cases, a constant amount of the drug present is handled per unit time. *A characteristic of zero-order disappearance from plasma* is that the plasma concentration falls by a constant amount regardless of the level at which the process starts. A plot of plasma concentrations versus time is linear on a linear graph but not on a semilogarithmic graph. Zero-order elimination in many cases is the result of capacity-limited metabolism due to saturation of metabolizing enzyme systems. Under such circumstances, a drug will exhibit apparent zero-order kinetics at high concentrations and first-order kinetics when concentrations have declined to lower levels and the metabolic system is no longer saturated. A notable example of this phenomenon is the elimination of ethanol and methanol.

Salicylate disposition exhibits saturation kinetics at levels in the high therapeutic range (Fig. 2–12). Salicylate elimination normally occurs by several parallel metabolic processes and renal clearance of unchanged drug. At low therapeutic doses, most of the drug is metabolized, and the contribution of renal excretion is small. As concentrations rise, the two quantitatively most important metabolic pathways become saturated. Decline of plasma salicylate concentrations takes on a character that is a mix of the simultaneous first-order and zero-order processes responsible for it. At toxic levels this "pseudo" half-life is as long as 25 hours. As concentrations fall into the lower range (approximately 10 mg/dl), the decline becomes a first-order process. Renal excretion of unchanged salicylate, which is pH dependent, is also quantitatively more important at high plasma levels.

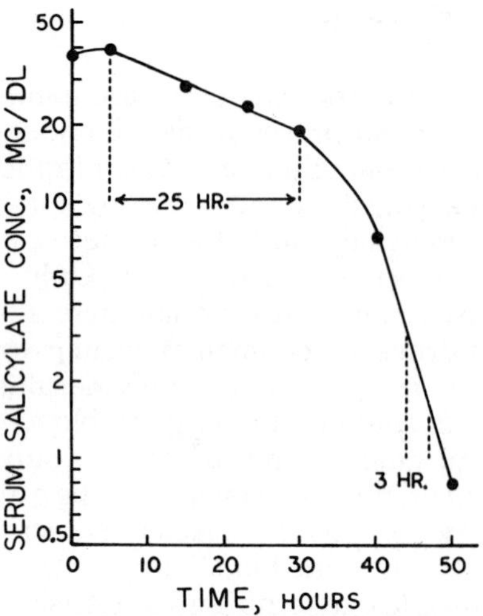

Figure 2–12. Elimination of salicylate by a boy aged 2 years, 9 months, after accidental ingestion of about 2.3 gm of aspirin, of which about 2 gm were absorbed. Serum concentrations are plotted as a function of time and show a 25-hour half-life at high levels and a 3-hour half-life at low blood levels. Zero-order or saturation kinetics prevailed when the concentration of the drug was greater than 10 mg/dl. Below that concentration, first-order kinetics took place. (Modified from Jusko WJ: Pharmacokinetics principles in pediatric pharmacology. Pediatr Clin North Am *19*:81, 1972.)

The half-life of a drug or toxin exhibiting first-order elimination can be obtained graphically from a semilogarithmic plot of the concentration data (Fig. 2–13). The slope of the line, equal to $-K_{el}/2.303$, represents the apparent first-order rate constant for elimination (K_{el}) and can be computed from the half-life ($T\frac{1}{2}$) by the following equation:

$$K_{el} = \frac{0.693}{T\frac{1}{2}}$$

A first-order process, as can be seen in Figure 2–14, is essentially complete after four or five half-lives.

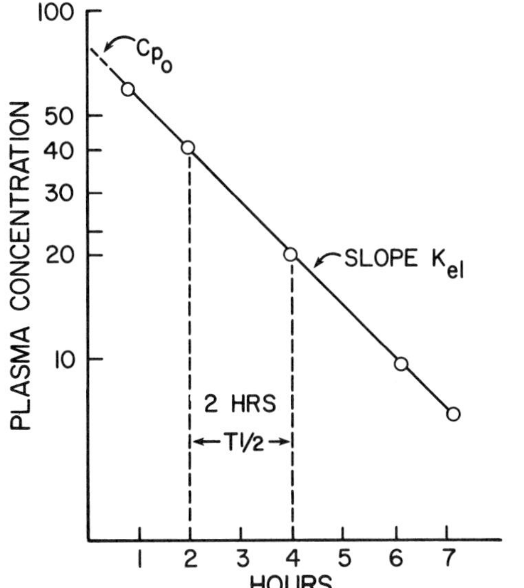

Figure 2–13. First-order elimination. A constant *fraction* of drug is eliminated in unit time.

The apparent volume of distribution (V_d), as noted earlier, is an expression of the extent to which the drug is distributed outside the blood or plasma compartment. It is the proportionality relating the amount of drug in the body and its plasma concentration. It does not represent any real volume and may be much larger than total body volume. It is the volume into which the drug would be dispersed if its concentration in the entire volume were the same as its plasma concentration. The apparent volume of distribution can be estimated from the following equation:

$$V_d = \frac{\text{dose}}{C_{Po}}$$

where C_{Po} is the concentration of drug in plasma immediately after the dose. C_{Po} can be obtained by back extrapolation of the plasma disappearance curve to the vertical axis, as shown in Figure 2–13.

In the least complex kinetic model, a drug confers on the body the characteristics of a single compartment (Fig. 2–15). That is, the drug is immediately distributed throughout the fluids and tissues it is able to penetrate. Because any drug requires some finite time for distribution, from a kinetic standpoint we consider a drug in a one-compartment model if distribution in the body is very rapid *relative* to its rates of absorption and excretion.

For practical application of kinetics, if useful approximations of drug disposition can be made by assuming a single-compartment model, it is worthwhile doing so because the mathematics become much easier. The data in Figure 2–16 simulate tissue and blood concentrations at various times after injection of a drug exhibiting one-compartment kinetics. Note that the decline of concentrations in each tissue is a single phase. Distribution is not necessarily uniform. Tissue concentrations may be higher or lower than those of blood, but they rapidly equilibrate and decline in parallel.

A multicompartment model is necessary to describe the disposition of most drugs (Fig. 2–17). This means that from a kinetic standpoint the drug is handled within the body as though it were moving between two or more separate compartments. Transfer processes between compartments are assumed to be first order and therefore describable by first-order rate constants (k). The volume of each

Figure 2–14. First-order elimination. Virtually all drug excretion is complete within 4 or 5 half-lives.

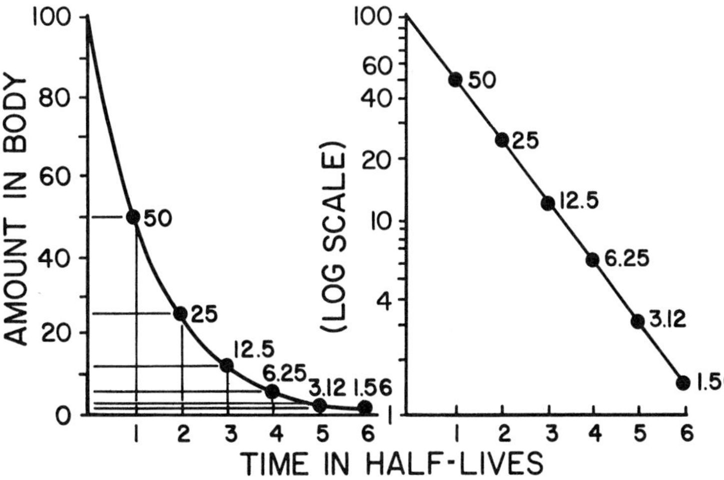

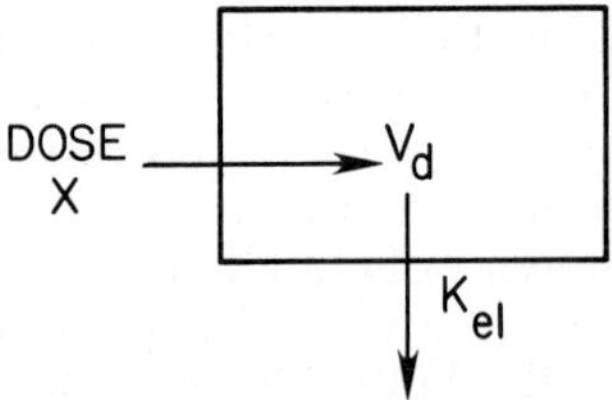

Figure 2–15. Single compartment drug elimination kinetic model.

compartment can be mathematically defined, and elimination is assumed to take place from the first, or central, compartment. Although these compartments cannot be defined anatomically, the central compartment probably consists of the plasma or blood volume and the extracellular fluid of the highly perfused organs, such as the liver, kidneys, lungs, and the heart. For those drugs able to penetrate the blood-brain barrier, it may also include the extracellular fluid of the brain. Since the major organs of excretion are included, the assumption of elimination from the central compartment seems reasonable.

The peripheral compartment (or compartments) is formed by the less well-perfused tissues or sites that the drug penetrates more slowly.

When a drug conferring on the body the characteristics of a two-compartment system is administered by intravenous injection, plasma concentration data plotted semilogarithmically yield a two-phase curve (Fig. 2–18). The first, more rapid phase represents primarily distribution of drug from the central compartment, although excretion processes are proceeding simultaneously. The

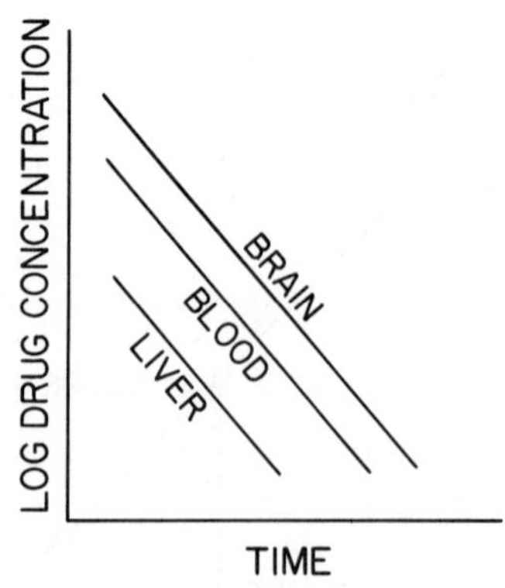

Figure 2–16. Drug elimination in a single compartment kinetic model. Note that log drug concentrations fall in parallel with time.

(first) distribution phase is approaching the (second) elimination phase as a baseline. Once distribution is essentially complete, the decline of plasma levels is determined mainly by excretion or elimination of drug from the central compartment. The plasma level curve can be described mathematically by the following equation:

$$C_p = Ae^{-\alpha t} + Be^{-\beta t}$$

where C_p is the plasma level at any time, t, after the drug injection. The terms A and B are the intercepts of the two phases, as indicated in Figure 2–18. The terms α and β can be computed from the half-lives as shown. These coefficients are related to, but not the same as, the intercompartmental and elimination rate constants of the model shown in Figure 2–17. These rate constants may be calculated, however, from the following equations.

$$k_{el} = \frac{A + B}{\frac{A}{\alpha} + \frac{B}{\beta}}$$

$$k_{21} = \frac{\alpha\beta}{k_{el}} = \frac{A_\beta + B_\alpha}{A + B}$$

$$k_{12} = \frac{AB}{(A + B)^2} \cdot \frac{(\beta - \alpha)^2}{k_{21}}$$

$$V_1 = \frac{\text{dose}}{A + B}$$

$$V_d\ (\text{area}) = \frac{\text{Dose}}{\beta \cdot (\text{area under plasma curve})} = \frac{\text{Dose}}{\beta \cdot \left(\frac{A}{\alpha} + \frac{B}{\beta}\right)}$$

$$V_2 = V_d - V_1$$

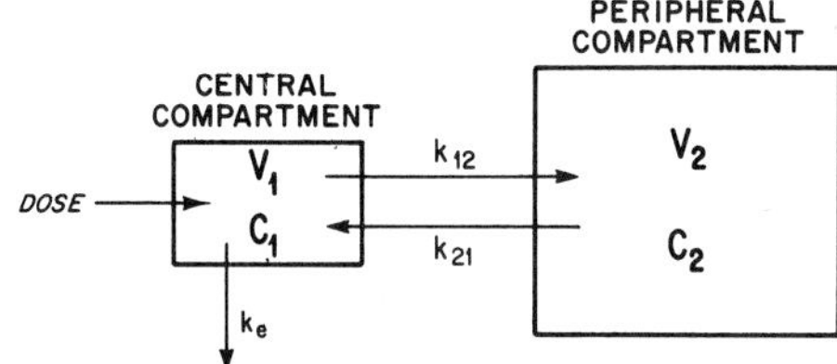

Figure 2–17. The two-compartment model. C_1 and C_2 represent drug concentrations in central and peripheral compartments. V_1 and V_2 represent apparent volumes of these compartments. K_{12} and k_{21} and first-order rate constants in drug transfer between central and peripheral compartments. K_e is the first-order rate constant for drug elimination from the central compartment. (From Greenblatt D, Koch-Weser J: Clinical pharmacokinetics. N Engl J Med *293*:702, 1975. Reprinted by permission.)

Concentrations of drug in the peripheral compartment will be rising during the distribution phase as drug moves from the blood into tissues. Once pseudoequilibrium occurs, concentrations in the two compartments decline in parallel (see Fig. 2–16). Again, concentrations in individual tissues will vary, and the peripheral compartment is actually a composite.

Clearance is an important kinetic parameter. It is an index of drug elimination independent of the amount of drug to be cleared. It is an apparent volume of blood (plasma or serum) from which drug can be completely extracted in a given period of time. When combined with the volume of distribution, it can indicate the rate at which the blood (plasma or serum) concentration is lowered by the processes of excretion (the half-life).

$$t_{1/2\beta} = \frac{\ln 2}{\beta} = \frac{0.693}{\beta}$$

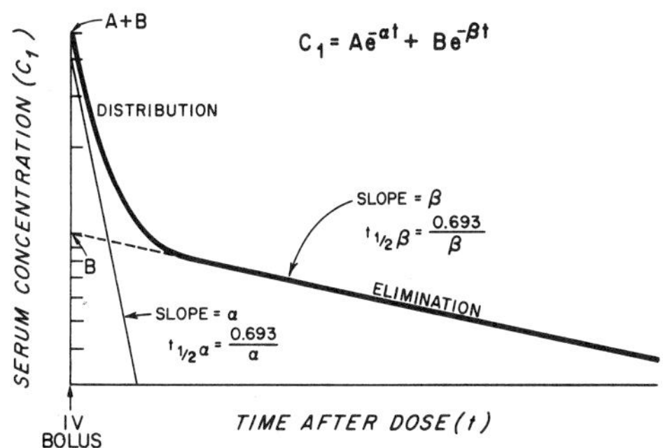

Figure 2–18. Graph of serum concentrations (C_1). Plotted on logarithmic scale, versus time (t) after a single intravenous bolus of a drug as predicted by the two-compartment model. (From Greenblatt D, Koch-Weser J: Clinical pharmacokinetics. N Engl J Med *293*:702, 1975. Reprinted by permission.)

Total clearance is the sum of clearances by the various organs of excretion. The extent to which the plasma concentration is reduced as it flows through the clearing organ is the extraction ratio (E):

$$E = \frac{C_A - C_V}{C_A}$$

where C_A is the inflow plasma concentration and C_V the outflow plasma concentration. If Q is the plasma flow to the clearing organ (ml/min), then the clearance (Cl) is determined by:

$$Cl = QE$$

It is usually not possible to measure organ clearance directly. Total clearance may be estimated from the following equations:

$$Cl = V_1 \cdot k_{el}$$

$$= \beta \cdot V_d\,(\text{area}) = \frac{0.693}{T\frac{1}{2}_\beta} \cdot V_d\,(\text{area})$$

The first equation is dependent on the selection of the proper kinetic model. The second equation is model independent. Rearranging the second equation gives:

$$T\tfrac{1}{2} = \frac{0.693}{Cl} \cdot V_d\,(\text{area})$$

which indicates that half-life is determined by both clearance and volume of distribution. Changes in half-life, therefore, may be less reliable indices of changes in ability to eliminate drugs. Half-life may be lengthened if liver or kidney disease causes a decrease in clearance by these organs. Also, the half-life of some drugs may be shortened if their volume of distribution is reduced. Volume of distribution and clearance are independent parameters, since they are determined by different physiologic factors and may vary independently of one another. In some cases, volume of distribution and clearance may change in such a way that there is little or no change in half-life. For example, in heart failure, there is simultaneous reduction in lidocaine clearance and volume of distribution so that plasma levels are increased, but there is little change in half-life to indicate the reduced clearance.

Consider again the following relationship:

$$Cl = QE$$

If the extraction ratio of a drug is high (the value of E approaches 1), then clearance becomes primarily a function of blood flow to the clearing organ. For drugs such as lidocaine with high hepatic extraction ratios, changes in hepatic blood flow have a corresponding effect on clearance. Important factors that may decrease hepatic blood flow are hepatic disease, volume depletion, congestive heart failure, shock, and the effects of drugs such as propranolol and general anesthetics. For drugs with low extraction ratios, clearance is uninfluenced by changes in flow over a wide range and is primarily related to the overall capacity of the liver to dispose of the drug, reflecting particularly the activity of drug metabolizing enzymes. For drugs with intermediate extraction ratios, clearance depends partly on flow and partly on the rate of drug metabolism.

The ability to enhance removal of drugs and toxins by use of extracorporeal devices, such as hemodialysis and hemoperfusion, is an important aspect of toxicology. Whether these techniques should be used depends on their ability to increase overall clearance significantly. The effectiveness of these methods in turn depends on the efficiency of the device and the extent of distribution of the drugs or toxins. Extensive distribution means that only a small fraction of total amount of drug in the body is in the central compartment, and the plasma concentrations are low. Since the device can remove drug only as it becomes available in the plasma, its ability to increase significantly total clearance of the drug may be limited. The use of kinetics to determine the effectiveness of dialysis or perfusion in removing toxins has been considered in detail elsewhere.[32]

Methanol, like salicylate (mentioned earlier), is a substance that exhibits saturation kinetics or zero-order elimination at all clinically important blood concentrations. Removal of substances across a hemodialyzer membrane is ordinarily a first-order or concentration-dependent process. Initially, failure to appreciate this led to an error in estimating the duration of dialysis required to lower methanol levels in an intoxicated patient to a safe range. Blood methanol data from the case are shown in Figure 2–19. The patient, a 64 year old alcoholic, was admitted to the hospital with a blood pH of 6.75, a blood pressure of 90/60 mm Hg, and a blood methanol of 130 mg per dl. While bicarbonate and ethanol therapy were instituted and preparations made for hemodialysis, blood methanol rose to 180 mg per dl. After 6 hours of dialysis, methanol concentration had dropped to approximately 90 mg per dl. Blood samples had been taken at several other time points prior to the 6-hour point, as indicated in Figure 2–19. Their analyses, however, were not available to the physician at that time. Since the methanol level had decreased by 90 mg per dl in 6 hours, the physician concluded that it was falling at the rate of 15 mg per dl each hour. He therefore instructed the dialysis team to continue dialysis for another 6 hours and then to stop. Since the removal of methanol by the dialyzer is in fact a first-order process, the methanol level, having decreased by half in the first 6 hours of dialysis, decreased by half again in the next 6 hours. This unfortunately did not lower it into a "safe" range, and valuable time was lost in treating the patient's intoxication.

Consider the data in Figures 2–10 and 2–20 from a kinetic standpoint. The logarithmic decline of phenobarbital concentrations is immediately evident (Fig. 2–20). The initial level of 47 mg per dl, together with knowledge of the average half-life (approximately

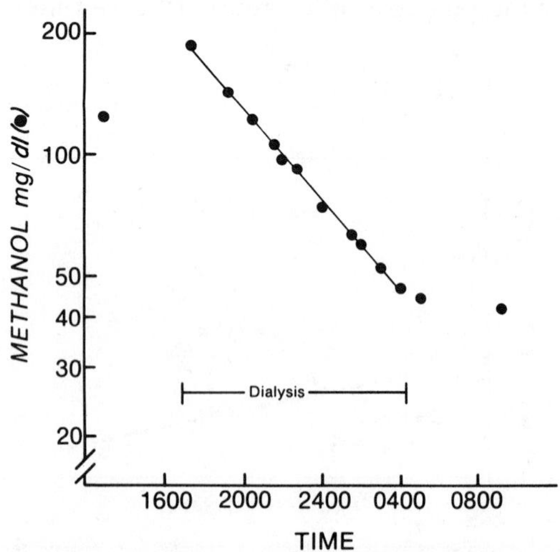

Figure 2–19. Blood methanol (mg/dl) in a patient undergoing hemodialysis. Note that after cessation of dialysis, blood levels failed to decline at the same rapid rate as during hemodialysis, indicating cessation of the first-order drug removal occurring with hemodialysis.

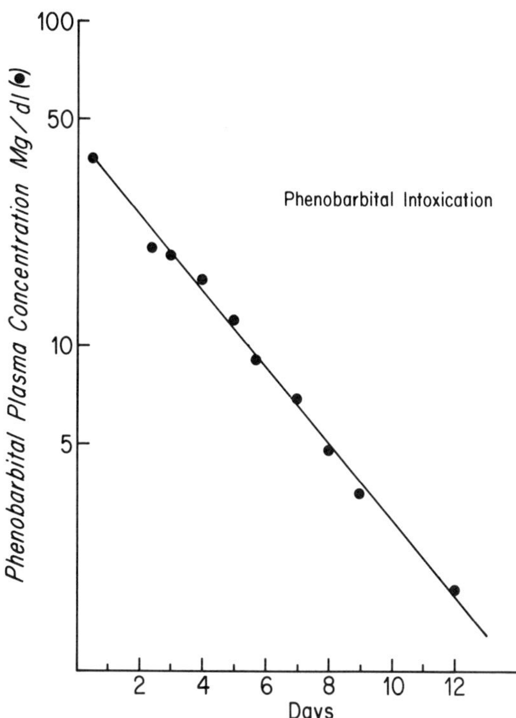

Figure 2–20. First-order drug elimination of phenobarbital in a severely intoxicated patient. Logarithmic decline of phenobarbital indicates that phenobarbital metabolism is not saturated.

80 hours) and therapeutic levels of phenobarbital, immediately indicates that the patient will be unconscious for 4 to 5 days, even accounting for the phenomenon of tolerance. This patient was not treated with dialysis or forced diuresis because an erroneous initial level of 16 mg per dl was reported from the hospital laboratory. The logarithmic decline indicates that even at these very high levels phenobarbital metabolism is not saturated. It also assures the physician that the long course and persistent coma are not related to continued or delayed absorption from the gastrointestinal tract. The influx of drug from any source would alter the first-order elimination phase.

Similar observations can be made of the glutethimide data in Figure 2–10. The persistent coma was not due to continuing glutethimide absorption or enterohepatic recycling of glutethimide, although the active metabolite may undergo such recycling to some extent. These cases illustrate the value and importance of relatively simple kinetic concepts.

TOLERANCE

Tolerance refers to an apparent state of decreased responsiveness to a pharmacologically active agent resulting from previous exposure to the agent. Increasing doses of the drug are required to produce the same effect. In the simplest context, there are at least two basic types of tolerance: dispositional tolerance and pharmacodynamic tolerance.

Dispositional tolerance, as the name implies, occurs as a result of a change in one or more aspect of drug disposition. The best documented instances of this involve an increase in rate of drug metabolism to inactive products. The essential feature is that concentrations of the drug at its site of action remain similar despite increasing doses as disposition is hastened. Common examples of dispositional tolerance are the enhanced metabolism of barbiturates and alcohol occurring with repeated administration. More rapid metabolism is in turn the result of metabolizing enzyme induction.

Pharmacodynamic tolerance results from a change in target systems such that response to a given concentration of drug is reduced. The dose must be increased to achieve the higher concentrations now required to produce the original level of response. Again, the best example of this is the tolerance that develops in the chronic alcoholic and opiate user. It is well appreciated that blood levels (and presumably brain levels) of alcohol that are associated with significant morbidity in the nonalcoholic person may be well tolerated by the chronic drinker.

Less well appreciated is the phenomenon of acute tolerance; that is, pharmacodynamic tolerance that appears over very short time periods, even within the course of the effects of a single dose. A variety of drugs produce some form of acute tolerance, and each may occur by a different cellular mechanism. A classic example is the rapidly decreasing response to administration of sympathomimetic amines, which act indirectly through release of norepinephrine. Repeated administration causes depletion of neurotransmitter stores. Responsiveness returns after repletion of stores by norepinephrine infusion.[33]

An excellent demonstration of acute tolerance to the hypnotic-anesthetic thiopental was described by Brand and associates.[34] Sur-

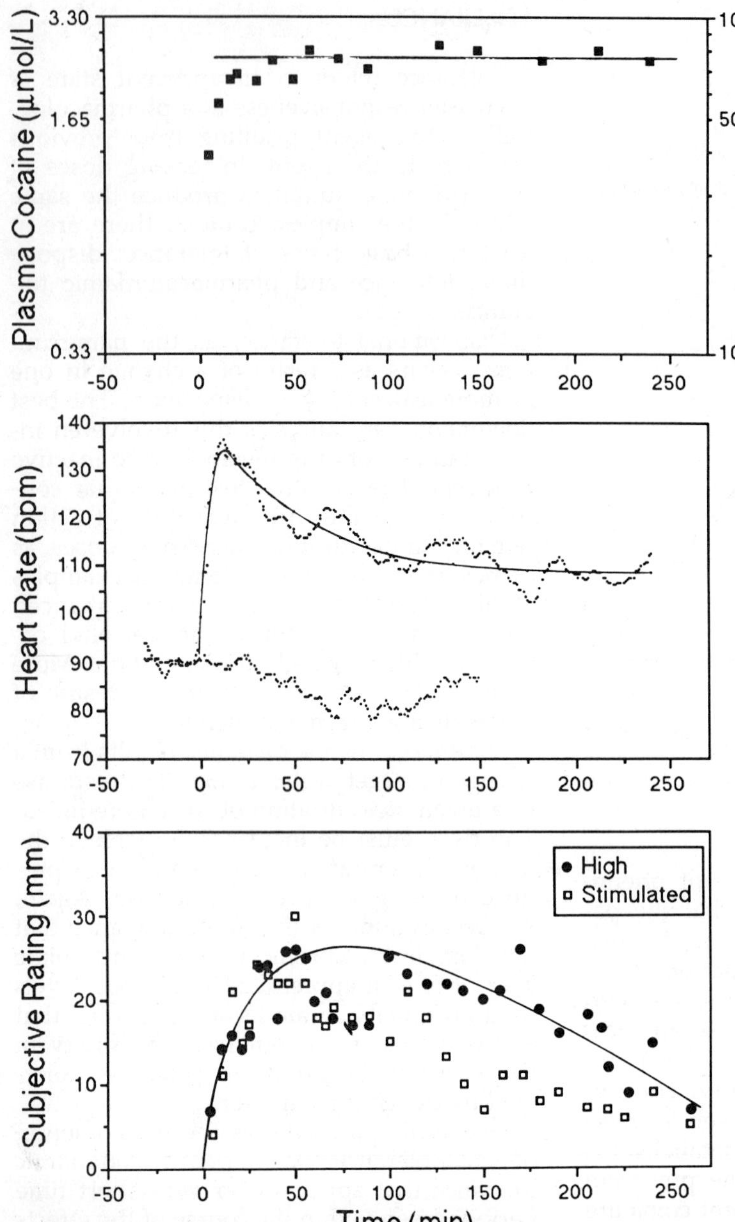

Figure 2–21. Acute tolerance to cocaine in humans. Graphs indicate that while plasma concentrations are held constant over a 4-hour period (top graph), the chronotropic effect (middle graph) indicates a diminishing response with time, as well as declining subjective effects (bottom graph) over this same period. (From Ambre J: Acute tolerance to cocaine in humans. Clin Pharmacol Ther *44*:1–8, 1988.)

gical patients were anesthetized with an intravenous injection of thiopental; enough was administered to produce a specifically selected EEG pattern associated with the desired level of surgical anesthesia. The chosen EEG pattern was then maintained by an infusion of thiopental controlled by a servo-apparatus that varied the infusion rate according to changes in the EEG activity. This resulted in maintenance of unconsciousness for relatively long periods of time, with the depth of unconsciousness precisely controlled and constant. It was found that the plasma level of thiopental producing the constant depth of anesthesia rose successively hour after hour.

The converse approach has also been used to demonstrate acute tolerance. When drug concentrations are held constant, changes in effect intensity are a reflection of changes in the drug level-effect relationship and allow direct determination of the rate of tolerance development. This technique was used by Ambre[35] to demonstrate acute tolerance to cardiac chronotropic and euphoric effects of cocaine in intravenous cocaine users (Fig. 2–21). The chronotropic effect declined to a stable intensity at a third of the initial response. The subjective effects appeared to dissipate or decline to a very low level after 4 hours despite identical cocaine plasma concentration.

The preceding example also displays another aspect of tolerance phenomena: that tolerance does not necessarily develop equally or at the same rate to all effects of the drug.

It has been demonstrated both in animals and in humans, with drugs such as alcohol, pentobarbital, paraldehyde, and trichloroethanol, that following administration of large doses, signs of intoxication disappear at concentrations that were associated with severe intoxication when the blood level was increasing.[36] It has also been observed that the degree of acute tolerance that occurs is directly related to the degree of central nervous system depression that was produced by the drug, that is, the size of the dose.[37] Acute tolerance would explain why the previously drug-naive patient whose plasma phenobarbital levels are shown in Figure 2–20 awakened when the phenobarbital level was 10 mg per dl, a level at which patients taking smaller doses may be in deep coma.[38]

The phenomena of chronic and acute pharmacodynamic tolerance must be considered in the interpretation of blood levels of drugs in the intoxicated patient. The value of blood level determinations in evaluation of the patient is not negated by the phenomenon of tolerance, but the interpretation is made more complex. Correlation of an intoxication score may still be possible,[39] but the variation limits are wider, and the scope of inference is more constricted. It is easy to see the complexity involved in relating concentrations of certain drugs to a particular level of drug effect.

References

1. Schanker LS, Jeffrey JJ: Active transport of foreign pyrimidines across intestinal epithelium. Nature *190*:727, 1961.
2. Waddell WJ, Butler TC: The distribution and excretion of phenobarbital. J Clin Invest *36*:1217, 1957.
3. Smith TW, Haber E, Yeatman L, Butler VP: Reversal of advanced digoxin intoxication with Fab fragments of digoxin-specific antibodies. N Engl J Med *294*:797–800, 1976.
4. Amdisen A: Serum level monitoring and clinical pharmacokinetics of lithium. Clin Pharmacokinet *2*:73, 1977.
5. Williams RT: Detoxication Mechanisms. The Metabolism of Drug and Allied Organic Compounds. New York, John Wiley & Sons, 1947.
6. Testa B, Jenner P: Drug Metabolism: Chemical and Biochemical Aspects. New York, Marcel Dekker, 1976.
7. Baud FJ, Galliot M, Astier A, Vu Bien D, Garnier R, Likforman J, Bismuth C: Treatment of ethylene glycol poisoning with intravenous 4-methylpyrazole. N Engl J Med *319*:97–100, 1988.
8. Vesell E: Polygenic factors controlling drug response. Med Clin North Am *58*:951, 1974.
9. Nebert DW, Jensen NM: The Ah locus: Genetic regulation of the metabolism of carcinogens, drugs and other environmental chemicals by cytochrome P-450-mediated mono-oxygenases. CRC Crit Rev Biochem *6*:401, 1979.
10. Stewart DJ, Inaba T, Tank BK, Kalow W: Hydrolysis of cocaine in human plasma by cholinesterase. Life Sci *20*:1557, 1977.
11. Sutfin TA, Jusko WJ: Compendium of active drug Metabolites. *In* Wilkinson GR, Rawlins DM (eds): Drug Metabolism and Disposition: Considerations in Clinical Pharmacology. Hingham, MA, MTP Press Limited, 1985.
12. Hansen AR, Kennedy KA, Ambre JJ, Fisher LJ: Glutethimide poisoning, a metabolite contributes to morbidity and mortality. N Engl J Med *292*:250, 1975.
13. Ambre JJ, Fischer LJ: Identification and activity of the hydroxy metabolite that accumulates in the plasma of humans intoxicated with glutethimide. Drug Metab Dispos *2*:151, 1974.
14. McMartin KE, Ambre JJ, Tephly TR: Methanol poisoning in human subjects; role for formic acid accumulation in the metabolic acidosis. Am J Med *68*:414, 1980.
15. Karch SB: Methsuximide overdose; delayed onset of profound coma. JAMA *223*:1463, 1973.
16. Mitchell JR, Thorgeirsson J, Potter WZ, Jollow DJ, Keiser H: Acetaminophen-induced hepatic injury: Protective role of glutathione in man and rationale for therapy. Clin Pharmacol Ther *16*:676, 1974.
17. Ambre JJ, Bures F, Haupt D, Graeff D, Deason K: Antipyrine metabolism in patients with lung cancer. J Med *8*:57, 1977.
18. Ayesh R, Idle J, Ritchie JC, Crothers MJ, Hetzel MR: Metabolic oxidation phenotypes as markers for susceptibility to lung cancer. Nature *312*:169–170, 1984.
19. Caldwell JH, Bush CA, Greenberger NJ: Interruption of the enterohepatic circulation of digitoxin by cholestyramine. J Clin Invest *50*:2638, 1971.
20. Plaa G: Biliary and other routes of excretion of drugs. *In* LaDu BN, Mandel HG, Way EL (eds): Fundamentals of Drug Metabolism and Drug Disposition. Baltimore, Williams & Wilkins, 1971, p 131.
21. Bernhard K, Just M, Vuillemier JP: Zur Bestimmung des zeitlichen Ablaufes in der leber stattfindender Detoxikationen durch Analyze fer Galle. Helv Physiol Acta *15*:177, 1957.
22. Butikofer EP, Cottier P, Inhof H, Keberle W, Riess W, Schmid K: Uber die Eliminierungsgeschwendikiet von glutethimid. Arch Exp Path Pharmak *244*:97, 1962.
23. Charyton C: The enterohepatic circulation in glutethimide intoxication. Clin Pharmacol Ther *11*:810, 1970.

24. Dayton PG, Israili ZH, Henderson JD: Elimination of drugs by passive diffusion from blood to intestinal lumen: Factors influencing nonbiliary excretion by the intestinal tract. Drug Metab Rev *14*:1193, 1983.
25. Boylan JJ, Egle JL, Guzelian PS: Cholestyramine: Use as a new therapeutic approach for chlordecone (Kepone) poisoning. Science *199*:893, 1978.
26. Cohn WJ, Boylan JJ, Blanke RV, Fariss MW, Howell JR, Guzelian PS: Treatment of chlordecone (Kepone) toxicity with cholestyramine. N Engl J Med *298*:243, 1978.
27. Boylan JJ, Cohn WJ, Egle JL, Blanke RV, Guzelian PS: Excretion of chlordecone by the gastrointestinal tract: Evidence for a nonbiliary mechanism. Clin Pharmacol Ther *25*:579, 1979.
28. Neuvonen PJ, Elonen E: Effect of activated charcoal on absorption and elimination of phenobarbital, carbamazepine and phenylbutazone in man. Eur J Clin Pharmacol *17*:51–57, 1980.
29. Berg MJ, Berlinger WG, Goldberg MJ, Spector R, Johnson GF: Acceleration of the body clearance of phenobarbital by oral activated charcoal. N Engl J Med *307*:642, 1982.
30. Levy G: Gastrointestinal clearance of drugs with activated charcoal. N Engl J Med *307*:676, 1982.
31. Hill JB: Salicylate intoxication. N Engl J Med *288*:1110, 1973.
32. Tilstone WJ, Winchester JF, Reavey PC: The use of pharmacokinetic principles in determining the effectiveness of removal of toxins from blood. Clin Pharmacokinet *4*:23, 1979.
33. Goldstein A, Aronow L, Kalman S: Principles of Drug Action. 2nd ed. New York, John Wiley & Sons, 1974, p 575.
34. Brand L, Mazzia V, Poznak AV, Burns JJ, Mark LC: Lack of correlation between electroencephalographic effects and plasma concentrations of thiopentone. Br J Anaesthesiol *33*:92, 1961.
35. Ambre JJ, Belknap SM, Nelson J, Ruo TI, Shin S-G, Atkinson AJ Jr: Acute tolerance to cocaine in humans. Clin Pharmacol Ther *44*:1–8, 1988.
36. Jaffe JH: Drug addiction and drug abuse. *In* Goodman LS, Gilman AG (eds): The Pharmacological Basis of Therapeutics. 6th ed. New York, Macmillan, 1980, p 539.
37. Jaffe JH, Martin WR: Opioid analgesics and antagonists. *In* Goodman LS, Gilman AG (eds): The Pharmacological Basis of Therapeutics. 6th ed. New York, Macmillan, 1980, p 513.
38. Sunshine I: Chemical evidence of tolerance to phenobarbital. J Lab Clin Med *50*:127, 1957.
39. McCarron MM, Schulze BW, Walberg CB, Thompson GA, Ansari A: Short-acting barbiturate overdosage: Correlation of intoxication score with serum barbiturate concentration. JAMA *248*:55–61, 1982.

CHAPTER 3

LABORATORY DIAGNOSIS AND DRUG TESTING

W. J. Tilstone, Ph.D.
D. G. Deutsch, Ph.D.

AIMS OF LABORATORY DIAGNOSIS

Drug testing of humans has many applications today. Socially, it is being used to regulate drug abuse in sport.[1] It is used in workplace monitoring as a combined social and health care measure, and it is used clinically in assessment of individuals who claim to be dependent on drugs.[2, 3] These are new and relevant extensions of traditional applications in therapeutic drug monitoring and the diagnosis and treatment of drug overdose.

Drug overdoses are a frequent cause of morbidity and mortality. Some 3 per cent of admissions to medical wards arise as a consequence of toxicity from drugs used as directed by physicians, and a further 3 per cent as a consequence of self-induced poisoning by drugs or chemicals.[4, 5] Laboratory aids are rarely required to identify the causal medication in the former instance, although they may be necessary to establish the extent of the consequences. The situation is markedly different in the case of self-poisoning.[6, 7]

The first objective of considering a resort to laboratory aids in diagnosis, therefore, is to establish the exact nature of the chemical or drug taken in overdose. This may be necessary for medicolegal or for clinical reasons. In the former case, drug assays on gastric washings, blood, and urine samples may be required. These can be done at leisure and do not require emergency services to be alerted. Similarly, with certain notable exceptions, emergency drug assays are infrequently necessary in conscious patients, or even in unconscious patients provided they have normal spontaneous respirations, normal reflexes, and adequate blood pressure. A list of drugs in which measurement of blood levels may be helpful in assessing the need for and progress of treatment is given in Table 3–1.

Before considering an emergency assay, it is important to appreciate the difficulty in interpreting single drug levels. This does not arise if diagnosis is the sole objective. Nevertheless, if a guide to the need for, or progress of, therapy is sought, several issues must be appreciated:

1. Tolerance may be present, thereby leading to possible inappropriate concern over high concentrations of drug.
2. Levels may be changing rapidly as a consequence of continued drug absorption. Thus assays within 4 hours of administration are frequently misleading.
3. The specificity of the assay must be known—is it measuring the parent drug only, or its active metabolites only, or a combination of drug and metabolites, including inactive metabolites?
4. Has an assay been performed to take into account concurrent alcohol administration?

INFLUENCE OF EPIDEMIOLOGIC ASPECTS

To be completely successful, laboratory diagnosis of the toxicologic patient demands a screen for every drug or likely poison, with detection limits well below those normally likely to be encountered in blood or urine, and with subsequent accurate quantification of levels. Such a goal is clearly unattainable; even to approach it would require an unacceptable deployment of resources. A certain degree of limitation is therefore necessary, and this is principally achieved by tailoring the service offered to match the most frequent clinical demands. The frequency of these demands is governed by two factors: the prevalence of the toxin, clearly related to prescription numbers of medicines and to geography for industrial and natural poisons, and to the clinical uses of the laboratory study. Thus, laboratory diagnosis would be sought more frequently when there was a suspicion of a particularly toxic substance such as paraquat, of a drug with a narrow therapeutic index such as lithium, or of a drug with a clear indication for a particular course of therapy, such as methanol.

Table 3–1. DRUGS FOR WHICH LABORATORY ASSAY IS ADVISABLE IN OVERDOSE

	INDICATOR FOR ASSAY
barbiturate	Severe CNS depression: therapy
glutethimide	Diagnosis and therapy
salicylate	Tinnitus/deafness/tachycardia: therapy
paracetamol	Diagnosis: urgent therapy
iron	Diagnosis: therapy
paraquat	Diagnosis and therapy
lithium	Diagnosis: therapy
methanol	Diagnosis: therapy
ethanol	Diagnosis
digoxin	Diagnosis: antibody therapy
theophylline	Diagnosis: therapy
ethylene glycol	Diagnosis: urgent therapy
tricyclics	Diagnosis

The laboratory investigation of the toxicologic patient differs markedly from laboratory adjuncts to diagnosis and therapy in other areas of medicine. Uniquely, the tests are performed with a low frequency, with a comparatively low through-put of samples, and are resistant to automation even when other indications are favorable. The only partial exception to this is in the use of systems established for therapeutic drug monitoring or for drug abuse programs. The contrasts between the toxicologist in the forensic laboratory, with fewer pressures of time but with the same requirement for analytic exactitude, and the hospital laboratory toxicologist are of note. The former has all the resources of classic analytic toxicology available, and the demand above all others placed upon him or her is identification and quantification of the poison. Toxicologists in the clinical setting have no value unless they can feed information appropriately to the team responsible for patient care. A major requirement of laboratory diagnosis of the toxicologic patient therefore is the "stat" test for a (fortunately) limited range of drugs, backed up with a "next day" service for a number of other compounds.

There is a certain conflict between this requirement for "stat" analyses and the relatively low frequency and painstaking multistep serial techniques that are so often used in drug analyses. Urban areas with a high concentration of population and therefore a sufficient number of poisoning cases to justify centralized facilities should have some advantages in this respect, although even here reliable ward tests, if only they were available, would have much to commend them.

In general, therefore, although the laboratory may be called on for analyses of drugs either as outlined in Table 3–1 or on a broader basis—reflecting, for example, drugs implicated in patient deaths as shown in Table 3–2—it could be argued that most of the requirements of laboratory diagnosis for the toxicologic patient could be handled by a relatively small battery of qualitative and quantitative tests. Fortunately, as will be seen later, modern techniques, particularly in the field of immunochemistry, make this more feasible than used to be the case.

EVALUATION OF LABORATORY TECHNIQUES

"Toxin screen" results are weighed heavily in the diagnosis and treatment of overdosed patients.[11] It is important, therefore, that clinical staff are aware of the analytic performance of the laboratories providing that screen or, alternatively, are able to make a good assessment of stat test procedures that may be offered to them for on-site use.

The laboratory techniques can be assessed according to the factors shown in Table 3–3. Any assay in the present context must be (1) adequately accurate, sensitive, specific, and reproducible; (2) capable of dealing with the likely workload; and (3) sufficiently rapid. The *accuracy* of the test may be defined as how close the reported value is to the true value, i.e., it is a measure of the correctness of a quantitative assessment. Related to this is the specificity of the test: in other words, its ability uniquely to identify compounds without cross-reactions from related or unrelated species. The *sensitivity* of the test is self-evident, and the reproducibility, or *precision,* of the test is a measure of how repeatable is the technique either within the laboratory or between laboratories. The key word in this evaluation is *adequate.* It may be felt that only completely accurate and specific tests are of value, but it should be remembered that some assays specific for groups of drugs rather than for individual members of the group—for example, barbiturates, benzodiazepines, or tricyclic antidepressants—may be of considerable help and that the confident, rapid identification of an unknown as being a tricyclic antidepressant may be of more help in treatment of the overdosed patient than would be a more lengthy laboratory evaluation showing that only amitriptyline at a particular concentration was present in blood.

The *through-put* of the assay—its ability to deal with the likely workload—should be carefully considered but is seldom a limitation in this field. Capital costs and running costs are always a problem and are often interrelated. In theory, a procedure such as gas chromatography–mass spectrophotometry would appear to offer sensitivity, accuracy, and specificity at the expense of a high capital cost and, when maintenance costs are included, higher-than-average running costs. However, a new generation of computer-operated instruments that are easy to operate and compact are now being introduced into a variety of laboratories. The capital expenditure for these gas chromatograph–mass spectrometers (GC-MS) is about the same as that for automated instruments (e.g., centrif-

Table 3–2. DRUGS IMPLICATED IN PATIENT DEATHS

US DRUG DEATHS *(Maryland, 1975–1980)*[8]	US NONDRUG DEATHS *(Maryland, 1975–1980)*[8]	US TRAUMA CENTER ADMISSIONS *(California)*[9]	DRUG DEATHS, ENGLAND *(1975–1984)*[10]
propoxyphene, 19.8	barbiturates, 24.8	amphetamines, 26.0	barbiturates, 26.5
tricyclics, 18.0	narcotics, 10.0	narcotics, 12.9	propoxyphene, 5.7
barbiturates, 18.0	benzodiazepines, 8.4	cocaine, 6.3	tricyclics, 5.2
narcotics, 8.7	phenytoin, 7.4	barbiturates, 0.9	salicylates, 5.0
phenothiazines, 4.8	phenothiazines, 7.2	salicylates, 0.6	acetaminophen, 4.1
ethchlorvynol, 3.3	lidocaine, 6.2	tricyclics, 0.3	
glutethimide, 3.3	propoxyphene, 5.7		

Numbers are percent of reported cases.
Narcotics include methadone and phencyclidine, but not cocaine.

Table 3–3. REQUIREMENTS OF DRUG ASSAY IN LABORATORY DIAGNOSIS

FEATURE	IMPORTANCE
Accuracy*	+ + +
Specific: groups of drugs	+ + +
individual drugs†	+ +
Rapid	+ + +
Reproducible‡	+ + +
Cost	+ +
Through-put	+

*In many cases, qualitative screen alone will suffice, but if quantitation is performed for diagnosis or to monitor progress, then accuracy is of paramount importance.

†Group of drugs probably more important, unless quantification is needed.

‡Within-laboratory reproducibility *must* be good. For comparison with published quantitative data, between-laboratory reproducibility should be high.

ugal analyzers) commonly used for immunoassays in therapeutic drug monitoring and toxicology. GC-MS is a relatively slow technique. Immunologic methods, by contrast, have a fairly high running cost and are extremely rapid.

Interrelating the areas of accuracy and precision is the question of complexity of the analytic technique. In general, it may be expected that specificity requires an increasing complexity of tests because of preliminary purification procedures. However, it is also a general finding that the more steps there are in a test, the less reliable is the outcome. This is sometimes known as Occam's razor, or the law of parsimony.

The clinician, therefore, should scrutinize critically the details of laboratory techniques offered in toxin screen procedures. These techniques must be as simple as possible consistent with preservation of specificity and accuracy. They should be sufficiently sensitive, bearing in mind that the overdosed patient will have higher blood levels of drugs than will be encountered in the normal therapeutic setting, and accuracy must always be sufficient such that no misclassification on the basis of blood levels will be made. The techniques must be sufficiently robust to allow comparable results to be obtained by different operators, thereby maintaining the integrity of the laboratory diagnostic procedure. Finally, the techniques must be sufficiently rapid to provide results that can be used during the time span of diagnosis and therapy for each patient.

METHODS FOR DRUGS AND OTHER SIMPLE ORGANICS

A drug assay has two criteria to satisfy: it must identify the drug or drugs and it must quantify them. In general, most of the techniques utilized go some way toward meeting both criteria.

Chromatographic Techniques. These are usually thought of as separation methods, and certainly classic column chromatography in its many variants as practiced in biochemistry laboratories is just that. The equivalent in toxicology laboratories is *thin-layer chromatography* (TLC). Generally performed on silica gel films coated on glass or plastic plates, the technique is simple, cheap, and, in experienced hands, reliable. It suffers from the drawbacks that it is qualitative only, and that separations depend on the activity of the stationary phase and the purity of the mobile phase. Therefore, in practice, reproducibility between operators and certainly between laboratories is less than might be hoped for. To a certain extent some of the ground lost by lack of reproducibility is recovered by the specificity engendered by the use of group-specific reagents to locate the compounds on the plate. Some of the specific reagents used are shown in Table 3–4. A limited degree of interlaboratory comparisons can be made by expressing results as R_f values, that is, the distance migrated by the solute compared with the distance migrated by the solvent. Some of the variation also can be taken out by intelligent use of standards, and in particular with mixtures being applied at both edges and in a central position in each plate run. The combination of R_f values obtained under these circumstances with group-specific reagents can give a rea-

Table 3–4. SOME TLC REAGENTS AND SPECIFICITY OF DETECTION

	DETECTS
mercurous nitrate	barbiturates
ferrichloride/potassium ferricyanide	analgesics (non-narcotic)
FPN*	phenothiazines
iodoplatinate	narcotic analgesics, tricyclic antidepressants
Dragendorff	alkaloids

*Ferrichloride, perchloric acid, nitric acid.

sonably rapid and reliable identification for most drugs. Toxi-Lab (Analytical Systems, Laguna Hills, CA 92653) and Stat-Tox (Biochemical Diagnostics, Edgewood, NY 11717) are two commercial TLC systems. The Toxi-Lab system, which comes with a compendium of colored chromatograms for most drugs, is relatively easy to use and is popular in smaller laboratories. Stat-Tox, a semi-automated system that spots the TLC plates after a urine specimen is passed through a column, is usually employed in laboratories that process large numbers of samples.

In contrast to TLC, *gas chromotography* (GC) offers greater sensitivity and considerably greater resolution of the components of complex mixtures and may be used very effectively to quantify compounds. A certain degree of capital expenditure is required, and the technique is limited by the need for the substances assayed to be volatile either in themselves or by means of formation of derivatives. The essential components are a temperature-controlled oven and a detector system, the specificity and sensitivity of the technique being very much determined by the latter (flame ionization, nitrogen/phosphorus, or electron capture detector). Within the temperature-controlled oven is a column containing the stationary phase onto which the separated components partition in the vapor phase as they are carried out along the column by an appropriate carrier gas. The stationary phase may be coated on fine, inert, support phase particles, as in conventional gas chromatography, or may be linked directly onto the walls of the tube in the case of capillary gas chromatography.

Assuming the requirement of volatility has been met, then excellent identification can be achieved from gas chromatography by judicious tailoring of stationary phase and temperature. Replicate analyses on different stationary phases or using different derivative formation will aid identification, as does the relative response to the various detectors available. The variations within the analytic system can be minimized by making use of internal standards—that is, the unknown mixture is chromatographed simultaneously with an added compound, which may be a member of the homologous series being investigated or may be a hydrocarbon.

A presentation of data analogous to that used in TLC is sometimes used: relative retention time or distance, in which the time lapse (or distance traveled on the chart recorder) from injection into the chromatographic system to appearance of the separated component at the detector is ratioed to the corresponding measure for the internal standard. Relative retention times so measured, under well-controlled conditions of the nature and loading of the stationary phase and of the temperature of the oven, are reproducible and certainly much better than is the case with R_f values. Table 3–5 compares the absolute and relative retention times for a mixture of hypnotic-sedative drugs analyzed by capillary gas chromatography and by a nitrogen-phosphorus detector. These drugs were extracted from serum with mephobarbital as the internal standard.

A better system for identification purposes is the use of Kovat's indices, in which the retention of the unknown is compared with that of two standards, usually hydrocarbons differing in chain length by one carbon and usually bracketing the retention time of the unknown. A number of equations are available for estimation of Kovat's indices, including

$$I = 100 \left[\frac{a - b}{c - d} \right] + 100\,d$$

where I is the retention index; a, b, and c are the logarithms of the retention distances of the unknown and the lower and higher hydrocarbon standards, respectively; and d is the number of carbon atoms in the low hydrocarbon standard. Kovat's indices are very reproducible between operators and indeed between laboratories. For example, excellent correlation was found in Kovat's indices for volatile bases in laboratory "A" using a capillary-based system, compared with those for the same stationary phase in a conventional GC in laboratory "B."[12] Identification "windows" can also be prepared by measuring the Kovat's indices for unknowns on two different stationary phases.[13] The only drawback at present to the use of Kovat's indices is their strange behavior in temperature-programmed runs, and this problem has yet to be overcome.

Quantitative techniques based on gas chromatography can be very accurate, reproducible, and sufficiently sensitive to deal with most drugs and toxins at overdose levels. For example, using a capillary gas chromatography system with a nitrogen-specific de-

Table 3–5. DAY-TO-DAY REPRODUCIBILITY OF ABSOLUTE (ART) AND RELATIVE (RRT) RETENTION TIMES

DRUG AND PEAK NO.	GAS CHROMATOGRAPHY			
	Mean ART (min) ± SD	*CV, %*	*Mean RRT ± SD*	*CV, %*
methyprylon, 1	7.02 ± 0.03	0.46	0.67 ± 0.010	0.77
butabarbital, 2	8.20 ± 0.04	0.50	0.78 ± 0.000	0.00
amobarbital, 3	8.71 ± 0.05	0.52	0.83 ± 0.010	0.62
pentobarbital, 4	8.95 ± 0.04	0.50	0.85 ± 0.000	0.00
secobarbital, 5	9.43 ± 0.05	0.49	0.89 ± 0.004	0.54
glutethimide, 6	10.11 ± 0.05	0.53	0.96 ± 0.000	0.00
carisoprodol, 7	10.23 ± 0.06	0.55	0.97 ± 0.000	0.00
mephobarbital, 8	10.54 ± 0.06	0.51	1.00 ± —	—
phenobarbital, 9	11.06 ± 0.06	0.54	1.05 ± 0.000	0.00
methaqualone, 10	12.82 ± 0.08	0.59	1.22 ± 0.000	0.00
diazepam, 11	14.99 ± 0.10	0.64	1.42 ± 0.003	0.27
nordiazepam, 12	15.52 ± 0.11	0.73	1.47 ± 0.003	0.21

N = nine each, determined over a 2-month period.
ART, absolute retention time; RRT, relative retention time.
(Adapted with permission from Deutsch DG, Bergert RJ: Evaluation of a benchtop capillary gas chromatograph–mass spectrometer for clinical toxicology. Clin Chem *31*:741, 1985.)

tector, a combination that enhances the positive response to the compound to be analyzed and minimizes background noise, picogram quantities of amphetamine can be detected.[14] Again, the use of internal standards with ratioing of the response from drug to that of internal standard minimizes most of the inherent system error and lends excellent reproducibility to the techniques. The equipment is also best utilized without down-time and without the need of alteration to different column or detector systems in one rig at different times.

Probably the best available method in the laboratory in terms of identification and sensitivity of detection is the combination of *gas chromatography with mass spectrometry* (GC-MS). This could certainly be regarded as the best reference method,[11] although historically it required expensive hardware. However, simpler, cheaper, more reliable benchtop devices, such as the Hewlett Packard Mass Selective Detector (MSD), are now available.

These benchtop GC-MS instruments give the best results for drugs when configured with a capillary column inserted directly into the ion source. With the MSD, the software programs on the computer cause the GC-MS to be highly automated, requiring little operator intervention. In addition to controlling the gas chromatograph and the autosampler, if installed, the computer program carries out such functions as autotuning, selective ion monitoring, total ion monitoring, background subtraction, and a library search for an unknown. This instrument comes with convenient software for internal standard method quantification and various formats for customizing reports. With the MSD the user has a choice of two library search routines (the 10-peak or probability-based matching, PBM) and a choice of various libraries. The most suitable library for the toxicology laboratory is that of Pfleger, Maurer, and Weber, which contains approximately 1700 drugs, poisons, and metabolites. All libraries must be customized to some extent by the user to include missing drugs, metabolites, endogenous urine and plasma compounds, and retention times. An example of using a combination of a case study and a literature search to customize the library is shown in Figure 3–1. In this figure, a mass spectrum obtained from a patient who ingested cocaine and one published by Ambre and associates for ecgonine methyl ester are compared.[15] The similarity of the two mass spectra suffices to allow one to add this metabolite, obtained from a peak resolved on a total ion chromatogram of a basic urine extract, to the library.

With the establishment of federal and state regulations for laboratory accreditation in workplace toxicology, cutoff levels for confirmation of some drugs in urine have been established as well as minimal levels for spiking of proficiency test specimens. Quantitative GC-MS confirmation is being instituted as a way to gauge the performance of laboratories on proficiency tests, although it is recognized that the results probably do not have any physiologic significance in samples

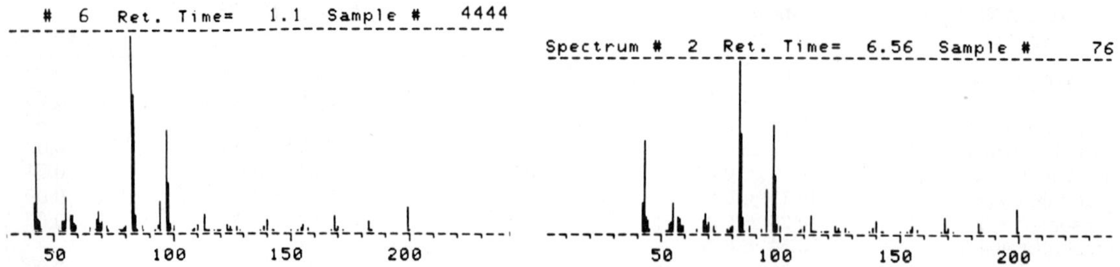

Figure 3–1. Mass spectrum of ecgonine methyl ester obtained by Ambre and associates[15] and in the authors' laboratory. (From Deutsch DG: Gas chromatography–mass spectrometry using table top instruments. *In* Deutsch DG: Analytical Aspects of Drug Testing. Vol. 100. Chemical Analysis Series. New York, John Wiley, 1989.)

of urine. The MSD comes with convenient packages for quantitation of drugs using the selective ion monitoring (SIM) mode of operation. The user has a choice of report formats when using the internal standard method, including automatically determining the ratios of selected analyte ions ("qualifiers") as a check for interfering substances. An example of a report containing this information is shown in Figure 3–2. The dimethyl derivative of 11-nor-delta-9-tetrahydrocannabinol-9-carboxylic acid (THC-COOH) and of trideuterated THC-COOH (the internal standard) were chromatographed and the ions for the metabolite (313, 357, and 372 amu) and internal standard (316, 360, and 375 amu) counted. When quantitation is performed using peak qualifiers, a calculated result will be reported only if the confirming ions are found in the proper retention time and if their ratios, relative to the quantitating ions, fall within an expected range.[16]

When using SIM, it has been pointed out by Foltz[17] that many factors must be considered regarding what constitutes a positive identification and accurate quantitation. These factors include the derivation and extraction procedures, the chromatography, the ionization process (which is restricted to electron ionization at present with the instruments described here), the number of ions monitored, and the uniqueness of the mass spectra.

As internal standards for GC/MS quantitation, it is generally accepted that, when available, stable isotope analogues are favored over unlabeled homologues or isomers. Although studies have not been performed for specific drugs of abuse comparing deuterium-labeled analogues to unlabeled homologues, there is substantial evidence that the former makes assays more precise, accurate, and specific, although a report to the contrary has been published.[18] While stable isotope analogues may also increase recoveries by serving as a carrier, they may lead to imprecision if the amount used is too large relative to the analyte.[19]

One of the more popular modern techniques is HPLC, originally an acronym for high pressure liquid chromatography but now meaning high *performance* liquid chromatography. The use of ion-pairing extraction and reverse phase systems with short, broad columns and low pressure systems can produce good and rapid resolution of most organic materials. Resolutions achieved are poorer than those from capillary column gas chromatography, but the limitation of volatility does not apply in liquid systems.

In contrast with the universal detection ability of the flame ionization detector in GC, there is a limitation of the detector side in HPLC, requiring that the substance either have good ultraviolet absorption or, even better, be fluorescent. In many cases—for example, benzodiazepines—there is little to choose between GC and HPLC in terms of adequate identification and adequate sensitivity for quantification. Two new HPLC detectors being evaluated for clinical and forensic toxicology are the ultraviolet photodiode array detector[20] and the mass spectrometer.[21] Both systems show great potential, since they provide the advantages of HPLC with the specificity of spectral analysis. When used in conjunction with computed spectral comparison of an unknown to drug libraries, these techniques are powerful tools for the identification of compounds.

Name Info: 494-1E
Misc Info:
Date : 26 Oct 87 9:39 pm

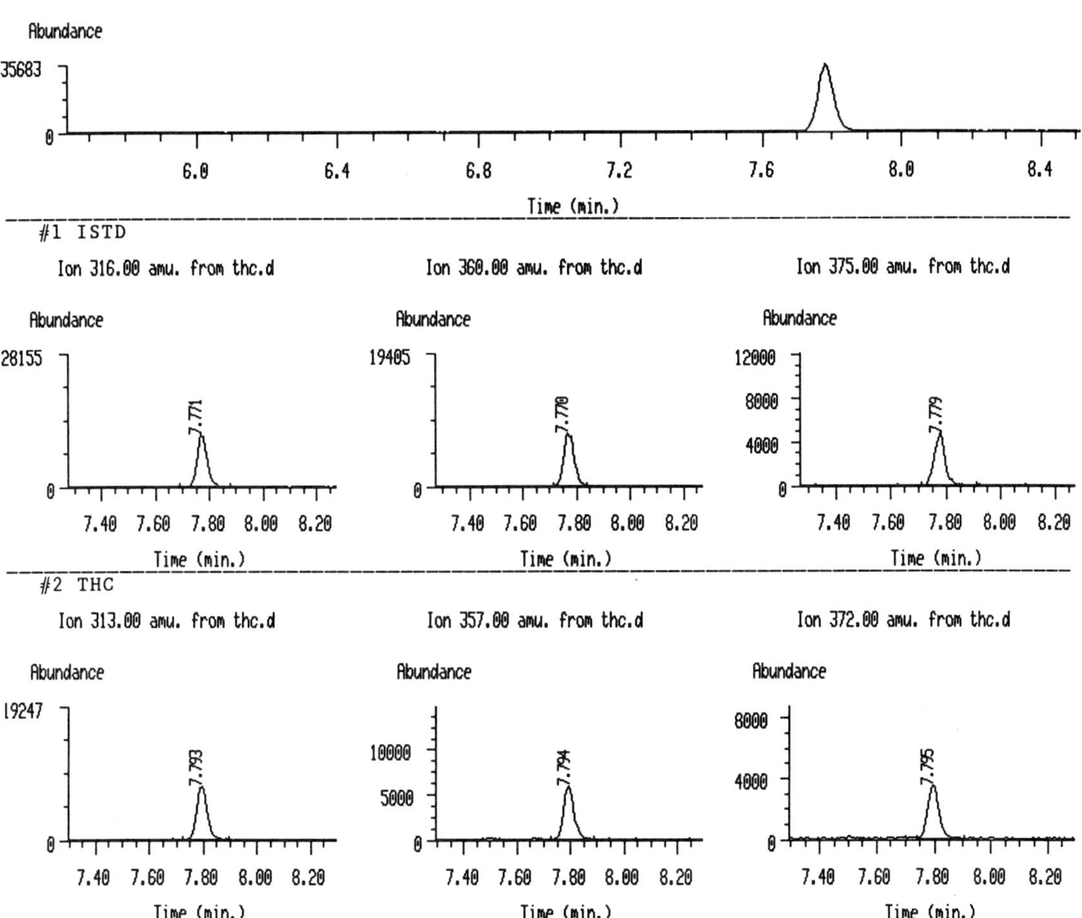

Thru-Put Systems, Inc.

THC ISTD and Ratio Report

Cal Inj Date : 26 Oct 87 21:39 Cal Operator : RODRIGUEZ TEMP 90-260,1/
Cal Date : 14 May 89 10:47 chemist Cal File: /chem/msd/THC.b/thc.d
Date : 26 Oct 87 21:39 Inst ID: msd
Data file: /chem/msd/THC.b/thc.d Tune Date: 14 May 89 10:18
Name Info: 494-1E
Misc Info:
Operator : RODRIGUEZ TEMP 90-260,1/30UL
Sequence index : 1
Als bottle num : 1
Replicate num : 1

COMPOUND	RT	MASS	AREA	AMT()	TARGET RANGE	RATIO
ISTD	7.77	316	296140	40.00		100.00
	7.77	360	199060		53.70 - 80.56	67.21
	7.78	375	123568		33.39 - 50.09	41.72
THC	7.79	313	214033	15.00		100.00
	7.79	357	157087		58.71 - 88.07	73.39
	7.80	372	93412		34.91 - 52.37	43.64

Figure 3–2. An example of graphic report format #6, the most commonly used format by TARGET users. (Reproduced with permission from Thru-Put Systems, Inc., Orlando, Florida.)

Spectrophotometric Techniques. These are much used in forensic toxicology; infrared spectrophotometry is used for identification of captured compounds, and ultraviolet, visible, and fluorescence spectrophotometry is used for quantification. In the clinical setting, infrared spectrophotometry does not have the sensitivity required to deal with biologic specimens and also demands a fairly high purity of form of presentation of sample. Ultraviolet and visible spectrophotometry have long been used for the quantification and partial identification of barbiturates, glutethimide, salicylate, paracetamol, and paraquat—the majority of the drugs of importance shown in Table 3–1. Nonetheless, there are major limitations to sensitivity and specificity that fail completely to offset the advantages of simplicity and the ability to be used for batch analyses. Similarly, colorimetric spot tests and crystal tests have even yet a role to play in forensic toxicology but are of little or no value in the clinical setting.

Immunologic Techniques. One of the major advances in laboratory diagnosis in recent years has been the application of immunologic techniques. It has been known for several decades that antibodies can recognize small organic molecules with a degree of specificity sufficient to differentiate between optical isomers.[22] However, use of antibodies is quantitative and qualitative assays of organic substances was delayed until the late 1950s and early 1960s with the introduction of radioimmunoassay (RIA) and other competitive binding techniques.[23] RIA offers immense sensitivity and potentially high specificity. Complete specificity, however, has not always been attained, and sensitivity on occasions has been disappointing. For example, gas chromatography offers better discrimination and equivalent sensitivity to RIA with regard to barbiturate analysis, but RIA far outstrips any other analytic technique for digoxin.[24]

A major drawback to RIA is the requirement for radiation-handling facilities and the possible inaccuracies introduced by chemical quenching of beta-iostopes when these are used to label competitor, or, alternatively, the short shelf-life of gamma-labeled competitors. These drawbacks in immunologic assays were all overcome with the introduction of enzyme-multiplied immunoassay techniques (EMITs). This is also a competitive immunologic procedure but uses the multiplying properties of enzymic reactions to give a simple spectrophotometric assay end-point.[25] EMIT is now well established in therapeutic drug monitoring, and it is sensitive and extremely rapid, of the order of a few minutes for each sample and less than 15 minutes for a batch. Limitations of sensitivity in some drug-screen settings have been encountered, particularly when cell lysis with turbidimetric measurements is used as the detector end-point. Spectrophotometric or spectrofluorometric analyses offer multiplication of sensitivity by a factor of at least 10 and show considerable promise for the future.

Immunologic techniques, therefore, have much to offer in both the qualitative and quantitative aspects of laboratory diagnosis of the toxicologic patient. Antibodies tailored to recognize *classes* of drugs—for example, barbiturates, tricyclic antidepressants, benzodiazepines, and phenothiazines—will give rapid qualitative results, and more specific antisera then can be used in a second stage EMIT or RIA analysis to identify and quantify the particular member of a group. Alternatively, the sample subsequently may be analyzed chromatographically with considerable gain in reliability and speed from knowledge of the class of drug.

Extraction Methods. Extractions are frequently used in the laboratory in identification and quantification of toxins, particularly drugs. The reasons for using extraction techniques are

- To purify the substance;
- To concentrate the substance; and
- To prepare the substance in the solvent vehicle utilized in the analytic technique—particularly so for TLC and GC, and GC-MS.

Purification is achieved usually by a one- or two-step extraction from the aqueous material into a suitable organic solvent. In single-step procedures, no further isolation is carried out, and the sample may be assayed directly—for example, extraction of benzodiazepines into low volumes of butyl acetate, followed by GC analyses on OV7—or may be concentrated and dried by addition of anhydrous sodium sulfate and evaporation. In two-stage procedures, the drugs are back-extracted into buffer at suitable pH and may be analyzed directly thereafter in the spectrophotometric techniques or re-extracted into suitable volumes of organic phase following pH adjustment.

The value of extraction for concentration is a frequently overlooked but important aspect of these procedures. For example, excretion of barbiturate in urine is often of the order of 0.1 μg per ml or less of urine. Urine samples, however, usually are available in fairly large volumes, thereby making available large absolute quantities of drug. Extraction into relatively small volumes of organic phase or into higher volumes followed by evaporation, therefore, will increase the concentration of drug to be analyzed in the organic phase by a factor of 10 to 100 without much difficulty. Occasionally problems are encountered in chromatography with impure solvents producing interfering substances when the organic phase is evaporated to low volume.

The third feature is that GC, GC-MS, and TLC, and in some cases HPLC, require the drug to be present in an organic phase, and this could be achieved in one step by solvent extraction. Not all analytic techniques have this requirement, and indeed it is contradicted in spectrophotometry. In addition, in an increasing number of HPLC assays drug in plasma is assayed following precipitation of proteins and injection of supernatant directly into the chromatographic apparatus.[26]

A simple scheme of direct solvent extraction is rapid and usually affords adequate purification but has the drawback that the nature of the drug or suspected drug must be known. Too often the analyst is searching for an unknown compound, and then certain constraints are applied, leading to a marked increase in the time required for the assay. Extraction techniques play an important role in group separation of organic nonvolatile compounds. The method generally followed consists of preparation of an acidic aqueous solution containing the drug either dissolved (bases) or finely precipitated (acids). The acidic aqueous solution is extracted with ether, which is then separated and re-extracted, first with sodium bicarbonate to remove strong acids such as salicylate and then with dilute sodium hydroxide to remove weak acids such as barbiturates. The ether phase will retain neutral drugs like methaqualone. The extracted acidic aqueous phase remaining from the first ether extraction will contain most of the basic compounds, such as the benzodiazepines, and can be rendered alkaline and re-extracted with ether. If morphine is suspected, however, the aqueous phase requires slightly different treatment, including salting out.

Solid phase extraction is now becoming popular as an alternative to liquid-liquid extraction. In solid phase extraction, a compound is partitioned between a solid phase adsorbent such as XAD-2 resin or diatomaceous earth, or a synthetic hydrophobic resin that contains, for example, a C8 group, and a liquid phase. Many manufacturers now produce solid phase sorbents for extraction (e.g., Bond Elute, Analytichem Int.; Prep cartridges, DuPont Company; Narc columns, J.T. Baker; Fisher PrepSep, Fisher Scientific; drug extraction columns from Biochemical Diagnostics, Applied Separations, and Worldwide Monitoring Corporation).

Many drugs, including morphine and related narcotics and the phenothiazines—that is, a large proportion of those encountered in the toxicologic setting—are extensively protein-bound either in their native form or as metabolites and demand a somewhat different approach to their extraction. Acidic hydrolysis and protein precipitation have been much used historically, but modern techniques utilize the enzyme *subtilisin carlsberg* to good effect, increasing the yield many times.[27]

Methods for Inorganics. Apart from lithium, lead, and iron, inorganics are seldom encountered in acute toxicology. Apart from iron, methods routinely used are mostly based on the equivalent of the spectrophotometric techniques used for drug molecules, but depending on energy changes in the elemental atomic conditions. Emission techniques—that is, flame photometry as used for serum sodium and potassium levels—were the earliest assay techniques but suffered from lack of sensitivity and specificity. The major method used now is atomic absorption, and assays with adequate sensitivity and speed of turnaround are available for quantification of these three main elements. Atomic absorption, however, is less suitable as a screening technique and is insufficiently sensitive for some other elemental analyses.[28]

Fortunately, in the clinical setting the screen for an unknown metal is almost never required, and confirmation of the presence or absence of a named metal can be achieved by simple application of the appropriate quantitative method. Metals such as cadmium are present at too low concentrations within body fluids and tissues for reliable quantification, even by atomic absorption utilizing the extreme sensitivity of flameless solid sampling devices, but atomic fluorescence seems to have much to offer in this field. Flameless sampling devices are also regularly used for analyses of mercury and of arsenic as its hydride and are reliable, sensitive, and accurate.

Qualitative assays will usually be spectrographic or utilize neutron activation analysis (NAA). Of these, NAA can be rapid, is extremely sensitive although not always more so than alternative technologies, and can be both qualitative and quantitative. The obvious major limitation to NAA is the requirement for the reactor to bombard the samples, which means that the mechanics of sample handling make this an unsuitable technique in the clinical context, and frequently it is made even less suitable by the requirement for a sufficient period of time to elapse to allow decay of interfering isotopes.

SAMPLE SELECTION FOR LABORATORY ANALYSIS

Blood and Blood Fractions. Frequently the body fluid offered for analysis in laboratory diagnosis of the toxicologic patient is blood, either serum or plasma. This fluid has the major advantage that concentrations therein directly reflect those at the site of action of the drug; therefore, quantitative anlaysis allows the clinician information that can be compared with a databank and used in differential diagnosis—for example, therapeutic and autopsy levels of barbiturates.[29] The fluid of choice probably would be serum, which is relatively clean, is easy to extract, and does not suffer from clot formation, which may interfere mechanically with apparatus and sometimes arises with old plasma samples. In the forensic setting, autopsy analyses frequently have to be carried out on whole blood, and the condition of the samples is often less than would be desired. Care should be taken in interpreting results, bearing in mind that drugs in general are not uniformly distributed between the cellular and fluid components of blood and that interconversion factors will be required.

Blood as a sample for laboratory analyses of drugs has one major drawback: concentrations are frequently low and, because sample size is limited, the absolute masses are in turn low. Blood, therefore, is not an ideal fluid for an unknown screen but is probably the sample of choice for a qualitative and quantitative analysis of one or a few specific drugs.

Urine. In contrast to blood, concentrations of drug in urine are frequently higher, and sample sizes are always much greater. Therefore, the job of the analyst is much simpler. The reason for the increased concentration of drugs in urine compared with blood is simply that renal clearances of drugs are usually greater than unity, and, given an average urine flow of approximately 1 ml per min, there will be a net increase in concentration of drug from plasma to urine. Extraction of 10- or 25-ml aliquots of urine into an 0.5-ml organic phase, therefore, will afford considerable enhancement of concentration as well as some degree of purification.

Purity of sample, however, is the major drawback with urine samples, since they also will contain all the metabolites of the drug as well as many other organic waste products. The possibility of interference in the assay from closely related (i.e., metabolites) or even unrelated compounds, therefore, is much higher with urine than with blood. In addition, urine suffers from the drawback that no direct, reproducible relationship exists between amounts or concentrations of drug in urine and those in plasma and therefore interpretation of quantitative urine data should not be depended upon.

Saliva. Saliva is becoming popular in therapeutic drug monitoring programs for drugs such as theophylline and procainamide. It affords simplicity of collection and the exciting feasibility of a reference fluid in which the concentration of drug closely reflects the unbound concentration of that drug in other body fluids, in contrast to plasma in which protein binding is an important governing factor. None of these advantages apply to investigation of the unconscious patient or in a forensic autopsy, since pure, uncontaminated, and sufficiently copious saliva samples cannot be obtained.

Tissues. In forensic autopsies, tissues such as kidney, liver, or brain are frequently offered for analyses and may be of some value. Their limitations in the clinical setting are obvious, and their preparation and extraction for drugs is more complex and time consuming than with blood or urine.

Timing of Samples. Interpretation of

quantitative measurements requires careful consideration of time relative to the taking of the dose of drug or poison. Assuming oral administration, then the plasma concentration–time curve will rise to a peak and decline. It is possible, therefore, that the same dose of drug in the same individual could show concentrations ranging from subtherapeutic to toxic, depending on the time relative to ingestion. In most instances, if an overdose has been taken then the patient will not be unconscious or toxic until sufficiently high blood/tissue drug levels have been achieved; in that sense, timing is of less critical importance. Continued monitoring of the patient's progress will require serial blood sampling, however, and this should be carried out on a time schedule such that the full pattern of the plasma concentration–time curve can be described adequately. Table 3–6 shows the approximate duration of detectability of drugs in urine.

Methods for Screening, Confirmation, and Quantification. Screening methods must be sufficiently sensitive, rapid, and of sufficient range. For the clinician to know that the patient is likely to have consumed a named drug in time for the information to be of assistance in therapy, a rapid turn-around is needed from the laboratory. The classic extraction and group separation techniques of forensic toxicology, therefore, are of limited value in the laboratory diagnosis of the toxicologic patient. Modification of the techniques used in cases of suspected alcohol- or drug-intoxicated drivers is a much better guide. In general, these utilize direct extraction into total acidic and basic fractions and analyses by a limited range of thin-layer and gas chromatographic techniques, backed up with a range of immunologic schemes. These are shown in Table 3–7, from which it can be seen that the major groups of drugs in terms of those encountered in poisoning are adequately covered.

Gas chromatography–mass spectrometry is frequently used in clinical toxicology (i.e., hospital or emergency room patients) for the confirmation or identification of un-derivatized drugs from acid or basic extracts of urine or serum.[30, 31] Usually the GC-MS is employed for confirmation of drugs detected by other screening procedures, such as immunoassay, thin layer chromatography, or gas chromatography. It is also used to identify compounds detected, but not identified, by other analytical methods, such as thin layer chromatography. Most conveniently, the same extraction procedures employed for TLC of drugs in urine has also been found to be suitable for the preparation of GC-MS samples. Therefore, by splitting the extract for TLC and GC-MS, GC-MS analysis may be completed in a timely manner for routine and emergency clinical toxicology.

For positive GC-MS identification of a drug, it is necessary to confirm that it has the correct retention time as well as to establish the similarity of the unknown spectrum, by visual inspection, to the library selected spectrum. At present, the benchtop systems do not, per se, have a search paradigm that includes retention in the calculation of match quality. However, with the MSD a user-contributed program (custom "macro") allows the retention time or retention index of the unknown to be compared with the retention time (retention index) of any drug match found by probability-based matching (PBM). Shown in Table 3–8 is a "short list" of the retention times and retention indices (calculated relative to mephobarbital as a standard) for the un-derivatized drugs most frequently confirmed by GC-MS in the laboratory of one of us (D.G.D.). The total turn-around for such screens with confirmation should be less than 2 hours.

Selection of Methods for Quantification. Quantification techniques can be divided into several categories. The GC method used in the screen can also be used for immediate quantification by reference to internal standards and standard curves. This will not have to be followed when a named drug is investigated, in which case a limited range of systems will be offered by the laboratory, including, in particular, immunologically based methods. When a centralized facility is offering a service to a large urban area, then immunologic techniques using group-specific antisera will play an important role in the screening. Most quantification will be carried out using these immunologic techniques, GC, HPLC, or GC-MS. Under these circumstances, confirmation of identity and quantitative assay should also be offered within 2 hours.

Quality assurance checks are vitally important in both screening and quantification and are very difficult to arrange because of the different nature of drug work from routine hematology or biochemistry. Probably the

Table 3–6. APPROXIMATE DURATION OF DETECTABILITY OF SELECTED DRUGS IN URINE

DRUG	APPROXIMATE DURATION OF DETECTABILITY*	LIMITS OF SENSITIVITY OF ANALYTIC TECHNIQUES (*μmol/L*)
amphetamine	48 hr	0.5 μg/ml
methamphetamine	48 hr	0.5 μg/ml
barbiturates		
Short-acting:	24 hr	
hexobarbital		1.0 μg/ml
pentobarbital		0.5 μg/ml
secobarbital		0.5 μg/ml
thiamylal		1.0 μg/ml
Intermediate-acting:	48–72 hr	
amobarbital		1.0 μg/ml
aprobarbital		1.5 μg/ml
butabarbital		0.5 μg/ml
butalbital		1.5 μg/ml
Long-acting:	≥ 7 days	
barbital		5.0 μg/ml
phenobarbital		1.0 μg/ml
benzodiazepines	3 days†	1.0 μg/ml
cocaine metabolites	2–3 days	
benzoylecgonine		0.5 μg/ml
ecgonine methyl ester		1.0 μg/ml
methadone	≈ 3 days	0.5 μg/ml
1,5-dimethyl-3,3-diphenyl-2-ethylidene pyrrolidine (metabolite of methadone)	≈ 3 days	0.5 μg/ml
codeine	48 hr	0.5 μg/ml
morphine		1.0 μg/ml
propoxyphene	6–48 hr	0.5 μg/ml
norpropoxyphene		1.5 μg/ml
cannabinoids (11-nor-9-tetra-hydrocannabinol-9-carboxylic acid)	3 days,‡ 5 days§ 10 days‖ 21–27 days¶	20 ng/ml
methaqualone	≥ 7 days	1.0 μg/ml
phencyclidine	≈ 8 days	0.5 μg/ml

*Interpretation of the duration of detectability must take into account many variables, such as drug metabolism and half-life; subject's physical condition, fluid balance, and state of hydration; and route and frequency of ingestion. These are general guidelines only.

†Using therapeutic dosages.

‡Single use.

§Moderate smoker (4 times per week).

‖Heavy smoker (smoking daily).

¶Chronic heavy smoker.

(From Report of Council on Scientific Affairs: Scientific issues in drug testing. JAMA *257*:3110–3114, 1987. Copyright 1987, American Medical Association.)

best approach would be the multilaboratory analyses of an authentic plasma or urine sample, with comparison to duplicate laboratory GC-MS analyses as the reference. Such materials are now becoming available as a result of proficiency testing programs that produce survey-validated samples. The Forensic Urine Drug Testing (FUDT) progam is jointly administered by the American Association of Clinical Chemistry (AACC) and the College of American Pathologists. It provides urine specimens containing the most commonly abused drugs and metabolites, as does a survey provided by the American Association of Bioanalysts. The College of American Pathologists also sponsors toxicology survey programs with both serum and urine specimens. In addition, the military and various states provide such programs.

Workplace Drug Testing. In recent years, workplace (employee) drug testing of urine and other nonclinical substance-abuse testing (athletic programs, the military, correctional facilities, etc.) have become widespread. In order not to jeopardize the livelihood and due process rights of the individuals being tested, laboratories must produce results that are scientifically and forensically defensible. Thus the needs of medical and workplace toxicology are somewhat different. For ex-

Table 3–7. SCHEME FOR DRUG SCREENING AND CONFIRMATION

TECHNIQUE	DRUGS DETECTED
Solvent extraction	Acids, bases
TLC	Barbiturates, narcotics, general bases
GC	
Direct extraction, OV7	Benzodiazepines*
OV17, Apiezon L	Barbiturates†
OV17	Bases†
Immunology & GC/MS	Wide range of "drug abuse" and toxic screen group, including benzodiazepines and narcotics

*Can be quantitative.
†In capillary work, cross-linked methylsilicone generally gives better speed and resolution.

ample, a patient in the emergency room may receive beneficial clinical treatment as a result of a STAT qualitative cocaine determination, whereas this result would probably not be useful legally. For a legal proceeding, in this example, in addition to use of the proper quality control procedures, the presence of cocaine or its metabolite, benzoylecgonine, would have to be confirmed by an independent method, probably GC-MS. Furthermore, the specimen would also have to be treated as evidence for possible court testimony.

Different programs also differ in the demands they place on optimal use of administrative policies. The selection of the population for testing is an often ignored requirement. The interaction between population surveyed, prevalence of drug, and positive predictive value of the tests used was addressed by the AMA Council on Scientific Affairs.[3] Thus for a test that is 90 per cent specific and has 99 per cent sensitivity, if the prevalence of use of target drug is 1 per cent, the predictive value is 9 per cent. That is, 9 per cent of all recorded positive results will be true-positives. The predictive value increases to 52 per cent at a 10 per cent prevalence.

Various states, the Federal Government, and the Department of Defense have established standards for certification of laboratories engaged in forensic drug testing of urine. These standards include such items as rigorous chain-of-custody procedures for collection and handling of specimens during testing and storage; laboratory security; definitive and confidential test results; extended storage for confirmed positives; documentation of all records, which may be used in court testimony; specific educational and experience requirements for laboratory personnel; proficiency testing programs; stringent quality assurance and quality control programs; and on-site laboratory inspection by regulatory agencies.

The Department of Health and Human Services (DHHS), for example, has established mandatory guidelines for laboratories that wish to be certified for workplace drug testing of federal employees.[32] These guidelines, for drug testing of urine, require an initial immunoassay screen and a GC-MS confirmation test, both performed at the same site. The cutoff levels for the initial screen by immunoassay and confirmation by GC-MS are shown in Table 3–9. Other programs may have different drug and cutoff level concentration requirements: for example, in New York State, a laboratory is licensed in forensic (workplace) toxicology assays for barbiturates, methadone, and oxazepam in addition to those required by the DHHS, in some cases with slightly different cutoff levels. Although an employee/applicant test result is reported qualitatively (positive or negative), quantitative GC-MS confirmation is used for the test samples and as a way to gauge the performance of laboratories on proficiency test samples. According to the DHHS guidelines, proficiency test specimens are spiked with concentration levels set at least 20 per cent above the cutoff limit for either the screen or the confirmation test, depending upon which is being evaluated.

The guidelines of the DHHS specify that immunoassay is the mandatory technique for screening. The military relies almost solely on the RIA while many private laboratories use the EMIT or the fluorescence polarization immunoassay (FPIA) of Abbott. For high-volume analysis, random or batch, automated chemistry type analyzers using EMIT reagents are preferred. These include the Cobas-Bio by Roche, the Hitachi 705 and 704 by Boehringer Mannheim Diagnostics, the Optimate by Ames, the Monarch by Instrumentation Laboratories, and many others. When the volume of samples is less, laboratories may use Syva's ETS system, which can test for six drugs on one sample, or Abbott's ADx, which can test for ten different drugs on one sample.

Many compounds are more effectively analyzed by GC-MS if they are first converted to

Table 3–8. LIST OF RETENTION TIMES AND LIBRARY LOCATIONS ON GC-MS

DRUG	ART	RRT	GC-MS LIBRARY LOCATION NUMBERS
acetaminophen	9.18	0.850	183, 115
acetaminophen metabolite	9.40	0.816	183, 115
amitriptyline	12.48	1.180	43
amphetamine	4.32	0.392	35, 186
amobarbital	9.22	0.871	378, 185, 25
aprobarbital			169, 184
butabarbital	8.82	0.834	387
butalbital	8.86	0.837	216, 213, 159, 67
caffeine	10.30	0.948	340, 59
carisoprodol (2)	7.86	0.743	376, 65
	10.36	0.979	376, 65
chlorodiazepoxide	14.32	1.354	360, 200, 23
cocaine	13.00	1.182	142, 191
cocaine metabolites (3)	7.14	0.641	391
(ecgonine methyl ester)	7.50	0.673	391
	7.86	0.716	391
codeine	13.80	1.282	192, 42
cotinine	9.16	0.848	394
desipramine	12.78	1.208	44
dextromethorphan	12.46	0.966	392
diazepam	13.92	1.316	361, 24, 218
diphenhydramine	10.58	0.980	86, 63, 383, 384,
diphenhydramine metabolites			383, 384, 385
doxepin (2)	12.56	1.187	388
	12.68	1.198	388
doxylamine	11.00	1.009	393
glutethimide	10.24	0.968	197, 28
imipramine	12.64	1.195	66
meperidine	9.72	0.900	114, 247, 195
methamphetamine			373
methadone	12.40	1.146	139, 202
methaqualone	12.28	1.161	386
methyprylon	7.92	0.747	9
mephobarbital (IS)	10.70	1.00	167, 316
meprobamate (2)	7.14	0.675	62, 201
	9.80	0.926	62, 201
nicotine	5.10	0.562	278, 56
nordiazepam	14.26	1.350	375
nortriptyline	12.58	1.189	47
nor-meperidine	9.96	0.920	248
pentazine	12.92	1.221	235
pentobarbital	9.40	0.888	206, 27
phencyclidine	10.56	0.994	208, 140
phenobarbital	10.98	1.038	158, 209
phenylpropanolamine	6.02	0.570	377
phenytoin	13.62	1.258	164, 196
propoxyphene	12.40	1.172	212, 22
propoxyphene metabolite	10.62	1.004	379, 380, 381, 382
secobarbital	9.76	0.922	214, 144

ART, absolute retention time; RRT, relative retention time.

(From Deutsch DG: Gas chromatography-mass spectrometry using table top instruments. *In* Deutsch DG: Analytical Aspects of Drug Testing. Vol 100, Chemical Analysis Series. New York, John Wiley, 1989.)

a derivative. Some of the GC-MS procedures for the more common drugs and metabolites have been reviewed.[33–36] The United States military has conducted drug screening for many years. Their methods, developed for the common drugs-of-abuse, are available in their standard operating procedure manuals (SOPM). For more recent information, one may also consult, for example, The Journal of Analytical Toxicology, which publishes many papers dealing with the development and evaluation of GC-MS procedures for drug confirmation. In addition to the journals and reference works cited, some GC-MS confirmation procedures may be found in a technical newsletter called *Toxi-Lab News*, pub-

Table 3–9. CUTOFF LEVELS FOR INITIAL SCREENING AND GC-MS CONFIRMATION

DRUG CLASS	CONCENTRATION (*ng/ml*) *Immunoassay Cutoff*	*GC-MS Cutoff*
Marijuana metabolites	100	
Delta-9-THC-9-COOH		15
Cocaine metabolites	300	
Benzoylecgonine		150
Opiate metabolites	300	
Morphine		300
Codeine		300
Amphetamines	1000	
Amphetamine		500
Methamphetamine		500
Phencyclidine	25	25

(Adapted from Alcohol, Drug Abuse, and Mental Health Administration: Mandatory guidelines for federal workplace drug testing program; Final guidelines; Notice. Fed Register *53*:11970, 1988.)

lished by Analytical Systems (Irvine, CA 92718). For example, one recent issue presented a procedure for sympathomimetic amines (phenylpropanolamines, pseudoephedrine, amphetamine, and methamphetamine) after derivatization with pentafluoropropionic anhydride, and another issue presented a procedure for six benzodiazepines after hydrolysis to their corresponding benzophenones. In addition, many manufacturers who produce solid phase sorbents for extraction frequently provide detailed procedures for extraction, derivatization and GC-MS analysis.

One of the most widely used procedures for derivatization of delta-9-THC-COOH involves treatment with iodomethane and tetramethylammonium hydroxide (TMAH) as the catalyst.[37, 38] The dimethyl derivative of 9-THC-COOH is monitored at 313, 357, and 372 amu whereas the trideuterated internal standard is usually monitored at 316 or 375 amu for quantitation (see Figure 3–2). The 9-THC-COOH glucuronide conjugate must be hydrolyzed before derivatization. Another procedure for 9-THC-COOH by GC-MS uses an adaptation of a method described by Foltz employing liquid-liquid or solid phase extraction.[17] The derivatizing agent is *N,O*-bis-(trimethylsilyl)-trifluoroacetamide + 1 per cent trimethylchloro-silane (BSTFA + TMCS), which yields the trimethylsilyl (TMS) derivative. This compound is monitored with the mass spectrometer at 371, 473, and 488 amu for 9-THC-COOH and at 374 or 491 amu for the trideuterated internal standard. A variety of other procedures are available for 9-THC-COOH in urine.

The most common method for GC-MS analysis of benzoylecgonine involves esterification producing the methyl, ethyl, or *n*-propyl derivative.[39] These can be formed by heating in the appropriate alcohol at acid pH, by heating with *N,N*-dimethylformamide di-*N*-alkylacetal, or, for the ethyl derivative, by using TMAH and ethyl iodide at room temperature. For quantitation and confirmation, deuterated benzoylecgonine is available as an internal standard from Merck Sharp & Dohme Isotopes or from the Research Triangle Institute. M/e values for GC-MS monitoring of propylbenzoylecgonine are 210, 272, and 331 amu, and 213, 275, and 334 amu for the deuterated internal standard. More recent methodology utilizes solid phase separation procedures and silylating reagents for derivatization.

One of the most common derivatization methods for the identification and quantitation of codeine and morphine by electron impact GC-MS employs acetylation.[40, 41] After hydrolysis of the glucuronide conjugate, a liquid-liquid extraction is performed and acetic anhydride is employed for acetylation. Nalorphine is used as an internal standard. The ion pair ratios 341 and 282 amu of acetylcodeine, 369 and 327 amu of diacetylmorphine, and 395 and 353 amu of diacetylnalorphine are monitored, and the ratios for an unknown must give a response within prescribed limits for positive identification. For quantitation of codeine and morphine, the ratios of 341:395 and 369:395 were employed, respectively. As reviewed by Paul and associates, many other methods for derivatization of morphine and codeine including silylation, pentafluorobenzylation, trifluoroacetylation, pentafluoro-propionylation, and heptafluorobutyrylation have been described.[40]

Amphetamine and methamphetamine may be converted to the trifluoroacetate derivative with trifluoroacetic anhydride (TFAA) using β-methylphenethylamine or phenylcyclohexylamine as the internal standard.

With the routine use of GC-MS instruments in more and more toxicology laboratories, one may expect to see a variety of new procedures developed that are simple and fast. It is hoped that GS-MS will become more available for patient care as a result of its development in the area of workplace drug testing.

Requirement for Hemoperfusion and Hemodialysis Monitoring. When hemoperfusion and hemodialysis are used to promote elimination of poisons, careful monitoring by the laboratory can be a useful adjunct. The simple principle of the laboratory back-up is confirmation that the active therapy is indeed removing drug from plasma. In many ways the requirements are similar to those already expounded—namely, accurate quantification, with rapid turn-around on properly chosen samples.

Quantification is at least as important in this context as in the comparison of blood level data with data banks in differential diagnosis. Thus, for example, an inaccurate assay that overestimated the extent of lowering of blood levels and did not match the change, if any, in the condition of the patient would mislead the clinician into thinking an otherwise unsuspected toxin also had been taken.

A knowledge of the disposition characteristics of the drug is also of vital importance, and it should be remembered that hemodialysis and hemoperfusion are best reserved for drugs with small volumes of distribution and low plasma protein binding—for example, theophylline. These techniques, with or without laboratory support, will be of little or no value in drugs with high volumes of distribution, such as digoxin, and will be of moderate use in drugs with moderate volumes of distribution.[42] This last group can cause some difficulties since there will be an early and rapid fall in blood levels upon institution of the active therapy because of drug redistribution. Without knowledge of the cause of this fall in blood levels, the clinician may feel that therapy is being more effective than is really the case, and the initial lowering is of course paid for by a rebound rise upon cessation of the active therapy.[42]

The final requirement for hemoperfusion and hemodialysis monitoring is that the samples must be taken frequently enough to adequately define the disposition curve of the drug and its new half-life.

References

1. Moss MS, Cowan DA: Drug abuse in sport. *In* Moffat AC (ed): Clarke's Isolation and Identification of Drugs. London, Pharmaceutical Press, 1986, p 87.
2. Editorial: Screening of drugs of abuse. Lancet 1:365, 1987.
3. Council on Scientific Affairs: Scientific issues in drug testing. JAMA *257*:3110, 1987.
4. Hutcheon AW, Lawson DH, Jick H: Hospital admissions due to adverse drug reactions. J Clin Pharmacol *3*:219, 1978.
5. Locket S: Overdose. Br J Hosp Med *19*:200, 1978.
6. Patel AR, Roy M, Wilson GM: Self-poisoning and alcohol. Lancet *2*:1099, 1972.
7. Lheureux P, Askenasi R: Specific treatment of benzodiazepine overdose. Hum Toxicol *7*:165, 1988.
8. Caplan YH, Ottinger WE, Crooks CR: Therapeutic and toxic drug concentrations in post mortem blood. A six year study in the State of Maryland. J Anal Toxicol *7*:225, 1983.
9. Bailey DN: Comprehensive toxicology screening in patients admitted to a university trauma center. J Anal Toxicol *10*:147, 1986.
10. Flanagan RJ, Widdop B, Ramsay JD, Loveland M: Analytical toxicology. Hum Toxicol *7*:489, 1988.
11. Ingelfinger JA, Isakson G, Shine D, Costello CE, Goldman P: Reliability of the toxic screen in drug overdose. Clin Pharmacol Ther *29*:570, 1981.
12. Stead AH, Moffat AC, Caddy B, Fish F, Scott D: A comparison of GLC retention indices on SCOT columns and on packed columns for a series of CNS stimulant drugs. J Chromatog *84*:392, 1973.
13. Caddy B, Kidd CMB, Leung SC: Identification of drugs using capillary gas chromatography. J Forensic Sci Soc *22*:3, 1982.
14. Caddy B, Fish F, Scott D: Chromatographic screening for drugs of abuse using capillary columns. Chromatographia *6*:293, 1973.
15. Ambre JJ, Ruo TI, Smith GL, Backes D, Smith CM: Ecgonine methyl ester, a major metabolite of cocaine. J Anal Toxicol *6*:26, 1982.
16. MSD Application Brief: GC-MS Confirmation of THC. Publication Number 23-5953-8069. Hewlett-Packard, 1987.
17. Foltz RL: Analysis of cannabinoids in physiological specimens by gas chromatography/mass spectrometry. *In* Baselt RC (ed): Advances in Analytical Toxicology. Vol 1. Foster City, CA, Biomedical Publications, 1984, pp 125–157.
18. Lee MG, Millard BJ: A comparison of unlabelled and labelled internal standards for quantification by single and multiple ion monitoring. Biomed Mass Spectrom *2*:78, 1975.
19. Garland WA, Barbalas MP: Applications to analytical chemistry: An evaluation of stable isotopes in mass spectral drug assays. J Clin Pharmacol *26*:412, 1986.
20. Hill DW, Langner KJ: Screening with high performance liquid chromatography. *In* Deutsch DG (ed): Analytical Aspects of Drug Testing. Vol 100, Chemical Analysis Series. New York, John Wiley & Sons, 1989.
21. Voyksner RD: High performance liquid chromatography/mass chromatography. *In* Deutsch DG (ed): Analytical Aspects of Drug Testing. Vol 100, Chemical Analysis Series. New York, John Wiley & Sons, 1989.
22. Bach JF: Antigens. *In* Bach JF (ed): Immunology. New York, John Wiley & Sons, 1978, p 113.
23. Yalow RS, Berson SA: Immunoassay of endogenous plasma insulin in man. J Clin Invest *39*:1157, 1960.
24. Evered DC, Chapman C, Hayter CJ: Measurement of plasma digoxin concentration by radioimmunoassay. Br Med J *3*:427, 1970.

25. Fletcher SM: Screening for drugs by EMIT. J Forensic Sci Soc *21*:327, 1981.
26. Groen-Terweij CP, Heemstra S, Kraak JC: Rapid determination of indomethacin and salicylic acid in serum by means of reversed-phase liquid chromatography. J Chromatog *181*:385, 1980.
27. Osselton MD: The release of basic drugs by the enzymic digestion of tissues in cases of poisoning. J Forensic Sci Soc *17*:189, 1977.
28. Friberg L, Nordberg GF, Vouk VB: Handbook on the Toxicology of Metals. Amsterdam, Elsevier, 1979.
29. Stead AH, Moffat AC: Interpretation of therapeutic, toxic and fatal phenobarbitone blood concentrations by use of concentration-response and toxicity probability curves. J Forensic Sci Soc *22*:47, 1982.
30. Deutsch DG, Bergert RJ: Evaluation of a benchtop capillary gas chromatograph–mass spectrometer for clinical toxicology. Clin Chem *31*:741, 1985.
31. Soo V, Bergert RJ, Deutsch DG: Screening and quantitation of hypnotic sedatives in serum by capillary gas chromatography with a nitrogen-phosphorus detector, and confirmation by capillary gas chromatography–mass spectrometry. Clin Chem *32*:325, 1986.
32. Alcohol, Drug Abuse, and Mental Health Administration: Mandatory guidelines for federal workplace drug testing program; Final guidelines; Notice. Fed Register 53:11970, 1988.
33. Deutsch DG: Gas chromatography/mass spectrometry using tabletop instruments. *In* Deutsch DG (ed): Analytical Aspects of Drug Testing. Vol 100, Chemical Analysis Series. New York, John Wiley & Sons, 1989.
34. Foltz FL, Fentiman AF, Foltz RB: GC/MS assays for abused drugs in body fluids. NIDA Research Monograph 32, DHHS Publication O (ADM) 80-1014. Washington, DC, Superintendent of Documents, 1980.
35. Mule SJ, Casella GA: Confirmation of marijuana, cocaine, morphine, codeine, amphetamine, methamphetamine, phencyclidine by GC/MS in urine following immunoassay screening. J Anal Toxicol *12*:102, 1988.
36. Drug analysis using GC/MS. Publication No. 23-5955-5391. Hewlett-Packard, 1987.
37. Whiting JD, Manders WW: The confirmation of a 9-carboxy-THC in urine by gas chromatography/mass spectrometry. Aviation Space Environ *54*:1031, 1983.
38. Abercrombie ML, Jewell JS: Evaluation of EMIT and RIA high volume test procedures for THC and metabolites in urine utilizing GC/MS confirmation. J Anal Toxicol *10*:178, 1986.
39. Wallace JE, Hamilton HE, King DE, Bason DJ, Schwertner HA, Harris SC: Gas-liquid chromatograpic determination of cocaine and benzoylecgonine in urine. Anal Chem *48*:34, 1976.
40. Paul BD, Mell LD Jr, Mitchell JM, Irving J, Novak AJ: Simultaneous identification and quantitation of codeine and morphine in urine by capillary gas chromatography and mass spectrometry. J Anal Tox *9*:222, 1985.
41. Strumpler RE: Detection of codeine and morphine following ingestion of poppy seeds. J Anal Toxicol *11*:97, 1987.
42. Tilstone WJ, Winchester JF, Reavey PC: Use of pharmacokinetic principles in determining the effectiveness of removal of toxins from blood. Clin Pharmacokinet *4*:23, 1979.

CHAPTER 4
CARDIAC DISTURBANCES

Neal L. Benowitz, M.D.
Nora Goldschlager, M.D.

Cardiovascular complications account for a substantial proportion of the morbidity and mortality of drug overdose. Drug- or toxin-induced cardiovascular syndromes include hypotension and circulatory shock, hypertension, arrhythmias, and pulmonary edema. This chapter will focus on disturbances of cardiac function, particularly circulatory failure, and arrhythmias. We will discuss pathophysiology, recognition of specific types of overdose, and principles of management.

HYPOTENSION AND CIRCULATORY SHOCK

Mechanisms

Hypotension occurs after overdosage with many different types of drugs. The mechanisms of hypotension are multiple, and hemodynamic patterns differ with different drugs in different stages of overdose and according to the presence and nature of underlying medical illness. Cardiac output may be reduced as a result of drug-induced myocardial depression, relative hypovolemia resulting from venous pooling, or true hypovolemia resulting from vascular injury and fluid loss from the vascular space. Peripheral vascular resistance may be reduced because of drug-induced vascular relaxation, adrenergic receptor blockade, or depression of central vasomotor tone. Myocardial and vascular dysfunction resulting from hypoxia, acidosis, and hypotension may complicate the picture.

The major importance of hypotension is that it warns the physician of possible circulatory insufficiency; blood pressure is also one of several indicators of response to treatment. The diagnosis of circulatory shock depends on evidence of tissue hypoperfusion. In previously healthy individuals, urine output is usually the most sensitive indicator of hypoperfusion. Lactic acidosis is biochemical evidence that a substantial amount of tissue is hypoperfused. In patients with underlying coronary artery or cerebrovascular disease, cardiac or cerebral dysfunction may limit the tolerable extent of hypotension.

Management

Hypotensive patients should be placed in an intensive care unit where vital signs, fluid intake and output, body weight, and other parameters of circulatory function can be monitored continuously. Because indirect measurements of arterial blood pressure are difficult to obtain and often do not reflect true intra-arterial pressure in hypotensive states, direct measurement of intra-arterial blood pressure is preferred.

If hypotension is present without signs of tissue hypoperfusion, fluids should be administered at sufficient rates to maintain urine output and to compensate for insensible losses; fluids should be of appropriate composition to provide electrolyte needs. In many patients with signs of hypoperfusion of tissues, correction of acid-base and electrolyte disturbances and modest fluid therapy are sufficient to increase perfusion to adequate levels. However, increased pulmonary vascular permeability complicates many cases of drug overdose, and fluid therapy may cause pulmonary edema. For this reason, fluids must be administered cautiously. A reasonably safe way to administer fluids is by short infusions of small volumes (100 to 200 ml) of normal saline solution. If the clinical response is inadequate and if there is no evidence of pulmonary edema, the short infusions should be repeated but should not exceed a total of 1000 to 2000 ml over 1 to 2 hours. Evidence of pulmonary edema includes worsening hypoxia, decreasing lung compliance (manifest by increasing pressure necessary to ventilate a patient with a given tidal volume), and appearance of pulmonary rales.

If shock persists despite fluid challenge, catheterization of the pulmonary artery and measurement of pulmonary capillary wedge pressure, cardiac output, and/or venous oxygen saturation are recommended to monitor subsequent fluid therapy and to optimize drug therapy. The goal of fluid therapy is to re-establish adequate tissue perfusion with as little effect as possible on the pulmonary capillary wedge pressure. As long as the pulmonary capillary wedge pressure remains low, further fluid can be administered. Although there are no published data in this regard, an end point of a mean pulmonary capillary wedge pressure of 8 to 12 torr in a person with previously normal cardiac function appears to be reasonable in light of the possibility of increased pulmonary vascular permeability. This is in contrast to treatment of hemorrhagic or cardiogenic shock in which a pulmonary capillary wedge pressure of 15 to 18 torr is often the end point. If evidence of tissue hypoperfusion persists when pulmonary capillary wedge pressures have been restored to "normal" or pulmonary edema is evident, pressor or inotropic agents should be administered to restore adequate perfusion. It should be noted that, in persons with chronic cardiac failure, higher pressures (up to 20 torr) may be necessary to maintain an adequate cardiac output, and fluid therapy must be managed more on the basis of clinical assessment of pulmonary edema than on filling pressures per se.

Hemodynamic monitoring aids in the selection of pressor and/or inotropic drugs. For example, if circulatory failure is associated with low or low-normal peripheral vascular resistance, pressor drugs with substantial direct vasoconstricting activity, such as norepinephrine and dopamine, should be selected. Normalization of vascular resistance is a useful end point for titration of infusion rate.

If vascular resistance is normal or high, and depressed cardiac output is the determining factor in circulatory failure, drugs or interventions that increase cardiac output should be selected. Isoproterenol is particularly useful when myocardial depression is associated with bradyarrhythmias, although it may be arrhythmogenic; dobutamine, a dopamine analogue with relatively selective inotropic activity and less arrhythmogenic potential, is useful when heart rate is already adequate. In some patients, the addition of the phosphodiesterase inhibitor amrinone to dobutamine or dopamine has resulted in hemodynamic improvement. Amrinone is both an inotropic and a vasodilating agent and should not be used when peripheral vascular resistance is low. When both myocardial depression and low vascular resistance are present, epinephrine or combinations of norepinephrine or dopamine and isoproterenol may be useful.

Primarily because of its renal vasodilating effect, dopamine has now become the pressor agent of choice in most cases of drug overdose, with the exception of overdose with drugs that have alpha-adrenergic receptor blocking effects, such as phenothiazines or tricyclic antidepressants, in which more selective alpha-adrenergic agonists, such as norepinephrine or phenylephrine, may be required.

Pressor therapy has potential risks: pressor-induced venoconstriction can increase venous return and worsen pulmonary edema, and arteriolar constriction can further reduce tissue perfusion. However, in studies of the effects of infusion of norepinephrine in patients who overdosed with sedative drugs, the positive effects of norepinephrine on cardiac output outweighed the vasoconstrictor effects, and blood pressure increased without an increase in vascular resistance.[1]

ARRHYTHMIAS

General Mechanisms

Many detailed reviews of the electrophysiology of arrhythmias have been published (see reference 2, for example). Three basic mechanisms are involved in the production and maintenance of arrhythmias: (1) abnormal impulse formation, (2) abnormal impulse conduction, and (3) triggered automaticity.

Abnormal Impulse Formation

The intrinsic firing rate of automatic tissues (those that can develop spontaneous diastolic depolarization) depends on certain characteristics of their action potentials: the slope of diastolic depolarization (phase 4), the duration, the refractory period, and the resting membrane and threshold potentials (see Chapter 95 on quinidine, Fig. 95–1).

Conditions or agents that increase the slope of phase 4, lower the threshold potential toward the resting potential, or raise the resting membrane potential so that it approaches the threshold potential result in an increase in the spontaneous firing rate of automatic tissue. Conversely, conditions or agents that decrease the rate of diastolic depolarization, raise the threshold potential toward 0, or lower the resting membrane potential so that it takes longer to reach threshold potential result in a decrease in the spontaneous firing rate.

Abnormal Impulse Conduction

Delays in, or block of, conduction of electrical impulses, together with differential refractoriness of myocardial tissues, may lead to re-entry tachyarrhythmias. Such arrhythmias are initiated by early impulses that encounter refractory tissue through which they cannot propagate because of their prematurity; thus, they travel down alternate slowly conducting pathways. If the impulses return to the area originally refractory but now excitable, the tissue is able to conduct them. This particular set of electrophysiologic circumstances (unilateral conduction delay and slow impulse transmission in alternate pathways) can lead to paroxysmal or sustained arrhythmias (Fig. 4–1).

Triggered Rhythms[3]

Certain arrhythmias may arise from cells and fibers that are normally quiescent but, when stimulated, develop delayed after-depolarizations that can then depolarize them for short periods of time. After-depolarizations reflect current fluxes that persist after an action potential, which, if they reach threshold, result in re-excitation of the cell or fiber. Affected fibers do not normally develop spontaneous phase 4 diastolic depolarization, nor is impulse conduction within them im-

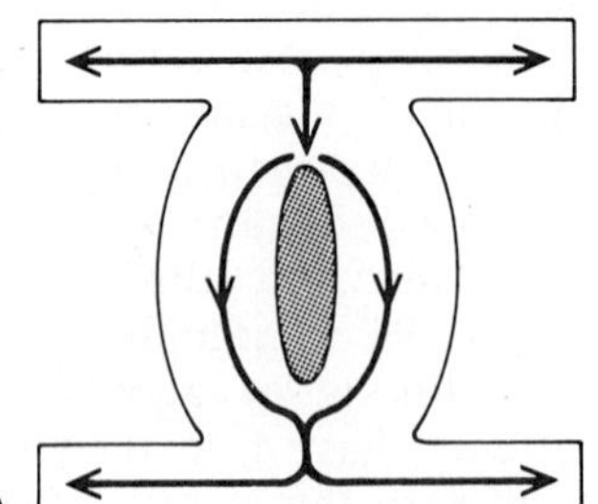

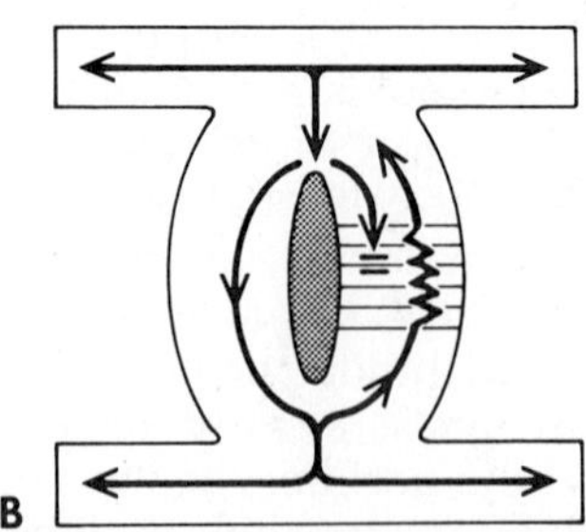

Figure 4–1. Drug-induced re-entry: Schema of Purkinje tissue or ventricular muscle through which impulse transmission occurs. *A,* Normal depolarization of a muscle segment. Impulses spread simultaneously down various conduction pathways to depolarize distal areas. Depolarization and repolarization proceed homogeneously. *B,* Re-entry. The hatched area represents a local area in which conduction is depressed, which might be produced by a membrane-depressant drug. An impulse traveling anterogradely in an area of depressed conduction is blocked (dark horizontal lines); impulses traveling in adjacent pathways, however, can pass through the area of conduction delay in retrograde fashion. If tissue proximal to the depressed area already repolarized and is now excitable, restimulation (re-entry) will occur.

paired, but when stimulated or "triggered," the fibers may become rhythmically active. In the experimental setting, triggered rhythms arise in the presence of stretch, hypoxia, digitalis, high concentrations of calcium, and low concentrations of potassium, and during catecholamine stimulation. Beta-blocking agents may antagonize triggered rhythms that are catecholamine-dependent, and calcium channel blocking agents such as verapamil may abolish those resulting from increased after-potential amplitude. Although it has not been proved that triggered rhythms are responsible for arrhythmias in patients, many rhythm disturbances, particularly if digitalis-induced, or occurring in association with a prolonged QTU interval, behave as though this were their underlying mechanism.

Arrhythmogenesis in Poisoned Patients

In the setting of drug overdose, cardiac arrhythmias can be caused by direct or indirect sympathomimetic effects, anticholinergic effects, the effects of altered central nervous system regulation of peripheral autonomic activity, and direct effects on myocardial membranes. Contributing factors to arrhythmogenesis during the course of drug overdose include hypotension, hypoxia, and disturbances in acid-base and electrolyte balance.

Sympathetic Influences

Because the action of many drugs involves the autonomic nervous system, it is useful to understand the effects of sympathetic and parasympathetic activity on cardiac electrophysiology. Beta-adrenergic stimulation accelerates spontaneous diastolic depolarization, thereby increasing the sinus rate; enhancement of automaticity in other pacemaker tissues (atrial, atrioventricular junctional, Purkinje) may result in accelerated ectopic rhythms.[4, 5] Beta-adrenergic stimulation also increases conduction velocity in slow (calcium-dependent) channel fibers, thus leading to more rapid sinoatrial and atrioventricular nodal conduction of impulses. The effect of catecholamines on fast (sodium-dependent) channel fibers such as normal Purkinje fibers is to accelerate repolarization and shorten the action potential duration and refractory period, although effects on conduction velocity are relatively negligible. Finally, beta-adrenergic stimulation enhances after-depolarization magnitude, thereby increasing the potential for triggered tachyarrhythmias.

Parasympathetic Influences

Parasympathetic stimulation slows the rate of spontaneous diastolic depolarization, resulting in slowing of the firing rates of pacemaker tissues.[6] Slowing of the sinus rate may result in the emergence of an escape rhythm originating in supraventricular, junctional, or ventricular tissue. Delay in impulse transmission through the atrioventricular node as a result of parasympathetic stimulation may produce atrioventricular block; this "vagotonic block" occurs in the presence of marked sinus slowing and usually takes the form of progressive delay in impulse conduction through the atrioventricular node (Figs. 4–2 and 4–3). The effects of cholinergic stimulation on ventricular conduction tissue include the raised electrical threshold necessary for induction of ventricular fibrillation, particularly in the presence of high sympathetic activity.[7]

An interesting arrhythmia resulting from increased parasympathetic tone has recently been recognized and is characterized by atrial tachyarrhythmias occurring during periods of high vagal tone, such as sleep, and is not found during exercise or stress.[8] Drugs such as digitalis or beta-adrenergic blocking agents tend to precipitate or worsen these arrhythmias. The underlying mechanism of their production is acetylcholine-mediated shortening and dispersion of atrial refractory periods, resulting in inhomogeneous atrial repolarization and depolarization sequences. Because this arrhythmia is benign and does not connote underlying heart disease, its recognition is important. Anticholinergic effects may also predispose to atrioventricular nodal re-entrant tachyarrhythmias via differential effects on nodal conduction velocity and refractoriness of re-entrant pathways.

Membrane Depression (For references, see Chapter 95, Quinidine)

In the drug-overdosed patient, a direct effect on myocardial membranes is another important mechanism contributing to arrhythmogenesis. Depressant effects on membrane responsiveness are exemplified by quinidine, which inhibits the fast sodium current, so that, for a given resting membrane potential, depolarization is associated with a reduced rate of voltage change and a reduced maximum achieved voltage. As a result, impulse conduction is slowed. In addition, membrane depressants shift the threshold potential toward 0, thus requiring stimuli of greater intensity to initiate the action potential. Additional effects of quinidine include prolongation of the action potential duration and refractory period, thus prolonging repolarization time. These electrophysiologic effects result in slowed repolarization and depolarization times, especially in His-Purkinje tissue. These events are reflected in the surface electrocardiogram as a prolongation of the QT interval and, in toxic doses, of the QRS duration. With severe intoxication, intraventricular block and asystole supervene, with inability to generate a response for any stimulus strength; this is manifested clinically by failure to respond to cardiac pacing at high-pacing stimulus voltage.

The basis for the arrhythmogenic effect of quinidine lies in its ability to produce disparate depolarization and repolarization times in His-Purkinje tissue and to delay impulse transmission. The production of unidirectional conduction block, and delay in impulse propagation in other areas, enables re-entry tachycardias to occur. In the case of quinidine and quinidine-like agents, a particular type of polymorphous ventricular tachycardia, termed "torsades de pointes," occurs (Fig. 4–4).

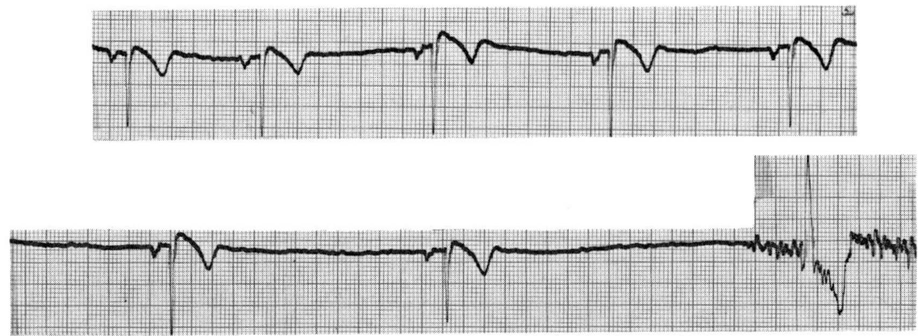

Figure 4–2. MCL1 tracing recorded during Ipecac-induced emesis in a patient with alleged barbiturate overdose. During the Valsalva maneuver of vomiting, marked slowing of sinus rate with prolongation of the PR interval occurs, resulting in a prolonged pause in rhythm terminated by a ventricular escape beat. Sinus slowing with or without concomitant atrioventricular block, such as depicted here, is due to hypervagotonia, and the arrhythmia is known as "vagotonic block." This has no prognostic significance for underlying heart disease. The arrhythmia is usually transient and requires no specific treatment.

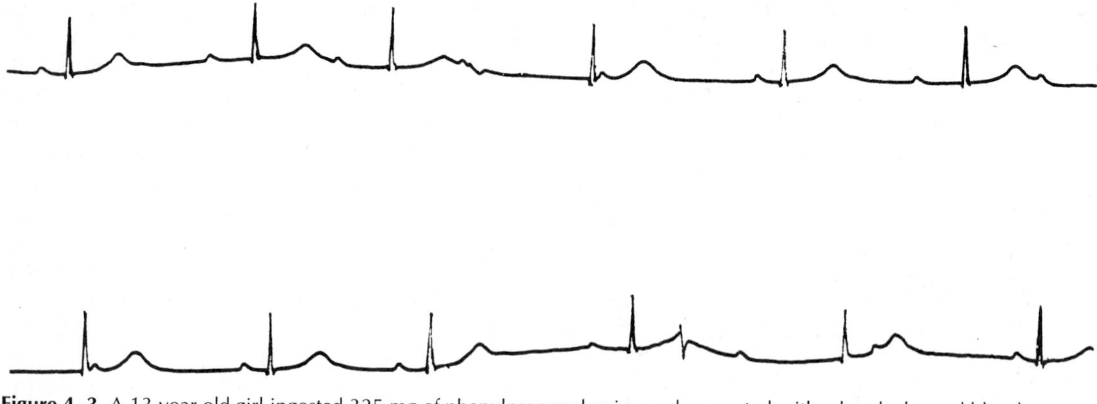

Figure 4–3. A 13 year old girl ingested 325 mg of phenylpropanolamine and presented with a headache and blood pressure of 130/100. The electrocardiogram showed sinus arrhythmia with Wenckebach-type atrioventricular block, reflecting surges of vagal tone. The vagal discharge is a reflex response to phenylpropanolamine-induced vasoconstriction and hypertension.[39a]

The arrhythmogenic effects of most drugs during overdose are best understood as the combination of autonomic influences, membrane depressant effects, and possibly triggered rhythms. Our analysis will attempt to categorize them in this way.

Management of Arrhythmias (Table 4–1)

Hypotension, hypoxia, and acid-base and electrolyte disturbances occurring during the course of drug overdose may contribute to arrhythmia production and should be corrected.

Supraventricular Arrhythmias

Sinus tachycardia and other supraventricular arrhythmias usually respond to supportive therapy, subsiding as the offending drug is excreted, but if they are associated with hemodynamic compromise, especially in patients with pre-existing coronary or cerebrovascular disease, specific therapy is warranted. Propranolol and physostigmine may be indicated for sympathomimetic and anticholinergic drug ingestions, respectively. However, with concomitant evidence of cardiac membrane depression, as occurs with overdose of tricyclic antidepressants, such an approach may itself be hazardous, as will be discussed. Digitalis, propranolol, esmolol, verapamil, or diltiazem may be useful in slowing a rapid ventricular response to atrial fibrillation or flutter, although these arrhythmias may be only transient. Electrical conversion is an acceptable alternative when arrhythmias are life threatening and fail to respond to pharmacologic treatment.

Ventricular Arrhythmias

Pharmacologic therapy for drug-induced ventricular irritability is similar to that employed in the setting of acute myocardial ischemia. An important exception exists in cases of overdose of membrane-depressant drugs like quinidine or tricyclic antidepressants; in these instances, similar agents such as procainamide and disopyramide are contraindicated, and lidocaine or phenytoin is the drug of choice. Selection of secondary drugs depends on the particular overdose; thus, propranolol might be indicated for sympathomimetic drug overdose, phenytoin for digitalis overdose, isoproterenol for polymorphous ventricular tachycardia with a long QT

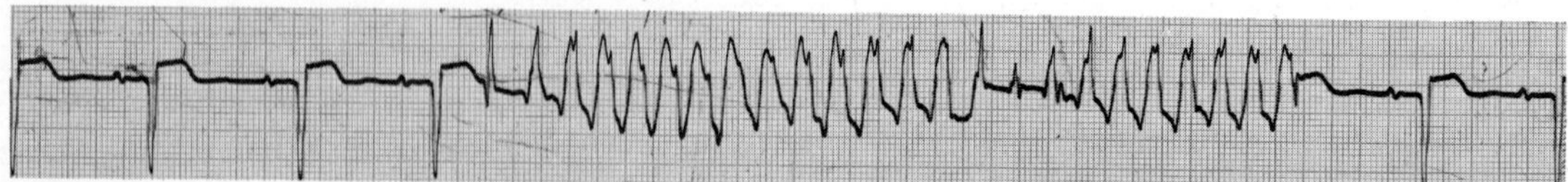

Figure 4–4. V_1 rhythm strip showing polymorphous ventricular tachycardia occurring abruptly and without warning. This particular arrhythmia is often referred to as "le torsades de pointes," reflecting a twisting of the QRS complexes around the electrocardiographic baseline. It occurs in association with prolongation of the QT interval from any cause (including idiopathic) and may also be seen in acute ischemic heart disease. In this tracing, the QT interval, measured from other leads, was 0.56 second.

Table 4–1. DRUG-RELATED ARRHYTHMIAS AND THEIR MANAGEMENT

TYPE	COMMENT	TREATMENT
Tachyarrhythmias		
All		Correct hypotension and acid-base and electrolyte disturbances
Sinus tachycardia	Usually can be made to vary with respiration, exercise, carotid sinus massage	No specific treatment indicated. If hemodynamic compromise, physostigmine, beta-blockade
Ectopic atrial tachycardia	If 2:1 atrioventricular conduction ratio, suspect digitalis toxicity	If hemodynamic compromise, physostigmine, beta-blockade, or calcium-channel blockade. If digitalis toxic, withdraw digitalis
Atrial flutter	Carotid sinus massage may produce sufficient atrioventricular block to discern atrial activity. If QRS rhythm is regular, suspect AV block, which might be due to digitalis toxicity and/or beta- and calcium entry blocker overdosage	Direct current cardioversion (low energy levels usually suffice); pace-termination; intravenous verapamil, esmolol, or propranolol will slow ventricular rate; digitalis and quinidine or procainamide
Atrial fibrillation	May appear to be regular at more rapid rates. Distinguish from multifocal atrial tachycardia by lack of defined atrial activity	Intravenous digitalis, verapamil, esmolol, and/or propranolol to slow ventricular response (if necessary). Direct current cardioversion if an accessory pathway is known or suspected and ventricular response is rapid
Junctional tachycardia	No variation in rate with respiration, exercise. Distinguish from sinus tachycardia with long PR interval or ventricular tachycardia (if QRS complex is wide). May be due to digitalis toxicity	If rate is rapid, beta-blockade, physostigmine,* pace-termination; direct current cardioversion
Ventricular ectopy (couplets, triplets, multiform complexes, sustained tachycardia, fibrillation)	If due to membrane-depressant drugs, other drugs in this class are to be avoided. If due to bradycardia, increase basic rate	Intravenous lidocaine, phenytoin, beta-blockade, bretylium; isoproterenol, magnesium and/or cardiac pacing if due to bradycardia or associated with long QT. Direct current cardioversion or defibrillation
Bradyarrhythmias		
Sinus bradycardia, including sinus arrest and sinoatrial block		No specific therapy. If hemodynamic decompensation, intravenous atropine, isoproterenol cardiac pacing
Vagotonic atrioventricular block	Atrioventricular block with varying PR intervals is associated with slowing of sinus rates. Seen in states with high vagal tone, including sleep	No specific therapy. Atropine, belladonna, theophylline, transdermal scopolamine, if sustained. Note: Atropine should not be administered if vagotonic rhythm is a reflex response to drug-induced hypertension, as it will aggravate the hypertension
Atrioventricular block Type I (Wenckebach)		If hemodynamic compromise, atropine, intravenous isoproterenol, cardiac pacing
Type II (Mobitz II) high degree or complete block	If atrial rate is increased by atropine or isoproterenol, increase in degree of atrioventricular block may occur	Cardiac pacing

*May be hazardous if associated with membrane-depressant drug overdose.

interval caused by quinidine-like drug overdose. Magnesium sulfate recently has been reported to control polymorphous ventricular tachycardia (with but not without long Q-T interval).[8a] Bretylium tosylate has been useful in the treatment of intractable ventricular arrhythmias occurring in the setting of acute ischemic heart disease, especially fibrillation unresponsive to defibrillation, and might be tried for similar arrhythmias occurring during drug overdose. Its use has a potential disadvantage of causing or worsening hypotension. It should be recalled that bretylium is a unique antiarrhythmic agent, being actually an antifibrillatory drug via increase in the threshold for ventricular fibrillation. As such, it might prevent ventricular fibrillation while failing to suppress ventricular ectopy. Sustained ventricular tachycardia and fibrillation require electrical conversion.

Wide Complex Tachycardia of Uncertain Origin

Occasionally the electrocardiogram shows a regular wide complex QRS rhythm without readily discernible atrial activity; the origin of the QRS rhythm may thus be uncertain. Rate alone is not a particularly useful criterion in distinguishing ventricular tachycardia from supraventricular tachycardia with intraventricular aberration, especially in the overdosed patient. QRS morphology, on the other hand, is often helpful. Ventricular tachycardia is suggested by very bizarre QRS complexes; rightward and superior deviation of the mean frontal plane QRS axis; qR, RR′, or R waves in leads aVr and V_1; rS or QS in leads aVL and V_6; or concordance (similarity) of QRS morphology in the precordial leads. Supraventricular tachycardia with intraventricular aberration is suggested by QRS morphology that closely resembles typical bundle branch block patterns. Past electrocardiograms with which to compare current ones may be helpful if they have shown a previously present bundle branch block pattern or ventricular premature complexes that resemble the present rhythm (Fig. 4–5).

The relationship of ventricular to atrial activity may afford another clue to the origin of the QRS rhythm. Establishing this relationship when atrial activity is not easily seen on the surface electrocardiogram often requires the placement of an electrode catheter in the esophagus or right atrium to register atrial electrical signals. The simultaneous recording of a surface electrocardiographic lead and intracardiac or intraesophageal electrogram will permit recognition of atrial activity. If this activity is occurring independent of (is dissociated from) the regular ventricular rhythm, the QRS rhythm is most likely ventricular tachycardia. If atrial activity is occurring irregularly at rates faster than the regular ventricular rhythm, the rhythm is ectopic atrial tachycardia or atrial fibrillation, depending on its rate, and is dissociated from the regular ventricular rhythm, which may then be junctional or ventricular in origin. If atrial activity is occurring at a rate that is a multiple of the QRS rate, atrial flutter is suggested. If a 1:1 relationship between atrial and ventricular activity is demonstrated, the direction of impulse transmission (atrioventricular or ventriculoatrial) is not known; only by changing the conduction ratios may the correct diagnosis be made. For example, if carotid sinus massage is applied in a patient with regular wide complex tachycardia and 1:1 atrioventricular relationship, and ventricular asystole occurs despite persistence of atrial activity, the rhythm was supraventricular in origin (Fig. 4–6). Some patients with hyperkalemia have a wide QRS complex rhythm without discernible P waves, in which the QRS complexes are nevertheless stimulated by the sinus node. This rhythm

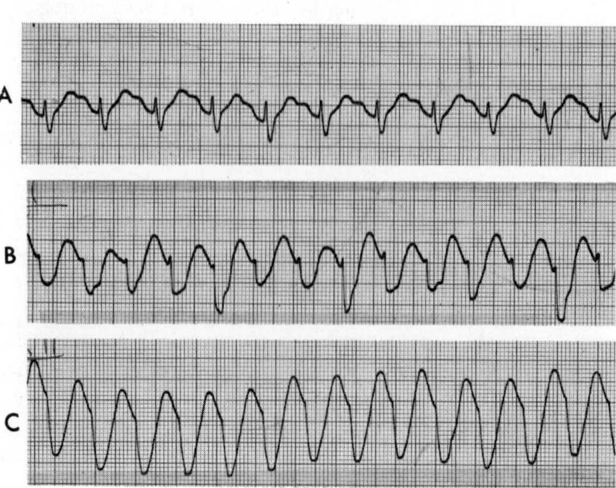

Figure 4–5. These lead 1 rhythm strips were obtained from a 40 year old woman who ingested 6 grams of amitriptyline (Elavil). In *A*, the rhythm is sinus with a long PR interval. In strips *B* and *C*, recorded within a 20-minute period, no P waves are seen, and the QRS complexes are broad and bizarre. Close scrutiny reveals that the QRS complexes in strips *B* and *C* resemble those in strip *A* except that they are more aberrant. The value of previously recorded tracings when evaluating a wide complex tachycardia, as in strip *C*, is illustrated by these electrocardiograms.

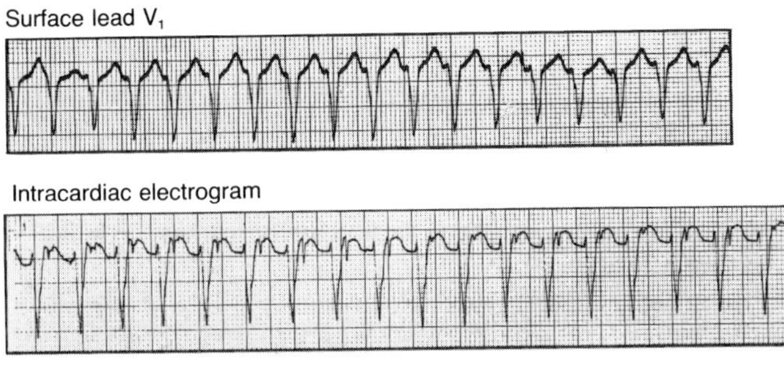

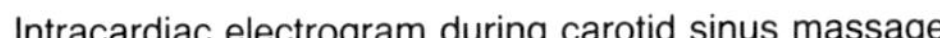

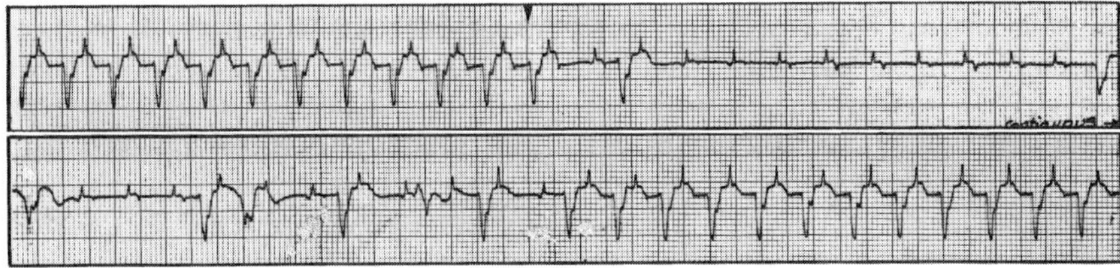

Figure 4–6. This 67 year old man with chronic obstructive pulmonary disease developed tachycardia during treatment with aminophylline. The surface electrocardiographic V_1 lead (top strip) shows a QRS duration of 0.12 second and no clearly discerned atrial activity. Intracardiac electrography (second strip) reveals a 1:1 relationship between ventricular (the broad, large deflections) and atrial (the sharp, small deflections) activity. The direction of impulse transmission is not known. Carotid sinus massage (lower two continuous strips) shows no change in atrial activity, while ventricular response is blocked, probably at the atrioventricular node. The change in the atrioventricular conduction ratio produced by carotid massage allows the diagnosis of atrial tachycardia to be made.

is termed *sinoventricular conduction*. The absence of P waves is due to hyperkalemia-related atrial arrest, and treatment of the hyperkalemia results in restoration of atrial muscle depolarization and appearance of P waves.

Management of hemodynamically significant wide complex tachycardia while the diagnosis is being established should include carotid sinus massage as a readily applied initial maneuver, but should be directed toward the potentially most life-threatening arrhythmia. Thus, intravenous lidocaine should be used for presumed ventricular tachycardia as the agent of first choice. When the nature of the overdose is unknown, however, direct current cardioversion may be the procedure of choice in order not to compound the problem of arrhythmia and hemodynamic instability, provided there is reasonable certainty that the rhythm is not sinus in origin. It is emphasized that failure to convert a wide complex tachycardia to another rhythm after direct current cardioversion should suggest that sinus tachycardia may indeed be present. It should also be recognized that certain antiarrhythmic agents, notably flecainide, can cause ventricular tachycardia refractory to cardioversion attempts.

Bradyarrhythmias

Bradyarrhythmias, particularly atrioventricular block, may occur unpredictably and may require temporary transvenous cardiac pacing. Before pacemaker insertion, transcutaneous pacing and pharmacologic therapy may be necessary in an attempt to maintain heart rate, blood pressure, and cardiac output. Intravenous administration of atropine should be tried to treat sinus or junctional bradycardia; intravenous administration of isoproterenol may be used for unresponsive sinus or junctional or ventricular bradycardias. These agents should be used with caution, however, because both may cause significant sinus or junctional tachycardia, and isoproterenol may cause ventricular extrasystolic activity, including ventricular tachycardia. Low doses of atropine (<0.5 mg) may cause paradoxic bradycardia.

Cardiac Pacing in Drug Overdose

Pacemaker-related difficulties encountered in drug-overdosed patients may be related to inability to sense a suboptimal intracardiac signal and/or to capture the ventricles. To be sensed properly by a pacemaker generator, an intracardiac signal must have certain characteristics: adequate amplitude, rapid rate of change of voltage, and optimal signal duration. In patients overdosed with agents that alter impulse conduction or cause or contribute to myocardial ischemia or failure, the intracardiac signal is often of too poor a quality to be sensed, leading to improper demand pacemaker function. The resulting earlier-than-expected pacing stimulus that follows unsensed spontaneous beats may cause repetitive ventricular rhythms, including ventricular tachycardia and fibrillation.

Another problem encountered in the drug-overdosed patient is failure of the pacing stimulus to depolarize sufficient amounts of myocardial tissue to cause ventricular activation, resulting in failure to pace.[9] This can come about as a result of myocardial inter- or intracellular edema or as a result of failure of pacing stimulus propagation due to hyperkalemia, hypoxia, acidosis, or membrane-depressant agents. The failure to pace may be total, with all pacing stimuli failing to depolarize the ventricles, or varying degrees of pacemaker exit block may be exhibited, including Wenckebach-type conduction (Fig. 4–7).

Because transcutaneous pacing is not effective over time, it should not be used except in emergencies and should be followed by transvenous pacing to ensure stable heart rate support.

Some patients in whom failure to pace is life-threatening may require cardiopulmonary bypass or intra-aortic balloon (triggering off the pacing stimulus) support to maintain circulatory function.

PULMONARY EDEMA

Pulmonary edema frequently complicates overdose with drugs such as narcotics, sedative-hypnotic drugs, and salicylates and sympathomimetic drugs. The pathophysiology of drug-induced pulmonary edema involves increased pulmonary capillary permeability, as evidenced by normal or low pulmonary capillary wedge pressures and pulmonary edema fluid with a protein concentration similar to that of plasma.[10, 11] In a series of 24 patients with pulmonary edema, those with drug-induced and other noncardiogenic pulmonary edema had pulmonary capillary wedge pressures of <20 mm Hg and ratios of edema fluid protein concentration to plasma protein concentration of >0.6.[11] Patients with hydrostatic or cardiogenic pulmonary edema had pulmonary capillary wedge pressures of >20 mm Hg and

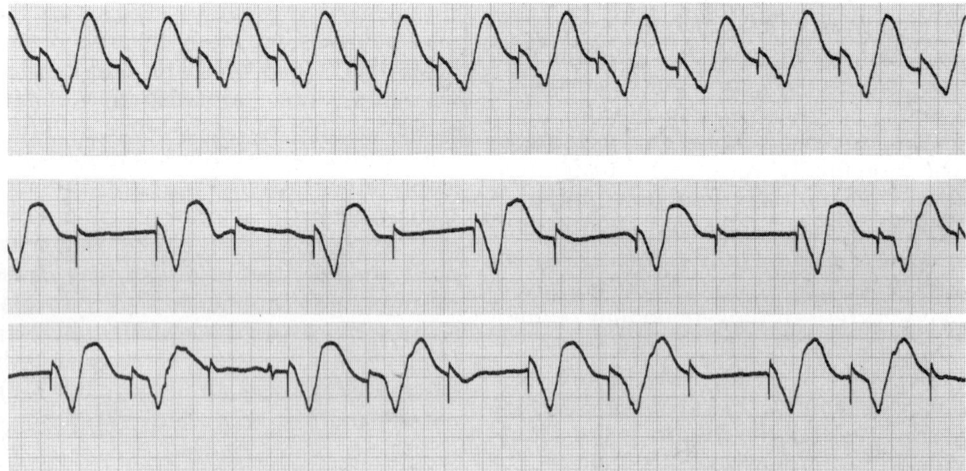

Figure 4–7. This 76 year old man had chronic congestive heart failure, recurrent ventricular tachycardia for which he was being treated with procainamide, paroxysmal atrioventricular block for which a transvenous pacing system had been implanted, and renal failure. He was admitted to the hospital with acute pulmonary edema. His serum potassium level was 5.0 mEq/L, and his serum procainamide level was 19 ng/ml. The top MCL1 rhythm strip shows a paced QRS rhythm with extremely wide QRS complexes; atrial activity is not discerned. The bottom two continuous MCL1 rhythm strips, recorded shortly after the top strip, show episodic failure of ventricular capture by the pacing stimuli, with a pattern suggesting Wenckebach block of the pacing stimuli. Because there was no evidence of pacemaker generator malfunction, the failure to capture in this clinical setting was considered to result from myocardial stimulation threshold elevation and failure of impulse conduction owing to the membrane-depressant effects of the procainamide. Treatment with low-dose isoproterenol and intravenous steroids was without effect, and the patient died.

ratios of edema fluid protein concentration to plasma protein concentration of <0.56.

The mechanisms by which sedative-hypnotic drugs produce capillary endothelial damage are still unknown. Depression of respiration may lead to hypoxemia, precapillary pulmonary hypertension, increased vascular permeability, and finally extravasation of fluid.[10] An analogy has been made to cases of pulmonary edema at high altitude, in which hypoxia produces a similar picture, which is rapidly reversed by oxygen therapy. Ethchlorvynol, when injected intravenously, is an example of a drug that directly injures the alveolar-capillary membrane.[12] Infused salicylate, possibly by effects on prostaglandin synthesis, increases microvascular permeability.[10] Pulsatile lymphatic activity is reduced and lymphatic drainage is retarded during barbiturate anesthesia.[13] This might also contribute to the net accumulation of fluid in the lung after drug overdose.

Neurogenic pulmonary edema, possibly mediated by massive sympathetic discharge, has been well described following brain injury and has been suggested to occur following overdoses of drugs such as narcotics and salicylates. Sympathomimetic drugs can cause pulmonary edema owing to severe hypertension. This is most common after intravenous administration. By the time such a patient is evaluated by the physician, blood pressure may be normal or even low, with evidence of hypovolemia due to sequestration of fluid into the lung and other extravascular sites. Direct depression of myocardial function by drugs may aggravate pulmonary edema caused by pulmonary capillary damage or, in the context of fluid therapy for hypotension, may result in cardiogenic pulmonary edema in the absence of pulmonary capillary damage.

Drug-induced pulmonary edema can be present on admission or may develop subsequently during the clinical course; in either case, it complicates management of shock states. Fluid filtration into the lung depends in part on pulmonary capillary pressure and, therefore, on left atrial pressure. A difficult clinical situation may arise in which intracardiac filling pressures adequate to maintain cardiac output may result in pulmonary transudation. Suggestions concerning fluid therapy and the use of pulmonary capillary wedge pressures have been discussed. Diuretics are not useful for drug-induced pulmonary edema because filling pressures are already normal or low, and further diuresis can potentiate hypotension. Infusions of albumin have been proposed to increase plasma oncotic pressure and to draw fluid from the lung. This is not rational because the protein content of the edema fluid is of similar composition to that of plasma, indicating that albumin passes through vascular endothelium as freely as water.

The use of mechanical ventilation with positive end-expiratory pressure (PEEP) is an important tool in the management of drug-induced pulmonary edema. Positive end-expiratory pressure increases functional residual capacity, reduces intrapulmonary shunting, and increases pulmonary compliance. Supplemental oxygen is usually necessary to maintain arterial PO_2 at 60 to 70 torr.

RECOGNITION AND MANAGEMENT OF CARDIAC DISTURBANCES CAUSED BY SPECIFIC DRUGS

Sedative-Hypnotic Drugs

Pathophysiology

Sedative-hypnotic drugs are involved in many or even the majority of cases of drug overdose. Although cardiac complications per se are uncommon, it is important to understand how this class of drugs might influence cardiovascular disturbances caused by co-ingested drugs. The major action of sedative-hypnotic drugs is on the central nervous system and results in reduced sympathetic and increased parasympathetic peripheral autonomic tone. Barbiturates have been shown to depress myocardial function in animals, but severe myocardial depression is uncommon in humans.[1, 14] Cardiac output is commonly reduced because of relative hypovolemia caused by increased venous capacitance and absolute hypovolemia due to fluid loss into tissues, the latter a consequence of increased vascular permeability.[15] Cardiac output and heart rate may be lower than normal as a result of hypothermia and reduced metabolic demands. As a consequence of inhibition of sympathetic function, heart rate is frequently less than expected for the degree of hypotension.

An important complication of sedative-hypnotic drug overdose is pulmonary edema, which results from increased pulmonary vascular permeability, as just discussed. As a consequence, hypoxia and metabolic acidosis develop, which may worsen myocardial performance and potentiate arrhythmias. Differences in clinical presentation of different sedative-hypnotic drugs are discussed in another review.[16]

General Management

The management of hypotension and shock due to sedative-hypnotic overdose includes judicious use of fluids and pressor drugs. Because venous pooling contributes to reduced cardiac output, the head-down leg-up (Trendelenburg) position may substantially increase venous return, cardiac output, and blood pressure. Infusion of modest amounts of colloid or crystalloid fluids is sufficient to correct hypovolemia and to increase cardiac output and tissue perfusion to adequate levels in many patients. Failure to achieve adequate tissue perfusion despite increased cardiac filling pressure or evidence of pulmonary edema is an indication for the use of pressor drugs, as discussed.

Table 4–2. CARDIAC DISTURBANCES DUE TO SYMPATHOMIMETIC DRUGS AND TOXINS

DRUGS	
Amphetamines	Delta-9-tetrahydrocannabinol
Cocaine	Lysergic acid diethylamide and other hallucinogens
Phencyclidine	Chloral hydrate*
Monoamine oxidase inhibitors	Ethanol
Phenylpropanolamine and other over-the-counter sympathomimetics	Hydrocarbon solvents* (such as toluene)
Theophylline	Freon* (and other fluorocarbon aerosols)
Caffeine	Sedative drug abstinence
CARDIOVASCULAR DISTURBANCES	
Sinus tachycardia	Ventricular tachycardia
Atrial tachycardia	Ventricular fibrillation
Sinus bradycardia**	Hypertension
Ventricular premature beats	Hypotension†
OTHER COMMON MANIFESTATIONS	
Dilated pupils‡	Tremor
Diaphoresis	Seizures
Fever	Hypokalemia
Excitement, anxiety, psychosis (often paranoid)§	Metabolic acidosis

*Sensitizes myocardium to catecholamines.
**Reflex response to vasoconstrictors such as phenylpropanolamine.
†Late manifestation, usually severe overdose.
‡Excepting phencyclidine and alcohols.
§Phencyclidine, alcohols, and solvents may cause ataxia, lethargy, or coma.

Sympathomimetic Drugs

General Considerations

As shown in Table 4–2, many drugs and toxins (as well as sedative-drug abstinence syndromes) are characterized by sympathetic overactivity. This typically results in sinus or atrial tachycardia (Fig. 4–8), hypertension, seizures and, after massive ingestions, cardiovascular collapse and respiratory arrest.[17,18] Occasionally, ventricular irritability and, rarely, ventricular fibrillation with death are observed.[18,19] Sympathomimetic drug-induced hypertension may result in pulmonary edema (although blood pressure may be normal or even low at the time of medical evaluation) or may be complicated by intracerebral hemorrhage.[20,21] Many sympathomimetic drugs, particularly amphetamine-like drugs and phencyclidine, produce muscular hyperactivity (fasciculations, myoclonus, convulsions) and hyperpyrexia, sometimes associated with rhabdomyolysis, acute renal failure, and disseminated intravascular coagulation.[22–24] Of note are studies of amphetamine and cocaine toxicity in conscious dogs that indicate that hyperpyrexia contributes significantly to death.[25] Pretreatment with pancuronium, which paralyzes the muscles that are the source of heat generation; diazepam, which prevents convulsions; and chlorpromazine, which sedated the animal, lessened the severity of the seizures and possibly also facilitated heat dissipation via peripheral alpha-adrenergic blockade. Environmental cooling substantially improved survival. In contrast, propranolol, which effectively blocked cardiovascular responses to amphetamines, or bicarbonate infusion, which reversed metabolic acidosis, did not improve survival.

Amphetamine-Like Drugs and Cocaine

Many amphetamine-like drugs are available as anorectic agents. Along with these, illicitly manufactured amphetamines and their derivatives and cocaine are widely abused, primarily for their euphoric effects.[19a] The euphoria is associated with central ner-

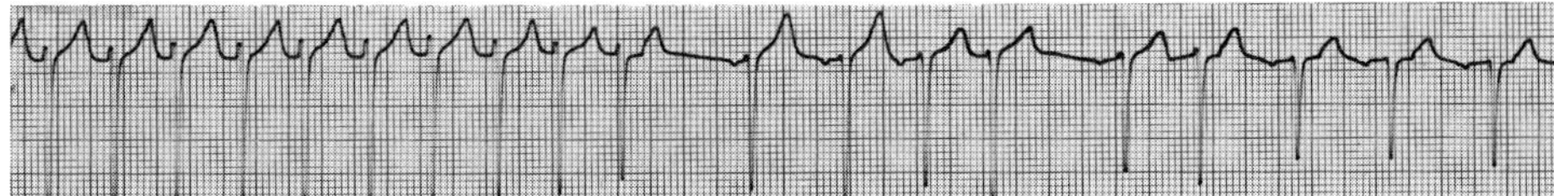

Figure 4–8. This 27 year old cocaine user was admitted to the coronary care unit for electrocardiographic monitoring after having had two syncopal spells. The MCL1 rhythm strip shows bursts of atrial tachycardia, which terminate spontaneously, and atrial premature beats, some of which are not conducted.

vous system and adrenomedullary sympathetic activation, producing typical sympathomimetic syndromes. However, tolerance to central nervous system effects develops rapidly, so the duration of euphoria is much shorter than the presence of the drug in the body. Repeated doses may result in accumulation of drug and cardiovascular toxicity at a time when the user is no longer euphoric.

Amphetamines displace and release catecholamines stored in neurons, directly stimulate postsynaptic adrenergic receptors, and may inhibit monoamine oxidase, the enzyme responsible for intraneuronal degradation of catecholamines. Cocaine in particular is a potent inhibitor of neuronal catecholamine uptake, which is a major route of detoxification for norepinephrine released from nerve endings or the adrenal medulla, or administered exogenously. Chronic administration of amphetamines and cocaine has also been reported to result in myocarditis and cardiomyopathy.[26, 27]

Cocaine intoxication has been associated with a number of additional cardiovascular complications, including acute myocardial infarction, myocardial necrosis, and dissecting aortic aneurysm.[27a] Myocardial infarction occurs as a consequence of increased myocardial work in the presence of fixed coronary artery disease, coronary vasospasm, or coronary thrombosis. Patchy myocardial necrosis with contraction band necrosis has been described after acute cocaine intoxication, believed to be a result of intense catecholamine stimulation of the heart.[27b] Fibrosis and chronic cardiomyopathy may ensue.

The management of amphetamine and cocaine drug toxicity depends on the specific manifestations (Table 4–3). Hypertension and tachycardia can be managed by alpha- and beta-adrenergic blocking agents or vasodilators such as sodium nitroprusside or rate-sparing calcium channel blockers or both. Because arrhythmias result primarily from beta-adrenergic stimulation, a beta-blocking agent is the drug of choice. Theoretically, a relatively specific beta-1 blocker such as metoprolol or esmolol would be preferred so as not to antagonize the beta-2-mediated arteriolar dilation that may be opposing alpha-mediated constriction. Thus beta-2 blockade could result in unopposed alpha effects and worsen hypertension.

Table 4–3. TREATMENT OF CARDIOVASCULAR COMPLICATIONS OF SYMPATHOMIMETIC DRUG POISONING

MANIFESTATION	TREATMENT
Tachyarrhythmias	Reduce environmental stimulation*
Sinus or atrial	None, propranolol, esmolol, verapamil
Ventricular	Propranolol, lidocaine, cardioversion, calcium channel blockers
Hypertension	Reduce environmental stimulation* Phentolamine Nitroprusside Beta-blocker (beta-1 specific if possible) if associated with tachycardia
Convulsions	Diazepam, phenytoin, phenobarbital
Hyperthermia	Stop seizures Pancuronium if seizures uncontrollable External cooling Chlorpromazine or haloperidol High inspired oxygen
Myocardial ischemia/ infarction	Nitrates, calcium channel blockers, thrombolysis
Cardiovascular collapse	Fluids (may require massive amounts in presence of hyperthermia) Pressors (unpredictable sensitivity)

*Especially phencyclidine and hydrocarbons.

Hyperpyrexia is potentially life threatening.[27c] Chlorpromazine or haloperidol may reverse hyperthermia[17] by central nervous or peripheral vascular actions, as discussed. While these drugs are known to lower the seizure threshold in some experimental seizure models, chlorpromazine seems to lessen the severity of seizures caused by sympathomimetic drugs. Seizures should be treated as rapidly and effectively as possible. Intravenous administration of diazepam is usually effective in terminating seizures, but then loading with phenobarbital and, if necessary, phenytoin should be accomplished.

If hyperthermia or severe metabolic acidosis complicates seizures or other evidence of muscular hyperactivity, external cooling and paralysis with pancuronium or curare are indicated. Even when muscular hyperactivity is prevented by paralysis, persistent seizure activity may cause brain injury.[28] Therefore, electroencephalograms should be monitored in paralyzed patients and seizures controlled with anticonvulsant drugs or general anesthesia, if necessary. Ventilation with high oxygen concentrations is indicated for all hyperthermic patients to meet the extreme metabolic demands of muscular hyperactivity and the effects of hyperthermia on metabolism in other body organs. Acute renal failure may result from hypovolemia, hypotension, and rhabdomyolysis with myoglobinuria and may be prevented by vigorous fluid replacement and use of mannitol and diuretics to increase urine flow and bicarbonate to alkalinize the urine.

Phencyclidine

The cardiovascular effects of phencyclidine resemble those of the amphetamines. In most cases, hypertension and tachycardia are present.[29, 30] Seizures are common, are often difficult to treat, and may be fatal.[31] However, unlike the patient who has ingested amphetamines, the phencyclidine-intoxicated patient usually appears ataxic, sedated, or even comatose. Blood pressure and heart rate are often quite labile and increase with environmental stimulation. With severe overdose, hypotension and respiratory depression occur.[32]

The mechanism of action of phencyclidine includes increased central nervous system–mediated sympathetic activity, potentiation of endogenous catecholamine actions; and direct vasoconstrictor effects, all of which are reversed by alpha-adrenergic-blocking agents.[33, 34] Neuronal uptake of norepinephrine may be inhibited, as it is with cocaine. The labile cardiovascular responses may be explained by increased sensitivity to endogenously released catecholamines.

Therapy of cardiovascular complications of phencyclidine consists of the use of alpha- and beta-adrenergic-blocking drugs and vasodilators, as discussed for amphetamines. Both nitroprusside and diazoxide have been used to treat phencyclidine-induced hypertension. Because phencyclidine enhances sensitivity to catecholamines, increased sensitivity to pressor drugs may be observed when these are used to treat hypotensive patients. Reducing environmental stimulation is helpful in minimizing toxicity. Diazepam is often given for sedation and haloperidol for extreme agitation.

Monoamine Oxidase Inhibitors

With the decreasing availability of electroconvulsive shock therapy, the use of monoamine oxidase (MAO) inhibitors alone and in combination with tricyclic antidepressants has been increasing. As a consequence, adverse reactions and poisoning with MAO inhibitors have become more frequent.

Clinical manifestations of MAO inhibitor toxicity resemble those of other sympathomimetic drugs: restlessness, hyperactivity, confusion or stupor, neuromuscular irritability, hypertension, seizures, and hyperpyrexia.[35–37] Hypertension, which most often occurs after ingestion of tyramine-containing foods or beverages or after taking other sympathomimetic drugs but also can occur after an overdose, may be severe, often is associated with severe headache, and has been associated with intracerebral hemorrhage. Hypotension can also occur after overdose.

Understanding the pathophysiology of MAO inhibitor reactions requires understanding of the role of MAO in the body. Monoamine oxidase is located within adrenergic neurons, where it metabolizes catecholamines and related monoamines, and in the gastrointestinal mucosa and liver, where it metabolizes dietary monoamines, such as tyramine. Inhibition of MAO within the adrenergic neuron results in accumulation of both active and relatively inactive (such as octopamine) monoamines. Octopamine and other relatively inactive monoamines act as false neurotransmitters in that they are released by neuronal stimulation into nerve endings where they do not effectively activate vascular receptors. As a consequence, MAO inhibitors when taken chronically may lower blood pressure. However, MAO inhibitors, by slowing metabolism, may also increase pressor responses to catecholamines released by other drugs. Most important in causing hypertension is that MAO inhibitors in the gut and liver increase the bioavailability of tyramine, which in turn releases catecholamines stored in adrenergic neurons. Ingestion of foods rich in tyramine can lead to massive catecholamine release and hypertensive crisis. Tranylcypromine is a MAO inhibitor that itself causes catecholamine release and, among the MAO inhibitor class of drugs, has been most commonly implicated in cardiovascular toxicity.[38] It is important also to recognize the potential interaction between meperidine (and possibly other narcotics) and MAO inhibitors. The combination has resulted in severe hypertension, hyperthermia, and seizures.[39] The mechanism is unknown. Therapy for MAO toxicity is similar to that of other sympathomimetic drugs.

Phenylpropanolamine and Other Over-the-Counter Sympathomimetic Drugs

Phenylpropanolamine, ephedrine, and many other over-the-counter decongestants and appetite-suppressant drugs have both direct and indirect (catecholamine-releasing) sympathomimetic effects. In most cases of overdose with cold or decongestant preparations, mild hypertension is observed that requires no specific therapy. After ingestion of predominantly vasoconstrictor drugs such as phenylpropanolamine, heart rate may be slow due to reflex slowing,[39a] or rapid due to co-ingested caffeine or anticholinergic antihistamines. After overdose and occasionally after therapeutic doses, severe hypertension occurs, sometimes associated with stroke, ventricular arrhythmias, or ST-T changes on the electrocardiogram and abnormally elevated myocardial creatine phosphokinase concentrations suggesting myocardial injury.[40–42] Unusual responsiveness to catecholamines may explain some of the exaggerated blood pressure response in some patients. In one such patient, pressor hypersensitivity to infused norepinephrine was documented that related to a previously unrecognized autonomic insufficiency state.[43]

Similar hypersensitivity to sympathomimetic drugs is expected in persons taking tricyclic antidepressants and the antihypertensive drug guanethidine, which block uptake and increase pressor sensitivity to released catecholamines, respectively.[44, 45] Antihistamines found in common cold preparations may contribute to sympathomimetic-induced hypertension by inhibiting vagally mediated cardiac deceleration, which normally serves to compensate for vasoconstrictor-mediated hypertension.

Amphetamine "look-alikes," containing phenylpropanolamine, ephedrine, or caffeine, are available without prescription. Several sudden deaths, presumably from arrhythmias, in the context of overdosage have been reported to the Food and Drug Administration.[46]

Management of overdose with phenylpropanolamine and related drugs includes careful monitoring of blood pressure and electrocardiogram. Management of hypertension, tachycardia, and arrhythmias is as discussed for amphetamines.

Theophylline and Caffeine

Cardiac toxicity of theophylline occurs in a different context from that of stimulant drugs. The most common circumstance is overdosage during therapy for obstructive airway disease, often as a result of hepatic dysfunction, which reduces the rate of theophylline metabolism. Accidental or suicidal overdosage often occurs in persons with underlying medical illnesses. The nature and severity of these medical conditions have a strong impact on the course and severity of cardiac toxicity.

The typical cardiovascular manifestations of theophylline overdose result from beta-adrenergic stimulation and include tachycardia and arrhythmias[47, 48] (Fig. 4–9). Hypotension (rather than hypertension as seen with most other sympathomimetic drugs) is seen in severe intoxications. Like amphetamines, theophylline causes systemic and local vascular catecholamine release but, in addition, at high concentrations, such as those seen in severe poisonings, may inhibit phosphodiesterase, an enzyme that degrades cyclic AMP, which, in turn, mediates beta-adrenergic actions. Theophylline also directly relaxes vascular smooth muscle. Convulsions typically occur with an overdose, and cardiac and respiratory arrest are causes of death.[47–49] Administration of theophylline via central venous catheters has been found to be particularly hazardous, resulting in several cases of cardiac arrest.[50] Management of cardiac toxicity due to theophylline in persons with chronic lung disease may be difficult. Beta-adrenergic blocking agents are logical and effective treatment for supraventricular and

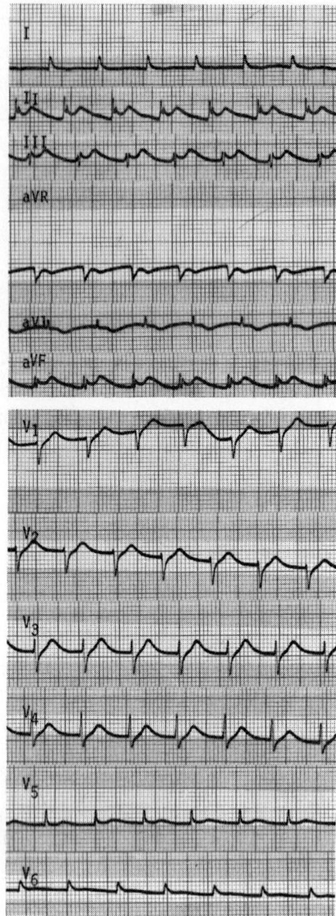

Figure 4–9. This 12-lead electrocardiogram was recorded from a 60 year old man with chronic obstructive pulmonary disease who ingested aminophylline and terbutaline in a suicide attempt. Peak theophylline concentration was 152 μg/ml. A narrow QRS tachycardia is present without discernible atrial activity, suggesting a junctional origin. J point and ST segment elevation are present in the inferolateral leads (II, III, aVF, V_5, and V_6). Serial enzyme determination failed to confirm myocardial infarction. The patient died 2 days later with refractory cardiovascular collapse.

ventricular arrhythmias,[51] but beta-blockers also may worsen airway obstruction. Relatively cardiospecific beta-blockers, such as esmolol or metoprolol, might be tried and the antiarrhythmic effects closely titrated against evidence of worsening airway obstruction.

Hypotension due to theophylline usually results from peripheral vasodilation, at least early in the course of overdose. However, in animals with prolonged beta sympathetic stimulation, myocarditis with reduced ventricular function has been observed;[52] a similar event may occur late in the course of theophylline overdose in humans. In addition, many older patients with chronic lung disease have ischemic heart disease. In the context of tachycardia and hypotension, myocardial perfusion may be inadequate and myocardial function impaired on that basis. Hypoxia caused by underlying lung disease, hypokalemia caused by sustained beta-adrenergic stimulation,[47, 53] and acidosis due to lung disease or convulsions may also contribute to hypotension.

Management of theophylline-induced hypotension includes correction of metabolic disturbances and arrhythmias and administration of fluids and pressor agents. If pressor drugs are to be used, it is useful to know the cardiac output and to be able to compute the systemic vascular resistance. If cardiac output is high and systemic vascular resistance is low, as is seen in many cases of theophylline overdose, administration of vasoconstrictors like norepinephrine and nonselective beta-adrenergic antagonists is indicated. If cardiac output is low despite adequate cardiac filling pressures and systemic vascular resistance is normal or high as occurs sometimes late in the case of theophylline overdose and in persons with pre-existing myocardial disease, inotropic agents like dobutamine might be selected.

In the presence of severe toxicity, particularly in a patient with serious underlying medical disease, the persistence of theophylline in the body and the time course of toxicity are quite prolonged, and acceleration of drug removal by hemoperfusion should be undertaken.[47, 48]

Caffeine is widely consumed in beverages such as coffee and colas, in over-the-counter stimulants, and in various other combination analgesic and cold medications. Caffeine has pharmacologic actions similar to those of theophylline. Caffeine potentiates effects of sympathomimetic drugs and might contribute to adverse cardiac events, including sudden death from amphetamine "look-alikes" as discussed earlier. Caffeine alone is thought to cause severe cardiac toxicity rarely, although cases of supraventricular tachycardias are reported.[54] There are reports of severe caffeine intoxication with tachyarrhythmias followed by cardiovascular collapse and death in children. We recently treated an adult following a massive ingestion of caffeine (No-Doz) who had sinus tachycardia with a rate of 190 beats per minute, hypokalemia, hyperglycemia, metabolic acidosis, and rhabdomyolysis (Fig. 4–10).

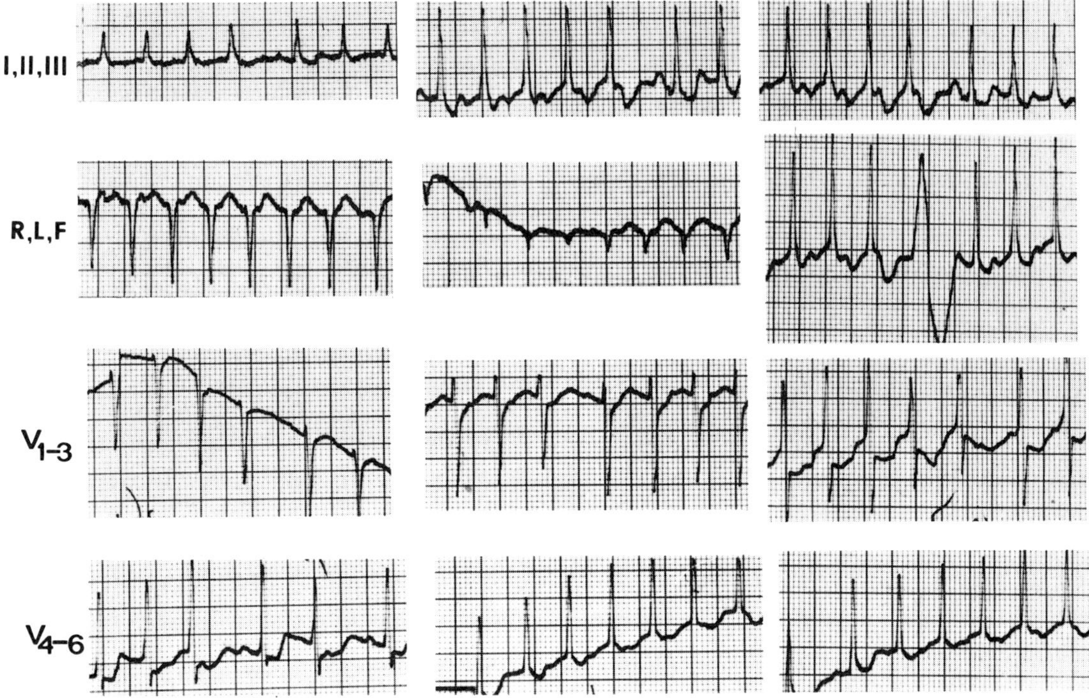

Figure 4–10. This 30 year old schizophrenic woman allegedly ingested the contents of four bottles of the over-the-counter preparation NoDoz, each containing 60 100-mg caffeine tablets. She was brought to the emergency room awake but mute and apparently hallucinating. Blood pressure was 112/74 mm Hg; heart rate, 180 to 200 beats/min; serum potassium, 2.2 mEq/L; and serum caffeine, 200 μg/ml.

This admission electrocardiogram shows a supraventricular tachycardia at a rate of about 180 to 190/min. The tachycardia is probably sinus in origin, judging from the P wave configurations. Atrioventricular nodal Wenckebach block is present and is probably the result of the tachycardia rate (and the inability of the atrioventricular node to respond) rather than to the pharmacologic effects of caffeine. Ventricular ectopic complexes are also present.

The patient was treated with potassium and fluids, with prompt initial slowing of the sinus rate to 150/min, then with gradual return to normal over the next 48 hours.

Delta-9-Tetrahydrocannabinol and Hallucinogens

The usual cardiovascular effects of delta-9 tetrahydrocannabinol (THC), the principal psychoactive component in marijuana and other cannabis products, are tachycardia, a slight increase in recumbent blood pressure, and, with large doses or in susceptible persons, orthostatic hypotension.[55] The effects of THC on heart rate result from central nervous system–mediated sympathetic activation and reduced parasympathetic activity, and from systemic release of catecholamines. Orthostatic hypotension results from impaired sympathetic reflex responses and, in particular, deficient venoconstriction.

Sinus tachycardia can reach rates of 140 to 150 beats per minute or higher and, manifested as palpitations, can contribute to the anxiety reaction occasionally reported by novice users or those consuming marijuana containing unusually large amounts of THC. In otherwise healthy persons, no specific treatment other than reassurance is necessary. Patients with ischemic heart disease are at greater risk from the effects of THC (as they are from those of all sympathomimetic drugs). The combination of (1) increased myocardial oxygen demand due to the tachycardia and increased myocardial contractility and (2) decreased myocardial oxygen delivery due to effects of carbon monoxide derived from marijuana smoke may aggravate the ischemia. For example, persons with angina pectoris are not able to exercise as long after smoking marijuana as they can when smoking tobacco or not smoking at all.[56] Ischemia combined with systemic release of catecholamines also might result in potentially severe arrhythmias.

Orthostatic dizziness is occasionally reported by recreational users of cannabis, particularly after eating larger than usual quantities of THC in cookies or brownies. Patients receiving THC as an adjunct to cancer chemotherapy may also exhibit orthostatic hypotension, particularly when they are dehydrated because of their disease. Hypotension responds well to placing the patient into the horizontal or Trendelenburg posture and administering fluids; administration of pressors is rarely necessary.

Lysergic acid diethylamide (LDS), psilocybin, and other hallucinogens commonly result in tachycardia and mild hypertension as part of a general sympathetic arousal syndrome.[57] Cardiovascular disturbances are rarely serious and require only supportive care.

Chloral Hydrate and Ethanol

Chloral hydrate overdose has been associated with supraventricular (mainly junctional) tachycardia, ventricular tachycardia (often polymorphous), and ventricular fibrillation.[58, 59] Chloral hydrate is metabolized to trichloroethanol, which is believed to produce the arrhythmias. Trichloroethanol as well as other alcohols releases catecholamines. Trichloroethanol also is believed to sensitize the myocardium to the effects of circulating catecholamine, an effect similar to that of hydrocarbon anesthetics, to be discussed.

Chronic alcoholics frequently are seen in emergency rooms with toxicologic problems. Chronic or acute cardiovascular disorders may appear as primary problems or may complicate other overdoses. Chronic alcoholism is well known to be associated with congestive cardiomyopathy and, less commonly, beriberi heart disease. Congestive cardiomyopathy with low cardiac output, pulmonary congestion, diverse arrhythmias and/or sudden death may result from the chronic toxic effects of ethanol.[60, 60a] Alcoholic cardiomyopathy is treated like other types of congestive failure.

Beriberi heart disease results from thiamine deficiency. The patient presents with high cardiac output manifested by tachycardia and wide pulse pressure, as well as peripheral neuritis. The heart may be enlarged, and dyspnea caused by pulmonary congestion, as well as neck vein engorgement and peripheral edema, may be present.[61] Prolonged QT interval, low QRS voltage, and T wave abnormalities may be present in the electrocardiogram. Decreased peripheral vascular resistance is responsible for the high cardiac output. Initial doses of thiamine occasionally result in pulmonary edema because of a sudden increase in vascular resistance combined with mobilization of edema fluid.

Heavy binge drinkers may present with a sudden onset of arrhythmias, particularly atrial fibrillation or flutter with rapid ventricular response but also atrial or junctional tachycardia and ventricular arrhythmias (this syndrome has been termed "holiday heart")[62] (Fig. 4–11). The arrhythmias may be due to preclinical cardiomyopathy, electrolyte abnormalities (including deficiency of potassium, phosphate, and/or magnesium), or early stages of alcohol withdrawal.

Abstinence from ethanol (and other sedative drugs) may be associated with intense sympathetic hyperactivity, hypertension, and many types of tachyarrhythmias, usually supraventricular but also ventricular arrhythmias, and sudden, unpredictable death.[63, 132]

Lidocaine, beta-adrenergic antagonists, and phenytoin have been used to treat arrhythmias caused by chloral hydrate and other alcohols. Beta-blockers, verapamil, or digitalis may be necessary to control the ventricular response rate in cases of alcohol-induced atrial fibrillation or flutter. Metabolic disturbances, particularly hypokalemia, hypophosphatemia, and hypomagnesemia, common in alcoholics, may contribute to arrhythmias and should be corrected.

Hydrocarbon Solvents and Fluorocarbon Aerosols

An epidemic of sudden deaths was associated with widespread abuse of solvents by inhalation in the late 1960s.[64] Witnesses reported that victims collapsed after sniffing glue, cleaning fluids, paint, or aerosol propellants (hair sprays, deodorant sprays, and frying pan lubricants) from plastic bags, becoming excited or panicky and then exercising. Animal studies have demonstrated that many solvents, including toluene, benzene, chloroform, trichloroethane, trichloroethylene, trichlorofluoroethane, and other fluoroalkenes (freons), potentiate arrhythmias due to infused epinephrine.[65] Thus doses of epinephrine that usually produce no arrhythmias may cause ventricular tachycardia or fibrillation after solvent or fluorocarbon exposure. Arrhythmias are also more easily produced in the presence of hypoxemia,[66]

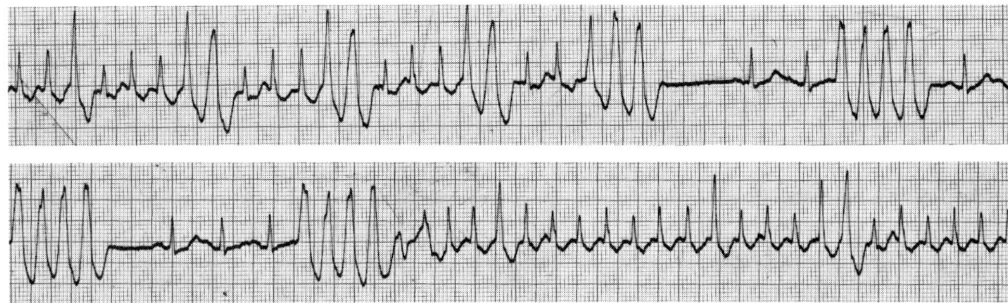

Figure 4–11. These two continuous lead 2 rhythm strips were recorded in a 48 year old alcoholic man admitted to the hospital after a syncopal spell preceded by palpitations. Sinus rhythm is interrupted by atrial tachycardia. Frequent premature ventricular complexes are also present, as well as bursts of ventricular tachycardia, which occasionally interrupt the atrial tachyarrhythmia. The rhythm was treated with intravenous lidocaine, which abolished the bursts of ventricular tachycardia but had no effect on the atrial arrhythmia. All arrhythmias resolved within 12 hours of admission. Work-up for organic heart disease was negative, and 24-hour ambulatory electrocardiographic monitoring prior to hospital discharge failed to reveal any rhythm abnormalities.

which might also be expected when breathing gases from a plastic bag.

Other animal studies have shown that solvent inhalation, even when normal oxygenation is maintained, may cause sinoatrial slowing followed by escape junctional or ventricular rhythms and subsequently asystole or ventricular fibrillation.[67] Possibly, the combination of depressed sinoatrial automaticity and myocardial sensitization to catecholamines, released by exercise or emotional stimuli, accounts for the fatal ventricular arrhythmias. Toluene sniffing in particular causes renal tubular dysfunction, as well as severe hypokalemia, hypophosphatemia, and metabolic acidosis, which might aggravate arrhythmias.[68] Ingestion of hydrocarbons is typically associated with pneumonitis and central nervous system depression; however, arrhythmias with electrocardiographic and enzyme changes, suggesting acute myocardial injury, have been reported.[69, 70] A recent case report described seizures and ventricular tachycardia in a 2 year old child after accidental exposure to nonfluorinated hydrocarbon aerosol propellants (isobutane and *N*-butane) used in a deodorant spray can.[70a]

Obviously, little can be done to treat victims of "sudden sniffing death." However, in persons who are intoxicated with solvents or fluorocarbons, steps can be taken to lessen the risk of arrhythmias, at least according to our current hypothesis of pathogenesis. Before evaluation at the hospital, patients should be advised to avoid strenuous exercise. In the hospital, patients can be placed in a quiet, nonthreatening environment and sedated if necessary. If hypoxic, oxygen should be administered and metabolic abnormalities corrected. Sympathomimetic drugs should be avoided. Ventricular arrhythmias are best treated with beta-blocking agents.

Sympathetic Inhibiting Drugs (Table 4–4)

(For references, see Chapter 91 on beta-blockers)

Beta-Adrenergic Receptor Blockers

Cardiac disturbances caused by beta-adrenergic receptor blockers result from both receptor blockade, which all drugs in this class demonstrate, and other actions such as mem-

Table 4–4. CARDIAC DISTURBANCES CAUSED BY SYMPATHETIC-INHIBITING DRUGS

DRUGS	
Propranolol and other beta-blockers	Reserpine
Methyldopa	Guanethidine
Clonidine	Prazosin
CARDIOVASCULAR DISTURBANCES	
Sinus bradycardia	Hypotension
Atrioventricular block	Cardiac failure*
OTHER COMMON MANIFESTATIONS	
Sedation†	Seizures§
Small pupils‡	Hyperkalemia
Diarrhea	Bronchoconstriction‖

*Usually in patients with underlying myocardial disease.

†Except guanethidine and prazosin.

‡Particularly clonidine and prazosin.

§Propranolol and other membrane-depressant beta-blockers; rarely clonidine.

‖Usually in patients with previous asthma.

brane depressant or sympathomimetic effects, which differ among drugs within the class. Beta-adrenergic blockade itself is associated with sinus bradycardia, atrioventricular block (usually first-degree) and the emergence of ectopic escape pacemakers in healthy hearts. In persons with underlying cardiac conduction disease, advanced atrioventricular block with slow ventricular rates can occur. In the presence of underlying myocardial disease in which contractility depends on sympathetic activity, beta-adrenergic receptor blockade can result in hypotension or cardiac failure, including shock or acute pulmonary edema and death.

In previously healthy persons, drugs such as propranolol, with membrane-depressant effects, can in large doses directly depress myocardial function and result in hypotension caused by reduced cardiac output. Drugs such as pindolol, with intrinsic sympathomimetic activity, can cause tachycardia and hypertension despite concurrent beta-blockade after an overdose.

Therapy is summarized in Table 4–5. Sinus bradycardia is usually well tolerated and requires no specific therapy. If sinus bradycardia results in hemodynamic compromise, atropine, isoproterenol, glucagon, or intracardiac pacing should be considered. Because of the competitive nature of drug-induced beta-blockade, extraordinary doses of isoproterenol may be required to increase heart rate. The dose may be limited by peripheral vasodilation and fall in blood pressure. Advanced atrioventricular block is an indication for intracardiac pacing.

Hypotension can usually be managed with fluids and correction of bradyarrhythmias. In the presence of myocardial depression, glucagon, which activates adenylate cyclase by a nonadrenergic mechanism, may enhance myocardial contractility and increase cardiac output. Epinephrine and dobutamine are potentially useful inotropic agents, although the doses may need to be higher than usual because of beta-blockade.

Table 4–5. TREATMENT OF CARDIOVASCULAR COMPLICATIONS OF SYMPATHETIC-INHIBITING DRUG POISONING

MANIFESTATION	TREATMENT
Bradyarrhythmias	
Sinus or atrial	None, atropine, isoproterenol, glucagon,* pacemaker
Junctional and ventricular	Isoproterenol, pacemaker, glucagon*
Ventricular tachyarrhythmias	Lidocaine, phenytoin, overdrive pacing
	Cardioversion
Hypotension	Trendelenburg position
	Treat bradyarrhythmias if present
	Fluids (hemodynamic monitoring advised with pre-existing cardiac disease)
	Glucagon, dobutamine* (if normal or high systemic vascular resistance)
	Dopamine, norepinephrine (if low systemic vascular resistance)
Hypertension†	Phentolamine, tolazoline
	Nitroprusside

*Particularly when related to beta-blocker overdose.
†Chlonidine, methyldopa, guanethidine; note hypertension is often *transient* and is followed by hypotension.

Sympatholytic Antihypertensive Drugs

Most patients who have ingested excessive doses of sympatholytic antihypertensive drugs have sinus bradycardia and hypotension when first seen. Drugs such as methyldopa, clonidine, and reserpine, which are active in the central nervous system, commonly cause sedation or coma. In addition, after an overdose of clonidine, miosis and respiratory depression resembling narcotic overdose can also be present.[71] However, after clonidine poisoning, hypotension and bradycardia are more prominent than respiratory depression. The reverse is true for narcotics. Clonidine, by direct alpha-adrenergic receptor agonist activity, and methyldopa, reserpine, and guanethidine, through systemic release of catecholamines, also have been associated with transient and sometimes severe hypertension.

In most cases, hypotension due to antihypertensive drug overdose is not severe and can be managed by the legs-up head-down position and intravenous fluids. When hypotension is severe in the presence of bradycardia, atropine, isoproterenol, or cardiac pacing will increase heart rate and cardiac output and may increase blood pressure. Although not often necessary, modest doses of dopamine and norepinephrine are usually effective. Hypertension resulting from clonidine or other sympatholytic drugs is best treated with the short-acting alpha-adrenergic receptor antagonist phentolamine and, if necessary, vasodilators such as nitroprusside. Oral nifedipine also has been effective. It should be recognized that the hypertensive phase is relatively brief, and its treatment should be tapered before the subsequent hypotensive effects become manifest.

Because clonidine exerts its hypotensive and sedating effects by actions on alpha-receptors in the brain, the use of centrally active alpha-blockers such as tolazoline has been recommended for clonidine overdose. Although tolazoline can reverse the effects of therapeutic doses of clonidine,[72] no benefit has been proved for its use in overdose. Because most clonidine-intoxicated patients do well with supportive care, we do not use tolazoline. Clonidine has been shown to reduce symptoms of narcotic withdrawal, so is used as an adjunct in this therapy.[73] (This explains recent epidemics of clonidine overdose in heroin addicts.) Conversely, in animals, high doses of naloxone reverse the hypotension and bradycardia due to clonidine[74] and might be expected to be of benefit in overdose cases in humans. However, the response to naloxone in people poisoned with clonidine is variable and should not be relied upon as the primary therapy for cardiovascular toxicity from this drug.[75]

Anticholinergic Drugs and Toxins
(Table 4–6)

The variety of anticholinergic drugs or toxins that may be ingested is too great to list each drug separately. In most cases, sinus or atrial tachycardia with mild hypertension occurs. Serious arrhythmias resulting from purely anticholinergic compounds are uncommon unless there is underlying ischemic heart disease. Thus by increasing myocardial oxygen demand owing to tachycardia, atropine has caused ventricular tachycardia and fibrillation in patients after myocardial infarction.[76] Many patients with anticholinergic signs have ingested antihistamine-sympathomimetic combinations or drugs such as tricyclic antidepressants or neuroleptics with both anticholinergic and membrane-depressant effects that result in more serious cardiovascular disturbances.

Table 4–6. CARDIAC DISTURBANCES CAUSED BY ANTICHOLINERGIC DRUGS AND TOXINS

DRUGS	
Atropine, belladonna, scopolamine	Tricyclic antidepressants
Antihistamines (including most over-the-counter hypnotics)	Plants (such as Jimson weed)
Propantheline	Mushrooms (such as *Amanita muscaria**)
CARDIAC DISTURBANCES	
Sinus tachycardia	Ventricular premature beats
Atrial tachycardia	Hypertension
OTHER COMMON MANIFESTATIONS	
Sedation	Dry mucous membranes
Delirium, coma	No sweating
Fever	Hypoactive or absent bowel sounds
Dry, flushed skin	Urinary retention
Dilated pupils	

*May have muscarinic as well as anticholinergic activity.

If treatment is necessary because of hypotension, organ ischemia, or severe hypertension due to anticholinergic drugs, the most specific therapy is administration of cholinesterase inhibitors. Physostigmine is most commonly used because it enters the brain and antagonizes the central nervous system and peripheral autonomic effects.[77] Alternatively, because anticholinergic drugs result in an imbalance between sympathetic and parasympathetic activity with a predominance of the former, propranolol also may be effective in treating supraventricular tachyarrhythmias. Both physostigmine and propranolol may be hazardous in persons with depressed atrioventricular conduction[78] (Fig. 4–12).

Cholinomimetic Toxins and Drugs
(Table 4–7)

The most common type of cholinomimetic poisoning is that due to ingestion of organophosphate or carbamate insecticides resulting in excess cholinesterase inhibition.[79] In recent years, a type of iatrogenic poisoning has occurred as a result of using physostigmine in the treatment of overdoses of tricyclic antidepressant and other anticholinergic drugs.

The cardiovascular effects of organophosphates are unpredictable and often change over the time course of the poisoning. Early in the course, acetylcholine stimulates nicotinic receptors at sympathetic ganglia and causes tachycardia and mild hypertension. Later it stimulates muscarinic receptors or blocks ganglionic transmission by hyperpolarization, resulting in bradycardia and hy-

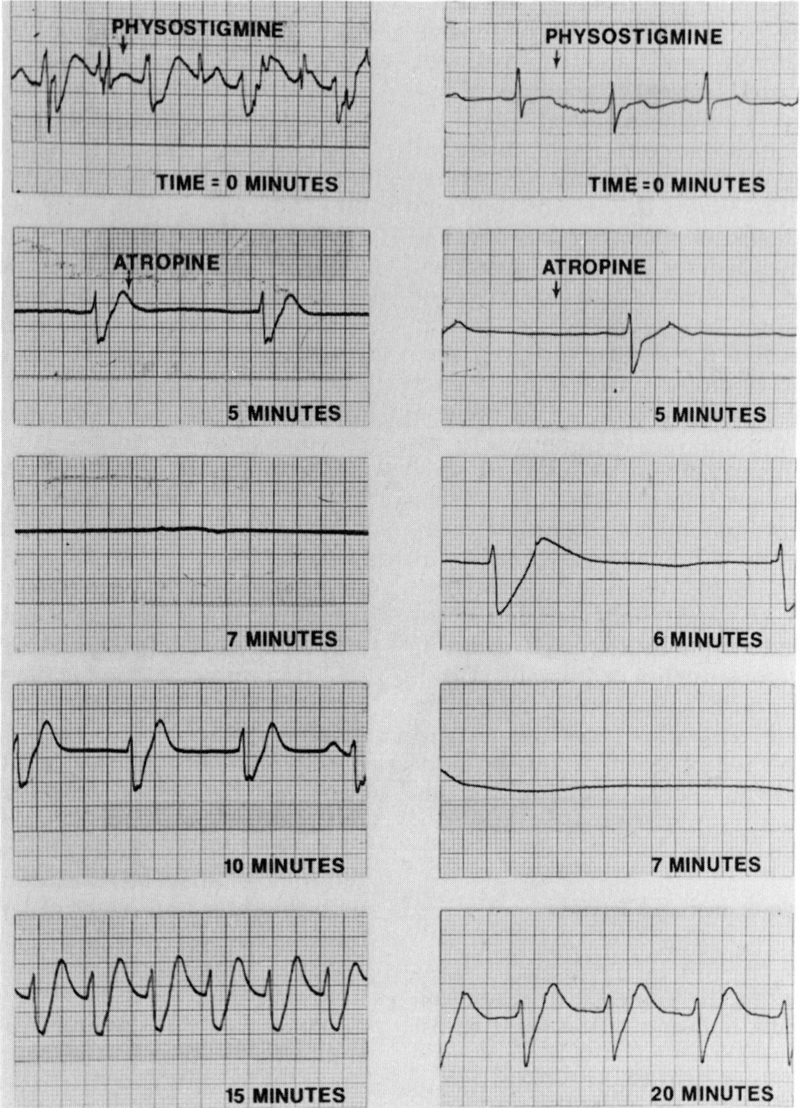

Figure 4–12. Case 1 (left panel) was a 32 year old man who had ingested 2300 mg of amitriptyline and who received physostigmine, 2 mg intravenously, for treatment of status epilepticus. Subsequently, junctional bradycardia developed that was unresponsive to atropine, and asystole occurred. Junctional rhythm was restored following treatment with epinephrine and bicarbonate. Sinus rhythm returned, the QRS narrowed over the next 12 hours, and the patient recovered fully.

Case 2 (right panel) was a 25 year old man who ingested 5000 mg of imipramine and 150 mg of propranolol. He received two doses of physostigmine, 2 mg intravenously, for recurrent motor seizures. After the second dose, sinus bradycardia developed that was unresponsive to atropine, and asystole occurred.[78] Following 10 minutes of closed chest cardiac massage and treatment with epinephrine and bicarbonate, sinus rhythm returned, although severe hypotension persisted. This patient's electrocardiogram and blood pressure eventually became normal but he died as a result of irreversible brain damage.

potension. The most common cardiac finding in organophosphate poisoning is sinus tachycardia.[79] However, in severe poisonings, advanced atrioventricular block, bradyarrhythmias with hypotension, and asystole may occur.[80]

Delayed ventricular tachycardia of the torsades de pointes type may occur for up to 5 days after acute intoxication with organophosphates.[80a] The mechanism is believed to be a persistent imbalance between sympathetic and parasympathetic influences on the heart, resulting in nonhomogenous repolarization (associated with a long Q-T interval)

Table 4–7. CARDIAC DISTURBANCES DUE TO CHOLINOMIMETIC DRUGS AND TOXINS

DRUGS	
Organophosphates	Pilocarpine
Carbamates	Neostigmine, pyridostigmine
Physostigmine	Nicotine
Bethanecol	
CARDIAC DISTURBANCES	
Sinus bradycardia	Ventricular tachycardia associated with Q-T interval prolongation†
Atrial or junctional or ventricular bradycardia	Hypotension
Atrioventricular block	Hypertension*
Sinus tachycardia*	Asystole
OTHER COMMON MANIFESTATIONS	
Pulmonary secretions and/or edema	Abdominal cramps
	Diarrhea
Small pupils	Fasciculations
Diaphoresis	Convulsions
Lacrimation	Muscle weakness and paralysis
Salivation	
Urinary frequency and/or incontinence	Respiratory failure

*May be seen in the early stages of cholinesterase inhibition and nicotine poisoning due to ganglionic stimulation.

†May be delayed up to several days after initial intoxication.

and a predisposition to ventricular arrhythmias. In patients with severe cardiac depression resulting from tricyclic antidepressant drugs, the use of physostigmine has resulted in loss of atrial activity, worsening of atrioventricular block, severe sinus or ventricular bradycardia, and/or asystole (Fig. 4–12).[78]

Bradyarrhythmias, if hemodynamically significant, can usually be effectively treated by administration of atropine. Atropine must compete with excess acetylcholine at the receptor site, and thus extremely large doses of atropine may be required. Doses should be increased until cholinergic signs such as salivation, diaphoresis, and bronchorrhea are reversed. When atropine is not effective, cardiac pacing is indicated. Sinus or atrial tachycardia causing hemodynamic compromise is a greater problem to treat because drugs such as propranolol that might slow the rate might also worsen bronchoconstriction or aggravate conduction disturbances later in the course of the overdose. Patients with clinical signs of cholinesterase inhibition or an abnormal electrocardiogram (including Q-T interval prolongation) should have continuous cardiac monitoring for the possibility of developing ventricular tachycardia. The ECG may remain abnormal for several days.[80a] Treatment of ventricular tachycardia is similar to that described for torsades de pointes previously, except that atropine also may be used to normalize autonomic influences on the heart. Pulmonary secretions (sometimes presenting as apparent acute pulmonary edema) or respiratory failure also may result in hypoxia and acidosis, which aggravate arrhythmias and hypotension; atropine is the treatment of choice for bronchorrhea. Pralidoxime (2-PAM) is often effective in reversing the neuromuscular blocking effects of organophosphates but has little effect on cardiovascular toxicity.

Membrane-Depressant Drugs and Toxins

(Tables 4–8, 4–9, and 4–10)

Type I Antiarrhythmic Drugs

Type IA, B, and C antiarrhythmic agents affect phase 0 (upstroke velocity of the action potential) and action potential durations to different degrees in different portions of the conduction system and in ventricular and atrial muscle. These differences will be reflected in varying effects on the electrocardiogram (Table 4–8).

Quinidine is the prototypical membrane-depressant drug. As discussed in the section on the mechanism of arrhythmogenesis, and in more detail in Chapter 95, quinidine and other type IA antiarrhythmic drugs (including procainamide and disopyramide) impede the fast sodium current across cardiac cell membranes and slow conduction, particularly in the His-Purkinje system. In toxic doses, slowed conduction is demonstrated by progressively marked QT prolongation, QRS widening, and/or atrioventricular block, with loss of atrial activity and slow ventricular rhythm (Fig. 4–13). Ventricular tachycardia and fibrillation may occur after therapeutic doses ("quinidine syncope"), as well as after overdose. Ventricular tachycardia in the presence of a long Q-T interval may be of the polymorphous ("torsades de pointes") type characterized by undulation of the QRS polarity about an isoelectric point (Fig. 4–14; see Fig. 4–4). The prolonged Q-T interval is believed to be caused by asynchronous repolarization of His-Purkinje fibers, which predisposes to ventricular arrhythmias, or possibly also by afterdepolarizations.

In addition to its electrophysiologic effects, quinidine in large doses depresses myocar-

Table 4–8. ELECTROPHYSIOLOGIC DIFFERENCES AMONG TYPE I ANTIARRHYTHMIC AGENTS

CLASS	CLASS NAME	EXAMPLES	DEPRESS PHASE 0 SODIUM CHANNEL BLOCKADE	PROLONG ACTION POTENTIAL DURATION	SYMPATHOLYTIC EFFECT	DEPRESS SLOW RESPONSE CALCIUM ENTRY BLOCKADE	DEPRESS PHASE 4 DEPOLARIZATION	PROLONGATION OF SURFACE ECG INTERVALS			
								PR	*QRS*	*QTc*	*JTc*
IA	Membrane anesthetics	quinidine procainamide disopyramide	2+	1+	0/+	0	1+	0/+	0/+	2+	2+
IB	Same	lidocaine tocainide mexiletine	2+	–	0	0	–	0	0	0	0
IC	Same	flecainide encainide propafenone	2+	0/–	0/+	0/+	1+	2+	2+	1+	0
II	Beta-blockers	propranolol acebutolol	0/+	0/–	2+	0	1+	0/+	0	0	0
III	—	bretylium amiodarone	1+	2+	1+	0	1+	1+	0	2+	2+
IV	Calcium blockers	verapamil diltiazem	0	1+	1+	2+	1+	0/+	0	0	0/+

Table 4–9. CARDIAC DISTURBANCES CAUSED BY MEMBRANE-DEPRESSANT DRUGS AND TOXINS

DRUGS	
quinidine	phenothiazines and related neuroleptics
procainamide	propranolol (and other membrane-depressant beta-blockers)*
disopyramide	
encainide	
flecainide	
tricyclic antidepressants	
CARDIAC EFFECTS AND DISTURBANCES	
QT interval prolongation†	Ventricular tachycardia (usually polymorphous)‡
Intraventricular conduction delay (QRS interval prolongation)	Ventricular fibrillation‡
Atrioventricular block	Asystole
Junctional or ventricular bradycardia	Hypotension
OTHER COMMON MANIFESTATIONS	
No syndromes about which one can generalize, although many agents in this group have anticholinergic effects.	

*Membrane depression seen with massive overdose; this is *not* a manifestation of beta-blockade.

†Among beta-blockers, only sotalol is reported to increase the QT interval. Flecainide and encainide usually do not increase the Q-T interval.

‡In the case of beta-blockers, usually occurs in association with bradyarrhythmia.

dial contractility and relaxes blood vessels, resulting in hypotension. In cases of massive overdose, this may produce shock. Disopyramide, and quinidine to a lesser extent, also has anticholinergic effects that may result in sinus tachycardia after a mild overdose. Similarly, overdoses of Type IC antiarrhythmic drugs—flecainide, encainide, and propafenone—may result in bradyarrhythmias, conduction delays, and depressed cardiac contractility with shock (see Chapter 97). These drugs may have a significant proarrhythmic action, causing ventricular tachycardia, even at therapeutic doses.[80b]

Therapeutic options for ventricular tachycardia due to quinidine or quinidine-like drugs include overdrive pacing, magnesium, lidocaine, phenytoin, isoproterenol, and bretylium. Isoproterenol increases the heart rate and shortens the Q-T interval and is recommended by some as the drug of choice, although the prospect of treating ventricular tachycardia with catecholamines is believed too hazardous by other clinicians. Treatment of conduction disturbances and hypotension is discussed in the section on tricyclic antidepressant toxicity.

Calcium Entry Blockers

The pathophysiology and management of calcium entry blocker poisoning are described in detail (with references) in Chapter 92. The primary electrophysiologic action of verapamil is to impede the calcium current responsible for depolarization of slow-response cardiac cells. Nifedipine acts preferentially on vascular smooth muscle, resulting in vasodilation. Diltiazem is similar to verapamil but produces less cardiac depression at therapeutic doses.

Serious toxicity can occur after therapeutic doses of calcium entry blockers in persons with presdisposing cardiac disease, and similar effects are seen in healthy people after an overdose. Verapamil- and diltiazem-induced depression of slow-response cardiac cells can result in sinus bradycardia or arrest and atrioventricular block, particularly in persons with underlying cardiac conduction disease. Inhibition of calcium entrance into the cell, which is necessary for muscular contraction, results in depression of myocardial contractility. This may cause worsening of

Table 4–10. TREATMENT OF CARDIOVASCULAR COMPLICATIONS OF MEMBRANE-DEPRESSANT DRUG POISONING

MANIFESTATION	TREATMENT
Arrhythmias	
Sinus tachycardia	None, esmolol or propranolol, physostigmine
Atrial tachycardia or fibrillation	Same as above plus verapamil, cardioversion
Ventricular premature beats and tachycardia	Magnesium, lidocaine, phenytoin, isoproterenol (with long Q-T only), bretylium Overdrive pacing
Bradyarrhythmias	Atropine Isoproterenol Pacemaker*
Hypotension	Fluids (hemodynamic monitoring advised in evidence of cardiac failure or myocardial depression) Treat bradyarrhythmias Dopamine, norepinephrine (low systemic vascular resistance) Dobutamine, isoproterenol (low cardiac output) Intra-aortic balloon pump or cardiopulmonary bypass (if intractable cardiogenic shock)

*May require higher than usual pacemaker voltage.

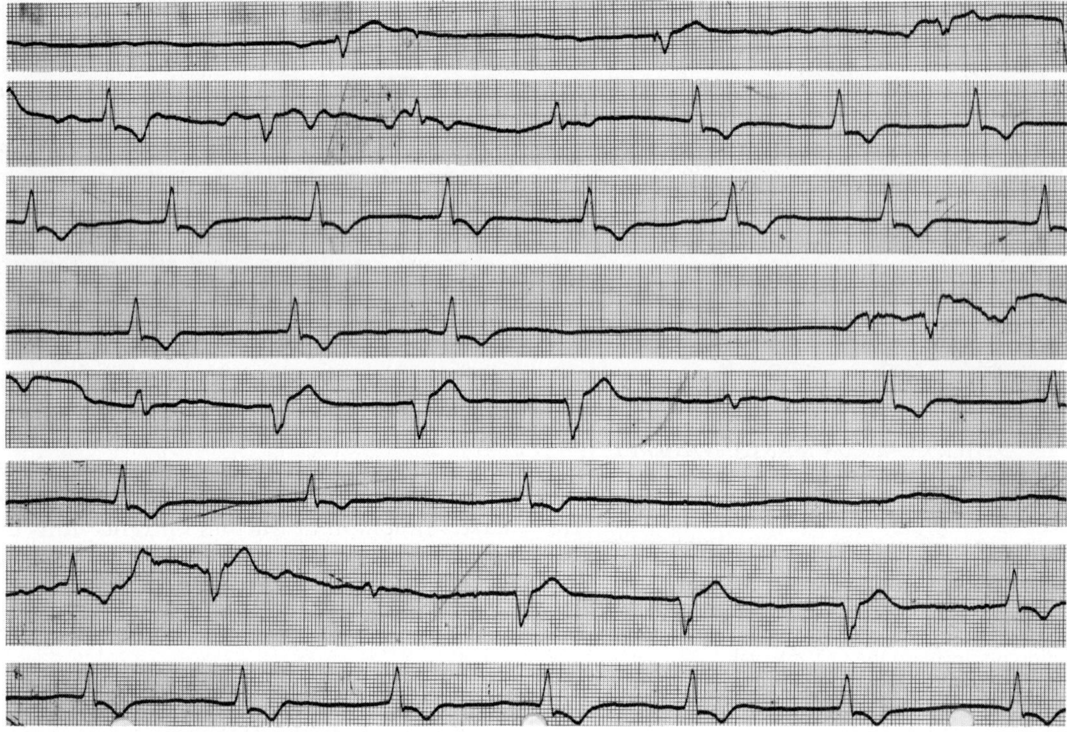

Figure 4–13. A 76 year old woman was admitted to the coronary care unit with syncopal spells. She had been taking digoxin and quinidine for congestive heart failure and ventricular arrhythmias. Serum levels of both these agents were in the toxic range (serum digoxin was 3.4 ng/ml and quinidine, 10 mg/ml). This continuously recorded V_1 rhythm strip demonstrates absence of atrial activity and prolonged pauses in QRS rhythm, which are terminated by different ventricular escape foci at different rates. Despite aggressive medical management, the patient died within 48 hours with electromechanical dissociation.

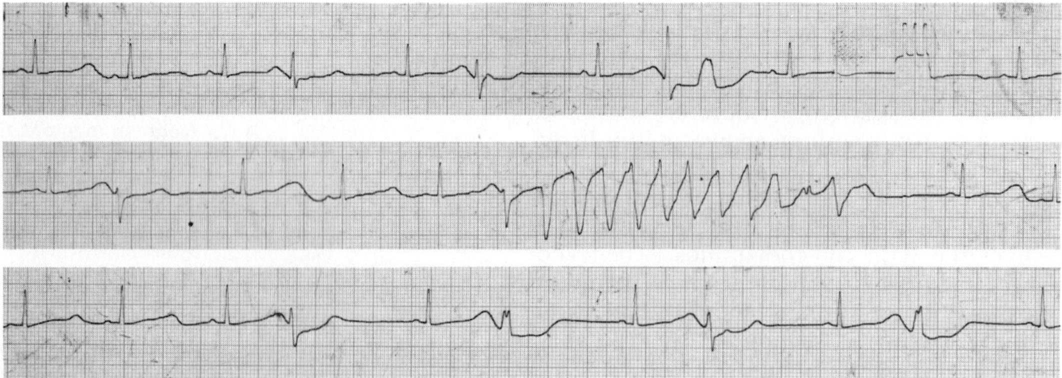

Figure 4–14. This 64 year old woman was begun on oral quinidine therapy for frequent premature ventricular beats associated with palpitations. These continuous lead 2 rhythm strips were recorded after the third 200-mg dose and show a markedly prolonged QT interval, frequent multiform ventricular ectopic beats, and a self-terminating burst of polymorphous ventricular tachycardia. The serum level of quinidine obtained after the recording of these tracings was 3.6 mg/ml. Quinidine was withdrawn, and oral procainamide substituted without further complications.

cardiac failure or hypotension or both, particularly in persons with underlying myocardial disease. In overdose, heart block, bradyarrhythmias, and hypotension may be expected. Nifedipine overdose usually results in hypotension without depressed cardiac conduction or contractility, although cardiac depression has occasionally been observed. Cardiac conduction and contractility are maintained because reflex sympathetic stimulation counterbalances the intrinsic myocardial depressant action.

In addition to supportive care, the use of calcium gluconate or calcium chloride is recommended, particularly for treatment of hypotension. It is noteworthy that calcium completely reverses the negative inotropic effects of calcium entry blockers and may partially reverse the electrophysiologic toxicity but appears to have no effect in reversing vasodilation.

Details on the efficacy and use of calcium in treatment of calcium entry blocker overdose are provided in Chapter 92.

Tricyclic Antidepressants and Antipsychotic Drugs

Tricyclic antidepressants account for more cardiac morbidity and mortality than any other class of drugs. Their mechanisms include a strong anticholinergic effect, inhibition of neuronal uptake of catecholamines, membrane depression, peripheral alpha-adrenergic blockade, and central nervous system–mediated inhibition of sympathetic reflexes. (For studies concerning mechanisms of toxicity, see reference 16.)

In mild and moderate cases of tricyclic antidepressant overdose, anticholinergic effects and increased circulating catecholamines result in supraventricular tachycardia, increased cardiac output, and normal or increased blood pressure.[83] In severe cases, impaired intracardiac conduction and depressed myocardial contractility predominate, and hypotension is observed.[84] Prolongation of the QRS duration is nearly universal in cases of serious tricyclic antidepressant toxicity. Bundle branch block, atrioventricular block, and slow ventricular rhythm and asystole may occur in the most severe poisonings (Fig. 4–15; see Figs. 4–5 and 4–12). Responsiveness to electrical stimulation is decreased so that pacing thresholds are often higher than normal; in extreme cases, the heart does not respond at all to pacing. Hypotension usually results from depressed cardiac output. Cardiac output may be reduced as a result of venous pooling with inadequate cardiac filling (associated with low pulmonary capillary wedge pressure), or in more severe poisoning to myocardial depression (with normal or high wedge pressure).[85]

Therapy for tricyclic antidepressant overdoses should be tailored to the particular cardiovascular disturbance. Sinus tachycardia and supraventricular arrhythmias, if associated wtih hemodynamic disturbances (either excessive hypertension or hypotension), can be controlled with physostigmine or propranolol. As noted, these drugs can depress cardiac conduction. They should be avoided, if possible, when membrane-depressant effects, manifest by the presence of a wide QRS interval, atrioventricular block, or the presence of a bradyarrhythmia, are present unless a temporary cardiac pacemaker is in place. Severe bradyarrhythmias and asystole have occurred after treatment with physostigmine[78] (see Fig. 4–12). Atropine also should be readily available to counteract the cholinergic effects of physostigmine.

Administration of either sodium bicarbonate or lactate or hyperventilation to correct acidemia and induce alkalemia reduces arrhythmias in animals and in humans[86, 87] (Fig. 4–15). The use of bicarbonate may be safer than hyperventilation because the hypocapnia due to the latter may lower the seizure threshold, and seizures are a common and serious complication of tricyclic antidepressant overdose. The mechanism of beneficial effects of alkali therapy is not proved, but most likely works by increasing extracellular sodium concentration, increasing extracellular pH and/or decreasing extracellular potassium concentration, all of which may improve membrane responsiveness and increases conduction velocity in fast-response (His-Purkinje) cells[87] (see Chapter 34).

After sodium bicarbonate, administration of lidocaine is the treatment of choice for ventricular arrhythmias. Phenytoin therapy has been reported in an uncontrolled study to improve intraventricular conduction,[88] but superior antiarrhythmic efficacy compared with lidocaine, or a more favorable outcome in patients treated with phenytoin, is unproved. Animal studies have shown no ben-

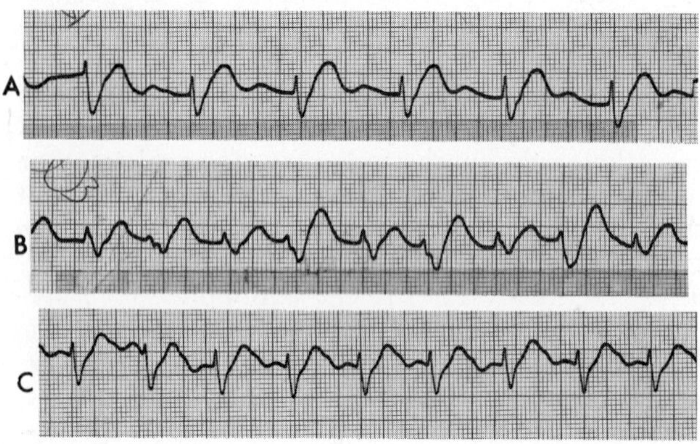

Figure 4–15. Lead II electrocardiograms recorded in a 40 year old woman who ingested 6 grams of amitriptyline (Elavil). The top strip *(A)*, recorded on admission, shows a wide QRS rhythm and markedly prolonged QTU interval; atrial activity is not clearly discernible. Strips *B* and *C* were recorded 30 and 60 minutes, respectively, after intravenous administration of 44 mEq of $NaHCO_3$. In *B*, the QRS rate has increased, and alternation of QRS complexes is present. The QT interval remains prolonged, but the U wave is less prominent, and the QRS duration of alternate complexes has narrowed. Atrial activity is still not readily seen. In *C*, P waves precede each QRS complex, and QRS duration remains prolonged, but the QT interval has shortened. This series of tracings suggests a supraventricular origin of the rhythm in strips *A* and *B*.

efit of phenytoin pretreatment in reducing cardiac toxicity from amitriptyline.[88a] Type IA or IC antiarrhythmic drugs (quinidine, procainamide, disopyramide, encainide, flecainide), which have additive membrane-depressant effects, should be avoided. Because of the possible role of excess catecholamine stimulation in causing ventricular arrhythmias, propranolol has been recommended,[89] but, as discussed earlier, may be hazardous in patients with bradycardia or atrioventricular block. Overdrive pacing has been used successfully to treat ventricular tachycardia caused by quinidine or long QT syndrome and would be expected to be useful in treating tricyclic antidepressant overdose as well.[90] Bretylium should be considered for refractory ventricular tachycardia or fibrillation, although it also might worsen the hypotension.

Because both tachycardia and intraventricular conduction delay are characteristic and ventricular tachycardia is not uncommon, the diagnostic problem of a wide complex tachycardia of uncertain origin is common. Diagnosis and treatment of this arrhythmia have been discussed in detail in an earlier section of this chapter.

Intracardiac pacing is indicated in patients with high-grade atrioventricular block. If intraventricular conduction is worsening (that is, if the QRS complex is widening) early in the clinical course, when the extent of ultimate myocardial depression is not yet known, prophylactic pacing is advised because of the chance of sudden deterioration. The presence of sinus or ventricular bradycardia rather than the usual supraventricular tachycardia indicates severe toxicity and warrants pacing as well. Bradyarrhythmias associated with reduced cardiac output and hypotension can be treated with isoproterenol until intracardiac pacing can be instituted.

Hypotension is common after a tricyclic antidepressant overdose. In many patients, hypotension can be managed successfully with fluids. If pressors are required, alpha-adrenergic agonists such as norepinephrine or dopamine are preferred. In the presence of selective alpha-blockade due to tricyclic antidepressants, the predominant effects of mixed alpha- and beta-agonists like epinephrine may be beta-mediated vasodilation and worsening of hypotension. Dobutamine may prove to be useful in managing myocardial depression with normal or increased vascular resistance. Profound cardiogenic shock resulting from tricyclic antidepressant overdose is often unresponsive to medical treatment and has a poor prognosis. In these cases, extracorporeal circulatory aids such as cardiopulmonary bypass or intra-aortic balloon pumping may be the only means of sustaining life until the body can eliminate the drug. The successful use of intra-aortic balloon pumping has been reported for drug intoxication associated with intractable shock.[91]

Phenothiazines and other antipsychotic drugs have pharmacologic properties similar to those of tricyclic antidepressants, but arrhythmias do not tend to be as difficult to control, and cardiogenic shock is uncommon. Hypotension caused by chlorpromazine is more likely due to peripheral alpha-adrenergic blockade and usually responds well to posture and intravenous fluids. Differences between tricyclic antidepressants and antipsychotic drugs probably reflect different potencies with respect to membrane actions and different concentrations in cardiac tissue. The tricyclic antidepressants and their potentially toxic demethylated and hydroxylated metabolites are concentrated in the myocardium to a much greater extent than are the phenothiazines.[92]

Miscellaneous Drugs and Toxins
(Table 4–11)

Digitalis

Mortality and major morbidity from digitalis overdose result from arrhythmias, heart block, and hyperkalemia.[93] Digitalis inhibits the sodium-potassium ATPase-dependent pump located on the cell membrane. In the therapeutic situation, this results in greater calcium movement into the cell, which is believed to account for increased myocardial contractility. After an overdose, disruption of sodium and potassium movement across membranes results in depressed conduction velocity, as described for membrane-depressant drugs. In addition, automaticity of previously nonautomatic tissue is enhanced, which is related to increased rate of diastolic depolarization and possibly to spontaneous after-depolarizations ("triggered" rhythms).[3] Digitalis also may increase sympathetic and parasympathetic neural activity. Sympathetic stimulation enhances automaticity and excitability, while parasympathetic stimulation further decreases conduction velocity. Thus, an overdose with digitalis is characterized by arrhythmias demonstrating both increased automaticity and depressed intracardiac conduction.

Tachyarrhythmias from digitalis intoxication typically include ectopic atrial tachycardia with atrioventricular block, atrioventricular junctional tachycardia, and ventricular tachycardia or fibrillation (Figs. 4–16 and 4–17). Ventricular arrhythmias are reported to occur more commonly in persons with underlying heart disease. Bradyarrhythmias include sinus bradycardia, sinoatrial block, second degree and complete atrioventricular block, atrial fibrillation or flutter with slow ventricular response, idioventricular rhythm, and asystole (Fig. 4–18). Severe hyperkalemia due to inhibition of sodium-potassium exchange in skeletal muscle can contribute to atrioventricular block and depressed myocardial excitability (Fig. 4–19).

Therapy for digitalis-induced arrhythmias is directed at the specific arrhythmia and normalization of serum potassium. Supraventricular arrhythmias often do not require specific treatment because the ventricular response is reasonably slow. If necessary, propranolol may be used to treat atrial tachycardia. Patients who have been taking diuretics chronically may be depleted of potassium, and supraventricular tachyarrhythmias may respond to potassium supplementation. However, potassium may depress atrioventricular conduction and, as described earlier, life-threatening hyperkalemia may be present.

The definitive treatment for life-threatening ventricular arrhythmia, heart block, or hyperkalemia is administration of digoxin-specific antibodies.[94] The antibodies bind free digoxin and may completely reverse digitalis toxicity within 15 to 30 minutes. Quinidine-like membrane-depressant drugs should be avoided. Phenytoin has been reported to be particularly effective in treating arrhythmias, as it may enhance atrioventricular conduction while depressing automaticity, but its effect is inconstant and unpredictable.[95] Lidocaine, propranolol, and esmolol also have been used to treat ventricular arrhythmias; the beta-blockers may also worsen conduction disturbances.

Sinus bradycardia and atrioventricular conduction block, in light of the vagal actions of digitalis, may respond to atropine. Isoproterenol is usually effective in treating bradyarrhythmias refractory to atropine but can result in increased ventricular excitability. If digoxin antibodies are not readily available, cardiac pacing is indicated in patients with complete atrioventricular block or second degree heart block, or when bradyarrhythmias result in hemodynamic compromise. Correction of hyperkalemia may in itself reverse atrioventricular block.

Because the course of toxicity after ingestion of most digitalis preparations lasts for several days, an attempt to accelerate removal of digitalis from the body should be considered. Techniques include repeated doses of cholestyramine or activated charcoal to interrupt enterohepatic recycling or hemoperfusion for digoxin, digitoxin, or both.[96, 97]

Opiates

Although toxicity from acute opiate overdose is primarily related to respiratory depression, opiates may have significant car-

Table 4–11. CARDIOVASCULAR DISTURBANCES—MISCELLANEOUS DRUGS AND TOXINS

DRUG/TOXIN	MECHANISMS OF ACTION	CARDIOVASCULAR DISTURBANCES	OTHER COMMON MANIFESTATIONS
Digitalis (including foxglove, oleander, lily of the valley)	Inhibits Na^+-K^+ ATPase-dependent pump, increases automaticity, after-depolarizations, decreases atrioventricular conduction velocity, increases vagal and ? sympathetic activity	Atrial tachycardia with atrioventricular block Junctional tachycardia Ventricular ectopy, tachycardia, fibrillation Sinus bradycardia* Sinoatrial block* High-grade atrioventricular block Slow ventricular response to atrial fibrillation or flutter Asystole	Nausea, vomiting Hypokalemia (with diuretic use) Hyperkalemia (severe intoxication)
Opiates	Central nervous system–mediated increase in parasympathetic and decrease in sympathetic tone	Bradycardia Atrial fibrillation Hypotension	Miosis Respiratory depression Coma Pulmonary edema
Lithium	Disturbed cardiac potassium metabolism	Sinus bradycardia ST-T abnormalities Ventricular ectopy	Tremor, ataxia Confusion, stupor, coma Neuromuscular irritability, convulsions Azotemia
Ergot derivatives	Constriction of vascular smooth muscle	Cardiac ischemia (angina, coronary spasm with possible myocardial infarction) Peripheral vasospasm Gangrene	Headache (reason for excessive use of ergots)
Carbon monoxide, hydrogen sulfide	Binds to hemoglobin, preferentially to oxygen, causing chemical asphyxia	Cardiac ischemia (electrocardiographic abnormalities, myocardial infarction) Hypotension	Headache Coma Metabolic acidosis (with normal P_{O_2}) Pulmonary edema
Cyanide	Binds to cytochrome oxidase, causing chemical asphyxia	Hypertension	
Arsenic	Interferes with cellular respiration	Cardiac ischemia Myocarditis ST-T abnormalities QT prolongation Polymorphous ventricular tachycardia Hypotension	Abdominal pain Vomiting, diarrhea Hepatitis Skin rash Renal failure Peripheral neuropathy (late)
Arsine	Hemolysis, anemia	Cardiac ischemia Peaked T waves Pulmonary edema	Chills, fever Hyperkalemia Hemoglobinuria Renal failure
Phosphorus	"Protoplasmic poison"	ST-T abnormalities QT prolongation Ventricular tachycardia/fibrillation Asystole Hypotension	Corrosive burns of skin and gastrointestinal tract Severe gastroenteritis "Smoking" luminescent vomitus and stool
Iron	Cellular membrane injury	ST-T wave abnormalities Hypovolemia Myocardial necrosis Hypotension	Nausea, vomiting, diarrhea Gastrointestinal bleeding Hyperglycemia Leukocytosis Metabolic acidosis Hepatic necrosis

Table 4–11. CARDIOVASCULAR DISTURBANCES—MISCELLANEOUS DRUGS AND TOXINS *Continued*

DRUG/TOXIN	MECHANISMS OF ACTION	CARDIOVASCULAR DISTURBANCES	OTHER COMMON MANIFESTATIONS
Fluoride	Hypocalcemia Hyperkalemia	Q-T interval prolongation Peaked T waves Ventricular fibrillation Sudden death	Nausea, vomiting, diarrhea Tetany, hyperreflexia Respiratory depression
Organic mercury (chronic)		ST-T abnormalities QT prolongation	Sore mouth, metallic taste, vomiting, diarrhea, tremor, dysarthria, ataxia
Lead		Chest pain Cardiac failure ST-T abnormalities Hypertension	Anorexia Abdominal pain, constipation Anemia Peripheral neuropathy Encephalopathy
Scorpion and spider venom	? Massive catecholamine release; myocarditis	Hypertension Tachycardia ST-T abnormalities QT prolongation Atrial and ventricular arrhythmias Pulmonary edema Hypotension	Pain at site of envenomation Anxiety Diaphoresis, fasciculations and/or muscle spasm Abdominal pain and rigidity† Paresthesias, convulsions‡
Ciguatera fish poisoning	Increased membrane sodium permeability	Bradycardia Hypotension	Paresthesias Abdominal pain, nausea, vomiting, diarrhea Respiratory depression
Emetine (syrup of ipecac)	Inhibition of protein synthesis Disrupts oxidative phosphorylation	ST wave abnormalities Q-T interval prolongation Cardiomyopathy (biventricular cardiac failure) Ventricular arrhythmias	Recurrent vomiting Cachexia Skeletal myopathy
Colchicine	Cellular microtubular toxin	Myocardial injury S-T segment abnormalities Hypovolemia Hypotension Pulmonary edema Sudden death	Nausea, vomiting, abdominal pain Respiratory failure Pancytopenia, leukopenia Coagulopathy Myopathy Polyneuropathy

*Occurrence variable depending on underlying autonomic nervous activity.
†Scorpion (poisonous species).
‡Black widow spider.

diac and vascular effects. They generally have little effect on the myocardium, although norpropoxyphene, a major metabolite of propoxyphene, may be cardiotoxic.[98] Central nervous system effects of narcotics result in increased vagal activity. Narcotics dilate peripheral veins and arterioles, presumably through a central nervous system–mediated effect on sympathetic tone. Consequently, hypotension and relative bradycardia are common. Arrhythmias have been observed in about 4 per cent of patients, most commonly atrial fibrillation.[99, 100] Prolongation of the QT interval and conduction disturbances have been described in heroin users, but the role of the narcotic per se in causing these disturbances has not been proved.[99, 101] Quinidine and procaine, as well as other local anesthetics, commonly adulterate heroin sold on the street and may themselves contribute to myocardial depression or even cardiac arrest.

Pulmonary edema is a common and serious complication of narcotic overdose and is noncardiogenic in origin.[102] Although pulmonary edema usually occurs after injection of narcotics, it may not become evident until naloxone has been administered. It is most likely that sudden reversal of narcotic-induced venodilation and venous pooling com-

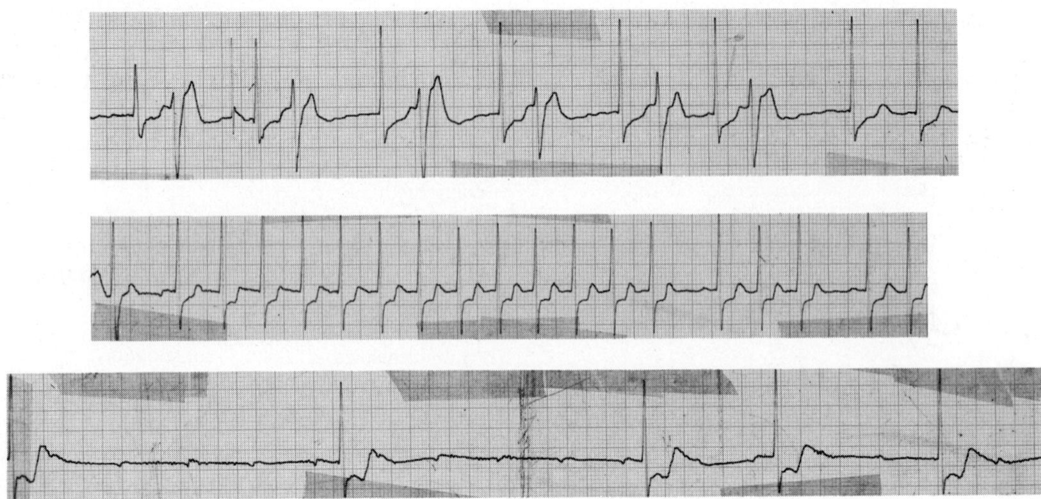

Figure 4–16. Three lead 2 rhythm strips were recorded over a period of several hours in a 30 year old patient who intentionally ingested 24.8 mg of digoxin. The top strip shows atrial fibrillation and R-on-T ventricular bigeminy. The middle strip shows a run of atrial tachycardia that terminates spontaneously to sinus rhythm and resumes immediately. The bottom strip illustrates high-degree atrioventricular block that, because of the morphology of the QRS complexes, is considered to be originating in the atrioventricular node or the His bundle. Because these rhythms all occurred and recurred within short periods of time, treatment was difficult and consisted only of transvenous cardiac pacing for bradyarrhythmias. All bradyarrhythmias disappeared by 22 hours, and all arrhythmias by 1 week.

bined with pulmonary capillary injury to the extent that fluid enters the lungs at relatively low cardiac filling pressures account for naloxone-induced pulmonary edema. Cases of recurrent hypotension and pulmonary edema, possibly due to coexistent cardiomyopathy, also have been reported.[103, 104]

Therapy for opiate overdose in general includes administration of naloxone (as described in Chapter 38). Usually, no specific therapy for arrhythmias is necessary. Naloxone has been reported to convert coarse atrial fibrillation to fine atrial fibrillation with a faster ventricular response rate than to normal sinus rhythm.[100] If atrial fibrillation with rapid ventricular response rate persists, digitalis, verapamil, or propranolol is indicated to slow the rate. The use of intermittent positive expiratory pressure is beneficial in the treatment of pulmonary edema, as discussed previously.

Lithium

Cardiac toxicity of lithium overdose has not been prominent, and no deaths due primarily to cardiovascular complications have been reported.[105, 106] Administration of lithium in usual therapeutic doses produces flattening or inversion of the T wave in nearly all patients. Sinus node disturbances, manifested by sinus bradycardia or sinoatrial block sometimes associated with ventricular ectopy, and junctional or ventricular escape rhythms have been reported in patients with lithium intoxication and during chronic therapy. Ventricular tachyarrhythmias in association with lithium therapy have been re-

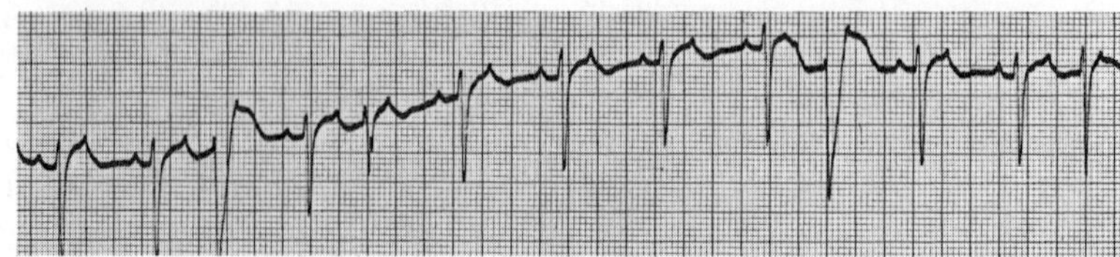

Figure 4–17. This 69 year old man was admitted to the hospital with acute congestive heart failure 7 weeks after having suffered an anterior wall myocardial infarction. This MCL1 rhythm strip was recorded after administration of 1.5 mg of intravenous digoxin over an 18-hour period. The atrial rate is somewhat irregular at about 150/minute. Periods of atrioventricular nodal Wenckebach block are present, with the second QRS complex of the period conducted aberrantly. Episodes of 2:1 atrioventricular block are also present. The serum digoxin level at this time was 4 ng/ml. The rhythm was restored to sinus after withdrawal of digoxin.

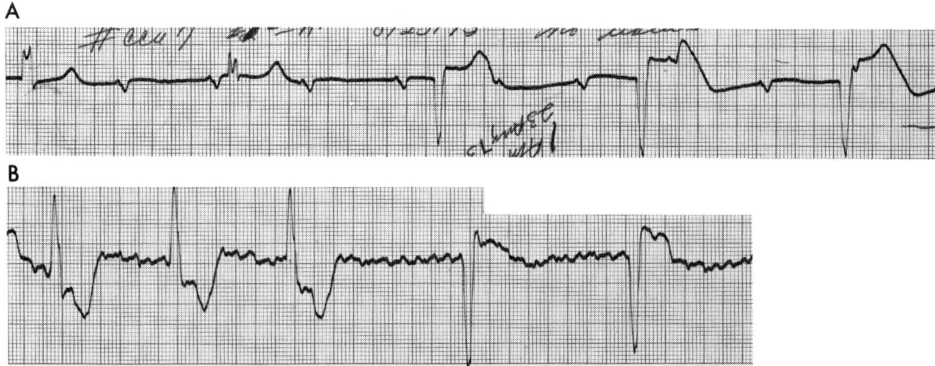

Figure 4–18. These two MCL1 rhythm strips depict examples of atrioventricular block in the setting of digitalis toxicity. In *A*, sinus rhythm and complete atrioventricular block are present. The QRS complexes are of two types: the first two have a right bundle branch block pattern and the last three have a left bundle branch block pattern; they occur at two different rates. The long duration of the QRS complexes as well as their very slow rate suggests that the origin of these escape beats is in the distal His-Purkinje system. In this situation, atropine may not result in improved atrioventricular conduction, and temporary cardiac pacing is often required.

In *B*, the atrial rhythm is fibrillation. High-grade atrioventricular block is present, as evidenced by the slow ventricular response. The QRS complexes have two morphologies: right and left bundle branch block patterns. The first three complexes occur at a near-regular rate, suggesting a ventricular escape focus. The last two complexes occur at a slower escape interval and rate, suggesting instability of the origin of the first three complexes and emergence of a yet more distal pacemaker. Again, atropine may not be of benefit in this situation, and cardiac pacing may be required.

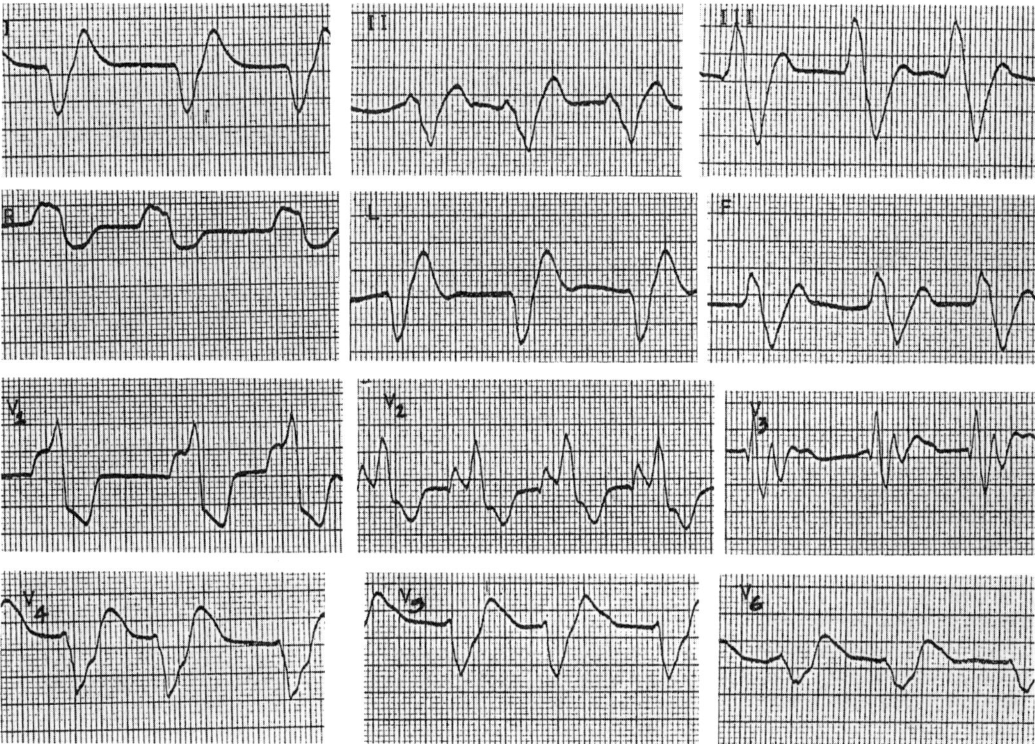

Figure 4–19. This 68 year old man was admitted to the hospital in moribund condition. He had long-standing congestive heart failure and was being treated with oral digoxin and diuretics. His serum potassium level on admission was 10.0 mEq/L, and his serum digoxin level was 5.2 ng/ml. He died shortly after this 12-lead electrocardiogram was obtained, with electromechanical dissociation. The electrocardiogram shows absence of discernible atrial activity and an irregular, wide, complex QRS rhythm having a right bundle branch block configuration. The markedly increased QRS duration suggests hyperkalemia, which in this patient may have been due in part to digitalis toxicity.

ported and are uncommon. Hypotension may complicate lithium overdose, but this appears to be related to dehydration or pulmonary complications in the course of prolonged coma rather than caused by direct cardiovascular toxicity. A mechanism for the cardiac effects of lithium has been suggested by animal studies. Lithium enters myocardial cells and displaces intracellular cations, predominantly potassium. Lithium then leaves the cell more slowly than does potassium and thereby disturbs the usual transmembrane ionic currents.

Treatment is directed toward the specific arrhythmia, as described in Table 4–1, and toward acceleration of lithium elimination, as discussed in Chapter 35.

Ergot Derivatives

Ergotamine and other ergot derivatives are widely used in the treatment of migraine headache and have resulted in significant cardiac and vascular toxicity. The basic action of ergot drugs is constriction of vascular smooth muscle (both alpha-adrenergic agonist and nonadrenergic effects), although many of the drugs also posess alpha-adrenergic receptor blocking activity.[107] Intense constriction of peripheral arteries, with resultant coolness, pallor, or cyanosis of the extremity, sometimes progressing to gangrene, is a typical manifestation of ergotism. There is intermittent claudication initially, and ischemic rest pain with progression of vasospasm. Hypertension is uncommon. In addition, ergot derivatives have been reported to worsen angina or cause myocardial infarction, presumably owing to coronary vasoconstriction in persons with underlying heart disease.[108, 109] Intravenous administration of ergonovine has been used diagnostically during cardiac catheterization to provoke coronary vasospasm.[110] We recently treated a patient who took excessive quantities of ergotamine tablets for severe migraine headaches; the patient had chest pain and diffuse ST segment elevation suggesting coronary vasospasm (Fig. 4–20).

Amphetamine-like drugs also can produce vascular spasm similar to that produced by ergot derivatives. In particular, 4-bromo-2,5-dimethoxyamphetamine injection has produced severe vascular insufficiency,[109a] and in one case (unpublished) resulted in bilateral lower extremity amputation.

Therapy for ergot-induced vasospasm includes anticoagulation with heparin, the use of direct vasodilators such as sodium nitroprusside for peripheral vasospasm,[111, 112] nitroglycerin for coronary vasospasm, and alpha-adrenergic blockers. Rapid dilation of vessels in an intensely vasoconstricted patient will result in relative hypovolemia and hypotension, so fluid replacement must be anticipated. If a specific vessel is affected, vasoconstrictors should be infused intra-arterially into that vessel so that maximal local vasodilation can be achieved without effecting excessive systemic hypotension. Nifedipine or other calcium channel blockers may also prove useful in treating ergot-induced coronary vasospasm. Other treatments with varying results have included anticoagulants, epidural anesthesia, low molecular weight dextran, hyperbaric oxygen, and surgical sympathectomy.

Chemical Asphyxiants

Carbon monoxide, hydrogen sulfide, and cyanide inhibit oxygen transport to or utilization of oxygen within tissues, resulting in tissue hypoxia. The usual presentation in severe cases of poisoning is coma or metabolic acidosis or both. Tachypnea (with evidence of respiratory alkalosis), tachycardia, and hypotension are common, although carbon monoxide poisoning in particular can be associated wtih hypertension.[113] Electrocardiographic changes, including T wave flattening or inversion, ST segment depression or elevation, and conduction disturbances, are frequently observed, and myocardial necrosis or infarction may occur.[114–117] Occasionally, premature ventricular contractions and atrial fibrillation are seen. Pulmonary edema may complicate acute carbon monoxide poisoning, and noncardiogenic versus cardiogenic edema resulting from myocardial damage must be differentiated. Even mild exposure to carbon monoxide can have significant effects in persons with underlying vascular disease. With carboxyhemoglobin concentrations as low as 3 per cent, the duration of exercise to the onset of chest pain in persons with angina pectoris, or leg pain in persons with intermittent claudication, is significantly reduced.[118] Therapy is directed toward improving tissue oxygenation, as described in other chapters. Of note is that electrocardiographic abnormalities after car-

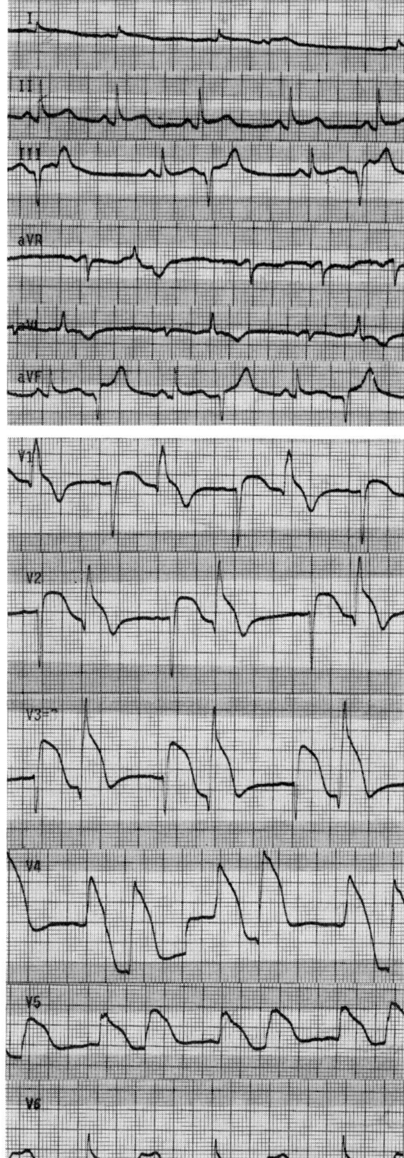

Figure 4–20. This 50 year old man was taking ergotamine for cluster headaches. When the headaches worsened, he ingested up to 10 mg/hr, developed severe substernal chest pain, and had an episode of syncope. This 12-lead electrocardiogram was recorded on admission to the coronary care unit. The rhythm is sinus with ventricular bigeminy; diffuse ST segment elevation is present, consistent with coronary artery spasm. Following large oral and intravenous doses of nitrates, chest pain and ST segment elevation resolved, but recurrent episodes of pain were associated with return of ST elevation, ventricular ectopy, and bursts of ventricular tachycardia. Myocardial infarction was not documented. Selective coronary arteriography documented coronary spasm during a spontaneous attack of chest pain. Pain and ST segment elevation resolved over 2 weeks coincidentally with oral nifedipine therapy.

bon monoxide poisoning may persist for days or even weeks after treatment, possibly due to focal myocardial injury.[113, 115] Mitral valve prolapse related to papillary muscle necrosis from carbon monoxide has been suggested on the basis of an unexpectedly higher incidence of prolapse found by echocardiography in one small series.[119]

Arsenic and Other Metals

Acute arsenic poisoning, by interfering with cellular respiration, may produce an electrocardiographic picture of myocardial ischemia and may be associated wtih focal myocardial hemorrhage,[120] although in patients who recover there are no cardiac symptoms. Acute and chronic arsenic poisoning can be associated with T wave changes and QT prolongation and with ventricular tachycardia and fibrillation.[121, 122] Recently, a patient with the torsades de pointes type of polymorphous ventricular tachycardia was reported.[122] Arsine gas, by causing massive hemolysis and severe anemia, also results in electrocardiographic abnormalities, most commonly peaked T waves (possibly related to hyperkalemia), but also there is evidence of myocardial ischemia (due to severe anemia and possibly myocardial effects of arsine).[123] Death from arsine exposure in patients who reach the hospital is often due to cardiac failure; pathology shows myocardial degeneration. Treatment should include correction of hyperkalemia, transfusion, and therapy of cardiac failure.

Elemental phosphorus and organic mercury poisonings have been associated with ST-T wave abnormalities, QT prolongation, and various arrhythmias (including ventricular tachycardia).[124–126] After elemental phosphorus ingestion, shock resulting from depressed myocardial contractility and abnormally low systemic vascular resistance occurs and is often difficult to treat.[125] Death in the early phase of phosphorus poisoning is due to shock, ventricular fibrillation, or asystole.

Although uncommon, chronic lead poisoning may be associated with myocarditis characterized by chest pain ("angina pectoris saturnina"), tachycardia, ventricular gallop, pulmonary congestion, hypertension, ST-T abnormalities, and premature ventricular contractions on the electrocardiogram. Autopsy of children dying from lead encephalopathy may show chronic myocarditis.[127] Clinical features usually subside after treatment with the chelating agent ethylenediaminetetra-acetic acid (EDTA).

Acute severe iron (and other heavy metal) poisoning causes shock owing to vasodilation and hypovolemia, the latter resulting from vascular damage and fluid loss. Myocardial injury and dysfunction may also contribute.[127a] Electrocardiographic abnormalities, including T wave inversion, may be present.[128]

Scorpions, Spiders, and Hymenoptera

Patients with poisonous scorpion stings typically show anxiety, profuse diaphoresis, and hypertension. Myocarditis, characterized by tachycardia, conduction abnormalities, ST-T abnormalities, including tall peaked T waves, QT prolongation, and atrial and ventricular arrhythmias, may be evident.[129] In severe poisoning, pulmonary edema, hypotension, and electrocardiographic changes suggesting myocardial infarction occur. Death is due to congestive heart failure or shock or both; sudden deaths presumably due to arrhythmias are also reported. The clinical and myocardial histologic manifestations of scorpion sting resemble those of massive catecholamine infusion, and urinary catecholamine excretion has been noted to be increased in scorpion sting victims. Although there is little published experience in this regard, the use of alpha- and beta-adrenergic blocking drugs for treatment of hypertension and arrhythmias would be logical. Treatment of cardiac failure and shock is supportive.

Labile blood pressure, atrial arrhythmias, and cardiovascular collapse are occasionally observed in patients after black widow spider bites.[130] Increased urinary catecholamine metabolite excretion also has suggested a role of excess catecholamines in this syndrome, and adrenergic blockers may be useful in management.

Hymenoptera (bees and wasps) stings are well known to cause anaphylaxis, manifested by hypotension, cyanosis, bronchospasm, and collapse in allergic patients. Occasionally, chest pain and myocardial infarction, probably resulting from profound hypotension, occur as well.[131]

References

1. Shubin H, Weil MH: The mechanism of shock following suicidal doses of barbiturate, narcotics and tranquilizing drugs, with observations on the effects of treatment. Am J Med *38*:853, 1965.
2. Singer DH, Baumgarten CM, Ten Eick RE: Cellular electrophysiology of ventricular and other dysrhythmias: Studies on diseased and ischemic heart. Progr Cardiovasc Dis *24*:97, 1981.
3. Rosen M: The links between basic and clinical cardiac electrophysiology. Circulation *77*:251–263, 1988.
4. Wit AL, Hoffman BF, Rosen MR: Electrophysiology and pharmacology of cardiac arrhythmias. IX. Cardiac electrophysiologic effects of beta-adrenergic stimulation and blockade. Am Heart J *90*:521, 665, 795, 1975.
5. Vargas G, Akhtar M, Damato AN: Electrophysiologic effects of isoproterenol on cardiac conduction system in man. Am Heart J *90*:25, 1975.
6. Martin P: The influence of the parasympathetic nervous system on atrioventricular conduction. Circ Res *41*:593, 1977.
7. Kolman BS, Verrier RL, Lown B: The effect of vagus nerve stimulation upon vulnerability of the canine ventricle. Role of sympathetic-parasympathetic interactions. Circulation *52*:578, 1975.
8. Coumel P, Leclercq JF, Attuel P, Lavallee JP, Flammang D: Autonomic influences in the genesis of atrial arrhythmias: Atrial fibrillation of vagal origin. *In* Narula OS (ed): Cardiac Arrhythmias: Electro-

physiology, Diagnosis, and Management. Williams & Wilkins, Baltimore, 1979, p 243.

8a. Tzivoni D, Banai S, Schuger C, et al: Treatment of torsade de pointes with magnesium sulfate. Circulation *77*:392–397, 1988.

9. Gay RJ, Brown DF: Pacemaker failure due to procainamide toxicity. Am J Cardiol *34*:728, 1974.

10. Staub NC: The pathogenesis of pulmonary edema. Progr Cardiovasc Dis *23*:53, 1980.

11. Fein A, Grossman RF, Jones JG, et al: The value of edema fluid protein measurement in patients with pulmonary edema. Am J Med *67*:32, 1979.

12. Glauser FL, Smith WR, Caldwell A, et al: Ethchlorvynol (Placidyl)-induced pulmonary edema. Ann Intern Med *84*:46, 1976.

13. Hall JG, Morris B, Woolley G: Intrinsic rhythmic propulsion of lymph in the unanaesthetized sheep. J Physiol (Lond) *180*:336, 1965.

14. Siegel JH: The myocardial contractile state and its role in the response to anesthesia and surgery. Anesthesiology *30*:519, 1969.

15. Shubin H, Weil MH: Shock associated with barbiturate intoxication. JAMA *215*:263, 1971.

16. Benowitz NL, Rosenberg J, Becker CE: Cardiopulmonary catastrophes in drug-overdosed patients. Med Clin North Am *63*:267, 1979.

17. Espelin DC, Done AK: Amphetamine poisoning. N Engl J Med *278*:1361, 1968.

18. Kalant A, Kalant OJ: Death in amphetamine users: Causes and rates. Can Med Assoc J *112*:299, 1975.

19. Benchimol A, Bartall H, Desser KB: Accelerated ventricular rhythm and cocaine abuse. Ann Intern Med *88*:519, 1978.

19a. Buchanan JF, Brown CR: "Designer drugs." A problem in clinical toxicology. Med Toxicol *3*:1–17, 1988.

20. Allred RJ, Ewer S: Fatal pulmonary edema following intravenous "freebase" cocaine use. Ann Emerg Med *10*:441, 1981.

21. Mangiardi JR, Daras M, Geller ME, et al: Cocaine-related intracranial hemorrhage. Report of nine cases and review. Acta Neurol Scand *77*:177–180, 1988.

22. Roth D, Alarcón MD, Fernandez MD, et al: Acute rhabdomyolysis associated with cocaine intoxication. N Engl J Med *319*:673–677, 1988.

23. Kendrick WC, Hull AR, Knochel JP: Rhabdomyolysis and shock after intravenous amphetamine administration. Ann Intern Med *86*:381, 1977.

24. Simpson DL, Rumack BH: Methylenedioxyamphetamine: Clinical description of overdose, death, and review of pharmacology. Arch Intern Med *141*:1507, 1981.

25. Catravas JD, Waters IW: Acute cocaine intoxication in the conscious dog: Studies on the mechanism of lethality. J Pharmacol Exp Ther *217*:350, 1981.

26. Smith HJ, Roche AHG, Jagusch MF, et al: Cardiomyopathy associated with amphetamine administration. Am Heart J *91*:792, 1976.

27. Wiener RS, Lockhart JT, Schwartz RG: Dilated cardiomyopathy and cocaine abuse. Report of two cases. Am J Med *81*:699–701, 1986.

27a. Cregler LL, Mark H: Medical complications of cocaine abuse. N Engl J Med *315*:1495–1500, 1986.

27b. Karch SB, Billingham ME: The pathology and etiology of cocaine-induced heart disease. Arch Pathol Lab Med *112*:225–230, 1988.

27c. Rosenberg J, Pentel P, Pond S, et al: Hyperthermia associated with drug intoxication. Crit Care Med *14*:964–969, 1986.

28. Meldrum BS, Vigouroux RA, Brierley JB: Systemic factors and epileptic brain damage. Arch Neurol *29*:82, 1973.

29. Burn RS, Lerner SE, Corrado R, et al: Phencyclidine—states of acute intoxication and fatalities. West J Med *123*:345, 1975.

30. Eastman JW, Cohen SN: Hypertensive crisis and death associated with phencyclidine poisoning. JAMA *231*:1270, 1975.

31. Kessler GF Jr, Demers LM, Berlin C, et al: Phencyclidine and fatal status epilepticus. N Engl J Med *291*:979, 1974.

32. Tong TG, Benowitz NL, Becker CE, et al: Phencyclidine poisoning. JAMA *234*:512, 1975.

33. Hitner H, DiGregorio GJ: Preliminary investigation of the peripheral sympathomimetic effects of phencyclidine. Arch Int Pharmacodyn *212*:36, 1974.

34. Ilett KF, Jarrott B, O'Donnell SR, et al: Mechanism of cardiovascular actions of 1-(Cl-phenylcyclohexyl)piperidine hydrochloride (phencyclidine). Br J Pharmacol Chemother *28*:73, 1966.

35. Blackwell B, Marley E, Price J: Hypertensive interactions between monoamine oxidase inhibitors and food stuffs. Br J Psychiatr *113*:349, 1967.

36. Linden CH, Rumack BH, Strehike C: Monoamine oxidase inhibitor overdose. Ann Emerg Med *13*:1137–1144, 1984.

37. Villiers JC: Intracranial hemorrhage in patients treated with monoamine oxidase inhibitors. Br J Psychiatr *112*:109, 1966.

38. Atkinson RM, Ditman KS: Tranylcypromine: A review. Clin Pharmacol Ther *6*:631, 1965.

39. Vigran IM: Dangerous potentiation of meperidine hydrochloride by pargyline hydrochloride. JAMA *187*:953, 1964.

39a. Woo OF, Benowitz NL, Bialy FW, Wengert JW: Atrioventricular conduction block caused by phenylpropanolamine. JAMA *253*:2646–2647, 1985.

40. Pentel P: Toxicity of over-the-counter stimulants. JAMA *252*:1898–1903, 1984.

41. Pentel PR, Mikell FL, Zavoral JH: Myocardial injury following phenylpropanolamine ingestion. Br Heart J *47*:51, 1982.

42. Kikta DG, Devereaux MW, Chandar K: Intracranial hemorrhages due to phenylpropanolamine. Stroke *16*:510–512, 1985.

43. Pentel P, Mikell F: Reaction of phenylpropanolamine/chlorpheniramine/belladonna compound on a woman with unrecognized autonomic dysfunction. Lancet *2*:274, 1984.

44. Boakes AJ, Laurence DR, Teoh PC, et al: Interactions between sympathomimetic amines and antidepressant agents in man. Br Med J *1*:311, 1973.

45. Ober KF, Wang RIH: Drug interactions with guanethidine. Clin Pharmacol Ther *14*:190, 1973.

46. Massey SR: Fake "speed" causes almost as much fear as the real thing. Wall Street Journal, Sept. 8, 1981.

47. Olson KR, Benowitz NL, Woo OF, Pond SM: Theophylline overdose: Acute single ingestion versus chronic repeated overmedication. Am J Emerg Med *3*:386–394, 1985.

48. Gaudreault P, Guay J: Theophylline poisoning. Pharmacological considerations and clinical management. Med Toxicol *1*:169–191, 1986.

49. Zwillich CW, Sutton FD, Neff TA, et al: Theophylline-induced seizures in adults: Correlation with serum concentrations. Ann Intern Med *82*:784, 1975.

50. Camarata SJ, Weil MH, Hanashiro PK, et al: Cardiac arrest in the critically ill. I. A study of predisposing causes in 132 patients. Circulation *44*:688, 1971.
51. Amin DN, Henry JA: Propranolol administration in theophylline overdose. Lancet *1*:520–521, 1985.
52. Wenzel DG: Drug-induced cardiomyopathies. J Pharm Sci *56*:1209, 1967.
53. Rosa RM, Silva P, Young JB, et al: Adrenergic modulation of extrarenal potassium disposal. N Engl J Med *302*:431, 1980.
54. Josephson GW, Stine RJ: Caffeine intoxication: A case of paroxysmal atrial tachycardia. JACEP *5*:776, 1976.
55. Benowitz NL, Jones RT: Cardiovascular and metabolic considerations in prolonged cannabinoid administration in man. J Clin Pharmacol *21*:214S, 1981.
56. Aronow WS, Cassidy J: Effect of marihuana and placebo-marihuana smoking on angina pectoris. N Engl J Med *291*:65, 1974.
57. Klock JC, Boerner U, Becker CE: Coma, hyperthermia and bleeding associated with massive LSD overdose. A report of 8 cases. West J Med *120*:183, 1974.
58. Marshall AJ: Cardiac arrhythmias caused by chloral hydrate. Br Med J *2*:994, 1977.
59. Bowyer K, Glasser SP: Chloral hydrate overdose and cardiac arrhythmias. Chest *77*:232, 1980.
60. Regan TJ, Haider B: Ethanol abuse and heart disease. Circulation *64*(Suppl III):III–14, 1981.
60a. Vikhert AM, Tsiplenkova VG, Cherpachenko NM: Alcoholic cardiomyopathy and sudden cardiac death. J Am Coll Cardiol *8*:3A–11A, 1986.
61. Robin E, Goldschlager N: Persistence of low cardiac output after relief of high output by thiamine in a case of alcoholic beriberi and cardiac myopathy. Am Heart J *80*:103, 1970.
62. Ettinger PO, Wu CF, de la Cruz C Jr, et al: Arrhythmias and the "holiday heart." Alcohol-associated cardiac rhythm disorders. Am Heart J *95*:555, 1978.
63. Abbasakoor A, Beanlands DC: Electrocardiographic changes during ethanol withdrawal. Ann NY Acad Sci *273*:364, 1976.
64. Bass M: Sudden sniffing death. JAMA *212*:2075, 1970.
65. Reinhardt CF, Mulin LS, Maxfield ME: Epinephrine-induced cardiac arrhythmia potential of some common industrial solvents. J Occup Med *15*:953, 1973.
66. Taylor GJ, Harris WS: Cardiac toxicity of aerosol propellants. JAMA *219*:33, 1972.
67. Flowers NC, Horan LG: Nonanoxic aerosol arrhythmias. JAMA *219*:33, 1972.
68. Streicher HZ, Gabow PA, Moss AH, et al: Syndromes of toluene sniffing in adults. Ann Intern Med *94*:758, 1981.
69. Steiner MH: Syndromes of kerosene poisoning in children. Am J Dis Child *74*:32, 1947.
70. James FW, Kaplan S, Benzing G III: Cardiac complications following hydrocarbon ingestion. Am J Dis Child *121*:431, 1971.
70a. Wason S, Gibler WB, Hassan M: Ventricular tachycardia associated with non-freon aerosol propellants. JAMA *256*:78–80, 1986.
71. Conner CS, Watanabe AS: Clonidine overdose: A review. Am J Hosp Pharm *36*:906, 1979.
72. Merguet P, Heimsoth V, Murata T, et al: Experimental study on the circulatory effects of 2-(2,6-dichlorophenylamino)-2-imidazoline-hydrochloride in man. Pharmacol Clin *1*:30, 1968.
73. Gold MS, Pottash ALC, Sweeney DR, et al: Efficacy of clonidine in opiate withdrawal: A study of thirty patients. Drug Alcohol Depend *6*:201, 1980.
74. Farsang C, Ramirez-Gonzalez MD, Mucci L, et al: Possible role of an endogenous opiate in the cardiovascular effects of central alpha adrenoceptor stimulation in spontaneously hypertensive rats. J Pharmacol Exp Ther *214*:203, 1980.
75. Banner W, Clawson L: Failure of narcan to reverse clonidine toxicity. Vet Hum Toxicol *23*:361, 1981.
76. Massumi RA, Mason DT, Amsterdam EA, et al: Ventricular fibrillation and tachycardia after intravenous atropine for treatment of bradycardias. N Engl J Med *287*:336, 1972.
77. Granacher RP, Baldessarini RJ: Physostigmine: Its use in acute anticholinergic syndrome with antidepressant and antiparkinson drugs. Arch Gen Psychiatr *32*:375, 1975.
78. Pentel P, Peterson CD: Asystole complicating physostigmine treatment due to organophosphate of tricyclic antidepressant overdose. Ann Emerg Med *9*:11, 1980.
79. Namba T, Nolte CT, Jackrel J, et al: Poisoning due to organophosphate insecticides: Acute and chronic manifestations. Am J Med *50*:475, 1971.
80. Namba T, Greenfield M, Grob D: Malathion poisoning: A fatal case with cardiac manifestations. Arch Environ Health *21*:533, 1970.
80a. Ludomirsky A, Klein HO, Sarelli P, et al: Q-T prolongation and polymorphous ("torsades de pointes") ventricular arrhythmias associated with organophosphorus insecticide poisoning. Am J Cardiol *49*:1654–1658, 1982.
80b. Winkelmann BR, Leinberger H: Life-threatening flecainide toxicity. A pharmacodynamic approach. Ann Intern Med *106*:807–814, 1987.
81. Epstein SE, Rosing DR: Verapamil: Its potential for causing serious complications in patients with hypertrophic cardiomyopathy. Circulation *64*:437, 1981.
82. Hariman RJ, Mangiardi LM, McAllister RG Jr, et al: Reversal of the cardiovascular effects of verapamil by calcium and sodium: Differences between electrophysiologic and hemodynamic responses. Circulation *59*:797, 1979.
83. Thorstrand C: Clinical features in poisonings by tricyclic antidepressants with special reference to the ECG. Acta Med Scand *199*:337, 1976.
84. Strom J, Madsen PS, Nielsen N, Sorensen MB: Acute self-poisoning with tricyclic antidepressants in 295 consecutive patients treated in an ICU. Acta Anaesthesiol Scand *28*:666–670, 1984.
85. Langou RA, Van Dyke C, Tahan SR, et al: Cardiovascular manifestions of tricyclic antidepressant overdose. Am Heart J *100*:458, 1980.
86. Nattel S, Mittleman M: Treatment of ventricular tachyarrhythmias resulting from amitriptyline toxicity in dogs. J Pharmacol Exp Ther *231*:430–435, 1984.
87. Pentel PR, Benowitz NL: Tricyclic antidepressant poisoning. Management of arrhythmias. Med Toxicol *1*:101–121, 1986.
88. Hagerman GA, Hanashiro PK: Reversal of tricyclic antidepressant-induced cardiac conduction abnormalities by phenytoin. Ann Emerg Med *10*:82, 1981.
88a. Callaham M, Schumaker H, Pentel P: Phenytoin prophylaxis of cardiotoxicity in experimental ami-

triptyline poisoning. J Pharmacol Exp Ther *245*:216–220, 1988.
89. Freeman JW, Loughhead MG: Beta blockade in the treatment of tricyclic antidepressant overdosage. Med J Aust *1*:1233, 1973.
90. Anderson JL, Mason JW: Successful treatment by overdrive pacing of recurrent quinidine syncope due to ventricular tachycardia. Am J Med *64*:715, 1978.
91. Shub C, Gau GT, Sidell PM, et al: The management of acute quinidine intoxication. Chest *73*:173, 1978.
92. Robinson DS, Barker E: Tricyclic antidepressant cardiotoxicity. JAMA *236*:2089, 1976.
93. Bigger JT Jr.: Digitalis toxicity. J Clin Pharmacol *25*:514–521, 1985.
94. Wenger TL, Butler VP Jr, Haber E, Smith TW: Treatment of 63 severely digitalis-toxic patients with digoxin-specific antibody fragments. J Am Coll Cardiol *5*:118A–123A, 1985.
95. Rumack BH, Wolfe RR, Gilfrich H: Phenytoin (diphenylhydantoin) treatment of massive digoxin overdose. Br Heart J *36*:405, 1974.
96. Cady WJ Rehder TL, Campbell J: Use of cholestyramine resin in the treatment of digitoxin toxicity. Am J Hosp Pharm *36*:92, 1979.
97. Pond S, Jacobs M, Marks J, et al: Treatment of digitoxin overdose with oral activated charcoal. Lancet *2*:1177, 1981.
98. Nickander R, Smits S: Some effects of a-D-propoxyphene (Darvon). Pharmacologist *15*:203, 1973.
99. Duberstein JL, Kaufman DM: A clinical study of an epidemic of heroin intoxication and heroin-induced pulmonary edema. Am J Med *51*:704, 1971.
100. Labi M: Paroxysmal atrial fibrillation of heroin intoxication. Ann Intern Med *71*:951, 1969.
101. Lipski J, Stimmel B, Donoso E: The effect of heroin and multiple drug abuse on the electrocardiogram. Am Heart J *86*:663, 1973.
102. Frand UI, Shim CS, Williams MH: Heroin-induced pulmonary edema: Sequential studies of pulmonary function. Ann Intern Med *77*:29, 1972.
103. Addington WW, Cugell DW, Bazley ES, et al: The pulmonary edema of heroin toxicity—an example of the stiff lung syndrome. Chest *62*:199, 1972.
104. Paranthaman SK, Khan F: Acute cardiomyopathy with recurrent pulmonary edema and hypotension following heroin overdosage. Chest *69*:117, 1976.
105. Brady HR, Horgan JH: Lithium and the heart. Unanswered questions. Chest *93*:166–169, 1988.
106. Tilkian AG, Schroeder JS, Kao JJ, et al: The cardiovascular effects of lithium in man. A review of the literature. Am J Med *61*:665, 1978.
107. Aellig WH, Berde B: Studies of the effect of natural and synthetic polypeptide type ergot compounds on a peripheral vascular bed. Br J Pharmacol *36*:561, 1969.
108. Snell NJC, Russell-Smith C, Coysh HL: Myocardial ischaemia in migraine sufferers taking ergotamine. Postgrad Med J *54*:37, 1978.
109. Goldfischer JD: Acute myocardial infarction secondary to ergot therapy. N Engl J Med *262*:860, 1960.
109a. Bowen JS, Davis GB, Kearney TE, Bardin J: Diffuse vascular spasm associated wtih 4-bromo-2,5-dimethoxyamphetamine ingestion. JAMA *249*:1473–1479, 1983.
110. Cipriano PR, Guthaner DF, Orlick AE, et al: The effects of ergonovine maleate on coronary arterial size. Circulation *59*:82, 1979.
111. Carliner NH, Denune DP, Firsch CS, et al: Sodium nitroprusside treatment of ergotamine-induced peripheral ischemia. JAMA *227*:308, 1974.
112. Skowronski GA, Tronson MD, Parkin WG: Successful treatment of ergotamine poisoning with sodium nitroprusside. Med J Aust *2*:8, 1979.
113. Whorton MD: Carbon monoxide intoxication: A review of 14 patients. JACEP *5*:505, 1976.
114. Anderson RF, Allensworth DC, deGroot WJ: Myocardial toxicity from carbon monoxide poisoning. Ann Intern Med *67*:1172, 1967.
115. Middleton GD, Ashby DW, Clark F: Delayed and long-lasting electrocardiographic changes in carbon-monoxide poisoning. Lancet *1*:12, 1961.
116. Cosby RS, Bergeron M: Electrocardiographic changes in carbon monoxide poisoning. Am J Cardiol *13*:93, 1963.
117. de Busk RF, Seidl LG: Attempted suicide by cyanide: A report of two cases. Calif Med *110*:394, 1969.
118. Aronow WS, Isabell MW: Carbon monoxide effect on exercise-induced angina pectoris. Ann Intern Med *79*:392, 1973.
119. Corya BC, Black MJ, McHenry PL: Echocardiographic findings after acute carbon monoxide poisoining. Br Heart J *38*:712, 1976.
120. Gousios AG, Adelson L: Electrocardiographic and radiographic findings in acute arsenic poisoning. Am J Med *26*:659, 1959.
121. Glazener FS, Ellis JG, Johnson PK: Electrocardiographic findings with arsenic poisoning. Calif Med *109*:158, 1968.
122. Goldsmith S, From AHL: Arsenic-induced atypical ventricular tachycardia. N Engl J Med *303*:1096, 1980.
123. Josephson CJ, Pinto SS, Petronella SJ: Arsine: Electrocardiographic changes produced in acute human poisoning. Arch Indust Hyg *4*:43, 1951.
124. Diaz-Rivera RS, Ramos-Morales F, Garcia-Palmieri MR, et al: The electrocardiographic changes in acute phosphorus poisoning in man. Am J Med Sci *241*:758, 1961.
125. Talley RC Linhart JW, Trevino AJ, et al: Acute elemental phosphorus poisoning in man: Cardiovascular toxicity. Am Heart J *84*:139, 1972.
126. Dahhan SS, Orfaly H: Electrocardiographic changes in mercury poisoning. Am J Cardiol *14*:178, 1964.
127. Kline TS: Myocardial changes in lead poisoning. J Dis Child *99*:48, 1960.
127a. Tenenbein M, Kopelow ML, deSa DJ: Myocardial failure and shock in iron poisoning. Hum Toxicol *7*:281–284, 1988.
128. Wallack MK, Winkelstein A: Acute iron intoxication in an adult. JAMA *29*:1333, 1974.
129. Gueron M, Yaron R: Cardiovascular manifestations of severe scorpion sting: Clinicopathologic correlations. Chest *57*:156, 1970.
130. Weitzmen S, Margulis G, Lehmann E: Uncommon cardiovascular manifestations and high catecholamine levels due to "black widow" bite. Am Heart J *93*:89, 1977.
131. Levine HD: Acute myocardial infarction following wasp sting: Report of two cases and critical survey of the literature. Am Heart J *91*:365, 1976.
132. Regan TJ, Ettinger PO, Lyons MM, Moschos CB, Weisse AB: Ethyl alcohol as a cardiac risk factor. Curr Prob Cardiol *2*:29, 1977.

CHAPTER 5

FLUIDS AND ELECTROLYTES I: GENERAL PRINCIPLES

Adult Fluid and Electrolyte Balance; Regulation of Volume and Tonicity and Management of Fluid Balance and Relative Hypovolemia

James F. Winchester, M.D.

Perhaps most critical for the management of poisoned patients is an understanding of fluid balance in normal human beings and the disturbances in it that poisoning creates. Clemmeson and Nilsson showed that adoption of conservative medical management of poisoned patients was associated with a far higher survival than the previously used "heroic" measures—an essential part of that management being care of the respiratory tract and proper management of fluid balance.[1] Before discussing the abnormalities of fluid and electrolyte balance in poisoned patients, normal fluid and electrolyte balance will be reviewed.

REGULATION OF BODY FLUID VOLUMES AND TONICITY

The body fluid, or whole body water, in an average 70-kg man consists of about 42 liters of water and is divided into two distinct subgroups: the intracellular fluid and the extracellular fluid (Fig. 5–1).

Except for bone, tissues that do not contain fat ("the lean body mass") are 60 to 85 per cent water, whereas muscle and gray matter of brain are the wettest tissues of the body (70 to 85 per cent water). Connective tissue and erythrocytes are the driest nonadipose tissues (60 per cent water). Fat tissue, on the other hand, contains 20 per cent water; therefore, an obese person contains by weight proportionately less water than a thin one. In obese individuals, whole body water falls closer to 40 per cent; in general, women contain more fat than men, so the water content of women is relatively less than that of men (Fig. 5–1).

The water content of the body is relatively high in infancy, falls to adult levels in late childhood, and then falls slowly but progressively with age. The sex difference in body water content develops at puberty and continues throughout life.

Intracellular water constitutes some 55 to 60 per cent of whole body water; excluding the relatively inaccessible bone water, total extracellular fluid water (plasma and interstitial and transcellular water) makes up the difference. For an average man, it accounts for 15 liters (or approximately 20 to 25 per cent of the body weight). The extravascular or interstitial fluid space accounts for 12 liters of the extracellular fluid, while 3 liters are present as plasma within the circulation. In an average young man, total blood volume is 6 to 8 per cent of body weight (70 ml/kg), which gives absolute values for blood and plasma volumes of 5 liters and 3 liters, respectively.

Intracellular and extracellular fluid compartments are separated by cell membranes that selectively control passage of ions and nutrients but are freely permeable to water; although ionic gradients may exist across cell membranes, movement of water will establish osmotic equilibrium, and any osmotic gradients will be rapidly corrected.

INTRACELLULAR FLUID COMPOSITION

The ionic composition of body fluids can be discussed in terms of chemical equivalents; concentrations of all ionic constituents are expressed as the sum of concentrations of the positive ions (cations) and negative ions (anions). As can be seen from Table 5–1, ionic balance is obligatory in order to

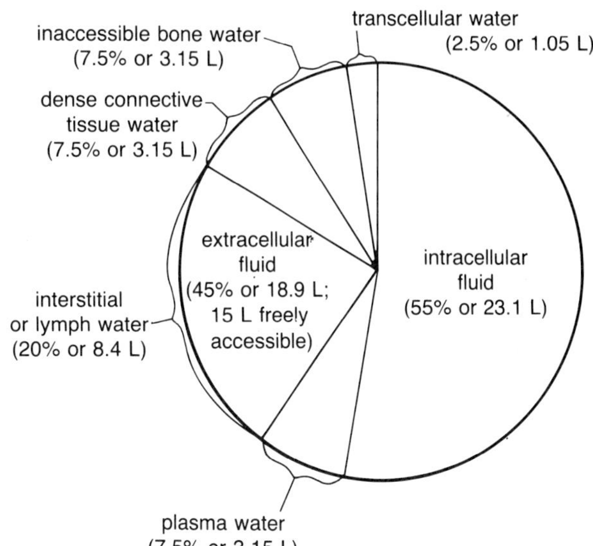

Figure 5–1. Distribution of whole body water in a 70-kg human adult. Men = 42 L; women = 35 L. Most values shown are for men.

maintain the electrical neutrality of the body fluids. It can be seen from Table 5–1 that the principal cations in extracellular fluid consist of sodium, potassium, calcium, and magnesium, whereas the principal cations in intracellular fluid are potassium and magnesium. On the other hand, the principal anions in extracellular fluid are chloride and bicarbonate, whereas the principal anions in intracellular fluid are phosphate, sulfate, and proteins.

Electrical neutrality is maintained in all body fluids by a balance of cations and anions, but in clinical practice it is usual to measure only plasma or serum sodium, potassium, chloride, and bicarbonate and assume that the rest of the cations and anions are balanced. A clinically useful guide to causes of metabolic acidosis may be reflected in change in the so-called "anion gap." Anion gap equals sodium (Na) minus chloride (Cl) plus bicarbonate (HCO_3), or, anion gap = Na − (Cl + HCO_3). The average normal value for the serum anion gap ranges from 8 to 16 mEq/L, with albumin contributing the greatest amount to the uncalculated anions that contribute to the anion gap (11 mEq/L) at an albumin concentration of 4 gm/dl. Anion gap is discussed in more detail in Chapter 7, but, in relation to poisoning, a negative or low anion gap may be seen in lithium and bromide intoxication; a normal anion gap may be seen in ingestion of anion exchange resins, calcium or magnesium salts, and carbonic anhydrase inhibitors, in poisoning with hydrochloric acid or other acids, and in sulfur ingestion; and an increased anion gap may be seen in salicylate poisoning, paraldehyde poisoning, methanol or ethylene glycol ingestion, or lactic acidosis. Table 5–1 also indi-

Table 5–1. NORMAL COMPOSITION OF BODY FLUIDS

	PLASMA *(mEq/L)*	INTERSTITIAL FLUID *(mEq/L)*	INTRACELLULAR FLUID *(mEq/L)*
Cations			
Na^+	142	144	11
K^+	4.5	4.0	164
Ca^{++}	5	2.5	2
Mg^{++}	3	1.5	28
Anions			
Cl^-	103	114	—
HCO_3^-	27	30	10
$PO_4^=$	2	2	105
$SO_4^=$	1	1	20
Proteins	16	0	65
Organic acids	6	5	5

cates that an increased anion gap may be seen with the failure of excretion of organic anions—phosphate and sulfate—such as is seen in renal failure.

The high intracellular–low extracellular concentration of potassium and the reverse for sodium favor movement of potassium out of and sodium into cells. Such ionic gradients are maintained by the presence of sodium-potassium pumps in the cell membrane and are critical in protecting cell volume. High concentrations of osmotically active anionic protein within cells, relative to the interstitial fluid, establish a Gibbs-Donnan equilibrium that increases the osmotic activity within the cell. Any movement of water into cells is prevented by the act of extrusion of sodium, while interference with the potassium-sodium pump mechanism results in cellular accumulation of sodium and chloride, with loss of potassium and resultant cellular edema.

Transcellular fluids are predominantly products of cell secretion. Composition of the fluids varies according to their cellular origin. Under physiologic conditions, secreted fluids tend to be recirculated or reabsorbed, but under pathologic (or treatment) conditions, failure to reabsorb continuously secreted fluids may lead to significant losses of volume and electrolytes, as seen with diarrhea, vomiting, and also nasogastric suction. The electrolyte composition of transcellular fluids is shown in Table 5–2. Drainage of intestinal fluids may result in considerable losses of chloride and bicarbonate (for instance, through small intestinal fistulas or extreme diarrhea as seen in cholera). Similarly, drainage of gastric and salivary juices may result in loss of considerable quantities of hydrogen ion, as well as chloride: Diarrhea produced by cholera will also result in massive sodium loss, as well as water, producing not only hypovolemia but also hyponatremia. "Third space" fluid loss refers to sequestration of fluids within cavities—pleural, pericardial, and intraperitoneal.

MOVEMENT OF WATER BETWEEN INTRACELLULAR AND EXTRACELLULAR FLUID SPACES: OSMOLARITY AND OSMOLALITY

Water moves freely across cell membranes, and an osmotic disequilibrium cannot be sustained. Distribution of total body water will then depend on the number of active particles in the intracellular and extracellular spaces. The osmotically driven "shifts" of body water will then adjust intracellular and extracellular osmolality to maintain osmotic neutrality. One osmole is the mass of a solute (or mixture of a solute) which, when dissolved in 1 liter, gives a solution that has an osmotic pressure of 22.4 atmospheres at 0°C. Osmolar concentrations are generally determined indirectly by measuring changes of the physical function of solutions, such as depression of the freezing point below that of water. Osmolality determined in this fashion (or osmoles/100 gm of plasma water) is obtained, and this term is to be preferred to the commonly misused term "osmolarity" (or osmoles/L of whole plasma), as well as being more appropriate to considering physiologic relationships.

In practice, plasma osmolality mainly reflects plasma sodium concentration, and it must be remembered that water added to or removed from any fluid compartment behaves as though it were added to or removed from whole body water; secondly, sodium added to or removed from extracellular fluid alters sodium concentration, as though it had been added to or removed from whole body water. Thirdly, sodium concentration in plasma does not necessarily reflect changes in extracellular fluid volume, since hypernatremia may exist with low, normal, or in-

Table 5–2. ELECTROLYTE COMPOSITION OF TRANSCELLULAR FLUIDS

	Na (mEq/L)	*K (mEq/L)*	*Cl (mEq/L)*	*HCO_3 (mEq/L)*
Saliva	33	20	34	0
Gastric juice	60	9	84	0
Bile	149	5	101	45
Pancreatic juice	141	5	77	92
Ileal fluid	129	11	116	29
Cecal fluid	80	21	48	22
Cerebrospinal fluid	141	3	127	23
Sweat	45	5	58	0

creased extracellular fluid. The same remarks apply to hyponatremia or normal serum sodium concentrations. Fourthly, changes in the volume of intracellular fluid and extracellular fluid are usually proportional (and in the same direction) with gain or loss of water, with intracellular and extracellular fluid volume changing in opposite directions with gains or losses of restricted solutes, such as sodium and potassium.

Other important solutes that contribute to plasma osmolality are glucose and blood urea nitrogen (BUN). Since sodium is accompanied by an approximately equal number of osmotically active anions, the ionic contribution of sodium to osmolality is twice its concentration in plasma. The following formula allows calculation of osmolality:

$$\text{Plasma osmolality} = 2\ \text{Na (mEq/L)} + \text{Glucose (mg/dl)}/18 + \text{BUN (mg/dl)}/2.8$$

The calculated osmolality generated by this formula under normal circumstances agrees well with the measured osmolality—measured by depression of freezing point. In certain circumstances, however, the difference between calculated and measured osmolality may be large and give rise to the so-called "osmolal gap." In clinical practice in toxicology, osmolal gaps are seen principally with ethylene glycol poisoning but also to a lesser extent with ethanol and methanol poisoning; treatment with mannitol or glycerol can also temporarily affect the plasma osmolality. Other major discrepancies between measured osmolality and calculated osmolality can indicate excessive quantities of protein or lipid in plasma, in addition to those unmeasured solutes previously mentioned.

CELLULAR RESPONSES TO REDISTRIBUTION OF FLUID

Changes in extracellular osmolality can bring about major swelling or contraction of cells, but the prime effects are seen in the brain. Hyponatremia induced in animals causes brain swelling initially, with diminishing changes within several hours. Correction of brain swelling is essentially complete at 24 hours, with the brain responding to extracellular hypotonicity by losing potassium and chloride. In hypernatremia in experimental animals, brain water is initially lost, with gains of sodium, potassium, and chloride being achieved by brain cells. Between 4 hours and several days, brain water content returns to normal, and an increased osmotic activity is sustained through the generation and accumulation of organic solutes such as amino acids. Hypoglycemia can also cause acute loss of brain water, with return to normal levels within a few hours principally because of changes in concentration of ions and organic solutes. Similarly, urea, mannitol, and glycerol remove water from brain but do not result in the generation of new intracellular organic molecules (idiogenic osmoles). For this reason, use of these latter compounds is not associated with effective adaptive changes in the regulation of intracellular volume of the brain, and consequently brain volume decreases.

REGULATION OF BODY FLUID VOLUMES AND DAILY FLUID BALANCE

Since sodium is the dominant cation of extracellular fluid, it is the critical determinant of extracellular fluid volume by virtue of its osmotic activity, and by virtue of its effect on renal sodium chloride reabsorption. It is the major determinant of renal water reabsorption. It is through the reabsorption of sodium and water that the kidney regulates extracellular fluid volume. The reabsorption of sodium by the kidney is an intensely finely regulated process for conservation of sodium and water, and also for its secondary effects on hydrogen ion excretion through bicarbonate reabsorption also linked to potassium secretion. A detailed discussion of sodium reabsorption by the kidney is beyond the scope of this text, but two major mechanisms in sodium homeostasis are worth discussing in relationship to diagnosis and management of intoxicated patients.

Sodium is freely filtered at the glomerulus and is reabsorbed isotonically at the proximal convoluted tubule, with 60 to 70 per cent of filtered sodium being proximally reabsorbed. Consequently, the glomerular filtrate volume is reduced by 60 to 70 per cent in the proximal tubule, providing substantial control of fluid balance. In the descending limb of the loop of Henle, the tubule is less permeable to sodium and urea but more permeable to water; consequently, the glomerular filtrate passing through the loop of Henle increases in sodium concentration, with consequent rises in osmolality. The thin ascending limb of the loop of Henle is permeable to sodium and urea but relatively impermeable to water, while in the thick ascending limb of the loop of Henle there is active transport of chloride, which also facilitates sodium reabsorption. Subsequently, the ascending limb of the loop of Henle accounts for 20 to 25 per cent of sodium reabsorption. In the distal nephron (the distal convoluted tubule and collecting duct), 5 to 10 per cent of sodium is reabsorbed, facilitating potassium secretion, and in part responsive to aldosterone.

Since the renal excretion of sodium is variable and under physiologic conditions is equal to sodium intake, the kidney must vary its excretion of sodium in the wide range encountered in human beings (1 to several hundred mEq every 24 hours). It follows that there are regulatory mechanisms governing sodium excretion. Glomerular filtration; physical factors such as postglomerular protein oncotic pressure, aldosterone, and antidiuretic hormone; and, finally, a natriuretic substance are all coordinated to maintain the balance of the extracellular fluid volume. It is well known that infusion of saline increases glomerular filtration rate and reduces renin excretion, thereby reducing aldosterone secretion; such physical forces favor natriuresis and release of a natriuretic substance, both of which will increase urinary sodium excretion. The reverse occurs when volume contraction is present and sodium is retained by the kidney. The daily water balance in human beings is maintained by the osmotic milieu and is shown in Table 5–3. As can be seen from this table, it is not surprising that the severely intoxicated patient who requires ventilation and gastric drainage quickly (within 24 hours) can have significant derangements of daily water balance if not given adequate replacement of the normal fluid intake in the form of beverages or food. However, compensatory mechanisms, principally through antidiuretic hormone secretion, are brought into play to conserve water, while reduction in renal blood flow will probably conserve sodium.

Antidiuretic hormone (ADH) is an octapeptide produced in the supraoptic and paraventricular nuclei of the hypothalamus. It is transported in the nerves from the hypothalamus to be stored in the posterior hypophysis and median eminence. In response to a variety of stimuli, ADH is released and alters the permeability of the late distal tubule and collecting duct to water; the renal tubular cell contains receptors for antidiuretic hormone. A resultant increase in the water permeability of the distal tubule and collecting duct occurs, and, if there is hypertonicity of the medullary interstitium (brought about by the countercurrent concentration mechanism in the loop of Henle), then water reabsorption occurs. The prime factor in producing ADH secretion is the plasma osmolality. It has been known since the late 1940s and early 1950s that a 1 per cent change in osmolality produces ADH secretion, and a 1 to 2 per cent change in osmolality initiates drinking. On the other hand, a 6 per cent change in the extracellular fluid volume is required to produce the same effect on ADH.

Table 5–3. DAILY WATER BALANCE IN HUMAN BEINGS

GAINS		LOSSES	
Beverages	1.2 L	Alimentary*	8.2 L secreted 0.2 L lost
Water with food	1.0 L	Renal	170.0 L secreted 1.5 L lost
Water of oxidation of food	0.3 L	Sweat	0.1 L lost (Can exceed 10.0 L/day)
		Lungs	1.0 L secreted 0.7 L lost
Total	2.5 L	Total	2.5 L

*Saliva	1.5 L
Gastric juice	2.5 L
Pancreatic juice	0.7 L
Bile	0.5 L
Intestine	3.0 L
Total	8.2 L

Table 5–4. DRUG-INDUCED ALTERATIONS IN ANTIDIURETIC HORMONE (ADH) RELEASE AND ACTIVITY

CENTRAL REDUCTION IN ADH SECRETION	PERIPHERAL REDUCTION IN ADH ACTIVITY
ethanol	lithium
phenytoin/diphenylhydantoin	demeclocycline
glucocorticoids	acetohexamide
chlorpromazine	tolazamide*
reserpine	glyburide*
morphine†	propoxyphene*
CENTRAL STIMULATION OF ADH RELEASE	amphotericin
clofibrate	methoxyflurane
chlorpropamide	colchicine
nicotine	vinblastine
vincristine	norepinephrine
cyclophosphamide	**PERIPHERAL ENHANCEMENT OF ADH ACTIVITY**
tolbutamide	chlorpropamide
carbamazepine	acetaminophen
acetylcholine	indomethacin
carbachol	
methacholine	
barbiturates	
meperidine	
prostaglandin E_1	
isoproterenol	

*Mechanism not fully elucidated; not due to reduction in ADH secretion
†Mechanism not fully elucidated; raises threshold for osmotically induced ADH secretion

Dehydration and hypernatremia lead to reduced renal perfusion and increased antidiuretic hormone secretion. The result is the excretion of small amounts of urine, low in sodium and highly concentrated. Replacement of free water corrects the problem in patients with pure insensible water loss. In the syndrome of diabetes insipidus, the problem of water loss arises either because of a central defect in antidiuretic hormone production or release, or because of renal insensitivity to antidiuretic hormone (nephrogenic diabetes insipidus), in which water is lost via the kidney. Because of the action of ADH on the most distal sites of the nephron, it is possible for the patient to retain sodium maximally but still excrete volumes of water equal to 10 to 50 per cent of the glomerular filtration rate. The loss of water in diabetes insipidus results in 10 to 15 liters of dilute urine occurring with a low total sodium excretion. The result is concentration of plasma and stimulation of the thirst mechanism, leading to ingestion of large quantities of water to replace water losses. Clinically, the picture is of polyuria and polydipsia, the latter also being induced by psychogenic polydipsia—a difficult syndrome to distinguish from central or nephrogenic diabetes insipidus unless ADH concentrations in plasma are known. Drugs known to have an effect on ADH status are shown in Table 5–4.

Detailed discussion of the factors involved in the production of hypernatremia or hyponatremia and hyperkalemia or hypokalemia is beyond the scope of this text. However, the principal disorders associated with abnormalities of these cations in poisoned patients are shown in Table 5–5. The management of derangements of both sodium and potassium is also outlined in Table 5–5.

ASSESSMENT AND MANAGEMENT OF FLUID AND ELECTROLYTE IMBALANCE

The most useful clinical guides to the assessment of fluid balance are the features of volume overload and volume of contraction. Volume overload is manifested by the presence of peripheral edema or ascites or both, or pleural effusions. In this respect, a useful reminder is that a 4 per cent increase in whole body water is required to produce a trace of peripheral edema. Other signs of volume overload are distended neck veins, normal skin turgor, and axillary sweat, and also the signs of congestive heart failure. On the other hand, volume contraction is manifested by the absence of peripheral edema, collapsed neck veins, diminished skin turgor, and absence of axillary sweat. Another important feature is that resting or orthostatic

Table 5–5. PRINCIPAL DISORDERS OF SODIUM AND POTASSIUM IN INTOXICATED PATIENTS

		DISORDER AND EXAMPLES	TREATMENT
Hypernatremia	Normal body Na	Drug-induced diabetes insipidus Sweating (salicylates, organophosphates)	Diuretics and water replacement
	High body Na	Steroids Hypertonic saline, NaCl, $NaHCO_3$ Saline emetics	Water replacement
	Low body Na	Osmotic diuretics (mannitol) Sweating (salicylates) Diarrhea (organophosphates, antibiotics)	Hypotonic saline
Hyponatremia	↓ ECF volume	Diuretics (tubular and osmotic) Rhabdomyolysis Steroid deficiencies Vomiting/diarrhea/pancreatitis	Isotonic saline
	↑ ECF volume (nonedematous)	Steroid deficiency Hypothyroidism Beer-drinker's hyponatremia Drugs (see Table 5–4)	Water restriction
	↑ ↑ ECF volume (edematous)	Drug-induced Hepatic, renal, cardiac failure ACE inhibitors	Water restriction
Hyperkalemia	↑ True K^+	Acidosis Arginine hydrochloride Digitalis intoxication Geophagia K-sparing diuretics Steroid deficiency NSAIDs Hemolysis Rhabdomyolysis Salt substitutes Penicillin-K β-Blockers Heparin	Correct Stop drug Glucose/insulin Ion exchange resins Dialysis
Hypokalemia	Without K^+ deficit	Respiratory alkalosis (salicylate or respirator induced)	Adequate K replacement
	With K^+ deficit	Nasogastric suction, vomiting Alcoholism Inadequate K replacement Laxative abuse Drug-induced diarrhea Excessive steroids Licorice abuse Osmotic diuretics (mannitol, glucose) Diuretics Carbenicillin/penicillin/aminoglycosides	Adequate K replacement

tachycardia and hypotension may be seen with volume contraction.

With an increased extracellular fluid volume, such as occurs in cirrhosis, nephrosis, or congestive heart failure, urinary sodium concentrations are low while urinary osmolality is high (or isotonic), and blood urea nitrogen is normal or high. Treatment in this setting requires sodium and water restriction.

In conditions of decreased extracellular fluid, as in nonrenal loss of sodium with gastrointestinal or skin losses, urinary sodium is low and urinary osmolality is high (or isotonic), whereas the BUN is normal or high. When renal loss of sodium is common, as with diuretics, renal disease, or Addison's disease, urinary sodium is high, urinary osmolality is isotonic, and the BUN is normal or high. Treatment of the latter two conditions requires judicious use of isotonic saline.

In normal extracellular fluid volume, as in

the syndrome of inappropriate ADH (SIADH) secretion, urine sodium is high, urine osmolality is high, and the BUN is low; the condition is treated best by water restriction.

In the intoxicated patient, especially those requiring ventilation and intravenous fluids, it is imperative that body weight be measured daily and that fluid intake and output be recorded accurately. Using these measurements, daily changes in fluid and electrolyte balance can be judged. It is stressed that in the absence of peripheral edema, certain drugs may produce pulmonary edema (see Chapter 10) or cerebral edema (see Chapter 11).

Day-to-day management of fluid electrolyte and caloric requirements will depend on the probable duration of coma; the total body deficits or excesses prior to institution of intravenous fluids; the likely therapeutic maneuvers to be used, such as forced diuresis and dialysis; and the intoxicating agents. In the absence of complicating factors, it is reasonable to assume a normal fluid electrolyte and caloric requirement for a 70-kg man, and this is defined as "basal" requirements, outlined in Table 5–6. For each increase of 0.1 unit in plasma pH, there is a reciprocal fall in plasma potassium of 0.6 mEq/L; the reverse also obtains with a reduction in serum pH. Such shifts are due to transfer of plasma potassium into and out of cells because of changes in pH. The daily basal fluid, electrolyte, and caloric requirements outlined in Table 5–6 do not take into account the potassium and bicarbonate required for forced diuresis, but these will be outlined in Chapter 8.

MANAGEMENT OF RELATIVE HYPOVOLEMIA IN POISONING

In acute poisoning due to barbiturate, opiate, and other sedative drugs, it is well recognized that an increase in the venous capacitance occurs, with a relative deficit of plasma volume. This often responds to augmentation of plasma volume by volume expansion and in some instances vasopressor drugs, with a consequent increase in cardiac output and mean blood pressure and fall in total peripheral vascular resistance. However, there may not be significant changes in central venous pressure, even with copious administration of fluids. The relative hypovolemia due to increased venous capacitance may also be compounded by decreased venous return and extravascular fluid loss. It is recommended in these circumstances that a flow-directed pulmonary arterial catheter (Swan-Ganz) be used to assess both central venous pressure and pulmonary capillary wedge pressure as guides to accurate fluid replacement.

In such circumstances, volume expansion using crystalloids may be disadvantageous in that crystalloids may reduce the osmotic-hydrostatic gradient, thereby increasing pulmonary capillary water. This occurrence has been implicated in the development of shock lung in severely hypotensive patients (see Chapter 10). In view of the adverse effects of crystalloid solutions, colloid solutions such as albumin and Plasmanate are best chosen for the treatment of relatively hypovolemic shock in those patients who might develop pulmonary edema. Plasma protein fractions or dextrans are suitable colloidal agents, while human protein solutions are available in various concentrations ranging from 5 to 25 per cent solutions; human albumin solutions contain between 130 and 160 mEq/L of sodium chloride.

Other colloidal expanders, such as dextran or hetastarch, are also available. Dextran solutions have the advantages of lowering blood viscosity and preventing red blood cell aggregation within the microcirculation in

Table 5–6. DAILY BASAL FLUID, ELECTROLYTE, AND CALORIC REQUIREMENTS

Water/Electrolyte Requirements	Basal Requirements	Metabolic Requirements
Water	1.5–2.0 L*	100 ml/100 Cal
Sodium	75 mEq	2–3 mEq/100 Cal
Potassium	60 mEq	2–3 mEq/100 Cal
Magnesium	8 mEq	—
Chloride	—	4–6 mEq/100 Cal
Caloric Requirements		
0–10 kg	100 Cal/kg	
11–20 kg	1000 Cal plus 50 Cal/kg over 10 kg	
>20 kg	1500 Cal plus 20 Cal/kg over 20 kg	

*Insensible losses (approximately 700 ml) plus volume equivalent to urine volume

low blood flow states, but volume replacement with large quantities of dextran may impair blood coagulation. In patients with poor cardiac function, it may result in transfer of extracellular fluid to the intravascular compartment and cause pulmonary edema by virtue of its powerful oncotic properties.

Persistent hypotension, despite adequate volume replacement, and elevated pulmonary capillary wedge pressure suggest myocardial dysfunction; recourse then must be made to drugs capable of improving myocardial performance, such as dopamine, dobutamine, and isoproterenol.

CALCULATION OF WATER EXCESS AND DEFICIT

Water excess:

Whole body water (actual weight [kg] × 0.6)
× serum Na (mEq/L)
= Desired body water (L)
× desired serum Na (mEq/L)

Example:

80 × 0.6 (i.e., 48 L) × 125
= Desired body water × 140
Desired body water = 42.8 L
i.e., excess water of 48 − 42.8 = 5.2 L

Water deficit:

$$\text{Desired whole body water (L)} = \text{Actual whole body water (actual weight [kg]} \times 0.6) \times \frac{\text{actual serum Na (mEq/L)}}{\text{desired serum Na (mEq/L)}}$$

Example:

$$42 \times \frac{150}{140} = 45\ \text{L},$$

i.e., 45 − 42 = 3 L to correct serum sodium

N.B. Serum sodium in hyponatremic states probably should not be corrected faster than 1 mEq/hr because of the risk of developing central pontine myelinolysis.[2]

References

1. Clemmeson C, Nilsson E: Therapeutic trends in the treatment of barbiturates poisoning: The Scandinavian method. Clin Pharmacol Ther *2*:220, 1961.
2. Ayus JC, Krothapalli RK, Arieff AI: Treatment of symptomatic hyponatremia and its relation to brain damage. N Engl J Med *317*:1190, 1987.

FURTHER READING

Campbell EJM, Dickinson CJ, Slater JDH: Clinical Physiology. Oxford and Edinburgh, Blackwell Scientific Publications, 1969.

Leaf A, Cotran RS: Renal Pathophysiology. 2nd ed. New York, Oxford University Press, 1980.

Pitts RF: Physiology of the Kidney and Body Fluids. 2nd ed. Chicago, Year Book Medical Publishers, 1968.

Schrier RW (ed): Renal and Electrolyte Disorders. 3rd ed. Boston, Little, Brown, 1986.

Thier SO: The kidney. *In* Smith LH, Thier SO (eds): Pathophysiology; The Biological Principles of Disease. Philadelphia, WB Saunders, 1981, p 799.

Levi M, Bichet DG, Berl T: Treatment of hypoosmolar and hyperosmolar states. *In* Suki WN, Massry SG (eds): Therapy of Renal Diseases and Related Disorders. Dordrecht, Martinus Nijhoff Publishing, 1984, p 1.

Buerkert J: The pathophysiologic bases for alterations in water balance. *In* Klahr S (ed): The Kidney and Body Fluids in Health and Disease. New York, Plenum Medical Book Company, 1984, p 149.

CHAPTER 6

FLUIDS AND ELECTROLYTES II: THE PEDIATRIC PATIENT

Thomas McKee, M.D.

A thorough understanding of pediatric fluids and electrolyte balance is necessary to provide optimal care in childhood poisoning. The general physiology of fluids and electrolytes, including body fluid composition and regulation, is reviewed in Chapter 5. In this chapter, pediatric body fluid composition and principles of maintenance fluids and electrolytes are reviewed, as well as evaluation and treatment of dehydration and other common pediatric electrolyte disorders.

BODY FLUID COMPOSITION

In the neonate, almost 80 per cent of body weight is composed of water. This drops to approximately 70 per cent by 6 months of age and to 60 per cent by age 1 year. Fluid requirements in pediatric patients are proportionately much greater than in adults. The relative daily turnover of fluids, as a percentage of total body water in infants, is much greater compared with older children and adults, placing these patients at greater risk from illnesses and conditions causing derangements in fluid status.

Total body water is divided into the extracellular fluid (ECF) and the intracellular fluid (ICF). At birth, the ECF is approximately 40 per cent of body weight, dropping to 30 per cent by age 1 year and 25 per cent by adolescence (Fig. 6–1). The ECF consists of blood plasma and interstitial fluid. The ICF increases from approximately 35 per cent at birth to 45 per cent by late childhood and adolescence. The remaining body water (approximately 2 per cent) is transcellular water, which is that body fluid not directly connected with either ICF or ECF, such as fluid within the gastrointestinal tract and cerebrospinal fluid (CSF).

Table 6–1. STANDARD BASAL CALORIES

AGE	WEIGHT *(Kg)*	CALORIC EXPENDITURE *(Cal/Kg/24 Hr)*
Neonate	2.5–4	50
1 week–6 months	3–8	65–70
6–12 months	8–12	50–60
1–2 years	10–15	45–50
2–5 years	15–20	45
5–10 years	20–35	40–45
10–16 years	35–60	25–40
Adult	70	15–20

(From Rowe PC (ed): The Harriet Lane Handbook. Chicago, Year Book Medical Publishers, 1987, p 231.)

The chemical composition of the intracellular and extracellular spaces in children is similar to that in adults. In the ECF, sodium is the predominant cation, and chloride and bicarbonate account for most of the anions. In the ICF, however, potassium is the major cation and negative charges are supplied mostly by phosphates, sulfates, and proteins. Under physiologic conditions, electrical neutrality is maintained within each space. The large concentration gradient of sodium and potassium between the intra- and extracellular spaces is maintained by the so-called "sodium pump." This is an active process dependent upon sodium-potassium-ATPase found in cell membranes.

MAINTENANCE REQUIREMENTS

Maintenance fluid and electrolyte requirements vary with the metabolic rate, which is expressed as caloric expenditure in kilocalories (kcal) per 24 hours. Estimates of basal metabolic rate may be obtained from standardized tables like Table 6–1. Normal activity in bed is thought to increase the basal metabolic rate by 20 to 30 per cent. Fever will increase the rate by 12 per cent for each °centigrade rise. When insensible fluid loss, obligatory renal and stool water losses, and the gain of water from indigenous metabolism are considered, maintenance water requirements are found to equal approximately 100 ml per 100 kcal.

Estimates of caloric requirements can also be made using the formula outlined in Table 6–2. Again, assuming 100 ml of H_2O is

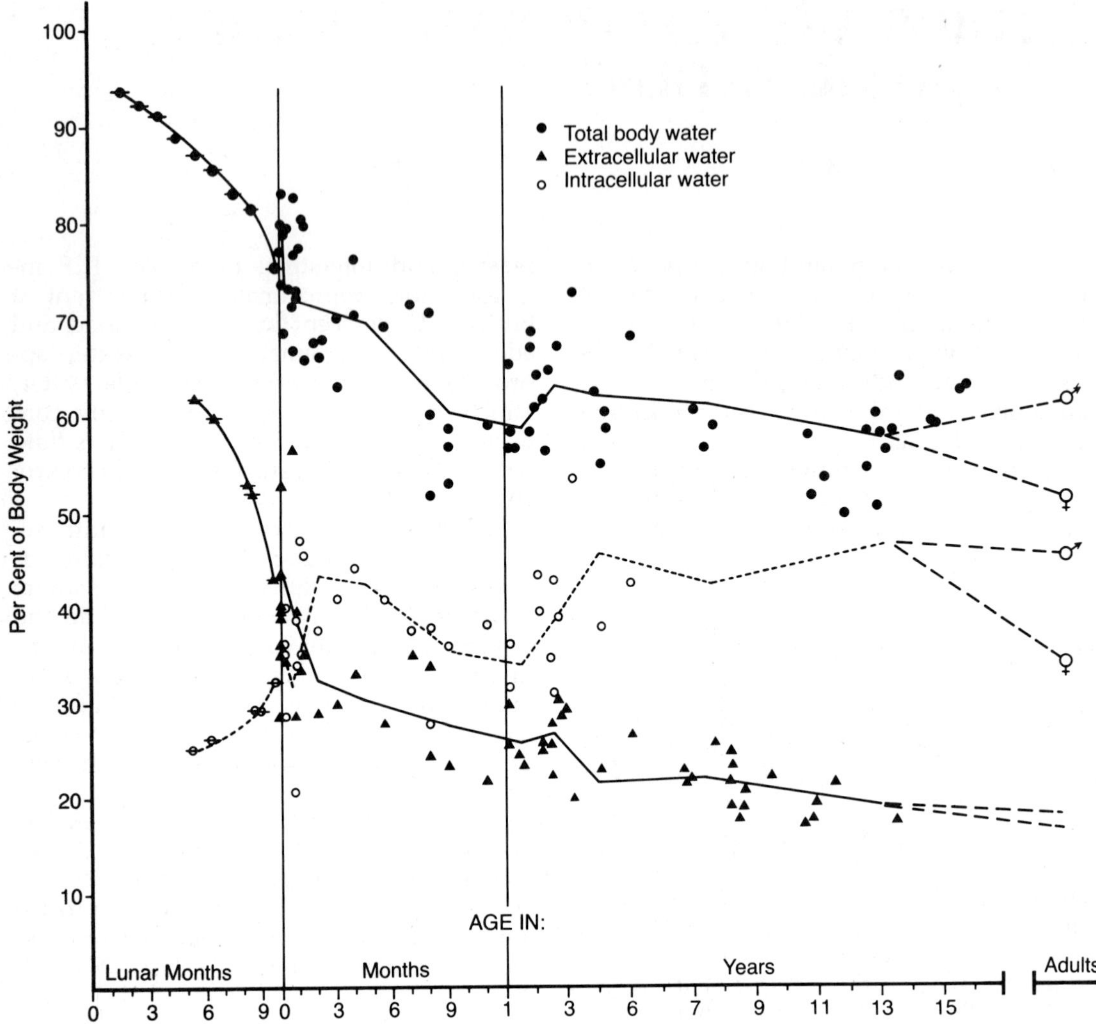

Figure 6–1. Body water compartments. (From Friis Hansen BJ: Body water compartments in children. Reproduced by permission of Pediatrics *28*:171, 1961.)

needed for every 100 kcal, maintenance fluid requirements are easily calculated. This method assumes that a child will have normal activity and no excessive requirements.

Sodium, potassium, and chloride are electrolytes necessary for the short-term administration of maintenance fluids. Daily sodium requirements are approximately 3 mEq per 100 kcal. Chloride requirements are similar to those of sodium. These elements are generally provided together as sodium chloride. Maintenance potassium requirements are approximately 2 mEq per 100 kcal. For short-term therapy, potassium is also usually administered in combination with chloride. A parenteral solution containing 30 mEq of sodium chloride and 20 mEq of potassium chloride per liter delivered at a maintenance rate will provide average daily requirements of sodium, potassium, and chloride. As in adults, parenteral fluids are usually administered as a solution containing 5 per cent dextrose to minimize endogenous protein breakdown.

Daily fluid and electrolyte requirements, of course, must be individualized. Maintenance requirements are decreased in many disease states. In anuric renal insufficiency, fluids should be reduced only to insensible losses (approximately 40 ml/100 kcal/day), and electrolytes, particularly potassium, should be reduced accordingly. Patients with inappropriate antidiuretic hormone secretion have an abnormally low urine output and

Table 6–2. CALORIC REQUIREMENTS

BODY WEIGHT (Kg)	CALORIC EXPENDITURE/DAY
Up to 10	100 kcal/kg
11–20	1000 kcal + 50 kcal/kg for each kg above 10 kg
Above 20	1500 kcal + 20 kcal/kg for each kg above 20 kg

(From Holliday MA, Segar WE: The maintenance need for water in parenteral fluid therapy. Pediatrics *19*:824, 1957.)

benefit from fluid restriction. Small children in highly humidified environments such as mist tents will have a reduced insensible water loss. Daily fluid and electrolyte requirements also will be reduced in hypometabolic states such as drug-induced coma.

More often, the acutely ill child will have abnormal fluid and electrolyte losses requiring an increase in maintenance requirements. As mentioned, fever can increase metabolic demands, and stressful situations such as major trauma, sepsis, and thermal injury can increase demands up to 30, 60, and 100 per cent, respectively. A hypermetabolic state is produced in certain intoxications, such as salicylate poisoning. Ongoing losses are often enteric in origin, secondary to infectious illness or surgery. Vomiting and diarrhea frequently accompany childhood poisonings and can significantly increase fluid and electrolyte losses. The composition of gastrointestinal fluids may be estimated from Table 6–3. The hypochloremic alkalosis resulting from gastric fluid loss is associated with renal potassium loss. Supplemental potassium chloride should be added to replacement fluids to prevent the development of hypokalemia in this situation. Excessive fluid and electrolyte losses also may be renal in origin, as is seen in diabetes mellitus, diabetes insipidus, adrenal insufficiency, or renal tubular abnormalities. Insensible fluid losses are increased in hyperthermia, and sodium chloride losses through sweat may be excessive in cystic fibrosis.

Whereas enteric and renal losses can be estimated or quantified by direct measurement, "third space" losses are more difficult to evaluate. These fluid losses occur within the body outside the vascular compartment and are not available for direct measurement. Fluid pooling within the peritoneal cavity in peritonitis or extravasated into the interstitial space in hypoproteinemic states is an example of a third space loss.

Occasionally, it is necessary to administer maintenance fluids at an accelerated rate to ensure adequate urinary output or enhance renal excretion of certain toxins. Most children with healthy cardiovascular systems will tolerate up to twice their normal maintenance fluid rate without problems. However, compensatory mechanisms may be limited in the acutely ill or poisoned child. In these situations, close monitoring is essential to prevent volume overload, cerebral edema, and iatrogenic electrolyte derangements.

FLUID AND ELECTROLYTE DEFICITS

Adequacy of hydration in pediatric patients is generally described by per cent of change in body weight. Any acute gain or loss of over 1 per cent of body weight is assumed to be the result of fluid gain or loss. For example, a child with gastroenteritis who has lost 10 per cent of body weight is said to be 10 per cent dehydrated. Of course, accurate pre- and post-illness weights are usually not available, so estimates must be made on clinical grounds. Such judgments are rough estimates only, as the severity of signs and symptoms will vary not only with the degree of dehydration, but also with the rate of fluid loss and the underlying tonicity of the plasma.

Deficits of less than 5 per cent are difficult

Table 6–3. COMPOSITION OF EXTERNAL ABNORMAL LOSSES

FLUID	Na	K (*mEq/L*)	Cl	PROTEIN (*Gm %*)
Gastric	20–80	5–20	100–150	—
Pancreatic	120–140	5–15	40–80	—
Small intestinal	100–140	5–15	90–130	—
Bile	120–140	5–15	80–120	—
Ileostomy	45–135	3–15	20–115	—
Diarrheal	10–90	10–80	10–110	—

(From Rowe PC (ed): Harriet Lane Handbook. Chicago, Year Book Medical Publishers, 1987, p 235.)

to detect clinically. A child who has mild, or 5 per cent, dehydration may have diminished skin turgor and thickened oral secretions. The anterior fontanel will be somewhat depressed in small infants. Other than for mild tachycardia, however, vital signs are stable. A child with moderate, or 10 per cent, dehydration appears acutely ill, with sunken eyes and, in infancy, a sunken fontanel. Skin turgor is diminished and mucous membranes are dry. Tachycardia is evident, but peripheral perfusion and blood pressure are maintained. A child with severe, or 15 per cent, dehydration usually appears "shocky." The extremities may be cool and poorly perfused, with thready or nonpalpable peripheral pulses. Skin turgor is poor; mucous membranes are dry. Such patients are often lethargic and respond poorly to stimulation. In these children, hemodynamic compensatory mechanisms are maximally stressed, and cardiovascular collapse may follow.

Dehydration is further classified according to the osmolality or tonicity of the plasma. Sodium is the most prevalent osmotically active particle in the extracellular fluid, and dehydration can be classified as hypotonic, isotonic, or hypertonic, based upon the measured serum sodium concentration. In isotonic dehydration, sodium and water have been lost from the ECF in approximately equal amounts. The resulting serum sodium levels range from 130 to 150 mEq per liter. The clinical changes seen with isotonic dehydration are those outlined above.

In hypotonic dehydration, there has been net loss of sodium in excess of water from the ECF, and the measured sodium is less than 130 mEq per liter. Such situations may occur in a child with isotonic dehydration whose deficits are partially replaced with a nonelectrolyte-containing solution. Clinical signs of hypotonic dehydration may be more severe than a similar degree of isotonic dehydration, because water will move from the ECF to the ICF to maintain osmotic equilibrium, further depleting the circulatory volume.

In hypernatremic dehydration, the serum sodium is greater than 150 mEq per liter. This condition results from loss of water in excess of sodium, which is seen in some diarrheal states, excessive insensible water loss, and diabetes insipidus. It also can occur from inappropriate fluid replacement with a solution containing excessive salt. The ECF is hypertonic compared with the ICF, so fluid moves from the ICF to the ECF. Thus, classic physical findings of dehydration are less pronounced than in isotonic or hypotonic dehydration. The cellular dehydration that occurs with this condition often gives what is described as a "doughy" consistency to the skin. Central nervous system signs and symptoms are often seen in hypernatremic states. Lethargy, irritability, and seizures are common.

TREATMENT OF DEHYDRATION

Fluid therapy must provide for maintenance requirements and ongoing losses in addition to the replacement of deficits. It is now well recognized that the oral route, when available, is preferred to provide fluids and electrolytes for maintenance therapy and replacement of moderate deficits. Solutions containing from 50 to 90 mEq per liter of sodium, 20 mEq per liter of potassium, and 20 grams per liter of glucose have been shown to be effective in treating most infants with mild or moderate dehydration secondary to enteric illness. For purposes of this chapter, however, discussion is limited to parenteral fluid therapy.

Of critical importance is the rapid restoration of adequate circulatory volume in patients who present with severe volume depletion and cardiovascular instability. This emergency phase of treatment should be accomplished with the rapid infusion of isotonic fluid, 20 ml/kg, to restore circulatory volume. If improvement in peripheral perfusion and blood pressure is not evident after an initial bolus, it should be repeated. Isotonic saline or lactated Ringer's solution is most often used for this purpose, though saline is preferred. In patients with severely impaired circulation, lactate may not be metabolized to bicarbonate, thus worsening acidosis. Five per cent albumin may also be used effectively to restore intravascular volume in the acute situation. Once hemodynamic stability has been achieved, further treatment will depend on the type of dehydration.

In isotonic dehydration, estimated fluid deficits are usually replaced over 24 to 36 hours. Many clinicians advocate replacing half the deficit within the first several hours, but in less critically ill patients, fluid deficits may be evenly replaced over 24 to 36 hours. Sodium and water losses are proportional in isotonic dehydration. Part of the sodium lost from the ECF moves to the ICF to compensate for intracellular potassium losses. Actual losses of sodium from the total body water are approximately 80 to 100 mEq per liter of fluid lost, or 8 to 10 mEq per kilogram in the small child with moderately severe dehydration. Daily maintenance sodium requirements and ongoing losses should be added to replacement solutions. Most children with isotonic dehydration can be successfully treated with a parenteral solution of approximately 75 mEq of sodium chloride per liter, or 0.5 per cent normal saline.

Fluid management of the child with hypotonic dehydration is similar to that of the isotonically dehydrated child. Estimated deficits and maintenance requirements are administered over 24 to 36 hours once hemodynamic stability has been achieved. The sodium deficit in the child with hypotonic dehydration, however, is greater than that of a child with a similar degree of isotonic dehydration. For replacement purposes, this extra sodium deficit can be calculated from the following formula:

$$(\text{Desired Na [sodium]} - \text{measured Na}) \times 0.6 \times \text{body weight (kg)}$$

(Six tenths of lean body weight approximates total body water, the fluid space in which sodium exerts an osmotic effect. Even though it is an extracellular cation, the concentration of sodium in the ECF will affect the water content in the ICF.) Initial therapy in hypotonic dehydration should begin with normal saline. Once serum sodium levels are greater than 130 mEq per liter, further replacement may be given with 0.5 per cent normal saline. Sodium deficits need not be corrected rapidly unless the patient exhibits neurologic symptoms associated with hyponatremia. Such symptoms rarely occur unless serum sodium is less than 120 mEq per liter. The amount of sodium needed to raise the serum level to 120 mEq per liter can be calculated from the formula and can be given as an infusion of 3 per cent saline (approximately 0.5 mEq Na/ml) over several hours if necessary. If the patient is actively seizing, then more rapid administration is indicated.

Although most children with isotonic or hypotonic dehydration will recover if given adequate fluid and sodium chloride, children with hypertonic dehydration (sodium greater than 150 mEq/L) present a difficult challenge. Children usually develop hypernatremic dehydration over a period of days, and osmotic equilibrium between the ECF and ICF is maintained by intracellular water loss and possibly by the formation of "idiogenic osmoles" in central nervous system cells. The estimated fluid deficit is predominately intracellular and should be replaced slowly over 48 hours or more. Rapid administration of fluid can create an osmotic gradient between the ECF and ICF, precipitating cerebral edema and convulsions. Sodium deficits are smaller than in isotonic dehydration and are usually replaced with 0.2 per cent saline. Once urine output is established, potassium chloride (30 to 40 mEq/L) is added, to correct intracellular potassium deficits and to increase the osmolality of the replacement fluid. The choice of fluid, however, is less important than the rate at which it is administered. The rate of lowering of serum sodium should not exceed 10 mEq per 24 hours. Frequent monitoring of serum sodium levels is necessary.

It should be stressed that these suggestions for parenteral fluid therapy are general guidelines only, based on gross estimations of body fluid deficits. The most complex calculations are no substitute for frequent clinical evaluation and close monitoring of the course of treatment.

OTHER DISORDERS OF SODIUM

Abnormalities of serum sodium also may be seen in the normovolemic or hypervolemic patient. Several of the more common disorders are reviewed.

The syndrome of inappropriate antidiuretic hormone secretion (SIADH) is the result of inappropriate secretion of the hormone vasopressin in the normovolemic patient, resulting in free water retention and hyponatremia. The diagnosis is made by demonstrating an inappropriately concentrated urine in the face of a dilute serum in the normovolemic patient. Symptoms rarely occur unless the serum sodium is less than 120 mEq per liter, and most patients are readily managed with fluid restriction. More rapid correction of serum sodium usually can be accomplished with the use of loop diuretics, such as furosemide, and volume replacement with sodium-containing solutions. SIADH is seen most often in pediatric patients with meningitis or other central nervous system pathology, although a number of other causes, including drugs, have been described (Table 6–4).

Dilutional hyponatremia may occur as the result of ingestion or administration of excessive free water in infants and small children. The infant's ability to excrete a large volume of free water is reduced compared with that in adults. Hyponatremia and seizures may be seen in infants less than 6 months of age who are fed dilute formulas and excessive amounts of water. Hyponatremia may also be seen with inappropriate administration of hypotonic parenteral fluids. In the euvolemic patient, simple fluid restriction and provision of adequate sodium chloride will suffice. The hypervolemic patient with hyponatremia is usually edematous and may also require diuresis in addition to sodium chloride replacement for correction.

Pseudohyponatremia occurs as the result of high concentrations of nonaqueous solids like lipids and proteins in the serum. These solids displace water and falsely appear to dilute the serum, although the physiologic concentration of sodium may be normal. A similar situation occurs with hyperglycemic states, in which serum sodium will be lowered 1.6 mEq per liter for every 100 mg per dl rise in glucose.

HYPERNATREMIA AND SALT POISONING

Hypernatremic states in the absence of dehydration are uncommon in children and usually result from the inappropriate administration or ingestion of excessive sodium. This may be seen with ingestion of table salt or from excessive administration of sodium bicarbonate, for example, following cardiac resuscitation. Free water deficits in hypernatremic states can be estimated from the following formula:

$$\text{Free water deficit (liters)} = \frac{0.6 \times \text{body wt (kg)} \times (1 - \text{measured Na})}{140}$$

The hypernatremic state should be gradually corrected using hypotonic fluid in a fashion similar to that described in treating hypertonic dehydration, lowering serum sodium by no more than 10 mEq per liter per day. Rapid correction may be associated with circulatory overload or create an osmotic gradient between the ICF and the ECF, precipitating cerebral edema.

Fatal salt poisoning has occurred in children following the inadvertent substitution of table salt for sugar in infant formulas and the administration of salt as an emetic. Symptoms are generally seen within hours of oral ingestion and include seizures, obtundation, coma, and cardiorespiratory arrest. Serum sodium levels may be greater than 180 mEq

Table 6–4. DISORDERS ASSOCIATED WITH EXCESSIVE ADH EFFECT

CNS: Infection, tumor, injury, vascular accidents, Guillain-Barré syndrome		
Drug-related:	acetaminophen (Tylenol)	morphine
	barbiturates	thiothixene (Navane)
	carbamazepine (Tegretol)	nicotine
	chlorpropamide	phenformin
	clofibrate	polymyxin B
	cyclophosphamide	thiazides
	amitriptyline (Elavil)	tolbutamide
	indomethacin	vincristine
	isoproterenol	
Endocrine: Myxedema, cortisol deficiency, pituitary stalk section		
Heart: Congestive heart failure, left atrial stretching, constrictive pericarditis		
Infections: Acute childhood infectious disorders, especially viral		
Liver: Cirrhosis, hepatic failure, portal hypertension		
Metabolic: Acute intermittent porphyria		
Pulmonary: Asthma, infections, emphysema, fibrosis, tumors, ventilation (CPAP)		
Renal: Changes in sodium handling by the kidney related to volume contraction and/or diuretic; hypoalbuminemia		
Surgery-related: Anesthesia or premedication, peritoneal reflexes, intracranial manipulation, postoperative pain		
Tumors: Duodenum, pancreas, salivary gland, thymus		

(From Gruskin AB, Baluarte HJ, Prebis MS, et al: Serum sodium abnormalities in children. Pediatr Clin North Am *29*:924, 1982.)

per liter. Such high levels of sodium will create a large osmotic gradient between the ECF and ICF, leading to extreme cellular dehydration and brain injury. Autopsy studies of children dying from salt poisoning have shown capillary and venous congestion of the central nervous system, subarachnoid and parenchymal hemorrhage, and dural sinus occlusion. In acute salt poisoning with serum sodium levels greater than 180 mEq per liter, removal of excess sodium chloride by means of dialysis will improve the outcome. Hemodialysis or peritoneal dialysis with a 4.25 per cent glucose solution can effectively lower sodium levels and limit the severity of symptoms.

DISORDERS OF POTASSIUM

As potassium is predominately an intracellular cation, measured serum potassium reflects only a small portion of total body stores. However, relatively small changes in serum potassium levels can have profound physiologic effects.

Hypokalemia (serum potassium of less than 2.5 mEq/L) can cause muscle weakness, renal tubular dysfunction, and electrocardiographic changes. T wave depression, U waves, and ST depression are seen with progressive hypokalemia. Low potassium states are seen with inadequate dietary intake or from excessive gastrointestinal or renal losses. Hypochloremic states from gastric losses or diuretic therapy will enhance renal potassium excretion. Potassium chloride can be given safely in concentrations of up to 40 mEq per liter in parenteral fluids. Higher concentrations should be given only when clearly indicated, in a monitored setting, to reduce the risk of hyperkalemia. In extreme circumstances, an infusion of 0.5 mEq per kg of potassium chloride over 30 to 60 minutes may be given to pediatric patients to correct severe potassium deficits. Such infusions should be administered only in an ICU setting with constant electrocardiographic monitoring.

Falsely elevated serum potassium levels are often seen as the result of hemolysis of red blood cells from blood collection in pediatric patients. True hyperkalemia (potassium levels greater than 5.5 mEq/L) may be precipitated by acidosis, administration of excessive potassium, adrenal insufficiency, massive cellular destruction, or renal failure. Signs and symptoms of hyperkalemia are predominantly cardiac. Electrophysiologic changes with increasing potassium levels include peaked T waves, first degree AV block, loss of P waves, widened QRS, sine wave formation, ventricular tachycardia or fibrillation, and asystole. If serum potassium levels are greater than 5.5 mEq per liter, all supplemental potassium should be discontinued. If levels are greater than 6.5 mEq per liter or ECG changes are present, immediate treatment to lower serum levels should be started (Table 6–5). Calcium given by slow intravenous push will temporarily counteract the electrophysiologic effects of hyperkalemia. This may cause bradycardia and should be used only in a monitored setting. Sodium bicarbonate given parenterally will raise the blood pH and cause potassium temporarily to move intracellularly. Similarly, glucose and insulin will cause a shift of potassium from the extracellular to the intracellular space. Lowering the body's potassium load can be accomplished by the oral or rectal administration of an exchange resin such as sodium polystyrene sulfonate (Kayexalate). Potassium is most effectively removed by dialysis.

CONCLUSION AND EXAMPLE: SALICYLATE POISONING

A wide spectrum of fluid and electrolyte derangements occurs in childhood poisonings. The patient's age and underlying state of health, the specific toxin and amount of exposure, and the magnitude and duration of resulting symptoms all affect fluid and electrolyte status. A prime example of the importance of early recognition and aggressive management of fluid and electrolyte disorders is seen in salicylate poisoning.

Salicylate intoxication (also see Chapter 51) is a complex poisoning, producing fever, central nervous system symptoms (lethargy, seizures, or coma), disorders of glucose metabolism, acid-base derangements, dehydration, and electrolyte abnormalities. Dehydration results from fever, increased metabolic demands, hyperventilation, vomiting, decreased oral intake, and obligatory renal water losses. Fluid deficits may be severe. Hypernatremia can be seen from the marked increase in insensible water loss. Hypokale-

Table 6–5. THERAPY FOR HYPERKALEMIA

DRUG	DOSE AND ROUTE	ONSET (DURATION)	MODE OF ACTION	COMMENTS
1. Calcium gluconate, 10% (100 mg/ml)	20 mg/kg IV over 5 min. May repeat × 2	Immediate (30–60 min)	Counteracts electrophysiologic effects of hyperkalemia	Monitor ECG for bradycardia. Stop infusion if heart rate < 100
2. Sodium bicarbonate, 7.5% (1 mEq/ml)	1–2 mEq/kg IV bolus or infusion over 20 min	20 min (1–4 hr)	Causes movement of K into cells	Assure adequate ventilation. Do not administer simultaneously with calcium gluconate: will precipitate
Glucose plus	1–2 gm/kg (5–10 ml of 20% dextrose)	15–30 min (3–6 hr)	Same	
Insulin	0.3 unit/gm of glucose. Administer by infusion together over 2 hr	15–30 min (3–6 hr)	Same	Monitor blood glucose
3. Sodium polystyrene sulfonate (Kayexalate)	1 gm/kg PO in 70% sorbitol or PR in 30% sorbitol every 6 hr		Removal of K from body	Removes 1 mEq of K/gm resin: 1 gm resin = 4.1 mEq Na. Watch for volume overload due to Na. Do not administer with Mg- or Al-containing antacids, since it may cause obstipation
4. Dialysis				Do not ignore 1, 2, and 3 while preparing for 4

(From Maxwell LG, Firush BA, McLean RH: Renal failure. *In* Rogers MC (ed): Textbook of Pediatric Intensive Care. Baltimore, Williams and Wilkins, 1987, p 1025.)

mia frequently results from obligatory urine losses and is further aggravated by iatrogenically induced metabolic alkalosis.

Parenteral fluid therapy in salicylate poisoning is directed toward replacement of deficits and enhancement of renal salicylate excretion. Fluid deficits should be estimated based on clinical presentation. Patients with severe dehydration should receive isotonic fluid as a bolus of 20 ml per kg to restore circulatory volume and urine output. Acidosis favors the intracellular movement of salicylate and should be treated with sodium bicarbonate. In addition, the renal elimination of salicylate is greatly enhanced by alkalinization of the urine. This may be accomplished by administering sodium bicarbonate as intermittent boluses (1 mEq/kg over several minutes) and by adding it to rehydrating fluids. Generally, 0.5 per cent normal saline with 1 ampule (44 mEq) of sodium bicarbonate added per liter will suffice. The amount of bicarbonate needed and the fluid rate should be adjusted to achieve a urine pH of 7.5 and a urinary output of 3 to 6 ml per kg per hr. It should be remembered that the addition of sodium bicarbonate can significantly increase the sodium load to the patient, producing or worsening hypernatremia. As in other hypernatremic states, serum sodium should be corrected gradually. Once urinary output is established, supplemental potassium chloride, 20 to 60 mEq per liter, should be added to correct potassium deficits. Overvigorous hydration can cause volume overload, cerebral edema, hypo- or hypernatremia, hypokalemia, hypocalcemia, or severe alkalosis. As with all critically ill patients, frequent clinical assessment and close monitoring of appropriate laboratory parameters is essential to provide optimal care.

References

1. Berkowitz ID, Rogers MC: Poisoning and the critically ill child. *In* Rogers MC (ed): Textbook of Pediatric Intensive Care. Baltimore, Williams and Wilkins, 1987, pp 1111–1178.

2. Finberg L, Kiley J, Luttrell CN: Mass accidental salt poisoning in infancy. JAMA *184*:187, 1963.
3. Finberg L, Kravath RE, Fleishman AR: Water and Electrolytes in Pediatrics. Philadelphia, WB Saunders, 1982.
4. Gruskin AB, Baluarte HJ, Prebis MS, et al: Serum sodium abnormalities in children. Pediatr Clin North Am *29*:294, 1982.
5. Robson AM: Parenteral fluid therapy. *In* Behrman RE, Vaughan VC (eds): Nelson Textbook of Pediatrics. Philadelphia, WB Saunders, 1983, pp 228–249.

CHAPTER 7
ACID-BASE BALANCE

James F. McAnally, M.D.

Perhaps nowhere in the practice of medicine is a knowledge of acid-base homeostasis more required than in the management of the poisoned or drug-overdosed patient. In this setting, the biochemical and physiologic data of the basic researcher are transformed into the diagnostic and therapeutic principles of the clinician.

In a poisoned patient, acid-base homeostasis may be disrupted by a variety of mechanisms. First, acid-base balance may be affected as a result of the toxic substance per se, i.e., the ingestion of strong inorganic acids causing metabolic acidosis. Second, acid-base homeostasis may be affected as a result of a metabolite of the toxic substance, e.g., formic acid, a metabolite of methanol, causing metabolic acidosis in methanol intoxication. Third, acid-base status may be affected as a result of the dysfunction or failure of various organ systems. Cardiac, respiratory, hepatic, and renal failure occur with substantial frequency in the poisoned or drug-overdosed patient, and damage of these organ systems often leads to aberrations in acid-base control. Last, acid-base homeostasis may be affected as a result of a therapeutic intervention, e.g., gastric lavage leading to metabolic alkalosis, or the use of potent cathartics leading to hyperchloremic metabolic acidosis. In addition, and especially in these critically ill patients, hemodialysis, may induce changes in pO_2, pCO_2 and bicarbonate not uncommonly, particularly with the use of acetate dialysate buffer.

Not only is it important to understand acid-base homeostasis in the treatment of the poisoned or overdosed patient, but also it is equally important in the diagnosis. All too often an adequate history is not available, or a history is obtained from an anxious and hysterical individual, thus confounding attempts to make an accurate diagnosis. In addition, the "classic" findings described in textbooks may be obscured by the ingestion of more than one substance. Results of toxicology screens and plasma drug levels often are unavailable. Despite these limitations, it is possible to make an early and accurate diagnosis, if one approaches the patient's history, physical findings, and laboratory data—especially the arterial blood gases, electrolytes, anion gap, and osmolal gap—in a logical sequence. Establishing an early diagnosis in these critically ill patients may lower the associated morbidity and mortality substantially.

BASIC CONCEPTS OF ACID-BASE HOMEOSTASIS

The pH of body fluids, especially the extracellular fluid, is maintained within a narrow range, predominantly owing to the participation and interplay of several regulatory systems. The most important of these are the lungs and central nervous system respiratory control center, the kidney, and the various body buffer systems. Of all the buffer systems, the most important is the bicarbonate–carbonic acid system. Unlike other systems, both variables, namely, extracellular bicarbonate and partial pressure of carbon dioxide or pCO_2, can be regulated independently.

The serum bicarbonate represents the metabolic component and is regulated in large part by renal mechanisms; the pCO_2 represents the respiratory component and is regulated in large part by the central nervous system respiratory center and pulmonary mechanisms.

Endogenous production of carbon dioxide leads to an increase in its concentration, which combines with water in various body fluids to form carbonic acid. Carbonic acid, in turn, readily dissociates according to the following equation to form hydrogen ion and bicarbonate:

$$CO_2 + H_2O \rightleftharpoons H_2CO_3 \rightleftharpoons H^+ + HCO_3^-$$

From this equation the Henderson-Hasselbalch equation is derived:

$$pH = pKa + \log \frac{[HCO_3^-]}{[pCO_2]}$$

Several terms involved in this equation should be understood: pH, or the negative logarithm of hydrogen ion concentration, is a reflection of plasma acidity and represents the balance between serum bicarbonate, the metabolic component, and the partial pressure of carbon dioxide, the respiratory component. The normal serum bicarbonate is approximately 24 to 28 mEq/L; the normal partial pressure carbon dioxide is 36 to 44 mm Hg.

Definitions

Acidemia-Alkalemia: The pH reflects the degree of plasma acidity. A pH of less than 7.36 is defined as acidemia, and a pH of greater than 7.44 is defined as alkalemia. Note that the pH does not provide information regarding the origin of disorder—that is, whether it is metabolic or respiratory—nor does it provide information regarding whether the physiologic compensatory response to the initial disorder is appropriate.

Acidosis and alkalosis refer to the pathophysiologic processes that, if left unopposed, can alter plasma acidity and thus change the plasma pH. If the initial change in bicarbonate or pCO_2 is severe enough to override the body's buffer and defense mechanisms, then acidemia or alkalemia will ensue. Note, however, that acidosis or alkalosis can be present without concomitant acidemia and alkalemia, respectively. For example, a patient with severe lactic metabolic acidosis secondary to hypotension and sepsis can have concomitant respiratory alkalosis secondary to the central nervous system effects of septicemia, and it may be severe enough to cause the pH to be normal or frankly alkalemic, despite the presence of metabolic acidosis.

Metabolic-Respiratory: A metabolic acid-base disorder refers to a disorder caused by a change in the serum bicarbonate. Metabolic acidosis can be defined as an acid-base disorder caused by a decrease in the serum bicarbonate level to less than 24 mEq/L. Metabolic alkalosis can be defined as an acid-base disorder caused by an increase in the serum bicarbonate level to greater than 28 mEq/L. A respiratory acid-base disorder refers to a disorder caused by a change in the pCO_2. Respiratory acidosis can be defined as an acid-base disorder caused by an increase in the pCO_2 of greater than 44 mm Hg. Respiratory alkalosis can be defined as an acid-base disorder caused by a decrease in the CO_2 of less than 36 mm Hg.

Regardless of the cause of the initial acid-base disorder, it sets into motion various defense mechanisms designed to minimize the ensuing change in pH. Metabolic acidosis leads to secondary hyperventilation and a decrease in the pCO_2, whereas metabolic alkalosis leads to secondary hypoventilation and increase in the pCO_2. Respiratory acidosis leads to increased renal reabsorption of bicarbonate and net acid excretion, which increases the serum bicarbonate, whereas respiratory alkalosis leads to an increase in renal excretion of bicarbonate, which decreases the serum bicarbonate.

These defense mechanisms possess the quality of appropriateness. They are physiologic responses that tend to be proportional to the magnitude of the initial disorder and tend to restore the pH toward normal, but never completely to normal. For example, a patient with mild respiratory acidosis would be expected to have a proportionately mild increase in the serum bicarbonate, whereas a patient with marked respiratory acidosis would be expected to have a proportionately marked increment in the serum bicarbonate. It would be inappropriate and unphysiologic for the patient with marked respiratory acidosis to have only a mild or no increase in the serum bicarbonate.

Simple/Mixed Acid-Base Disorders: A simple acid-base disorder can be defined as a single acid-base disorder with its appropriate accompanying secondary physiologic response. A response outside the predicted range would be inappropriate and would imply the coexistence of another primary disorder. A mixed acid-base disorder can be defined as the coexistence of two or more primary acid-base disorders. Knowledge of the formulas that predict the expected secondary response allows one to establish the diagnosis of mixed acid-base disorders. Since none of the causes of acid-base disorders are mutually exclusive, it is not surprising that mixed acid-base disorders occur with considerable frequency, especially in critically ill patients, such as the poisoned or drug-overdosed patient. Common examples of the occurrence of mixed acid-base disorders in poisoning include salicylate poisoning leading to both metabolic acidosis and respiratory alkalosis and ethanol poisoning leading to the development of lactic acidosis and metabolic acidosis as well as to respiratory acidosis secondary to its central nervous system–depressing effects. A detailed review of the subject has been provided by Narins and Emmett.[1]

METABOLIC ACIDOSIS

Metabolic acidosis is defined as an acid-base disturbance characterized by a decrease in a subject's serum bicarbonate level to less than 24 mEq/L. Usually, but not always, this fall in bicarbonate is associated with a fall in pH to less than 7.36 and thus results in acidemia. In general, metabolic acidosis develops by one of the following mechanisms: (1) loss of extracellular bicarbonate greater than extracellular chloride, e.g., diarrhea, renal tubular acidosis; (2) gain of hydrogen ion either exogenously or endogenously and subsequent consumption of extracellular bicarbonate, e.g., methanol ingestion, lactic acidosis; (3) failure to excrete the daily acid load, or renal failure; or (4) dilution of extracellular bicarbonate.

As a result of the initial fall in the serum bicarbonate level and subsequent acidemia, secondary mechanisms are initiated that prevent drastic changes in the pH and tend to return the pH toward normal. These mechanisms include extracellular buffering, intracellular buffering, the renal excretion of the acid load, and the respiratory compensatory response. Bicarbonate is the most important extracellular buffer. Initially, following an acid load, extracellular bicarbonate will immediately buffer almost the entire acid load, mEq for mEq. After several hours intracellular buffers also participate in the defense of pH and will buffer approximately 55 to 60 per cent of the acid load.[2] The excess extracellular hydrogen ion enters the cell and is exchanged for intracellular sodium and potassium. However, metabolic disorders tend to cause a greater shift of intracellular potassium to the extracellular space than do respiratory disorders.[3] In addition, changes in serum bicarbonate can cause shifts of potassium without concomitant changes in pH.[4] Lastly, because organic acid anions (ketoacids, lactic acid) can enter the cell with the excess hydrogen ion whereas chloride cannot, organic acidosis does not cause significant potassium redistribution as compared with mineral acidoses, such as with hydrochloric acid.[5–7] Although these mechanisms act in concert to minimize drastic changes in the pH, only the kidney possesses the ability to generate new bicarbonate by excreting the excess hydrogen ion. This process begins early but takes several days and occurs by way of an increase in both ammonium excretion and titratable acidity.[8]

The initial fall in pH stimulates ventilation as part of the respiratory compensatory response. This response appears to be mediated by peripheral chemoreceptors[9, 10] and by medullary receptors in the central nervous system that respond to changes in cerebral interstitial pH.[11, 12] A characteristic of this degree of ventilation is an increase in tidal volume rather than respiratory rate. Although this respiratory response occurs within minutes to hours, the maximum ventilatory response to metabolic acidosis may take 12 to 24 hours.[13] This is probably related to the slow movement of hydrogen ions across the relatively impermeable blood-brain barrier. This protective effect lasts only several days, probably because the reduction in pCO_2 lowers renal bicarbonate reabsorption and results in an inappropriate bicarbonate loss.[14]

The secondary hyperventilation should be considered as a secondary physiologic response to an initial aberration in homeostasis and thus should be proportional to the initial fall in serum bicarbonate. Albert and associates[15] have described mathematically the appropriate pCO_2 response for any degree of metabolic acidosis as

$$pCO_2 = 1.5\ (HCO_3) + 8$$

This formula defines the predictable relationship between the pCO_2 and bicarbonate for any degree of metabolic acidosis. From the clinical standpoint, a pCO_2 response outside the predicted range would be inappropriate and would imply the presence of a second primary disturbance (mixed acid-base disturbance). For example, a patient with severe metabolic acidosis and a serum bicarbonate of 10 mEq/L would be expected to have a pCO_2 of approximately 23 mm Hg. A pCO_2 significantly greater than 23 mm Hg would be inappropriately elevated and would, therefore, constitute concomitant respiratory acidosis along with metabolic acidosis. Likewise, a pCO_2 significantly less than 23 mm Hg would constitute concomitant respiratory alkalosis along with metabolic acidosis.

Causes

Metabolic acidosis can be divided into two general categories, based on the presence or absence of an elevated anion gap.[16, 17]

$$\text{Anion gap} = \text{serum Na} - (\text{serum Cl} + \text{serum } HCO_3)$$

The anion gap represents other unmeasured anions not accounted for by chloride and bicarbonate, such as plasma proteins and albumin, in order to maintain electric neutrality. The normal anion gap is 12 ± 2 mEq/L, with a range of 8 to 16 mEq/L.[18]

Elevated Anion Gap Metabolic Acidosis

Metabolic acidosis with an elevated anion gap results from the accumulation of organic and inorganic acids and subsequent fall in extracellular bicarbonate. The causes of elevated anion gap metabolic acidosis are listed in Table 7–1. The mere presence of an elevated anion gap has prognostic significance. Patients with an elevated anion gap have a greater frequency and severity of multiple electrolyte disorders, a greater frequency of admission to the ICU, and, more important, a greater mortality rate compared with patients with a normal anion gap.[19]

Table 7–1. CAUSES OF ELEVATED ANION GAP METABOLIC ACIDOSIS

Causes
Renal failure
Lactic acidosis
Ketoacidosis
Diabetic ketoacidosis
Alcohol ketoacidosis
Starvation
Isopropanol
Salicylate intoxication
Methanol intoxication
Ethylene glycol intoxication
Paraldehyde
Toluene
Miscellaneous causes
Formaldehyde
Ibuprofen
Rhabdomyolysis
Inborn errors of metabolism

It has been assumed that elevated anion gap acidosis is associated with readily identifiable increases in organic acids. However, Gabow and colleagues demonstrated that this relationship most often occurs only when the anion gap is greater than 30 mEq/L.[20] In patients with an anion gap of between 20 and 29 mEq/L, 29 per cent had no identifiable organic acidosis. The clinician, therefore, should be cautious in equating an elevated anion gap with an easily identifiable organic acidosis. Furthermore, measured organic anions contribute on average only 62 per cent of the increase in the anion gap. Changes in other charged substances, such as protein, phosphate, potassium, and calcium as well as the presence of D-lactic acid, 2-hydroxybutyric acidosis, and other organic acids, may account for this discrepancy.[20] Although it is common practice to equate elevated anion gap acidosis with lactic acidosis in the absence of positive ketones, renal failure, and drug intoxication, lactic acidosis was confirmed biochemically in only 43 per cent of the cases in which it was clinically suspected.[20]

The degree to which the anion gap is elevated can be helpful in identifying the specific cause of the metabolic acidosis. Solvent ingestion and salicylate ingestion usually are associated with anion gaps in the range of 15 to 20 mEq/L, whereas ethylene glycol ingestion, methanol ingestion, and lactic acidosis are often associated with anion gaps of greater than 35 mEq/L.[18]

Although metabolic acidosis is the most

common cause of elevated anion gap, it may also be present in metabolic alkalosis. Possible mechanisms for this include the coexistence of an elevated anion gap acidosis and metabolic alkalosis (mixed metabolic disorder) (see later), alkalemia-induced increase in lactic acid production, and an increase in the negative charges of plasma protein.[18] Other causes of an elevated anion gap include dehydration and therapy with sodium salts of strong acids and certain antibiotics.[16, 18]

Occasionally, organic acidosis, such as ketoacidosis, may be associated with normal anion gap metabolic acidosis if organic acid excretion and catabolism equal the rate of organic acid production.[21–23]

In elevated anion gap metabolic acidosis, the fall in the serum bicarbonate level is usually directly proportional to the rise in the anion gap because of the principle of electroneutrality. This simple reciprocal stoichiometric relationship assumes that the excess organic acids are buffered, mEq for mEq, by extracellular bicarbonate. Therefore, examining the relationship between the fall in serum bicarbonate and the rise in the anion gap allows for the diagnosis of mixed metabolic disorders. A decrement in serum bicarbonate greater than the increment in the anion gap suggests another mechanism causing a decrease in serum bicarbonate other than the elevated anion gap acidosis, such as hyperchloremic metabolic acidosis, and constitutes a mixed elevated anion gap–normal anion gap acidosis. On the other hand, an increment in the anion gap greater than the decrement in serum bicarbonate suggests another mechanism causing an increase in serum bicarbonate, such as metabolic alkalosis, and constitutes mixed elevated anion gap metabolic acidosis–metabolic alkalosis.

In prolonged metabolic acidosis, the excess hydrogen ion is buffered to a large degree by intracellular buffers, leaving the anionic counterparts in the extracellular space, and thus the increase in the anion gap may exceed the decrease in serum bicarbonate. Studies have shown that in lactic acidosis the ratio of change in the anion gap to change in the serum bicarbonate is approximately 1.6 to 1.[24] Furthermore, hypochloremia may occur in patients with elevated anion gap metabolic acidosis without an unrecognized metabolic alkalosis, presumably secondary to expansion of the extracellular space that occurs with release of cellular cations during the process of intracellular buffering.[25] Exercise-induced lactic acidosis, as well as seizure-induced lactic acidosis, however, is not associated with hypochloremia, and the increase in anion gap is proportional to the decrease in serum bicarbonate.[26, 27] Therefore, early in the development of elevated anion gap metabolic acidosis this reciprocal stoichiometry may hold. However, over time, with greater participation of intracellular buffers and cationic shifts, the increase in the anion gap may exceed the decrease in serum bicarbonate without a hidden metabolic alkalosis.

The clinician, therefore, should be aware of the potential presence of not only mixed metabolic–respiratory acid-base disorders but also mixed metabolic disorders, especially in the poisoned or drug overdosed patient.

Calculation of the *osmolal gap* also may be helpful in establishing the differential diagnosis of elevated anion gap acidosis. The osmolal gap can be defined as the difference between the measured and calculated plasma osmolality.

$$\text{Serum osmolality} = 1.86\,[\text{Na}] + \frac{\text{Blood glucose}}{18} + \frac{\text{BUN}}{2.8}$$

If the measured osmolality exceeds the calculated osmolality by 10 mOsm or more, then the presence of other osmotically active substances should be strongly considered.[28] Common causes of elevated osmolal gap include ethanol, methanol, ethylene glycol, isopropanol, mannitol, ethyl ether, acetone, paraldehyde, trichloroethane, lactic acidosis, ketoacidosis, and chronic renal failure.[18, 29]

Renal Failure

Acute renal failure (ARF) and chronic renal failure (CRF) are common causes of elevated anion gap acidosis. Unlike other causes of elevated anion gap metabolic acidosis which develop as a result of an increase exogenous or endogenous acid load, the metabolic acidosis of renal failure develops as a result of the inability to excrete the acid load presented. The organic anions that contribute to the elevated anion gap are mainly sulfate, phosphate, and other unmeasured organic anions. In chronic renal failure, the anion gap is usually normal until the glomerular filtration rate (GFR) falls to less than 30 ml/min. Below that level the anion gap increases to 17 to 23 mEq/L.[18] Occasionally, when tubulointerstitial disease occurs concomitantly with glomerular disease, hyperchloremic metabolic acidosis may also be present.

Numerous drugs and other intoxicants, such as analgesics, lithium, lead, and so on, may lead to the development of CRF,[30–32] but the drugs and intoxicants that cause acute renal failure often provoke life-threatening clinical situations.

Poisoning and drug intoxication should always be considered in a differential diagnosis of unexplained ARF. Although ARF may be associated with an elevated anion gap in the range of 16 to 29 mEq/L,[18] greater increases may be present in the poisoned or drug-overdosed patient. This may occur as a result of increased acid production secondary to hypotension, from sepsis, or from the catabolic effects of tissue injury. Greater increases in the anion gap may result from the effects of the ingested substances, such as aspirin, on intermediary oxidative metabolism and also from the effects of the ingested substances on renal function per se. Ethylene glycol and toluene can not only cause ARF, but also can elevate the anion gap independent of ARF. If tubular damage leads to the development of hyperchloremic metabolic acidosis along with elevated anion gap metabolic acidosis, then the potential for mixed metabolic acidosis exists.

A variety of mechanisms can result in ARF: (1) acute tubular necrosis due to direct toxic effect, e.g., mercury, arsenic, and other heavy metals; (2) intrarenal obstruction secondary to inordinate consumption of sulfate or secondary to oxalate deposition from ethylene glycol; (3) vasculitis secondary to amphetamine or cocaine abuse; (4) acute tubular necrosis due to myoglobinuria secondary to coma from a variety of agents, such as ethanol, heroin, glutethimide, and barbiturates, or secondary to intoxications producing seizures; (5) acute tubular necrosis due to toxic-ischemic injury from nonsteroidal anti-inflammatory agents; and (6) bilateral cortical necrosis due to arsenic.

Lactic Acidosis

Lactic acidosis is one of the most common causes of elevated anion gap acidosis in hospitalized patients.[20, 33] Often anion gaps are greater than 35 mEq/L and can range from 18 to 67 mEq/L.[18] As noted, the diagnosis of lactic acidosis was confirmed biochemically in only 43 per cent of the cases in which it was suspected clinically.[20] Consequently, biochemical confirmation should be obtained when the diagnosis of lactic acidosis has important consequences.

Lactic acid represents a metabolic endproduct. It exists in equilibrium with pyruvate, from which it is generated by reduction. Redox conditions, such as hypoxemia, volume depletion, and hypotension, increase the reduced NADH:oxidized NAD ratio, which favors the formation of lactic acid. The only metabolic fate of lactic acid is conversion back to pyruvate, which in turn is converted to glucose via the Cori cycle or to carbon dioxide and water via the Krebs cycle. The conversion of lactic acid back to pyruvate releases the extracellular bicarbonate buffer that was initially consumed during the generation of lactic acidosis. The normal serum lactic acid level is approximately 1.0 mEq/L, with a range of 0.5 to 1.5 mEq/L.

Lactic acidosis can develop as a result of increased production or decreased catabolism of lactic acid or from a variety of miscellaneous reasons. Most cases of lactic acidosis display components of both. Increased production of lactic acid may occur with an increased production of pyruvate, with little change in the normal lactate to pyruvate ratio of 0:1. However, most cases of increased production of lactic acid result from anaerobic metabolism when cellular delivery of oxygen or cellular utilization of oxygen is impaired, resulting in anaerobic glycolysis and increased production.

Lactic acidosis is an unfortunate yet common clinical feature of the severely poisoned or drug-overdosed patient. It may occur alone or be superimposed on another form of acidosis, such as alcohol ketoacidosis, methanol intoxication, and salicylate poisoning. Pathophysiologic mechanisms that lead to the development of lactic acidosis include (1) drug-related hypotension, as from central nervous system sedative-hypnotics; (2) drug-related seizures, as from cocaine, theophylline; (3) drug-related respiratory failure or aspiration pneumonia with a subsequent pO_2 of less than 35 mm Hg, as with paraquat and heroin; (4) drug-related hepatic failure, as with carbon tetrachloride and paracetamol; or (5) as a result of the specific effects of the ingested substance on lactic acid metabolism, as with cyanide. Table 7–2 lists the causes of lactic acidosis in the poisoned or drug-overdosed patient.

The clinical picture of lactic acidosis is profound. Common presentations include weakness, anorexia, impaired mentation often associated with hypotension, tachycardia, and hyperventilation. Blood lactate levels are uniformly elevated, and the greater the blood lactate level the worse the prognosis.[34]

Early in the development of lactic acidosis, the fall in serum bicarbonate is associated with a concomitant rise in the anion gap.[26, 27] When intracellular buffers begin to participate in the handling of excess generated hydrogen ion, the increase in anion gap may exceed the fall in serum bicarbonate.[24]

Although respiratory acid-base disorders, especially respiratory alkalosis, may occur with lactic acidosis, the majority of patients with lactic acidosis manifest a pCO_2 within the 95 per cent predicted confidence limits for metabolic acidosis.[35] Another laboratory feature of lactic acidosis is hyperphosphatemia in the absence of renal failure. A serum phosphate to serum creatinine ratio of greater than 3 strongly suggests the presence of lactic acidosis.[36] Hyperuricemia also may occur with lactic acidosis, since lactate and urate compete for the same secretory mechanism in the renal tubule. Although hyperkalemia may occur during lactic acidosis, its presence is related to an increase in potassium production or to a decrease in potassium excretion, rather than intracellular potassium shifting to the extracellular space.[37]

Drug-Induced Lactic Acidosis. Ethanol intoxication is a common cause of lactic acidosis.[38, 39] However, no correlation between plasma lactate levels and ethanol levels exists.[39] Several factors may contribute to the elevated lactic acid levels seen in ethanol abusers. As a result of the oxidation of ethanol to acetaldehyde and then to acetate, the NADH:NAD ratio increases, thus favoring the conversion of pyruvate to lactate. Ethanol also can inhibit the utilization of lactate for glucose formation.[38] Additional factors that can contribute to the development of lactic acidosis in ethanol abusers are thiamine deficiency,[40] severe hepatic dysfunction,[41] and seizures.[27]

Table 7–2. CAUSES OF LACTIC ACIDOSIS IN POISONING

Drug-associated hypotension	
Drug-associated seizures	
Drug-associated respiratory failure ($pO_2 < 35$)	
Drug-associated hepatic/renal failure	
Specific ingestions:	
ethanol	papaverine
biguanides	paracetamol
methanol	chloramphenicol
ethylene glycol	strychnine
aspirin	nalidixic acid
isoniazid	fructose
iron	sorbitol/xylitol
cyanide	epinephrine/norepinephrine
nitroprusside	carbon monoxide
streptozotocin	

The biguanide derivatives, such as phenformin, buformin, and metformin, are well-recognized causes of lactic acidosis. Prior to being taken off the commercial market, phenformin, an oral hypoglycemic agent, was a common cause of lactic acidosis in the diabetic patient.[42, 43] Predisposing factors to the development of phenformin-associated lactic acidosis include age, ethanol abuse, cardiopulmonary disease, hepatic disease, and renal failure.[42] Studies have suggested that the lactic acidosis occurs as a result of inhibition of lactate utilization as well as an increase in lactate production.[44] Furthermore, the elevated anion gap metabolic acidosis of the biguanides may be a mixed lactic-ketoacidosis, since alteration of cellular redox and an increased NADH:NAD ratio result not only in an increased lactate pyruvate ratio, but also an increased β-hydroxybutyrate:acetoacetate ratio, shifting ketone formation to the undetectable β-hydroxybutyrate form.[45]

Lactic acidosis has also been reported in methanol intoxication,[46, 47] although the major cause for the development of metabolic acidosis in this setting is formic acid production.[48] Proposed mechanisms include decreased hepatic uptake and increased hepatic production of lactate during profound acidemia, the increased NADH:NAD ratio as a result of the metabolism of methanol to formic acid, and the associated hypotension and subsequent tissue hypoxia.

Similarly, while glycolic acid is the major etiologic factor in the development of metabolic acidosis in ethylene glycol intoxication,[48] lactic acidosis also has been reported in severe ethylene glycol intoxication.[49, 50] Proposed mechanisms include tissue hypoxia secondary to cardiovascular collapse, seizures, renal failure, and concomitant ethanol ingestion.

Salicylate intoxication also may be associated with lactic acidosis, which may be related to salicylate's ability to uncouple oxidative metabolism, leading to increased production of lactic acids, ketoacids, and other organic acids.[42, 51]

Acetaminophen (paracetamol) poisoning is another cause of lactic acidosis. The lactic acidosis may occur in two distinct periods:[52] (1) Transient elevated lactic acid levels may occur within 15 hours of the ingestion, before the development of hepatic necrosis, in over 55 per cent of patients.[51, 52] This metabolic acidosis is usually transient, remits spontaneously, and is relatively unimportant from a clinical standpoint.[53] Furthermore, there is a direct correlation between the plasma acetaminophen concentration and the lactic acid concentration, which suggests that the early form of lactic acidosis may be due to the direct effect of acetaminophen on hepatic lactate uptake.[54] (2) The second phase occurs with the onset of hepatic failure.[55] It has been demonstrated that acetaminophen poisoning is associated with a decrease in hepatic lactate clearance, as well as an increase in the peripheral production of lactic acid.[56] Since acetaminophen and related compounds are frequent causes of drug overdose, they should be considered in the differential diagnosis of a patient who presents with lactic acidosis of unknown etiology.

Isoniazid overdose also may cause lactic acidosis. This has been reported most often in children as a result of accidental ingestion or in adults as a result of suicide attempts. The lactic acidosis is most likely due to increased lactic acid production secondary to seizures.[57]

Carbon monoxide is another cause of drug-induced lactic acidosis,[42] most often in the setting of smoke inhalation.[58] In carbon monoxide poisoning, carboxyhemoglobin production increases and results in oxygen being more tightly bound to hemoglobin. This leads to reduced tissue oxygen delivery, tissue hypoxia, and subsequent anaerobic metabolism and the development of lactic acidosis.

Fructose and other similar sugars also can be associated with lactic acidosis, since 30 per cent of fructose is converted to lactic acid, which may be enhanced by anaerobic conditions, liver disease, and concomitant ingestion of ethanol.[42]

Cyanide poisoning may be associated with the development of lactic acidosis.[42] Poisoning may occur as a suicide attempt or accidentally.[59] Cyanide inhibits electron transport and cellular oxidative metabolism, thus leading to anaerobic glycolysis. The severity of the lactic acidosis is directly proportional to the blood cyanide level. Common clinical presentations include the odor of bitter almonds, pulmonary edema, and severe metabolic acidosis.[42] In a similar fashion, sodium nitroprusside, which is metabolized to cyanide, also has been associated with lactic acidosis, especially with prolonged infusion rates of greater than 10 μg/kg/min.[60]

Cocaine poisoning may lead to the development of metabolic acidosis.[61] Although plasma lactate levels were not directly measured in the study of Jonsson and colleagues, the elevated anion gap metabolic acidosis was most likely due to lactic acidosis. Because of the increased prevalence of the use of cocaine and its derivatives, the clinician should consider cocaine poisoning in the differential diagnosis of patients with unexplained lactic acidosis. Although the pathogenesis of the lactic acidosis is not clear, it is most likely secondary to cocaine-related seizures and hypoxemia secondary to respiratory failure. Concomitant respiratory acidosis also may be present. Furthermore, cocaine can cause severe vasoconstriction, leading to anaerobic metabolism and increased lactic acid production. Similarly, a large amount of epinephrine, self-administered intravenously, has led to severe lactic acidosis.[62] Lactic acidosis also has been reported to be a complication of pheochromocytoma, presumably through increased vasoconstriction and increased glycolysis.[63]

Miscellaneous causes of drug-induced lactic acidosis include iron intoxication, streptozotocin poisoning, papaverine, strychnine, lye, chloramphenicol, nalidixic acid, sorbitol, and xylitol.[33, 42]

Treatment. Attention should be directed primarily at the underlying cause of the lactic acidosis. In addition, cardiovascular function, hypovolemia, hypoxemia, and ventilatory status should be improved. Although intravenous sodium bicarbonate has been standard therapy for this profoundly life-threatening condition, controversy exists regarding its use in the treatment of lactic acidosis.[64–67] (See treatment of metabolic acidosis.)

Dichloroacetate, which stimulates pyruvate dehydrogenase, the enzyme that catalyzes the oxidation of lactate to pyruvate, may also be helpful in the treatment of lactic acidosis.[68] Hemodialysis and peritoneal dialysis with bicarbonate buffer may be indicated in the treatment of lactic acidosis associated with volume overload or renal failure.

Ketoacidosis. Since alcohol ketoacidosis is a common clinical entity with potential for serious acid-base and electrolyte disturbances[69] and is part of the differential diagnosis of elevated anion gap metabolic acidosis in the alcoholic patient, a discussion of this subject is warranted.

Although the pathogenesis of alcohol ketoacidosis is not clear, several factors have been implicated. Depleted glycogen storage, poor caloric intake, and alcohol's direct suppression of gluconeogenesis[38] can lead to hypoglycemia. Hypoglycemia and the often concomitant volume depletion suppress insulin release and stimulate the secretion of glucagon, both of which are important factors in the development of ketosis.[70] Additionally, alcohol can directly stimulate lipolysis,[71] and its metabolism to acetaldehyde and ultimately to acetate allows for increased acetate availability for ketone production.[70, 72] The metabolism of alcohol also increases the NADH:NAD ratio, which in turn favors the conversion of acetoacetate to β-hydroxybutyrate; an increased β-hydroxybutyrate to acetoacetate ratio is a characteristic feature of alcohol ketoacidosis.

Clinically, alcohol ketoacidosis may occur at any age. There may be an individual predisposition toward its development.[70] Patients have a history of poor caloric intake, nausea, vomiting, and abdominal pain, often following a recent episode of binge drinking.[73–75] Ethanol levels are either low or undetectable. Mental status changes may be present, as well as evidence of chronic liver disease. Variable degrees of acidemia are seen, with the average anion gap being 25 mEq/L and the average plasma pH 7.16.[73] The nitroprusside reaction that detects only acetoacetate may be negative or only faintly positive, since the majority of ketone products are in the form of β-hydroxybutyrate. This syndrome may go unrecognized. Lactic acidosis also may be concomitant but usually occurs only as a result of a severe coexisting process, such as hypotension, sepsis, gastrointestinal bleeding, or ethanol intoxication.[39] Furthermore, in some patients with acute ethanol intoxication, alcohol ketoacidosis was not demonstrated, perhaps because of continued caloric intake in the form of ethanol.[39]

Although elevated anion gap metabolic acidosis is the most common acid-base disturbance encountered in alcohol ketoacidosis, the clinician should be aware of the potential for mixed acid-base disorders. Metabolic alkalosis may occur as a result of vomiting associated with volume depletion and hypokalemia.[72] Likewise, acute and chronic respiratory alkalosis may occur as a result of decompensated liver disease, alcohol withdrawal syndrome, and sepsis.

Blood glucose concentrations are usually normal but can be low in as many as 25 per cent of patients.[76] The presence of significant hyperglycemia raises the possibility of coexistent diabetes mellitus. Other electrolyte disturbances that may occur in this syndrome include hypokalemia, hypophosphatemia, hypomagnesemia, and hypocalcemia.

Treatment. Treatment consists of volume resuscitation with glucose-containing solutions, which usually reverses the ketosis within hours. Concomitant electrolyte abnormalities also should be corrected. The administration of sodium bicarbonate is rarely necessary and should be reserved for those patients with severe acidemia in whom adverse hemodynamic effects are present. Insulin is rarely necessary and in fact may be dangerous.

Isopropanol. Isopropanol is a clear, colorless aliphatic alcohol with a characteristic odor. It is found in a variety of solvent and cleaning products, often in combination with methanol, ethylene glycol, or ethanol.[77, 78] The most frequent source of isopropanol is rubbing alcohol, in which it is the main constituent. Ingestion may occur accidentally, often by children, or it may occur deliberately by adult alcoholics for use as a more potent substitute for ethanol. As little as 20 ml has been reported to cause symptoms; the lethal dose is approximately 150 to 240 ml of 100 per cent isopropanol.[79] Isopropanol is rapidly absorbed within 30 minutes, and approximately 80 per cent is metabolized to acetone by hepatic alcohol dehydrogenase and then excreted by the kidney. The remaining 20 per cent is excreted unchanged in urine.[80]

The clinical picture of isopropanol is similar

to that of ethanol, but in general it is more severe since isopropanol is approximately two times as potent. Isopropanol is a central nervous system and myocardial depressant. Common presentations include lethargy, stupor, and coma accompanied by hemodynamic disturbances such as hypotension, arrhythmia, and hemorrhagic gastritis. The clinical signs and systems, especially hypotension, are better prognostic indicators than is an isolated plasma level.[77]

Isopropanol ingestion leads to acetonemia and acetonuria, usually without hyperglycemia. Elevated anion gap metabolic acidosis rarely develops and, if present, is most often related to the presence of lactic acidosis secondary to concomitant ingestion of ethanol or secondary to hypotension and tissue hypoxia. Another cause for elevated anion gap metabolic acidosis may be related to the coingestion of adulterants known to cause elevated anion gap metabolic acidosis, such as methanol or ethylene glycol. The presence of a markedly elevated anion gap metabolic acidosis in the setting of isopropanol ingestion should alert the clinician to this possibility. In addition, since isopropanol can cause central nervous system disturbances ranging from lethargy to coma, one should also consider the potential for concomitant respiratory acid-base disturbances.

Isopropanol, like methanol, ethylene glycol, and ethanol, can also cause an elevated osmolal gap. For every 100 mg/dl of isopropanol, the serum osmolality increases by approximately 17 mOsm/L, and for every 100 mg/dl of acetone, the serum osmolality increases by 18 mOsm/L.[81]

Treatment. Treatment of isopropanol ingestion is largely supportive and consists of gastric lavage, preservation of vital signs—especially a patent airway, and maintenance of fluid and electrolyte balance. Early hemodialysis should be considered, especially with hypotension, coma, and serum levels greater than 400 mg/dl.[77, 82]

Miscellaneous causes of ketoacidosis include salbutamol, which can cause hyperglycemia as well as ketoacidosis in both normal subjects and diabetics,[83] and diazoxide.[84]

Salicylate Intoxication. Salicylate intoxication represents a significant cause of drug-induced morbidity and mortality.[81, 85–87] Salicylate intoxication can be classified into one of the following categories: (1) acute intoxication in children secondary to accidental ingestion or in young adults secondary to suicide attempts, with a mortality rate of approximately 1 to 2 per cent; death is often preceded by neurologic features and profound metabolic acidosis; and (2) chronic intoxication in older adults and occasionally in children, in whom there is often a delay in diagnosis and an associated mortality rate of approximately 25 per cent.[85, 86] The toxic dose is approximately 200 to 300 mg/kg.

Following oral intake, acetylsalicylic acid is rapidly absorbed, and approximately 40 per cent is converted to salicylic acid.[88] In usual therapeutic doses, approximately 90 per cent of ingested drug is protein bound,[89] but in toxic doses, plasma concentration exceeds binding and results in a greater percentage of the drug, unbound or free. Salicylic acid is excreted by renal mechanisms and depends on glomerular filtration rate, urine pH, and urine flow rate.[88]

Salicylate intoxication can produce a variety of complex acid-base disturbances.[90] Salicylate directly stimulates the central medullary respiratory center, leading to hypocapnia and respiratory alkalosis early in the course of intoxication. Later, elevated anion gap metabolic acidosis also may develop. The anion gap is usually less than 20 mEq/L, with a range of 10 to 34 mEq/L.[18] The pathogenesis of the elevated anion gap metabolic acidosis is not clear, although several mechanisms may be involved. By virtue of its ability to uncouple oxidative metabolism, salicylic acid stimulates the production of lactic acid, ketoacids, and other organic acids. Ketone products may be found in 25 per cent of the cases.[86] Respiratory alkalosis, which is a prominent feature of salicylate intoxication, promotes lactate production, this additionally may play a role in elevating the anion gap.[91] Lastly, salicylic acid, a weak acid, can increase the anion gap directly. A blood salicylate level of 100 mg/dl increases the anion gap by approximately 7.3 mEq/L.[92]

Since these two properties of salicylate are not mutually exclusive, mixed acid-base disturbances are common in salicylate intoxication. In a study of adults with significant salicylate ingestion, a mixed elevated anion gap metabolic acidosis–respiratory alkalosis occurred in 57 per cent of patients. In another 30 per cent of the patients, simple respiratory alkalosis occurred. In only 10 per cent of adults with significant salicylate intoxication did pure elevated anion gap metabolic acidosis occur.[90] Respiratory acidosis also may occur in salicylate intoxication, especially in patients with a history of chronic obstructive lung disease or pulmonary edema, and especially if salicylates are ingested along with central nervous system depressants.[90] In children under the age of 6 years, elevated anion gap metabolic acidosis is the predominant acid-base disturbance.[93]

The importance of recognizing the potential for complex acid-base disorders in salicylate intoxication cannot be overemphasized, since unrecognized cases have a substantial morbidity and mortality.[86] Therefore, salicylate intoxication should be considered in the patient with unexplained respiratory alkalosis, especially if combined with elevated anion gap metabolic acidosis. In summary, the older the patient, the smaller the ingested dose, and the earlier the patient is seen by medical personnel, the greater is the tendency toward the development of respiratory alkalosis. On the other hand, the younger the patient, the greater the dose ingested, and the later the patient is seen by medical personnel, the tendency is greater for the development of elevated anion gap metabolic acidosis.

Acetylsalicylic acid is the most common form of salicylate responsible for intoxication. The clinical picture consists of nausea, vomiting, hyperventilation, tinnitus, coma, asterixis, and seizures. Cardiogenic and noncardiogenic pulmonary edema may occur, the latter especially in elderly patients and in smokers.[94] In addition to the acid-base disturbances, other common laboratory features are hyperglycemia, ketonemia, and hypouricemia,[86, 90] abnormal liver function studies and abnormal bleeding time,[95] and proteinuria.[94] The diagnosis of salicylate intoxication can be made rapidly by a urine ferric chloride test or a Phenistix test or by obtaining a plasma salicylate level.

Treatment. The treatment of salicylate intoxication is largely supportive including maintenance of vital signs and adequate ventilation, cleansing of the gastrointestinal tract and maintenance of volume and electrolyte balance. Arterial blood gases, serum electrolytes, urine pH, and plasma salicylate levels should be monitored carefully. Salicylate exists in both ionized and un-ionized form. The un-ionized form freely penetrates cell membranes and at the renal tubular level is reabsorbed, whereas the ionized form does not readily penetrate cells and remains trapped in the tubular lumen. With a pKa of 3, most of the drug is ionized at alkaline pH. Although forced alkaline diuresis has long been recommended to enhance salicylate excretion, recent studies have suggested that urinary alkalization alone may be as effective as forced alkaline diuresis without the associated risk of volume overload, pulmonary edema, and electrolyte disturbances.[96] Carbonic anhydrase inhibitors, although effective, may lead to worsening of the metabolic acidosis and should be avoided.[97] Hemodialysis is indicated, especially with volume overload, coma, or renal failure, or hemodynamic instability associated with a plasma salicylate level of greater than 70 to 80 mg. Hemodialysis not only will remove the offending agent, but also will correct the volume overload and metabolic acidosis.[98]

Methanol. Methanol is a widely used solvent found in a variety of compounds, including paints, antifreeze, windshield fluid, photocopy fluid, and bootleg whiskey. It has been proposed as a substitute fuel for gasoline, which may increase the number of intoxications.

Methanol intoxication may occur sporadically and also in epidemics, especially in prisons with illicit whiskey as the source.[99, 100] The minimal lethal dose is 30 ml of absolute methanol.[101]

Methanol itself is nontoxic, but it is metabolized by hepatic alcohol dehydrogenase to the toxic compounds formaldehyde and formic acid. Formic acid is subsequently oxidized to CO_2 and water via a folate-dependent mechanism. It has been suggested that the folate acid deficiency commonly seen in alcohol abusers may enhance and prolong the formic acidosis.[102] Because the metabolism of methanol to formaldehyde and formic acid occurs slowly over a period of 12 to 18 hours, a latent period exists from the time of ingestion until formic acid accumulates and subsequent clinical signs and symptoms develop.[99, 100]

Methanol ingestion may lead to a serious and life-threatening metabolic acidosis, with extremely elevated anion gaps—frequently greater than 35 and occasionally greater than 50—usually developing 12 to 18 hours after ingestion.[18, 103] Controversy has existed regarding the cause of the elevated anion gap metabolic acidosis in methanol intoxication.[46, 47, 102–104] Several studies have demonstrated that the decrement in serum bicarbonate and the increment in the anion gap is explained by the accumulation of formic acid, especially in the early stages of methanol intoxication.[102, 104, 105] Other studies have shown that although the fall in serum bicarbonate and rise in the anion gap correlated with the plasma formate concentration, not all the fall in serum bicarbonate could be accounted for by the formic acid level. This has led to speculation that lactic acid and other organic acids may contribute to the elevated anion gap metabolic acidosis.[106]

Lactic acidosis has been reported to occur in methanol poisoning. It has been proposed that the oxidation of methanol to formic acid leads to an increased NADH:NAD ratio that in turn favors the conversion of pyruvate to lactate.[46, 47] Furthermore, formic acid has been reported to stimulate anaerobic glycolysis by inhibiting mitochondrial oxidative metabolism.[105] Concomitant ethanol ingestion or administration also may lead to the development of lactic acidosis.[46, 47] Significant lactic acidosis may occur in the later stages of methanol intoxication secondary to multiple organ failure and tissue hypoxia, which occurs commonly in methanol intoxication. With severe acidemia, lactic acidosis may result from decreased hepatic lactate utilization.[107]

Although elevated anion gap metabolic acidosis is the most common acid-base disturbance encountered in methanol intoxication, the absence of an elevated anion gap acidosis has been reported.[108, 109] This has been attributed to prior ethanol ingestion, or therapeutic administration of ethanol, which inhibits the metabolism of methanol and thus prevents the accumulation of formic acid.

In summary, the elevated anion gap metabolic acidosis encountered in methanol intoxication is multifactorial in etiology and depends on several variables, including the dose ingested, the time of presentation from ingestion, concomitant ingestion or administration of ethanol, and the presence of organ failure. The earliest presentations, especially those associated with small amounts of methanol ingestion, may be associated with little or no elevated anion gap metabolic acidosis.[100] Presentations 12 to 18 hours following ingestion of methanol are most often associated with elevated formic acid levels, whereas later presentations, especially in the presence of multiple organ failure, hypoxemia, and perhaps the administration of ethanol, may be associated with variable degrees of lactic acidosis.

Although elevated anion gap metabolic acidosis is the most common acid-base disturbance encountered in methanol intoxication, the absence of an elevated anion gap acidosis has been reported.[108, 109] This has been attributed to prior ethanol ingestion, or therapeutic administration of ethanol, which inhibits the metabolism of methanol and thus prevents the accumulation of formic acid.

The clinical picture of methanol intoxication consists of a variety of central nervous system manifestations, including confusion, drowsiness, ataxia, and in the later stages coma, often accompanied by a hyperemic optic disk and visual impairment.[99] Nausea, vomiting, and abdominal pain are also common. The abdominal pain has been associated with an elevated serum amylase presumably secondary to pancreatitis,[99] although an elevated amylase also may be a nonspecific finding in acidemic states,[110] and concomitant ingestion of ethanol also may be operative in the elevated serum amylase. In addition, an elevated amylase of the salivary type has been reported in methanol intoxication.[111]

In addition to the elevated anion gap metabolic acidosis, methanol intoxication may be associated with an elevated osmolal gap.[28, 112] The increased osmolal gap can range from 37 to 125 mOsm/L, and for each 100 mg/dl increment in plasma methanol concentration the serum osmolality increases by approximately 34 mOsm/L.[113] Concomitant ingestion or administration of ethanol may increase the osmolal gap to a greater degree than the anion gap, since ethanol prevents the metabolism of methanol to formic acid. Thus early presentations of methanol intoxication may be associated with a greater increase in the osmolal gap than anion gap, whereas later presentations may be associated with little or no osmolal gap yet marked increases in the anion gap. Lastly, although methanol and formic acid do not directly affect respiration, associated cerebral edema and other central nervous system damage may lead to respiratory acid-base disorders.

Treatment. The cornerstone of therapy is the administration of sodium bicarbonate to correct profound acidemia, ethanol to prevent the metabolism of methanol, folic acid to enhance formate oxidation, and bicarbonate hemodialysis to correct the profound acidemia and enhance the removal of toxic compounds.[114, 115] The clinician should also be alert to the acid-base disturbances related to these therapeutic interventions.

The mortality from methanol intoxication is approximately 20 per cent and is related to the duration and severity of the metabolic acidosis and the magnitude of the serum formic acid levels.[114, 115] The prognosis correlates poorly with the initial methanol level.[116]

Ethylene Glycol. Ethylene glycol is a colorless, odorless, intoxicating, water-soluble substance with a warm, sweet taste that contributes to its popularity among debilitated alcoholics.[49, 117] It is found in a variety of commercial products, including paints, lacquers, and plastics, and is the major component of antifreeze. Unlike methanol intoxication, which can occur in epidemics, ethylene glycol intoxication usually occurs sporadically in debilitated alcoholics who drink it in combination with or as a substitute for ethanol, in adults who imbibe it as a suicide attempt, and rarely in children who ingest it by accident. The fatal dose is 100 ml.[49]

Ethylene glycol is nontoxic, but its metabolites are extremely toxic. It is rapidly absorbed following oral ingestion and is metabolized by hepatic alcohol dehydrogenase to glycoaldehyde, which in turn is rapidly oxidized to glycolic acid. Glycolic acid is further oxidized to glyoxylic acid, which can be converted to formic acid, glycine, or oxalic acid.[118]

Ethylene glycol intoxication, like methanol intoxication, can lead to a serious, life-threatening elevated anion gap metabolic acidosis, with anion gaps ranging from 11 to 58 mEq/L and the majority greater than 35 mEq/L.[18] Some controversy exists regarding the etiology of the elevated anion gap metabolic acidosis.[113] It has been shown experimentally that the fall in serum bicarbonate was due to buffering of the excess glycolic acid, whereas the fall in serum bicarbonate was proportionate to the rise in glycolic acid.[119] Likewise, in humans, it has been shown that glycolic acid levels correlated with elevation of the anion gap and contributed to over 95 per cent of the anion gap, yet small increases in lactic acid and β-hydroxybutyrate were also demonstrated.[118]

Although lactic acidosis has been reported as an important component of the elevated anion gap metabolic acidosis in ethylene glycol intoxication, on closer scrutiny lactic acidosis usually occurs in the later stages of the intoxication and appears to be related more to hypotension, seizures, concomitant consumption or administration of ethanol, and multiple organ failure rather than being a direct consequence of ethylene glycol ingestion, as has been reported.[49, 50]

In addition to the elevated anion gap metabolic acidosis, hyperchloremic metabolic acidosis also may occur secondary to either diarrhea or proximal renal tubular dysfunction.[120] Likewise, ethylene glycol intoxication may be associated with hyperchloremic metabolic acidosis owing to concomitant bromide poisoning, since bromide will be measured as chloride via a colorimetric method and thus will spuriously decrease the anion gap, preventing the expected increased anion gap due to ethylene glycol.[121] Additionally, since vomiting may occur in ethylene glycol intoxication, the clinician should be alert to the presence of metabolic alkalosis and mixed elevated anion gap metabolic alkalosis. Furthermore, respiratory acid-base disorders may occur, especially in central nervous system depression and cardiopulmonary failure.[49, 117]

The clinical features of ethylene glycol intoxication have been divided into three stages.[49, 117] The first stage resembles ethanol intoxication and may be accompanied at the beginning by significant anion gap metabolic acidosis. Neurologic manifestations are predominant and are usually seen 30 minutes to 12 hours following ingestion. Common presentations include nausea, vomiting, seizures, and coma. The second stage is seen 12 to 24 hours after ingestion and consists predominantly of cardiorespiratory manifestations, including dyspnea, tachycardia, hyperventilation, hypertension, pulmonary edema, and congestive heart failure. The third stage is seen 24 to 72 hours after ingestion and consists predominantly of ARF.

Like methanol, ethylene glycol may be associated with an increased osmolal gap.[28, 112] For each 100-mg/dl increment in ethylene glycol plasma concentration, the serum osmolality increases by 17 mOsm/L.[112] Since the osmolal gap depends on significant plasma levels of ethylene glycol, early in the course of intoxication the osmolal gap may be significantly elevated. Late in the course of intoxication, when the majority of ethylene glycol has been metabolized to its toxic compounds, the osmolal gap may be normal, although significant elevated anion gap metabolic acidosis would be present.

In addition to elevated anion gap metabolic acidosis and osmolal gap, other laboratory features of ethylene glycol intoxication include hypocalcemia often leading to tetany, leukocytosis in the absence of sepsis, proteinuria, hematuria, pyuria, and profound crystalluria.[117, 122] Examination of the urinary sediment demonstrates calcium oxalate monohydrate crystals and calcium oxalate dihydrate crystals. Since crystalluria depends on the formation of oxalic acid and its subsequent precipitation with calcium, it may be absent at the time of admission and, therefore, repetitive microscopic analysis of the urine should be performed in order to establish the diagnosis of ethylene glycol intoxication.[123]

The diagnosis of ethylene glycol intoxication rests on a high index of suspicion in the appropriate clinical setting. Since ethylene glycol is rapidly metabolized, ethylene glycol levels may be unreliable as a diagnostic tool. Determination of glycolic acid, the major metabolite of ethylene glycol and the predominant cause for the metabolic acidosis, has been reported to be valuable in the diagnosis and management of intoxicated patients.[124] Unfortunately, glycolic acid determinations are not readily available in most hospitals. Therefore, a high index of suspicion must be mounted; an elevated anion gap metabolic acidosis, an elevated osmolal gap, and the presence of calcium oxalate monohydrate and dihydrate crystals on microscopic examination of the urine are strong clues to the diagnosis.[123]

Clinical toxicity depends on production of glycolic acid and the development of metabolic acidosis, as well as deposition of calcium oxalate in various organ systems including kidney, brain and myocardium.[113]

Treatment. The treatment of ethylene glycol intoxication consists of administration of sodium bicarbonate to correct profound acidemia, ethanol administration to inhibit the metabolism of ethylene glycol, and bicarbonate hemodialysis to enhance removal of ethylene glycol and glycolic acid, as well as other metabolites, and to correct the profound acidemia and often-present volume overload.[118, 120, 125, 126]

Paraldehyde. Paraldehyde is a colorless, pungent liquid that has been used in medicine for many years and on occasion can lead to elevated anion gap metabolic acidosis, especially when consumed in excessive quantities by chronic alcoholics.[16, 127, 128] Paraldehyde is metabolized predominantly to acetaldehyde and acetic acid and ultimately to carbon dioxide and water. Prolonged storage and exposure to sunlight can increase the decomposition of paraldehyde.

The genesis of the elevated anion gap metabolic acidosis is not well defined. Acetic acid levels do not totally correlate with the elevated anion gap.[127] Since oxidation of paraldehyde increases the NADH:NAD ratio, which in turn favors the conversion of acetoacetate to β-hydroxybutyrate, it is possible that the elevated anion gap metabolic acidosis can be explained by β-hydroxybutyric acidosis and also that cases of paraldehyde-induced elevated anion gap metabolic acidosis may have been simply undiagnosed alcohol ketoacidosis.[16] In addition, paraldehyde also can cause a false-positive ketone reaction, because it reacts with nitroprusside to give a positive reaction.[129]

The clinical presentation of paraldehyde intoxication is usually that of a chronic alcoholic presenting with abdominal pain, central nervous system depression, and the odor of paraldehyde on the breath.[16] In addition to the elevated anion gap metabolic acidosis, laboratory studies demonstrate marked leukocytosis in the absence of obvious causes.[16] Furthermore, in large quantities paraldehyde may cause an elevated osmolal gap.[29]

Renal tubular acidosis may also occur, thus leading to the development of hyperchloremic metabolic acidosis.[130] Uremic metabolic acidosis secondary to acute renal failure may be a complication. As with other intoxications, respiratory acid-base disorders may occur secondary to the development of pulmonary edema.[131] The diagnosis of paraldehyde ingestion rests on the exclusion of other causes of elevated anion gap metabolic acidosis. Treatment is largely supportive.

Toluene. Toluene is a colorless liquid used as an industrial solvent and found in a variety of substances, including model glues, paint thinner, and transmission fluid. Acute exposure occurs by deliberate inhalation for its euphoric properties, whereas chronic exposure occurs via inhalation at the work site.[132] The organic acids responsible for the elevated anion gap are unknown; however, toluene is metabolized to benzoic acid and hippuric acid, and an accumulation of hippuric acids and other organic acids may be responsible for the elevated anion gap metabolic acidosis.[18, 133] In addition, elevated anion gap metabolic acidosis may occur secondary to hepatic and renal failure, which are complications of toluene intoxication.[133] Lastly, in addition to the elevated anion gap metabolic acidosis, toluene exposure can lead to type I distal renal tubular acidosis[132, 134, 135] and type II proximal renal tubular acidosis associated with Fanconi's syndrome.[136]

Miscellaneous Causes of Elevated Anion Gap Metabolic Acidosis

Formaldehyde. Formaldehyde ingestion has been reported to cause life-threatening metabolic acidosis with an anion gap of 32.5 mEq/L and a pH of 6.7, presumably secondary to its metabolism to formic acid. Formic acid levels directly correlated with the fall in serum bicarbonate.[137]

Ibuprofen. Acute ibuprofen overdose has been reported to cause elevated anion gap metabolic acidosis in the absence of hypotension and ARF. Although lactic acid and ketoacid levels were not measured, the investigators speculated that the elevated anion gap metabolic acidosis was related to the accumulation of large amounts of ibuprofen and its metabolites in the serum. Ibuprofen and both its metabolites are weak acids and thus may contribute to the elevated anion gap.[138]

Rhabdomyolysis. Rhabdomyolysis is a rather common complication of poisoning and drug overdose and may occur as a result of a direct effect of the intoxicant, as a result of drug-induced seizures, e.g., cocaine, theophylline, and phencyclidine, or as a result of prolonged coma, e.g., ethanol, barbiturates, glutethimide. Elevated anion gap metabolic acidosis presumably occurs owing to the release of intracellular organic acid anions with the destruction of skeletal muscles.[139, 140]

Inborn Errors of Metabolism. The inborn errors of metabolism, including type I glycogen storage disease, maple syrup urine disease, isovaleric acidemia, propionic acidemia, and methylmalonic acidemia, may lead to an elevated anion gap metabolic acidosis.[141]

Normal Anion Gap Metabolic Acidosis

Metabolic acidosis with a normal anion gap (hyperchloremic metabolic acidosis) results from one of three mechanisms: (1) loss of fluid, with a bicarbonate concentration greater than the chloride concentration, (2) the addition of acids, with chloride as the associated anion, and (3) transient dilution of extracellular bicarbonate with nonbicarbonate solutions. In general, in normal anion gap metabolic acidosis, the principle of electroneutrality is maintained, and thus the fall in serum bicarbonate is associated with a proportionate rise in the serum chloride. For example, in diarrhea, bicarbonate loss is greater than chloride loss and thus hyperchloremia develops. Furthermore, the associated sodium and potassium losses lead to extracellular volume contraction, which in turn stimulates the renal retention of sodium with chloride rather than bicarbonate because of the increased availability of chloride, thus leading to the development of hyperchloremic metabolic acidosis.

Normal anion gap metabolic acidosis can be divided into hypokalemic and hyperkalemic forms. Examples of hypokalemic normal anion gap metabolic acidosis include diarrhea, laxative abuse, and renal tubular acidosis, whereas examples of hyperkalemic normal anion gap metabolic acidosis include obstructive nephropathy, type IV renal tubular acidosis, and occasionally diabetic ketoacidosis. Table 7–3 lists the causes of normal anion gap metabolic acidosis.

Diarrhea is the most common cause of

Table 7–3. CAUSES OF NORMAL ANION GAP METABOLIC ACIDOSIS

Diarrhea
Ureterosigmoidostomy/obstructed ileal conduit
Small bowel/pancreatic drainage
Anion exchange resins
Renal tubular acidosis
Primary hyperparathyroidism
Parenteral alimentation
Posthypocapnic state
Recovery phase of diabetic ketoacidosis
Dilution acidosis
Miscellaneous ingestions
Sulfur
Chlorine
Hydrochloric acid
Ammonium chloride
Calcium chloride
Magnesium chloride
Lysine hydrochloride
Arginine hydrochloride

normal anion gap metabolic acidosis. In poisoning or drug intoxication, numerous ingested substances can lead to diarrhea, such as colchicine, inordinate consumption of alcohol, various antibiotics and cholestyramine, an anion exchange resin exchanging chloride for bicarbonate at the level of the gut.[142] Although not usually considered a drug intoxication, covert laxative abuse should be considered in the patient with unexplained normal anion gap metabolic acidosis. Clues to this diagnosis include a neuropsychiatric history and a preoccupation with body image and bowel habits. Occasionally, patients may also induce vomiting or ingest concomitant analgesic preparations, leading to the development of renal failure and associated renal tubular acidosis.[143] Since carthartics are often used in the management of poisoning and drug intoxication, the associated diarrhea may also lead to significant hyperchloremic metabolic acidosis.

Renal tubular acidosis (RTA) represents a diverse group of functional disorders that have in common an inability to acidify the urine appropriately. Type I (distal) renal tubular acidosis is a disorder that results from the inability of the distal tubule and collecting duct to secrete hydrogen ion normally, thus leading to impaired urine acidification. Urine pH is usually greater than 5.5, and fractional excretion of bicarbonate is less than 5 per cent.[144, 145] The causes of drug-related Type I RTA are listed in Table 7–4.

Type II (proximal) renal tubular acidosis is mainly a disorder of the proximal tubule that results from defective reclamation of filtered bicarbonate load, leading to urinary bicarbonate loss. Urine pH is usually greater than 5.5 but can be less than 5.5, especially with systemic acidosis. The fractional excretion of bicarbonate is greater than 15 per cent.[144, 145] In addition to hypokalemic normal anion gap metabolic acidosis, patients with Type II renal tubular acidosis also may develop aminoaciduria, phosphaturia, glycosuria, and uricosuria (Fanconi syndrome). Table 7–4 lists the causes of drug-related Type II RTA.

Type IV renal tubular acidosis is a disorder of the distal tubule and collecting duct. It results from inability to secrete hydrogen ion and potassium normally, thus leading to the development of hyperkalemia and metabolic acidosis. Type IV renal tubular acidosis is probably not a single pathophysiologic disorder but rather represents a heterogeneous group of disorders, including primary aldosterone deficiency (primary adrenal insufficiency or isolated aldosterone deficiency), secondary or hyporeninemic hypoaldosteronism (diabetes mellitus, tubular interstitial disease), beta-blockers, and mineralocorticoid-resistant hyperkalemia (obstructive nephropathy and some forms of interstitial nephritis).[147, 148] Table 7–4 lists the causes of drug-related Type IV RTA.

Table 7–4. CAUSES OF DRUG-RELATED RENAL TUBULAR ACIDOSIS

TYPE I[146]
Amphotericin
Lithium
Toluene
Vitamin D
Analgesics
Cyclamates
TYPE II[145]
Outdated tetracycline
Carbonic anhydrase inhibitors
Cadmium
Mercury
Lead
Uranium
Toluene
Mafenide acetate
6-Mercaptopurine
Methyl-5-chrome
Streptozotocin
TYPE IV
Amiloride
Spironolactone
Lithium[149]
Triamterene[147, 148]
Nonsteroidal anti-inflammatory agents[150]
Angiotensin-converting enzyme inhibitors[151]
Cyclosporine[152]
β-Blockers

Ingestion of elemental sulfur, as well as the sulfur-containing amino acids methionine, cystine, and cysteine, can lead to the development of normal anion gap metabolic acidosis. Although the metabolism of sulfur leads to sulfuric acid and the potential for elevated anion gap acidosis, the sulfate anion undergoes rapid renal excretion, thus leading to the development of normal anion gap metabolic acidosis.[153]

Chlorine gas inhalation can occur from exposure to household cleaning agents and water chlorination systems and through industrial accidents. It may lead to the development of normal anion gap metabolic acidosis.[154] The exact mechanism for the development of the metabolic acidosis is not clear but may be related to the fact that chlorine combines with tissue water to form hydrochloric acid. Other intoxications that can lead to the development of normal anion gap metabolic acidosis include those from hydrochloric acid, ammonium chloride, lysine hydrochloride, arginine hydrochloride, calcium chloride, and magnesium chloride.

Although not considered in the setting of poisoning or drug intoxication, other causes of normal anion gap metabolic acidosis include small bowel or pancreatic drainage, ureterosigmoidostomy, obstructed ileal loop conduit, primary hyperparathyroidism, parenteral alimentation, posthypocapnic metabolic acidosis, the recovery phase of diabetic ketoacidosis, and dilution acidosis.

Recently the utility of the urinary anion gap in the differential diagnosis of normal anion gap metabolic acidosis has been demonstrated.[155] Since ammonium is an unmeasured cation usually accompanied by chloride, the urine anion gap becomes progressively negative as the rate of ammonium excretion increases. Since some patients with diarrhea may have a urine pH of greater than 5.5, it may be difficult to distinguish the normal anion gap metabolic acidosis of diarrhea from that of renal tubular acidosis. A negative anion gap suggests the presence of ammonium and thus appropriate urinary acidification, whereas a positive anion gap suggests impaired ammonium excretion and therefore distal renal tubular acidosis.[155]

Clinical Features and Consequences of Metabolic Acidosis

The clinical features and consequences of metabolic acidosis, especially those encountered in the poisoned and drug-overdosed patient, depend in large part on the specific cause of the intoxication. However, metabolic acidosis and acidemia per se may have significant clinical sequelae that depend on the magnitude and the rate of development of the metabolic acidosis and acidemia.

The cardiovascular effects of metabolic acidosis and acidemia are the most important and most life-threatening. Acidemia directly impairs myocardial contractility, yet indirectly has a positive inotropic effect by stimulating catecholamine release.[156] However, as the pH falls to less than 7.20, the negative inotropic effects become predominant. The heart rate increases as the pH falls, presumably secondary to the release of catecholamines. A fall of the pH to less than 7.10 however, may cause the heart rate also to fall. Acidemia may predispose to life-threatening ventricular arrhythmias.[157] Profound acidemia leads to arterial vasodilatation and venoconstriction, which increases central blood volume; combined with the negative inotropic effects, this leads to the development of pulmonary edema.

The hemodynamic consequences of acidemia can lead to a life-threatening vicious circle. As acidemia progresses, myocardial contractility becomes further impaired and cardiac output declines when central blood volume increases. The decline in cardiac output leads to further tissue hypoxia, generating lactic acidosis, which results in increasing acidemia, further impairment of myocardial contractility, and shock.

The pulmonary effects of acidemia include a change in respiratory pattern, with an increase in tidal volume and in the rate of respiration. Acidemia via the Bohr effect leads to a shift to the right of the oxyhemoglobin dissociation curve.[155]

The neurologic side effects of acidemia include a spectrum of consciousness from confusion to coma, which presumably relates to changes in the cerebrospinal fluid pH. Respiratory acidosis tends to have a greater effect than metabolic acidosis. Other factors leading to the development of neurologic symptoms include changes in serum osmolality as well as the specific underlying disease process or intoxication. Gastrointestinal side effects include abdominal pain, nausea, and vomiting, especially with ketoacidosis.

Although hyperkalemia is a common finding in acidemia, formulas that relate the serum potassium to pH may be oversimplified. Changes in serum potassium depend on the form of the acidosis, i.e., metabolic versus respiratory; the specific type of metabolic acidosis, i.e., mineral versus organic; as well as other factors, including changes in serum osmolality and changes in plasma insulin, aldosterone, and catecholamines.[158] Acidemia also displaces bound calcium, leading to an increase in ionized calcium.

Treatment of Metabolic Acidosis

The clinician should primarily tend to the treatment of the underlying cause of the metabolic acidosis. However, attention should also be paid to the metabolic acidosis and acidemia per se. Factors to consider include not only the magnitude of the metabolic acidosis, but also the rate with which it develops. For example, treatment of a patient with mild elevated anion gap metabolic acidosis secondary to lactic acidosis, and in the postictal state stable from the neurologic and hemodynamic standpoints, would be quite different from treatment of a patient with severe metabolic acidosis secondary to ethylene glycol poisoning with cardiovascular collapse, developing renal failure, and ongoing generation of organic acids.

Recently, controversy has surfaced about the use of sodium bicarbonate in the treatment of metabolic acidosis.[64, 65] Proponents of the use of bicarbonate recommend that it should be administered to maintain a blood pH of greater than 7.20, since a systemic pH of less than 7.20 is associated with adverse hemodynamic effects, including reduced cardiac output, impaired cardiac contractility, venoconstriction, arterial vasodilatation and arrhythmias.[64] Critics of this approach have argued that the administration of sodium bicarbonate not only is not helpful but also may in fact be detrimental.[65] This is based on experimental models of lactic acidosis[66] and the observation that in lactic acidosis associated with certain malignancies, alkali administration increases lactic acid production.[67] Because of this controversy, as well as known side effects of sodium bicarbonate, it seems prudent to use sodium bicarbonate judiciously in the treatment of metabolic acidosis. Consideration should be given to the underlying etiology of the metabolic acidosis, its severity, the rate at which the metabolic acidosis develops, and the clinical condition of the patient. At present, sodium bicarbonate administration should be reserved for patients with significant acidemia: a pH of less than 7.20 and HCO_3 less than 10 to 12 mEq/L, associated with hemodynamic instability.

Although several formulas have been suggested to express the bicarbonate deficit, based on a patient's body weight and the volume distribution of bicarbonate, these formulas at best should be used only as guides and should by no means be substitutes for careful clinical monitoring since they do not take into account the rate of generation of the acidosis nor the volume of distribution of bicarbonate. The volume of distribution of bicarbonate is not constant. Acidemia increases the volume of distribution of bicarbonate[159]—at a pH of 7.10, the volume of distribution of bicarbonate is approximately 80 per cent of total body weight.

The administration of sodium bicarbonate is not without complication. Because rapid bolus administration may be dangerous, it is recommended that large amounts of sodium bicarbonate be infused slowly over 30 to 60 minutes. Overshoot alkalosis occurs when the organic acids generated (lactic acid, ketoacids under severe reductive conditions) are oxidized to bicarbonate in a patient who is receiving large quantities of exogenous bicarbonate.

Sodium bicarbonate administration also may cause hypokalemia and hypocalcemia, with the attendant risk of producing cardiac arrhythmias. Large amounts of sodium bicarbonate may lead to volume overload, especially in the patient with hemodynamic compromise or pre-existing cardiovascular disease. If volume overload precludes the use of sodium bicarbonate, then hemodialysis or peritoneal dialysis should be considered, to correct not only the volume overload but also the acid-base disturbance.

METABOLIC ALKALOSIS

Metabolic alkalosis is an acid-base disturbance characterized by an increase in the serum bicarbonate to greater than 28 mEq/L. Usually, but not always, this increase in bicarbonate is associated with an increase in pH to greater than 7.40. Metabolic alkalosis represents one of the most common acid-base disturbances encountered in the hospitalized patient[160] and is also associated with significant morbidity and mortality.[161]

In general, metabolic alkalosis develops by one of the following mechanisms: (1) net gain of extracellular bicarbonate or one of its precursors, (2) net loss of hydrogen ion from the extracellular space, or (3) loss of fluid containing chloride greater than bicarbonate from the extracellular space. The metabolic alkalosis generated is maintained by a variety of factors, including (1) decreased glomerular filtration rate (GFR), (2) decreased real or effective extracellular volume, (3) hypokalemia, (4) hypochloremia, (5) hypercapnia, and (6) increased mineralocorticoid effect.[162, 163]

As a result of the initial increase in serum bicarbonate and subsequent alkalemia, secondary mechanisms are initiated that prevent drastic changes in pH and tend to return the pH toward normal. These mechanisms include extracellular and intracellular buffering, the renal excretion of the excess alkali, and the respiratory compensatory response. The excess extracellular bicarbonate is buffered by the addition of hydrogen ion to the extracellular space, which is derived from phosphate and proteins and from an increase in lactic acid production.

The initial rise in pH depresses the central and peripheral chemoreceptors and leads to hypoventilation and hypercapnia, which minimizes the initial increase in pH. The respiratory response, however, is not as predictable as it is in metabolic acidosis and is limited by the development of hypoxemia, which occurs as a result of the hypoventilation. As pO_2 falls below 70 to 80 mm Hg, the ensuing hypoxemia serves to stimulate ventilation,[164] which, therefore, counterbalances the effects of metabolic alkalosis. As a result, the respiratory response to metabolic alkalosis tends to be more variable. Rarely does the pCO_2 increase to greater than 55 to 60 mm Hg in response to the development of simple metabolic alkalosis. Furthermore, since the hypoxemia that develops is secondary to hypoventilation, as opposed to ventilation-perfusion, mismatching, diffusion abnormalities, or anatomic shunting, the alveolar-arterial oxygen gradient is normal.

In general, the pCO_2 rises 0.5 to 0.7 mm Hg for each 1.0 mEq/L increase in serum bicarbonate. From the clinical standpoint, a pCO_2 response outside the predicted range would be inappropriate and would imply the presence of a second primary disturbance or mixed acid-base disturbance. A pCO_2 less than predicted suggests the concomitant presence of respiratory alkalosis along with metabolic alkalosis, whereas a pCO_2 response greater than predicted suggests the concomitant presence of respiratory acidosis along with the metabolic alkalosis.

Causes

Metabolic alkalosis can be classified into three general categories: (1) sodium chloride–responsive metabolic alkalosis, (2) sodium chloride–resistant metabolic alkalosis, and (3) alkalosis of miscellaneous causes.

In sodium chloride–responsive metabolic alkalosis, a decrease in real or effective extracellular volume and hypochloremia are present, which serve to stimulate avid renal reabsorption of sodium chloride, resulting in a urine chloride of less than 10 mEq/L. Occasionally, however, the urine chloride may be greater than 20 mEq/L if the patient is taking diuretics and the kidney is under their pharmacologic influence. Patients with sodium chloride–responsive metabolic alkalosis demonstrate hypovolemia; correction of the volume depletion and the hypochloremia will correct the metabolic alkalosis.

In sodium chloride–resistant metabolic alkalosis, extracellular volume is normal to increased, due to an increase in mineralocorticoid activity. As a result, there is an increase in distal reabsorption of sodium and an increase in potassium and hydrogen ion excretion. A characteristic finding in sodium chloride–resistant metabolic alkalosis is a urine chloride level of greater than 20 mEq/L. Patients with sodium chloride–resistant metabolic alkalosis do not demonstrate signs of hypovolemia, and administration of sodium chloride does not correct the metabolic alkalosis. Treatment is directed at inhibiting the effects of the excess mineralocorticoid activity. Several miscellaneous causes of metabolic alkalosis do not fall into the aforementioned categories. Table 7–5 summarizes the causes of metabolic alkalosis.

Metabolic Alkalosis in Poisoning and Drug Overdose

Although metabolic alkalosis is a common acid-base disorder in the hospitalized patient, it is an uncommon primary disorder in the poisoned patient. However, it may develop in specific instances as well as in the form of a mixed acid-base disorder, often as a result of therapeutic intervention.

Sodium chloride–responsive metabolic alkalosis may occur in the poisoned or drug-overdosed patient. Numerous drugs and poisons can induce vomiting, either on the basis of stimulation of central nervous system centers or because of local irritation at the level of the stomach. In addition, induction of vomiting and gastric lavage are often indicated in the therapeutic management of the poisoned patient. In vomiting, hydrochloric acid is lost, thus, metabolic alkalosis is gen-

Table 7–5. CAUSES OF METABOLIC ALKALOSIS

SODIUM CHLORIDE–RESPONSIVE
Vomiting
Villous adenoma
Congenital chloride diarrhea
Diuretics
Posthypercapnia
Cystic fibrosis
SODIUM CHLORIDE–RESISTANT
Cushing's syndrome
Primary aldosteronism
Bartter's syndrome
Adrenogenital syndrome
Liddle's syndrome
Renal artery stenosis
Licorice ingestion
Chewing tobacco
Carbonoxolone
Capreomycin
Gentamicin
Severe potassium depletion
MISCELLANEOUS
Bicarbonate administration
Overshoot alkalosis
Bicarbonate precursor administration
Antacids–sodium polystyrene in renal failure
Milk-alkali syndrome
Penicillin, carbenicillin, ticarcillin
Nonparathyroid hypercalcemia
Poststarvation refeeding
Hypomagnesemia

erated and maintained by the concomitant volume depletion, hypochloremia, and hyperaldosteronism. Surreptitious vomiting and bulimarexia should be considered in patients with unexplained hypokalemic sodium chloride–responsive metabolic alkalosis.[165, 166] Although the exact prevalence of bulimarexia is not known, it is not uncommon in the college age population.[165] Often, because of an unrealistic concern for body weight and distorted body image, these patients will also abuse laxatives and diuretics and thus compound the potential for acid-base and electrolyte disturbances.

Diuretics such as thiazides, ethacrynic acid, furosemide, and bumetanide are probably the most common cause of metabolic alkalosis. Generally, diuretics are not considered as part of the spectrum of poisoning and drug overdose; however, they can be abused in a surreptitious fashion, leading to significant acid-base and electrolyte disturbances.[167] This syndrome has been most often described in women, especially those in the health care profession who are preoccupied with body image and weight control. In addition, in the absence of urine and plasma diuretic levels, this syndrome may be indistinguishable from Bartter's syndrome. Loss of sodium, potassium, and chloride leads to the generation of metabolic alkalosis and the accompanying volume depletion. Secondary aldosteronism leads to the maintenance of the metabolic alkalosis.

Other causes of sodium chloride–responsive metabolic alkalosis include villous adenoma, congenital chloride diarrhea, cystic fibrosis, and posthypercapnia.

Sodium chloride–resistant metabolic alkalosis also may occur in the poisoned or drug-overdosed patient. Drug-induced Bartter's syndrome has been reported following long-term administration of capreomycin, viomycin, and gentamicin.[168] Imported licorice and certain chewing tobaccos contain high quantities of glycyrrhizic acid, which possesses potent mineralocorticoid activity and can lead to metabolic alkalosis. Similarly, carbonoxolone, an agent used in the treatment of peptic ulcer disease, also can cause metabolic alkalosis. Exogenous steroid ingestion could also lead to sodium chloride–resistant metabolic alkalosis. Other causes include Cushing's syndrome, primary hyperaldosteronism, Bartter's syndrome, Liddle's syndrome, adrenogenital syndrome, renal artery stenosis, and severe total body potassium depletion.

Miscellaneous causes of metabolic alkalosis also can be encountered in the poisoned or drug-overdosed patient. Sodium bicarbonate ingestion, either in the form of tablets or baking soda, does not usually cause metabolic alkalosis since the kidney will respond appropriately and excrete the excess alkali. However, if the kidney's ability to excrete excess alkali is impaired or renal failure is present, then metabolic alkalosis may occur. Additionally, in the treatment of the poisoned patient, when organic acidosis occurs as a consequence and sodium bicarbonate is administered therapeutically, the clinician should be alert to the potential for overshoot alkalosis, since organic acids, such as ketoacids and lactic acid, can be converted back to bicarbonate.

Metabolic alkalosis also can occur when bicarbonate precursors, such as citrate, acetate, lactate, and gluconate, are administered. When oxidative metabolism is normal, these organic anions can be metabolized to bicarbonate. Whole blood contains 17 mEq/L of citrate, and packed red blood cells contain 5 mEq/L of citrate, thus in the volume-depleted patient who requires a significant number of blood transfusions, metabolic alkalosis could develop. Similarly, volume expanders, such as plasmatein, proteinate, and hyperalimentation fluid, which contain large quantities of acetate in the range of 40 to 50 mEq/L, may lead to metabolic alkalosis. Additionally, severe metabolic alkalosis has been reported with the use of regional citrate as an alternative to heparin anticoagulation for hemodialysis[169] and plasmapheresis in patients with glomerulonephritis who use replacement fluids containing large quantities of citrate as a preservative.[170]

Although orally administered antacids do not usually cause metabolic alkalosis, these are not without systemic side effects and are associated with increases in urine pH and bicarbonate excretion and a decrease in net acid excretion despite normal serum bicarbonate levels.[171] Metabolic alkalosis may occur in patients with end-stage renal disease ingesting "nonabsorbable" antacids, such as aluminum hydroxide or magnesium hydroxide, along with a cationic resin like sodium polystyrene sulfonate.[172] In this situation, the resin binds the cationic moiety—namely, aluminum or magnesium—and this renders the alkali more absorbable. If renal function is normal, there will be minimal or no change in acid-base homeostasis; however, when renal function is impaired, metabolic alkalosis can occur. Likewise, metabolic alkalosis can occur in patients with chronic renal failure following inordinate consumption of oral sodium bicarbonate in the form of baking soda.

Another instance when orally administered antacids can lead to the development of metabolic alkalosis is the milk-alkali syndrome. Patients ingest large quantities of calcium and absorbable alkali, particularly calcium carbonate, resulting in hypercalcemia, metabolic alkalosis, and renal impairment.[173] The chronic consumption of calcium-containing antacids leading to hypercalcemic metabolic alkalosis and renal failure is a well-recognized syndrome. It may also occur as an acute syndrome and, therefore, should be considered in the differential diagnosis of the patient with unexplained hypercalcemia, renal failure, and metabolic alkalosis. Since calcium carbonate is used frequently in chronic renal failure to control hyperphosphatemia, to treat osteoporosis, and to prevent peptic ulcer disease, it is quite possible that the incidence of milk-alkali syndrome will increase.[174] Metabolic alkalosis is generated as the result of the gastrointestinal absorption of orally administered alkali and is maintained by the development of renal failure, which precludes the excretion of the absorbed bicarbonate, and by the effects of hypercalcemia on bicarbonate reabsorption. Hypercalcemia increases tubular bicarbonate reabsorption directly and indirectly by suppressing parathyroid hormone, which normally causes a decrease in bicarbonate reabsorption.

Another cause of drug-induced metabolic alkalosis is the administration of large doses of sodium carbenicillin, penicillin, and ticarcillin. The penicillin combinations acting as impermeant anions in the distal tubule along with an increased sodium load to the distal tubule, act as potent stimuli for the excretion of potassium and hydrogen ion, leading to hypokalemic metabolic alkalosis.[175] Two miscellaneous causes of metabolic alkalosis are nonparathyroid hypercalcemia and poststarvation refeeding.

Finally, metabolic alkalosis may occur as a direct result of a therapeutic intervention, such as inordinate administration of sodium bicarbonate, alkaline diuresis, gastric lavage, bicarbonate dialysis, and so on.

Features

The features of metabolic alkalosis are in large part related to the specific cause; however, alkalemia per se has its serious side effects. Neuromuscular irritability is significantly enhanced in the presence of metabolic alkalosis, and this can be manifested as seizures, tetany, delirium, and hyperreflexia. Cardiac arrhythmias may occur in the digitalized patient secondary to increased sensitivity to digitalis, as well as in the nondigitalized patient.

In addition, as noted, there is a slight increase in the anion gap secondary to a mild increase in intracellular lactic acid generation, as well as, perhaps, an increase in plasma protein equivalency. Metabolic alkalosis also shifts the oxyhemoglobin dissociation curve to the left, rendering oxygen less available to tissues.

The concomitant presence of other electrolyte disturbances, such as hypokalemia, hypocalcemia, and a decrease in ionized calcium, hypomagnesemia, hypophosphatemia, and hypoxemia, can further complicate the clinical picture of metabolic alkalosis.

Treatment

The primary treatment of metabolic alkalosis is to identify and treat the underlying cause. In sodium chloride–responsive metabolic alkalosis, volume expansion in the form of saline and correction of hypochloremia will correct the metabolic alkalosis. Recently it has been suggested that chloride repletion can correct sodium chloride–responsive metabolic alkalosis, independent of changes in plasma volume or in glomerular filtration rate.[176] In addition, other electrolyte abnormalities, such as hypokalemia and hypomagnesemia, should be corrected. In sodium chloride–resistant metabolic alkalosis, inhibition of the excess mineralocorticoid activity will correct the metabolic alkalosis.

Occasionally, some clinical situations preclude this simplistic approach to the treatment of metabolic alkalosis. In patients with metabolic alkalosis who are volume overloaded, as in congestive heart failure, the use of acetazolamide, a carbonic acid anhydrase inhibitor, may be helpful, since acetazolamide will lead to enhanced renal bicarbonate excretion. In the patient with gastric alkalosis in whom continued vasogastric suction or protracted vomiting occurs, the use of cimetidine, which reduces hydrochloric acid secretion, can be useful.

In the patient with renal failure who has significant metabolic alkalosis, use of a dialysate with a low bicarbonate or low acetate concentration and a high chloride concentration can be useful.[177]

RESPIRATORY ACIDOSIS

Respiratory acidosis can be defined as an acid-base disturbance characterized by an increase in the pCO_2 to greater than 44 mm Hg. In general, respiratory acidosis develops because of a decrease in alveolar ventilation and rarely because of an increase in CO_2 production, especially in a patient with already compromised pulmonary function. As a result of the increase in pCO_2 and subsequent acidemia, secondary mechanisms are initiated that attempt to prevent drastic changes in pH and tend to return the pH toward normal.

Intracellular buffering, via red cell hemoglobin, phosphate, and protein, exchange intracellular sodium and potassium for the excess extracellular hydrogen ion. In addition, hypercapnia leads to an increase in renal hydrogen ion secretion and net acid excretion, as well as an increase in bicarbonate reclamation. Although this response begins early, the maximum effect takes several days.

In general, in acute respiratory acidosis, for each 10 mm Hg rise in the pCO_2, the serum bicarbonate level increases by 1 to 2 mEq/L. In chronic respiratory acidosis, for every 10 mm Hg rise in pCO_2, the bicarbonate level increases by 3 to 4 mEq/L. A serum bicarbonate level greater than predicted for the increment in pCO_2 would imply the coexistence of metabolic alkalosis as well as respiratory acidosis, and likewise, a serum bicarbonate less than predicted for the increment in pCO_2 would imply the existence of metabolic acidosis as well as respiratory acidosis.

Respiratory acidosis is one of the most commonly encountered acid-base disturbances in the poisoned or drug-overdosed patient. It may occur as a result of a specific drug ingested, or from complications of poisoning, such as coma leading to aspiration pneumonia or laryngeal edema secondary to corrosive poisoning. Table 7–6 lists the numerous potential causes for respiratory acidosis.

Features

The features of respiratory acidosis result in large part from both the increase in pCO_2 and the associated hypoxemia. Altered states of consciousness are quite common, as are abnormal ventilatory patterns, tachycardia and arrhythmias, diaphoresis, visual disturbances, headache, delirium, and coma. Many of the central nervous system effects are related to the increase in cerebral blood flow secondary to hypercapnia and subsequent increase in cerebral spinal fluid pressure. As in metabolic acidosis, the subsequent acidemia can have significant adverse hemodynamic effects.

Treatment

The treatment of respiratory acidosis is directed primarily at improving ventilation.

Table 7–6. CAUSES OF RESPIRATORY ACIDOSIS

CENTRAL CAUSES	
Drugs	
Opiates	Sedatives
Ethanol	Methanol
Barbiturates	Ethylene glycol
Anesthetics	
CNS Lesions	
Trauma	Infection
Tumor	Vascular accidents
NEUROMUSCULAR CAUSES	
Guillain-Barré syndrome	Botulism
Myasthenia gravis	Hypokalemia
Aminoglycoside toxicity	Pickwickian syndrome
Primary hypoventilation	
THORACIC-PULMONARY CAUSES	
Pneumonia	Smoke inhalation
Pulmonary embolism	Pneumothorax
Pulmonary edema	Chronic obstructive lung disease
Aspiration pneumonia	
AIRWAY OBSTRUCTION	
Foreign body	
Epiglottal/laryngeal edema (e.g., phencyclidine poisoning)	
Bronchoconstriction	

RESPIRATORY ALKALOSIS

Respiratory alkalosis is an acid-base disturbance characterized by a decrease in the pCO_2 to less than 36 mm Hg. In general, respiratory alkalosis develops as a result of an increase in the rate of alveolar ventilation. As a result of the decrease in pCO_2 and subsequent alkalemia, several mechanisms are initiated that prevent drastic changes in pH. Intracellular hydrogen ions exit to the extracellular space to exchange for sodium and potassium and neutralize the excess bicarbonate, thus minimizing the increase in pCO_2.

In addition, in response to respiratory alkalosis, the kidney decreases net acid excretion and bicarbonate reabsorption, thus tending to return the pH toward normal. As in respiratory acidosis, even though this mechanism begins early the maximal response does not occur for several days.

In acute respiratory alkalosis, the serum bicarbonate level falls by approximately 1 to 3 mEq/L for each 10 mm Hg fall in pCO_2, whereas in chronic respiratory alkalosis, the serum bicarbonate falls by approximately 3 to 5 mEq/L for each 10 mm Hg fall in pCO_2. A serum bicarbonate that is greater than predicted by this formula would imply the concomitant presence of metabolic alkalosis as well as respiratory alkalosis, whereas a serum bicarbonate less than predicted by the formula would imply the concomitant presence of metabolic acidosis as well as respiratory alkalosis. Furthermore, rarely will the serum bicarbonate fall less than 14 to 16 mEq/L as a compensatory mechanism for respiratory alkalosis. In addition, respiratory alkalosis was the most common acid-base disorder encountered in over 8000 arterial blood gas samples from the intensive care unit. It was observed that the greater the degree of hypocapnia and alkalemia, the worse the prognosis.[178]

Table 7–7 lists the causes of respiratory alkalosis, which occurs frequently in the poisoned or drug-overdosed patient. Salicylate ingestion is the most common cause of respiratory alkalosis in this setting. Other causes may be secondary to one of the complications of the drug ingestion, that is, cerebral edema, hepatic failure, sepsis, or mechanical ventilation.

Features

Like metabolic alkalosis, the main features of respiratory alkalosis are related to neuromuscular irritability and manifest as circumoral and digital paresthesias, carpopedal spasm, tetany, seizures, and altered states of consciousness. Many of these symptoms may be related to the effect of pCO_2 on cerebral blood flow, with significant hypocapnia lead-

Table 7–7. CAUSES OF RESPIRATORY ALKALOSIS

GENERAL
Anxiety
Salicylates
Brain stem lesions
Encephalitis and meningitis
Metabolic encephalopathy
Pregnancy
Tumors
Pain
Fever
Thyrotoxicosis
PERIPHERAL
Hypotension
Hypoxemia
Pneumonia
Congestive heart failure
Interstitial lung disease
Pulmonary embolism
MISCELLANEOUS
Mechanical ventilation
Sepsis
Cirrhosis

ing to a decrease in cerebral blood flow. Likewise, some of the effects may be related to alkalemia and its effects on ionized calcium, as well as on serum potassium. In addition, respiratory alkalosis and alkalemia may be associated with a small increase in the anion gap secondary to increased lactic acid production due to increased tissue anaerobic glycolysis.

Treatment

The treatment of respiratory alkalosis, as in other disorders, should be directed primarily at the underlying cause, as well as the magnitude of the respiratory alkalosis. When severe enough and associated with morbid complications, administering a rebreathing mask, or, if a patient is on a mechanical ventilator, increasing the dead space can increase the pCO_2 and decrease the degree of alkalemia.

MIXED ACID-BASE DISORDERS

A mixed acid-base disorder is defined as the presence of two or more primary acid-base disorders. The clinician should be aware of the possibility of mixed metabolic disorders. In view of the numerous potential aberrations in acid-base homeostasis that may occur in the poisoned or drug-overdosed patient, either as a result of the intoxicating substance or a therapeutic intervention, it is not surprising that mixed acid-base disorders occur with considerable frequency in these critically ill patients. Often the diagnosis of a mixed acid-base disorder can be strongly suspected based on the history and physical examination. However, only the knowledge of predicted compensatory response allows the clinician to establish the presence of a mixed acid-base disorder. This cannot be overemphasized, since the systemic pH in mixed acid-base disorders can range from life-threatening to normal values, and thus the presence of another acid-base disorder may be overlooked. Examples of mixed acid-base disorders that may occur in the poisoned or drug-overdosed patient follow.

METABOLIC ACIDOSIS–RESPIRATORY ACIDOSIS

A common example of mixed metabolic acidosis–respiratory acidosis is the aftermath of cardiopulmonary arrest. With respiratory and cardiovascular failure, lactic acidosis will develop because of hypoxemia and decreased tissue profusion. The subsequent respiratory failure leads to the retention of CO_2. Methanol and ethylene glycol also can cause mixed metabolic acidosis–respiratory acidosis. As noted, the metabolic acidosis most likely is due to the production of metabolites of these substances, namely formic acid and glyoxalic acid, and lactic acidosis to a lesser degree, whereas the respiratory acidosis may occur in the later stages of these intoxications because of respiratory central depression or aspiration pneumonia. Another common example of a mixed acid-base disorder that may occur in poisoned or drug overdosed patients is following the ingestion of central nervous system depressants, such as sedative-hypnotics and barbiturates. Depression of the respiratory central control mechanisms ensues, hypotension develops, oxygen utilization at the cell level decreases, culminating in lactic acidosis.

Another example of a mixed acid-base disorder is after the ingestion of agents that may cause the development of pulmonary edema, such as heroin and paraquat. If the resultant pulmonary edema is severe enough to impair ventilation, it may cause respiratory acidosis. If combined with significant hypoxemia, this can generate lactic acidosis.

METABOLIC ACIDOSIS–RESPIRATORY ALKALOSIS

Mixed metabolic acidosis–respiratory alkalosis also may occur in the setting of poison or drug overdose. Perhaps the most common cause for this acid-base disorder is salicylate intoxication. Metabolic acidosis develops as a result of the effects of salicylic acid on intermediary oxidative metabolism, and respiratory alkalosis develops from the stimulatory effects of salicylate on the central respiratory centers.

Severe liver disease also can cause mixed metabolic acidosis–respiratory alkalosis. Metabolic acidosis may develop as a result of decreased lactic acid uptake by the liver or from accelerated lactic acid production in the severe acidemic state. A remote cause is as a result of uremic acidosis in a patient with concomitant acute renal failure. The respiratory alkalosis of severe liver disease develops because of the stimulatory effects of ammonia and other biogenic amines on the respiratory center, as well as hypoxemia leading to ventilation perfusion mismatching, and the presence of hypoventilation because of diaphragmatic elevation. Agents such as carbon tetrachloride, acetaminophen, and other acute hepatic toxins may be associated with a mixed acid-base disorder.

METABOLIC ALKALOSIS–RESPIRATORY ACIDOSIS

This is an uncommon mixed acid-base disturbance in poison or drug overdose but could occur in a patient with chronic obstructive lung disease who develops metabolic alkalosis as a result of vomiting. The severe hypokalemia and hypophosphatemia that may occur in metabolic alkalosis can also lead to respiratory weakness and eventual respiratory muscle paralysis, thus generating respiratory acidosis.

METABOLIC ALKALOSIS–RESPIRATORY ALKALOSIS

Although metabolic alkalosis–respiratory alkalosis is a rather common mixed acid-base disturbance, especially in critically ill surgical patients, it is rare in poisoning.

MIXED METABOLIC DISORDERS

Mixed High Anion Gap Acidosis

As noted, a variety of organic acidoses may occur simultaneously, such as methanol and lactic acidosis, ketoacidosis, and lactic acidosis. The clinician should suspect the presence of this disorder when an increment in the anion gap exceeds the increase in the measured organic anion.

Mixed Elevated Anion Gap–Hyperchloremic Metabolic Acidosis

Here the decrement in the serum bicarbonate is greater than the increase in the anion gap. A poison or drug overdose or any intoxicant leading to severe diarrhea will result in hyperchloremic acidosis. If severe enough, hemodynamic compromise, the generation of lactic acidosis, and an elevated anion gap acidosis will occur. A similar picture can occur with a poison or drug that leads to interstitial renal disease, in which hyperchloremic acidosis may occur as a result of renal tubular acidosis; with a subsequent decline of the GFR, elevated anion gap acidosis occurs as a result of the retention of sulfate, phosphate, and other organic anions.

Mixed Elevated Anion Gap Metabolic Acidosis–Metabolic Alkalosis

This mixed acid-base disorder may occur in a patient who develops elevated anion gap acidosis and vomiting as a result of the intoxication. Examination of the anion gap will lead to the diagnosis of a mixed acid-base disorder. In this setting, the anion gap will be greater than the fall in serum bicarbonate; occasionally, the serum bicarbonate may be within the range of normal, despite the presence of this disorder.

References

1. Narins RG, Emmett M: Simple and mixed acid base disorders: A practical approach. Medicine *59*:161, 1980.
2. Androgue HJ, Brensilver J, Cohen JJ, Madias NE: Influence of steady state alterations in acid-base equilibrium on the fate of administered bicarbonate in the dog. J Clin Invest *71*:867, 1983.
3. Androgue HJ, Madias NE: Changes in plasma potassium concentration during acute acid-base disturbances. Am J Med *71*:456, 1981.
4. Fraley DS, Adler S: Isohydric regulation of plasma potassium by bicarbonate in the rat. Kidney Int *9*:333, 1976.
5. Oster JR, Perez GO, Vaamonde CA: Relationship between blood pH and K and phosphorus during acute metabolic acidosis. Am J Physiol *235*:F345, 1978.
6. Fulop M: Serum potassium in lactic acidosis and ketoacidosis. N Engl J Med *300*:1087, 1979.
7. Perez GO, Oster JR, Vaamonde CA: Serum potassium concentration in acidemic states. Nephron *27*:233, 1981.
8. Tizianello A, Deferrari G, Garibotto G, Roboudo C, Acquarone N, Ghiggeri GM: Renal ammoniagenesis in early stages of metabolic acidosis in man. J Clin Invest *69*:240, 1982.
9. Mitchell RA, Carman CT, Severinghaus JW, Richardson BW, Singer MM, Shnider S: Stability of cerebrospinal fluid pH in chronic acid-base disturbances in blood. J Appl Physiol *20*:443, 1965.
10. Berger AJ, Mitchell RA, Severinghaus JR: Regulation of respiration (third of three parts). N Engl J Med *297*:194, 1977.
11. Fencl V, Miller TB, Poppenheimer JR: Studies on the respiratory response to disturbances of acid-

base balance with deductions concerning the ionic composition of cerebral interstitial fluid. Am J Physiol *210*:459, 1966.
12. Keahny WD, Jackson JT: Respiratory response to HCl in dogs after carotid body denervation. J Appl Physiol *46*:1138, 1979.
13. Pierce NF, Fedson DS, Brigham KL: The ventilatory response to acute base deficit in humans: Time course during development and correction of metabolic acidosis. Ann Intern Med *72*:633, 1970.
14. Madias NE, Schwartz WB, Cohen JJ: The maladaptive renal response to secondary hypocapnia during chronic HCl acidosis in the dog. J Clin Invest *60*:1393, 1977.
15. Albert MD, Dell RB, Winters RW: Quantitative displacement of acid-base equilibrium in metabolic acidosis. Ann Intern Med *66*:312, 1967.
16. Emmett M, Narins RG: Clinical use of the anion gap. Medicine *56*:38, 1977.
17. Oh MS, Carrol HJ: The anion gap. N Engl J Med *297*:814, 1977.
18. Gabow PA: Disorders associated with an altered anion gap. Nephrology Forum. Kidney Int *27*:472, 1985.
19. Brenner BE: Clinical significance of the elevated anion gap. Am J Med *79*:289, 1985.
20. Gabow PA, Kaehny WD, Fennessey PV, Goodman SI, Gross PA, Schrier RW: Diagnostic importance of an increased serum anion gap. N Engl J Med *303*:854, 1980.
21. Androgue HJ, Wilson H, Boyd AE III: Plasma acid-base patterns in diabetic ketoacidosis. N Engl J Med *307*:1603, 1982.
22. Oh MS, Banerji MA, Carroll HJ: The mechanism of hyperchloremic acidosis during the recovery phase of diabetic ketoacidosis. Diabetes *30*:310, 1981.
23. Gamblin GT, Ashburn RW, Kemp DG, Beuttel SC: Diabetic ketoacidosis presenting with a normal anion gap. Am J Med *80*:758–760, 1986.
24. Oh MS, Carroll HJ, Goldstein DA, Fern IA: Hyperchloremic acidosis during the recovery phase of diabetic ketosis. Ann Intern Med *89*:925, 1978.
25. Madias NE, Homer SM, Johns CA, Cohen JJ: Hypochloremia as a consequence of anion gap metabolic acidosis. J Lab Clin Med *104*:15, 1984.
26. Osnes JB, Hermansen L: Acid-base balance after maximal exercise of short duration. J Appl Physiol *32*:59, 1972.
27. Orringer CE, Eustace JC, Wunsch CD, Gardner L: Natural history of lactic acidosis after grand-mal seizures: A model for the study of anion gap acidosis not associated with hyperkalemia. N Engl J Med *297*:796, 1977.
28. Gennari JF: Serum osmolality: Uses and limitations. N Engl J Med *310*:102, 1984.
29. Glasser L, Sternglanz PD, Cambie J, Robinson A: Serum osmolality and its application to drug overdose. Am J Clin Pathol *680*:695, 1973.
30. Schreiner GE, McAnally JF, Winchester JF: Analgesic nephropathy revisited. Arch Intern Med *141*:349, 1981.
31. Hestbech J, Hanson HE, Amdison A, Olsen E: Chronic renal lesions following long-term treatment with lithium. Kidney Int *12*:205, 1977.
32. Wedeen RP: Occupational renal disease. Am J Kidney Dis *3*:241, 1984.
33. Madias NE: Lactic acidosis. Nephrology Forum. Kidney Int *29*:752, 1986.
34. Luft D, Deichsel G, Schmolling RM, Stein W, Eggstein M: Definition of clinically relevant lactic acidosis in patients with internal diseases. Am J Clin Pathol *80*:484, 1983.
35. Fulop M: Ventilatory response in patients with acute lactic acidosis. Crit Care Med *10*:173, 1982.
36. O'Connor LR, Klein KL, Bethune JE: Hyperphosphatemia in lactic acidosis. N Engl J Med *297*:707, 1977.
37. Fulop M: Serum potassium in lactic acidosis and ketoacidosis. N Engl J Med *300*:1087, 1979.
38. Kreisberg RA, Owen WC, Siegal AM: Ethanol-induced hyperlacticacidemia; Inhibition of lactate utilization. J Clin Invest *50*:166, 1971.
39. Fulop M, Bock J, Ben-Ezra J, Antony M, Danzig J, Gage J: Plasma lactate and β-hydroxybutyrate levels in patients with acute ethanol intoxication. Am J Med *80*:191, 1986.
40. Campbell CH: The severe lactic acidosis of thiamine deficiency: Acute pernicious or fulminating beriberi. Lancet *2*:446, 1984.
41. Heinig RE, Clark EF, Waterhouse C: Lactic acidosis and liver disease. Arch Intern Med *139*:1229, 1979.
42. Kreisberg RA, Wood BC: Drug and chemical-induced metabolic acidosis. Clin Endocrinol Metab *12*:391–411, 1983.
43. Misbin RI: Phenformin-associated lactic acidosis: Pathogenesis and treatment. Ann Intern Med *87*:591, 1977.
44. Searle GL, Siperstein MD: Lactic acidosis associated with phenformin therapy. Diabetes *24*:741, 1975.
45. Fulop N, Hoberman HD: Phenformin-associated metabolic acidosis. Diabetes *25*:292, 1976.
46. Smith SR, Smith SJM, Buckley BM: Combined formate and lactate acidosis in methanol poisoning. Lancet *2*:1295, 1981.
47. Smith SR, Smith SJM, Buckley BM: Lactate and formate in methanol poisoning. Lancet *1*:561, 1982.
48. Jacobson D, McMarin KE: Methanol and ethylene glycol poisonings: Mechanisms of toxicity, clinical course, diagnosis and treatment. Med Toxicol *1*:309, 1986.
49. Parry MF, Wallach R: Ethylene glycol poisoning. Am J Med *57*:143, 1974.
50. Gabow PA, Clay K, Sullivan JB, Lepott R: Organic acids in ethylene glycol intoxication. Ann Intern Med *105*:16, 1986.
51. Hill JB: Salicylate intoxication. N Engl J Med *228*:1110, 1973.
52. Gray TA, Buckley BM, Vale JA: Hyperlactataemia and metabolic acidosis following paracetamol overdose. Q J Med *246*:811, 1987.
53. Zezulka A, Wright N: Severe metabolic acidosis in paracetamol poisoning. Br Med J *285*:851, 1982.
54. Caldwell J, Woods HF: Metabolic consequences of the short-term exposure of the liver to paracetamol. Clin Sci Mol Med *55*:10P, 1978.
55. Record CO, Chase RA, Williams R, Appleton D: Disturbances in lactate metabolism in patients with liver damage due to paracetamol overdosage. Metabolism *30*:638, 1981.
56. Record CO, Iles RA, Cohen RD, Williams R: Acid-base and metabolic disturbance in fulminant hepatic failure. Gut *16*:144, 1975.
57. Chin L, Sievers ML, Herner RN, Picchion AL: Convulsions as the etiology of lactic acidosis in acute isoniazid toxicity in dogs. Toxicol Appl Pharmacol *49*:377, 1979.
58. Buehler JH, Berns AS, Webster JR: Lactic acidosis from carboxyhemoglobinemia after smoke inhalation. Ann Intern Med *82*:803, 1975.

59. Graham DL, Laman D, Theodore J, Robin ED: Acute cyanide poisoning complicated by lactic acidosis and pulmonary edema. Arch Intern Med *137*:1051, 1977.
60. Humphruy SH, Nash DA: Lactic acidosis complicating sodium nitroprusside. Ann Intern Med *88*:58, 1978.
61. Jonsson S, O'Meara M, Young JB: Acute cocaine poisoning; Importance of treated seizures and acidosis. Am J Med *75*:1061, 1983.
62. Kolendorf K, Moller BB: Lactic acidosis in epinephrine poisoning. Acta Med Scand *196*:465, 1974.
63. Bornemann N, Hill SE, Kid GS II: Lactic acidosis and pheochromocytoma. Ann Intern Med *105*:880, 1986.
64. Narins RG, Cohen JJ: Bicarbonate therapy for organic acidosis: The case for its continued use. Ann Intern Med *106*:615, 1987.
65. Stacpoole PW: Lactic acidosis: The case against bicarbonate therapy (editorial). Ann Intern Med *105*:276, 1986.
66. Arieff AI, Leach W, Park R, Lazarowitz UC: Systemic effects of $NaHCO_3$ in experimental lactic acidosis in dogs. Am J Physiol *242*:F586, 1982.
67. Fraley DS, Adler S, Bruns FJ, Zeh B: Stimulation of lactate production by administration of bicarbonate in a patient with a solid neoplasm and lactic acidosis. N Engl J Med *303*:1100, 1980.
68. Stacpoole PW, Harman EN, Curry SH, Baumgartner TG, Misbin RI: Treatment of lactic acidosis with dichloroacetate. N Engl J Med *309*:390, 1983.
69. Oster JR, Epstein M: Acid-base aspects of ketoacidosis. Am J Nephrol *4*:137, 1984.
70. Cahill GJ Jr: Ketosis. Nephrology Forum. Kidney Int *20*:416, 1981.
71. Lefevre HA, Adler H, Liber C: Effect of ethanol on ketone metabolism. J Clin Invest *49*:1775, 1970.
72. Halperin ML, Hammeke M, Josse RG, Jungas RL: Metabolic acidosis in the alcoholic: A pathophysiological approach. Metabolism *32*:308, 1983.
73. Levy LJ, Duga J, Girjis M, Gordon EE: Ketoacidosis associated with alcoholism in nondiabetic subjects. Ann Intern Med *78*:213, 1973.
74. Fullop M, Hoberman HD: Alcoholic ketosis. Diabetes *24*:785, 1975.
75. Cooperman MT, Danidoff F, Sark R, Palotta J: Clinical studies of alcoholic ketoacidosis. Diabetes *23*:433, 1974.
76. Felig P, Havel RJ, Smith LH: Metabolism and nutrition. *In* Smith LH Jr, Thier SO (eds): Pathophysiology: The Biological Principles of Disease. Philadelphia, WB Saunders, 1981, p 479.
77. Lacouture PG, Wason S, Abrams A, Lovejoy FH Jr: Acute isopropyl alcohol intoxication: Diagnosis and management. Am J Med *75*:680, 1983.
78. Kelner M, Bailey DN: Isopropanol ingestion: Interpretation of blood concentrations and clinical findings. J Toxicol Clin Toxicol *20*:497, 1983.
79. Lehman AJ, Chase HF: The acute and chronic toxicity of isopropyl alcohol. J Lab Clin Med *29*:561, 1944.
80. Litowitz T: The alcohols: Ethanol, methanol, isopropanol, and ethyl glycol. Pediatr Clin North Am *33*:311, 1983.
81. Garella S: Extracorporeal techniques in the treatment of exogenous intoxications. Nephrology Forum. Kidney Int *33*:735, 1988.
82. Winchester JF, Gelfand MC, Knepshield JH, Schreiner GE: Dialysis and hemoperfusion of poisons and drugs—update. Trans Am Soc Artif Intern Organs *23*:762, 1977.
83. Thomas DJB, Gill B, Brown T, Stubbs WA: Salbutamol-induced diabetic ketoacidosis. Br Med J *123*:438, 1977.
84. Updike SJ, Harrington AR: Acute diabetic ketoacidosis. A complication of intravenous diazoxide treatment of refractory hypertension. N Engl J Med *280*:768, 1969.
85. Proudfoot AT: Toxicity of salicylates. Am J Med Antipyretic-Analgesics Symposium *75*:99, 1983.
86. Anderson RJ, Potts DE, Gabow PA, Rumack BH, Schrier RW: Unrecognized adult salicylate intoxication. Ann Intern Med *85*:745, 1976.
87. McGuigan MA: A two year review of salicylate deaths in Ontario. Arch Intern Med *147*:510, 1987.
88. Flower RJ, Moncada S, Vane JR: Analgesic-antipyretic and anti-inflammatory agents. Drugs employed in the treatment of gout. *In* Goodman A, Gilman LS, Rall TW, Murad F (eds): The Pharmacological Basis of Therapeutics. 7th ed. New York, Macmillan, 1985, p 674.
89. Wosilait WD: Theoretical analysis of the binding of salicylates by human serum albumin: The relationship between free and bound drug and therapeutic levels. Eur J Clin Pharmacol *9*:285, 1976.
90. Gabow PA, Anderson RJ, Potts DE, Schrier RW: Acid-base disturbances in the salicylate-intoxicated adult. Arch Intern Med *138*:1481, 1978.
91. Eichenholz A, Mulhausen RO, Redleaf PS: The nature of acid-base disturbances in salicylate intoxication. Metabolism *12*:164, 1963.
92. Kaehny WD, Gabow PA: Pathogenesis in management of metabolic acidosis and alkalosis. *In* Schrier R (ed): Renal and Electrolyte Disturbances. 3rd ed. Boston, Little, Brown, 1986, p 141.
93. Winter SRW, White JS, Hughes MC: Disturbances of acid-base equilibrium and salicylate intoxication. Pediatrics *23*:260, 1959.
94. Heffner JE, Sahn SA: Salicylate-induced pulmonary edema. Ann Intern Med *95*:405, 1981.
95. Temple AW: Acute and chronic effects of aspirin toxicity and their treatment. Arch Intern Med *141*:364, 1981.
96. Prescott LF, Balali-Mood M, Critchley JAJH, Johnstone AF, Proudfoot AT: Diuresis or urinary alkalinisation for salicylate poisoning? Br Med J *285*:1383, 1983.
97. Cowan RA, Hartnell GG, Lowdell CP, Mclean-Bair DI, Leak AM: Metabolic acidosis induced by carbonic anhydrase inhibitors and salicylates in patients with normal renal function. Br Med J *289*:347, 1984.
98. Winchester JF, Gelfand MC, Helliwell M, Val JA, Goulding R, Schreiner GE: Extracorporeal treatment for salicylate or acetaminophen poisoning—is there a role? Arch Intern Med *141*:370, 1971.
99. Bennett IL Jr, Cary FH, Mitchell GL, Cooper MN: Acute methyl alcohol poisoning. A review based on experience in an outbreak of 323 cases. Medicine *32*:431, 1953.
100. Swartz RD, Millman RP, Billy JE, Bondar MP, et al: Epidemic methanol poisoning; Clinical and biochemical analysis of a recent episode. Medicine *60*:373, 1981.
101. Gonda A, Gault H, Churchill D, Hollomby D: Hemodialysis for methanol intoxication. Am J Med *64*:749, 1978.
102. McMartin KE, Ambre JJ, Tephly TR: Methanol

poisoning in human subjects; Role for formic acid accumulation in the metabolic acidosis. Am J Med *68*:414, 1980.
103. Pappas S, Silverman M: Treatment of methanol poisoning with ethanol and hemodialysis. Can Med Assoc J *126*:391, 1982.
104. Clay KL, Murphy RC, Watkins WD: Experimental methanol toxicity in primates: Analysis of metabolic acidosis. Toxicol Appl Pharmacol *34*:49, 1975.
105. Sejersted OM, Jacobsen D, Ovrebo S, Jansen H: Formate concentration in plasma from patients poisoned with methanol. Acta Med Scand *213*:105, 1983.
106. McMartin KE, Makar AB, Martin G, Palese M, Tephly TR: Methanol poisoning. I. The role of formic acid in the development of metabolic acidosis in the monkey and the reversal by 4-methylpyrazole. Biochem Med *13*:319, 1975.
107. Lloyd MH, Iles RA, Simpson BR, Strunin JM, Layton JM, Cohen RD: The effect of stimulated metabolic acidosis on intracellular pH and lactate metabolism in the isolated perfused rat liver. Clin Sci Mol Med *45*:543, 1973.
108. Palmisano J, Gruver C, Adams MD: Absence of anion gap metabolic acidosis in severe methanol poisoning: A case report and review of the literature. Am J Kidney Dis *9*:441, 1987.
109. Martensson E, Olofsson U, Heath A: Clinical and metabolic features of ethanol-methanol poisoning in chronic alcoholics. Lancet *1*:327, 1988.
110. Eckfeldt JH, Leatherman JW, Levitt MD: High prevalence of hyperamylasemia in patients with acidemia. Ann Intern Med *104*:362, 1986.
111. Eckfeldt JH, Kershaw MJ: Hyperamylasemia following methyl alcohol intoxication. Arch Intern Med *146*:193, 1986.
112. Jacobsen D, Bredesen JE, Eide I, Ostburg J: Anion and osmolal gaps in the diagnosis of methanol and ethylene glycol poisoning. Acta Med Scand *212*:17, 1982.
113. Jacobsen D, McMartin KE: Methanol and ethylene glycol poisoning: Mechanisms and toxicity, medical course, diagnosis, and treatment. Med Toxicol *1*:309, 1986.
114. Jacobsen D, Jansen H, Wiik-Larsen E, Bredesen JH, Halvorsen S: Studies on methanol poisoning. Acta Med Scand *212*:5, 1982.
115. Osterloh JD, Pond SM, Grady S, Becker CE: Serum formate concentrations in methanol intoxications as a criterion for hemodialysis. Ann Intern Med *104*:200, 1986.
116. Editorial: Methanol poisoning. Lancet *1*:910, 1983.
117. Frommer JP, Agus JC: Acute ethylene glycol intoxication. Am J Nephrol *2*:1, 1982.
118. Jacobsen D, Ovrebo S, Ostborg J, Sejersted LM: Glycolate causes the acidosis of ethylene glycol poisoning and is effectively removed by hemodialysis. Acta Med Scand *216*:409, 1984.
119. Clay KL, Murphy RC: On the metabolic acidosis of ethylene glycol intoxication. Toxicol Appl Pharmacol *39*:39, 1977.
120. Sabatini S: Severe metabolic acidosis in an intoxicated patient. Am J Nephrol *8*:323, 1988.
121. Heckerling PS: Ethylene glycol poisoning with a normal anion gap due to occult bromide intoxication. Ann Emerg Med *16*:1384, 1987.
122. Berman LB, Schreiner JE, Feys J: The nephrotoxic lesion of ethylene glycol. Ann Intern Med *46*:611, 1957.
123. Jacobsen D, Hewlett P, Webb R, Brown ST, Ordinaro AT, McMartin KE: Ethylene glycol intoxication: Evaluation of kinetics and crystalluria. Am J Med *84*:145, 1988.
124. Hewlett P, McMartin KE: Ethylene glycol poisoning: The value of glycolic acid determinations for diagnosis and treatment. Clin Toxicol *24*:389, 1986.
125. Schreiner GE, Maher JF, Marc-Aurele J, Knowlan D, Alvo M: Ethylene glycol—Two indications for hemodialysis. Trans Am Soc Artif Intern Organs *5*:81, 1959.
126. Jacobsen D, Bostby N, Bredesen JE: Studies on ethylene glycol poisoning. Acta Med Scand *212*:11, 1982.
127. Beier LS, Pitts WH, Gonick HC: Metabolic acidosis occurring during paraldehyde intoxication. Ann Intern Med *58*:155, 1963.
128. Gutman RA, Burnell JM: Paraldehyde acidosis. Am J Med *42*:435, 1967.
129. Hadden JH, Metzner RJ: Pseudoketosis and hyperacetaldehydemia in paraldehyde acidosis. Am J Med *47*:642, 1969.
130. Elkinton JR: Renal tubular acidosis with organic aciduria during paraldehyde ingestion. Am J Med *23*:977, 1957.
131. Mountan R: Noncardiac pulmonary edema following the administration of parenteral paraldehyde. Chest *82*:371, 1982.
132. Streicher HZ, Gabow PA, Moss AH, Kono D, Kaehny WD: Syndrome of toluene sniffing in adults. Ann Intern Med *94*:758, 1981.
133. Fischman CM, Oster JR: Toxic effects of toluene. A new cause of high anion gap metabolic acidosis. JAMA *241*:1713, 1979.
134. Taher SM, Anderson RJ, McCartney R, Popobtzer MM, Schrier RW: Renal tubular acidosis associated with toluene sniffing. N Engl J Med *290*:765, 1974.
135. Batlle DC, Sabatini S, Kurtzman NA: On the mechanism of toluene-induced renal tubular acidosis. Nephron *49*:210, 1988.
136. Moss AH, Gabow PA, Kaehny WD, Goodman SI, Haut LL, Haussler MR: Fanconi's syndrome and distal renal tubular acidosis after glue sniffing. Ann Intern Med *92*:69, 1980.
137. Eells JT, McMartin KE, Black K, Viragotha V, Tisdell RH, Tephly TR: Formaldehyde poisoning—Rapid metabolism and formic acid. JAMA *246*:1237, 1981.
138. Linden CH, Townsend PL: Metabolic acidosis after acute ibuprofen overdosage. J Pediatr *111*:922, 1987.
139. Gabow PA, Kaehny WD, Keleher SP: The spectrum of rhabdomyolysis. Medicine *61*:141, 1982.
140. McCarron DA, Elliott WC, Rose JJ, Bennett WM: Severe metabolic acidosis secondary to rhabdomyolysis. Am J Med *67*:905, 1976.
141. Cohen JJ: Methylmalonic acidemia. Kidney Int *15*:311, 1979.
142. Kleinman PK: Cholestyramine and metabolic acidosis (letter). N Engl J Med *290*:861, 1974.
143. Finn R, Waincoat JS: Laxan nephropathy. Lancet *1*:1202, 1975.
144. Kurtzman NA: Renal tubular acidosis: A constellation of syndromes. Hosp Prac *22*:173, 1987.
145. Glassock RJ, Feinstein EI, Tannen R, Blau R, Koss M: Metabolic acidosis in a young woman. Am J Nephrol *4*:58, 1984.
146. Sebastian A, Morris RC: Renal tubular acidosis. Clin Nephrol *7*:216, 1977.
147. DeFronzo RA: Hyperkalemia and hyporeninemic hypoaldosteronism. Kidney Int *17*:118, 1980.

148. Halperin ML, Goldstein MB, Richardson RM, Stinebaugh BJ: Distal renal tubular acidosis: A pathophysiological approach. Am J Nephrol *5*:1, 1985.
149. Batlle DC, Gaviri AN, Grupp M, Arruda JA, Wynn J, Kurtzman NA: Distal nephron function in patients receiving chronic lithium therapy. Kidney Int *21*:477, 1982.
150. Garell AS, Matarese RA: Renal effects of prostaglandins and clinical adverse effects of nonsteroidal anti-inflammatory agents. Medicine *63*:165, 1984.
151. Sakemi T, Ohchi N, Sanai T, Rikitake O, Maeda T: Captopril-induced metabolic acidosis with hyperkalemia. Am J Nephrol *8*:245, 1988.
152. Adu D, Turney J, Michael J, Arruda JA, Wynn J, Kutzman NA: Hyperkalemia in cyclosporine-treated renal allograft recipients. Lancet *2*:370, 1983.
153. Blum JE, Coe FL: Metabolic acidosis after sulfur ingestion. N Engl J Med *297*:869, 1977.
154. Szerlip HM, Singer I: Hyperchloremic metabolic acidosis after chlorine inhalation. Am J Med *77*:581, 1984.
155. Batlle DC, Hizon M, Kohen E, Gutterman C, Gupta R: The use of the urinary anion gap in the diagnosis of hyperchloremic metabolic acidosis. N Engl J Med *318*:594, 1988.
156. Mitchel JH, Wildenthal K, Johnson RL: The effects of acid-base disturbances on cardiovascular and pulmonary function. Kidney Int *1*:375, 1972.
157. Gerst PH: Increased susceptibility of the heart to ventricular fibrillation during metabolic acidosis. Circ Res *19*:63, 1966.
158. Androgue HJ, Lederer ED, Suki WN, Eknoyan G: Determinants of plasma potassium levels in diabetic ketoacidosis. Medicine *65*:163, 1986.
159. Garella S, Dana CL, Chazan JA: Severity of metabolic acidosis as a determinant of bicarbonate requirements. N Engl J Med *289*:121, 1973.
160. Hodgkin JE, Soeprono FF, Chand M: Incidence of metabolic alkalemia in hospitalized patients. Crit Care Med *8*:725–728, 1980.
161. Wilson RF, Gibson D, Percival AK: Severe alkalosis in a critically ill surgical patient. Arch Surg *105*:197, 1972.
162. Seldin DW, Rector FC: The generation and maintenance of metabolic alkalosis. Kidney Int *1*:306, 1972.
163. Sabatini S, Kurtzman NA: The maintenance of metabolic alkalosis. Factors which decrease bicarbonate excretion. Kidney Int *25*:357, 1984.
164. Weil JV, Byrne-Quine J, Sadal E, Friesen WO, Underhil B, Fille JF, Grover RF: Hypoxic ventilatory drive in normal man. J Clin Invest *49*:1061, 1970.
165. Harris RT: Bulimarexia and related serious disorders with medical complications. Ann Intern Med *99*:800, 1983.
166. Oster JR: The binge-purge syndrome: A common albeit unappreciated cause of acid-base and fluid-electrolyte disturbances. South Med J *80*:58, 1987.
167. Jameson RL, Ross JC, Kempcson RL, Sufit CR, Parker TE: Surreptitous diuretic ingestion and pseudo-Bartter syndrome. Am J Med *73*:142, 1982.
168. Steiner RW, Omachi AS: A Bartter's-like syndrome from capreomycin and a similar gentamicin tubulopathy. Am J Kidney Dis *7*:245, 1986.
169. Kelleher SP, Schulman G: Severe metabolic alkalosis complicating regional citrate hemodialysis. Am J Kidney Dis *9*:235, 1987.
170. Pearl DG, Rosenthal MH: Metabolic alkalosis due to plasmaphoresis. Am J Med *79*:391, 1985.
171. Stemmer CT, Oster JR, Vaamonde CA, Perez JO, Rogers AI: Effect of routine doses of antacid on renal acidification. Lancet *2*:3, 1986.
172. Madias NE, Levey AS: Metabolic alkalosis due to absorption of "nonabsorbable" antacids. Am J Med *74*:155, 1983.
173. Orwall ES: The milk-alkali syndrome: Current concepts. Ann Intern Med *97*:242, 1982.
174. Kapsner P, Langsdor FL, Marcus R, Craener FB, Hoffman AR: Milk-alkali syndrome in patients treated with calcium carbonate after cardiac transplantation. Arch Intern Med *146*:1965, 1986.
175. Lipner HI, Ruzany R, Dasgupta M, Lief PD, Bank N: The behavior of carbenicillin as a nonreabsorbable anion. J Lab Clin Med *86*:183, 1975.
176. Rosen RA, Julian BA, Dubovasky EV, Gallo JH, Luke RG: On the mechanism by which chloride corrects metabolic alkalosis in man. Am J Med *84*:449, 1988.
177. Swartz RD, Rubin JE, Brown RS, Yager HM, Steinman TI, Frazier HS: Correction of post operative metabolic alkalosis and renal failure by hemodialysis. Ann Intern Med *86*:52, 1977.
178. Mazzara JT, Ayres SM, Grace WJ: Extreme hypocapnia in the critically ill patient. Am J Med *56*:450, 1974.

CHAPTER 8
ACTIVE METHODS FOR DETOXIFICATION

James F. Winchester, M.D.

The overall mortality rate from poisoning in hospitalized patients is low (less than 1 per cent of admitted patients), a result that has been obtained by the use of intensive supportive care and the abandonment of analeptic drugs and of the injudicious use of active treatment methods.[1] However, in certain groups of patients severe poisoning contributes to a high mortality, especially those poisoned with narcotic agents to a degree that produces deep coma; those poisoned with drugs for which significant quantities of the intoxicant are metabolized to more noxious substances, such as the conversion of methanol to formaldehyde and ethylene glycol to oxalic acid; and also those poisoned with agents known to produce delayed toxicity, such as paraquat and related compounds. The purposes of this chapter are to outline the place of oral sorbents in the management of poisoning; to discuss briefly the physical characteristics of forced diuresis, hemodialysis, and hemoperfusion; and to enumerate specific criteria that should allow the clinician rationally to judge when these techniques should be used. In addition, other techniques for solute removal, such as hemofiltration, continuous arteriovenous hemo filtration (CAVH), plasmapheresis, and exchange blood transfusion as well as the use of specific antibodies to drugs will be discussed briefly.

The 1987 annual report of the American Association of Poison Control Centers National Data Collection System (AAPCC)[2] recorded 1,166,940 poisonings, with 397 deaths and 3631 patients suffering from major effects of poisoning. Since 63 centers report to the AAPCC with a population base of 137.5 million, the number of poisonings in the United States is probably close to 2 million. Initial decontamination (dilution, emesis, gastric lavage, activated charcoal, and cathartics) was used in the vast majority (940,912) of the reported cases. Antidotes were used in 10,274 cases, and measures to enhance drug or poison elimination in 3666 instances;[2] 3139 patients underwent alkalinization or acidification with or without diuresis, 310 patients had hemodialysis, 33 had peritoneal dialysis, 124 had charcoal hemoperfusion, 35 had resin hemoperfusion, and 25 had exchange transfusion. Analysis of poisonings for which dialysis or hemoperfusion was employed in the 1986 AAPCC report[3] is shown in Table 8–1.[4]

ORAL SORBENTS

In modern toxicology, the use of oral sorbents (particularly activated charcoal) has a definite role in strongly binding certain poisons, reducing their absorption, and contributing to their active elimination from the gastrointestinal tract, with or without concomitant use of cathartics. (The use of oral

Table 8–1. POISONS FOR WHICH HEMOPERFUSION OR DIALYSIS WERE EMPLOYED IN THE 1986 AAPCC REPORT

POISON	HEMOPERFUSION	DIALYSIS
acetaminophen	1	9
aspirin	1	25
barbiturate	9	13
boric acid	0	5
cardiac glycosides	1	6
cyclic antidepressants	20	8
ethanol	4	10
formaldehyde	0	6
glycols	0	41
isopropanol	0	7
lithium	0	39
methanol	0	31
mushrooms	3	5
phenothiazines	3	5
theophylline	30	15

Total cases: 297 hemodialysis, 99 charcoal, and 23 resin hemoperfusion.

Note: many cases multiple ingestions.

(Reproduced by permission of Litovitz TL, Martin TG, Schmitz B: 1986 Annual Report of the American Association of Poison Control Centers National Data Collection System. Am J Emerg Med 5:405, 1987.)

sorbents in poisoning is discussed in Chapter 1.) Curtailment of enterohepatic circulation by sorbents is possible for the following drugs, with hastening of the elimination half-time: chlordecone (cholestyramine),[5] salicylate (charcoal),[6] phenobarbital (charcoal),[7] β-methyldigoxin (charcoal),[8] and theophylline (charcoal).[9] In paraquat poisoning, oral sorbents in the form of diatomaceous earths (fuller's earth or bentonite) are the mainstay of treatment to prevent gastrointestinal absorption of paraquat, thereby preventing its active accumulation in the lung.[10] Arising from the known physical process of adsorption, the technique of hemoperfusion of recirculated blood over sorbent particles has been introduced for the treatment of severely intoxicated patients with poisoning due to specific agents.

FORCED DIURESIS

Most drugs are weak acids or bases and in solutions exist both as nonionized or ionized species. The nonionized molecules are usually lipid soluble and diffuse across the cell membrane by the process known as *nonionic diffusion*. The ionized form, in contrast, is usually unable to penetrate lipid membranes.[11, 12]

Excretion of drugs by the kidney also depends on the ionization state of the specific drug or its metabolites and involves three main processes. The first is glomerular filtration. In the glomerular tufts, drugs that are not bound to albumin are ultrafiltered, depending on the degree of protein binding, whereas drugs that are strongly bound to albumin are retained by the glomerulus.

The second process whereby drugs are excreted by the kidney is tubular secretion at the proximal convoluted tubule. This takes place through transport systems that carry drugs from plasma to urine. There is one transport system for acidic drugs and another for basic drugs. Tubular epithelium can also secrete free drug and drug bound to protein-binding sites. As free drug is removed by the tubular cells, there is rapid breakdown of the circulating drug-protein complex in the plasma. Examples of drugs that compete for proximal secretion are acidic drugs like probenecid, which can be used to reduce the elimination of penicillins and to prolong their half-life in the body. Little is known, however, of competitive interplay among basic drugs.

The third process by which drugs are excreted by the kidney is passive tubular reabsorption. This process involves a bidirectional movement of drugs across the tubular epithelium of the nephron; however, as water and electrolytes are progressively reabsorbed from the tubular fluid (as it passes through the loop of Henle and the collecting system), a favorable concentration gradient is created for net absorption of dissolved materials back into the blood stream. This reabsorption requires little energy and is limited to lipid-soluble drugs and the nonionized fraction of those drugs that are weak electrolytes and that undergo partial ionization at physiologic pH. Increasing the pH of tubular fluid increases the degree of ionization of weak acids and reduces passive tubular free drug absorption by lowering its nonionic diffusion, whereas the reverse applies to weak bases. The dissociation of a weak acid or base is determined by its dissociation constant (pK_a) and the pH gradient across the tubular membrane.

The ratio of nonionized to ionized drug can be calculated from the Henderson-Hasselbalch equation. At a pK_a equal to the pH, the concentrations of nonionized drug and ionized drug are equal (see Chapter 2). Elimination of weak acids by the kidney is increased in the range 3.0 to 7.5, while for weak bases elimination is increased in acid urine if their pK_a is 7.5 to 10.5. This is illustrated in Figure 8–1.

For drugs to respond to pH manipulation of the urine, they must first satisfy the following criteria: (1) the drug is predominantly eliminated in the unchanged form via the kidneys, (2) the drug is a weak electrolyte with a pK_a in the appropriate acidic or basic pK_a range seen in Figure 8–1, and (3) the drug is distributed mainly to the extracellular fluid compartment and is minimally protein bound. A representative listing of pK_a values for various drugs is shown in Table 8–2. It is inappropriate to manipulate pH and attempt forced diuresis when the drug is mainly eliminated from the circulation by hepatic or tissue metabolism, is strongly protein bound, or has a large volume of distribution and is highly lipid soluble.

As can be seen from Figure 8–1, phenobarbital (pK_a 7.2) and thiopental (pK_a 7.6) have similar dissociation constants. How-

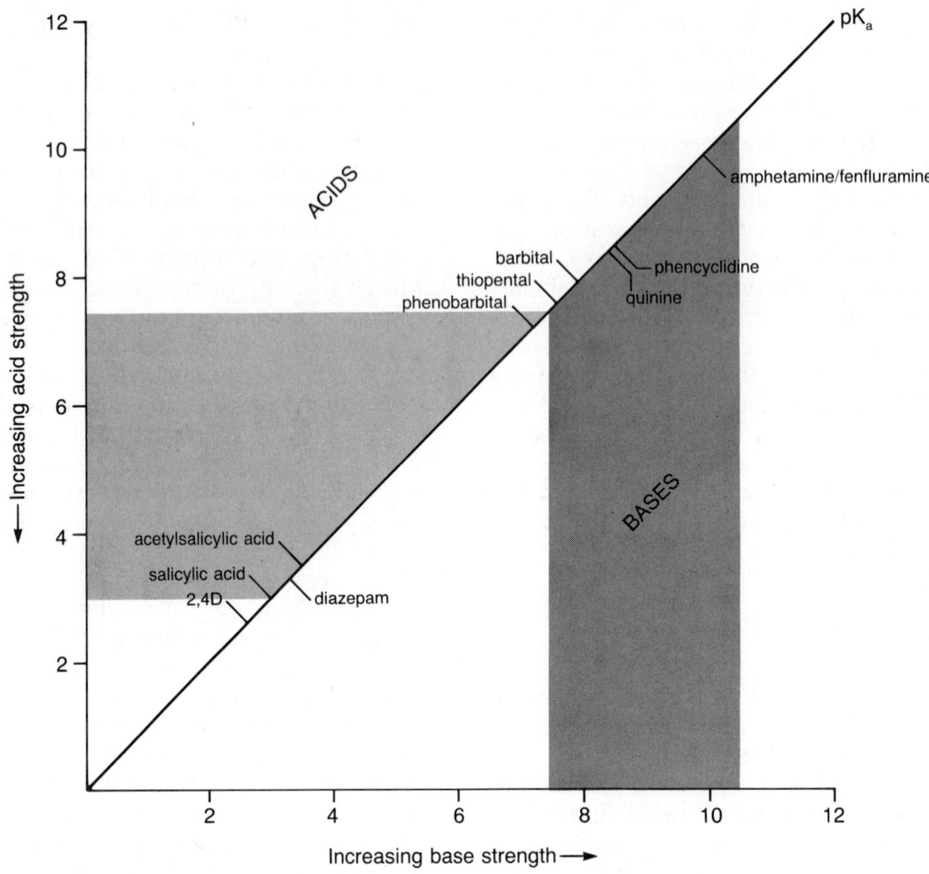

Figure 8–1. Dissociation constants (pK$_a$) for several drugs. Shaded areas represent urinary pH limits that allow increased excretion of drugs shown.

ever, their lipid solubility is quite different; as measured by the methylene chloride–water partition coefficient, phenobarbital has a coefficient of 3, whereas thiopental has a partition coefficient of about 80. This means that while 25 to 50 per cent of a dose of phenobarbital is excreted unmetabolized in the urine—and this can be even higher in a large overdose—the renal excretion of thiopental, unchanged in the urine, is less than 1 per cent. Therefore, it is clear that forced alkaline diuresis is of no value in the treatment of overdosage with thiopental or other highly lipid-soluble drugs.

Although no fatalities have been recorded, the use of forced diuresis may be complicated by the development of hyponatremia and water intoxication, pulmonary edema, cerebral edema, hypokalemia, and either alkalinemia or acidemia secondary to the use of alkaline or acidic agents, respectively, in promoting the diuresis. For these reasons, any commitment to the use of forced diuresis must be accompanied by close vigilance and measurement of urinary pH, at least hourly, and of electrolytes every 1 to 2 hours initially and frequently thereafter.

The advantages of alkalinization of urine in salicylate poisoning can be illustrated by the following facts: salicylic acid has a pK$_a$ of 3.0; therefore, at urinary pH 3.0, the ratio of salicylate (ionized) to salicylic acid (nonionized) is 1:1. At a urine pH of 7.0, this ratio rises to 10,000:1. When the pH is raised to 7.4, the ratio is increased to about 25,000:1. It is not surprising that the elimination half-time for salicylate is greatly prolonged when the urinary pH is less than 7.4. Blood acidemia also increases the amount of nonionized and diffusible salicylic acid and enhances its accumulation within the cerebral tissue.[12]

Urinary alkalinization by systemic bicarbonate and a saline-glucose fluid-induced diuresis increases the ratio of ionized salicylate to nonionized salicylic acid in the renal tubule; consequently, "ion trapping" of salicy-

Table 8–2. DISSOCIATION CONSTANTS (pK_a) FOR VARIOUS DRUGS

ACIDS		BASES	
Drug	*pK_a*	*Drug*	*pK_a*
acetazolamide	7.2	allopurinol	9.4
acetylsalicylic acid	3.49	amiloride	7.2
amobarbital	7.7	amitriptyline	9.4
barbital	7.91	amphetamine	9.9
boric acid	9.24	atropine	9.8
chlorpropamide	4.8	chlorpheniramine	9.2
2,4-dichlorophenoxy-		chlorpromazine	9.3
acetic acid	2.6	clonidine	8.25
ethosuximide	9.3	codeine	8.2
furosemide	3.8	diazepam	3.3
hydrochlorothiazide	7.9	diphenhydramine	8.3
indomethacin	4.5	phenytoin	8.3
methotrexate	5.5	ephedrine	9.36
pentobarbital	8.2	fenfluramine	9.9
phenobarbital	7.2	haloperidol	8.7
probenecid	3.4	hydralazine	7.1
salicylic acid	3.0	imipramine	9.5
sulfadiazine	6.48	ketamine	7.5
theophylline	8.75	lidocaine	7.9
thiopental	7.6	meperidine	8.7
tolbutamide	5.3	methadone	8.6
valproate sodium	4.8	morphine	8.05
		naloxone	7.94
		nortriptyline	9.73
		pentazocine	9.0
		phencyclidine	8.5
		procainamide	9.2
		procaine	8.8
		quinidine	8.4
		quinine	8.4
		reserpine	6.6
		triamterene	6.2

late occurs in the tubular lumen. Accompanying these changes, potassium shifts into cells as blood pH rises, and potassium excretion is enhanced by alkaline diuresis: Consequently, the serum potassium concentrations will fall.[13] It is, therefore, essential to replace potassium in such situations. The opposite effect occurs with the induction of acidemia. Every rise in pH of 0.1 unit in the blood is accompanied by a fall in plasma potassium of 0.6 mEq per L, with identical but reciprocal changes occurring with falls of pH.[13] Therefore, in forced acid diuresis, careful attention must also be paid to the measurement of plasma potassium.

It has also been shown that in moderate salicylate poisoning, the same quantity of salicylate was excreted in the urine when identical quantities of sodium bicarbonate were administered with or without "forced" diuresis.[14] Such a measure avoided the risk of copious fluid administration (6 L) and illustrates the importance of ion trapping alone in moderate salicylate poisoning (32.8 to 46.7 mg/dl plasma concentrations at the start of therapy).[14]

In moderate-to-severe salicylate poisoning, examination of the Done nomogram[15] for estimating the severity of poisoning in relation to time of ingestion of salicylate should allow for the adoption of forced alkaline diuresis. It may be necessary to resort to dialysis or hemoperfusion when the levels of salicylate exceed 130 mg per dl at 6 hours after ingestion or exceed the extrapolated initial level of 160 mg per dl or when there is an unresponsive acidosis or development of renal failure. When other measures have failed, persistence of the manifestations of salicylate poisoning, with progressive deterioration, is another indication for consideration of dialysis.

GUIDELINES TO THE TECHNIQUES OF FORCED ALKALINE OR FORCED ACID DIURESIS

For both types of diuresis, it is wise to measure baseline electrolytes and arterial and urinary pH as well as drug levels in the blood. It is also preferable to place a bladder catheter in the patient because urine flow rates should be accurately assessed. Where appropriate, a flow-directed pulmonary arterial line (Swan-Ganz line) should be used to assess the dangers of fluid overload during the intravenous infusion of fluids. The latter is necessary since there may be impairment of renal or cardiac function. In the presence of hypotension with a high pulmonary capillary wedge pressure, forced diuresis is contraindicated.

ALKALINE DIURESIS

The urinary pH should be maintained within the range of 7.5 to 8.5 by the adjustment of the amount of bicarbonate administered. The diuresis can be initiated by using furosemide or osmotic diuretic agents like mannitol or urea. The use of mannitol as the diuretic agent may be associated with hyponatremia and hyperosmolality in patients with acute barbiturate or salicylate poisoning. Theoretically, if hemodialysis were subsequently used in patients in whom diuresis was maintained by high-dose mannitol therapy, the dialysis disequilibrium syndrome might be induced. For this reason, it is recommended that the total dose of mannitol not exceed 300 gm. In practice, however, it is rare to use such high doses of mannitol, and the usual clinical case of salicylate poisoning may be treated by doses of between 20 and 100 gm of mannitol.

In salicylate poisoning, frequently some degree of dehydration is present before initiation of treatment, so 1 L of 5 per cent dextrose containing 25 mEq per L of bicarbonate and 75 mEq per L of sodium and appropriate levels of potassium judged on the initial serum potassium level should also be given. In the presence of severe acidosis, however, the bicarbonate supplements should be increased and adjusted to maintain the urinary pH in the optimal range. Such solutions are best administered for 1 to 2 hours until volume expansion occurs. Thereafter, in the adult, 500 ml per hour of 5 per cent dextrose in half-normal saline containing 20 to 35 mEq of bicarbonate should be given until the salicylate level falls to the therapeutic range (30 to 35 mg/dl). The goal of treatment is to maintain a urine flow of 300 to 500 ml per hour, and either mannitol or boluses of furosemide, 20 mg, may be required to maintain the diuresis; 10 to 20 mEq of potassium per L of infused fluid may also be required.

Alkaline diuresis is suitable for the following drugs: phenobarbital, when the plasma level exceeds 10 mg per dl; barbital, when the plasma level exceeds 10 mg per dl; and salicylates, when the plasma level exceeds 50 mg per dl (relative to time of ingestion). Forced alkaline diuresis has also been shown to be of benefit in the treatment of (2,4-dichlorophenoxy)acetic acid (2,4-D) poisoning.[16]

ACID DIURESIS

One liter of 5 per cent dextrose in normal saline per hour is given in the first 1 or 2 hours, with added arginine or lysine hydrochloride (10 gm given intravenously over 30 minutes). Thereafter, 5 per cent dextrose in normal saline is given every 2 hours. Ammonium chloride, 4 gm every 2 hours, should be administered orally, or in the patient who cannot tolerate a nasogastric or duodenal tube, a 1 to 2 per cent solution of ammonium chloride in normal saline should be given intravenously. With either technique the dose is adjusted to maintain a urinary pH of 5.5 to 6.5. Plasma potassium should be monitored frequently. Urinary pH should be measured at least hourly. Forced acid diuresis can increase the excretion of amphetamines,[17, 18] fenfluramine,[19, 20] phencyclidine,[21, 22] and quinine.[23, 24] Acid diuresis may or may not be indicated in the management of poisoning with these agents (see each specific chapter for indications). Ascorbic acid (1 gm every 6 hours in adults) can also be administered orally to acidify the urine.

WATER AND CHLORIDE DIURESIS

It is clear that chloride loading (especially ammonium chloride) increases the excretion of bromides; bromide excretion can be further increased with administration of mannitol or loop diuretics. On the other hand, lithium excretion is not further enhanced by ammonium chloride, water, saline, or loop diuretics (furosemide, ethacrynic acid) administration. Bicarbonate, acetazolamide, urea, and aminophylline may increase lithium excretion in volunteers with normal renal function; the evidence, however, is inconclusive, and there is no good evidence in lithium-intoxicated patients that forced diuresis (after correction of fluid deficits) is of benefit.

DIALYTIC TECHNIQUES FOR REMOVING POISONS

The term *dialysis* was coined in 1854 by Thomas Graham, Professor of Physic, in Glasgow, Scotland, to describe the transfer of solute across a semipermeable membrane (in this case, parchment).[25] Graham predicted that dialysis would be used for the treatment of medical conditions. Not until 1913, however, did the concept of removing diffusible substances from blood stimulate Abel, Rowntree, and Turner to construct the first hemodialyzer.[26] This was a hollow fiber dialyzer constructed with collodion as the hollow fiber membrane enclosed in a glass cylinder through which dialysate passed. It was used in animals for the removal of toxic substances, one of which was salicylate. The clinically usable artificial kidney designed by Kolff was introduced in 1944.[27] In 1951, Doolan and his colleagues attempted to remove aspirin from an intoxicated patient.[28] However, this first clinical application of dialysis in poisoning was not successful because of technical problems with the dialyzer. In 1955 Schreiner and colleagues used hemodialysis successfully in a patient poisoned with aspirin.[29] Since that time, many substances have been reported to be removed by hemodialysis and peritoneal dialysis, and exhaustive reviews of the state of the art of dialysis in poisoning have been published.[30–35]

Prior to discussion of dialysis in specific drug poisoning, it is worthwhile to consider the basic principles of dialysis, factors favoring drug removal with dialysis, and the potential problems associated with dialysis in poisoned patients.

PRINCIPLES OF DIALYSIS

Various forms of dialytic techniques are available in modern therapeutics: *peritoneal dialysis* and *hemodialysis* utilizing artificial semipermeable membranes, with either aqueous dialysate or lipid-containing dialysate (soybean oil). Direct extensions of hemodialysis have used the principle of *ultrafiltration*, whereby drug removal is increased by the process of "solvent drag." Drug removal may also be increased by *hemofiltration* or *CAVH*. Both of these are modifications of hemodialysis that utilize in the former the passage of high volumes of diluted blood, ultrafiltered at a high rate, through membranes that have a pore structure larger than conventional dialysis membranes,[36] or in the latter ultrafiltration at a slow rate throughout 24 hours without the use of dialysate.[37]

Solute (or drug) removal by dialysis has numerous determinants but involves principally the juxtaposition of a replaceable stream of blood and an appropriate rinsing solution, or dialysate. In peritoneal dialysis, the blood supply is in the capillary bed supplying the peritoneum; in hemodialysis, blood is supplied through the dialysis circuit by a blood pump. Drug removal depends not only on drug characteristics but also on physical factors of the specific dialyzer used.

These factors governing drug removal[38] depend on solute (or drug) size, its lipid-water partition coefficient (or lipid solubility), the degree to which it is protein bound, its volume of distribution, and the maintenance of a concentration gradient. The physical factors governing drug removal by the dialyzer itself depend on blood flow rate through the dialyzer, dialysate flow rate, dialyzer surface area, and the characteristics of the specific membrane chosen. To illustrate the effect of dialysis on these important points, it is worthwhile discussing analysis of two markedly different drugs—lithium and amitriptyline.

Lithium, the lightest cation known, is not lipid soluble, is freely distributed in whole body water, and does not have any degree of plasma protein binding. Its apparent volume of distribution equates to about 0.8 L per kg of body weight. Because it is not present in dialysate, there is a continual concentration gradient across either the peritoneal membrane or across an artificial semipermeable membrane. Consequently, lithium is one of the most highly dialyzable drugs; its clearance from blood is proportional to blood flow rate, dialysate flow rate, and dialyzer surface area. Because of its low molecular weight, its removal rate by different dialyzer membranes does not depend on the pore characteristics, since its clearance by the membrane is proportional to that of sodium. On the other hand, amitriptyline is of larger molecular weight, is somewhat lipid soluble, and is 96.4 per cent bound to serum albumin in plasma. Its apparent volume of distribution is also extremely large (8.3 L/kg of body weight). Although this drug is also not found in dialysate, with a consequent high concentration gradient possible, it is very poorly dialyzable in view of its characteristics just noted.

For drugs that are diffusible across semipermeable membranes under the usual operating conditions, the solute removal rate for small molecules is predominantly flow limited; in other words, clearance increases with increase in blood flow rate. For larger solutes, the rate of diffusion across the membrane is less, concentration gradients across the membrane remain high, and increasing flow rates have a smaller effect on drug clearance rates. In short, drug removal is limited by the membrane area times the permeability. Clearances reach a plateau above a blood flow rate of 200 to 300 ml per minute. For larger drugs, therefore, the removal rate can be increased by increasing the surface area, a situation similar to removal of larger uremic solutes. For this reason, also, in uremic patients treated with a variety of drugs, which are usually greater than 300 daltons, it is to be expected that drug accumulation occurs even in the face of dialysis, which is more effective for removal of small solutes.[39]

DIALYSANCE, OR CLEARANCE

Dialysance (D) is the traditional term used for solute removal by dialysate, which is given by the following formula:

$$D = Q_b \frac{(B_i - B_o)}{(B_i - D_i)} \text{ or } = Q_d \frac{(D_o - D_i)}{(B_i - D_i)}$$

where Q_b and Q_d are flow rates of blood and dialysate, respectively; B_i and B_o are blood concentrations entering and leaving the dialyzer; and D_i and D_o are the dialysate inlet and outlet concentrations. Dialysance takes into account the concentration of drug in the dialysate. However, when the concentration of drug in dialysate is negligible (i.e., when the dialysate does not come into further contact with the dialyzer in the process known as "single pass dialysis," such as used in hollow fiber and flat plate modern dialyzers), then such a formula gives the *clearance* of solute from the blood.

$$\text{Clearance equals } Q_b \frac{A - V}{A}$$

where A is arterial, or inlet concentration, V is venous, or outlet concentration, of drug going through the dialyzer, and Q_b is blood flow rate through the dialyzer. The ratio A−V/A also equates to the drug *extraction ratio* across the dialyzer, and this will be dealt with in some detail in the following section.

FACTORS GOVERNING DRUG REMOVAL WITH DIALYSIS

Drug removal rates with dialysis can be calculated from in vitro experiments. Unfortunately, most experiments quoted in the literature have used aqueous solutions containing drugs, thereby overestimating the effect of dialysis on drug removal, since the experiments failed to take account of the significant influence of plasma protein binding. One must therefore be careful in assessing dialyzability from such experimental results. Classically, it is assumed that the plasma concentrations are representative of whole blood concentrations, and blood flow rates have been used for calculations of clearances on the assumption that blood represents the volume from which the solute diffuses to the dialysate. It has recently been pointed out, however, that not only are drugs removable from red cells but also that failure to use the whole blood flow rate through dialyzers (or hemoperfusion devices) can introduce considerable errors into calculation of clearances.[40] While the volume of distribution of drugs and their lipid solubility are extremely important in relation to drug removal with dialysis, it is also important to consider the intercompartmental transfer of drugs from tissues into plasma and its influence on drug removal rates;[41] the influence of this factor on drug removal for most drugs is unknown and will not be discussed further.

While plasma protein binding is an important factor and the degree of protein binding depends upon plasma protein concentrations and solute concentrations, it must be pointed out that some solutes do not saturate binding sites at the usual pharmacologic concentrations, while others demonstrate an increase in the ultrafilterable fraction at very high drug levels; this is seen with salicylate poisoning and renders salicylate an ideal dialyzable drug.[42]

Lipid solubility of drugs also governs their removal by dialysis. Removal of ethchlorvynol and glutethimide, as examples of highly lipid-soluble drugs, has been shown to be low with aqueous dialysis; this rate is increased by the use of lipid dialysis, which allows partitioning of these drugs in lipid globules within the dialysate. However, with modern dialysis and with large surface area dialyzers, this technique has fallen into disfavor. In addition, lipid-soluble drugs are more readily removed with activated charcoal or resin hemoperfusion; these techniques will be discussed later.

Ultrafiltration dialysis is the term used to describe aqueous hemodialysis, with hydrostatic ultrafiltration of water through the semipermeable membrane. This process is known to increase solvent drag of solute, thereby making its clearance higher than at a degree at which no ultrafiltration occurs. This type of dialysis has been suggested for treating poisoning with agents such as paraquat,[43] but with conventional hemodialyzer membranes the degree of increase in clearance is rather small. The clearance of solutes by the process of ultrafiltration, however, is greatly enhanced if the membrane has larger pores, such as those introduced by Henderson and colleagues.[36] Although these large-pore membranes were not specifically introduced for poisoning therapy, it is known that removal of solutes ranging from 64 (urea) up to 1500 (vitamin B_{12}) daltons is identical; therefore, this type of treatment theoretically should allow higher clearance rates for rather large molecular weight drugs. CAVH, using similar large-pore membranes, relies on ultrafiltration for solute and fluid removal and will be discussed in a following section.

It thus can be appreciated that peritoneal dialysis is the least effective method for removing drugs compared with hemodialysis and hemofiltration in view of the slower dialysate transit times within the abdominal cavity. Peritoneal dialysis should therefore be used for treating only dialyzable poisons if the other methods are unavailable. Certain drugs have been shown to increase peritoneal clearances of various solutes by inducing changes in vascular permeability,[44, 45] but this method has not been used in human clinical poisoning.

PERITONEAL DIALYSIS

This technique uses the instillation of sterile, preheated, commercially available dialysate solutions (2 L) into the abdominal cavity of the poisoned patient, using a semirigid peritoneal catheter placed 4 to 5 inches below the umbilicus under local anesthesia. The peritoneal dialysate is changed, usually hourly, with the dialysate "dwelling" within the peritoneal cavity for about 30 minutes, after which it is drained and discarded. As pointed out earlier, this technique is less efficient than hemodialysis, but in certain situations it is of some use. In hypothermic patients, the instillation of preheated solutions into the abdominal cavity can rapidly reverse the hypothermia; theoretically, equilibration across the gastrointestinal wall may influence removal of ingested drugs before equilibration with body stores is achieved.

HEMODIALYSIS

Hemodialysis requires the passage of anticoagulated (heparinized) blood through dialyzer lines and dialyzers consisting of semipermeable membranes through which dialysate is brought into juxtaposition with blood on the other side of the semipermeable membrane. Dialyzers are available as flat plate or hollow fiber models. Blood is usually pumped through the dialyzer lines with a roller pump. Blood is derived from an arteriovenous shunt placed in the arm or leg, or more commonly in modern toxicology, blood is derived from two venous catheters or a double-lumen venous catheter placed in the inferior vena cava through the femoral veins. Blood flows can be adjusted, depending on the patient's blood pressure and whole blood clotting time, or activated clotting time must be maintained within limits by adjusting heparin dosage. CAVH requires either a plastic arteriovenous shunt (giving enough pressure to maintain ultrafiltration without a blood pump) or an arteriovenous catheter and blood pump to maintain continuous ultrafiltration and drug removal. CAVH has been used in the treatment of paraquat poisoning because of the continuous nature of drug removal.[37]

In the hypotensive patient who requires dopamine or dobutamine for blood pressure control, these drugs must be placed distal to the dialyzer. Requirements of these catecholamines may increase during dialysis, since they are readily removed through the hemodialyzer membrane. Lipid hemodialysis requires the addition of quantities of soybean oil to aqueous dialysate to form an emulsion, but as previously noted, utilization of modern hemodialyzers and hemodialyzer apparatus largely outweighs the benefits of lipid hemodialysis. "Single-pass" dialysis systems are the most efficient methods for removing drugs (or other solutes) because they maintain a constant concentration gradient, enhancing drug removal.

Dialysate regeneration apparatus in which the dialysate is regenerated using a sorbent system (the REDY system) may be used in the treatment of poisoned patients. However, it must be pointed out that the sorbent system may theoretically become saturated with drug, and removal rates will decrease over time for certain drugs.[46]

CRITERIA FOR CONSIDERATION OF HEMODIALYSIS IN POISONING

The decision whether a patient should undergo active drug removal is not always easily made, and it is certainly not the purpose of this discussion to suggest that every patient suffering from poisoning of an extractable drug undergo hemodialysis. *The prime consideration in the decision is based on the clinical features of poisoning; hemodialysis or hemoperfusion should be considered in general if the patient's condition progressively deteriorates despite intensive supportive therapy.*

The use of active drug-removing techniques has engendered a great deal of controversy. Some clinicians are conservative[47–51] in their approach, while others are more aggressive.[32, 52–55] Appraisal of each viewpoint, however, reveals little difference and may be explained by patient spectrum[48] and geographic area. Both groups are however very close in their use of interventional techniques in specific poisons as well as for specific clinical indications.[49, 57] Supportive therapy includes appropriate fluid balance, correction of acid-base abnormalities, dopamine infusion, and forced diuresis.

Suggested clinical criteria are outlined in Table 8–3. These criteria should be used along with the plasma concentrations of common drugs (Table 8–4), above which hemodialysis or hemoperfusion should be considered. Table 8–5 lists the reported dialyzable drugs; please note that many of these reports[32] are anecdotal and uncritical, and it is suggested that dialysis be reserved for only those drugs that are not placed in parentheses in Table 8–5. For further discussion of specific agents, see the appropriate chapter.

SORBENT HEMOPERFUSION

The process of hemoperfusion, by which anticoagulated blood is passed through a column containing sorbent particles, was introduced by Muirhead and Reid in 1948 for the investigation of removal of uremic toxins using a mixed ion exchange resin in animals.[58] Following this study, Schreiner in 1958 employed a lactated anion exchange resin column for two 15-minute periods in a patient with pentobarbital poisoning but did not achieve a great deal of drug removal.[59] Both the early resin studies and others were complicated by pyrogenic reactions, electrolyte disturbances, and hemolysis. It was not until 1964 that Yatzidis presented work showing that in vitro a column containing 200 gm of activated charcoal particles could absorb from plasma considerable quantities of barbital, phenobarbital, and pentobarbital

Table 8–3. CLINICAL CONSIDERATIONS FOR HEMODIALYSIS OR HEMOPERFUSION IN POISONING

1. Progressive deterioration despite intensive supportive therapy.
2. Severe intoxication with depression of midbrain function leading to hypoventilation, hypothermia, and hypotension.
3. Development of complications of coma, such as pneumonia or septicemia, and underlying conditions predisposing to such complications (e.g., obstructive airway disease).
4. Impairment of normal drug excretory function in the presence of hepatic, cardiac, or renal insufficiency.
5. Intoxication with agents with metabolic and/or delayed effects, e.g., methanol, ethylene glycol, and paraquat.
6. Intoxication with an extractable drug or poison, which can be removed at a rate exceeding endogenous elimination by liver or kidney.

Table 8–4. PLASMA CONCENTRATION* OF COMMON POISONS IN EXCESS OF WHICH HEMODIALYSIS (HD) OR HEMOPERFUSION (HP) SHOULD BE CONSIDERED

DRUG	SERUM CONCENTRATION (μg/mL)	(mmol/L)	METHOD OF CHOICE
phenobarbital	100	430	HP>HD
other barbiturates	50	200	HP
glutethimide	40	160	HP
methaqualone	40	160	HP
salicylates	800	5000	HD
theophylline	400	2200	HP>HD
paraquat	0.1	0.5	HP>HD
methanol	50		HD
trichloroethanol	50	335	HP>HD
meprobamate	100	460	HP

*Suggested concentrations only: Clinical condition may warrant intervention at lower concentrations, e.g., in mixed intoxications.

as well as salicylic acid and glutethimide.[60] The first clinical study in 1965 by Yatzidis and associates demonstrated that two patients with barbiturate poisoning and severe intoxication recovered consciousness after three and five hemoperfusions, each lasting 1 hour.[61] With early hemoperfusion devices, transient side effects were seen, such as facial flushing, dyspnea, and burning sensations as well as platelet depletion and reduction of fibrinogen concentrations.

It was also demonstrated in animals that particle embolization from the surface of the charcoal particles occurred. Specially prepared activated charcoal coated with polymer solutions[62, 63] has abolished this phenomenon. Clinical use of uncoated activated charcoal hemoperfusion is associated with a greater reduction in platelet counts than use of coated charcoal; coated charcoal gives an average platelet loss of about 30 per cent.[64] Arising from the work of Rosenbaum and associates,[65] nonionic resins became available for the treatment of drug intoxication. Early devices utilized XAD-2 resin, a polystyrene Amberlite resin, but this was superseded by the introduction of a more efficient compound, XAD-4, also a polystyrene Amberlite compound. These resins had been shown to be most effective for removal of lipid-soluble drugs, with drug clearance rates from blood often exceeding those achieved by charcoal hemoperfusion. Resin hemoperfusion devices are no longer available in the United States. A list of the clinically available hemoperfusion devices and the contained sorbents is shown in Table 8–6.

Hemoperfusion relies on the physical process of drug adsorption for its efficiency, and in many instances drug removal in terms of clearance is far better achieved with it than with hemodialysis, peritoneal dialysis, or forced diuresis. With activated charcoal, drugs are often so tightly bound with Van der Waals' forces as to be unextractable from the sorbent. On the other hand, with the resin preparations the drug is tightly but not irreversibly bound within the resin bead matrix and can be eluted with organic solvents. "Activation" of carbon is the formation induced by chemical or physical processes of pores within the carbon structure; pores are divided into macropores and micropores—the latter are principally responsible for drug uptake and have a size of 20 angstroms, which varies with the selection of starting material. Water- and lipid-soluble substances with molecular weights ranging from 113 to 40,000 daltons are well adsorbed, although substances at the higher molecular weights are adsorbed less efficiently to charcoal when a coating polymer solution is used.[66]

A typical hemoperfusion circuit for treatment of drug intoxication is shown in Figure 8–2; in general, hemoperfusion is instituted with a column (Fig. 8–3) that contains between 100 and 300 gm of activated charcoal or 650 gm (wet weight) of polystyrene resin. Most devices are flushed with saline prior to use (since most come already sterilized), and blood is withdrawn through an arteriovenous shunt or venovenous shunt, as in hemodialysis, using a blood pump. Blood flow rates are graduated, depending upon the clinical condition of the patient, but the most efficient drug removal is achieved with blood flow rates of approximately 300 ml per minute. Pressure devices can detect interior rises in pressure, which serve as an index of

Table 8–5. DRUGS AND CHEMICALS REMOVED WITH VARIOUS DIALYTIC TECHNIQUES

BARBITURATES

amobarbital
aprobarbital
barbital
butabarbital
cyclobarbital
pentobarbital
phenobarbital
quinalbital
(secobarbital)

NONBARBITURATE HYPNOTICS, SEDATIVES, TRANQUILIZERS, ANTICONVULSANTS

carbamazepine
carbromal
chloral hydrate
(chlordiazepoxide)
(diazepam)
(diphenylhydantoin)
(diphenylhydramine)
ethiamate
ethchlorvynol
ethosuximide
gallamine
glutethimide
(heroin)
meprobamate
(methaqualone)
methsuximide
methyprylon
paraldehyde
primidone
valproic acid

ANTIDEPRESSANTS

(amitriptyline)
amphetamines
(imipramine)
isocarboxazid
MAO inhibitors
(pargyline)
(phenelzine)
tranylcypromine
(tricyclics)

ALCOHOLS

ethanol
ethylene glycol
isopropanol
methanol

ANALGESICS, ANTIRHEUMATICS

acetaminophen
acetophenetidin
acetylsalicylic acid
colchicine
methylsalicylate
(d-propoxyphene)
salicylic acid

ANTIMICROBIALS/ ANTICANCER

amikacin
dibekacin
fosfomycin
gentamicin
kanamycin
neomycin
netilmicin
sisomicin
streptomycin
tobramycin
(vancomycin)

bacitracin
colistin

ampicillin
amoxicillin
azlocillin
carbenicillin
clavulinic acid
(cloxacillin)
(floxacillin)
mecillinam
mezlocillin
(nafcillin)
penicillin
peperacillin
temocillin
ticarcillin

(cefaclor)
cefadroxil
cefamandole
cefazolin
cefixime
cefmenoxime
(cefonicid)
(cefoperazone)
ceforanide
(cefotaxime)
(cefotetan)
cefotiam
cefoxitin
cefroxadine
cefsulodin
ceftazidime
(ceftriaxone)
cefuroxime
cephacetrile
cephalexin
cephaloridine
cephalothin
(cephapirin)
cephradine

aztreonam
cilastin
imipinem
moxalactam

(chloramphenicol)
ciprofloxacin

ANTIMICROBIALS/ ANTICANCER

(clindamycin)
(erythromycin)
metronidazole
nitrofurantoin
ornidazole
sulfonamides
tetracycline
tinidazole

isoniazid
cycloserine
ethambutol
5-fluorocytosine

acyclovir
amantadine
(chloroquine)
quinine

(azathioprine)
bredinin
cyclophosphamide
5-fluorouracil
(methotrexate)

CARDIOVASCULAR AGENTS

acebutolol
atenolol
bretylium
captopril
(diazoxide)
(digoxin)
(lidocaine)
metoprolol
methyldopa
(ouabain)
N-acetylprocainamide
nadolol
practolol
procainamide
propranolol
(quinidine)
sotalol
tocainide

METALS, INORGANICS

(aluminum)*
arsenic
(copper)*
(iron)*
lead
lithium
(magnesium)
(mercury)*
potassium
phosphate
sodium
strontium
(tin)
(zinc)

( ) = Not well removed; ( )* = removed with chelating agent

Table 8–5. DRUGS AND CHEMICALS REMOVED WITH VARIOUS DIALYTIC TECHNIQUES *Continued*

METALS, INORGANICS *(Continued)*	SOLVENTS, GASES	PLANTS, ANIMALS, HERBICIDES, INSECTICIDES
	acetone	
bromide	camphor	alkyl phosphate
chloride	carbon monoxide	amanitin
iodide	(carbon tetrachloride)	demeton sulfoxide
fluoride	(eucalyptus oil)	dimethoate
	thiols	diquat
MISCELLANEOUS	toluene	methylmercury complex
	trichloroethylene	(organophosphates)
acipimox		paraquat
aminophylline		snake bite
aniline		sodium chlorate
borates		potassium chlorate
boric acid		
(chlorpropamide)		
chromic acid		
cimetidine		
dinitro-*o*-cresol		
folic acid		
mannitol		
methylprednisolone		
potassium dichromate		
sodium citrate		
theophylline		
thiocyanate		
ranitidine		

( ) = Not well removed; ( )* = removed with chelating agent.

thrombosis occurring inside the device. With the resin preparations, greater falls in platelet counts were observed.

Table 8–7 shows that the plasma-drug extraction ratios for many drugs are greater with hemoperfusion than with hemodialysis. Removal of lipid-soluble drugs, such as glutethimide and methaqualone, is far more efficient with XAD-4 resin hemoperfusion than with activated charcoal.

Table 8–8 lists representative drugs that have been reported to be removed by various types of hemoperfusion; again, it cannot be overstated that many of these reports are anecdotal,[32] but critical review of drug removal rates indicates that those drugs not

Table 8–6. AVAILABLE HEMOPERFUSION DEVICES

MANUFACTURER	DEVICE	SORBENT TYPE	AMOUNT OF SORBENT	POLYMER COATING
Bioencapsulation Technology	DiaKart	Petroleum-based charcoal	70 gm	collodion
Clark	Biocompatible system	Charcoal	50, 100, 250 ml	heparinized polymer
Erika	Hemocart or Alukart	Petroleum-based charcoal	60 or 155 gm	collodion
Gambro	Adsorba	Norit	100 or 300 gm	cellulose acetate
Organon-Teknika	Hemopur 260	Norit-extruded charcoal	250 gm	cellulose acetate
Smith and Nephew*	Hemocol or Haemocol	Sutcliffe Speakman charcoal	100 to 300 gm	acrylic hydrogel
Extracorporeal*	XR-004	XAD-4 resin	350 gm	none

*No longer available in the United States.

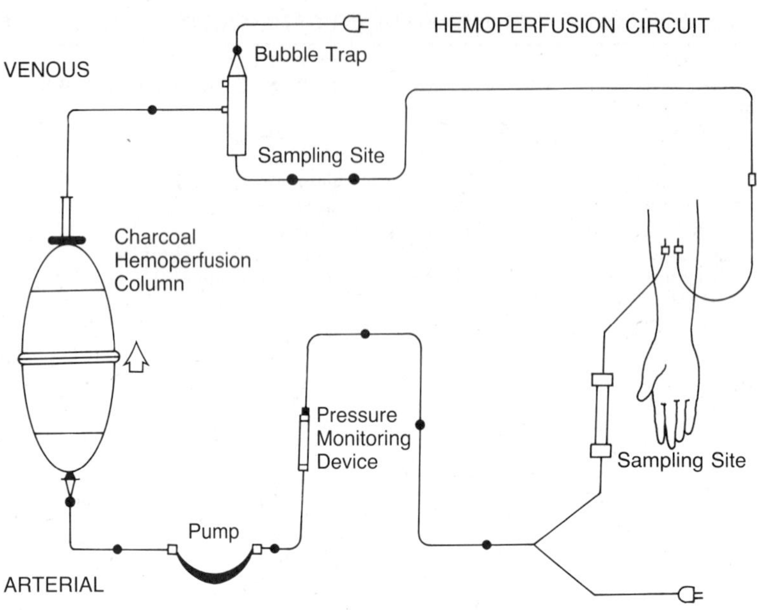

Figure 8–2. Clinical hemoperfusion circuit. (From Gelfand MC, Winchester JF, Knepshield JH, et al: Charcoal hemoperfusion in severe drug overdosage. Trans Am Soc Artif Intern Organs 23:599, 1977, with permission of copyright holder.)

enclosed in parentheses are most efficiently removed.

Criteria for Consideration of Hemoperfusion in Poisoning

The criteria outlined in Tables 8–3 and 8–4 for hemodialysis also apply to hemoperfusion. However, in certain situations one is preferred over the other, so Table 8–9 is provided as a guide in choosing either hemoperfusion or hemodialysis.

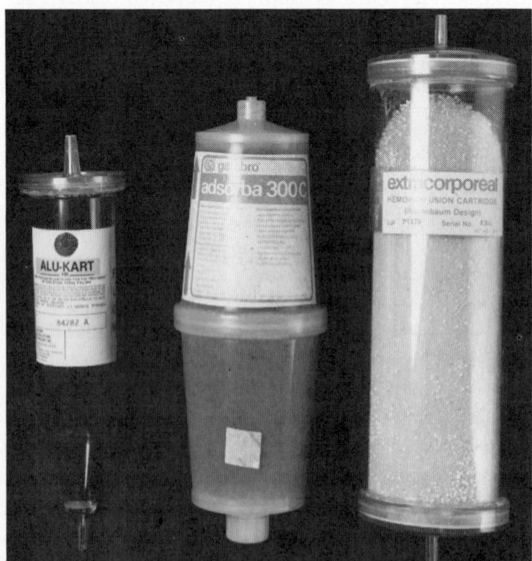

Figure 8–3. Three hemoperfusion devices. The two columns on the left contain coated activated charcoal, and the column on the right contains XAD-4 Amberlite resin (the latter is no longer available in the United States). For full description, see Table 8–6.

Complications of Hemoperfusion

The principal side effect of hemoperfusion with charcoal or resin preparations is platelet depletion. Most studies of hemoperfusion in humans show an average loss of 30 per cent of platelets with coated or uncoated charcoal or resin preparations.[64] Occasionally, however, a higher drop in platelet count can occur, which may give rise to clinical bleeding problems.[67] Other side effects noted are reductions in serum calcium and serum glucose and transient falls in white blood cell counts, all of which are usually mild and can be managed clinically.[68] In addition, with the recirculation of blood in the extracorporeal circuit, there is also a mild reduction of 1 to 2 degrees in body temperature, and frequent body temperatures should be taken in deeply comatose patients.[68] Although hypotension as a consequence of circulation of blood in the extracorporeal circuit is an infrequent phenomenon in drug overdosage, pressor agents like dopamine for hypotensive comatose patients should be administered distal to the sorbent devices, since they are also adsorbed by the sorbent preparations.[69] The

Table 8–7. PLASMA DRUG EXTRACTION RATIOS WITH DIFFERENT DEVICES*

	STANDARD HEMODIALYSIS	COATED OR UNCOATED CHARCOAL HEMOPERFUSION	XAD-2 OR XAD-4 RESIN HEMOPERFUSION
acetaminophen	0.4	0.5	0.7
amobarbital	0.26	0.3	0.9
acetylsalicylic acid	0.5	0.5	—
carbromal	0.31	0.55	1.0
digoxin	0.2	0.3 to 0.6	0.4
ethchlorvynol	0.32	0.7	1.0
glutethimide	0.16	0.65	0.8
paraquat	0.5	0.6	0.9†
phenobarbital	0.27	0.5	0.85
theophylline	0.5	0.7	0.75
tricyclics	0.35	0.35	0.8

*Calculated for blood flow rate of 200 ml per minute.
†Ion exchange resin.

Table 8–8. DRUGS AND CHEMICALS REMOVED WITH HEMOPERFUSION

BARBITURATES

amobarbital
butabarbital
hexabarbital
pentobarbital
phenobarbital
quinalbital
secobarbital
thiopental
vinalbital

NONBARBITURATE HYPNOTICS, SEDATIVES, TRANQUILIZERS

carbamazepine
carbromal
chloral hydrate
chlorpromazine
(diazepam)
diphenhydramine
ethchlorvynol
glutethimide
meprobamate
methaqualone
methsuximide
methyprylon
promazine
promethazine

ANALGESICS, ANTIRHEUMATICS

acetaminophen
acetylsalicylic acid
colchicine
d-propoxyphene
methylsalicylate
phenybutazone
salicylic acid

ANTIMICROBIALS/ ANTICANCER

(adriamycin)
ampicillin
carmustine
chloramphenicol
chloroquine
clindamycin
dapsone
doxorubicin
gentamicin
isoniazid
methotrexate
thiabendazole

ANTIDEPRESSANTS

(amitriptyline)
(imipramine)
(tricyclics)

PLANTS, ANIMALS, HERBICIDES, INSECTICIDES

amanitin
chlordane
demeton sulfoxide
dimethoate
diquat
methylparathion
nitrostigmine
organophosphates
phalloidin
polychlorinated biphenyls
paraquat
parathion

CARDIOVASCULAR AGENTS

digoxin
diltiazem
(disopyramide)
metoprolol
N-acetylprocainamide
procainamide
quinidine

METAL, INORGANICS

(aluminum)*
(iron)*

MISCELLANEOUS

aminophylline
caffeine
cimetidine
(fluoroacetamide)
(phencyclidine)
phenols
(podophyllin)
theophylline

SOLVENTS, GASES

carbon tetrachloride
ethylene oxide
trichloroethanol

( ) = Not well removed; ( )* = removed with chelating agent.

Table 8–9. CHOICE OF HEMODIALYSIS OR HEMOPERFUSION FOR CERTAIN DRUGS

HEMODIALYSIS	HEMOPERFUSION
lithium	lipid-soluble drugs
bromide	barbiturates
ethanol	nonbarbiturate hypnotics,
methanol	sedatives, and tranquilizers
ethylene glycol	digitalis glycosides
salicylates	

observed falls in platelet concentrations have usually returned to normal limits within 24 to 48 hours following a single hemoperfusion. Such falls are far outweighed by the clinical benefits to be obtained.

INFLUENCE OF ACTIVE DRUG REMOVAL PROCEDURES ON DRUG ELIMINATION RATES

In barbiturate poisoning, forced diuresis has not been conclusively shown to alter duration of coma or overall mortality; in one large study of forced diuresis in barbiturate poisoning, mortality was reduced from 3.5 to 2.4 per cent, but if deaths in the most severely affected groups were excluded, mortality with diuresis was 2.1 per cent compared with 2.6 per cent without diuresis, results that may not be significantly different.[70] Peritoneal dialysis is not substantially more effective than diuresis, since peritoneal clearance of most drugs is usually less than 10 ml per minute. However, as mentioned, pharmacologic agents or albumin added to dialysate may increase drug removal rates, although it has not been confirmed that peritoneal dialysis shortens coma time or substantially increases total clearance of barbiturates.[71]

Schreiner has pointed out that any procedure used in poisoning treatment must be demonstrated to have a greater effect on drug elimination than that which occurs spontaneously.[72] In human beings, the spontaneous half-life of barbiturates in barbiturate poisoning ranges from 37 to 96 hours, and hemodialysis does seem to have some effect on this, with reported rates of drug half-life ranging from 3.6 to 9.7 hours.[71] Hemoperfusion, on the other hand, has been shown in animals to reduce mortality in barbiturate,[73, 74] salicylate,[74] and paraquat[75] poisoning and to reduce coma time in barbiturate-poisoned dogs.[73] In humans, in comparison with standard supportive therapy, hemoperfusion also appears to shorten coma time,[55, 68] but no controlled studies have been undertaken. For further discussion of specific agents see the appropriate chapter.

To obtain accurate documentation of the effects on drug elimination rates, recourse must be made to animal experiments in relationship to the effects of hemodialysis or hemoperfusion; most work has in fact centered on hemoperfusion.[76–79] Using appropriate pharmacokinetic models, it has been shown that hemoperfusion increases drug elimination rates in animals intoxicated with acetaminophen,[76] amobarbital,[77] ethchlorvynol,[80] doxorubicin (Adriamycin),[81] digoxin,[79] and digitoxin.[82] In all these experiments, as well as in clinical experience, it has been observed that "rebound" of drug concentration occurs following hemoperfusion as drug redistributes from tissues into the plasma following its removal from the plasma compartment. This is consistent with pharmacokinetic handling of drugs after their removal from the central compartment[78] but clinically may return the patient to coma: for instance, as occurs after hemoperfusion for glutethimide poisoning.[68, 83]

Intermittent hemoperfusion has two major advantages: reduction in blood concentrations and reduction in the hematologic side effects of prolonged hemoperfusion. Replacement of saturated devices with fresh devices is not usually necessary but is another positive aspect of short intermittent hemoperfusion. Any rebound in plasma drug concentrations released from tissue can be reduced with further hemoperfusion (e.g., paraquat[84] and glutethimide[83]). Review of pharmacokinetic data[85–88] not unexpectedly has shown that hemodialysis and hemoperfusion enhance drug elimination for only specific drugs. In humans, in view of the difficulties in conducting controlled prospective clinical trials,[89] reduction in coma time or overall mortality has not conclusively been demonstrated, although it has been suggested by retrospective studies.[90] In the severely hypothermic patient, hemoperfusion can be combined with hemodialysis for blood warming.

Systemic hemoperfusion or exchange transfusion for drug removal from systemic circulation appears promising for anticancer drugs.[91–94]

PLASMA EXCHANGE AND EXCHANGE BLOOD TRANSFUSION

Both these techniques have been used infrequently in the treatment of poisoning. Plasma exchange or plasmapheresis involves the removal of the patient's plasma by means of centrifugal or filtration devices, with substitution of fresh plasma; exchange blood transfusion involves the removal of a quantity of blood and its replacement with an identical quantity of fresh whole blood. Plasma exchange involves a 3- to 4-L exchange of plasma in a 4-hour treatment period; therefore, the total maximal quantity of drug removed will be its concentration times the volume of plasma removed. This technique, therefore, is most applicable to strongly protein-bound drugs that are not well removed with hemodialysis. (Examples are chromic acid and chromate poisoning.[95]) The effectiveness of plasmapheresis in various poisonings has been reported anecdotally, but at present the role of plasmapheresis is unclear. Exchange blood transfusion has also been used infrequently in the treatment of poisoning, principally when hemolysis and methemoglobinemia have complicated the poisoning (for example, sodium chlorate poisoning[96]), while plasma exchange with subsequent plasma perfusion over sorbents has been used in a variety of poisons.[97]

HEMOPERFUSION AND HEMODIALYSIS WITH CHELATING AGENTS

In dialysis patients, aluminum intoxication with refractory bone disease or dialysis dementia can be treated with deferoxamine in conjunction with dialysis (continuous ambulatory peritoneal dialysis[98] or hemodialysis[99]) or hemoperfusion[100, 101] for removal of the deferoxamine-aluminum complex. Clinical improvement in the osteomalacic component of renal osteodystrophy,[102, 103] encephalopathy,[104] and anemia[105] has been reported.

Although less common, iron overload is recognized in dialysis patients[106] and has also been treated by deferoxamine in conjunction with dialysis,[107, 108] hemofiltration,[109] or hemoperfusion,[107] especially since in hemoglobinopathy subjects long-term iron deposition responsible for cardiomyopathy, diabetes, and other complications may improve with chelation therapy.[110–112]

Heavy metals and their salts are not removed efficiently by dialysis or hemoperfusion alone.[113–115] During hemodialysis, metal removal may be enhanced with certain chelating agents, such as *n*-acetylcysteine[116] or cysteine.[117] On the other hand, removal of mercury[113] and thallium[114, 115] by hemoperfusion appears modest at best. Development of chelating microspheres[118] or chelate-metal groups for adsorption[117, 119] may eventually prove useful clinically for heavy metal removal.

IMMUNOPHARMACOLOGY AS AN ACTIVE TREATMENT METHOD IN POISONING

An antibody is composed of two Fab fragments and an Fc fragment. Fab fragments retain the binding sites of the antibodies and have a molecular weight of about 50,000 daltons. By appropriately binding the drug to a hapten, an antibody response can be mounted, and antibody fractions can be subjected to splitting to obtain Fab fragments. When injected, these Fab fragments combine with specific antigens (drug) with a high degree of specificity to neutralize their toxic effects. In potentially fatal cases of glycoside poisoning, such procedures have resulted in a response far greater than that obtained with conventional therapy.[120, 121] In the presence of renal failure, however, for drugs that depend on renal elimination, the effectiveness of Fab fragment administration may be minimized.

Poisoning treated by immunopharmacology is presently limited to digoxin poisoning. In digoxin poisoning the elimination half-time of digoxin in anephric patients can be substantially reduced with the addition of hemoperfusion.[122] Potentially fatal cases of digoxin poisoning have been treated successfully by Fab antibody fragments,[120, 121] but failures have also been reported,[123, 124] and the cost of treatment averages $1680 (range of $175 to $7000).[123] Immobilized antibody on hemoperfusion devices may offer an alternative.[125] In dialysis patients (in whom vascular access facilitates interventional therapy) a judgment to use either hemoperfusion or Fab antibody fragments is required.

Problems with immunopharmacology have been reviewed by Colburn.[126] For further discussion see Chapter 15. It is likely that in the future drugs with a high toxicity ratio and poor removal rate with hemodialysis or hemoperfusion (e.g., tricyclic antidepressants)[127] or drugs with delayed effects (e.g., paraquat) may be treated by such methods.[126]

References

1. Clemmesen C, Nilsson E: Therapeutic trends in the treatment of barbiturate poisoning: The Scandinavian method. Clin Pharmacol Ther *2*:220, 1961.
2. Litovitz TL, Schmitz BF, Matyunas N, Martin TG: The 1987 Annual Report of the American Association of Poison Control Centers National Data Collection System. Am J Emerg Med *6*:479, 1988.
3. Litovitz TL, Martin TG, Schmitz B: 1986 Annual Report of the American Association of Poison Control Centers National Data Collection System. Am J Emerg Med *5*:405, 1987.
4. Litovitz TL, Veltri JC: The role of hemoperfusion and hemodialysis in toxicology. Am J Emerg Med *6*:80, 1988.
5. Cohn WJ, Boylan JJ, Blanke RV, Fariss MW, Howell JR, Guzelian PS: Treatment of chlordecone (kepone) toxicity with cholestyramine. N Engl J Med *298*:243, 1978.
6. Hillman RJ, Prescott LF: Treatment of salicylate poisoning with repetitive oral charcoal. Br Med J *291*:1472, 1985.
7. Boldy DA, Vale JA, Prescott LF: Treatment of phenobarbitone poisoning with repeated oral administration of activated charcoal. Q J Med *61*:997, 1986.
8. Belz GG: Plasma concentrations of intravenous B-methyl-digoxin with and without oral charcoal. Klin Wochenschr *52*:749, 1974.
9. Sintek C, Hendeles L, Weinberger M: Inhibition of theophylline absorption by activated charcoal. J Pediatr *94*:314, 1979.
10. Smith LL, Wright A, Wyatt I, Rose MS: Effective treatment for paraquat poisoning in rats and its relevance to treatment of paraquat poisoning in man. Br Med J *4*:569, 1974.
11. Pitts RF: Physiology of the Kidney and Body Fluids. 2nd ed. Chicago, Year Book Medical Publishers, 1968.
12. Mayer SE, Melman KL, Gilman AG: Introduction: The dynamics of drug absorption, distribution and elimination. *In* Gilman AG, Goodman LS, Gilman A (eds): The Pharmacological Basis of Therapeutics. 6th ed. New York, Macmillan, 1981, p 1.
13. Gabow PA, Peterson LN: Disorders of potassium metabolism. *In* Schrier RW (ed): Renal and Electrolyte Disorders. 2nd ed. Boston, Little, Brown & Co, 1980, p 183.
14. Prescott LF, Balali-Mood M, Critchley JA, Johnstone, AF, Proudfoot, AT: Diuresis or urinary alkalinization in salicylate poisoning? Br Med J *285*:1383–1386, 1982.
15. Done AK: Salicylate intoxication: Significance of measurements of salicylate in blood in cases of acute ingestion. Pediatrics *26*:800, 1960.
16. Hayes WJ: Toxicology of Pesticides. Baltimore, Williams & Wilkins, 1975, p 131.
17. Beckett AH, Rowland M, Turner P: Influence of urinary pH on excretion of amphetamine. Lancet *1*:303, 1965.
18. Astatoor AM, Galman BR, Johnson JR, Milne JD: The excretion of dexamphetamine and its derivatives. Br J Pharmacol Chemother *24*:293, 1965.
19. Beckett AH, Brookes LG: The absorption and urinary excretion in man of fenfluramine and its main metabolite. J Pharm Pharmacol *19*(Suppl 1):41S, 1967.
20. Von Muhlendahl KE, Krienke EG: Fenfluramine poisoning. Clin Toxicol *14*:97, 1979.
21. Done AK, Aronow R, Micelli JN: The pharmacokinetics of phencyclidine in overdosage and its treatment. Natl Inst Drug Abuse Res Monogr Ser *21*:210, 1978.
22. Aronow R, Micelli JN, Done AK: Clinical observations during phencyclidine and treatment based on ion-tapping. Natl Inst Drug Abuse Res Monogr Ser *21*:218, 1978.
23. Haag HB, Larson PS, Schwartz JJ: The effect of urinary pH on the elimination of quinine in man. J Pharmacol Exp Ther *79*:136, 1943.
24. Sabto JK, Pierce RM, West RH, Gurr FW: Hemodialysis, peritoneal dialysis, plasmapheresis and forced diuresis for the treatment of quinine overdose. Clin Nephrol *16*:264, 1981.
25. Graham T: Bakerian lecture on osmotic force. Phil Trans Roy Soc London, 1854, p 177.
26. Abel JJ, Rowntree LG, Turner BB: On the removal of diffusible substances from the circulating blood by means of dialysis. Trans Assoc Am Phys *28*:51, 1913.
27. Kolff WJ, Berk HT: Artificial kidney: Dialyzer with great area. Acta Med Scand *117*:121, 1944.
28. Doolan PD, Walsh WP, Kyle LH, Wishinsky H: Acetylsalicylic acid intoxication: A proposed method of treatment. JAMA *146*:105, 1951.
29. Schreiner GE, Berman LB, Griffin J, Feys J: Specific therapy for salicylism. N Engl J Med *253*:213, 1955.
30. Seyffart G: Poison Index. Bad Homburg, West Germany, Fresenius Foundation, 1977.
31. Maher JF, Schreiner GE: The dialysis of poisons and drugs. Trans Am Soc Artif Intern Organs *13*:369, 1967.
32. Winchester JF, Gelfand MC, Knepshield JH, Schreiner GE: Dialysis and hemoperfusion of poisons and drugs—Update. Trans Am Soc Artif Intern Organs *23*:762, 1977.
33. Takki S, Gambertoglio JG, Honda DH, Tozer TN: Pharmacokinetic evaluation of hemodialysis in acute drug overdose. J Pharmacokinet Biopharm *6*:427, 1976.
34. Pond S, Rosenberg J, Benowitz NL, Takki S: Pharmacokinetics of haemoperfusion in drug overdose. Clin Pharmacokinet *4*:329, 1979.
35. De Broe ME, Verpooten BA, Van Haesebrouck B: Recent experience with prolonged hemoperfusion-hemodialysis treatment. Artif Organs *3*:188, 1979.
36. Henderson LW, Silverstein MAE, Ford CA, Lysaght MJ: Clinical response to maintenance hemodiafiltration. Kidney Int *7*:S52, 1975.
37. Pond SM, Johnston SC, Schoof DD, Hampson EC, Bowles M, Wright DM, Petrie JJ: Repeated hemoperfusion and continuous arteriovenous hemofiltration in a paraquat poisoned patient. J Toxicol Clin Toxicol *25*:305, 1987.
38. Maher JF: Principles of dialysis and dialysis of drugs. Am J Med *62*:475, 1977.

39. Bennett WM, Singer I, Golper T, Feig P, Coggins CJ: Guidelines for drug therapy in renal failure. Ann Intern Med *86*:754, 1977.
40. Gibson TP, Matusik E, Nelson LE, Briggs WA: Artificial kidneys and clearance calculations. Clin Pharmacol Ther *20*:720, 1976.
41. Gibson TP, Atkinson AJ: Effect of changes in intercompartment rate constants on drug removal during hemoperfusion. J Pharm Sci *67*:1178, 1978.
42. Flower RJ, Moncada S, Vane JR: Analgesics—antipyretics and anti-inflammatory agents: Drugs employed in the treatment of gout. *In* Gilman AG, Goodman LS, Gilman A (eds): The Pharmacological Basis of Therapeutics. 6th ed. New York, Macmillan, 1981, p 682.
43. Fairshter RD, Rosen SM, Smith WR, Glauser FL, McRae DM, Wilson AF: Paraquat poisoning. New aspects of therapy. Q J Med *45*:180, 1976.
44. Hirszel P, Maher JF: Pharmacologic alteration of peritoneal transport rates. *In* Nolph KD (ed): Peritoneal Dialysis, 3rd ed. Norwall, Mass, Kluwer Academic Publishers, 1989, p 184.
45. Carozzi S, Lamperi S: Intraperitoneal (IP) verapamil in CAPD patients with ultrafiltration (UF) loss. *In* La Greca G, Chiaramonte S, Fabris A, Feriani M, Ronco C (eds): Peritoneal Dialysis. Milan, Italy, Wichtig Editore, 1988, p 53.
46. Whalen JE, Richards CJ, Ambre J: Inadequate removal of methanol and formate using the sorbent based regeneration hemodialysis delivery system. Clin Nephrol *11*:318, 1979.
47. Chazan JA, Garella S: Glutethimide intoxication: A prospective study of 70 patients treated conservatively without hemodialysis. Arch Intern Med *128*:215, 1971.
48. Lorch JA, Garella S: Hemoperfusion to treat intoxications. Ann Intern Med *91*:301, 1979.
49. Garella S: Nephrology forum: Extracorporeal techniques in the treatment of exogenous intoxications. Kidney Int *33*:735, 1988.
50. Garella S, Lorch JA: Hemoperfusion for poisoning: Who needs it? *In* Schreiner GE, Winchester JF (eds): Controversies in Nephrology, Volume 2. Washington DC, Georgetown Nephrology Press, 1980, p 219.
51. De Broe ME, Bismuth C, De Groot G, Heath A, Okonek S, Ritz DR, Verpooten GA, Volans GN, Widdop B: Haemoperfusion: A useful therapy for a severely poisoned patient? Hum Toxicol *5*:11, 1986.
52. Schreiner GE, Berman LB, Griffin J, Feys J: Specific therapy for salicylism. N Engl J Med *253*:213, 1955.
53. Maher JF, Schreiner GE: Editorial review: The dialysis of poisons. Trans Am Soc Artif Intern Organs *9*:385, 1963.
54. Gelfand MC, Winchester JF, Knepshield JH: Hemoperfusion is indicated in severe drug overdosage. *In* Schreiner GE, Winchester JF (eds): Controversies in Nephrology, Volume 2. Washington DC, Georgetown Nephrology Press, 1980, p 210.
55. Vale JA, Rees AJ, Widdop B, Goulding R: Use of charcoal haemoperfusion in the management of severely poisoned patients. Br Med J *1*:5, 1975.
56. Maher JF (in discussion of): Hemoperfusion for poisoning—is it really necessary? *In* Schreiner GE, Winchester JF (eds): Controversies in Nephrology, Volume 2. Washington DC, Georgetown Nephrology Press, 1980, p 228.
57. Winchester JF: Active methods for detoxification: Oral sorbents, forced diuresis, hemoperfusion, and hemodialysis. *In* Haddad LM, Winchester JF (eds): Clinical Management of Poisoning and Drug Overdose. Philadelphia, WB Saunders, 1983, p 154.
58. Muirhead EE, Reid AF: Resin artificial kidney. J Lab Clin Med *33*:841, 1948.
59. Schreiner GE: The role of hemodialysis (artificial kidney) in acute poisoning. Arch Intern Med *102*:896, 1958.
60. Yatzidis H: A convenient haemoperfusion microapparatus over charcoal for the treatment of endogenous and exogenous intoxications. Its use as artificial kidney. Proc Eur Dial Transplant Assoc *1*:83, 1964.
61. Yatzidis H, Voudiclari S, Oreopoulos D, Tsaparas D, Triantaphyllidis D, Gavras C, Stavroulaki A: Treatment of severe barbiturate poisoning. Lancet *2*:216, 1965.
62. Chang TMS: Artificial Cells. Springfield, Il, Charles C Thomas, 1972.
63. Fennimore J, Munro GD: Design and development of the Smith and Nephew column. *In* Williams R, Murray-Lyon IM (eds): Artificial Liver Support. London, Pitman, 1975, p 330.
64. Winchester JF: Haemostatic changes induced by adsorbent haemoperfusion. *In* Kenedi RM, Courtney JM, Gaylor JDS, Gilchrist T (eds): Artificial Organs. London, Macmillan, 1977, p 280.
65. Rosenbaum JL, Kramer MS, Raja R: Resin hemoperfusion for acute drug intoxication. Arch Intern Med *136*:263, 1976.
66. Denti E, Luboz MP, Tessore V: Adsorption characteristics of celulose acetate coated charcoals. J Biomed Mater Res *9*:143, 1975.
67. Winchester JF, Forbes CD, Lang S, Courtney JM, Prentice CRM: Platelet function regulating agents—Experimental data relevant to renal disease. *In* Mitchell JRA, Domenet JG (eds): Thromboembolism—A New Approach to Therapy. New York, Academic Press, 1977, p 83.
68. Gelfand MC, Winchester JF, Knepshield JH, Hanson KM, Cohan SL, Strauch BS, Geoly KL, Kennedy AC, Schreiner GE: Charcoal hemoperfusion in severe drug overdosage. Trans Am Soc Artif Intern Organs *23*:599, 1977.
69. Horres CR, Hill JB, Ellis FW: The adsorption of sympathomimetic agents by activated carbon hemoperfusion. Trans Am Soc Artif Intern Organs *22*:425, 1976.
70. Myschetzky A, Lassen NA: Forced diuresis in treatment of acute barbiturate poisoning. *In* Matthew H (ed): Acute Barbiturate Poisoning. Amsterdam, Excerpta Medica, 1971, p 194.
71. Hadden J, Johnson K, Smith S, Price L, Giardana E: Acute barbiturate intoxication: Concepts in management. JAMA *209*:893, 1969.
72. Schreiner GE: Dialysis of poison and drugs—Annual review. Trans Am Soc Artif Intern Organs *16*:544, 1970.
73. Medd RK, Widdop B, Braithwaite RA, Rees AJ, Goulding B: Comparison of haemoperfusion and haemodialysis in the therapy of barbiturate intoxication in drugs. Arch Toxicol *31*:163, 1973.
74. Hill JB, Palaia FL, McAdams JL, Palmer PJ, Maret SM: Efficacy of activated charcoal hemoperfusion in removing lethal doses of barbiturates and salicylates from the blood of rats and dogs. Clin Chem *22*:754, 1976.
75. Widdop B, Medd RK, Braithwaite RA, Vale JA:

Haemoperfusion in the treatment of paraquat poisoning. Proc Eur Soc Artif Organs *1*:244, 1975.

76. Winchester JF, Tilstone WJ, Edwards RO, Gilchrist T, Kennedy AC: Hemoperfusion for enhanced drug elimination—A kinetic analysis in paracetamol poisoning. Trans Am Soc Artif Intern Organs *20A*:358, 1974.
77. Winchester JF, Gelfand MC, Tilstone WJ: Hemoperfusion in drug intoxication: Clinical and laboratory aspects. Drug Metab Rev *8*:69, 1978.
78. Tilstone WJ, Winchester JF, Reavey PC: The use of pharmacokinetic principles in determining the effectiveness of removal of toxins from blood. Clin Pharmacokinet *4*:23, 1979.
79. Gibson TP, Lucas SV, Nelson HA, Atkinson AJ, Okita GT, Ivanovich P: Hemoperfusion removal of digoxin from dogs. J Lab Clin Med *91*:673, 1978.
80. Zmuda MD: Resin hemoperfusion in dogs intoxicated with ethchlorvynol (Placidyl). Kidney Int *17*:303, 1980.
81. Winchester JF, Rahman A, Tilstone WJ, Kessler A, Mortensen L, Schreiner GE, Schein PS: Sorbent removal of Adriamycin in vitro and in vivo. Cancer Treat Rep *63*:1787, 1979.
82. Shah G, Nelson HA, Atkinson AJ, Okita GT, Ivanovich P, Gibson TP: Effect of hemoperfusion on the pharmacokinetics of digitoxin in dogs. J Lab Clin Med *93*:370, 1979.
83. Rosenbaum JL, Winsten S, Kramer MS, Moros J, Raja R: Resin hemoperfusion in the treatment of drug intoxication. Trans Am Soc Artif Intern Organs *16*:134, 1970.
84. Okonek S, Baldamus CA, Hofman A, Schuster CJ, Bechstein PD, Zoller S: Two survivors of severe paraquat intoxication by "continuous hemoperfusion." Klin Wochenshr *57*:957, 1979.
85. Verpooten GA, De Broe ME: Combined hemoperfusion-hemodialysis in severe poisoning: Kinetics of drug extraction. Resuscitation *11*:275, 1984.
86. Cutler RE, Forland SC, St John Hammond PG, Evans RJ: Extracorporeal removal of drugs and poisons by hemodialysis and hemoperfusion. Ann Rev Pharmacol Toxicol *27*:169, 1987.
87. Farrell PC: Commentary: Acute drug intoxication and extracorporeal intervention. ASAIO J *3*:39, 1980.
88. Guenzet J, Bourin M, Laurent D, Aminou T: Theoretical study of haemoperfusion: Drugs obeying a one compartment model. Methods Find Exp Clin Pharmacol *7*:259, 1985.
89. Uldall PR: Controlled trial of resin hemoperfusion for the treatment of drug overdose at Toronto Western Hospital (TWH). Trans Am Soc Artif Intern Organs. *28*:676, 1982.
90. Hampel G, Crome P, Widdop B, Goulding R: Experience with fixed-bed charcoal haemoperfusion in the treatment of severe drug intoxication. Arch Toxicol *45*:133, 1980.
91. Oldfield EH, Dedrick RL, Yeager RL, Clark WC, DeVroom HL, Chatterji DC, Doppman JL: Reduced systemic drug exposure by continuous intra-arterial chemotherapy with hemoperfusion of regional venous drainage. J Neurosurg *163*:726, 1985.
92. Molina R, Fabian C, Cowley B Jr: Use of charcoal hemoperfusion with sequential hemodialysis to reduce serum methotrexate levels in a patient with acute renal insufficiency. Am J Med *82*:350, 1987.
93. Frappaz D, Bouffet E, Biron P: Methotrexate poisoning: Value of exchange transfusion. Pediatrie *42*:257, 1987.
94. Relling MV, Stapleton FB, Ochs J, Jones DP, Meyer W, Wainer IW, Crom WR, McKay CP, Evans WE: Removal of methotrexate, leucovorin, and their metabolites by combined hemodialysis and hemoperfusion. Cancer *62*:884, 1988.
95. Hubner W, Borber H, Iffland R, Heller A, Niehues B, Grosser KD: Erfolgreiche therapeutische Plasmapherese nach Intoxikation mit einer mehrfach letalen Dosis Kaliumbichromat 9. Tagg Dtsch Osterr Ges Intern Intensivmedizin, Linz, Osterr, 1977.
96. Seyffart G: Plasmapheresis in treatment of acute intoxication. Trans Am Soc Artif Intern Organs *28*:673, 1982.
97. Berning T, Krummener T, Glaser J: Plasma perfusion in life-threatening exogenous poisoning. Schweiz Med Wochenschr *117*:1368, 1987.
98. Schwartz RD: Deferoxamine and aluminum removal. Am J Kidney Dis *6*:358, 1985.
99. Brown DJ, Dawborn JK, Ham KN, Xipell JM: Treatment of dialysis osteomalacia with desferrioxamine. Lancet *2*:343, 1982.
100. Chang TMS, Barre P: Effect of desferrioxamine on removal of aluminum and iron by coated charcoal haemoperfusion and haemodialysis. Lancet *2*:1051, 1983.
101. Hakim RM, Schulman JM, Lazarus JM: Hemoperfusion in the treatment of aluminum (Al) and iron (Fe) induced bone disease. Abstr Am Soc Nephrol *18*:65a, 1985.
102. Andress DL, Maloney NA, Endres DB, Sherrard DJ: Aluminum-associated bone disease in chronic renal failure: High prevalence in a long-term dialysis population. J Bone Miner Res *1*:391, 1986.
103. Malluche H, Smith AJ, Abreo K, Fauyere MC: The use of deferoxamine in the management of aluminum accumulation in bone in patients with renal failure. N Engl J Med *311*:140, 1984.
104. Payton CD, Junor BJR, Fell G: Successful treatment of aluminum encephalopathy by intraperitoneal desferrioxamine. Lancet *1*:1132, 1984.
105. Tielemans C, Collart F, Wens R, Smeyers-Verbeeke J, van Hooff I, Dratwa M, Verbeelen D: Improvement in anemia with deferoxamine in hemodialysis patients with aluminum-induced bone disease. Clin Nephrol *24*:237, 1985.
106. Bregman H, Gelfand MC, Winchester JF, Manz HJ, Knepshield JH, Schreiner GE: Iron overload-associated myopathy in patients on maintenance haemodialysis. A histocompatibility linked disorder. Lancet *2*:882, 1980.
107. Winchester JF: Management of iron overload. Semin Nephrol *4*(Suppl 1):22, 1986.
108. Falk RJ, Mattern WD, Lamanna RW, Gitelman HJ, Parker NC, Cross RE, Rastall JR: Iron removal during continuous ambulatory peritoneal dialysis using deferoxamine. Kidney Int *24*:110, 1983.
109. McCarthy JT, Libertin CR, Mitchell JC III, Fairbanks VF: Hemosiderosis in a dialysis patient. Treatment with hemofiltration and deferoxamine chelation therapy. Mayo Clin Proc *57*:439, 1982.
110. Rahko PS, Salerni R, Uretsky BF: Successful reversal by chelation therapy of congestive cardiomyopathy due to iron overload. J Am Coll Cardiol *8*:436, 1986.
111. Marcus RE, Davies SC, Bantock HM, Underwood SR, Walton S, Huehns ER: Desferrioxamine to improve cardiac function in iron overloaded patients with thalassemia major. Lancet *1*:392, 1984.
112. Wolfe L, Olivieri N, Sallan D, Colan S, Rose V,

Propper R, Freedman M, Nathan DG: Prevention of cardiac disease by subcutaneous deferoxamine in patients with thalassemia major. N Engl J Med *312*:1600, 1985.
113. Worth DP, Davison AM, Lewins AM, Ledgerwood MJ, Taylor A: Haemodialysis and charcoal haemoperfusion in acute inorganic mercury poisoning. Postgrad Med J *60*:636, 1984.
114. De Backer W, Zachee P, Verpooten GA, Maes RA: Thallium intoxication treated with combined hemoperfusion-haemodialysis. J Toxicol Clin Toxicol *19*:259–264, 1982.
115. De Groot G, van Heijst AN, van Kesteren RG, Maes RA: An evaluation of the efficacy of charcoal haemoperfusion in the treatment of three cases of acute thallium poisoning. Arch Toxicol *57*:61, 1985.
116. Lund ME, Banner W, Clarkson TW, Berlin M: Treatment of acute methylmercury ingestion by hemodialysis with n-acetylcysteine (Mucomyst) infusion and 2,3-dimercaptopropane sulfonate. J Toxicol Clin Toxicol *22*:31, 1984.
117. Al-Abassi AH, Kostyniak PJ, Clarkson TW: An extracorporeal complexing hemodialysis system for the treatment of methylmercury poisoning. III. Clinical applications. J Pharmacol Exp Ther *207*:249, 1978.
118. Margel S: A novel approach for heavy metal poisoning treatment, a model. Mercury poisoning by means of chelating microspheres; hemoperfusion and oral administration. J Med Chem *24*:1263, 1981.
119. Banner W, Koch M, Capin DM, Hopf SB, Chang S, Tong TG: Experimental chelation therapy in chromium, lead and boron intoxication with n-acetylcysteine and other compounds. Toxicol Appl Pharmacol *83*:142, 1986.
120. Smolarz A, Roesch E, Lenz E, Neubert H, Abshagen P: Digoxin specific antibody (Fab) fragments in 34 cases of severe digitalis intoxication. Clin Toxicol *83*:769, 1985.
121. Shumaik GM, Wu AW, Ping AC: Oleander poisoning: Treatment with digoxin-specific antibody fragments. Ann Emerg Med *17*:723, 1988.
122. Hoy WE, Gibson TP, Rivero AJ, Jain JK, Talley TT, Bayer RM, Montondo DF, Freeman RB: XAD-4 resin hemoperfusion for digitoxic patients with renal failure. Kidney Int *23*:79, 1983.
123. Martiny SS, Phelps SJ, Massey KL: Treatment of severe digitalis intoxication with digoxin-specific antibody fragments: A clinical review. Crit Care Med *16*:629, 1988.
124. Rose SR, Gorman RL, McDaniel J: Fatal digoxin poisoning: An unsuccessful resuscitation with use of digoxin-immune Fab. Am J Emerg Med *5*:509, 1987.
125. Savin H, Marcus L, Margel S, Ofarim M, Ravid M: Treatment of adverse digitalis effects by hemoperfusion through columns containing antidigoxin antibodies bound to agarose polyacrolein microsphere beads. Am Heart J *113*:1078, 1987.
126. Colburn WA: Specific antibodies and Fab fragments to alter the pharmacokinetics and reverse the pharmacologic/toxicologic effects of drugs. Drug Metab Rev *11*:223, 1980.
127. Heath A, Wickstrom I, Martensson E, Ahlmen J: Treatment of antidepressant poisoning with resin hemoperfusion. Hum Toxicol *1*:361, 1982.

CHAPTER 9
RENAL CONSIDERATIONS

A. Acute Renal Failure

John F. Maher, M.D.

An abrupt loss of renal function may complicate medical or surgical shock or follow exposure to a variety of poisons or overdosage of certain drugs. Following such intoxications, the most frequently observed clinical syndromes are tubular necrosis secondary to aminoglycoside antibiotic usage, acute drug-hypersensitive interstitial nephritis, and postischemic acute renal failure induced by hemodynamic complications of various intoxicants.

Acute renal failure indicates a rapid loss of renal function that is usually severe, potentially lethal, and gradually reverses spontaneously after several days or weeks. Most patients manifest oliguria—i.e., a urine volume below 500 ml per day in the absence of maximum urinary concentration. In some pa-

The opinions or assertions contained herein are the private views of the author and should not be construed as official or as necessarily reflecting the views of the Uniformed Services University of the Health Sciences or Department of Defense. There is no objection to its presentation and/or publication.

tients, particularly those with milder lesions, the urine volume is not decreased.[1] Renal failure induces progressive increments in plasma concentrations of phosphate, potassium, and hydrogen ion and nitrogenous metabolites such as creatinine and urea. The inability to excrete water, sodium, and drugs complicates the clinical course unless these are administered in carefully measured quantities. Partial correction of biochemical abnormalities by dialysis is often required to prevent overt uremia and such problems as potassium cardiotoxicity. Nevertheless, despite dialysis the mortality in patients with acute renal failure approaches 50 per cent because of the severity of the initial insult and such complications as infection and hemorrhage.[2,3] The mortality is higher in patients with oliguria or with lesions that are irreversible or improve spontaneously only after a long interval.

The annual incidence of acute renal failure severe enough to require dialysis is 30 per million population.[4] Milder cases are much more frequent. Hospitalized patients are at much higher risk for acute renal failure because they are exposed to organic iodides, aminoglycosides, surgical shock, and other risk factors.[5]

DIFFERENTIAL DIAGNOSIS

Acute renal failure must be distinguished from azotemia due to prerenal and postrenal causes. In prerenal failure the perfusion of the kidney is decreased, but significant ischemic structural damage has not occurred. Renal function improves promptly on restoration of blood flow. Because renal blood flow varies directly with cardiac output, heart failure induces renal ischemia. Such renal hypoperfusion is usually only modest, however, because very severe decrements in cardiac output are not compatible with survival. On the other hand, severe renal ischemia may accompany a loss of perfusion volume, as occurs with hemorrhage or with sodium depletion. With prerenal failure the urine typically has a low volume and a very low sodium concentration. The urinary concentration of any solute such as creatinine that is filtered and not reabsorbed is very high relative to the plasma concentration. The urinary specific gravity and osmolality are also likely to be high, but these parameters often do not achieve maximum levels in salt-depleted patients.[6] When salt depletion results from urinary losses due to intrinsic renal disease, adrenal insufficiency, or diuretics, the urinary sodium concentration may be high despite overt depletion, and the diagnosis is recognized only because of such systemic evidence of extracellular fluid depletion as postural hypotension and tachycardia.

Because the decrease in volume that results from dehydration is spread over the total volume of body water, the hemodynamic effects are less prominent, and severe renal ischemia is not as pronounced as with extracellular fluid depletion. In dehydrated patients the urine should be maximally concentrated, and the fall in solute excretion is usually less pronounced. A modest degree of proteinuria may accompany dehydration or sodium depletion, but the urine sediment is characteristically normal except for some hyaline casts.

When acute renal failure complicates glomerulonephritis, the daily urine volume may be below 100 ml, and the urine sodium concentration is often very low, mimicking prerenal failure.[7] The urine sediment, however, shows hematuria, red cell casts, and leukocytes, reflecting the acute glomerular injury.

With tubular necrosis or severe acute interstitial nephritis, acute renal failure is usually accompanied by oliguria with high urine sodium and low osmolar and nitrogenous solute concentrations. Occasionally, patients with nonoliguric acute renal failure manifest specific tubular abnormalities such as renal tubular acidosis or glycosuria. The urine sediment contains renal tubular cells, often a few red or white blood cells, and an abundance of casts. Increased excretion of *N*-acetylglucosaminidase is an early sign of renal tubular epithelial injury, and a sensitive sign of toxic or ischemic impairment of renal tubular function is increased excretion of β_2-microglobulin.[8]

Patients with acute urinary obstruction frequently have a dramatic fall in urinary volume to complete anuria, unlike those with chronic obstructive uropathy, who are usually polyuric. If residual urine is obtained, it may show blood or crystals, or it may have no sediment and may be poorly concentrated with a high sodium concentration reflecting prior tubular injury.

Differentiating these lesions is often impossible without assessing the response to hemodynamic manipulations designed to improve renal perfusion, such as saline or blood infusion or digitalization. In patients with total anuria despite a normal perfusion pressure, urologic evaluation must be considered. Some nephrotoxins can cause total anuria,[9] however, and instrumentation should be avoided when an obvious cause is present. When perfusion and drainage of the kidney are normal, the cause of acute renal failure may be differentiated by the medical history, but renal biopsy to establish the diagnosis and prognosis and to direct specific therapy may be required as well.[10]

PATHOLOGY OF TOXIC ACUTE RENAL FAILURE

When renal perfusion and urinary drainage are adequate, several types of pathologic lesions that may have ischemic or toxic causes should be considered as potential causes of acute renal failure. These lesions include acute interstitial nephritis, acute glomerulonephritis, vasculitis, tubular necrosis, cortical necrosis, and acute intrarenal urinary obstruction.

Acute Interstitial Nephritis

An acute diffuse interstitial nephritis can result from hypersensitivity to a variety of drugs or to certain bacterial antigens. The lesion does not depend on high dosage and often follows a second exposure to a given drug. Drugs that induce this lesion[11] are listed in Table 9–1. Most cases follow exposure to antibiotics or antirheumatic drugs. In some of the isolated reports it is not clear that the lesion began with tubular injury that became inapparent by the time of renal biopsy, compared with the overt interstitial inflammation. The kidneys become enlarged and diffusely infiltrated by lymphocytes, plasma cells, and sometimes eosinophils.[12] With increased diagnostic awareness, this entity is now being recognized in milder forms that may show only modest morphologic and functional changes. Extreme swelling of the kidney suggests that increased interstitial pressure may play a pathogenetic role, but ischemia may make a more important contribution to the functional abnormalities. The extensive leukocytic infiltration may be recognized by diffuse renal uptake of radiogallium-labeled leukocytes. The recognition of immunoglobulin deposition at the tubular basement membrane suggests an immunologic mechanism, at least for penicillin nephritis.

Table 9–1. DRUGS ASSOCIATED WITH ACUTE HYPERSENSITIVITY AND INTERSTITIAL NEPHRITIS

Penicillins	Allopurinol
Sulfonamides	Nonsteroidal analgesics
Polymyxins	Azathioprine
Rifampin	Gold
Cephalosporins	Phenazone
Cotrimoxazole	Phenindione
Bismuth	Phenytoin
Para-amino salicylates	Glafenine
Thiazides	Erythromycin
Furosemide	Captopril
Cimetidine	

Most frequently, acute interstitial nephritis has been associated with hypersensitivity to the penicillins, especially methicillin and ampicillin, but also nafcillin, oxacillin, carbenicillin, and penicillin G.[13, 14] Hemagglutinating antibodies to ampicillin and an intense immune response to penicillin, with a penicilloyl haptene and gamma globulin in tissue, occur. Irreversible damage occurs rarely. A similar pathologic entity occurs infrequently with cephalosporin therapy.

Acute interstitial nephritis can complicate tuberculostatic treatment with rifampin. Nephrotoxicity most often follows interrupted therapy and may be heralded by a febrile flulike syndrome.[10] Allopurinol-hypersensitive interstitial nephritis may similarly present with such features of serum sickness as adenopathy, fever, jaundice, and malaise. Rifampin-dependent antibodies have been demonstrated in plasma, but immune globulin complement and fibrinogen are not found in renal tissue. Some proximal tubular necrosis may accompany the interstitial nephritis.

Acute renal failure complicating nonsteroidal anti-inflammatory drug therapy is infrequent, occurring about once every 4000 treatment days. In addition to an interstitial infiltrate, the kidneys may show glomerular podocyte fusion, and patients may manifest the nephrotic syndrome. Although the renal failure is usually mild, disproportionate hyperkalemia can occur and may be lethal.[15] Nonsteroidal analgesic drug toxicity accounts for more than 5 per cent of cases of acute renal failure, a higher incidence occurring in those predisposed by diuretic use, sodium depletion, heart failure, or advanced age.[16, 17]

Sulfonamide hypersensitivity may cause a diffuse interstitial nephritis as described above or focal granulomatous interstitial lesions that show necrosis with giant cells, neutrophils, eosinophils, and mononuclear cells and similar granulomas in the bone marrow and lungs.[18] Diffuse or focal glomerular lesions with a granulomatous necrotizing arteritis reminiscent of the lesions of bacterial endocarditis occur rarely. Acute hypersensitivity arteritis involving large vessels is rarely seen with sulfonamide exposure.

Acute Glomerulonephritis

Most cases of oliguric renal failure due to acute glomerulonephritis, of either the immune complex deposition or antiglomerular basement membrane type, are unrelated to nephrotoxin exposure. Severe proliferation of glomerular cells with an inflammatory infiltrate occurs with or without necrosis. In nephritic patients with antiglomerular basement membrane antibodies a high frequency of exposure to industrial solvents has been recognized. Both this type of immunologically mediated lesion and immune complex glomerulonephritis may also follow exposure to engine fuels and to pesticides.[19] Extracapillary glomerulonephritis with immune deposits can be induced by penicillamine or by substituted benzidines.

Acute Renal Vasculitis

Occasionally, drugs precipitate vasculitis. A syndrome resembling polyarteritis nodosa may complicate sulfonamide therapy. Other drugs that may induce an acute arteritis involving the kidney include penicillin, thiazides, phenytoin, phenylbutazone, propylthiouracil, and iodides.[20, 21] Acute necrotizing arteritis has also been recognized recently, complicating illicit intravenous use of amphetamines.[22]

Acute Tubular Necrosis

Many nephrotoxins can cause tubular necrosis, either by inducing ischemia with or without myohemoglobinuria or by direct tubular injury. Although toxic ischemic tubular necrosis may be indistinguishable from that due to nontoxic causes, direct tubular toxins can sometimes be recognized when the injury is localized to a specific tubular segment or when characteristic inclusion bodies or crystals are present.

Pathogenesis of Acute Renal Failure

Tubular injury due to varied causes may induce abnormalities that lead to dramatic renal functional decrements. Blood is shunted away from the outer renal cortex with relative preservation of medullary blood flow. In the pathogenesis of acute renal failure considerable controversy has focused on whether renal hemodynamic or tubulointerstitial factors contribute more importantly.[23] Renal tubular epithelial injury, an essential pathogenetic ingredient that may be inapparent by light microscopy, impairs sodium reabsorption by that nephron, leading to sodium loss. Such increased distal delivery of sodium, sensed by the macula densa, stimulates renin-mediated vasoconstriction, decreasing glomerular filtration in that nephron, which spreads to other nephrons, thereby preventing severe sodium depletion until healing can occur.[24] A final common pathway in the development of acute renal failure is preglomerular vasoconstriction with renal cortical ischemia.[25] Factors that stimulate the renin-angiotensin system prior to nephrotoxin exposure or to ischemic insults exaggerate renal failure, whereas suppression of renal renin decreases the severity of renal failure for any given extent of tubular injury.[26] This fact provides a rationale for using mannitol before vascular surgery and for avoiding salt depletion by diet or diuretics in such clinical situations. Blockade of thromboxane or leukotrienes purportedly also ameliorates ischemic acute renal failure.[27] Once renal failure is established, however, restoration of renal plasma flow by volume loading or vasodilators will not restore renal function and urinary volume. Factors such as a decreased glomerular capillary filtration coefficient, tubular obstruction, and back leak of tubular fluid as well as prolonged vasoconstriction may contribute to the maintenance of acute renal failure.[25, 28] At the cellular level, mechanisms of toxicity include phospholipase activation, production of free radicals and lipid peroxidases, calcium entry, and loss of the high-energy phosphate pool.[29]

Heavy Metal Intoxication. Intoxication by mercury is usually suicidal but may result from inadvertent ingestion, inhalation of mercury vapors, overdosage of ingested or injected organic mercurials, or dermal absorption of ammoniated mercury. Mercury rapidly binds to plasma proteins. During subsequent renal excretion, some mercury concentrates in tubular epithelium, which has a high binding affinity and where it can persist for weeks. By combining with sulfhydryl groups of protein in the mitochondrial membrane, mercury causes mitochondrial disintegration, necrosis of nuclei, and loss of renal tubular epithelial enzyme activity.[30] Such tubular necrosis becomes manifest as glycosuria, proteinuria, hematuria, renal tubular cyturia with casts, and severe oliguria. When exposure is minimal, proximal tubular dysfunction and proteinuria may be the only signs. Other heavy metals that can induce acute renal failure include arsenic, a notorious culprit in toxic homicides and a component of fertilizers and pigments. The pathologic changes and clinical signs of arsenic toxicity are similar to those of mercury poisoning. Bismuth, once in popular use for antisyphilitic therapy, also causes acute renal failure. The kidneys excrete bismuth and selectively concentrate it in the proximal tubules, where it causes degeneration and necrosis. Characteristic inclusion bodies can be recognized in the nuclei and cytoplasm of the proximal tubule. Nephrotoxicity has also been demonstrated with excessive exposure to antimony, copper, silver, chromium, iron, silicon, gold, uranium, and platinum.[10] Acute toxicity complicating chelate therapy may indicate direct renal injury or may be related to mobilization of tissue stores of trace metals. Renal injury is the major toxic danger limiting the use of the potent antitumor agent cis-dichlorodiammine-platinum.[31] Some cisplatinum is metabolized and concentrated in tissues including the kidney. Necrosis of the proximal tubules occurs in about 50 per cent of patients who are given a therapeutic course, increasing in frequency and severity with higher and repetitive doses and decreasing with prehydration, slow infusions, and mannitol diuresis. An early sign of such renal injury is hypomagnesemia complicating polyuria. Platinum entry into the cell can be blocked by organic bases.

Iodinated Radiocontrast Media. Nephrotoxicity is the most important hazard of iodinated contrast media used for radiography of the vasculature, gallbladder, and kidney. Postulated pathogenetic mechanisms include direct cellular toxicity, intrarenal osmotic effects, uricosuria with obstructive crystalluria, precipitation of Tamm-Horsfall protein following antecedent dehydration, direct depression of renal blood flow and glomerular filtration rate, and idiosyncratic reactions.[32] Nephrotoxicity is more likely with increased dose and iodide content of the agent or when more iodide is delivered to the kidney (for example, in cholecystography in patients with hepatic failure) or when renal elimination of the organic iodide is delayed by pre-existing renal ischemia or renal failure.[33] Proximal tubular vacuolization, glomerular hypercellularity, and interstitial hemorrhage may occur, and with severe damage there may be bilateral cortical necrosis or medullary necrosis. With angiography the incidence of acute renal failure may be as high as 12 per cent, whereas with pyelography and cholecystography the incidence is less than 0.2 per cent. Patients with myeloma, diabetes, proteinuria, hypoalbuminemia, hyperuricemia, hypertension, or pre-existing renal insufficiency and elderly patients are more prone to renal injury.[34]

Antibiotic Nephrotoxicity. Nephrotoxicity is the major problem complicating antibiotic therapy, especially in patients with underlying renal disease. Amid the hemodynamic effects of sepsis or the renal functional changes of acute pyelonephritis, the diagnosis can be difficult in the individual case. Nevertheless, characteristic nephrotoxic signs of numerous antibiotics have been recognized. The severity and frequency of nephrotoxicity vary considerably among the different antibiotics, some of which have a narrow margin of safety and many of which are excreted by the kidney and consequently are retained in patients with renal failure.[35]

The aminoglycoside antibiotics are noted for ototoxicity and nephrotoxicity, which are most severe with neomycin and least severe with streptomycin.[36] Although first gentamicin and later tobramycin and amikacin were heralded as less toxic than kanamycin, their liberal use makes aminoglycoside exposure the most frequent cause of acute renal failure in hospital practice today. Proteinuria and a decreased glomerular filtration rate, often preceded by enzymuria and saluresis, occur in about 20 per cent of patients receiving 2.0 mg per kg of aminoglycosides daily for more than a week. The nephrotoxicity of aminoglycosides correlates with the dose and duration of treatment, advanced age, prior renal dysfunction, diuretic use, and dehydration. Nephrotoxicity may be anticipated when high plasma concentrations precede subsequent doses and depends most directly on renal cortical concentrations when the elimination half-life exceeds 100 hours.[37] During transcellular absorptive transport, gentamicin accumulates in tubular epithelium, which then manifests increased numbers of lysosomes containing whorled inclusions.[38] Necrosis is most prominent in the proximal convoluted tubules. After tubular functional abnormalities occur, renal blood flow and glomerular filtration rate decrease progressively, aggravated by renal retention of the aminoglycoside. Depending on the dose, progressive oliguria begins insidiously, usually during the second week of exposure. Toxicity is more likely with extracellular fluid depletion, advanced age, prior renal dysfunction, and concurrent exposure to other nephrotoxins. The number of amino groups in the aminoglycoside molecule correlates with toxicity and possibly with renal tissue protein binding.[39] Accordingly, the newer aminoglycoside congeners such as netilmicin may prove less toxic, unless excessive doses are used.

The polymyxins, a closely related group of polypeptide antibiotics, have nephrotoxic properties of varying severity. Tubular necrosis is likely to complicate polymyxin B therapy when the dose exceeds 3 mg per kg per day or when underlying renal dysfunction is present. Similar complications occur in as many as 20 per cent of patients treated with sodium colistimethate.[40]

Dose-related toxicity occurs frequently with high intrarenal concentrations of cephaloridine due to its toxic polymers that cause injury by polymerization and covalent bonding in tubular epithelium, damaging first the brush border and then causing coagulative necrosis.[41] Cephalothin and other later generation cephalosporin congeners recently introduced are much less toxic, but with excessive doses, pre-existing renal insufficiency, blockade of tubular secretion (e.g., by probenecid), hypersensitivity, advanced age, or concurrent use of other nephrotoxins, qualitatively similar changes occur, inducing reversible renal failure.[42]

The development of soluble sulfonamides and drug mixtures decreased the frequency of nephrotoxicity but did not eliminate it. Tubular necrosis and crystalline precipitates still occur occasionally with sulfonamide administration, including the trimethoprim-sulfonamide mixture and such derivatives as acetazolamide.[10]

Although massive doses of tetracyclines acutely depress the glomerular filtration rate in animals, no such effects are seen in humans except for the occurrence of renal failure after fluid volume depletion, for example, from vomiting or in cirrhotic patients treated by demeclocycline.[43] Fluid volume depletion in the latter situation may result from the hemodynamic effects of impaired water conservation. The tetracyclines do impair amino acid incorporation into protein, however, causing a negative nitrogen balance and aggravating azotemia, hyperphosphatemia, and acidosis.

Antifungal therapy with the insoluble polyene antibiotic amphotericin B is often limited by dose-dependent and potentially reversible nephrotoxicity, often heralded by tubular acidosis and manifesting as progressive renal failure secondary to tubular necrosis and interstitial calcification.

Pigment Nephropathy. Myoglobinuria or hemolysis with hemoglobinuria causing acute renal failure occasionally complicates a wide variety of drug intoxications such as quinine use, heroin abuse, or massive doses of ethanol. Rhabdomyolysis associated with acute renal failure has especially been a problem among phencyclidine users.[44] Glycerol-induced acute renal failure is a classic experimental model that involves hemolysis, myohemoglobinuria, and osmotically induced hypovolemia. Acute renal failure rarely has complicated the clinical intravenous use of glycerol to reduce cerebral edema. Other chemicals that have caused hemoglobinuric acute renal failure include aniline, arsine, benzene, cresol, hydralazine, methyl chloride, nitrofurantoin, phenol, quinidine, sodium chlorate, and triamterene.

In patients with pre-existing renal impairment, large doses of phenazopyridine can cause pigmented urinary casts and crystals with skin pigmentation and acute renal failure accompanying degenerative changes in the collecting duct epithelium.

Other Toxic Causes of Tubular Necrosis. The halogenated hydrocarbons such as carbon tetrachloride and trichloroethylene are industrial chemicals that induce renal tubular necrosis with or without concurrent hepatic necrosis. Varied glycols also cause acute renal failure through a variety of mechanisms, often involving hemolysis and shock. With ethylene glycol, the most frequent culprit among such compounds, marked destruction of the tubular epithelium and complete anuria result from widespread precipitation of its metabolite, oxalate. Tubular necrosis may also follow exposure to the anticoagulant hexadimethrine bromide, to carbamazepine, a drug used for trigeminal neuralgia, and to the cancer chemotherapeutic drug streptozocin. Nephrotoxic insecticides include DDT, chlordane, biphenyl, and parathion.

Ischemic Tubular Necrosis Unrelated to Toxins. Acute tubular necrosis occasionally follows shock, especially if it is profound or prolonged, in such clinical situations as postsurgical, traumatic, postpartum, hemorrhagic, or septic shock or a combination of these with or without concurrent nephrotoxin exposure. The necrosis is usually patchy, may be unimpressive in comparison with the functional abnormalities, and is often associated with hemoglobin casts. Less frequently, these clinical insults are followed by patchy or even diffuse bilateral cortical necrosis. Nephrotoxins may account for up to half of the cases of acute renal failure, the others being attributed to nontoxic ischemia. This causal distribution varies geographically and by diagnostic criteria, a large fraction of cases having multiple potential causes.

Toxic Renal Ischemia

In selected patients, such as those with congestive heart failure or systemic lupus erythematosus, the vasodilator prostaglandins such as prostaglandin E_2 (PGE_2) compensate for renin-mediated renal vasoconstriction. When prostaglandin synthetase is inhibited in these patients, for example by indomethacin, renal plasma flow promptly decreases, causing overt azotemia but with no renal histologic alterations.[45] Renal failure promptly abates on drug withdrawal and recurs on rechallenge. Ischemia may also contribute to the pathogenesis of chronic interstitial fibrosis that is occasionally recognized in such patients. Reversible acute renal failure may also occur with ergot, with norepinephrine, and with overzealous use of or hypersensitivity responses to such antihypertensive drugs as captopril or minoxidil. Captopril, by reducing angiotensin-mediated high glomerular pressure in selected patients, greatly reduces the glomerular filtration rate.[46] Immunosuppressive therapy with cyclosporin A is also limited by ischemic nephrotoxicity. Increments in plasma creatinine concentrations usually reverse, but with high doses overt acute renal failure may be fatal.[47] The kidneys show glomerular thromboses and vacuolar degeneration of the proximal tubules.

Acute Intrarenal Crystalline Obstruction

Intrarenal obstructive uropathy, often abrupt in onset and accompanied by painful hematuria, may occur with certain drugs. Toxic crystallization of the drug itself is best exemplified by sulfonamide intoxication and correlates with the dose and duration of the drug, the heterocyclic ring substitution of the sulfonamide, and its solubility. Acute oxalate nephrocalcinosis may result from the metabolism of ethylene glycol or methoxyflurane, but the nephrotoxicity of this anesthetic is related more to injury by fluoride.[48] Moreover, chemotherapy of lymphoproliferative disease or uricosuric therapy may be complicated by massive intraluminal or urinary precipitation of uric acid. Methotrexate and its 7-hydroxy(OH) metabolite may also precipitate acutely in the renal parenchmya when given in high dose.[49] Mithramycin may cause tubular necrosis, but other toxic cancer chemotherapeutic drugs such as doxarubicin and methyl CCNU cause a more chronic progressive interstitial nephritis.[50] Obstruction of a solitary ureter by a necrotic papilla, for example, complicating analgesic excess is a rare cause of anuria.

CLINICAL COURSE

The course of acute renal failure is usually divided into an early phase, which may be dominated by the manifestations of the precipitating insult, and the oliguric phase, which induces acute uremia, diuresis, and late recovery.

Early Insult Phase

Acute renal failure may begin abruptly, as exemplified by situations involving trauma, an incompatible transfusion, or exposure to a severe nephrotoxin such as mercury or ethylene glycol. Under such circumstances, the obvious anuria is usually overshadowed by such findings as shock, pain, and acute insults to other organs. Provided that severe hyperkalemia is not present, these associated problems must have therapeutic priority for the first few hours. In other conditions, for example, following exposure to halogenated hydrocarbons, acute renal failure often begins somewhat insidiously and may be overlooked for as long as several days. When precipitated by an overdosage of toxins eliminated by the kidney such as aminoglycosides, the renal functional impairment contributes to further accumulation of the toxin; severe renal failure may develop during the course of a few days, culminating in anuria. Extracellular fluid volume expansion can sometimes prevent oliguria, and a trial of diuretics and vasodilator therapy can be justified if the patient is not fluid depleted. Clinically, a specific effect of calcium channel blockers or of magnesium in preventing cellular injury has not been proved.

Oliguric Phase

After an interval that usually lasts only a few hours, acute renal failure is no longer reversible by manipulation of extrarenal factors. Thereafter, most patients are oliguric. The urine volume is typically about 200 ml per day and varies somewhat with the osmotic and water loads. Only an occasional patient is totally anuric after hemodynamic factors are optimal. Unless there is another obvious explanation, totally anuric patients should always be evaluated for urinary or renal arterial obstruction. Oliguria may persist for only a few hours or up to several weeks but typically lasts for about 10 days unless it is caused by more slowly reversible lesions such as cortical necrosis or acute glomerulonephritis.[40] As many as 25 per cent or more of all patients with acute renal failure are nonoliguric,[1] urine volume being fixed at a value somewhat above 500 ml per day but still insufficient for metabolic needs and responding little to osmotic and water loads. Although such volumes are in the normal range, osmolar excretion remains far below normal. Nonoliguric acute renal failure often reflects a milder lesion, occurs more often following nephrotoxin exposure than after ischemia, and generally has a better prognosis than oliguria.

Urinary Findings

Characteristically, urinary composition differs little from that of the plasma in patients with acute renal failure. Osmolality is usually below 350 mOsm per kg of water, sodium concentration typically exceeds 30 mEq per liter, and the urine-to-plasma ratio of a freely filtered, nonreabsorbed solute such as creatinine is often only 3 or 4 to 1. Accordingly, the fraction of filtered water that is excreted (i.e., escapes reabsorption) is one-third or one-fourth, and the fractional excretion of sodium is also high, often exceeding one-tenth, unlike such values in good health, which typically are below one one-hundredth. Moreover, these data indicate that in the typical patient with oliguric acute renal failure the glomerular filtration rate is less than 1.0 ml per minute.

Proteinuria in acute renal failure may occur in a high concentration but rarely occurs in large quantity. Glycosuria also occurs, often reflecting glomerulotubular imbalance, but the presence of many nephrotoxins such as mercury may indicate proximal tubular injury as well. The urinary sediment typically shows renal tubular cells, hyaline, granular, and cellular casts, leukocytes, and erythrocytes, reflecting epithelial injury. Abnormalities of the sediment are often most severe at the onset of oliguria and again at the onset of diuresis.

Accumulation of Toxic Metabolites

Because of the marked decline in renal elimination rates, solutes entering body fluids exogenously or from endogenous metabolism accumulate unless they are eliminated adequately by nonrenal routes. Of major concern are hydrogen ions, potassium, phosphate, and the nitrogenous products of protein metabolism. Although urea is not very toxic, its accumulation rate reflects the rate of protein catabolism and the release of more toxic solutes. Given that an anuric patient catabolizes 1.0 gm of protein per kg daily from endogenous and exogenous sources, that most of this protein becomes urea, and that about 16 per cent of protein by weight is nitrogen, approximately 10 gm of urea nitrogen would accumulate daily. Distributed into 40 liters of total body water, the increment in plasma urea nitrogen concentration would be 25 mg per dl per day.[51] Because the protein catabolic rate is often reduced and some metabolite nitrogen is eliminated by extrarenal routes, the average rate of urea nitrogen accumulation is frequently somewhat lower.[52] Patients that accumulate urea nitrogen more rapidly have increased protein catabolism, which may suggest occult infection if another source of catabolism is not obvious. As plasma urea concentrations increase, the extrarenal elimination rate increases and appetite decreases, so that accumulation rates are lower. A decrease in the plasma urea increment may be an early sign of diuresis.

Serum creatinine, which derives from rather constant nonenzymatic metabolism of muscle, increases by 1.0 to 2.0 mg per dl per day in oliguric patients. In patients with acute renal failure complicating rhabdomyolysis, the daily increment in serum creatinine is higher because of the increased release of creatine from muscle that is converted by hydrolysis to creatinine. Since diet has little influence on creatinine but definite influence on urea accumulation, serum creatinine can be a better guide to the severity of renal impairment but not necessarily to uremic toxicity.

Numerous other organic compounds accumulate in body fluids of patients with acute renal failure.[53] These include uric acid, which rarely induces symptoms, guanidines, phenols, indoles, amines, certain amino acids, myoinositol, various hormones, organic acids, and incompletely defined middle molecules.

Hyperkalemia

Potassium cardiotoxicity is the major early threat to life in the untreated, uncomplicated, anuric patient. Potassium released from cell water, glycogen breakdown, and exogenous sources accumulates in plasma at an average rate of 0.3 to 0.5 mEq per liter per day but can increase as rapidly as 3.0 mEq per liter per day after extensive trauma or with administration of drugs or foods that have a high potassium content. Since even a small volume of urine can contribute importantly to potassium elimination in patients with intact aldosterone-mediated distal tubular cation exchange, anuric patients are at greater risk. Because acidosis shifts potassium extracellularly, patients in such toxic states as ethylene glycol poisoning that cause severe metabolic acidosis and those prone to acute respiratory acidosis—for example, acidosis due to chest injuries—are especially susceptible to hyperkalemia. Few if any symptoms precede severe potassium cardiotoxicity. Occasionally, weakness of muscles including those involved in respiration, apprehension, or anesthesia precedes overt cardiotoxicity. With serum potassium concentrations below 6.5 mEq per liter, the electrocardiogram may be normal unless there is concurrent hyponatremia, hypocalcemia, acidosis, or cellular depletion of potassium, factors that aggravate potassium intoxication. Thereafter, progressive changes beginning with increased T-wave amplitude and culminating in cardiac arrest correlate with increments in extracellular potassium concentration.[54] The following signs are typical of potassium intoxication:

1. Progressive T-wave elevation reflects altered repolarization.
2. Depressed atrial conduction broadens and flattens the P wave.
3. Atrioventricular conduction block prolongs the P-R interval.
4. Gross intraventricular conduction defects induce progressive decrease of R-wave amplitude and widening of the QRS complex, occasionally with a bundle branch pattern.
5. Cardiac arrest eventually occurs unless escape mechanisms cause ectopic rhythms, which in themselves may lead to ventricular fibrillation.

Salt and Water Balance

Oliguria affects water balance considerably. Although insensible water loss averages close to 1000 ml per day, an insensible gain of water due to water derived from metabolism and release of preformed cellular water averages about 500 ml per day. The uncomplicated anuric patient thus has a daily need of only 500 ml of water per day. Fever increases insensible water loss by about 10 per cent per degree Fahrenheit but often increases metabolic production of water as well. Water loss from the lungs is accelerated by increased ventilation unless the air is humidified. An excess amount of salt and water may be required to offset the effective loss of volume sequestered by the injured tissues, but this amount may return to the circulation before diuresis occurs. In the absence of losses of other body fluids (e.g., from the gastrointestinal tract or drainage of serous cavities that are isosmotic), there is no appreciable loss of sodium. Accordingly, excess water administration causing dilution of body fluids is the most frequent cause of hyponatremia in the oliguric patient. When hyponatremia is misinterpreted as sodium loss and treated with sodium administration, pulmonary edema and severe hypertension may occur from the resultant extracellular shift of fluid. Similarly, total body chloride should remain constant in the uncomplicated oliguric patient, and a decreased plasma chloride concentration suggests water excess.

Hydrogen Ion Balance

Protein catabolism releases hydrogen ions that normally depend on eventual elimination by the kidney. The daily load of hydrogen ion averages about 60 mEq per day, retention of which causes a decrement in the concentration of the plasma buffer, bicarbonate, of about 2.0 mEq per liter per day. Associated lactic acidosis or other acid base abnormalities will change the rate of accumulation. Although overtly well tolerated, even mild acidosis can contribute to uremic bone disease, aggravate potassium intoxication, affect intermediary metabolism, and increase the work of breathing. Obviously, severe acidosis causes overt symptoms, notably Kussmaul's respirations, a finding that is often misinterpreted as dyspnea. The hemodynamic effects of acidosis including myocardial depression also argue for its prevention and control.

Divalent Ion Abnormalities

In patients with acute renal failure phosphate accumulates rapidly in extracellular fluid. In high concentrations, phosphate complexes with calcium, precipitating the product that depletes extracellular calcium, thereby stimulating parathyroid hormone secretion, which releases calcium from bone. With concurrent deficiency of dihydroxyvitamin D, any lag in or insufficiency of parathyroid hormone-mediated calcium release or excessive phosphate accumulation results in persistent hypocalcemia. Although hypocalcemia may contribute to neuromuscular irritability, it rarely is the primary or sole explanation for the twitching or convulsions that are sometimes seen in these patients. Magnesium also accumulates in oliguric patients but not to levels high enough to cause central nervous system depression unless there is also an exogenous source. The accumulation of sulfate in plasma correlates with the rate of acid production but does not cause symptoms per se.

Symptoms of Acute Renal Failure

Few if any symptoms are attributable to acute renal injury in the majority of patients. Occasionally, flank pain occurs, and dysuria or tenesmus rarely heralds the onset of oliguria. Thereafter, oliguria, about which most patients do not complain, is often the only manifestation until accumulation of uremic toxins induces symptoms. After a lag of a few days anorexia and nausea may occur, followed by hiccups and vomiting; with more severe uremia, hematemesis and sometimes bloody diarrhea may occur.[54] Abdominal pain mimicking a surgical abdomen occurs occasionally; sometimes this is related to ileus and is responsive to control of uremia. Serum amylase concentration increases because of impaired renal elimination. Although pancreatitis is a frequent late sign of uremia, it does not account for either the abdominal pain or the increased amylase levels seen in most patients treated for acute renal failure.

Lethargy and decreased mental concentration are also early symptoms of acute uremia. Unless azotemia is controlled, these symptoms progress to stupor and eventually coma. Characteristically, there is concurrent neuromuscular irritability manifested by twitching and, when uremia is severe, occasionally by asterixis and convulsions. When neuromuscular irritability is more severe than other symptoms, associated problems such as dilutional hyponatremia or sepsis should be sought.

Dermal signs of uremia, including pruritus, are infrequent in patients with acute renal failure, unlike those with chronic uremia. When present, superimposed problems such as drug reactions should be suspected. Despite clear evidence of early abnormalities in calcium metabolism, symptomatic bone disease is not a problem in patients with acute renal failure that reverses within a few weeks.

Salt and water retention in patients with acute renal failure contributes to the high incidence of cardiovascular abnormalities, namely, dyspnea, edema, and hypertension. Uremic pneumonitis, a proteinaceous hilar pulmonary infiltrate, is frequently precipitated by salt and water excess. The hyperventilation characteristic of acidosis helps maintain clear peripheral lung fields. Myocardial dysfunction may result from a variety of the biochemical abnormalities characteristic of uremia but is often precipitated by acute hypertension and anemia. The serositis of uremia not only may affect the distribution of extracellular fluid but may also induce acute pleurisy or pericarditis with or without effusions, which may be hemorrhagic.[55] Clinically apparent pericarditis should be considered a serious and late manifestation of acute uremia, indicating a need for more intensive therapy, but echocardiographic evidence of minimal accumulation of pericardial fluid is not as ominous. Overt pericarditis frequently causes chest pain unless the patient's sensorium is blunted by drugs or uremia.

Hematologic abnormalities of acute uremia include a bleeding diathesis attributed to abnormal platelet function, anemia, and impaired neutrophil chemotaxis contributing to the high rate of infection. The anemia of renal failure, often aggravated by bleeding, results from a combination of marrow suppression resulting from lack of erythropoietin and circulating inhibitors and from hemolysis due primarily to toxins in plasma. Often the onset is delayed for several days, and the anemia persists for weeks after the uremia has abated. Although dialysis can improve platelet function, bleeding is rarely if ever an isolated justification for initiating dialysis.

Complications

The major complications of acute renal failure are bleeding, infection, and drug intoxication. The high incidence of bleeding is related not only to the hemorrhagic diathesis and the use of anticoagulant drugs but also to the frequent occurrence of erosive and inflammatory lesions. Hemorrhagic gastritis, bloody diarrhea, hemopericardium, and intracranial bleeding are occasionally preterminal events.

Infections complicate the course of acute renal failure in about half of the patients and may result in septicemia, a leading cause of morbidity and mortality. Both gram-positive and gram-negative infections occur frequently in the respiratory tract, operative sites, and urinary tract. The high incidence of infection may be related to altered defense mechanisms and disruption of normal anatomic barriers by indwelling tubing of varied types. Despite overt infection, many patients do not manifest fever because uremia depresses the normal body temperature. Moreover, since there are often other explanations for leukocytosis such as traumatic tissue injury and adrenal steroid therapy, the diagnosis may be difficult.

Drug intoxications of various types contribute to the morbidity and mortality of patients with acute renal failure. Most frequent among severe drug intoxications are digitalis excess, sedative accumulation, and antibiotic toxicity.

The Diuretic Phase

After a variable interval but usually in the second week of oliguria, diuresis begins. This change is ordinarily obvious shortly after it commences and does not require repetitive bladder catheterizations or other invasive techniques to be recognized. The urine volume increases by 50 per cent of the previous day's volume until it reaches 3 to 4 liters per day, except in patients with less common lesions such as oliguric glomerulonephritis or cortical necrosis, in whom improvement is much slower. Typically, the urine is dilute with a high sodium concentration. Despite the onset of diuresis, azotemia may continue to become worse for a few days, uremic symptoms may persist, and the patient continues at risk for several potentially lethal complications. After the daily urine volume exceeds 2 liters, azotemia ordinarily begins to improve. Blood urea nitrogen and serum creatinine concentrations approach normal values about 5 to 7 days thereafter as the glomerular filtration rate increases gradually. At this time, wound healing, the response to infection, appetite, and general well-being often improve dramatically, but anemia persists. The increased urine volume can be explained by osmotic diuresis due to excess extracellular fluid and retained urea, but impaired tubular transport maxima can also be demonstrated. Prolonged or massive diuresis usually attributed to excessive replacement of salt and water may contribute to such electrolyte disturbances as potassium depletion. The urine volume usually returns to normal when the patient has reached a body weight that is sufficiently decreased to account for loss of lean body mass of about 0.2 kg per day of oliguria.

Prognosis

Before modern concepts of renal therapeutics were established, the mortality due to acute renal failure was as high as 90 per cent. About 30 years ago the survival rate increased to about 50 per cent coincident with an improved understanding of fluid and electrolyte homeostasis in acute renal failure, control of factors exaggerating catabolism, and availability of dialysis. Despite further refinements in nutritional and antibiotic therapy and in dialysis techniques, the survival rate has not improved in the past three decades. Fewer patients die of hyperkalemia, uncontrolled uremia, and salt and water excess, but death now is most often due to infection, hemorrhage, or the underlying problem that precipitated acute renal failure.[3] It is generally accepted that many of the milder lesions that induce acute renal failure such as transfusion reactions have become more preventable and are less frequently seen, whereas oliguria now more often occurs as a complication of extensive surgical procedures or severe infections and in older patients who often have serious associated morbidity, factors that contribute to the persistently high mortality. The probability of surviving the acute episode has been shown to correlate inversely with age, male sex, severity of the injury (reflected by the number of transfusions), failure of other organs, particularly the heart, and type of surgery (notably cardiac).[56]

Recovery Phase

During the second or third week of diuresis while the urine volume remains rather constant at about 3 liters per day, the glomerular filtration rate rises rapidly from as low as 6 to 8 liters per day to 60 to 80 liters per day. This rate is consistent with greater modification of the filtrate by the tubules, coincident with their regeneration. Reconstitution of the normal tubular structure takes many weeks and includes regeneration of normal brush borders and intracellular organelles. During the next few months the concentrating capacity for total solutes increases and there are further increases in clearance values, correlating with the return to normal of the tubular structure as evaluated by electron microscopy.

LONG-TERM EFFECTS

Glomerular filtration rate and urinary osmolar concentration reach maximal values after 1 or 2 years. In most patients renal function will be entirely normal 5 to 10 years after acute tubular necrosis.[57] Some patients have a modest, persistent impairment of filtration rate or tubular transport maxima that is clinically insignificant. Interstitial fibrosis is evident in a few patients evaluated several years after an episode of acute renal failure, and in these instances renal function may deteriorate gradually after previously reaching acceptable values. The long-term prognosis depends in large part on the histopathology and the etiology of the acute renal failure.[58]

TREATMENT

Appropriate management of the patient with acute renal failure requires careful monitoring and control of fluid and electrolyte balance while maintaining nutrition as well as possible and avoiding undue loading with precursors of uremic toxins. When such conservative measures cannot maintain well-being, early and frequent use of dialysis is advisable.

Prophylaxis

Since tubular necrosis occurs most often in predictable clinical settings, anticipation can frequently prevent the problem. Prompt and adequate repletion of blood and body fluid volumes in patients with surgical, thermal, or traumatic losses may prevent postischemic tubular necrosis. Since arterial blood pressure may return to normal owing to intense vasoconstriction, it is often necessary to ensure that venous pressure has also been increased to normal to be certain that blood volume has been adequately replenished. Proper treatment of cardiogenic and septic shock and of such problems as toxemia of pregnancy may also reduce the incidence of tubular necrosis in these clinical settings. Acute renal failure will also be prevented by monitoring carefully the dosage of such potential nephrotoxins as aminoglycoside antibiotics and iodinated radiographic contrast media. Once the clinical circumstance of an ischemic episode or nephrotoxin exposure has occurred or is inevitable, however, renal function may still be preserved by the use of mannitol. A loading dose of 0.5 gm per kg can be given intravenously; if diuresis occurs, this dose should be followed by a sustaining infusion of dilute mannitol. Mannitol can reduce endothelial cell swelling, which may contribute to the no-reflow phenomenon that follows ischemia,[59] and it can decrease plasma renin activity, enhance removal of some toxins, and minimize intratubular precipitation. Continuation of mannitol infusion in the unresponsively oliguric patient may lead to dilutional hyponatremia and pulmonary edema, however, and is ill advised. Potent diuretics such as furosemide can also prevent acute renal failure under certain circumstances. Too often, however, furosemide is administered in high doses to patients who are already volume depleted and without adequate fluid infusion, and the focus is on urine volume rather than on hemodynamics. Under such circumstances, acute renal failure may be precipitated or aggravated rather than prevented. Moreover, furosemide aggravates certain types of injuries such as cephalosporin toxicity, possibly by affecting tubular transport.[60] However, if the patient is adequately hydrated or if saline is given concurrently, a trial of furosemide (10 to 15 mg/kg/h) with dopamine (3 μg/kg/min) can be justified in those patients with renal ischemia in the first 24 hours because this regimen has often induced diuresis.[61] Provided that extracellular fluid volume is maintained, diuretics may reduce vasoconstriction and clear tubular obstruction.

Fluids and Electrolytes

Unless body weight is monitored, it is very difficult to maintain fluid balance in patients with acute renal failure. Patients with established oliguria should receive about 500 ml of electrolyte-free fluid daily to maintain fluid balance. Because of catabolism and insufficient nutrition, a weight loss of about 0.2 kg daily should be anticipated. Weight gain must be interpreted as a result of excess fluid administration. A volume of water equal to the urine volume can be added to the daily allotment, and losses due to vomiting, diarrhea, or drainage fluid can be replaced by isotonic sodium solutions. Under certain circumstances, patients may sequester fluid because of localized injury. To achieve a normal circulating volume, it may be necessary to overload the patient intentionally, cognizant that once sequestered fluid is mobilized it must be removed. Thirst is an unreliable guide to the state of hydration, even in alert patients, because of several factors including decreased salivary flow, which correlates with increased plasma osmolality. The physician can knowingly overhydrate some hemodynamically stable oliguric patients by 200 to 400 ml daily for a few days in anticipation of ultrafiltration dialysis.

Sodium should be given only to replace overt losses. Since hyponatremia results most often from excess water intake, hyponatremia is not an indication for sodium administration. In general, when supplemental sodium is required bicarbonate is the preferred salt because it enhances buffering of acidosis. In calculating balance, the sodium content of medications should not be ignored, and, of course, in patients who are able to eat the salt in food must be considered as well.

Once diuresis occurs, salt and water intake must be increased accordingly. By simply continuing to administer a fluid volume equal to net insensible fluid loss plus the measured urine volume, fluid balance can be maintained. Prescribing the fluid intake based on the previous day's volume under circumstances of increasing diuresis results in an appropriate negative fluid balance. For patients who are overtly edematous a lower intake is appropriate. The sodium content of this liberalized intake should be about 50 mEq per liter to avoid overt imbalance. Often, diuretic patients require potassium supplements.

Management of Hyperkalemia

Despite modern treatment, hyperkalemia is still potentially lethal. Prevention of severe hyperkalemia requires careful monitoring of the intake of potassium in foods, notably meat and fruit, and in drugs, control of acidosis, lowering of the catabolic rate by providing adequate calories, and treatment of infection and trauma. Provision of at least 100 gm of glucose daily will help to maintain glycogen stores, preventing release of potassium. Once hyperkalemia occurs, additional glucose intake can lower serum potassium concentrations provided that there is adequate insulin and capacity for glycogen storage. Because of these uncertainties, it may be preferable in those patients who can tolerate additional sodium to treat severe hyperkalemia by administration of hypertonic sodium bicarbonate. Not only does sodium rapidly antagonize the physiologic effects of potassium, but by improving acidemia, bicarbonate also decreases hyperkalemia, shifting potassium intracellularly, thereby improving the extracellular-intracellular concentration ratio, a determinant of toxicity. Daily control of hyperkalemia in oliguric patients should include the use of an ion exchange resin. Although this resin adds sodium, control of hyperkalemia ordinarily has priority over sodium balance. By enema, 30 to 50 gm of sodium polystyrene sulfonate (Kayexalate) in a hypertonic sugar solution can lower the serum potassium level within an hour, but by mouth, even with an osmotic laxative, the effect may be delayed for a day or more. Accordingly, ion exchange resins should be used orally to prevent, not to treat, severe hyperkalemia and should be initiated as soon as the serum potassium concentration exceeds normal.

Emergency treatment of potassium intoxication should be instituted for patients with serum potassium concentrations of above 7.0 mEq per liter with electrocardiographic abnormalities. Early signs such as modest increases in T-wave amplitude can usually be managed conservatively. When widened QRS complexes have little or no antecedent P waves, however, there may be only a few minutes before cardiac arrest occurs. Calcium salts or sodium bicarbonate will improve the electrocardiographic picture within a few seconds. Such emergency treatment must be followed by a more sustained therapy, usually dialysis. Both hemodialysis and peritoneal dialysis rapidly correct hyperkalemia, removing some potassium but primarily correcting the associated electrolyte abnormalities that aggravate potassium intoxication, e.g., by safely providing bicarbonate in large quantities. Rapid correction of hyperkalemia may precipitate digitalis intoxication in patients whose dosage has not been monitored carefully and kept to a minimum.

Control of Acidosis

Management of acidosis requires limitation of protein catabolism and provision of adequate buffer, such as bicarbonate. Because cellular destruction releases potassium, magnesium, and phosphate as well as hydrogen ion, provision of adequate nutrition, treatment of infection, and care of wounds by decreasing the rate of cell breakdown also help to control these electrolyte abnormalities. Uncontrolled hyperphosphatemia with resultant hypocalcemia promptly stimulates parathyroid hormone secretion, which may mediate cerebral uptake of calcium,[62] contributing to uremic abnormalities. Uremic acidosis may be aggravated by associated respiratory, lactic, or ketoacidosis, each of which should be appropriately treated. When bicarbonate concentrations cannot be maintained above 15 mMol per liter or when the hydrogen ion concentration exceeds 50 nanoequivalents per liter despite conservative measures, correction of acid base balance by dialysis must be considered. Dialysis is effective not because large quantities of hydrogen ion are removed, but because buffer is provided safely. Because rapid correction can be dangerous, it is better to prevent severe acidosis than to treat it late.

Nutrition

Because of uremic anorexia and increased catabolism associated with the precipitating causes of acute renal failure and with some of the complications, malnutrition can develop rapidly in such patients. Glucose should be provided to reduce endogenous protein catabolism. In patients restricted to parenteral alimentation, limited fluid tolerance may allow an intake of only 100 gm per day unless hyperalimentation is carried out using a central vein or excess fluid is removed artificially. Oral nutrition is preferable when possible. The caloric intake should be high but protein should be restricted, and in patients with anorexia it may be difficult to achieve an intake of 2000 calories per day. Protein intake should be restricted to below 1.0 gm per kg per day unless dialysis is employed frequently. The protein should be of high biologic value or, on a more restricted diet, it should be supplemented with essential amino acids. The keto analogues of essential amino acids have also been used as nutritional supplements. Should acute renal failure persist for more than a few days, supplementary water-soluble vitamins may be advisable. Hyperalimentation has been recommended in patients with postsurgical acute renal failure.[63] Although a high caloric intake using glucose, lipid, and amino acid solutions may be commendable, most authorities are not convinced that anabolism can be achieved safely or that the course of acute renal failure is abbreviated by such therapy.[64] Not only are potassium, phosphorus, and nitrogenous supplements potentially dangerous, but the complications of indwelling cannulae in central veins may add to the risk. Nevertheless, in catabolic patients undergoing frequent dialysis, such therapy may promote wound healing and resistance to infection. Anabolic androgens have been used in the past, but their value is not clearly established.

TREATMENT OF SPECIFIC COMPLICATIONS

Control of uremia by dialysis and by restricted intake of toxins and their precursors can prevent many of the complications of acute renal failure. Hypertension and congestive heart failure are most likely caused by salt and water excess, which should improve with ultrafiltration dialysis. Antihypertensives and digitalis should not be used when control of salt and water balance can prevent these problems. Heart failure may be precipitated by pericarditis with effusion, which is an indication for more intensive dialysis and occasionally for emergency pericardiocentesis. The central nervous system signs of uremia should indicate a need for dialysis rather than symptomatic therapy, but therapy of severe anxiety is sometimes needed. Nausea and vomiting can temporarily be treated symptomatically if dialysis is not otherwise required. Anemia is preferably left untreated unless symptoms or active bleeding indicate a need for transfusion. Because anemia is related more to shortened red cell survival than to impaired production, it is not anticipated that erythropoietin would correct it completely. Except for control of uremia, specific therapy for hemorrhagic diathesis and impaired leukocyte function is usually not helpful. Hyperuricemia should be attributed to renal retention of uric acid, not overproduction. Allopurinol is ordinarily not advisable unless gouty arthritis has occurred.

PHARMACOKINETICS

Because the metabolism and elimination of many drugs are impaired in patients with renal failure, precise adjustment of the dose is often required. The incidence of drug reactions is high in uremic patients, not only because of decreased elimination of the drug and its metabolites but also because of alterations in drug metabolic rates, changes in protein binding and distribution volumes, drug-associated metabolic loads, synergism of drug toxicity and metabolic abnormalities, and increased target organ susceptibility. The drugs that most frequently cause toxicity are cardiovascular drugs such as digoxin, such antibiotics as the aminoglycosides and tetracyclines, and the sedative-tranquilizer drugs. Because of potential inaccuracies in dosage calculation, pharmacologic recommendations for patients with renal failure include the following:

1. In patients with acute renal failure, restrict drug use to definite indications.
2. When established, follow a previously determined regimen for dosage of a given drug in oliguric patients.[65, 66, 67]
3. The proper dose may be estimated roughly by formulas that use an assay of renal function factored by the renal contribution to normal elimination. Remember that when renal function declines acutely, serum creatinine concentration does not reflect the severity of functional loss until an equilibrium concentration is reached.
4. If available, drug assays should be used to measure blood levels periodically.

5. Careful clinical monitoring for effectiveness and toxicity of an administered drug is mandatory for all patients with acute renal failure.

THE ROLE OF DIALYSIS

Some patients with acute renal failure, notably those who are not oliguric and have low rates of catabolism, can be managed successfully with minimal or no use of dialysis. Early use of dialysis is recommended, however, to prevent overt uremia and minimize the occurrence of complications. When acute renal failure has been precipitated by certain nephrotoxins, their removal by dialysis within the first few hours or days may abort or shorten the clinical course. Sometimes a chelating agent is required to mobilize the toxin to make it accessible for dialysis.[68] The early and frequent use of dialysis allows a more liberal fluid and nutrient intake and improves well-being. Although death from hemorrhage and infection can be prevented,[69] mortality has not been decreased convincingly by liberal use of dialysis. Most centers prefer to maintain concentrations of plasma urea nitrogen and creatinine below 100 and 10 mg per dl, respectively, even though this may require daily dialysis in the catabolic, oliguric patient and may precipitate the need for one or more dialyses in the patient with milder lesions. The development of resistant hyperkalemia, severe fluid overload, or uncontrolled acidosis is a more urgent indication for dialysis. Overt symptomatic uremia with severe central nervous system or gastrointestinal manifestations or pericarditis is considered a late indication for dialysis treatment.

For many patients, peritoneal dialysis can control acute uremia adequately. It may be preferable to extracorporeal hemodialysis when the hemodynamics are unstable or when anticoagulants are especially dangerous, and it is often less disruptive of intensive care unit management and of the schedule of other patients requiring chronic maintenance hemodialysis. Hemodialysis is often preferred for certain patients with recent abdominal surgery, e.g., those with aortic grafts or abdominal drains. The higher rate of transport of low molecular weight toxins favors the use of hemodialysis for removal of exogenous toxins or for management of patients with increased rates of catabolism.

Continuous arteriovenous ultrafiltration has also been recommended because hemodynamic stability is greater than during intermittent hemofiltration or hemodialysis.[70] Despite the use of more permeable membranes or continuous slow hemodialysis sufficient to maintain nitrogenous metabolites at concentrations in serum half those usually achieved by dialysis, the mortality remains above 50 per cent.[70, 71, 72]

Prevention of acute renal failure is preferable to the most intensive treatment.

References

1. Anderson RJ, Linas SL, Berns AS, Henrich WL, Miller TR, Gabow PA, Schrier RW: Nonoliguric acute renal failure. N Engl J Med *288*:695, 1977.
2. Merrill JP: Acute renal failure. *In* Drukker W, Parsons FM, Maher JF (eds): Replacement of Renal Function by Dialysis. The Hague, Martinus Nijhoff, 1978, p 322.
3. Maher JF, Schreiner GE: Cause of death in acute renal failure. Arch Intern Med *110*:493, 1962.
4. Wing AJ, Broyer M, Brunner FP, Brynger H, Challah S, Donckerwolcke RA, Gretz N, Jacobs C, Kramer P, Selwood NH: Combined report on regular dialysis and transplantation in Europe, XIII, 1982. Proc Eur Dial Transplant Assoc *20*:5, 1983.
5. Hou S, Bushinsky DA, Wish JB, Cohen JJ, Harrington, JT: Hospital-acquired renal insufficiency: A prospective study. Am J Med *74*:243, 1983.
6. Meroney WH, Rubini ME, Blythe WB: The effect of antecedent diet on urine-concentrating ability. Ann Intern Med *48*:562, 1958.
7. Schreiner GE, Rakowski TA, Argy WP Jr, Marc-Aurele J, Maher JF, Bauer H: Natural history of oliguric glomerulonephritis. *In* Kincaid-Smith P, Mathew TH, Becker EL (eds): Glomerulonephritis: Morphology, Natural History and Treatment. New York, John Wiley and Sons, 1972, p 711.
8. Tack ED, Perlman JM, Robson AM: Renal injury in sick newborn infants: A prospective evaluation using urinary β_2 microglobulin concentrations. Pediatrics *81*:432, 1988.
9. Schreiner GE, Maher JF: Toxic nephropathy. Am J Med *38*:409, 1965.
10. Mustonen J, Pasternack A, Helin H, Pystynen S, Twominen T: Renal biopsy in acute renal failure. Am J Med *4*:27, 1984.
11. Maher JF: Clinicopathologic spectrum of drug nephrotoxicity. Adv Intern Med *30*:295, 1984.
12. Heptinstall RH: Interstitial nephritis: A brief review. Am J Pathol *83*:214, 1976.
13. Linton A, Clark WR, Driedgere AA, Turnbull DI, Lindsay RM: Acute interstitial nephritis due to drugs. Review of the literature with a report of nine cases. Ann Intern Med *93*:735, 1980.
14. Adler SG, Cohen AH, Border WA: Hypersensitivity phenomena and the kidney: Role of drugs and environmental agents. Am J Kidney Dis *5*:75, 1985.

15. Corwin HL, Bonventre JV: Renal insufficiency associated with nonsteroidal anti-inflammatory agents. Am J Kidney Dis *4*:147, 1984.
16. Henrich WL: Nephrotoxicity of nonsteroidal antiinflammatory agents. Am J Kidney Dis *3*:478, 1983.
17. Kleinknecht D, Landais P, Goldfarb B: Analgesic and nonsteroidal anti-inflammatory drug-associated acute renal failure: A prospective collaborative study. Clin Nephrol *25*:275, 1986.
18. French AJ: Hypersensitivity in the pathogenesis of the histopathologic changes associated with sulfonamide chemotherapy. Am J Pathol *22*:679, 1946.
19. Zimmerman SW, Groehler K, Beirne GJ: Hydrocarbon exposure and chronic glomerulonephritis. Lancet *2*:199, 1975.
20. Heptinstall RH: Pathology of the Kidney. 2nd ed. Boston, Little, Brown & Co., 1974.
21. Burry HC: Drug induced nephropathies. Proc R Soc Med *66*:897, 1973.
22. Citron BP, Halpern M, McCarron M: Necrotizing angiitis associated with drug abuse. N Engl J Med *283*:1003, 1970.
23. Oken DE: Modern concepts of the role of nephrotoxic agents in the pathogenesis of acute renal failure. Prog Biochem Pharmacol *7*:219, 1972.
24. Thurau K, Boylan J: Acute renal success. The unexpected logic of oliguria in acute renal failure. Am J Med *61*:308, 1976.
25. Stein JH, Sorkin MI: Pathophysiology of a vasomotor and nephrotoxic model of acute renal failure in the dog. Kidney Int *10*:586, 1976.
26. DiBona GF, McDonald FD, Flamenbaum W, Dammin GJ, Oken DE: Maintenance of renal function in salt-loaded rats despite severe tubular necrosis induced by $HgCl_2$. Nephron *8*:205, 1971.
27. Badr KF, Kelley VE, Rennke HG, Brenner BM: Roles of thromboxane A_2 and leukotrienes in endotoxin-induced acute renal failure. Kidney Int *30*:474, 1986.
28. Myers B, Moran SM: Hemodynamically mediated acute renal failure. N Engl J Med *314*:97, 1986.
29. Humes HD, Jackson NM, O'Connor RP, Hunt DA, White MD: Pathogenetic mechanisms of nephrotoxicity: Insights into cyclosporine nephrotoxicity. Transplant Proc *17*(Suppl 1):S51, 1985.
30. Cuppage FE, Tate A: Repair of the nephron following injury with mercuric chloride. Am J Pathol *51*:405, 1967.
31. Madias NE, Harrington JE: Platinum nephrotoxicity. Am J Med *65*:307, 1978.
32. Mudge GH: Uricosuric action of cholecystographic agents: A possible factor in nephrotoxicity. N Engl J Med *284*:929, 1971.
33. Gomes AS, Baker JD, Martin-Paredo V, Dixon SM, Takiff H, Machleder HI, Moore WS: Acute renal dysfunction after major arteriography. Am J Roentgenol *145*:1249, 1985.
34. Byrd L, Sherman RL: Radiocontrast-induced acute renal failure: A clinical and pathophysiologic review. Medicine *58*:270, 1979.
35. Appel GB, Neu HC: The nephrotoxicity of antimicrobial agents. N Engl J Med *296*:663, 1977.
36. Luft FC, Block R, Sloan RS, Yum MN, Costello R, Maxwell DR: Comparative nephrotoxicity of aminoglycoside antibiotics in rats. J Infect Dis *138*:541, 1978.
37. Smith CR, Moore RD, Lietman PS: Studies of risk factors for aminoglycoside nephrotoxicity. Am J Kidney Dis *8*:308, 1986.
38. Humes HD, Weinberg JM, Knauss TC: Clinical and pathophysiologic aspects of aminoglycoside toxicity. Am J Kidney Dis *2*:5, 1982.
39. Cronin RE: Aminoglycoside nephrotoxicity: Pathogenesis and prevention. Clin Nephrol *11*:251, 1979.
40. Koch-Weser J, Sidel VW, Federman EB, Kanarek P, Finer DC, Eaton AE: Adverse effects of sodium colistimethate. Manifestations and specific reaction rates during 317 courses of therapy. Ann Intern Med *72*:857, 1970.
41. Boyd JF, Butcher BT, Stewart GT: The nephrotoxicity and histology of cephaloridine and its polymers in rats. Br J Exp Pathol *52*:503, 1971.
42. Verma S, Kieff E: Cephalexin related nephropathy. JAMA *234*:618, 1975.
43. Clausen G, Nagy Z, Szaloy L, Aukland K: Mechanisms in acute oliguric renal failure induced by tetracycline infusion. Scand J Clin Lab Invest *35*:625, 1975.
44. Patel R, Connor G: A review of thirty cases of rhabdomyolysis-associated acute renal failure among phencyclidine users. J Toxicol Clin Toxicol *23*:547, 1985–1986.
45. Kimberly RP, Gill JR Jr, Bowden RE, Keiser HR, Plotz PH: Elevated urinary prostaglandins and the effects of aspirin on renal function in lupus erythematosus. Ann Intern Med *89*:336, 1978.
46. Hricik DE, Browning PJ, Kopelman R, Goorno WE, Madias NE, Pzau VJ: Captopril-induced functional renal insufficiency in patients with bilateral renal-artery stenosis or renal-artery stenosis in a solitary kidney. N Engl J Med *308*:373, 1983.
47. Atkinson K, Gibbs JC, Hages J, Ralston M, Dodds AJ, Concannon AJ, Naidoo D: Cyclosporin A associated nephrotoxicity in the first 100 days after allogenic bone marrow transplantation: Three distinct syndromes. Br J Haematol *54*:59, 1983.
48. Mazze RI: Fluorinated anaesthetic nephrotoxicity: An update. Can Anaesth Soc J *31*(Suppl):S16, 1984.
49. Ahmad S, Shen F, Bleyer WA: Methotrexate-induced renal failure and ineffectiveness of peritoneal dialysis. Arch Intern Med *138*:1146, 1978.
50. Raymond JR: Nephrotoxicities of antineoplastic and immunosuppressive agents. Curr Probl Cancer *8*:1, 1984.
51. Maher JF, Schreiner GE: Metabolic problems related to prolonged dialytic maintenance of life in oliguria. JAMA *176*:399, 1961.
52. Gotch FA, Sargent JA, Keen JL, Lee M: Individualized quantified dialysis therapy of uremia. Proc Clin Dial Transplant Forum *4*:27, 1974.
53. Bergström J, Fürst P: Uraemic toxins. *In* Drukker W, Parsons FM, Maher JF (eds): Replacement of Renal Function by Dialysis. The Hague, Martinus Nijhoff, 1978, p 334.
54. Schreiner GE, Maher JF: Uremia: Biochemistry, Pathogenesis and Treatment. Springfield, IL, Charles C Thomas, 1961, p 487.
55. Maher JF: Uremic pleuritis. Am J Kidney Dis *10*:19, 1987.
56. Cioffi WG, Ashikaga T, Gamelli RL: Probability of surviving postoperative acute renal failure. Ann Surg *200*:205, 1984.
57. Lewers DT, Mathew TH, Maher JF, et al: Long-term follow-up of renal function and histology after acute tubular necrosis. Ann Intern Med *73*:523, 1970.
58. Bonomini V, Stefoni S, Vangelista A: Long-term patient and renal prognosis in acute renal failure. Nephron *36*:169, 1984.
59. Flores J, Dibona GH, Leaf A: Role of cell swelling in

ischemic renal damage and the protective effect of hypertonic solute. J Clin Invest *51*:118, 1972.
60. Barza M: The nephrotoxicity of cephalosporins: An overview. J Infect Dis *137*:560, 1978.
61. Graziani G, Cantaluppi A, Caseti S, Citterio A, Scalamonga A, Aroldi A, Silenzio R, Brancaccio D, Ponticelli C: Dopamine and furosemide in oliguric acute renal failure. Nephron *37*:39, 1984.
62. Arieff AI, Massry SG: Calcium metabolism of brain in acute renal failure. Effects of uremia, hemodialysis and parathyroid hormones. J Clin Invest *53*:387, 1974.
63. Abel RM, Beck CH, Abbott WM, Ryan JA Jr, Barnett GO, Fischer JE: Improved survival from acute renal failure after treatment with intravenous essential L-amino acids and glucose. Results of a prospective double blind study. N Engl J Med *288*:695, 1973.
64. Feinstein EI, Kopple JD, Silberman H, Massry SG: Total parenteral nutrition with high or low nitrogen intakes in patients with acute renal failure. Kidney Int *26*(Suppl 16):S319, 1983.
65. Anderson RJ, Bennett WM, Gambertoglio JG, Schrier RW: Fate of drugs in renal failure. *In* Brenner BM, Rector FC Jr (eds): The Kidney. Philadelphia, W.B. Saunders Co., 1981, p 2659.
66. Maher JF: Pharmacologic aspects of regular dialysis treatment. *In* Drukker W, Parsons FM, Maher JF (eds): Replacement of Renal Function by Dialysis. 2nd ed. The Hague, Martinus Nijhoff, 1983, p 749.
67. Bennett WM, Aronoff GR, Morrison G, Golper TA, Pulliam J, Wolfson M, Singer I: Drug prescribing in renal failure: Dosing guidelines for adults. Am J Kidney Dis *3*:155, 1983.
68. Kostyniak PJ: Mobilization and removal of methylmercury in the dog during extracorporeal complexing hemodialysis with 2,3-dimercaptosuccinic acid (DMSA). J Pharmacol Exp Ther *221*:63, 1982.
69. Gillum DM, Dixon BS, Yanover MJ, Kelleher SP, Shapiro MD, Benedetti RG, Dillingham MA, Paller MS, Goldberg JP, Tomford RC, Gordon JA, Unger JP: The role of intensive dialysis in acute renal failure. Clin Nephrol *25*:249, 1986.
70. Paganani E, Suhoza K, Swann S, Golding L, Nakamoto S: Continuous renal replacement therapy in patients with acute renal dysfunction undergoing intraaortic balloon pump and/or left ventricular device support. Am Soc Artif Intern Organs *32*:414, 1986.
71. Sigler MH, Teehan BP: Solute transport in continuous hemodialysis: A new treatment for acute renal failure. Kidney Int *32*:562, 1987.
72. Ronco C, Brendolan A, Bragantini L, Chiaramonte S, Feriani M, Fabris A, Dell'Aquila R, LaGreca G, Milan M: Continuous arteriovenous hemofiltration with AN 69S membrane; procedures and experience. Kidney Int *33*(Suppl 24):S150, 1988.

B. Chronic Drug Nephropathy

George E. Schreiner, M.D., FACP, FRCPS (Glas)
Carlos Rotellar, M.D.

Chronic drug nephrotoxicity is defined as a persistent and progressive functional or structural defect in the kidney (nephropathy) produced by a chemical or biologic product that is inhaled, ingested, injected, or otherwise absorbed into the body.

The term *nephrotoxicity*, or toxic nephropathy, also has been used, by extension, for the renal effects of normal blood constituents circulating in abnormal concentrations.[1] Thus, there is hypercalcemic, hypokalemic (kaliopenic), hyperuricemic (gouty), and hypomagnesemic nephropathy.

GENERAL CONSIDERATIONS

Unlike the case with acute toxic nephropathy, the diagnosis of chronic disease caused by drugs is often difficult to establish unless it is noted following acute disease or shows a characteristic lesion. Often only a subtle effect occurs in the presence of the organic disease for which the drug was taken. The patient may be unaware of exposure; for example, lead in drinking water, inhalation, unusual drug prescription, and so on. The patient may have forgotten the drug ingestion, which could have occurred years before. More often, multiple toxic drugs in the history or multiple etiologies render it difficult to establish a cause-and-effect relationship except by markedly circumstantial evidence. Often the association is either made by epidemiologic studies or remains simply a suspicion until a cluster of anecdotal reports appears.

Classification

The involvement of multiple disciplines, each with its own approach and specialized terminology, has engendered some confusion in the problem of drug nephropathy. Thus, the pharmacologist tends to focus on the drug, the pathologist on the lesion, and the clinician on the syndrome. We shall try to synthesize these varied points of view by

Table 9–2. SOME MECHANISMS OF INDIRECT NEPHROTOXICITY

AGENTS	MECHANISM
Ethylene glycol, methoxyflurane	Via oxalic acid
Phencyclidine (PCP) and amphetamines	Via rhabdomyolysis
Methysergide	Via retroperitoneal fibrosis
Ergot alkaloids	Via severe arteriolar constriction
Heroin	Via lead, staphylococcus and fungal toxin, or other contaminants of illicit use
Chemotherapy of hematopoietic neoplasms and uricosuric drugs	Via obstruction with uric acid crystals, intra- or extrarenal
Vitamin D + milk + alkali + vitamin D analogue	Nephrocalcinosis and lithiasis
Diphenyl and some pesticides	Via cysts and dysplasia
Mushroom and colchicine poisoning	Via diarrhea and fluid loss
Aniline, *p*-phenetidine, and a host of drugs, foods, and industrial agents	Via methemoglobin formation
Phenacetin and oxidant drugs	Only in G6PD-deficient patients

(From Berkow R (ed): The Merck Manual of Diagnosis and Therapy. 15th ed. West Point, PA, Merck Sharp & Dohme Research Laboratories, Copyright 1987, p 1606. Used with permission.)

presenting four classifications of drug nephropathy: (1) by syndrome, (2) by lesion, (3) by evolution of the disease, and (4) by agent (Tables 9–2 through 9–6).

PATHOGENETIC CONSIDERATIONS

The fundamental question is, "Why kidney?" Why is drug nephropathy such an important part of understanding adverse reactions to drugs? Why is the list of nephrotoxins so long (Table 9–7)? Why is drug nephropathy an evergrowing disease, as the human chemical environment escalates in complexity? Both general and specific answers to these questions exist. Kidney lesions and malfunctions are readily diagnosed by means of the urine. Function tests are varied and accurate. Nephrology is based on elaborate knowledge of basic physiology and cell biology. Renal biopsy treated by light immunofluorescent techniques, electron microscopy, and microenzymology gives clinical access to the most sophisticated developments in disease morphology.

The kidneys, weighing a few hundred grams, receive a fifth to a quarter of the cardiac output and thus have one of the highest blood flows per gram of cellular tissue. Therefore, they have available an enormous "first-pass" sample for all drugs and chemical agents received parenterally and a disproportionately large "second-pass" sample of drugs received enterally. The kidneys have a very high oxygen consumption and,

Table 9–3. CLASSIFICATION OF DRUG NEPHROPATHY BY SYNDROME

Ischemic syndromes—vasculitides, sclerosis, papillary and cortical necrosis, etc.
TID (tubulointerstitial disease)
Nephritis syndrome
Nephrotic syndrome
Specific tubular syndromes—Fanconi syndrome, tubular acidosis, aminoaciduria, nephrogenic diabetes insipidus, glycosuria, etc.
Crystal deposition—nephrocalcinosis, oxalosis, urate, etc.
Obstructive syndromes—intra- and extrarenal
Cysts
Neoplasm—renal, pelvic, ureteral, and bladder

Table 9–4. CLASSIFICATION OF DRUG NEPHROPATHY BY LESION

TIN (tubulointerstitial nephritis)
Glomerulonephritis—focal, diffuse, membranous
Lipoid nephrosis—minimal change glomerulonephritis, focal segmental glomerulosclerosis
Crystal deposition—cortex, medulla, proximal/distal tubule
Vascular disease—infarction, necrosis, sclerosis, vasculitis
Papillary (medullary) and cortical necrosis
Granulomatous disease
Periureteral fibrosis
Cysts
Neoplasms

Table 9–5. CLASSIFICATION OF DRUG NEPHROPATHY BY EVOLUTION

Postacute tubular necrosis—acute lesions with failure to recover
Postcortical necrosis—patchy or diffuse
Postmedullary necrosis—amputation and calcification of papillae
Progressive renal failure, leading to end stage renal disease
Progressive nephrotic syndrome
Specific tubular syndromes
Vascular disease—hypertension and renal insufficiency
Obstructive disease—dilation, atrophy, etc.
Cystic disease—symptomatic, or by imaging
Neoplastic disease—asymptomatic, or imaging of metastases

Table 9–6. CLASSIFICATION OF DRUG NEPHROPATHY BY AGENT

Diagnostic agents—e.g., iodinated contrast agents
Antibiotics—e.g., sulfonamides, amphotericin, etc.
Other therapeutic agents—e.g., analgesics, antiepileptics, chemotherapy, cimetidine, furosemide, etc.
Physical agents—e.g., radiation, heat stroke, etc.
Heavy metals—e.g., mercury, lead, etc.
Solvents—halogenated hydrocarbons, glycols, etc.
Pesticides and agricultural chemicals—e.g., biphenyls
Other environmental agents—occupational, water, air, ice, etc.
Biologicals & nephroallergens—e.g., venoms, poison oak, mushroom, fungi, etc.
Sulfhydryl drugs—D-penicillamine, thiopronine, captopril, methimazole
Miscellaneous—e.g., aniline and others, myoglobinuria

therefore, are highly susceptible to agents producing vasoconstriction and anoxia; they also have a vascular "rete mirabile," which acts as the basis for the countercurrent concentration mechanism, resulting in hypertonicity of the interstitium proceeding in the direction of the medulla. Thus, the distribution of compounds within the interstitial areas of the kidneys may result in high local concentrations much in excess of blood concentrations (Table 9–8).

Drugs excreted by the kidney may involve mechanisms of (a) filtration at the glomerulus, (b) nonionic diffusion, (c) active tubular reabsorption, (d) active tubular secretion, and (e) passive movement with water. These mechanisms can result in localized high concentrations on either the intraluminal border or peritubular capillary border. Active drug reabsorption and secretion may involve membrane binding, receptor sites, carrier proteins, enzyme systems, cell energetics, and the opportunity to interact with intracellular organelles. The kidney, a very active endocrine organ both in the manufacture of hormones and in its regulation by hormones, has a number of receptor sites with which some drugs act by competing directly for physiologic receptors (for example, spironolactone for aldosterone). Some cells of the kidney (e.g., tubule brush border) are extremely rich in sulfhydryl groups and are therefore susceptible to binding by heavy metals and other reactive agents, whereas other cells of the kidney seem to be particularly susceptible to coupling with drugs containing free sulfhydryl groups. This property has been used to deliver active drugs to the tubules (for instance, ethacrynic acid) and

Table 9–7. TOXIC NEPHROPATHY; PARTIAL LIST OF NEPHROTOXINS

Metals: Mercury (organic and inorganic), bismuth, uranium, cadmium, chromium and chromic acid, lead, gold, arsine and arsenic, iron, silver, antimony, copper, thallium, beryllium, manganese and lithium
Solvents: Carbon tetrachloride, tetrachloroethylene, methyl cellosolve, methanol, methyl chloroform, polyvinyl alcohol, and miscellaneous solvents
Glycols: Ethylene glycol, ethylene glycol dinitrite, propylene glycol, ethylene dichloride, diethylene glycol, xylitol, and glycerol
Environmental pollutants increasing xenobiotic metabolizing enzymes: 3,4-Benzo(a)pyrene, chlorinated dibenzodioxins (TCDD), dichlorodiphenyl trichloroethane (DDT), 3-methylcholanthrene (3MCA), polybrominated biphenyls (PBBs), polychlorinated biphenyls (PCBs), and hexachlorobenzene
Aminoglycoside antibiotics: Gentamicin, tobramycin, amikacin, netilmicin, kanamycin, neomycin, streptomycin
Other antibiotics: Sulfonamides, ampicillin, methicillin, colistin, cephaloridine, cephazolin, cephamandole, guanylureidopenicillin (BLP 1654), amphotericin, vancomycin, bacitracin, polymyxin, tetracycline, puromycin
Anesthetic agents: Methoxyflurane and halothane
Diagnostic agents: Bunamiodyl, iopanoic acid, sodium and meglumine salts of diatrizoate, iothalamate, metrizoate
Other therapeutic agents: Tridione, Paradione, mephenytoin, phenindione, levambusol, probenecid, allopurinol, carbo-amide, lithium, perchlorate, furosemide, cimetidine
Analgesic and antiarthritis agents: Aspirin and other salicylates, indomethacin, phenacetin, acetaminophen, phenylbutazone, ibuprofen, mefenamic acid, and probably all nonsteroidal anti-inflammatory agents
Sulfhydryl drugs: D-penicillamine, thiopronine, captopril, methimazole
Physical agents: Radiation, heat stroke, electroshock, and rhabdomyolysis
Miscellaneous chemicals: Carbon monoxide, snake venom, mushroom poisoning, spider venom, nephroallergens, cresol, aniline, EDTA, renacidin, cyclophosphamide, and all agents that produce methemoglobin
Abnormal concentrations of physiologic substances: Hypercalcemia, hyperuricemia, hypokalemia, hypomagnesemia, hyperxanthinemia

Table 9–8. INTRARENAL DISTRIBUTION OF SUSPECT ANALGESIC

	CONCENTRATION				INTRACELLULAR DISTRIBUTION IN PAPILLA
	Plasma	*Cortex*	*Papilla*	*Urine*	
Phenacetin (dog)	1	1	1	1	+
Paracetamol (dog)	1	1.5	4	16	+
Acetaminophen conjugates (dog)	1	1	5	95	0
Salicylate (rabbit)	1	6	13	90	+
Inulin (dog)	1	1.5	8	100	0

(Modified from Duggin CG: Mechanism of the development of analgesic nephropathy. Kidney Int *18*:553, 1980.)

may be responsible for the rather unique toxicities of drugs that have in common a reactive sulfhydryl group, such as D-penicillamine, thioproline, captopril, pyrithioxin, and methimazole.[2]

Some drug reactions occur by an immunologic or hypersensitivity mechanism. The large renal blood flow can deliver immune complexes preferentially to the kidney as well as to cross-reacting antibodies. Furthermore, the human kidney contains both a C_3 receptor,[3] on the epithelial side of the glomerulus at a site appropriate for the development of segmental sclerosis, and a receptor for the Fc fragment of IgG in the interstitium in humans and animals.[4] Furthermore, renal mesangium contains a structural phagocyte uniquely situated to sample the capillary lumen and capable of making I protein and processing antigen for presentation to T lymphocytes; it is, therefore, capable of initiating an immune response.

With the highest surface area of endothelium relative to weight, the kidney is uniquely situated for a plethora of reactions that occur at vascular and endothelial surfaces. Only recently has it been realized that the kidney is extremely active in affecting the biotransformation of drugs; in some cases, because of its huge blood flow, the kidney approaches or exceeds the liver in metabolic capacity. The biotransformation of organic compounds can be divided into oxidative, reductive, and hydrolytic steps as well as conjugation. Oxidative reactions are to our present knowledge largely catalyzed by the cytochrome P-450–dependent, mixed function oxidase system, consisting of aromatic and aliphatic hydroxylation, dealkylation, and epioxidations. Kidney tissue also performs reduction reactions, such as the conversion of aldehydes and ketones to alcohol. The hydrolysis of esters and amides is usually enzyme-catalyzed and can be performed by the rich load of renal enzymes, while epoxide hydrase activity is also known to be present in the kidney. The well-known conjugative reactions, which usually involve combining drug or metabolite with carbohydrate or amino acid, result in the formation of glucuronides, sulfates, and hippurates. Renal enzymes have been shown to form glucuronides, while sulfate esters and glutathione form conjugates. In the conjugative metabolism of phenols, the kidney makes a significant contribution to total metabolite production.

It is unfortunate that medical students have learned these reactions under the term *detoxification,* since in many examples both metabolites and conjugates are more toxic than the parent compound, or they may have compartmental distribution lending themselves to toxicity in specific compartments, such as the renal papilla. A detailed review of drug metabolism in the kidney has been recently published by Anders.[5]

In addition, as listed in Table 9-2, many agents cause nephrotoxicity indirectly.

SOME SPECIFIC CAUSES OF NEPHROTOXICITY

1. Drugs Containing an Available Sulfhydryl Group

Although the kidney is rich in sulfhydryl groups, particularly in the brush border of the proximal tubule, structures in the glomerulus appear to have an affinity for drugs containing an available sulfhydryl group. Thus, similar toxic reactions, with proteinuria often progressing to the nephrotic syndrome, have been reported with D-penicillamine, thioproline, captopril, pyrithioxin, and methimazole.[2]

D,1 and D-penicillamine (beta-dimethylcysteine) has had a broad-ranging therapeutic usefulness in rheumatoid arthritis, scleroderma, hepatolenticular degeneration of Wilson's disease, divalent metal intoxication, cystinuria, macroglobulinemia, cold agglutinin syndrome, chronic hepatitis, and biliary cirrhosis. It has been used successfully to treat acrodynia (from mercury) and will protect fetal rats from brain damage caused by methyl mercury chloride. Both the racemic mixture and the D-isomer were found to be toxic after being introduced into therapeutic use, and some fatal cases of nephrotic syndrome have been reported.[6–10]

Increased glomerular permeability occurs in 7 to 10 per cent of patients with rheumatoid arthritis receiving D-penicillamine, which frequently progresses to a frank nephrotic syndrome; usually this occurs within the first year of treatment but may develop after several years.[2] There may be a special relationship with high doses[10] and with previous nephrotoxicity from gold compounds.[11] Most cases have regressed, with the disappearance of the proteinuria 6 to 12 months after the drug is withdrawn, but some cases of proteinuria have been chronic. The predominant renal lesion is a membranous glomerulonephritis with deposits that are only modestly electron dense; they are usually segmental and subepithelial and may be seen together with granular deposits of IgG and C_3.[12] Other reported lesions include renal amyloidosis, minimal change disease (lipoid nephrosis), focal glomerulonephritis, proliferative extracapillary glomerulonephritis, Goodpasture's syndrome, renal angiitis, and renal angiitis without glomerular involvement.[13]

In Wistar rats, proteinuria, nuclear proliferation, and hypertrophy of the mesangium can be produced by oral administration of 1 to 2 gm/kg/24 hr of D-penicillamine.[14]

Captopril is an angiotensin-converting enzyme inhibitor widely heralded as a specific therapy for hypertension. Shortly after its limited clinical trial was begun, scattered reports of proteinuria and nephrotic syndrome were seen.[15] The Squibb data indicated an occurrence of proteinuria in 34 (1.2 per cent) of 2937 patients treated for hypertension for periods ranging from 3 to 12 months.[15] Seven had a clinical nephrotic syndrome, and four of these regressed after withdrawal. Of 23 renal biopsies, membranous glomerulonephritis was observed in 10.[2] It has been shown that the side effects of captopril are dose dependent.

Thioproline has been used for rheumatoid arthritis, and in one study proteinuria was noted in 4 of 20 patients treated with this new agent.[16] Of two patients treated for cystinuria, one developed nephrotic syndrome.[17] One case of nephrotic syndrome associated with a membranous glomerulonephritis and granular deposition of IgG and C_3 was reported after 8 months of treatment with *pyrithioxin*.[2] The nephrotic syndrome has been reported in three patients treated with *methimazole*,[2] one of whom had mesangial hypertrophy.

Nephrotic syndrome has been produced in rats given the antiepileptic drug trimethadione and has also been seen clinically with a wide variety of drugs, including Paradione, mephenytoin, probenecid, phenindione, phenylbutazone, levambutol, tolbutamide, carbutamide, diclofenac, fenclofenac, ethosuximide, and lithium carbonate.[2] Perchlorate has also produced nephrotic syndrome in the course of its use for thyrotoxicosis.[18]

2. Heavy Metal Nephrotoxicity

Mercury has become a major pollutant in industrial societies, principally because it is prevalent in the effluent of paper mills and other manufacturing processes and can form an insoluble salt in the sediment of rivers, streams, and shallow water basins. Biotransformation to more soluble and toxic forms can be performed by marine life and fish, and mercury thus can enter the food chain and has indeed been found in increased amounts in the flesh of tuna, swordfish, marine birds, and other life a great distance from the source of pollution. Clinical experience of nephrotoxicity has occurred largely with bichloride of mercury, merbromin, mercurial diuretics, and related compounds.[19]

The nephrotic syndrome has been reported after the use of mercurial diuretics,[20] mercuric chloride in calomel and teething powder, the mercury salt of fulminic acid,[21] and ammoniated mercury ointment,[22] paint additives,[23] and teething powders containing mercury.[24] It has also been reported from the use of protiodide mercury in the treatment of verruca plana, or flat wart.[25] Nephrotic syndrome is still being reported from chronic ingestion of calomel-containing laxatives. Among the rare causes are workers handling mercury or exposed to its vapors, children playing with a broken thermometer, inhalation from a Miller-Abbott tube, and use by African women of skin-lightening creams containing mercury.[26] In general, a membranous glomerulonephritis with IgG and C_3 deposits is the most frequently observed lesion. The deposits are generally granular, although linear deposits have been reported.[26]

Mercury and other heavy metals, like gold, bind readily to —SH groups in the proximal tubule and also to tubular basement membrane and indeed may be found on electron microscopy in cellular components. However, more recent opinion is that many heavy metal–induced nephropathies are immunologically mediated. Such a mechanism is suspected because the heavy metals are rarely found in subepithelial deposits in the glomerulus.

Druet and associates have observed a biphasic course of glomerulonephritis induced in brown Norway rats by prolonged low doses of mercuric chloride.[27]

A linear and smooth pattern of fixation of antirat IgG antiserum along the glomerular basement membrane (GBM) is characteristic of an anti-GBM type of glomerulonephritis and was observed at day 15 when the rats were first examined. Later, the pattern had become granular and characteristic of an immune complex glomerulonephritis.

Fillastre and colleagues hypothesized that they too initially could modify a component of the glomerular basement membrane, rendering it antigenic with subsequent formation of immune complexes either in situ or in the circulation.[2] Similar biphasic glomerulonephritis has been observed in New Zealand rabbits.[28] There are data to suggest that a genetic predisposition of immune-mediated, drug-induced glomerulonephritis is possible. Only some strains of animals are susceptible; Wooley and associates estimate that the relative risk of proteinuria during treatment of rheumatoid arthritis by oral thiomalate is increased 32 times in human beings who have HLA-DRw_3 antigens on tissue typing.[28]

Besides mercury and gold, other metals reported to produce nephrotoxicity and often nephrotic syndrome[19] are bismuth, uranium, cadmium, chromium and chromic acid, lead, arsine and arsenic, iron, silver, antimony, copper, thallium, beryllium, magnesium, and lithium.

Gold nephropathy may become more prominent in the near future because of the recent introduction of effective oral gold-containing salts for the treatment of rheumatoid arthritis. Mild transient proteinuria has been reported in about 10 per cent of patients with rheumatoid arthritis treated with gold salts.[29] Membranous glomerulonephritis is the most frequently observed lesion. Diffuse granular deposits of IgG, IgM, and C_3 may occur. X-ray studies and electron microanalysis demonstrate the presence of gold mainly in the proximal tubular epithelium and in podocytes, mesangium, and interstitial macrophages. Gold, however, is not found in the subepithelial deposits, which suggests that small deposits are immunologically mediated.[2] A membranous glomerulonephritis has been induced in Wistar rats following repeated injections of low doses of the oral preparation of sodium thiomalate.[30]

3. Cyclosporin A Nephrotoxicity

Cyclosporin A (CyA) is an immunomodulating drug used in the prevention of transplant rejection and in clinical research protocols for the treatment of some autoimmune diseases (e.g., idiopathic nephrotic syndrome, uveitis, diabetes mellitus). Chronic nephrotoxicity is the most frequent and important side effect of CyA therapy. In kidney transplant patients, it is difficult to differentiate between allograft rejection and CyA toxicity, since the clinical presentation is so similar. However, some histologic features suggest CyA toxicity, including tubular cell vacuolization, diffuse interstitial fibrosis with little cellular infiltration or patchy areas of focal interstitial fibrosis surrounding atrophic tubules, and obliterating arteriolopathy. The clearest evidence of chronic nephrotoxicity from CyA is the observation of renal disease in patients with nonrenal transplants, such as heart or liver, or in patients treated for autoimmune diseases.[31, 32] In such patients nephrotoxicity may be dose related, since low doses may not be associated with renal impairment.

4. Analgesic Nephropathy

Analgesics, particularly the mixed analgesics containing salicylates, caffeine, phenacetin, and/or acetaminophen, are among the most widely used and abused over-the-counter medications. The medical world was alerted to a potential relationship between cumulative abuse of these agents and the development of a chronic tubular interstitial disease and renal papillary necrosis by the timely studies of Spuhler and Zollinger in 1953.[33]

A curious feature of analgesic nephropathy is the great geographic variation. Analgesic nephropathy accounts for from 18 to 30 per cent of uremic patients in some geographic areas versus 1 to 3 per cent in other areas.[34–37] Of course, vast differences exist in the per capita consumption of analgesics: of the major reporting nations, Australia and Denmark have the highest rate and the United States and Canada the lowest.[34–37] In many countries, consumption of analgesics is increasing at a rate exceeding the growth of the population.[36, 37] Other reasons for variations include genetic influences, high temperatures, and dehydration. In Australia, it has been demonstrated that presentation to a hospital of patients with this disease is commoner in the summer than in the winter and that the disease has acute exacerbations during episodes of dehydration.[35]

We completed a retrospective study of analgesic intake in the dialysis population of our affiliated dialysis centers in Washington, DC. A carefully constructed questionnaire was administered by nonbiased observers to 277 patients receiving long-term hemodialysis. The questionnaire was designed to elicit demographic data, type of renal disease, and pattern of analgesic consumption. Only 8 of 277 patients (2.8 per cent) met the criteria for excessive analgesic intake, defined as more than six tablets per day or more than 1 gram a day producing a cumulative dose greater than 1 kilogram. The drugs consumed were predominantly phenacetin, acetaminophen, or aspirin, and ingestion existed for at least 1 year in the period before the institution of maintenance hemodialysis. Of patients who met the criteria for analgesic abuse, one had diabetic nephropathy and one had systemic lupus erythematosus. This percentage (2.8 per cent) is in remarkable agreement with the 2.5 per cent analgesic nephropathy in dialysis patients reported in the European Dialysis and Transplant Registry. This figure again was true in 1976, with 9000 patients, and dropped to 1.4 per cent in 1977 among 47,000 patients. It is also in agreement with the 2.5 per cent reported by Gault and Wilson in Canada.[37]

Pathogenetic Considerations

Mixed analgesic nephropathy was initially wrongly labeled as phenacetin nephritis. This is unlikely, since phenacetin is relatively nonreactive and, as shown in Table 9–8, is not concentrated in cortex, papilla, or medulla. The suspected drugs in analgesic nephropathy are acetaminophen, aspirin, and phenacetin, because there is little or no evidence that the antihistamines, codeine, aminopyrine, barbiturates, steroids, and many other agents often found in complex mixed formulations of analgesic powders or tablets contribute significantly to nephrotoxicity. Of these suspect agents, acetaminophen undergoes glomerular filtration and is passively reabsorbed by the tubules. It becomes concentrated in the renal medulla during antidiuresis to a concentration five to seven times that found in the cortex and plasma. Phenacetin per se does not achieve a concentration in the medulla greater than that in the cortex or plasma. Aspirin and salicylate undergo proximal renal tubular secretion by the organic ion secretory system; both are reabsorbed in the distal nephron by nonionic passive diffusion and are concentrated by the countercurrent mechanism.

All three—aspirin, phenacetin, and acetaminophen—are distributed within the intracellular compartment of the medulla. Acetaminophen depletes cellular glutathione in the kidney and becomes metabolized to a very reactive intermediate, by both an NADPH-dependent and an NADPH-independent mechanism. This intermediate subsequently binds covalently to cellular protein macromolecules when glutathione is reduced. The half-life of acetaminophen covalently bound to protein in the medulla is in the range of 120 hours.[38] Glutathione exists in kidney cells in two pools, one confined to the cell membrane and the other intracellular, presumably attached to organelles.[38] Aspirin can acetylate kidney protein, but the implication of this for nephrotoxicity is not known. However, aspirin is to some extent a prostaglandin synthetase inhibitor and may induce renal vasoconstriction. Insulin and PAH clearances in patients with analgesic nephropathy were reduced upon rechallenge with aspirin alone.[39]

Since aspirin is an inhibitor of prostaglandin synthetase, a hypothesis for the mechanism of analgesic nephropathy is shown in outline form in Figure 9–1 and graphically in Figure 9–2. It has been shown by Prescott[40] and Mitchell and associates[41] that liver glutathione may be replenished by circulating sulfhydryl compounds such as mercaptamine (cysteamine), methionine, cysteine, and *N*-acetylcysteine, particularly if given within the first 12 hours after acetaminophen. They can sufficiently replenish glutathione to prevent covalent binding in the liver and thus prevent hepatotoxicity and cell death. We have hypothesized that the reactive metabolites of acetaminophen deplete intrarenal glutathione. The cellular toxicity, therefore, is generated by covalent binding of these reactive metabolites to intracellular protein in organelles and may relate to the depletion of glutathione in one of the two pools, membrane or intracellular. Theoretically, this could be prevented by continuous replenishment of bound glutathione from sulfhydryl-containing compounds in plasma. These, however, must be delivered via the blood flow, which is rather poor in the medullary area of the kidney. Furthermore, perfusion in selective vascular beds in the kidney appears to be under the control of a balance between vasoconstrictor substances, such as angiotensin, and vasodilator substances, such as the vasodilator derivatives of arachidonic acid. Aspirin, by inhibiting prostaglandin synthetase, would result in preponderance of vasoconstriction. This would reduce the filtered load of any solute at the arterial end of the capillary, by reducing the blood flow portion of the formula for filtered load. With impairment of the mechanism for repletion, glutathione depletion in the renal cell theoretically becomes more possible and the incidence of covalent binding more frequent, with resulting cell injury or cell death, but this requires blood levels generally in excess of 100 mg/dl.

Chronic administration of therapeutic doses of aspirin to large numbers of patients with rheumatoid arthritis is not accompanied by any exceptional incidence of nephrotoxicity. Similarly, very few clinical cases of nephropathy have been reported in the United States from the extensive sales of the formulation of Tylenol, which contains acetaminophen alone. In two recent retrospective studies,[42, 43] it has been suggested that long-term daily use of acetaminophen alone *may be* associated with an increased risk of chronic renal disease. However, these are retrospective studies and are based on patients' recollection of their analgesic abuse. It is clear that further studies are necessary to evaluate this problem. Sandler and associates also suggested that the daily use of aspirin alone does not increase such a risk.[42] We have recently seen a physician who has taken one aspirin daily for several years as part of the Harvard Coronary Study, in whom the addition of acetaminophen for jogging aches and pains resulted in a reversible analgesic nephropathy. By any reckoning, the majority of cases result from combinations of salicylate and acetaminophen (itself derived from the first-pass circulation of phenacetin to the liver). In these cases, the proposed hypothesis for synergism may be operative.[43]

Clinical Considerations

Analgesic nephropathy should be suspected if one or more of the following conditions are elicited from the patient's history or from clinical observation:

- renal disease and peptic ulcer,
- renal disease and drug-prone neurosis,
- renal disease and headache or arthritis or depression, distortion of a papilla on

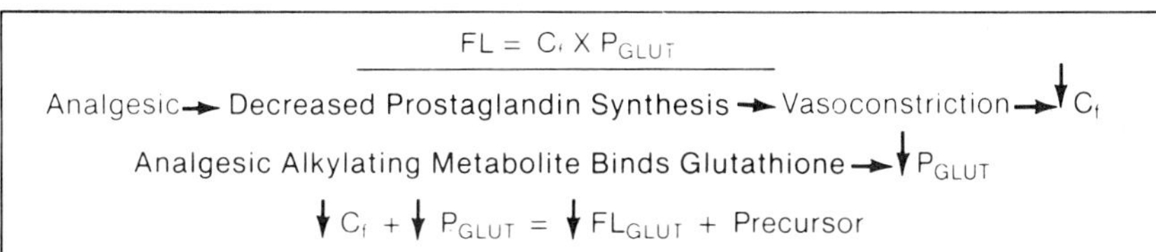

Figure 9–1. Hypothetical mechanism for analgesic nephropathy. Clearance of filtered substance is C_f; plasma concentration of glutathione, P_{GLUT}; and filtered load, FL. (From Schreiner GE, McAnally JF, Winchester JF: Clinical analgesic nephropathy. Arch Intern Med *141*:349, 1981. Copyright 1981, American Medical Association.)

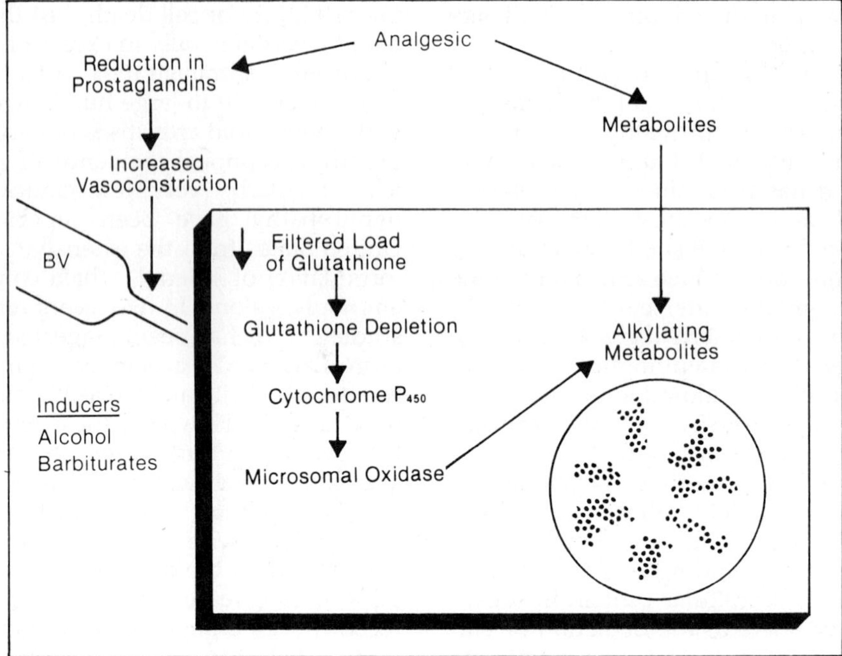

Figure 9–2. Cell model to show mechanism for analgesic renal cytotoxicity. BV, blood vessel. (From Schreiner GE, McAnally JF, Winchester JF: Clinical analgesic nephropathy. Arch Intern Med *141*:349, 1981. Copyright 1981, American Medical Association.)

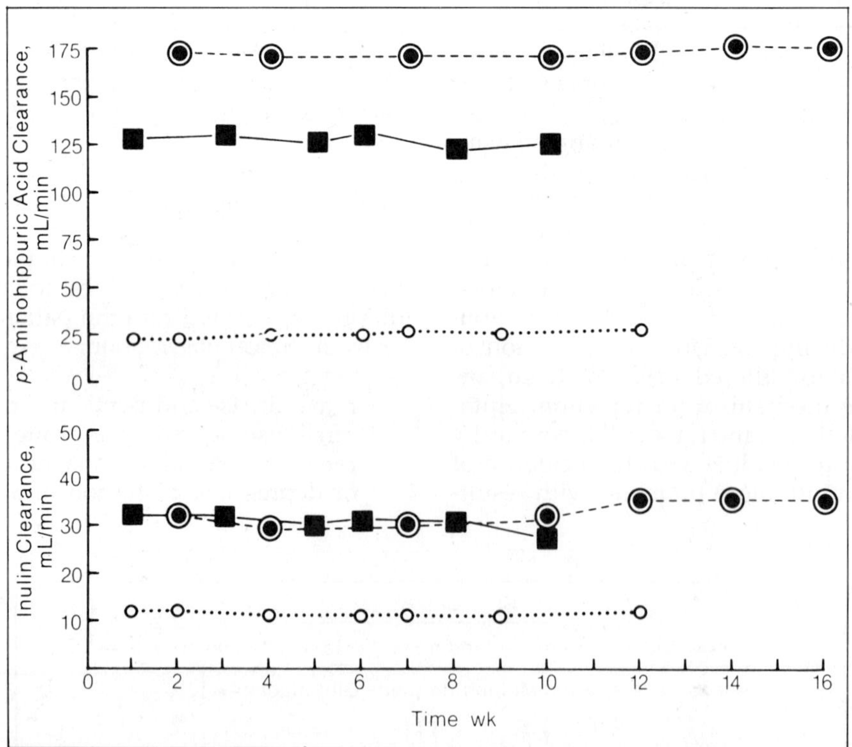

Figure 9–3. Serial clearance of *p*-aminohippuric acid and inulin in three patients with analgesic nephropathy observed in the metabolic ward after analgesic withdrawal. (From Schreiner GE, McAnally JF, Winchester JF: Clinical analgesic nephropathy. Arch Intern Med *141*:349, 1981. Copyright 1981, American Medical Association.)

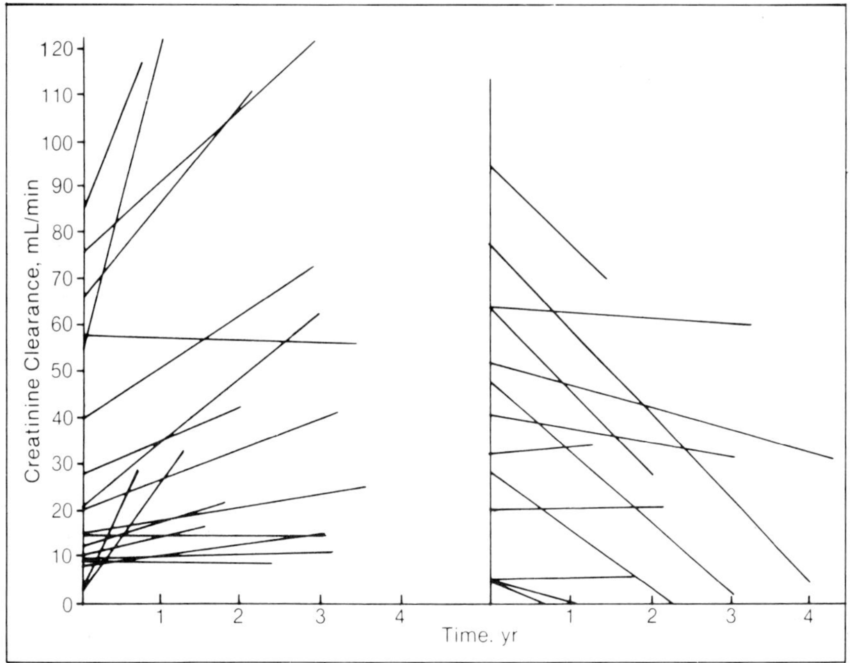

Figure 9–4. Filtration rates in patients who continued and in those who ceased ingestion of analgesics. (From Schreiner GE, McAnally JF, Winchester JF: Clinical analgesic nephropathy. Arch Intern Med *141*:349, 1981. Copyright 1981, American Medical Association.)

an intravenous pyelogram (ring sign), or nephrocalcinosis,

- a history of recurrent and excessive drug purchase or ingestion or the finding of an acetaminophen metabolite (*N*-acetyl-*p*-amino phenol, or NAPAP) in random urine samples, or
- pigmentation of the lips, skin, or liver on biopsy or autopsy.

Patients with analgesic nephropathy are most often middle-aged women with histories of psychiatric disorders, frequent headaches, backaches, or other arthralgias. Inves-

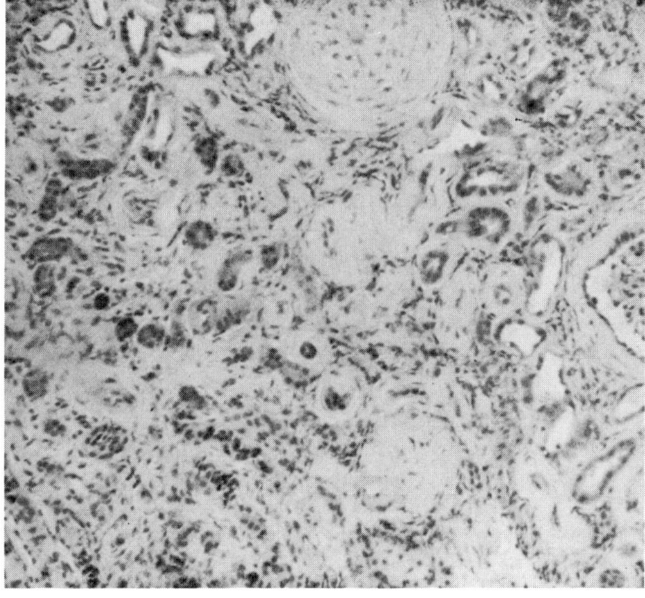

Figure 9–5. Interstitial nephritis of analgesic nephropathy (hematoxylin-eosin). (From Schreiner GE, McAnally JF, Winchester JF: Clinical analgesic nephropathy. Arch Intern Med *141*:349, 1981. Copyright 1981, American Medical Association.)

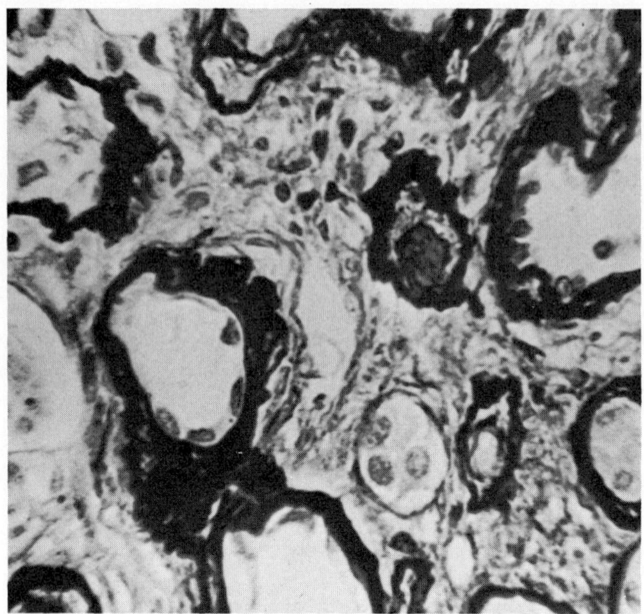

Figure 9–6. Thickened tubular basement membrane in renal biopsy specimen of patient with analgesic nephropathy (silver methenamine). (From Schreiner GE, McAnally JF, Winchester JF: Clinical analgesic nephropathy. Arch Intern Med *141*:349, 1981. Copyright 1981, American Medical Association.)

tigation may show an anemia often out of proportion to the azotemia, if present; pyuria, with or without positive urine cultures; and papillary distortion or papillary necrosis or calyceal dilatation on intravenous urograms. These defects appear to be most frequent on the lower left side. Evidence is accumulating that analgesic abuse also may be associated with malignant lesions of the urinary tract, particularly epitheliomas of the renal pelvis and tumors of the bladder. Dubach and associates, in their prospective study, found that patients being monitored for metabolite (NAPAP) often lied in both directions.[44] That is, some patients denied taking analgesics though the metabolite was

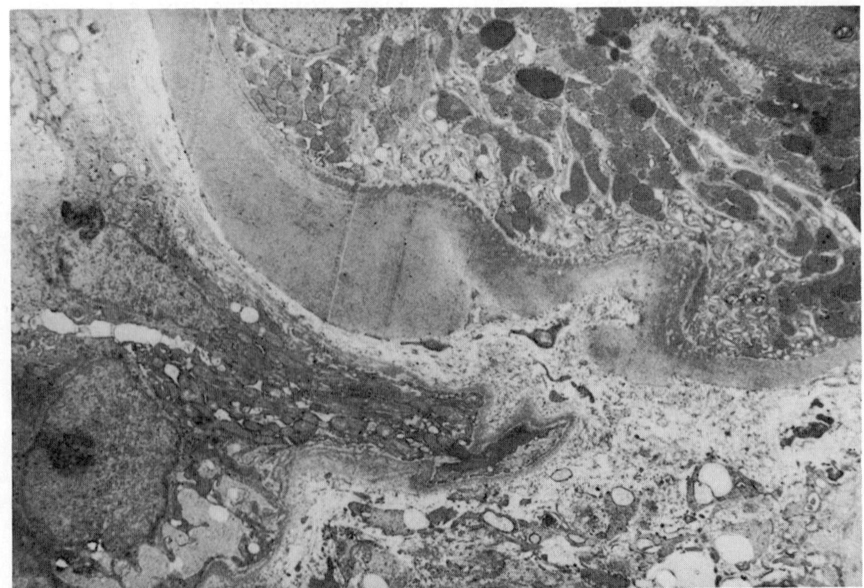

Figure 9–7. Electron photomicrograph of thickened tubular basement membrane in analgesic nephropathy. (From Schreiner GE, McAnally JF, Winchester JF: Clinical analgesic nephropathy. Arch Intern Med *141*:349, 1981. Copyright 1981, American Medical Association.)

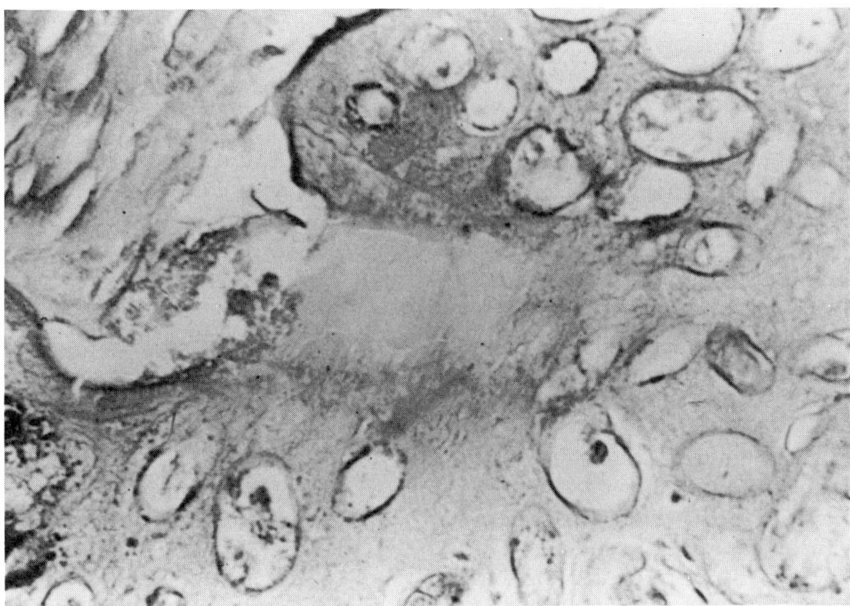

Figure 9–8. Excreted papilla showing ghosts of collecting ducts. Tissue was passed in urine by patient. (From Schreiner GE, McAnally JF, Winchester JF: Clinical analgesic nephropathy. Arch Intern Med *141*:349, 1981. Copyright 1981, American Medical Association.)

found in their urine, while other patients denied having stopped ingestion but nonetheless their urine showed no metabolites.

Treatment

The prime treatment of mixed analgesic nephropathy is to discover the basis for it and to persuade the patient to withdraw the analgesic or substitute another. This may be quite difficult to accomplish in a habituated patient. A patient with intolerable or recurrent symptoms like headache generally will revert to analgesics despite medical advice. The substitution of an analgesic substance acting on the central nervous system, which in animal studies does not worsen the disease, may be successful. Codeine is an example. Another practical step is to find the precise mechanism of the headache and use an alternate therapeutic approach. Migraine, for example, may yield to beta-blockers such as propranolol, to phenytoin when an abnormal electroencephalogram is present, or to drugs preventing platelet aggregation. The abnormalities of acidosis, dehydration, and specific electrolyte depletion should, of course, be corrected. Any obstructive lesions, such as a tumor, stone, or sloughed papilla, should be removed by either cystoscopy or surgery. Hypertension, metabolic acidosis, and drug-induced anemias should be corrected. Long-term observation should be continued to monitor patients for the increased incidence of tumor formation.

In patients whose infection and dehydration were corrected and who had very low creatinine clearances, my colleagues and I found that improvement did not occur with monitored withdrawal of the mixed analgesic tablets, as shown in Figure 9–3. However, in patients with less severely damaged kidneys and with abuse of acetaminophen-derived drugs, Linton found a significant difference in the course of renal function over a 4-year period among those who continued and those who ceased ingestion of analgesics.[45] These data are shown in Figure 9–4.

Pathophysiology of Analgesic Nephropathy

The functional defects in analgesic nephropathy are principally related to loss of efficiency of the countercurrent concentration mechanisms, with lowering of the specific gravities after dehydration, and, more precisely, a decreased maximal osmotic urine/plasma (U/P) ratio. This sensitive test reflects the integrity of the countercurrent system. If two vasa rectae in a papilla have interposing fibrous tissue or edema, they become less efficient as an ion exchange device, as would happen if the wall of a heat exchanger were thickened. Maximum concentration is thus impaired. A decline in the glomerular filtration rate associated with an increase in plasma creatinine may be a late reversible or irreversible feature of analgesic nephropathy. Histologic evidence from biopsy specimens usually shows interstitial nephritis with evidence of either acute healing or scarred tubular or medullary necrosis.

Papillary necrosis, the most dramatic form of analgesic nephropathy, has been reported in experimental animals and humans after use of a wide variety of drugs, including aspirin, antipyrine, acetaminophen, phenylbutazone, indomethacin, diclofenac, and phenacetin. Most analgesic drugs and most of the nonsteroidal anti-inflammatory drugs can produce microscopic foci of necrosis in animal species with large, prolonged doses. On light microscopy the most frequent lesion is an interstitial nephritis with or without cellular infiltration, as shown in Figure 9–5. A particular feature is a nodular or irregular thickening of the tubular basement membrane, as shown in Figure 9–6. This is even more prominent on electron microscopy, as seen in Figure 9–7. Unique to NSAIDs is the combination of interstitial nephritis and lipoid nephrosis. This has been described after fenoprofen therapy.[46] T cells dominated B cells in the infiltrate seen on biopsy in a ratio of 4:1, and the suppressor/inducer T cell ratio was 3:1. Corticosteroids induced a remission with restoration of foot processes. Any tissue passed in the urine should be carefully examined microscopically. Ghosts of tubules may be found in a sloughed papilla visible in Figure 9–8. Radiographic findings in the patient who passed this papilla include a positive ring sign in the left lower pole.

Chronic renal disease resulting from the multiplicity of drugs outlined in this chapter often may be overlooked in the clinical setting. In addition, the list of drugs responsible for disease is continually growing. Therefore, the clinician should report suspected agents to the proper authorities in order to enlarge the body of evidence incriminating such agents in the pathogenesis of renal disease to prevent further occurrences.

References

1. Schreiner GE, Maher JF: Toxic nephropathy. Am J Med *38*:409, 1965.
2. Fillastre JP, Mery JP, Morrell MJL, Confer A, Bodin M: Drug-induced glomerulonephritis. Proceedings, VIIIth International Congress on Nephrology, Athens. Karger, Basel, 1981, p 49.
3. Gelfand MC, Shin ML, Magle RB, Green I, Frank MN: The glomerular complement receptor in immunologically mediated renal glomerular injury. N Engl J Med *295*:10, 1976.
4. Schreiner GE, Kiely J-M, Cotran RS, Unanue ER: Characterization of glomerular cells in the rat expressing Ia determinants and manifesting genetically restricted interactions with lymphocytes. J Clin Invest *68*:920, 1981.
5. Anders MW: Metabolism of drugs by the kidney. Kidney Int *18*:736, 1980.
6. Javett SN, Kaplan B: Acrodynia treated with D-penicillamine. Am J Dis Child *115*:71, 1968.
7. Nakamura K, Suzuki A, Murita C: Preventive effects of penicillamine on the brain defect of fetal rats poisoned transplacentally with methyl mercury. Life Sci *6*:2321, 1967.
8. Sternlieb I, Sheinberg IH: Penicillamine therapy for hepatolenticular degeneration. JAMA *189*:748, 1964.
9. Yonis IZ, Karp M: Chelating agents in Wilson's disease. Lancet *2*:689, 1963.
10. Stein HB, Patterson AC, Offer RC, Atkins CJ, Teufel A, Robinson HS: Adverse effects of D-penicillamine on rheumatoid arthritis. Ann Intern Med *92*:24, 1980.
11. Billingsley LM, Stevens MB: Penicillamine proteinuria: A sequel to gold nephropathy. Arthritis Rheum *22*:594, 1977.
12. Gartner HB: Membranous glomerulonephritis—prototype of an immune complex glomerulonephritis. I.G. Fisher, Stuttgart, 1980, p 136.
13. Falck HM, Tornroth T, Coch B, Magelies O: Fatal renal vasculitis and minimal-change glomerulonephritis complicating treatment with penicillamine—report on 2 cases. Acta Med Scand *205*:133, 1970.
14. Batsford SR, Auerbach R, Riede UN, Sandritter W, Kluther R: Effects of D-penicillamine administration to rats and induction of renal changes: Preliminary communication. Clin Nephrol *7*:394, 1976.
15. Pigott PV: Side effects induced by captopril; Multicenter results. Communication, Captopril Satellite Symposium, 8th European Congress on Cardiology, Paris, June, 1980.
16. Amor B, Mery R, DeGery A: La tiopronine, nouvel antirumatismal à action lente dans la polyarthrite rhumatoide. Rev Rhum Mal Osteoartic *47*:157, 1980.
17. Reveillaud RJ, Blanc G, Daudon M: Syndrome néphrotique et troubles cutanés survenus au cours du traitement de deux cas de lithiase cystinique par l'alpha-mercapto-propionyl-glycine. J Urol Nephrol (Paris) *84*:663, 1978.
18. Lee RE, Vernier RL, Ulstrom RA: Nephrotic syndrome as a complication of perchloric treatment of thyroid toxicosis. N Engl J Med *264*:1221, 1961.
19. Schreiner GE: Toxic nephropathy due to drugs, solvents and metals. *In* Edwards KDG (ed): Drugs Affecting Kidney Function and Metabolism. Progress in Biochemical Pharmacology. Vol 7. Basel, Karger, 1972, p 248.

20. Burston J, Darmady EM, Stranack F: Nephrosis due to mercurial diuretics. Br Med J *1*:1277, 1958.
21. Freeman RB, Maher JF, Schreiner GE, Mostofi FK: Renal tubular necrosis due to nephrotoxicity of organic mercurial diuretics. Ann Intern Med *57*:34, 1962.
22. Riva G: Zur Frage der cronischen Quecksilbernephrose. Helv Med Acta *12*:539, 1945.
23. Becker CG, Becker EL, Maher JF, Schreiner GE: Nephrotic syndrome after contact with mercury. Arch Intern Med *110*:178, 1962.
24. Wilson BK, Thompson MD, Holzel A: Mercury nephrosis in young children with special reference to teething powders containing mercury. Br Med J *1*:358, 1972.
25. Warren DE: Nephrotic syndrome used by protiodide of mercury. Arch Dermatol *91*:240, 1965.
26. Lindquist KL, McKeen WJ, Shaba JK, Nantulya V: Immunofluorescence in electron microscopic studies of kidney biopsies in patients with nephrotic syndrome, possibly induced by skin lightening creams containing mercury. E Africa Med J *51*:168, 1974.
27. Druet P, Ayed K, Bariety J, Bernardin JF, Druet E, Girard JF, Hinglais N, Sapen C: Experimental immune glomerulonephritis induced in the rat by mercuric chloride. Adv Nephrol *8*:321, 1979.
28. Wooley PH, Griffin J, Panayi GS, Batcheolor JR, Welsch KL, Gibson TJ: HLA-DR antigens and toxic reaction to sodium oral thiomalate and D-penicillamine in patients with rheumatoid arthritis. N Engl J Med *303*:300, 1980.
29. Empire Rheumatism Council: Gold therapy in rheumatoid arthritis. Ann Rheum Dis *30*:315, 1961.
30. Nagia H, Alexander F, Berabus JL: Gold nephropathy in rats, a light and electron microscopic study. Exp Molec Pathol *15*:354, 1971.
31. Myers BD, Sibley R, Newton L, Tomlanovich SJ, Boshkos C, Stinson E, Luetscher JA, Whitney DJ, Krasny D, Coplon NS, Perlthon MG: The long-term course of cyclosporine-associated chronic nephropathy. Kidney Int *33*:590–600, 1988.
32. Palestine AG, Austin HA III, Balow JE, Antonovych TT, Sabnis SG, Preuss HG, Nussenblat RB: Renal histopathologic alterations in patients treated with cyclosporine for uveitis. N Engl J Med *314*:1293–1298, 1986.
33. Spuhler O, Zollinger HU: Die chronischinterstitielle Nephritis. Z Klin Med *151*:1, 1953.
34. Schreiner GE, McAnally JF, Winchester JF: Clinical analgesic nephropathy. Arch Intern Med *141*:349, 1981.
35. Nanra RS, Kincaid-Smith P: Chronic effect of analgesics on the kidney. *In* Edwards KDG (ed): Drugs Affecting Kidney Function and Metabolism. Progress in Biochemical Pharmacology. Vol 7. Basel, Karger, 1972, p 285.
36. Duggin CG: Mechanism of the development of analgesic nephropathy. Kidney Int *18*:553, 1980.
37. Gault MH, Wilson DR: Analgesic nephropathy in Canada: Clinical syndrome management. Kidney Int *13*:58, 1978.
38. Sugara R, Meister A: Glutathione turnover in the kidney: Considerations relating to the delta glutamyl cycle and the transport of amino acids. Proc Natl Acad Sci USA *71*:2969, 1974.
39. Schreiner GE: The nephrotoxicity of analgesic abuse. Ann Intern Med *57*:1047, 1962.
40. Prescott LF: The nephrotoxicity and hepatotoxicity of antipyretic analgesics. Br J Clin Pharmacol *7*:453, 1979.
41. Mitchell JR, Thorgeirsson SS, Potter WZ, Jollow JW, Keiser H: Hepatic injury: Protective role of glutathione in man and rationale for therapy. Clin Pharmacol Ther *16*:676, 1974.
42. Sandler DP, Smith JC, Weinberg CR, Buckalew VM, Dennis VW, Blythe WB, Burges WP: Analgesic use and chronic renal disease. N Engl J Med *143*:1238–1243, 1989.
43. Segasothy M, Suleiman AB, Puvaneswary M, Rohano A: Paracetamol: A cause for analgesic nephropathy and end-stage renal disease. Nephron *50*:50–54, 1988.
44. Dubach VC, Rosnel B, Levy PS, Baumeler HR, Muller A, Peyer A, Ehrengsperger T, Ettlin C: Epidemiological study in Switzerland. Kidney Int *13*:41, 1978.
45. Linton AL: Renal disease due to analgesics. Can Med Assoc J *107*:749, 1972.
46. Stachura I, Jayakumar S, Bourke E: T and B lymphocyte subsets in fenoprofen nephropathy. Am J Med *75*:9–15, 1983.

CHAPTER 10
MANAGEMENT OF RESPIRATORY COMPLICATIONS

Angelo M. Taveira Da Silva, M.D.

Self-medication with hypnotic-sedative drugs is a major cause of death in the 15- to 34-year-old population.[1–4] Once a patient has self-administered a large dose of a drug, the therapeutic options are limited. The absorption of the drug may be prevented by the use of emetics, adsorbents, or cathartics. Antidotes, if available, may be used. As the drug reaches the blood stream, its removal by means of forced diuresis, hemodialysis, or hemoperfusion may be an option, or the patient may be supported until the drug is metabolized. This requires intensive cardiopulmonary therapy.

Most of the commonly used drugs can depress the circulatory system and cause shock. Depression of the respiratory system is also common, therefore mechanical respiratory support is frequently required. Because the altered state of consciousness, acidosis, and hypoxia impair lung defense mechanisms against noxious agents, severe pulmonary infections may result.[5, 6] Aspiration of secretions or gastric contents or both is also likely to occur. Finally, shock, excessive fluid administration, and a direct "toxic" effect of these drugs on the lungs may lead to acute respiratory failure or the adult respiratory distress syndrome (ARDS).

Adequate respiratory care of the patient with drug overdose is essential to prevent complications and provide respiratory support. These measures will provide time for normal drug elimination mechanisms and therapeutic measures to enhance elimination of drugs.

The respiratory care required by the intoxicated victim may vary from close observation to the most advanced forms of respiratory support, including mechanical ventilation and positive end-expiratory pressure (PEEP).

In the next two sections of this chapter we will discuss the effects of the most commonly abused drugs on the respiratory system and the pathophysiology of respiratory failure and ARDS associated with drug intoxication. A systematic approach to the management of patients with poisoning and drug overdose will be discussed, including airway care of the patient with altered mental status and treatment of ARDS and other pulmonary complications.

RESPIRATORY EFFECTS OF POISONS AND DRUGS

Of the drugs directly affecting the respiratory system, two main categories must be considered (see Table 10–1). (1) Drugs like alcohol and hypnotic-sedatives may produce coma and also depress respiration. The result is impairment of the lung defense mechanisms, such as coughing, gag reflex, activity of the ciliated bronchial mucosa cells, and alveolar macrophage function. Respiratory depression results in alveolar hypoventilation, with hypercapnic respiratory acidemia and hypoxemia. In severe cases, respiratory arrest occurs. In addition to these effects, narcotics and some sedatives—for example, ethchlorvynol—may cause ARDS and lead to severe hypoxemic respiratory failure. (2) Another group of drugs, including analgesics such as salicylates and propoxyphene, radiographic contrast media, colchicine, nitrofurantoin, and thiazides, also cause severe respiratory failure. Whereas in barbiturate overdose pulmonary edema most likely results from overhydration of the patient, the second group of drugs produces ARDS by direct damage to the alveolocapillary membrane.

Generally, the remainder of the frequently abused drugs compromise respiratory function only because they alter the victim's mental state and make aspiration of oral secretions and gastric contents more likely. Other drugs may cause renal failure, hepatic failure, cardiac failure, and autonomic imbalance, leading to fluid balance abnormalities,

Table 10–1. RESPIRATORY EFFECTS OF POISONS AND DRUGS

CLASS OF DRUG	AGENT	RESPIRATORY DEPRESSION OR APNEA[a]	PULMONARY EDEMA (ARDS)[a]	OTHER EFFECTS[a]
Narcotics	Heroin	Yes (7–10)	Yes (11, 12, 16, 19–22, 26, 27, 29, 30)	Chronic users have pulmonary function abnormalities (13–15, 17, 18, 127)
	Morphine	Yes (7–10)	Yes (31)	
	Codeine	Yes (7–10)	Yes (37, 38)	
	Methadone	Yes (35)	Yes (28, 32–36)	
	Pentazocine	Yes (39)	?	
	Diphenoxylate	Yes (40)	?	
Hypnotic-sedatives	Barbiturates	Yes (56, 58, 60, 130)	Yes (56, 58, 60, 61)	Alkaline diuresis used for treatment of barbiturate overdose may play a role in the pathophysiology of pulmonary edema
	Glutethimide	Yes (56, 82)	Yes (80–83)	
	Methaqualone	Yes (56, 130)	Yes (87)	
	Ethanol	Yes (130)	Yes (130)	
	Ethchlorvynol	Yes (56, 84, 85)	Yes (84, 85)	
	Chloral hydrate	Yes (56, 130)	Not reported	
	Methyprylon	Yes (56, 130)	Not reported	
	Nitrazepam	Yes (63, 64)	Not reported	Sleep apnea (74)
	Chlordiazepoxide	Yes (65)	Yes (79)	
	Diazepam	Yes (66, 71)	Not reported	Sleep apnea (75)
	Meprobamate	Yes (56, 75, 130)	Yes (75)	
	Midazolam	Yes (71, 72)	Not reported	—
Anesthetics	Halothane	Yes (90, 91)	Yes (90, 91)	—
	Cocaine	Yes (119)	Yes (124, 125)	Myocardial infarction strokes, pneumothorax (119, 120–123, 126)
	Ketamine	Yes (92)	No	—
Neuromuscular blockers	D-tubocurarine	Yes (130)	No	—
	Pancuronium bromide	Yes (94, 179)	No	—
	Succinylcholine	Yes (130)	No	—
	Gallamine	Yes (93)	No	—
Antipsychotic drugs	Isocarboxazid	Yes } (56, 117)	Yes } (114-116)	Severe cardiovascular toxicity may play a role in the pathophysiology of pulmonary edema
	Phenelzine	Yes	Yes	
	Amitriptyline	Yes	Yes	
	Nortriptyline	Yes	Yes	
	Imipramine	Yes	Yes	
	Doxepin	Yes	Yes	
	Phenothiazines	No	No	

Table continued on page 200

pulmonary edema and acute respiratory failure.

Narcotics

Morphine and its derivatives depress respiration, particularly in patients with underlying lung disease.[7] Tidal volume, respiratory rate, and the ventilatory response to carbon dioxide and hypoxic gas mixtures are depressed.[8–10] Heroin also causes a fulminant but rapidly reversible form of pulmonary edema[11] (Fig. 10–1). In a review of fatalities associated with the use of narcotics in New York City, pulmonary edema was observed at autopsy in all cases.[12] In addition to pulmonary edema, narcotic addicts and abusers present a gamut of pulmonary pathology. This includes pneumonias, bacterial endocarditis with septic pulmonary emboli, and pulmonary granulomatosis, fibrosis, and arteritis, which may lead to pulmonary hypertension.[13, 14] Pulmonary function in narcotic addicts is frequently abnormal, even though recovery may occur with time. Abnormal lung scans,[15] roentgenograms,[16] and diffusion capacity for carbon monoxide (DLCO)[17] have been reported in such patients. The DLCO is the test that is most frequently abnormal; however, it usually returns to normal after discontinuation of the drug.[18]

Pulmonary edema due to heroin usually has a rapid onset, sometimes occurring hours

Table 10–1. RESPIRATORY EFFECTS OF POISONS AND DRUGS *Continued*

CLASS OF DRUG	AGENT	RESPIRATORY DEPRESSION OR APNEA[a]	PULMONARY EDEMA (ARDS)[a]	OTHER EFFECTS[a]
Cholinergic agonists and cytotoxins	Mushroom poisoning	Yes (168, 169)	No	Severe bronchospasm may occur
Anticholinesterases	Parathion Malathion	Yes (130, 157, 158, 161)	No	Severe bronchospasm may occur
Antimuscarinics	Atropine Belladonna alkaloids	Yes (130)	No	—
Sympathicomimetic drugs	Epinephrine and amphetamines	Yes (56, 131, 132, 136)	Yes (89, 131, 132)	—
Psychedelics	LSD	No	No	—
	Phencyclidine	Yes (135, 138)	No	—
Analgesics	Propoxyphene	Yes (105)	Yes (106–108)	
	Salicylates	No	Yes (97, 99, 100, 103)	
	Acetaminophen	No	No	Acetaminophen causes hepatorenal failure, thus fluid overload and pulmonary edema may occur
Intravenous contrast agents	Methylglucamine iothalamate	No	Yes (141)	—
	Sodium iothalamate	No	Yes (139)	—
	Meglumine diatrizoate	No	Yes (139, 141)	—
	Ethiodized oil	No	Yes (142)	—
Miscellaneous	Nitrofurantoin	No	Yes (170)	—
	Colchicine	No	Yes (172)	—
	Disopyramide	No	Yes (173)	—
	Hydrochlorothiazide	No	Yes (171)	—
	Insulin	Yes (hypoglycemic coma)	Yes (174)	—
Herbicides	Paraquat	No	Yes (145, 146, 148)	Causes rapidly progressing pulmonary fibrosis (152, 153)
Smoke inhalation	Carbon monoxide	Yes (166, 167)	—	—
Hydrocarbons	Aliphatic	No	Yes	—
	Gasoline	No	Yes (163, 164)	—
	Kerosene	No	Yes	—

[a]Reference numbers are given in parentheses.

after respiratory depression has already subsided.[19] Improvement is also rapid—within 24 to 48 hours—but a lag period has been reported by Stern and associates.[20] Therefore, a narcotic overdose victim should rarely be discharged before the end of 24 hours of hospitalization. The prevalence of pulmonary edema in patients with heroin overdose is probably 90 per cent or more,[21, 22] and it is important to remember that, since patients may be found unconscious in various positions, the pulmonary edema may be unilateral or may have an unusual localization. In chronic narcotic users the prevalence of episodes of pulmonary edema is lower, probably not more than 5 to 20 per cent.[23, 24] Considerable variability may be encountered because of the relative potency of the product available in the streets at a given time.[12, 13]

Cardiac arrhythmias occur with heroin-induced pulmonary edema.[25, 26] There is no evidence that heart failure plays a role in the pathophysiology of pulmonary edema. In a review of 149 cases of heroin overdose, 71 patients (48 per cent) developed pulmonary edema. Mean arterial blood gases in 39 of

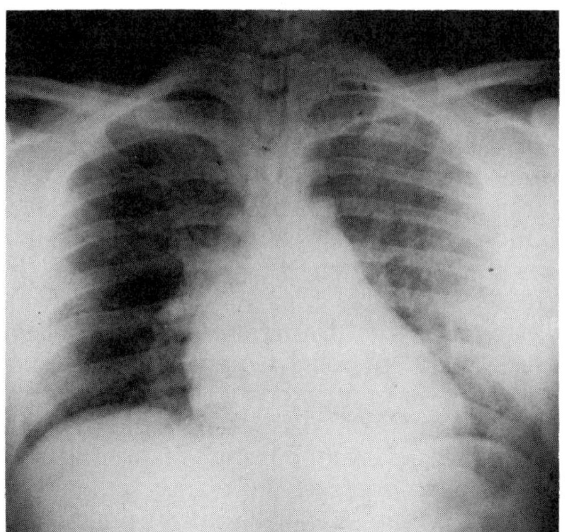

Figure 10–1. Heroin-induced pulmonary edema in a 30 year old man. Note the predominance of infiltrates in the left lung.

the 71 patients showed a PaO_2 of 50 mm Hg, a $PaCO_2$ of 53 mm Hg, and a pH of 7.22. All 13 fatalities had pulmonary edema, and six patients had atrial fibrillation. Hemodynamic measurements showed a high cardiac index of 4.1 $L/m/m^2$, a slight elevation of pulmonary artery pressure (32/12 mm Hg), and a normal pulmonary capillary wedge pressure (PCWP) of 8 mm Hg.[26] Cardiac output in heroin-induced pulmonary edema has been reported to be depressed[19–27] or elevated.[26, 27] Significant elevations of PCWP have not been reported. Excess lung water with a low central venous pressure was reported in a case of narcotic-induced pulmonary edema.[28] Left ventricular failure and an acute cardiomyopathy-like syndrome have also been reported in heroin overdose.[29] Pulmonary edema associated with this condition responds to diuretics and digitalis.

Pulmonary function abnormalities were reported in 16 patients with heroin-induced pulmonary edema.[30] The mean PaO_2 was 37 mm Hg, the $PaCO_2$ was 56 mm Hg, and the pH, 7.15. Chest roentgenograms showed bilateral alveolar infiltrates. The vital capacity (VC) was decreased to 46 per cent of predicted normal and the DLCO to 53 per cent. The alveolar-arterial oxygen gradient ($A\text{-}a/O_2$) was increased, and the dynamic compliance (Cdyn) decreased. Hypoxemia was also present in those patients without overt pulmonary edema. Recovery of the VC and Cdyn was slow, and impairment of DLCO persisted for many weeks.

Pulmonary edema has been reported also after abuse or overdose of other opiates besides heroin. The first case of narcotic-induced pulmonary edema was reported by Osler in 1880 in a patient who had been poisoned with morphine.[31] Methadone, a narcotic currently used to treat narcotic addicts, causes pulmonary edema. The clinical presentation is similar to that of heroin overdose. Progression is slower, but return to normal pulmonary function may take weeks.[32] In general, clinical recovery is slow.[33, 34] In 81 cases of methadone overdose, four patients developed pulmonary edema, and all of them survived. Unless associated with the ingestion of other drugs, methadone pulmonary dysfunction is probably not as severe as that resulting from heroin abuse.[35] However, as little as 80 mg can cause pulmonary edema, and 6 or more hours may elapse between ingestion and development of signs and symptoms of pulmonary edema.[36] Codeine, when ingested, causes pulmonary edema within 2 to 3 hours.[37] The inhalation of codeine (or heroin) may rapidly produce acute pulmonary edema and death.[38] Other opiate derivatives such as pentazocine and diphenoxylate cause severe respiratory depression and also have the potential to induce acute pulmonary edema.[39, 40]

Pathophysiology of Narcotic-Induced Pulmonary Edema

The pathophysiology of narcotic-induced pulmonary edema is obscure. Some authors have suggested that it is an idiosyncratic reaction to the drug, whereas others claim that inert particulate matter contained in the street product produces microembolization and causes pulmonary edema.[11, 14] The protein content of the edematous fluid has been measured in several studies. The fluid is rich in protein, and its composition approaches that of plasma.[11, 32, 41] Katz and associates compared the protein content of edematous fluid in patients with narcotic overdose pulmonary edema with that of pulmonary edema resulting from left ventricular failure.[41] In narcotic-induced pulmonary edema, the fluid protein content was within 98.3 ± 10 per cent of the plasma protein, whereas in cardiogenic pulmonary edema a lower value of 40 ± 8 per cent was observed. These findings are similar to those reported in other forms of noncardiogenic pulmonary edema.[42, 43] These observations indicate that this form of pulmonary edema is due to alveolocapillary membrane damage or a capillary leak syndrome leading to increased permeability of the lung vessels, interstitial edema, and eventually alveolar flooding. The fact that this form of pulmonary edema can resolve so rapidly indicates that the capillary damage or leak is rapidly reversible.

It is believed that hypoxemia plays an important role in the pathogenesis of narcotic-induced pulmonary edema.[44, 45] Similarities to high-altitude pulmonary edema have been established. Either through central neurogenic mechanisms or directly at the vascular level, acute hypoxemia may induce severe pulmonary, arterial, capillary, or venous constriction, thus increasing the pulmonary vascular pressure.[46, 47] In addition, sudden release of catecholamines or other mediators like histamine and bradykinin would increase both the vascular pressure and the permeability of the pulmonary vessels, leading to pulmonary edema.[48–50]

Some experimental evidence substantiates this theory. First, increased intracranial pressure causes an increase in pulmonary artery pressure (PAP) and pulmonary edema.[51–53] Studies in human subjects have demonstrated that marked increases in PAP and systemic and pulmonary vascular resistance, occurring simultaneously with elevation in intracranial pressure, are followed by pulmonary edema.[54] Hypoxemia, hypercapnia, and acidosis may precipitate the release of bradykinin and other mediators, producing pulmonary edema.[55] An increase in intracranial pressure caused by hypoxemia (resulting from the respiratory depression) and the release of catecholamines and other mediators, by producing severe pulmonary vasoconstriction, are the most likely causes of this form of pulmonary edema. Once pulmonary edema has occurred, the marked loss of plasma into the lungs would lower the vascular pressures. Therefore, hemodynamic measurements done at this stage would not demonstrate an increase in vascular pressures.

Hypnotics and Sedatives

This group of drugs includes the drugs often implicated in suicide attempts and drug-related deaths. Besides causing coma, circulatory shock, and respiratory depression, they may also precipitate noncardiogenic pulmonary edema.[56] Hypotension is frequent in these patients and cardiac output is usually depressed, whereas plasma volume is reduced, probably because of increased capillary permeability and redistribution of extracellular fluid.[57] Systemic vascular resistance is either normal or increased, and the heart rate is less than expected for the magnitude of hypotension observed.[56–58] A relative hypovolemia exists, and this state of shock itself may lead to "shock lung," or ARDS, a condition characterized by severe hypoxemic respiratory failure and an increase in extravascular lung water.[59] Administration of intravenous fluids as part of the treatment of circulatory shock and as a means of enhancing renal elimination of the toxic drug is at least in part responsible for the frequent occurrence of pulmonary edema. Whereas a normal subject would have no difficulty in eliminating the administered fluids, patients with hypnotic-sedative overdose do. This suggests that damage to the alveolocapillary membrane has occurred (Fig. 10–2).

In a review of 185 patients with barbiturate intoxication, pulmonary infection was found to be the major cause of morbidity and mortality.[60] Pneumonias are usually due to aspiration of oral or gastric secretions or both. Aspiration is common because in patients in coma, clearance of tracheal bronchial secretions is abnormal.[5, 6] In addition, macrophage and leukocyte functions are impaired by hypercapnia, acidosis, hypoxia, and alcohol intake.[5, 6] Pneumonia was particularly frequent in patients requiring endotracheal intubation (35 to 96 per cent). Although not as common, fluid overload and pulmonary edema are the next most serious complications.[60, 61] Close monitoring of central venous pressure or PCWP is mandatory, particularly because elimination of these drugs by forced diuresis is frequently carried out.

Benzodiazepines are a group of drugs widely used as anxiolytics, hypnotics, and anticonvulsants and preoperatively in patients undergoing invasive diagnostic and therapeutic procedures.[62] These drugs have a wide margin of safety, but in patients with cardiorespiratory disorders, hypotension, and shock, cardiorespiratory depression and apnea may occur.[63–66] Apnea is more likely to occur if narcotics and alcohol are given con-

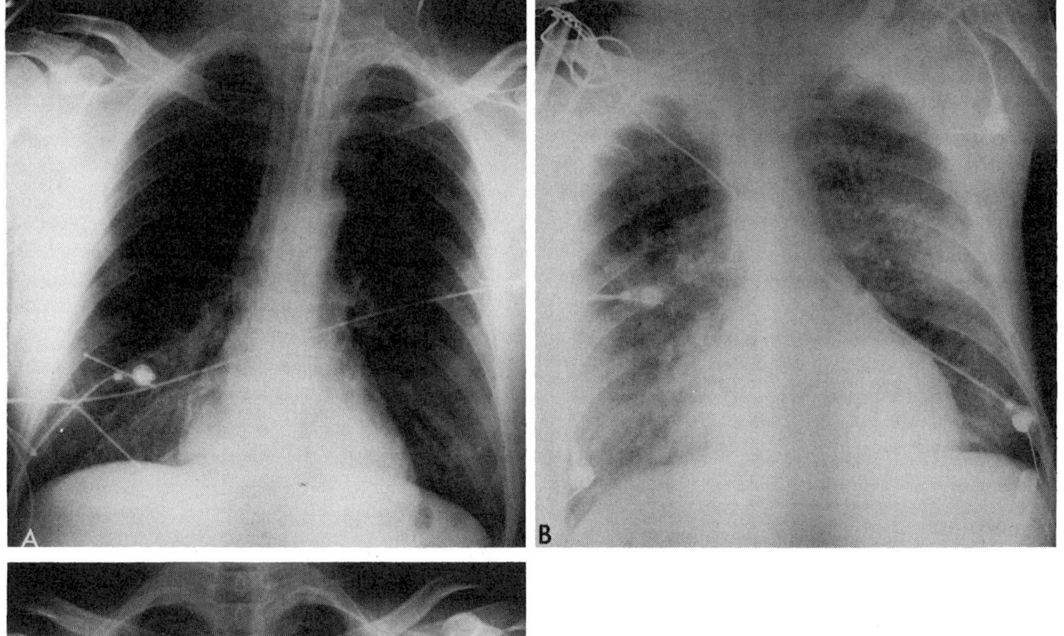

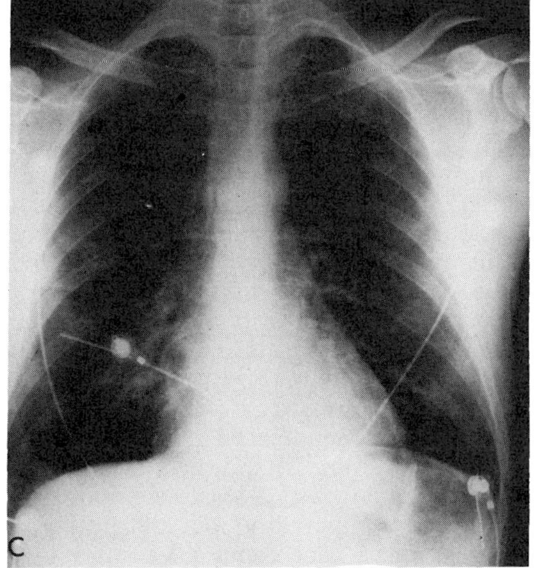

Figure 10–2. Barbiturate overdose in a 52 year old man. A, The patient is intubated and a nasogastric tube and CVP catheter have been inserted. The lung fields are clear. B, Fluid replacement and alkaline diuresis resulted in acute pulmonary edema and severe respiratory failure (PaO_2 = 100 mm Hg on 50 per cent FiO_2). C, Two days later: the bilateral infiltrates have cleared and the patient was successfully extubated.

currently.[67] Apnea may occur in as many as 20 per cent of all patients receiving the new short-acting benzodiazepine midazolam by the intravenous route.[62]

Diazepam has been shown to decrease alveolar ventilation, increase arterial pCO_2, and impair the ventilatory response to CO_2.[68, 69] Blood pressure and stroke volume are also decreased.[70] Other benzodiazepines such as midazolam exert similar effects, decreasing the ventilatory response to CO_2 as well as other indexes of central respiratory drive.[71] These effects are more pronounced in patients with chronic obstructive lung disease (COLD), and recovery may take longer to occur.[69, 72] In another study, midazolam decreased the tidal volume by 39 per cent and minute ventilation by 17 per cent. Respirations became shallow and fast.[72] Midazolam can cause shock in patients with hypovolemia.[73] Benzodiazepines can increase the number and severity of obstructive episodes in patients with obstructive sleep apnea because they have an inhibitory effect on genioglossal muscle activity.[74, 75]

The cardiorespiratory depressant effects of benzodiazepines are exerted centrally,[76] and a potential site of action for these effects seems to be the ventral surface of the medulla oblongata.[77] The specific benzodiazepine antagonist RO-15-1788 (Flumanezil) is capable of reversing these cardiorespiratory depressant effects of benzodiazepines.[78]

Acute pulmonary edema has been reported after intravenous injections of chlordiazepoxide.[79]

Glutethimide is a hypnotic-sedative that has more serious side effects. The cardiovascular depression is severe and is in part due to the strong anticholinergic properties of the drug. Gastrointestinal absorption is slow, and the drug's metabolic products are secreted from the bile into the intestine, where reabsorption occurs. Shock, apnea, and mydriasis dominate the clinical picture of acute intoxication. Cerebral and pulmonary edema are common at autopsy.[80–83] Management of patients with glutethimide overdose is extremely difficult and has prompted the view that this drug should be withdrawn from the market.

Ethchlorvynol overdoses are not common but are particularly dangerous because of the duration of coma.[56] Intravenous administration of ethchlorvynol causes severe acute pulmonary edema that may be fatal.[84, 85] In dogs, doses of 12 to 80 mg per kg given intravenously cause hypotension and pulmonary edema. Severe fluid loss through the lungs with hemoconcentration may occur after overdose with this drug. Hemoperfusion with Amberlite resin is effective in removing ethchlorvynol.[86] Charcoal hemoperfusion is also effective.

Methaqualone is a frequently abused drug and can produce pulmonary edema.[56, 87] Respiratory depression is usually mild. Meprobamate causes hypotension and pulmonary edema, but Amberlite resin hemoperfusion is quite effective in removing it from the body.[56, 88] Chloral hydrate and methyprylon overdoses are rare and simulate barbiturate intoxication.

Anesthetics and Curare

Accidental or suicidal administration of anesthetics and curarizing agents may be fatal. Epinephrine, which is used during anesthesia, has been reported to cause severe pulmonary edema.[89] The accidental intravenous administration of halothane has been reported to cause fatal acute pulmonary edema.[90] Halothane abuse occurs in hospital personnel, and its inhalation has been reported to cause arrhythmias and pulmonary edema resulting in death.[91] Ketamine, gallamine, D-tubocurarine, and pancuronium have the potential to cause respiratory arrest and death.[92–94]

Analgesics

Salicylates are commonly used drugs. Intoxication may occur in accidental or suicidal overdoses or during salicylate therapy. Pulmonary edema was reported in patients with rheumatic fever undergoing salicylate therapy. However, it was difficult to tell whether the edema was a result of the salicylates or of left ventricular failure. Salicylates cause mixed metabolic acidosis–respiratory alkalosis (adults), metabolic acidosis (children), and, at times, pulmonary edema.[95–104] Accidental ingestion of 6.5 gm or more of aspirin for several days caused acute pulmonary edema in a previously healthy 32 year old man.[95] Ingestion of salicylates for toothache caused severe ARDS in a 37 year old woman who required mechanical ventilation and PEEP.[97] Unrecognized toxicity is particularly serious in elderly patients, in whom the mortality may reach 25 per cent.[96] Salicylate overdose is common in children and may even occur after topical application of salicylate-containing compounds on the gums of teething infants.[101, 102]

The pathophysiology of salicylate-induced pulmonary edema has been studied. Cardiac output is preserved, and the PCWP is either normal or low.[97, 100, 103] Severe hypovolemia caused by pulmonary loss of protein-rich fluid has also been reported. Urinary losses of protein also may be significant. Administration of colloid rather than crystalloid solutions may be necessary to treat shock.[103] Available data indicate that this form of pulmonary edema is due to a direct toxic effect on the alveolocapillary membrane. In a sheep model, salicylates increased lung lymph flow, transvascular flux of protein, and lung water. Direct damage to capillaries, mediated by prostaglandins or other vasoactive substances, is probably responsible for this form of pulmonary edema.[99, 100]

Propoxyphene, a narcotic analgesic structurally related to methadone, causes respiratory depression and pulmonary edema.[105–108] Respiratory arrest may occur with doses above 180 mg. Three cases of acute pulmonary edema, two fatal, were reported after ingestion of doses between 1.6 and 3.5 gm. However, pulmonary edema has occurred after ingestion of just 455 mg. Propoxyphene is a commonly abused drug and in addition to respiratory depression and pulmonary edema causes psychotic reactions and addiction. Evidence of direct myocardial toxicity has been demonstrated.[107] Therefore, even though pulmonary edema has been attributed to diffuse capillary lung damage, myocardial dysfunction may play a role.

Acetaminophen is an analgesic widely abused, particularly in the United Kingdom and the United States.[109] The ingestion of a few grams may cause fulminant hepatic failure and acute tubular necrosis.[110–113] Pulmonary complications are only secondary and may be infectious in nature due to prolonged hepatic coma or to fluid overload resulting from hepatorenal failure and injudicious fluid administration (Fig. 10–3).

Tricyclic Antidepressants and Antipsychotic Drugs

Tricyclic antidepressants are extremely toxic drugs with a low safety margin, and they may have severe cardiovascular effects resulting in shock and death. The large volume of distribution and the slow absorption of these drugs may account for sudden death days after ingestion. Pulmonary edema has been reported in tricyclic antidepressant overdose.[114–116] Fluid overload and myocardial depression are certainly contributing factors, as are marantic endocarditis and widespread arterial thrombosis. In one review of 40 cases, 16 patients required mechanical ventilation and 2 succumbed.[115] Life-threatening overdose should be considered when there is widening of the QRS interval on the electrocardiogram or when the blood level of the drug is more than 1000 ng per ml[117] (Figs. 10–4 and 10–5).

Cocaine and Other Central Nervous System Stimulant Drugs

This group of drugs includes cocaine, amphetamine and its derivatives, phencyclidine (PCP), lysergic acid diethylamide (LSD), and methylphenidate.[56] Most of these drugs have significant cardiovascular effects owing to their sympathomimetic actions. Tachycardia, hypertension, arrhythmias, shock, and respiratory arrest occur with severe overdose. Approximately 20 million Americans have used cocaine and 5 million use it regularly.[118] Recently, the recreational use of cocaine has been associated with an increasing number of reports of respiratory and cardiovascular toxicity.[119] Acute myocardial infarction, cardiac arrhythmias, rupture of the aorta, and cerebrovascular accidents have been reported.[120–123] Some of the patients suffering acute myocardial infarction had normal coronary circulation. The intravenous injection of cocaine freebase as well as its inhalation can precipitate acute pulmonary edema and

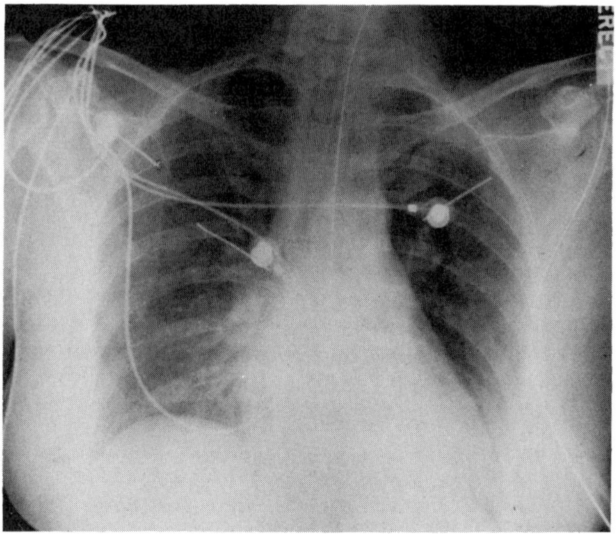

Figure 10–3. Acetaminophen overdose and pulmonary edema (ARDS) in a 40 year old woman.

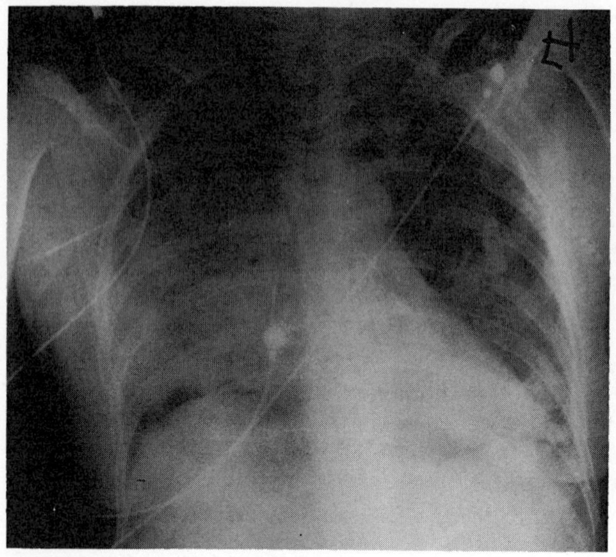

Figure 10–4. Tricyclic antidepressant overdose in a 37 year old woman. Bilateral pulmonary edema and a right pneumothorax secondary to subclavian vein puncture for insertion of a CVP line are seen.

shock.[124, 125] We have seen a fatal case of a young woman who presented in shock complicated by pulmonary edema and severe cardiorespiratory failure. Although the patient was in shock, the cardiac output was 8 liters per minute and the PCWP was normal, ruling out the presence of cardiogenic shock. Therefore, it seems that cocaine may cause not only acute myocardial infarction and cardiogenic pulmonary edema but also noncardiogenic pulmonary edema (ARDS) (Fig. 10–6).

Other pulmonary complications of cocaine abuse are pneumothorax and pneumomediastinum.[119, 126] These complications are believed to result from the deep inspirations followed by Valsalva maneuvers performed by the victims during smoking or inhalation of freebase vapors. Repeated inhalation of cocaine freebase results in lung function abnormalities, particularly a decrease in lung diffusion capacity.[119, 127] Recently, Patel et al.[128] have described a case of bronchiolitis obliterans in a patient known to be a cocaine user. Good response to treatment with corticosteroids was observed. Cocaine has also been reported to cause seizures and respiratory arrest, particularly when it is injected intravenously or inhaled as freebase. Doses that are known to be in the life-threatening range cause death by respiratory failure, and in experimental animals cocaine may compromise respiratory function before affecting the cardiovascular system.[129, 130]

In experimental animals Jain and associates (Fed Proc *46*:402, 1987) have reported that the intravenous injection of cocaine in cumulative doses produces a decrease in tidal volume and apnea. The mechanism and site of action of these effects is presumably central, but the precise location is unknown.

Hyperpyrexia, rhabdomyolysis with disseminated intravascular coagulation, and renal failure have been reported with amphetamine use.[131] Noncardiogenic pulmonary edema may occur; however, with hypertension and cardiac arrhythmias a cardiovascular role must be considered.[131–133] A combination

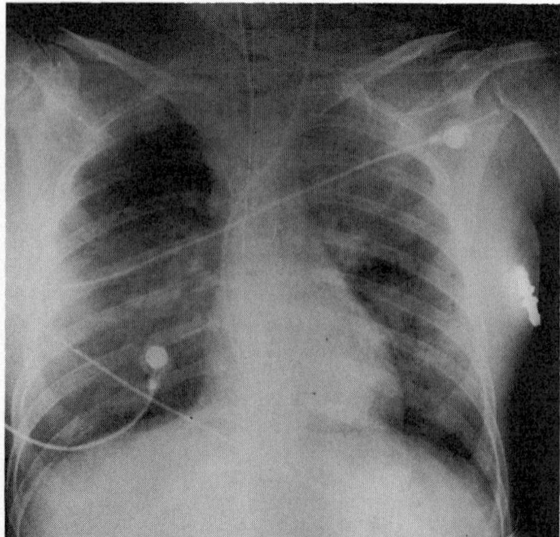

Figure 10–5. Tricyclic antidepressant overdose and severe ARDS in a 22 year old woman. On 50 per cent FiO_2, a PEEP of 12 cm H_2O, and a PaO_2 of 84 mm Hg, the cardiac output was 5.7 L/min and the PCWP was 12 mm Hg.

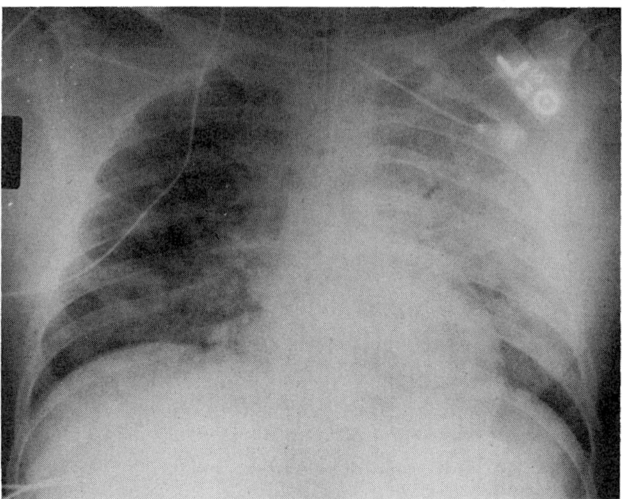

Figure 10–6. Cocaine overdose and noncardiogenic pulmonary edema (ARDS) in a 30 year old woman. The cardiac output was 8.8 L/min, and the PCWP was 2.5 mm Hg. Note the bilateral pulmonary infiltrates predominating on the left side.

of cocaine and epinephrine is particularly dangerous because cocaine blocks neuronal catecholamine uptake. PCP stimulates the central nervous and cardiovascular systems but depresses respiration.[134–138] Calcium-antagonist drugs like verapamil may become useful in the treatment of the vascular spasms produced by some of these drugs.[138]

Roentgenographic Intravenous Contrast Media

Noncardiogenic pulmonary edema may occur after intravenous administration of radiographic contrast products. No suicidal or accidental administration of these products has been reported. Several cases of pulmonary edema after injection of methylglucamine iothalamate and meglumine diatrizoate have been reported.[139–141] Severe respiratory failure may occur, and mechanical ventilation and PEEP may be required. Hemodynamic measurements show a high cardiac output, low PCWP, and systemic hypotension. The edematous fluid is rich in protein, and marked hemoconcentration occurs as a result of massive leakage of plasma into the lungs. Among the possible mechanisms involved are activation of complement fraction by the contrast product and the sudden increase in osmolality that is observed after intravenous administration of these agents.

Lymphangiographic contrast media are also known to cause ARDS, both in human beings and in animals.[142] As in the fat embolism syndrome, capillary injury may be due to release of fatty acids in the circulation. Fatty acids are known to be capable of inducing severe respiratory failure when instilled into the trachea or injected into the pulmonary artery.

Insecticides and Herbicides

Among these compounds, paraquat is the most likely to cause severe respiratory failure and death.[143–145] Paraquat is a potent herbicide. When ingested, 10 to 20 ml of the 20 per cent solution is usually lethal.[143–148] The substance can cause mouth ulcerations, pseudomembrane formation, and esophageal perforation.[149, 150] Transcutaneous absorption has been documented,[151–153] especially if skin is damaged, e.g., in the presence of skin ulceration. Absorption of small amounts is compatible with survival, but continuous skin absorption due to improper use of sprays may cause death. For further discussion of the potential lethality of dermal absorption of paraquat, see Chapter 69. After ingestion, if blood levels are higher than 2 mg per liter at 4 hours, death is the rule. Unless paraquat is rapidly removed from the body by hemoperfusion, death occurs even with lower blood levels. With very high levels, the fatality rate is 100 per cent. In these cases the clinical picture is one of acute pulmonary edema (Fig. 10–7), followed by rapidly progressive lung fibrosis, inability to oxygenate the patient, and a respiratory death.

The lung is the target organ because paraquat concentrations in this organ reach a level

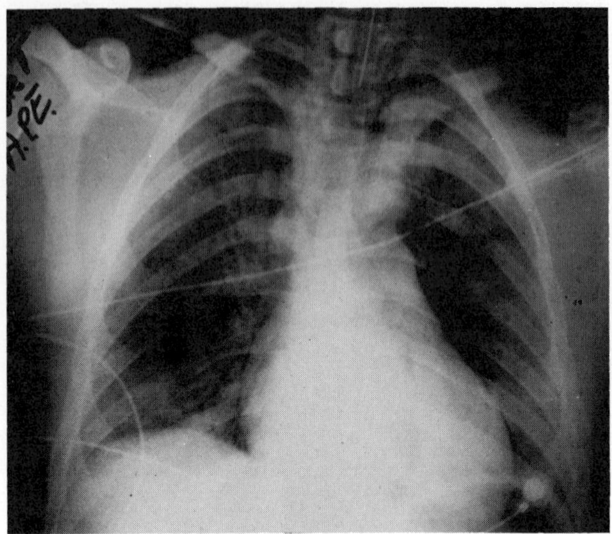

Figure 10–7. Paraquat overdose in a 21 year old man. Bilateral pulmonary infiltrates are evident. While the patient was breathing room air, the PaO_2 was 75 mm Hg. The patient died with intractable respiratory failure.

50 times greater than that in blood. Depending on the amount of paraquat accumulated in the lungs, either a fulminant form of pulmonary edema or rapidly progressing pulmonary fibrosis will develop. Intra-alveolar fibrosis with small airway involvement, medial hypertrophy of the pulmonary arterioles, and fibrosis and destruction of these vessels have been described. Evidence of endothelial cell damage is suggested by a report documenting an increase in serum angiotensin-converting enzyme (ACE) levels after exposure to paraquat.[154]

The mechanism of action of paraquat has been reviewed.[143, 146, 147, 153] Paraquat interferes with the ability of the lung to handle superoxide radicals. Therefore, paraquat enhances oxygen toxicity.[155] Conversely, after paraquat poisoning oxygen may cause and contribute to further lung damage. Serial pulmonary function studies in patients with paraquat poisoning have shown that lung volumes are decreased, but initially arterial blood gas measurements may be normal. An increase in the A-a/O_2 gradient and an abnormal DLCO measurement are always present. An increase in shunting caused by development of very low ventilation-perfusion ratio units occurs terminally, making oxygenation of the patient virtually impossible even on 100 per cent oxygen.

Parathion and malathion are organophosphate compounds that inactivate acetylcholinesterase.[130, 156] Exposure to or inhalation of these substances causes miosis, conjunctival congestion, rhinorrhea, bronchoconstriction, bronchorrhea, and nausea, vomiting, and diarrhea. Coma, seizures, respiratory failure, and respiratory paralysis are followed by death.

Central respiratory depression is a major cause of toxicity produced by some organophosphate compounds.[157–159] Acute toxicity caused by these compounds seems to be due to a loss of central respiratory drive resulting from disruptions of normal patterned activity in respiratory-related unit discharge.[160, 161] Recent studies by Gillis et al.[162] indicate that the intermediate area of the ventral surface of the medulla oblongata is the most sensitive site for responses elicited by cholinesterase inhibition. The respiratory effects observed following application of cholinesterase inhibitors to this area consist of an initial stimulatory response characterized by an increase in tidal volume, followed by apnea. These respiratory depressant effects are counteracted by atropine.

Treatment of organophosphate poisoning consists of administering large doses of atropine, which acts as a physiologic antidote, and pralidoxime (PAM), the specific cholinesterase reactivator, which serves as a specific antidote (see Chapter 68). In addition, mechanical ventilation and intensive cardiorespiratory support are necessary.

Hydrocarbon insecticides can cause severe pneumonitis if they are aspirated into the lungs.[163] The intravenous administration of these compounds also causes a severe form of noncardiogenic pulmonary edema.[164] For discussion of hydrocarbon-induced lung disease, see Chapter 76.

Carbon Monoxide

Carbon monoxide (CO) accounts for over 2000 accidental or suicidal deaths yearly due to poisoning. The affinity of carbon monoxide for hemoglobin (Hb) is about 200 times greater than that of oxygen. Indeed, at concentrations of 0.1 per cent carbon monoxide, hemoglobin becomes 70 per cent saturated, and victims become comatose. Grand mal seizures, shock, and death will follow. The symptomatology is insidious. First, intellectual impairment may be observed (at COHb concentrations of 5 to 10 per cent) followed by headaches, dyspnea, and a feeling of drunkenness (COHb 10 to 40 per cent). Because of this altered state of consciousness accidental victims of carbon monoxide poisoning are not always capable of seeking help. The most common cause of accidental poisoning with carbon monoxide is fires. The incomplete combustion of materials in confined spaces generates toxic levels of this gas. Carbon monoxide poisoning, however, has been reported in open spaces in subjects standing near smoldering fires. Besides decreasing the oxygen-carrying capacity of hemoglobin, carbon monoxide shifts the hemoglobin dissociation curve to the left, resulting in increased affinity of hemoglobin for oxygen. It also inhibits oxidative metabolism by interfering with cytochrome systems throughout the body.[165, 166] When COHb reaches 50 per cent, permanent brain damage may occur. The diagnosis is established by measurement of COHb or oxyhemoglobin. The level of COHb correlates well with the dose of smoke inhaled by fire victims.[167]

Treatment of carbon monoxide poisoning consists of speeding the elimination of this gas by the administration of 100 per cent oxygen, which decreases the half-life of COHb by a factor of 4. When very high levels of COHb are present, treatment in a hyperbaric oxygen chamber is recommended. If this is not available, endotracheal intubation and mechanical ventilation with 100 per cent oxygen should first be initiated. This treatment should be continued until COHb is reduced to less than 5 per cent and the patient is asymptomatic. Subsequent referral to an HBO center may be indicated. Carbon monoxide poisoning is discussed further in Chapter 74.

Mushrooms

Ingestion of some mushrooms of the *Amanita* genus causes effects similar to those observed in patients intoxicated with organophosphates. Various toxins are present in these plants.[168, 169] In most instances, parasympathetic stimulation or an anticholinergic effect is observed. Amanitin, a cytotoxin, is the most potent toxin found in mushrooms. It causes hepatic and renal failure and is responsible for most of the fatalities observed.

Miscellaneous Drugs

Nitrofurantoin may cause various types of pulmonary toxicity, including pulmonary edema.[170] Idiosyncratic reactions to hydrochlorothiazide were responsible for two cases of pulmonary edema.[171] Colchicine, a drug used to treat acute gout, can cause ARDS.[172] Disopyramide, an antiarrhythmic drug, also has been reported to cause fatal pulmonary edema in three patients without previous cardiac disease.[173] Hypoglycemia secondary to insulin administration or ethanol intoxication also may cause pulmonary edema.[174] The list of drugs potentially capable of causing lung damage is large, and among these is the ever-increasing number of chemotherapeutic agents used in the treatment of malignant disease.[175, 176] This subject is discussed in Chapter 55.

TREATMENT OF THE ADULT RESPIRATORY DISTRESS SYNDROME, RESPIRATORY INSUFFICIENCY, AND ARREST

General Principles of Management

Patients with suicidal or accidental intoxication either die at home or are brought to the hospital emergency department. When seen at the hospital, their condition may vary from profound coma with circulatory shock and apnea to a normal state of consciousness and vital signs. One should not be deceived by the lack of clinical signs and, based on these findings, discard the history of drug overdose as untrue. Therefore, history-taking, physical examination, intravenous access, toxic screening of gastric contents, urine, and blood, and appropriate measures to remove unabsorbed drug must be carried out when appropriate. If the patient is not fully alert, induction of emesis may lead to aspiration of gastric contents. The resulting chemical pneumonitis may unnecessarily worsen the prognosis of a patient with a relatively mild intoxication.

Airway Care of the Intoxicated Patient

If a poisoned patient is comatose, the upper airway must be protected (Table 10–2). Indeed, the upper airway defense mechanisms against aspiration of oral secretions and gastric contents are impaired in these patients. Gastric motility is decreased by many drugs, and thus it is likely that victims of poisoning or drug overdose will have a full stomach. Oral intubation with an endotracheal (ET) tube having an inside diameter of at least 8 mm is recommended. Tubes of this size or larger will permit the passage of a fiberoptic bronchoscope, which may be required to (1) remove foreign bodies and food particles (aspiration), (2) assess the upper airway (fire victims, inhalation of toxic gases), and (3) remove secretions (atelectasis). Nasotracheal intubation may be difficult because it is more time-consuming, needs a spontaneously breathing cooperative patient, and may trigger gastric reflux, vomiting, and aspiration of gastric contents. Airway protection by means of an endotracheal tube with administration of a humidified gas mixture containing a concentration of oxygen that will ensure a pO_2 of 70 mm Hg or more is recommended. If the patient has had respiratory arrest or has respiratory failure, mechanical ventilation is added. Respiratory failure is another indication for endotracheal intubation (Table 10–3). Patients with seizures or who are severely agitated (due to PCP overdose, alcohol withdrawal, and so on) may also need endotracheal intubation, particularly because they will require heavy sedation, which then may cause respiratory depression. In these circumstances, rapid sequence intubation is recommended. This procedure is needed in order to decrease the risks of aspiration of gastric contents. In general, the patient is oxygenated with 100 per cent oxygen for 5 minutes, and this is followed by rapid administration of succinylcholine, morphine (or fentanyl), and diazepam (or midazolam). These drugs, however, blunt the upper airway reflexes and may cause vomiting at a time when the upper airway is being stimulated by a foreign body (i.e., a laryngoscope or ET tube). Thus, aspiration may result. After the drugs have been given, an assistant performs the Selick maneuver by applying pressure against the cricoid cartilage, causing occlusion of the esophagus. Mask ventilation is avoided because it may trigger aspiration.

Table 10–2. INDICATIONS FOR ENDOTRACHEAL INTUBATION

Respiratory arrest
Deep coma (stage IV)
Mechanical ventilation
Seizures
Gastric lavage in an unresponsive, unconscious patient
Severe hypoxemia and/or acute respiratory acidosis
Emergency bronchoscopy

Table 10–3. INDICATIONS FOR MECHANICAL VENTILATION

Respiratory arrest
Severe hypoxemia
Alveolar hypoventilation and respiratory acidosis
Seizures requiring the use of diazepam or barbiturates
Administration of curarizing agents
Shock
Vital capacity < 15 ml/kg
Tidal volume < 5 ml/kg
Negative inspiratory force < 25 cm H_2O
$PaO_2 < 70$ mm Hg on an $FiO_2 > 50$ per cent
A-a/O_2 on 100 per cent $FiO_2 > 350$ mm Hg
Shunt > 15 per cent

After the muscle relaxant (i.e., succinylcholine) takes effect, laryngoscopy and intubation are performed, the cuff of the tube is inflated, ventilation is begun, and the Selick maneuver is discontinued.

Another indication for endotracheal intubation is gastric lavage, particularly if lavage is to be undertaken in a patient who is lethargic or unconscious. In these instances, because the risk of aspiration is great, the airway must be protected. Endotracheal intubation of victims of poisoning or drug overdose is at times difficult and should be performed only by an experienced physician.

Among some of the immediate complications of endotracheal intubation are (1) bleeding, (2) ablation of a tooth, (3) intubation of the esophagus, and (4) intubation of the right main stem bronchus (Fig. 10–8). Laryngeal and tracheal damage may result from traumatic intubation. Constant motion of the tube caused by a patient's restlessness and high cuff pressures may lead to tracheal mucosal damage and eventual stenosis. The use of low-pressure, high-volume cuffs has minimized this problem.[177]

Once the proper position of the tube has been ascertained, the patient's tidal volume and minute ventilation can be measured and the presence of hypoventilation detected. Preferably, arterial blood gases should be determined and oxygen given to maintain the PaO_2 above 70 mm Hg. If blood gas measurements cannot be obtained immediately, 100 per cent oxygen administration is recommended. If the patient is apneic or has a slow and shallow respiratory pattern, mechanical ventilation should be initiated.

General Principles of Mechanical Ventilation in the Intoxicated Patient

When the victim of drug intoxication has bradypnea and low tidal volume or when arterial blood gases show an elevated $PaCO_2$, hypoventilation is present. In these circumstances, intravenous naloxone should be administered. The dose is 0.4 mg, and it may be repeated one or two times.[178] A prompt response will occur in patients with opiate intoxication, consisting of arousal and an increase in the rate and depth of breathing, with normalization of the $PaCO_2$. Patients with narcotic overdose may later develop pulmonary edema.[19, 20] There is no evidence that naloxone will prevent this complication of opiate overdose.

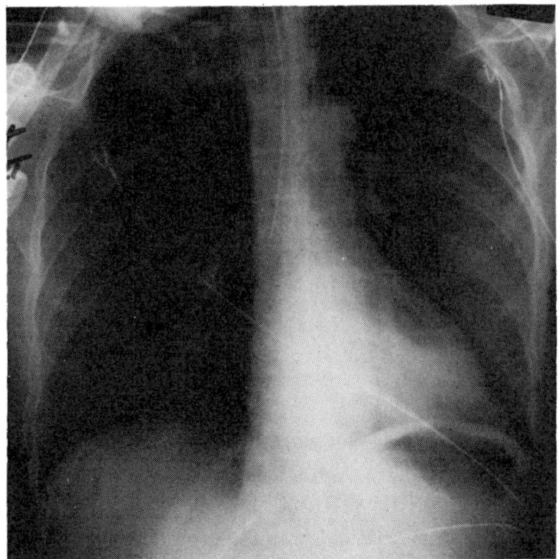

Figure 10–8. Multiple drug overdose in a 52 year old man. The endotracheal tube tip is in the right main stem bronchus.

The indications for mechanical ventilation in overdosed patients (see Table 10–3) are as follows: (1) lack of spontaneous respirations, (2) alveolar hypoventilation, (3) hypoxemia with or without alveolar hypoventilation requiring 50 per cent or more oxygen to maintain a PaO_2 of at least 70 mm Hg, (4) bilateral pulmonary infiltrates on the chest roentgenogram, (5) seizures requiring the use of intravenous diazepam or barbiturates, (6) administration of sedatives and curarizing agents during intubation, (7) aspiration of gastric contents, and (8) shock.

Unless the patient is known to have chronic obstructive lung disease (COLD) and has chronic hypercapnia, we recommend the following respirator settings: tidal volume should be between 12 and 15 ml per kg of ideal body weight, the respiratory rate between 10 and 12, and the inspired oxygen fraction (FiO_2) 100 per cent. Arterial blood gases should be checked 15 to 20 minutes after beginning mechanical ventilation. The objective of mechanical ventilation is to achieve a PaO_2 of 70 mm Hg or more at a FiO_2 below 50 per cent and to maintain a normal pH (7.36 to 7.45) unless otherwise indicated. In a patient with COLD, this may entail keeping the $PaCO_2$ around 50 mm Hg by either decreasing the respirator rate or adding mechanical dead space. With severe metabolic acidosis, it may be necessary to hyperventilate the patient to a $PaCO_2$ of 20 or 30 mm Hg in order to obtain a normal pH, at least until the acidosis is corrected. In a patient with tricyclic antidepressant poisoning, an alkaline pH is indicated.

In patients who are agitated, are having seizures, or have tachypnea secondary to severe respiratory distress, efficient mechanical ventilation may be difficult to achieve. In these instances, the use of sedatives and curarizing drugs may be required. We commonly use diazepam or morphine sulfate in small doses every hour, or pancuronium bromide. Pancuronium is given first as a test dose of 0.01 mg per kg. If no arrhythmias occur, then an intravenous loading dose of 0.07 mg per kg is given.[179] Doses of 1 to 2 mg are then repeated hourly if required.

Treatment of the Adult Respiratory Distress Syndrome

ARDS is a condition characterized by diffuse injury to the alveolocapillary membrane of the lung, resulting in a breakdown of the normal mechanisms regulating transvascular flux of plasma in this organ.[59, 180] The lung reacts to injury uniformly; regardless of the etiology of ARDS, the early pathologic abnormalities are the same. There is an increase in lung water, aggregation of platelets and leukocytes in the capillaries, proliferation of alveolar type II cells, disruption of the alveolar type I cells, endothelial cell damage, and, at a later stage, alveolar flooding, hyaline membrane formation, loss of vascular bed, and fibrosis.[181] This syndrome is associated with shock, particularly septic shock, fat embolism, aspiration of toxic gases or liquids, including gastric contents, and drug overdose.

Various mechanisms have been invoked. The central or neurogenic theory postulates that a centrally mediated pulmonary vasoconstriction causes pulmonary edema and initiates the sequence of severe lung damage.[46] Saldeen has described the so-called microembolism syndrome as the cause of ARDS.[182] Tissue injury leads to platelet aggregation and trapping in the lung.[183] Vasoactive substances are released and contribute to further lung damage.[48, 49, 53, 55] Jacob and associates have reported activation of C5a complement fraction by endotoxin and other noxious stimuli, leading to lung leukostasis and subsequent release of proteolytic enzymes that attack the endothelial cell, producing capillary injury.[184] The multifactorial causes of ARDS indicate that several mechanisms are at work. At times the noxious agent is blood borne and acts from within the capillaries (septic shock, fat emboli), whereas in other instances the substance is inhaled and literally produces a lung "burn." It would be simplistic to assume that activation of a complement fraction is the cause of ARDS in all the above conditions.

Drug overdose causes severe respiratory failure. Usually this form of ARDS is reversible within a few days. The reason might be that the most significant lesion is a self-limited capillary leak syndrome. An excess of extravascular lung water is always observed in ARDS.[59] However, it is likely that in drug-induced ARDS, progression into more severe pathologic forms, including fibrosis, does not occur. Exceptions to this rule are intoxications with paraquat and cancer chemotherapeutic agents such as bleomycin. Here, progression to fibrosis is the rule.[148, 153, 175, 176] Other drugs such as amphetamines, PCP, and tricyclic antidepressants have the potential to cause serious cardiac dysfunction. Therefore, pulmonary edema may be due to left ventricular failure.

The great majority of the drugs discussed in the first section of this chapter are capable of causing pulmonary edema of a self-limited nature. Through unknown mechanisms they can suddenly increase the permeability of the lung capillaries to plasma and red cells. The fluid loss may be so massive that hypovolemic shock may occur.[85, 103] The edematous fluid is protein rich, proving that permeability to plasma proteins is increased. Lymphatic flow is increased, and, again, the protein content of this fluid is high. Interference with lymphatic flow by drugs has not been documented, with the possible exception of barbiturates.[56]

The forces that regulate fluid exchange in the lungs have been the subject of several reviews.[185–187] The equation defining these forces states that $Qf = K(Pmv - Ppmv) - \rho(\pi mv - \pi pmv)$, where Qf is the transvascular flux of fluid conductance, Pmv and Ppmv are respectively the microvascular and perimicrovascular hydrostatic pressures, ρ is a correction term for the effective osmotic pressure of solutes such that it is equal to 0 for electrolytes and 1 for protein, and πmv and πpmv are the microvascular and perimicrovascular osmotic pressures.

A similar but more complex equation defines the transvascular flow of protein. Increase in fluid filtration secondary to an increase in the Pmv − Ppmv gradient is the cause of the so-called cardiogenic pulmonary edema that is due to cardiac failure. If the capillary wall is intact, pressures above 24 mm Hg are necessary to produce lung edema.[188] However, Guyton and Lindsey showed that if the plasma osmotic pressure was decreased by protein depletion (πmv), pulmonary edema occurred at a much lower microvascular pressure.[188] As fluid accumulates in the lung interstitium, πpmv falls and acts as a negative feedback. When the capillary barrier is disrupted, this mechanism does not work; ρ will be less than 1, and the edematous fluid will contain large molecular weight proteins. Any increase in microvascular hydrostatic pressure or PCWP will worsen the situation. An increase in lymph flow protects the lung from fluid accumulation. Lymph flow may increase fivefold. This protective mechanism may not be sufficient to clear fluid from the lungs; therefore, interstitial edema occurs. As πpmv increases, edema will decrease. However, by that time alveolar flooding, which is an "all or nothing" phenomenon, may already have developed. Increased permeability to fluid and protein through lung capillaries or veins is the cause of ARDS in patients with drug overdose. Fluid overload, heart failure, and shock may play additional roles.

The lungs of patients with "shock lung" or noncardiogenic pulmonary edema due to drug overdose contain an excessive amount of water, and alveoli are either flooded or unstable with a tendency to collapse. The lungs are heavy and stiff and have decreased compliance and resting lung volume or functional residual capacity.[189, 190] Breathing at these low lung volumes requires large inspiratory pressures, hence the work of breathing is increased. Lack of ventilation of flooded or collapsed alveoli results in low ventilation/perfusion ($\dot{V}/\dot{Q}$) ratios, venous admixture, and hypoxemia (shuntlike effect). Increased oxygen concentrations may improve the PaO_2 somewhat, but oxygen toxicity will occur when patients are exposed to more than 50 per cent FiO_2 for prolonged periods of time.[191]

Treatment of ARDS in Patients with Drug Overdose

Drug-intoxicated patients with ARDS are in critical condition and their prognosis is often grave. Their management is difficult at best. The treatment of ARDS in the setting of drug intoxication can be summarized as follows: Even if the patient is alert and breathing spontaneously, mechanical ventilation is needed for hypoxemia requiring more than 50 per cent FiO_2, a respiratory rate above 30 per minute, a vital capacity of less than 15 ml per kg, a tidal volume of less than 5 ml per kg, and an alveolar to arterial oxygen gradient (A-a/O_2) on 100 per cent oxygen above 350 mm Hg[189, 190] (see Table 10–3). The A-a/O_2 can be calculated by subtracting the PaO_2 from the alveolar oxygen tension (PAO_2). PAO_2 can be derived from the simplified alveolar air equation for 100 per cent oxygen breathing: $PAO_2 = (PB - 47 \text{ mm Hg}) - PaCO_2$, where PB is the barometric pressure in millimeters of mercury and 47 is the water vapor pressure at 37° Celsius.

Mechanical ventilation is begun at a frequency of 10 to 12 per minute, a net tidal volume of 12 to 15 ml per kg, and 100 per cent FiO_2. Blood gases are measured 15 to 20 minutes later and the severity of impairment of oxygen exchange assessed by calculating again the A-a/O_2 gradient. As a general rule, for each 20 mm Hg of gradient there is a 1 per cent shunt, the normal figure being 5 per cent. Frequently, it is observed that gas exchange improves somewhat on the respirator; however, high oxygen concentrations are still required. At this time the patient should be started on PEEP, usually starting with 5 cm of water. PEEP increases functional residual capacity (FRC) and PaO_2 and decreases the A-a/O_2 and venous admixture.[189, 190] In addition, perfusion to areas of low $\dot{V}/\dot{Q}$ ratio is decreased by PEEP, thus improving the PaO_2.[192] The objectives of using PEEP are (1) to recruit unstable and collapsed alveoli and therefore increase FRC, (2) to decrease venous admixture (shunt) and improve PaO_2, (3) to allow a decrease in FiO_2 to nontoxic levels, and (4) to prevent further alveolar collapse and closure.

Following oxygenation and recruitment and expansion of the alveoli the patient should be gently dehydrated. Analysis of the modified Starling equation for the lung capillaries shows that, everything else remaining constant, transvascular flux of fluid will be less when Pmv is low. Ideally, as long as cardiac output is not compromised, PCWP should be kept low by judicious use of diuretics or fluid restriction. For various reasons (antidiuretic hormone [ADH] release, and so on), patients on respirators have a tendency to retain fluids.[193] Fluid intake should be limited to 20 ml per kg in 24 hours plus nonurinary losses, and urinary output should be kept at 1 ml per kg per hr. Unfortunately, patients with drug intoxication are frequently in shock or require forced diuresis for the purpose of drug elimination. This need is usually translated into administration of as much as 500 ml of fluids per hour. The situation is further complicated by the fact that mechanical ventilation and PEEP compromise cardiovascular function.[194–196] Compromise occurs through several mechanisms: (1) a decrease in the venous return because the intrathoracic pressure is now positive throughout the respiratory cycle, (2) an increase in pulmonary vascular resistance by action on the alveolar vessels and therefore an increase of right ventricular work, (3) an increase in the mediastinal and pericardial pressure, which interferes with the filling of the left ventricle, and (4) a shift of the intraventricular septum to the left because of the right ventricular strain, thus decreasing left ventricular compliance and stroke volume.

Regardless of the mechanism, a drop in cardiac output with PEEP, though accompanied by an increase in PaO_2, may result in less oxygen being available for cellular metabolism. The availability of oxygen, given by the product of cardiac output in liters times the arterial oxygen content in milliliters per 100 ml of blood ($O_2Av = CO \times 10 \times CaO_2$), is the crucial parameter to be followed as PEEP is increased. If no blood pressure and urinary output changes are observed with a PEEP of 5 to 8 cm H_2O and it is possible to increase significantly the PaO_2 to the point where the FiO_2 may be decreased to 50 per cent or less, nothing else is necessary.

Remember that there is no specific treatment for this form of ARDS, and therapy involves keeping the patient alive to allow time for the lung to heal. However, if the blood pressure or urinary output drops, if adequate PaO_2 at a low FiO_2 is not achieved, if the patient is in shock, or if large volumes of fluids are being administered, a Swan-Ganz catheter should be inserted to monitor PCWP and cardiac output.[197] With this information it is possible to assess the effect of PEEP on the cardiac output and stop when it falls. In addition, the measurement of PCWP will give information about the patient's fluid status.

What should be the approach to the patient who has a low cardiac output initially or in whom it drops with the use of PEEP? In drug-overdosed patients normal response mechanisms to positive-pressure breathing may be impaired.[156, 189, 198] In addition, some types of drugs produce a true hypovolemia as a result of massive volume loss into the lungs. Fluids may be given to a patient with low PCWP in a shock state undergoing mechanical ventilation and PEEP. Cardiac output will increase; however, gas exchange may worsen.

There is great controversy about how far to go in terms of fluid challenge and what fluids to give. With a leaky capillary syndrome, colloids may also leak into the interstitium of the lung, exacerbating edema by pulling fluid out of the vessels.[185, 187] With some types of drug intoxication, data indicate that the protein loss is so severe that colloids may have to be given.[103] A conservative approach is recommended. In a patient who is in shock or in whom the cardiac output drops with PEEP, fluid challenges must be given; however, it is not advisable to raise the PCWP above normal even though data suggest that hypervolemic animals better tolerate mechanical ventilation.[199] Since most of these forms of ARDS are self-limited, an increase in PEEP to very high values (super-PEEP) is not recommended, even if that means having an FiO_2 above 50 per cent for 12 or 24 hours.[200]

Lowering the PCWP, if hemodynamically tolerated, will decrease pulmonary edema. This effect may be achieved in two ways. One is by use of diuretics, and the other is by use of vasodilators such as nitroprusside.[197, 201] The difference between the two approaches is that the first may decrease the cardiac output and compromise renal function, whereas the latter will increase cardiac output. An increase in cardiac output may be accompanied by worsening of shunt because of preferential perfusion of poorly ventilated areas.[202] The concurrent rise in central venous blood saturation could minimize the changes in PaO_2. In a hemodynamically stable patient, these two methods are likely to decrease lung water and improve lung function.[197]

Although the use of vasopressors has been associated with a higher mortality in patients with drug intoxication, these data may not apply to dopamine. This drug can improve splanchnic circulation, decrease muscle blood flow, and increase cardiac output. Therefore, when the PCWP is high or normal, diuresis or restriction of fluids or both are recommended as cardiac function is supported with dopamine.[197] In some situations (phenothiazine or tricyclic antidepressant overdose), levarterenol is preferable to dopamine.[114]

Once the objectives are achieved and the patient is well oxygenated at an FiO_2 of less than 50 per cent and is otherwise stable, attention must be directed to weaning him or her from the ventilator. Meanwhile, the pH should be kept within normal limits, and acidosis and alkalosis should be corrected by improving perfusion and oxygenation, by dialyzing the severely ill patient (those with metabolic acidosis), or by adjusting minute ventilation or dead space or both. Intermittent mandatory ventilation (IMV) may be used as soon as patients have spontaneous respirations, and the rate should be slowly decreased while arterial blood gases are monitored. With a vital capacity of 10 ml per kg or more, a tidal volume of 5 ml per kg or more, a negative inspiratory force of 25 cm H_2O or more, and a minute ventilation of less than 10 liters per minute, a patient should be able to breathe spontaneously.[203]

PEEP is the last thing to be discontinued. It is my practice to ascend by increments of 3 cm H_2O and descend by the same amount, at the same time monitoring the patient and following respiratory parameters and blood gas measurements. A sudden drop in PEEP may cause an abrupt drop in PaO_2.[189–191, 194]

It is important to keep in mind that PEEP affects the measurements of PCWP.[197] The Swan-Ganz catheter tip must be located in lung zone III below the level of the left atrium where both pulmonary arterial and venous pressures are larger than the airway's pressure. When PEEP is above 15 cm H_2O, the correlation between PCWP and left atrial pressure is less than optimal.[204, 205] Therefore, chest radiographs and cardiac output must be followed carefully.

After the patient has been weaned from the respirator and PEEP, extubation should follow, provided that the patient is alert, has an effective cough, and is capable of swallowing.

Besides the cardiovascular complications of mechanical ventilation (MV) and PEEP, an increase in the incidence of barotrauma (pneumomediastinum, subcutaneous emphysema, and pneumothorax) has been noted in these patients.[211] A pneumothorax in a patient on MV and PEEP requires immediate placement of a chest tube. MV and PEEP also cause release of ADH, sodium and water retention, abnormal liver function tests, and increased intracranial pressure.[190, 207]

Only occasionally does a patient with drug overdose require a tracheostomy. Frequently, the endotracheal tube is needed for just a few days. It is safer to keep it in place for 2 weeks or longer than to proceed with a tracheostomy.[208] The complications of prolonged endotracheal intubation are multiple and vary from lip or tongue pressure ulcers to laryngeal damage and tracheal stenosis. The latter is the most serious. By keeping the endotracheal tube cuff pressure below 25 mm Hg, keeping the tube properly anchored, using swivel adaptors, and keeping the patient calm by means of sedatives, these risks can be minimized.

Aspiration Pneumonia

Aspiration pneumonia is one of the most serious complications of drug overdose (Fig. 10–9). Because of altered mental status and impairment of lung defense mechanisms, the patient is in a perfect setting for pulmonary infections.[5, 6] The etiology of these pneumonias depends on the nature of the patient's mouth flora. Commonly, the oropharynx is colonized with aerobic organisms like *Streptococcus pneumoniae* and *Staphyloccus aureus.* Aspiration of oral secretions outside the hospital or nursing home environment produces anaerobic or gram-positive *(Pneumococcus)* pneumonia; therefore, penicillin is the antibiotic of choice.[209] It is now known that hospitalized, institutionalized, and debilitated patients develop changes in their mouth flora that result in a significant overgrowth of gram-negative organisms.[210–213] Therefore, the treatment must include antibiotics that are effective against these organisms.

Aspirated bacteria, aerobic or anaerobic,

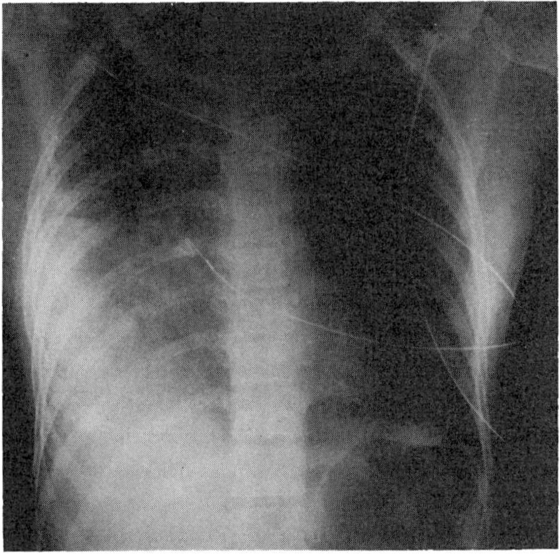

Figure 10–9. Barbiturate overdose and aspiration pneumonia involving the right lower lobe in a 15 year old boy.

may cause either abscess, empyema, or pneumonia. Acute bronchial obstruction may be produced by solid particles in the tracheobronchial tree that cause atelectasis and infection. Finally, aspiration of gastric contents produces a chemical pneumonitis and respiratory failure with severe hypoxemia, requiring mechanical ventilation and PEEP.[214–216] This form of aspiration pneumonia is quite common in the drug-intoxicated victim. It may occur spontaneously, during cardiopulmonary resuscitation resulting from gastric distension, during emesis induction, during attempts to pass a nasogastric tube, and during endotracheal intubation. The pathology of this condition, known by the eponym Mendelson's syndrome, is similar to that of ARDS except that bronchiolar damage is much more severe and bronchiolitis obliterans often results. Increase in lung water (pulmonary edema) is observed, and the edematous fluid is as rich in protein as the plasma. Decreased lung compliance, FRC, and hypoxemia follow owing to edema and alveolar instability and collapse. Tachycardia, hypotension, wheezing, and dyspnea are common.

Aspiration of water or saline solutions can also cause dyspnea and hypoxemia. However, this condition subsides rapidly. Aspiration of food particles without acid causes a hemorrhagic pneumonia and a granulomatous reaction in the lung. Hypercapnia is seen more commonly with this condition than with aspiration of acid.[216, 217] Although the pH of the gastric fluid was for a long time believed to be a critical factor in the development of this condition, Schwartz and associates recently demonstrated that gastric contents with a pH of 5.9 produced as severe a chemical pneumonitis as that induced by fluid at a pH of 1.8.[217] In both instances, the presence of food particles worsens the severity of the pneumonia. The role of infection in this form of aspiration pneumonia is unclear. Once the lung is damaged, it probably becomes more susceptible to infections. Unlike the situation in aspiration of oral secretions in nonhospitalized patients, in whom gram-positive organisms and anaerobes predominate, in aspiration of gastric contents the infection is hospital acquired and therefore may be gram-negative. It is important to keep in mind that an endotracheal tube does not ensure against silent aspiration, although it usually prevents massive aspiration.

The treatment of aspiration pneumonia consists of administration of antibiotics, oxygen, and mechanical ventilation. For aspiration that occurs outside the hospital, the drugs of choice are still penicillin and clindamycin. In those patients in whom colonization with gram-negative organisms is likely, we recommend (1) a cephalosporin and an aminoglycoside; *or* (2) ticarcillin and an aminoglycoside; *or* (3) a third-generation cephalosporin alone, such as ceftazidine or cefoperazone; *or* (4) Timentin (ticarcillin and potassium clavulanate); *or* (5) imipenem (Primaxin). Once the organism is identified, one can then narrow the antibiotic coverage to the most effective, less toxic, and less expensive drug.

In cases of aspiration of gastric contents, endotracheal suction may be helpful in removing secretions and aspirated material. The patient should be immediately intubated with a large (No. 8 or 9 French) endotracheal tube. A bronchoscopy should be performed if there is a question of aspiration of large particulate matter. Corticosteroids in large doses have been recommended to treat this condition, but no evidence suggests that corticosteroids are in any way helpful. In the doses recommended (30 mg per kg), they are expensive, cause glucose intolerance, and may increase the chances for infection.[215, 216] Recent studies indicate that not only do corticosteroids not decrease the prevalence of ARDS in septic patients but also they may actually delay or prevent recovery from ARDS and increase mortality.[218] High doses of corticosteroids do not affect the outcome of patients with ARDS.[219]

Prophylactic antibiotics are frequently administered immediately after aspiration.[216] In a review of 50 cases of gastric content aspiration, Bynum and Pierce could not demonstrate any benefit from use of prophylactic antibiotics.[215] Nosocomial pneumonia with gram-negative organisms usually occurred when improvement from the initial chemical pneumonitis was already evident. This was interpreted as representing infection; therefore, only at this time, after appropriate cultures, should antibiotic therapy be initiated.

The cornerstone of the treatment of gastric content aspiration is ventilatory support. Mechanical ventilation and PEEP not only keep the patient alive but do it without use of excessive concentrations of oxygen. Mechanical ventilation itself may help the lung to heal, and, although this is controversial, it is generally agreed that the patient should be managed like any other case of ARDS.[216] Close monitoring of fluid balance, cardiac output, and PCWP is necessary, particularly if the patient requires high levels of PEEP. Even with optimal therapy, mortality ranges from 28 to 60 per cent.

Other Complications

Besides pneumonia, other complications are common in patients with drug overdose, particularly those with severe intoxication requiring endotracheal intubation and mechanical ventilation. Among these complications are atelectasis due to secretions or intubation of the right main stem bronchus (Fig. 10–10), pneumothorax (see Fig. 10–4), pulmonary edema resulting from fluid overload (see Fig. 10–2), and traumatic intubation involving damage to the vocal cords, epistaxis, hemoptysis, and tracheal stenosis.

Jay and associates reviewed the respiratory complications of 195 patients with drug overdose admitted to a medical intensive care unit, of whom 77 per cent (a high percentage) were intubated.[220] Traumatic intubation and right main stem bronchus intubation were documented in 10.7 per cent of the patients. Aspiration was reported in 10.8 per cent, and aspiration of gastric contents (24 per cent) was observed only in intubated patients. Dislodgement or obstruction of the tube, postextubation upper airways obstruction, and subglottic stenosis occurred in about 10 per cent of all intubated patients. Three cases of pneumothorax were described. Nine patients died, eight from progressive respiratory insufficiency. At autopsy, all had pulmonary edema. The high prevalence of complications secondary to endotracheal intubation (32 per cent) has to be attributed to the use of tubes fitted with high-pressure, low-compliance cuffs. In addition, almost half the patients were in deep coma, and prophylactic intubation was undertaken for that reason.

Our experience is considerably different. Of 131 patients admitted to the intensive care unit in a 3-year period, 33 required endotracheal intubation (25 per cent), and only 20 required mechanical ventilation (15 per cent). Of the 33 intubated patients, four had pulmonary edema. There were six cases of pneumonia, seven of atelectasis, one of pneumothorax, two of intubation of the right main stem bronchus, and one of severe subglottic edema due to traumatic intubation. There were no cases of tracheal stenosis. Overall, 33 intubated patients experienced 11 complications. However, only a few of the complications (two of atelectasis, two of right main stem bronchus intubation, one of pneumothorax, and one of subglottic edema) could be attributed to the intubation and mechanical ventilation. Pneumonia, including one case of gastric contents aspiration, occurred in four nonintubated patients. Two patients developed atelectasis and pulmonary emboli, respectively. Only four patients died: one with paraquat overdose, and the others with

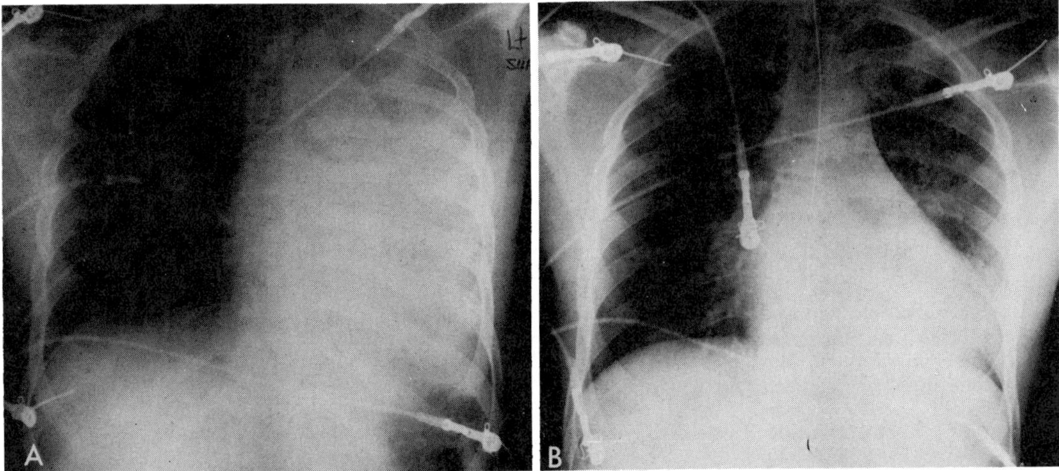

Figure 10–10. *A*, Complete atelectasis of the left lung secondary to intubation of the right main stem bronchus in a patient with barbiturate overdose. *B*, The endotracheal tube has been pulled up, and the left lung is now re-expanded.

tricyclic antidepressant, cocaine, and salicylate overdoses, respectively. Our data indicate that the complications of endotracheal intubation and mechanical ventilation in these patients are now much less frequent than previously reported, in part because of better facilities, better nursing care, and the availability of endotracheal tubes fitted with high-compliance, low-pressure cuffs.[177]

References

1. Vital Statistics of United States. Washington DC, US National Center for Health Statistics, 1977.
2. Finkle BS, et al: A national assessment of propoxyphene in post mortem medical investigation. J Forensic Sci *21*:706, 1976.
3. National Academy of Sciences: Sleeping pills, insomnia and medical practice. Washington DC, National Academy of Sciences, 1979, p 67.
4. US Department of Health, Education, and Welfare, Public Hearing on Propoxyphene, April 6, 1979. Statement of Robert H. Furman, MD, based on DAWN reports and IMS New Prescription Audits for 1977.
5. Newhouse M, Sanchis J, Bienenstock J: Lung defense mechanisms. N Engl J Med *295*:990, 1976.
6. Brayton RG, Stokes PE, Schwartz MS, Louria DB: Effect of alcohol and various diseases on leukocyte mobilization, phagocytosis and intracellular bacterial killing. N Engl J Med *282*:123, 1970.
7. Wilson RH, Hoseth W, Dempsey ME: Respiratory acidosis. I. Effects of decreasing respiratory minute volume in patients with severe chronic pulmonary emphysema, with specific reference to oxygen, morphine and barbiturates. Am J Med *17*:464, 1954.
8. Dripps RD, Comroe JG: The immediate effect of morphine administered intravenously and intramuscularly upon the respiration of normal man. Anesthesiology *6*:462, 1945.
9. Weil JV, McCullough RE, Kline JS, Sodal I: Diminished response to hypoxia and hypercapnia after morphine in normal man. N Engl J Med *292*:1103, 1975.
10. Santiago TV, Johnson J, Riley DJ, Edelman NH: Effects of morphine on ventilatory response to exercise. J Appl Physiol *47*:112, 1979.
11. Silber R, Clerkin EP: Pulmonary edema in acute heroin poisoning. Am J Med *27*:187, 1959.
12. Helpern M, Rho YM: Deaths from narcotism in New York City. Incidence, circumstances and postmortem findings. NY State J Med *66*:2391, 1966.
13. Louria DB, Hensle T, Rose J: The major medical complications of heroin addiction. Ann Intern Med *67*:1, 1967.
14. Sapira JD: The narcotic addict as a medical patient. Am J Med *45*:555, 1968.
15. Spiritus EM, Wilson AF, Berke RA: Lung scans in asymptomatic heroin addicts. Am Rev Respir Dis *108*:994, 1973.
16. Stern WZ: Roentgenographic aspects of narcotic addiction. JAMA *236*:963, 1976.
17. Camargo G, Colp CH: Pulmonary function studies in ex-heroin users. Chest *67*:331, 1975.
18. Overland ES, Nolan AJ, Hopewell PC: Alteration of pulmonary function in intravenous drug abusers. Am J Med *68*:231, 1980.
19. Steinberg AD, Karliner J: The clinical spectrum of heroin pulmonary edema. Arch Intern Med *122*:122, 1968.
20. Stern WZ, Spear WP, Jacobson HG: The roentgen findings in acute heroin intoxication. Am J Roentgenol *103*:522, 1968.
21. Lynch K, Greenbaum EG, O'Loughlin BJ: Pulmonary edema in heroin overdose. Radiology *94*:377, 1970.
22. Morrison WJ, Wetherill S, Zyroff J: The acute pulmonary edema of heroin intoxication. Radiology *97*:347, 1970.
23. Jaffe RB, Koschmann EB: Intravenous drug abuse. Pulmonary, cardiac and vascular complications. Am J Roentgenol *109*:107, 1970.
24. Joseph WL, Fletcher HS, Giordano JM, Adkins PC: Pulmonary and cardiovascular implications of drug addiction. Ann Thorac Surg *15*:263, 1973.
25. Gann D, Mansour N, Crosby DJ: Atrial fibrillation and pulmonary edema in acute heroin intoxication. Ariz Med *28*:672, 1971.
26. Duberstein JL, Kaufman DM: A clinical study of an epidemic of heroin-induced pulmonary edema. Am J Med *51*:704, 1971.
27. Bertona G, Domenighetti G, Reigner PH, Perret CP: Intoxication massive a l'heroine. Schweiz Med Wschr *109*:1854, 1979.
28. Presant S, Knoght L, Klassen G: Methadone-induced pulmonary edema. Can Med Assoc J *113*:966, 1975.
29. Paranthaman SK, Kahn F: Acute cardiomyopathy with recurrent pulmonary edema and hypotension following heroin overdose. Chest *69*:117, 1976.
30. Frand UI, Shim CS, Williams MH: Heroin-induced pulmonary edema. Ann Intern Med *77*:29, 1972.
31. Osler W: Oedema of the left lung in morphia poisoning. Montreal Gen Hosp Rep *1*:291, 1880.
32. Frand UI, Shim CS, Williams MH: Methadone-induced pulmonary edema. Ann Intern Med *76*:975, 1972.
33. Zyroff J, Slovis TL, Nagler J: Pulmonary edema induced by oral methadone. Radiology *112*:567, 1974.
34. Sokolowski JW: Case report. Methadone-induced pulmonary edema. Clin Notes Respir Dis *13*:15, 1974.
35. Persky VW, Goldfrank LR: Methadone overdoses in a New York City hospital. J Am Coll Emerg Phys *5*:111, 1976.
36. Kjeldgaard JM, Hahn GW, Heckenlively JR, Genton E: Methadone-induced pulmonary edema. JAMA *218*:882, 1971.
37. Sklar J, Timms RM: Codeine-induced pulmonary edema. Chest *72*:230, 1977.
38. Hirsch CS, Adelson L: Acute fatal intranasal narcotism. Hum Pathol *3*:71, 1972.
39. Reichenberg S, Pobirs F: Severe respiratory depression following Talwin. Am Rev Respir Dis *107*:280, 1973.
40. Rainier-Pope CR: Lomotil poisoning. South Afr Med J *48*:39, 1974.
41. Katz S, Aberman A, Frand UI, Stein IM, Fulop M: Heroin pulmonary edema. Evidence for increased capillary permeability. Am Rev Respir Dis *106*:472, 1972.
42. Gelb AF, Klein E: Hemodynamic and alveolar pro-

tein studies in non-cardiac pulmonary edema. Am Rev Respir Dis *114*:831, 1976.
43. Raskin MM: Pulmonary edema of acute overdose reaction and near-drowning: Some radiographic and physiologic comparisons. South Med J *69*:1063, 1976.
44. Overland ES, Sveringhaus JW: Non-cardiac pulmonary edema. Adv Intern Med *23*:307, 1978.
45. Hultgren HN, Grover RF, Hartley LH: Abnormal circulatory responses to high altitude in subjects with a previous history of high-altitude pulmonary edema. Circulation *44*:759, 1971.
46. Moss G: The role of the central nervous system in shock: The centroneurogenic mechanism of the respiratory distress syndrome. Crit Care Med *2*:181, 1974.
47. Fishman AP: Hypoxia of the pulmonary circulation. How and where it acts. Circ Res *38*:221, 1976.
48. Pietra GG, Szidon JP, Leventhal MM, Fishman AP: Histamine and interstitial pulmonary edema in the dog. Circ Res *29*:323, 1971.
49. Pietra GG, Szidon JP, Carpenter HA, Fishman AP: Bronchial venular leakage during endotoxin shock. Am J Pathol *77*:387, 1974.
50. Malik AB, Van der Zee H: Lung vascular permeability following progressive pulmonary embolization. J Appl Physiol *45*:590, 1978.
51. Bowers RE, McKean CR, Park BE, Brigham KL: Increased pulmonary vascular permeability follows intracranial hypertension in sheep. Am Rev Respir Dis *119*:637, 1979.
52. Maron MB, Dawson CA: Pulmonary venoconstriction caused by elevated cerebrospinal fluid pressure in the dog. J Appl Physiol *49*:73, 1980.
53. Van der Zee H, Malik AB, Lee BC, Hakim TS: Lung fluid and protein exchange during intracranial hypertension and role of sympathetic mechanisms. J Appl Physiol *48*:273, 1980.
54. Wray NP, Nicotra MB: Pathogenesis of neurogenic pulmonary edema. Am Rev Respir Dis *118*:783, 1978.
55. O'Brodovich HM, Stalcup AS, Mei Pang L, Lipset JS, Mellins RB: Bradykinin production and increased pulmonary endothelial permeability during acute respiratory failure in anesthetized sheep. J Clin Invest *67*:514, 1981.
56. Benowitz NL, Rosenberg J, Becker CE: Cardiopulmonary catastrophes in drug-overdosed patients. Med Clin North Am *63*:267, 1979.
57. Shubin H, Weil MH: The mechanism of shock following suicidal doses of barbiturates, narcotics and tranquilizer drugs with observations on the effects of treatment. Am J Med *38*:853, 1965.
58. Thorstrand C: Cardiovascular effects of poisoning by hypnotic and tricyclic antidepressant drugs. Acta Med Scand *198*(Suppl):583, 1975.
59. Murray J: Mechanisms of acute respiratory failure. Am Rev Respir Dis *115*:1071, 1977.
60. Goodman JM, Bischel MD, Wagers PW, Barbour BH: Barbiturate intoxication. Morbidity and mortality. West J Med *124*:179, 1976.
61. Clemmesen C, Lassen NA: Treatment of circulatory shock in narcotic poisoning. Danish Med Bull *10*:100, 1963.
62. Reves JG, Fragen RJ, Vinik HR, Greenblatt DJ: Midazolam: Pharmacology and uses. Anesthesiology *62*:310, 1985.
63. Clark TJH, Collins JV, Tang D: Respiratory depression caused by nitrazepam in patients with respiratory failure. Lancet *2*:737, 1971.
64. Model DG: Nitrazepam-induced respiratory depression in chronic obstructive lung disease. Br J Dis Chest *67*:128, 1973.
65. Model DG, Berry DJ: Effects of chlordiazepoxide in respiratory failure due to chronic bronchitis. Lancet *2*:869, 1974.
66. Brauninger G, Ravin M: Respiratory arrest following intravenous valium. Ann Ophthalmol *6*:805, 1974.
67. Kanto J, Sjovall S, Vuori A: Effect of different kinds of premedication on the induction properties of midazolam. Br J Anaesth *54*:507, 1982.
68. Catchlove RFH, Kafer ER: The effect of diazepam on the ventilatory response to carbon dioxide on steady state gas exchange. Anesthesiology *39*:9, 1971.
69. Catchlove RFH, Kafer ER: The effects of diazepam on respiration in patients with chronic obstructive pulmonary disease. Anesthesiology *34*:14, 1971.
70. Rao S, Sherbaniuk RW, Prasad K, Lee JK, Sproule BJ: Cardiopulmonary effects of diazepam. Clin Pharmacol Ther *14*:182, 1973.
71. Forster A, Gardaz JP, Suter PM, Gemperle M: Respiratory depression by midazolam and diazepam. Anesthesiology *53*:494, 1980.
72. Gross JB, Zebrowki ME, Carel WD, Gardner S, Smith TC: Time course of ventilatory depression after thiopental and midazolam in normal subjects and in patients with chronic obstructive lung disease. Anesthesiology *58*:540, 1983.
73. Adams P, Gelman S, Reves JG, Greenblatt DJ, Alvis JM, Bradley E: Midazolam pharmacodynamics and pharmacokinetics during acute hypovolemia. Anesthesiology *63*:140, 1985.
74. Mendelson WB, Garnett D, Gillin JC: Flurazepam-induced sleep apnea syndrome in a patient with insomnia and mild sleep related respiratory changes. J Nerv Ment Dis *169*:261, 1981.
75. Leiter JC, Knuth SL, Krol RC, Bartlett D: The effect of diazepam on genioglossal muscle activity in normal subjects. Am Rev Respir Dis *132*:136, 1985.
76. Al-Khudairi D, Askitopoulou H, Whitwam JG: Acute tolerance to the central respiratory effects of midazolam in the dog. Anesthesiology *54*:953, 1982.
77. Gillis RA, Namath IJ, Easington C, Abraham TP, Quest JA, Hamosh P, Taveira DA Silva AM: Drug interaction with aminobutyric acid/benzodiazepine receptors at the ventral surface of the medulla results in pronounced changes in cardiorespiratory activity. J Pharmacol Exp Ther *248*:863, 1989.
78. O'Sullivan GE, Wade DN: Flumazenil in the management of acute drug overdose with benzodiazepines and other agents. Clin Pharmacol Ther *42*:254, 1987.
79. Richman S, Harris RD: Acute pulmonary edema associated with librium abuse. Radiology *103*:57, 1972.
80. Afifi AA, Sacks ST, Liu VY, et al: Cumulative prognostic index for patients with barbiturate, glutethimide, and meprobamate intoxication. N Engl J Med *285*:1497, 1971.
81. Arieff AL, Friedman EA: Coma following nonnarcotic drug overdose: Management of 208 patients. Am J Med Sci *266*:405, 1973.
82. Chazan JA, Garella S: Glutethimide intoxication: A prospective study of 70 patients treated conservatively without hemodialysis. Arch Intern Med *128*:215, 1971.
83. Wright N, Roscoe P: Acute glutethimide poisoning:

Conservative management of 31 patients. JAMA *214:*1704, 1970.
84. Glauser FL, Smith WR, Caldwell A, Hoshkiko M, Dolan GS, Baer H, Olsher N: Ethchlorvynol (Placidyl)-induced pulmonary edema. Ann Intern Med *84:*46, 1976.
85. Payne CB, Kerr HD, Diaconis JN: Pathophysiologic effects of intravenous ethchlorvynol (Placidyl) in man following acute pulmonary edema. Md State Med J *26:*69, 1977.
86. Lynn RI, Honig CL, Jatlow PI, Klinger, AS: Resin hemoperfusion for treatment of ethchlorvynol overdose. Ann Intern Med *91:*549, 1979.
87. Oh TE, Gordon TP, Burden PW: Unilateral pulmonary edema and "Mandrax" poisoning. Anaesthesia *33:*719, 1978.
88. Hoy WE, Rivero A, Marin MG, Rieders F: Resin hemoperfusion for treatment of a massive meprobamate overdose. Ann Intern Med *93:*455, 1980.
89. Woldorf NM, Pastore PN: Extreme epinephrine sensitivity with a general anesthesia. Arch Otolaryngol *96:*272, 1972.
90. Franks CR, Hudson PM, Rees AJ, Searle JF: Accidental intravenous halothane. Guy's Hosp Rep *123:*89, 1974.
91. Spencer JD, Raasch FO, Trefny FA: Halothane abuse in hospital personnel. JAMA *235:*1034, 1976.
92. Lockhart CH, Jenkins JJ: Ketamine-induced apnea in patients with increased intracranial pressure. Anesthesiology *37:*92, 1972.
93. McLaughlin AP, Altwein JE, Kessler WO, Gittes RF: Hazards of gallamine administration in patients with renal failure. J Urol *108:*515, 1972.
94. Dykes MH: Evaluation of a muscle relaxant: Pancuronium bromide (Pavulon). JAMA *225:*745, 1973.
95. Granville-Grossman KL, Sergeant HGS: Pulmonary edema due to salicylate intoxication. Lancet *1:*575, 1960.
96. Hill JB: Salicylate intoxication. N Engl J Med *288:*1110, 1973.
97. Hernicek G, Skelton J, Miller WC: Pulmonary edema and salicylate overdose. JAMA *230:*866, 1974.
98. Anderson RJ, Potts DE, Gabow PA, Rumack BH, Schrier RW: Unrecognized adult salicylate intoxication. Ann Intern Med *85:*745, 1976.
99. Bowers RE, Brigham KL, Owen PJ: Salicylate pulmonary edema: The mechanism in sheep and review of the clinical literature. Am Rev Respir Dis *115:*261, 1977.
100. Thomas C, Gullmer HG: Adult respiratory distress syndrome in salicylate intoxication. Lancet *1:*1294, 1979.
101. Kahn A, Blum D: Fatal respiratory distress syndrome and salicylate intoxication in a two year old. Lancet *2:*1131, 1979.
102. Paynter AS, Alexander FW: Salicylate intoxication caused by teething ointment. Lancet *2:*1132, 1979.
103. Hormaechea E, Carlson RW, Rogove H, et al: Hypovolemia, pulmonary edema and protein changes in severe salicylate poisoning. Am J Med *66:*1046, 1979.
104. Gabow PA, Anderson RJ, Potts DE, Schrier RW: Acid base disturbances in the salicylate-intoxicated adult. Arch Intern Med *138:*1481, 1978.
105. Tennant FS: Complications of propoxyphene abuse. Arch Intern Med *132:*191, 1973.
106. Fisch HP, Wands J, Yeung J, Davis PJ: Pulmonary edema and disseminated intravascular coagulation after intravenous abuse of D-propoxyphene (Darvon). South Med J *65:*493, 1972.
107. Ogbuihi S, Bohn G, Audick W: Fatal case of propoxyphene overdose. Morphological and toxicological findings. Z Rechtsmed *84:*161, 1980.
108. Bogartz LJ, Miller WC: Pulmonary edema associated with propoxyphene intoxication. JAMA *215:*259, 1971.
109. Proudfoot AT, Wright N: Acute paracetamol poisoning. Br Med J *3:*557, 1970.
110. Prescott LF, Park J, Sutherland GR, Smith IJ: Cysteamine, methionine and penicillamine in the treatment of paracetamol poisoning. Lancet *2:*109, 1976.
111. Ambre J, Alexander M: Liver toxicity after acetaminophen ingestion. Inadequacy of the dose estimate as an index of risk. JAMA *238:*500, 1977.
112. Ferguson DR, Snyder SK, Cameron AJ: Hepatotoxicity in acetaminophen poisoning. Mayo Clin Proc *52:*246, 1977.
113. Ameer B, Greenblatt DJ: Acetaminophen. Ann Intern Med *87:*202, 1977.
114. Callaham M: Tricyclic antidepressant overdose. J Am Coll Emerg Phys *8:*413, 1979.
115. Lindstrom FD, Floodmark O, Gustafsson B: Respiratory distress syndrome and thrombotic, nonbacterial endocarditis after amitriptyline overdose. Acta Med Scand *202:*203, 1977.
116. Marshall A, Moore K: Pulmonary disease after amitriptyline overdose. Br Med J *1:*716, 1973.
117. Biggs JT, Spiker DG, Petit JM, Ziegler VE: Tricyclic antidepressant overdose. JAMA *238:*135, 1977.
118. Schnoll SH, Daghestani AM, Hansen TR: Cocaine dependence. Resident Staff Physician *30:*24, 1984.
119. Cregler LL, Mark H: Medical complications of cocaine abuse. N Engl J Med *315:*1495, 1986.
120. Isner JM, Estes M, Thompson PD, Constanzo-Nordin MR, Subramanian R, Miller G, Katsar G, Sweeney K, Sturner WQ: Acute cardiac events temporally related to cocaine abuse. N Engl J Med *315:*1438, 1986.
121. Wehbie CS, Vidaillet HJ, Navetta FI, Peter RH: Acute myocardial infarction associated with initial cocaine use. South Med J *80:*933, 1987.
122. Haines JD, Sexter S: Acute myocardial infarction associated with cocaine abuse. South Med J *80:*1326, 1987.
123. Wojak JC, Flamm ES: Intracranial hemorrhage and cocaine use. Stroke *18:*712, 1987.
124. Allred RJ, Ewer S: Fatal pulmonary edema following intravenous "freebase" cocaine use. Ann Emerg Med *10:*441, 1981.
125. Goldenberg SP, Zeldis SM: Fatal acute congestive heart failure in a patient with idiopathic hemochromatosis and cocaine use. Chest *92:*374, 1987.
126. Wiener MD, Putnam CE: Pain in the chest in a user of cocaine. JAMA *258:*2087, 1987.
127. Glassroth J, Adams GD, Schnoll S: The impact of substance abuse on the respiratory system. Chest *91:*596, 1987.
128. Patel RC, Dutta D, Schonfeld SA: Free-base cocaine use associated with bronchiolitis obliterans organizing pneumonia. Ann Intern Med *107:*186, 1987.
129. Steinhaus JE, Tatum AL: An experimental study of cocaine intoxication and its treatment. J Pharmacol Exp Ther *100:*351, 1950.
130. Gilman AG, Goodman LS, Rall TW, et al (eds): The Pharmacological Basis of Therapeutics, 7th ed. New York, Macmillan, 1985.
131. Kendrick WC, Hull AR, Knochel JP: Rhabdomyol-

ysis and shock after intravenous amphetamine administration. Ann Intern Med *86:*381, 1977.
132. Shamsie SJ, Barriga C: The hazards of use of monoamine oxidase inhibitors in disturbed adolescents. Can Med Assoc J *104:*715, 1971.
133. Gary NE, Saidi P: Methamphetamine intoxication. A speedy new treatment. Am J Med *64:*537, 1978.
134. Cohen S: Angel dust. JAMA *238:*515, 1977.
135. Stillman R, Peterson RC: The paradox of phencyclidine. Ann Intern Med *90:*428, 1979.
136. Khantzian EJ, McKenna GJ: Acute toxic and withdrawal reactions associated with drug use and abuse. Ann Intern Med *90:*361, 1979.
137. Louria DB: Lysergic acid diethylamide. N Engl J Med *278:*435, 1968.
138. Altura BT, Altura BM: Phencyclidine, lysergic acid diethylamide, and mescaline: Cerebral artery spasms and hallucinogenic activity. Science *212:*1051, 1981.
139. Greganti MA, Flowers WM: Acute pulmonary edema after the intravenous administration of contrast media. Radiology *123:*583, 1979.
140. Chamberlin WH, Stockman GD, Wray NP: Shock and non-cardiogenic pulmonary edema following meglumine diatrizoate for intravenous pyelography. Am J Med *67:*684, 1979.
141. McLennan BL, Kassner EG, Becker JA: Overdose of excretory urography: Toxic cause of death. Radiology *105:*383, 1972.
142. Silvestri RC, Huseby JS, Rughani I, et al: Respiratory distress syndrome from lymphangiography contrast medium. Am Rev Respir Dis *122:*543, 1980.
143. Fairshter RD, Wilson AF: Paraquat poisoning. Am J Med *59:*751, 1975.
144. Paraquat poisoning (editorial). Lancet *1:*1057, 1976.
145. Cooke NJ, Flenley DC, Mathew H: Paraquat poisoning. Q J Med *42:*683, 1973.
146. Raffin TA, Robin ED, Pickersgill J, et al: Paraquat ingestion and pulmonary injury. West J Med *128:*26, 1978.
147. Proudfoot AT, Stewart MS: Paraquat poisoning: Significance of plasma-paraquat concentrations. Lancet *2:*330, 1979.
148. Smith P, Heath D: Paraquat lung: A reappraisal. Thorax *29:*643, 1974.
149. Ackrill P, Hasleton PS, Ralston AJ: Oesophageal perforation due to paraquat. Br Med J *1:*1252, 1978.
150. Stephens DS, Walker DH, Schaffner W, et al: Pseudodiphtheria: Prominent pharyngeal membrane associated with fatal paraquat ingestion. Ann Intern Med *94:*202, 1981.
151. Jaros F: Acute percutaneous paraquat poisoning. Lancet *1:*275, 1978.
152. Newhouse M, McEvoy D, Rosenthal D: Percutaneous paraquat absorption. Arch Dermatol *114:*1516, 1978.
153. Levin PH, Kaff LJ, Rose AG, Ferguson AD: Pulmonary effects of contact exposure to paraquat: A clinical and experimental study. Thorax *34:*150, 1979.
154. Hollinger MA, Patwell SW, Zuckerman JE, et al: Effect of paraquat on serum angiotensin-converting enzyme. Am Rev Respir Dis *121:*795, 1980.
155. Fisher HK, Clements JA, Wright RR: Enhancement of oxygen toxicity by the herbicide paraquat. Am Rev Respir Dis *107:*246, 1973.
156. Wyckoff DW, Davies JE, Barquet A, Davis JH: Diagnostic and therapeutic problems of parathion poisonings. Ann Intern Med *68:*875, 1968.
157. DeCandole CA, Douglas WW, Evans CL, Holmes R, Spencer KEV, Torrance RW, Wilson KM: The failure of respiration in death by anticholinesterase poisoning. Br J Pharmacol *8:*466, 1953.
158. Krivoy WA, Hart ER, Marazzi AS: Further analysis of the actions of DFP and curare on the respiratory center. J Pharmacol Exp Ther *103:*351, 1951.
159. Anzueto A, Berdine GG, Moore GT, Gleiser C, Johnson D, White CD, Johanson WG: Pathophysiology of soman intoxication in primates. Toxicol Appl Pharmacol *86:*56, 1986.
160. Ricket DL, Foster RE, Glenn JF, Gregory WT, Randolph TC, Traub RK: Acute Sarin toxicity: Comparison of central nervous system and neuromuscular effects. Neurosci Abstr *8:*558, 1982.
161. Ricket DL: Differentiation of peripheral and central actions of soman-produced respiratory arrest. Research News Letter of the U.S. Army Medical Research and Development Command, April 1983, p. 7.
162. Gillis RA, Walton DP, Quest JA, Namath I, Hamosh P, Dretchen KL: Cardiorespiratory effects produced by activation of cholinergic muscarinic receptors on the ventral surface of the medulla. J Pharmacol Exp Ther *247:*765, 1988.
163. Eade NR, Taussig LM, Marks MI: Hydrocarbon pneumonitis. Pediatrics *54:*351, 1974.
164. Neeld EM, Limacher MC: Chemical pneumonitis after intravenous injection of hydrocarbon. Radiology *129:*36, 1978.
165. Chance B, Erecinska M, Wagner M: Mitochondrial responses to carbon monoxide toxicity. Ann NY Acad Sci *174:*193, 1970.
166. Urboretti J: Carbon monoxide poisoning. Prog Clin Biol Res *51:*355, 1981.
167. Zawacki BE, Jung RC, Joyce J, Rincon E: Smoke, burns and the natural history of inhalation injury in fire victims: A correlation of experimental and clinical data. Ann Surg *185:*100, 1977.
168. McCormick DJ, Avbel AJ, Gibbons RB: Non-lethal mushroom poisoning. Ann Intern Med *90:*332, 1979.
169. Mitchel DH: Amanita mushroom poisoning. Annu Rev Med *31:*51, 1980.
170. Murray MJ, Kronenberg R: Pulmonary reactions simulating cardiac pulmonary edema caused by nitrofurantoin. N Engl J Med *273:*1185, 1965.
171. Steinberg AD: Pulmonary edema following ingestion of hydrochlorothiazide. JAMA *204:*167, 1968.
172. Hill RN, Spragg RC, Wedel MK, Moser KM: Adult respiratory distress syndrome associated with colchicine intoxication. Ann Intern Med *83:*523, 1975.
173. Hayler AM, Holt DW, Volans GN: Fatal overdosage with disopyramide. Lancet *1:*968, 1978.
174. Baruh S, Sherman L: Hypoglycemia, a cause of pulmonary edema. J Nat Med Assoc *67:*200, 1975.
175. Rosenow EC: The spectrum of drug-induced lung disease. Ann Intern Med *77:*977, 1972.
176. Weiss RB, Muggia FM: Cytotoxic drug-induced pulmonary disease: Update 1980. Am J Med *68:*259, 1980.
177. Lewis FR, Schlobohm RM, Thomas AN: Prevention of complications from prolonged tracheal intubation. Am J Surg *135:*452, 1978.
178. Martin WR: Naloxone. Ann Intern Med *85:*765, 1976.
179. Roizen MF, Feeley TW: Pancuronium bromide. Ann Intern Med *88:*64, 1978.
180. Hopewell PC, Murray JF: The adult respiratory distress syndrome. Annu Rev Med *27:*343, 1976.

181. Bachofen M, Weibel ER: Alterations of the gas exchange apparatus in adult respiratory insufficiency associated with septicemia. Am Rev Respir Dis *116:*589, 1977.
182. Saldeen T: Microembolism syndrome. Microvasc Res *11:*227, 1976.
183. Schneider RC, Zapol WM, Carvalho A: Platelet consumption and sequestration in severe acute respiratory failure. Am Rev Respir Dis *122:*445, 1980.
184. Jacob HS, Craddock PR, Hammerschmidt DE, Moldow CF: Complement-induced granulocyte aggregation. An unsuspected mechanism of disease. N Engl J Med *302:*789, 1980.
185. Staub NC: Pathogenesis of pulmonary edema. Am Rev Respir Dis *109:*358, 1974.
186. Staub NC: Pulmonary edema. Physiol Rev *54:*678, 1974.
187. Staub NC: Pulmonary edema. Physiological approaches to management. Chest *74:*559, 1978.
188. Guyton AC, Lindsey AW: Effect of elevated left atrial pressure and decreased plasma protein concentration on the development of pulmonary edema. Circ Res *7:*649, 1959.
189. Pontoppidan H, Geffin B, Lowenstein E: Acute respiratory failure in the adult. N Engl J Med *287:*690, 1972.
190. Pontoppidan H, Wilson RS, Rie MA, Schneider RC: Respiratory intensive care. Anesthesiology *47:*96, 1977.
191. Briscoe WA, Smith JP, Bergofsky E, King TKS: Catastrophic pulmonary failure. Am J Med *60:*248, 1976.
192. Dantzker DR, Brook CJ, Dehart P, Lynch JP, Weg LG: Ventilation-perfusion distributions in the adult respiratory distress syndrome. Am Rev Respir Dis *120:*1039, 1979.
193. Sladen A, Laver MB, Pontoppidan H: Pulmonary complications and water retention in prolonged mechanical ventilation. N Engl J Med *279:*448, 1968.
194. Falke KJ, Pontoppidan H, Kumar A, Leith DE, Geffin BG, Laver MB: Ventilation with end-expiratory pressure in acute lung disease. J Clin Invest *51:*2315, 1972.
195. Powers SR, Dutton RE: Correlation of positive end-expiratory pressure with cardiovascular performance. Crit Care Med *3:*64, 1975.
196. Cassidy SS, Mitchell JH: Effects of positive pressure breathing on right and left ventricular preload and afterload. Fed Proc *40:*2178, 1981.
197. Broaddus VC, Berthiaume Y, Biondi JW, Mathay MA: Hemodynamic management of the adult respiratory distress syndrome. J Intensive Care Med *2:*190, 1987.
198. Scharf SM, Ingram RH: Influence of abdominal pressure and sympathetic vasoconstriction on the cardiovascular response to positive end-expiratory pressure. Am Rev Respir Dis *116:*661, 1977.
199. Sykes MK, Adams AP, Finlay WEI, et al: The effects of variations in end-expiratory inflation pressure on cardiorespiratory function in normo-, hypo-, and hypervolaemic dogs. Br J Anaesth *42:*669, 1970.
200. Kirby RR, Downs JB, Civetta JM, et al: High level positive end-expiratory pressure (PEEP) in acute respiratory insufficiency. Chest *67:*156, 1975.
201. Prewitt RM, McCarthy J, Wood LDH: Treatment of acute low pressure pulmonary edema in dogs. J Clin Invest *67:*409, 1981.
202. Lynch JP, Mhyre JG, Dantzker DR: Influence of cardiac output on intrapulmonary shunt. J Appl Physiol *46:*315, 1979.
203. Sahn SA, Lakshminarayan S, Petty TL: Weaning from mechanical ventilation. JAMA *235:*2208, 1976.
204. Lozman J, Powers SR, Older T, Dutton RE, Roy RJ, English M, Marco D, Eckert C: Correlation of pulmonary wedge and left atrial pressures. A study in the patient receiving positive end-expiratory pressure ventilation. Arch Surg *109:*270, 1974.
205. Tooker J, Huseby J, Butler J: The effect of Swan-Ganz catheter height on the wedge pressure-left atrial pressure relationship in edema during positive-pressure ventilation. Am Rev Respir Dis *117:*721, 1978.
206. Cullen DJ, Caldera DL: The incidence of ventilator-induced pulmonary barotrauma in critically ill patients. Anesthesiology *50:*185, 1979.
207. Powers SR: The use of positive end-expiratory pressure (PEEP) for respiratory support. Surg Clin North Am *54:*1125, 1974.
208. Stauffer JL, Olson DE, Petty TL: Complications and consequences of endotracheal intubation and tracheostomy. A prospective study of 150 critically ill adult patients. Am J Med *70:*65, 1981.
209. Bartlett JG, Gorbach SL, Finegold SM: Bacteriology of aspiration pneumonia. Am J Med *56:*202, 1974.
210. Johanson WG, Pierce AK, Sanford JP, Thomas GD: Nosocomial respiratory infections with gram-negative bacilli: The significance of colonization of respiratory tract. Ann Intern Med *77:*701, 1972.
211. Lorber B, Swenson RM: Bacteriology of aspiration pneumonia. A prospective study of community and hospital acquired cases. Ann Intern Med *81:*329, 1974.
212. Valenti WM, Trudell RG, Bentley DW: Factors predisposing to oropharyngeal colonization with gram-negative bacilli in the aged. N Engl J Med *298:*1108, 1978.
213. LaForce FM: Hospital-acquired gram-negative rod pneumonias: An overview. Am J Med *70:*664, 1981.
214. Mendelson CL: The aspiration of stomach contents into the lungs during obstetric anesthesia. Am J Obstet Gynecol *52:*191, 1946.
215. Bynum LJ, Pierce AK: Pulmonary aspiration of gastric contents. Am Rev Respir Dis *114:*1129, 1976.
216. Wynne JW, Modell JH: Respiratory aspiration of stomach contents. Ann Intern Med *87:*466, 1977.
217. Schwartz DJ, Wynne JW, Gibbs CP, Hood CI, Kuck EJ: The pulmonary consequences of aspiration of gastric contents at pH values greater than 2.5. Am Rev Respir Dis *121:*119, 1980.
218. Bone RC, Fisher CJ, Clemmer TP, Slotman GJ, Metz CA: Early methylprednisolone treatment for septic syndrome and the adult respiratory distress syndrome. Chest *92:*1032, 1987.
219. Bernard GR, Luce JL, Sprung CL, Rinaldo JE, Tate RM, Sibbald WJ, Kariman K, Higgins S, Bradley R, Metz CA, Harris TR, Brigham KL: High-dose corticosteroids in patients with the adult respiratory distress syndrome. N Engl J Med *317:*1565, 1987.
220. Jay SJ, Johanson WG, Pierce AK: Respiratory complications of overdose with sedative drugs. Am Rev Respir Dis *112:*591, 1975.

CHAPTER 11
CENTRAL NERVOUS SYSTEM DISTURBANCES AND BRAIN DEATH

Stanley L. Cohan, M.D., Ph.D.

A. Central Nervous System Disturbances

Central nervous system dysfunction is a prominent feature of most intoxications. Although coma may be the major neurologic manifestation of severe intoxication, less pronounced alterations in the level of consciousness, as well as behavioral changes, may be important clinical features of patients with lesser degrees of intoxication or may serve as signs of impending life-threatening coma early in the clinical course of severe intoxication. Recognition that behavioral disturbances may be secondary to encephalopathy before coma supervenes may be a critical factor in making an early diagnosis of intoxication and initiating therapy before the patient's status becomes more precarious. The same is to be said of the lethargic patient. A suspicion of intoxication may allow appropriate diagnosis before the patient becomes comatose or before autonomic dysfunction leads to worsening of the patient's status and prognosis.

This chapter identifies the features of the neurologic examination that raise the suspicion of intoxication to the clinician. Where appropriate, the characteristic patterns of neurologic abnormalities produced by certain poisons, particularly drugs, are described. With increased availability of toxicologic laboratory diagnosis, a false sense of security may be created and the clinician see less need to use these signs to make a qualitative diagnosis. Toxicology laboratories are not available in all hospitals and clinics, excessive delays in producing laboratory results, and analytic errors or inability to make a toxicologic diagnosis all are reasons for physicians not to become overly dependent on the laboratory. These signs may be extremely important, particularly in creating the suspicion that poisoning is responsible for the patient's neurologic impairment.

The most important areas of systematic neurologic assessment in evaluation of an intoxicated patient are the level of consciousness, the presence or absence of thought or behavioral disturbances, spontaneous motor activity, motor tone and reflex motor activity, respiratory pattern, pupillary reflexes, and extraocular motor function.[1] Approaching a patient in this systematic manner should allow the clinician to establish whether encephalopathy is present and whether a likelihood exists that intoxication is responsible for it.

A word of caution is in order. *The presence of an intoxicating agent does not necessarily account for the patient's neurologic status.* An example is the patient who develops severe hypotension as a result of a barbiturate overdose and in whom continued coma is the result of ischemic brain damage rather than the central effects of the barbiturate. A patient may be in coma as a result of severe hepatic failure due to poisoning with acetaminophen; although coma with acetaminophen alone does not occur, poisoning with acetaminophen–narcotic drug combinations initially may produce central nervous system depression. A patient may be severely intoxicated with alcohol, but persistence of altered mental state and even threat of permanent brain damage may be the result of head trauma sustained from a fall during an earlier phase of the intoxication.

Differentiation between altered mental status that is caused by the direct effect of a poison or one caused by indirect effects at times may be extremely difficult, particularly in the early stages of patient management, and can compromise the physician's ability to provide an accurate prognosis for recovery of normal brain function. This difficulty is magnified by an absence of accurate data on the relationship between blood concentration and the central nervous system (CNS) toxic effects of many drugs and the unavailability of rapid, accurate determination of blood concentrations of many of the most commonly encountered intoxicants. With time, of course, some distinction may be made, particularly if a patient remains encephalopathic despite the absence of significant amounts of residual drug or poison.

As mentioned, any drug or poison in sufficiently high dose can lead to loss of consciousness. In some cases, global brain hypoxia may be responsible, as in carbon monoxide poisoning. Other causes are a drug or poison directly suppressing respiration, either through neuromuscular blockade as with botulism, or tetanus toxins and curare-like drugs, or a drug or poison directly suppressing respiratory centers within the brain, as in barbiturate or glutethimide poisoning. In a similar manner, drugs that produce hypotension, severe bradycardia, or both may produce coma as a result of global central nervous system ischemia rather than as a direct effect of the intoxicant on brain function. Many drugs and poisons will cause loss of consciousness as a result of their direct toxic effect upon the brain; this may take place at several sites within the brain. Drugs like barbiturates and benzodiazepines may produce coma by directly suppressing the activity of neurons of the cerebral cortex[2] by mimicking the effects of inhibitory neurotransmitters. However, the central gray reticular core of the brain stem, from the hypothalamus to the midpontine region, contains neuronal groups—the reticular activating system—which project to and activate the cerebral cortex or maintain the wakeful state.[3–5] Some patients lose consciousness largely because of suppression of this reticular activating system.

Patients can be in coma from many different causes. Assessment of the patient's level of consciousness alone is not sufficient to determine the cause or the locus of impairment within the CNS but must be combined with an appraisal of other modalities of brain function,[1] evaluation of which may add importantly to the understanding of the status of patients in whom drug overdose is suspected. *Autonomic dysfunction* manifested by pupillary abnormalities, inappropriate sudomotor activity, cardiac rhythm disturbances, and blood pressure abnormalities is an essential feature of the neurologic assessment of the encephalopathic patient. Drugs with potent anticholinergic activity, such as the tricyclic antidepressants and atropine-like compounds, may influence pupillary size and cardiac rhythm in such a way as to raise the suspicion of their presence in a comatose patient in whom there is no history of drug ingestion or in whom it has not been possible to determine what substances were ingested. The selective vulnerability of the autonomic nervous system to certain drugs or poisons sometimes allows for differentiation between an anatomic cause for coma, such as brain stem or global cerebral ischemic stroke, and drug intoxication.

Evaluation of *extraocular muscle function* is also an important part of the evaluation of the comatose patient, because it allows assessment of brain stem function. In patients who are in coma as a result of structural damage to the brain stem, extraocular function is likely to be abnormal because of the close anatomic relationship among the extraocular motor nerves, their nuclei, the medial longitudinal fasciculus (which integrates conjugate eye movements), and the reticular activating system of the brain stem. Extraocular paresis is not invariably the result of structural damage to the brain stem, however, because certain drugs, such as phenytoin, carbamazepine, ethchlorvynol, and barbiturates, and neuromuscular toxins, such as botulism toxin, pavulon, and curare, may interfere with extraocular muscle function. Comatose patients with extraocular paresis who do not have other evidence of brain stem dysfunction should be considered as candidates for a diagnosis of intoxication.

Examination of the *skeletal motor system* in a comatose patient usually will reveal abnormalities in tone and reflex activity, but such an examination is frequently of little assistance in determining whether a patient is in coma as a result of intoxication; it is of value in deciding whether a patient is improving or deteriorating clinically. Flaccidity and hypoactive or absent tendon reflexes are commonly encountered in poisoned patients, but hypertonus and hyperreflexia are seen in some patients, and thus these motor findings are not, in themselves, reliable guides as to whether the patient has a toxic encephalopathy or structural brain damage.

Equally important is the *neurologic assessment* of the patient who is not in coma but instead is either alert or lethargic or excessively sleepy. What clues in the neurologic examination of these patients will suggest the presence of encephalopathy? If the features of encephalopathy are present, what features suggest the possibility of intoxication? Many patients will be in a state of agitation or excitement. When confusion, hallucinations, delusions, seizures, disorientation, tremulousness, aggressiveness, diaphoresis, tachycardia, or hypertension is present, the possibility of acute intoxication must be seriously considered. This acute confusional state may be considered delirium. Although delirium is not invariably the result of intoxication—meningoencephalitis, sepsis, and postictal state being other important considerations—intoxication should be a diagnostic consideration in every case in which delirium is encountered. Delirium may also be a feature of drug withdrawal, the delirium tremens of ethanol being the best known, but withdrawal from chronic use of many pharmacologic agents, such as benzodiazepines, ethchlorvynol, barbiturates, meprobamate, and neuroleptics, also may be responsible.[6-10] Other abnormalities may be observed in the neurologic examination to strengthen the clinical impression that the agitated patient or the patient with lethargy has been intoxicated. Many patients may have nystagmus as a result of cerebellar or vestibular dysfunction, or pupils may be inappropriately dilated, as in cocaine or amphetamine intoxication, or constricted, as in opiate intoxication. The patient may have tremor, ataxia, Babinski reflexes, or frontal release signs, such as a snout reflex. Although these findings in themselves certainly do not allow a diagnosis of brain intoxication to be made, when they are combined with altered mental status one can infer that the altered behavior or mental status is the result of encephalopathy; prominent among the causes for such encephalopathies are intoxication and drug withdrawal.

Seizure activity, frequently in the form of generalized, major motor seizures (grand mal), may be an important feature of the clinical presentation of intoxicated patients. Sympathomimetic drugs like cocaine, tricyclic antidepressants, amphetamines, theophylline, and aminophylline[11-18] may cause major motor seizures themselves or, at lower doses, increase the likelihood of seizure breakthrough in patients who already have a seizure disorder. Seizures are also seen in phencyclidine intoxication. Seizure rarely occurs in opiate overdose[19] and in some cases really may be due to another contaminant in the opiate or secondary to opiate-induced cerebral hypoxia. Ethanol also can lower the seizure threshold in epileptic patients and probably increases the epileptogenicity of cocaine.

Penicillin, cephalosporin, and beta-lactam *antibiotics* can produce encephalopathy, including seizure activity in some patients.[20-22] This may seriously confound diagnosis and treatment, since many of these patients are being treated for disorders such as sepsis or meningoencephalitis, which also can produce severe encephalopathy.

Lidocaine, a sodium channel blocker, has potential anticonvulsant properties, but at high doses can produce generalized convulsions.[23] This effect may not readily be attributable to lidocaine in some patients who are being treated for severe ventricular arrhythmia, which itself could produce seizures secondary to global cerebral ischemia or embolic cerebral cortical ischemia. Drug withdrawal, particularly from barbiturates, benzodiazepines, and ethanol, also can produce seizures.

However, many patients with pre-existent seizure disorders present with seizures or the encephalopathic picture of postictal state because withdrawal has led to blood and brain anticonvulsant levels falling into the subtherapeutic range, thus disinhibiting seizure discharge.

The electroencephalogram may be of assistance in patient evaluation; it could establish the presence of seizure disorder as well as demonstrate patterns that may support the diagnosis of intoxication or help differentiate metabolic effects, such as those seen in association with hypoxia, ischemia, and hepatic or renal failure, and those effects generally associated with drug-induced encephalopathy.

The remainder of this chapter discusses the clinical features that characterize poisoning of patients by specific agents.

BARBITURATES

The barbiturates exert their pharmacologic effects primarily upon the CNS, acting as suppressors of neuronal activity.[2, 24] They act in part by suppression of oxidative metabolism and more importantly by producing pre- or postsynaptic inhibitory neurotransmission.[25-30] Barbiturates promote hyperpolarization, thus reducing neuronal excitability, by increasing chloride conductance. There is a barbiturate receptor site on the gamma-aminobutyric acid (GABA) receptor supramolecular complex. GABA is the near-ubiquitous inhibitory neurotransmitter of the CNS that hyperpolarizes by increasing chloride conductance.[31, 32] Barbiturates act pharmacologically by facilitating this inhibitory GABAergic effect.[6] The barbiturates are commonly used as hypnotics and anticonvulsants. Thus they are in common usage and are readily available.

Acute intoxication presents lethargy, clumsiness, and slurred, thickened speech. While the patient is still awake, nystagmus may be present. If the ingested dose of medication is sufficiently high, coma will supervene, with associated hypotonia, hyporeflexia, and Babinski reflexes. Because of suppression of brain stem autonomic function, severe hypoventilation, hypotension, and bradycardia may occur. The pupils may react sluggishly to light but generally will be in midposition. Although oculocephalic reflexes and caloric responses may be preserved, they are absent in many patients.[1] *The preservation of pupillary reflexes in a comatose patient with extraocular motor palsy always should raise the suspicion of barbiturate intoxication.*

Although acute intoxication and coma are usually results of suicide attempts or gestures, chronic intoxication may occur in individuals who are habitual abusers of barbiturates, or in those who use barbiturates, particularly phenobarbital, for the treatment of epilepsy. In these patients may be seen the gradual development of difficulty with memory, increased sleepiness, slowness of speech, nystagmus, dysarthria, and ataxia.

It is believed that acute or chronic barbiturate intoxication will not permanently damage the central nervous system; however, hypotension, bradycardia, and hypoxia secondary to direct suppression of respiratory drive may lead to brain damage, resulting, in the mildest cases, in delay in regaining consciousness. In the severest cases, brain death caused by anoxic and ischemic cell death and possibly cerebral edema may occur.

Barbiturate withdrawal may be seen following cessation of drug use in epileptics or chronic barbiturate abusers. Patients may be agitated, confused, tremulous, combative, and disoriented, with incomprehensible speech. In addition, patients may develop withdrawal seizures and may develop status epilepticus, especially patients who have epilepsy for which they have been taking phenobarbital or primidone, which has phenobarbital as its major degradation product. Such seizure activity can be notoriously difficult to treat, although success has been reported with ethosuximide.[6] Many patients in withdrawal become psychotic, displaying paranoid delusions and hallucinations readily mistaken for functional psychosis. When present, seizures should alert the physician to an organic basis for the psychotic behavior and raise the suspicion of barbiturate withdrawal; however, differentiation from delirium tremens or withdrawal from other drugs such as ethchlorvynol, methaqualone, meprobamate, benzodiazepines, or amphetamine can be extremely difficult.

OTHER SEDATIVES

Although now less commonly seen in overdose cases than in the past, chloral hydrate, meprobamate, ethchlorvynol, and methaqualone may still be encountered as overdose agents. Each of these compounds is a potent central nervous system depressant. Lesser degrees of CNS intoxication result in lethargy, confusion, dysarthria, and gait ataxia. At higher doses, hypotonia, coma, and hypoventilation leading to apnea may be seen. In addition, each of these compounds may produce ophthalmoplegia. Chloral hydrate intoxication may also result in pinpoint pupils, thus resembling opiate intoxication.

Withdrawal from any of these drugs may result in acute confusional states with delirium and, particularly in the case of chloral hydrate and meprobamate, generalized convulsions.

OPIATES

Opiate intoxication is manifested primarily in the central nervous system, in which inhibition of autonomic function can be prominent. Although opiates generally suppress CNS function, respiratory suppression, even in less than toxic doses, is a prominent effect and is the usual cause of death from overdose. Following acute intoxication, slurred speech, lethargy, and clumsiness are seen, but at sufficiently high doses coma will supervene. Comatose patients almost always have markedly constricted pupils (however, an exceptional case may have midposition or even dilated pupils), shallow and irregular respiration, and even apnea, which often precedes cardiac asystole. The patient is flaccid and generally without tendon reflexes but may have Babinski reflexes and frontal release signs early in the progress of coma. Extraocular motor paralysis may be present, but oculocephalic or caloric responses can be elicited in many patients.

Generalized seizures are uncommon[19] and may be caused more by hypoxia or the presence of other epileptogenic contaminants than by direct effects of opiates.

The presence of pinpoint pupils, flaccid quadriplegia, apnea, and extraocular motor paralysis sometimes may be mistaken for infarction or hemorrhage in the brain stem. Although historically the two conditions should readily be separated, one obviously does not always have the advantage of a history. Parenteral administration of an opiate antagonist such as naloxone should allow differentiation of these two syndromes. Caution must be noted in the use of naloxone. Although this antagonist is preferable to nalorphone because it has no agonist activity, it has a comparatively short half-life and may have to be readministered frequently or else the patient, if unattended, again may develop coma and become apneic. Obviously, this is not a cause for concern if the patient has been intubated and is receiving assisted ventilation. This problem may be alleviated if the longer-acting opiate antagonist naltrexone is available.

Although a patient who reaches the hospital alive after opiate ingestion may survive and have no neurologic sequelae, several complications may lead to brain damage. Patients may have brain damage from sustained hypoxemia, hypotension, and acidosis prior to securing an airway. Patients may also incur aspiration of stomach contents into the trachea. This is particularly a problem in heroin addicts,[33] who sometimes aspirate milk given by other addicts in the belief that this is an effective means of overdose treatment. Patients with opiate overdose also may develop pulmonary edema, further complicating adequate brain oxygenation.[33, 34] An additional source of irreversible brain damage in the heroin addict may be mycotic cerebral embolization as a result of endocarditis, so that the patient may develop embolic infarction, brain abscess, meningitis, or even mycotic aneurysm and hemorrhage. Lastly, anoxic-ischemic damage may explain prolonged coma or continued obtundation when one would have anticipated the patient's regaining consciousness.

Opiate withdrawal also can produce prominent abnormalities, with insomnia, restlessness, yawning, tremulousness, confusion, agitation, piloerection ("turkey skin"), pupillary dilation, diaphoresis, nausea, abdominal pain, and diarrhea. Although this is most commonly seen in the addict withdrawing "cold turkey," features of physiologic dependence may be seen in withdrawal in any patient who has received opiates for a prolonged period of time. This is a particular problem to neonates whose mothers are heroin or methadone users.[35, 36] These drugs readily cross the placenta, and the fetus may develop biologic dependence. Withdrawal ensues generally within 24 to 36 hours after birth. The neonates become restless and agitated, with frequent yawning, sneezing, crying, tremulousness, vomiting, diarrhea, and, in some cases, generalized convulsions.

GLUTETHIMIDE

Although frequently discussed in conjunction with the barbiturates, this drug deserves separate consideration. Unlike the barbiturates, there is a poor correlation between plasma levels of glutethimide and the clinical state.[37]

Although such observations are usually attributed to a drug having a larger volume of distribution—that is, strong tissue-binding—it is likely that metabolites of glutethimide contribute to the clinical features of intoxication, particularly the prolonged period of unconsciousness frequently observed after glutethimide is taken in larger doses.

At one time it was suggested that an erratic or recurrent intestinal absorption of glutethimide was responsible for the biphasic mental status changes seen after overdose, such as patients regaining consciousness and relapsing into coma without having ingested additional drugs.[1] A 4-OH derivative of glutethimide has been identified that may explain some of the unusual features of glutethimide poisoning.[38, 39] In animal studies it has been demonstrated that the 4-OH derivative is twice as lethal as glutethimide.[38] Furthermore, the depth of coma correlates better with the sum of glutethimide and 4-OH metabolite concentrations in the blood.[37]

A frequently abused drug in the past, glutethimide has poisoning features in common with barbiturate overdose: lethargy, dysarthria, ataxia, nystagmus, occasional extraocular paresis, and eventually respiratory suppression and coma.

BENZODIAZEPINES

As a group of drugs, the benzodiazepines produce effects on the central nervous system that vary little from one compound to the next, although significant differences in potency certainly exist. Most of these drugs have anxiety-relieving, sedative, and hypnotic qualities as well as varying degrees of anticonvulsant potency and spasmolytic effect on skeletal muscle. These drugs are widely prescribed, thus availability is a major reason for their common use in intentional as well as accidental overdose.

The benzodiazepines are indirect agonists of gamma-aminobutyric acid (GABA),[40–44] a widely distributed, largely presynaptic inhibitory neurotransmitter within the central nervous system. The GABA receptor is a supramolecular complex that contains a benzodiazepine receptor site that facilitates GABAergic action. This property is responsible for the CNS-depressing potential of these drugs. In low doses, many of these compounds allay anxiety, but at higher doses, dysarthria, confusion, sedation, lethargy, and eventually marked suppression of the level of consciousness leading to coma may occur as a result of depression of the reticular activating system of the midbrain. In addition to impairment of consciousness, ataxia and particularly nystagmus are seen. Effects on pupillary function are negligible, and extraocular muscle paresis rarely occurs. Respiratory depression and marked hypotension and bradycardia may occur, particularly in older patients. Patients often develop apnea after intravenous diazepam for status epilepticus; thus, caution is advised when using diazepam in this fashion.

Although few deaths are actually proved to result from benzodiazepine overdose, they do occur, particularly with concomitant use of alcohol, barbiturates, or opiates.[45, 46]

The benzodiazepines have an enterohepatic circulation[44] that can lead to delayed secondary peaks in plasma concentration, prolonging the duration of intoxication. Concurrent use with ethanol also may prolong the duration of intoxication.

It has become increasingly apparent that chronic abuse of benzodiazepines is common, with the attendant problems of the development of tolerance and withdrawal following cessation of their use.[47, 48] Thus patients may be seen with severe anxiety, irritability, tremulousness, agitation, depression, insomnia, and acute psychosis. Some of the benzodiazepines are potent anticonvulsants; it is not surprising that benzodiazepine withdrawal can be associated with seizures, which on rare occasions can evolve into severe repetitive generalized convulsions, or status epilepticus.

TRICYCLIC ANTIDEPRESSANT DRUGS

The tricyclic antidepressants are widely employed in the treatment of affective disorders and also have been found useful in the treatment of some patients with the narcolepsy-cataplexy syndrome.

Because most of the people with access to the tricyclics are depressed, the likelihood of their being used in suicide attempts is high, with very significant potential for life-threatening toxicity. However, the incidence of significant toxic effects in patients treated under controlled conditions is also high. In the Boston Collaborative Drug Surveillance Program, 4.6 per cent of patients developed acute psychosis, hallucinations, disorientation, and agitation, as well as autonomic abnormalities.[49]

The spectrum of neurologic abnormalities seen in patients intoxicated with the tricyclic antidepressants is a result primarily of their autonomic effects. By blocking the reuptake of biogenic amines,[50–52] these drugs facilitate the actions of noradrenergic and serotonergic neurons. The drugs also have prominent anticholinergic properties,[53–55] blocking the action of the parasympathetic nervous system.

In patients who are mildly intoxicated, autonomic side effects include dry mouth and pharynx, dry skin or diaphoresis, hyperthermia, urinary hesitancy or retention, and constipation. In some patients, hypertension also may be seen. As mentioned, acute confusional state, restlessness, agitation, and psychosis with hallucinations all may be seen. A patient with psychosis and the combination of prominent sympathetic nervous system hyperactivity and prominent anticholinergic features should raise the suspicion of tricyclic antidepressant as well as amphetamine or cocaine intoxication. In doses sufficient to produce coma, the presence of severe tachycardia and other rhythm disturbances should suggest strongly the possibility of tricyclic overdose, particularly if associated with pupillary dilation, hyperthermia, and hyperreflexia. Deepening coma is associated with respiratory depression, hypotension, and in some cases extraocular muscle paralysis, hallucinations, and eventually flaccidity and areflexia. In patients reaching the hospital alive, clearly the greatest threat to survival is cardiac toxicity.[56, 57] Recent evidence suggests that the depression in consciousness produced by the tricyclic antidepressants is due also to an anticholinergic mechanism.[58, 59]

Generalized seizures are a major potential side effect of all the tricyclic antidepressants.[11, 13, 17, 60] The mortality rate associated with seizures in such patients may be as high as 10 percent.[17] Although most seizures in these patients are brief and require no anticonvulsant medications, patients may have repetitive seizures or status epilepticus and may greatly increase the cardiovascular morbidity of tricyclic overdose.[17] The epileptogenicity of the tricyclic drugs may derive from their inhibition of conductance through the chloride channel of the GABA receptor, GABAergic mechanisms for seizure prevention depending upon increased chloride conductance.[61] It is not surprising that benzodiazepines, which are GABA agonists, are the drugs of choice for the treatment of seizures in tricyclic antidepressant intoxication.[17]

The simultaneous use of alcohol or sedatives may have an additive effect, thus significantly increasing the risk in the patient intoxicated with the tricyclic antidepressants. Because the tricyclic antidepressants may influence cardiac output, producing hypotension as well as respiratory depression, ischemic anoxic damage to the brain is a serious potential complication of overdose and may lead to severe permanent morbidity even if the patient survives the overdose.

AMPHETAMINE AND RELATED DRUGS

Amphetamine, methamphetamine, dextroamphetamine, and related compounds have potent sympathomimetic effects, exerted by their enhancement of catecholamine release and inhibition of their reuptake by catecholaminergic neurons.[62–65] Although the accepted clinical indications for their use have been narrowed, they still find wide illicit use and are still used in treatment of narcolepsy[66, 67] and some hyperactive children.[68]

Amphetamines have prominent stimulating effects; thus, intoxicated patients are energetic, euphoric, aggressive, and fast talking. When they are taken in sufficient doses, patients may not sleep for days at a time. This insomniac property leads to their extensive abuse by students and by individuals whose occupations require long periods of wakefulness.

The prominent sympathomimetic features of these drugs produce dry mouth, mydriasis, and reduced pupillary accommodation leading to difficulty with near vision. Patients develop tremor and marked hyperreflexia, as well as tachycardia and hypertension. At sufficiently high doses, marked agitation, delirium, hallucinations, seizures, or coma may occur. In the comatose patient, hyperreflexia, pupillary dilation, hypertension, and tachycardia are suggestive of amphetamine overdose, but differentiation may be difficult from patients intoxicated with the tricyclic antidepressants or other sympathomimetics, which may produce a similar autonomic picture because of their facilitation of noradrenergic activity and their prominent inhibition of parasympathetic nervous system function (antimuscarinic effect). Chronic abuse may lead to a syndrome indistinguishable from paranoid schizophrenia.[69, 70]

COCAINE

Cocaine is a potent sympathomimetic compound that appears to exert its sympathetic potentiation by blocking presynaptic reuptake of norepinephrine.[62, 71, 72] In low doses, cocaine acts clinically as a stimulant, with attendant increase in motor activity, frequently a sense of increased strength, and the production of euphoria. Undoubtedly these features are among the major reasons for the explosive increase in its popularity as a substance of abuse.[73, 74] Toxic side effects of cocaine include hyperpyrexia, hypertension, and tachycardia.[75] More serious cardiac complications include intractable arrhythmias and myocardial infarction.[76] Seizures are among the commonly observed serious neurologic complications of cocaine abuse.[14, 16, 18, 19, 75, 77] Diazepam appears to reduce cocaine-induced seizures effectively and the attendant mortality.[78] In experimental models, cocaine can promote epileptogenicity even at "subconvulsive" doses.[79] Neurologic and psychiatric complications are the primary presentations for patients who are hospitalized because of cocaine intoxication.[19] Seizures are the most common major neurologic complication, with focal cerebral infarction,[14, 80] syncope, and severe headache[19] frequently seen. Psychosis manifested by hallucinations, severe anxiety, agitation, and depression are commonly observed serious complications.[14] Furthermore, there is poor correlation between amount used, route of administration or prior use of cocaine, and the occurrence of these serious neuropsychiatric side effects.[14, 19]

Even passive exposure of young children to volatile free-based cocaine has resulted in seizures, lethargy, and ataxia.[81] Seizures also have been produced in neonates receiving cocaine in breast-fed milk.[82]

At sufficiently high doses, cocaine, independent of its epileptogenicity, suppresses the reticular activating system, producing coma and death. Among the less serious side effects of cocaine use are tremor, confusion, irritability, hyperthermia, mydriasis, sweating, palpitations, insomnia, and excoriation of the skin. The subjective effects of cocaine, as described by drug abuse patients, are so reminiscent of amphetamine[83] and related compounds that it is not certain there are any significant differences in affect or mood by the latter drugs, except that the time course of action of cocaine, particularly free-base or crack, is significantly shorter.[84, 85] Cocaine may act as a mood elevator secondary to central norepinephrine potentiation. In patients who use cocaine chronically, intoxication may be similar in appearance to that of acute, undifferentiated schizophrenia.[69]

ANTIDOPAMINERGICS

Antidopaminergics are the most important antipsychotic agents and are therefore available to patients in whom there is higher risk of overdose. These drugs include phenothiazines, such as chlorpromazine, thioridazine, fluphenazine, trifluperazine, and perphenazine, and the butyrophenones haloperidol and loxapine. Because of their antidopaminergic effects, these drugs can produce the features of parkinsonism, with rigidity, hypokinesia, and tremor, particularly in chronically intoxicated patients. In acute intoxication, lethargy, somnolence, occasionally coma, and, on rare occasion, seizures are seen. Although death as a result of overdose is extremely rare, the duration of coma, when it does occur, can be long and is largely the result of the large volume of distribution of these drugs, reflecting the avid binding to dopamine receptors within the brain and thus their slow rate of removal by excretion and hepatic degradation.

ANTICHOLINESTERASES

Anticholinesterases inhibit the hydrolysis of acetylcholine and thus produce symptoms of excessive parasympathetic activity and skeletal neuromuscular hyperirritability. The reversible competitive cholinesterase inhibitors that do not enter the central nervous system include pyridostigmine and neostigmine, which are used in the treatment of myasthenia gravis, as well as the short-acting drug edrophonium. The toxic effects of these drugs are restricted to the peripheral nervous system. Physostigmine, a competitive, reversible anticholinesterase that enters the brain, and the noncompetitive lipid-soluble anticholinesterase organophosphate insecticides have potent central nervous system effects.[86–89]

Pupillary constriction, excessive sweating, bradycardia, hypotension, bronchospasm, and excessive pulmonary secretions, as well as gastrointestinal hypermotility, are among the important peripheral parasympathetic effects, which, when present, should raise the suspicion of anticholinesterase poisoning. These drugs also affect nicotinic cholinergic function (skeletal muscle) and, as a result of excessive cholinergic activity, fasciculations and eventually increasing neuromuscular weakness produce paralysis of the extremities and respiratory muscles. When combined with the muscarinic toxicity that produces airway obstruction, respiratory muscle failure and severe hypoxia may occur from anticholinesterase neuromuscular toxicity.

Physostigmine and the centrally active organophosphates may also produce severe alteration in brain function, including confusion, lethargy, central depression of respiration, seizures, and coma.

The presence of coma, with or without seizure, in a patient with small pupils, bradycardia, and skeletal muscle fasciculation strongly suggests anticholinesterase poisoning.

ANTICHOLINERGIC DRUGS

Anticholinergic drugs, which generally interfere with the interaction between acetylcholine and its receptors, may have striking effects on central nervous system function when they are able to enter the brain, as well as prominent inhibitory effects on the parasympathetic nervous system peripherally. Atropine, which was commonly used for the treatment of heart block prior to the advent of cardiac pacemaker insertion, produces pupillary dilation, dryness of mucous membranes, and increased heart rate at low doses. It produces dry, hot skin, fever, and encephalopathy in cardiac patients when used in excessive doses and also confusion, agitation, and psychosis that could be accompanied by hallucinations.[90–94]

Although atropine intoxication is no longer commonly encountered, toxicity due to centrally acting anticholinergics such as benztropine and trihexphenidyl is still occasionally seen. Although their use in the treatment of parkinsonism has greatly diminished, they are still used in the treatment of neuroleptic-induced tardive dyskinesia and bradykinesia.[94, 95] Recently, scopolamine has become popular for the treatment of motion sickness. When used in excessive doses, or when the dosage is increased too rapidly, confusion, lethargy, lightheadedness, agitation, and hallucinations may be seen. In severe overdose, coma may occur. This is consistent with the observation that the coma seen in tricyclic antidepressant overdose may be due to an anticholinergic effect, since the coma has been reported reversed with centrally acting physostigmine.[59]

SALICYLATES

Salicylate poisoning is commonly seen in both children and adults. Many patients, especially elderly individuals with chronic illness, can be severely intoxicated from chronic drug use. In intoxicated patients, lassitude, lightheadedness, and tinnitus are among the earliest complaints, with the tinnitus sometimes going on to complete deafness. Salicylates act directly on central nervous system respiratory centers to increase respiratory drive, which in turn produces respiratory alkalosis—this, in part, being responsible for the complaints of paresthesia of the digits and the carpopedal spasm sometimes observed.

Patients may develop agitation, confusion, hyperactivity, and combativeness and may become psychotic with hallucinations, seizures, and coma.[96, 97]

As has been frequently described, the respiratory alkalosis of salicylate intoxication has an associated metabolic acidosis. Severe acidosis significantly worsens the neurologic prognosis in such patients,[97, 98] since acidemia promotes an increase in the dissociated fraction of salicylate that enters the brain, thus increasing the cytotoxic potential of the drug. One way in which acidemia may occur is when the patient is taking other drugs such as barbiturates, which are CNS depressants, thus decreasing the respiratory drive produced by salicylates. Once a patient with salicylate poisoning becomes comatose, hyperventilation and an invariably abnormal acid-base balance are major clues to salicylism. In addition, if the patient is acidemic, the possibility of polydrug intoxication must be considered. Correction of the acidemia is essential to prevent further increases in salicylate levels within the brain.

ACETAMINOPHEN (PARACETAMOL) AND PHENACETIN

These commonly employed analgesics have been incriminated increasingly in drug overdose and in parts of Europe have become a leading cause of death due to overdose. Their ready availability as nonprescription drugs increases the opportunity for their improper use.

Many deaths in acute ingestion result from hepatic necrosis and intractable hepatic encephalopathy, with attendant autonomic nervous system dysfunction producing severe hypotension and respiratory failure. In severe intoxication, hepatic encephalopathy first makes its appearance several days after ingestion. The hepatic encephalopathy is heralded by lethargy, slurred speech, tremulousness, nystagmus, asterixis, and coma.

Once these patients develop coma owing to hepatic failure, the prognosis for survival is poor despite the institution of aggressive hepatic failure management. Once acetaminophen- or phenacetin-induced hepatic failure results in deep coma, there is virtually no chance of the patient regaining consciousness.[99] This only serves to emphasize the importance of introducing sulfhydryl-containing compounds and perhaps utilizing extracorporeal means for lowering plasma concentration of these drugs.[100, 101]

In addition to the toxic encephalopathy produced by hepatic failure, cerebral hemorrhage and subdural hematoma also may be present because of the bleeding disorder resulting from hepatic failure.

DIGITALIS

Although the major manifestations of digitalis poisoning are in cardiovascular function, striking central nervous system effects may be present and include nausea and vomiting, headache, lethargy, agitation, confusion, delirium, and hallucinations; signs of acute diffuse brain dysfunction may occur, as may seizures. Paresthesias and pain may also occur in the face and extremities. Visual symptoms are also prominent features of digitalis intoxication, particularly chromatopsia (usually with yellow vision). Halos, scotomata, and occasionally diplopia are also described most commonly, but not exclusively.[102, 103]

MARIJUANA

A series of psychoactive compounds called cannabinoids are present in the *Cannabis sativa* plant, of which Δ-9-tetrahydrocannabinol is probably the most potent. Cannabis generally produces a state of euphoria and relaxation but also impairment of short-term memory. Time span perception frequently is distorted, and individuals report that only several minutes seem to have been a much longer time span.[104–106] Although visual perceptions may not be distorted, they may have an unreal quality, and, when combined with the possibility of impaired judgment and coordination,[107, 108] operation of an automobile or other machinery can be dangerous, particularly when its use is combined with alcohol,[109, 110] which frequently occurs. In most cases, mood changes or levels of activity or other signs of CNS alteration are unlikely to be sufficiently characteristic to suggest alone that an individual is intoxicated.

Under less common circumstances, very large amounts of cannabis are administered with striking psychologic effects, including frank organic psychotic reactions that include severe anxiety, confusion, delusions, and hallucinations.[111, 112] When combined with tachycardia and increased systolic blood pressure, cannabis may be considered as a possible cause of organic psychosis, but this is in no way characteristic of cannabis, since a variety of sympathomimetic agents like amphetamines and cocaine can produce the same picture. Marked conjunctival erythema may be of diagnostic help, since it is so characteristic of cannabis intoxication.

Withdrawal syndromes following cessation of chronic cannabis use are not usually encountered, although irritability and restlessness have been reported by individuals who have ceased regular marijuana usage.

LYSERGIC ACID DIETHYLAMIDE

One of the best-known psychedelic compounds, lysergic acid diethylamide (LSD), is capable of producing striking alterations in perception, with heightened spiritual or religious feelings and experiences.[113–115] These subjective effects are not limited to LSD; patients have reported similar experiences with the use of psilocybin, mescaline, and STP (2,-5-dimethyoxy-4-methylamphetamine). Although the use of LSD seems to have diminished, intoxication as a result of use of this compound may still be seen. The syndrome consists of particularly severe anxiety or panic reactions, in which individuals experience frightening feelings. On occasion, patients may have acute organic psychoses, with paranoid ideation and vivid hallucinations. Such patients frequently resemble acute schizophrenic patients.[116]

PHENCYCLIDINE

Phencyclidine (PCP), after many years of popularity, has become somewhat less common as a drug of abuse.

Originally employed as an anesthetic, this use was soon abandoned because PCP produced acute postoperative psychosis in some patients. Smoked, snorted, or injected, PCP has a wide range of effects on the central nervous system, and the acutely intoxicated patient may present confusion, severe agitation, paranoia, striking distortion of perceptions, bizarre behavior, hallucinations, seizures, or coma.

At lower doses, confusion, ataxia, and nystagmus may be the presenting symptoms. Although these features characterize intoxication with a large group of drugs, severe, sustained, or intermittent muscle hypertonus may strongly suggest PCP as the responsible compound, especially when associated with hyperthermia and cutaneous erythema. In more severe cases of PCP intoxication, severe depression in the level of consciousness may produce coma, respiratory depression, and death.[117–119]

Withdrawal from PCP may be associated with depression, tremors, twitches, and seizures.

Although seizures have been reported frequently in association with PCP use,[19] there are recent reports that it has anticonvulsant properties.[120] The recent demonstration that PCP blocks facilitative glutamate receptors in rat hippocampus[121] is consistent with potential anticonvulsant properties.

METHANOL

Methyl alcohol poisoning can result in the rapid development of coma and death without preceding lethargy, confusion, somnolence, or dysarthria—all frequently encountered signs in patients with moderate CNS intoxication resulting from other drugs. Patients may complain, however, of severe headache, abdominal pain, dyspnea, vertigo, and visual loss, the latter being a very important clue to making a diagnosis of methanol poisoning. Methanol is metabolized into formic acid and formaldehyde; these compounds are responsible for the signs and symptoms of methanol poisoning. The presence of acidosis, important in the diagnosis, and hyperemia of the optic discs also should suggest methanol intoxication. Many patients are blind or have serious visual impairment, probably secondary to destruction of the retina by formaldehyde. In addition to coma, severely intoxicated patients may have apnea, muscle rigidity, and generalized convulsions.[122–125]

ETHYL ALCOHOL

Ethanol is undoubtedly the most commonly employed intoxicant. Its use is socially acceptable and is actually part of certain social circumstances. Only age restricts availability, and even this barrier to use is diminished by its presence and ready access in most homes in the Western world. Ethanol is a CNS depressant but may produce seemingly paradoxic stimulation, really the result of the dysinhibiting effects of depression of portions of the central nervous system. Ethanol depresses both cortical and reticular activating system neurons,[126, 127] thus providing several sites of inhibition that may result in depression of level of consciousness.

Mildly intoxicated patients may be talkative and expansive. However, since ethanol use may lead to reduced inhibition of impulses and feelings, some individuals may become aggressive or abusive. At higher levels of intoxication, confusion, disorientation, dysarthria, ataxia (initially for fine motor coordination but later in truncal and gait control), lethargy, and even coma may occur.[128, 129] Although the majority of people with ethanol intoxication can safely "sleep it off," serious complications—including hypotension, aspiration pneumonia, and direct respiratory depression leading to hypoxic brain damage—may occur.[130]

Of great danger to patients is simultaneous use of ethanol and other drugs,[131] particularly barbiturates, benzodiazepines, and opiates. This problem is commonly observed in both suicide attempts and recreational uses of ethanol. Severe respiratory depression and hypotension associated with cortical and brain stem reticulum suppression, resulting from the additive effects of ethanol and other drugs, may be fatal. *Ethanol use always should be ascertained in any intoxicated patient, since its presence so greatly increases the risk of serious brain injury or death resulting from intoxication with other drugs.*

Because of ataxia and sometimes because of ethanol-induced aggressive behavior, patients who ingest alcohol acutely or chronically may sustain serious head injury. Subdural hematoma, particularly in chronic alcoholics, may be present and not appreciated clinically because the ethanol intoxication is assumed to be the cause of altered mental status.

The nutritional deficiency so commonly found in chronic alcoholics may result in hypovitaminosis. Inadequate brain stores of thiamine may result in acute psychosis, manifested by an acute confusional delirium state that can have extremely serious consequences if not appreciated clinically, with resultant permanent brain damage and even death. The presence of prominent nystagmus and the development of extraocular paresis should suggest thiamine deficiency as the cause of the psychosis (Wernicke's encephalopathy).

Lastly, ethanol withdrawal can also produce an acute psychosis, with confusion; rapid, incoherent or mumbled speech; marked tremulousness; vivid hallucinations; and seizures. Again, failure to recognize ethanol withdrawal (delirium tremens) can result in death. Seizures in an ethanol user are not always indicative of delirium tremens, since patients who have a seizure disorder or a clinically latent seizure focus also may have seizures following ethanol use.

HEAVY METALS

Lead

Except under conditions of intoxication, lead is present in the central nervous system in small quantities. Thus, there is little likelihood of observing effects of acute lead intoxication on the central nervous system. When it does occur, musculoskeletal weakness is the major manifestation. Lead intoxication occurs more commonly after chronic exposure, and the portion of the nervous system affected appears to be largely determined by age. In adults, a pure motor neuropathy,[132] sometimes simulating amyotrophic lateral sclerosis, is seen.[133] The greatest danger is to children in whom lead intoxication can produce severe encephalopathy. Since the syndrome is frequently seen in young children who may have difficulty describing their symptoms, the presentation is often vague and may result in a missed diagnosis unless there is a high index of suspicion of lead intoxication. Irritability with frequent crying, restlessness, deterioration in speech and motor skills, and headache when elicitable, are all important clues to the diagnosis of lead encephalopathy in children. Seizures, opisthotonos, obtundation, and eventually coma may be seen in more advanced cases, reflecting cerebral edema, necrosis, and hemorrhage, at least in part due to the damaging effects of lead on CNS blood vessels as well as subsequent blood-brain barrier alterations.[134–137]

Although most lead intoxication has been the result of exposure to air pollution from auto emission, lead in paints, or illicitly produced alcohol, patients also have developed severe CNS syndromes from direct exposure to tetraethyl and tetramethyl lead in gasoline. Thus accidental drinking of gasoline or the use of gasoline as a cooking fuel may also result in acute lead poisoning manifested by confusion, agitation, anxiety, anorexia, nausea, vomiting, headache, and weakness.

Mercury

Although acute mercury intoxication may produce CNS dysfunction, this is uncommon. The most striking features of nervous system damage occur in chronic exposure, as when industrial waste enters the food chain. In chronic mercury poisoning are seen mood swings, hyperirritability, agitation, insomnia, confusion, ataxia, and tremors of extremities, all of a cerebellar type, and also vasomotor instability with alternating cutaneous hyperemia and pallor.[135–141]

Arsenic

Arsenic intoxication generally arises from chronic exposure caused by industrial or environmental pollution. An exception to this is in individuals receiving arsenicals for the treatment of parasitism. Arsenic characteristically produces peripheral neuropathy. I have seen one patient with peripheral neuropathy and dementia who had a lifelong occupational exposure to arsenic. When the central nervous system is affected, as after oral ingestion of arsenic, headache, confusion, seizures, and coma may be seen.[142]

CARBON MONOXIDE

Carbon monoxide poisoning in the United States most commonly results from excessive exposure to automobile exhaust. Patients may arrive in the emergency room in coma or with less severe depression in levels of consciousness subsequent to being resuscitated, without apparent brain damage but with residual symptoms of headache, lightheadedness, or confusion. However, some patients suffer permanent neurologic damage, particularly to the basal ganglia and hippocampus, producing a parkinson-like syndrome of rigidity, tremor, and bradykinesia as well as memory loss, disorientation, or other features of dementia.[143–145]

In addition, some patients with severe carbon monoxide poisoning may make a seemingly unremarkable recovery only to deteriorate neurologically several weeks later.[146–148] These patients may present features of diffuse cerebral dysfunction, such as confusion, agitation, and disorientation, and may deteriorate to a state of akinetic mutism and rigidity, spasticity, and urinary incontinence. Although striking, this syndrome of delayed neurologic deterioration is rare; the majority of patients either die of asphyxia or make an uneventful recovery.[149, 150]

CYANIDE

Cyanide poisoning results from binding to and inactivation of cytochrome oxidase in mitochondria. Most experimental evidence suggests that there is neuronal sparing and that central nervous system white matter is the major site of damage[151–153] in the absence of hypoxia or ischemia.[153, 154] It has been suggested that the selective vulnerability of white matter to cyanide may be the result of the lower levels of cytochrome oxidase in white than in gray matter.[155]

If taken in large enough doses by humans, rapid loss of consciousness, convulsions, and death will occur within several minutes. At lower doses, confusion and agitation may be followed by the development of ataxia, flushed skin, and eventually coma and seizures.

Chronic intoxication also may occur, and it has been suggested that the optic atrophy seen in some alcoholics who smoke (toxic amblyopia) is due to chronic cyanide poisoning, possibly resulting from vitamin B_{12} deficiency. Cassava root is also a source of cyanide, which can lead to chronic intoxication when ingested and which produces optic atrophy, deafness, and weakness of the extremities.

Amygdalin use also may result in cyanide poisoning; in one case it resulted in transient extraocular muscle paralysis.[156]

Cyanide and thiocyanate may both accumulate when sodium nitroprusside is used chronically in the treatment of hypertension, since these are both products of drug degradation. Confusion, disorientation, and frank psychosis, all reversible with cessation or decrease in drug dosage, may occur.

References

1. Plum F, Posner, JB: The Diagnosis of Stupor and Coma. 3rd ed. Philadelphia, FA Davis, 1980.
2. Quastel JH: Effects of anesthetics, depressants, and tranquilizers on brain metabolism. *In* Elliott KAC, Page IH, Quastel JH (eds): Neurochemistry: The Chemistry of Brain and Nerve. 2nd ed. Springfield, IL, Charles C Thomas, 1962.
3. Moruzzi G, Magoun HW: Brain stem reticular formation and activation of the EEG. Electroencephalogr Clin Neurophysiol *1*:455, 1949.
4. Magoun HW: The Waking Brain. 2nd ed. Springfield, IL, Charles C Thomas, 1963.
5. Moruzzi G: The sleep-waking cycle. Rev Physiol *64*:1, 1972.
6. Sandoval MR, Palermo-Neto J: GABAergic influences on phenobarbital withdrawal–induced convulsions. Gen Pharmacol *17*:431, 1986.
7. Ghadririan AM, Gauthier S, Wong T: Convulsions in patients abruptly withdrawn from clonazepam while receiving neuroleptic medication. Am J Psychiatr *144*:686, 1987.
8. Theodore WH, Porter RJ, Raubertas RF: Seizures during barbiturate withdrawal: Relation to blood level. Ann Neurol *22*:644, 1987.
9. Young GP, Roves C, Murphy C, Dailey RH: Intravenous phenobarbital for alcohol withdrawal and convulsions. Ann Emerg Med *16*:847, 1987.
10. Wilson MA, Gallagher DW: Ro 15-1788–induced seizures in rats continually exposed to diazepam for long periods. Epilep Res *2*:14, 1988.
11. Peterson SL, Trzeciakowski JP, St. Mary JS: Chronic but not acute treatment with antidepressants enhances the electroconvulsive seizure response in rats. Neuropharmacology *24*:941, 1985.

12. Czuczwar SJ, Turski WA, Ikonomidou C, Turski L: Aminophylline and CGS 8216 reverse the protective action of diazepam against electroconvulsions in mice. Epilepsia *26*:693, 1985.
13. Edward JG, Long SK, Sedgwick EM, Wheal HV: Antidepressants and convulsive seizures: Clinical electroencephalographic, and pharmacologic aspects. Clin Neuropharmacol *9*:329, 1986.
14. Lowenstein DH, Massa SM, Rowbotham MC, et al: Acute neurologic and psychiatric complications associated with cocaine abuse. Am J Med *83*:841, 1987.
15. Blake KV, Massey KL, Hendeles L, et al: Relative efficacy of phenytoin and phenobarbital for the prevention of theophylline-induced seizures in mice. Ann Emerg Med *17*:1024, 1988.
16. Choy-Kwong M, Lipton RB: Seizures in hospitalized cocaine abusers. Neurology *39*:425, 1989.
17. Ellison DW, Pentel PR: Clinical features and consequences of seizures due to cyclic antidepressant overdose. Am J Emerg Med *7*:5, 1989.
18. Schwartz RH: Seizures associated with smoking crack—a survey of adolescent crack smokers. West J Med *150*:213, 1989.
19. Aldredge BK, Lowenstein DH, Simon RP: Seizures associated with recreational drug abuse. Neurology *39*:1037, 1989.
20. Cho I, Berton JM, Hopkins L: Moxalactam myoclonus, seizures and encephalopathy. Drug Intell Clin Pharm *20*:223, 1986.
21. Tse CS, Madura AJ, Vera FH: Suspected cefonicid-induced seizure (letter). Clin Pharm *5*:629, 1986.
22. Williams PD, Bennett DB, Comereski CR: Animal model for evaluating the convulsive liability of beta-lactam antibiotics. Antimicrob Agents Chemother *32*:758, 1988.
23. Forrence E, Covinsky JO, Mullen C: A seizure induced by concurrent lidocaine-tocainide therapy—is it just a case of additive toxicity? Drug Intel Clin Pharm *20*:56, 1986.
24. Smith AR: Barbiturate protection in cerebral hypoxia. Anesthesiology *47*:285, 1977.
25. Polc P, Heafely W: Effects of two benzodiazepines, phenobarbitone and baclofen, on synaptic transmission in the cat cuneate nucleus. Naunym Schmiedebergs Arch Pharmacol *294*:121, 1976.
26. Cutler RWP, Markowitz D, Dudzinsky DS: The effect of barbiturates on (3H)GABA transport in rat cerebral cortex slices. Brain Res *81*:189, 1974.
27. Sutton I, Simmonds MA: Effects of acute and chronic pentobarbitone on the γ-aminobutyric acid system in rat brain. Biochem Pharmacol *23*:1801, 1974.
28. Ransom BR, Barker JL: Pentobarbital selectivity enhances GABA-mediated post-synaptic inhibition in tissue cultured mouse spinal neurons. Brain Res *114*:530, 1976.
29. Nicoll RA: Pentobarbital: Differential postsynaptic actions on sympathetic ganglion cells. Science *199*:451, 1978.
30. Norton PRE: The effects of drugs on barbiturate withdrawal. Convulsions in the rat. J Pharmacol *22*:763, 1970.
31. Cohan S: Central nervous system disturbances. *In* Haddad LM, Winchester JF (eds): Clinical Management of Poisoning and Drug Overdose. Philadelphia, WB Saunders, 1983.
32. Braunwald E, Isselbaeher KJ, Petersdorf RG, Wilson JD, Martin JB, Fauci AS: Harrison's Principles of Internal Medicine. 11th ed. New York, McGraw-Hill, 1987.
33. Duberstein JL, Kaufman DM: A clinical study of an epidemic of heroin intoxication and heroin-induced pulmonary edema. Am J Med *51*:704, 1971.
34. Steinberg AD, Karliner JS: The clinical spectrum of heroin-induced pulmonary edema. Arch Intern Med *122*:122, 1968.
35. Zelson C, Lee SJ, Casalino M: Neonatal narcotic addiction: Comparative effects of maternal intake of heroin and methadone. N Engl J Med *289*:1226, 1973.
36. Stimmel B, Adamson K: Narcotic dependency in pregnancy. Methadone maintenance compared to use of street drugs. JAMA *235*:1121, 1976.
37. Curry SH, Riddall D, Gordon JS, et al: Disposition of glutethimide in man. Clin Pharmacol Ther *12*:849, 1971.
38. Hansen AR, Kennedy KA, Ambre JJ, et al: Glutethimide poisoning. A metabolite contributes to morbidity and mortality. N Engl J Med *292*:250, 1975.
39. Crow JW, Lain P, Bochner F, Azarnoff DL: Glutethimide and 4-OH glutethimide: Pharmacokinetics and effect on performance in man. Clin Pharmacol Ther *22*:458, 1977.
40. Costa E, Guidotti A, Mao CC, Suria A: New concepts on the mechanism of action of benzodiazepines. Life Sci *17*:167, 1975.
41. Haefley W, Kulcsar A, Mohler H, et al: Possible involvement of GABA in the central actions of benzodiazepines. *In* Costa E, Greengard P (eds): Mechanisms of Action of Benzodiazepines. New York, Raven Press, 1975, p 131.
42. Snyder SH, Enna SJ, Young AB: Brain mechanisms associated with therapeutic actions of benzodiazepines: Focus on neurotransmitters. Am J Psychiat *134*:662, 1977.
43. Bloom FE: Neural mechanisms of benzodiazepine actions. Am J Psychiat *134*:669, 1977.
44. Costa E, Guidotti A, Toffano G: Molecular mechanisms mediating the action of diazepam on GABA receptors. Br J Psychiat *133*:239, 1978.
45. Mendelson WB, Goodwin DW, Hill SY, Reichman JD: The morning after: Residual EEG effects of triazolam and flurazepam alone and in combination with alcohol. Curr Ther Res *19*:155, 1976.
46. Ascione FJ: Benzodiazepines with alcohol. Drug Ther *9*, 1978.
47. Greenblatt DJ, Shader RI: Benzodiazepines. N Engl J Med *291*:1239, 1974.
48. Misra PC: Nitrazepam (Magadon) dependence. Br J Psychiat *126*:81, 1975.
49. Boston Collaborative Drug Surveillance Program: Adverse reactions to the tricyclic-antidepressant drugs. Lancet *1*:529, 1972.
50. Schildkraut JJ: Current status of the catecholamine hypothesis of the affective disorders. *In* Lipton MA, DiMascio A, Killarn K (eds): Psychopharmacology: A Generation of Progress. New York, Raven Press, 1978, p 1223.
51. van Praag HM: Amine hypotheses of affective disorders. *In* Iversen LL, Iversen SD, Snyder S (eds): Handbook of Psychopharmacology. Vol 13. New York, Plenum Press, 1978, p 187.
52. Murphy DL, Campbell I, Costa JL: Current status of the indoleamine hypothesis of the affective disorders. *In* Lipton MA, DiMascio A, Killarn K (eds): Psychopharmacology: A Generation of Progress. New York, Raven Press, 1978, p 1235.

53. Richelson E, Diventz-Romero S: Blockade by psychotic drugs on muscarinic acetylcholine receptors in cultured nerve cells. Biol Psychiat *12*:711, 1977.
54. Blackwell B, Stefopoulos A, Enders P: Anticholinergic activity of two tricyclic antidepressants. Am J Psychiat *135*:722, 1978.
55. Baldessarini RJ, Gelenberg AJ: Use of physostigmine in antidepressant-induced intoxication. Am J Psychiat *136*:1608, 1979.
56. Jefferson JW: A review of the cardiovascular effects and toxicity of tricyclic antidepressants. Psychosom Med *37*:160, 1975.
57. Burrows GD, Vohra J, Hunt D, et al: Cardiac effects of different tricyclic antidepressant drugs. Br J Psychiat *129*:335, 1976.
58. Granacher RP, Baldessarini RJ: Physostigmine. Its use in acute anticholinergic syndrome with antidepressant and antiparkinson drugs. Arch Gen Psychiat *32*:375, 1975.
59. Nattel S, Bayne L, Ruedy J: Physostigmine in coma due to drug overdose. Clin Pharmacol Ther *25*:97, 1979.
60. Markowitz JC, Brown RP: Seizures with neuroleptics and antidepressants Gen Hosp Psychiat *9*:135, 1987.
61. Malatynska E, Knapp RJ, Ikeda M, Yamamura HI: Antidepressants and seizure-interactions at the GABA receptor chloride-ionophore complex. Life Sci *43*:303, 1988.
62. Burns HL, Rand JM: The actions of sympathomimetic amines in animals treated with reserpine. J Physiol *144*:314, 1958.
63. Trendelenberg U, Muskus A, Fleming WW, DeLaSerra BGA: Effects of cocaine denervation and decentralization on the response of the nictitating membrane to various sympathomimetic amines. J Pharmacol Exp Ther *138*:181, 1962.
64. Glowinski J, Axelrod J: The effects of drugs on the uptake, release and metabolism of H3-norepinephrine in the rat brain. J Pharmacol Exp Ther *149*:43, 1965.
65. Axelrod J: Amphetamine metabolism, physiological disposition and its effects on catecholamine storage. *In* Costa E, Garattini S (eds): International Symposium on Amphetamine and Related Compounds. New York, Raven Press, 1970, p 207.
66. Baekeland F: Pentobarbital and dextroamphetamine in the sleep cycle in man. Psychopharmacologia *11*:338, 1967.
67. Rechtschaffen A, Maron L: The effect of amphetamine in the sleep cycle. Electroencephalogr Clin Neurophysiol *16*:438, 1964.
68. Lasagna L, Epstein LC: The use of amphetamines in the treatment of hyperkinetic children. *In* Costa E, Garattini S (eds): International Symposium on Amphetamine and Related Compounds. New York, Raven Press, 1970, p 849.
69. Connel PH: Clinical aspects of amphetamine dependence. *In* Wilson CWM (ed): The Pharmacological and Epidemiological Aspects of Adolescent Drug Dependence. London, Pergamon Press, 1968.
70. Griffith JD, Cavanaugh JH, Oates JA: Psychosis induced by the administration of D-amphetamine to human volunteers. *In* Efon DH (ed): Psychomimetic Drugs. New York, Raven Press, 1970, p 897.
71. Hertting G, Axelrod J, Whitby LG: Effect of drugs on the uptake of noradrenaline by heart and spleen. J Pharmacol Exp Ther *1343*:146, 1961.
72. Muscholl E: Effect of cocaine and related drugs on the uptake and metabolism of H3-norepinephrine. Br J Pharmacol Chemother *16*:352, 1961.
73. Colliver J: A decade of DAWN: Cocaine related cases, 1976–1985. Washington, DC, National Institute on Drug Abuse, Division of Epidemiological and Statistical Publication, 1987.
74. Cocaine Client Admissions 1976–1985. DHHS publication No. ADM87–1528. National Institute on Drug Abuse, Division of Epidemiological and Statistical Publication. Washington, DC, Government Printing Office, 1987.
75. Campbell BG: Cocaine abuse with hyperthermia, seizures and fatal complications. Med J Aust *149*:387, 1988.
76. Ruitchie JM, Greene NM: Local anesthetics. *In* Gilman AG, Goodman LS, Gilman A (eds): The Pharmacologic Basis of Therapeutics. 6th ed. New York, Macmillan, 1980, p 307.
77. Schwartz RH, Estroff T, Hoffmann NG: Seizures and syncope in adolescent cocaine abusers. Am J Med *85*:462, 1988.
78. Derlet RW, Albertson TE: Diazepam in the prevention of seizures and death in cocaine-intoxicated rats. Ann Emerg Med *18*:542, 1987.
79. Stripling JS, Gramlich CA, Cunningham MG: Effect of cocaine and lidocaine on the development of kindled seizures. Pharmacol Biochem Behav *32*:463, 1989.
80. Klonoff DC, Andrews KBT, Obana WG: Stroke associated with cocaine use. Arch Neurol *46*:989, 1989.
81. Bateman DA, Heagarty MC: Passive freebase cocaine (crack) inhalation by infants and toddlers. Am J Dis Child *143*:27, 1987.
82. Chaney NE, Franke J, Wadlington WB: Cocaine convulsions in a breast-fed baby. J Pediatr *112*:123, 1988.
83. Fischman MW, Schuster CR, Rosenkov L, et al: Cardiovascular and subjective effects of intravenous cocaine administration in humans. Arch Gen Psychiat *33*:983, 1976.
84. VanDyke C, Jatlow P, Ungerer J, et al: Oral cocaine: Plasma concentrations and central effects. Science *200*:211, 1978.
85. Javaid JL, Fischman MW, Schuster CR, et al: Cocaine plasma concentration: Relation to physiological and subjective effects in humans. Science *202*:227, 1978.
86. Holmstedt B: Pharmacology of organophosphorus cholinesterase inhibitors. Pharmacol Rev *11*:567, 1959.
87. Grob D: Anticholinesterase intoxication in man and its treatment. *In* Koelle GB (ed): Cholinesterase and Anticholinesterase Agents. Handbuch der Experimentellen Pharmakologie. Vol 15. Berlin, Springer-Verlag, 1963, p 989.
88. Gaines TB: Acute toxicity of pesticides. Toxicol Appl Pharmacol *14*:515, 1969.
89. Wills JH: Toxicity of anticholinesterases and treatment of poisoning. *In* Karacaman AG (ed): Anticholinesterase Agents. International Encyclopedia of Pharmacology and Therapeutics. Oxford, Pergamon Press, 1970, p 355.
90. Parfitt DN: An outbreak of anticholinesterases and treatment of poisoning. J Neurol Neurosurg Psychiat *10*:85, 1949.
91. Grossier VW: Atropine poisoning: Two cases. Ann Intern Med *44*:1020, 1956.
92. Alexander E, Morris DP, Eslick RL: Atropine poisoning. N Engl J Med *234*:258, 1956.

93. Ketchum JS, Sidell FR, Crowell EB Jr, et al: Atropine, scopolamine and ditran: Comparative pharmacology and antagonists in man. Psychopharmacologia *28*:121, 1973.
94. Cunningham RW, Harned BK, Clark MC, et al: The pharmacology of 3-(*N*-piperidyl)-1-phenyl-1-cyclohexyl-1 propanol HCl (Artane) and related compounds: New antispasmodic agents. J Pharmacol Exp Ther *96*:151, 1949.
95. Baldessarini RJ: The "neuroleptic" antipsychotic drugs. Neurologic side effects. Postgrad Med *65*:123, 1979.
96. Anderson RJ, Potts DE, Gabow PA, et al: Unrecognized adult salicylate intoxication. Arch Intern Med *138*:481, 1978.
97. Gabow PA, Anderson JR, Potts DE, et al: Acid-base disturbances in the salicylate-intoxicated adult. Arch Intern Med *138*:1481, 1978.
98. Hill JB: Salicylate intoxication. N Engl J Med *288*:1110, 1973.
99. Cohan SL, Winchester JF, Gelfand MC: Treatment of intoxication with charcoal hemadsorption. Drug Metab Rev *13*:681, 1978.
100. Prescott LF, Part J, Sutherland GR, et al: Cysteamine, methionine, and penicillamine in the treatment of paracetamol poisoning. Lancet *2*:109, 1976.
101. Winchester JF, Edwards RO, Tilstone WJ, Woodcock BG: Activated charcoal hemoperfusion and experimental acetaminophen poisoning. Toxicol Appl Pharmacol *31*:120, 1975.
102. Beller GA, Smith TW, Abelman WH, et al: Digitalis intoxication. A prospective clinical study with serum level correlations. N Engl J Med *284*:989, 1971.
103. Smith TW, Haber E: Medical progress: Digitalis. N Engl J Med *289*:1125, 1973.
104. Melges FT, Tinklenberg JR, Hollister LE, et al: Temporal disintegration and depersonalization during marijuana intoxication. Arch Gen Psychiat *23*:204, 1970.
105. Hollister LE: Marijuana in man: Three years later. Science *172*:21, 1971.
106. Jones RT: Marijuana-induced "high:" influence on expectation, setting and previous drug experience. Pharmacol Rev *23*:359, 1971.
107. Evans MA, Martz R, Brown DJ, et al: Impairment of performance with low performance with low doses of marijuana. Clin Pharmacol Ther *14*:936, 1973.
108. Klonoff H: Marijuana and driving in real-life situations. Science *186*:317, 1974.
109. Rafaelson OJ, Bech P, Christiansen J, et al: Cannabis and alcohol: Effects on simulated car driving. Science *179*:920, 1973.
110. Belgrave BE, Bird KD, Chester GB, et al: The effect of (-)trans-Δ9-tetrahydrocannabinol, alone and in combination with ethanol, on human performance. Psychopharmacology *62*:53, 1979.
111. Chopra GS, Smith JW: Psychotic reactions following cannabis use in East Indians. Arch Gen Psychiat *30*:24, 1974.
112. Thacore VR, Shukla SRP: Cannabis psychosis and paranoid schizophrenia. Arch Gen Psychiat *30*:24, 1974.
113. Freedman DX: The use and abuse of LSD. Arch Gen Psychiat *18*:300, 1968.
114. Cohen S: Psychotomimetic agents. Ann Rev Pharmacol *7*:301, 1967.
115. Freedman DX: The psychopharmacology of hallucinogenic agents. Annu Rev Med *20*:409, 1969.
116. Bowers MB Jr: Acute psychosis induced by psychomimetic drug abuse. Arch Gen Psychiat *27*:437, 1972.
117. Domino EF: Neurobiology of phencyclidine and update. *In* Petersen RC, Stillman RC (eds): PCP (Phencyclidine) Abuse: An Appraisal. DHEW Publication (ADM)(78–728). Washington, DC, National Institute of Drug Abuse, 1978, p 18.
118. Petersen RC, Stillman RC: Phencyclidine: An Overview. *In* Petersen RC, Stillman RC (eds): PCP (Phencyclidine) Abuse: An Appraisal. DHEW Publication (ADM)(78–728). Washington, DC, National Institute of Drug Abuse, 1978, p 1.
119. Siegel RK: Phencyclidine and ketamine intoxication: A study of four populations of recreational users. *In* Petersen RC, Stillman RC (eds): PCP (Phencyclidine) Abuse: An Appraisal. DHEW Publication (ADM)(78–728). Washington, DC, National Institute of Drug Abuse, 1978, p 1.
120. Buterbaugh GG, Michelson HB: Anticonvulsant properties of phencyclidine and ketamine. National Institute Drug Abuse Res Monogr *64*:67, 1986.
121. Leander JD, Rathbun RC, Zimmerman DM: Anticonvulsant effects of phencyclidine-like drugs: relation to N-methyl-D-aspartic acid antagonism. Brain Res *454*:368, 1988.
122. Cooper JR, Kini MM: Biochemical aspects of methanol poisoning. Biochem Pharmacol *11*:405, 1962.
123. Kolvusalo M: Methanol. *In* Tremoliers J (ed): Alcohols and Derivatives. Vol 2. International Encyclopedia of Pharmacology and Therapeutics. Oxford, Pergamon Press, 1970, p 465.
124. Guggenheim MA, Couch JR, Weinberger W: Motor dysfunction as a permanent complication of methanol ingestion. Arch Neurol *24*:550, 1971.
125. Clay KL, Murphy RC, Watkins WD: Experimental methanol toxicity in the primate: Analysis of metabolic acidosis. Toxicol Appl Pharmacol *34*:49, 1975.
126. Israel Y, Rosenmann E, Hein S, et al: Effects of alcohol on the nerve cell. *In* Israel Y, Mordoues J (eds): Biological Basis of Alcoholism. New York, John Wiley & Sons, 1971, p 53.
127. Himwich HE, Callison DA: The effects of alcohol on evoked potentials of various parts of the central nervous system of the cat. *In* Kissin B, Begleiter H (eds): The Biology of Alcoholism. Vol 2: Physiology and Behavior. New York, Plenum Press, 1972, p 67.
128. Newman HW: Acute Alcoholic Intoxication: A Critical Review. Stanford, CA, Stanford University Press, 1941.
129. Morgan R, Cagan EJ: Acute alcohol intoxication, the disulfiram reaction, and methyl alcohol intoxication. *In* Kissin B, Begleiter H (eds): The Biology of Alcoholism. Vol 3: Clinical Pathology. New York, Plenum Press, 1974, p 163.
130. Johnston RE, Reier CE: Acute respiratory effects of ethanol in man. Clin Pharmacol Ther *14*:501, 1973.
131. Kissin B: Interactions of ethyl alcohol and other drugs. *In* Kissin B, Begleiter H (eds): The Biology of Alcoholism. Vol 3: Clinical Pathology. New York, Plenum Press, 1974, p 109.
132. Catton MJ, Harrison MJG, Fullerton PM, et al: Subclinical neuropathy in lead workers. Br Med J *2*:80, 1980.
133. Conrad S: Lead concentration in skeletal muscle in amyotrophic lateral sclerosis patients and control subjects. J Neurol Neurosurg Psychiat *41*:1001, 1978.

134. Sanford HN: Lead poisoning in young children. Postgrad Med *17*:162, 1955.
135. Byers RK: Lead poisoning. Review of literature and report on 45 cases. Pediatrics *23*:585, 1959.
136. Smith HD, Boehner RL, Corney T, et al: The sequela of pica with and without lead poisoning. Am J Dis Child *105*:609, 1963.
137. Popoff N, Weinberg S, Feigin I: Pathologic observations in lead encephalopathy. Neurology *13*:101, 1963.
138. McAlpine D, Shukuro A: Minimata disease. An unusual neurologic disorder caused by contaminated fish. Lancet *2*:629, 1958.
139. Koos BJ, Longo L: Mercury toxicity in pregnant women, fetus and newborn infant. Am J Obstet Gynecol *126*:390, 1976.
140. Langlof GD, Chaffin DB, Whittle HP, et al: Effects of industrial mercury exposure on urinary mercury, EMG and psychomotor functions. *In* Brown SS (ed): Clinical Chemistry and Chemical Toxicology of Metals. Amsterdam, Elsevier, 1977, p 213.
141. Clarkson TW: Mercury poisoning. *In* Brown SS (ed): Clinical Chemistry and Chemical Toxicology of Metals. Amsterdam, Elsevier, 1977, p 189.
142. Jenkins RB: Inorganic arsenic and the nervous system. Brain *89*:479, 1966.
143. Grinkler RR: Parkinsonism following carbon monoxide poisoning. J Nerv Ment Dis *64*:18, 1926.
144. Gordon EB: Carbon-monoxide encephalopathy. Br Med J *1*:1232, 1965.
145. Bour H, Tutin M, Pasquier P: The central nervous system and carbon monoxide poisoning. 1. Clinical data with reference to 20 fatal cases. Prog Brain Res *24*:1, 1967.
146. Courville CB: The process of demyelination in the central nervous system. IV: Demyelination as a delayed residual of carbon monoxide asphyxia. J Nerv Ment Dis *125*:534, 1957.
147. Garland H, Pearce J: Neurological complications of carbon monoxide poisoning. Q J Med *36*:445, 1967.
148. Plum F, Posner JB, Hain RF: Delayed neurological deterioration after anoxia. Arch Intern Med *110*:18, 1962.
149. Shillito FH, Drinker CK, Shaughnessy TJ: The problem of nervous and mental sequelae in carbon monoxide poisoning. JAMA *106*:669, 1936.
150. Meigs JW, Hughes JPW: Acute carbon monoxide poisoning. Arch Indust Hyg Occup Med *6*:344, 1952.
151. Ferrar A: Experimental toxic encephalomyelopathy (diffuse sclerosis) following subcutaneous injections of potassium cyanide. Psychiatr Q *7*:267, 1933.
152. Hurst EW: Experimental demyelination in the central nervous system. Part I, The encephalopathy produced by sodium cyanide. Aust J Exp Biol Med Sci *18*:201, 1940.
153. Levine S, Stypulkowski W: Experimental cyanide encephalopathy. Arch Pathol *67*:306, 1959.
154. Brierly JB, Prior PF, Alverly J, et al: Cyanide intoxication in *Macaca mulatta*. Physiology and neuropathological aspects. J Neurol Sci *31*:133, 1977.
155. Wald G, Allen DW: The equilibrium between cytochrome oxidase and carbon monoxide. J Gen Physiol *40*:593, 1957.
156. Smith FP, Butler TP, Cohan S, et al: Laetrile toxicity: A report of two patients. Cancer Treat Rep *62*:169, 1978.

B. Brain Death

The topic of brain death must be included in any comprehensive discussion of poisonings, since severe intoxication results in brain death, and certain drugs by their action can simulate brain death to the extent that a diagnosis of brain death may be made erroneously in an otherwise salvageable patient. Additionally, the question of organ donation from brain-dead poisoned patients is so frequently raised that this topic has become one of concern in modern medicine. This chapter will discuss the diagnosis of brain death and outline pitfalls in making such a diagnosis.

The development of respiratory and vasopressor support methods now permits the maintenance of patients, despite brain destruction that formerly would have resulted in their deaths. Before the advent of modern ventilatory and cardiovascular support methods, patient death was thought of as cessation of respiration and heart beat. Originally, life support techniques were designed and intended for preservation of vital body functions through a transient period of life-threatening disease. Because physicians and patients' families are commonly faced with the difficult decision of whether or not to terminate support systems because the patients cannot survive, will never regain consciousness, and can never maintain body support without mechanical assistance because their brains are destroyed, there has occurred a redirection in thought, and death is now frequently equated with brain destruction or "brain death." The President's Commission for the Study of Ethical Problems in Medicine and Biomedical and Behavioral Research and the Task Force for the Determination of Brain Death in Children states that "an individual who has sustained irreversible cessation of circulatory and respiratory functions, *or* irreversible cessation of all functions of the *entire* brain, including the brain stem, is dead."[1]

Although total brain destruction may not be the sole criterion upon which the decision to discontinue extraordinary methods of care is based, it is the determining factor in many cases. First, the decision to discontinue life support techniques in a patient with total brain destruction would be consistent with the belief of many individuals that support of cardiac and pulmonary function in a person whose brain will never function again is unacceptable. This is regardless of the issue of whether a patient with "brain death" is dead or alive. Second, the decision to discontinue supportive care in a patient with total brain destruction tacitly recognizes that all body functions would cease spontaneously in every such patient, leading to death soon after.

Organ transplantation has increased our need to understand the relationship between brain destruction and viability of the individual. Although we may desire to improve or save the life of a human being in need of organ replacement, we cannot do so at the expense of depriving another human being of life. The legal and moral arguments that surround the issue of whether or not an individual is "dead" once his or her brain is destroyed raise many emotions.[1–3] Instead, we should recognize that we are making a decision that expresses our belief that it is not morally wrong to remove a vital organ from a human being whose brain is functionally irreversibly destroyed to preserve the life of a sensate human being, recognizing that removal of vital organs from such donors has not deprived them of the opportunity of independent survival or resumption of brain function.

To approach these problems clinically, we first must ask ourselves if we have the ability to determine whether total destruction, to be referred to as "brain death," has occurred.[3] We must subsequently demonstrate that patients with brain death may be suitable candidates for removal of organs or discontinuation of artificial life support systems, and that making these decisions does not deprive a salvageable human being of the opportunity to survive.

DIAGNOSIS OF BRAIN DEATH

Currently, in at least two clinical circumstances it is necessary to ascertain whether all brain function has permanently ceased. First when major mechanical and pharmacologic life support methods are being used to sustain the patient, determination of the occurrence of irreversible cessation of brain function may be critical in deciding whether or not these life support systems are to be discontinued. This is not to suggest that evidence of brain destruction must be present for physicians to discontinue supportive care. The second circumstance in which irreversible cessation of brain function must be determined is when human organs are to be removed for the purpose of transplantation. In these cases, it is desirable that the transplantable organs have been maintained with adequate blood flow and oxygenation to preserve their viability. When the potential donor is presumed to have irreversible total destruction of brain function, we must be certain that organ removal would not deprive the donor of the opportunity of surviving and regaining brain function—that is, that organ removal has not altered the outlook for patient survival. Progress has been made in establishing reliable criteria for brain death.[1–10]

A starting point in recognizing brain death is an understanding of coma, a state in which the individual is totally unresponsive to any external or internal stimulus, except perhaps in a reflex manner—the latter type of response not necessarily requiring the integrity of brain structures mediating the conscious state.[11–13] This is essentially the definition of coma provided by Plum and Posner.[14] However, many patients in coma appear to have brain death, and thus we must determine what additional features must be present in the unresponsive patient to be certain that brain death has occurred. What criteria are necessary to show that cerebral hemispheric and brain stem function have permanently ceased? The cause of cessation of brain function must be determined, and it must be sufficient to account for the patient's neurologic status.[1, 2] Recovery of brain function must not be possible, and there must be an appropriate length of observation of the absence of brain function.[1, 2] Criteria have been developed that incorporate features of the neurologic examination, respiration, and confirmatory tests of electrophysiologic activity of the brain and cerebral blood flow.[1, 2, 7–9] The patient should be apneic if brain death has occurred. The neurologic examination should reveal that the patient is unresponsive to any stimulus and that there are no reflex responses indicative of continued brain function. These include absence of corneal and snout reflexes, absence of pupillary response to bright light, absence of spontaneous eye movements or eye movements in response to head turning (oculocephalic response) or to irrigation of the ear with ice water ("cold calorics" or the oculovestibular response), absence of gag reflexes, and absence of spontaneous swallowing or tongue or facial movements. These features of the neurologic examination are part of current brain death criteria in use.[1, 2, 9]

Opinion is still divided about whether the patient's brain should have no electric activity, a "flat" electroencephalogram (EEG) being a requirement for the diagnosis of brain death.[1–9, 15–24] Most currently accepted criteria emphasize that the diagnosis of brain death is based upon clinical evidence of a permanent cessation of brain function[2, 3, 9] and that additional laboratory tests may be employed when needed. Although the presence of an isoelectric EEG figures prominently in many published criteria of brain death, persistence of EEG activity has been observed, despite all clinical criteria of brain death having been met and cerebral blood flow being absent for up to 2 weeks.[2, 5, 6, 25, 26] Furthermore, EEG changes, or absence thereof, are not necessarily a reliable indication of brain stem function.[25, 26] In the pediatric age group, and particularly in asphyxiated neonates, an initially flat EEG has been observed in neurologically viable patients.[6] Lastly, drugs, such as barbiturates and benzodiazepines, and hypothermia may produce flat EEG.[4, 18, 27–31]

Some criteria require demonstration of absence of cerebral blood flow.[32] Although the absence of cerebral blood flow is incompatible with brain survival, persistence of blood flow has been seen in patients with definite brain death.[33, 34] With the most commonly used method of measuring cerebral blood flow, radionuclide scintigraphy, cerebral blood flow up to 24 per cent of normal cerebral blood flow may be present but undetected.[35, 36] The use of Doppler techniques, to demonstrate loss of intracerebral blood flow, although still experimental, appears to predict brain death reliably.[37–39] This methodology may become extremely important in the neonatal and early infant groups, in which there is concern for the reliability and predictability of the neurologic examination and EEG.[1, 2, 6, 10, 40, 41] The presence of normal middle cerebral artery flow by transcranial Doppler may indicate preservation of the cerebral hemispheres despite absence of brain stem reflexes.[38] The typical pattern in patients with brain death is brief, "sharply contoured" forward flow during systole, and absent or reversed flow direction during diastole,[38] a pattern that can also be seen with marked increase in intracranial pressure prior to onset of cerebral death.[38] It has been suggested recently that absence of spontaneous esophageal motility is a reliable determinant of lower brain stem destruction.[42]

Some criteria employ the somatosensory (SSEP) and auditory (BAEP) evoked potentials as confirmatory tests.[6, 7, 43, 48] These tests are particularly useful in neonates and in ruling out drug effects in patients in whom clinical examination and EEG suggest cessation of cerebral cortical function. The BAEP change seen with ensuing brain death is prolongation of interpeak latencies or complete loss of the brain stem components (peaks III, IV, and V).[44–45] However, hypothermia may affect interpeak latencies and mimic ensuing brain death.[45] In addition, the combination of barbiturates and lidocaine, commonly employed in the intensive care setting, also may prolong interpeak latencies of brain stem waves. There is evidence to suggest that BAEPs cannot reliably diagnose "brain stem" death in the neonate.[46, 47] Lastly, BAEP cannot assess brain stem function below the level of the eighth cranial nerve, a problem addressed by the measurement of esophageal motility that assesses function of the distal medulla.[42]

All studies demonstrate that cortical SSEPs reliably predict eventual brain death,[43, 48–50] and probably disappear before EEG loss[50]; and their loss is a more serious prognostic indicator than EEG loss.[50] Although the loss of the cortical response of the SSEP points to cortical destruction, it cannot be used alone to prove brain death, since brain stem function may still be present. This problem may be solved by addition of BAEP determination[44, 45] or a short latency SSEP measured at the C2 level.[48] One could also require the absence of response by the nervous system to certain pharmacologic agents, such as absence of tachycardia in response to atropine, an effect requiring brain stem function.[51]

DRUG EFFECTS SIMULATING BRAIN DEATH

It is essential that the physical and physiologic features of a patient evaluated for brain death be shown not to result from reversible causes; it is particularly important to rule out drug effects. Examples of drugs that may mimic features of brain death include curare-like neuromuscular blocking drugs and other blocking agents, such as the aminoglycoside antibiotics; drugs that act centrally to depress consciousness and suppress respiration, including barbiturates, opiates, and benzodiazepines; drugs that can suppress brain stem reflexes, such as meprobamate, barbiturates, phenytoin, ethchlorvynol, benzodiazepines, and tricyclic antidepressants; neuromuscular blocking agents; and drugs like the barbiturates that can suppress the electroencephalogram. All must be excluded as significant contributors to the clinical picture before a diagnosis of brain death can be made confidently.

Respiration also can be suppressed by hypocapnia after prolonged hyperventilation on a respirator. Thus, one must be certain that an apneic patient has a pCO_2 sufficiently high to serve as a potential respiratory stimulus, particularly since comatose patients are generally less responsive to respiratory stimulation by CO_2.[14] It is generally agreed that a pCO_2 of 50 to 60 mm Hg must be reached to be certain that apnea is present,[52] but it has recently been demonstrated that one cannot predict the rate of rise in pCO_2 during apnea,[53] and if pre-apnea hyperventilation is excessive, then a pCO_2 in the 50 to 60 mm Hg range may not be reached during apnea, thus necessitating actual measurement of pCO_2 before and after completion of apnea testing and placing the patient back on assisted ventilation until the pCO_2 values return from the laboratory.

BRAIN DEATH CRITERIA

Various criteria have been developed and tested to determine whether brain death can be diagnosed reliably. With progress in pediatric and particularly neonatal intensive care over the past few years, it has become clear that separate criteria are required for neonates, infants, children, and adults.[1, 2, 6–8, 10] The Harvard criteria,[54] applicable to adults, included complete lack of neurologic response to any form of stimulation, no spontaneous movement, apnea after respiratory support had been discontinued for 3 minutes, fixed dilated pupils, and absent oculocephalic, oculovestibular, corneal, pharyngeal, and postural (decorticate or decerebrate) reflexes. Additionally, an isoelectric electroencephalogram in the absence of hypothermia or drugs that will depress it, observed on two occasions at least 24 hours apart, was also considered of great confirmatory value. To be valid, these criteria, in every case in which they were applied, had to identify a patient in whom return of brain function would never be observed and who could not survive systemically.

A collaborative study involving 503 adult patients with suspected brain death determined that the Harvard criteria were completely reliable, since no patient fulfilling the criteria survived.[55] However, these standards were too strict, since the majority of patients who died did not fulfill all the criteria. Thus if the Harvard criteria were used to select organ donors for transplantation, it is readily apparent that too great a number of potential organ donors, in whom removal of an organ would not have altered survival, would not have qualified.

The United States Collaborative Study of Cerebral Death modified the Harvard criteria by shortening the period of time that the criteria for brain death had to be fulfilled from 24 hours to 6 hours. Patients who (1) were without purposive response to any stimulus, (2) were apneic for 6 hours or more, (3) had fixed dilated pupils; no oculocephalic, oculovestibular, snout, gag, corneal, or ciliospinal reflexes; and no cough or swallowing movements for 30 minutes, and (4) had an isoelectric EEG fulfilled the criteria for brain death. If any of these criteria were missing, evidence of absent cerebral blood flow was necessary for a diagnosis of brain death. Using these criteria, accuracy remained 100 per cent, but the number of patients fulfilling the criteria increased by tenfold. Such criteria subsequently increased the number of potential organ transplant donors and potentially reduced the number of patients who would continue to receive supportive care.

The Canadian Congress Committee on Brain Death requires that the patient be unarousable and respirator-dependent, and that apnea testing reveal no spontaneous respiration.[9] Reversible causes of coma, such as drugs, hypothermia, and shock, must be absent, and the patient's status must be the result of a disease process capable of producing death. A second assessment should be performed 2 to 24 hours later. These clinical criteria, properly applied by qualified people, are felt to be sufficient to establish brain death and remove the need for confirmatory electrophysiologic testing, angiography, or cerebral blood flow measurements.

The President's Commission[1] requires evidence of irreversible cessation of function of the entire brain—requiring, as in the Canadian Congress, that the proposed cause be capable of producing irreversible cessation of brain function, that there be no possibility of recovery, that there be an appropriate duration of observation, that core body temperature be sufficiently high (more than 32°C, or 90°F) and that drugs, including neuromuscular blocking agents, which can mimic brain death and/or produce an isoelectric EEG, not be present. Parenthetically, the neuromuscular blocking effects of severe Guillain-Barré disease can also mimic brain death clinically.[55]

Whereas these criteria may suffice for adults and children over the age of 5 years, the President's Commission recognized that results of studies of brain death in younger children made evident the need for separate criteria for the diagnosis of brain death.[1] It has been assumed that the brains of young children are more resistant to permanent damage by certain insults, although this has not been documented,[56, 57] and that the cause of impaired function, particularly in neonates, may not be determined reliably. The clinical assessment may be difficult and the reliability of confirmatory tests, particularly the EEG, is not established.[1, 2, 41] The Task Force for the Determination of Brain Death in Children has developed criteria for establishing "irreversible cessation of all functions of the entire brain, including the brain stem."[2] As in adult criteria, there must be loss of consciousness, apnea, no evidence of brain stem function on clinical examination, no hypothermia or hypotension for a patient of that age, flaccid quadriplegia, and no evidence of metabolic disease or intoxication that could mimic brain death. The application of criteria varies with patient age:

- In patients 7 days to 2 months old, there must be two clinical examinations and two EEGs separated by 48 hours.
- In patients 2 months to 1 year old, there must be two clinical examinations and two EEGs separated by 24 hours, but only one examination and one EEG are required if a concomitant radionuclide cerebral angiogram demonstrates "no flow."
- In patients more than 1 year old, in whom the cause is known to be irreversible, clinical observation for 12 hours, and no EEG, is sufficient. When irreversibility is difficult to establish, such as after hypoxia or ischemia, clinical observation should be for at least 24 hours, unless the EEG is flat or there is no flow on radionuclide cerebral angiography.

Because electroencephalographic and clinical assessment may be made unreliable by hypothermia, intoxication, or severe hypotension, evoked responses have been employed as additional confirmatory tests.[58] The Children's Hospital of Boston criteria state that absence of BAEP is unequivocal evidence of brain death[7]; this must be challenged, since there are well-documented cases of brain stem destruction, with preservation of cerebral cortex, so-called "brain stem death," in which auditory evoked responses are absent.[44] As mentioned, there may be preservation of brain stem function distal to the region of the brain stem evaluated by auditory evoked responses.[42] It must be emphasized that current criteria for the diagnosis of brain death demand that there be irreversible cessation of function of the *entire* brain.[1, 2, 9] An apparent solution to the problem is that many patients with "brain stem death" have preservation of electroencephalographic activity,[34] and even in patients with brain stem destruction who have received drugs that suppress the EEG, cerebral blood flow, as measured by radionuclide angiography[35] or transcranial Doppler[37–39] will be present if the cerebral cortex has not been destroyed. Of studies reported thus far, there have been no cases of patients with absent cerebral blood flow surviving, or of absent cerebral blood flow returning on serial studies in the same patient.[37–39]

The use of transcranial Doppler,[37–39] radionuclide angiography,[35, 36] and most recently xenon-enhanced computed tomography[59] should supplant traditional contrast cerebral angiography, employed as a confirmatory test in some early criteria of brain death.[32] The disadvantages of contrast cerebral angiography are that it could further damage brain, as well as damaging organs that may be used for transplantation.

One may argue that the criteria of brain

death are too stringent and that EEG criteria alone would be sufficient, in the absence of hypothermia[60, 61] or drug intoxication, provided the methods for recording the EEG are sufficiently reliable. In reviewing several series,[13, 17, 22, 62] it is clear that adult patients with a single isoelectric EEG, recorded for 10 to 30 minutes, will not recover provided they are not hypothermic or intoxicated. However, the Harvard criteria,[52] the Swedish criteria,[32] and the criteria of the United States Collaborative Study[55] all have been previously and successfully tested.

INCORPORATED APPROACH TO DIAGNOSIS OF BRAIN DEATH

It should be possible to incorporate features of several sets of criteria of brain death that maintain a high degree of accuracy in diagnosis, permit accurate assessment of the maximum number of patients, exclude procedures that may be harmful to the patients' organs, and are within the capabilities of most, if not all, hospitals.

It is evident that separate criteria for establishment of the diagnosis of brain death are considered desirable for children and adults,[1, 2] although the results of some studies argue that adult criteria can be applied reliably to children over 3 months of age.[8] There are no reports of children, beyond the neonatal age group, who fulfill adult criteria for brain death who survived.[8] What is clear is that there are no reliable criteria for diagnosis of brain death in neonates less than 7 days of age,[2] and the situation is worse in premature neonates. Nevertheless, it is possible to incorporate features of several criteria of brain death, present objections notwithstanding, and employ guidelines which, although perhaps prolonging the period of mechanical and pharmacologic support of a brain-dead patient, have the advantage of assuring against unintentional termination of care in a patient owing to a mistaken diagnosis of brain death:

1. The patient must be unresponsive to any stimulus except for the presence of spinal reflexes, which may persist despite brain death.
2. The patient must have apnea in the absence of drugs or hypocapnia that suppresses respiration centrally, or neuromuscular blocking agents that interfere with respiration peripherally.
3. Neurologic examination must reveal absence of pupillary responses and oculocephalic, oculovestibular, corneal, gag, and snout reflexes. The patient must not have spontaneous swallowing or facial movements.
4. Toxic and metabolic causes of unresponsiveness, presence of sedation, hypnotic and paralytic agents, hypothermia, and shock must all be ruled out as contributing factors.

These are criteria that can be applied to all age groups but the minimal period of observation of patients should vary with age and cause of unresponsiveness.

5. For children 7 days to 2 months of age: patients should fulfill the clinical criteria of brain death for 48 hours and have two isoelectric EEGs 48 hours apart.

   For children 2 months to 1 year of age: 24 hours of observation and two isoelectric EEGs 24 hours apart or a single examination and isoelectric EEG if a concomitant radionuclide angiogram shows no cerebral blood flow.

   For children 1 year of age and older: adult criteria can be applied, with clinical criteria alone being sufficient, with continuous demonstration of no cerebral or brain stem function for 12 hours.

6. If electroencephalography is to be used, its execution and interpretation should follow the guidelines of the American Electroencephalographic Society, and the patient must have an isoelectric EEG for 30 minutes.[17, 54, 55, 63, 64] In the adult, a clinically brain dead patient who is not hypothermic or intoxicated by drugs known to suppress the EEG, a 30-minute isoelectric EEG is sufficient to confirm the diagnosis. This is justified in light of the observation of the Ad Hoc Committee of the American Electroencephalographic Society for EEG criteria for determination of cerebral death,[63] in which study of the outcome of 16,665 patients with isoelectric EEGs revealed return of electroencephalographic activity in only three patients, each of whom was intoxicated by drugs.

The second safeguard of the proposed protocol is to rule out drug effects. A number of drugs can produce electrocerebral silence, including barbiturates,[4, 28, 29–31] diazepam,[18, 31] methaqualone,[18, 30, 65] lidocaine, trichloroethylene,[66] meprobamate,[27, 30, 31] and succinylcholine.[67] Each of these should be excluded, if possible, by toxicologic evaluation of urine or serum or both. In addition, many other drugs can produce coma and respiratory depression without producing an isoelectric EEG, again pointing to the need for toxicologic evaluation of the patient in whom the diagnosis of brain death is considered. Lastly, apnea in the absence of hypocapnia and in the absence of the use of neuromuscular blocking, curare-like drugs or aminoglycosides, which may interfere with the neuromuscular response to respiratory drive, is an essential feature of the protocol to reduce the chance of spurious diagnosis of brain death.

The use of SSEP to evaluate cortical destruction, BAEP to evaluate brain stem destruction, and cerebral blood flow when the age of the patient and the presence of drugs, hypothermia, or shock cast doubt on the reliability of the clinical examination or EEG may be extremely helpful adjuncts to establish the diagnosis of brain death, when employed in the appropriate situation, by qualified personnel.

In summary, the need has arisen for accurate assessment of the presence of brain death in unresponsive patients. This requirement is partly the result of the use of modern life support systems. The certain diagnosis of cerebral death may be required, in some circumstances, to discontinue these support systems. It is also necessary to be certain that brain death has occurred before removing organs for transplantation. It is now possible to make a reliable diagnosis of brain death by several sets of criteria that require unresponsiveness, apnea, absence of cerebral or brain stem reflexes, an isoelectric EEG, absence of intoxication or hypothermia, and in some cases absence of cerebral blood flow or evoked responses. *It cannot be overemphasized that in the comatose poisoned patient, no avenue should be left unexplored to rule out the possible simulation of brain death by drugs, prior to the determination of brain death.*

References

1. Report of the Medical Consultants on the Diagnosis of Death to President's Commission on the Study of Ethical Problems in Medical and Biomedical and Behavioral Research: Guidelines for the determination of death. JAMA *246*:2184, 1981.
2. Guidelines for the determination of brain death in children. Neurology *37*:1077, 1987.
3. Bernat JL: Ethical and legal aspects of the emergency management of brain death and organ retrieval. Emerg Clin North Am *5*:661, 1987.
4. Mollaret P, Bertrand I, Mollaret H: Coma depasse et necroses nerveuses centrales massives. Rev Neurol (Paris) *101*:116, 1959.
5. Mollaret P, Boulon M: Le coma depasse. Rev Neurol *101*:3, 1959.
6. Drake B, Ashwal S, Schneider S: Determination of cerebral death in the pediatric intensive care unit. Pediatrics *78*:107, 1986.
7. Chrone RK, Bresnan MJ, Erga G, Fischer EG, Treves ST, Weiss EC: Determination of brain death. Ad hoc committee on brain death, The Children's Hospital, Boston. J Pediatr *110*:15, 1987.
8. Alvarez LA, Moshe SL, Belman AL, Maytal J, Resnick TJ, Keilson M: EEG and brain death determination in children. Neurology *38*:227, 1988.
9. Canadian Congress Committee on Brain Death: Death and brain death: A new formulation for Canadian medicine. Can Med Assoc J *138*:405, 1988.
10. Freeman JM, Ferry PC: New brain death guidelines in children: Further confusion. Pediatrics *81*:301, 1988.
11. Becker DP, Robert CM, Nelson JR: An evaluation of the definition of cerebral death. Neurology (Minneap) 20:459–462, 1970.
12. Ivan LP: Spinal reflexes in cerebral death. Neurology (Minneap) *23*:650, 1973.
13. Jorgensen EO: EEG without detectable cortical activity and cranial nerve areflexia as parameters of brain death. Electroenceph Clin Neurophysiol *36*:70, 1974.
14. Plum F, Posner JB: Diagnosis of Stupor and Coma. 3rd ed. Philadelphia, FA Davis, 1980, p 317.
15. Conference of Royal Colleges and Faculties of the United Kingdom: Diagnosis of brain death. Lancet *1*:1069, 1976.
16. Jennett B, Gleave J, Wilson P: Brain death in three neurosurgical units. Br Med J *282*:533, 1981.
17. Korein J, Maccario M: On the diagnosis of cerebral death: A prospective study on 55 patients to define irreversible coma. Clin Electroenceph *2*:178, 1971.
18. Cohan S: Brain death. *In* Haddad LM, Winchester JF (eds): Clinical Management of Poisoning and Drug Overdose. Philadelphia, WB Saunders, 1983.
19. Searle J, Collins C: A brain-death protocol. Lancet *1*:641, 1980.
20. Bennet DR: Brain death. Lancet *1*:107, 1981.
21. Jennett B: The brain death debate. Lancet *1*:107, 1981.
22. Legg NJ, Prior PF: Brain death. Lancet *1*:107, 1981.
23. Pallis C, MacGillivray B: Brain death. Lancet *1*:223, 1981.
24. Paul R: The brain death debate. Lancet *1*:502, 1981.
25. Ashwal S, Schneider S: Failure of electroencephalography to diagnose brain death in comatose patients. Ann Neurol *6*:512, 1979.
26. Grigg MM, Kelly MA, Celesia GC, Ghobrial MW, Ross ER: Electroencephalographic activity after brain death. Arch Neurol *44*:948, 1987.
27. Silverman D, Saunders MG, Schwab RS, Masland RL: Cerebral death and the electroencephalogram. Report of the Ad Hoc Committee of the American Electroencephalographic Society on EEG criteria for

determination of cerebral death. JAMA *209*:1505, 1969.
28. Jorgensen EO: The EEG during severe barbiturate intoxication. Acta Neurol Scand *46*(Suppl 43):281, 1970.
29. Kirshbaum RF, Carollo VJ: Reversible iso-electric EEG in barbiturate coma. JAMA *212*:1215, 1970.
30. Mellerio F: EEG changes during acute intoxication with trichloroethylene. Electroenceph Clin Neurophysiol *29*:101, 1970.
31. Powner DJ: Drug-associated isoelectric EEGs. A hazard in brain-death certification. JAMA *236*:1123, 1976.
32. Ingvar DH, Widen L: Brain death: Summary of a symposium. Lakatidningen *69*:3804, 1972.
33. Altman DI, Perlman JM, Powers WJ, Herscovitch P, Dodson WE, Raichle ME, Volpe JJ: Exuberant brain stem blood flow despite clinical and pathological evidence for brain stem and cerebral necrosis in an asphyxiated newborn infant. Ann Neurol *20*:409, 1986.
34. Ogata J, Imakita M, Yutani C, Miyamoto S, Kikuchi H. Primary brainstem death: A clinico-pathological study. J Neurol Neurosurg Psychiat *51*:646, 1988.
35. Goodman JM, Heck LL, Moore B: Confirmation of brain death with portable isotope angiography. A review of 204 consecutive cases. Neurosurgery *16*:492, 1985.
36. Korein J, Braunstein P, Kricheff I: Radioisotope bolus technique for evaluation of critical deficit of cerebral flow. Ann Neurol *2*:195, 1977.
37. Kirkham FJ, Levin SD, Padeychee TS, Kyme MC, Neville BGR, Gosling RG: Transcranial pulsed Doppler ultrasound findings in brainstem death. J Neurol Neurosurg Psychiat *50*:1504, 1987.
38. Ropper AH, Kehne SM, Wechsler L: Transcranial Doppler in brain death. Neurology *37*:1733, 1987.
39. Hassler W, Steinmetz H, Gawlowski J: Transcranial Doppler ultrasonography in raised intracranial circulatory arrest. J Neurosurg *68*:745, 1988.
40. Brierly JB, Grahm DI, Adams JH: Neocortical death after cardiac arrest: A clinical neurophysiological report of two cases. Lancet 2:560, 1975.
41. Vernon DD, Holtzman BH: Brain death: Considerations for pediatrics. J Clin Neurophysiol 3:251, 1986.
42. Evans JM: Lower esophageal contractility as an indicator of brain death. Br Med J *295*:270, 1987.
43. Chiappa KH, Young RR, Goldie WD: Origins of the components of human short-latency somatosensory evoked responses (SERS). Neurology *29*:598, 1979.
44. Kaga K, Takamori A, Mizutani T, Nagai T, Marsh RR. The auditory pathology of brain death as revealed by auditory evoked potentials. Ann Neurol *18*:360, 1985.
45. Garcia-Larrea L, Bertrand O, Artru F, Pernier J, Maugiere F: Brain-stem monitoring. II Preterminal BAEP changes observed until brain death in deeply comatose patients. Electroencephalogr Clin Neurophysiol *68*:446, 1987.
46. Dear PR, Godfrey DJ: Neonatal auditory brainstem response cannot reliably diagnose brainstem death. Arch Dis Child *60*:17, 1985.
47. Boyd SG, Harden A: Neonatal auditory brainstem response cannot reliably diagnose brainstem death (letter). Arch Dis Child *60*:396, 1985.
48. Stöhr M, Riffel B, Trost E, Ullrich A: Short-latency somatosensory evoked potentials in brain-stem death. J Neurol *234*:211, 1987.
49. Buchner H, Ferbert A, Hacke W: Serial recording of median nerve stimulated subcortical somatosensory evoked potentials (SEPs) in developing brain death. Electroenceph Clin Neurophysiol *69*:14, 1988.
50. Ganes T, Lundar T: EEG and evoked potentials in comatose patients with severe brain damage. Electroenceph Clin Neurophysiol *69*:6, 1988.
51. Walker AE: Cerebral Death. 2nd ed. Baltimore, Urban and Schwarzenberg, 1981, p 23.
52. Ropper A, Kennedy S, Russel L: Apnea testing in the diagnosis of brain death. J Neurosurg *55*:942, 1981.
53. Van Donselaor C, Meerwaldt JD, Van Gijn J: Apnoea testing to confirm brain death in clinical practice. J Neurol Neurosurg Psychiat *49*:1071, 1986.
54. A definition of irreversible coma. Report of the Ad Hoc Committee of the Harvard Medical School to Examine the Definition of Brain Death. JAMA *205*:337, 1968.
55. Langendorf FG, Mallin JF, Masdeu JC, Moshe SL, Lipton RB: Fulminant Guillain-Barré syndrome simulating brain death. Electroenceph Clin Neurophysiol *64*:74, 1986.
56. Schwartz JA, Baxter J, Brill DR: Diagnosis of brain death in children by radionuclide cerebral imaging. Pediatrics *73*:14, 1984.
57. Moshe SL, Alvarez LA: Diagnosis of brain death in children. J Clin Neurophysiol *3*:239, 1983.
58. Lutschg J, Pfenninger J, Ludin HP, Vassella F: Brain–stem auditory evoked potentials and early somatosensory evoked potentials in neurointensively treated comatose children. Am J Dis Child *137*:421, 1983.
59. Dorby JM, Yonas H, Gur D, Latchaw RE: Xenon-enhanced computed tomography in brain death. Arch Neurol *44*:551, 1987.
60. Pearcy WC, Virtue RW: The electroencephalogram in hypothermia with circulatory arrest. Anesthesiology *20*:341, 1959.
61. Tentler RL, Sadove M, Becka DR: Electroencephalographic evidence of cortical "death" followed by full recovery; Protective action of hypothermia. JAMA *164*:166, 1957.
62. Kimura J, Gerber HW, McCormick WF: The isoelectric electroencephalogram: Significance in establishing death in patients maintained on mechanical respirators. Arch Intern Med *121*:511, 1968.
63. Guideline Three: minimal technical standards for EEG recording in suspected cerebral death. J Clin Neurophysiol 3:12, 1986.
64. American Electrophysiologic Society: Guideline in EEG 1–7 (revised 1985). J Clin Neurophysiol 3:12, 1986.
65. Haider I, Oswald I: Electroencephalographic investigation in acute drug poisoning. Electroenceph Clin Neurophysiol *29*:105, 1970.
66. Mellerio F: EEG changes during acute intoxication with trichloroethylene. Electroenceph Clin Neurophysiol *29*:101, 1970.
67. Tyson RN: Simulation of cerebral death by succinylcholine sensitivity. Arch Neurol *30*:409, 1974.

CHAPTER 12
GASTROINTESTINAL EFFECTS OF POISONING

Williamson B. Strum, M.D.

The effect of poisoning on the gastrointestinal tract is a consequence of the interaction of specific chemical agents (xenobiotics) on a susceptible tissue. In certain ways, the gastrointestinal tissue is uniquely resistant; in other ways, it is vulnerable to certain poisons. To understand the gastrointestinal tissue response to poisons, an awareness of certain decisive aspects of its epithelial structure, cell renewal characteristics, and specific functions is required. Although the gastrointestinal tract is lined throughout with an epithelium of entodermal origin, both the structure and function vary considerably from esophagus to colon. This chapter begins with a concise assessment of the essential features of epithelial cell structure, cell kinetics, and function as they occur in human beings and as they relate to poisoning.

GASTROINTESTINAL EPITHELIAL CELL STRUCTURE

Esophagus

The epithelium of the esophagus differs strikingly from the epithelium found elsewhere in the gastrointestinal tract.[1] The esophagus is lined with stratified squamous cells that are similar to the squamous cell covering of the skin except for the absence of a keratin surface and cells of skin appendages (hair, nails, and sweat glands). Mucus is secreted from small superficial glands, identical in appearance to the cardiac glands of the stomach, located beneath the epithelial surface at the levels of the cricoid cartilage and the esophagogastric junction. The mucus provides a protective and lubricant surface to facilitate the passage of food from the mouth into the stomach. The proliferating zone is the layer of polygonal cells in the basal portion of the epithelium. The squamous epithelial cell lining of the esophagus is a protective coating of cells for the underlying tissue.

Stomach

The stomach has an epithelial cell lining, 0.5 mm thick. The epithelium is characterized by a uniform surface with shallow pits (foveolae gastricae), below which are gastric glands. The epithelium lining the surface and pits consists of surface mucous cells uniform throughout the stomach. Differences in the underlying glands permit histologic separation of three distinct gastric regions: the cardia, body (body and fundus), and pyloric antrum.[1]

The cardia is the first 1 to 3 cm of gastric epithelium distal to the esophagogastric junction. The cardia epithelium is composed of columnar mucous cells lining the surface and pits and mucus-secreting cells in the glands, and undifferentiated neck cells. As a rule, parietal, chief, and endocrine cells are absent. A characteristic feature is the presence of one or more dilated cystic glands.

The epithelial cell lining of the body and fundus is more complex and accounts for approximately 80 per cent of the remaining stomach. In addition to the surface and pit mucous cells, mucous neck cells, and undifferentiated neck cells, the glands contain parietal (oxyntic) cells, chief (zymogen) cells, mucous cells, and endocrine cells. The parietal cells are located in the mid to upper half of the glands and secrete hydrochloric acid and intrinsic factor. Electron microscopy reveals that the cytoplasm is packed with mitochondria and contains a secretory canaliculi system with a microvillous lining. The chief cells are located in the deepest portion of the glands, and their cytoplasm contains pepsinogen granules, precursors of the proteolytic enzyme pepsin. The mucous cells of the glands also secrete mucus and pepsinogens. The endocrine cell population of this region includes argentaffin and argyrophilic cells that are scattered singly or in small clusters in the midzone of the glands. The argentaffin cells secrete serotonin and histamine. The endocrine cells are thought to have their embryologic origin from the neural crest. The undifferentiated neck cells are thought to be multipotential proliferating cells from which the other cell types are derived.

The epithelium of the pyloric antrum occupies a triangular area in the distal fifth of the stomach. The architecture of the epithelium differs from that of the body in that the pits are deeper and the glands shorter but more extensively coiled. The cell population differs in that parietal cells are less frequent and chief cells are rarely seen at all; gastrin-secreting (G) cells are added to the endocrine cell types. The gastrin-secreting cells are found most frequently in the midportion of the glands; these cells are able to synthesize DNA and to replicate through mitosis.

Small Intestine

The small intestine is composed of the duodenum, jejunum, and ileum. It is about 280 cm in length and 4 cm in internal diameter.[1] However, the surface area is much greater than these measurements suggest because the surface is extensively folded and contains numerous finger-like projections called villi. Villi are visible under the microscope at low power and have been estimated to number 25 million.[2] The length and shape of the villi change in the three portions of the intestine; they are longest and broadest in the duodenum and shortest and most finger-like in the ileum. The villi project from cryptlike glands. The number of cells that compose the crypts (of Lieberkühn) does not differ in the three regions of the bowel. In fact, the basic structure of the epithelium is the same throughout the small intestine.

The epithelial cell lining is a single layer of columnar cells, 40–50 μm in height, which make up the cover of the villi and the crypts. The villous epithelium is composed of absorptive, goblet, and a few endocrine cells. The crypt epithelium is composed of undifferentiated goblet, endocrine, and Paneth cells. Of particular interest to the toxicologist are the undifferentiated proliferating cells of the crypts and the absorptive cells of the villi. Because of the great proliferative activity of the undifferentiating crypt cells, the intestinal epithelium is particularly susceptible to damage by mitotic inhibitors that interfere with normal cell growth. This subject will be discussed further, in the next section on epithelial cell proliferation. Since the major function of the small intestine is the digestion and absorption of nutrients and this function also can be poisoned by a variety of agents, the highly specialized role of the absorptive cells will be further discussed.

The absorptive cells are distinguished by a surface brush border that is a complex organelle containing hydrolytic enzymes, receptors, and other proteins involved in transport and contraction. The brush border is a membranous sheet, 6.0 nm wide, which has on the luminal side a carbohydrate-rich layer known as the glycocalyx (fuzzy coat).[3] Filamentous structures, thought to be actin, are attached to the inner aspect of the brush border membrane. These fibrils extend into the region of the terminal web, where they intertwine and form attachments to each other so that the contractions of the filaments shorten the microvilli. Mitotic figures are never seen in the villous epithelium. All the recognized brush border enzymes are hydrolases that degrade polymeric substances in the human. These enzymes include disaccharidases, peptidases, phosphatases, and others (see Table 12–3). Other nonenzymatic proteins, such as the receptors for intrinsic factor-B_{12} complex, are also found in the brush border.

Colon

The colon is composed of several anatomically distinct regions: cecum, ascending colon, transverse colon, descending colon, sigmoid colon, and rectum. The basic architecture of the epithelial lining is the same throughout.[1] The epithelial lining differs from that of the small bowel in that villi are absent; therefore, the absorptive surface is flat. However, numerous straight tubular crypts, up to 0.7 mm in depth, are present. The crypts are lined with three main cell types: proliferating differentiated cells, mucus-secreting goblet cells, and absorptive cells. The absorptive cells vary from the similar cells of the small intestine, and the microvilli are much less abundant. Paneth cells are seen occasionally in the proximal colon. Of particular interest to the toxicologist are the proliferating cells and the absorptive cells, which are subject to damage from internal and external toxins.

GASTROINTESTINAL EPITHELIAL CELL RENEWAL

A number of agents, including chemotherapeutic drugs used in the treatment of cancer and other diseases of proliferating tissues, are poisonous to the rapidly dividing cells of the gastrointestinal epithelium. An understanding of how these agents adversely affect the gastrointestinal epithelium requires a general appreciation of the kinetics of epithelial cell growth. It is beyond the scope of this chapter to review the subject in great detail, and a brief overview with emphasis on the epithelium of the small intestine should suffice. A number of excellent reviews[4–12] from which these comments are derived are available for the reader who desires more information.

Cell Cycle. The cell cycle in human intestine is the most rapid of all cycles in normal tissue and is the reason for the intestine being exquisitely sensitive to a variety of poisons. The events of cell proliferation are studied by mitotic counting, which identifies the cells in mitosis, and by autoradiography, using tritiated thymidine to label cells entering DNA synthesis. Concomitant estimation of the *mitotic index* (percentage of cells undergoing mitosis), and the *DNA synthesis index* (percentage of cells involved in DNA synthesis), provides a more dynamic picture of the cell cycle than either alone. The phases of the cell cycle are identified by serial examination of the epithelium at intervals after labeling. Baserga defines the cell cycle as the period between the midpoint of mitosis and the midpoint of the subsequent mitosis in one daughter cell, including the cellular and biochemical events that regulate cell growth.[4] Tissues grow primarily through an increase in the number of cells. Occasionally, tissues grow by increasing the amount of intracellular substance. In either case, cells also must increase in mass, and all cell components double their mass before mitosis.

Cycling cells go through various phases. The G_1 (initial growth) phase is the most variable period of the cell cycle, and its duration largely determines the rate of cell proliferation. In general, rapidly growing populations of the intestine consist of cells with G_1 periods shorter than those of slowly growing cells. Some rapidly proliferating cell lines do not even have a G_1 period. The S (synthesis) phase is the period during which DNA replicates and chromosomal proteins are laid down on the newly synthesized DNA. The G_2 phase is the interval between completion of DNA synthesis and mitosis.

Many biochemical events that apply specifically to certain phases of the cell cycle (cell cycle-specific) have been described. These events seem to occur only in proliferating cells and are absent or undetectable in nongrowing cells. A number of enzymes that are strictly related to DNA synthesis increase in activity during the S phase. These enzymes include thymidine kinase, DNA polymerase, dihydrofolate reductase, and ribonucleotide reductase. DNA replication occurs only during a discrete and brief period (S phase) of the intestinal cell cycle. The sequence of events and the position of the key enzymatic steps in the sequence are outlined in Table 12–1.

From the standpoint of cell proliferation, the intestinal epithelium contains a mixture of two cell populations: (1) Cells that are continuously dividing, i.e., going from one mitosis to the next in a short time. After mitosis, these cells go through the G_1 phase, the S phase, and the G_2 phase and then back into mitosis. Since they regularly traverse the cell cycle, they are called cycling cells. In the intestine they are represented by rapidly proliferating cells of the crypt epithelium. (2) Cells that leave the cell cycle after a certain number of divisions and differentiate; these cells are destined to die without dividing

Table 12–1. THE KEY METABOLIC STEPS INVOLVED IN THE CELL CYCLE

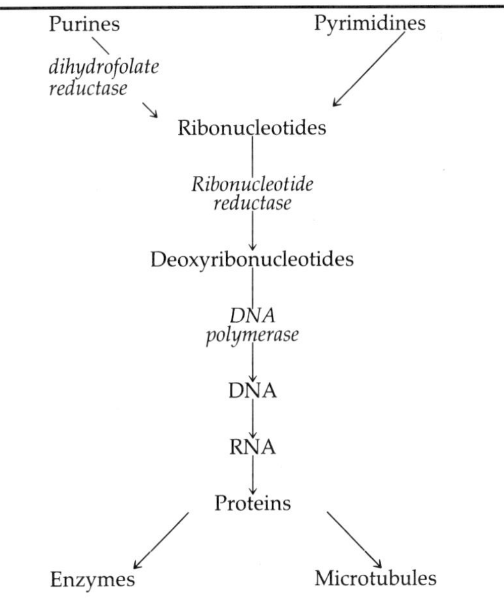

Metabolic poisons interrupt the pathway by enzyme inhibition or substrate alteration, resulting in injury or death to the cell.

again. Absorptive cells of the villous epithelium are an example of this class of nondividing, mature cells. Absorptive cells migrate onto the villus after at least two divisions within the crypt and, having lost the ability to incorporate thymidine, undergo further mitosis. Differentiation into a mature columnar cell is accompanied by the appearance of enzymes necessary for the primary function of nutrient digestion. Cell migration is more rapid in the ileum than the jejunum as a result of the decreasing aboral gradient of villous height, down the small intestine.

A third class of cells seen in most normal tissue leaves the cycle temporarily and remains in a dormant state until environmental conditions stimulate re-entry into the cell cycle. Some stem cells belong to this third group, since they do not cycle until tissue depletion causes them to re-enter the cycle and proliferate in order to replenish the tissue. These cells are called G_0 cells.

Normal intestinal epithelial tissue growth depends on (1) the cell-cycle time, (2) the growth fraction, and (3) the rate of cell loss. The *cell-cycle time* in cycling cells refers to the interval between mitosis—the shorter the interval, the faster cells are produced. The *growth fraction* refers to the fraction of cycling cells; when all the cells participate in the process of cell renewal, the growth fraction equals 1, and the cell-cycle time equals the turnover time. The larger the fraction of cycling cells in a population, the faster the increase in cell number. The *rate of cell loss* in the cell population refers to the fraction of cells that dies or migrates to other tissues. The cell-cycle time and the growth fraction determine the number of cells produced per unit of time, and the rate of cell loss determines the number of cells lost per unit of time. In the adult intestine in which cell proliferation is rapid yet growth has ceased, the number of cells produced per unit of time is equal to the number that die—the tissue is in a steady state. Measurement of DNA exfoliated into the intestinal lumen can be used to determine the rate of cell renewal since, under these steady-state conditions, cell loss from the villous tip is balanced by cell birth at the crypt base.

Cell division in enteric epithelium is restricted to the base of the crypts of Lieberkühn, where cells have high activities of the enzymes of nucleic acid synthesis. The complete cell cycle in human intestine lasts approximately 24 hours. The M phase of actual mitosis occupies only a brief part (about 1 hour). DNA synthesis is confined to a discrete period (S phase) lasting 6 to 11 hours, but RNA and proteins are actively elaborated throughout the S phase and during the premitotic (G_2) and postmitotic (G_1) periods.

Table 12–2. TURNOVER TIME OF HUMAN GASTROINTESTINAL EPITHELIAL CELLS

SITE	METHOD	TURNOVER TIME[a] *(days)*	REFERENCES
Esophagus (rodent)[b]	labeling	7–10	8
Stomach[c]	labeling	2–6	9, 10
Duodenum	mitotic counting	2	11
	labeling	5–6	9
Jejunum	labeling	5	12
Ileum	labeling	3	13
Colon	labeling	4–8	14

[a]Turnover time refers to the surface epithelium; Paneth cells, argentaffin cells, chief cells, and parietal cells renew more slowly, estimated on the order of weeks.

[b]Comparable data in humans are not available, but human esophageal epithelial renewal is probably much slower, estimated on the order of weeks to months.

[c]The glandular portion of the stomach renews itself more slowly than the surface epithelium.

The epithelial surface of the gastrointestinal tract is in a constant state of renewal. As described, the renewal process can be divided into three phases: replication, migration, and differentiation. The epithelium has the fastest rate of turnover for any normal tissue of the body. Enteric epithelium is completely replaced in 3 to 6 days. The constant turnover of the epithelium is maintained by a delicate balance between cell population in the proliferative zones and cell loss from the differentiated regions. This rate of turnover is so rapid that cells do not normally enter the prolonged interphase (G_0) found in other, more slowly renewing tissue. The turnover time, or epithelial cell renewal time, for each organ of the gastrointestinal tract is shown in Table 12–2.

GASTROINTESTINAL EPITHELIAL CELL FUNCTION

The functions of gastrointestinal epithelium are numerous, and a complete discussion is beyond the scope of this chapter. However, selected functions bear a relationship to poisoning and have been chosen for discussion.

$$H_2O \longrightarrow OH^- + H^+ \longrightarrow H^+$$

$$HCO_3^- \longleftarrow HCO_3^- \xleftarrow[\text{anhydrase}]{\text{carbonic}} OH^- + CO_2$$

(Reaction 1)

Esophagus

The function of the esophagus is to transport food from the mouth and pharynx to the stomach. The normal process of swallowing is a function of the underlying muscular coats and occurs in a peristaltic manner requiring 5 to 7 seconds. The role of the epithelium is to protect the underlying tissue.

Gastric Acid Secretion

Hydrochloric acid is secreted into the gastric lumen by parietal cells.[15] The process requires energy, which is derived from hydrolysis of adenosine triphosphate (ATP). As mentioned, the parietal cell is well endowed with mitochondria that generate the high energy phosphate bonds of ATP during aerobic metabolism. For each H^+ secreted, a molecule of CO_2 derived from arterial blood or epithelial cell metabolism is converted to HCO_3^-, which ultimately enters the interstitial fluid. Parietal cells contain a high concentration of carbonic anhydrase, which catalyzes the conversion (Reaction 1). The H^+ concentration in gastric juice is 3 million times greater than that in blood tissue, and the maximum concentration is between 140 and 160 mM. In addition to H^+, the other principal cations are Na^+ (137 mM) and K^+ (17 mM). There is an inverse relationship between the concentration of H^+ and Na^+; the concentration of K^+ is relatively stable. The principal anion is Cl^- (166 mM). In the fasting state, acid secretion has a circadian rhythm, with a peak at 6 PM to 1 AM and a valley from 5 AM to 11 AM; periods of achlorhydria are not uncommon.

Acid secretion is regulated by three major endogenous chemicals: acetylcholine, gastrin, and histamine.[15] A diagram of the interrelationship of these secretagogues is presented in Reaction 2.

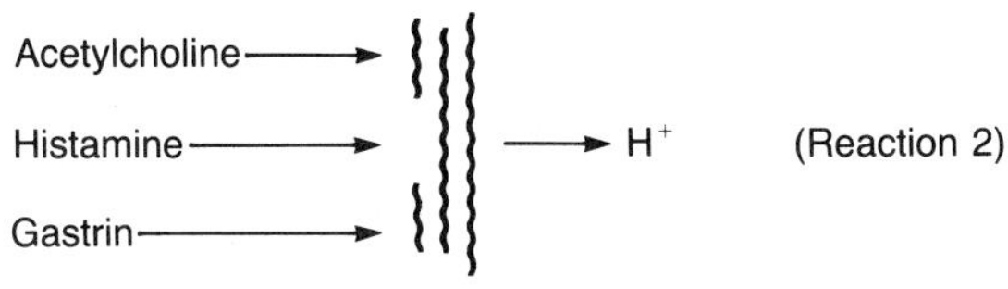

Parietal cell receptors

Acetylcholine release at the neuroeffector site of the parietal cell can be initiated by vagal efferent nerves and local nerves. Acetylcholine causes direct stimulation of acid secretion and the effect is potentiated by histamine. The effect of acetylcholine can be mimicked by cholinomimetic drugs such as carbachol and inhibited by muscarinic antagonists such as atropine at the neuroeffector site.

Gastrin occurs in two major forms: big gastrin, or G34, and little gastrin, or G17, which are distinguished by the number of amino acid residues. On a molar basis, little gastrin is six times more potent than big gastrin. Pharmacologically, the effect can be reproduced with the five-terminal amino acid synthetic peptide, pentagastrin. The highest concentration and total amount of gastrin are in the G cells of antral glands. Appreciable amounts of gastrin are also found normally in the epithelium of the duodenal bulb, where the concentration is about 10 to 20 per cent of that in antral epithelium. Antral gastrin is 90 to 95 per cent little gastrin, and duodenal gastrin is about 50 per cent big gastrin. After meals, the predominant form of gastrin in plasma is big gastrin, comprising 60 to 70 per cent of the total gastrin, although little gastrin remains the main stimulant of acid secretion. The predominance of big gastrin in the plasma is accounted for by the slower removal—a T½ of about 50 minutes contrasted to a T½ of about 6 minutes for little gastrin. Gastrin causes direct stimulation of acid secretion, and the effect is potentiated by histamine.

Histamine is abundantly present in most tissues of the body, and the gastric mucosa is not excepted. Histamine originates from mast cells, which are especially numerous around small blood vessels and basophils. Histidine decarboxylase, present in gastric endocrine cells of rats, but not of people, can convert histidine to histamine. However, this enzyme has not been found in any human tissue, and the mechanism of human biosynthesis of histamine is not known. Nor is it known whether mast cells or basophils are more important to histamine release or how release occurs. Nevertheless, the appearance of histamine H_2-antagonists, such as cimetidine, confirms that histamine is involved in all or most forms of acid secretion.[15] H_2-antagonists inhibit acid secretion stimulated not only by histamine but also by a variety of other agents, including gastrin, caffeine, and insulin. It is hypothesized that histamine is released constantly and sensitizes the parietal cells to other stimuli. Therefore, when the effect of histamine is blocked by H_2-antagonists, acid secretion in response to other stimuli is inhibited.

In reality, the physiology and biochemistry of acid secretion are much more complex than suggested by this brief overview. A general presentation has been provided to give at least the major concepts regarding endogenous stimulation of acid secretion and to provide some background for an appreciation of the effects on the stomach of various chemicals, including drugs, and of strong acids and alkalis.

Digestion and Absorption

Virtually all food enters the gastrointestinal tract in polymeric form and requires enzymatic digestion to hydrolyze the subunits to monomers that can be absorbed by specific transport systems. These digestive enzymes originate primarily from the stomach chief cells, pancreas, and small intestinal absorptive cells. Absorptive cells of the small intestinal epithelium have a highly specific brush border on which many enzymes reside. Brush border enzymes are all hydrolases that degrade substances in the lumen of the intestine.[16, 18] These enzymes include disaccharidases, peptidases, and phosphatases and are shown in Table 12–3. The enzymes hydrolyze their substrates outside the cell, so at least some part of the protein faces the external surface of the membrane. The surface exposure of these enzymes renders them susceptible to damage from poisons within

Table 12–3. HUMAN BRUSH BORDER ENZYMES

ENZYME	PRINCIPAL SUBSTRATE	PRODUCTS
Peptidases		
Oligopeptidases	Oligopeptides	Peptides
Dipeptidases	Dipeptides	Amino acids
Folate conjugase	Folate polyglutamate	Folate monoglutamate
Enterokinase	Trypsinogen	Trypsin
Carbohydrases		
Glucoamylase	α-Dextrins, maltose, maltotriose*	Glucose, oligosaccharides
Isomaltase (α-dextrinase)	α-Dextrins	Glucose, oligosaccharides
Lactase	Lactose	Glucose, galactose
Sucrase	Sucrose, maltose, maltotriose	Glucose, fructose
Trehalase	Trehalose	Glucose
Others		
Alkaline phosphatase		
Guanylate cyclase		

*α-Dextrins, maltose, and maltotriose are products of starch digestion that originate in the intestinal lumen from pancreatic amylase hydrolysis.

the lumen of the intestinal tract, including drugs, but also from infectious organisms, foreign antigens and pancreatic proteases. The proteolytic digestion of the surface enzymes leads to a rapid turnover of some of these proteins and reduces the half-life to 4 to 6 hours. Therefore, the maintenance of activity of some brush border enzymes requires several cycles of protein synthesis during the approximately 5-day lifespan of jejunal cells.[3]

Absorption of dietary nutrients follows their digestion from polymers to monomers. Complex starches are digested to hexoses, proteins to dipeptides and amino acids, and vitamin complexes to free vitamins.[15–17] These monomers are then absorbed by specific carrier-mediated mechanisms. Sodium-dependent active transport systems have been described for glucose and galactose, amino acids and peptides, pteroylglutamate, vitamin C, biotin, bile salts, riboflavin, thiamine, and other water-soluble organic substrates.[18] It is hypothesized that the sodium gradient across the intestinal absorptive cell membrane is the driving force for active transport. The carrier systems for these nutrients have not been isolated in humans but are thought to be represented by integral proteins situated in the lipid membrane of the brush border. For a membrane protein to have a carrier function, it must be able to orient to the internal and external surfaces of the cell. As with the surface orientation of brush border digestive enzymes, it is the external orientation that is most susceptible to toxic injury from ingested poisons.

Lipids do not appear to require a membrane protein for absorption. Following digestion of dietary neutral fat (triglycerides) to long-chain fatty acids and monoglycerides by pancreatic lipase, the monomers as well as cholesterol are solubilized in bile salts to form micelles. Micellar formation requires bile salts at a concentration of 2 mM or higher. The concentration of bile salts in the duodenum after gallbladder contraction averages 2 to 10 mM under normal circumstances. Long-chain fatty acids, monoglycerides, and cholesterol are absorbed by diffusion when the molecules by chance collide with the absorptive cell membrane. Fat absorption then is diminished by factors that interrupt the formation of micelles or alter the absorptive membrane.[19]

Colon Function

The functions of the colon mediated by the epithelium include (1) absorption of water and electrolytes, and (2) secretion of potassium. The storage and discharge functions of the colon depend on the motor activity and may be altered by poisons affecting the autonomic nervous system. They will not be considered here. The fact that colonic epithelium has a much more decisive role than intestinal motility in controlling stool water excretion has been discovered in recent years.[20]

Colonic epithelium is confronted with about 1500 ml of water, 200 mEq of sodium, 5 mEq of potassium, 120 mEq of chloride, and 60 mEq of bicarbonate for absorption per 24 hours. A normal stool contains about 100 to 150 ml of water, 5 mEq of sodium, 9 to 13 mEq of potassium, 2 mEq of chloride, and 3 mEq of bicarbonate, thus indicating the net absorption of water, sodium, chloride, and bicarbonate and the net secretion of potassium. A variety of agents can alter fluid and electrolyte movement. These agents exert their effect by different mechanisms: (a) decrease in electrolyte absorption; (b) stimulation of active electrolyte secretion; (c) increase in mucosal permeability; (d) increase in mucosal cyclic AMP levels; and (e) alteration of the mucosal morphology. Water and electrolyte movement are affected by pH, osmolality, and ions (bile acids, sulfates, hydroxy fatty acids) but not by glucose, amino acid, or bicarbonate. Mucosal cyclic AMP may affect water and electrolyte movement. A number of hormones clearly affect water and electrolyte movement, including aldosterone, 9-α-fluorohydrocortisone, and antidiuretic hormone. Pentagastrin, glucagon, angiotensin, and prostaglandins E_3 and $F_2\alpha$ have not altered water and electrolyte movement.

The absorption of bile acids by colonic epithelium is a special situation.[21] In healthy adults, a bile acid pool of 2 to 4 grams recycles through the enterohepatic circulation 6 to 8 times per day. Each cycle results in the release of 0.2 to 0.6 gram of bile acids into the proximal small intestine after each meal. More than 90 per cent of the bile acids secreted are reabsorbed by ionic, nonionic, and active transport systems within the small intestine. The remaining 0.4 to 0.8 gram of bile acid reaches the colon per 24 hours, where 30 to 40 per cent is absorbed by nonionic diffusion, and 0.3 to 0.6 gram is lost in the feces per 24 hours. Dihydroxy bile acids—chenodeoxycholic acid and deoxycholic acid—have cathartic properties. Water and sodium secretion results from perfusion of the colon with a dihydroxy bile acid at a concentration above 3 mM. Diarrhea is a serious consequence of bile salt malabsorption from ileal disease and is a potential side effect of chenodeoxycholic acid therapy when given for the dissolution of cholesterol gallstones. The mechanism may involve cyclic AMP as bile acids activate adenyl cyclase.

INHIBITORS OF CELL GROWTH

Chemotherapeutic agents serve as a model for gastrointestinal toxicity. These agents exert their poisonous effect on gastrointestinal epithelium by a number of mechanisms, each of which results in interference with cell proliferation without reducing the normal rate of cell death. Thus, the steady state is interrupted. Chemotherapeutic poisons are discussed in detail in Chapter 55, therefore only the specific features of these poisons that affect the gastrointestinal epithelium will be described. A list of chemotherapeutic agents that are potentially poisonous to the gastrointestinal epithelium is presented in Table 12–4. The table includes the mechanism of action, cell-cycle specificity, metabolic activation requirements, nature of gastrointestinal toxicity, excretion mechanisms, and treatment alternatives. It is of special interest to take one well-studied example from the list of agents for more detailed review. Amethopterin is a good example for this purpose since intestinal toxicity from this drug is a major limitation in its use.

Amethopterin, or methotrexate (4-amino-10-methylpteroylglutamic acid), is a folate antagonist that has been effective in the treatment of acute leukemia, choriocarcinoma, lymphomas, Wegener granulomatosis, certain solid tumors, and severe psoriasis.[23, 24] Recent results with high-dose amethopterin in the treatment of osteogenic sarcoma and lung and breast cancer[25] have encouraged the hope that improved amethopterin therapy of other solid tumors may be possible.

The chemotherapeutic usefulness of amethopterin appears to be referable to two separate effects of the drug at the molecular level: (1) inhibition of intracellular dihydrofolate reductase (the enzyme responsible for the reduction of pteroylglutamate or dihydrofolate to tetrahydrofolate) (Reaction 3), which, in turn, leads to decreased synthesis of certain metabolites (thymidylate, inosinate, methionine, serine, histidine) that serve as precursors of DNA, RNA, and protein; and (2) inhibition of the transport of 5-methyl-tetrahydrofolate into cells. The effect of this metabolic block on DNA synthesis is illustrated in Reaction 3.

Toxicity toward the nonmalignant proliferating cells of the intestinal epithelium is a major limitation in the therapeutic use of amethopterin. Efforts to circumvent this undesirable side effect have utilized *reduced* folate derivatives (e.g., 5-formyltetrahydrofolate and 5-methyltetrahydrofolate) as "rescue agents,"[24] enzymatic cleavage of the drug,[26] and removal of the drug by hemodialysis and charcoal filtration,[27] although the latter method appears to be of limited value.[28] Studies of amethopterin toxicity to the small intestine in mice have shown that amethopterin accumulates in intestinal mucosa and appears to be transported into cells by a carrier-mediated system; the drug reaches much higher levels in the intestine, compared with tumor cells, and has a substantially longer duration of inhibition of DNA synthesis.[29] Amethopterin doses of greater than 3 mg/kg or concentrations in plasma of 5×10^{-9} M inhibit DNA synthesis in the intestine,[30] and cell death occurs when inhibition of DNA synthesis lasts for more than 25 to 30 hours.[29] In humans, plasma levels of amethopterin of approximately 1×10^{-6} M for more than 48 hours lead to appreciable toxicity.[31] Intestinal toxicity, at least in mice, appears to be related to the duration of inhibition of DNA synthesis, which reflects the persistence of exchangeable amethopterin levels in tissue adequate for complete inhi-

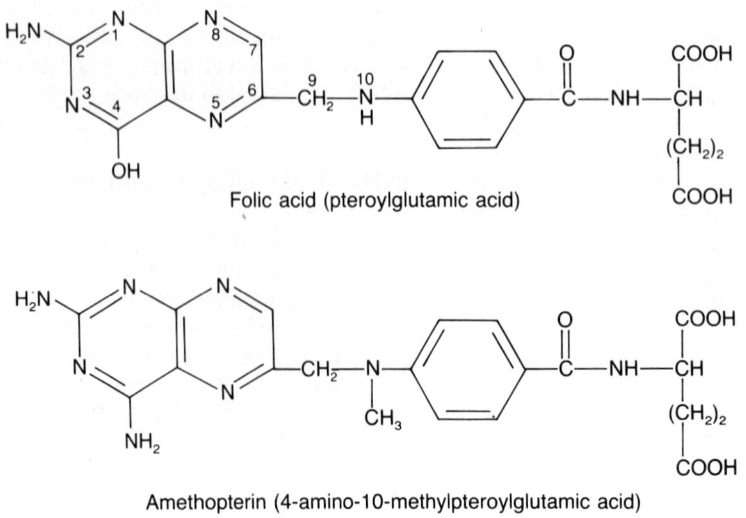

Folic acid (pteroylglutamic acid)

(Reaction 3)

Amethopterin (4-amino-10-methylpteroylglutamic acid)

Table 12–4. CHEMOTHERAPEUTIC AGENTS WITH PROMINENT GASTROINTESTINAL TOXICITY

DRUG	ROUTE OF ADMINISTRATION	MECHANISM OF ACTION	CELL CYCLE–SPECIFIC	ACTIVATION	GASTROINTESTINAL TOXICITY		DEACTIVATION	TREATMENT
					Acute	*Delayed*		
ALKYLATING AGENTS								
cyclophosphamide (Cytoxan)	PO/IV	Alkylates DNA	No	Converted to active intermediates in liver (and plasma)	Nausea and vomiting, pain, bleeding, jaundice		Excreted in urine as a metabolite	High fluid intake
mechlorethamine (nitrogen mustard; Mustargen)	IV	Alkylates DNA	No	None	Nausea and vomitng	Sore throat, bleeding	Metabolized rapidly	Prochlorperazine, 10–20 mg, barbiturate prior to administration
busulfan (Myleran)	PO	Alkylates DNA	No	None	Pain, sore throat, bleeding	Bleeding		High fluid intake
carmustine (BCNU, BiCNU)	IV	Alkylates DNA	No	None	Mouth, lip, and throat sores			
chlorambucil (Leukeran)	PO				Pain, mouth and throat sores	Sore throat, bleeding		High fluid intake
cisplatin (Platinol)	IV	Alkylates DNA	No	None	Pain, sore throat, nausea, and vomiting			High fluid intake
estramustine (Emcyt, Estacyt)	PO	Alkylates DNA in cells with estrogen receptors	No	None	Pain, nausea and vomiting	Diarrhea, bleeding		
lomustine (CeeNu, CCNU)	PO				Mouth, lip, and throat sores	Sore throat, bleeding		Cessation
melphalan (Alkeran, phenylalanine, mustard)	PO	Alkylates DNA	No	None	Diarrhea, jaundice, bleeding, unsteadiness	Sore throat, bleeding		Cessation
streptozotocin (Zanosar)	IV	Alkylates DNA	No	None	Sore throat and mouth, lip, throat; diarrhea, jaundice	Sore throat, bleeding		High fluid intake
ANTIMETABOLITES								
cytarabine hydrochloride (arabinosylcytosine; Cytosar-U)	IV	Inhibits DNA polymerase	Yes	None	Sore throat, bleeding, jaundice			Cessation
floxuridine (FUDR)	IV				Nausea, vomiting, mouth sores	Diarrhea, pain, bleeding	Metabolized in liver	Cessation
fluorouracil (5-FU, FU, Adrucil)	IV	Competitive inhibition of thymidine synthetase	Yes	None	Nausea	Oral and GI ulceration, stomatitis and diarrhea	Metabolized in liver	Cessation

Table continued on following page

Table 12–4. CHEMOTHERAPEUTIC AGENTS WITH PROMINENT GASTROINTESTINAL TOXICITY *Continued*

DRUG	ROUTE OF ADMINISTRATION	MECHANISM OF ACTION	CELL CYCLE–SPECIFIC	ACTIVATION	GASTROINTESTINAL TOXICITY *Acute*	GASTROINTESTINAL TOXICITY *Delayed*	DEACTIVATION	TREATMENT
mercaptopurine (6-MP, Purinethol)	PO	Inhibits enzymes of purine metabolism	Yes	Converted to 5′-phosphate ribonucleotides; toxicity increased by xanthine oxidase allopurinol	Occasional nausea and vomiting	Occasional hepatic damage	Metabolized in liver and excreted in urine	Cessation
methotrexate (amethopterin; Mexate, MTX)	PO/IV	Competitive inhibition of dihydrofolate reductase	Yes	None	Occasional diarrhea, hepatic necrosis	Oral and GI ulceration, cirrhosis	Excreted in urine and bile	Leucovorin; $NaHCO_3$; hemodialysis
thioguanine (6-TG)		Inhibits enzymes of purine metabolism	Yes	Converted to 5′-phosphate ribonucleotides	Occasional nausea and vomitng	Mouth sores, diarrhea	Metabolized and excreted in urine	Cessation
PLANT ALKALOIDS								
vinblastine sulfate (Velban)	IV	Binds microtubular protein	Yes	None	Nausea and vomiting, anorexia, diarrhea	Constipation, paralytic ileus, stomatitis	Secreted in bile	Prophylactic laxatives
vincristine sulfate (Oncovin)	IV	Binds microtubular protein	Yes	None		Constipation, paralytic ileus	Secreted in bile	Prophylactic laxatives
ANTIBIOTICS								
doxorubicin (Adriamycin)	IV	Intercalates DNA base pairs	No	None	Pain, mouth, lip, and throat sores	Nausea, vomiting		
bleomycin (Blenoxane)	IV/IM	Causes scission of DNA	Yes	None	Nausea	Bone marrow depression, cardiotoxicity, alopecia, stomatitis	Metabolized in liver	Cessation; hemodialysis
dactinomycin (actinomycin D; Cosmegen)	IV	Forms complex with DNA that inhibits RNA synthesis	No	None	Nausea and vomiting	Stomatitis	Unknown	Cessation
daunorubicin	IV	Intercalates DNA base pairs	No	None	Nausea and vomiting	Stomatitis, oral ulcers, diarrhea, bleeding	Excreted in urine and bile	Cessation
mitomycin C (Mutamycin)	IV	Alkylates DNA and RNA	No	Cleaved to aziridine ring	Nausea and vomiting, hepatotoxicity	Sore throat, bleeding	Excreted in urine	Cessation
plicamycin (Mithramycin, Mithracin)		Binds DNA	No	None	Nausea and vomiting	Sore throat, bleeding	Metabolized by liver and other tissues and excreted in urine	Cessation

OTHER SYNTHETIC AGENTS								
dacarbazine (DTIC-Dome; DIC)	IV	Purine analogue with alkylating properties	No	None	Nausea and vomiting	Sore throat, bleeding	Excreted in urine	May subside after several days of therapy
hydroxyurea (Hydrea)	PO	Inhibits ribonucleoside diphosphate reductase	Yes	None	Mild nausea and vomiting	Nausea, vomiting, abdominal pain	Excreted in urine	Cessation
mitotane (o.p′-DDD; Lysodren)	PO	Inhibits adrenal steroid synthesis	No	None	Nausea and vomiting	Nausea, vomiting, diarrhea	Excreted in urine and bile	Cessation
procarbazine hydrochloride (methylhydrazine; ibenzmethyzin; Matulane, Natulan)	PO	Inhibition of DNA, RNA and protein synthesis	No	None	Nausea and vomiting	Pain, nausea, vomiting	Metabolized and excreted in urine	Administer drug in gradually escalating doses
prednisone (Deltasone, Meticorten, Orasone)	PO	Lymphocytolytic and interacts with glucocorticoid receptors	No	Converted to prednisone in tumor cells	Bleeding, pain, burning	Pain, nausea, vomiting		Cessation
tamoxifen (Nolvadex)	PO	Estrogen antagonist		None	None	None		High fluid intake
asparaginase (Elspar)	IV	Hydrolysis of serum aspargine, thus depriving leukemia cells of this essential amino acid		None	Pain, nausea, vomiting	Pain, nausea, vomiting, jaundice		High fluid intake
etoposide (VP-16, VePesid)	IV	Podophyllum derivative	Yes	None	Mouth, lip, and throat sores	Diarrhea		Cessation

bition of dihydrofolate reductase. Consequently, both the duration of exposure and suprathreshold concentrations of drug, rather than the peak levels of drug achieved, are responsible for the intestinal toxicity.[32]

In humans, amethopterin is well absorbed from the gastrointestinal tract, and its toxicity via the oral route is no greater than when it is administered parenterally. Absorption appears to occur by a saturable mechanism. After intravenous injection, amethopterin disappearance from plasma is triphasic. The initial half-life (distribution) is 0.65 to 0.85 hr; the second half-life (clearance) is 2 to 3.5 hr; and the third (enterohepatic circulation) is 9 to 12 hr. The terminal half-life, which is perpetuated by the enterohepatic circulation, is responsible for the majority of intestinal toxicity.[32] Amethopterin is concentrated 4- to 8-fold in the liver and further concentrated 200-fold in bile to that of plasma concentrations. The amount of drug secreted in bile after intravenous administration of 30 mg/m^2 is 5 to 10 per cent per 24 hr. Fifty to 70 per cent of the drug binds to albumin and lesser amounts (0 to 17 per cent) to protein in interstitial fluids.[33] The mechanisms by which amethopterin enters normal intestinal epithelial cells are not fully characterized but energy-coupled, carrier-mediated, and passive systems operate in different cell types.

Amethopterin is metabolized to polyglutamates by the liver and probably other organs and to other metabolites by tissue and intestinal bacterial enzymes. Metabolites account for up to a third of the total plasma levels during the terminal plasma disappearance of high-dose therapy. Since the terminal phase of amethopterin disappearance determines the severity of amethopterin toxicity, then metabolism, as well as the enterohepatic circulation, may be important in the origin of this toxicity.[32] Amethopterin excretion occurs primarily by renal glomerular filtration (110 $ml/min/m^2$), and at high concentrations the drug is actively secreted by tubular cells. One to 2 per cent of the drug is excreted in stool, indicating that most of the drug secreted in bile is reabsorbed by the intestinal mucosa. The fecal excretion rises as the amethopterin dosage increases, as predicted by the limitations of the absorptive mechanisms.[32]

The interaction of chemotherapeutic agents with other drugs is a critical factor in the poison potential. Amethopterin interacts with a variety of other drugs, as described in vivo and in vitro using human tumor cells, including the following ways: displacement from plasma albumin (salicylate, sulfisoxazole), decrease in renal tubular transport (probenecid, salicylate, other organic acids), decrease in human leukemia cell uptake (cephalothin, hydrocortisone), and inhibition of intestinal absorption (oral broad-spectrum nonabsorbable antibiotics).[32]

The intestinal response to subtoxic doses of amethopterin is characterized by a decrease in the number of mitoses in the crypts, which is detectable within 3 hours and returns to normal within 96 hours; the villous pattern and epithelial length remain normal.[34] Toxic doses lead to a sustained reduction in mitoses with loss of surface absorptive cells without replacement cells. This desquamation of the epithelial cell lining is associated with extensive leukocytic infiltration of the lamina propria. Eventually, large areas of ulceration develop, and bleeding occurs. The mucositis may involve the tongue, buccal mucosa, esophagus, stomach, small intestine, or colon. The pathology is not specific for amethopterin and may be seen with a variety of poisonous or otherwise noxious agents, a fact that contributes to the intestine's notoriety for its limited response to injury. Experimental data indicate important time- and concentration-dependent relationships that may be specific for different organs. The critical time and plasma concentration thresholds for gastrointestinal epithelium are approximately 42 hours and 2×10^{-8} M, respectively, both of which must be exceeded for toxicity to occur. The severity of toxicity is more closely associated with the duration of amethopterin exposure beyond the time threshold than the magnitude above the concentration threshold.[32]

Gastrointestinal symptoms include nausea, vomiting, abdominal pain, diarrhea, and, in severe cases, hematemesis and melena. An assessment of the toxicity must bear in mind toxicity to other organs and toxicity from other agents that may be in combined use with amethopterin. The rapidly dividing cells of the bone marrow have a short cell-cycle time like that of intestinal epithelium and are frequent recipients of amethopterin toxicity.

Prevention. The use of amethopterin and other powerful chemotherapeutic agents should be limited to physicians who are specifically trained in their use and to institutions prepared to deal with the complications of toxicity. Experienced staff, trained laboratory personnel, intensive care facilities, and renal dialysis should be available. The hazards of potent cytotoxic therapy are too numerous for use outside specialized centers.

The example of amethopterin therapy can be carried further to illustrate how prevention of toxicity can be accomplished. Extremely high initial plasma concentrations of amethopterin of 10^{-4} to 10^{-3} M may occur, especially following high-dose therapy used for osteogenic sarcoma or lung or breast cancer. Plasma levels of amethopterin are determined by a dihydrofolate reductase inhibition assay. Patients destined to have toxicity can be suspected by 24 hours and identified definitively by 3 to 4 days.[35] Thus, at 4 days all patients with plasma levels of amethopterin greater than 2×10^{-7} M are expected to have serious toxicity, and those with lower levels are not. This finding has led to earlier and more aggressive use of antidotes in patients with slow plasma disappearance of this drug.

Treatment. Outlines for treatment of intestinal toxicity from chemotherapeutic agents in wide use are included in Table 12–4. To continue with the illustration of amethopterin toxicity, the effects of this drug can be offset by leucovorin (5-formyltetrahydrofolate, folinic acid), 15 mg IV q 3 to 6 h, for 72 hours or longer if needed.[25] In fact, this antidote is frequently administered as a part of the treatment protocol and has acquired the distinguished term *rescue therapy*. The use of leucovorin rescue is guided by the plasma levels of amethopterin. In addition, patients are well hydrated, and urine is alkalinized by infusion of $NaHCO_3$, 45 mEq q 6 h, to increase the solubility of amethopterin and to facilitate its excretion by the kidney. Renal dialysis may be needed by patients in whom glomerular filtration rate is reduced for any reason; in patients treated with high-dose amethopterin, the drug actually may precipitate in renal tubules and lead to obstructive nephropathy. This latter complication is usually reversible following alkalinization of the urine and temporary dialysis. Nausea and vomiting resulting from amethopterin, or other chemotherapeutic agents, may be relieved by prochlorperazine, 10 mg PO tid, or delta-9-tetrahydrocannabinol, 15 mg PO tid.[36] Despite leucovorin "rescue," amethopterin has been implicated as a cause of death in a recent review of anticancer drug–associated deaths.[28]

This example of treatment of toxicity from amethopterin, a widely used but potentially lethal drug, illustrates the complexities involved in the assessment and treatment of poisoning from drugs used therapeutically and exemplifies the multitude of measures that may be available and needed in patients receiving chemotherapeutic poisons. Treatment of toxicity on a recurring basis preferably should be managed by physicians who are trained in oncology and who are knowledgeable in treatment of poisonous side effects of cancer chemotherapy. The importance of prevention of toxicity, if at all possible, cannot be overemphasized.

CHEMICAL POISONS

Chemical injury to the gastrointestinal tract involves a variety of agents, including heavy metals, especially iron, lead, arsenic, and mercury; laxatives; colchicine; nonsteroidal anti-inflammatory drugs (NSAIDs); Lomotil; acids and alkalis (Fig. 12–1); lithium and

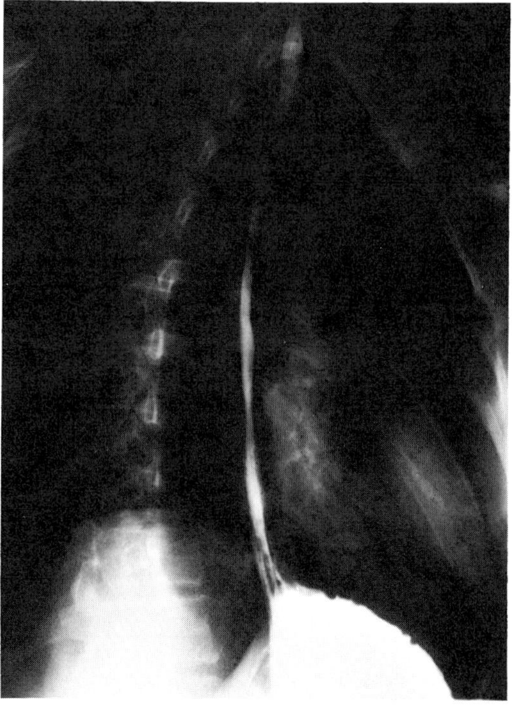

Figure 12–1. Lye stricture of the esophagus. This patient ingested lye accidentally as a child. She had persistent dysphagia, and a colon interposition was performed in early adulthood. (Courtesy of Dr. L. Goldberger.)

fluoride; bacterial, plant, and mushroom toxins; phosphorous; radiation injury; and miscellaneous drugs.

Laxatives and certain drugs that injure the esophagus will be discussed here. The other agents are discussed in specific chapters.

Laxative Abuse

Acute Laxative Poisoning

Excess ingestion of laxatives may result in acute or chronic poisoning. Cases of acute poisoning are usually accidental, but occasionally laxatives are used in suicide attempts. Most laxatives have a wide margin of safety, and large doses must be consumed to be fatal. A classification of laxatives and representative examples for each group are presented in Table 12–5.

Acute poisoning may lead to watery or bloody diarrhea (with accompanying water and electrolyte abnormalities), abdominal and rectal pain, vomiting, and respiratory and circulatory failure. The diagnosis is usually apparent from the history. The severity of magnesium intoxication can be assessed by serum magnesium levels; toxicity begins at levels of 4 mEq/L and worsens as the concentration rises.

Table 12–5. CLASSIFICATION OF LAXATIVES* AND REPRESENTATIVE EXAMPLES†

Stimulant (or Irritant)
Ricinoleic acid (castor oil)
Dehydrocholic acids (Decholin)
Bisacodyl (Dulcolax)
Phenolphthalein (Ex-Lax; Correctol)
Oxyphenisatin (Lavema)‡
Aloe
Cascara sagrada
Senna (Senokot)
Danthron (Modane)
Stool Softener
Dioctyl sodium sulfosuccinate (DSS)
Dioctyl calcium sulfosuccinate (Surfak)
Kondremul
Saline
Magnesium hydroxide (milk of magnesia)
Magnesium sulfate
Sodium sulfate
Sodium phosphate (Fleet Phospho-Soda)
Sodium chloride
Bulk
Psyllium seed derivatives (Konsyl, Metamucil, LA formula, Effersyllium, Serutan, Hydrocil)
Bran products
Lubricant
Mineral oil (Agoral)

*Based on the report of the FDA panel on laxatives and antidiarrheal, anti-emetic, and emetic products.[37]

†Over 100 laxatives are listed in the 1988 Physicians' Desk Reference and Physicians' Desk Reference for Nonprescription Drugs.

‡Withdrawn from distribution by the FDA because of its association with chronic active hepatitis.

Treatment

1. An airway is established and respirations are maintained.

2. Intravenous fluids are given to restore or maintain hydration, replenish electrolytes, and facilitate kidney perfusion.

3. Calcium gluconate, 10 per cent, 1 ml/kg IV, is given as an antidote for magnesium intoxication. In patients with renal insufficiency, hemodialysis may be necessary.

4. The laxative is diluted with oral tap water, 250 to 500 ml, and removed by emesis or gastric lavage. The comparative efficacy of emesis versus lavage is controversial for the removal of poisons, but emesis is preferred over gastric lavage in the conscious patient. Both emesis and lavage are safe and effective in removing approximately 30 per cent of stomach contents.

5. Emesis is induced with syrup of ipecac, 15 ml orally, followed by half a glass of water. The ipecac is repeated in 30 minutes if vomiting has not occurred. Table salt in water is not a suitable or safe emetic. Sodium chloride solutions lead to an excessive rise in plasma sodium and may be fatal.

6. Activated charcoal (Nuchar C, Norit A) is an effective adsorbent for many laxatives, is nontoxic, has few contraindications, and should be used routinely in poisoned patients.

Chronic Laxative Abuse

Chronic laxative abuse occcurs in three forms. One is the constipated patient in whom laxatives are taken chronically and wittingly. Another is the bulimic patient who uses laxatives for weight loss, and the third is the surreptitious laxative abuser.

Cathartic colon is a consequence of prolonged laxative abuse. Clinically, the abnormality is discovered by barium enema and is primarily a radiologic diagnosis (Fig. 12–2). Almost all cases occur in patients who have taken irritant laxatives for 15 or more years. The major historical features are chronic constipation and laxative use. Diarrhea, fever, and blood in the stool are not seen with cathartic colon. The rectal mucosa is not friable, and proctosigmoidoscopy is normal. If the laxative taken contained anthracene derivatives, such as cascara, aloes, and senna, melanosis coli may be present. The earliest and mildest changes are found in the cecum and ileocecal valve; these appear shortened and atrophic. More extensive changes are associated with a tubular colon with diminished or absent haustrations, which may extend to the distal descending colon (Fig. 12–2). Ulcerations and rigidity are absent. The differential diagnosis of the radiologic findings includes inflammatory bowel disease (chronic ulcerative colitis and Crohn's disease) and amebiasis, but the diagnosis of cathartic colon can usually be made without difficulty. Systemic effects of chronic laxative abuse result from the increased fecal loss of sodium and potassium.[39] The patients may present to the emergency department with potassium depletion, muscle weakness, metabolic alkalosis, hyperaldosteronism, and chronic thirst. Cessation of excessive use is usually satisfactory treatment. Most of the laxatives in the stimulant category are too irritating for harmless, continuous use and should be avoided.

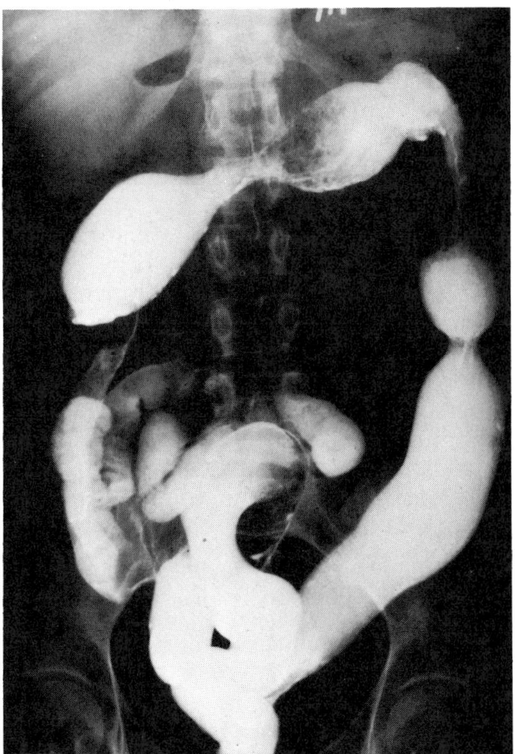

Figure 12–2. Cathartic colon from chronic laxative abuse. This patient, a 53 year old woman, had taken laxatives daily for the preceding 30 years for relief of chronic constipation. (Courtesy of Dr. L. Goldberger.)

The second and emerging group of laxative abusers are patients with bulimia, especially women aged 12 to 25 years, who binge-eat and then use cathartics in an effort to lose or control weight.[40–44] This disorder is usually practiced in secrecy and may present only in the form of one of its complications. An estimated 10 to 15 per cent of adolescent girls and young women have anorexia nervosa or bulimia, and up to 19 per cent of college women have bulimia. Bulimia is distinct from anorexia and is characterized by secretive binge-eating followed by various methods of purging, including cathartics, diuretics, and self-induced vomiting. An intense preoccupation with food is common to both syndromes. Persons who are in occupations for which thinness is considered a virtue or necessity, e.g., models, actors and actresses, jockeys, dancers, wrestlers, gymnasts, etc., are at risk as well. These patients may develop severe metabolic disturbances and ventricular tachyarrhythmias. Sudden death may occur and may be heralded by prolongation of the Q-T interval.[45] Very careful heart and electrocardiographic monitoring is essential for these patients. Long-term therapy with medical, psychologic, and nutritional professionals may be required.

The third and most trying group with chronic laxative abuse are those people who use laxatives surreptitiously and present with diarrhea of unknown cause or with metabolic abnormalities related to long-term laxative misuse.[46] A key feature of the disorder is denial by the patient that he or she takes the laxative, and this denial may continue well beyond the time that prima facie evidence has proven the point. Although clinical clues abound to alert the physician of laxative abuse, patients often attract at least an initial medical work-up designed to rule out infectious, inflammatory, metabolic, and neoplastic diseases before abusive behavior is considered. These studies usually include stool for bacterial culture, ova and parasite examinations, proctosigmoidoscopy, and barium radiographs, all of which may be within normal limits. Metabolic abnormalities showing dehydration and hypokalemia are common but are seen in many diarrheal illnesses and are not specific.

It is less labor intensive and costly to examine a patient's blood and urine for signs of laxatives than to launch into a barrage of additional tests looking for occult malabsorptive diseases and exotic tumors with secretory hormone production if there is any lingering doubt about the patient's veracity. A very simple examination is accomplished by alkalinizing stool with sodium hydroxide; if phenolphthalein, a common ingredient in over-the-counter laxatives, is present the stool will turn bright red. Urine containing aloes will turn red if alkalinized. Clinical laboratories offer a laxative abuse screen of urine for bisacodyl and danthron. The proctosigmoidoscopy itself may be diagnostic by showing a darkened-to-black mucosa. Mucosal pigmentation results from melanin accumulation in macrophages in the lamina propria and may begin within 4 months of chronic laxative abuse. The trained sigmoidoscopist can detect color changes at an early stage. Pigmentation is seen most often with anthracene derivatives, including cascara, aloes, and senna. The barium enema may be abnormal as well. The characteristic features are shown in Figure 12–2.

If neither stool, urine, proctosigmoidoscopy, nor barium enema are abnormal and the diagnosis is still suspect, the patient should be admitted to hospital for further evaluation. A room search is indicated, but it should be performed by an impartial participant and with the patient's consent in order to avoid an invasion of privacy. If the suspicion is well grounded but nothing is found, the symptoms should improve while the patient is under direct observation. Meanwhile, a stool collection can be obtained while the patient fasts and receives intravenous glucose and fluids. A large volume of 500 to 1000 ml or more suggests a secretory diarrhea, and the stool is evaluated for sodium, potassium, and osmolality. In secretory diarrhea the osmolality is accounted for by twice the sodium plus potassium concentration and may be simulated by secretagogue laxatives like senna, bisacodyl, and phenolphthalein. An osmotic diarrhea is characterized by a wide ion gap that may be caused by magnesium, sulfate, or other laxative ions, and these can be quantified in the stool.

Laxatives by nature are not addictive. Persons who use them surreptitiously have a serious psychologic condition, usually anxiety or depression or both. The psychologic category most specific for this entity is chronic factitious disease with physical symptoms, also known as Munchausen's syndrome. The apparent goal of the patient is to assume the role of a patient. There is usually no other secondary gain as there is in persons who are malingering. The physician must realize that recognizing laxative abuse is only half the battle. These patients may prove very difficult to treat and may continue to use laxatives while under continued medical care.

Table 12–6. COMMON AGENTS THAT HAVE AN ACID- OR ALKALI-LIKE EFFECT

CORROSIVE	USE	COMMON NAMES
Acids		
sulfuric	Industrial	Oil of vitriol
nitric	Industrial	Aquafortis
hydrochloric	Industrial	Muriatic acid
hydrofluoric	Industrial	
oxalic	Industrial, bleach	Ethandioic acid
carbolic	Antiseptic	Phenol
lactic	Antiseptic, industrial	
silver nitrate	Antiseptic	
iodine	Antiseptic	
ammonium chloride	Antiseptic	Anchlor
boric	Antiseptic, industrial	Borofax
mercuric chloride	Antiseptic	
Alkalis		
sodium hydroxide	Drain cleaner	Lye, Dran-O
potassium hydroxide	To make soap, paint remover	Potash
sodium hypochlorite	Bleach	Clorox, soda lye
sodium bicarbonate	Baking powder, non-phosphate detergent	Baking soda
potassium carbonate	Industrial	
ammonia water	Detergent	
calcium oxide	Building material	Lime

Drug-Induced Esophageal Injury

Chemical injury to the esophagus from drugs is more common than generally supposed.[47] The drugs implicated in esophageal damage include antibiotics (tetracycline, doxycycline, clindamycin, and lincomycin), 5-fluorouracil, anti-inflammatory agents (aspirin, indocin, phenylbutazone), oral potassium supplements, emepronium bromide, iron, quinidine, carbachol, ascorbic acid, cromolyn inhalant, and cimetidine. The mechanism of injury appears to be a direct corrosion, either through acid or alkali effect (Table 12–6). Tetracycline and doxycycline are known to be highly acidic in solution. Although the injury is more likely in patients with mechanical or peristaltic abnormalities, drug injury may occur in a normal esophagus.

The most common symptoms are chest pain and dysphagia. In patients with an underlying esophageal disease, the symptoms may be mistaken for the primary disease. The pathology varies from diffuse inflammation to ulceration or necrotizing esophagitis and hemorrhage. Perforation and stricture have occurred as complications. Treatment includes cessation of the offending drug and management of the complications. Recognition of this disorder is critical since the disease is usually reversible if discovered early. Caustic alkali (Chapter 65) and acid (Chapter 66) ingestions are discussed later in greater detail.

POISONING OF DIGESTIVE-ABSORPTIVE FUNCTION

Interference of nutrient digestion and absorption results from the toxic effect of a wide variety of exogenous agents. Not only do these agents interfere with nutrient absorption but often they also affect the absorption of therapeutic drugs. The mechanisms leading to maldigestion and malabsorption include (1) alteration of environmental pH, (2) chemical binding of nutrients, (3) inhibition of digestive enzymes and inhibition of transport processes requiring membrane proteins, and (4) direct toxic injury to the epithelium. The steps involved in digestion and absorption of most nutrients have already been reviewed in the section on Gastrointestinal Epithelial Cell Function.

The most-studied toxin of the small intestine is gluten.[48, 49] Gluten-sensitive enteropathy or celiac sprue is a nonallergic sensitivity to wheat, specifically the gliadin fraction of wheat protein. The enteropathy is characterized by flattening of the villi, cuboidal epithelial cells in disarray, elongation of the crypts, and inflammation of the lamina propria. The results of these changes, at their worst, include malabsorption of fat, protein, carbohydrate, salt, water, minerals, and water-soluble and fat-soluble vitamins. Selective malabsorption of individual food components may occur; for example, iron deficiency anemia secondary to iron malabsorption may be the presenting feature of the enteropathy. Epithelial cells arising from the crypts do not become susceptible to the cytotoxic process characteristic of the disease

Table 12–7. COMMONLY USED DRUGS THAT INHIBIT DIGESTIVE-ABSORPTIVE MECHANISMS

DRUG	NUTRIENT MALABSORBED	PUTATIVE MECHANISMS
Neomycin	Fat, cholesterol, fat-soluble vitamins	Precipitates fatty acids and bile acids[50]
	Glucose, amino acids, B_{12}, minerals	Histologic damage
Colchicine	Fat, glucose, B_{12}	Inhibits mitotic spindle[51]
Ethanol	Fat, glucose, amino acids, vitamins, minerals	Alters physical properties of the membrane. Inhibits Na^+, K^+, ATPase; stimulates cAMP[52]
p-Aminosalicylic acid	Fat, cholesterol, folate, B_{12}	Unknown[53]
Dilantin	Folate	Inhibits folate conjugase[54]
		Alkalinizes intestinal contents[55]
Folate antagonists (methotrexate, aminopterin, trimethoprim)	Folate	Inhibit folate transport[56, 57]
		Inhibit cell proliferation[41]
Oral contraceptives	Folate	Inhibit folate conjugase[58]
Sulfasalazine	Folate	Inhibits folate transport[59, 60]
Biguanides	Glucose, amino acids, folate, B_{12}	Inhibit oxidative phosphorylation[61]
Aluminum hydroxide antacids	Phosphate, vitamin A	Intraluminal formation of insoluble complexes[62]
Anion exchange resins (cholestyramine, colestipol)	Water- and fat-soluble vitamins, bile salts, oxalate	Intraluminal binding[60, 63]
Cimetidine	B_{12} bound to food	Inhibits gastric acid and intrinsic factor secretion[64]

until they cross the crypt-villous junction and become mature (see the normal epithelial cell cycle in the section on Gastrointestinal Epithelial Cell Renewal). In other words, the absorptive cells must be exposed to gluten in the intestinal lumen.

The pathophysiologic mechanism underlying gluten-sensitive enteropathy is not known for certain, but two main theories exist: (1) cells at the crypt-villous junction show one or more surface antigens, including gluten, and become targets of a local immunologic effector mechanism; and (2) the absorptive cell is deficient in a peptidase or protease. As a result, gluten digestion is impaired, allowing accumulation of gluten or its particular digestive products, with resulting tissue toxicity. Gluten-sensitive enteropathy occurs only in susceptible persons, and the enteropathy subsides on a gluten-free diet. The reaction of the susceptible intestine to gluten represents the relatively limited pathologic response of the intestine to injury.

Numerous drugs affect adversely the digestion and absorption of nutrients. The most commonly used drugs for which reasonable evidence exists for their adverse effect are shown in Table 12–7. Removal of the drugs from the patient's treatment program and restoration of nutrient deficiencies are usually sufficient treatment.

References

1. Whitehead R: Mucosal Biopsy of the Gastrointestinal Tract. Philadelphia, WB Saunders, 1979.
2. Crane RK: Intestinal structure and function related to toxicology. Environ Health Perspect *33*:3, 1979.
3. Alpers DH, Seetharam B: Pathophysiology of diseases involving intestinal brush-border proteins. N Engl J Med *296*:1047, 1977.
4. Baserga R: The cell cycle. N Engl J Med *304*:453, 1981.
5. Williamson RCN: Intestinal adaptations. N Engl J Med *298*:1393, 1978.
6. Eastwood GL: Gastrointestinal epithelial reviews. Gastroenterology *72*:962, 1977.
7. Willems G: Factors controlling cell proliferation in gastroduodenal mucosa. Prog Gastroenterol *3*:29, 1977.
8. Leblond CP, Greulich RC, Pereira JPM: Relationship of cell formation and cell migration in the renewal of stratified squamous epithelium. Adv Biol Skin 5, 1964.
9. MacDonald WC, Trier JS, Everett NB: Cell proliferation and migration in the stomach, duodenum, and rectum of man: Radioautographic studies. Gastroenterology *46*:405, 1964.
10. Lipkin M, Sherlock P, Bell B: Cell proliferation kinetics in the gastrointestinal tract of man. II. Renewal in stomach, ileum, colon, and rectum. Gastroenterology *45*:721, 1963.
11. Bertalanffy FD, Nagy KP: Mitotic activity and renewal of the epithelial cells of human duodenum. Acta Anat *45*:362, 1961.
12. Shorter RG, Moertel CG, Titus JL, et al: Cell kinetics in the jejunum and rectum of man. Am J Dig Dis *9*:760, 1964.
13. Lipkin M, Bell B, Sherlock P: Cell proliferation kinetics in the gastrointestinal tract of man. I. Cell renewal of colon and rectum. J Clin Invest *42*:767, 1963.
14. Cole JW, McKalen A: Observations of cell renewal in human rectal mucosa in vivo with thymidine-H^3. Gastroenterology *41*:122, 1961.
15. Grossman MI: Control of gastric secretion. In Sleisenger MH, Fordtran JS (eds): Gastrointestinal Disease. Philadelphia, WB Saunders, 1978, p 640.
16. Sleisenger MH, Kim YS: Protein digestion and absorption. N Engl J Med *300*:659, 1979.
17. Gray GM: Carbohydrate digestion and absorption. N Engl J Med *292*:1225, 1975.
18. Crane RK: Digestion and absorption: Water-soluble organics. Gastrointest Physiol II, *12*:325, 1977.
19. Henn RM, Isenberg JI, Maxwell V, et al: Inhibition of gastric acid secretion by cimetidine in patients with duodenal ulcer. N Engl J Med *293*:371, 1975.
20. Powell DW: Muscle or mucosa: The site of action of antidiarrheal opiates? Gastroenterology *80*:406, 1981.
21. Hofmann AF: Enterohepatic circulation of bile acids. In Sleisenger MH, Fordtran JS (eds): Gastrointestinal Disease. Philadelphia, WB Saunders, 1978, p 92.
22. Weinstein GD: Methotrexate. Ann Intern Med *86*:199, 1977.
23. Chabner BA, Myers CE, Coleman N, Johns DG: The clinical pharmacology of antineoplastic agents. N Engl J Med *292*:1107, 1975.
24. Johns DG, Bertino JR: Folate antagonists. In Holland JF, Frei E, III (eds): Cancer Medicine. Philadelphia, Lea & Febiger, 1973, p 739.
25. Jaffee N, Frei E, III, Traggis D, et al: Adjuvant methotrexate and citrovorum factor treatment of osteogenic sarcoma. N Engl J Med *7*:994, 1974.
26. Chabner BA, Johns DG, Bertino JR: Enzymatic cleavage of methotrexate provides a method for prevention of drug toxicity. Nature *293*:395, 1972.
27. Djerassi I, Ciesielka W, Kim SJ: Removal of methotrexate by filtration-absorption using charcoal filters or by hemodialysis. Cancer Treat Reports *61*:751, 1977.
28. Winchester JF, Rahman A, Tilstone WJ, Breeman H, Mortensen LM, Gelfand MC, Schein PS, Schreiner GE: Will hemoperfusion be useful for cancer chemotherapeutic drug removal? Clin Toxicol *17*:557, 1980.
29. Sirotnak FM, Moccio DM: Pharmacokinetic basis of differences in methotrexate sensitivity of normal proliferative tissue in the mouse. Cancer Res *40*:1230, 1980.
30. Chabner BA, Young RC: Threshold methotrexate concentrations for in vivo inhibition of DNA synthesis in normal and tumorous target tissue. J Clin Invest *52*:1804, 1973.
31. Frei E III, Jaffee N, Tattersall M, et al: New approaches to cancer chemotherapy with methotrexate. N Engl J Med *292*:846, 1975.
32. Bleyer WA: The clinical pharmacology of methotrexate. Cancer *41*:36, 1978.

33. Liegler DG, Henderson ES, Hahn MS, et al: The effect of organic acids on renal clearance of methotrexate in man. Clin Pharmacol Ther *10*:849, 1969.
34. Trier JS: Morphologic alterations induced by methotrexate in the mucosa of human proximal intestine. Gastroenterology *42*:295, 1962.
35. Stoller RG, Hande K, Jacobs SA, et al: Use of plasma pharmacokinetics to predict and prevent methotrexate toxicity. N Engl J Med *297*:630, 1977.
36. Sallan SE, Cronin C, Zelen M, et al: Antiemetics in patients receiving chemotherapy for cancer. N Engl J Med *302*:135, 1980.
37. Food and Drug Administration: Over-the-Counter Drugs, 1975. Proposal to establish monographs for OTC laxative, antidiarrheal, emetic, and antiemetic products. Fed Regist *40*:12902, 1975.
38. Binder HJ: Pharmacology of laxatives. Annu Rev Pharmacol Toxicol *17*:355, 1977.
39. Cummings JH: Laxative abuse. Gut *15*:758, 1974.
40. Drossman DA, Ontjes DA, Heizer WD: Anorexia nervosa. Gastroenterology *77*:1115–1131, 1979.
41. Schwabe AD, Lippe BM, Chang J, Pops MA, Yager J: Anorexia nervosa. Ann Intern Med *94*:371–381, 1981.
42. Harris RT: Bulimarexia and related serious eating disorders with medical complications. Ann Intern Med *99*:800–807, 1983.
43. Diamond GA: Eating disorders. Ann Intern Med *105*:790–794, 1986.
44. Health and Public Policy Committee, American College of Physicians: Eating disorders: Anorexia nervosa and bulimia. Ann Intern Med *105*:790–794, 1986.
45. Isner J, Roberts WC, Heymsfield SB, Yager J: Anorexia nervosa and sudden death. Ann Intern Med *102*:49–52, 1985.
46. Case Records of the Massachusetts General Hospital (Case 47–1985). N Engl J Med *313*:1341–1346, 1985.
47. Collins FJ, Mathews HR, Baker SE et al: Drug-induced esophageal injury. Br Med J *1*:1673, 1979.
48. Trier JS: Celiac sprue and refractory sprue. Gastroenterology *75*:307, 1978.
49. Katz SI, Hall RP, Lowley TJ, et al: Dermatitis herpetiformis: The skin and the gut. Ann Intern Med *93*:857, 1980.
50. Longstreth GF, Newcomer AD: Drug-induced malabsorption. Mayo Clin Proc *50*:284, 1975.
51. Stemmerman GN, Hayoshi T: Colchicine intoxication: A reappraisal of its pathology based on a study of three fatal cases. Hum Pathol *2*:321, 1971.
52. Wilson FA, Hoyumpa AM Jr: Ethanol and small intestinal transport. Gastroenterology *7*:387, 1979.
53. Longstreth GF, Newcomer AD, Westbrook P: Paraaminosalicylic acid–induced malabsorption. Dig Dis *17*:731, 1972.
54. Rosenberg IH: Absorption and malabsorption of folates. Clin Haematol *507*:589, 1976.
55. Benn A, Swan CJ, Cooke WT, et al: Effect of intraluminal pH on the absorption of pteroylmonoglutamic acid. Br Med J *10*:148, 1971.
56. Strum WB: A pH-dependent, carrier-mediated transport system for the folate analog, amethopterin, in rat jejunum. J Pharmacol Exp Ther *203*:640, 1977.
57. Strum WB: Enzymatic reduction and methylation of folate following pH-dependent, carrier-mediated transport in rat jejunum. Biochim Biophys Acta *554*:249, 1979.
58. Streiff RR: Folate deficiency and oral contraceptives. JAMA *214*:105, 1970.
59. Franklin JL, Rosenberg IH: Impaired folic acid absorption in inflammatory bowel disease: Effects of salicylazosulfapyridine (Azulfidine). Gastroenterology *64*:517, 1973.
60. Strum WB: Characteristics of the transport of pteroylglutamate and amethopterin in rat jejunum. J Pharmacol Exp Ther *216*:329, 1981.
61. Berchtold P, Dahlquist A, Gustafson A, et al: Effects of a biguanide (metformin) on vitamin B_{12} and folic acid absorption and intestinal enzyme activity. Scand J Gastroenterol *6*:751, 1971.
62. Spencer H, Lender M: Adverse effects of aluminum-containing antacids on mineral metabolism. Gastroenterology *76*:603, 1979.
63. Hofmann AF, Poley JR: Cholestyramine treatment of diarrhea associated with ileal resection. N Engl J Med *281*:397, 1969.
64. Steinberg WM, King CE, Toskes PP: Malabsorption of protein-bound cobalamin but not unbound cobalamin during cimetidine administration. Dig Dis Sci *25*:1980.

CHAPTER 13
CHEMICAL HEPATIC INJURY

Hyman J. Zimmerman, M.D.

Poisonous doses of any of a huge number of chemical and biologic agents can lead to hepatic injury.[1–9] Some hepatotoxins are plant or fungal products. Some are minerals. Many are industrial products, byproducts, or wastes (Table 13–1).

Hepatotoxic agents may be encountered at home or at work (Table 13–2). Toxic exposure to some agents has occurred only in industry (e.g., trinitrotoluene); to others only in the home (e.g., acetaminophen, poisonous mushrooms); and to some, in both settings (e.g., carbon tetrachloride).

Occupational exposure to hepatotoxic agents has long been a worrisome cause of hepatic injury. Indeed, a variety of agents with experimentally proved hepatotoxic potential (Table 13–3) has been employed in numerous industries (Table 13–4). Improved industrial hygiene in recent years, however, apparently has led to a reduced incidence of acute toxic liver damage.[2] The risk of chronic hepatic disease remains to be monitored and evaluated.[9]

Household poisonings are today, by far, the most frequent cause of acute hepatic injury. The poisoning may result from the accidental or suicidal intake of a known toxin (carbon tetrachloride, acetaminophen); from the inhalation of haloalkane solvent as the result of careless use, accident, or "solvent sniffing"; or from the ingestion of natural toxins or synthetic chemicals that are contaminants of food or drink.

Table 13–1. HEPATOTOXIC AGENTS

ORGANIC
Natural
Plants
Mycotoxins
Bacterial toxins
Synthetic
Nonmedicinal
Medicinal
INORGANIC
Metals and metalloids
Hydrazine derivatives
Iodides

Table 13–2. CIRCUMSTANCES OF EXPOSURE TO CHEMICAL HEPATIC INJURY

TOXICOLOGIC
Occupational
Domestic
Accidental or suicidal
Ingestion as food or contaminant
Drug abuse—solvent sniffing
—ingestion or injection
PHARMACEUTICAL
Iatrogenic
Self-medication

HEPATOTOXIC AGENTS

All agents that can produce hepatic injury might be defined as hepatotoxins. It is essential, however, to distinguish agents that are *true* toxins from those whose hepatotoxic effects are idiosyncrasy-dependent toxins. Those that can produce dose-dependent hepatic injury in humans and in experimental animals are considered to be *true* (intrinsic, predictable) hepatotoxins, whereas agents that produce hepatic injury only in unusually susceptible humans, seemingly not dose-dependent, are designated *idiosyncrasy*-dependent (nonpredictable) hepatotoxins. This chapter is concerned with true hepatotoxins. Indeed, hepatic injury due to a medicinal agent is usually a therapeutic misadventure resulting from individual susceptibility (idiosyncrasy).* Accordingly, most forms of drug-induced liver damage are not included in this discussion. Reference is made to the few drugs that, in overdose, do lead to important hepatic injury.

A large number of chemicals are found in the home as components of household products (Table 13–5) or as pesticides (Table 13–6).[10–12] In addition, some of the agents encountered in industry (see Table 13–3) may find their way into the home. Chemicals employed in industry or in research laboratories may be "borrowed" for use in the household.[12] The presence of these in the home, often in unlabeled containers and in the absence of the discipline of the occupa-

*In an appendix at the end of this chapter, a table lists drugs that lead to hepatic injury as therapeutic misadventures.

Table 13–3. PARTIAL LIST OF AGENTS LIKELY TO BE ENCOUNTERED OCCUPATIONALLY, WITH INDICATION OF HEPATOTOXIC EFFECTS IN EXPERIMENTAL ANIMALS AND HUMANS

	EXPERIMENTAL ANIMALS	HUMANS		EXPERIMENTAL ANIMALS	HUMANS
alcohols and glycols	±	±	chloronitroaromatic compounds	+	+
aldehydes, acetals, ketones	±	±	cycloparaffins	±	0
alkanes	±	0	dioxin	+	+
amines, aliphatic	±	0	diphenyl oxide	+	+
aromatic	+	+	esters	±	0
aromatic compounds			ethers	±	0
benzene	±	±	furans	±	±
cymene	+	±	halogenated aromatic compounds*	+	+
mesitylene	+	0			
naphthalene	+	±	halogenated paraffins†	+	+
pseudocumene	+	0	nitroaromatic compounds‡	+	+
p-terbutyltoluene	+	±	nitroparaffins		
toluene	±	±	nitroethane	+	0
tetralin	+	0	nitromethane	+	0
xylene	+	+	1-nitropropane	+	0
carbon disulfide	+	+	2-nitropropane	+	0
chloronitroparaffins	+	0	nitroso compounds	+	+
			pesticides*	±	±

0, none known; ± slight or equivocal; +, definite.

*Chlorinated biphenyls, naphthalenes, pesticides, and a variety of other chloro, bromo, or iodo compounds.

†Toxic potential depends on firmness of the carbon-halogen bond, which in turn depends on the atomic number of the halogen—the higher, the more toxic. Also depends on the number of halogens.

‡Includes trinitrotoluene, dinitrobenzene, nitrobenzene, and so on. Susceptibility varies. See Table 13–6.

(From Zimmerman HJ: Hepatotoxicity: Adverse Effects of Drugs and Other Chemicals on the Liver. New York, Appleton-Century-Crofts, 1978, with permission of the copyright holder.)

Table 13–4. SOME OCCUPATIONS THAT ENTAIL EXPOSURE TO HEPATOTOXIC CHEMICALS

Airplane dope makers
Airplane pilots (insecticide sprayers)
Airplane hangar employees
Artificial pearl makers
Burnishers
Cement (rubber, plastic) makers
Cementers (rubber)
Chemical industry workers
Chemists
Chlorinated rubber makers
Cobblers
Color makers
Degreasers
Dry cleaners
Dye makers
Dyers
Electrical transformer and condenser makers
Electroplaters
Enamel makers and enamelers
Extracters, oil and fats
Fillers (plastics)
Fire extinguisher makers
Galvanizers
Garage workers
Gardeners (insecticides)
Gas (illuminating) workers
Glass (safety) makers
Glue workers
Ink makers
Insecticide makers
Insulaters (wire)
Lacquer makers and lacquerers
Leather workers
Linoleum makers
Lithographers
Paint remover makers and users
Painters, paint makers
Paraffin workers
Perfume makers
Petroleum refiners
Pharmaceutical workers
Photographic material workers
Polish (metal) makers and users
Printers
Pyroxylen-plastics workers
Rayon makers
Refrigerator workers
Resins (synthetic) makers
Rubber workers
Scourers (metal)
Shoe factory workers
Soap makers
Spreaders (rubber works)
Straw hat makers
Tapers (airplanes)
Thermometer makers
Tobacco denicotinizers
Varnish makers and users
Varnish removers
Waterproofers
Wax makers

(From Zimmerman HJ: Hepatotoxicity: Adverse Effects of Drugs and Other Chemicals on the Liver. New York, Appleton-Century-Crofts, 1978, with permission of the copyright holder.)

Table 13–5. HOUSEHOLD PRODUCTS THAT MIGHT BE HEPATOTOXIC

PRODUCT	TOXIC AGENT
Antifreeze	chlorobenzene
Carburetor cleaner	chlorobenzene
Christmas tree lights (bubbling)	methylene chloride
Dry cleaning fluids	chlorinated aliphatic compounds
Drugs hepatotoxic in overdose	acetaminophen aspirin ethanol ferrous salts phenylbutazone
Furniture polishes and waxes	antimony (trivalent) nitrobenzene cellosolve
Moth balls	chlorobenzenes
Paint products	
brush cleaners	cresols
paints	arsenic (trivalent)
plasticizers, lacquers, resins	varied
removers, paint, wax, etc.	chlorinated aliphatic compounds
Pesticides	see Table 13–6
Plastic menders, greasers, plasticizers, glues	ethylenedichloride, phthalates
Shoe cleaners	aniline nitrobenzene
Spray repellent	vinyl chloride
Stamping inks	phenol
Toilet bowl blocks	paradichlorobenzene

Any unknown product should be considered potentially hepatotoxic and all halogenated ones should be considered hepatotoxic until otherwise determined.

tional setting, may set the stage for accidental intoxication.

Household Products. The household products likely to contain hepatotoxic chemicals are those used for cleaning of clothes and furniture and for paint removal. Chloroalkane solvents are the likely toxic agents (see Table 13–5). The chloroalkanes used today, however, are less toxic than carbon tetrachloride, which was used widely in the past; they include ethylene dichloride, tetrachlorethylene, trichlorethylene, and methyl chloroform.[10] Polishes for furniture, floors, and shoes are likely to contain nitrobenzene and antimony trichloride.[10] These agents have a potential for producing hepatic injury.[2] Despite the potential toxicity of some household products, the number of reported instances of serious injury attributable to them seems very low.

Pesticides. Little evidence exists that hepatic injury has occurred as the result of exposure to pesticides being used as such. Organochlorine insecticides, herbicides,* fungicides, copper salts, or compounds of trivalent arsenic can lead to hepatic injury, but only on ingestion (Table 13–6). Indeed, ingestion of rodenticides containing phosphorus, by accident or with suicidal intent, has led to numerous instances of severe hepatic injury.[13–15] Rare instances of liver damage caused by accidental ingestion of rodenticides containing thallium[16] or warfarin[17] also have been recorded. In general, however, acute hepatic injury due to pesticides, even as the result of ingestion, has been very rare.[2]

Rare instances of gross contamination of food[11] or water[18–22] by pesticides have been described, but for the most part no recognized hepatic injury has resulted. There are, however, several reports of chronic hepatic disease attributed to toxic levels of trivalent arsenic in well water, presumably derived from use of arsenical insecticides.[19–22]

Hexachlorobenzene (HCB) in wheat was responsible for an epidemic of severe liver disease in Turkey over 30 years ago. The HCB had been added as a fungicide to wheat intended for use as seed grain. Diversion of the seed grain to use as food led to ingestion of toxic amounts of HCB and the subsequent

*The herbicide 2,4,5-T is subject to regular contamination, during manufacture or processing, by the highly toxic chlorinated dibenzodioxins.[11] It seems reasonable to ascribe the hepatotoxic effects of the herbicide to the contaminant.

Table 13–6. SPECIFIC USES OF VARIOUS POTENTIALLY HEPATOTOXIC PESTICIDES

	Halogen Compounds	*As*	*Cu*	*Dioxins**	*P, Th, Warfarin*
Fumigants	+	−	−	−	−
Fungicides	+	+	+	−	−
Herbicides	+	−	−	+	−
Insecticides	+	+	+	−	−
Rodenticides	−	+	−	−	+

As, inorganic arsenic derivatives; *Cu,* copper compounds; *P,* white allomorph of phosphorus; *Th,* thallium compounds.

*Dioxins present in herbicides as contaminants.

Table 13–7. HEPATOTOXIC AGENTS FOUND IN NATURE

	RELEVANCE*		
	Experimental	*Human*	*Veterinary*
PLANTS	+	−	+
Albitocin	+	+	−
Cycasin	+	+	−
Hypoglycin A	+	−	+
Icterogenin	+	−	+
Indospicine	+	−	+
Lantana	+	+	−
Mushrooms (amanitins, phalloidins)	+	−	+
Ngaione	+	±	−
Nutmeg	+	+	+
Pyrrolizidine alkaloids	+	±	−
Safrole	+	+	+
Tannic acid			
MYCOTOXINS	+	+	+
Aflatoxins	+	±	+
Cyclochloritine	+	+	−
Ethanol	+	±	−
Griseofulvin	+	−	+
Ipomeamarone	+	±	+
Luteoskyrin	+	±	+
Ochratoxin	+	±	+
Sterigmatocystin	+	−	+
Sporidesmin	+	+	−
Tetracycline			

*Considered of human relevance if human hepatic injury has been attributed to the agent on the basis of evidence (+) or suspicion (±). Considered of veterinary relevance if disease in livestock is attributed to the agent.

epidemic of a syndrome resembling porphyria cutanea tarda, accompanied by severe liver disease and characterized by a mortality rate above 10 per cent.

Accidental contamination of food by industrial chemicals can lead to domestic hepatotoxicity. A prime example is the epidemic of cholestatic jaundice in Epping, England ("Epping jaundice"), caused by the contamination of flour by a leaking container of 4,4′-diaminodiphenylmethane (methylenedianiline).[25] Similar injury by this chemical agent also has been occupationally acquired.[26–28] Somewhat similar to Epping jaundice but far more disastrous was the recent epidemic of "toxic oil syndrome" caused by contaminated cooking oil.[29]

Polychlorinated biphenyls (PCBs) also have been implicated as causes of hepatic disease.[30, 31] Prior to and during World War II, serious subacute hepatic necrosis occurred in patients occupationally exposed to chloronaphthalene-chlorinated biphenyl mixtures.[32–39] However, these agents under ordinary circumstances would not be found in the home except as components of electrical appliances and household fixtures, and as pollutants of food and water.[2] Although the hazard of hepatotoxicity from the general pollution of the food chain and water by PCBs is entirely speculative, specific contamination of food can lead to hepatic disease. Indeed, in 1968 hepatic disease developed in 11 per cent of more than 1000 persons in Japan who had ingested food prepared in cooking oil contaminated with PCBs.*[31] Contamination of animal feed with polybrominated biphenyls in Michigan several years ago was associated with appearance of hepatic injury in animals ingesting the feed and in human beings, although of minimal degree, presumably as a result of ingesting the contaminated meat.[40]

Natural Hepatotoxins. A large number of poisonous botanic and microbiologic products exist.[1–9] Many include hepatic injury in their repertoire of toxic effects (Table 13–7). These are discussed in a subsequent section dealing with foods as hepatotoxins.

MODES OF EXPOSURE

Exposure to hepatotoxins may be the product of careless use of a volatile agent. It also

*There is evidence that the contaminating PCB mixture also contained small amounts of polychlorinated dibenzofurane (PCDFs). The PCDFs rather than the PCBs may have been responsible for the disease.[2]

may be mediated by ingestion of the toxins as the result of ignorance, accident, or suicidal intent, or of food contaminated by toxic agents.[2] Exposure also may be a byproduct of a form of drug abuse, such as "solvent sniffing"[41] or even, conceivably, cocaine use[42] (Table 13–8).

The number of occupations that permit exposure to hepatotoxic agents is large. The list includes the manufacture of munitions, rubber, rocket fuels, cosmetics and perfumes, processed foods, paints, insecticides, herbicides, pharmaceuticals, and, of course, chemical products (see Table 13–4). The risk, however, is largely hypothetic, and there is little evidence today of acute hepatic injury due to occupational exposure to hepatotoxic agents. Chronic hepatic injury, however, has been documented to result from occupational exposure to toxic chemicals.[10, 43] Evaluation of its extent, frequency, and importance awaits appropriate epidemiologic studies.

Careless Use or Accidental Ingestion of Toxic Agents

Many instances of poisoning from exposure to *carbon tetrachloride* (CCl_4) have been the result of use of this volatile solvent as a dry cleaning agent in a poorly ventilated room, particularly by alcoholics.[2, 44] Alcohol potentiates the toxicity of CCl_4,[46–48] and drinkers are often careless with its use. Formerly a solvent with many domestic uses, this toxin is rarely found in the home, yet its availability as an industrial and laboratory reagent may permit both occupational and household exposure.[2] Inadvertent ingestion of CCl_4 also has led to devastating hepatotoxic events. Carbon tetrachloride has been mistaken for a potable beverage, most often by alcoholics.

Ingestion of a variety of other toxic substances found in the home can occur. Large doses of chlorinated pesticides and fungicides are hepatotoxic for experimental animals, but hepatotoxic accidents from their ingestion by humans are rare. Nevertheless, instances of serious hepatic injury resulting from ingestion of DDT,[48] chlordane,[49] and paraquat[50, 51] have been reported. Also, children have ingested other pesticides containing white phosphorus,[14–16] thallium compounds,[17, 52] copper compounds,[53] and warfarin.[18]

Suicide and Homicide by Hepatotoxic Agents

Homicide by poisoning is an ancient practice. History and fiction provide many ex-

Table 13–8. EXAMPLES OF HEPATOTOXICITY OF HOME PRODUCTS

AGENT	EXPOSURE	LESION *Necrosis*	*Fat*	*Other*
Toxic Chemicals				
Carbon tetrachloride, et al	Careless use			
Halogen compounds	Accident/suicide Sniffing	CZ	+	–
Phosphorus	Accident/suicide	PZ	4+	
4,4′Methylenedianiline	Food contamination (Epping jaundice)	–	–	Cholestatic jaundice
Rapeseed oil and aniline	Toxic oil syndrome	+		Cholestatic jaundice
Hexachlorobenzene	Fungistatic—in wheat	CZ	+	Toxic porphyria
Drugs				
Acetaminophen	Suicide	CZ	–	–
Ferrous sulfate	Accident	PZ	–	–
Phenylbutazone	Accident	+	+	–
Cocaine	Abuse	+	–	Mallory bodies
Ethanol	Abuse	+	+	
Trichlorethylene	Abuse	CZ	+	
Halothane	"Sniffing"			
Toxic Foods				
Mushrooms	Food	CZ	4+	–
Senecio, pyrrolizidine alkaloid, and other plants	Food, bush tea	CZ	–	Veno-occlusive disease
Mycotoxins (aflatoxins)	Food	+	4+	Carcinoma

CZ, centrizonal; *PZ*, peripheral zonal.

amples of arsenic poisoning.[54] Purposeful *arsenic* poisoning, however, is of more than historic interest; instances of deliberate poisoning still occur.[2] The dramatic clinical features of poisoning by inorganic arsenic, which include dementia, neuropathy, skin changes, and other systemic manifestations, may overshadow the hepatic disease, but the liver damage is an important part of the toxicity.

A major cause of hepatic injury in the home is attempted suicide. Most agents taken with suicidal intent are not hepatotoxic. Suicide by ingestion of *white phosphorus*, however, continues to be an important entity in some parts of the world.[14–16] Indeed, 70 per cent of cases of phosphorus poisoning are the result of deliberate suicidal intent; the remainder are the result of accidental ingestion, usually by children.[16]

Ingestion of huge doses of *acetaminophen* is today a popular means of attempting suicide in America and to a lesser degree in other countries.[55, 56] This agent, a weak and nontoxic analgesic and antipyretic in single therapeutic doses, becomes a potent hepatotoxin in large overdoses.[55, 56] In patients with enhanced susceptibility, e.g., alcoholics, even modest, therapeutically intended doses may lead to hepatic injury.[57]

Abuse of Euphorigenic Hepatotoxic Agents

It has become increasingly clear that *alcohol* per se is a hepatotoxin; it is largely responsible for liver disease of alcoholics, perhaps abetted by the usual accompanying malnutrition.[58] Other forms of drug abuse can lead to hepatic injury. Hepatic injury occurs in "sniffers" of trichlorethylene[41, 59] and even of halothane.[60] The hepatic injury resembles that of CCl_4 poisoning. The recent demonstration that *cocaine* is hepatotoxic for mice[42] and the report of human hepatic disease attributed to cocaine use[61] suggests that that drug of abuse should be added to the list of those threatening the liver.

Foods as Hepatotoxins

Natural Toxins as Food or Contaminants. Hepatotoxic mushrooms may be mistaken for edible ones. Also, poisonous plants of the *Senecio, Heliotropium, Crotolaria*, and related species may be eaten as contaminants of foods, or as medicinal decoctions, because their toxic effects are not appreciated. The unripened fruit of the *Blighia sapida* tree, on ingestion by Jamaican infants, leads to *Jamaican vomiting sickness*. The fruit of the *Cycad* tree, found on Guam, contains a potent hepatotoxin that can lead to hepatic injury when eaten. The most important of the natural hepatotoxins appear to be the mycotoxins, of which the aflatoxin group has attracted the greatest attention.[2]

Poisonous mushrooms, and the fatalities they cause, have been known since the fifth century B.C.[62, 63] Several hundred deaths per year are still attributable to these plants, especially in Europe. Fatal mushroom poisoning is relatively rare in North America. While there are many genera and thousand of species of mushrooms, the number of poisonous species is relatively small. Virtually all fatal poisonings are due to the ingestion of *Amanita phalloides* or the closely related *A. verna* or *A. virosa*.[64–67]

Poisonous mushrooms remain a significant cause of hepatotoxicity in the home. The amount ingested need not be great. The content of toxin in *A. phalloides* is so great and the toxic peptides are so potent that a single mushroom has been estimated to contain a fatal dose.[65–67] The clinical syndrome is described in a later section of this chapter.

Pyrrolizidine alkaloids (PAs) also are important household hepatotoxins in some parts of the world.[68–73] More than 100 alkaloids have been identified in the more than 200 plants that have been studied.[68, 69] The total number of PA-bearing plants is about 10 times as great. The best known genera are *Crotolaria, Heliotropium*, and *Senecio*.[70, 71] The hepatic injury produced by the PAs consists of centrizonal necrosis and damage to the small branches of the hepatic veins, producing the syndrome of veno-occlusive disease (VOD). The picture may be that of relatively acute or subacute hepatic failure, with ascites and slight jaundice, and a mortality rate of approximately 20 per cent; or the syndrome may be one of prolonged chronic insufficiency with severe ascites.[3, 68–73] While PA toxicity is far more likely to be encountered in the Third World, the toxic plants are found in many other areas.[68, 69] Indeed, cases have occurred in the United States, and it is clear that these hepatotoxins can be bought in some natural food stores.[74, 75]

Cycasin, found in the cycad nut, is a potent experimental hepatotoxin and hepatocarcinogen.[76] In chemical structure and in the effects on the liver of its aglycone, cycasin (methylazoxymethanol) resembles dimethylnitrosamine. Despite the known human ingestion of cycad nuts, evidence that cycasin causes human liver disease has been scant, perhaps because the populations that eat the cycad nut have learned to process the fruit in a manner that removes the toxin.[77] Nevertheless, a recent report from Japan described a small epidemic of acute hepatic injury attributable to the ingestion of cycad nuts,[78] and this toxic plant warrants being included among the domestic hepatotoxins.

Hypoglycin A, a compound found in the unripened fruit (called akee) of the *Blighia sapida* tree in Jamaica, clearly warrants listing with the domestic hepatotoxins. Ingestion of the unripe fruit, especially if poorly cooked, leads to an acute fatty liver with severe hypoglycemia and a syndrome (Jamaican vomiting sickness) that can be fatal, if untreated. This entity resembles Reye's syndrome. It seems particularly likely to occur in winter, when food is scarce.[9]

Tannic acid is a known experimental hepatotoxin, especially when administered parenterally.[1, 79, 80] Human toxicity has resulted from its use for the treatment of burns and, in barium sulfate suspensions, for colonic roentgenography. Despite the toxicity of tannic acid when fed to experimental animals or when ingested by grazing livestock,[2] there had been no evidence that oral intake of tannic acid had ever led to human disease until a recent report described a patient whose eccentricity led to the ingestion of a half-pound of tea every 3 to 4 days.[81] These large amounts of dried tea were presumed to be responsible for the hepatic injury that she developed.[81]

Other botanic hepatotoxins are sufficiently numerous and potent to warrant the concern that as yet unrecognized opportunities for human exposure may exist.[2] Safrole, hydroxysafrole, and isosafrole are hepatotoxic and, in large doses, hepatocarcinogenic for experimental animals.[82–84] Despite having been barred from use in soft drinks, safrole remains available in substances sold in natural food shops.[84] Indeed, a large variety of herbal products sold in these shops contain botanic agents of diverse and obscure chemical nature, with rare reports of some apparently being hepatotoxic.[84]

Mycotoxins include a large number of compounds of diverse chemical nature (see Table 13–7) that are produced as metabolites by a number of different mycotic species.[2, 5, 7, 85] Many are known to cause hepatic injury in experimental animals, and some may possibly cause human liver disease. Instances of acute disease attributed to aflatoxins (AFs) have been reported from several parts of the world. In Uganda, fatal hepatic necrosis occurred in a 15 year old boy who was found to have eaten food with a very high content of AF.[86] Groups in Thailand,[87] New Zealand,[88] Czechoslovakia,[89] and the United States[90] have demonstrated AFs in the livers of patients dying of Reye's syndrome, the lesions of which resemble closely the acute fatty liver produced in the monkey[91] and other animals[92] by AFs. A report of 106 fatal instances of hepatic disease among 397 individuals who became ill after eating maize containing very large amounts of AF also suggests that acute aflatoxicosis can occur in human beings.[93]

Chronic disease is readily produced in experimental animals given food contaminated by AFs.[2] It has been difficult, however, to prove that humans develop chronic liver disease as the result of ingesting AF-contaminated food, and the possible role of AF in causing "cryptogenic cirrhosis" in tropical areas remains to be established. Nevertheless, epidemiologic studies demonstrate the opportunity for cirrhosis to be produced in humans and also support the view that these agents are hepatocarcinogenic or cocarcinogenic for human beings.[94, 95]

In general, the hazard of mycotoxin contamination of foods has seemed to apply particularly to tropical parts of the world. The mycotoxins are produced in grains, cereals, nuts, and rice under conditions of temperature and moisture provided best by the tropics.[95] Evidence that AF contamination can occur even in temperate climates, however, is provided by reports of AF in the liver of a patient with Reye's syndrome in Minnesota[90] and of AF in corn harvested in Iowa.[96]

Chemical Contaminants of Foods. Toxic chemicals may be found in food as accidental contaminants.[2] Classic examples are the cases of cholestatic jaundice (Epping jaundice) that involved 84 people who had eaten bread baked from flour accidentally and heavily contaminated by methylenedianiline (4,4′-

diamindiphenylmethane),[26] the epidemic of Yusho that involved over 1000 Japanese who had eaten rice prepared in oil contaminated by PCBs,[31] and the devastating epidemic of severe liver disease and toxic porphyria involving over 3000 Turkish Kurds who had ingested wheat treated with the fungicide hexachlorobenzene.[24, 25]

A dramatic recent example of the phenomenon is the "epidemic toxic oil syndrome" due to use of cooking oil containing rapeseed oil contaminated with aniline.[97–100] The hepatic injury includes severe cholestatic disease as well as veno-occlusive injury. There are also extensive vascular lesions of other organs. The mortality rate has been approximately 20 per cent.

Nitrites and nitrates added to foods as preservatives have posed hypothetic hazards of potential hepatotoxicity and carcinogenicity.[101–106] The potential toxicity of nitrites in foods was first noted as hepatic necrosis among sheep and mink that had been fed herring meal preserved with nitrite.[105] The hepatic injury was found to have been caused by dimethylnitrosamine (DMN), which had been formed by reaction of the nitrite with secondary amines in the fish. Subsequent studies have shown that nitrites may be present in plant food products as the result of enzymatic reduction of nitrates from the soil, and in meat and fish products to which nitrites have been added as preservatives and colorants.[102–104] These may react with dimethylamine and other alkylamines that occur in fish, fishmeal, and other fish products; in cereals and tea; and in some drugs. The reaction can occur nonenzymatically at the acid pH of the gastric juice.[103] Formation of DMN also can occur by reaction of nitrites with dimethylamine produced by intestinal bacteria. Furthermore, some foods and alcoholic beverages have been found to contain measurable amounts of nitrosamines.[106] The magnitude of the human hazard of nitrites and nitrosamines in food and drink is unknown and has been the subject of controversy. Nevertheless, there is no doubt that DMN and other nitrosamines are potent experimental hepatotoxins and carcinogens, and that the ingestion of nitrites and secondary amines as well as nitrite-preserved feed can produce hepatic injury in experimental animals.

MORPHOLOGIC TYPES OF CHEMICAL HEPATIC INJURY

Chemical injury in human beings can lead to acute, subacute, or chronic hepatic disease (Table 13–9). A single, relatively heavy exposure may lead to acute disease, whereas repeated exposure of lesser intensity may lead to subacute or chronic liver disease.

Acute

Chemical injury may be mainly *cytotoxic,* involving overt damage to hepatocytes, mainly *cholestatic,* involving arrested bile flow, or *mixed* (Table 13–9). Some relationship exists between the type of hepatotoxin and the form of injury. Most true toxins produce mainly cytotoxic injury; only a few produce mainly cholestatic injury (Table 13–9). Many of the drugs that produce hepatic damage in humans as an idiosyncratic reaction produce mainly cholestatic injury, others produce cytotoxic injury, and some produce the mixed pattern (see appendix at the end of this chapter).

Cytotoxic Injury. This includes degeneration, necrosis, and steatosis of hepatocytes. *Necrosis* may be zonal or diffuse. That produced by true toxins is often zonal (Fig. 13–1), whereas the necrosis due to idiosyncrasy-dependent hepatic injury, in most instances, is not zonal.[2] The zonal necrosis produced by some hepatotoxins is in the central zone (zone 3) of the lobule; fewer agents lead to peripheral zone (zone 1) necrosis. Midzonal necrosis is most uncommon. The necrosis produced by carbon tetrachloride, acetaminophen, mushroom poisoning, and many other toxins is centrizonal; that produced by phosphorus and ferrous salts is in the peripheral zone.

The zonality appears to be related to the mechanism of injury. The centrizonal necrosis produced by carbon tetrachloride (Fig. 13–2) and acetaminophen, for example, appears to be a consequence of the centrizonal concentration of the enzyme system responsible for conversion of these agents to hepatotoxic metabolites. The necrosis in the peripheral zone produced by allyl formate has been attributed to the location in that zone of the enzyme system that converts the compound to its toxic metabolites.[2] The basis for

Table 13–9. MORPHOLOGIC TYPES OF HEPATIC INJURY

TYPE OF INJURY	AGENT OR COMMENT
ACUTE	
Parenchymal	
Cytotoxic	
Necrosis	
Zonal: central	carbon tetrachloride, acetaminophen, ngaione
mild	phosphorus, iron
peripheral	trinitrotoluene, some drugs
Massive	some drugs
Diffuse, focal	large number of agents—see text
Degeneration: ballooning, acidophilic bodies	
Steatosis	
Microvesicular	aspirin, tetracycline, phosphorus
Macrovesicular	ethanol, many agents
Cholestatic	see Table 13–10
Vascular (hepatic veins and branches)	
Hepatic venule injury (VOD)	pyrrolizidine alkaloids
Peliosis hepatis	anabolic and contraceptive steroids, vinyl chloride*
SUBACUTE	
Subacute hepatic necrosis	trinitrotoluene, tetrachloroethane
Subacute veno-occlusive disease	pyrrolizidine alkaloids
CHRONIC	
Parenchymal	
Cirrhosis	
Macronodular	carbon tetrachloride
Micronodular	carbon tetrachloride, aflatoxin
Congestive ("cardiac" type)	pyrrolizidine alkaloids
Biliary	chlorpromazine and a few other drugs
Steatosis	ethanol†, methotrexate
Chronic necroinflammatory disease	drugs
Neoplasm	
Carcinoma	
Hepatocellular	aflatoxin, vinyl chloride, and many other chemicals
Cholangiocellular	rare
Adenoma	anabolic and contraceptive steroids
Sarcoma	dimethylnitrosamine
Angiosarcoma	vinylchloride, Thorotrast, inorganic arsenicals
VASCULAR	
Veno-occlusive disease	pyrrolizidine alkaloids
Peliosis hepatitis	anabolic and contraceptive steroids, vinyl chloride
Hepatic vein thrombosis	contraceptive steroids

*Other agents (e.g., phalloidin) can produce lesions experimentally.
†Also leads to degenerative lesion called "alcoholic hyaline" or "Mallory body."

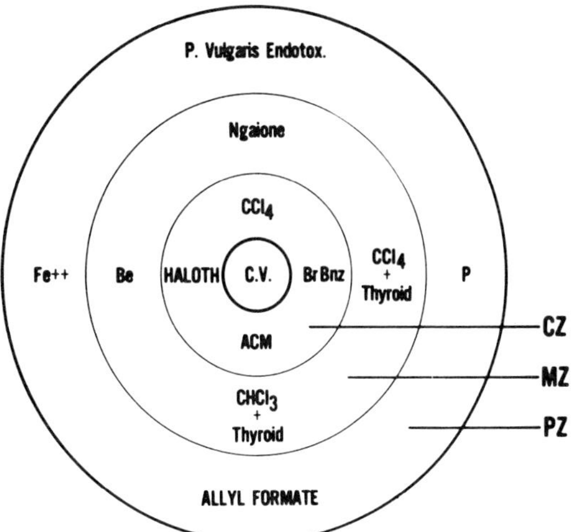

Figure 13–1. Types of zonal necrosis, containing examples of etiologic agents for each. ACM, acetaminophen; Be, beryllium; Br Bnz, bromobenzene; C.V., central vein; Fe^{++}, ferrous ion; HALOTH, halothane; P, white phosphorus; P. Vulgaris Endotox., *Proteus vulgaris* endotoxin. (From Zimmerman HJ: Hepatotoxicity. Adverse Effects of Drugs and Other Chemicals on the Liver. New York, Appleton-Century Crofts, 1978.)

the peripheral zone necrosis of phosphorus and ferrous salts is not clear.

Steatosis can be produced by a large number of toxic agents. Two main types can occur. Some agents (e.g., tetracycline, hypoglycin A) produce microvesicular steatosis—that is, the droplets are small, there are many in each hepatocyte, and the nucleus remains in the center of the cell. Other substances (e.g., ethanol, methotrexate) lead to macrovesicular steatosis—individual large, fat droplets within each cell displace the nucleus to the periphery.

Necrosis and *steatosis* comprise the lesion produced by some agents. With some (e.g., CCl_4), the necrosis is more prominent; and with others (e.g., toxic mushrooms, phosphorus), the steatosis predominates.

Cholestatic Injury. Some agents lead to hepatic injury characterized mainly by ar-

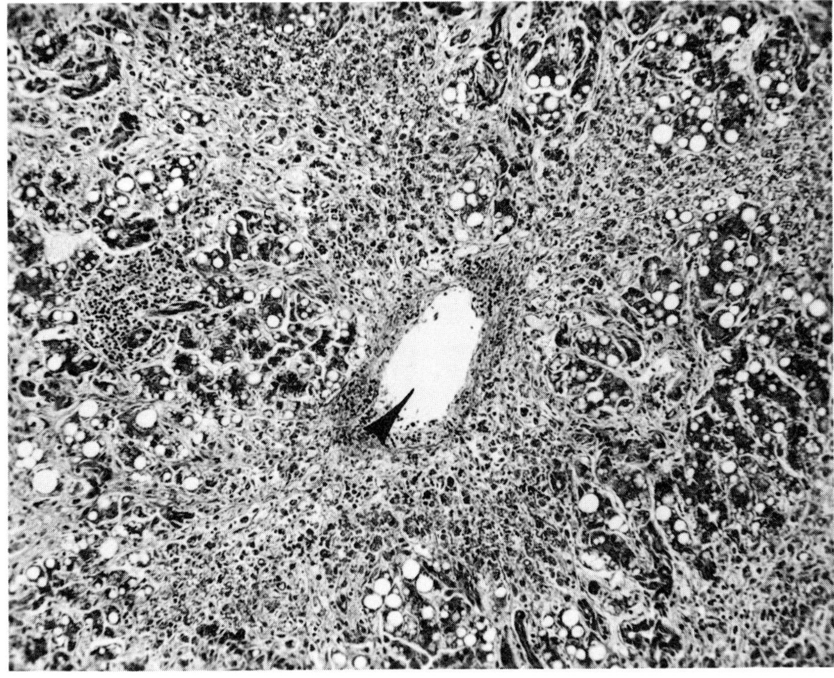

Figure 13–2. Fatal centrizonal necrosis in CCl_4 poisoning. Arrow in central vein. H & E × 80. AFIP No. 72–8406. (Courtesy of Dr. Kamal G. Ishak.)

Table 13–10. AGENTS THAT CAUSE CHOLESTASIS

	CHOLESTATIC EFFECT				
	Experimental	*Grazing Animals*	*Occupational*	*Drug*	COMMENT
Intrinsic Hepatotoxin					
NATURAL					
Bile acids	+	−	−	+	Especially lithocholate
Cytochalasin B	+	−	−	−	
Endotoxin	+	−	−	−	?Responsible for jaundice in neonates with infection
Icterogenin	+	+	−	−	
Rifampicin	+	−	−	+	Acts at both sites
Sporidesmin	+	+	−	−	In some species
SYNTHETIC					
α-Naphthylisothiocyanate	+	−	−	−	
4,4-Diaminodiphenylmethane	+	−	+	−	Cause of Epping jaundice
Paraquat	−	−	−	−	
Steroids					
C-17 anabolic	+	−	−	+	
Oral contraceptive	+	−	−	+	
Rapeseed oil and ajmaline	+	−	−	−	Food contaminant

rested bile flow with little or no parenchymal damage. This is particularly true of some drugs, but cholestasis-producing chemicals also can be found among natural hepatotoxins, among synthetic industrial compounds, and even among the secondary bile acids (Table 13–10).

Chronic

The forms of chronic hepatic disease attributable to chemical injury are listed in Table 13–9. A few warrant special comment.

Cirrhosis. Chronic or repeated chemical injury can lead to necrosis, fibrosis, nodular regeneration, and the pseudolobule development that produces the distortion of hepatic architecture that is cirrhosis. It may be the consequence of prolonged and repeated parenchymal injury, the result of subacute hepatic necrosis, or, rarely, the sequel to a single episode of necrosis. In general, a single bout of zonal necrosis in experimental animals (e.g., CCl_4 poisoning), even when extensive, is followed by complete histologic restitution in surviving animals, and cirrhosis does not develop. Given repeatedly to experimental animals at intervals too short to permit recovery from each dose, a toxin such as carbon tetrachloride can lead to cirrhosis.[107]

Table 13–11. TOXIC AGENTS KNOWN TO CAUSE CIRRHOSIS IN EXPERIMENTAL ANIMALS

acetone	manganese
aflatoxins	mushroom toxins
arsenicals	nitrosamines
azocompounds	pyridine
bromobenzene	pyrrolizidine alkaloids
carbutamide	safrole
cadmium	selenium
CCl_4	stilbamidine
chlorinated biphenyls	tetrachloroethane
chloronaphthalene	thioacetamide
DDT	Thorotrast
dioxins	trinitrotoluene
ethionine	trypan blue
galactosamine	vinyl chloride
indospicine	

Some of the toxic agents that can lead to experimental cirrhosis are listed in Table 13–11. Among them are toxins to which there has been human exposure. Nevertheless, relatively few convincing examples of chemical poisoning have led to human cirrhosis. Drug-induced idiosyncratic hepatic injury that apparently can lead to cirrhosis is identified in the appendix at the end of this chapter.

Hepatoportal Sclerosis. Selective deposition of collagen in the space of Disse accompanied by periportal sclerosing fibrosis can lead to portal hypertension, a lesion that has been dubbed "hepatoportal sclerosis."[108] Also called "noncirrhotic portal hypertension," it has been attributed to chronic exposure to inorganic arsenicals or vinyl chloride.[109–111] Another form of noncirrhotic portal hypertension results from fibrosis in the centrilobular zone as a result of the toxic effects of prolonged intake of large overdoses of vitamin A.[112]

Veno-Occlusive Disease (VOD). A form

Table 13–12. SALIENT FEATURES OF SYNDROMES OF ACUTE TOXIC HEPATIC INJURY*

	CCl_4	PHOSPHORUS	TOXIC MUSHROOMS	ACETAMINOPHEN
Phase I (1st 24 hr)				
GI: Diarrhea	±	+†	+	±
Vomiting	±	+†	+	−
Pain	±	+	−	−
Hemorrhage	−	+	−	−
Shock	−	+	±	±
Asymptomatic latent period	−	−	+ (1st 12 hr)	± (12–96 hr)
Phase II (24–72 hr)				
Asymptomatic period	±	+	+	+
Jaundice	+	−	−	−
CNS	−	−	+	−
Phase III (48–72 hr)				
Hepatic failure	+	+	+	+
Jaundice	4+	4 +	4 +	+
Renal failure	+	+	+	±
Hemorrhagic phenomena	+	+	+	+
Hepatic lesion	+	4 +	4 +	±
necrosis	CZ(4 +)	PZ(+)	CZ(+)	CZ(4 +)
Death	10–20%	30–40%	>50%	15%

*Syndrome of poisoning by iron and copper salts similar.
†Phosphorescent appearance and garlic odor to vomitus and feces.
CZ, central zone; PZ, peripheral zone.
(From Zimmerman HJ: Hepatotoxicity: Adverse Effects of Drugs and Other Chemicals on the Liver. New York, Appleton-Century-Crofts, 1978, with permission of the copyright holder.)

of chronic hepatic disease resembling the hepatic change of prolonged right heart failure *(cardiac cirrhosis)* results from ingestion of pyrrolizidine alkaloids. These agents can lead to central necrosis and occlusion of hepatic venules, hence the designation VOD.[68–71] A similar lesion has been produced by reactions to several drugs used in cancer chemotherapy and by x-ray injury (radiation hepatitis). Thrombosis of the hepatic veins, which leads to a somewhat similar histologic picture, can result from the thrombogenic effect of the estrogenic component of oral contraceptives. This lesion and VOD can lead to the Budd-Chiari syndrome.[2] The syndrome may present as acute disease with abdominal pain, acutely evolving ascites and edema, mild jaundice, and aminotransferase levels sufficiently high to reflect necrosis; or it may present as chronic disease with severe ascites, edema, and portal hypertension.

Peliosis Hepatis. This curious lesion consists of blood-filled lacunae of varying size. It appears in human beings as a complication of the administration of anabolic and contraceptive steroids[113] and after prolonged occupational exposure to vinyl chloride.[111] It also has been produced in experimental animals by administration of lasiocarpine[114] and phalloidin.[115] The lesion has been ascribed to injury of sinusoidal supporting membranes.

SYNDROMES OF TOXIC HEPATIC INJURY

Acute

Liver disease, often accompanied by renal failure, dominates the syndrome of poisoning caused by some agents (Table 13–12). In the syndrome produced by others, the hepatic injury may be only one facet of systemic injury (Table 13–13). The acute injury produced by most agents is hepatocellular in character.

Acute hepatic failure, usually accompanied by renal failure, is the dominant feature of poisoning due to chlorinated hydrocarbons, white phosphorus, and poisonous mushrooms (Table 13–13). It is usually preceded by neurologic and gastrointestinal manifestations. The syndrome of acetaminophen poisoning is similar, but the hepatic failure is not preceded by the neurologic manifestation.[2]

Severe hepatic injury also results from the intake of toxic doses of iron and copper

Table 13–13. RELATIVE IMPORTANCE OF HEPATIC INJURY IN SEVERAL FORMS OF ACUTE TOXICITY

Toxicity Manifested Chiefly with or without Renal Injury
Carbon tetrachloride and other chlorinated hydrocarbons
Phosphorus (white)
Mushrooms; mycotoxins; cycasin etc.; natural toxins
Acetaminophen
Ferrous and copper salts in high dose
Toxicity Manifested by Systemic Effects with Hepatic Injury Only One Facet
Arsenic (inorganic)
Thallium salts
Insecticides
Hypoglycin A
Borates

compounds. However, the liver damage is usually only one facet, though a serious one, of the total systemic toxicity.

Significant hepatic injury, as part of a syndrome that is dominated by the extrahepatic manifestations of toxicity, is caused by a number of other toxic agents. Thallium poisoning, for example, leads to severe hepatic steatosis, but the manifestations of the liver injury are overshadowed by neurologic and systemic features of the poisoning.[17, 52] This is also true of the fatty liver of borate poisoning.[116]

A form of hepatic injury resembling that of Reye's syndrome may be caused by toxic agents.[117] Reye's syndrome is a curious, acute illness of children characterized by microvesicular hepatic steatosis and encephalopathy. It is usually considered to be of viral origin, or due to the interaction of virus and chemical toxin. Nevertheless, a similar hepatic lesion is produced by some toxic agents—e.g., parenteral tetracycline[2] and hypoglycin A.[9] Most important is the evidence that aspirin in large doses,[118] or even in the therapeutic doses given children with acute viral illness,[119, 120] may precipitate Reye's syndrome.

Acute cholestatic jaundice is a rare manifestation of poisoning, although it is a characteristic syndrome resulting from the adverse effects of some medicinal agents (see Table 13–10). The foregoing material has described the production of cholestatic injury in humans by 4,4'-diaminodiphenylmethane (methylenedianiline): as a contaminant of bread,[26] by occupational exposure,[27–29] by poisonous intake of paraquat,[51] and by the mixture of rapeseed oil and aniline (toxic oil syndrome).[97–100]

SPECIAL SYNDROMES OF HEPATOTOXICITY

Acute Hepatic and Renal Failure

Carbon Tetrachloride (CCl_4) Poisoning

A half century ago, the usual setting for CCl_4 poisoning was the hepatic injury induced by use of the agent as a vermifuge. Since abandonment of the practice, almost all cases have been the result of industrial or domestic accidents.[44] Exclusion of this solvent from most of its former industrial uses, increased caution in its use, and removal of it from the list of readily available household cleaning agents have minimized opportunities for exposure to this toxin.[121] Nevertheless, instances of toxicity continue to be reported.[2]

Exposure in industry to acute intoxicating doses has occurred by inhalation, as in the cleaning of large vats without proper aeration or as the result of exposure to heavy fumes in other closed settings. In the home, ingestion by mistake and inhalation in a poorly ventilated small room have been the common modes of intoxication.[2, 122–124]

Most instances of CCl_4 poisoning have occurred in alcoholics, who are more vulnerable than others to the toxic effects of this agent and likely to be more careless with its use.[2, 44, 47] Alcoholics exposed to an atmospheric concentration that led to no apparent hepatic injury in simultaneously exposed nonalcoholic individuals have been severely poisoned. Ingestion of CCl_4 mistaken for a potable beverage has led to instances of hepatic injury in alcoholics. The nonalcoholic, although less likely to develop CCl_4 hepatotoxicity, is not immune.

Histopathology. Centrizonal hepatic necrosis is characteristic, as is necrosis of renal tubular epithelium. The lungs usually show edema, an alveolar pseudomembrane, and thickened fibrotic alveolar walls with epithelial cell proliferation—a change perhaps secondary to renal failure rather than to CCl_4 per se.[125] "Focal pancreatitis" similar to that seen in association with other forms of renal failure also is seen in fatal CCl_4 poisoning, but true pancreatitis also occurs.[122–124]

Clinical Features. The syndrome consists of hepatic and renal failure, usually preceded by transitory neurologic and gastrointestinal symptoms, and in some patients complicated in the late phases by cardiac failure and pulmonary edema. Immediately after exposure to the agent, dizziness, headache, visual disturbances, and confusion are usual, reflecting the anesthetic properties of haloalkanes.[2, 44, 122–124] Indeed, a small proportion of the deaths from CCl_4 poisoning are "anesthetic" deaths. Nausea, vomiting, abdominal pain, and diarrhea also occur during the first 24 hours, especially after ingestion of the toxin; to a lesser degree they may also occur after inhalation. Both neurologic and gastrointestinal symptoms, however, may be mistaken for symptoms of the acute and chronic alcoholism so characteristic of victims of CCl_4 poisoning.

Evidence of hepatic diseases usually follows the exposure by 2 to 4 days but may be observed as early as 24 hours after. Jaundice develops in about half the cases of poisoning. Severe cases develop ascites and hepatic coma, often accompanied by hemorrhagic phenomena. The jaundice is hepatocellular in type and usually rapid in its evolution. The rapidity of increase of the bilirubin levels probably reflects the rapid progression of hepatic injury and loss of excretory function. Increased production of bilirubin by hemolysis[123] and perhaps by known destruction of cytochrome P-450[126] also might contribute to the hyperbilirubinemia. It is probable that the renal injury induced by this toxin also contributes to the rapid intensification of the depth of jaundice by interference with renal excretion of the bilirubin.

Renal failure usually begins a few days after the hepatic damage becomes manifest and reaches a peak in the second week. It may be heralded by the oliguria that is usually noted between the second and fourth day after exposure, presumably mainly of prerenal origin. Continued oliguria or anuria beyond the early phase and mounting azotemia during the first and second week indicate the presence of tubular necrosis. Renal failure has been the cause of death in a majority of fatal cases.[2, 44, 122–124]

Pulmonary edema is observed in most patients who survive for more than 1 week.[125] Cardiac failure, which is seen in the second week or beyond, has been ascribed to the administration of excess amounts of fluid in the treatment of azotemia, and to the sodium retention incident to the renal failure. Nevertheless, toxic effects of CCl_4 on the myocardium may be inferred from the tendency of early acute poisoning to produce ventricular arrhythmias and might contribute to the heart failure.[44, 123, 124]

Laboratory Features. Anemia is common, as is a moderate degree of neutrophilic leukocytosis.[123] The urine usually contains protein, erythrocytes, leukocytes, and epithelial cells, as well as hyaline, epithelial, granular, or, rarely, even red blood cell casts. The blood urea nitrogen (BUN) and total nonprotein nitrogen (NPN) may be elevated early in the episode as a manifestation of extrarenal azotemia secondary to nausea, vomiting, and dehydration or of early renal tubular necrosis. Toward the end of the first week, frank azotemia secondary to tubular necrosis develops. Although the BUN, NPN, and creatinine levels are all elevated, the severe liver damage may lead to a disproportionately modest degree of elevation of BUN relative to the level of NPN and creatinine.[2]

Biochemical manifestations of hepatic injury include the striking elevation of a number of serum enzymes. Serum levels of AST (GOT) may be increased 10- to 100-fold,[2] and there is a reported instance of a 700-fold elevation to 27,000 Karmen units.[127] Values for ALT (GPT) and a number of other enzymes also reach very high levels.[2] Values for alkaline phosphatase are elevated to only a modest degree.

Laboratory evidence of impaired coagulation includes hypoprothrombinemia as well as decreased levels of plasma clotting factors. There is evidence of increased fibrinolysis in experimental CCl_4 toxicity.[128]

Prognosis. Prior to the era of hemodialysis, the case fatality rate was estimated to be approximately 25 per cent.[2] About one fourth of those who died had died in hepatic failure, usually during the first or early part of the second week of illness; about three fourths of the fatal cases had died in renal failure, usually during the second week or later.[122] The current availability of hemodialysis has improved the outlook for patients with severe renal failure.

Treatment. Management is mainly supportive, as in other forms of acute hepatic failure. Careful attention to fluid and electrolyte balance, attending to dehydration during the first day or two, and judicious replenishment thereafter, with care to avoid overloading with fluids, is important. Multiple small feedings rich in carbohydrate provide a means of maintaining caloric intake. If azotemia is slight or absent, a standard intake of protein (1 gm/kg) seems permissible. It is wise to restrict protein, however, in patients with mounting azotemia. An elevated value for the BUN beyond the fourth day seems a reasonable basis for reduction of protein intake to 0.25 gm/kg/24 hr, if hemodialysis is not available. Reduction of protein also is in order, of course, if asterixis or other evidence of hepatic encephalopathy develops. If available, alternate-day hemodialysis should be substituted for the protein restriction unless the latter seems required for the management of hepatic encephalopathy. In this setting of acute hepatorenal failure, when hyperammonemia and azotemia are both troubling, the recently considered substitution of keto-analogues of amino acids for dietary protein should be useful, if available.[114]

Other Haloaliphatic Compounds

A number of other chlorinated, brominated, and iodinated aliphatic hydrocarbons, depending on their structure, can induce similar hepatic injury and the same syndrome after sufficiently heavy, acute exposure.[2, 44, 123] Trichlorethylene, as a result of accidental industrial exposure[130] or as the result of "sniffing,"[41] can lead to a similar syndrome—usually of lesser severity than that of CCl_4. Chloroform toxicity, formerly an iatrogenic disease and now a potential but virtually unheard of laboratory accident, also would lead to a similar syndrome upon accidental ingestion or inhalation.[123] Carbon tetrabromide has been reported to produce a syndrome similar to that of CCl_4 poisoning as the result of exposure in the laboratory.[131] Tetrachlorethane, a potent occupational hepatotoxin, in the past has caused subacute hepatic disease in industrially exposed humans; less commonly, this exposure has led to acute disease (discussed in a later section). Ingestion or inhalation of a high concentration, however, would lead to acute disease similar to that induced by CCl_4.[123]

Phosphorus Poisoning

This is relatively rare today.[2] Large groups of cases, however, have been described from Latin America.[15, 16] Before the outlawing in 1942 of the use of white phosphorus as a constituent of firecrackers and matches, poisoning was much commoner.[116] Cases that have occurred since then have been the result of ingestion of rat or roach poison or firecracker contents, by accident or with suicidal intent. Despite its relative infrequency, phosphorus poisoning remains an important form of intoxication as one of the classic syndromes of hepatotoxicity with a high (>50 per cent) mortality.[2]

Histopathology. The characteristic lesion is fatty metamorphosis. It may involve the entire lobule, but it begins or is most prominent in the periportal area. Necrosis, which usually accompanies the steatosis, is also most prominent in the peripheral zone.

Renal tubular necrosis is regularly seen in fatal cases. Droplets of fat also engorge the renal tubules that have not undergone necrosis and are seen also in the myocardium.[14, 16]

Clinical Features. The clinical picture has been characterized[132] as consisting of three stages (see Table 13–12). An immediate acute toxic stage that consists of severe gastrointestinal and neurologic symptoms, often accompanied by vascular collapse, is followed by a second symptom-free period. The third stage is characterized by hepatic and renal failure and serious neurologic abnormalities.

The first stage reflects the immediate, severe, irritative effects of phosphorus on the gastrointestinal tract. Nausea, vomiting, abdominal pain, and, at times, diarrhea dominate the picture. Hematemesis occurs in about 30 per cent of patients, presumably a reflection of acute gastric and duodenal ulceration. Thirst is extreme; shock, convulsions, and coma are frequent. The vomitus and feces are characteristically phosphorescent and have a strong odor of garlic, which also may be detected on the breath.[14, 16] This acute phase is brief, with a duration of 8 to 24 hours. Approximately one fourth of patients die during this stage. About one third recover; the remainder go on to the third stage with or without going through the second, asymptomatic stage.

The second stage classically has been described as a symptom-free or latent period of 1 to 3 days.[132] Some investigators, however, have emphasized the merging of the first with the third stage and have minimized the benign aspects of the asymptomatic stage.[14]

The third stage is characterized by hepatic failure, renal insufficiency, and recurrent involvement of the central nervous system. Jaundice occurs in the majority of patients who reach this stage. In most reported cases the jaundice becomes apparent between 3 and 5 days after poisoning. It is usually preceded by rapidly increasing hepatomegaly. Renal failure may be noted as early as the first or as late as the fourth day after ingestion of the toxin.[14]

Restlessness, delirium, and "toxic psychosis" occur during the first stage and often progress to coma. Indeed, this is the usual sequence in the 25 per cent of patients who die early in the course. Early coma apparently reflects the neurotoxicity of phosphorus; that which occurs later results from the hepatorenal failure.

Laboratory Features. The jaundice of phosphorus poisoning is hepatocellular in type. The urine contains bilirubin and urobilinogen and has been said to show leucine and tyrosine crystals. The leukocyte level is normal or low, and anemia is not usual.[14]

Serum enzyme levels are only moderately elevated.[2] In experimental poisoning, values for the AST (SGOT) and ALT (SGPT) are usually elevated only two- to sixfold.[133] Higher values may be seen, but they are usually far lower than those of severe CCl_4 poisoning. The development of shock presumably accounts for higher levels in some patients. Abnormal coagulation parameters and a hemorrhagic tendency are usual.[133]

Diagnosis. This is based on a history of ingestion of roach powder, rat poison, firecracker contents, or other material containing white phosphorus. Phosphorescence of the vomitus and stools and the garlic odor of these and the breath provide diagnostic clues. In a patient with hepatic and renal failure preceded by violent gastrointestinal complaints, these clues may lead to the diagnosis when the history has been incomplete.[14, 16, 132]

Prognosis. Large doses of phosphorus, ingestion of the poison in a liquid medium, and late treatment appear to be associated with a high mortality.[14] A mortality of 15 per cent has been recorded for patients who had ingested less than 0.8 gm, and of more than 90 per cent for those who had taken 1.5 gm or more. Ingestion of phosphorus without liquid has been reported to lead to a lower mortality rate (25 per cent) than that associated with ingestion of the agent in water, rum, beer, or wine (50 to 90 per cent). In general, jaundice, azotemia, shock, and convulsions early in the course appear to augur a poor prognosis.[14]

Treatment. The most important aspect of management is early (within 5 hours) gavage; this has appeared to decrease the mortality rate. The use of potassium permanganate to convert the elemental phosphorus to harmless oxidation products has been recommended on theoretic grounds,[134] but there is scant evidence of benefit. Hepatic and renal failure probably should be treated in a manner similar to that recommended for CCl_4 poisoning. Glucocorticoid therapy seems to be of no value.[15] Exchange transfusion has been credited with benefit.[15, 135] Extracorporeal perfusion employing a charcoal column, accordingly, may be useful.

Mushroom Poisoning

The poisonous *Amanita phalloides* and related species produce hepatic and renal failure. This form of mushroom poisoning has been called mycetismus choleriformis to distinguish it from mycetismus nervosus, the muscarine poisoning of *Amanita muscaria*. The latter produces no hepatic lesions.[136]

Hepatotoxic mushroom poisoning in the United States is usually the result of ingestion of *Amanita verna* (or *virosa*), whereas in Europe it is usually the result of ingestion of *Amanita phalloides*.[2, 64, 136, 137] The responsible mushroom, which grows in all parts of the country, may be found from early June until the first frost. Young forms, which are the most poisonous, are also most likely to be mistaken for edible mushrooms.[67] The toxicity results from the presence in the mushroom of thermostable toxins (amatoxins and phallotoxins).[66] These substances together produce a syndrome of hepatorenal failure that somewhat resembles that caused by CCl_4 and white phosphorus.

Histopathology. The hepatic lesion produced by mushroom poisoning is steatosis and centrizonal necrosis. Degenerative changes of the gastrointestinal tract, kidney, heart, and central nervous system also occur.[62, 65, 66, 136–140] Fatal cases often show severe steatosis and variable degrees of necrosis.[138–144] The relative degree of hepatic fat and necrosis seems to vary from case to case. In biopsy specimens from nonfatal cases, Wepler and Opitz have found necrosis without steatosis and have suggested that the necrosis and steatosis are of independent pathogenesis.[139] Indeed, in experimental animals, phallotoxins produce only necrosis, and amatoxins cause mainly steatosis.[136] The balance between necrosis and steatosis, accordingly, may be governed by the relative roles played by the two toxins.

Clinical Features. The syndrome consists of extremely severe gastrointestinal symptoms, neurologic abnormalities, and collapse, usually followed by jaundice and renal failure. A latent period of 6 to 15 hours after ingestion of the poisonous mushrooms precedes the first symptoms. Thereafter come severe spasm and abdominal pain, vomiting—at times bloodstreaked, and diarrhea. These symptoms usually are promptly followed by cyanosis and shock. Within 1 or 2 days, hepatocellular jaundice and azotemia are noted. Central nervous system damage, as indicated by confusion, delirium, coma, and convulsions, may occur during the first 3 days after ingestion.[62, 63, 66, 138–141] Electrocardiographic evidence of myocardial involvement may include bundle branch block and premature ventricular beats.[137]

Laboratory Features. Anemia, presumably hemolytic, may occur, or it may be obscured by the extreme dehydration. The biochemical reflections of the liver damage resemble those of CCl_4 poisoning. Aminotransferase values are strikingly elevated in some patients[141–145] and only modestly elevated in others.[139] Hyperbilirubinemia is characteristic. The coagulation abnormalities have attracted considerable attention.[142, 143, 146, 147] A reduction of the prothrombin complex below 30 per cent has an adverse prognostic significance, but even patients with these values may recover.[145] The suggestion that disseminated intravascular coagulation is an important part of the syndrome is controversial.[142, 146]

Prognosis. The outlook is poor. Thirty to ninety per cent of the patients in the reported series have died.[143, 144] Death within 4 to 8 days results from hepatic failure, severe dehydration and collapse, or central nervous system complications. Death may occur during the first 48 hours as a result of the choleriform diarrhea.

Treatment. The management is similar to that of other forms of acute hepatorenal failure. As renal failure evolves, carefully limited fluid and electrolyte replacement and restriction of protein intake are in order. Renal failure may require treatment with hemo- or peritoneal dialysis. Impressions of benefit from glucocorticoid therapy are controversial,[144, 147] although experimental lysosomal injury by phalloidin can be blunted by hydrocortisone.[148] Early hemodialysis or hemoperfusion has been suggested as treatment for removal of the circulating toxins (see Chapter 8).

A number of studies have reported that the administration of cytochrome C,[149] thioctic acid,[147] or an "antitoxin principle" from milk thistle (silybin, formerly silymarin)[158] after ingestion of mushroom toxins can prevent or ameliorate the hepatotoxic syndrome in animals, and these have been recommended for human use,[152] but the claims remain to be clinically validated.[150]

Acetaminophen Toxicity

Acetaminophen poisoning is discussed in Chapter 50. The hepatic injury and the clinical syndrome of acute acetaminophen poisoning resemble somewhat those of CCl_4, phosphorus, and hepatotoxic mushroom poisoning, in that there are also three phases (see Table 13–12). The first consists of the acute gastrointestinal symptoms of the irritative effects of the large dose of drug. In the second, the symptoms abate. In the third, there is overt hepatic injury.[2]

Most instances of acetaminophen-induced hepatic injury are the result of a single intake of a large overdose. In 80 per cent of cases, the individual has taken at least 15 gm of the drug and in most of the remainder, 6 to 15 gm. A number of instances have now been reported however, in which doses in the therapeutic range (2.5 to 4 gm/24 hr) have appeared to produce hepatic injury in patients whose susceptibility was enhanced by alcoholism or other factors.[153]

Iron Salts[154, 155]

Acute hepatic necrosis can result from ingestion of large amounts of ferrous sulfate. Indeed, accidental intake of ferrous sulfate tablets has been one of the most frequent causes of poisoning in children. The resulting syndrome resembles that described for CCl_4, phosphorus, mushroom, and acetaminophen poisoning, in that there are three phases. Shortly after ingestion evidence of severe gastrointestinal injury is seen, with nausea, vomiting, diarrhea, and often melena. Shock is frequent. Usually, if the patient does not die during this phase, symptoms may abate for a short period, followed within 1 to 3 days by the third phase in which evidence of hepatic injury, jaundice, elevated aminotransferase levels, and striking hypoprothrombinemia appear.

The necrosis is periportal and accompanied by steatosis. Striking degrees of hyperferremia are seen, and a heavy tissue overload of iron would be expected. Accordingly, it is curious that some fatal cases may show little or no iron in the liver by staining.

Treatment consists of efforts to remove iron from the stomach by gavage and from the tissues by intravenous administration of the chelator deferoxamine. In addition, the supportive measures for hepatic failure already described should be followed.

Copper Poisoning[53, 156, 157]

The clinical features of copper poisoning are similar to those of ferrous sulfate overdose. Ingestion of toxic amounts (1 to 10 gm) is usually accidental; it may be with suicidal intent in adults. Hepatotoxic effects also have been ascribed to the absorption of copper ion from sites of local application of cupric sulfate as an astringent antiseptic.

Copper salts produce gastrointestinal erosions, centrizonal hepatic necrosis, and renal tubular necrosis. Jaundice is the result of the hepatic injury, enhanced by the hemolysis produced by high blood copper levels.

The course resembles that of the other forms of acute hepatorenal failure (see Table 13–12). Severe nausea, vomiting, diarrhea, and abdominal pain, accompanied by a metallic taste, characterize the first few hours after ingestion. During this phase shock may develop. Hepatic injury is manifested by jaundice, high aminotransferase levels, and hepatomegaly by the second or third day after ingestion.

Treatment is directed at removing excess copper and providing support. Penicillamine, the chelator employed to treat the copper overload of Wilson's disease, has been credited with benefit in enhancing copper excretion and leading to clinical improvement. Glucocorticoid therapy has been alleged to be of benefit.

Acute Necrosis Due to Insecticide Poisoning

A number of insecticides are chlorinated hydrocarbons. Some are hepatotoxic for experimental animals and in large doses for human beings. Specifically, isolated instances of ingestion of large amounts of DDT (approximately 6 gm)[48] and of paraquat (approximately 20 gm)[50] have led to centrizonal hepatic necrosis and a clinical syndrome of hepatic failure resembling carbon tetrachloride poisoning. Paraquat poisoning also has been reported to lead to selective destruction of bile ducts.[51]

ACUTE HEPATIC INJURY AS A FEATURE OF SYSTEMIC TOXICITY

Poisonous doses of a number of agents can lead to serious injury accompanied by liver damage that is a relatively minor facet of the syndrome (see Table 13–13). Large doses of inorganic arsenicals, thallium salts, borates, and several insecticides lead to neurologic, muscular, renal, and gastrointestinal manifestations that may indeed be responsible for a fatal outcome.[116] Hepatic injury is a regular feature of the intoxication but plays only a contributory role in determining the gravity of the syndrome.

Inorganic arsenic, in the trivalent state, is a strong protoplasmic poison with a long tradition of use as a homicidal or suicidal agent. Large doses ($>$3 gm) can cause death in 1 to 3 days. Hepatic injury is a regular feature but is eclipsed by the gastrointestinal, neurologic, and vascular effects. Severe nausea, vomiting, diarrhea, depression of the central nervous system, and vascular collapse dominate the clinical picture.[116] Necrosis of capillary walls is apparently responsible for congestion, edema, and hemorrhagic necrosis of gastric and intestinal mucosa.[22] The liver shows severe steatosis and varying degrees of necrosis.

Descriptions of the zonality of arsenic-induced necrosis have differed.[1, 157] Von Glahn and associates have emphasized periportal necrosis in experimental animals.[158] Other investigators have emphasized centrizonal predominance of the necrosis, perhaps as the result of shock.[1] Jaundice and other evidence of hepatic failure in arsenic poisoning are rare and can be recognized only among patients who survive for a few days. That the hepatic injury is significant, however, is clear from the histologic findings in acute poisoning and the cirrhotogenic effects of prolonged exposure to arsenic.

Acute Cholestatic Hepatic Injury

Almost all forms of acute hepatic injury in humans caused by true toxins involve the hepatic parenchyma and produce hepatocellular jaundice. Interesting exceptions include the cholestasis produced by 4-4′-diaminodiphenylmethane (methylenedianiline), the cause of Epping jaundice,[26] the "toxic oil syndrome," and the ductal destruction produced by paraquat poisoning.[51] However, there is no doubt that other experimental toxins (see Table 13–10) can produce a cholestatic type of jaundice[2] by selective injury of the canaliculi or bile ducts or by an effect on the hepatocyte.

Epping jaundice refers to an epidemic of toxic hepatic injury that involved 84 persons in Epping, England, who had eaten bread made from flour contaminated with aromatic amine.[26] Methylenedianiline, employed in industry as a hardener for epoxy resin, had spilled from a plastic container on the floor of a van that was also carrying flour. The compound had apparently seeped into the flour. Subsequent to this report, a syndrome similar to that of Epping jaundice has been reported to result from occupational exposure to this aromatic amine.[27–29] The clinical picture consisted of cholestatic jaundice preceded or accompanied by abdominal pain, fever, and chills. Onset in 60 per cent of the cases was abrupt, with severe abdominal pain. In the remainder the illness was more insidious.

The cholestatic nature of the jaundice has been evident in the prominence of itching, the histologic predominance of bile stasis and portal inflammatory infiltration, accompanied by only slight parenchymal injury in most cases, and by the only moderately elevated aminotransferase values. Alkaline phosphatase values, however, also have been only moderately elevated, and a number of patients showed some hepatocellular injury. The pattern of jaundice, accordingly, appears to have been of a mixed cholestatic-hepatocellular type, as seen with a number of drugs. Indeed, Epping jaundice is a form of hepatic injury very similar to that caused by many drugs and accompanied by clinical (fever, chills, rash) and laboratory (eosinophilia) features considered to be hallmarks of hypersensitivity.[2] Yet, unlike the drugs that are considered to cause hepatic injury as the result of hypersensitivity, 4,4′-diaminodiphenylmethane is a true (intrinsic) toxin. It produces similar hepatic injury in experimental animals.[26, 29]

The cholestatic injury of the toxic oil syndrome resembles that of Epping jaundice. The systemic manifestations that reflect vascular, pulmonary, and other extrahepatic injury tend to overshadow the hepatic lesion.

Subacute Hepatic Injury

Several syndromes of subacute hepatic disease may be caused by toxic agents. One form has been the subacute hepatic necrosis seen as a result of prolonged exposure to industrial hepatotoxins (Table 13–14). Another is the veno-occlusive disease (VOD) caused by ingestion of pyrrolizidine alkaloids (PAs).[2]

Subacute Hepatic Necrosis (SHN)

This form of toxic hepatic injury was a major problem for industrial medicine during both World Wars. Most attention was directed to the liver disease caused by prolonged exposure to trinitrotoluene (TNT),[158, 159] tetrachloroethane (TCE),[160, 161] and chloronaphthalene-PCB (CNP-PCB) mixtures.[162, 163] Dinitrobenzene (DNB)[159] and dimethylnitrosamine[164] also have been found to cause SHN, although they are of less clinical importance because of reduced occupational exposure to these agents and the small number of cases

Table 13–14. HEPATOTOXICITY OF TRINITROTOLUENE (TNT), TETRACHLOROETHANE (TCE), AND CHLORONAPHTHALENE-POLYCHLORINATED BIPHENYL (CNP-PCB) MIXTURE

	TNT*	TCE	CNP-PCB
Occupational Injury			
Acute necrosis	+	+	+
Massive	+	+	+
Zonal (central)	−	+	+
Fat	±	+	+
Subacute necrosis and cirrhosis	+	+	+
Delayed-onset	+	+	+
Case fatality rate	25%	16%	50%
Associated features			
Dermatitis	+	+	+
Blood			
Methemoglobinemia	+	−	−
Aplastic anemia	+	−	−
Monocytosis (early)	−	+	−

*Dinitrobenzene toxicity produces a similar syndrome.

observed. Fortunately, SHN as a form of industrial hepatotoxicity has virtually disappeared. Nevertheless, as a classic syndrome of the past and one that might reappear in another setting, it warrants description. Little difference appeared among the syndromes of hepatic disease caused by TNT, TCE, CNP-PCB mixtures (Table 13–14), and DNB. The two nitro derivatives, especially TNT, however, were prone to lead to aplastic anemia and methemoglobinemia in addition to hepatic disease.

The *syndrome* of SHN caused by these agents was a smoldering illness characterized by the delayed onset of jaundice. With the appearance of jaundice, a syndrome of grave prognostic import, characterized by ascites and progressive hepatic insufficiency, was set in motion. Death occurred in some patients within 1 to 4 months, although others survived this phase and achieved at least clinical recovery. Some were later found or assumed to have developed macronodular cirrhosis.

The liver disease caused by these agents was serious. The estimated case fatality rates ranged from 17 to 50 per cent. In patients with a relatively brief course (1 month or less), the syndrome was that of acute hepatic failure rather than SHN. Indeed, approximately half of the fatal cases of TNT-induced liver disease died of acute hepatic failure. Many patients had less severe disease characterized only by jaundice and hepatomegaly with ultimate clinical recovery.

Trinitrotoluene (TNT) Poisoning. The severe hepatic disease caused by TNT was recorded among workers in munitions factories during the two World Wars. The incidence among exposed workers was low, estimated to be 5 per cent or less.[164, 165] Susceptibility seemed greater among workers with direct manual contact with the agent, especially those with grease on the skin. Women seemed far more susceptible than men. Individual differences, beyond the differential exposure and caution at work, also appeared to account for apparent striking differences in susceptibility. Indeed, the very low incidence, analogous to that of idiosyncratic reactions to some drugs, suggests that a metabolic aberration permitting conversion to toxic metabolites may have accounted for the uncommon susceptibility.

Clinical features were those of acute or subacute hepatic necrosis. Onset of illness was usually delayed for 1 to 4 months (at times even longer) from initial exposure. Indeed, in some instances illness did not appear until days or weeks after cessation of exposure to TNT. Early symptoms consisted of fatigue, weakness, anorexia, and nausea. Some patients had overt methemoglobinemia, as manifested by cyanosis, but many patients developed jaundice without having shown cyanosis. Jaundice usually followed the digestive complaints by several weeks.

Prognosis was grim. Death occurred in about 25 per cent of the approximately 500 cases that occurred in Great Britain during World War I. Approximately half the fatal cases developed acute hepatic failure and died in hepatic coma within 5 to 30 days of the appearance of jaundice. The others had a more prolonged (1 to 3 months) downhill course, characterized by persistent jaundice and the development of ascites and portal hypertension. Among surviving patients, some were found to have cirrhosis at a later date. Many, however, seemed to have returned to normal health.

The histologic picture ranged from massive hepatic necrosis, in patients who survived only a few days, to varying degrees of fibrosis and architectural distortion accompanying the necrosis in patients who survived for weeks or months. The latter lesion has been called toxic cirrhosis, subacute yellow or red atrophy, subacute necrosis, or submassive necrosis.[159]

There were also extrahepatic manifestations of TNT toxicity. Erythematous dermal plaques and methemoglobinemia were common but quite independent of hepatic injury and posed no threat to survival. Methemoglobinemia was far more common than hepatic injury and, of course, reversible. Aplastic anemia, a somewhat more common result of exposure to TNT than was hepatic injury, was usually fatal.[164, 165]

Treatment of TNT-induced injury consisted of prompt withdrawal from exposure upon the recognition of hepatic injury. Despite the observation that some patients showed progression of liver disease or even its first appearance after withdrawal, many instances of liver damage appeared to have been aborted by cessation of exposure to the agent. Prevention of hazardous exposure is by far the most important approach to this form of injury. Indeed, proper preventive measures have virtually wiped out TNT toxicity.

Tetrachloroethane (TCE) Toxicity. The syndrome of hepatic injury produced by exposure to this highly toxic chloroalkane resembled that of TNT-induced hepatic disease. A delayed onset of a few to many weeks was also characteristic. Toxic exposure, apparently, was most often by inhalation, although ingestion or percutaneous absorption also can lead to toxicity. Susceptibility appeared to have been enhanced among alcoholics and women.[160, 161]

Premonitory symptoms resembled those of TNT toxicity; digestive complaints (anorexia, nausea, vomiting) were common. Neurologic symptoms (dizziness, headache, paresthesias) were also prominent, but presumably were evidences of "anesthetic" effects of TCE vapor rather than of early hepatic damage. Indeed, jaundice was in some instances the first evidence of toxicity; in others, it appeared after weeks of premonitory symptoms. The appearance of jaundice ushered in the syndrome of SHN or of acute hepatic failure.[161]

The prognosis of SHN caused by exposure to TCE was probably almost as grave as exposure to TNT. In one series, a 15 per cent case fatality rate was recorded.[160] However, attention to early cases of jaundice and prompt withdrawal from exposure apparently helped abort hepatic injury at milder levels. Among the clues to early injury, the digestive complaints and a curious hematologic abnormality—increased numbers of circulating large monocytes—appeared to be helpful.[161]

Chloronaphthalene-PCB Toxicity. Hepatic injury acquired as the result of industrial exposure to these compounds usually has been subacute or chronic, at times acute. During World War II, it was a serious entity with a grave prognosis.[163] Toxicity due to the ingestion of food heavily contaminated by PCBs ("Yusho poisoning") has been mentioned in an earlier section.[31]

The clinical syndrome of this type of industrial poisoning also resembles that of TNT toxicity. It appeared as early as 7 weeks after beginning exposure or as late as many months. Toxic exposure of cases described during World War II appeared to have resulted from inhalation of toxic fumes released by the melting of the chloroaromatic agent during the soldering of electrical materials.[163]

Initial symptoms among reported cases usually included fatigue, anorexia, and nausea, sometimes accompanied by edema of the face and hands. The complaints were usually followed by jaundice. In some instances, severe abdominal pain occurred, perhaps a manifestation of the acute pancreatitis that can accompany the hepatic injury.[156] The appearance of jaundice often signaled the beginning of a downhill course, either as fulminant disease with death in less than 2 weeks or as SHN with death in 1 to 3 months.

It appears that the subacute hepatic necrosis attributed to PCBs was the result of a toxic "cocktail" containing mixtures of several PCBs, the toxic chloronaphthalenes, and probably the ultratoxic tetrachlordibenzofurans and tetrachlordibenzodioxins.[30]

Veno-Occlusive Disease

This condition is caused by the ingestion of pyrrolizidine alkaloids (PAs). Ingestion of plants containing PAs had led to a number of epidemics of liver disease among humans in various parts of the world and, in retrospect, these plants can be recognized as having been a scourge of livestock as far back as the nineteenth and perhaps even the eighteenth centuries.[69] Epidemic liver disease due to ingestion of PAs has been reported recently from India[73] and Afghanistan.[74]

Focus on PA poisoning of humans came with the description of Bras and his associates in the 1950s of a syndrome in children characterized by abdominal distention, hepatomegaly, ascites, and edema.[70, 71] They named the syndrome veno-occlusive disease (VOD) because they were able to attribute the centrilobular hepatic congestion, congestive cirrhosis, and clinical features to the regularly demonstrable occlusion of the hepatic venules.

Cultural practices, economic circumstances, and the plants involved determine the mode of exposure to the PAs.[69, 72] Drinking "bush tea," a decoction of *Senecio jacobae* taken as a folk remedy for acute illness, has been responsible for the VOD of Jamaican children. Cases in South Africa have appeared to be the result of ingestion of *Senecio*-contaminated bread. Those in Central Asia appeared to have resulted from the ingestion of cereal grain contaminated by seeds of *Heliotropium lasiocarpium*. A recent epidemic of VOD in central India was due to the ingestion of cereal contaminated by seeds of a species of *Crotolaria*, and the epidemic in Afghanistan was attributed to the ingestion of wheat contaminated by a species of *Heliotropium*.

Exposure to PAs has occurred in the United States. Preparations containing the toxic alkaloids can be obtained in some of the natural food stores.[74, 75] Also, pharmacies in New Mexico, Arizona, and Texas contain a variety of preparations that are home remedies for pharyngitis and that contain pyrrolizidine alkaloids.[74]

Veno-occlusive disease can also be produced by drugs employed in the treatment of neoplastic diseases.[166] Radiation to the liver can also lead to this change.[167] The curious cholestatic injury of the toxic syndrome has in some instances been accompanied by veno-occlusive changes.

Predisposing factors to the development of VOD have appeared to be malnutrition and childhood. Among the Jamaican patients, the majority have been young children, usually beyond the age of 1 year.[70, 71] Relatively few adults have been involved. That susceptibility to toxic effects of the alkaloid is not limited to children, however, is demonstrated by reports of epidemics of subacute and chronic VOD in other parts of the world that have involved various age groups or even been predominantly among adults.[69, 72, 73] The greater tendency for acute VOD to be seen among children is presumably related to the manner in which the toxic agent has been taken, namely, as bush tea. Nutrition appears relevant in that the incidence of VOD in a given area has been greater among the poor. Whether this relates to the effects of protein deprivation on conversion of pyrrolizidine alkaloids to toxic metabolites or to the increased likelihood that the impoverished ingest contaminated foods is unclear. Perhaps both factors play a role. Experimental attempts to clarify the role of nutrition in the toxicity of the alkaloids also have led to inconclusive results.[68, 69, 168] The adverse effects of some alkaloids are enhanced, and those of others inhibited, by protein deprivation.

Clinical Features.[69, 71, 73] Veno-occlusive disease may present as acute, subacute, or chronic illness. In all three forms there is hepatomegaly, ascites and edema, and "collagenous" occlusion of the small branches of the hepatic vein. The clinical features result from the interference with hepatic flow and can lead to the Budd-Chiari syndrome.

Acute VOD generally refers to cases with abrupt onset of hepatomegaly and ascites and may be accompanied by modest degrees of jaundice. These cases usually have a relatively short course with fatal outcome or complete recovery within 2 to 8 weeks. However, almost half the patients undergo transition to subacute or chronic VOD. Onset of acute VOD is usually marked by gnawing or colicky epigastric pain that usually precedes the first evidence of ascites by a few days. Jaundice occurs only in one fifth of the patients, and vomiting and diarrhea are variably present. The average duration of the acute form in the cases of Stuart and Bras[71] was 4 weeks, but instances with rapid development of hepatic failure and death within 1 week have been recorded. A fatal outcome or recovery as late as 4 months after onset also has been observed. Acute VOD has been attributed to a single ingestion of the toxic alkaloids or to their ingestion over a brief period of time.

Subacute VOD consists of a syndrome lasting for many months and manifested mainly by persistent hepatomegaly and varying degree of ascites but by few other complaints. The course is punctuated by acute episodes similar to those of acute VOD. Subacute VOD may develop by transition from the acute form or may be the result of the ingestion of small amounts of toxic substances over a prolonged period.

Chronic VOD includes cirrhosis. The cirrhosis resembles that of other types of the Budd-Chiari syndrome and of "cardiac" cirrhosis. Similar to subacute VOD, the course of the chronic form can be punctuated by acute injury. Chronic VOD may be either a sequel to the acute form or may be the result of ingestion of the toxic alkaloid over a prolonged period of time.

Morphologic Features. Histologic changes consist of collagenous, fibrotic partial or total occlusion of the efferent (central and sublobular) veins. In the acute form of the syndrome, there is centrilobular hepatic necrosis and sinusoidal dilation.[69, 71] In the subacute and chronic forms, there is central fibrosis and bridging between central veins, leading to a form of cirrhosis similar to cardiac cirrhosis and to the cirrhosis of the classic Budd-Chiari syndrome. This "nonportal" cirrhosis, caused by PA toxicity, apparently accounts for one third of the cirrhosis seen in Jamaica.[69] Megalocytosis is a characteristic fea-

Table 13–15. CLASSIFICATION OF HEPATOTOXIC DRUGS AND MAJOR CHARACTERISTICS OF EACH GROUP

CATEGORY OF AGENT	INCIDENCE	EXPERIMENTAL REPRODUCIBILITY	DOSE-DEPENDENT	MECHANISM	HISTOLOGIC LESION	EXAMPLES
Intrinsic toxicity	High	Yes	Yes			
Direct				Direct physicochemical distortion and destruction of basis of cell metabolism	Necrosis (zonal)	CCl_4, $CHCl_3$
Indirect						
Cytotoxic				Interference with specific metabolic pathway leads to structural injury	Steatosis or Necrosis	Tetracycline Oncotherapeutic drugs, etc.
Cholestatic				Interference with hepatic excretory pathways leads to cholestasis	Bilirubin casts	C-17 alkylated steroids
Host idiosyncrasy	Low	No	No			
Hypersensitivity*				Drug allergy	Necrosis or Cholestasis	Phenytoin, PAS, HALO CPZ, PBZ
Metabolic abnormality				Production of hepatotoxic metabolites (aberrant metabolism of drug)	Necrosis or Cholestasis	INH, IPRO ?Oral hypoglycemic agents

*Intrinsic toxicity may participate in injury.
PAS, Paraminosalicylate; HALO, halothane; CPZ, chlorpromazine; PBZ, phenylbutazone; INH, isoniazid; IPRO, Iproniazid.

ture of clinical and experimental pyrrolizidine alkaloid poisoning. This refers to the presence of huge hepatocytes, presumed to result from the interference with the multiplication of the hepatocytes by the toxic effect of the alkaloid.[169]

Prognosis and Treatment. The prognosis of VOD has been well studied. The acute form is characterized by a rapidly fatal course in 15 to 20 per cent of patients, and by apparently complete recovery in about 25 per cent of patients. Approximately one sixth of the patients with the acute disease undergo transition into the subacute or chronic form and succumb to the illness within 1 to 3 years. In one fourth of the patients whose follow-up has been possible, there has been transition to chronic disease with little progression during the years of follow-up, and the presence of apparently inactive cirrhosis with varying evidences of portal hypertension. Transition from acute disease to cirrhosis may occur with extraordinary rapidity in VOD. Indeed, a period as brief as 3 months may intervene between onset of the syndrome and fully established cirrhosis. Death in the acute phase is often due to liver failure. In the chronic phase, it appears to be usually the result of portal hypertension.[70, 71]

Treatment of this condition consists of prevention. Adequate education with regard to the use of folk remedies containing these toxic alkaloids and public health measures to insure minimal chances of contamination of wheat or cereals by the seeds of toxic plants are obviously essential steps. Nevertheless, the combination of famine and availability of plants, the toxicity of which is not appreciated, will lead to epidemics such as those described in India[72] and Afghanistan.[73] It is also clear that education to prevent PA toxicity in the United States is also in order.

Chronic Hepatic Injury

A single episode of acute hepatic injury seemingly rarely leads to chronic disease. I am aware of no evidence showing that the severe necrosis of white phosphorus or of toxic mushroom poisoning leaves a residue of cirrhosis after recovery from the acute episode. The picture with carbon tetrachloride (CCl_4) poisoning, however, is more complex. Although single necrotizing doses given to animals do not usually lead to cirrhosis as a sequel,[107] they have been reported to do so in humans.[156] Since alcoholism is a predisposing factor in poisoning of humans by CCl_4, the presence of cirrhosis in a patient recovered from acute toxicity would not nec-

Table 13–16. HISTOLOGIC TYPES OF ACUTE HEPATIC INJURY AND ASSOCIATED BIOCHEMICAL AND CLINICAL ASPECTS

HISTOLOGIC LESION	BIOCHEMICAL ABNORMALITIES OF SERUM*			CLINICAL SYNDROME†	EXAMPLES‡
	Aminotransferases	*Alkaline Phosphatase*	*Cholesterol*		
Cytotoxic					
Necrosis					
Zonal	8–500 ×	1–2 ×	N, ↓	Hepatic and renal failure	CCl_4, ACM, HALO
Diffuse	8–200 ×	1–2 ×	N, ↓	Severe hepatitis	INH, α-Methyldopa
Steatosis					
Microvesicular	5–20 ×	1–2 ×	N, ↓	FLP, RS	Tetra, VPA
Macrovesicular	1–5 ×	1–2 ×	N, ↓	Resembles AFL	MTX
Cholestasis					
Hepatocanalicular	1–8 ×	3–10 ×	↑	Resembles EHOJ	CPZ, EE
Canalicular	1–5 ×	1–3 ×	N, ↑	Resembles EHOJ	Anabolic and contraceptive steroids
Mixed (mixture of cytotoxic and cholestatic)	Variable	Variable	N, ↑	Resembles hepatitis or EHOJ	PBZ, PAS, sulfonamides

*Degree of abnormality indicated as fold increase; N indicates normal; ↑ indicates elevated values; ↓ indicates depressed values.

†AFL, Alcoholic fatty liver; EHOJ, extrahepatic obstructive jaundice; FLP, fatty liver of pregnancy; RS, Reye's syndrome.

‡ACM, Acetaminophen; CPZ, chlorpromazine; EE, erythromycin estolate; HALO, halothane; INH, isoniazid; MTX, methotrexate; PAS, para-aminosalicylic acid; PBZ, phenylbutazone; Tetra, tetracycline; VPA, valproic acid.

Table 13–17. CHRONIC HEPATIC LESIONS CAUSED BY MEDICINAL AGENTS

Lesion	Agents
1. Chronic necroinflammatory disease (Chronic active hepatitis) (CAH)	oxyphenisatin, α-methyldopa, isoniazid, nitrofurantoin, dantrolene, sulfonamides, perhexiline maleate[b], propylthiouracil, aspirin[a], acetaminophen[a]
2. Steatosis	methotrexate, glucocorticoid, L-asparaginase, and a variety of oncotherapeutic drugs
3. Phospholipidosis	Coralgil[c], amiodarone, perhexiline
4. Vascular lesions	
Peliosis hepatis	anabolic and contraceptive steroids
Hepatic vein thrombosis[d]	contraceptive steroids
Veno-occlusive disease[d]	thioguanine, urethane
5. Granulomas	allopurinol, halothane, hydralazine, penicillin, phenylbutazone, quinidine, sulfonamides, sulfonylureas, methyldopa, carbamazepine
6. Cirrhosis	
Micronodular type	ethanol, methotrexate, inorganic arsenic
Macronodular type	drugs that lead to chronic active hepatitis and subacute hepatic necrosis
"Primary biliary" type	chlorpromazine, organic arsenical, tolbutamide, thiobendazole
Congestive type	drugs that lead to hepatic vein thrombosis and veno-occlusive disease[d]
7. Noncirrhotic portal hypertension	vinyl chloride, inorganic arsenic
Hepatoportal sclerosis	vitamin A overdoses
Centrilobular fibrosis	alcoholic hepatitis
8. Neoplasms	
Adenoma and hepatocellular carcinoma	contraceptive and anabolic steroids
Cholangiocarcinoma, angiosarcoma	Thorotrast, vinyl chloride, inorganic arsenic

*Causative role in lesion is in doubt; [b]Perhexiline leads to lesion with features of both CAH and alcoholic liver disease; [c]4,4'-Diethylaminoethoxyhexestrol, an amphiphilic compound used to treat coronary disease in Japan; [d]Can cause Budd-Chiari syndrome.

Table 13–18. TYPES OF ACUTE HEPATIC INJURY CAUSED BY DRUGS IN VARIOUS THERAPEUTIC CATEGORIES

	CYTOTOXIC (HEPATOCELLULAR) AND MIXED[b]	CHOLESTATIC AND MIXED[b]	SOME CYTOTOXIC AND SOME CHOLESTATIC[c]
Anesthetics[a]	enflurane fluroxene halothane isoflurane?[j] methoxyflurane		
Neuropsychotropics	amineptine clozapine cocaine famoxitine hydrazides (all) maprotiline metopimazine[j] methylphenidate molindone tranylcypromine tricyclics (most) zimelidine	CPZ et al, PZs haloperidol trimipramine	chlordiazepoxide diazepam mianserin trazodone tricyclics (some)
Anticonvulsants	phenytoin progabide valproate		carbamazpeine phenobarbital
Analgesic, anti-inflammatory, anti–muscle spasm, antigout agents	acetaminophen chlorzoxazone clomatacine dantrolene diclofenac fenclozic acid glafenine ibuprofen indomethacin salicylates pirprofen tolmetin zoxazolamine	benoxaprofen diflunisal penicillamine propoxyphene	allopurinol[d] gold compounds naproxen phenylbutazone[d] piroxicam sulindac
Hormonal derivatives and drugs used in endocrine disease	acetohexamide carbutamide cyclofenil glipizide metahexamide propylthiouracil[d] tamoxifen diethylstilbesterol	carbimazole chlorpropamide[d] tolazemide[d] tolbutamide[d] methimazole methylthiouracil anabolic and contraceptive steroids danazol	thiouracil
Antimicrobials	amodiaquine amphotericin B antimonials clindamycin hycanthone hydroxystilbamidine idoxyuridine isoniazid ketoconazole mebendazole mepacrine metronidazole novobiocin PAS[h] penicillin (very rare) rifampicin sulfonamides[d] sulfones tetracycline[e] thiosemicarbazone	carbenicillin–clavulinic acid erythromycin estolate[g] griseofulvin organic arsenicals thiobendazole xenelamine	cephalosporins chloramphenicol nitrofurantoin[d] penicillins[h] TAO[h] SMZ–TMP sulfadoxine-pyrimethamine

Table 13–18. TYPES OF ACUTE HEPATIC INJURY CAUSED BY DRUGS IN VARIOUS THERAPEUTIC CATEGORIES
Continued

	CYTOTOXIC (HEPATOCELLULAR) AND MIXED[b]	CHOLESTATIC AND MIXED[b]	SOME CYTOTOXIC AND SOME CHOLESTATIC[c]
Drugs used to treat cardiovascular disease	amiodarone[e, f, k]	ajmaline	amrinone
	aprindin	captopril	disopyramide
	benziodarone	chlorthalidone	
	diltiazem	coumadin	
	α-methyldopa	phenindione	
	mexiletine	prajmaline	
	hydralazine[d]	propafenone	
	dihydralazine	quinethazone	
	nicotinic acid	thiazides	
	nifedipine	verapamil	
	papaverine		
	perhexiline m.[e, f, k]		
	procainamide[d]		
	pyridinol carbamate		
	quinidine[d]		
	suloctidil		
	ticrynafen		
	tocainamide		
Antineoplastic[i] and immunosuppressive	asparaginase[e, f]	aminoglutethimide	azathioprine
	cis-platinum	busulfan	
	cyclophosphamide	floxuridine	
	dacarbazine		
	DES		
	doxorubicin		
	etoposide		
	fluorouracil		
	indicine-*N*-oxide		
	methotrexate[f]		
	N-methyl-formamide		
	mithramycin		
	6-MP		
	nitrosoureas		
	tamoxifen		
	thioguanine		
	vincristine		
Miscellaneous (including analgesics)	disulfiram	propoxyphene	cimetidine
	iodide ion	rapeseed oil–amiline	ranitidine
	oxyphenisatin	methylene dianiline	etretinate
	phenazopyridine		
	salizopyridine		
	tannic acid		
	vitamin A		
	PABA		

[a]Hepatic injury produced by volatile anesthetic agents is always cytotoxic.
[b]Mixed forms of injury are categorized according to the predominant injury as cytotoxic or cholestatic.
[c]Refers to agents that are inconsistent in the form of injury produced, with some instances having been cholestatic and others cytotoxic.
[d]Can cause granulomas.
[e]Microvesicular steatosis. Valproate injury also includes necrosis in some cases.
[f]Macrovesicular steatosis.
[g]Also E-ethylsuccinate and E-proprionate.
[h]Semisynthetic penicillins.
[i]Some of these agents alone or as combinations lead to veno-occlusive disease.
[j]One credible case reported.
[k]Also leads to phospholipidosis and changes resembling alcoholic liver disease.

essarily or even probably be a sequel to the bout of acute injury.

Cirrhosis can result from the syndrome of subacute hepatic necrosis (SHN). Indeed, SHN may be regarded as consisting of continued smoldering necrosis, paralleled by increasing degrees of fibrosis, architectural distortion, and regeneration—that is, cirrhosis. The terms "toxic cirrhosis" and "active postnecrotic cirrhosis" have been applied to this lesion. In cases of recovery from the phase of subacute necrosis, which have followed removal from exposure to the offending agent, a residual macronodular scarring has been described.[156]

Cirrhosis also may develop more slowly as the result of prolonged subtle injury. Examples are provided by cases of cirrhosis in refrigeration engineers, workers in dry cleaning plants exposed to chlorinated hydrocarbons,[44] and vintners exposed to inorganic arsenicals.[170]

Hepatoportal sclerosis is the term recently applied to a curious portal and periportal fibrosis and deposition of collagen in the space of Disse, with consequent portal hypertension.[108] It has been attributed to prolonged exposure to vinyl chloride[111] and to inorganic compounds of arsenic.[109, 110] Also referred to as noncirrhotic portal hypertension, it consists of portal and periportal fibrosis, as seen by light microscopy, and of collagen fibrils in the space of Disse, as seen by electron microscopy. This curious deposition of fibrous material is held accountable for the development of portal hypertension. The lesion leads to no clinical manifestations until the varices, collateral venous pattern, and splenomegaly become evident.

Neoplasms should be included among the delayed results of exposure to toxins. Many toxic synthetic chemicals and some botanic toxins can produce hepatocellular carcinoma in experimental animals, but cancer of the liver in humans has never been proved to be the result of toxic exposure. Aflatoxins, however, have been implicated epidemiologically in hepatic carcinogenesis, and, of course, the virus of virus B hepatitis has been shown to be involved in hepatic carcinogenesis. Recent evidence has implicated industrial exposure to vinyl chloride in the etiology of angiosarcoma.

CONCLUDING COMMENTS

Acute, subacute, and chronic hepatic disease may result from domestic and occupational exposure to hepatotoxic agents. The classic syndromes of acute and subacute hepatic injury are today more likely to have resulted from accidental or suicidally motivated exposure to hepatotoxins in the home than from occupational exposure. Chronic hepatic disease may result from occupational exposure. Knowledge of the syndromes and circumstances of exposure to the toxic agent permits prevention.

APPENDIX
DRUGS AS THE CAUSE OF HEPATIC INJURY

A large number of drugs can produce hepatic injury as therapeutic misadventures. Some of these drugs are intrinsic hepatotoxins. Others produce the injury as the result of a special vulnerability of the exposed individual (idiosyncrasy). There are several types of intrinsic hepatotoxins and at least two categories of idiosyncrasy (Table 13–15). The hepatic injury may be acute or chronic. The forms of acute injury are shown and defined in Table 13–16 and of chronic injury in Table 13–17. Table 13–18 contains a list, by pharmacologic category, of a large number of drugs with an indication of the type of hepatic injury each is likely to produce.

References

1. Rouiller C: Experimental toxic injury of the liver. *In* Rouiller C (ed): The Liver. Vol II. New York, Academic Press, 1964, p 335.
2. Zimmerman HJ: Hepatoxicity; The Adverse Effects of Drugs and Other Chemicals on the Liver. New York, Appleton-Century Crofts, 1978.
3. Klaassen CD, Amadur TO, Doull J (eds): Casarett and Doull's Toxicology. 3rd ed. New York, Macmillan, 1986.
4. Kraybill HR: The toxicology and epidemiology of natural hepatotoxin exposure. Isr J Med Sci *10*:416, 1974.
5. Crampton RF, Charlesworth FA: Occurrence of natural toxins in food. Br Med Bull *31*:209, 1975.
6. Wogan GN: Mycotoxins and liver injury. *In* Gall EA, Mostofi FK (eds): International Academy of

Pathology Monograph. Baltimore, Williams & Wilkins, 1973, p 161.
7. Farber E, Fisher MM (eds): Toxic Injury of the Liver. New York, Marcel Dekker, 1979.
8. Tanaka K, Kean EA, Johnson B: Jamaican vomiting sickness. Biochemical investigation of two cases. N Engl J Med *295*:461, 1976.
9. Tamburro CH, Greenberg RA: Identification of human toxicity and carcinogenicity by ethylene derivates. *In* Holmstedt B, Lauwerys R, Mercier M, Roberford M (eds): Mechanisms of Toxicity and Hazard Evaluation. Amsterdam, Elsevier/North Holland Biomedical Press, 1980, p 319.
10. Arena JM: Poisoning: Toxicology—Symptoms—Treatment. 4th ed. Springfield, IL, Charles C Thomas, 1979.
11. Murphy SD: Toxic effects of pesticides. *In* Klaassen CD, Amadur TO, Doull J (eds): Casarett and Doull's Toxicology: The Basic Science of Poisons. 3rd ed. New York, Macmillan, 1986, pp 519–581.
12. Goulding R: Chemical hazards in the home. Br Med Bull *31*:191, 1975.
13. Diaz-Rivera RS, Collazo PJ, Pons ER, Torregrosa MV: Acute phosphorus poisoning in man. A study of 56 cases. Medicine *29*:269, 1950.
14. Marin GA, Montoya CA, Sierra JL, Senior JR: Evaluation of corticosteroid and exchange-transfusion treatment of acute yellow phosphorus intoxication. N Engl J Med *284*:125, 1971.
15. Salfedler K, Doehnert HR, Doehnert G, et al: Fatal phosphorus poisoning. A study of forty-five autopsy cases. Beitr Pathol *147*:321, 1972.
16. Fischl J: Aminoaciduria in thallium poisoning. Am J Med Sci *251*:40, 1966.
17. Mogilner B, Freeman J, Blashor Y, Pincus R: Reye's syndrome in three Israeli children. Possible relationship to warfarin toxicity. Isr J Med Sci *10*:1117, 1974.
18. Chlordane contamination of a municipal water system—Tennessee. Morbid Mortal Weekly Rep *25*:117, 1976.
19. Halmost T, Berki E: Maj cirrhosis es vesel aescoval jaro chronicus arsen mer gezes. Orv Hetil *99*:1835, 1958.
20. Pataky L, Lusztig G: Arsenic cirrhosis of the liver in several members of a family. Z Gesamte Inn Med *13*:668, 1958.
21. Rosenberg HG: Systemic arterial disease and chronic arsenicism in infants. Arch Pathol *97*:360, 1974.
22. Feinglass EJ: Arsenic intoxication from well water in the United States. N Engl J Med *288*:828, 1973.
23. Schmid R: Cutaneous porphyria in Turkey. N Engl J Med *263*:397, 1960.
24. Peters HA: Hexachlorobenzene poisoning in Turkey. Fed Proc *35*:2400, 1976.
25. Kopelman H, Scheuer P, Williams R: The liver lesion in Epping jaundice. Q J Med *35*:553, 1966.
26. McGill DB, Motto JD: An industrial outbreak of toxic hepatitis due to methylenedianiline. N Engl J Med *291*:278, 1974.
27. Williams SV, Bryan JA, Burk JR, Wolf FS: Toxic hepatitis and methylenedianiline. N Engl J Med *291*:1256, 1974.
28. Bastian PG: Occupational hepatitis caused by methylenedianiline. Med J Aust *141*:533, 1984.
29. Posada M, Castro M, Kilbourne EM, et al: Toxic oil syndrome: Case report associated with the Ith oil refinery in Sevilla. Food Chem Toxicol *25*:87, 1987.
30. Kimbrough RD: The toxicity of polychlorinated polycyclic compounds and related chemicals. CRC Crit Rev Toxicol *2*:445, 1974.
31. Kuratsune M, Yoshimura T, Matsuzaka J, Yamaguchi A: Epidemiologic study of oil contaminated with a commercial brand of polychlorinated biphenyls. Environ Health Perspect *1*:119, 1972.
32. Flinn FB, Jarvik NE: Actions of certain chlorinated naphthalenes on the liver. Proc Soc Exp Biol Med *35*:118, 1936.
33. Drinker CK, Warren MF, Bennett GA: Problem of possible systemic effects from certain chlorinated hydrocarbons. J Industr Hyg Toxicol *19*:283, 1937.
34. Flinn FB, Jarvik NE: Liver disease caused by chlorinated naphthalene. Am J Hyg *27*:19, 1938.
35. Greenburg L, Meyers MR, Smith AR: The systemic effects resulting from exposure to certain chlorinated hydrocarbons. J Industr Hyg Toxicol *21*:29, 1939.
36. McLetchie NGB, Robertson D: Chlorinated naphthalene poisoning. Br Med J *1*:691, 1942.
37. Greenburg L: Chlorinated naphthalenes and diphenyls. Industr Med *12*:520, 1943.
38. Collier E: Poisoning by chlorinated naphthalene. Lancet *1*:72, 1943.
39. Cotter LH: Pentachlorinated naphthalenes in industry. JAMA *125*:273, 1944.
40. Anderson HA, Jolstein EC, Daum SM, Sarkozi L, Selikoff IJ: Liver function tests among Michigan and Wisconsin dairy farmers. Environ Health Perspect *23*:333, 1978.
41. Baerg RD, Kimberg DV: Centrilobular hepatic necrosis and acute renal failure in "solvent sniffers." Ann Intern Med *73*:712, 1970.
42. Kloss MW, Rosen GM, Rauchman EJ: Cocaine-mediated hepatotoxicity. A critical review. Biochem Pharmacol *33*:169, 1984.
43. Maroni M, Columbi A, Antonini C, Foa V: Health effects of long-term occupational exposure to polychlorinated biphenyls. *In* Holmstedt B, Lauwerys R, Mercier M, Roberfroid M (eds): Mechanisms of Toxicity and Hazard Evaluation. Amsterdam, Elsevier/North Holland Biomedical Press, 1980, p 351.
44. Hardin BL Jr: Carbon tetrachloride poisoning—review. Industr Med Surg *23*:93, 1954.
45. Plaa GL: Toxic responses of the liver. *In* Klaassen CD, Amadur MD, Doull J (eds): Casarett and Doull's Toxicology; The Basic Science of Poisons. 3rd ed. New York, Macmillan, 1986, pp 286–309.
46. Strubelt O: Alcohol potentiation of liver injury. Fund Appl Toxicol *4*:144, 1978.
47. Zimmerman HJ: Effects of alcohol on other hepatotoxins; Alcoholism. Clin Exp Res *10*:3, 1986.
48. Smith NJ: Death following accidental ingestion of DDT. JAMA *136*:439, 1948.
49. Schubert WK: Liver disease in infancy and childhood. *In* Schubert WK: Diseases of the Liver. 4th ed. Philadelphia, JB Lippincott, 1975, p 1173.
50. Bullivant CM: Accidental poisoning by paraquat. Report of two cases in man. Br Med J *1*:1272, 1966.
51. Mullick FG, Ishak KG, Makibir R, Stromeyer FW: Hepatic injury associated with paraquat toxicity in humans. Liver *1*:209, 1981.
52. Editorial: Thallium. Lancet *2*:564, 1974.
53. Chutlani HR: Acute sulfate poisoning. Am J Med *39*:849, 1965.
54. Doull J, Bruce MC: Origins and scope of toxicology. *In* Klaassen CD, Amadur MO, Doull J (eds): Casarett and Doull's Toxicology: The Basic Science of

Poisons. 3rd ed. New York, Macmillan, 1986, pp 3–10.
55. Volans GN: Self-poisoning and suicide due to paracetamol. J Intern Med Res *4*:7, 1976.
56. Rumack BH, Peterson RC, Koch GG, Amara IA: Acetaminophen overdose: 662 cases with evaluation of oral acetylcysteine treatment. Arch Intern Med *141*:380, 1987.
57. Seeff LB, Cuccherini BA, Zimmerman HJ, et al: Acetaminophen hepatotoxicity in alcoholics. A therapeutic misadventure. Ann Intern Med *104*:399–404, 1986.
58. Leiber CS: Alcohol, protein metabolism and liver injury. Gastroenterology *79*:373, 1980.
59. Clearfield JR: Hepatoreneal toxicity from sniffing spot remover (trichloroethylene). Am J Dig Dis *15*:851, 1970.
60. Tucker SC, Patterson TE: Hepatitis and halothane sniffing. Ann Intern Med *80*:667, 1974.
61. Perino LE, Warren GH, Levine JS: Cocaine-induced hepatotoxicity in humans. Gastroenterology *93*:176, 1987.
62. Ford WW: The toxins and anti-toxins of poisonous mushrooms *(Amanita phalloides)*. J Infect Dis *3*:191, 1906.
63. Larcan A: Actualites sur l'intoxication phalloidienne. Agressologie *16*:257, 1975.
64. Editorial: Death-cap poisoning. Lancet *2*:1320, 1972.
65. Kingsbury JJ: Poisonous Plants of the United States and Canada. 3rd ed. Englewood Cliffs, NJ, Prentice Hall, 1964, p 88.
66. Wieland T: Poisonous principles of mushrooms of the genus *Amanita*. Science *159*:946, 1968.
67. Litten W: The most poisonous mushrooms. Sci Am *232*:91, 1975.
68. Bull LB, Culvenor CCJ, Dick AT: The Pyrrolizidine Alkaloids. New York, John Wiley, 1968, p 249.
69. McLean EK: The toxic actions of pyrrolizidine *(Senecio)* alkaloids. Pharmacol Rev *22*:429, 1970.
70. Bras G, Jelliffe DB, Stuart KL: Veno-occlusive disease of the liver with non-portal type of cirrhosis occurring in Jamaica. Arch Pathol *57*:285, 1954.
71. Stuart KL, Bras G: Veno-occlusive disease of the liver. Q J Med *26*:291, 1957.
72. Mohabbat O, Younos M, Merzad AA, Srivastava RN, Sediq CG, Aram GN: An outbreak of hepatic veno-occlusive disease in northwestern Afghanistan. Lancet *2*:269, 1976.
73. Tandon BN, Tandon RK, Randon HD, Narndranathan M, Joshi YK: An epidemic of veno-occlusive disease of liver in central India. Lancet *2*:271, 1976.
74. Huxtable R: New aspects of the toxicology and pharmacology of pyrralizidine alkaloids. Gen Pharmacol *10*:159, 1979.
75. Stillman HE, Huxtable R, Comroe P, et al: Hepatic veno-occlusive disease due to pyrrolizidine poisoning in Arizona. Gastroenterology *73*:349, 1977.
76. Laquer GL, Spatz M: Toxicology of cycasin. Cancer Res *28*:2262, 1968.
77. Magee PN: Liver carcinogens in the human environment. *In* Liver Cancer. IARC Scientific Publication No. 1, WHO. Lyon, International Agency for Research on Cancer, 1971, p 110.
78. Fukunishi R: Acute hepatic lesions induced by cycasin. Acta Pathol *23*:639, 1973.
79. Korpassy B: The hepatocarcinogenicity of tannic acid. Cancer Res *19*:501, 1959.
80. Editorial: Toxicity of tannic acid. Lancet *2*:34, 1966.
81. Murphy KL: Liver dysfunction and tea eating. Med J Aust *2*:428, 1975.
82. Hall RL: Toxicants occurring naturally in spices and flavors. *In* Toxicants Occurring Naturally in Foods. Publication 1354. Washington, DC, National Academy of Sciences, National Research Council, 1966, p 164.
83. Homburger F, Kelley TK Jr, Friedler G, Russfield AB: Toxic and possible carcinogenic effect of 4-allyl-1,2-methylenedioxynbenzene (safrole) in rats on deficient diets. Med Exp *4*:1, 1961.
84. Segelman AB, Segelman FP, Karline J, Sofia D: Sassafras and herb tea. Potential health hazards. JAMA *263*:477, 1976.
85. Wogan GN: Mycotoxins. Annu Rev Pharmacol *15*:437, 1975.
86. Serck-Hansen A: Aflatoxin-induced fatal hepatitis? Arch Environ Health *20*:729, 1970.
87. Shank RC, Bourgeois CH, Neschamaras N, Chandavimol P: Aflatoxins in autopsy specimens from Thai children with an acute disease of unknown etiology. Food Cosmet Toxicol *9*:501, 1971.
88. Becroft DMO, Webster DR: Aflatoxins and Reye's disease. Br Med J *2*:117, 1972.
89. Dvorackova I, Zilkova J, Brodsky F, Cerman J: Aflatoxin and liver damage with encephalopathy. Sb Ved Pr Lek Fak Karlovy Univ *15*:521, 1972.
90. Chaves-Carballo E, Ellefson RD, Gomez MR: An aflatoxin in the liver of a patient with Reye-Johnson syndrome. Mayo Clin Proc *51*:47, 1976.
91. Bourgeois CH, Shank RC, Grossman RA, et al: Acute aflatoxin B1 toxicity in the macaque and its similarities to Reye's syndrome. Lab Invest *24*:206, 1971.
92. Rogers AE: Toxicity and carcinogenicity of aflatoxins in experimental animals. *In* Pollack JD (ed): Reye's Syndrome. New York, Grune & Stratton, 1974, p 135.
93. Krishnamarchan K, Nagarjan V, Bhat RV, Tilak TBG: Hepatitis due to aflatoxicosis. An outbreak in Western India. Lancet *1*:1061, 1975.
94. Wogan GN: Aflatoxins and their relationship to hepatocellular carcinoma. *In* Okuda K, Peters RL (eds): Hepatocellular Carcinoma. New York, John Wiley, 1976, p 25.
95. Goldblatt LA (ed): Aflatoxin—Scientific Background, Control and Implications. New York, Academic Press, 1969.
96. Lillehoj EB, Fennell DI, Kwolek WF: *Aspergillus flavus* and aflatoxin in Iowa corn before harvest. Science *193*:495, 1976.
97. Noriega RA: Toxic epidemic syndrome, Spain, 1981. Lancet *2*:697, 1982.
98. Tabuenca JM: Toxic-allergic syndrome caused by ingestion of rapeseed oil derivatives with aniline. Lancet *2*:567, 1981.
99. Soliz-Herruzo JA, Castellanos G, Colina F, et al: Hepatopatia en el sindrome toxia por consumo ve aceita adulterado en el area de Madrid, 1981. Gastroenterol Hepatol *5*:113, 1982.
100. Kilbourne E, Rigau-Perez JG, Heath CW, et al: Clinical epidemiology of toxic oil syndrome. Manifestation of a new illness. N Engl J Med *309*:1408, 1983.
101. Lloyd AG, Drake JJP: Problems posed by essential food preservatives. Br Med Bull *31*:214, 1975.
102. Shirley RL: Nutritional and physiological effects of nitrates, nitrites, and nitrosamines. BioScience *25*:790, 1975.
103. Asahina S, Friedman NAA, Arnold E, et al: Acute synergistic toxicity and hepatic necrosis following

oral administration of sodium nitrite and secondary amines to mice. Cancer Res *31*:1201, 1971.
104. Klubes P, Jondorf WR: Dimethylnitrosamine formation from sodium nitrite and dimethylamine by bacterial flora of rat intestine. Res Com Chem Pathol Pharmacol *2*:24, 1971.
105. Ender F, Havre GN, Madsen R, Ceh L, Helgebostad A: Studies on conditions under which *N*-nitrosodiumethylamine is formed in herring meal produced by nitrite-preserved herring. The risk of using nitrite. Z Tierphysiol Tiernaebr Futtermilk *22*:181, 1967.
106. White JW Jr: Relative significance of dietary sources of nitrate and nitrite. J Agric Food Chem *23*:886, 1975.
107. Cameron GR, Karunaratne WAE, Thomas JE: Massive necrosis ("toxin infarction") of the liver following intra-portal administration of poisons. J Pathol Bacteriol *44*:297, 1937.
108. Mikkelsen WP, Edmondson HA, Peters RL, Redeker AG, Reynolds TP: Extra- and intrahepatic portal hypertension without cirrhosis (hepato-portal sclerosis). Ann Surg *162*:202, 1965.
109. Zeegen R, Stransfield AG, Dawson AM, Hunt AH: Prolonged survival after portal decompression of patients with non-cirrhotic intrahepatic portal hypertension. Gut *11*:610, 1970.
110. Neale G, Azzopardi JG: Chronic arsenical poisoning and non-cirrhotic portal hypertension—A case for diagnosis. Br Med J *4*:725, 1971.
111. Popper H, Thomas LB: Alternations of liver and spleen among workers exposed to vinyl chloride. Ann NY Acad Sci *246*:172, 1975.
112. Russell RM, Boyer JL, Bagheri SA, Huban Z: Hepatic injury from chronic hypervitaminosis A resulting in portal hypertension and ascites. N Engl J Med *291*:435, 1974.
113. Bagheri SA, Boyer JL: Peliosis hepatis associated with androgenic-anabolic steroid therapy. A severe form of hepatic injury. Ann Intern Med *81*:610, 1974.
114. Allen JR, Carstens LA: Monocrotaline-induced Budd-Chiari syndrome in monkeys. Am J Dig Dis *16*:111, 1971.
115. Tuchweber B, Kovacs K, Khandehar JD, Gorg BD: Peliosis-like changes induced by phalloidin in the rat liver: A light and electron microscopic study. J Med (Basel) *4*:327, 1973.
116. von Oettingen WF: Poisoning. A Guide to Clinical Diagnosis and Treatment. Philadelphia, WB Saunders, 1958.
117. Pollack JD (ed): Reye's Syndrome. New York, Grune & Stratton, 1974.
118. Starko KM, Mullick FG: Hepatic and cerebral pathology in children with fatal salicylate intoxication: Further evidence for a causal relation between salicylate and Reye's syndrome. Lancet *1*:326, 1983.
119. Remington PL, Rowley D, McGee H, Hall WN, Monto AS: Decreasing trends in Reye syndrome and aspirin use in Michigan, 1979 to 1984. Pediatrics *77*:93, 1986.
120. Barrett MJ, Hurwitz ES, Schonberger LB, Rogers MF: Changing epidemiology of Reye syndrome in the United States. Pediatrics *77*:598, 1986.
121. Hamilton A, Hardy HL: Industrial Toxicology. 3rd ed. Acton, MA, Publishing Science Group, 1974.
122. Jennings RB: Fatal fulminant acute carbon tetrachloride poisoning. Arch Pathol *59*:269, 1955.
123. von Oettingen WF: The Halogenated Hydrocarbons of Industrial and Toxicological Importance. Amsterdam, Elsevier, 1964.
124. Moon HD: The pathology of fatal carbon tetrachloride poisoning with special reference to the histogenesis of the hepatic and renal lesions. Am J Pathol *26*:1041, 1950.
125. Pearce WJ: Nature and agenesis of pulmonary alterations in carbon tetrachloride poisoning. Arch Pathol *55*:203, 1953.
126. Recknagel RO, Gelnde EA Jr: Carbon tetrachloride hepatotoxicity: An example of lethal cleavage. CRC Crit Rev Toxicol *2*:263, 1973.
127. Wroblewski F: Clinical significance of alterations in transaminase activities in serum and other body fluids. Adv Clin Chem *1*:313, 1958.
128. Tygtat GN, Collen D, Oei LS, Van Damme B: Fibrinogen metabolism in healthy dogs and in dogs with CCl_4-induced liver damage and with portal vein occlusion. Thromb Diath Hemorr *28*:320, 1972.
129. Maddrey WC, Weber FL, Coulter AW, Chura CM, Chapanis NP, Walser M: Effects of keto analogues of essential amino acids in portal-systemic encephalopathy. Gastroenterology *71*:190, 1976.
130. DeFalque RJ: Pharmacology and toxicology of trichlorethylene: A critical review of the world literature. Clin Pharmacol Ther *2*:665, 1960.
131. Van Haaften AB: Acute tetrabromoethane (acetylenetetrabromide) intoxication in man. Am Industr Hyg Assoc J *30*:251, 1969.
132. Rubitsky HJ, Myerson RM: Acute phosphorus poisoning. Arch Intern Med *83*:164, 1949.
133. Ghostal AK, Porta EA, Hartroft WS: The role of lipoperoxidation in the pathogenesis of fatty liver by phosphorus poisoning in rats. Am J Pathol *54*:275, 1969.
134. Brewer E, Haggerty RJ: Toxic hazards. Rat poisons. II. Phosphorus. N Engl J Med *258*:147, 1958.
135. Rodrigues-Iturbe B: Acute yellow phosphorus poisoning. N Engl J Med *284*:157, 1971.
136. Wieland T, Wieland O: The toxic peptides of *Amanita* species. Microbiol Toxins *8*:249, 1972.
137. Frimmer M: Toxic cyclopeptides of the toadstool *Amanita phalloides* and related species. Naunyn Schmiedebergs Arch Pharmakol *269*:152, 1971.
138. Larcan A, Lamarche M, Laprevote-Heully MC, Lambert H, Patret JL: Bases physiopathologiques due traitement de l'intoxication phalloidienne. Resultats cliniques. Agressologie *16*:319, 1975.
139. Wepler W, Opitz K: Histologic changes in the liver biopsy in *Amanita phalloides* intoxication. Hum Pathol *3*:249, 1972.
140. Panner BJ, Hanss RJ: Hepatic injury in mushroom poisoning: Electron microscopic observations on two nonfatal cases. Arch Pathol *87*:35, 1969.
141. Trad J, Paraf A, Opolon R, Rollen A: Syndrome paraphalloidien avec ictere grave du à "Lepiota Helveola" (Sensu Lato). Sem Hôp Paris *46*:2163, 1970.
142. Meili EO, Frick PG, Straub PW: Coagulation changes during massive hepatic necrosis due to *Amanita phalloides* poisoning. With special reference to antihemophilic globulin. Helv Med Acta *35*:304, 1969.
143. Herold R, Straub PW: Acute hepatic necrosis of hepatitis and mushroom poisoning. The value of coagulation tests in their differentiation, prognostic assessment and pathogenesis. Helv Med Acta *37*:5, 1978.
144. Gaultier M, Benhamou J-P, Caroli J, DeBray C,

Leger L: Les hepatites phalloidiennes. Presse Med *76*:575, 1968.
145. Kisilevsky R: Hepatic nuclear and nucleolar changes in *Amanita* poisoning. Arch Pathol *97*:253, 1974.
146. Rake MO, Flute PT, Pannell G, Williams R: Intravascular coagulation in acute hepatic necrosis. Lancet *1*:533, 1970.
147. Menache D, Gullin MC, Rueff B: Etudes de l'hemostate au cours des hepatites phalloidiennes. Probl Reanim *5*:499, 1969.
148. Zulik R, Bako F, Budavari J: Death-cap poisoning. Lancet *2*:228, 1972.
149. Dolara P, Buiatta E, Geddes M: Hydrocortisone protection of phalloidin-induced rat liver lysosome damage. Pharmacol Res Comm *3*:1, 1971.
150. Skarabel F, Ditrich P: Death-cap poisoning. Lancet *1*:767, 1973.
151. Floersheim GL: Treatment of human amatoxin poisoning. Myths and advances in therapy. Med Toxicol *2*:1, 1987.
152. Floersheim GL: Neue Gesichtspunkte zur Therapie von Vergiftungen durch den grunen Knollenblatterpilz *(Amanita phalloides)*. Schweiz Med Wschr *102*:901, 1972.
153. Seeff LB, Cuccherini BA, Zimmerman HJ, et al: Acetaminophen hepatotoxicity in alcoholics. A therapeutic misadventure. Ann Intern Med *104*:399, 1986.
154. Luongo MA, Bjornson SS: The liver in ferrous sulfate poisoning. A report of three fatal cases in children and an experimental study. N Engl J Med *251*:995, 1954.
155. Robotham JL, Troxler RF, Lietman PS: Iron poisoning: Another energy crisis. Lancet *2*:664, 1974.
156. Hammond PB, Beliles RP: Metals. *In* Klaassen CD, Amadur TO, Doull J (eds): Casarett and Doull's Toxicology: The Basic Science of Poisons. 2nd ed. New York, Macmillan, 1980, p 409.
157. Klatskin G: Drug-induced hepatic injury. *In* Schaffner F, Sherlock S, Leevy CM (eds): The Liver and Its Diseases. New York, Intercontinental Medical Book Corporation, 1974, p 173.
158. Von Glahn WC, Flinn FB, Keim WF Jr: Effect of certain arsenates on the liver. Arch Pathol *25*:488, 1938.
159. Miller J, Rutherford H: Discussion of atrophy of the liver. Br Med J *2*:581, 1920.
160. Bridge JC, Swanston C, Lane RE, Davie TB: Discussion on trinitrotoluene poisoning. Proc R Soc Med *35*:19, 1942.
161. Gurney R: Tetrachlorethane intoxication. Early recognition of liver damage and means of prevention. Gastroenterology *1*:1112, 1943.
162. Gurney R: Useful procedures in the early diagnosis of liver damage following exposure to the chlorinated hydrocarbons. NY State J Med *47*:2566, 1947.
163. Strauss N: Hepato-toxic effects following occupational exposure to Halowax (chlorinated hydrocarbons). Rev Gastroenterol *11*:381, 1944.
164. Barnes JM, Magee PN: Some toxic properties of dimethyl-nitrosamine. Br J Industr Med *11*:167, 1954.
165. Marltand HS: Tri-nitro-toluene poisoning. JAMA *68*:835, 1917.
166. Zimmerman HJ: Hepatotoxic effects of oncotherapeutic agents. Progr Liver Dis *8*:621, 1986.
167. Reed GB, Cox AJ: The human liver after radiation injury. A form of veno-occlusive disease. Am J Pathol *48*:597, 1966.
168. Jago M: Factors affecting the chronic hepatotoxicity of pyrrolizidine and alkaloid poisoning. Am J Pathol *105*:1, 1971.
169. Jago MV: The development of the hepatic megalocytosis of chronic pyrrolizidine alkaloid poisoning. Am J Pathol *56*:405, 1969.
170. Luchtrath H: Cirrhosis of the liver in chronic arsenical poisoning. German Med Mon *2*:127, 1972.

CHAPTER 14
HEMATOLOGIC CONSEQUENCES OF POISONING AND ANTICOAGULANTS

A. Hematologic Consequences of Poisoning

Joseph M. Brandwein, M.D.,
Armand Keating, M.D.

A number of toxic substances as well as therapeutic drugs are known to have adverse effects on quantitative or functional aspects of blood cells. The major mechanisms of such effects are outlined in Table 14–1. Marrow production may be impaired by inhibition of hemoglobin synthesis, resulting in sideroblastic anemia, and by other direct inhibitory effects on marrow production, which in most cases are poorly understood. Many agents

Table 14–1. MECHANISMS OF ADVERSE HEMATOLOGIC EFFECTS OF DRUGS AND TOXINS

	EXAMPLE	
	Therapeutic Agent	*Nontherapeutic Agent*
Alterations in Marrow Production		
Sideroblastic anemia	isoniazid	lead
Other marrow-toxic effects of ethanol		
Marrow aplasia	chloramphenicol	benzene
Red cell aplasia	chloramphenicol	
Megaloblastic anemia	nitrous oxide	ethanol
Hemolysis		
Oxidant-induced	dapsone	naphthalene
Immune-mediated	penicillin	
Other mechanisms		arsine
Decreased Oxygen-Carrying Capacity		
Methemoglobinemia	dapsone	nitrites
Carbon monoxide		
Alterations in Platelet Function	acetylsalicylic acid	ethanol
Increased Platelet Destruction		
Immune	quinidine	tonic water (quinine)
Nonimmune	mitomycin	
Neutropenia		
Dose-related	phenothiazines	
Idiosyncratic	aminopyrine	
Coagulation Abnormalities	moxalactam	snake venoms

act as oxidants, which, depending on their precise mechanism of action or severity, may lead to methemoglobinemia, hemolysis, or both. Other toxins cause hemolysis by different mechanisms. Some agents, such as alcohol or lead, have more than one effect on blood cells and will therefore be covered in more than one section. Mechanisms relating to effects on the coagulation are reviewed in Part B of this chapter. The marrow-suppressive effects of cytotoxic agents used in cancer chemotherapy will not be discussed.

AGENTS TOXIC TO BONE MARROW

Impairment in Hemoglobin Synthesis

Lead. Lead poisoning is an occupational hazard for painters (particularly those involved in the removal of paint by power-sanding), smelter workers, welders, printers, and those involved in the manufacture of storage batteries.[1] It is also seen in children exposed to lead-contaminated paint and house dust.[2] In addition to its hematologic effects, lead poisoning also affects the neurologic, renal, and musculoskeletal systems.

Chronic lead poisoning results in sideroblastic anemia and is manifested by hypochromic microcytic red cells with prominent basophilic stippling. The major mechanism responsible for the anemia is an impairment of both heme and globin synthesis. The two major enzymatic steps inhibited by lead are aminolevulinic acid (ALA) dehydrase and ferrochelatase. Although ALA dehydrase activity is markedly inhibited in chronic lead poisoning, excess baseline enzyme activity prevents significant impairment of heme synthesis.[3] Inhibition of this enzyme results in excess ALA appearing in the urine at blood lead levels above 40 μg/dl. Urinary ALA is thus a sensitive indicator of lead poisoning.[4]

Ferrochelatase, the last step in heme synthesis, is a mitochondrial enzyme that incorporates iron into the porphyrin ring. Lead appears to impair this step indirectly by inhibiting the transfer of iron into mitochondria.[5] This results in an accumulation of iron in the mitochondrial membrane and of protoporphyrin in the cytoplasm. The former results in the appearance of ringed sideroblasts in the bone marrow, seen on iron staining with Prussian blue. Other features of sideroblastic anemia (a population of hypochromic microcytic red cells, erythroid hyperplasia, and increased marrow hemosiderin) are also seen.

The decreased heme level releases ALA synthetase, resulting in a further increase in porphyrin production. This is seen as a markedly increased free erythrocyte protoporphyrin (FEP), up to 200 times greater than normal.[2] Other intermediates of heme synthesis are also increased but to a lesser extent, probably related to inhibitory effects of lead on other enzymes in the pathway, including uroporphyrin decarboxylase and coproporphyrin oxidase.[6] Porphobilinogen levels, however, are normal.[2]

Both α and β globin chain syntheses are decreased,[7] because of impairment of amino acid transport by lead.[8] The decreased heme synthesis also inhibits the initiation of globin chain synthesis—this latter mechanism is also seen in other conditions associated with decreased heme production, such as iron deficiency.[2]

Other hematologic manifestations of lead poisoning are described in the section on hemolysis.

Ethanol. Chronic alcohol abuse may produce a sideroblastic anemia, with a population of circulating hypochromic microcytic red cells and an increase in ringed sideroblasts in the bone marrow. Alcohol inhibits the conversion of pyridoxine to pyridoxal-phosphate, the coenzyme required by ALA synthetase.[2] This impairs heme synthesis and also inhibits globin synthesis by activation of a heme-controlled repressor. The sideroblastic changes generally do not respond to pyridoxine administration but do reverse within 2 weeks of abstention from drinking.[9]

Therapeutic Agents. The most common cause of drug-induced sideroblastic anemia is isoniazid (INH). Other antituberculous drugs, including cycloserine, pyrazinamide, and ethionamide,[10] have been less commonly implicated. These drugs appear to inhibit the ALA synthetase step, possibly by preventing pyridoxal-phosphate formation. The classic sideroblastic changes that are seen rapidly reverse with cessation of the offending drug or with pyridoxine administration.[2]

Dose-dependent erythroid suppression by chloramphenicol (see later) may progress to a sideroblastic anemia upon prolonged use at high doses. This effect rapidly reverses with cessation of the drug.[2]

Other Direct Marrow Suppressive Effects of Ethanol

Ethanol has other direct toxic effects on bone marrow. Vacuolization of marrow precursors appears with acute and chronic alcohol abuse. It occurs predominantly in proerythroblasts and appears within 5 to 7 days of ingesting 200 to 400 grams of ethanol.[11] The vacuoles generally disappear within 7 days of abstinence. Identical changes appear with chloramphenicol, but the latter is associated with severe erythroid suppression.[11]

Chronic heavy alcohol use results in a generalized decrease in marrow cellularity. Macrocytosis, with or without anemia, occurs in chronic alcoholics, independent of folate deficiency or associated liver disease. Macrocytes are round and have an increased mean corpuscular volume, generally in the 100 to 110 FL range. This change often persists for up to 4 months with abstention.[12] Anemia, if present, is generally mild unless complicated by folate deficiency or bleeding. Abstinence is rapidly followed by reticulocytosis in uncomplicated ethanol-induced marrow suppression.

Thrombocytopenia has been reported in up to 80 per cent of patients admitted for alcohol withdrawal.[13] Ethanol directly suppresses platelet production, despite adequate megakaryocytes, suggesting that ineffective thrombopoiesis is a major factor. The mechanism of suppression is unclear, but it occurs independently of folate deficiency. In addition, a reduction in platelet survival of over 50 per cent occurs with high blood alcohol levels[14]—again, the mechanism is unknown. Abstinence is accompanied by a rebound thrombocytosis in the absence of complicating factors like hypersplenism or folate deficiency.

Leukopenia associated with granulocytopenia has been described in 8 per cent of alcoholics[15] but is more common in association with infection, particularly pneumococcal sepsis. Deaths increase significantly in such patients. Bone marrows in these patients are hypocellular, with markedly decreased mature myeloid activity. There is evidence that ethanol may inhibit granulopoietic factors.[16] Ethanol at concentrations often seen in blood can suppress granulocyte colony growth in culture.[16] Other factors, such as granulocyte margination, hypersplenism, and folate deficiency, may exacerbate granulocytopenia in these patients. Ethanol also causes impaired neutrophil adhesion, chemotaxis,[15] and migration,[11] contributing to an increased frequency of bacterial infections in chronic alcoholics.[17]

Marrow Aplasia

Benzene. Benzene is a lipophilic hydrocarbon used as a solvent in the manufacture of dyes, enamels, varnishes, rubber, waterproof fabrics, and leather goods. It is also often present in variable amounts in paint removers and degreasers. Benzene poisoning was a major occupational hazard in North America earlier in the century, but its use has been markedly curtailed since the 1940s. It is a recognized cause of dose-dependent marrow aplasia. Inhalation of concentrations greater than 100 ppm causes some degree of marrow suppression in almost half of individuals, while concentrations greater than 300 ppm are estimated to carry a 3 to 4 per cent risk of subjects' developing aplastic anemia. National occupational standards for benzene have been lowered further since September 1987, to levels below 1 ppm.[18]

Once established, aplastic anemia progresses in up to 90 per cent of cases, but recovery over a 10-year period appears to occur in many individuals.[19] However, severe aplasia is associated with a 50 per cent mortality over the first 6 months, primarily due to infection and bleeding.[2]

In many cases, dysplastic islands of marrow are seen. Some individuals develop increasing dysplasia over the ensuing months and years, eventually transforming their disease to a refractory anemia with excess blasts and subsequently terminating in acute myeloid leukemia (AML). The incidence of AML in chronic benzene poisoning has been estimated at up to 20 times that of the general population.[20] An unusually high incidence of erythroleukemia (FAB-M6) is seen in these patients.[2]

Benzene is highly concentrated in marrow fat, from where it likely enters membrane lipids of adjacent hematopoietic cells.[21] The mechanism of marrow damage is unclear but may be mediated by catechol derivatives,[21] arene oxides,[22] or other metabolites. Marrow depletion begins in the periphery (long bones), and replacement by fat proceeds centripetally.

Trinitrotoluene (TNT). TNT is a nitro-substituted benzene derivative. Workers in the explosives industry who are heavily exposed to TNT have developed fatal marrow aplasia.[23] As with benzene, marrow recovery can occur after exposure is stopped.[2] Other hematologic effects of TNT are described later.

Arsenic. Inorganic arsenic is used in the manufacture of insecticides, glass, ceramics, paint, weed killers, and other products. Chronic exposure, either by ingestion or inhalation, may cause pancytopenia with basophilic stippling of red cells and eosinophilia. The bone marrow shows widespread cell death, as well as megaloblastoid and various other dyserythropoietic changes.[24] Changes to this point are reversible with cessation of exposure.[2] However, with continued exposure severe irreversible marrow aplasia may ensue.

Arsenic impairs DNA synthesis and also inhibits absorption and utilization of folic acid.[25] The most widely used screening test of chronic poisoning is measurement of levels in hair, nails, and urine. Numerous other organ systems (gastrointestinal, CNS, skin, kidneys) may also be affected. Hematologic effects of acute arsine poisoning are described later.

Other Toxins. Various insecticides, including DDT[26] and pentachlorophenol,[27] have been implicated as causing aplastic anemia. Toluene (methylbenzene) appears to be innocuous at usual occupational levels but may cause marrow aplasia with excessive glue inhalation.[28] Lindane (benzene hexachloride) is another insecticide that has been implicated in a number of cases of aplastic anemia.[29]

Therapeutic Agents (Table 14–2). The most common cause of drug-induced aplastic anemia is chloramphenicol. The risk is estimated at 1 in 30,000 and is unrelated to dose or duration of administration.[30] It has occurred after as little as 2 grams of the drug and has also been reported after topical ocular use.[31] Mortality is 50 per cent within 1 year; only about 10 per cent recover.[2] Acute myeloid leukemia has developed a number of years later in about 4 per cent of affected patients. Allogeneic bone marrow transplantation with grafts from HLA-matched siblings has been curative.

The risk of marrow aplasia with use of

Table 14–2. THERAPEUTIC AGENTS IMPLICATED AS CAUSING APLASTIC ANEMIA

acetazolamide	phenytoin
acetylsalicylic acid	phenylbutazone
chloramphenicol	potassium perchlorate
chlordiazepoxide	primidone
chlorothiazide	prochlorperazine
chlorpheniramine	pyrimethamine
chlorpromazine	quinacrine hydrochloride
chlorpropamide	salicylamide
epinephrine	streptomycin
gold salts	sulfonamides
mepazine	tolbutamide
mephenytoin	trimethadione
meprobamate	

phenylbutazone, an anti-inflammatory drug, has been estimated at four times that of the general population.[18] As with chloramphenicol, aplastic anemia from phenylbutazone is unrelated to dose and sometimes occurs after brief exposure.

Gold therapy results in reversible marrow suppression in 5 per cent of patients, while about 1 per cent develop irreversible aplastic anemia.[18] The latter is again independent of dose, and mortality is in the range of 80 per cent.[2] *N*-Acetylcysteine with plasmapheresis and corticosteroids has been reported to be successful in the treatment of aplastic anemia caused by this drug.[32]

Pancytopenia and aplastic anemia have been reported in patients receiving various anticonvulsants, including diphenylhydantoin and trimethadione. The former may be due to an inherited defect in arene oxide metabolism.[2]

Acetazolamide has been used as a diuretic and for the treatment of glaucoma and severe metabolic acidosis. A number of cases have been reported in association with ophthalmic administration.[33, 34] Aplasia usually develops within the first few weeks of therapy, progresses rapidly, and is often fatal. Other carbonic anhydrase inhibitors also have been reported to cause aplasia.[34]

Isolated Erythrosuppression

Various medications have been reported to cause an isolated decrease in marrow erythropoiesis. Chloramphenicol commonly causes selective dose-dependent erythroid suppression, associated with vacuolation of proerythroblasts. This is thought to be related to mitochondrial damage.[35] Rapid reversal occurs following cessation of use and is in no way related to the idiosyncratic aplastic anemia.

Drugs implicated as the cause of isolated pure red cell aplasia are also associated with aplastic anemia. They include diphenylhydantoin,[18] isoniazid,[36] chlorpropamide,[37] and carbonic anhydrase inhibitors.[38]

Megaloblastic Anemia

Therapeutic Agents. Anticonvulsants, particularly diphenylhydantoin, phenobarbital, and primidone, are capable of causing mild megaloblastic changes, associated with low serum folate levels.[2] The mechanism is unclear, but it may be related to impairment of intestinal absorption of folate[39] or to induction of hepatic microsomal enzymes leading to increased folate catabolism.[2]

Prolonged use of oral contraceptives also may occasionally lead to megaloblastic anemia, possibly related to an increase in folate metabolism.[2]

Brief exposure to the anesthetic agent nitrous oxide can cause megaloblastic changes in the marrow. The mechanism appears to be inhibition of the methyltransferase enzyme,[40] a vitamin B_{12}–dependent reaction. Nitrous oxide oxidizes B_{12}, preventing methylcobalamin formation. The result is a reduction in *N*–5,10–methylene tetrahydrofolate (THF), vital to thymidylate synthesis, thus impairing DNA synthesis. The effect of nitrous oxide can be prevented by folinic acid administration.[41]

Ethanol. Folate deficiency with resulting megaloblastic anemia is extremely common in chronic alcoholics. The major reason is decreased dietary folate intake due to poor nutrition. However, ethanol also has a direct antifolate effect related to interruption of the enterohepatic circulation of folate compounds,[42] to intestinal folate malabsorption, and because of increased urinary folate excretion.[40]

TOXIC AGENTS CAUSING HEMOLYSIS

Oxidant-Induced

A number of agents are capable of generating oxygen-free radicals that can disrupt red cell integrity. Normal red cells are able to overcome the toxic effects of free radicals primarily via generation of NADPH by the hexose monophosphate shunt. This generates glutathione, which in turn reduces oxygen-free radicals. In individuals with deficient antioxidant mechanisms—most commonly glucose-6-phosphate dehydrogenase (G6PD) deficiency—exposure to certain oxidant compounds at low levels may result in the irreversible oxidation of thiols of hemoglobin.[43] This results in hemoglobin denaturation and Heinz body formation with subsequent hemolysis. Oxidation of red cell membrane thiols may contribute to membrane damage and hemolysis. Even in normal individuals, massive exposure to oxidant agents may result in hemolysis.

Toxins. Naphthalene, used as a moth repellent and synthetic intermediate,[44] forms metabolites that act as oxidants. Ingestion or inhalation can result in massive hemolysis in G6PD-deficient subjects: hemolysis in normal individuals occurs only with exposure to very high levels.[45] Some of the agents in high doses, described later in the section on methemoglobinemia, are also capable of causing oxidative hemolysis in individuals with normal G6PD levels. These include various aromatic nitro and amino compounds (aniline, toluidine, trinitrotoluene), chlorates, and copper.[1]

Ingestion of inorganic copper sulfate results in intravascular hemolysis as well as renal and hepatic damage, which may be fatal.[46] Studies have shown that copper sulfate inhibits G6PD and increases oxidation of NADPH.[47] This results in oxidative damage to membrane components and subsequent hemolysis. Methemoglobinemia may also be seen.[1] A high copper content in tap water has been implicated as a cause of hemolysis during hemodialysis.

Fava beans (vicia fava), although harmless to normal individuals, may cause severe acute intravascular hemolysis in subjects with G6PD deficiency. It is a common staple in Mediterranean regions, an endemic area of G6PD deficiency. Hemolysis occurs within hours of ingestion and may be accompanied by fever, chills, headache, and back pain; in severe cases, hypovolemic shock and death may ensue.[48] Jaundice and hematuria occur over the next few days, with Heinz bodies found in red cells. The toxins implicated appear to be the reducing agents vicine and convicine, pyrimidine derivatives that induce formation of oxygen-free radicals.[49]

Therapeutic Agents. A number of oxidants are well recognized as a cause of Heinz body hemolytic anemia when given at therapeutic doses to G6PD-deficient subjects; these are listed in Table 14–3. At toxic doses, these agents are also capable of overwhelming red cell antioxidant mechanisms in normal subjects and causing Heinz body hemolytic anemia. Sulfones (of which dapsone is the most commonly used) may induce Heinz body formation in normal subjects even at therapeutic doses, but the drop in hemoglobin is generally mild. However, at toxic doses severe hemolytic anemia may result.[50]

Antibody-Related

A wide variety of therapeutic agents are capable of initiating hemolysis via immune mechanisms. All are reversible with discontinuation of the offending drug. Hemolysis generally falls into three categories:

Hapten Mechanism. This process involves binding of the drug to the red cell membrane, resulting in the binding of specific antibodies, usually IgG, directed against the drug–membrane protein complex. Affected red cells are then cleared by macrophages in the spleen. The most common offending drug is penicillin, particularly when used at high doses.[51] Other antibiotics implicated rarely include cephalothin[52] and streptomycin.[53]

Immune Complex Mechanism. In this mechanism, the drug first binds to a preformed antibody, usually IgM, in the plasma. The complex then attaches to the red cell surface, resulting in complement binding and activation. Erythrocyte destruction is intravascular, resulting in hemoglobinemia and hemoglobinuria. However, some extravascular destruction may also occur, mediated by splenic and hepatic macrophages recognizing C3b-coated red cells.[51] The anti-C3 Coombs test is positive. The most common

Table 14–3. THERAPEUTIC AGENTS CAUSING HEINZ BODY HEMOLYTIC ANEMIA

acetanilid	primaquine
dapsone	sulfacetamide
methylene blue	sulfanilamide
nalidixic acid	sulfapyridine
niridazole	sulfamethoxazole
nitrofurantoin	trinitrotoluene
pamaquine	
pentaquine	
phenylhydrazine	

drugs involved are quinine and quinidine, as well as various sulfonamides.

Autoantibody Induction Mechanism. This is most commonly related to methyldopa. This drug, by an unknown mechanism, induces formation of an IgG antibody that binds to the red cell surface. This occurs in 15 to 20 per cent of patients, resulting in a positive anti-IgG Coombs test. In most patients this is innocuous, but in less than 1 per cent of patients an immune hemolytic anemia results, due to splenic sequestration and destruction.[51]

Other Causes

Arsine. Arsine is a colorless gas produced by the addition of acid to metals containing arsenic trioxide. This may occur accidentally during smelting, galvanizing, soldering, etching, and lead plating and in the microchip processing industry.[1] Intravascular hemolysis occurs within 12 hours after inhaling arsine fumes, accompanied by abdominal pain, nausea, dyspnea, and hypovolemic shock that may be fatal.[54] If the patient survives, massive hemoglobinuria with acute renal failure may still ensue. The overall mortality is 25 per cent.[54]

Arsine has a strong affinity for sulfhydryl groups. This may impair the red cell sodium-potassium pump, resulting in sodium and water influx, osmotic swelling, and hemolysis.[55] Blood arsenic levels are generally markedly elevated. Treatment includes vigorous hydration and, if plasma hemoglobin is markedly elevated, exchange transfusion.[1]

Chronic exposure to low levels of arsine gas may result in a chronic low-grade hemolysis. This has been reported to occur during the cyanide extraction of gold.[1]

Hemolytic Plant Toxins. Ricin is a toxic protein found in castor beans; abrin is a similar protein found in tropical jequirity beans.[56] Ingestion of a single bean of either species results in massive intravascular hemolysis owing to the direct toxic action of these two proteins.[56] Saponins are potent hemolysins found in the corn cockle and bouncing bet plants. Ingestion may lead to massive fatal intravascular hemolysis.[57]

Venoms. The brown recluse spider of the southern United States and South America releases a venom that appears to have a direct lytic effect on red cells.[58] Bites may be insignificant or may lead to extensive local tissue necrosis and ulceration requiring skin grafting.[59] Intravascular hemolysis, if it occurs, generally subsides within one week;[59] transfusion may be required in severe cases.[1]

Lead. In addition to its effects on hemoglobin synthesis, lead strongly inhibits the enzyme pyrimidine-5′-nucleotidase.[60] This enzyme is important in the degradation of ribosomal RNA. The consequence of its inhibition is the presence of coarse basophilic stippling in erythrocytes, along with a hemolytic anemia.[60]

TOXINS CAUSING A DECREASED OXYGEN-CARRYING CAPACITY

Methemoglobinemia

Methemoglobin is hemoglobin in which the iron is metabolized to the ferric (3+) state, rendering it unable to complex with molecular oxygen. Under normal conditions, small amounts of methemoglobin are constantly being formed and are reduced to the functional (Fe2+) state mainly by NADH, a reaction catalyzed by methemoglobin reductase (cytochrome b5 reductase or diaphorase I). An NADPH-dependent methemoglobin reductase (diaphorase II) plays a lesser role in maintaining reduced hemoglobin.[2] Normally, methemoglobin levels are maintained at less than 3 per cent. An increase in the blood level above 15 gm/L results in cyanosis that is unresponsive to 100 per cent oxygen and a maroon-brown color to the blood. Concentrations above 30 to 40 per cent are associated with signs and symptoms of hypoxia, including dyspnea, tachycardia, and headache. Higher levels cause metabolic acidosis, cardiac arrhythmias, and seizures;[2] levels greater than 70 per cent are uniformly fatal without treatment.[61]

Nitrites. The most prevalent toxins producing methemoglobinemia are nitrites. These agents rapidly oxidize heme iron because of their high oxidation potential.[43] Some, such as amyl, butyl, and isobutyl nitrites, have been used as recreational agents along with various intoxicants[61] and have led to methemoglobinemia. Others, such as nitrites or bismuth subnitrate, can be converted to nitrites by gut or skin bacteria and then absorbed. Nitrates have been found as contaminants of well water[62] and have been used as topical ointments (silver nitrate) in the treatment of burns.[63] Both have been associated with the development of severe methemoglobinemia.

Anilines. Aniline and related compounds (toluidine, nitrobenzenes) are used in the synthesis of aniline dyes, paints, rubber, plastics, fungicides, and pharmaceutical products. These agents induce methemoglobin formation and, as mentioned earlier, may subsequently cause extensive hemolysis.[64] Aniline easily penetrates skin and has been associated with many instances of accidental exposure[65] and attempted suicide,[2] with resulting severe, sometimes fatal methemoglobinemia. Absorption of aniline from diapers marked with aniline-containing ink has resulted in cases of severe methemoglobinemia in newborn nurseries.[66]

Chlorates. Sodium chlorate and potassium chlorate have been used in toothpastes and mouthwashes and are also used in matches and weed killers.[67] They are potent oxidants, and accidental or intentional ingestion has resulted in fatal methemoglobinemia as well as in hemolysis.[68] They are also toxic to the gastrointestinal tract, liver, and kidney.[67]

Therapeutic Agents. Nitroglycerin has been reported to cause methemoglobinemia when given intravenously during cardiopulmonary bypass.[1] Dapsone causes mild methemoglobinemia at therapeutic doses in most patients—this may be life-threatening with acute poisoning and require methylene blue treatment.[69] Phenacetin[1] and antimalarial agents[70] also have been reported to cause methemoglobinemia.

Treatment of severe methemoglobinemia includes supportive measures (intravenous fluids, oxygen) and prompt removal of the suspected agent from the gastrointestinal tract or skin. Methylene blue increases the rate of methemoglobin reduction via the NADPH-dependent methemoglobin reductase and is indicated for methemoglobin levels of over 30 per cent.[2] Methemoglobin levels are generally brought below 10 per cent within 30 minutes.[61] However, it is not useful in methemoglobinemia caused by chlorates;[2, 67] exchange transfusion has been advocated by some workers in this instance.[68, 71]

Carbon Monoxide

Carbon monoxide binds to hemoglobin, forming carboxyhemoglobin, with an affinity several hundred times greater than that of oxygen. This decreases hemoglobin oxygen saturation and also shifts the oxygen hemoglobin dissociation curve to the left, decreasing the unloading of the remaining oxygen to tissues. Carbon monoxide also binds to cytochromes, thereby worsening tissue hypoxia.

Carbon monoxide is produced by the incomplete combustion of hydrocarbon compounds and is produced by automobiles, coal-burning stoves and industries, tobacco smoke, and smoke from fires. Chronic low-level exposure may cause persistent headaches, nausea, and mild polycythemia.[72] Higher levels lead to vomiting, altered mental status, cardiac arrhythmias, seizures, and death.[2]

Treatment includes 100 per cent oxygen and, in severe cases, hyperbaric oxygen. The half-life of carboxyhemoglobin is 6 hours at room air, 1.5 hours with 100 per cent oxygen, and 23 minutes at three atmospheres of pressure.[2]

TOXINS CAUSING ALTERATION IN PLATELET FUNCTION

Ethanol. In addition to its effects on platelet counts, ethanol has variable effects on platelet function. Exposure to ethanol in vitro causes impaired secondary platelet aggregation in response to collagen, epinephrine, and ADP.[73] Numerous platelet metabolic changes in response to ethanol have been identified. Clinically, ethanol exposure may prolong the bleeding time and potentiates the bleeding time prolongation produced by aspirin.[54] On the other hand, the acute alcohol withdrawal period may be associated with an increased tendency to platelet aggregation compared with normal subjects.[74] This may partially explain an increased tendency to cerebral thrombosis and venous thromboembolism in heavy drinkers.[14]

Therapeutic Agents. Some medications causing alterations in platelet function are listed in Table 14–4. Acetylsalicylic acid and nonsteroidal anti-inflammatory agents prolong the bleeding time by inhibition of cyclooxygenase, thereby inhibiting platelet prostaglandin synthesis and abrogating the platelet release reaction. This leads to a significantly increased bleeding tendency in patients with underlying hemostatic defects or

Table 14–4. THERAPEUTIC AGENTS CAUSING IMPAIRED PLATELET FUNCTION

Cyclo-oxygenase inhibitors	acetylsalicylic acid (ASA) nonsteroidal anti-inflammatory agents
Drugs that increase cyclic AMP	dipyridamole methylxanthines (aminophylline)
Antimicrobials	penicillins cephalosporins nitrofurantoin
Membrane-stabilizing agents	tricyclic antidepressants phenothiazines halothane
Others	heparin dextrans hydroxychloroquine clofibrate ticlopidine furosemide vasodilators (nitroprusside, nitroglycerin)

undergoing cardiac surgery but is probably of little significance in normal individuals.[75]

A number of penicillins and cephalosporins inhibit platelet aggregation and can result in clinically significant bleeding. A major mechanism appears to be interference of platelet binding by various agonists, including ADP and von Willebrand's factor. Specific drugs implicated include cephalothin, penicillin, carbenicillin, ticarcillin, piperacillin, and moxalactam.[75]

TOXINS CAUSING INCREASED PLATELET DESTRUCTION

Immune-Mediated Toxins

Over 50 different therapeutic agents have been found to cause immunologic platelet destruction. The best known are quinine and quinidine. Thrombocytopenia may occur after days or years of exposure, but the patient has always ingested either the medication or a quinine-containing beverage (e.g., tonic water, mixer) within the past 24 hours.[76] The latter has evoked the term "cocktail purpura." Thrombocytopenia is often severe, with extensive purpura and possibly serious hemorrhage. Cessation of exposure is followed by platelet count recovery within 3 to 14 days.[76]

Other medications commonly associated with immune thrombocytopenia include heparin, sulfamonides and their derivatives, and gold salts. This topic is discussed in detail in the standard textbooks of hematology.[76, 77]

Nonimmune Toxins

Thrombotic thrombocytopenic purpura (TTP) and the closely-related entity, hemolytic uremic syndrome (HUS) have been described in patients receiving mitomycin and (less commonly) other chemotherapeutic agents, such as cisplatin.[78] It has also been reported in association with the use of oral contraceptives, cyclosporin A, penicillamine, and penicillin.[79] However, in some of these the effect of the drug is difficult to separate from that of the underlying disease (collagen vascular, infection), which also may trigger the syndrome.

TOXINS CAUSING AGRANULOCYTOSIS

A large number of medications have been associated with isolated severe neutropenia. Phenothiazines, carbamazepine, and other agents appear to cause nonimmune, dose-related myelosuppression, but on an idiosyncratic basis.[80] Most drugs, however, appear to cause nondose-related severe neutropenia via immune mechanisms—this is what is commonly referred to as drug-induced agranulocytosis.

Drug-induced agranulocytosis has a mortality rate in the range of 20 per cent, mainly owing to infection.[81] Onset is often abrupt, with the neutrophil count dropping to zero within days. The bone marrow may show an apparent "maturation arrest" in which late granulocyte precursors are absent, or it may show a virtual absence of all stages of maturation. The mechanisms are analogous to those described for immune hemolysis. Some (e.g., aminopyrine) form immune complexes with antibody, which then deposit on the neutrophil surface, activating the complement cascade.[80] Others (e.g., penicillin) bind to the neutrophil surface and induce IgG antibody binding.[82] The latter process usually has a less abrupt onset than does the immune complex mechanism.

Treatment is generally supportive, with empiric use of broad-spectrum antibiotics for fever. Neutrophil recovery generally occurs within 2 weeks of cessation of the offending drug.

A list of classes of drugs associated with neutropenia is given in Table 14–5. More detailed lists of individual drugs with references are provided elsewhere.[80]

DISSEMINATED INTRAVASCULAR COAGULATION

Disseminated intravascular coagulation (DIC) is characterized by the presence of fibrin in the microcirculation, fibrinolysis, and the presence of schistocytes (burr cells or helmet cells), which represent red cells damaged by passage through the partially thrombosed microvasculature.[1, 40] In addition, thrombocytopenia of varying degrees due to the formation of platelet aggregates (consequent on release of procoagulant substances into the blood) produces the picture of microangiopathic hemolytic anemia along with thrombocytopenia. The condition is most commonly seen in association with gram-negative sepsis, transfusion reactions, shock, cancer, obstetric complications, burns, liver disease, and poisoning.[1, 40]

With regard to poisoning, on a worldwide basis snakebite[1] is probably the most common cause of disseminated intravascular coagulation. Cyclopeptide mushroom poisoning also can cause DIC. Drug-induced DIC fortunately is fairly rare but has been noted in overdoses of phencyclidine, lysergic acid diethylamide (LSD), bromisoval, and colchicine and in pennyroyal oil intoxication.

The cardinal manifestation of acute DIC is bleeding,[1, 40] often of abrupt onset, which may present as petechiae, ecchymoses, bleeding from venipuncture sites or from around indwelling intravenous catheters, hematuria, nasal hemorrhage, gastrointestional bleeding, or the like.

The diagnosis is based upon the laboratory findings, particularly the plasma fibrinogen level, PTT, prothrombin time, platelet count, thrombin time, and estimates of the fibrin degradation products.

The cornerstone of therapy is *treatment of the underlying condition*[1, 40] that precipitated the disseminated intravascular coagulation. The administration of heparin, fresh frozen plasma, platelet transfusions, and other modalities is supportive in nature. For a thorough discussion of this entity and its management, consult a textbook of hematology, such as that of Wintrobe and associates.[40]

Table 14–5. CLASSES OF DRUGS COMMONLY CAUSING IDIOSYNCRATIC NEUTROPENIA

CLASS	EXAMPLES
Analgesics	aminopyrine
Antibiotics	penicillins, sulfonamides, cephalothin, isoniazid, chloramphenicol
Anticonvulsants	phenytoin
Antiarthritics	gold salts, phenylbutazone
Cardiovascular	captopril, procainamide, disopyramide
Antithyroid	propylthiouracil, methimazole
Phenothiazines	chlorpromazine, prochlorperazine, thioridazine
Antihistamines	cimetidine
Hypoglycemics	chlorpropamide
Miscellaneous	allopurinol penicillamine

References

1. Wilson AJ, Mielke CH: Hematologic consequences of poisoning. *In* Haddad LM, Winchester JF (eds): Clinical Management of Poisoning and Drug Overdose. Philadelphia, WB Saunders, 1983, pp 886–905.
2. Jandl JH: Blood; Textbook of Hematology. Boston, Little, Brown, 1987.
3. Piomelli S: *In* Nathan DG, Oski FA (eds): Hematology of Infancy and Childhood. Philadelphia, WB Saunders, 1981, p 392.
4. Selander S, Cramer K: Interrelationships between lead in blood, lead in urine and ALA in urine during lead work. Br J Industr Med *27*:28, 1970.
5. Flatmark T, Romslo I: Energy dependent accumulation of iron by isolated rat liver mitochondria. J Biol Chem *250*:6433, 1975.
6. Goldberg A: Lead poisoning and haem biosynthesis. Br J Haematol *23*:521, 1972.
7. White JM, Harvey DT: Defective synthesis of alpha and beta globin chains in lead poisoning. Nature *236*:71, 1972.
8. Piddington SK, White JM: The effect of lead on total globin and α- and β-chain synthesis, in vitro and in vivo. Br J Haematol *27*:415, 1974.
9. Lindenbaum J, Roman MJ: Nutritional anemia in alcoholism. Am J Clin Nutr *33*:2727, 1980.

10. Bottomley SS: Sideroblastic anemia. Clin Haematol *11*:389, 1982.
11. Colman N, Herbert V: Hematologic complications of alcoholism: Overview. Semin Hematol *17*:164, 1980.
12. Wu A, Chanarin I, Levi AJ: Macrocytosis of chronic alcoholism. Lancet *1*:829, 1974.
13. Cowan DH, Hines JD: Thrombocytopenia of severe alcoholism. Ann Intern Med *74*:37, 1971.
14. Girard DE, Kumar KL, McAfee JH: Hematologic effects of acute and chronic alcohol abuse. Hematol Oncol Clin North Am *1*:321, 1987.
15. Lin YK: Effects of alcohol on granulocytes and lymphocytes. Semin Hematol *17*:130, 1980.
16. Imperia PS, Chikkappa G, Phillips PG: Mechanism of inhibition of granulopoiesis by ethanol. Proc Soc Exp Biol Med *175*:219, 1984.
17. Adams HG, Jordan C: Infections in the alcoholic. Med Clin North Am *68*:179, 1984.
18. Rinsky RA, Smith AB, Hornung R, Filloon TG, Young RJ, Okun AH, Landrigan PJ: Benzene and leukemia—an epidemiologic risk assessment. N Engl J Med *316*:1044, 1987.
19. Hernberg S, Savilahti M, Ahlman K, Asp S: Prognostic aspects of benzene poisoning. Br J Industr Med *23*:204, 1966.
20. Viglioni EC, Saita G: Benzene and leukemia. N Engl J Med *271*:872, 1964.
21. Rickert DE, Baker TS, Bus JS, Barrow CS, Irons RD: Benzene disposition in the rat after exposure by inhalation. Toxicol Appl Pharmacol *49*:417, 1979.
22. Jerina DM, Daly JW: Arene oxides: A new aspect of drug metabolism. Science *185*:573, 1974.
23. Crawford MAD: Aplastic anemia due to trinitrotoluene intoxication. Br Med J *2*:430, 1954.
24. Westhoff DD, Samaha RJ, Barnes A Jr: Arsenic intoxication as a cause of megaloblastic anemia. Blood *45*:241, 1975.
25. Van Tongeren JHM, Kunst A, Majoor CLH, Schillings PHM: Folic acid deficiency in chronic arsenic poisoning. Lancet *1*:784, 1965.
26. Sanchez-Medal L, Castonedo JP, Garcia-Rajas F: Insecticides and aplastic anemia. N Engl J Med *269*:1365, 1963.
27. Roberts HJ: Aplastic anemia due to pentochlorophenol. N Engl J Med *305*:1650, 1981.
28. Roodman GD, Reese EP Jr, Cardamone JM: Aplastic anemia associated with rubber cement used by a marathon runner. Arch Intern Med *140*:703, 1980.
29. West I: Lindane and hematologic reactions. Arch Environ Health *15*:97, 1967.
30. Cone TE, Abelson SM: Aplastic anemia following two days of chloramphenicol therapy. J Pediatr *41*:340, 1952.
31. Fraunfelder FT, Bagby GC Jr, Kelly DJ: Fatal aplastic anemia following topical administration of ophthalmic chloramphenicol. Am J Ophthalmol *93*:356, 1982.
32. Hansen RM, Csuka ME, McCarty DJ, Saryan LA: Gold-induced aplastic anemia. Complete response to corticosteroids, plasmapharesis and *N*-acetylcysteine infusion. J Rheumatol *12*:794, 1985.
33. Rentiers PK, Johnston AC, Buskard N: Severe aplastic anemia as a complication of acetazolamide therapy. Can J Ophthalmol *5*:337, 1970.
34. Wisch N, Fischbein FI, Siegel R, Glass JL, Leopold I: Aplastic anemia resulting from the use of carbonic anhydrase inhibitors. Am J Ophthalmol *75*:130, 1973.
35. Yunis AA: Chloramphenicol-induced bone marrow suppression. Semin Hematol *10*:225, 1973.
36. Goodman SB, Block MH: A case of red cell aplasia occurring as a result of antituberculosis therapy. Blood *24*:616, 1964.
37. Recker RR, Hynes HE: Pure red blood cell aplasia associated with chlorpropamide therapy. Arch Intern Med *123*:445, 1969.
38. Krivoy N, Ben-Arieh Y, Carter A, Alroy G: Methazolamide-induced hepatitis and pure RBC aplasia. Arch Intern Med *141*:1229, 1981.
39. Dahlke MB, Mertens-Roster E: Malabsorption of folic acid due to diphenylhydantoin. Blood *30*:341, 1967.
40. Wintrobe MM, Lee GR, Boggs DR, Bithell TC, Foerster J, Athens JW, Lukens JN: Clinical Hematology. 8th ed. Philadelphia, Lea and Febiger, 1981.
41. Amos RJ, Amess JA, Nancekievill DG, Rees GM: Prevention of nitrous oxide–induced megaloblastic changes in bone marrow using folinic acid. Br J Anaesthesiol *56*:103, 1984.
42. Weir DG, McGing PG, Scott JM: Folate metabolism, the enterohepatic circulation and alcohol. Biochem Pharmacol *34*:1, 1985.
43. Allen DW, Jandl JH: Oxidative hemolysis and precipitation of hemoglobin. II: Role of thiols in oxidant drug reaction. J Clin Invest *40*:454, 1961.
44. Dreisbach RH: *In* Handbook of Poisoning. 11th ed. Los Altos, CA, Lange Medical Publications, 1983, p 211.
45. Valaes T, Doxiadis SA, Fessas P: Acute hemolysis due to naphthalene inhalation. J Pediatr *63*:905, 1963.
46. Thirumalaikolundusubramanian P, Chandramohan M, Johnson ES: Copper sulphate poisoning. J Indian Med Assoc *82*:6, 1984.
47. Fairbanks VF: Copper sulfate–induced hemolytic anemia. Arch Intern Med *120*:428, 1967.
48. Jandl JH: *In* Blood; Textbook of Hematology. Boston, Little, Brown, 1987, p 335.
49. Chevion M, Novak T, Glaser G, Mager J: The chemistry of favism-inducing compounds. The properties of isouramil and divicine and their reaction with glutathione. Eur J Biochem *127*:405, 1982.
50. Cream JJ, Scott TL: Anemia in dermatitis herpetiformis. The role of dapsone-induced hemolysis and malabsorption. Br J Dermatol *82*:333, 1970.
51. Packman CH, Leddy JP: Drug-related immunologic injury of erythrocytes. *In* Williams WJ, Beutler E, Erslev AJ, Lichtman MA (eds): Hematology. 3rd ed. New York, McGraw-Hill, 1983, p 647.
52. Gralnick HR, McGinnis MH, Elton W, McCurdy P: Hemolytic anemia associated with cephalothin. JAMA *217*:1193, 1971.
53. Martinez L, Letona J, Barbolla L, Frieyro E, Bouza E, Gilsanz F, Fernandez MN: Immune haemolytic anaemia and renal failure induced by streptomycin. Br J Haematol *35*:561, 1977.
54. Fowler BA, Weissberg JB: Arsine poisoning. N Engl J Med *291*:1171, 1974.
55. Levinsky WJ, Smalley RV, Hillger PN: Arsine hemolysis. Arch Environ Health *20*:436, 1970.
56. Dreisbach RH (ed): Handbook of Poisoning. 11th ed. Los Altos, CA, Lange Medical Publications, 1983, p 541.
57. Altschul S von R: Drugs and Foods from Little-Known Plants. Cambridge, MA, Harvard University Press, 1973.
58. Denny WF, Dillaha CJ, Morgan PN: Hemotoxic effect of *Loxosceles reclusus* venom: In vivo and in vitro studies. J Lab Clin Med *64*:291, 1964.
59. Wasserman GS, Siegel C: Loxoscelism (brown re-

cluse spider bites): A review of the literature. Clin Toxicol *14*:353, 1979.
60. Valentine WN, Paglia DE, Fink K, Madokaro G: Lead poisoning—association with hemolytic anemia, basophilic stippling, erythrocyte pyrimidine 5′-nucleotidase deficiency, and intraerythrocytic accumulation of pyrimidines. J Clin Invest *58*:926, 1976.
61. Jandl JH: *In* Blood: Textbook of Hematology. Boston, Little, Brown, 1987, p 436.
62. Bucklin R, Myint MK: Fatal methemoglobinemia due to well water nitrates. Ann Intern Med *52*:703, 1960.
63. Strauch B, Buch W, Grey W, Laub D: Successful treatment of hemoglobinemia secondary to silver nitrate therapy. N Engl J Med *281*:257, 1969.
64. Dreisbach RH (ed): *In* Handbook of Poisoning. 11th ed. Los Altos, CA, Lange Medical Publications, 1983, p 153.
65. Kewney TE, Manoguerra AS, Dunford JV: Chemically induced methemoglobinemia from aniline poisoning. West J Med *140*:282, 1984.
66. Ramsay DHE, Harvey CC: Marking-ink poisoning. An outbreak of methaemoglobin cyanosis in newborn babies. Lancet *1*:910, 1959.
67. Dreisbach RH (ed): *In* Handbook of Poisoning. 11th ed. Los Altos, CA, Lange Medical Publications, 1983, p 407.
68. Lee DBN, Brown DL, Baker LRI, et al: Haematological complications of chlorate poisoning. Br Med J *2*:31, 1970.
69. Bolin G, Brodin B, Hilden J-O, Martensson J: Acute dapsone intoxication. Clin Toxicol *22*:537, 1984–85.
70. Cohen RJ, Sachs JR, Wicker DJ, Conrad ME: Methemoglobinemia provoked by malarial chemoprophylaxis in Vietnam. N Engl J Med *279*:1127, 1968.
71. Steffen C, Seitz R: Severe chlorate poisoning: Report of a case. Arch Toxicol *48*:281, 1981.
72. Ersler AJ: *In* Williams WJ, Beutler E, Erslev AJ, Lechtman MA (eds): Hematology. 3rd ed. New York, McGraw-Hill, 1983, p 673.
73. Hant MJ, Cowan DH: The effect of ethanol on hemostatic properties of human blood platelets. Am J Med *52*:22, 1974.
74. Hillbom M, Muuronen A, Lowbeer C, Anggard E, Beving H, Kangasaho M: Platelet thromboxane formation and bleeding time is influenced by ethanol withdrawal but not by cigarette smoking. Thromb Haemost *53*:419, 1985.
75. Carvalho ACA, Koneti Rao A: *In* Colman RW, Hirsh J, Marder VJ, Salzman EW (eds): Hemostasis and Thrombosis. 2nd ed. Philadelphia, JB Lippincott, 1987, p 750.
76. Jandl JH: Disorders of platelets. *In* Blood; Textbook of Hematology. Boston, Little, Brown, 1987, p 1041.
77. Aster RH: Thrombocytopenia. *In* Williams WJ, Beutler E, Erslev AJ, Lechtman MA (eds): Hematology. 3rd ed. New York, McGraw-Hill, 1983, p 1298.
78. Byrnes JJ, Moake JL: Thrombotic thrombocytopenic purpura and the hemolytic-uremic syndrome: Evolving concepts of pathogenesis and therapy. Clin Haematol *15*:413, 1986.
79. Eisenstadt RS, Calman RW, Marder VJ: Thrombotic Thrombocytic Purpura. *In* Colman RW, et al (eds): Hemostasis and Thrombosis. 2nd ed. Philadelphia, JB Lippincott, 1987, p 1016.
80. Finch SC: Neutropenia. *In* Williams WJ, Beutler E, Erslev AJ, Lichtman MA (eds): Hematology. 3rd ed. New York, McGraw-Hill, 1983, p 773.
81. Arnebom P, Palblad J: Drug-induced neutropenia in the Stockholm region, 1973–75: Frequency and causes. Acta Med Scand *204*:283, 1978.
82. Murphy MF, Riordan T, Minchinton RM, Chapman JF, Amess JA, Shaw EJ, Waters AH: Demonstration of an immune-mediated mechanism of penicillin-induced neutropenia and thrombocytopenia. Br J Haematol *55*:155, 1983.

B. Anticoagulants

Andre Schuh, M.D., Armand Keating, M.D.

Intravascular thrombosis is associated with significant morbidity and mortality. For more than 40 years, anticoagulants have been used both to treat and to prevent thrombosis and its extension, thereby reducing both morbidity and mortality. When properly used and monitored, such therapy can usually achieve this goal without inducing serious bleeding. However, the risk of hemorrhage may be greatly increased in certain situations:

- excessive amounts of anticoagulants may be administered inadvertently or intentionally;[1]
- a variety of comorbid factors or drug interactions may adversely influence a patient's response to anticoagulants;[2]
- even stable, well-controlled anticoagulation may be inappropriate in a patient involved in trauma[3] or requiring surgery.[4]

In such cases, the rapid and appropriate management of drug-induced coagulopathy may be lifesaving.

Drug-induced disorders of blood coagulation may be caused by oral anticoagulants and the related anticoagulant rodenticides, by heparin, and by defibrinogenating enzymes such as ancrod. These agents will be discussed in turn. Heparin and ancrod are most often, but not always, administered only to hospitalized patients. The most common drug-induced coagulopathy seen in the emergency setting, therefore, will be the result of oral anticoagulant use.

Other drugs that may be associated with

hemorrhage include antiplatelet agents and fibrinolytic (thrombolytic) agents. These drugs are discussed elsewhere.

ORAL ANTICOAGULANTS

Oral anticoagulants are small, organic compounds, structurally similar to vitamin K, and act as vitamin K antagonists. All are synthesized derivatives of either hydroxycoumarin or indanedione. The former include ethyl biscoumacetate (Tromexan), bishydroxycoumarin (Dicumarol), phenprocoumon (Liquamar), acenocoumarin (Sintrom), and sodium warfarin (Coumadin, Panwarfin). The latter include phenindione, diphenadione, and anisindione. Anticoagulant rodenticides are also coumarin or indanedione derivatives (see later). Because of its favorable pharmacokinetics and the absence of significant direct toxicity, sodium warfarin is by far the most widely used oral anticoagulant.[2,7]

Indications for Use

Warfarin use may be short-term or long-term. Long-term use may be indicated for treatment of ischemic cerebrovascular disease, deep vein thrombosis and pulmonary embolism, ischemic heart disease or myocardial infarction, the prevention of systemic embolization with atrial fibrillation, valvular heart disease, thrombogenic prosthetic heart valves, or recurrent arterial embolization from a persistent cardiac source.[17,28] Short-term use may be indicated prophylactically for prevention of venous thromboembolism in high-risk surgery—particularly hip surgery—and for short-term treatment after myocardial infarction.[17,28] Less usual indications may include peripheral vascular disease and experimental therapy in some types of malignancy.[55]

Warfarin ingestion may also be inadvertent or surreptitious.[1,56]

Contraindications

Contraindications to oral anticoagulants include pre-existing or coexisting abnormalities of blood coagulation, active bleeding, recent or imminent surgery of the central nervous system or eye, diagnostic or therapeutic procedures with potential for uncontrollable bleeding including lumbar puncture, malignant hypertension, peptic ulceration, pregnancy, threatened abortion, intrauterine device, cerebrovascular hemorrhage, and bacterial endocarditis. Relative contraindications include thrombocytopenia, pericarditis, pericardial effusions, and unreliability of the patient or of patient supervision. Breast-feeding is not a contraindication to warfarin therapy.[5,6]

Mechanism of Action

Warfarin and other vitamin K antagonists inhibit the hepatic vitamin K–dependent post-translational gamma-carboxylation of amino-terminal glutamic acid residues of the vitamin K–dependent coagulation factors II, VII, IX, and X[8] and of anticoagulant proteins C[9,10] and S.[11,12] Normally, the presence of γ-carboxyglutamate residues enables these proteins to bind calcium, thereby facilitating their binding to phospholipids, a process that is required for their effective participation in coagulation.[13] In the presence of vitamin K antagonists, however, γ-carboxylation does not occur, resulting in the synthesis of biologically inactive but immunologically detectable forms of the vitamin K–dependent proteins.[8] However, the subsequent metabolism of these proteins is not affected. Therefore, following the institution of oral anticoagulant therapy, the activities of the various vitamin K–dependent factors fall according to the half-life of each factor.

Pharmacology

Warfarin has excellent bioavailability with almost complete absorption from the GI tract.[14] Maximal concentration in plasma is reached within 1 hour.[14] At therapeutic doses, 99 per cent of warfarin sodium is bound to albumin, with only the small remaining free fraction being therapeutically active.[7] Metabolism of warfarin is by hepatic microsomal enzymes, with metabolites appearing in urine and stool.[15] Overall, the mean half-life of warfarin in human beings is 35 hours, and its duration of action may be up to 5 days.[14] However, the absorption of warfarin is influenced by diet and drugs,

Table 14–6. RECOMMENDED THERAPEUTIC RANGES OF INR AND PT RATIO IN ORAL ANTICOAGULANT THERAPY[16, 17]

CLINICAL INDICATION	INR	PT RATIO*
Prophylaxis—venous thromboembolism (high-risk surgery)	2.0–2.5	1.3–1.4
Prophylaxis—venous thromboembolism (hip surgery)	2.3–3.0	1.3–1.5
Treatment of deep vein thrombosis or pulmonary embolism	2.0–3.0	1.3–1.5
To prevent systemic embolization in patients with atrial fibrillation, valvular heart disease, tissue heart valves, or acute myocardial infarction	2.0–3.0	1.3–1.5
Mechanical prosthetic heart valves, recurrent systemic embolism	3.0–4.5	1.5–2.0

*Using relatively insensitive rabbit brain thromboplastin in common use.

and its protein binding and transport, and subsequent metabolism and excretion, are modified by drugs and disease (see later). Moreover, warfarin pharmacodynamics are altered by a variety of factors, including disease and vitamin K intake, absorption, and metabolism (see later). Therefore, the anticoagulant effect of warfarin may vary greatly among patients and temporally within individual patients.

Monitoring

Optimal anticoagulant control is achieved when the antithrombotic effect is maximized while the risk of bleeding is minimized. Since this goal may be difficult to achieve or maintain because of the marked inter- and intraindividual variability in warfarin anticoagulant effect, frequent monitoring of warfarin action is essential for optimal anticoagulant control.

Oral anticoagulant therapy is usually monitored by the one-stage prothrombin time (PT) or less commonly by the thrombotest. Conventional teaching states that anticoagulation is adequate if the PT is increased to 1.5 to 2.5 times normal. This rule is misleading, however, and may result in over-anticoagulation. In recent years it has become clear that there is marked variation in the responsiveness of the PT to reduction in the vitamin K–dependent coagulation factors, depending on which commercially available thromboplastin reagent is used in the PT assay.[7, 17] In other words, some thromboplastins are much more sensitive than others to warfarin action and produce a much larger change in the PT for the same degree of anticoagulation. A more sensitive thromboplastin may allow finer titration of anticoagulant effect. However, the therapeutic PT ratio must be individualized for each commercial reagent. Standardization of PT results would eliminate this confusion. The international normalized ratio (INR) has been introduced to standardize the PT ratio by normalizing the test ratio with a correction factor that compares the relative sensitivity of the commercial thromboplastin used to that of the WHO Primary International Reference Thromboplastin (IRP). The INR is the PT ratio that would be observed if the thromboplastin used were the IRP instead of the commercial reagent actually used.[17] The use of the INR, therefore, allows the same therapeutic anticoagulation guidelines to be applied to PT results derived using thromboplastins of varying sensitivity. Recommended therapeutic ranges of INR and PT ratio are listed in Table 14–6.

The implications of the foregoing discussion for emergency management are obvious. In the absence of an INR result, the PT ratio can be interpreted only if the therapeutic range for the specific thromboplastin used is known. For example, a PT of 28s implies over-anticoagulation if an insensitive thromboplastin is used, but it is in the therapeutic range if a sensitive thromboplastin is used. Conversely, a PT of 17s is in the therapeutic range if an insensitive reagent is used but is subtherapeutic if a sensitive reagent is used. Such confusion is especially likely to arise if all laboratories in one area do not use the same thromboplastin, or if a commonly used laboratory switches to a new thromboplastin of different sensitivity.

Interactions of Oral Anticoagulants with Drugs and Comorbid Conditions

Optimal anticoagulant control may be complicated by numerous anticoagulant interactions. As mentioned previously, both the pharmacokinetics and pharmacodynamics of warfarin action may be altered by a large variety of drugs and comorbid factors. Consequently, alteration of anticoagulant control should be anticipated in patients receiving oral anticoagulants who undergo medication changes or changes in clinical status. Conversely, sudden loss of anticoagulant control or bleeding in a previously stable patient should stimulate the search for drug or comorbid factor interactions.

Drugs are thought to interact with oral anticoagulants and/or increase the risk of hemorrhage by altering one or more of the following:

- drug absorption
- protein binding
- receptor site affinity
- metabolism and excretion
- additional parameters of the hemostatic mechanism[15]

Potential interactions of oral anticoagulants with drugs are listed in Table 14–7 and with comorbid conditions in Table 14–8.

A few points deserve special mention. Choice of an analgesic may be problematic in patients receiving oral anticoagulants. Aspirin not only potentiates the warfarin effect but also has marked antiplatelet action, the combination of which may predispose to bleeding. Similarly, numerous nonsteroidal anti-inflammatory drugs—most notably phenylbutazone and congeners—have also been reported to potentiate warfarin action and also have antiplatelet action. Although some caution against acetaminophen in this setting,[24] this drug is probably the safest analgesic in patients receiving oral anticoagulants.[19, 15]

Table 14–7. INTERACTIONS OF ORAL ANTICOAGULANTS WITH DRUGS[2, 14, 15, 18, 19]

INCREASED PROTHROMBIN TIME	
Common	***Also Reported***
anabolic steroids	acetaminophen
acetylsalicylic acid	allopurinol
cimetidine	amiodarone
clofibrate	azapropazone
disulfiram	cephalosporins (third-generation)
glucagon	chloral hydrate
heparin	chloramphenicol
metronidazole	chlorpropamide
phenylbutazone (and congeners)	diazoxide
sulfinpyrazone	diflunisal
trimethoprim-sulfamethoxazole	ethacrynic acid
	indomethacin
	MAO inhibitors
	mefenamic acid
	methyldopa
	methylphenidate
	nalidixic acid
	nortryptiline
	phenyramidol
	phenytoin
	PTU
	quinidine/quinine
	sulfonamides (and other antibiotics, with vitamin K deficiency)
	sulindac
	thyroxine
DECREASED PROTHROMBIN TIME	
Common	***Also Reported***
barbiturates	allopurinol
cholestyramine	carbamazepine
contraceptive steroids	griseofulvin
diuretics	haloperidol
ethchlorvynol	paraldehyde
glutethimide	6-mercaptopurine
rifampin	
vitamin K	

Complications

Nonhematologic complications of warfarin include hypersensitivity reactions, skin necrosis,[111] alopecia, and purple toes.[112] The main hematologic complication of warfarin is hemorrhage.

Hemorrhagic Complications

Incidence

The rate of hemorrhage and the clinical and laboratory risk factors predisposing to bleeding have been addressed by several studies.[15, 25–28] Results of a recent review of hemorrhage in 22 published reports of long-term oral anticoagulation[28] are listed in Table 14–9.

Predisposing Factors

Overall, the bleeding rate of oral anticoagulant therapy is influenced by several factors:

- the intensity of anticoagulation, either intentional or inadvertent;[29–31]
- the underlying clinical disorder for which anticoagulant therapy is used [with bleeding occurring most frequently in ischemic cerebrovascular disease and venous thromboembolism[28] (Table 14–9)];
- age, with bleeding occurring more commonly in the elderly;[15, 25]
- the presence of adverse drug interactions

Table 14–8. INTERACTIONS OF ORAL ANTICOAGULANTS WITH COMORBID CONDITIONS[2, 14, 15, 20–23]

INCREASED PROTHROMBIN TIME
- Hepatic disease, acute and chronic
- Hypermetabolic states—hyperthyroidism
  —fever
- Congestive heart failure
- Old age
- Vitamin K deficiency
  - decreased intake
  - TPN
  - biliary obstruction
  - malabsorption
  - liver disease
  - drug-related:
    - broad spectrum antibiotics plus decreased vitamin K intake
    - third-generation cephalosporins
    - megadoses of vitamins A and E

DECREASED PROTHROMBIN TIME
- Hereditary resistance
- Hypometabolic states
- Nephrotic syndrome
- Hypoalbuminemia
- Pregnancy

or comorbid factors such as clinical states potentiating warfarin action (see earlier), pre-existing hemorrhagic diathesis, malignancy,[28] recent surgery,[28] trauma,[3] or pre-existing potential bleeding sites (e.g., surgical wound, peptic ulcer, recent cerebral hemorrhage, carcinoma of colon);[15]
- the simultaneous use of aspirin (but not of dipyridamole);[28]
- patient reliability (e.g., increased bleeding in alcoholics not due to ethanol-warfarin drug interaction but rather to unreliability of drug intake).

Sites of Hemorrhage

Most commonly, oral anticoagulant-induced bleeding is minor and consists of bruising, hematuria, epistaxis, conjunctival hemorrhage, minor gastrointestinal bleeding,[15] bleeding from wounds and sites of trauma, and vaginal bleeding.[25] More serious major or fatal bleeding is most commonly gastrointestinal, intracranial,[15] vaginal, retroperitoneal, or related to a wound or site of trauma,[25] although a large variety of other sites of bleeding have been reported (Table 14–10). Intracranial bleeding occurs most frequently in patients receiving oral anticoagulants for cerebrovascular disease[28] and most commonly presents as a subdural hematoma,[32] often unassociated with head trauma. Fatal gastrointestinal bleeding is most commonly from a peptic ulcer,[15] although any gastrointestinal lesion may be a potential source of major bleeding. Overall, a bleeding lesion can be identified in about two thirds of cases of oral anticoagulant-related hemorrhage.

Bleeding after warfarin overdose is similar to that seen with anticoagulant therapy: ecchymoses, hematuria, uterine/vaginal bleeding, gastrointestinal bleeding, epistaxis, spontaneous hematomas, gingival bleeding, hemoptysis, and hematemesis occur in order of decreasing frequency following warfarin overdose.[1]

In the emergency setting, bleeding (often serious) may also occur in the anticoagulated patient as a result of phlebotomy, establishment of central venous access, arterial puncture, urinary catheterization, endotracheal intubation, intramuscular injection, and so on. Bleeding of this sort is almost always potentially avoidable.

Management of Excessive Anticoagulation and Bleeding in Patients on Oral Anticoagulants and After Anticoagulant Overdose

Several clinical situations should be considered. In all cases, possible drug interactions and a bleeding site should be sought.

Elevated PT, Bleeding Absent

If a patient is found on follow-up to have

Table 14–9. INCIDENCE OF HEMORRHAGE DURING LONG-TERM ORAL ANTICOAGULANT THERAPY[28]

INDICATION FOR ANTICOAGULATION	NUMBER OF PATIENTS	BLEEDING (%)			
		Total	*Minor†*	*Major**	*Fatal*
Ischemic cerebrovascular disease	588	28.7	21.8	7.0	4.8
Prosthetic heart valves	405	5.7	3.2	2.5	1.7
Atrial fibrillation	302	15.2	14.2	0.01	0.3
Ischemic heart disease	1890	19.1	10.5	4.7	1.0
Venous thromboembolism	159	22.6	14.5	8.2	0.8

*Intracranial, retroperitoneal, fatal, or resulting in hospitalization or transfusion.
†Other gastrointestinal bleeding, epistaxis, hematuria, ecchymosis, hemoptysis.

Table 14–10. LESS COMMON SITES OF HEMORRHAGE IN PATIENTS ON ORAL ANTICOAGULANTS

RESPIRATORY	larynx, oropharynx[33]
	interstitial pulmonary hemorrhage[15]
	hemothorax[34]
CARDIAC	hemopericardium[35, 36]
NEUROLOGIC	intracerebral[28, 32, 43]
	subarachnoid[37]
	spinal—epidural[38]
	—subdural[39]
	nerve palsies and compartment syndromes
	—femoral nerve[40]
	—carpal tunnel[41, 42]
	—lower limb palsies[44]
ENDOCRINE	adrenal[45]
	ovarian[46]
SKIN AND SOFT TISSUE	hemorrhagic skin infarction[47]
MUSCULOSKELETAL	rectus abdominis[48]
	hemarthrosis[49]
	compartment syndrome[42]
	iliacus syndrome[50]
INTRA-ABDOMINAL	hemorrhagic pancreatitis[51]
	intramural bowel hematoma[52, 53]
	intraperitoneal[43]
RETROPERITONEAL[25]	spontaneous renal rupture[54]

a PT slightly outside the therapeutic range but is not bleeding and has been taking the oral anticoagulant as directed, the drug should be omitted for 24 to 48 hours. The patient should be followed closely, and the PT should be repeated serially. Additionally, the patient should be questioned about any changes in medication that might have resulted in loss of control.

If the PT is grossly prolonged and the patient is not bleeding, a small dose of vitamin K_1 (2 to 2.5 mg) may be given orally or subcutaneously in addition to stopping the anticoagulant, checking for drug interactions, and repeating the PT serially. This will ensure rapid correction of the abnormal PT but will not make the patient refractory to subsequent re-anticoagulation, which would result if a larger dose of vitamin K_1 were given.

PT Therapeutic, Bleeding Present

If bleeding occurs when the PT is in the therapeutic range, an underlying source or cause of bleeding should be sought. Contributing medications should be considered. If bleeding in this situation is severe, anticoagulation should be reversed (see later) while the cause of bleeding is identified.

Elevated PT, Bleeding Present (or Serious Trauma or Imminent Surgery)

If bleeding occurs and the PT is excessively prolonged, the oral anticoagulant should be stopped. If bleeding is minor, vitamin K_1 in a dose of 10 mg can be administered intravenously. This will alter the PT within 4 to 6 hours and will likely correct the PT within 12 to 24 hours. A dose of more than 25 mg will make the patient refractory to further anticoagulation for a few days.

If bleeding is potentially life threatening, the coagulation defect should be fully reversed more rapidly; in addition to stopping the anticoagulant and administering vitamin K_1 in a dose of 10 mg intravenously, vitamin K–dependent coagulation factors should be replaced quickly. This can usually be achieved by administering 4 to 6 units (1000 to 1500 ml) of stored plasma (SP) or, if this is not available, fresh frozen plasma (FFP). In the absence of significant blood loss, such a large volume may be a problem in patients with poor cardiac status or renal failure and may necessitate monitoring of central pressures. Alternatively, and if hemorrhage is immediately life threatening (e.g., massive intracranial hemorrhage), the vitamin K–dependent factors can be replaced more quickly with prothrombin complex/factor IX concentrate. Most hemorrhagic episodes caused by warfarin can be managed without the use of concentrates, and their use should be minimized because they are associated with hepatitis,[57] HIV infection,[58] thromboembolism,[59] and myocardial infarction.[60] Coumarin anticoagulation cannot be reversed with cryoprecipitate.

Anticoagulated patients requiring imminent surgery or involved in serious trauma should be rapidly reversed as outlined earlier.

Oral Anticoagulant Overdose

Anticoagulation and bleeding associated with warfarin overdose are managed as just outlined, with a few variations. In the acute overdose, emesis should be induced with ipecac in the unanticoagulated patient. However, patients who present already anticoagulated should rather undergo gastric lavage with a large orogastric tube.[61] Acute management with vitamin K_1 (10 mg intravenously) and plasma is identical to that outlined previously. However, if large amounts of warfarin have been consumed, a single injection of vitamin K_1 will be inadequate. Because the half-life of vitamin K_1 after intravenous injection is only 1.7 hours[62] whereas the half-life of warfarin is 35 hours, and the minimum effective plasma concentration of vitamin K_1 required to drive coagulation factor synthesis varies with the degree of warfarin poisoning,[62–64] vitamin K_1 should be repeated (10 mg IV) every 4 to 6 hours until the PT is stable in the normal range.

Vitamin K Preparations

Several other points should be considered. To reverse warfarin, vitamin K should be given only in the K_1 form (phylloquinone, phytonedione, Aquamephyton, Mephyton). Vitamin K_3 (menaquinone-0, menadione, Synkayvite, Hykinone) is ineffective in reversing coumarin anticoagulants and should not be used for this purpose.[65, 66] To reverse coumarin urgently, vitamin K_1 should be given intravenously. However, if given quickly, vitamin K_1 may cause cardiovascular collapse and even death.[67–70] Therefore, it should be diluted in 0.9 per cent NaCl or 5 per cent dextrose in water and be given slowly at a rate of 0.5 mg/min.[67]

Precautions in the Anticoagulated Patient

In the emergency setting, care must be taken to avoid inducing bleeding in the anticoagulated patient. Antiplatelet agents and other interacting drugs should be avoided, as should intramuscular injections. Arterial puncture should be performed only in a location that can be compressed easily to minimize bleeding (e.g., radial artery preferable to femoral artery). Similarly, to minimize bleeding, central venous access is more safely established via an internal jugular approach than by the subclavian route.

ANTICOAGULANT RODENTICIDES

Warfarin has been used for more than 40 years as a chronic-acting rodenticide. The subsequent development of warfarin resistance by rodents,[71] however, has prompted the development of new coumarin and indanedione derivatives with greater anticoagulant activity even in the presence of warfarin resistance.[72] Rodenticide 4-hydroxy-coumarin derivatives include difenacoum, bromodiolone, and brodifacoum. Indanedione derivatives include diphacinone, pindone, and chlorphacinone. Collectively, both groups are termed "superwarfarins."

Numerous commercially available rodenticides contain one of these superwarfarins in concentrations ranging from 0.005 to 2 per cent.[61] However, some rodenticides contain acute-acting poisons such as strychnine or arsenic. Therefore, it is extremely important to verify the content of the rodenticides consumed when first assessing a poisoned patient.

Anticoagulant rodenticides have the same mechanism of action as do the oral anticoagulants used clinically in humans (see earlier). However, important pharmacokinetic and pharmacodynamic differences exist between these rodenticides and their human counterparts: Superwarfarins are more lipophilic and have a greater volume of distribution and longer half-life. For example, in rats, brodifacoum has a half-life of 156 hours and a volume of distribution of 1.0 L/kg.[78] The equivalent values for warfarin are 37 hours and 0.1 L/kg, respectively. In dogs, brodifacoum is reported to have a half-life of approximately 120 days.[73] Additionally, the chemical potency of superwarfarins is felt to be increased as a result of binding to lipophilic liver sites. In rats, brodifacoum levels in the liver are 20 times greater than in the serum.[74] Moreover, on a molar basis, difenacoum and brodifacoum have roughly a 100-fold greater effect on gamma-carboxylation of glutamic acid residues than does warfarin.[73]

Bleeding complications of rodenticide poisoning are identical to those described for warfarin[1] (see earlier). It is not surprising, however, that superwarfarin poisoning is characterized by very prolonged and refractory anticoagulation. In published cases, despite daily (or up to four times daily) vitamin K_1 administration, the time required for the

PT to stabilize in the normal range without further vitamin K_1 being required was 51 days for brodifacoum,[73] 42 days for difenacoum,[75] over 2 months for bromodiolone,[76] and over 45 days for chlorphacinone,[77] in the absence of further ingestion.

Ingestion of small amounts of superwarfarin (e.g., 25 gm of 0.005 per cent concentration) likely requires no treatment. However, if ingestion is of a concentration exceeding 0.005 per cent or of an amount exceeding 25 gm of a 0.005 per cent concentration acutely, or a lesser amount consumed chronically over several days, treatment will be necessary.[61] The chemical composition of the rodenticides should be verified. In acute poisoning the stomach should be emptied by induced emesis (in the unanticoagulated patient) or by gastric lavage (in the anticoagulated patient). Vitamin K_1 (10 mg IV) should be given and repeated every 6 hours intravenously until the PT is within or close to the normal range. Oral vitamin K_1 may then be substituted and should be continued until the PT remains normal after vitamin K_1 is withdrawn (likely longer than 1.5 months). The replacement of vitamin K–dependent coagulation factors with plasma or plasma fractions should be as outlined for warfarin earlier. Phenobarbital (100 to 200 mg daily) has been used in this setting in an attempt to enhance metabolism of coumarin anticoagulants by inducing hepatic microsomal enzymes.[74] However, this is unproved therapy at present.

HEPARIN

Heparin is a naturally occurring, highly sulfated glycosaminoglycan of varying molecular weight, consisting of chains of alternating sulfated and nonsulfated uronic acid and glucosamine residues linked to a protein backbone.[79] Heparin is distributed widely throughout the animal kingdom, and in mammals is found in a variety of tissues. Commercial heparin is usually prepared from bovine or porcine lung or intestinal mucosa.

Indications for Use

Heparin may be used prophylactically in low doses for the prevention of venous thrombosis and pulmonary embolism in certain surgical patients at risk and in hospitalized patients, such as those who are immobilized, are convalescing from myocardial infarction, or have congestive heart failure. Low dose heparin also may be used to maintain patency of venous and arterial catheters. Heparin also may be used in larger doses to prevent further thrombosis and embolism (both venous and arterial) in patients with established thrombosis, acute myocardial infarction, stroke-in-evolution, and atrial fibrillation with embolization, and to prevent clotting during cardiac bypass, ECMO, hemodialysis, and plasmapheresis. Heparin also may be used in certain types of disseminated intravascular coagulation. Finally, heparin may be used as a warfarin replacement during pregnancy.

Contraindications

Contraindications to heparin include preexisting abnormalities of coagulation (e.g., hemophilia), thrombocytopenia, previous severe heparin-induced thrombocytopenia with or without thrombosis, known hypersensitivity to heparin, surgery of the brain, eye, and spinal cord (including lumbar puncture), peptic ulcer disease, severe hypertension, threatened abortion, and bacterial endocarditis.

Mechanism of Action

Heparin inhibits coagulation by several mechanisms. At therapeutic concentrations, its main action is to enhance markedly the effect of antithrombin III in the inhibition of the activated clotting factors IXa, Xa, XIa, XIIa, and thrombin.[7] At higher heparin concentrations, an additional effect is the acceleration of inhibition of thrombin by heparin cofactor II.[7] Additionally, heparin also may inhibit the activation of thrombin by factor Xa via a mechanism independent of antithrombin III or heparin cofactor II.[80] Finally, heparin also may have an effect on platelets, either by causing thrombocytopenia (see later)[81] or by inhibiting platelet function.[82]

Monitoring

Tests used to monitor heparin therapy include several global tests of blood coagulation of which the activated partial thromboplastin time (APTT) is most commonly employed. Specific heparin levels also can be measured. Low-dose heparin therapy usually requires no monitoring. For full heparinization, however, the APTT should be adjusted to 1.5 to 2 times control (or the patient's pretreatment APTT).[7] If the heparin level is used, it should be maintained between 0.3 and 0.5 U/ml.[7]

Pharmacology

Heparin has a half-life of 1 to 1.5 hours and a volume of distribution of 0.06 L/kg in humans. However, the elimination half-life varies with the dose administered[83] and is prolonged in hepatic[84] and renal[85] disease. Heparin has high affinity for binding proteins and significant electronegativity.[86] It is primarily (90 per cent) metabolized in the liver. Less than 10 per cent is recovered unchanged in the urine.[86]

Complications

Nonhematologic complications of heparin include osteoporosis,[87] hypersensitivity reactions, hyperkalemia secondary to aldosterone suppression, and, more rarely, alopecia, priapism, and rebound hyperlipidemia following heparin discontinuation.

Hematologic complications include hemorrhage and thrombocytopenia (see later). The former may be aggravated by the latter. Rarely, heparin-induced thrombocytopenia is associated with arterial thrombosis.

Hemorrhagic Complications

Bleeding is the most important complication of heparin therapy. It occurs much more frequently when heparin is given in large doses therapeutically than when low-dose heparin is used prophylactically. Heparin-associated hemorrhage is likely related to its anticoagulant effect. However, bleeding may also be related in part to heparin-induced platelet dysfunction or thrombocytopenia[7] (see later).

Incidence

Reported rates of major bleeding (see definition, Table 14–9) with therapeutic (high-dose) heparin are quite variable: intermittent intravenous injection, 9 to 33 per cent; continuous intravenous infusion, 0 to 15 per cent; subcutaneous injection, 3 to 4 per cent.[28] Low-dose prophylactic subcutaneous heparin usually results in bleeding in less than 2 per cent of cases.[88]

Risk Factors for Hemorrhage

1. Intensity of anticoagulation or heparin dose. Although there is a suggestion that bleeding is more likely to occur when anticoagulation is prolonged excessively, as measured by an in vitro test, this relationship is not proved for either intermittent injection or continuous infusion.[7, 28] However, there may be a relationship between the dose of heparin used per 24 hours and the rate of bleeding.[7]
2. Age.[90]
3. Female sex (especially elderly women).[89]
4. Comorbid factors:[28]
   - recent surgery (especially within 14 days)
   - intramuscular injections
   - trauma
   - defective hemostasis prior to heparin
   - uremia
   - associated platelet function defects
   - occult bleeding lesion
   - thrombocytopenia
   - ? alcoholism[86]
5. Aspirin therapy (in therapeutic heparin). In low-dose heparin prophylaxis, addition of aspirin probably does not increase risk of bleeding. Vigilance is necessary, however.[28]

Management of Hemorrhage Due to Heparin Therapy

Excessive anticoagulation with heparin in the absence of bleeding can be easily managed by stopping the drug for one or more half-lives and then restarting it at a lower dose.

If serious bleeding occurs, the anticoagulation effect of heparin should be reversed with protamine sulfate, a strongly basic drug that combines with heparin and neutralizes it. One milligram of protamine neutralizes 100 units of heparin. The amount of protamine required depends on the time elapsed since the heparin injection, because the half-life of heparin is 60 to 90 minutes. Therefore, within minutes of a heparin injection, a full neutralizing dose should be given. For every 60 minutes elapsed from the time of the heparin injection, the protamine dose should be halved. Protamine should be given slowly intravenously over 10 minutes, since rapid infusion may cause hypotension. Since the half-life of protamine is shorter than that of heparin, a patient initially fully reversed with protamine may subsequently become re-anticoagulated (heparin rebound phenomenon) and may require additional protamine.

Factors predisposing to hemorrhage should be sought. Intramuscular injections and potentially dangerous invasive procedures, such as obtaining central venous access or arterial puncture, should be avoided if possible. If unavoidable, such procedures should be performed in locations that are easily compressed to minimize bleeding (e.g., radial artery favored over femoral artery; internal jugular approach favored over subclavian approach). Heparin anticoagulation cannot be reversed by the infusion of plasma or plasma fractions.

Heparin-Induced Thrombocytopenia

Heparin/platelet interactions are either common or idiosyncratic. Common interactions include a minor fall in platelet count following intravenous heparin injection,[91] which may be artifactual and is of no clinical significance, and an inhibition of platelet function, which varies with the molecular weight of the heparin used,[7, 92] prolongs the bleeding time,[82] and may contribute to heparin-related bleeding.[7] In contrast, heparin-induced thrombocytopenia is an immune-mediated idiosyncratic reaction. The frequency of this entity is apparently decreasing. Pooled series suggest a frequency of 15.6 per cent for bovine heparin and 5.8 per cent for porcine heparin.[81] More recently, however, a frequency of approximately 1 per cent is cited.[93] Thrombocytopenia typically appears 5 to 10 days after the start of heparin therapy and may occur sooner if the patient is subsequently rechallenged with heparin. At the time of thrombocytopenia, heparin-dependent platelet antibodies are present in the serum.[93] Heparin-induced thrombocytopenia on its own is of minor clinical significance as it rarely leads to bleeding, even though the platelet count may drop below 20 $\times 10^9$/L.[93] However, a small subset of patients with heparin-induced thrombocytopenia (less than 1 per cent of patients receiving heparin) will develop arterial thrombosis that may lead to death or major morbidity.[81] This serious complication may be related to heparin-dependent immune-mediated endothelial damage.[93] Heparin-induced thrombocytopenia should be recognized and managed early, to avoid devastating thrombotic consequences.

Management may be difficult. Heparin should be discontinued in patients who develop severe thrombocytopenia or who develop thrombocytopenia with acute thrombosis. If oral anticoagulation has already been started, it should be continued. However, patients with documented pulmonary embolism or who are at high risk of embolism (e.g., acute proximal vein thrombosis), in whom oral anticoagulation has not been started, require alternative therapy such as anticoagulation with ancrod or caval interruption.[81] In moderate thrombocytopenia, oral anticoagulation should be started and heparin should be continued cautiously for the shortest time possible (about 3 days) while the platelet count is monitored carefully.

A patient who has had a previous episode of severe heparin-induced thrombocytopenia with or without thrombosis should probably not be re-exposed to heparin, although thrombocytopenia may not invariably recur following re-exposure.

ANCROD

Ancrod (Arvin, Arwin, Venacil) is a defibrinogenating, thrombin-like enzyme purified from the venom of the Malayan pit viper, *Agkistrodon rhodostoma.* Its use as an antithrombotic agent arose from the observation that the blood of victims bitten by this snake was incoagulable due to marked hypofibrinogenemia, but that this defect did not cause much bleeding.[94, 95] In addition to its anticoagulant action, ancrod also reduces blood viscosity.[96] Batroxopin (Defibrase, Reptilase), a similar enzyme from the venom of *Bothrops atrox,* has been used variously in humans.[97] Crotalase (Defibrizyme) from *Crotalus adamanteus* has not been used in humans. The following discussion is limited to ancrod.

Indications[98, 99]

Ancrod has been used in clinical conditions for which oral anticoagulants or heparin may be indicated and also in conditions in which reduced blood viscosity may be desirable in addition to anticoagulation. Therapeutic uses have included venous and arterial thrombosis, pulmonary embolism, myocardial infarction, peripheral vascular disease, ischemic stroke, prosthetic heart valves, priapism, sickle cell crisis, and renal transplant rejection. Ancrod has also been used prophylactically to prevent thrombosis in patients undergoing hip surgery. Other possible uses include anticoagulation for hemodialysis or cardiac bypass. Ancrod may be most useful in situations in which therapy with conventional anticoagulants is problematic, unsuccessful, or contraindicated (e.g., ongoing thrombosis despite oral anticoagulants and heparin, heparin-induced thrombocytopenia with or without arterial thrombosis, as an outpatient anticoagulant in a TPN patient with no gut, and so on).

Contraindications

Contraindications to ancrod are essentially identical to those noted for heparin. In addition, it has been suggested that ancrod not be used earlier than 72 hours following surgery or extensive soft tissue trauma.[98] Ancrod should not be used in pregnancy.

Mechanism of Action

The anticoagulant action of ancrod occurs via a proteolytic effect on circulating fibrinogen. Unlike thrombin, which produces both fibrinopeptides A and B, ancrod cleaves only the A-fibrinopeptides from fibrinogen and then progressively digests the fibrinogen Aα chain.[100] Ancrod does not activate factor XIII[100] and does not affect factors V, VIII, IX, or X.[101] Since the fibrin produced is not cross-linked (lack of factor XIII action) and contains degraded α-chains, it is susceptible to fibrinolysis.[15] The net result of ancrod action is rapid and profound hypofibrinogenemia with resultant anticoagulation. Defibrinogenation also results in a decrease in blood viscosity.[96]

Monitoring

Ancrod action is monitored by following the fibrinogen level itself, or by using the fibrinogen titer as a guide. A fibrinogen level of 50 mg/dl (0.5 gm/L) or a titer of 1:2 or less is considered satisfactory.[15]

Pharmacology

Ancrod is given intravenously or subcutaneously. Following intravenous injection of radiolabeled ancrod, the extravascular/intravascular distribution ratio is 1.7 and elimination follows a multiexponential function. Initially, the half-life is 3 to 5 hours, but after several days the label disappears with a terminal half-life of 11.5 days.[102] Catabolism may be intravascular, with breakdown products appearing in the urine. In addition, ancrod is inactivated by forming enzyme/antiprotease complexes which are then removed from the circulation by the reticuloendothelial system.[103, 104] Ancrod rapidly produces hypofibrinogenemia. Following ancrod withdrawal, fibrinogen slowly returns to normal in days to weeks.[105] In fever, infection, or malignancy, fibrinogen levels may return to normal much more quickly (acute-phase response).

Following ancrod administration, resistance to defibrinogenation develops in a minority of patients. This is probably due to the development of inactivating antibodies.[106]

Complications

Nonhematologic complications include rare allergic reactions and impaired wound healing, which occurs in animals[107] but is not confirmed in humans.[98] The main hematologic complication is bleeding. Risk factors for hemorrhage are similar to those for heparin-related bleeding (see earlier) (e.g., recent surgery, antiplatelet agents). The incidence of hemorrhage is low, occurring in only 0 to 5 per cent of patients.[97, 108] Moreover, in two studies the rate of bleeding with ancrod was significantly lower than in concomitantly studied patients who received heparin[109] or streptokinase.[110]

Emergency Reversal of Ancrod Anticoagulation

Should serious bleeding occur, or should the ancrod-anticoagulated patient require urgent surgery or be involved in trauma, anticoagulation can be easily reversed. Ancrod should be discontinued. Fibrinogen can be replaced with plasma (e.g., 4 U/1000 ml) or cryoprecipitate. The fibrinogen level assay should be repeated following the replacement. Additionally, in an emergency, circulating ancrod can be quickly neutralized with an antiancrod antivenom (e.g., Arvin Antidote). This preparation may cause anaphylaxis and delayed serum sickness. The manufacturer's instructions regarding test doses should be reviewed, and care should be exercised in its use.

References

1. O'Reilly RA, Aggeler PM: Covert anticoagulant ingestion: Study of 25 patients and review of the world literature. Medicine *55:*389, 1976.
2. O'Reilly RA: Vitamin K and the oral anticoagulant drugs. Annu Rev Med *27:*245, 1976.
3. O'Mara K, Mavichak V: Trauma and oral anticoagulants. Ann Emerg Med *12:*700, 1983.
4. Cade JF, Hunt D, Stubbs KP: Guidelines for the management of oral anticoagulant therapy in patients undergoing surgery. Med J Aust *2:*292, 1979.
5. Orme MLE, Lewis PJ, De Swiet M, Serlin MJ, Sibeon R, Baty JD, Breckenridge AM: May mothers given warfarin breast feed their infants? Br Med J *1:*1564, 1977.
6. De Swiet, Lewis PJ: Excretion of anticoagulants in human milk. N Engl J Med *297:*1471, 1977.
7. Hirsh J: Mechanism of action and monitoring of anticoagulants. Semin Thromb Hemost *12:*1, 1986.
8. Suttie JW: Oral anticoagulant therapy: The biosynthetic basis. Semin Hematol *14:*365, 1977.
9. Stenflo J: A new vitamin K–dependent protein. J Biol Chem *251:*355, 1976.
10. Kisiel W, Caufield WM, Ericsson LH, Davie EW: Anticoagulant properties of bovine plasma protein C following activation by thrombin. Biochemistry *16:*5824, 1977.
11. Di Scipio RG, Davie EW: Characterization of protein S, a γ-carboxyglutamic acid–containing protein from bovine and human plasma. Biochemistry *18:*899, 1979.
12. Walker FJ: Regulation of activated protein C by protein S. J Biol Chem *256:*11128, 1981.
13. Esmon CT, Suttie JW, Jackson CM: The functional significance of vitamin K action. Difference in phospholipid between normal and abnormal prothrombin. J Biol Chem *250:*4095, 1975.
14. Breckenridge AM: Oral anticoagulant drugs: Pharmacokinetic aspects. Semin Hematol *15:*19, 1978.
15. Mackie MJ, Douglas AS: Drug-induced disorders of coagulation. *In* Ratnoff OD, Forbes CD (eds): Disorder of Hemostatis. New York, Grune and Stratton, 1984, pp 485–510.
16. American College of Chest Physicians and the National Heart, Lung, and Blood Institute National Conference on Antithrombotic Therapy. Chest 89 (Suppl):*1S,* 1986.
17. Hirsh J: Is the dose of warfarin prescribed by American physicians unnecessarily high? Arch Intern Med *147:*769, 1987.
18. Williams JRB, Griffin JP, Parkins A: Effect of concomitantly administered drugs on control of long-term anticoagulant therapy. Q J Med *45:*63, 1976.
19. Hansten PD (ed): Oral anticoagulant drug interactions. *In* Clinical Drug Interactions. 4th ed. London, Henry Kimpton, 1979, pp 33–68.
20. Corrigan JJ, Marcus FL: Coagulopathy associated with vitamin E ingestion. JAMA *230:*1300, 1974.
21. Schrogie JJ: Coagulopathy and fat-soluble vitamins. JAMA *232:*19, 1975.
22. Husted S, Anderson F: The influence of age on the response to oral anticoagulants. Br J Clin Pharmacol *4:*559, 1977.
23. Shepherd AMM, Hewick DS, Moreland TA, Stevenson IH: Age as a determinant of sensitivity to warfarin. Br J Clin Pharmacol *4:*315, 1977.
24. Antlitz AM, Mead JA Jr, Tolentino MA: Potentiation of oral anticoagulation by acetaminophen. Curr Ther Res *10:*501, 1968.
25. Coon WW, Willis PW III: Hemorrhagic complications of anticoagulant therapy. Arch Intern Med *133:*386, 1974.
26. Pastor BH, Resnick ME, Rodman T: Serious hemorrhagic complications of anticoagulant therapy. JAMA *180:*747, 1962.
27. Mosley DH, Schatz IJ, Breneman GM: Long-term anticoagulant therapy. Complications and control in a review of 978 cases. JAMA *186:*914, 1963.
28. Levine MN, Hirsh J: Hemorrhagic complications of anticoagulant therapy. Semin Thromb Hemost *12:*39, 1986.
29. Forfar JC: A 7-year analysis of hemorrhage in patients on long-term anticoagulant treatment. Br Heart J *42:*128, 1979.
30. Hull R, Hirsh J, Jay R, Carter C, England C, Gent M, Turpie AGG, McLoughlin D, Dodd P, Thomas M, Raskob G, Ochelford P: Different intensities of oral anticoagulant therapy in the treatment of proximal-venous thrombosis. N Engl J Med *307:*1676, 1982.
31. Moschos CB, Wong PCY, Sise HS: Controlled study of the effective level of long-term anticoagulation. JAMA *190:*799, 1964.
32. Iizuka J: Intracranial and intraspinal hematomas associated with anticoagulant therapy. Neurochirurgia (Stuttg) *15:*15, 1972.
33. Gooder P, Henry R: Impending asphyxia induced by anticoagulant therapy. J Laryngol Otol *94:*347, 1980.
34. Simon HB, Paggett WM, Desanctis RW: Hemothorax as a complication of anticoagulant therapy in the presence of pulmonary infarction. JAMA *208:*1830, 1969.
35. Fell SC, Rubin IL, Enselberg CD, et al: Anticoagulant-induced hemopericardium with tamponade: Its occurrence in the absence of myocardial infarction or pericarditis. N Engl J Med *272:*670, 1965.
36. Aarseth S, Lange HF: The influence of anticoagulant drugs on the occurrence of cardiac rupture and hemopericardium following heart infarction. I. A study of 89 cases of hemopericardium (81 of them cardiac ruptures). Am Heart J *56:*250, 1958.
37. Vinters HV, Barnatt HVM, Kaufmann JCE: Subdural hematoma of the spinal cord and wide-spread subarachnoid hemorrhage complicating anticoagulant therapy. Stroke *11:*459, 1980.

38. Harik SI, Raichle ME, Reis DJ: Spontaneously remitting spinal epidural hematomas in a patient on anticoagulants. N Engl J Med *284*:1355, 1971.
39. Russell N, Maroun FB, Jacob JC: Spinal subdural hematoma in association with anticoagulant therapy. Can Sci Neurol *8*:87, 1981.
40. Spiegel PG, Meltzer JL: Femoral nerve neuropathy secondary to anticoagulation. J Bone Joint Surg *56*:2, 1974.
41. Hartwell SW, Kurtay M: Carpal tunnel compression caused by hematoma associated with anticoagulant therapy. Cleveland Clin Q *33*:127, 1966.
42. Luce EA, Sutrell JW, Wilgis ES, et al: Compression neuropathy following brachial arterial puncture in anticoagulated patients. J Trauma *16*:9, 1976.
43. Silverstein A: Complications of anticoagulation therapy. Arch Intern Med *139*:217, 1979.
44. Lange LS: Lower limb palsies with hypoprothrombinemia. Br Med J *2*:93, 1966.
45. O'Connell TX, Aston SJ: Acute adrenal hemorrhage complicating anticoagulant therapy. Surg Gynecol Obstet *139*:355, 1974.
46. Honore LH: Ovarian hemorrhage. A complication of long-term anticoagulant therapy. West J Med *132*:460, 1980.
47. Everett ED, Overholt EL: Hemorrhagic skin infarction secondary to anticoagulants. Arch Dermatol *100*:588, 1969.
48. Borkovich KH, Stafford ES: Acute anemia and abdominal tumour due to hemorrhage in rectus abdominis sheath following anticoagulant therapy. Arch Intern Med *117*:103, 1966.
49. McLaughlin GE, McCarthy DJ, Segal BL: Hemarthrosis complicating anticoagulant therapy. JAMA *196*:1020, 1966.
50. Fearn CB: Iliacus hematoma syndrome as a complication of anticoagulant therapy. Br Med J *4*:97, 1968.
51. Larsen RR, Sawyer RB, Sawyer KC, et al: Hemorrhagic pancreatitis complicating anticoagulant therapy. NY State J Med *62*:2397, 1962.
52. Herbert DC: Anticoagulant therapy and the acute abdomen. Br J Surg *55*:353, 1968.
53. Sullivan WG, Gordon WC: Intramural intestinal hemorrhage complicating anticoagulant therapy. Am Surg *35*:234, 1969.
54. Luna I, Leadbetter RL, Gilbert DR: Spontaneous rupture of the kidney: A complication of anticoagulation. Report of two cases. J Urol *109*:788, 1973.
55. Zacharski LR, Henderson WG, Rickles FR, et al: Rationale and experimental design for the VA cooperative study of anticoagulants (warfarin) in the treatment of cancer. Cancer *44*:732, 1979.
56. Bowie EJW, Todd M, Thompson JH Jr, et al: Anticoagulant malingerers (the dicoumarol eaters). Am J Med *39*:855, 1965.
57. Hellerstein LJ, Deykin D: Hepatitis after Konyne administration. N Engl J Med *284*:1039, 1971.
58. Evatt BL, Ramsey RB, Lawrence DN, et al: The acquired immunodeficiency syndrome in patients with hemophilia. Ann Intern Med *100*:499, 1984.
59. Blatt PM, Lundblad RL, Kingdon HL, et al: Thrombogenic materials in prothrombin complex concentrates. Ann Intern Med *81*:766, 1974.
60. Fuerth JH, Mahrer P: Myocardial infarction after factor IX therapy. JAMA *245*:1455, 1981.
61. Katona B, Wason S: Anticoagulant rodenticides. Clin Toxicol Rev *8*:12, 1986.
62. Park BK, Scott AK, Wilson AC, Haynes BP, Breckenridge AM: Plasma disposition of vitamin K_1 in relation to anticoagulant poisoning. Br J Clin Pharmacol *18*:655, 1984.
63. Shearer MJ, Barkhan P: Vitamin K_1 and therapy of massive warfarin overdose. Lancet *i*:266, 1979.
64. Bjornsson TD, Blashke TF: Vitamin K_1 disposition and therapy of warfarin overdose. Lancet *ii*:846, 1978.
65. Udall JA: Don't use the wrong vitamin K. West J Med *112*:65, 1970.
66. Douglas AS, Brown A: Effect of vitamin K preparations on hypoprothrombinemia induced by dicumarol and tromexan. Br Med J *1*:412, 1952.
67. Lefrere JJ, Girot R: Acute cardiovascular collapse during intravenous vitamin K_1 injection. Thromb Haemostas *58*:790, 1987.
68. Rich CE, Drage CN: Severe complications of intravenous phytonadione therapy. Two cases with one fatality. Postgrad Med *72*:303, 1982.
69. Barash P, Kitahata LM, Mandel S: Acute cardiovascular collapse after intravenous phytonadione. Anesth Analg *55*:304, 1976.
70. Pelletier G, Attali P, Ink O: Arrest cardiorespiratoire apres injection intraveineuse de vitamine K_1. Gastroenterol Clin Biol *10*:615, 1986.
71. Hermodson MA, Suttie JW, Link KP: Warfarin resistance in the rat. Fed Proc *28*:386, 1969.
72. Hadler MR, Shadbolt RS: Novel 4-hydroxycoumarin anticoagulants active against resistant rats. Nature *253*:275, 1975.
73. Klass EM, Lipton RA: Human ingestion of a "superwarfarin" rodenticide resulting in a prolonged anticoagulant effect. JAMA *252*:3004, 1984.
74. Jones EC, Growe GH, Naiman SC: Prolonged anticoagulation in rat poisoning. JAMA *252*:3005, 1984.
75. Barlow AM, Gay AL, Park BK: Difenacoum (Neosorexa) poisoning. Br Med J *285*:541, 1982.
76. Greeff MC, Mashile O, MacDougall LG: "Superwarfarin" (Bromodiolone) poisoning in two children resulting in prolonged anticoagulation. Lancet *ii*:1269, 1987.
77. Murdoch DA: Prolonged anticoagulation in chlorphacinone poisoning. Lancet *i*:355, 1983.
78. Bachmann KA, Sullivan TJ: Dispositional and pharmacodynamic characteristics of brodifacoum in warfarin sensitive rats. Pharmacology *27*:281, 1983.
79. Yurt RW, Leid RW, Austen KF, Silbert JE: Native heparin from rat peritoneal mast cell. J Biol Chem *253*:6687, 1978.
80. Ofosu FA, Blajchman MA, Hirsh J: The inhibition of heparin of the intrinsic pathway activation of factor X in the absence of antithrombin III. Thromb Res *23*:331, 1981.
81. King DJ, Kelton JG: Heparin-associated thrombocytopenia. Ann Intern Med *100*:535, 1984.
82. Heiden D, Rodvien R, Mielke CH Jr: Heparin bleeding due to qualitative platelet dysfunction. Angiology *30*:645, 1978.
83. Estes JW, Poulin PF: Pharmacokinetics of heparin. Thromb Diathes Haemorrh *33*:26, 1974.
84. Teien AN: Heparin elimination in patients with liver cirrhosis. Thromb Haemostas *38*:701, 1977.
85. Perry PJ, Herron GR, King JC: Heparin half-life in normal and impaired renal function. Clin Pharmacol Ther *16*:514, 1974.
86. Colucci R, Lovejoy FH Jr.: Heparin. Clin Toxicol Rev *8*:7, 1986.
87. Avioli LV: Heparin-induced osteopenia: An appraisal. Adv Exp Med Biol *52*:375, 1975.

88. Hirsh J: Effectiveness of anticoagulants. Semin Thromb Hemostats *12*:21, 1986.
89. Jick H, Slone D, Borda IT, Shapiro S: Efficacy and toxicity of heparin in relation to age and sex. N Engl J Med *279*:284, 1968.
90. Mant MJ, O'Brien BD, Thong KL, Hammond GW, Birtwhistle RV, Grace MG: Haemorrhagic complications of heparin therapy. Lancet *i*:1133, 1977.
91. Davey MG, Lander H: Effect of injected heparin on platelet levels in man. J Clin Pathol *21*:55, 1968.
92. Salzman EW, Deykin D, Shapiro RM: Effect of heparin and heparin fractions on platelet aggregation. J Clin Invest *65*:64, 1980.
93. Cines DB, Tomaski A, Tannenbaum S: Immune endothelial-cell injury in heparin-associated thrombocytopenia. N Engl J Med *316*:581, 1987.
94. Reid HA, Chan KE, Thean PC: Prolonged coagulation defect (defibrination syndrome) in Malayan viper bite. Lancet *i*:621, 1963.
95. Reid HA, Chan KE, Thean PC: Clinical effects of bites by Malayan viper *(Agkistrodon rhodostoma)*. Lancet *i*:617, 1963.
96. Ehrly AM: Influence of Arvin on the flow properties of blood. Biorheology *10*:453, 1973.
97. Latallo ZS: Retrospective study on complications and adverse effects of treatments with thrombin-like enzymes. A multi-centre trial. Thromb Haemostas *50*:604, 1983.
98. Sharp AA: Clinical use of Arvin. Thromb Diath Haemorrh *45*(suppl):69, 1971.
99. Latallo ZS: Report of the task force on clinical use of snake venom enzymes. Thromb Haemostas *39*:768, 1978.
100. Pizzo SV, Schwartz ML, Hill RL, McKee PA: Mechanism of ancrod anticoagulation: A direct proteolytic effect of fibrin. J Clin Invest *51*:2841, 1972.
101. Bell WR, Bolton G, Pitney WR: The effect of Arvin on blood coagulation factors. Br J Haematol *15*:589, 1968.
102. Regoeczi E, Bell WR: *In vivo* behaviour of the coagulant enzyme from *Agkistrodon rhodostoma* venom: Studies using ^{125}I-Arvin. Br J Haematol *16*:573, 1969.
103. Pitney WR, Regoeczi E: Inactivation of Arvin by plasma proteins. Br J Haematol *19*:67, 1970.
104. Ashford A, Bunn DRG: The effect of Arvin on reticuloendothelial activity in rabbits. Br J Pharmacol *40*:37, 1970.
105. Bell WR, Pitney WR, Goodwin JF: The concept of therapeutic defibrination in the treatment of thrombotic disease. Lancet *i*:490, 1968.
106. Sapru RP, Moza AK, Kuman M, Ganguly NK: Antibodies to Arvin following prolonged intravenous therapy. Thromb Res *7*:635, 1975.
107. Holt FJL, Holloway V, Raghupati N, Calnan JS: The effect of a fibrinolytic agent (Arvin) on wound healing and collagen formation. Clin Sci *38*:9P, 1970.
108. Pitney WR: Clinical experience with Arvin. Thromb Diath Haemorrh *38*(suppl):81, 1969.
109. Davies JA, Merrick MV, Sharp AA: Controlled trial of Ancrod and heparin in treatment of deep-vein thrombosis of the lower limb. Lancet *i*:113, 1972.
110. Tibbutt DA, Williams EW, Walker MW: Controlled trial of Ancrod and streptokinase in the treatment of deep vein thrombosis of the lower limb. Br J Haematol *27*:407, 1974.
111. McGehee WG, Kotz TA, Epstein DJ, Rapaport SI: Coumarin necrosis associated with hereditary protein C deficiency. Ann Intern Med *100*:59, 1984.
112. Feder W, Anerback R: Purple toes, an uncommon sequela of oral coumarin therapy. Ann Intern Med *55*:911, 1961.

CHAPTER 15
IMMUNOLOGIC CONSEQUENCES OF POISONING

John B. Sullivan, Jr., M.D.

Immunotoxicology is the study of alterations of the immune system by xenobiotics: drugs, biologicals, and chemicals. Clinically, immunotoxic manifestations may be indicated by infections, autoimmunity, allergy, hypersensitivity reactions, and, in some cases, cancer. Autoimmune responses and hypersensitivity reactions to drugs and chemicals are the most widely recognized types of immune alterations. Clinical manifestations may range from dermatitis, fever, hepatitis, glomerulonephritis, and arthralgias to hemolytic anemia, thrombocytopenia, neutropenia, and anaphylaxis. A variety of organ systems are targets for immunotoxins, particularly the blood-forming elements, liver, kidneys, skin, heart, and muscle tissue.

The discipline of immunotoxicology is concerned with three broad areas:

1. The effects of drugs and chemicals on the

immune system and the resulting disease or enhancement of immune functions,

2. The utilization of immunoassays for detection of and quantifying drugs,
3. The use of antibodies and antibody fragments as therapeutic agents to reverse the effects of drugs or toxins.

The complex activity of the immune system with its various components provides multiple targets for disruption by immunotoxicants (Fig. 15–1). Alterations in the immune system may become clinically evident or, as in some cases, may be subclinical or not evident at all. The fact that chemicals produce immune dysfunction is historically recognized.[1] Benzene exposure has been identified as a cause of aplastic anemia since the 19th century.[2] Benzene is also a known cause of bone marrow depression and is strongly associated with acute myelogenous leukemia as well as other forms of cancer.[2] Chronic arsenic exposure is associated with leukemia and respiratory and skin cancer.[3, 4] Procainamide-induced systemic lupus syndrome and drugs of abuse–related impairment of host resistance to infection are other well-known examples of immune alterations. In addition to drugs, many environmental contaminants have been demonstrated to depress function of cell- and humoral-mediated immunity. An accidental exposure in 1973 of Michigan residents to farm products contaminated with polybrominated biphenyls (PBBs) produced early insight into clinical as well as laboratory immunotoxicity.[1]

Immunotoxicity has been blamed for a variety of environmental diseases; multiple chemical sensitivities (MCS) has received particularly strong attention.[5] The syndrome of MCS has been alluded to as the environmental disease of the 1980s. MCS is a syndrome said to be caused by low-level exposure to environmental chemical contaminants in the home or workplace that results in immune

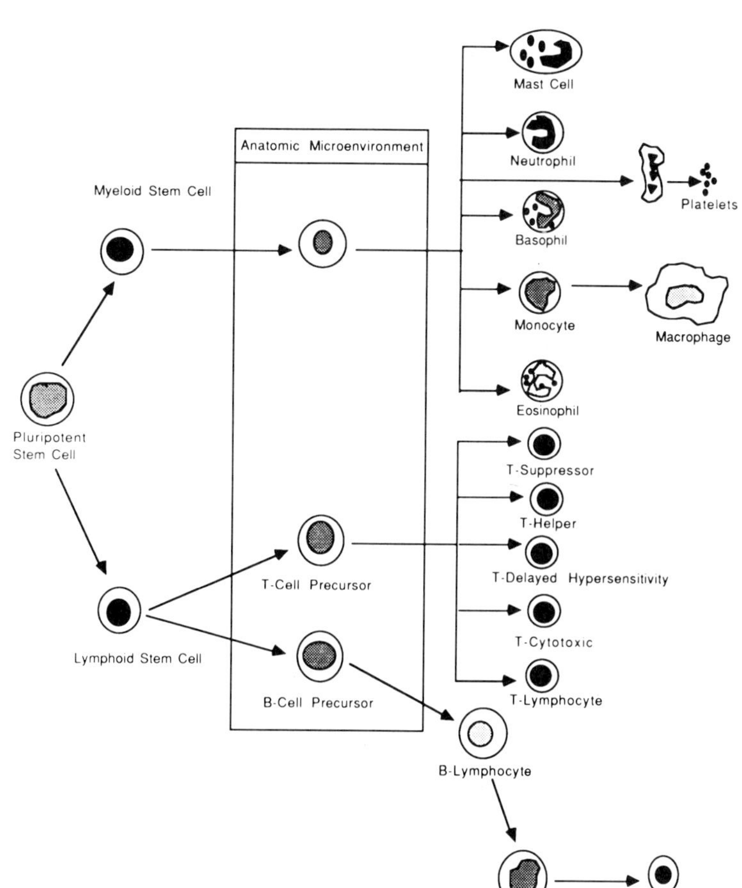

Figure 15–1. The immune system.

Table 15–1. CLINICAL IMMUNOTOXIC SYNDROMES

Dermatitis
Asthma
Pneumonitis
Pyoderma
Anaphylaxis
Viral infections
Neoplasms
Hepatitis
Lupus syndromes
Delayed hypersensitivity reactions
Serum sickness
Bacterial pneumonias
Hemolytic anemias
Aplastic anemia
Thrombocytopenia
Bone marrow suppression

system alteration.[5] Presently there is little scientific evidence to support immune alteration as a cause of this syndrome in the majority of people.[6] However, the eventual effects of exposures to pesticides, formaldehyde, and other low-level pollutants in the work and home environment remain to be established. It has now been demonstrated that human IgG, IgM, and IgE antibodies are formed in vivo to the formaldehyde–human serum albumin conjugate in some patients who became symptomatic following chronic exposure to low concentrations of formaldehyde vapors.[7]

Animal studies, in addition to limited human studies, have demonstrated that immune system alteration can occur following exposure from a wide variety of environmental chemicals and from many commonly used drugs. The list of immunotoxic disease states is impressive (Table 15–1). Resulting health effects and clinical spectrum of disease depends on the route of exposure, duration of exposure, dose, and host factors (Fig. 15–2). Diagnosing immunologic disorders requires the use of standard clinical immunologic tests and components as well as more unusual tests requiring specialized laboratories to examine both the humoral- and cell-mediated immune functions. Host resistance to disease is the ultimate test of an intact immune system.

THE NORMAL IMMUNE SYSTEM

The normal immune system is a complex defensive network consisting of the following functions:[8]

1. Encounter between antigen and lymphocyte
2. Recognition of the antigen by the immune system
3. Lymphocyte activation
4. Amplification of immune response
5. Discrimination: self versus nonself
6. Regulation and control over the immune response

Antigen Encounter and Lymphocyte Function

A heterogeneous group of cells, including monocytes, macrophages, and cells in lymph nodes, spleen, liver, and virtually every other tissue, capture and break down invading microorganisms and foreign material into smaller antigenic fragments.[8] These antigens are taken up onto the surfaces of these cells where they encounter circulating lymphocytes. An antigen is a unique and foreign molecule that elicits the immune response. Typically, antigens are high-molecular-weight proteins. Another important aspect of the normally functioning immune system is memory, or anamnestic response. A normal immune system will recognize an antigen to which it has previously been exposed and will produce a secondary response by T cells, B cells, and macrophages. The immune system has two main divisions: humoral-mediated and cellular-mediated. Humoral immunity arises from the production of antibody by the plasma cells, or B lymphocytes. Cellular immunity arises from T cell lymphocytes, macrophages, and natural killer (NK) cells. The immune system originates from developing lymphoid tissue in embryogenesis. Pluripotent stem cells in bone marrow give rise to three specific cell lines[8–10] (see Fig. 15–1): (1) thymus-dependent cells, or T cells, (2) bursa-dependent cells, or B cells, and (3) macrophages. The stem cell gives rise to progenitor cell lines prior to specialization into three distinctive cell populations. Stem cells are induced to differentiate by specific anatomic microenvironments. These hematopoietic-inducing environments stimulate arriving stem cells to differentiate. Stem cells arriving in the thymus are acted upon by humoral factors (thymosin) to develop into T cells. The main functions of T lymphocytes are to assist B cells to form antibody, to recognize and kill viral infected cells, to ac-

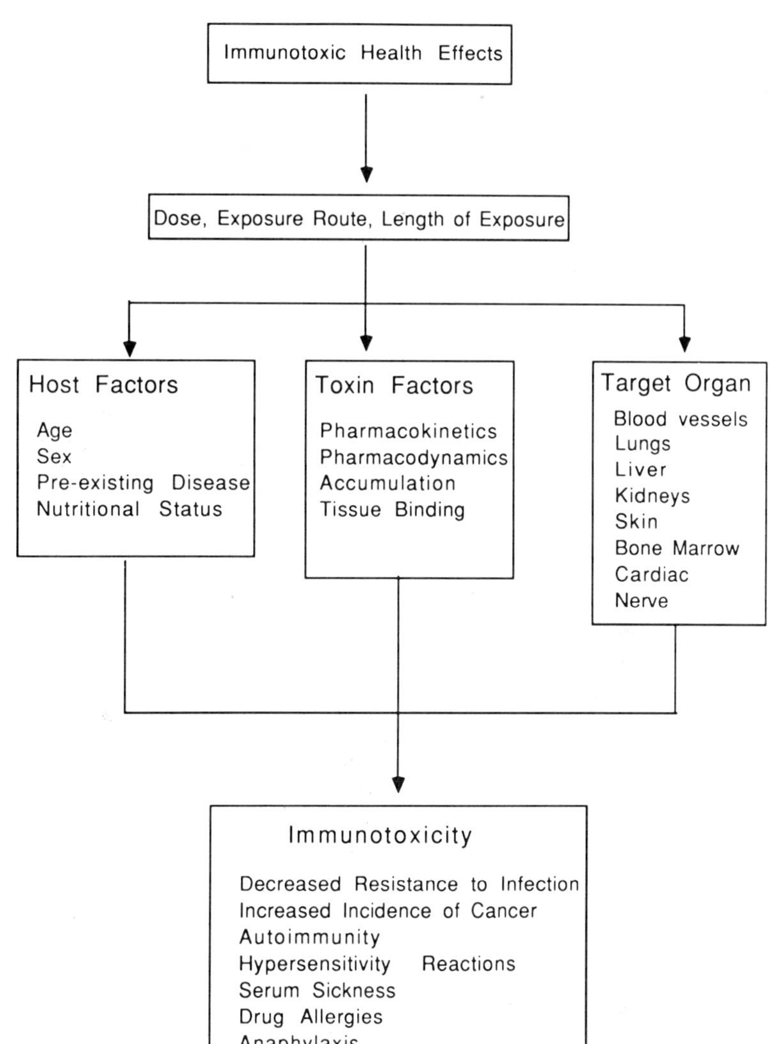

Figure 15–2. Immunotoxic disease states.

tivate phagocytosis, and to control the overall immune response in general.[11] Resulting B cells are responsible for antibody- or humoral-induced immunity. No anatomic microenvironment similar to the thymus has been located in the human body for the site of B cell differentiation. However, B cell precursors are found in fetal liver, placenta, and adult bone marrow. The B cell obtained its name from the anatomic region in the chick embryo for B cell differentiation, the bursa of Fabricius.

The third cell line, macrophages, is responsible for phagocytosis of foreign particles. The mechanism of phagocytosis is critical for a normally functioning immune system. A portion of the phagocytosed material remains on the macrophage cell surface and is presented to the T cells and B cells. This presentation of antigen to the other cell lines is crucial for maximum immune response to occur.

Humoral-Mediated Immunity (HMI)

Electrophoretically, five major classes of human immunoglobulins can be separated.[12] These classes are IgM, IgA, IgG, IgE, and IgD. Each immunoglobulin class is synthesized by a separate population of B cells. Immature B cells have no surface antigen and are uncommitted to any antibody production. When stimulated by antigens, these cells differentiate into antibody producers. These antibody-producing B cells are recognized by the presence of cell surface immunoglobulins. Memory B cells are responsible for the secondary humoral immune response. B cells also have surface receptors for the activated third component of complement (C_3 receptor). Antibodies, due to their polyclonal and polyvalent features, are able to recognize a multiplicity of antigens. This function is essential for the organism to be able to recognize the vast array of foreign antigens. Maximum antibody response requires the presence and involvement of T cells. Subpopulations of T cells, particularly "helper" and "suppressor" T cells, are critical for normal immune regulation.[8, 11] The cooperation of both T cell helpers and B cells is critical for the production of IgG, IgA, and IgE antibody classes. Without T cell helpers, some B cells will differentiate upon antigenic stimulation to produce IGM antibody only.

The role of macrophages in antibody production is also important. Antigen that presents itself to the human immune system is taken up by macrophages and processed. The antigen is combined with an immune response–associated mucoprotein that is a product of genes linked to the major histocompatibility complex (MHC).[13] The combination of macrophage-processed antigen and immune-associated mucoprotein is then presented to the T cell by the macrophage. This process stimulates immune recognition by the cell and differentiation of the T cell into a helper population.[11, 14] Activation of T cells thus requires both antigen recognition and immune-associated compatibility.

Cell-Mediated Immunity (CMI)

T cell lymphocytes develop in the thymus gland where they acquire their antigen receptors and divide into subpopulations of cells with distinctive functions[8] (see Fig. 15–1). These subpopulations of T cells are recognized by their different cell surface markers.[14] One subset cell, T helper cells, assists B cells in producing antibody to antigens. To accomplish this antibody production both the T cell and the B cell must recognize different portions of the antigens. T helper cells also assist cytotoxic lymphocytes in destroying virus-infected cells and allogeneic grafts. Helper cells also release lymphokines that activate macrophages (Table 15–2). T helper cells recognize antigen in association with special molecules associated with the major histocompability complex (MHC).[8, 13, 14] The MHC is a cluster of genes possessed by all mammals, which influence immune functions by aiding recognition and signaling between cells of the immune system. Thus T cell recognition of antigen is different from that of B cells, and this dual antigen-recognition function is crucial for proper immune function.

T suppressor cells regulate actions of B cells and other T cells through the release of specific soluble factors.[10, 11, 15] T cytotoxic cells are lymphocytes that destroy viral infected cells and allogeneic cells, which they recognize by interaction with Class I MHC antigens. T delayed hypersensitivity cells (T-D) bring macrophages and other inflammatory cells to areas where delayed hypersensitivity reactions occur.[10, 14]

Immune System Activation Function

The T cell that encounters specific antigen is stimulated to multiply (blastogenic transformation) into a T cell clone line that secretes soluble mediators (lymphokines) and begins a variety of immunologic events.[15] Since antibody formation requires the encounter of a T cell receptor with antigen, the presentation of antigen to the T cell is the initial critical step in the eventual development of antibody. Thus antibody functions can be indirectly influenced by T lymphocyte dysfunctions.

Amplifications and Host Defense Function

Following the encounter, recognition, and T cell activation phases, the immune response balloons into a myriad of events in-

Table 15–2. T CELL LYMPHOKINES

Interferon
Migration-inhibition factor
Transfer factor
Macrophage-activating factor
Lymphotoxin
Chemotactic factor
Blastogenic factor
Lymph node permeability factor
Skin-reactive factors
Macrophage-activating factors

tended to provide host defense against foreign antigens and infections. T cells secrete their biologic mediators to ensure an amplified response to the initial antigen encounter.[15] These mediators enhance bone marrow production of granulocytes, eosinophils, mast cells, and macrophages in addition to influencing other cell responses to the antigen.

Macrophage Function

The third cell line critical to normal immune function, the macrophage, originates from progenitor cells in the bone marrow. Macrophages and monocytes represent different stages of development within the same cell line.[16] These precursor cells mature first into promonocytes and then monocytes. The monocytes circulate in the blood to organs and tissues where they become macrophages.[16] Blood-borne monocytes replace tissue macrophages as needed. Macrophages provide tissue defense against mechanical injuries, chemicals, drugs, toxins, infectious agents, and neoplastic cells.[15] Macrophage dysfunction can lead to both decreased resistance to infection and cancer and increased local tissue damage because of the effects of their cellular products.[14–16] Macrophage function can be altered by many environmental chemicals, gases, and particulate fibers.[17] Macrophages are similar to polymorphonuclear leukocytes in that they contain a variety of cytoplasmic enzymes, possess phagocytic abilities, adhere to plastic surfaces as well as to microbes, share similar cell surface receptors for the F(c) portion of IgG, and have cytotoxic activity against tumor cell lines.[18] Normal macrophages, as well as polymorphonuclear leukocytes, express cytotoxic action against antibody-coated tumor cells, bacteria, and other antibody-coated particles by phagocytosis. Part of the cytotoxic activity of these cells is their ability to generate a myeloperoxidase-dependent reactive oxygen species.[18] Stimulation of macrophages produces an augmentation of cytotoxic and phagocytic activity, as well as cytotoxic-related enzymes released from the cells. Macrophages also produce a number of immunoregulator products, which include interferon, lymphocyte-activating factor, prostaglandins, and colony-stimulating factor.[18] The interaction of macrophages with foreign target cells does not depend on specifically recognized antigenicity.

Host Resistance Function

The control and eradication of acute bacterial infections with organisms such as *Staphylococcus* and *Streptococcus* are mediated by the production of antibody. Antibodies attach to the bacteria and enhance phagocytosis and killing of these microorganisms. Granulocytes and macrophages accumulate in the area of infection because of complement activity and opsonization. Infections like those produced by *Mycobacterium tuberculosis* and *Listeria monocytogenes* are chronic in nature because these organisms are intercellular pathogens that can multiply within the phagocytes and escape antibody. The cell-mediated function of the immune system enhances macrophage killing of these intercellular pathogens through lymphokine production. The cell-mediated system also generates the lymphokine interferon, which sends a signal to adjacent cells to produce an antiviral protein that blocks virus replication.[18]

Primary immunodeficiency is associated with an increased incidence of both infections and neoplasia. Cell-mediated responses are important in cancer cell surveillance and growth limitation of spontaneously arising cancers. Alteration of the immune system thus can result in an increased risk of neoplasia. The mechanism of neoplastic cell killing involves cytotoxic cells, antibody-dependent cytotoxic T-cells, and natural killer cells.[19] Cytotoxic T cells are generated by specific antigens in tissue grafts and transplants. Macrophages are both antigen-specific and nonspecific mediators of neoplastic cell cytolysis. They serve as effector cells in antibody-dependent cytotoxicity and as direct cytotoxic cells. Natural killer cells are a subpopulation of T cells with neoplastic cell cytotoxic activity.[14] Natural killer cells, devoid of the cell surface markers that are present on both B cells and T cells, can spontaneously lyse cancer cells in vitro.[18]

Control and Regulation of Immune Response

To maintain normal health, the immune system must be kept under constraints to ensure recognition of normal tissue and to not mount attacks upon it.[8, 14, 19] There is always some formation of antibody with low avidity to autologous tissues; however, the function of immune tolerance is not to allow for self-recognition.[19] Diseases of autoimmunity can result from failure of this immune tolerance. The immune response is also regulated by the elimination of antigen. As antigen supplies diminish, the immune response subsides. Thus, the activity of antibody regulates the activity of immune cells.

Immunologic Tolerance

Immunologic tolerance refers to a nonreactivity to antigens by the immune system.[19] Both B cell and T cell tolerance can occur. B cell tolerance may develop through four mechanisms:[19]

(1) Immature B cells that encounter antigen for the first time in a low concentration may produce tolerance through abortion of the B cell line that would have normally developed at high antigen concentration.
(2) Repeated antigenic stimulation with an immunizing dose of T-independent antigen may slowly remove all mature B cells in the clonal line.
(3) Absence of T cell help may cause the B cell not to respond normally to the antigen.
(4) Antibody-forming cell blockade can occur if high concentrations of antigen block the cell surface receptors and interfere with antibody secretion.[19]

T cell tolerance may develop by three mechanisms:[19]

(1) Immature T cells may be aborted in a manner similar to that of the B cell clone. However, since there are many subsets of T cells, tolerance may develop to only one of these populations.
(2) Subsets of T cells may be functionally deleted and provide some level of immune tolerance.
(3) T cell suppressors can suppress the normal function of both T cells and B cells.[19]

Tolerance to self is an important basic immune function. Tolerance to foreign antigens can result in a decreased host resistance or hypersensitivity reaction.

ANATOMIC CONSIDERATIONS OF THE IMMUNE SYSTEM

Spleen

The spleen is the major filter for bloodborne antigens and infections as well as the major site of the immune response to foreign antigens. In addition to these tasks, the spleen also functions as a site of extramedullary hematopoiesis. The two basic anatomic components of the spleen are the capsule and the trabeculae. The trabeculae form poorly demarcated areas within the spleen. These demarcated areas contain splenic nodules (white pulp) and splenic sinuses (red pulp). These areas are named for their appearance in a freshly sectioned organ. The two histologic regions of the spleen, red pulp and white pulp, represent functional immune areas. Most of the splenic pulp is red. The white pulp is irregularly scattered throughout the organ. Red pulp contains reticular cells, phagocytic cells, and circulating blood elements. White pulp consists of a dense population of lymphocytes. The spleen has no afferent lymphatics; thus, any antigen that enters the spleen must do so through the blood vessels.

Thymus

Not a true lymphatic organ, the thymus is bilobular and located in association with the great vessels at the base of the heart. The thymus reaches a size of 10 to 15 gm at birth and 30 to 40 gm by puberty. After puberty it involutes. Each of the two lobes of the thymus is subdivided into several smaller lobules. Each lobule consists of an outer cortex and an inner medulla. Thymocytes are concentrated in the cortical areas. The thymus also produces thymic humoral factor (THF), necessary for regulation of lymphoiesis in all lymphoid tissues.

Lymph Nodes

There are 500 to 600 lymph nodes in the body. They may be individually located or occur in certain anatomic groups along the course of blood vessels. Lymph nodes produce lymph and lymphocytes. Lymph nodes are divided into three structural histologic areas: cortex, paracortex, and medulla. Lymph flow arrives into the nodes by afferent vessels, which also carry foreign antigens to the nodes. Efferent lymph vessels carry lymph-containing antibodies, lymphokines, and lymphocytes produced in response to antigenic stimulation. The cortex, site of B cell depot, is usually a thin rim of tissue and lymphocytes. Upon antigenic stimulation, the cortex proliferates into germinal sensors containing dense populations of lymphocytes, which differentiate into antibody-producing cells. In the dense portion of the germinal centers, the lymphocytes are actively dividing. The paracortex, between the cortex and the medulla, is a T cell site and a major area of T cell and macrophage interaction. The medulla of the node is composed of cords and sinuses that serve to filter particulate matter from lymph. The medullary cords also contain lymphocytes, and, upon antigenic stimulation, these lymphocytes produce antibody.

Liver

The normal adult liver weighs between 1400 and 1600 gm and consists of a left lobe, right lobe, and two rudimentary lobes, the caudate and quadrate. The right lobe makes up the majority of the liver's mass. Histologically, the liver consists of lobules. Each lobule has a central hepatic vein from which cords of hepatocytes concentrically radiate as spokes from a wheel. The outer boundaries of these lobules are demarcated by a combination of hepatic artery, portal vein, and bile duct. This combination is referred to as the portal triad. The walls of hepatocytes, which form the masses of liver lobules, are penetrated by vascular sinusoids lined by endothelial cells and special reticuloendothelial cells, called Kupffer cells, which have immune system function. Intrahepatic circulation of blood is basically through both the portal vein system and the hepatic artery. Sixty per cent of hepatic blood flow is through the portal vein. The liver thus plays a pronounced role in host resistance mechanisms and antigen detection.

CLINICAL IMMUNOTOXICITY

Laboratory Assessment

A variety of in vitro and in vivo immunologic assay systems are available to investigate the effects of chemicals and drugs on the immune system. Information concerning immunotoxic effects of drugs and chemicals can be used to extrapolate risk to humans in some instances. The sensitivity of the immune system to xenobiotics is a function of its complexity. The immune system is highly regulated, and many of the cells undergo rapid proliferation. Therefore, any toxic injury or dysfunction will be amplified as an alteration and inspected within an established assay. Immune alterations can be expressed as an enhancement or suppression of the immune function, or no demonstrable effect. Immune enhancement could result in autoimmunity, hypersensitivity disease, or allergy states. Immune depression can result in increased incidence of infections or decreased surveillance of neoplasia. The immune cells can be easily isolated and their functions studied in in vitro assay systems. Antibodies can be isolated and quantified.

The functional components of the immune system are available for study with respect to the impact of drugs and chemicals. The immune response to xenobiotics can be quantified and isolated to either the humoral or cell-mediated arm. However, no single immune function can be used to ascertain the immunotoxicity of a chemical or drug. A battery of tests is required.[19–21] In general, assessment of the immune system includes an evaluation of immunopathology, cell-mediated function, and humoral-mediated function, along with host resistance and macrophage function. Immunotoxicity testing is conducted both in vitro and in vivo. So far, a rate model and a mouse model have been developed. The mouse has been selected as the prime test animal by the National Toxicology Program. The National Institute of Public Health and Environmental Hygiene (NIPHEH) in the Netherlands uses the rat model for testing.[20]

Health effects of immune depression will present differently, depending on which aspect of the immune system is affected. T cell dysfunctions are associated with viral infections and opportunistic organisms like fungi and intracellular organisms. B cell dysfunction is associated with increased bacterial infections. Recurrent pyogenic infections from staphylococcus or streptococcus and fungal skin infections may be due to interference with phagocytosis. Complement dysfunction is associated with increased infection from bacteria. The National Toxicology Program (NTP) at the National Institute of Environmental Health Services (NIEHS) has been conducting immunologic assays on a priority list of environmental chemicals since 1979.[20, 22] The overall purpose of these tests was eventually to develop a sensitive and reproducible screening panel to detect subtle immune dysfunctions following exposures to select chemicals in animals and humans. The NTP immunotoxicology assay system consists of a tiered approach.[19, 20, 22] Tier I testing (Table 15–3) is a limited screen, including assays for cell-mediated immunity (CMI) and humoral-mediated immunity (HMI), as well as immunopathology. Tier II is a confirmatory testing battery that specifically identifies the immune lesion[19, 20, 22] (Table 15–4).

Tier I Immunotoxicity Assay

Tier I testing provides high sensitivity for detection of immunotoxicants, but it lacks the specificity of the Tier II assay. As listed in Table 15–3, the basic testing panel scrutinizes the immune system in immunopathology, cell-mediated immunity, humoral-mediated immunity, and nonspecific immunity.[19–22]

Tier I screening also can be used in clinical evaluation of humans. If the Tier I screen is negative, then there is reasonable confidence that a drug or chemical is not immunotoxic under the conditions of the assay system (Fig. 15–3). Assay-designed appropriate controls and data analysis are important considerations in routine testing of drugs and chemicals for immunotoxicity. Selection of controls is critical. Animals of the same strain, birth rate, and weight as the exposed group should be used in the control population. In some cases, a positive control (immunosuppression) group should be included. Assay variation should be within the 95 per cent confidence interval.

Complete blood counts with cell differentials help screen for the neutropenias and lymphopenias commonly seen from immunosuppressive drugs and chemicals, although a normal CBC and differential do not exclude immunotoxicity. Hemoglobin concentration and total RBC count are also part of this battery. The weights of lymphoid organs are an important part of immunotoxicology screening. The individual organ weights are usually compared in an organ-to-body weight ratio. Alteration of these normal ratios serves as an indicator of immunotoxicity and immune dysfunction. The organs typically studied are the thymus, spleen, and lymph nodes. Occasionally, such events as severe stress and weight loss of the animal and general chemical toxicity can alter

Table 15–3. TIER I ASSAY SYSTEM

1. IMMUNOPATHOLOGY
   - Hematology: CBC with differential count
   - Organ weights: Spleen, liver, thymus, kidneys, adrenals
   - Histology: Spleen, thymus, lymph node, cellularity of the bone marrow and spleen
2. CELL-MEDIATED IMMUNITY
   - Lymphocyte blastogenesis in response to mitogens (phytohemagglutinin, CON-A, and LPS)
   - Mixed leukocyte response (MLR) against allogeneic leukocytes
3. HUMORAL-MEDIATED IMMUNITY
   - Antibody plaque-forming cell reponse to sheep erythrocytes (IgM) or specific antibody concentrations, LPS mitogen response
4. NONSPECIFIC IMMUNITY
   - Natural killer cell function

Table 15–4. TIER II TESTING

1. IMMUNOPATHOLOGY
   - Quantification and per cent of splenic B cells, T cells, and macrophages present in organ histologic examinations
2. HUMORAL-MEDIATED IMMUNITY
   - Primary antibody response (IgM) to T-independent antigen (LPS) and secondary antibody response (IgG) to sheep erythrocytes
3. CELL-MEDIATED IMMUNITY
   - Cytotoxic T lymphocyte cytolysis function
   - Delayed hypersensitivity response
   - Quantitation of lymphokines
   - Antibody-dependent cellular cytotoxicity
4. NONSPECIFIC IMMUNITY
   - Macrophage function and phagocytosis
   - Bactericidal activity by phagocytes
   - Tumor cell cytolysis
   - NBT reduction in granulocytes
5. HOST RESISTANCE
   - Synergetic tumor cells
   - Bacterial models (*Listeria monocytogenes, Streptococcus* species)
   - Viral models (influenza)
   - Parasite models (*Plasmodium yoellii*)

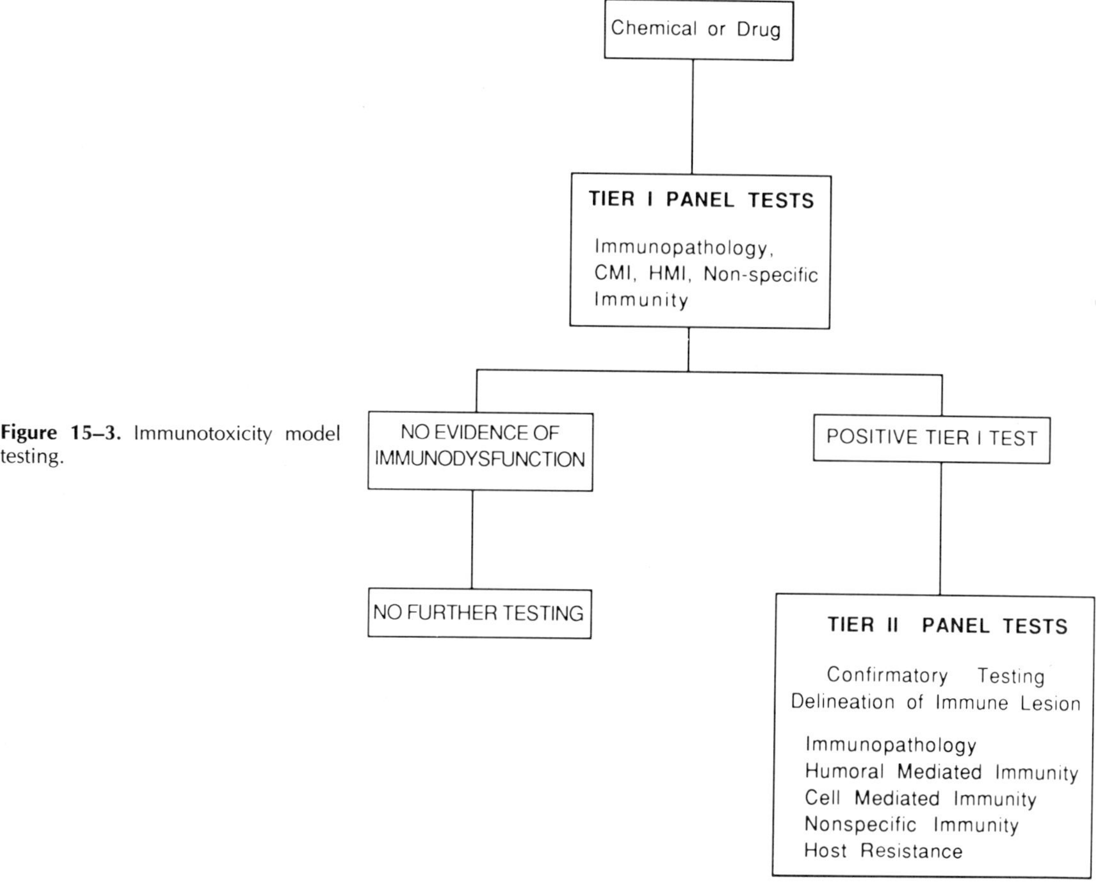

Figure 15–3. Immunotoxicity model testing.

thymus weight. In addition to the weights of organs, cellularity and histology of the spleen, thymus, lymph nodes, and bone marrow are useful in assaying for immunotoxicity. Circulating B cells temporarily reside in the splenic follicles and peripheral regions of the spleen's white pulp, as well as in the follicles and the medulla of lymph nodes. T cells reside temporarily in the periarteriolar lymphocyte sheath of the spleen. A decrease in the paracortical areas of the spleen is due to a toxic effect on the T cells. A decrease in splenic-to-body weight ratio, along with alteration of the histology and cellularity of specific anatomic areas, indicates an alteration of the normal immune system and either T lymphocyte or B lymphocyte depletion from an immunotoxin.

Splenic histology is an important component in determining the nature of the organ weight change. Lack of germinal centers in the spleen occurs from any immunotoxin and also results in decreased antibody production. Following the introduction of an antigenic stimulus, the splenic germinal centers should increase in numbers if the immune system is functioning normally. The induction of cell-mediated immunity normally results in a proliferation of cells in the paracortex of lymph node tissue. Chemicals and drugs that alter cell-mediated immunity will produce paracortical cellular hypoplasia.

In the thymus, the cortex, rather than the medulla, seems to be the target for immunotoxins. Medullary areas of the thymus contain immunoincompetent T cells. The thymic cortical areas contain immature T cells with varying degrees of immunocompetency. Thymus weight reduction correlates well with alteration of cell-mediated immune system competency by drugs and chemicals. Cellularity and histology of the bone marrow are also important to assess in immunotoxicity testing, because the pluripotent stem cells arise from the marrow and eventually develop into the mature immune cells. Quantitative measurement of stem cell proliferation can be ascertained using the colony growth of various hematopoietic cells.[21] Assays for the colony growth of B cells (CFU-B) and T cells (CFU-T) have been developed.[21] Because of their rapid proliferation, bone marrow hematopoietic cells are especially vulnerable to immunotoxins. Additional useful tests include serum proteins and quantitative protein electrophoresis, clinical chemistries, liver function tests, and other organ weights and histology, such as the kidneys, heart, adrenal glands, and liver.

In a normally functioning cell-mediated immunity, sensitized T cells must proliferate by undergoing blastogenesis in response to antigens. T cell response to the blastogenic antigens, Con-A or phytohemagglutin (PHA), is usually assessed.[21, 23] Mixed leukocyte response (MLR) is a particularly sensitive indicator for the effects of chemicals on cell-mediated immunity.[21, 23] Natural killer (NK) cells are a lymphocyte subpopulation possessing natural cytotoxicity against various neoplastic cell lines as well as infectious agents.[18, 24] Natural killer cell activity is quantified from mouse spleen using a ^{51}Cr-recluse assay.[24] Humoral-mediated response is assessed via enumeration of antibody-producing cells following immunization with antigen.[25] Sheep red blood cells are employed as the antigen, since cooperation of other immune cell populations, including B cells, T helper cells, and macrophages is required for antigen processing, as well as for production of interleukin 1.[26] T cells aid in both antigen recognition and B cell proliferation and differentiation through the release of soluble mediators.[15, 21]

Tier II Immunotoxicity Assay

Tier I testing consists of a general screening panel of immune assays. Tier II testing is a comprehensive evaluation which includes in depth analysis of HMI and CMI functions, as well as host resistance (Table 15–4). Tier II tests are restricted to confirmation of the initial screening or to delineating the mechanism of immune dysfunction. Tier II assays are more detailed in their location of the actual immune alteration and include more comprehensive immunopathology: examination of macrophage phagocytosis, bactericidal activity, macrophage enzyme levels, and macrophage cytolysis of tumor cells; quantification of T cell subpopulations using monoclonal antibodies; host resistance to infections and tumors; quantification of lymphokines; granulocyte function by nitro blue tetrazolium (NBT) testing; and bone marrow examinations.

Delayed hypersensitivity response and cytotoxic T lymphocyte response are included in Tier II testing and are performed when T cell dysfunction is detected in the Tier I assay. Tier II assays are conducted only if Tier I screening demonstrates immune dysfunction. Nonspecific immunity testing for Tier II involves evaluations of macrophage function, including phagocytic ability.[19, 21]

Since the most clinically relevant endpoint for immune dysfunction is altered host resistance, infection models are included in Tier II testing (Table 15–5). Host-resistant assays include infectious agents as well as tumor cells. Agents used are listed in Table 15–5.[27]

Comprehensive two-tiered testing panels have been developed by NTP for evaluation of environmental chemicals in mice. The sensitivity (dose-response) and reproducibility of the assays, in particular Tier I, have been documented extensively. The immune system represents a sensitive immunotoxicologic environment amenable for testing chemicals and drugs. Extrapolation of these results to

Table 15–5. HOST DEFENSE TESTING

TESTING METHOD OR AGENT	IMMUNE COMPONENT TESTED
Listeria monocytogenes	T cell sensitization with macrophage activation
Streptococcus species	Induction of opsonizing antibody, enhancement of phagocytosis, and intracellular killing. Also tests PMNs and complement. T dependent antibody
PYB6 tumor (fibrosarcoma)	Resistance to tumor growth reflects intactness of cell-mediated immunity and natural killer cell function
Metastatic pulmonary tumor	Resistance to tumor spread reflects competence of macrophage and natural killer cell functions
Mouse malaria (*Plasmodium yoellii*)	Parasitemia clearing is dependent on specific antibody production, as well as on normal T cell and macrophage functioning
Influenza virus	Evaluates non-T cell–mediated defense involving antibody and interferon

humans can be difficult. Clinical immunotoxicity from environmental chemicals is not as well documented as immunotoxicity resulting from some of the therapeutic drugs.

MEDICAL IMMUNOTOXICOLOGY

Although vast amounts of information documenting the immunotoxic effects of chemicals and drugs exist at subclinical doses in animal test models, these test results are difficult to extrapolate to humans. There are, however, many examples of human immunotoxic syndromes produced by chemicals at low environmental concentrations and by drugs in therapeutic doses (see Table 15–1). Chemicals such as benzene, arsenic, mercury, beryllium, platinum, chloromethyl ethers, ethylene oxide, formaldehyde, and polyhalogenated aromatic hydrocarbons are known to produce human health effects through immunologic mechanisms. Drugs such as procainamide, chloramphenicol, salicylates, gold salts, nonsteroidal anti-inflammatory agents, penicillins, carbamazepine, phenytoin, and nitrofurantoin are known to produce human diseases ranging from acute anaphylaxis, dermatitis, vasculitis, glomerulonephritis, and bone marrow suppression to drug-induced lupus erythematosus, erythema multiforme, hypersensitivity pulmonary disease, and neutropenia. Drugs of abuse also have been documented to produce alteration of the immune system with respect to host defense mechanisms.

Detecting of immune system effects and documenting causation of an immune alteration by xenobiotics require careful analysis of the clinical situation in which exposure occurred, a thorough history and physical examination, and sometimes sophisticated clinical immunologic laboratory testing. Not all patients will present with easily documented end-organ immunotoxicity, such as glomerulonephritis, pneumonitis, asthma, dermatologic lesions and exanthems, or hepatitis from well-known exposure sources.

Because of the established body of knowledge available, the following classes of chemicals will be reviewed relative to their associated human immunotoxicity.

Metals

Heavy metals have been steadily increasing in our environment since the Industrial Revolution. Inorganic arsenic, lead, mercury, cadmium, chromium, nickel, and others are present as environmental contaminants from a variety of occupational and industrial processes. For over a century, it has been known that lead exposure could produce infertility in women and that spouses of men exposed in the workplace could experience reproductive difficulties.[28] Most human metal exposure is occupationally related, and many of these metals are known immunotoxicants.[29, 30] Chronic exposure to most metals results in bioaccumulation owing to their relatively slow elimination half-life. Many of the metals to which humans are exposed occupationally and environmentally are documented to be immunotoxic in animal models at subclinical doses (Table 15–6).

Nephritis from inorganic lead, mercury,

Table 15–6. METAL IMMUNOTOXICITY

METAL	ANIMAL STUDIES
Lead, lead compounds, and tetraethyl lead	Enhanced mitogen response, decreased resistance to endotoxins, decreased serum immunoglobulins, decreased complement, impaired phagocytosis, decreased lysozyme activity
Mercury, methyl mercury, mercuric chloride	Decreased antibody production
Arsenic, Arsenite	Enhanced antibody production as well as decreased antibody production
Chromium	Decreased antibody titer to T1 phage sensitization
Magnesium	Decreased antibody response to sheep RBCs
Cadmium and cadmium compounds	Decreased circulating antibody, decreased host resistance to endotoxin, decrease in number of antibody-forming spleen cells
Beryllium	Hypersensitivity reactions, immune inflammatory response
Platinum	Decreased antibody titer to sheep RBC sensitization
Nickel, nickel chloride, nickel acetate	Decreased host resistance, decreased antibody formation, decreased phagocytosis
Cobalt sulfate	Decreased host resistance
Selenium	Immune system enhancement

(From Descotes J: Biphenyls: 1. Polybrominated biphenyls. *In* Descotes J (ed): Immunotoxicology of Drugs and Chemicals. New York, Elsevier, 1986.)

and cadmium is mediated via an immune mechanism.[29–31] This immunologically mediated glomerulonephritis is secondary to glomerular basement membrane (GBM) deposition of anti-GBM antibodies. Clinically, patients usually present with proteinuria and occasionally nephrotic syndrome without renal insufficiency. It is interesting that metal-induced glomerulonephritis does not appear to be dose related.[29–31] Immune glomerulonephritis can occur in up to 10 per cent of patients receiving gold salt therapy for rheumatoid arthritis.[31]

Cadmium exposure has been reported to produce renal tubular lesions as well as glomerulonephritis.[31] Animal models have demonstrated IgG glomerular deposits in the basement membrane as well as antibodies directed against GBM glycoproteins following chronic cadmium exposure.[31] In addition, cadmium has been shown to suppress antibody formation in animal models.[32] Epidemiologically, cadmium exposure and respiratory cancer have been linked.[29–31]

Lead is known to reduce host resistance to infection as well to interfere with reproductive functions.[28, 29] However, immunotoxicity in humans has not been well documented. One study in 12 children examined the effect of blood lead concentration on major immunoglobulin concentrations, total complement, C_3 component of complement, or the antigenic response to tetanus toxoid and failed to demonstrate any correlation.[33, 34]

Sensitizing metals produce a variety of dermal and respiratory problems, ranging from rashes to occupationally induced asthma.[35, 36] Chromium, beryllium, and platinum are particularly potent sensitizing metals that produce a variety of hypersensitivity pulmonary diseases as well as dermal lesions in exposed humans.[35, 36] Chromium compounds can produce both corrosive and irritating effects clinically following dermal exposure.[37] The dermatotoxicity consists of skin ulceration, dermatitis, and nasal septum ulceration.[37] Chromium is a shiny, white metal that is nontoxic in the elemental state. Chromium salts, trioxides, and chromic acid are strong irritants and oxidants and have been known to produce glomerulonephritis.[31, 37] Chronic inhalation of chromium dust can produce asthma and reactive airway disease.[23]

Beryllium, one of the rare metals, was described as being toxic as early as the 1930s.[38, 39] Control of environmental air concentrations of beryllium has been demonstrated to control disease in workers. Current exposure occurs in alloy workers, beryllium extraction, microelectronics manufacturing, and the aerospace and nuclear energy technologies. Beryllium in all forms has been shown to cause human disease through inhalation. Acute beryllium inhalation can cause a direct toxic effect on mucous membranes of the tracheobronchial tree, resulting in inflammation and necrosis. Chronic exposure to beryllium can result in both pulmonary and systemic granulomatous disease. Immunotoxicity from beryllium exposure is thought to occur through a sensitization process that is antibody mediated.[38, 39] Blastogenic transformation of lymphocytes occurs in the presence of beryllium sulfate in tissue cultures from patients with chronic berylliosis, but not in human controls.[38, 39] Dermal lesions caused by beryllium occur through inhalation and through direct contact. Nodular granulomatous, noncaseating lesions have been documented in workers with inhalational exposure only. Direct skin contact produces a hypersensitivity dermatitis. Beryllium is thus a potent sensitizing metal that can produce pulmonary and dermal disease via immunologic mechanisms not fully understood. Epidemiologic data suggest an association between beryllium and lung cancer in some workers.

Nickel and nickel compounds (nickel, nickel carbonyl, nickel sulfate, nickel hydroxide, and nickel carbonate) can produce human skin and pulmonary disease and are associated with both lung and nasal cancer in exposed human populations.[40] Workers who chronically inhale high concentrations of nickel may present with asthma. In addition, high environmental exposure to nickel can cause nasal septum necrosis.[41] Nickel carbonyl is a potent toxin whose syndrome of toxicity can be delayed for hours after exposure. Nickel carbonyl can produce a severe, delayed pulmonary distress syndrome consisting of pneumonitis and cerebral edema. Nickel carbonyl is metabolized in the body to Ni^{++} and carbon monoxide.[41] Nickel carbonyl is a known animal teratogen. Nickel is also a known cause of allergic contact dermatitis.[41] Nickel has been reported to be a stimulus for lymphocyte blastogenesis transformation in human lymphocytes and has been shown to directly bind to lymphocyte cell surface membranes.[40]

Chronic exposure to manganese compounds can result in increased pulmonary infections as well as the neurologic effects of parkinsonism.[41] Inhalational exposure to manganese dioxide can reduce host defense mechanisms of the lungs and may result in pulmonary inflammation and impairment of pulmonary macrophages.[41]

Chronic arsenic exposure has adverse hematologic effects with resulting disturbance of erythropoiesis.[29, 30] Lymphatic cancers and leukemia also have been associated with chronic arsenic exposure.[29, 30] Arsenic-related dermatologic lesions include eczematous dermatitis, follicular dermatitis, and hyperkeratosis. Arsenic is also associated with basal cell and squamous cell skin cancers. An increased incidence of respiratory cancers that are arsenic related has been reported in epidemiologic studies of smelter workers.[42, 43]

Selenium is a unique metal in that it may enhance the immune response, which has been demonstrated in animal models. It is of interest to note that the metals that are considered to be primary irritants and human sensitizers are also those associated with human carcinogenesis.[44]

Halogenated Polyaromatic Hydrocarbons

These compounds include polychlorinated biphenyls, phenols, chlorinated dibenzo-*p*-dioxins, dibenzofurans, hexachlorobenzene, pentachlorophenol, and polybrominated biphenyls.[45] The general classification of these chemicals is as follows:

Polychlorinated biphenyls (PCB)
Polybrominated biphenyls (PBB)
Polychlorinated dibenzo-*p*-dioxins (PCDD)
Polychlorinated dibenzofurans (PCDF)

PCBs were produced in the United States under the name Aroclor, which was a mixture of 209 congeners of PCBs.[46] These congeners differ in chlorination and were identified by a number following the Aroclor trade name; the number also identified the percentage of chlorination.[47] The production of PCBs in the United States was suspended in 1977. About half the PCBs produced between 1966 and 1974 were used in transformers.[46] Even though PCBs in transformers are being replaced, a significant number of transformers still contain large quantities, so transformer maintenance and repair personnel are the most exposed. PCBs are inert compounds and are virtually resistant to environmental degradation. Thus they tend to accumulate in the environment. Human exposure occurs via inhalation or ingestion of foods. The high lipid solubility of these compounds allows for them to accumulate up the food chain.[47] Toxic effects of PCBs have included chloracne, ocular irritation, arthritis, gastrointestinal symptoms, and hepatotoxicity.

An incident in Michigan in 1973, involving the contamination of dairy cattle feed with polybrominated biphenyls highlighted the concern over these compounds.[1] Local farmers and Michigan residents who consumed these contaminated dairy products were subjects of close investigation. PBBs were detected in the plasma of many residents. Immunologic investigations demonstrated that 34 per cent of farm residents and 59 per cent of PBB manufacturing workers had reduced T lymphocyte numbers.[48] B cell and T cell lymphocyte blastogenesis was reduced in exposed farmers and workers, compared with controls. In the Michigan population, T cells and B cells were normal, compared with controls.[48] Two occurrences of rice oil contamination have been extensively studied. These human exposures occurred in Japan in 1968 and in Taiwan in 1979.[47]

These incidents have generated great concern over polyhalogenated compounds. As an additional concern, polychlorinated dibenzofurans were found to be contaminants of PCBs. PBBs were used as flame retardants in fire extinguishers. Immunotoxicology studies with animals have demonstrated potent effects of these chemicals on the thymus, host resistance, cell-mediated immunity, and humoral mediated immunity (Table 15–7).

In humans, it has been difficult to assess the immunologic health effects of PCBs, dibenzodioxins, and dibenzofurans. Chloracne, a recognized dermatologic effect of PCB exposure in workers, is probably the best described toxicity of the compounds, along with hepatotoxicity.[47] Although animal studies have proved the carcinogenicity of PCBs, there is no conclusive evidence that exposure to PCBs results in an increased incidence of cancer in humans.[47] Small short-term epidemiologic studies of capacitor manufacturing workers exposed to PCBs have not indicated

Table 15–7. POLYHALOGENATED AROMATIC HYDROCARBON IMMUNOTOXICITY

CHEMICAL	ANIMAL STUDIES
2,3,7,8-Tetrachlorodibenzofuran-(TCDF)	Decreased thymus to body weight ratio, impaired CMI, impaired HMI, decrease in splenic B cells, decrease in granulocyte and macrophage colony-forming units in bone marrow (CFU-GM)
1,2,3,6,7,8-Hexachlorodibenzo-*p*-dioxin (HCDD)	Dose-related suppression of T cells, suppression of antibody response to sheep RBCs, depressed HMI
2,3,7,8-Tetrachlorodibenzo-*p*-dioxin (TCDD)	Severe thymic atrophy with histologic cortical lymphoid depletion, depressed CMI in mice and rats, depressed host resistance, suppression of cytotoxic T cell formation, suppression of B cell formation
Polybrominated Biphenyls (PBB)	Decreased host resistance in dairy cattle, thymic atrophy in cattle and laboratory animals, species-variable immune effects, depressed HMI and CMI, decreased serum immunoglobulins

any increased incidence in cancer.[46] Other epidemiologic studies have also failed to demonstrate an increased incidence of cancer in exposed humans.[49–51] In the 1979 incident in Taiwan, over 200 people were exposed to PCBs as a contaminant of rice oil. Chang studied the delayed immune response in 30 patients from the Taiwan incident and compared their response with 50 controls.[47] His findings documented that dermal lesions appeared to correlate with whole blood PCB concentrations. He also demonstrated decreased IgM and decreased IgA but no effect on IgG. In addition, there was a decrease in the percentage of T lymphocytes and T lymphocyte helper cells, as well as a suppression of delayed hypersensitivity to antigens.[47]

Health effects of long-term exposure to 2,3,7,8-tetrachlorodibenzo-*p*-dioxin (TCDD) have been reported following various spills or contaminations that lead to human exposure. In 1971, sludge oil contaminated with TCDD was sprayed on dirt roads at various sites in eastern Missouri.[52] In 1983, 12 years later, one of the nine residential sites where TCDD spraying had occurred was studied for human health effects. The area chosen had TCDD concentrations in surrounding soil ranging from 39 to 1100 parts per billion. The mobile homes in the area had inside dust concentrations above 1 part per billion. The study included 155 exposed individuals. There was no increase in the number of usual medical complaints above the control population in the study nor any incidences of chloracne or increased incidence of cancer. Nor was there any increased incidence of spontaneous abortions, reproductive problems, or congenital malformations. Gross liver function tests of all exposed individuals were normal; however, subclinical hepatotoxicity was suggested by some of the assays, particularly higher mean urinary uroporphyrin concentrations in exposed persons and correlation of serum levels of five liver enzymes—AST, ALT, GGTP, alkaline phosphatase, and alanine aminopeptidase—with years of residence at the contaminated site. Immunologic evaluation of the exposed individuals revealed an elevated incidence of anergy and relative anergy, compared with controls. T cell surface marker analyses demonstrated statistically significant decreases in percentages of T_3, T_4, and T_{11} cells in the exposed group. The number of non–T lymphocytes in peripheral blood samples was elevated in the exposed group. There was no significant difference in T lymphocyte proliferative response to mitogen stimulation nor cytotoxic T cell activity in either of the groups. Overall, the exposed group had a nonstatistically significant increased frequency of abnormal T cell subsets, as well as a nonstatistically significant abnormality in T cell function.[52] The presence of in vitro immune alterations in the exposed population with the absence of overt clinical signs and symptoms of immune deficiency points to a subclinical immunotoxicity from TCDD following prolonged exposure.

Another study of individuals exposed to TCDD for 10 years who lived or worked near contaminated areas in Missouri showed no difference in the study population compared with the control group in delayed hypersensitivity, T cell subsets, and cytotoxic T cell proliferation assays.[53] Another study reported health effects of TCDD in children following an environmental accident near Seveso, Italy, in 1976.[54] The exposed children totaled approximately 1500 and ranged in age from 6 to 10 years. Immunologic parameters were not studied, but liver function tests showed alterations in alanine aminotransferase and γ-glutamyltransferase.

An immunologic investigation of 55 transformer repairmen with high adipose concentrations of PCBs has been reported.[46] These workers were exposed predominantly to Aroclor 1260 and some to Aroclor 1242. Physical examinations and immunologic evaluations were performed. Delayed hypersensitivity, evaluated with an intradermal injection of mumps and tricophytin antigens, was not different from the nonexposed controls. There was no incidence of chloracne in this study.

Thus while animal studies have supported the immunotoxicity of PCBs, human studies to date have been questionable in terms of immunologic health effects.

Pesticides and Insecticides

Pesticides and insecticides include cholinesterase-inhibiting as well as noncholinesterase-inhibiting compounds. Cholinesterase inhibitors are classified as organophosphates or carbamates. Noncholinesterase insecticides include organochlorines, paraquat, fumigants, pyrethroids, and phenolic derivatives. Knowledge of the immunotoxicity of pesticides in humans is very limited. Animal studies demonstrate wide-ranging immunologic dysfunctions following exposures (Table 15–8). Animal toxicity studies have demonstrated atrophy of lymphoid tissues, as well as CMI and HMI immunosuppression induced by a variety of pesticides.

Human exposure to pesticides is widespread as a result of home spraying, agricultural use, and industrial use. Bioaccumulation of chlorinated pesticides in the adipose tissue of humans is well documented. These pesticides can be detected in serum as well as adipose tissue in a range of parts per million concentrations.[55] DDT and its metabolite DDE are detected in the adipose tissue and serum of nonexposed individuals owing to bioaccumulation through the normal food chain. Other pesticides found in the adipose tissue and serum of the general population include benzene hexachloride and its isomers, lindane, chlordane, heptachlor, heptachlor epoxide, and dieldrin. Their presence in the normal general population creates a confounding factor in studies of immunotoxicity involving human exposures. Their presence in the adipose tissue and serum at low parts per million and parts per billion does not appear to constitute an immunologic health risk in terms of altered host defense in the general population. The concentrations of these particular pesticides in humans are sometimes used to support the argument for the disease constellation of "multiple chemical sensitivities (MCS)." Patients with MCS

Table 15–8. PESTICIDE IMMUNOTOXICITY

PESTICIDE/ INSECTICIDE	ANIMAL STUDY
Chlordane	Defect in delayed hypersensitivity, enhancement of CMI as measured by CON-A and PHA mitogen response
DDT	Decrease in lymphoid organ weights, decreased antibody response to antigens, increased delayed hypersensitivity to tuberculin and BSA, decreased neutrophil chemotaxis
Dieldrin	Decreased antibody response, decreased host resistance to infectious agents
Heptachlor	Decreased lymphoid organ weights
Lindane	Increased immunoglobulin concentrations, decrease in T lymphocyte proliferative response to PHA
Benzene hexachloride	Decrease in neutrophil chemotaxis
Parathion	Decreased lymphoid organ weight
Methyl parathion	Decrease in neutrophil chemotaxis
Malathion	Decrease in lymphoid organ weight, decrease in lymphocyte proliferative response to PHA

(From Descotes J: Biphenyls: 1. Polybrominated biphenyls. *In* Descotes J (ed): Immunotoxicology of Drugs and Chemicals. New York, Elsevier, 1986.)

have wide-ranging symptoms that do not fit any immunosuppressive syndrome. Frequently, people who are diagnosed as having MCS have symptoms of fatigue, headache, nausea, and a variety of neurologic and neurobehavorial complaints; in the majority of cases, no objective immunotoxicity can be demonstrated.

Documented human effects from pesticides include allergic skin reactions. Autoimmunity in humans has been suggested.[48] Studies of human leukocyte functions in vitro have shown definite alterations following pesticide exposure.[56] Cultures of human lymphocytes undergoing PHA mitogen blastogenic stimulation in the presence of pesticides showed some inhibition.[56] Carbamates inhibited lymphocyte PHA stimulation 10 per cent, organophosphates by 11 to 18 per cent, and organochlorine pesticides (BHC, endrin, DDT) by 11 to 17 per cent in this study. Lymphocyte stimulation as well as rosette formation in response to PHA when human T cells are exposed to sheep RBCs is a characteristic of T lymphocytes. DDT was a potent inhibitor of in vitro human erythrocyte rosette formation. In the same study, DDT did not alter neutrophil chemotaxis. However, methyl parathion and benzyl benzoate did inhibit PMN chemotaxis.[56]

Studies with lindane have shown inhibiting effects on human lymphocyte PHA mitogenesis. Lindane was found to alter T lymphocyte membrane-associated events leading to mitogen activation by PHA.[57]

Other studies have shown defects in chemotaxis, NBT reduction by phagocytes, and phagocytosis in occupationally exposed workers.[48] In addition, the incidence of infectious episodes was higher in these workers.[58] In contrast, children exposed to DDT did not show alteration in antibody titers to diphtheria immunization.[59]

Immunologic Sensitizers and Irritants of the Lung and Skin

Immunologic hypersensitivity can result from numerous environmental chemicals as well as drugs (Table 15–9). These chemicals and environmental contaminants produce immunotoxicity by these mechanisms:

(1) They are directly antigenic by themselves.
(2) They haptenize with serum proteins to form immunogens.
(3) They covalently bind to macromolecules present in the target organ areas of the lung, gastrointestinal tract, or skin.[23]

Hypersensitivity disease involving the lung and skin is a common occupational health problem that results in increased costs through lost work time, decreased productivity, and increased worker compensation benefits, medical care, and litigation. Dermatitis, asthma, and reactive airway disease are the most common clinical problems seen in occupational exposures involving sensitizing and irritant chemicals.

Occupational immunologic lung disease may take the form of asthma, hypersensitivity pneumonitis, or fibrotic lung disease. Reactive hypersensitivity of the airways that is nonimmunologically mediated is also a result of exposure to irritant chemicals. Chemicals that produce irritant effects on the airways may act in both immunologic and nonimmunologic ways. Bronchospasm and cough to some degree is the usual clinical outcome. Stimulation of subepithelial vagal receptors by chemicals inhaled as vapors or dusts can induce this clinical syndrome.[60] Commonly involved chemicals are

formaldehyde	1,4-dioxane
ammonia	chlorinated solvents
nitrous oxide	inorganic acids
chlorine	inorganic bases
bromine	alcohols
sulfur dioxide	nitromethane
ozone	phosgene

Certain metals are allergenic in humans, resulting in both dermal and pulmonary lesions. The dual property of allergenicity and carcinogenicity of certain metals in animals and humans has been noted.[44] The presence of both allergenicity and carcinogenicity has been demonstrated in 15 metals. Arsenic, beryillium, chromium, and nickel are accepted as both animal and human carcinogens as well as potent sensitizing agents. Metals that are carcinogenic in animals or humans are also allergenic.[60]

Occupational Asthma

Chemically induced asthma can be by one of three mechanisms: (1) direct effect on airways, (2) IgE-mediated, or (3) irritant effect

Table 15–9. CHEMICALS THAT PRODUCE HYPERSENSITIVITY DISEASE

TYPE I (ASTHMA, ANAPHYLAXIS)	TYPE II (CYTOTOXIC ANTIBODY-MEDIATED)
ethanolamine	gold salts
formaldehyde	sulfonamides
ammonia	chlorpromazine
metal dusts	methyldopa
platinum salts	propranolol
phthalic anhydrides	practolol
diisocyanates	quinidine
trimetallic anhydrides	procainamide
ethylenediamine	hydralazine
chloramine	isoniazid
polyvinylchloride	penicillamine
acrylamide	methicillin
monoethanolamine	cephalothin
ammonium thioglycolate	**TYPE III (SERUM SICKNESS)**
piperazine hydrochloride	horse serum (antivenin)
nickel sulfate	penicillin
dichloroamine	phenytoin
wood dust	sulfonamides
enzymes	thiazides
proteins	thiouracils
aspirin	cephalosporins
penicillin	
TYPE IV (CONTACT DERMATITIS AND DELAYED)	
beryllium salts	benzoic acid
cosmetics	dichromate
formaldehyde	ethylenediamine
mercury bichloride	cleaning agents with ammonia
pyrethrin insecticides	alprenolol
organophosphate insecticides	quinidine
nickel sulfate	neomycin
resins	ethanolamines
zirconium salts	diphenhydramine topical
chromium salts	benzocaine
toluene diisocyanate	

on airways. Between 2 and 15 per cent of all asthma in industrialized countries is due to industrial and occupational chemical exposure.[23] Allergy-mediated asthma has been documented to occur from many different sources, including chemicals, vegetable matter, and proteins. Repeated exposure to the offending agent is required to produce sensitization. Once this IgE-mediated problem occurs, any exposure to minute amounts can precipitate bronchospasm. Sensitizing environmental contaminants and chemicals act as haptens by combining with proteins present in mucosal surfaces or by combining to albumin and other serum proteins. Following repeated exposure, IgE antibodies form against this hapten complex. Trimellitic anhydride and toluene isocyanate are well known precipitators of allergic asthma.[61] Trimellitic anhydride, a component of resin-curing agents, is an example of a chemical that produces asthma. Trimellitic anhydride may produce an asthmatic syndrome, an irritant syndrome, and a sensitivity pneumonitis syndrome. The biotechnology industry is an occupational source of exposure to a variety of proteins, peptides, and chemicals that can result in IgE-mediated asthma. This includes enzymes such as papain, pepsin, alkaline phosphatase, glucose oxidase, peroxidase, ribonuclease; acrylamide monomers and aliphatic amines; chemicals used to haptenize drugs to albumin molecules, such as carbodiimides; toluene diisocyanate, glutaraldehyde, and phenylenediamine. Nickel sulfate exposure has been demonstrated to produce a positive inhalational challenge test as well as antibody formation.[36] Platinum workers can experience not only pulmonary sensitization with development of specific IgE and asthma, but also conjunctivitis and rhinitis.[36]

Formaldehyde exposure is widespread due to its presence in many commonly used products, including fabrics, wood products and particle board, and carpets. It is a direct upper airway and respiratory irritant at concentrations ranging from 1 to 3 parts per million.[62] Recognition of the health effects from low-level formaldehyde exposure has recently resulted in a lowering of the previous standard of 3 ppm to 1 ppm. A variety of health effects, including respiratory irritation, ocular irritation, headache, and cough, can occur at formaldehyde concentrations of between 0.05 and 1 ppm. Human antibodies to the hapten complex of formaldehyde and human albumin recently have been demonstrated.[7] Clinical cases of documented health effects, including asthma, rhinitis, and flu symptoms, have been associated with the presence of anti-formaldehyde–human serum albumin IgG, IgM, and IgE.[7] Reports of immune system alterations in certain T cell subpopulations also have been documented following formaldehyde exposure.[7] Incidents of asthma from formaldehyde exposure have been documented; however, formaldehyde-induced asthma remains rare.[63] Instead, formaldehyde deposits mainly in the moist mucous membranes of the upper airway and produces a direct, nonimmunologic irritant effect on the respiratory system.

Decomposition products are other chemical sources of respiratory irritants and asthma: polyvinyl chloride decomposition products; acetylene gas and metal oxides from welding fumes; heating of polyurethanes; and phosgene, a product of heated chlorinated aliphatic solvents like trichloroethylene, methylene chloride, and trichloroethane.

Hypersensitivity Pneumonitis

This disease can be acute or chronic in onset. Chemically induced acute hypersensitivity pneumonitis presents with fever, chills, nonproductive cough, chest pain, and dyspnea and usually resolves in 24 hours.[36] Chronic pneumonitis from an immunologic etiology occurs following a chronic or subchronic exposure to low concentrations of chemicals. Fever, chronic cough, fatigue, weight loss, and shortness of breath are the clinical manifestations. Permanent pulmonary damage with fibrosis can occur unless the exposure is terminated. Many compounds and agents can produce hypersensitivity pulmonary disease. The most common chemical causes are anhydrides, beryllium, and isocyanates.[36] Metal oxide fumes produce a "fume fever" syndrome with similar clinical findings.

Reactive Airway Dysfunction

A one-time exposure or multiple pulmonary exposure to certain irritant chemicals can result in reactive airway disease manifested by chronic cough, bronchospasm, chest tightness, and shortness of breath on re-exposure to the same or other irritating chemical.[64] Chemicals that produce direct effects on the pulmonary airways usually do so via release of histamine from mast cells instead of an immunologic mechanism. Dust and cotton are known to produce a nonantigenic release of histamine that can result in cough and bronchospasm. A number of chemicals have been associated with reactive airway disease: nitromethane, uranium hexafluoride, chlorinated solvents, decomposition products, spray paint, acids, and sealants.[64]

Diagnosis can be made using the following criteria:[64]

1. Absence of prior pulmonary disease
2. Symptom onset after chemical exposure
3. Chemical has an irritant quality
4. Symptom onset within 24 hours of exposure
5. Symptoms persisting for 3 months
6. Symptoms include cough, wheezing, dyspnea
7. Pulmonary function tests show obstruction
8. Methacholine challenge test is positive
9. Other pulmonary disease is ruled out

Reactive airway disease is a nonimmunologic clinical problem.

Immunology-Associated Fibrotic Lung Disease

Fibrotic pulmonary disease associated with immunologic abnormalities is known to occur as a result of the chronic inhalation of dusts and manufactured fiberogenic materials, including asbestos, mica, graphite, silica, and beryllium. The release of lysosomal enzymes from macrophages occurs as a result of the phagocytosis of these manufactured fiberogenics. Pulmonary fibrosis is a result of chronic exposure. In addition, other immunologic abnormalities occur as a result of human exposure to these fibers.

Patients with silicosis have been found to have elevated circulating immune complexes, including antinuclear antibody and rheumatoid factor.[69] No direct correlation between severity of disease and the presence of immune complexes is documented. In addition, patients with silicosis have documented increased immunoglobulins with increased secretory IgA.[36]

Asbestos-related lung disease has a number of immunologic features. Asbestos fibers activate both classic and alternate complement pathways.[36] The activity of natural killer cells and antibody-dependent cellular cytotoxicity (K cells) has been demonstrated to be depressed in patients with asbestosis.[65–67] In addition, asbestosis is associated with a decrease in the number of T cells, increased immune complexes, and increased serum immunoglobulin concentrations.[36]

Beryllium inhalation produces a delayed hypersensitivity syndrome with an interstitial granulomatous process. Dermal granulomas also can be a result of pulmonary exposure. Patients with berylliosis have been noted to have increased lymphocyte transformation in in vitro studies. Biopsies of dermal lesions in patients with pulmonary berylliosis have demonstrated noncaseating granulomas.[38]

Hypersensitivity Skin Disease

Dermatitis can be caused by a wide variety of chemicals as well as drugs. Dermatitis from environmental exposures can be immunologic or non-immunologic. Human skin disease secondary to contact from irritant and sensitizing chemicals is usually occupationally related. Mechanisms of exposure include (1) dermal contact with chemicals in the vapor phase, liquids, or solids. Examples are chemicals containing formaldehyde, phenols, amines, metals, acids, alkalis, and other irritant chemicals; and (2) systemic exposure via inhalation of airborne chemicals, either volatilized or carried on particles of dust via contaminated ventilation systems. Examples of this are nickel dermatitis and berylliosis.

Rashes may thus appear in a variety of areas, including exposed surfaces of the neck, arms, legs, face, and hands. Frequently, chemicals or fiberogenic materials such as fiber glass accumulate in work clothes and are in chronic contact with the skin. Soluble chemicals in vapor phase may dissolve in the sweat present on skin surfaces. Clinical symptoms of airborne dermal irritants are itching, a burning sensation, and ocular irritation. Rashes may be evident, and their clinical picture may vary from true urticarial lesions to papular or maculopapular lesions. These airborne dermatoses have been subdivided into allergic contact dermatitis, nonimmunologic urticarial rash, phototoxic contact dermatitis, photoallergic contact dermatitis, nonallergic contact dermatitis, and acne venenata.[68] Common contact allergens found in industry include:

- epoxy resins and components;
- organic amines;
- methacrylates;
- chromates and dichromates;
- nickel, gold, platinum, arsenic, beryllium
- chemical accelerators and antioxidants;
- phthalic acids and anhydrides;
- formaldehyde, glutaraldehyde, acrolein;
- carbonless copy paper.

The more commonly recognized contact urticarial rashes are to formaldehyde and nickel in occupational environments.[68, 69] Nickel dermatitis can occur either by direct dermal exposure or via systemic exposure.[70] Patients with sensitivity to nickel can have chronic eczema.

Dermatitis from airborne dusts and particulates can appear underneath clothing if particulates can penetrate fabric or remain trapped in clothing. Fiber glass dermatitis is an example. Contact dermatitis from corrosive chemicals such as cement, acids, and alkalis is in reality a chemical burn. Carbonless paper has recently been recognized as a source of human health effects, including dermal and pulmonary irritation.[71] Carbonless paper products contain a variety of irritating inks as well as formaldehyde.

The diagnosis of contact dermal allergy can be difficult to make since many chemicals produce dermatitis via direct contact, nonimmunological methods. Patch testing to prove the existence of cell-mediated immunologic dermatitis should be performed only by a dermatologist with competence in this area. False-negative and false-positive results of patch testing are encountered frequently.[72]

Drug Allergies, Hypersensitivity, and Autoimmunity

Drugs are not complete antigens by virtue of their molecular size. To be a complete immunogen, the molecular weight of the drug must be larger than 5000 daltons. For this reason, antibodies, large proteins such as streptokinase, insulin, and F(ab) fragments can produce an immune response. To be immunogenic, the drug must form a covalent bond with a large protein carrier, and this unique hapten must be recognized as being unusual by the immune system. The immune system may then respond by forming polyclonal antibodies to the drug-protein combination at a variety of antigenic sites around this complex. Because most drugs are incapable of forming a covalent bond with macromolecules, the possibility of a reactive metabolite must be entertained. The formation of epoxides, anhydrides, quinones, oxazelones and other reactive drug metabolites could account for the protein binding and immunogen formation.[73]

Drug hypersensitivity reactions can be classified according to the traditional four types of hypersensitivity mechanisms:[73]

Type I: Anaphylaxis, urticarial reactions, angioedema (IgE-mediated)

Type II: Cytotoxic reactions involving complement

Type III: Immune complex disease, serum sickness

Type IV: Cell-mediated reactions

Frequently, drugs may act by more than one of these mechanisms to produce a hypersensitivity syndrome. The route of absorption of a drug appears to have an influence on clinical allergic manifestations. Anaphylaxis may be less common with parenteral administration of drugs than with oral administration.[74]

Vehicles for drug dissolution, preservatives, and incipients administered with drugs are sometimes responsible for either allergic reactions or act as adjuvants to stimulate the development of allergic reactions. The presence of sulfiting agents in drugs is a well-known cause of allergic reactions in sulfite-sensitive individuals. Sulfites and metasulfites are used in a wide variety of drugs, food products, and beverages as preservatives and antibacterial agents. These include sulfur dioxide, sodium sulfite, sodium bisulfite, potassium bisulfite, and potassium metabisulfite.[75] Clinical cases of bronchospasm and respiratory distress are reported in patients receiving sulfite-containing isoetharine bronchodilator via inhalation.[75–77] An asthmatic patient is described who developed acute bronchospasm, diffuse pruritus, and skin erythema following the intravenous administration of sulfite-containing metoclopramide.[76]

Many preparations of epinephrine, phenylephrine, dexamethasone, lidocaine, aminoglycosides, isoetharine, isoproterenol, and dopamine contain sulfiting agents. The route of administration of these sulfite-containing drugs bears an important relationship to the development of an allergic reaction. It is interesting that there are no reports of allergic reactions following the subcutaneous or intramuscular administration of sulfite-containing medications.[75–77] Investigators have shown that the subcutaneous administration of 10 mg of sulfite to six sulfite-sensitive individuals did not produce an allergic reaction.[78] This dose was ten times the amount of sulfites present in epinephrine solution and yet resulted in no reaction.[75] Apparently, the inhalational and intravenous routes of administration of sulfite-containing drugs are required for allergic reactions.

Drug Hypersensitivity

Drug-related immunologic reactions present as anaphylaxis, bronchospasm, serum sickness, febrile reactions, thrombocytopenia, agranulocytosis, neutropenia, and a variety of rashes. Lymphadenopathy, hepatosplenomegaly, and hepatitis also may be present in autoimmune syndromes. Multiple organ systems may be affected. Common target organs of drug-related immunotoxic reactions are the liver, skin, blood elements, lungs, heart, nervous system, and muscle. These reactions may be IgE mediated, a reaction of the drug with tissues initiating cell-mediated cytotoxicity, or antigen-antibody complexes may be formed following the haptenization of a drug with a larger macromolecule via enzymatic action, which then reacts with complement. The incidence of an acute allergic reaction from a particular drug occurring in a patient without previous exposure to the drug is less than 3 per cent and most likely is closer to less than 1 per cent.[79] Allergic drug reactions constitute about 6 per cent of adverse drug reactions in hospitalized patients.[79] The most common manifestation of these drug allergies is skin rash. These rashes can be urticarial, morbilliform, maculopapular, or erythematous.

Anaphylaxis (Type I, IgE-Mediated). This is an acute, potentially lethal reaction characterized by hypotension, angioedema, bronchospasm, cardiovascular collapse, urticaria, diffuse dermal erythema, pruritus, and laryngeal edema. The onset is usually within minutes, but it can be delayed for up to 2 hours. A result of these reactions is a massive loss of intravascular volume into the interstitial tissues, which exacerbates hypotension. Anaphylaxis has a mortality rate of approximately 10 per cent. Penicillin is the most common cause of drug-induced anaphylaxis. However, many other drugs are also causes. Urticarial reactions to certain drugs may be the only manifestation of IgE-related allergies. Sulfonamides, ampicillin, hydralazine, quinidine, barbiturates, opiates, aminoglycosides, and various sedative-hypnotic drugs have been implicated as causes of acute urticarial reactions.

Serum Sickness (Type III). This is produced by antigen excess causing increased circulating antigen-antibody complexes. Clinical manifestations include fever, arthralgias, urticarial rash, maculopapular rash, vasculitis, or nephritis. The most commonly associated drug is heterologous horse serum, such as is present in antivenin for treatment of snake envenomations. The use of antivenin is associated with an approximate 75 per cent incidence of serum sickness reactions. Drugs recognized to produce serum sickness reactions include penicillins, sulfonamides, thiouracils, phenytoin, cephalosporins, and thiazide diuretics.[74]

Rashes and Dermatitis. Dermatitis is the most common clinical reaction to a wide number of pharmaceuticals. Drug-induced rashes can be maculopapular, urticarial, diffuse erythematous, or morbilliform. Topical application of drugs has resulted in allergic contact dermatitis and eczema. This is a T cell–mediated delayed hypersensitivity reaction. Common skin sensitizers are benzocaine, formaldehyde, bacitracin, neomycin, antihistamines, amines, platinum, nickel, and sulfonamides.

Photoallergic reactions of the skin occur following exposure to certain drugs used either orally or dermally. A photoallergic reaction begins following exposure to certain lengths of ultraviolet radiation in sunlight. Erythematous reactions like a sunburn with vesicle formation are common. Drugs associated with these adverse reactions are oxsoralen, thiazide diuretics, chlordiazepoxide, chlorpromazine, tetracycline, and doxycycline.[79]

Hematologic Reactions (Types II and III). The destruction of formed blood elements by immunologic mechanisms can lead to thrombocytopenia, hemolytic anemia, neutropenia, aplastic anemia, or agranulocytosis. Fever, fatigue, infection, and malaise are the clinical symptoms and signs that result. The actual hematologic lesion may be in the peripheal blood or in the bone marrow, thus affecting the hematopoietic generation of blood cells. Direct cellular cytotoxic reactions are more common than immunologically mediated destruction of these cells.

Thrombocytopenia is probably the most common immunologically mediated hemopathy. Many drugs are known to be associated with or causes of thrombocytopenia[77] (Table 15–10).

Two immunologic reactions may occur in drug-induced thrombocytopenia: Type II and Type III. Drugs that act as haptens (Type II) combine with platelets to form an immunogen. Antibodies are then formed that combine to this immunogen. The second mechanism (Type III) of drug-induced thrombocytopenia involves the formation of a drug-protein hapten that is nonspecifically absorbed to platelets. Antibodies formed to the drug-protein complex initiate complement activation, and the platelets are destroyed by cytotoxic activities or phagocytosis.[73] Clinical manifestations include petechiae, ecchymosis, and, rarely, gastrointestinal bleeding, hemoptysis, and intracranial bleeding. Examination of the bone marrow shows normal megakaryocytes. Following discontinuation of the insulting drug, platelet counts usually return to normal in 2 to 3 weeks. Readministration of the drug can produce rapid onset of thrombocytopenia. Some in vitro tests are available to help determine whether a certain drug has produced thrombocytopenia.[69, 80]

Table 15–10. DRUGS ASSOCIATED WITH THROMBOCYTOPENIA

carbamazepine	methyldopa
gold salts	quinidine
acetaminophen	aspirin
actazolamide	cephalothin
imipramine	digitoxin
chloramphenicol	isoniazid
phenytoin	penicillamine
quinine	procainamide
levodopa	opiates
rifampin	spironolactone
thiazides	sulfonamides
	sulfonylureas

Drug-induced hemolytic anemia from an immunologic cause is mainly a result of Type II and Type III immunologic reactions. Hemolytic anemia is associated with a number of drugs[73] (Table 15–11).

The most common mechanism responsible for drug-induced hemolytic anemia is an immune complex reaction in which the erythrocyte binds to a drug-protein complex to which an antibody has been generated. The binding of the drug-protein complex by the erythrocyte includes the red cell as a target for the antibody and subsequent activation of the complement system. The patient with sensitized erythrocytes may experience a sudden onset of intravascular hemolysis following exposure to the drug. Hemoglobinuria may compromise renal function. The antibody is usually an IgM and can be detected by laboratory testing. A direct positive Coombs test may be present in patients with drug-induced hemolysis from an immunology-mediated mechanism. Penicillin and cephalosporins bind to erythrocytes and can induce IgG antibodies.

Drugs can induce agranulocytosis by immunologic mechanisms. Chloramphenicol-induced bone marrow depression is a well-known phenomenon. Other drugs implicated in agranulocytosis include phenylbutazone, sulfonamides, phenothiazines, gold salts, thiouracils, antihistamines, anticonvulsants, indomethacin, antidepressants, barbiturates, semisynthetic penicillins, and thiouracils.[74] Agranulocytosis may be clinically recognized between the second and eighth week of drug therapy.[74] Patients usually present with fever and secondary infection. The polymorphonuclear count is usually found to be less then 1000 per mm^3. The discontinuation of the drug is followed by reversal of the agranulocytosis and recovery of the patient in the majority of cases.[74] Both the bone marrow and the peripheral granulocytes are involved with maturational arrest of bone marrow stem cells as well as peripheral destruction. Re-exposure to the causative drug may induce sudden leukopenia with concomitant chills, fever, arthralgia, and shock.[74] Immunologic mechanisms involved are thought to be Types II and III.

Table 15–11. DRUGS ASSOCIATED WITH HEMOLYTIC ANEMIAS

phenytoin	sulfonamides
quinidine	tetracycline
rifampin	sulfonylureas
phenacetin	isoniazid
alpha-methyldopa	ibuprofen
quinine	cis-platin
penicillin	cephalosporins

Drug-Induced Autoimmunity

Clinical manifestations of drug-induced autoimmunity include systemic lupus erythematosus, scleroderma, and Sjögren's syndrome. Immunopathology can result in nephritis, hepatitis, hemolytic anemia, polyarthritis, myalgia, alveolitis, fever, lymphadenopathy, dermatitis, leukopenia, and other blood dyscrasias.[74] Symptom onset usually occurs following several weeks or months of therapy. Systemic lupus erythematosus (SLE) is probably the best-known manifestation of autoimmunity secondary to drug therapy. The drugs most commonly associated with SLE are procainamide, isoniazid, and hydralazine.[74] Other drugs associated with a lupus-like syndrome are methyldopa, antimalarials, thiouracils, tetracycline, practolol and other beta-receptor blocking drugs, phenytoin, and penicillamine.[79] Adverse reactions to the combination drug pyrimethamine-sulfadoxine (Fansidar) have included erythema multiforme, Stevens-Johnson syndrome, and toxic epidermal necrolysis.[81] Practolol has been associated with connective tissue disease similar to Sjögren's syndrome. Autoantibodies to beta$_2$-adrenergic drug receptors have been found in a few patients with autonomic abnormalities.[82] Interstitial nephritis and polymyositis have been reported following institution of cimetidine therapy.[83] Allergic reactions to cisplatinum, including asthma and anaphylaxis, have been reported.[84]

Drug-induced lupus, manifested by antinuclear antibodies and clinical symptoms, occurs in two thirds of patients taking procainamide over several weeks to months. Approximately 10 per cent of patients taking hydralazine develop lupus syndrome. Up to 20 per cent of patients taking isoniazid will develop antinuclear antibodies during therapy.[74] Serum complement concentrations usually remain normal in drug-induced lupus syndromes. Clinical symptomatology includes arthralgias, pleuritic pain, adenopathy, fever, rash, and hepatosplenomegaly.[79] In addition to elevated antinuclear-antibody titers, the laboratory findings may include eosinophilia, anemia, and leukopenia along with an elevated erythrocyte sedimentation rate. Discontinuation of the drug usually results in disappearance of clinical symptoms.

Immunologically, drug-induced hepatitis may be manifested by hepatocellular injury, necrosis, and cholestasis associated with fever, rashes, fatigue as well lymphadenopathy, and eosinophilia. Many drugs produce relatively asymptomatic rises in hepatic enzymes. This is true of ranitidine as well as oral contraceptives. Terminating use of the suspected drug offender usually results in clearing of symptoms as well as reversal of hepatic dysfunction. Chlorpromazine was one of the initial drugs to be suspected as a cause of allergic hepatitis.[74] Other phenothiazines and chlordiazepoxide also have been associated with cholestatic jaundice.[74] Halothane has been known to induce a severe, life-threatening hepatitis with hepatocellular necrosis in previously exposed individuals. Studies have demonstrated that patients with halothane hepatitis have antibodies of the IgG variety, which react with halothane-carrier conjugates in livers of previously exposed animals or humans.[85] Other drugs associated with allergic hepatitis include phenytoin, penicillamine, sulfonamides, and methyldopa. A liver biopsy may aid in the diagnosis if an eosinophilic infiltrate is present. Otherwise, the liver biopsy histology is not discernible from viral hepatitis–induced hepatocellular necrosis.

Clinical Diagnosis of Drug-Induced Hypersensitivity

Diagnosing a drug-related or drug-caused hypersensitivity disorder is based on the following criteria:[85]

- The reaction occurs following repeat or multiple exposures to the drug in question.
- There is at least a 7-day or greater lag time in the appearance of symptoms, which suggests that a period of sensitization and antibody formation to the drug has occurred.
- Clinical symptoms may include fever, arthralgia, hepatitis, nephritis, and malaise, as well as a blood picture of eosinophilia.
- The reaction is independent of the dose.
- Symptoms abate on termination of the drug unless a drug-related auto-immune disorder is produced by the drug.
- Symptoms return on readministration of the drug.
- The most specific test to demonstrate hypersensitivity is finding specific antibodies or sensitized T cells that react with the drug, drug metabolites, or a drug-serum protein hapten combination. However, this is not always possible to obtain.

Currently, procedures used to detect drug-related antibodies include radioallergsorbent tests (RAST) and enzyme-linked immunosorbent assays (ELISA).[85] These tests can detect the presence of IgG, IgM, IgE, IgA, and IgD antibodies. The detection of drug-induced T cell sensitization is by way of the lymphocyte transformation (LT) test. This involves incubating lymphocytes of patients suspected of drug allergy along with the drug and examining the specimen for lymphocyte blastogenesis.[85]

"Multiple Chemical Sensitivities"

Many of the chemicals and drugs that are documented to produce immune suppression and alteration in animal models have not been adequately assessed for similar effects in humans. However, an increasing number of people have a diverse variety of medical complaints originating from environmental exposures, which are termed "multiple chemical sensitivities." The "syndrome" of multiple chemical sensitivities (MCS) is thought to arise from exposure to the many low-level chemical pollutants in the work and home environment that act as immunotoxins to alter the immune system.[5] Controversy over MCS as a real disease has raged for the past several years.

The MCS syndrome is stated to be an immunologic dysfunction by "clinical ecology" groups.[86] Patients proclaiming to have MCS generally complain of a vague syndrome consisting of neurobehavioral disorders, memory disturbance, abdominal pains, pain in the extremities, fatigue, headache, myalgias, and skin discolorations. Generally, no organ pathology or objective signs of disease can be found in these individuals, and no conclusive evidence of disease is present.[86a, b] Occasionally patients are discovered to have autoimmune disease or other pathology as a basis for their clinical complaints.

Many MCS patients have visited "clinical ecologists" who have performed unsophisticated provocative challenge tests on them in closed booths. Surveys of these challenge tests indicate the subjective nature of their end-point measurements and thus invite objective skepticism of their validity. However, by means of these uncontrolled and irreproducible tests, some patients are led to believe that they have contracted an immunologic illness from their environmental exposures. Many individuals so diagnosed by clinical ecologists seek legal compensation for injury based on unscientific studies with unvalidated conclusions. The only logical and ethical approach to patients with alleged MCS is to perform rational clinical and laboratory evaluation of their immune functions and present the patients with objective data to identify causes of their medical complaints. Psychiatric intervention may be necessary because of the hysteria, depression, and anxiety resulting from the patient's inability to work and live in a normal environment. Many people spend large sums of money in building special rooms and houses to separate themselves from the "contaminated" environment. In many situations, these people feel that they are forced to terminate their employment owing to continuing exposures.

Drugs of Abuse

The chronic abuse of alcohol, narcotics, and other substances has been documented to result in a number of clinical immunologic problems in human addict populations.[87–91] The increased susceptibility of alcoholics to pneumonia and other infections is well known. In addition to alcohol, other substances of abuse such as phencyclidine, cocaine, marijuana, and amphetamine have been associated with immune system alterations in animal models as well as in humans. The lifestyles and other habits of drug addicts also may be partially responsible for some of the immune system pathology, particularly the lifestyles of chronic intravenous drug abusers.

Drug abusers in general may have a variety of immune dysfunctions that may be silently present or obvious as clinical immunopathology.[92] Opportunistic infections, increased T helper lymphocytes, and decreased numbers of T suppressor lymphocytes have been documented in polydrug abusers.[93] Circulating immune complexes also may be found in polydrug abusers.[92] There is an apparent enhancement of humoral-mediated immunity in drug abusers, manifested by increased serum concentrations of IgG and IgM.[94] Drug abusers also have been found to have an increased risk of cancer, increased T suppressor function, increased IgG, and anergy to skin tests.[95] Intravenous drug abuse is the second leading cause of the acquired immunodeficiency syndrome (AIDS).

Narcotic abusers have a higher incidence of endocarditis and septicemia as well as increased serum concentrations of IgA, IgG, and IgM.[96–100] One clinical study demonstrated circulating immune complexes in up to 55 per cent of heroin addicts.[99] In patients who have died from heroin-associated pulmonary edema, pulmonary deposits of C_3 complement, IgM, IgG, and IgA have been found at autopsy.[94] Cell-mediated immunity, mitogen stimulation of T cells, and phagocytosis have not been found to be abnormal in narcotic addicts.[101] Immunologically induced thrombocytopenic purpura has been documented in some narcotic abusers.[87] Some chronic intravenous narcotic addicts have been found to have elevated platelet-reactive IgG titers.[87]

Phencyclidine (PCP) has been found to act as an immunodepressant in vitro and binds to lymphocyte subpopulations of both T cells and B cells.[102] In a biologic assay, PCP caused a depression in antibody production as well as cellular immunity depression.[102]

Controversy surrounds the immune effects of marijuana use. Some investigators have discovered decreased mitogen stimulation of lymphocytes, decreased lymphocyte numbers, and impaired mixed lymphocyte culture response.[92] Other investigators found normal mitogen responses in marijuana users.[92] Cocaine is known to have an adverse effect on nonspecific human cellular defense.[103] Fatal cerebral mucormycosis associated with pronounced lymphopenia has been reported in intravenous amphetamine abusers.[88] Mucormycosis is an opportunistic fungus that can infect immunosuppressed individuals and is most likely introduced via intravenous use of needles.

CHEMICALLY INDUCED DISORDERS OF PHAGOCYTES

The pulmonary system is assaulted by a variety of vapors, metals, fumes, fibers, and particles, which macrophages are responsible for removing or neutralizing. Pulmonary host defense macrophages are found in interstitial tissues of the alveoli or free in the alveolar luminal surface. The ability of the macrophage system to effectively clear particles from the lung is an important defense function. The effectiveness and efficiency of phagocytosis and the lytic functions by pulmonary macrophages dictate the ultimate level of host protection. Any chemical or particulate matter that interferes with either the absolute macrophage number or basic functions can produce pulmonary susceptibility to damage. Macrophage elimination of particles involves the following steps:[17]

1. Chemotaxis
2. Opsonization by complement and antibody
3. Attachment of particle to phagocyte
4. Phagocytosis of particle
5. Formation of primary lysosome
6. Fusion with secondary lysosome
7. Destruction of particle

Because of the number of sensitive functions performed by macrophages, interruption of normal pulmonary host defense can occur if any one event is interfered with by an environmental pollutant. A variety of environmental pollutants have been found to stimulate increased numbers of macrophages in the pulmonary environment: lead oxide (PbO), nickel chloride ($NiCl_2$), nickel oxide (NiO), cadmium chloride ($CdCl_2$), carbon monoxide, quartz crystals, tobacco smoke, and a variety of environmental dusts.[17] Some environmental contaminants do the opposite and reduce the absolute number of free pulmonary macrophages: silica, chrysotile asbestos, cadmium fumes, acrolein from products of combustion, manganese dioxide (MnO_2), some lead oxides (Pb_2O_3), and antimony fumes.[17]

The ultimate fate of the macrophage that ingests particles entering the respiratory system depends on whether the cell can destroy the particle or whether the particle destroys the cell. If the macrophage is killed, the toxin is then released into the lung environment to promote further damage. In some situations, macrophage viability is affected but cell lysis does not occur.

Phagocytic functions of macrophages can be directly affected by a range of environmental chemicals and contaminants. Acute exposure of macrophages to ozone (O_3) or nitrous oxide (NO_2) can decrease phagocytic ability.[17, 104] Other chemicals directly impairing macrophage phagocytic functions include nickel chloride ($NiCL_2$), cadmium, nickel, copper, mercury, zinc, platinum, vanadium oxides (V_2O_5), and cadmium oxide (CdO). The shape, size, chemical composition, and surface area of the inhaled particles determine ultimate macrophage dysfunction.

The capacity of macrophages to combat viral infections is depressed by certain environmental chemicals. Interferon production by macrophages is depressed after exposure to ozone, automobile exhaust, and NO_2.[17] Alteration of macrophage lysosomal enzymes and release of these enzymes as well as other biologically active substances is promoted by some environmental contaminants. These substances include prostaglandins, collagenase, elastase, plasminogen-activating factor, and lytic enzymes. Asbestos and silica particles stimulate the release of lysosomal enzymes, which subsequently elicit inflammatory processes with tissue destruction and fibrosis of the lungs. The macrophage particle contents are then released and the cycle is repeated.[17, 104] Thus a number of environmental metals, as well as vapors and pollutants, can reduce pulmonary host defense against both bacterial and viral infections by affecting macrophage immune functions.

CLINICAL EVALUATION FOR IMMUNOTOXICITY

Clinical evaluation of the immune system can involve much expense and unnecessary testing. The clinical utility of exhaustive immunologic testing has been questioned.[105] Patients with suspected immunotoxicity can be diagnostically screened to examine humoral-mediated immunity (HMI), cell-mediated immunity (CMI), phagocyte function, complement function, and autoimmunity. The evaluation of the patient should include a careful history and physical examination, with particular attention to the classic signs and symptoms of immune disorders. These include pyogenic infections that recur after antibiotic therapy, infections from opportunistic microorganisms, and some neoplasias (Table 15–12). These infections may take the form of dermal abscesses or pneumonias from a variety of microbial sources.

Because of the complexity of the immune system, with its multiple cellular, humoral, and host defense functions, clinical assessment can be difficult. A large number of laboratory tests can provide detailed evaluations of HMI, CMI, complement, and phagocyte functioning. However, these tests are not required in the great majority of clinical immunologic evaluations. It is possible to have insight into immune lesions, though, by combining a number of in vitro and in vivo testing procedures. However, the ultimate end-point in determining proper functioning of the immune system is an intact host defense. Because of the dynamic nature of the immune system, test results will provide information only about a particular area of the immune system at one particular time. Also, it is difficult to distinguish immune dysfunctions that occur as a result of disease secondary to the immune lesion from those that are a result of the initial lesion.

Immunodeficiencies are categorized as primary and secondary. Primary immunodeficiencies usually present at an early age. Secondary or acquired immunodeficiencies may occur at any age and have a variety of etiologies. Physical examination should include evaluation of host defense mechanisms, such as normal pulmonary function studies, intact dermal barrier, presence of cancers, or use of immunosuppressive drugs and drugs of abuse. Clinical evaluation for drug- or chemical-induced immune dysfunction can be frustrating and difficult to make a causal connection to the xenobiotic in question or even to discover the immune lesion. Part of the problem in making a toxic causation argument involving an environmental chemical is that humans are exposed to low levels of multiple chemicals in their everyday work and home environments.

Table 15–12. CLINICAL INFECTIONS AND DISEASE FROM IMMUNE DYSFUNCTION

T CELL DYSFUNCTION	B CELL DYSFUNCTION
Epstein-Barr virus	Recurrent bacterial skin infection
Herpes simplex virus	*Streptococcus pneumoniae*
Herpes zoster virus	*Haemophilus influenzae*
Cytomegalovirus	Bacterial conjunctivitis
Mycobacteria	Bacterial pneumonia
Candida albicans	*Giardia lamblia*
Cryptococcus neoformans	
Pneumocystis carinii	
Toxoplasma gondii	
Cryptosporidium	
Lymphomas	

Screening for Clinical Immunologic Defects

The evaluation of immunotoxicity in a patient parallels the tier testing of chemicals, using first a screening panel and then secondary, more specific tests as needed. The screening panel of tests for evaluation of immune function in a patient should be performed before more elaborate and expensive testing is undertaken. Eight immunologic tests have been critiqued by the World Health Organization's (WHO) immunology sections.[105] WHO recommended that these diagnostic tests be performed before any more elaborate and expensive tests are conducted in evaluation of the immune system. These initial tests plus other useful screens include the following (Fig. 15–4):

1. Protein electrophoresis
2. Immunoelectrophoresis
3. CBC with absolute lymphocyte and neutrophil counts
4. Quantitative immunoglobulins
5. Skin testing for delayed hypersensitivity
6. Complement function tests CH_{50}, C_3, C_4
7. Autoantibodies (antinuclear, anti-DNA, rheumatoid factor)
8. Isoantibody titers
9. Common viral titers (Epstein-Barr, CMV)

A variety of other in-depth confirmatory immunologic tests can be performed beyond this initial screening (Figs. 15–5 and 15–6). The judicious use of these tests and their proper interpretation are essential in the evaluation of possible immune disorders.[106]

Immunoglobulin Quantitation and Protein Electrophoresis

These tests are easily obtained and give direct information concerning the absence of an immunoglobulin class.[106] The three major immunoglobulins measured are IgG, IgM, and IgA. IgE can be measured if allergies are part of the clinical syndrome. Hypogamma-

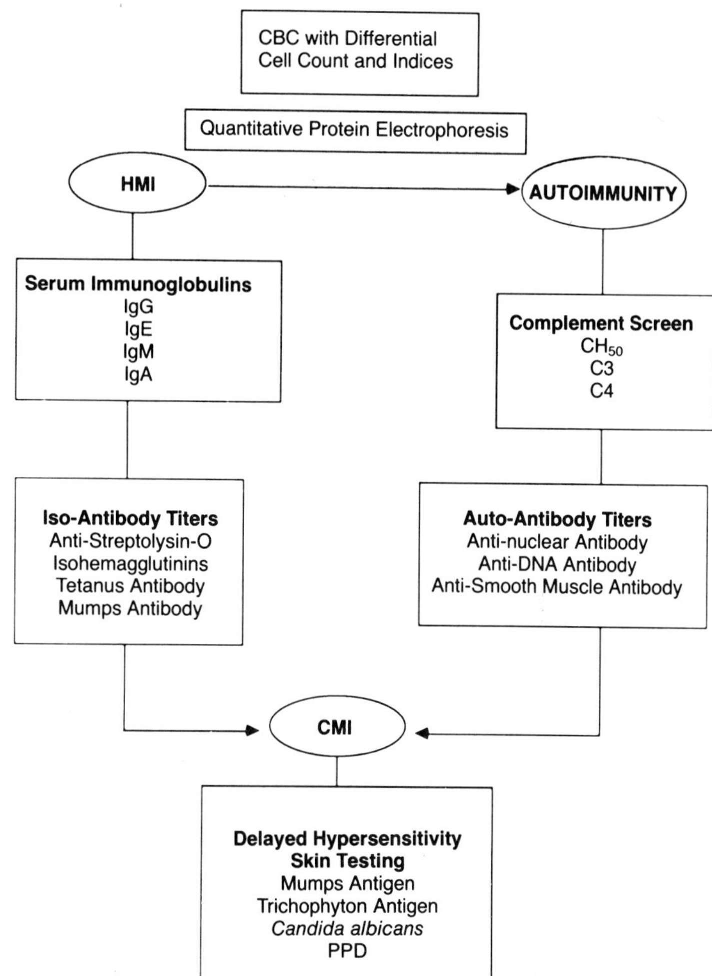

Figure 15–4. Clinical immunotoxicity screening tests.

globulinemias are usually the result of a secondary immune deficiency. The most frequent immunoglobulin deficiency is IgA, and in 50 per cent of these cases the patient is clinically asymptomatic.[107]

Secretory IgA is a mucosal barrier defense mechanism, and its assay is separate from the measurement of regular IgA.[107] Examination of the protein electrophoretic pattern can indicate quickly whether a patient has normal concentrations of immunoglobulins, hypogammaglobulinemia, or dysgammaglobulinemia.

Immunoelectrophoresis

Immunoelectrophoresis identifies the major immunoglobulin classes as well as immunoproliferative disorders. Measurement of total specific IgE is rarely useful or needed in most immunology investigations. Instead, IgE determination should be reserved for investigation of allergic syndromes when elevation of IgE would be diagnostic in separating the disease from non-IgE–mediated allergic phenomena.[105, 106]

Cell-Mediated Immunity

Cell-mediated immunity defects are recognized by clinical symptoms of infections associated with common CMI functions. These functions are related to killing of intracellular pathogens, delayed hypersensitivity reactions to recognized antigens, tumor cell rejection, contact dermatitis, and tissue injury from autoimmunity. Diagnostic evaluation of cell-mediated immunity involves both

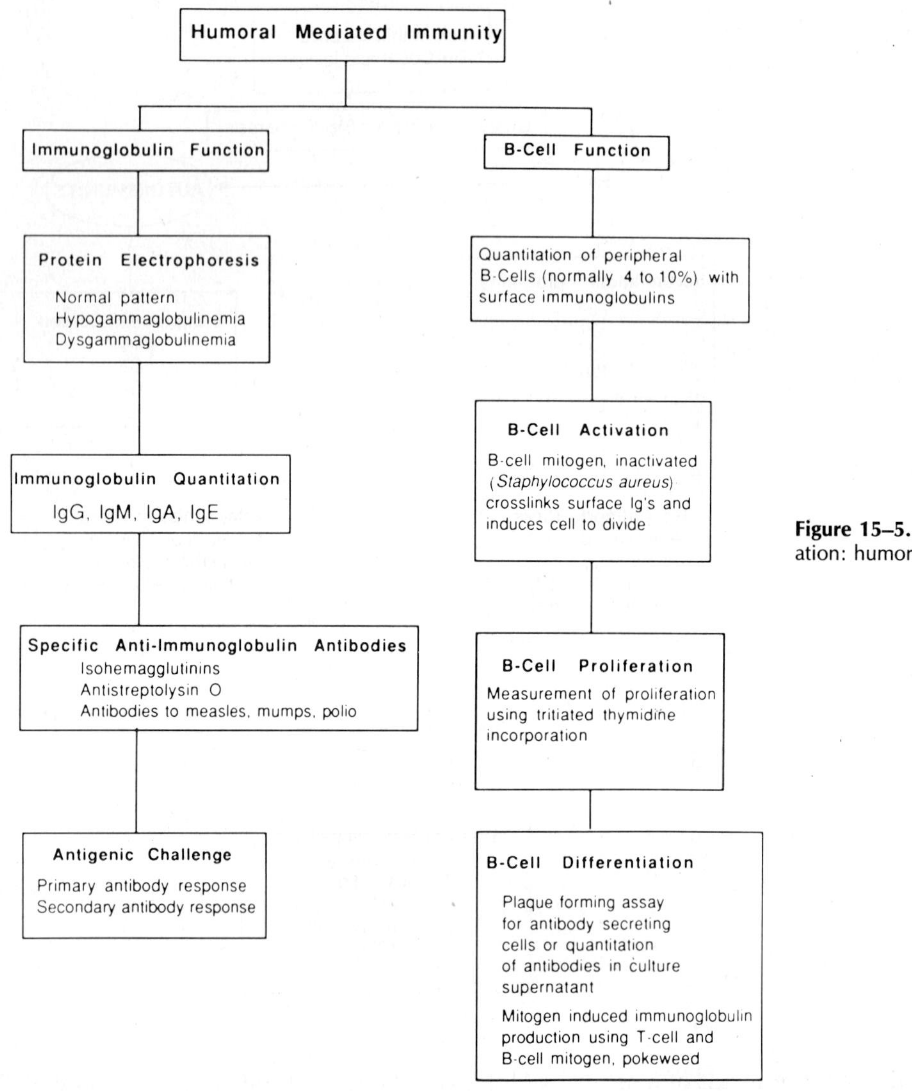

Figure 15–5. Immunotoxicity evaluation: humoral-mediated immunity.

in vivo and in vitro testing procedures (Fig. 15–6). Defects are seen usually as an increase in infections with agents such as viruses, intercellular pathogens, and fungi. Cell-mediated immunity of a patient can be evaluated by the following:

Peripheral lymphocyte count
Skin tests for delayed hypersensitivity
Quantitation of T cell subsets
T cell response to mitogens
Lymphokine release
Mixed lymphocyte reaction (MLR)
Generation of cytotoxic T cells
T cell helper/suppressor function
Natural killer cell function
Antibody-dependent cell cytotoxicity (ADCC)

Lymphocyte Count

Any significant decrease in the number of T lymphocytes will result in a lymphopenia in peripheral blood smears since they make up approximately 75 to 85 per cent of the peripheral blood lymphocyte population. The absolute lymphocyte count should exceed 1500. Determination of the number of T cells in peripheral blood is also performed by using the sheep erythrocyte rosette formation method.[106] Another, more sophisticated method for enumerating T cells involves the use of fluorescent-labeled monoclonal antibodies directed against mature T cells.[106]

Delayed Hypersensitivity

Skin tests to measure delayed hypersensitivity can be performed with common anti-

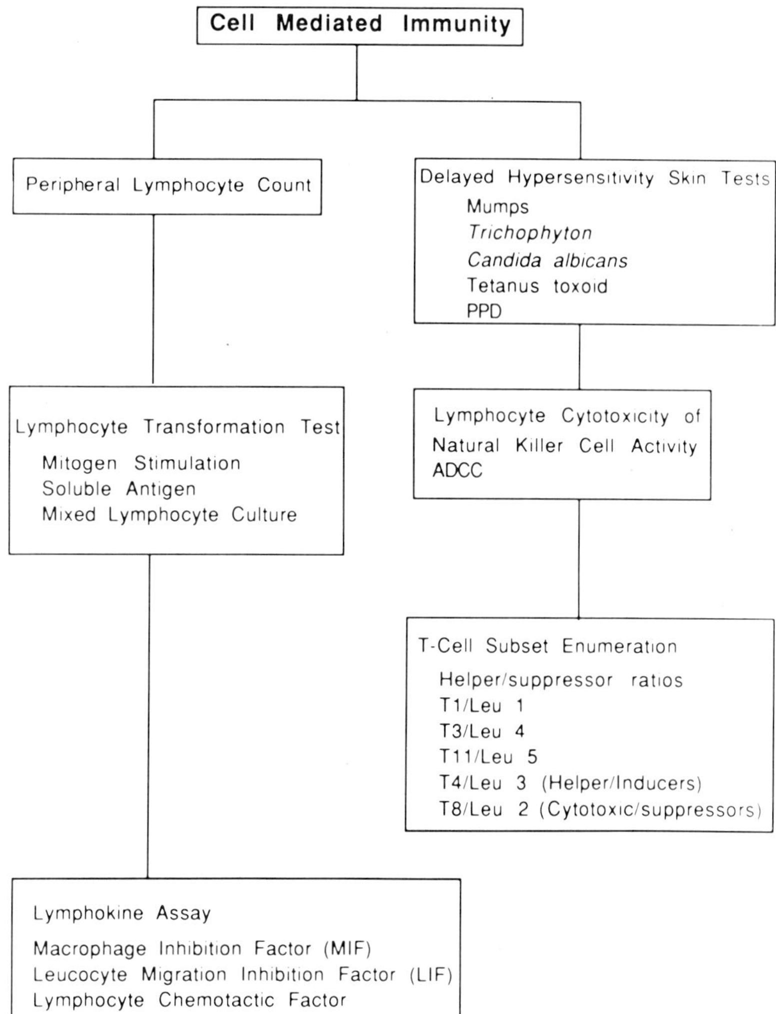

Figure 15–6. Immunotoxicity evaluation: cell-mediated immunity.

gens. An erythematous dermal reaction and induration greater than 10 mm in diameter, at 24, 48, or 72 hours after intradermal injection of 0.1 ml of the antigen into the volar surface of the forearm, indicates that a complex series of cell-mediated events occurred: the antigen was recognized by lymphocytes and processed appropriately, helper/inducer T cells were activated, lymphokines were secreted, and recruitment of nonsensitized lymphocytes to the antigen deposition area occurred.[105, 106] Development of a positive skin test depends on previous antigen exposure; commonly employed skin tests are mumps, tetanus toxoid, trichophyton, purified protein derivative (PPD), and *Candida albicans*. A positive skin test for delayed hypersensitivity indicates a normally functioning cell-mediated immune system, and 95 per cent of the normal population will react to three of five skin tests.[108] Standardization of skin test antigens has been a problem; lack of standardized reagents may complicate the skin test. This should be checked before applying any skin tests. Also, a negative result may indicate an inproperly administered test and not an immune defect.

Delayed hypersensitivity skin tests are useful in surveying the functioning of CMI. Over 90 per cent of normal adults will react to one or more of the common skin test antigens by 48 hours (*Candida albicans*, trichophyton, tetanus toxoid, mumps, streptokinase-streptodornase, coccidioidin).[106] The skin tests are checked at 24, 48, and 72 hours. A positive reaction consists of 5 mm or more of erythema and induration by 24 to 48 hours.[106] A positive delayed hypersensitivity skin test indicates an intact and normally functioning cell-mediated immune system.

Autoantibodies

Measurement of autoantibodies can be useful in diagnosing mixed connective tissue disease, chronic active hepatitis, and systemic lupus. The commonly measured autoantibodies are antibodies against nuclei, smooth muscle, DNA, and thyroid tissue. Antimitochondrial antibodies are characteristic of primary biliary cirrhosis.[106]

Antiviral Titers

Certain antiviral titers, such as Epstein-Barr virus and hepatitis A and B, may be useful in delineating a chronic viral infection from disease that is thought to be an immune dysfunction from an environmental chemical source. In addition, many autoimmune diseases and chronic inflammatory states may be misdiagnosed as an immunotoxicity from xenobiotics. Complete and detailed testing of the immune system can be entertained if an abnormality is demonstrated in the initial screening (see later sections). However, these detailed tests are uncommonly required if sound clinical judgment is employed in evaluating a suspected immune dysfunction.

Isoantibodies

Normally, humans have antibodies that are formed against common antigens to which everyone is exposed. These antibodies occur as a normal response and can be quantified: isohemagglutinins, antistreptolysin-O, antibodies to measles, mumps, and polio, and tetanus toxoid immunizations.[105, 106]

Antigenic Challenge

The primary and secondary immune response to an antigen can be determined in humans in some situations. Evaluation of the primary immune response requires an antigen to which the person has never been exposed. This can produce some problems and introduce risk to the patient. The secondary immune response is easier to evaluate and can be as easy as administration of tetanus toxoid and measuring antibody titers. However, the primary immune response is usually the most sensitive to immunosuppressants.

T Cell Subsets and Helper: Cytotoxic/Suppressor Functions

In some situations, quantitation of T cell subpopulations may be indicated. This can be accomplished using monoclonal antibodies directed against specific T cell surface receptors.[106] Helper and suppressor cells can be enumerated in peripheral blood using monoclonal antibody assays that are commercially available. Actual helper/suppressor cell function is assessed using in vitro antibody plaque-forming assays.[109] The most common monoclonal antibodies for the identification and quantitation of T cell subsets are the Leu and OK series.[110] T helper cells, which comprise about 50 to 60 per cent of the T lymphocyte population, have surface membrane receptors for the Fc portion of IgM antibody. T suppressor cells have receptors for the Fc region of IgG antibody, and these cells make up 25 to 35 per cent of the T lymphocyte population. Helper T cells also have OKT4 and Leu-3 antigens, whereas cytotoxic/suppressor T cells have OKT8 and Leu-2 surface antigens.[110] The normal helper:suppressor ratio is 1.8 to 2.2. Patients with acquired immunodeficiency syndrome (AIDS) may have helper/suppressor ratios of less than 1.0;[110] however, a low ratio is not diagnostic of AIDS and can occur in other conditions.

Phagocytes

For proper functioning of the immune system, especially the HMI, the participation of nonimmune cells and complement is critical to protect effectively the host against infectious agents. Both the complement system and phagocytes must function normally for antibody to provide host defense. Phagocytes are divided into neutrophils and macrophages (monocytes). A complete evaluation of phagocyte functions includes the following tests: neutrophil count in peripheral blood; nitroblue tetrazolium reduction; chemotaxis; phagocytosis; and killing ability. However, not all these tests are needed in screening for abnormalities. The absolute neutrophil count should be obtained by Wright's stain of a peripheral blood smear. This may reveal any neutrophil morphologic abnormalities. A PMN count of less than 1000 per mm^3 is associated with an increased risk of infection. There are many causes of neutropenia, including infections, drugs, and familial factors. Neutropenia that is drug- or chemical-induced may be due to peripheral PMN destruction from an autoimmunity or to depression of granulocyte formation in the bone marrow.

Critical functions of neutrophils are chemotaxis, phagocytosis, and killing of ingested microbial agents. Interference with any one of these functions can produce clinical disease. PMN chemotaxis is typically determined using the Boyden chamber in vitro and the Rebuck skin window technique in vivo.[111] Ingestion and oxidative killing functions of neutrophils can be measured using the nitroblue tetrazolium reduction test.[112] It is a limited test and is most useful for the diagnosis of chronic granulomatous disease. Another test of phagocytosis is the elicitation of chemiluminescence, which is counted in a scintillation counter.[112] It is based on the instability of the superoxide ion that activates luminol in the assay system after superoxide dissociation. The extracellular release of β-glucuronidase can be used to determine PMN degranulation.[112]

Complement

The complement system can be screened by most clinical laboratories by quantifying C_3 (alternate complement pathway), C_4 (classical pathway), and CH_{50} (total complement). The measurement of CH_{50} is most useful for monitoring immune complex diseases like glomerulonephritis or systemic lupus.[105, 106] The complement system consists of the alternate and classical pathways. Deficiencies in selected complement components can present with different disease patterns. Indications for assaying complement function are repeated infections by pyogenic bacteria, systemic bacterial infections, or suspected autoimmune disease. Some of the clinical syndromes associated with inappropriate activation of complement include recurring angioedema, chronic urticaria, palpable purpura, arthralgias, cutaneous vasculitides, unexplained fever, nephritis, and arthritides.[113]

A screening method for proper complement function involves quantification of total hemolytic complement (CH_{50}), C_3, and C_4. Most clinical laboratories can measure C_3 and C_4. Reduced serum concentration of the C_4, a component of the classical pathway, is a sensitive indicator of a low-level activation of the complement system. C_3 usually has a high serum concentration, and its measurement provides information about the alternate complement pathway. A normal C_4 with a low concentration of C_3 indicates alternate pathway activation of the complement system.[110] The overall functioning of the complement system is best screened for by the CH_{50} measurement, which reflects the amount of serum necessary to lyse 50 per cent of a suspension of sheep erythrocytes coated with anti-red cell antibody.[110] Low C_3, C_4, and CH_{50} are associated with classical pathway activation. Normal C_3 and C_4 with a low CH_{50} suggest a deficiency of one of the other complement components.

Other complement components are not necessary in general screening situations. However, they are available to be measured and include C_1 esterase; C_1, C_2, C_5, and C_6 through C_9; and C1q binding.

Activation of the complement system and the presence of autoantibodies indicate immune complex diseases and autoimmunity. Positive results for immune complexes, the presence of certain autoantibodies, and complement system activation should encourage the clinician to search for end-organ pathology in specific organ systems involved in the clinical syndrome. Negative results in the immune complex assays for complement and autoantibodies are helpful in ruling out a humoral-mediated cause of clinical disease.

SUMMARY

How far should the clinician proceed in the evaluation of a suspected immune dysfunction? Many elaborate in vivo and in vitro tests are available to assess the immune system. Many of these tests require specialized laboratories; some are still research tools, and they can be expensive. Clinical judgment must take the place of random testing from which no diagnostic or therapeutic decision can be reached. A basic history of toxic or environmental exposure, a careful physical examination, and appropriate use of screening immunologic tests can be useful in guiding the clinician in the evaluation of patients with suspected immunotoxicities. Ruling out other causes, such as collagen vascular disease, autoimmunity, and neoplasia, is essential. A screening battery of general clinical tests as well as a screening panel of immunology tests should precede a full laboratory evaluation of the immune system. If these screening tests are abnormal, then consultation should be sought, and more specific immunologic tests can be performed.

References

1. Bekesi JG, Holland JF, Anderson HA, Fischbein AS, Rom W, Wolff MS, Selikoff IJ: Lymphocyte function of Michigan dairy farmers exposed to polybrominated biphenyls. Science *199*:1207–1209, 1978.
2. Aksoy M: Benzene as a leukemogenic and carcinogenic agent. Am J Ind Med *8*:9–20, 1985.
3. Kjeldsberg CR, Ward HP: Leukemia in arsenic poisoning. Ann Intern Med *77*:935–937, 1972.
4. Welch K, Higgins I, Oh M, Burchfiel C: Arsenic exposure, smoking, and respiratory cancer in copper smelter workers. Arch Environ Health *37*:325–335, 1982.
5. Cullen MR: The worker with multiple chemical sensitivities: An overview. Occup Med 2:655–662, 1987.
6. Terr AI: Multiple chemical sensitivities—Immunologic critique of clinical ecology theories and practice. Occup Med 2:655–662, 1987.
7. Thrasher JD, Broughton A, Micevich P: Antibodies and immune profiles of individuals occupationally exposed to formaldehyde: Six case reports. Am J Ind Med *14*:479–488, 1988.
8. Nossal GJV: Current concepts: Immunology. The basic components of the immune system. N Engl J Med *316*:1320–1325, 1987.
9. Graziano FM, Bell C: The normal immune response and what can go wrong. Med Clin North Am *69*:439–452, 1985.
10. Roitt IM, Brostoff J, Male DK: Cells involved in the immune response. *In* Roitt IM, Brostoff J, Male DK (eds): Immunology. St. Louis, CV Mosby, 1985, pp 2.1–2.15.
11. Reinherz EL, Schlossman SF: Current concepts in immunology: Regulation of the immune response–inducer and suppressor T-lymphocyte subsets in human beings. N Engl J Med *303*:370–380, 1980.
12. Roitt IM, Brostoff J, Male DK: Antibody structure and function. *In* Roitt IM, Brostoff J, Male DK (eds): Immunology. St. Louis, CV Mosby, 1985, pp 5.1–5.9.
13. Roitt IM, Brostoff J, Male DK: Major histocompatibility complex. *In* Roitt IM, Brostoff J, Male DK (eds): Immunology. St. Louis, CV Mosby, 1985, pp 4.1–4.11.
14. Flier JS, Underhill LH: The human T-cell receptor: Structure and function. N Engl J Med *312*:1100–1111, 1985.
15. Fudenberg HH, Whitten HD: Immunostimulation: Synthetic and biological modulators of immunity. Annu Rev Pharmacol Toxicol *24*:147–174, 1984.
16. Adams DO, Hamilton TA: The cell biology of macrophage activation. Annu Rev Immunol 2:283–318, 1984.
17. Gardner DE: Alterations in macrophage functions by environmental chemicals. Environ Health Perspec *55*:343–358, 1984.
18. Herberman RB, Ortaldo JR: Natural killer cells: Their role in defenses against disease. Science *214*:24–30, 1982.
19. Dean JH, Murray MJ, Ward EC: Toxic responses of the immune system. *In* Klaassen CD, Amdur MO, Doull J (eds): Casarett and Doull's Toxicology: The Basic Science of Poisons. New York, Macmillan, 1986, pp 245–285.
20. Dean JH, Vos JG: An introduction to immunotoxicology assessment. *In* Descotes J (ed): Immunotoxicology of Drugs and Chemicals. New York, Elsevier, 1986, pp 3–18.
21. Luster MI, Dean JH, Moore JA: Evaluation of immune functions in toxicology. *In* Hayes AW (ed): Principles and Methods of Toxicology. New York, Raven Press, 1982, pp 561–586.
22. Dean JH, Padarathsingh ML, Jerrells TR: Assessment of immunobiological effects induced by chemicals, drugs or food additives. I. Tier testing and screening approach. Drug Chem Toxicol 2:5–17, 1979.
23. Luster MI, Dean JH: Immunological hypersensitivity resulting from environmental or occupational exposure to chemicals: A state-of-the-art workshop summary. Fund Appl Toxicol 2:327–330, 1982.
24. Herberman RB: Immunologic mechanisms of host resistance to tumors. *In* Dean JH, Luster MI, Munson AE, Amos H (eds): Immunotoxicology and Immunopharmacology. New York, Raven Press, 1985, pp 69–77.
25. Cunningham AJ: A method of increased sensitivity for detecting single antibody forming cells. Nature *20*:1106–1107, 1965.
26. Reynolds CW, Herberman RB: In vitro augmentation of rat natural killer (NK) cell activity. J Immunol *126*:1581–1585, 1981.
27. Dean JH, Luster MI, Boorman GA, Leubke RW, Lauer LD: Application of tumor, bacterial and parasite susceptibility assays to study immune alterations induced by environmental chemicals. Environ Health Perspect *43*:81–88, 1982.
28. Cullen MR, Kayne RD, Robins JM: Endocrine and reproductive dysfunction in men associated with occupational inorganic lead intoxication. Arch Environ Health *39*:431–440, 1984.
29. Koller LD: Review/Commentary: Immunotoxicology of heavy metals. Int J Immunopharmacol 2:269–279, 1980.
30. Koller LD: Effects of environmental contaminants on the immune system. Adv Vet Sci Comp Med *23*:267–295, 1979.
31. Druet P, Bernard A, Hirsch F, Weening JJ, Gengoux P, Mahieu P, Birkeland S: Immunologically mediated glomerulonephritis induced by heavy metals. Arch Toxicol *50*:187–194, 1982.
32. Koller LD, Exon JH, Roan JG: Antibody suppression by cadmium. Arch Environ Health *30*:598–601, 1975.
33. Reigart JR, Graber CD: Evaluation of the humoral immune response of children with low level lead exposure. Bull Environ Contam Toxicol *16*:112–117, 1976.
34. Sachs HK: Intercurrent infection in lead poisoning. Am J Dis Child *132*:315–316, 1978.

35. Lam S, Chan-Yeung M: Occupational asthma: Natural history, evaluation and management. Occup Med 2:373–381, 1987.
36. Grammer LC: Occupational immunologic lung disease. *In* Patterson R (ed): Allergic Diseases: Diagnosis and Management. Philadelphia, JB Lippincott, 1985, pp 691–708.
37. Royle H: Toxicity of chromic acid in the chromium plating industry (2). Environ Res *10*:141–163, 1975.
38. Sprince NL, Kazemi H: Beryllium disease. *In* Rom WN (ed): Environmental and Occupational Medicine. Boston, Little, Brown, 1983, pp 481–490.
39. Krivanek N, Reeves AL: The effect of chemical forms of beryllium on the production of the immunologic response. Am Ind Hyg Assoc J *33*:45–52, 1972.
40. Sunderman FW: A review of the metabolism and toxicology of nickel. Ann Clin Lab Sci *7*:377–398, 1977.
41. Smith TJ, Blough S: Chromium, manganese, nickel, and other elements. *In* Rom WN (ed): Environmental and Occupational Medicine. Boston, Little, Brown, 1983, pp 491–510.
42. Enterline PE, Marsh GM: Cancer among workers exposed to arsenic and other substances in a copper smelter. Am J Epidemiol *116*:895–911, 1982.
43. Pershagen G: Lung cancer mortality among men living near an arsenic-emitting smelter. Am J Epidemiol *122*:684–694, 1985.
44. Eisenbud M: Carcinogenicity and allergenicity (letter). Science *236*:1613, 1987; also *237*:964, 1987.
45. Luster MI, Rosenthal GJ: The immunosuppressive influence of industrial and environmental xenobiotics. TIPS 408–412, 1986.
46. Emmett EA, Maroni M, Schmith JM, Levin BK, Jefferys J: Studies of transformer repair workers exposed to PCBs: 1. Study design, PCB concentrations, questionnaire, and clinical examination results. Am J Ind Med *13*:415–427, 1988.
47. Kimbrough RD: Human health effects of polychlorinated biphenyls (PCBs) and polybrominated biphenyls (PBBs). Annu Rev Pharmacol Toxicol *27*:87–111, 1987.
48. Descotes J: Biphenyls: 1. Polybrominated biphenyls. *In* Descotes J (ed): Immunotoxicology of Drugs and Chemicals. New York, Elsevier, 1986, p 342.
49. Evans RG, Webb KB, Knutsen AP, Roodman ST, Roberts DW, Bagby JR, Garrett WA, Andrews JS: A medical follow-up of the health effects of long-term exposure to 2,3,7,8-tetrachlorodibenzo-*p*-dioxin. Arch Environ Health *43*:273–278, 1988.
50. Stehr-Green PA, Burse VW, Welty E: Human exposure to polychlorinated biphenyls at toxic waste sites: Investigations in the United States. Arch Environ Health *43*:420–424, 1988.
51. Brown DP: Mortality of workers exposed to polychlorinated biphenyls—an update. Arch Environ Health *42*:333–339, 1987.
52. Hoffman RE, Stehr-Green PA, Webb KB, Evans RG, Knutsen AP, Schramm WF, Staake JL, Gibson BB, Steinberg KK: Health effects of long-term exposure to 2,3,7,8-tetrachlorodibenzo-*p*-dioxin. JAMA *255*:2031–2038, 1986.
53. Webb K, Evans RG, Stehr P, Ayres SM: Pilot study on health effects of environmental 2,3,7,8-TCDD in Missouri. Am J Ind Med *11*:685–691, 1987.
54. Mocarelli P, Marocchi A, Brambilla P, Gerthoux P, Young DS, Mantel N: Clinical laboratory manifestations of exposure to dioxin in children: A six-year study of the effects of an environmental disaster near Seveso, Italy. JAMA *256*:2687–2695, 1986.
55. Hayes WJ: Pesticides Studied in Man. Baltimore, Williams & Wilkins, 1982, p 202.
56. Lee TP, Moscati R, Park BH: Effects of pesticides on human leukocyte functions. Res Comm Chem Pathol Pharmacol *23*:597–609, 1979.
57. Roux F, Treich I, Brun C, Desoize B, Fournier E: Effect of lindane on human lymphocyte responses to phytohemagglutinin. Biochem Pharmacol *28*: 2419–2426, 1979.
58. Hermanowicz A, Nawarska Z, Borys D, et al: The neutrophil function and infectious disease in workers occupationally exposed to organochlorine insecticides. Int Arch Occup Environ Health *50*:329, 1982.
59. Costa M, Schvartsman S: Antibody titers and blood levels of DDT after diphtheric immunization in children. Acta Pharmacol Toxicol *41*:249, 1977.
60. Aaronson DW, Rosenberg M: Occupational immunologic lung disease. *In* Patterson R (ed): Allergic Diseases: Diagnosis and Management. Philadelphia, JB Lippincott, 1985, pp 253–303.
61. Zeiss CR, Wolkonsky P, Chacon R, Tuntland PA, Levitz D, Prunzansky JJ, Patterson R: Syndromes in workers exposed to trimellitic anhydride. Ann Intern Med *98*:8–12, 1983.
62. Alexandersson R, Kolmodin-Hedman B, Hedenstierna G: Exposure to formaldehyde: Effects on pulmonary function. Arch Environ Health *37*:279–284, 1982.
63. Burge PS, Harries MG, Lam WK, O'Brien IM, Patchett PA: Occupational asthma due to formaldehyde. Thorax *40*:255–260, 1985.
64. Brooks SM, Weiss MA, Bernstein IL: Reactive airways dysfunction syndrome (RADS): Persistent asthma syndrome after high level irritant exposures. Chest *88*:376–384, 1985.
65. Doll NJ, Stankus RP, Hughes J, Weill H, Gupta RC, Rodriguez M, Jones RN, Alspaugh MA, Salvaggio JE: Immune complexes and autoantibodies in silicosis. J Allergy Clin Immunol *68*:281–285, 1981.
66. Kubota M, Kagamimori S, Yokoyama K, Okada A: Reduced killer cell activity of lymphocytes from patients with asbestosis. Br J Ind Med *42*:276–280, 1985.
67. Barbers RG, Oishi J: Effects of in vitro asbestos exposure on natural killer and antibody-dependent cellular cytotoxicity. Environ Res *43*:217–226, 1987.
68. Lachapelle JM: The concept of industrial airborne irritant or allergic contact dermatitis. *In* Maibach HI (ed): Occupational and Industrial Dermatology. 1987, pp. 179–189.
69. Lindskov R: Contact urticaria to formaldehyde. Contact Derm *8*:333–334, 1982.
70. Menne T, Kaaber K, Tjell JC: Treatment of nickel dermatitis. Ann Clin Lab Sci *10*:160–164, 1980.
71. LaMarte FP, Merchant JA, Casale TB: Acute systemic reactions to carbonless copy paper associated with histamine release. JAMA *260*:242–243, 1988.
72. Calnan CD: The use and abuse of patch tests. *In* Maibach HI (ed): Occupational and Industrial Dermatology. 1987, pp 28–31.
73. DeSwarte RD: Drug allergy. *In* Patterson R (ed): Allergic Diseases: Diagnosis and Management. Philadelphia, JB Lippincott, 1985, pp 505–661.
74. Parker CW: Allergic reactions in man. Pharmacol Rev *34*:85–103, 1982.

75. Dalton-Bunnow MF: Review of sulfite sensitivity. Am J Hosp Pharm *42*:2220–2226, 1985.
76. Dalton-Bunnow MF: Sulfite content of drug products. Am J Hosp Pharm *42*:2196–2201, 1985.
77. Riggs BS, Harchelroad FP, Poole C: Allergic reaction to sulfiting agents. Ann Emerg Med *15*:129–131, 1986.
78. Goldfarb G, Simon R: Provocation of sulfite-sensitive asthma. J Allergy Clin Immunol *73*:135, 1984.
79. VanArsdel PP: Drug allergy, an update. Med Clin North Am *65*:1039–1103, 1981.
80. Mayer K: Immunohematology. *In* Grieco MH, Meriney DK (eds): Immunodiagnosis for Clinicians: Interpretation of Immunoassays. Chicago, Year Book Medical Publishers, 1983, pp 187–199.
81. Leads from the MMWR. Adverse reactions to fansidar and updated recommendations for its use in the prevention of malaria. JAMA *253*:483, 1985.
82. Fraser CM, Venter JC, Kaliner M: Autonomic abnormalities and autoantibodies to beta-adrenergic receptors. N Engl J Med *305*:1165–1170, 1981.
83. Watson AJS, Dalbow MH, Stachura I, Fragola JA, Rubin MF, Watson RM, Bourke E: Immunologic studies in cimetidine-induced nephropathy and polymyositis. N Engl J Med *308*:142–145, 1983.
84. Von Hoff DD, Slavik M, Muggia FM: Allergic reactions to cis-platinum. Lancet *1*:90, 1976.
85. Pohl LR, Satoh H, Christ DD, Kenna JG: The immunologic and metabolic basis of drug hypersensitivities. Annu Rev Pharmacol *28*:367–387, 1988.
86. Levin AS, Byers VS: Environmental illness: A disorder of immune regulation. Occup Med 2:669–681, 1987.
86a. American College of Physicians: Clinical ecology—position paper. Ann Intern Med *111*:168, 1989.
86b. Kahn E, Letz G: Clinical ecology: Environmental medicine or unsubstantiated theory? Ann Intern Med *111*:104, 1989.
87. Savona S, Nardi MA, Lennette ET, Karpatkin S: Thrombocytopenic purpura in narcotics addicts. Ann Intern Med *102*:737–741, 1985.
88. Micozzi MS, Wetli CV: Intravenous amphetamine abuse, primary cerebral mucormycosis, and acquired immunodeficiency. J Forensic Sci *30*:504–510, 1985.
89. Gluckman SJ, Kvorak VC, MacGregor RR: Host defenses during prolonged alcohol consumption in a controlled environment. Arch Intern Med *137*:1539–1543, 1977.
90. Smith WR, Glauser FL, Dearden LC, Wells ID, Novey HS, McRae DM, Reid JS, Newcomb KA: Deposits of immunoglobulin and complement in the pulmonary tissue of patients with "heroin lung." Chest *73*:471–476, 1978.
91. Newell GR, Adams SC, Mansell PWA, Hersh EM: Toxicity, immunosuppressive effects and carcinogenic potential of volatile nitrites: Possible relationship to Kaposi's sarcoma. Pharmacotherapy *4*:284–291, 1984.
92. Descotes J: Immunotoxicity of addictive chemicals. *In* Descotes J (ed): Immunotoxicology of Drugs and Chemicals. New York, Elsevier, 1986, pp 363–370.
93. Moll B, Emeson E, Smoll C, et al: Inverted ratio of inducer to suppressor T-lymphocyte subsets in drug abusers with opportunistic infections. Clin Immunol Immunopathol *25*:417–423, 1982.
94. Cushman P: Persistent increased immunoglobulin M in treated narcotic addiction. J Allergy Clin Immunol *52*:122–128, 1973.
95. Harris P, Garret D: Susceptibility of addicts to infection and neoplasia. N Engl J Med *287*:310, 1972.
96. Briggs J, McKerron C, Souhani R, et al: Severe systemic infections complicating "mainline" heroin addiction. Lancet *2*:1227–1231, 1967.
97. Dryer N, Fields B: Heroin-associated infective endocarditis—A report of 28 cases. Ann Intern Med *78*:699–720, 1973.
98. Cushman P: Hyperimmunoglobulinemia in heroin addiction. Am J Epidemiol *99*:218–224, 1974.
99. Ortona L, Laghi V, Cauda R: Immune functions in heroin addicts. N Engl J Med *300*:45, 1979.
100. Blanck R, Ream N, Deegan M: Immunoglobulins in heroin users. Am J Epidemiol *111*:81–86, 1980.
101. Nickerson D, Williams R, Boxmeyer M, et al: Increased opsonic capacity of serum in chronic heroin addiction. Ann Intern Med *72*:671–677. 1970.
102. Khansari N, Whitten HD, Fudenberg HH: Phencyclidine-induced immunodepression. Science *225*:76–78, 1984.
103. Welch W: Effect of cocaine on non-specific human cellular host defences. Res Comm Subst Abuse *4*:1, 1983.
104. Descotes J (ed): Immunotoxicology of Drugs and Chemicals. New York, Elsevier, 1986, p 359–362.
105. Report of IUIS/WHO Working Group: Use and abuse of laboratory tests in clinical immunology: Critical considerations of eight widely used diagnostic procedures. Clin Exp Immunol *46*:662–674, 1981.
106. deShazo RD, Lopez M, Salvaggio JE: Use and interpretation of diagnostic immunologic laboratory tests. JAMA *258*:3011–3031, 1987.
107. Virella G: Diagnostic evaluation of humoral immunity. *In* Virella G, Goust JM, Fudenberg HH, Patrick CC (eds): Introduction to Medical Immunology. New York, Marcel Dekker, 1986, pp 247–265.
108. Patrick CC, Goust JM, Virella G: Diagnostic evaluation of cell-mediated immunity. *In* Virella G, Goust JM, Fudenberg HH, Patrick CC (eds): Introduction to Medical Immunology. New York, Marcel Dekker, 1986, pp 265–283.
109. Cunningham-Rundles C, Cunningham-Rundles WF: Immunodeficiency disorders. *In* Grieco MH, Meriney DK (eds): Immunodiagnosis for Clinicians: Interpretation of Immunoassays. Chicago, Year Book Medical Publishers, 1983, pp 336–365.
110. Katz P: Clinical and laboratory evaluation of the immune system. Med Clin North Am *69*:453–464, 1985.
111. Virella G: Diagnostic evaluation of phagocyte function. *In* Virella G, Goust JM, Fudenberg HH, Patrick CC (eds): Introduction to Medical Immunology. New York, Marcel Dekker, 1986, pp 283–301.
112. Grieco MH: Immunologic assays of cellular function. *In* Grieco MH, Meriney DK (eds): Immunodiagnosis for Clinicians: Interpretation of Immunoassays. Chicago, Year Book Medical Publishers, 1983, pp 40–59.
113. Rosenfeld SI: Interpretation of complement and immune complex assays. *In* Grieco MH, Meriney DK (eds): Immunodiagnosis for Clinicians: Interpretation of Immunoassays. Chicago, Year Book Medical Publishers, 1983, pp 161–187.

CHAPTER 16
DERMATOLOGIC TOXICITY

Susanne Freeman, M.D.
Howard I. Maibach, M.D.

The skin forms an effective two-way barrier that controls the loss of chemicals from the body as well as the absorption of many foreign chemicals into the body. However, many chemicals do enter via the skin and some, when specifically applied to the skin, have been found to be sufficiently well absorbed to produce systemic toxicity.

Many drugs for topical use on the skin and mucous membranes are capable of producing systemic side effects whose occurrence and severity depend largely on factors that affect the absorption of topically applied drugs. These factors are (1) the integrity of the barrier, (2) the physicochemical properties of the substance, (3) occlusion, (4) the vehicle containing the drug, (5) the site of application, (6) age, (7) temperature, and (8) metabolism.

The Integrity of the Barrier. The stratum corneum layer of the epidermis is the skin's main barrier to transepidermal absorption (Fig. 16–1). Follicular orifices and sweat gland ducts may provide additional pathways for absorption. Anything that alters the structure or function of the stratum corneum will affect epidermal absorption. The integrity of this barrier, with resultant increase in percutaneous absorption, is reduced by any inflammatory process of the skin, such as any form of dermatitis or psoriasis. Similarly, removal of the stratum corneum by stripping or damage by alkalis, acids, and soap, will increase percutaneous absorption.

The Physicochemical Properties of the Substance. Absorption decreases with increasing molecular size. It is affected by the relative water/lipid solubility of the drug and the relative solubility of the drug in its vehicle, compared with its solubility in the stratum corneum.

Occlusion. The penetration of topical drugs may be increased by a factor of 10 or more through use of an occlusive covering. This is because of increased H_2O retention in the stratum corneum, increased blood flow,

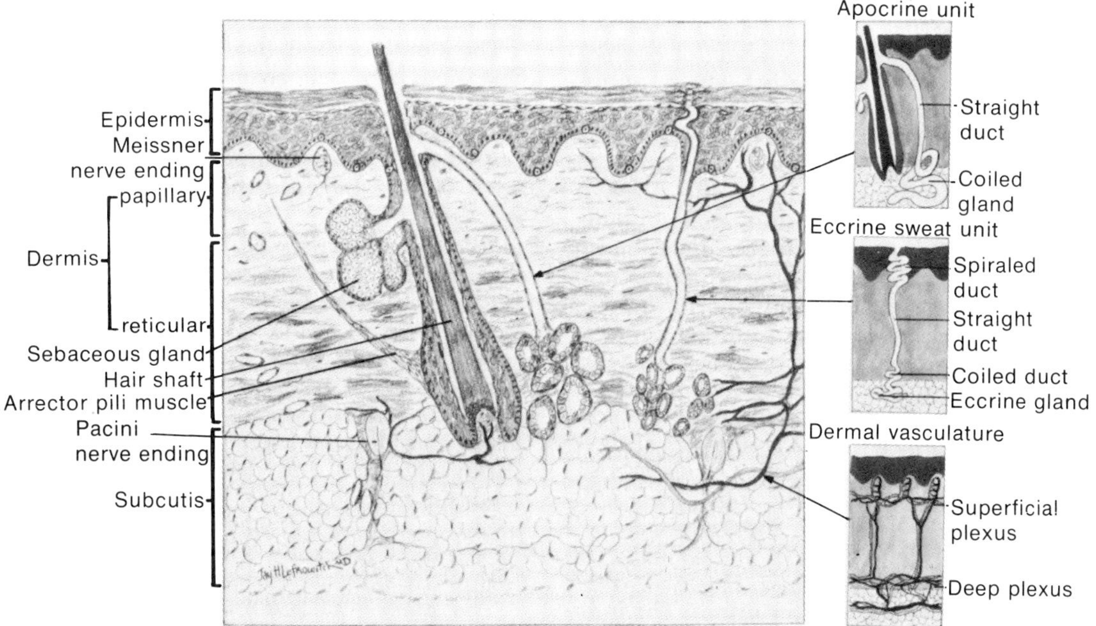

Figure 16–1. Diagram of skin structure. (From Arnold HL, Odom RB, James W: Andrews' Diseases of the Skin. 8th ed. Philadelphia, WB Saunders, 1989.)

increased temperature, and increased surface area after prolonged occlusion (skin wrinkling).

The Vehicle Containing the Drug

1. The greater the affinity of a vehicle for the drug it contains, the less the percutaneous absorption of the drug.

2. Physical properties of vehicles, especially the degree of occlusion they produce, affect percutaneous absorption (e.g., greases), as just noted.

3. Structural or chemical damage to the barrier layer can be caused by the vehicle used; vehicles such as dimethyl sulfoxide cause greatly increased percutaneous absorption.

4. In general, a higher concentration of the drug in its vehicle enhances penetration.

Site of Application. Regional differences in permeability of skin largely depend on the thickness of the intact stratum corneum. According to the findings of a study by Feldman and Maibach, the highest total absorption of hydrocortisone is that from the scrotum, followed (in decreasing order) by absorption from the forehead, scalp, back, forearms, palms, and plantar surfaces.[1]

Age. The greatest toxicologic response to topical administration has been seen in the infant. The preterm infant does not have intact barrier function and hence is more susceptible to systemic toxicity from topically applied drugs.[2, 3]

A normal full-term infant probably has a fully developed stratum corneum with complete barrier function.[4] Yet, according to Wester and colleagues, topical application of the same amount of a compound to both adult and neonate results in a 2.7 times greater systemic availability in the infant.[5] This is because the ratio of surface area to body weight in the neonate is three times that in the adult. Therefore, given an equal area of application of a drug onto skin of neonates and adults, the proportion absorbed per kilogram of body weight is much more in babies.

Temperature. Increased skin temperature usually enhances penetration.

Metabolism. Like the liver, the skin is capable of metabolizing drugs and foreign substances. It contains many of the enzyme systems of the liver, and its metabolizing potential has been estimated to be about 2 per cent that of the liver.[6]

Systemic Side Effects Caused by Topically Applied Drugs and Cosmetics. Topically applied drugs and cosmetics can cause allergic or irritant contact dermatitis. However, this type of side effect, usually limited to the skin, is outside the scope of the present article. The reader is referred to the textbooks of Cronin[7] and Fisher[8] for references to contact dermatitis. Systemic side effects from topically applied chemicals can sometimes result from either a toxic (irritant) reaction or a hypersensitivity reaction. The latter can be an anaphylactic type of reaction, which is the extreme manifestation of the contact urticaria syndrome.[9] Many topical drugs and cosmetics reportedly have caused anaphylactic reactions.

Although anaphylactic reactions to topical medicaments are uncommon, their potentially serious nature warrants attention.

However, reports of toxic (as distinct from allergic) reactions to applied drugs and cosmetics are more numerous; these include many medicaments that have been safely used for many years, but that can be toxic under special circumstances.

TOPICALLY APPLIED DRUGS AND COSMETICS CAUSING SYSTEMIC SIDE EFFECTS

Antibiotics

Chloramphenicol. Oral administration of chloramphenicol may lead to aplastic anemia.[10] A case of marrow aplasia with a fatal outcome after topical application of chloramphenicol in eye ointment was described by Abrams and colleagues.[11] There have been three earlier reports of bone marrow aplasia after the use of chloramphenicol-containing eye drops.

Clindamycin. Topical clindamycin is widely used in the treatment of acne vulgaris. It is estimated that 4 to 5 per cent of clindamycin hydrochloride is absorbed systemically.[12] The degree of absorption largely depends on the vehicle, ranging from 0.13 per cent (acetone) to 13.92 per cent (DMSO).[13] Several cases of diarrhea associated with topical clindamycin have been reported.[14–16]

Pseudomembranous colitis is a well-recognized side effect of systemic administration of clindamycin. A case of pseudomembranous colitis after topical administration has been reported by Milstone and colleagues.[17] They conclude that all patients receiving topical clindamycin should be warned to discontinue therapy and consult their physician if intestinal symptoms occur.

Gentamicin. Ototoxicity is a well-known hazard of systemic gentamicin administration. However, topical application to large thermal injuries of the skin has similarly caused ototoxic effects, ranging from mild-to-severe hearing loss, with an associated decrease of vestibular function.[18] In the two patients described, serum levels of gentamicin measured were 1.0 to 3.0 μg/ml and 3.3 to 4.3 μg/ml, respectively. Drake described a woman who developed tinnitus each time she treated her paronychia with gentamicin sulfate cream 0.1%.[19] Use of gentamicin ear drops may also be associated with ototoxic reactions.[20]

Neomycin. Just as ototoxicity is a well-known hazard of parenteral neomycin administration, so has deafness been reported after almost any form of local treatment, including treatment of skin infections and burns,[21–23] application as an aerosol for inhalation, instillation into cavities,[24] irrigation of large wounds,[25] and use of neomycin-containing eardrops.[26] Kellerhals reported 13 cases of inner ear damage in which the use of eardrops containing neomycin and polymycin was incriminated.[27] All cases had perforated tympanic membranes and Kellerhals concluded that these drops (and also those containing chloromycetin, colistin, and polymycin) should not be used in such cases for periods longer than 10 days.

Antihistamines

Diphenylpyraline Hydrochloride. Diphenylpyraline hydrochloride has been used topically in Germany for the treatment of eczematous and other itching dermatoses. Symptomatic psychosis has been observed in 12 patients, 9 of whom were children. The amounts of the active drug applied ranged from 225 to 1350 mg. The first symptoms of intoxication were psychomotor restlessness in all cases, usually within 24 hours. Other symptoms included disorientation and optic and acoustic hallucinations. All symptoms disappeared 4 days after discontinuation of the topical medication.[28]

Promethazine. Block and Beysovec reported a 16 month old boy weighing 11.5 kg who was treated with 2 per cent promethazine cream for generalized eczema.[29] After approximately 15 to 20 gm of the cream had been applied, the child fell asleep. He woke a few hours later with abnormal behavior, loss of balance, inability to focus, irritability, drowsiness, and failure to recognize his mother. One day later all symptoms had spontaneously disappeared. A diagnosis of promethazine toxicity through percutaneous absorption was made. Known symptoms of promethazine toxicity include disorientation, hallucinations, hyperactivity, convulsions, and coma.

Antimicrobials

Boric Acid. The toxicity of this mildly bacteriostatic substance is dealt with in Chapter 104.[30] Undoubtedly the use of borates should be abandoned because of their limited therapeutic value and high toxicity. In recent times, few cases of borate intoxication have been published, probably due to its disappearing use.

Castellani's Solution. Castellani's solution (or paint) is an old medicament mainly used for the local treatment of fungal skin infections. It contains boric acid 5.0, fuchsin 5.0, resorcinol 100.0, water 705.0, phenol 40.0 (90 per cent), acetone 50.0, and spirit 100.0.

Lundell and Nordman reported a case in which two applications of Castellani's solution severely poisoned a 6 week old boy, who became cyanotic with 41 per cent methemoglobin.[31] They state that this case demonstrates that the application of Castellani's to napkin eruptions and other areas where absorption is rapid may cause serious complications.

Another case report states that hours after the application of Castellani's paint to the entire body surface except the face of a 6 week old infant for severe seborrheic eczema, the child became drowsy and had shallow breathing.[32] Phenol was detected in the urine of four of 16 children treated with Castellani's paint.[32]

Hexachlorophene. Hexachlorophene had been extensively used in hospital nurseries, mainly for reducing the incidence of staphylococcal infections among newborn infants.[33] In addition, it had been an ingredient of many medical preparations, cosmetics, and other consumer goods.

Hexachlorophene readily penetrates damaged skin, and its absorption through intact skin has also been demonstrated.[34–36]

In 1972 in France, as a result of the accidental addition of 6.3 per cent of hexachlorophene to batches of baby talcum powder, 204 babies fell ill and 36 died from respiratory arrest.[37, 38] This report was followed by animal experiments with hexachlorophene confirming that the drug is neurotoxic. Consequently, in 1972, the US Food and Drug Administration banned hexachlorophene to prescription use only or as a surgical scrub and hand wash for health care personnel. Hexachlorophene was excluded from cosmetics except as a preservative in levels not exceeding 0.1 per cent.

Because of the high absorption through damaged skin and its proven neurotoxicity, hexachlorophene is contraindicated for the treatment of burns or application to otherwise damaged skin. Premature infants are also at risk. The safety of hexachlorophene for routine bathing of babies is still controversial. Plueckhahn and colleagues[39] and Hopkins[40] have reviewed the benefits and risks of hexachlorophene.

4-Homosulfanilamide (Sulfamylon acetate). 4-H-S is a topical sulfonamide that was used for the treatment of large burns. It has been largely replaced at present by silver sulfadiazine. Sulfamylon is a carbonic anhydrase inhibitor. It caused hyperchloremic metabolic acidosis through percutaneous absorption in patients whose extensive burns were treated by topical application.[41, 42] Reversible pulmonary complications[43] and methemoglobinuria[44] also have been reported.

Iodine and Povidone Iodine. Povidone-iodine (Betadine) is a water-soluble iodine complex that retains the broad-range microbicidal activity of iodine without the undesirable effects of iodine tincture.

However, toxicity still occurs from povidone iodine percutaneously absorbed, mainly when it is used on large areas of burned skin or on neonates. This subject is dealt with comprehensively in Chapter 63.[45]

Phenol (Carbolic Acid). Phenol is no longer widely used as a skin antiseptic, but in dilutions of 0.5 to 2.0 per cent it is sometimes prescribed as an antipruritic in topical medicaments, and it is used for phenol face peels.

It has been shown that as much as 25 per cent of phenol is absorbed from 2 ml of a solution of 2.5 gm of phenol per liter of water applied to the skin of the forearm and left on for 60 minutes.[46] The toxic dose for adults has been estimated to be 8 to 15 gm.

Phenol-induced ochronosis has been reported in patients who for many years treated leg ulcers with wet dressings containing phenol.[47]

There are several case reports in the literature of fatal reactions to percutaneously absorbed phenol. One was caused by accidental spillage of phenol,[48] one was due to treatment of burns with a phenol-containing preparation,[49] and another to the application of phenol to wounds.[50] A 1 day old child died after application of 2 per cent phenol to the umbilicus.[51]

Several cases of sudden death or intra- or postoperative complications have been reported after phenol face peels.[52]

Major cardiac arrhythmias were noted in 10 of 43 patients during phenol face peels.[53] However, this item is rather controversial, and some feel that when the procedure is done over more than 1 hour, and when the dose applied is carefully monitored, phenol face peels are not risky.[54, 55] Poisoning from phenol ingestion is discussed in Chapter 89.[56]

Resorcinol. Resorcinol is used for its keratolytic properties in the treatment of acne vulgaris. It is also a constituent of the antifungal agent, Castellani's solution. Formerly, leg ulcers were treated with external applications of resorcinol-containing applications.

Resorcinol can penetrate human skin. It has an antithyroid activity similar to that of methyl thiouracil, although it is chemically unrelated to any of the known groups of antithyroid drugs. Consequently, several cases of myxedema caused by percutaneous absorption of resorcinol, especially from ulcerated surfaces, have been described.[57, 58]

Methemoglobinemia in children, caused by absorption of resorcinol applied to wounds, has been reported.[59, 60] Cunningham reported a case in which an ointment containing 12.5 per cent resorcinol applied to the napkin area of an infant produced cyanosis, hemolytic anemia, and hemoglobinemia.[61] In the literature are seven cases of acute poisoning in babies as a consequences of topical resorcinol application, in some instances to limited areas; five fatalities were recorded.

A case of severe poisoning of a 6 week old infant due to two application of Castellani's paint has been described.[62]

Although the use of resorcinol in young

children and for leg ulcers should be avoided, topical resorcinol, when used for acne vulgaris, appears to be safe.[63]

Silver Sulfadiazine. Sulfadiazine silver cream is widely used for the topical treatment of burns. Intended primarily for the control of *Pseudomonas* infections, this bactericidal agent acts on the cell membranes and cell walls of a variety of gram positive and gram negative bacteria, as well as on yeasts. Its relative freedom from appreciable side effects has contributed to its popularity.

Absorption of sulfonamide from burns to 17 to 46 per cent of the body area that were treated with sulfadiazine silver showed that 20 to 25 per cent of the daily topical dose could be accounted for as conjugated sulfonamide. Unconjugated drug represented from 35 per cent to 95 per cent of the total output. Total plasma sulfonamide concentration did not exceed 10 μg/ml.[64]

There is one report of nephrotic syndrome following topical therapy.[65] Several investigators have reported leukopenia during treatment with silver sulfadiazine.[66–68] Current evidence suggests a causal relationship of silver sulfadiazine with leukopenia, although the mechanism of this reaction is unknown. Examination of bone marrow aspirates shows hyperplasia with no evidence of maturation arrest. The drug presumably affects the white blood cells peripherally.[68] The sulfadiazine-induced leukopenia is at its nadir within 2 to 4 days of starting therapy. The leukocyte count returns to normal levels within 2 to 3 days, and recovery is not affected by continuation of therapy. The erythrocyte count is not affected.

Triclocarban (Trichlorocarbanilide, TCC). Triclocarban is a bacteriostatic agent used as an antimicrobial in toilet soap since 1956.

The percutaneous absorption has been studied by Scharpf and colleagues. They showed that, after a simple shower employing a whole body lather with approximately 6 gm of soap containing 2 per cent TCC, about 0.23 per cent of the applied dose of TCC was recovered in feces after 6 days and 0.16 per cent of the dose in the urine after 2 days.[70] At all sampling times, blood levels of radioactivity were below the detection limit of 10 parts per billion.

There have been several reports of methemoglobinemia presumably induced by topical TCC in neonates.[71, 72]

Arsenic

The toxicity of ingested or inhaled arsenic is discussed Chapter 59.[73] Fowler's solution, long used orally in the treatment of psoriasis, contained arsenic. Arsenical keratoses and malignancies are well-recognized long-term reactions to this.

Carmustine (BCNU)

Topical carmustine (BCNU) has been used for the treatment of mycosis fungoides, lymphomatoid papulosis, and parapsoriasis en plaques.[75] Percutaneous absorption of BCNU has been demonstrated in humans.[76] Zackheim and colleagues treated 91 patients who had mycosis fungoides and related disorders with topical BCNU.[75] Mild-to-moderate reversible bone marrow depression occurred in three patients. Their data suggest that hematologic toxicity arises primarily from the shorter intensive schedules; the prolonged use of up to 100 mg per week appears to be safe. Although an occasional mild elevation in the blood urea nitrogen or serum glutamic oxaloacetic transaminase (SGOT) level was noted in patients treated with courses exceeding 600 mg, no such changes were seen with lower doses. No long-term harmful effects on the hematopoietic system or internal organs were apparent.

Camphor

Camphor is a pleasant-smelling cyclic ketone of the hydroaromatic terpene group. When rubbed on the skin, camphor is a rubefacient but produces a feeling of coolness if not vigorously applied. It is an ingredient of a large number of over-the-counter remedies (with a camphor content of 1 to 20 per cent), taken especially for symptomatic relief of "chest congestion" and "muscle aches," but its effectiveness is rather dubious.

Camphor is readily absorbed from all sites of administration, including topical application to the skin.

The compound is classified as a Class IV chemical, i.e., a very toxic substance. Hundreds of cases of intoxications have been reported, usually in children after accidental ingestion.[77, 78]

Cosmetic Agents

Henna Dye and *p*-Phenylenediamine. The use of a henna dye is traditional in Islamic communities. The dye is used on nails, skin, and hair by married women, and traditionally it is also used by the main participants in marriage ceremonies, when the bridegroom and best man also apply henna to their hands.

Henna consists of the dried leaves of *Lawsonia alba* (family Lythraceae), a shrub cultivated in North Africa, India, and Sri Lanka. The coloring matter, lawsone, is a hydroxynaphthoquinone, and this is associated with fats, resin, and henna-tannin in the leaf. Dyeing hair or skin with powdered henna is a somewhat lengthy procedure; to speed up this process, Sudanese women mix a "black powder" with henna, which accelerates the fixing process of the dye to a matter of minutes. This black powder is paraphenylenediamine. The combination of henna and black powder is particularly toxic, and over 20 cases of such toxicity, some fatal, have been noted in Khartoum alone in a 2-year period. Initial symptoms are those of angioneurotic edema, with massive edema of the face, lips, glottis, pharynx, neck, and bronchi. These occur within hours of the application of the dye-mixture to the skin. The symptoms may then progress on the second day to anuria and acute renal failure, with death occurring on the third day. Dialysis has helped some patients, but others have died from renal tubular necrosis.[79] Whether this toxicity is due to *p*-phenylenediamine per se (probably grossly impure) or whether its toxicity is potentiated in its combination with henna powder is unknown. Systemic administration of the black powder leads to similar symptoms, and several deaths due to ingestion with suicidal intent have been reported.[80, 81]

Diethyltoluamide

This has been used as an insect repellent since 1957. Although diethyltoluamide has an overall low incidence of toxic effects, prolonged use in children has been discouraged because of reports of toxic encephalopathy.[82, 83] In one case, the bedding, nightclothes, and skin of a 3.5 year old girl were sprayed daily for 2 weeks with a total amount of 180 ml of 15 per cent diethyltoluamide. Shaking and crying spells, slurred speech, and confusion developed. Improvement occurred after vigorous medical treatment including anticonvulsants. In another report, one of two children displaying signs of severe toxic enencephalopathy died after prolonged hospitalization. At autopsy, edema of the brain and congestion of the meninges were found.

Dimethyl Sulfoxide

The toxicology of topical dimethyl sulfoxide (DMSO) has been investigated by Kligman.[84] In this study, 9 ml of 90 per cent dimethyl sulfoxide were applied twice daily to the entire trunk of 20 healthy volunteers for 3 weeks. The following laboratory tests were done: complete blood count, urinalysis, blood sedimentation rate, and SGOT, BUN, and fasting blood sugar determinations. At the end of the study, all laboratory values had remained normal. Except for the appearance of such cutaneous signs as erythema, scaling, contact urticaria, and stinging and burning sensations, the drug was tolerated well by all but two individuals, who developed systemic symptoms. In one, a toxic reaction developed on the 12th day, characterized by a diffuse erythematous and scaling rash accompanied by severe abdominal cramps; the other had a similar rash and complained of nausea, chills, and chest pains. These signs, however, abated in spite of continued administration of the drug.

To investigate possible side effects of *chronic* exposure to dimethyl sulfoxide, another 20 volunteers were painted with 9 ml of 90 per cent dimethyl sulfoxide over the entire trunk, once daily for a period of 26 weeks.

Neither clinical nor laboratory investigations showed adverse effects of the drug. However, most subjects did experience the well-known DMSO-induced, disagreeable oyster-like breath odor, to which they eventually became insensitive. One fatality due to a hypersensitivity reaction has been reported.[85]

Dinitrochlorobenzene (DNCB)

Dinitrochlorobenzene (DNCB), a potent contact allergen, has been used with some success for the treatment of recalcitrant alopecia areata; today however, its use has been discouraged because suspicion has been aroused that DNCB may be mutagenic. Another drawback for its use is its ability to potentiate epicutaneous sensitization to nonrelated allergens.[86] DNCB is absorbed in substantial amounts through the skin, and about 50 per cent of the applied dose is ultimately recoverable in the urine.[87]

A possible systemic reaction to DNCB has been reported: a 25 year old man was treated with 0.1 per cent DNCB in an absorbent ointment base for alopecia areata after prior sensitization.[88] After 2 months of daily applications, the patient experienced generalized urticaria, pruritus, and dyspepsia; discontinuing the drug led to cessation of all symptoms, which recurred after reintroduction of DNCB therapy.

Ethyl Alcohol

Twenty-eight children with alcohol intoxication from percutaneous absorption were described by Gimenez and colleagues from Buenos Aires, Argentina.[89] Apparently, in that area it is (or was) a popular procedure to apply alcohol-soaked cloths to the abdomens of babies as a home remedy for disturbances of the gastrointestinal tract, such as cramps, pain, vomiting, and diarrhea, or because of crying, excitability, and irritability.

The children were of both sexes and ranged in age from 1 year to 33 months (mean: 12 months, 27 days). Alcohol-soaked cloths had been applied on the babies' abdomens under rubber panties, and the number of applications varied from one to three. It was estimated that each application contained approximately 40 ml of ethanol. Medical consultation took place from 1 to 23 hours after application. Alcoholic breath and abdominal erythema were valuable clues to the diagnosis.

All 28 children showed some degree of CNS depression, 24 showed miosis; 15, hypoglycemia; 5, convulsions; and 5, respiratory depression. Two died. Eleven patients showed a blood alcohol level of from 0.6 to 1.49 gm per cent. One of the two who died had an autopsy: the findings were consistent with ethyl alcohol intoxication.

More recently, a case was reported of acute ethanol intoxication in a preterm infant weighing 1800 gm, because of local application of alcohol-soaked compresses on the legs as a treatment for puncture hematomas.[90]

Topically applied ethanol in tar gel[91] and beer-containing shampoo[92] has caused Antabuse-like effects in patients on disulfiram for alcoholism, through percutaneous absorption.

Fumaric Acid Monoethyl Ester

The effect of systemically or topically administered fumaric acid monoethyl ester (ethyl fumarate) on psoriasis was studied by Dubiel and Happle in six patients.[93] Two patients who had been treated with locally applied ointments consisting of 3 per cent or 5 per cent ethyl fumarate in petrolatum developed symptoms of renal toxicity.

Local Anesthetics

Benzocaine. Methemoglobinemia has been reported following the topical application of benzocaine to both skin and mucous membranes.[94–98] However, this is an uncommon occurrence;[99] most cases occurred in infants.

Lidocaine. Lidocaine hydrochloride is widely used for both topical and local injection anesthesia. When the drug is applied to mucous membranes, blood levels simulate those resulting from intravenous injection.[100] Serum lidocaine concentrations higher than 6 μg/ml are associated with toxicity.[101] The signs are central nervous system stimulation followed by depression and, later, inhibition of cardiovascular function. Systemic toxicity from viscous lidocaine applied to the oral cavity in two children has been described.[102, 103] In one, the mother had been applying lidocaine hydrochloride, 2 per cent solution, to her infant's gums with her finger five to six times daily for a week; the child experienced two generalized seizures within an hour. Urine examined by thin layer chromatography revealed a large amount of lidocaine, and a blood level of 10 μg/ml was determined.[103] The other child had a seizure after having received 227.8 mg/kg of oral viscous lidocaine for stomatitis herpetica over a 24-hour period. In this case, however, ingestion and resorption from the gastrointestinal tract may have contributed to the clinical picture.

It has been suggested that for pediatric patients viscous lidocaine should be applied with an oral swab to individual lesions, thus limiting buccal absorption by decreasing the surface area exposed to lidocaine.[102]

Mercurials

The toxicology of mercury is dealt with comprehensively in Chapter 56.[104] With a few exceptions, the use of mercury in medicine is considered to be outdated. However, attention should be paid to the possibility of mercurial poisoning even today, as mercury may still be present in many drugs. In many countries mercury may be present even in over-the-counter remedies, often without mention on the label.

Although there are considerable differences between various mercurials regarding the rate of absorption through the skin, all mercurial preparations are a potential hazard and may cause intoxication. Metallic mercury is readily absorbed through intact skin; absorption of ammoniated mercury chloride in psoriatic patients was demonstrated by Bork and associates.[105]

Young examined 70 psoriatic patients treated with an ointment containing ammoniated mercury before, during and after treatment. Symptoms and signs of mercurial poisoning could be detected in 33 of them.[106]

Nephrotic syndrome has been reported in a 24 year old man using an ammoniated mercury–containing ointment for psoriasis.[107, 108] Nephrotic syndrome resulting from topical mercury also was reported by Lyons and associates.[109]

There have been two case reports of children who died following treatment of an omphalocele with merbromin (an organic mercurial antiseptic).[110, 111]

In view of the risks of both systemic side effects and contact allergic reactions to mercurials, there seems to be no justification for continuing the use of these drugs in dermatologic therapy.

Monobenzone

Monobenzone (monobenzyl ether of hydroquinone) is used topically by patients with extensive vitiligo to depigment their remaining normally pigmented skin. A patient who had been applying the drug for 1 year had an anterior linear deposition of pigment on both corneas. Of 11 patients with vitiligo who were using monobenzone, acquired conjuctival melanosis occurred in two patients and pingueculae in three.[112]

2-Naphthol (β-Naphthol)

2-Naphthol is used in peeling pastes for the treatment of acne; between 5 per cent and 10 per cent of a cutaneous dose has been recovered from the urine.[113, 114]

The extensive application of 2-naphthol ointments has been responsible for systemic side effects, including vomiting, and death has occurred.[115, 116] Hemels concludes that 2-naphthol–containing pastes should be applied only for short periods of time and to a limited area not exceeding 150 cm^2.[114]

Pesticides, Insecticides, and Herbicides

Agricultural Chemicals. In recent years, it has become clear that the skin is a major portal of entry for certain agricultural chemicals. A full review is beyond this chapter's scope. Certain generalizations are noteworthy: some chemicals, such as paraquat, are minimally absorbed, whereas others, such as carbaryl, are extensively absorbed. Absorption is dose and surface dependent. References relevant to the general area are Feldman and Maibach[117] and Wester et al.[118]

Lindane. Lindane (gamma-benzene hexachloride) is widely used in the treatment of scabies and pediculosis, usually in a 1 per cent lotion applied to the entire body and left on for 24 hours (in the case of scabies). The percutaneous absorption of the drug has been studied.[117, 119, 120] The general toxicology is discussed in Chapter 68 of this book.[121]

Intoxication from excessive topical therapeutic application of lindane has been documented.[122–124] The issue of possible toxic reactions to a single therapeutic application of lindane, notably central nervous system toxicity, has not been settled yet.[122, 125–129]

Most authorities seem to agree that the benefits to be derived from the use of lindane as a scabicide and pediculicide outweigh the risks involved.[128–131] The risk of toxicity appears minimal when lindane is used properly according to directions.

Solomon and associates, in their review of lindane toxicity, give the following observations and recommendations:[128]

(1) lindane should not be applied after a hot bath,

(2) the regime of application for 24 hours may be unnecessarily long; 8 to 12 hours may be sufficient,[130]

(3) a concentration weaker than 1.0 per cent may suffice, particularly for badly excoriated patients,

(4) lindane 1 per cent should be used with extreme caution if at all in pregnant women, very small infants, and people with massively excoriated skin. Rassmussen does not agree on this point.[130]

(5) lindane treatment should not be repeated within 8 days, and then only if necessary.

Malathion. The detailed toxicology of malathion is discussed in Chapter 68.[132] Malathion is used in the treatment of lice; a single application of 0.5 per cent in a solution is customary. Used in this way, it is generally safe. Ramu and associates reported four children with an intoxication following hair washing with a solution containing 50 per cent malathion in xylene for the purpose of louse control.[133] Malathion is also a weak but definite skin sensitizer.[134]

Podophyllum

The toxicity of podophyllum was reviewed in 1982 and 1983.[135, 136]

Although there have been a significant number of case reports describing serious neurologic illness or death following the application of podophyllum, these are generally related to its use in widespread lesions. Twenty per cent podophyllum in tincture of benzoin is still indicated for isolated venereal warts.[137] Its use is contraindicated in pregnancy.[138] Following application, it should be washed off after a specific period of time.

Salicylic Acid

The general toxicology of salicylates is discussed in Chapter 51, including its absorption through the skin.[139] Salicylic acid is widely used in dermatology as a topical application for its keratolytic properties. Cases of salicylate poisoning after topical use of salicylic acid have been reported several times. Taylor and Halprin used 6 per cent salicylic acid in a gel base under plastic suit occlusion in adults with extensive psoriasis.[140] During their 5-day study, serum salicylate never exceeded 5 mg/dl, and no patient developed toxicity. However, toxicity was noted by von Weiss and Lever; they found serum salicylate levels ranging from 46 to 64 mg/dl.[141] Salicylic acid therapy for extensive lesions may be especially dangerous for children. An unpublished review revealed 13 deaths associated with the widespread use of salicylic acid preparations, and all but three occurred in children.[142] This compound should not be used on large areas (more than 25 per cent) of the skin of a child.[141]

Von Weiss and Lever reported on three adults with extensive psoriasis who were treated six times daily with an ointment containing 3 per cent or 6 per cent salicylic acid. Between the second and fourth days, symptoms of salicylism developed in all three patients.[141] The levels of salicylic acid in the serum ranged from 46 to 64 mg/dl. Within one day after discontinuation of the ointment, the symptoms had largely disappeared. The serum salicylic acid in the serum decreased to zero within a few days.

The same investigators also recorded 13 deaths resulting from intoxication with salicylic acid following the application of salicylic ointment to the skin, which were reported in the medical literature up to 1964, and several nonfatal intoxications. The 13 deaths included 3 patients with psoriasis, 5 cases of scabies, 3 of dermatitis, 1 of lupus vulgaris, and 1 of congenital ichthyosiform erythroderma. Ten of the fatal cases occurred in children, three of them being under 3 years of age.

The most dramatic account in the literature is that of two plantation workers in Bougainville, in the Solomon Islands, who were painted twice a day with an alcoholic solution of 20 per cent salicylic acid for tinea imbricata involving about 50 per cent of the body. The victims were comatose within 6 hours and dead within 28 hours.[143]

Wechselberg reported a 3 month old baby with scaly erythroderma who was treated in a hospital with 1 per cent salicylic acid in soft paraffin. After 10 days, the child began to vomit and lose weight. Later, hyperpnea developed and an increasing somnolence.

When the treatment was stopped, the child recovered rapidly.[144]

Recently, a case was described of salicylic acid intoxication leading to coma in an adult patient with psoriasis, who had been treated with 20 per cent salicylic acid in petrolatum.[145]

Selenium Sulfide

Ransone and colleagues reported a case of systemic selenium toxicity in a woman who had been shampooing her hair two or three times weekly for 8 months with selenium sulfide suspension.[146]

Silver Nitrate

Ternberg and Luce observed fatal methemoglobinemia in a 3 year old girl suffering from burns involving 82 per cent of the body surface, who was treated with silver nitrate solution.[147]

Another complication of the use of silver nitrate in the treatment of large burns is electrolyte disturbance, especially in children. Because of the hypotonicity of the silver nitrate dressings, hyponatremia, hypokalemia, and hyperchloremia may develop.[148, 149] Also, loss of other water-soluble minerals and vitamins may occur. Postmortem examinations of patients treated with silver nitrate have revealed that silver has been deposited in internal organs, showing that absorption of silver from topical preparations does occur.[150] The excessive use of silver-containing drugs has led to local and systemic argyria[151] and to renal damage involving the glomeruli with proteinuria.[152]

Steroids

Corticosteroids. It has been amply documented that topically applied glucocorticosteroids are absorbed through the skin.[153] Systemic absorption in quantities sufficient to replace endogenous production is not uncommon. However, iatrogenic Cushing's syndrome resulting from the use of topical steroids is rare. Pascher summarized the relevant data of 12 cases.[154]

Systemic side effects of topical corticosteroids occur more frequently in children than in adults[155] and in patients with liver disease because of retarded degradation of the drug.[156] The two main causes of systemic side effects are hypercorticism leading to an iatrogenic Cushing's syndrome and suppression of the hypothalamic-pituitary-adrenal axis.[157]

It is not easy to provide data on "safe" uses of topical corticosteroids, but for the potent corticosteroid clobetasol-17-propionate 0.05 per cent, the dose is recommended to be limited to 45 gm per week.[158]

Sex Hormones. ***Estrogens.*** Topical application of estrogen-containing preparations may lead to resorption of these hormones and systemic estrogenic effects.

Beas and colleagues reported on seven children with pseudoprecocious puberty caused by an ointment containing estrogens.[159] The common factor found in every patient was the use of the same ointment for treatment or prevention of ammoniacal dermatitis for a period of 2 to 18 months, with two to ten daily applications. Endocrinologic and radiologic studies had excluded other possible causes of sexual precocity. The most important clinical signs were intense pigmentation of the mammary areolae, the linea alba, and the genitals; mammary enlargement; and the presence of pubic hair. Three female patients also had vaginal discharge and bleeding. Estrogenic contamination of the ointment was suspected and confirmed by a biologic test of the vaginal opening of castrated female guinea pigs. After discontinuation of the incriminated topical drug, all symptoms progressively disappeared in every patient.

Pseudoprecocious puberty also has been observed in young girls after contact with hair lotions and other substances containing estrogens.[160–162] Such contact has led to gynecomastia in young boys.[163, 164] Gynecomastia in a 70 year old man from exposure to 0.01 per cent dienestrol cream used by his wife for atrophic vaginitis and as a lubricant before intercourse has been reported.[165]

Estrogen cream for the treatment of baldness also has caused gynecomastia, which was persistent in the reported case.[166] In adult men, both oral and topical administration of estrogens may result first in pigmentation of the areolae and then in gynecomastia.[167, 168]

Tars

Coal Tar. A case of methemoglobinemia has been reported in an infant following the 5-day application of an ointment containing 2.5 per cent crude coal tar and 5 per cent benzocaine to about half the body surface.[169]

Dithranol. Dithranol has been used since 1916 for the treatment of psoriasis. Although it causes irritant dermatitis and discoloration of the skin, its use is generally considered to be devoid of systemic side effects.[170, 171]

Comment

This chapter summarizes literature citations and the basic aspects of percutaneous penetration. The purpose is to alert the reader to the potential for systemic toxicity from topical exposure. Demonstrating causality (rather than association) requires careful documentation. Combining knowledge of the inherent molecular and animal toxicology, cutaneous penetration, and metabolism with the literature of adverse human reactions permits a more precise determination of causality. In each example presented here, the original citations combined with the further documentation should permit more discriminate causality judgments.

Acknowledgment

We drew heavily upon the very useful studies of J. P. Nater and A. C. de Groot in Chapter 16 of Unwanted Effects of Cosmetics and Drugs Used in Dermatology, 2nd edition, Amsterdam, Elsevier, 1985.

References

1. Feldman RJ, Maibach HI: Regional variation in percutaneous penetration of 14C cortisol in man. J Invest Dermatol *48*:181, 1967.
2. Nachman RL, Esterly NB: Increased skin permeability in pre-term infants. J Pediatr *89*:628–632, 1971.
3. Greaves SJ, Ferry DG, McQueen EG, et al: Serial hexachlorophene blood levels in the premature infant. NZ Med J *81*:334–336, 1975.
4. Rasmussen JE: Percutaneous absorption in children. *In* Dobson RL (ed): 1979 Year Book of Dermatology. Chicago, Year Book Medical Publishers, 1979, pp 15–38.
5. Wester RC, Noonan PK, Cole MP, Maibach HI: Percutaneous absorption of testosterone in the newborn rhesus monkey: Comparison to the adult. Pediatr Res *11*:737–739, 1977.
6. Pannatier A, Jenner B, Testa B, et al: The skin as a drug-metabolizing organ. Drug Melab Rev *8*:319–343, 1978.
7. Cronin E: Contact Dermatitis. Edinburgh, Churchill Livingstone, 1980.
8. Fisher AE: Contact Dermatitis. 3rd ed. Philadelphia, Lea and Febiger, 1986.
9. Von Krogh G, Maibach HI: The contact urticaria syndrome. *In* Marzulli FN, Maibach HI (eds): Dermatotoxicology. Washington, DC, Hemisphere Publishing Corporation. 3rd ed. 1987, p 341.
10. Wilson AJ, Mielke CH: Hematological consequences of poisoning. *In* Haddad LM, Winchester JF (eds): Clinical Management of Poisoning and Drug Overdose. Philadelphia, WB Saunders, 1983, p 893.
11. Abrams SM, Degnan TJ, Vinciguerra V: Marrow aplasia following topical application of chloramphenicol eye ointment. Arch Intern Med *140*:576, 1980.
12. Barza M, Goldstein JA, Kane A, et al: Systemic absorption of clindamycin hydrochloride after topical application. J Am Acad Dermatol *7*:208, 1982.
13. Franz TJ: On the bioavailability of topical formulations of clindamycin hydrochloride. J Am Acad Dermatol *9*:66, 1983.
14. Stoughton RB: Topical antibiotics for acne vulgaris: Current usage. Arch Dermatol *115*:486, 1979.
15. Voron DA: Systemic absorption of topical clindamycin. Arch Dermatol *114*:798, 1978.
16. Becker LE, Bergstresser PR, Whiting DA, et al: Topical clindamycin therapy for acne vulgaris: A cooperative clinical study. Arch Dermatol *117*:482, 1981.
17. Milstone EB, McDonald AJ, Scholhamer CF: Pseudomembranous colitis after topical application of clindamycin. Arch Dermatol *117*:154, 1981.
18. Dayal VS, Smith EL, McCain WG: Cochlear and vestibular gentamicin toxicity: A clinical study of systemic and topical usage. Arch Otolaryngol *100*:338, 1974.
19. Drake TE: Reaction to gentamicin sulfate cream. Arch Dermatol *110*:638, 1974.
20. Mittelman H: Ototoxicity of "ototopical" antibiotics: Past, present, and future. Trans Am Acad Ophthalmol Otolaryngol *76*:1432, 1972.
21. Friedmann I: Aerosols containing neomycin. Lancet *1*:1662, 1977.
22. Anonymous: Warning on aerosols containing neomycin. Lancet *1*:1115, 1977.
23. Bamford MFM, Jones LF: Deafness and biochemical imbalance after burns treatment with topical antibiotics in young children. Arch Dis Child *53*:326, 1978.
24. Masur H, Whelton PK, Whelton A: Neomycin toxicity revisited. Arch Surg *3*:822, 1976.
25. Kelly DR, Nilo EN, Berggren RB: Deafness after topical neomycin wound irrigation. N Engl J Med *280*:1338, 1969.
26. Goffinet M: A propos de la toxicite cliniquement presumable de certaintes gouttes otiques. Acta Otorhinolaryngol Belg *31*:585, 1977.
27. Kellerhals B: Horschaden durch ototoxische Ohrtropfen. Ergebnisse einer Umfrage. HNO (Berl) *26*:49, 1978.
28. Cammann R, Hennecke H, Beier R: Symptomatische Psychosen nach Kolton-Gelee-Applikation. Psychiat Neurol Med Psychol *23*:426, 1971.
29. Bloch R, Beysovec L: Promethazine toxicity through

percutaneous absorption. Contin Practice *9*:28, 1982.
30. Done AK: Borates. *In* Haddad LM, Winchester JF (eds): Clinical Management of Poisoning and Drug Overdose. Philadelphia, WB Saunders, 1983, p 929.
31. Lundell E, Nordman R: A case of infantile poisoning by topical application of Castellani's solution. Ann Clin Res *5*:404, 1973.
32. Rogers SCF, Burrows D, Neill D: Percutaneous absorption of phenol and methyl alcohol in Magenta Paint B.P.C. Br J Dermatol *98*:559, 1978.
33. Haddad LM: Miscellany. *In* Haddad LM, Winchester JF (eds): Clinical Management of Poisoning and Drug Overdose. Philadelphia, WB Saunders, 1983, p 963.
34. Tyrala EE, Hillman LS, Hillman RE, Dodson WE: Clinical pharmacology of hexachlorophene in newborn infants. J Pediatr *91*:481, 1977.
35. Curley A, Hawk RE, Kimbrough RD, Nathenson G, Finberg L: Dermal absorption of hexachlorophene infants. Lancet *2*:296, 1971.
36. Alder VD, Burman D, Coroner-Beryl D, Gillespie WA: Absorption of hexachlorophene from infant's skin. Lancet *2*:384, 1972.
37. Pines WI: Hexachlorophene: Why FDA concluded that hexachlorophene was too potent and too dangerous to be used as it once was? FDA Consumer *6*:24, 1972.
38. Editorial: Hexachlorophene today. Lancet *1*:500, 1982.
39. Plueckhahn VC, Ballard BA, Banis JM, Collins RB, Flett PT: Hexachlorophene preparations in infant antiseptic skin care: Benefit, risks and the future. Med J Aust *2*:555, 1978.
40. Hopkins J: Hexachlorophene: More bad news than good. Food Cosmet Toxicol *17*:410, 1979.
41. Otten H, Plempel M: Antibiotika und Chemotherapeutika in Einzeldarstellungen. Chemotherapeutika mit breitem Wirkungsbereich. Sulfonamide. *In* Otten H, Plempel M, Siegenthaler G (eds): Antibiotika-Fibel. Stuttgart, Thieme Verlag, 1975, p 110–145.
42. Liebman PR, Kennelly MM, Hirsch EF: Hypercarbia and acidosis associated with carbonic anhydrase inhibition: A hazard of topical mafenide acetate use in renal failure. Burns *8*:395, 1982.
43. Albert TA, Lewis NS, Warpeha RL: Late pulmonary complications with use of mafenide acetate. J Burn Care Rehabil *3*:375, 1982.
44. Ohlgisser M, Adler MN, Ben-Dov B, Taitelman U, Birkhan HJ, Bursztein S: Methemoglobinaemia induced by mafenide acetate in children. A report of two cases. Br J Anaesth *50*:299, 1978.
45. Mofenson HC, Caraccio TR, Greensher J: Iodine. *In* Haddad LM, Winchester JF (eds): Clinical Management of Poisoning and Drug Overdose. Philadelphia, WB Saunders, 1983, p 697.
46. Baranowski-Dutkiewicz B: Skin absorption of phenol from aqueous solutions in men. Int Arch Occup Environ Health *49*:99, 1981.
47. Cullison D, Abele DC, O'Quinn JL: Localized exogenous ochronosis. Report of a case and review of the literature. J Am Acad Dermatol *8*:882, 1983.
48. Johnstone RT: Occupational Medicine and Industrial Hygiene. St. Louis, CV Mosby, 1948, p 216.
49. Cronin TD, Brauer RO: Death due to phenol contained in Foille®. JAMA *139*:777, 1949.
50. Deichmann WB: Local and systemic effects following skin contact with phenol—a review of the literature. J Industr Hyg *31*:146, 1949.
51. Von Hinkel GK, Kitzel HW: Phenolvergiftungen bei Neugeborenen durch kutane Resorption. Dtsch Gesundh-Wes *23*:240, 1968.
52. Del Pizzo A, Tanski EL: Chemical face peeling—Malignant therapy for benign disease? (editorial). Plast Reconstr Surg *66*:121, 1980.
53. Truppman ES, Ellerby JD: Major electrocardiographic changes during chemical face peeling. Plast Reconstr Surg *63*:44, 1979.
54. Tromovitch TA: Safety of chemical face peels (letter). J Am Acad Dermatol *7*:137, 1982.
55. Baker TJ: The voice of polite dissent. Plast Reconstr Surg *63*:262, 1979.
56. Haddad LM: Phenol, dinotrophenol and pentachlorophene. *In* Haddad LM, Winchester JF (eds): Clinical Management of Poisoning and Drug Overdose. Philadelphia, WB Saunders, 1983, p 810.
57. Berthezene F, Fournier M, Bernier E, Mornex R: L'hypothyroidie induite par la resorcine. Lyon Med *230*:319, 1973.
58. Thomas AE, Gisburn MA: Exogenous ochronosis and myxoedema from resorcinol. Br J Dermatol *73*:378, 1961.
59. Flandin C, Rabeau H, Ukrainczyk M: Intolerance à la resorcine. Test cutane. Soc Dermatol Syph *12*:1804, 1953.
60. Murray MC: An analysis of sixty cases of drug poisoning. Arch Pediatr *43*:193, 1926.
61. Cunningham AA: Resorcinol poisoning. Arch Dis Child *31*:173, 1956.
62. Lundell E, Nordman R: A case of infantile poisoning by topical application of Castellani's solution. Ann Clin Res *5*:404, 1973.
63. Yeung D, Kanto S, Nacht S, Gans EH: Percutaneous absorption, blood levels and urinary excretion of resorcinol applied topically in humans. Int J Dermatol 22:321, 1983.
64. Gabrilove JL, Luria M: Persistent gynecomastia resulting from scalp inunction of estradiol: A model for persistent gynecomastia. Arch Dermatol *114*:1672, 1978.
65. Owens CJ, Yarbrough DR, Brackett NR: Nephrotic syndrome following topically applied sulfadiazine therapy. Arch Intern Med *134*:332, 1974.
66. Chan CK, Jarrett F, Moylan JA: Acute leukopenia as an allergic reaction to silver sulfadiazine in burn patients. J Trauma *16*:395, 1976.
67. Jarrett F, Ellerbe S, Demling R: Acute leukopenia during topical burn therapy with silver sulfadiazine. Am J Surg *135*:818, 1978.
68. Fraser GL, Beaulieu JT: Leukopenia secondary to sulfadiazine silver. JAMA *241*:1928, 1979.
69. Haddad LM, Winchester JF (eds): Clinical Management of Poisoning and Drug Overdose. Philadelphia, WB Saunders, 1983.
70. Scharpf LG, Hill ID, Maibach HI: Percutaneous penetration and disposition of tricarban in man. Arch Environ Hlth *30*:7, 1975.
71. Fisch RO, Berglund EB, Bridge AG, Finley PR, Quie PG: On triclocarban and methemoglobinemia. *Quoted in* Marzulli F, Maibach H: Dermatotoxicology. 3rd Ed. Washington, DC, Hemisphere Press, 1985.
72. Ponte C, Richard J, Bonte C, Lequien P, Lacombe A: Methemoglobinemies chez le nouveau-né. Discussion du role etiologique du trichlorcarbanilide. Ann Pediatr *21*:359, 1974.
73. Robertson WO: Arsenic and other heavy metals. *In* Haddad LM, Winchester JF (eds): Clinical Manage-

ment of Poisoning and Drug Overdose. Philadelphia, WB Saunders, 1983, p 656.
74. Connell JF Jr, Rousselot LM: Povidone-iodine; Extensive surgical evaluation of a new antiseptic. Am J Surg *108*:849, 1964.
75. Zackheim HS, Epstein EH Jr, McNutt NS: Topical carmustine (BCNU) for mycosis fungoides and related disorders: A 10-year experience. J Am Acad Dermatol *9*:363, 1983.
76. Zackheim HS, Feldman RJ, Lindsay C, Maibach HI: Percutaneous absorption of 1,3-bis(2-chloroethyl)-1-nitrosurea (BCNU, carmustine) in mycosis fungoides. Br J Dermatol *97*:65, 1977.
77. Committee on Drugs: Camphor—Who needs it? Pediatrics *62*:404, 1978.
78. Gossweiler B: Kampfervergiftungen heute. Schweiz Rundschau Med (PRAXIS) *71*:1475, 1982.
79. D'Arcy PF: Fatalities with the use of a henna dye. Pharm Int *3*:217, 1982.
80. El-Ansary EH, Ahmed MEK, Clague HW: Systemic toxicity of paraphenylenediamine. Lancet *1*:1341, 1983.
81. Cronin E: Immediate-type hypersensitivity to henna. Contact Derm *5*:198, 1980.
82. Grybowksy J, Weinstein D, Ordway N: Toxic encephalopathy apparently related to the use of an insect repellent. N Engl J Med *264*:289, 1961.
83. Zadicoff C: Toxic encephalopathy associated with use of insect repellent. J Pediatr *95*:140, 1979.
84. Kligman AM: Dimethyl sulfoxide—Part 2. JAMA *193*:151, 1965.
85. Bennett CC: Dimethyl sulfoxide. JAMA *244*:2768, 1980.
86. De Groot AC, Nater JP, Bleumink K, de Jong MCJM: Does DNCB therapy potentiate epicutaneous sensitization to non-related contact allergens? Clin Exp Dermatol *6*:139, 1981.
87. Feldman RJ, Maibach HI: Absorption of some organic compounds through the skin in man. J Invest Dermatol *54*:399, 1970.
88. McDaniel DH, Blatchley DM, Welton WA: Adverse systemic reaction to dinitrichlorobenzene (letter). Arch Dermatol *118*:371, 1982.
89. Gimenez ER, Vallejo NE, Roy E, Lis M, Izurieta EM, Rossi S, Capuccio M: Percutaneous alcohol intoxication. Clin Toxicol *1*:39, 1968.
90. Castot A, Garnier R, Lanfranchi E, et al: Effets systematiques indesirables des medicaments appliques sur la peau chez l'enfant. Therapie *35*:423, 1980.
91. Ellis CN, Mitchell AJ, Beardsley GR Jr: Tar gel interaction with disulfiram. Arch Dermatol *115*:1367, 1979.
92. Stoll D, King LE Jr: Disulfiram—alcohol skin reaction to beer-containing shampoo (letter). JAMA *244*:2045, 1980.
93. Dubiel W, Happle R: Behandlungsversuch mit Fumarsäuremonoäthylester bei Psoriasis vulgaris. Z Hautkr *47*:545, 1972.
94. Haggerty RJ: Blue baby due to methemoglobinemia. N Engl J Med *267*:13303, 1962.
95. Meynadier J, Peyron J-L: Resorption transcutanée des médicaments. Rev Pract (Paris) *32*:41, 1982.
96. Steinberg JB, Zepernick RGL: Methemoglobinemia during anesthesia. J Pediatr *61*:885, 1962.
97. Adriani J, Zepernick R: Summary of methemoglobinemia: Study of child receiving benzocaine. Letter to the Commissioner in OTC, Volume 060150: *Quoted in* Marzulli F, Maibach H: Dermatotoxicology. 3rd Ed. Washington, DC, Hemisphere Press, 1985.
98. Olson ML, McEvoy GK: Methemoglobinemia induced by local anesthetics. Am J Hosp Pharm *38*:89, 1981.
99. AMA Drug Evaluations. 3rd Ed. Littleton, MA, Publishing Sciences Group, 1977, p 269.
100. Adriani J, Zepernick R: Clinical effectiveness of drugs used for topical anesthesia. JAMA *118*:711, 1964.
101. Seldon R, Sasahara AA: Central nervous system toxicity induced by lidocaine. JAMA *202*:908, 1967.
102. Giard MJ, Uden DL, Whitelock DJ: Seizures induced by oral viscous lidocaine. Clin Pharm *2*:110, 1983.
103. Mofenson HC, Caraccio TR, Miller H, Greensher J: Lidocaine toxicity from topical mucosal application. Clin Pediatr *22*:190, 1983.
104. Aronow R: Mercury. *In* Haddad LM, Winchester JF (eds): Clinical Management of Poisoning and Drug Overdose. Philadelphia, WB Saunders, 1983, p 637.
105. Bork K, Morsches B, Holzmann H: Zum Problem der Quecksilber-Resorption aus weisser Prazipatatsalbe. Arch Dermatol Forsch *248*:137, 1973.
106. Young E: Ammoniated mercury poisoning. Br J Dermatol *72*:449, 1960.
107. Silverberg DS, McCall JT, Hunt JC: Nephrotic syndrome with use of ammoniated mercury. Arch Intern Med *120*:581, 1967.
108. Turk JL, Baker H: Nephrotic syndrome due to ammoniated mercury. Br J Dermatol *80*:623, 1968.
109. Lyons TJ, Christer CN, Larsen FS: Ammoniated mercury ointment and the nephrotic syndrome. Minn Med *58*:383, 1975.
110. Stanley-Brown EG, Frank JE: Mercury poisoning from application to omphalocele (letter). JAMA *216*:2144, 1971.
111. Clark JA, Kasselberg AG, Glick AD, O'Neill JA Jr: Mercury poisoning from merbromin (Mercurochrome) therapy of omphalocele. Clin Pediatr *21*:445, 1982.
112. Hedges TR III, Kenyon KR, Hanninen LA, Mosher DB: Corneal and conjunctival effects of monobenzone in patients with vitiligo. Arch Ophthalmol *101*:64, 1983.
113. Harkness RA, Beveridge GW: Isolation of β-naphthol from urine after its application to skin. Nature (Lond) *211*:413, 1966.
114. Hemels HGWM: Percutaneous absorption and distribution of β-naphthol in man. Br J Dermatol *87*:614, 1972.
115. Osol A, Farrar GE Jr: The Dispensary of the United States of America. 24th ed. Philadelphia, JB Lippincott, 1947.
116. Merck Index. 9th ed. Rahway, NJ, Merck and Company, Inc, 1976, p 291.
117. Feldmann R, Maibach H: Percutaneous penetration of some pesticides and herbicides in man. Toxicol Appl Pharmacol *28*:126–132, 1974.
118. Wester R, Maibach H, Bucks D, Aufrere M: In vivo percutaneous absorption of paraquat from hand, leg and forearm of humans. J Toxicol Environ Health *14*:759–762, 1984.
119. Ginsburg CM, Lowry W, Reisch JS: Absorption of lindane (gamma benzene hexachloride) in infants and children. J Pediatr *91*:998, 1977.
120. Hosler J, Tschanz C, Higuite C, et al: Topical application of lindane cream (Kwell) and antipyrine metabolism. J Invest Dermatol *74*:51, 1980.

121. Haddad LM: The carbamate, organochlorine, and botanical insecticides; Insect repellents. *In* Haddad LM, Winchester JF (eds): Clinical Management of Poisoning and Drug Overdose. Philadelphia, WB Saunders, 1983, p 711.
122. Lee B, Groth P: Scabies: Transcutaneous poisoning during treatment. Pediatrics *59*:643, 1977.
123. Telch J, Jarvis DA: Acute intoxication with lindane (gamma benzene hexachloride). Can Med Assoc J *126*:662, 1982.
124. Davies JE, Dedhia HV, Morgade C, et al: Lindane poisonings. Arch Dermatol *119*:142, 1983.
125. Gamma benzene hexachloride (Kwell) and other products alert. FDA Drug Bulletin: *6*:28, 1976.
126. Matsuoka LY: Convulsions following application of gamma benzene hexachloride. J Am Acad Dermatol *5*:98, 1981.
127. Pramanik AK, Hansen RC: Transcutaneous gamma benzene hexachloride absorption and toxicity in infants and children. Arch Dermatol *115*:1224, 1979.
128. Solomon LM, Fahrner L, West DP: Gamma benzene hexachloride toxicity. A review. Arch Dermatol *113*:353, 1977.
129. Shacter B: Treatment of scabies and pediculosis with lindane preparations: An evaluation. J Am Acad Dermatol *5*:517, 1981.
130. Rasmussen JE: The problem of lindane. J Am Acad Dermatol *5*:507, 1981.
131. Kramer MS, Hutchinson TA, Rudnick SA, et al: Operational criteria for adverse drug reactions in evaluating suspected toxicity of a popular scabicide. Clin Pharmacol Ther *27*:149, 1980.
132. Haddad LM: The organophosphate insecticides. *In* Haddad LM, Winchester JF (eds): Clinical Management of Poisoning and Drug Overdose. Philadelphia, WB Saunders, 1983, p 704.
133. Ramu A, Slonim EA, Egal F: Hyperglycemia in acute malathion poisoning. Israel J Med Sci *9*:631, 1973.
134. Milby TH, Epstein WL: Allergic sensitivity to malathion. Arch Environ Health *9*:434, 1964.
135. Haddad LM: Miscellany. *In* Haddad LM, Winchester JF (eds): Clinical Management of Poisoning and Drug Overdose. Philadelphia, WB Saunders, 1983, p 965.
136. Cassidy DE, Drewry J, Fanning JP: Podophyllum toxicity: A report of a fatal case and a review of the literature. J Toxicol Clin Toxicol *19*:35, 1982.
137. Chamberlain MJ, Reynolds AL, Yeoman WB: Toxic effect of podophyllum application in pregnancy. Br Med J *3*:391, 1972.
138. Karol KD, Conner CS, Watanabe AS, Murphey KJL: Podophyllum: Suspected teratogenicity from topical application. Clin Toxicol *16*:283, 1980.
139. Proudfoot AT: Salicylates and salicylamide. *In* Haddad LM, Winchester JF (eds): Clinical Management of Poisoning and Drug Overdose. Philadelphia, WB Saunders, 1983, p 575.
140. Taylor JR, Halprin K: Percutaneous absorption of salicylic acid. Arch Dermatol *106*:740, 1975.
141. Von Weiss JF, Lever WF: Percutaneous salicylic acid intoxication in psoriasis. Arch Dermatol *90*:614, 1964.
142. United States Department of Health, Education and Welfare, Food and Drug Administration, OTC Antimicrobial II Advisory Panel. Quoted by Rasmussen JE: Percutaneous absorption in children. *In* Dobson RL (ed): Year Book of Dermatology. Chicago, Year Book Medical Publishers, 1979, p 28.
143. Lindsey CP: Two cases of fatal salicylate poisoning after topical application of an antifungal solution. Med J Aust *1*:353, 1968.
144. Wechselberg K: Salizylsaure—Vergiftung durch perkutane Resorption 1%-iger Salizylvaseline. Anaesth Prax *4*:103, 1969.
145. Treguer G, Le Bihan G, Coloignier M, Le Roux P, Bernard JP: Intoxication salicylee par application locale de vaseline salicylee à 20% chez un psoriasique. Nouv Presse Med *9*:192, 1980.
146. Ransone JW, Scott NM, Knoblock EC: Selenium sulfide intoxication. N Engl J Med *9*:631, 1973.
147. Ternberg JL, Luce E: Methemoglobinemia: A complication of the silver nitrate treatment of burns. Surgery *63*:328, 1968.
148. Editorial: Burns and silver nitrate. JAMA *193*:230, 1965.
149. Connely DM: Silver nitrate—ideal burn wound therapy? NY State J Med *70*:1642, 1970.
150. Bader KF: Organ deposition of silver following silver nitrate therapy of burns. Plast Reconstr Surg *37*:550, 1966.
151. Marshall JP, Schneider RP: Systemic argyria secondary to topical silver nitrate. Arch Dermatol *113*:1072, 1977.
152. Zech P, Colon S, Labeeuw R, Blanc-Brunat N, Richard P, Porol M: Syndrome nephrotique avec depot d'argent dans les membranes glomerulaires au cours d'une argyrie. Nouv Presse Med *2*:161, 1973.
153. Feldmann RJ, Maibach HI: Penetration of 14C-hydrocortisone through normal skin. Arch Dermatol *91*:661, 1965.
154. Pascher F: Systemic reactions to topically applied drugs. Int J Dermatol *17*:768, 1978.
155. Feiwell M, James VHT, Barnett ES: Effect of potent topical steroids on plasma-cortisol levels of infants and children with eczema. Lancet *1*:485, 1969.
156. Burton TT, Cunliffe WJ, Holti G, Wright W: Complications of topical corticosteroid therapy in patients with liver disease. Br J Dermatol *9(Suppl 10)*:22, 1974.
157. May PH, Stern EJ, Ryter RJ, Hirsch FS, Michel B, Levy RP: Cushing syndrome from percutaneous absorption of triamcinolone cream. Arch Intern Med *136*:612, 1976.
158. Van der Harst LCA, Smeenk G, Burger PM, Van der Rhee JH, Polano MK: Waardebepaling en risicoschatting van de uitwendige behandeling met clobetasol-17-propionaat (Dermovate). Ned T Geneesk *122*:219, 1978.
159. Beas F, Vargas L, Spada RP, Merchak N: Pseudoprecocious puberty in infants caused by a dermal ointment containing estrogens. J Pediatr *75*:127, 1969.
160. Bertaggia A: A case of precocious puberty in a girl following the use of an estrogen preparation on the skin. Pediatria (Napoli) *76*:579, 1968.
161. Landolt R, Murset G: Vorzeitige Pubertatsmerkmale als Folge unbeabsichtigter Ostrogenverabreichung. Schweiz Med Wschr *98*:638, 1968.
162. Ramos AS, Bower BF: Pseudosexual precocity due to cosmetics ingestion. JAMA *207*:369, 1969.
163. Stoppelman MRH, Van Valkenburg RA: Pigmentaties en gynecomastie ten gevolge van het gebruik van stilboestrol bevattend haarewater bij kinderen. Ned T Geneesk *99*:3925, 1955.
164. Edidin DV, Levitsky LL: Prepubertal gynecomastia associated with estrogen-containing hair cream. Am J Dis Child *136*:587, 1982.

165. DiRaimondo CV, Roach AC, Meador CK: Gynecomastia from exposure to vaginal estrogen cream (letter). N Engl J Med *302*:1089, 1980.
166. Gabrilove JL, Luria M: Persistent gynecomastia resulting from scalp inunction of estradiol: A model for persistent gynecomastia. Arch Dermatol *114*:1672, 1978.
167. Bazex A, Salvader R, Dupre A, Christol B: Gynecomastie et hyperpigmentation areolaire apres oestrogenotherapie locale antiseborrheque. Bull Soc Franc Dermatol Syph *74*:466, 1967.
168. Goebel M: Mamillenhypertrophie mit Pigmentierung nach lokaler Oestrogentherapie im Kindesalter. Hautarzt *20*:521, 1969.
169. Goluboff N, MacFadyen DJ: Methemoglobinemia in an infant. J Pediatr *47*:222, 1955.
170. Gay MW, Moore WJ, Morgan JM, Montes LF: Anthralin toxicity. Arch Dermatol *105*:213, 1972.
171. Farber EM, Harris DR: Hospital treatment of psoriasis. Arch Dermatol *101*:381, 1970.

CHAPTER 17
CHEMICAL AND DRUG INJURY TO THE EYE

Peter A. Campochiaro, M.D.
J.A. Fogle, M.D.
Daniel A. Spyker, Ph.D., M.D.

Emergency department and primary care medical personnel usually represent the first contact for patients with eye-related problems due to chemical and drug toxicity. As such, they must be able to recognize such problems, initiate treatment when needed, and make appropriate referrals to an ophthalmologist. The goal of this chapter is to provide guidelines for the recognition and management of three types of problems: (1) ocular problems due to local chemical or drug exposure, (2) ocular problems due to systemic chemical or drug exposure, and (3) systemic problems due to ocular or periocular drug exposure.

The ocular insult of greatest emergency is surface assault with chemicals, particularly alkalis and acids. Precise identification of a particular agent is often difficult in the setting of accidental injury. Since straightforward first aid, namely lavage, is relatively safe, such first aid should be started *immediately,* and questions related to identification of the agent may be asked once lavage is under way. Devastating ocular damage may result from treatment delay measured in seconds.

Ocular complaints stemming from systemic exposure to drugs or toxins can usually be handled with more deliberation with regard to specific causes after initial management of the acute poisoning has been started. Systemic problems due to ocular or periocular drugs may on rare occasions be acute and life-threatening, but more often they are indolent and difficult to recognize.

Ocular responses to toxic substances evoke diverse symptoms, among them the following: pain, irritation, lacrimation, photophobia, visual disturbance (e.g., altered colors, refractive change), visual decrease, and blindness. Such symptoms correlate with effects on particular eye structures. Surface damage leading to epithelial injury or loss may cause pain, irritation, and reflex lacrimation. The opacification of critical refractive structures such as the cornea and the lens leads to visual decrease. Destruction or closure of the anterior chamber angle may lead to an acute increase in intraocular pressure (glaucoma), with attendant pain. Influences on ciliary muscle innervation may affect the capacity to focus, leading to a decrease in visual perception. Injury to ciliary body vasculature may lead to secondary deficiency of lens and corneal nutrition. Damage to critical retinal structures or to optic nerve fibers may alter perception, decrease vision, and lead to blindness. Influences may be instantaneous or accrue over long intervals.

Table 17–1 organizes some common agents of eye injury based on their clinical effects. More extensive tables have been collected by Grant[1] and Fraunfelder.[2]

Complete destruction of the globe may follow overwhelming topical injury before any saving steps are possible. Any injury less grave will benefit from appropriate steps taken at the scene or in the emergency department. When there is *any doubt* about the assessment or management of an ocular injury or complaint, an ophthalmologist should be consulted. *Irrigation of chemically damaged eyes should never await the advice or arrival of a consultant.* Rescue squads, poison centers, emergency department staff, and lay people should know this fact.

Table 17–1. EFFECTS OF SELECTED TOXINS

Pain and/or lacrimation, photophobia
- *Surface damage*
  - Thermal (sunlamp)
  - Ultraviolet light (welding arc, sunlamp)
  - Caustics (acids, alkalis)
  - Solvents (alcohols, toluene)
  - Surfactants/detergents (benzalkonium chloride, soap)
  - Lacrimators (mace)

Severe pain (headache, nausea)
- *Acute glaucoma*
  - Sympathomimetics (ephedrine, phenylpropanolamine, nicotine) in susceptible individuals
  - Parasympatholytics (atropine, Jimson weed) in susceptible individuals
  - Caustic or thermal injury with anterior segment shrinkage
- *Surface damage* (see above)

Decreased vision
- *Surface damage* (blur, photophobia)
- *Cataract* (blur)
  - Infrared light
  - Electric shock
  - Ionizing radiation
  - Corticosteroids (topical, systemic)
  - Busulfan (Myleran)
  - Chlorpromazine (Thorazine)
  - Intraocular foreign body (copper, iron)
- *Altered accommodation* (blur)
  - Sedative-hypnotics (ethanol, barbiturates, benzodiazepines)
  - Parasympathomimetics (pilocarpine, organophosphates)
  - Parasympatholytics (atropine, Jimson weed)
- *Retinal and retinal pigment epithelium degeneration* (decreased vision, visual field defects, dyschromatopsia, ± pigmentary retinopathy)
  - Solar retinopathy
  - Chloroquine, hydroxychloroquine
  - Clofazimine
  - Thioridazine (Mellaril)
  - Quinine
  - Metals
  - Deferoxamine

The first section in this chapter contains our recommendations for treatment of surface eye exposures—those exposures for which *rapid management steps must be taken.* The second section outlines relevant ocular anatomy and physiology. The last section deals with selected local and systemic toxic agents.

No emergency department that cares for eye injuries should be without Grant's Toxicology of the Eye[1] and Fraunfelder's Drug-Induced Ocular Side Effects and Drug Interactions.[2] A useful reference for neuro-ophthalmologic toxins is Walsh and Hoyt's Clinical Neuro-Ophthalmology.[3]

TREATMENT FOR SURFACE EXPOSURE

Figure 17–1 summarizes treatment recommendations for eye surface exposure.

On-Site Treatment: Irrigation

Irrigation of the eye provides the greatest opportunity to reduce damage from surface exposure to chemicals. *Time* so outweighs other considerations that the most accessible and plentiful bland irrigants should be used. Water or physiologic saline solutions are first choices. Dilution and flushing begun as soon as possible after injury and continued throughout emergency department treatment is especially critical following caustic exposure. DO NOT use neutralizing solutions and do not delay on-site irrigation for transport to a hospital.

Workplaces and laboratories often supply small squeeze bottles of irrigant, clipped to a wall mount, for emergency eye treatment. These are inadequate for all but the most trivial insults. Showers with large pull-rings or commodious sinks must be provided where there is genuine risk. Anyone at risk should wear eye protection and should be drilled in irrigation techniques. Persons working outdoors should irrigate with hoses, spigots, or whatever is available to flush the eyes. Jumping into a pond or pool is undesirable as a treatment for ocular injury because pain brings blepharospasm (forced closure of the lids), which protects the

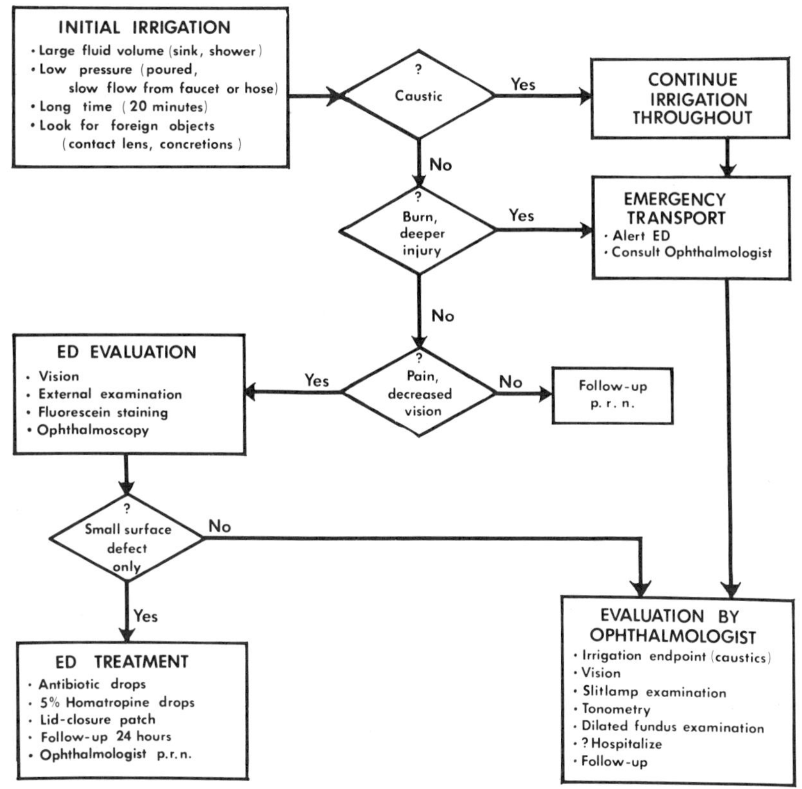

Figure 17–1. Protocol for managing eye surface exposures, emphasizing importance of irrigation and ophthalmologic consultation.

contaminated surface from the water. The distraught victim, who will need assistance in keeping the lids apart, should not become isolated from such assistance. Assistance is also important in identifying and recovering foreign objects, such as contact lenses. Twenty to thirty minutes of effective irrigation should be begun on site and should not be interrupted by other events, including transport to the emergency department.

For minor eye exposures, to such agents as dog repellent, insecticides, and so on, 20 minutes of irrigation may be all that is necessary.

Transport

Continued irrigation en route to the emergency department is desirable for any serious ocular chemical injury and mandatory for any caustic exposure. The transport vehicle should have topical anesthetic available to facilitate effective irrigation to the surface and all recessed parts of the eye. Lid retractors or other aids to lid manipulation are necessary. Figure 17–2 shows standard retractors and an easy-to-fashion substitute.

Emergency Department Evaluation

Once in the emergency department, irrigation should continue without interruption for caustic injuries. A decision should then be made, on the basis of all available facts in the history, about the need for further irrigation.

Irrigation in the emergency department can be expedited by having available several suspended bottles of normal saline with sterile tubing. Topical anesthetic and lid retractors (e.g., Desmarres retractors), used with flexible intravenous tubing, allow the fluid to be directed on to the eye comfortably and precisely for as long as is required (Fig. 17–3). Measurement of visual acuity or inspection of the eye for contact lenses or other extraneous materials should not delay transition to emergency department irrigation. Swab the fornices if necessary to remove adherent debris *during* irrigation. Evert or

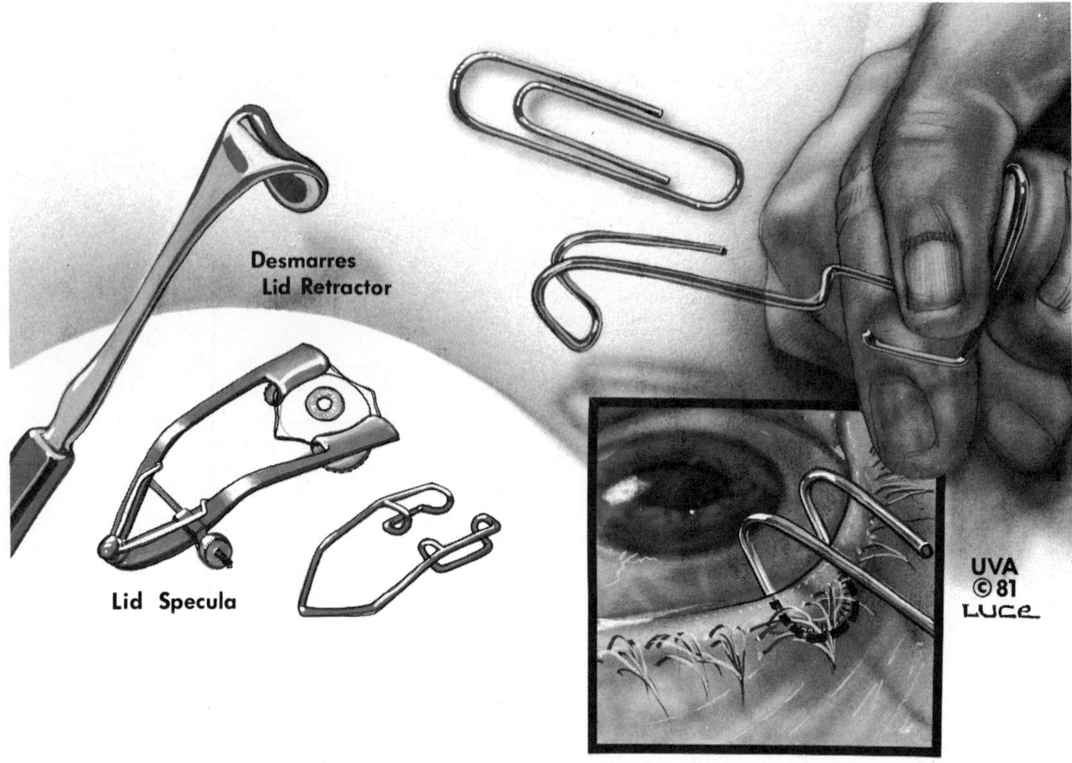

Figure 17–2. Devices for holding lids apart, including Desmarres retractor (allows active manipulation), specula (free-standing, may require 7th nerve block), and retractor improvised from a paper clip.

doubly evert the upper lids to provide proper access to the superior cul-de-sac (Fig. 17–4). Try to avoid pressure on the globe during these maneuvers. If both eyes are injured, simultaneous irrigation is essential. In selected cases, 7th nerve block to counteract blepharospasm may be considered. Intravenous acetazolamide (Diamox), 500 mg, is used in patients with severe caustic injuries to blunt the ocular hypertensive effects of shrinkage of the anterior segment.

If a victim of tear gas, solvent, or surfactant injury appears in the emergency department without benefit of previous irrigation, 30 minutes of effective irrigation should be provided.

Emergency department evaluation of caustic, thermal, or mechanical (e.g., explosive) injuries may require an ophthalmologist (see later section, When To Consult). Following irrigation, in persons with less serious injuries, visual acuity should be tested, the surface of the globe should be stained with fluorescein to search for external defects, and the fundus is examined. If there is any doubt about the gravity of an injury or if extensive denudation of the surface is clearly present, an ophthalmologist should see the patient.

Emergency Department Treatment

Small epithelial defects may be appropriately treated by instilling an antibiotic (e.g., neosporin, sulfacetamide, gentamicin) and homatropine 5 per cent eye drops and applying an eye patch sufficiently snug to *keep the lid closed*. The patient should be told that the patch is *not* intended to exclude light but to minimize lid movement, a disturbance to healing. A history of narrow-angle glaucoma should be sought before routinely using cycloplegic eye drops such as homatropine. The patch should be removed in 24 hours, either in the emergency department or by the ophthalmologist. Adequate healing without infection and with resolution of symptoms must be ensured.

When to Stop Irrigation

Visual acuity testing and fundus examination must await adequate irrigation. The end-

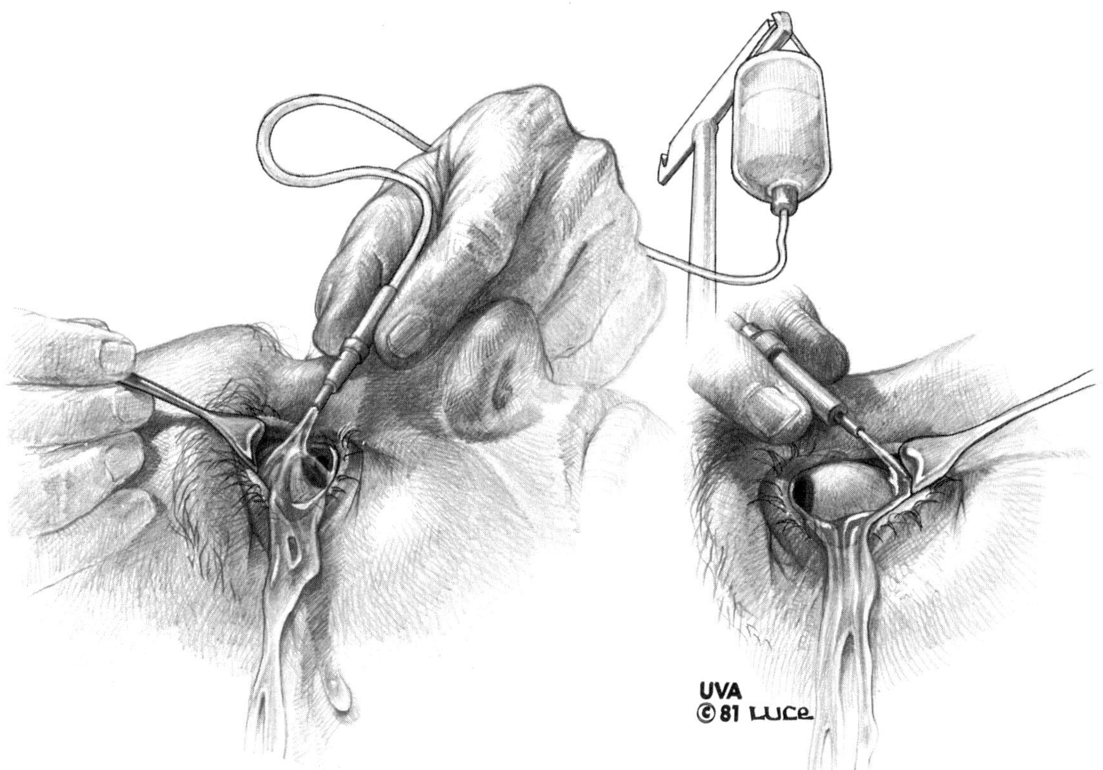

Figure 17–3. Suggested technique for surface irrigation using IV solution and Desmarres retractor.

point of irrigation for caustic injuries depends on the nature of the substance and the extent of exposure. For acid burns, pH measurements may be taken from the globe surface, using standard testing papers. In an acid burn, a pH of around 7, following 30 to 60 minutes of irrigation, is an end-point. Since alkaline agents produce deeper injuries and substances may persist in tissue as reservoirs, surface pH is less useful as an indicator in such injuries. Irrigation in alkali injuries should continue until an ophthalmologist decides that further irrigation is probably fruitless. Such a decision may be based in part on pH assessment, but the nature of the chemical and the appearance of the eye contribute significantly to the decision. Irrigation in alkali injuries may continue for hours, through multiple bottles of solutions.

When to Consult

An ophthalmologist should see all patients with caustic alkali injuries because informed

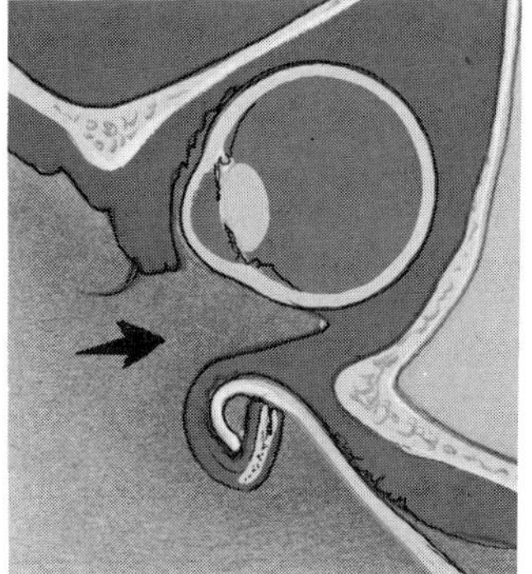

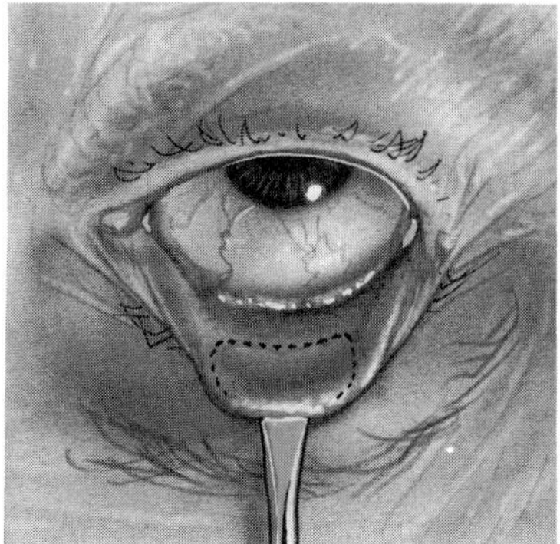

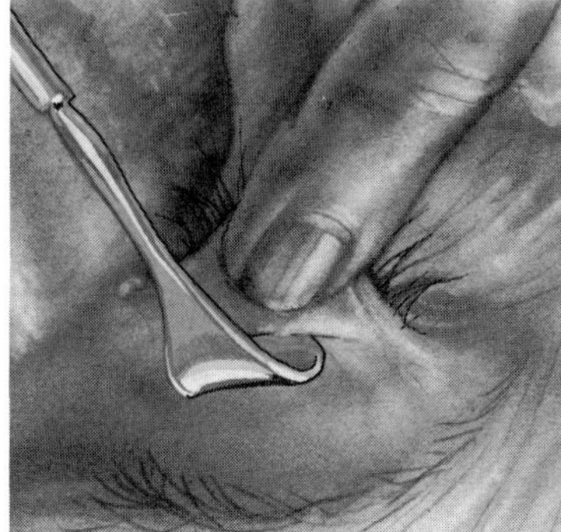

Figure 17–4. Flipping the lid (eversion) and further extension with the lid retractor (double eversion) permit optimal access to the superior cul de sac for inspection and irrigation of the upper globe.

decisions must be made regarding the extent of initial damage, duration of irrigation, and need for hospital admission. The need for consultation should be anticipated and a consulting ophthalmologist identified, so that patient evaluation may be expedited. Until the ophthalmologist arrives and only after adequate irrigation, saline-moistened gauze squares should be placed over the closed lids.

Following adequate irrigation, chemical burns are usually treated with lubricant ointments and lid closure sufficient to protect the damaged surface and encourage healing. Because ointments may interfere with early wound healing and may obscure facets of damage of interest to the ophthalmologist, antibiotic *drops* preferentially should be used by the emergency department staff. Atropine drops should be used for cycloplegia, but, again, an ophthalmologist should see the patient first, if possible, to establish baselines for judging abnormality. The use of topical corticosteroids and anticollagenase drugs will depend on details of the ophthalmologic examination.[4–6] The ophthalmologist will also consider the use of topical chelating rinses (e.g., 0.01 M NaEDTA) to remove damaging concretions that cannot be safely removed by mechanical means. Anterior chamber drainage or irrigation is a dangerous and controversial means of depleting intraocular alkali and should be done, if at all, only by an ophthalmologist.[4]

Ostensibly mild alkali burns, after initially gratifying surface healing, may have delayed effects, with spontaneous epithelial breakdown and stromal melting occurring weeks after the initial injury.[6, 7] Therefore, close ophthalmologic follow-up must be ensured.

RELEVANT OCULAR ANATOMY

The Ocular Surface

The *ocular surface*[7, 8] consists of the tear film, the conjunctiva, and the cornea. This first line of defense receives the brunt of surface injury. Both the conjunctiva and the cornea have squamous epithelial surfaces about five to six cells thick. A cementing basement membrane separates the columnar basal epithelial cells from the underlying tissues, which consist, in the conjunctiva, of fibrovascular stroma and in the cornea, of a dense matrix of collagen. Surface cells desquamate following their migration from the generative basal layers, giving a cell a lifespan of about a week.

The coating of the conjunctival and corneal epithelial surfaces is mucin, secreted by goblet cells nestled within the conjunctival epithelium. The mucinous component of the tear film decreases the surface tension of the aqueous tears sufficiently to discourage tear film disruption between blinks. Aqueous lacrimal fluid is provided by accessory lacrimal glands situated within the forniceal conjunctiva. Aqueous tears are also provided by the main lacrimal gland, usually as part of a reflex arc triggered by surface disturbance. Autonomic nerves stimulate the tear gland itself. Modified sebaceous glands within the tarsal plates of the eyelid contribute a lipid layer to the tear film, probably reducing tear evaporation between blinks. Alterations in the quantity or the quality of any of the three components of the tear film may affect tear function and, hence, epithelial cell safety. Critical to tear function is the role of the eyelids in blinking, effecting renewal of tear film and drainage of debris toward the nasolacrimal duct.

The corneal stroma consists of collagen and ground substance. The cornea is approximately 80 per cent water, and corneal permeability depends to a large degree on the integrity of the surface cell layers and the lipid solubility or water solubility of a given substance. Degradation of corneal collagen and associated mucoproteins leads to tissue disarray and loss of clarity as well as decreased tissue strength.

In humans, the innervation of the cornea is probably limited to afferent (sensory) nerves of the first branch of the trigeminal nerve. Smaller nerve branches ramify from larger nerves at the limbus, and raw nerve endings extend up into the epithelium to within one or two cells from the surface. Hence, considerable discomfort may result from trivial surface injury.

The level of hydration of the corneal stroma ensures a proper relationship of the collagen fibrils that allows light to pass through this macroscopically clear tissue. The monolayer of cells on the back of the cornea, the endothelium, acts as a barrier to fluid flow into the stroma. Damage to the endothelial layer leads to imbibition of aqueous fluid into the corneal stroma, with resultant swelling and reduction in transparency.

Corneal wounds can be repaired by fibroblast-like activity of the stromal keratocytes, with associated contributions from the epithelial and endothelial cell layers. Damage to the corneal epithelial cells can be repaired by sliding of adjacent cells, followed by mitotic regeneration of cells. When many corneal epithelial cells are lost, reconstitution of the surface must come from sliding of conjunctival epithelial cells, which differ in certain biochemical ways from corneal epithelial cells.[9] Extensive epithelial damage to the ocular surface can be nonhealing if physical, metabolic, and topographic factors are not ideal. Such a poor healing surface leaves the stroma vulnerable to infection, inflammation, and enzymatic degradation. A damaged ocular surface must be protected from drying and, as much as possible, from infection. A good tear film and complete lid coverage are critical. Residual disturbances from chemicals or other foreign material must be minimized.

Anterior Segment

The term *anterior segment* refers to the ocular surface components described in the preceding section, the aqueous outflow channels, the anterior uvea including the iris and ciliary body, the lens, and the anterior vitreous.

Aqueous humor derives from the blood in the ciliary processes behind the iris and peripheral to the lens. The fluid exits from the eye through the trabecular pores, which are endothelialized channels surrounding the anterior chamber, coursing eventually into episcleral veins. Physical plugging or damage to these outflow channels, as from thermal shrinkage, can lead to an elevated intraocular pressure.

The iris is a portion of the anterior uvea and, like the choroid, is heavily pigmented and vascular. The iris moves in response to sympathetic influences on its dilator muscle and parasympathetic influences on its sphincter muscle. Agents capable of mimetic or lytic autonomic influences therefore can influence pupillary size.

Parasympatholytic and parasympathomimetic influences can alter the shape of the lens by acting on the ciliary muscle. For example, atropine paralyzes the ciliary muscle and hence decreases focusing capacity for near objects. On the other hand, acetylcholine-like agents cause the focusing muscle to act, the result being a "spasm of accommodation." The ciliary muscle is able to exert such influences on lens shape by means of the zonular fibers, which extend from the ciliary processes to the lens capsule about the lens equator. Contraction of the circular ciliary muscle normally decreases zonular tension and allows the lens to assume a thicker shape with a shorter focal distance.

The ciliary processes contain an epithelium that actively aids in the derivation of aqueous fluid from the blood. Damage to this epithelium and to the vessels themselves may result in an eye that is too soft and has poorly nourished anterior structures such as the endothelium of the cornea and the epithelium of the lens.

The lens is transparent and has two convex surfaces. The lens coating is its capsule, secreted by the lens epithelium. Epithelial cells become elongated at the lens equator (the lens periphery), forming lens fibers, which become serially compacted toward the firm lens center, the nucleus. With age, these fibers lose their nuclei and organelles and become quite densely packed. This tight packing of lens protein results in an increasing index of refraction toward the lens center. The epithelial cells, in addition to evolving into fibers that make up the lens cortex, help to maintain an appropriate ionic equilibrium within the lens.[10] The aqueous humor provides oxygen, glucose, amino acids, and other nutrients and provides the necessary turnover of metabolites. Damage to the lens epithelium, directly or by interference with aqueous production, can result in a spectrum of derangements that are commonly associated with lens opacity (cataracts).

The vitreous gel consists of collagen and hyaluronic acid. The vitreous body does not play a critical part in most toxic reactions in the eye, except for the *severe* inflammatory effects of intraocular copper.[5, 11, 12]

Posterior Segment

The *posterior segment* includes the posterior portion of the vitreous, the retina, the choroid, and the optic nerve.

The choroid is a pigmented vascular layer between the retina and the sclera. Its inner layer, the choriocapillaris, provides oxygen and nutrients to the outer retinal layers and the retinal pigment epithelium.

The retina has a high level of metabolic activity, and oxygen deprivation, resulting either from a compromised retinal or choroidal blood supply or other blood abnormality, leads to suboptimal function. The retinal pigment epithelium has numerous functions that help to maintain the photoreceptors and are therefore required for normal vision.

Visual stimuli are converted to electrical activity in the photoreceptors. This activity is propagated through the other retinal layers, which help to encode spatial and temporal parameters of the stimuli. These stimuli are delivered to the innermost cell layer of the retina, the ganglion cell layer, which generates the impulses that pass through the optic nerve to the brain. Synapses occur in the lateral geniculate body on neurons that send axons to the occipital cortex, where the impulses are decoded into images.

AGENTS OF INJURY

Lists of specific agents of harm are available in comprehensive reference books, which no medical library should lack. Mention has been made of the indispensible reference by Grant.[1] The most inclusive of reference books is of little help if effective assessment of a specific injury cannot be made.

Radiant Energy

Nonionizing and ionizing radiant energy causes several types of injury to the eye. Instances that may result in a *sudden* complaint are more limited in number.

Ultraviolet Light. Chronic exposure to *ultraviolet light* can result in indolent lesions of the surface, such as pinguecula and pterygia, in which conjunctival and corneal collagen degenerates. The relationship of a lifetime of ultraviolet exposure to the development of cataract has been postulated. Accumulation in the lens nucleus of photoinduced pigments with age is associated with increased lens opacity.[14]

Most *acute* damage from ultraviolet light is inflicted on the ocular surface, specifically the epithelial cells. Damage of this kind brings a person to an emergency department with complaints of decreased vision, photophobia, and significant pain. It was demonstrated decades ago that a particular type of epithelial derangement can be induced by ultraviolet light. The corneal epithelium contains chromophores, such as nucleic acids, which absorb most of the ultraviolet energy (wavelengths of less then 295 nm) near the surface of the eye.[14] Up to a point, free radical scavengers protect the cells from photodamage. Overexposure to these wavelengths of light results in cell loosening and disturbances of maturation.[15] Sloughing of superficial epithelium results, with exposure of raw nerve endings and development of a gritty and often painful sensation. Because of the pathophysiology of this damage, there may be a lag of as much as 24 hours between exposure and development of symptoms. The patient describes photophobia and, owing to the irregular surface, decreased vision (acute photokerato-conjunctivitis). Appropriate management includes lubricant drops and lid closure, accomplished either with taping or firm patching. Generally speaking, both eyes must be treated this way to ensure good lid coverage for a period of 12 to 24 hours, allowing time for reconstitution of the epithelial cover.

Some persons are administered photosensitizing agents for various symptoms ranging from anxiety to psoriasis. Some of these materials may accumulate in the ocular structures, such as the lens, potentiating photodamage.[14] However, it is unlikely that acute visual complaints arising from this type of photodamage will appear. Prophylaxis with sunglasses capable of filtering ultraviolet light is wise.

Visible Light. Although ultraviolet radiation is absorbed mainly by the corneal epithelium and somewhat by the lens, *visible light* preferentially is absorbed by the photoreceptors (rods and cones) and by melanin within the retinal pigment epithelium. Absorption of excessive light energy in the visual range causes *thermal* damage. Laser and xenon arc photocoagulation use this principle to destroy certain chorioretinal lesions. Sungazing or allied experiences accomplish the same thing.

Solar retinopathy typically follows a history of exposure to bright light for even a short period of time. Vision decreases to the 20/50 to 20/100 level and in most instances gradually recovers to normal levels. With time, a remnant lesion consisting of pigment disturbance in the fovea may develop. In the acute phase, careful study of the fovea reveals some edema, which resolves. The early use of high-dose systemic corticosteroids in the amelioration of this acute condition has not proved effective, although anecdotal descriptions ascribe some benefit.[16] Generally speaking, solar retinopathy should be given time to recover to the best level possible, often about 6 weeks.

The photosensitive pigments that capture visible light reside in the outer segments, encased in lamellae resembling discs. There is a constant turnover, somewhat light-dark dependent, for both rods and cones. In rods, the inner segments produce photosensitive pigment that is incorporated into discs that move down the extent of the outer segment and are then shed and phagocytized by the retinal pigment epithelium. It has been shown in experimental animals and in clinical studies of certain retinal dystrophies that prolonged exposure to visible light energy disturbs this steady-state mechanism, resulting in severe structural abnormality of the photoreceptors.[14]

Infrared Light. *Light* of the *infrared* wavelength may impart significant thermal energy to appropriate absorptive tissues; in the eye, the damage occurs mainly to the lens and the retina. Mention has already been made of solar retinopathy, in which absorption of light in the visible and infrared spectra gives rise to coagulative damage to the retinal pigment epithelium and adjacent choroid and outer layers. In addition, particular types of anterior cortical cataracts ("glassblower's" cataract) are caused by the absorption of heat by the iris pigment epithelium, a tissue physically intimate with the anterior lens surface. In addition, cataracts can form in the posterior lens if the infrared radiation is sufficiently intense to cause more generalized thermal damage. Acute damage to the retina evokes sharp complaints because this energy is intensely focused by the cornea and the lens is toward the fovea, the area where decreased function is immediately noticed.

Public health measures in industry, such as the enforced use of goggles and heat shields, have significantly decreased the risk of thermal cataracts. Acute retinal burns, however, may occur outside of industry and are fairly commonplace. Prophylaxis is the linchpin to management.

Electricity. *Electric shock* can cause thermal damage basically to all parts of the eye, and, generally speaking, damage to the rest of the patient will be correspondingly significant. In the event of thermal damage to an ocular surface, attempts should be made to protect the eye from further physical damage and infection until an ophthalmologist can be consulted. Such protection can often be accomplished with the use of standard metal eye shields and lightly applied saline-soaked sterile pads.

In patients with less acute damage, lesions can begin developing in the lens, leading during the course of weeks and months to cortical cataracts—so-called electric cataracts. Apparently, there is damage to the equatorial fiber-generating complex, with interruption of normal elongation of cells.[14]

Ionizing Radiation. High energy *ionizing radiation* (e.g., radiotherapy treatments) can damage an eye severely, in a manner analogous to radiation dermatitis. The conjunctiva initially becomes swollen and injected, and the surface cells of the cornea and conjunctiva are acutely damaged, with ensuing discomfort. In the weeks following injury, epithelial repair is faulty, with persisting defects and risk of infection. Along with this, direct damage to the lacrimal gland, the accessory lacrimal glands, and the mucus-producing cells of the conjunctival epithelium leads to a dry eye state, abetting the patient's discomfort and risk.

Artificial tears, either drops or ointments, must be used often, every half-hour in severe cases. Erythromycin or similar prophylactic topical antibiotics should be used daily. Lid closure, by tape or tarsorrhaphy, may be required if adequate wetting is not possible. Atropine is often the most effective cycloplegic agent, given as a 1 per cent drop once or twice a day. It reduces light sensitivity from an inflamed anterior segment. If the patient has a history of narrow angle glaucoma, or if the clinician suspects it because of the apparent shallowness of the anterior chamber, then such dilating agents should be withheld. An ophthalmologic consultation should be obtained quickly. Steroids should be avoided in these cases unless their use is specifically monitored by an ophthalmologist, because the poorly protected surface is subject to enzymatic degradation of collagen and eventual corneal perforation. The use of steroids, which inhibit wound healing, in an ocular condition in which normal mechanisms are already abridged can make matters worse.

Damage to the metabolic activities of the lens and retina can result (respectively) in cataract, severe retinal degeneration, and consequent loss of sight.

Microwaves. Despite experimental evidence in animals and anecdotal evidence in humans, the role of *microwaves* in the development of human ocular pathology is not clear. Available evidence suggests that the principal tissue interaction is one of tissue warming.

INJURY FROM TOPICAL EXPOSURE

Surface injuries generally feature acute discomfort as the premier symptom because the highly innervated epithelium is both delicate and vulnerable. Fortunately, the injured epithelium regenerates quickly, provided the injury is limited to the surface cells. There may be immediate or delayed effects of injury because damage-evoking delayed cell slough is common and is similar to injury from ultraviolet exposure.[4, 6, 7]

Caustics

Burns by alkalis and acids comprise the most dreaded class of ocular injury resulting from chemical exposure, because devastating eye damage may occur in seconds from a trivial quantity of caustic. Concomitant thermal damage may result pari passu from the heat of reaction in the tissues.

It should be clear that a momentary and perhaps solitary lapse in industrial, laboratory, or domestic use of caustics can result in a lifetime of decreased vision or blindness. This should be kept in mind whenever these materials are used or *stored.*

Alkali. Any chemical capable of generating a *high pH* in solution can cause irreversible injury with sufficient *concentration* and *duration of exposure.*[17, 18] Experimental studies in animals have disclosed certain discriminating factors regarding critical pH (over 11.5) and cation type, but in practice one should assume the worst case initially and take *immediate* steps to dilute and remove the alkaline substance and to nullify any thermal response.

Alkali injuries are especially damaging to the corneal structure because the cationic portions bind at high pH with collagen and mucoproteins.[1, 17–19] Defilement of the strength and order of this tissue leads to many early and long-term postinjury problems, including faulty epithelial adherence and corneal perforation.[6, 18–21] Damage to conjunctival epithelium and episcleral blood vessels may confound healing.[7] Inflammatory response to this devastation leads to enzymatic degradation of the eye wall.

Access to the corneal stroma by the chemical depends on its degree of lipid solubility. The heat of reaction alone can coagulate the epithelium and reduce its barrier effect, but experimental studies imply a gradation of penetrability among the alkalis, ammonia having the greatest penetrating capability. Calcium hydroxide penetrates less than sodium hydroxide because the formation of soap precipitates at the surface may limit deeper effects. The more severe the penetration of such a caustic agent, the less pain there may be as corneal nerves are destroyed.

Household cleaners commonly feature alkaline substances that, if misused, can lead to morbid injury. First among these are particulate and liquid drain cleaners, ammonia, and cement/plaster material containing calcium oxide (unslaked lime). Calcium hydroxide, when hydrated, exudes a harmful thermal reaction. Further, there may be proteinaceous concretions of the substance resting under the lids, with continuous discharge of calcium hydroxide. Alkali bound within the stroma may also slowly dissipate and prolong the exposure. Naturally, should irrigation cease before such reservoirs are eliminated, the damage will inexorably proceed.

Because of the heat of reaction to be expected, specific efforts to neutralize a high pH may be counterproductive. Such efforts may also waste valuable time because specific neutralizing solutions may not be at hand. Abundant and rapidly poured water or physiologic saline is preferred. Alkali, once within the deep stroma and aqueous humor, is ineffectively diluted by short courses of irrigation. Alkali burns, therefore, require *prolonged irrigation.*

Aside from surface damage, alkali injuries may damage deeper structures because of significant penetration.[1, 20] Destruction of the chamber angle, as by tissue shrinkage, may lead to glaucoma, whereas destruction of the ciliary body may yield an eye that is too "soft" (or hypotensive). Lye burns typically cause a rapid depletion of anterior segment ascorbate, suggesting nutritional depletion of the anterior segment and poor healing capability. Supplementation with topical and systemic ascorbate seems beneficial in rabbits; human studies are underway.[20, 22, 23] Direct damage to the lens epithelium and lens protein may result in an early cataract; hypotony may lead to delayed cataract formation. Severe alkali injuries, despite early irrigation, may lead to irretrievable visual loss. Everyone should be aware of the value of prevention and of rapid lavage.

Acids. Acid burns, generally speaking, cause less morbidity than alkali burns because the reaction between acids and the surface epithelium is more limiting.[1, 24] Owing to less rapid and effective penetration of the cornea, deeper damage is less likely, and the formation of reservoirs of injurious substance deep in the tissues is less of a problem.

Burns involving a moderate degree of acidity (greater than a pH of 2.5) are more surface-limited. Remnant epithelium usually effects rapid repair. When the epithelium has been traumatized, either mechanically or thermally, or when an ion is particularly lipid soluble (e.g., sulfurous), then deeper (stromal) damage may ensue. High concentration and extremely low pH (below pH 2) of a variety of acids may render the epithelium worthless as a barrier.[1, 24, 25] Deeper injury to the stroma, endothelium, uveal structures, and lens can lead to a result resembling that of an alkali burn. The most feared acidic agents include sulfuric, hydrochloric, nitric, phosphoric, and chromic acids and liquid sulfur dioxide.[4] Battery acid (sulfuric) burns are probably the most common eye burns.

Solvents. Organic solvents (e.g., ethyl alcohol, methyl alcohol, toluene, acetone, butanol), being common in laboratories and in industry, are responsible for numerous splash and vapor injuries to the external eye. Because of their fat solubility, they inflict epithelial injuries and damage to the nerve endings, with resultant pain. Heated solvents can cause additional thermal damage involving protein denaturation and potential destruction of the globe. Lavage at the scene is critical, and ophthalmologic care should follow.

War Gas. Vesicant war gases can cause significant immediate *and* delayed ocular damage. The major risk now exists in industrial settings and in the chemotherapeutic use of alkylating agents. Reviews of the range of ocular damage were provided at the time of World War II.[26, 27]

Surfactants and Detergents. Surfactants lower the surface tension of water and promote wetting. A given molecule contains both polar and nonpolar portions. Surfactants promote the dispersion, for example, of fats in water. Cationic, anionic, and nonionic surfactants exhibit decreasing ocular surface toxicity, in that order.[1] Although nonionic surfactants, by comparison, have the least surface toxicity, some of them have anesthetic properties and may therefore cause a delay in irrigation.[28] Concentrated benzalkonium chloride is a well-known cationic surfactant capable of causing significant anterior segment damage. Modest exposure, quickly rinsed, will likely result in epithelial injury and pain but good recovery. Household soaps and shampoos typically contain anionic surfactants. As with the cationic agents, severe discomfort resulting from cell lysis and nerve irritation may follow the slightest splash, which mandates quick lavage to minimize injury.

Lacrimatory Agents. The stimulation of corneal nerve endings by any means generates reflex lacrimation. Agents have been developed that, when administered in measured concentration, stimulate these nerves but produce minimal tissue damage. Naturally, elevated concentrations and prolonged exposure cause tissue damage of varying degree. For example, the accidental exposure to formaldehyde vapors may cause simply irritation with tearing, but when the vapors are concentrated, prolonged ocular surface inflammation may result, with development of corneal opacity. The same can occur with tear gas. The effects of smog are widespread, though it does not typically lead to permanent damage.

Common tear gases (chloroacetophenone, orthochlorobenzylidene malononitrile) can of course result in significant eye trauma owing to the mechanical force of discharge. Aerosolized agents, mixed with solvents, may adhere to the ocular surface. This is the rationale for lavage in cases of tear gas exposure. These S_N2 alkylating agents work quickly to promote the tearing reflex, possibly by an effect on sulfhydryl enzymes. The effect is reversed quickly with clearing of the vapor except when exposure is prolonged. In the latter case, damaged cells may become irritated, and treatment of the epithelial injury may be required. If cell damage is great, the deeper stroma may be injured, leading to possible eventual vascularization and opacity.[30–32]

Autonomic Agents. Topical agents used for eye examinations (dilating drops) and for therapeutic purposes (miotics for glaucoma) may result in alarming symptoms when used by mistake. A naturally occurring parasympatholytic agent is the hyoscyamine found in jimson weed, a seed from which, landing in the cul-de-sac of the harvester's eye, can induce a dilated pupil and paralysis of accommodation.[1, 33]

Pupillary and ciliary muscle responses to autonomic agents will eventually decline and usually require no treatment. The danger of indiscriminate pupillary dilatation is that acute angle-closure glaucoma may be triggered in the susceptible individual. Nausea and severe headache or eye ache in the setting of pharmacologic mydriasis should suggest acute angle-closure glaucoma.

Miscellaneous. Many topical fluids, powders, and vapors may damage the eye, particularly its vulnerable surface. Pain and decreased vision will quickly bring problems to light. The physician also should know the specific danger of topical corticosteroids. The temptation to treat irritated eyes with steroid drops should be tempered by the facts that long-term use promotes posterior subcapsular cataract formation,[41, 42] and some humans develop a drug-related, nonpainful *glaucoma* resulting in blindness if steroids are maintained for months or years.[43–45]

Certain plants produce well-known toxic reactions in the ocular surface. Saponins interact with superficial cholesterols and lipids in corneal and conjunctival epithelium. Self-limited pain and photophobia result from trivial to moderate exposure, whereas a more severe stromal keratitis may follow serious exposure.[1] Juices from *Dieffenbachia exotica* and, especially, *Dieffenbachia picta* contain an irritating protein that produces effects on the cornea according to the stringency of exposure.[1] Treatment consists of lavage and nonspecific measures used to counteract surface damage (lubrication, cycloplegia, lid closure). An ophthalmologist should be consulted if there is *any* alarm.

Fine hairs from plants and animals (e.g., caterpillar hairs) may become implanted in the ocular surface and cause an inflammatory response in excess of that to be expected from mechanical irritation alone. Recognition and physical removal are critical. An ophthalmologist should be consulted in suspected cases.

TOXICITY FROM SYSTEMIC AGENTS

A multitude of visual complaints, ranging from "wavy" vision to dyschromatopsia (disturbed color vision) accompany the use of many common pharmaceuticals, including digitalis, autonomic drugs, and sedative-hypnotic agents. The pathogenesis of many of these symptoms is poorly understood, and cessation or adjustment of medication by and large leads to resolution, or at least stabilization. Of greater interest are those many instances when significant visual loss of a potentially more permanent nature occurs. Such visual loss may result from cataract formation or toxic influences on retinal or optic nerve elements. Typically, symptoms are less acute and are accompanied by less pain with systematically active toxins compared with topically active ones. Cessation of exposure may lead to resolution, stabilization, or progressive damage. Aside from this first step, which depends on recognition of the exposure, treatment of eye damage due to systemic toxins is less tangible than the approach to topical exposures.

Corneal Opacities[33–40]

Corneal changes have been noted in association with drug treatment with amiodarone,[34, 35] chloroquine,[36] clofazimine,[37] and chlorpromazine.[38–40] These changes consist of granular deposits at the level of the corneal epithelium that often become linear in configuration with time and finally advance to a whorl of vortex-like patterns. In general, these changes are not associated with visual impairment, are rarely the cause of even mild symptomatology, and regress when the drugs are withdrawn. However, each of these drugs has been implicated in more serious eye disease, and therefore the corneal changes may serve as a reminder of the possibility of other ocular changes (see later).

Cataract Formation

Substances related to cataract formation include corticosteroids, busulfan, chlorpromazine, and intraocular metals, among many. Generally, lens opacity sufficient to cause symptoms develops slowly, and such patients infrequently appear in the emergency department with poor vision as their only complaint.

Steroids.[41, 42] The typical lens changes resulting from chronic, moderate-to-large dose, systemic steroid therapy occur in the posterior subcapsular zone. Although it is recognized that steroid derivatives do accumulate within the *N*-crystallins of the lens,[46–48] the exact pathophysiology of the lens opacity remains obscure.

Busulfan.[49] The alkylating agent busulfan induces, in time, posterior subcapsular changes in the lens. The mechanism may relate to interference in the development of cortical fibers at the lens equator, a process that requires cell mitosis.

Chlorpromazine.[38–40] Antipsychotic medication exceeding a daily dosage of 0.5 gm for extended periods may cause anterior subcapsular lens opacities.

Intraocular Metals.[1, 5, 11, 12] A common source of visual morbidity in industrial settings is the occurrence of intraocular metallic foreign bodies. Operators of machines with rapidly moving parts, particularly those involving metal hitting on metal, are at significant risk and should never be without safety glasses. Depending on the size of the foreign body and the nature of the injury, patients may present acutely with a clear history of a projectile injury, or they may present days, weeks, or months later completely unaware of any association of their problem with a previous event that seemed insignificant at the time. Any foreign body that penetrates or passes through the lens can cause a cataract, although in some instances it may remain localized and not affect vision. Metallic foreign bodies, regardless of any changes due to mechanical damage may also result in lens changes due to ion deposition. Such deposition is particularly prominent in the case of copper foreign bodies, which may cause anterior capsular discoloration, more significant as an announcement that such a foreign body is present than as a lens opacity. Similar capsular deposition can occur in the systemic copper excess seen in patients with Wilson's disease. Iron foreign bodies may result in a dark discoloration of the iris (heterochromia) in addition to lens changes, which are also signals of the potential for more serious sequelae (see below).

Retinal and Retinal Pigment Epithelial Degeneration

Retinal and retinal pigment epithelial degeneration, often irreversible, can occur with chloroquine, hydroxychloroquine, clofazimine, thioridazine, quinine, intraocular metals, and deferoxamine, among many agents. Dyschromatopsia may occur with a variety of agents, perhaps most commonly with digitalis. Oral contraceptives may damage the retina indirectly by promoting vascular occlusions.[50] Peripheral retinal blood vessels of the premature infant are easily damaged by high oxygen concentrations in the blood, and such damage may lead to retinal injury through progressive hemorrhage and scarring.[51, 52]

Chloroquine, Hydroxychloroquine.[36, 53–68] These antimalarial drugs (4-aminoquinoline derivatives) are commonly used in the treatment of collagen vascular diseases, for which the dosage far exceeds that used for malaria. As retinopathy has become recognized as a significant potential problem,[36, 53–68] recommended doses have been adjusted downward. Doses of 250 mg per day for chloroquine and 400 mg per day for hydroxychloroquine are commonly considered safe[62] but are not safe for all patients.[63] It is now felt that the dosage should be determined based on lean body mass (4 mg/kg/day for chloroquine and 6.5 mg/kg/day for hydroxychloroquine) with adjustments made for altered liver or renal function.[64] Even with appropriate dosage adjustments the risk with hydroxychloroquine may be less than that with chloroquine.[68]

The earliest ophthalmoscopic sign of chloroquine and hydroxychloroquine retinopathy is loss of the foveal reflex. This is followed by pigmentary changes in the macula, typically progressing to a pigmented ring surrounding the fovea ("bull's eye lesion") and sometimes accompanied by pigment flecks in the midperiphery. Fluorescein angiography is a sensitive way to detect early pigmentary alterations, but visual complaints may develop prior to development of any visible changes.[65] The most common complaint is difficulty in reading, which with further questioning can usually be related to paracentral scotomas.[62] Light flashes and streaks and other entopic phenomena may also be present.[62] Any patient who is on chloroquine or hydroxychloroquine and presents with visual complaints should be seen by an ophthalmologist for a detailed investigation of the central visual field. This can be done with an Amsler grid,[66, 67] static perimetry,[65] or tangent screen examination using a red test object.[62] Documented appearance of paracentral scotomas during therapy with these is generally felt to be an indication to stop or at least decrease the dosage. It has been stated that relative scotomas often resolve after drug cessation, whereas absolute scotomas frequently persist.[67] Patients with more advanced disease, manifested by pigmentary retinopathy, tend to remain stable once the drug is stopped, but occasionally the retinal disease progresses.[55, 56]

The pathogenesis of chloroquine and hydroxychloroquine retinopathy has not been fully elucidated. Chloroquine binds strongly with melanin, and therefore high concentrations occur in the retinal pigment epithelium and choroid and persist for years.[59] It is unclear, however, whether this high concentration plays any role in the development of retinopathy.[69, 70] Ultrastructural studies demonstrate the most striking change to be the presence of membranous cytoplasmic bodies (which most authors believe to be degenerative forms of lysosomes) in retinal ganglion cells and, to a lesser extent, in other retinal neurons and retinal pigment epithelium.[69–72] In the monkey, photoreceptor degeneration precedes degeneration of the retinal pigment epithelium.[72] It has been postulated that direct retinotoxic effects may occur by altered protein synthesis and/or by alteration of lysosomes.[69–72]

Clofazimine.[37] Clofazimine is a red phenazine dye that is used to treat dapsone-resistant leprosy, psoriasis, pyoderma gangrenosum, and discoid lupus. It has been reported to cause whorl-like corneal opacities and bull's-eye retinopathy, similar to the signs seen in association with chloroquine usage.[37]

Thioridazine.[73–79] Thioridazine (Mellaril) is a piperidyl phenothiazine used in the treatment of schizophrenia. It causes a pigmentary retinopathy that is dose-dependent. Doses up to 800 mg per day are usually accepted as safe, but with higher doses, even for a few months, patients may experience blurred vision.[73–75] If the drug is stopped, vision may return to normal, but if continued, coarse black pigmentary stippling occurs throughout the posterior fundus, usually in association with a further decline in vision. The pigmentary changes are not reversible and often become associated with large patches of atrophy. Even at this stage, improvement in vision can occur if the drug is stopped, though this is not always the case.[73–75]

Phenothiazines bind to melanin, resulting in high concentrations in the retinal pigment epithelium and choroid.[76, 77] As with chloroquine, however, it is unclear if the melanin binding plays any role in retinal toxicity because chlorpromazine, which has a greater affinity for melanin than thioridazine,[76, 77] is much less toxic. On the other hand, piperidyl chlorophenothiazine (NP-207), like thioridazine, but unlike chlorpromazine, has a piperidyl side chain and is even more toxic than thioridazine.[78] It may be that the presence of a piperidyl side chain is the key to retinal toxicity. Inhibition of oxidative phosphorylation in photoreceptors has been suggested to play a potential role in development of toxicity.[79]

Quinine.[80–85] Quinine is a cinchona alkaloid that is used in the treatment of malaria and nocturnal cramps. Retinal and systemic toxicity usually occur after an overdose,[80, 81] however, there is one report of toxicity occurring in a patient taking a standard dose of 300 mg per day for 1 week.[82] Toxicity is usually heralded by the acute onset of severe loss of vision, often accompanied by tinnitus, deafness, vertigo, nausea, vomiting, and abdominal pain. In severe cases, respiratory depression can be fatal.[83] Over the next few days, vision often improves to a variable extent, and arteriolar narrowing and optic atrophy become evident. It has been suggested that vascular constriction plays a role in the retinal toxicity, but the preponderance of evidence supports the occurrence of direct toxicity to retinal neurons and the retinal pigment epithelium.[84] Treatment should be directed toward decreasing quinine levels as quickly as possible and consists of gastric lavage if the patient is seen early enough, followed by forced diuresis and urinary acidification by administering ammonium chloride, 1 gm qid, or ascorbic acid, 500 mg q 4 h.[85]

Metals.[86, 88] Occult intraocular metallic foreign bodies can cause changes in the anterior segment (see above) but are more significant if they cause changes in the posterior segment. Compounds containing iron result in iron deposition throughout the eye, a process called siderosis. This results in progressive visual field constriction and loss of central visual acuity. Abnormalities in the electroretinogram may precede visual loss, and the electroretinogram may even be extinguished with good central vision remaining.[86] The fundus may show generalized pigment atrophy or pigment proliferation, resulting in pigmented flecks throughout the retinal periphery.[86] When suspected, the diagnosis can be confirmed by skull x-rays or a CT scan of the eye. Treatment consists of surgery to remove the foreign body.

Copper foreign bodies result in deposition of copper in ocular tissues. Unlike iron, copper appears to be well tolerated by the retina and retinal pigment epithelium and does not cause progressive visual loss. It can, however, cause significant vitreous inflammation, which, when severe, can simulate endophthalmitis and necessitate surgery.[87]

Deferoxamine.[88–91] Deferoxamine is an iron chelating agent used in the treatment of systemic iron overload, most often in patients who require frequent blood transfusions. Its use has been associated with acute loss of central vision,[88–91] night blindness,[88, 89] and color vision abnormalities.[88, 89] Ophthalmoscopic findings include retinal pigmentary changes and optic atrophy.[88–91] These effects are dose-dependent, and vision loss is at least partially reversible on discontinuation of the drug.[88–91] Histopathology in one case demonstrated ultrastructural abnormalities that were most prominent in the retinal pigment epithelium.[91]

Digitalis.[92] A usually reversible effect on photoreceptors may lead to altered color perception (yellow vision).[92]

Toxic Optic Neuropathy

The optic nerve is particularly vulnerable to toxic assault. It consists of axons that travel a significant distance and are dependent on axonal transport for maintenance of structure and function. There are many substances (both drugs and industrial toxins) that alter this critical function or others and adversely affect optic nerve function in an isolated manner or as part of a more generalized neuropathy. Toxic optic neuropathies usually result in decreased visual acuity due to central or cecocentral scotomas, often associated with color vision abnormalities. These neuropathies may be anterior (associated with optic disc swelling) or retrobulbar (no disc swelling). When chronic, both types result in optic atrophy. Some drugs that are particularly prone to cause optic nerve dysfunction are ethambutol, isoniazid, ethchlorvynol, chloramphenicol, disulfiram, and iodochlorohydroxyquine. Industrial and domestic toxins that have a particular propensity to cause optic nerve disease are methanol, carbon disulfide, carbon tetrachloride, chlorodinitrobenzene, and toluene. "Tobacco amblyopia" is a peculiar, multifaceted entity of interest to the emergency department worker.

Ethambutol.[93–99] Ethambutol is a drug used in tuberculosis that has been associated with anterior and retrobulbar forms of toxic optic neuropathy.[93–98] Toxicity appears to be dose-related and is rare with a dosage below 15 mg per kg per day. It usually presents with a derangement in color vision followed by decreased central vision and visual field defects. Drug withdrawal usually results in visual improvement, and dibencoside (coenzyme B) may provide additional benefit.[99]

Isoniazid.[98, 100] Isoniazid is one of the mainstays of antituberculous therapy and, like ethambutol, has been associated with anterior and retrobulbar toxic optic neuropathy. The relationship of optic nerve disease to peripheral neuropathy, a well-established complication of isoniazid therapy, is unclear, but both appear to be responsive to pyridoxine (25 to 100 mg daily).[98, 100]

Ethchlorvynol.[101, 102] Decreased vision, on the basis of toxic optic neuropathy, has been reported with prolonged use of this sedative-hypnotic.[101, 102] Visual improvement occurs after drug withdrawal and vitamin B supplements.[102]

Chloramphenicol.[103–105] Several cases of anterior toxic optic neuropathy have been reported, usually in patients treated for prolonged periods for chronic infections.[103–105] The condition usually presents after several months of treatment with decreased vision due to central scotoma, and optic discs that are mildly swollen and hyperemic. Early recognition and drug withdrawal result in variable improvement.

Disulfiram.[106, 107] Disulfiram (Antabuse) is used industrially as a seed disinfectant and fungicide and clinically as a drug for treatment of chronic alcohol addiction. Several well-documented cases of retrobulbar optic neuropathy have been associated with its use, presenting as rapid loss of vision with central or cecocentral scotomas and temporal pallor of the optic discs. Visual improvement occurs after the drug is stopped.[106, 107]

Iodochlorohydroxyquine.[96, 98, 108–110] This drug, a halogenated hydroxyquinoline, remains a common antiamebiasis therapeutic agent in some parts of the world and may be purchased over-the-counter for traveler's diarrhea. It can cause a sudden, widespread demyelinating process that includes the optic nerves. In Japan, the clinical term *subacute myelo-opticoneuropathy* (SMON) arose to describe this idiosyncratic response. Leopold suggests a course of zinc supplementation.[96]

Amiodarone.[111] Optic disc swelling and hemorrhages without significant visual decline have recently been reported in two patients receiving amiodarone.[111] Decreased dosage led to resolution in one patient, but further study is needed to determine if amiodarone can cause an optic neuropathy.

Tobacco Amblyopia.[96, 97, 112] The entity "tobacco-alcohol amblyopia" ("alcohol-nutritional amblyopia") occurs most often in ardent pipe smokers, especially those with significant alcohol intake. Such individuals may present to an emergency department with the complaint of bilaterally progressive visual loss, and no obvious toxic history or physical signs may be ascertained. Testing may reveal bilateral cecocentral scotomas. Cyanide (CN) in inhaled smoke may be a toxic factor. Poor nutrition, especially associated with vitamin B_{12} deficiency, is often found, and the amblyopia may develop on a nutritional basis alone. One theory suggests an abnormality in sulfur metabolism in these patients, resulting in poor detoxification of CN.[112] A regimen for treatment includes a 3-week course of weekly intramuscular hydroxycobalamin (1000 mg) and oral thiamine (300 mg).[96]

Industrial Toxins

Methanol.[13, 98, 113] Methyl alcohol poisoning leads to profound systemic acidosis and a swelling of the retinal nerve fibers and their ganglion cells, resulting in ganglion cell death. Optic disc swelling may occur and is difficult to differentiate from that occurring with increased intracranial pressure. Part of the reason for the systemic toxicity relates to the oxidation of methanol, via alcohol dehydrogenase, to formic acid, with a decrease in serum bicarbonate. Ocular symptoms generally develop within 24 hours of ingestion and probably stem from interference with axoplasmic flow.[13] Blindness develops in a significant number of cases, and persisting torpor of the pupillary light reflex is a poor prognostic sign. The earliest clinical change may be a visual field defect, connecting fixation with the physiologic blind spot (cecocentral), and vision may improve or deteriorate from there. Good visual recovery may slowly unfold in patients with mild intoxications. Varying degrees of disc pallor develop within months.

Carbon Disulfide.[3, 114] Carbon disulfide is a volatile liquid used in the rubber and rayon industries. Chronic inhalation of its vapors has been associated with retrobulbar optic neuropathy manifested by decreased vision, central scotomas, and optic disc pallor.[114]

Carbon Tetrachloride.[3, 115–117] Carbon tetrachloride is a volatile liquid widely used in industry and homes as a cleaning agent. There are several case reports linking chronic inhalation of its vapors to visual loss, presumably from optic neuropathy.

Chlorodinitrobenzene.[3, 118] Chlorodinitrobenzene is a yellow crystalline solid used in combination with dinitrobenzene in an explosive mixture. Chronic exposure in munitions workers has been associated with retrobulbar optic neuropathy.

Toluene.[119] Toluene and a related compound, vinyl benzene, have been implicated in reversible toxic optic neuropathy after chronic industrial exposure.

SYSTEMIC TOXICITY FROM LOCAL EXPOSURE

The rationale behind periocular injection and topical application of drugs is to provide therapeutic levels in the eye while limiting systemic exposure. In general, this approach has definite advantages in terms of decreasing toxicity; however, it does not completely eliminate it. This section strives to point out some examples of toxicity of potential importance to the emergency department physician.

Periocular Injections[120–123]

Retrobulbar injection of local anesthetics is used to eliminate pain and motility for ocular surgery and procedures such as panretinal photocoagulation. It is frequently used in outpatient settings and is occasionally complicated by intravascular[120] or intraoptic nerve sheath injection.[120–122] Depending on the dose injected, this procedure may result in a range of symptoms from altered mental status to seizures, loss of consciousness, or respiratory depression.[120–123] Diagnosis is usually straightforward because of the temporal relationship of the symptoms to the injection, but management is of critical importance because of the potentially life-threatening nature of the problem. Emergency department physicians are frequently called on to assist in this management. The key is maintenance of the airway, which requires insertion of an oral airway and mask insufflation followed by intubation unless spontaneous respirations resume quickly. Extubation is usually possible after a brief period of assisted ventilation. Bupivacaine, because of its longer half-life, is more dangerous than lidocaine, and should be avoided in outpatient settings.[123]

Topical Drugs

Timoptic.[124–129] Timoptic is a nonselective beta-blocker used in the treatment of glaucoma. It has been demonstrated to exacerbate bronchospasm in patients with asthma and chronic obstructive pulmonary disease[124–126] and also may worsen congestive heart failure.[127] Infants may be at particular risk; apneic spells[128] and severe bradycardia[129] have been reported in these patients. As is the case with systemic beta-blockers, depression, anxiety, and confusion are sometimes seen in association with topical therapy with timoptic.[124] Betoptic, a selective β blocker, is felt to be associated with fewer systemic side effects but has also been noted to exacerbate pulmonary obstructive disease[130, 131] and congestive heart failure.[132]

Phenylephrine.[133–135] When used in a concentration of 10 per cent, this drug has been associated with hypertensive reactions in elderly people with cardiovascular disease,[133] patients with drug-induced sympathetic denervation,[134] and infants.[135]

Anticholinergics[1, 136, 137]

Cyclopentolate, atropine, and scopolamine have been associated with episodes of dysarthria, ataxia, hallucinations, mood changes, and/or disorientation.[1, 136, 137] Such reactions are characteristically associated with an increased pulse rate and normal blood pressure. Symptoms occur 20 to 60 minutes after drop application and may last 2 to 4 hours.

References

1. Grant WM: Toxicology of the Eye. 3rd ed. Springfield, IL, Charles C Thomas, 1986.
2. Fraunfelder FT: Drug-Induced Ocular Side Effects and Drug Interactions. 2nd ed. Philadelphia, Lea & Febiger, 1982.
3. Miller NR: Walsh and Hoyt's Clinical Neuro-Ophthalmology. 4th ed. Baltimore, Williams & Wilkins, 1982.
4. Ralph RA: Chemical burns of the eye. *In* Duane T (ed): Clinical Ophthalmology. Vol 4. Hagerstown, MD, Harper & Row, 1980.
5. Paton D, Goldberg MF: Management of Ocular Injuries. Philadelphia, W.B. Saunders, 1976.
6. Thoft RA, Dohlman CH: Chemical and thermal burns of the eye. *In* Freeman HM (ed): Ocular Trauma. New York, Appleton-Century-Crofts, 1979.
7. Thoft RA, Friend J, Kenyon KR: Ocular surface response to trauma. Int Ophthalmol Clin *19:*111, 1979.
8. Kenyon KR: Anatomy and pathology of the ocular surface. Int Ophthalmol Clin *19:*3, 1979.
9. Friend J: Biochemistry of ocular surface epithelium. Int Ophthalmol Clin *19:*73, 1979.
10. Duncan G: Role of membranes in controlling ion and water movements in the lens. *In* CIBA Foundation Symposium: The Human Lens—in Relation to Cataract. Amsterdam, Elsevier-Excepta Medica, 1963.
11. Neubauer H: Management of nonmagnetic intraocular foreign bodies. *In* Freeman HM (ed): Ocular Trauma. New York, Appleton-Century-Crofts, 1979.
12. Rosenthal AR, Appleton B, Hopkins JL: Intraocular copper foreign bodies. Am J Ophthalmol *78:*671, 1974.
13. Hayreh MS, Hayreh SS, Baumbach GS, Caucilla P, Martin-Amat G, Tephly TR, McMartin KE, Makar AB: Methyl alcohol poisoning. III. Ocular toxicity. Arch Ophthalmol *95:*1851, 1977.
14. Lerman S: Radiant Energy and the Eye. New York, Macmillan, 1980.

15. Buschke W, Friedenwald JS, Moses SG: Effects of ultraviolet irradiation on corneal epithelium: Mitosis, nuclear fragmentation, post-traumatic cell movements, loss of tissue cohesion. J Cell Comp Physiol *26:*147, 1945.
16. Ewald R: Solar retinopathy. *In* Fraunfelder F, Roy F (eds): Current Ocular Therapy. Philadelphia, W.B. Saunders, 1980.
17. Hughes WF, Jr: Alkali burns to the eye. I. Review of literature and summary of present knowledge. Arch Ophthalmol *35:*423, 1946.
18. Hughes WF, Jr: Alkali burns of the eye. II. Clinical and pathological course. Arch Ophthalmol *36:*189, 1946.
19. Grant WM, Kern HL: Action of alkalies on the corneal stroma. Arch Ophthalmol *54:*931, 1955.
20. Pfister RR, Friend J, Dohlman CH: The anterior segment of rabbits after alkali burns: Metabolic and histologic alterations. Arch Ophthalmol *86:*189, 1971.
21. Stanley J: Strong alkali burns to the eye. N Engl J Med *273:*1265, 1965.
22. Pfister RR, Paterson CA: Additional clinical and morphological observations on the favorable effect of ascorbate in experimental ocular alkali burns. Invest Ophthalmol Vis Sci *16:*478, 1977.
23. Pfister RR, Paterson CA, Hayes SA: Topical ascorbate decreases the incidence of corneal ulceration after experimental alkali burns. Invest Ophthalmol Vis Sci *17:*1019, 1978.
24. Friedenwald JS, Hughes WF, Herrmann H: Acid-base tolerance of the cornea. Arch Ophthalmol *31:*279, 1944.
25. Friedenwald JS, Hughes WF, Jr, Herrman H: Acid-burns of the eye. Arch Ophthalmol *35:*98, 1946.
26. Mann I, Pirie A, Pullinger BD: An experimental and clinical study of the reaction of the anterior segment of the eye to chemical injury, with special reference to chemical warfare agents. Br J Ophthalmol (Suppl) *13:*1, 1948.
27. Maumenee AE, Scholz RO: The histopathology of the ocular lesions produced by the sulfur and nitrogen mustards. Bull Johns Hopkins Hosp *82:*121, 1948.
28. Martin G, Draize JH, Kelley EA: Local anesthesia in eye mucosa produced by surfactants in cosmetic formulations. Proc Sci Sect Toilet Goods Assoc *37:*2, 1962.
29. Jaffe NS: Photochemical air pollutants and their effect on men and animals. I. General characteristics and community concentrations. Arch Environ Health *15:*782, 1967.
30. Levine RA, Stahl CJ: Eye injury caused by tear-gas weapons. Am J Ophthalmol *65:*497, 1968.
31. Sanford JP: Medical aspects of riot control (harassing) agents. Ann Rev Med *27:*421, 1976.
32. Thatcher DB, Blaug SM, Hyndiuk RA, Watzke RC: Ocular effects of chemical mace in the rabbit. Clin Med *78:*11, 1971.
33. Goldey JA, Dick DA, Porter WL: Cornpicker's pupil: A clinical note regarding mydriasis from Jimson weed dust (stramonium). Ohio State Med J *62:*921, 1966.
34. Watillon M, Lavergne G, Weekers JF: Lesions corneenes au cours du traitement par le cordarone (chlorhydrate d'amiodarone). Bull Soc Belge Ophthalmol *150:*715, 1968.
35. Orlando RG, Dangel ME, Schaal SF: Clinical experience and grading of amiodarone keratopathy. Ophthalmology *91:*1184, 1984.
36. Hobbs HE, Eadie SP, Somerville F: Ocular lesions after treatment with chloroquine. Br J Ophthalmol *45:*284, 1961.
37. Craythorn JM, Swartz M, Creel DJ: Clofazimine-induced bull's-eye retinopathy. Retina *6:*50, 1986.
38. Zelickson AS, Zeller HC: A new and unusual reaction to chlorpromazine. JAMA *188:*394, 1964.
39. Barsa J, Newton J, Saunders J: Lenticular and corneal opacities during phenothiazine therapy. JAMA *193:*10, 1965.
40. Siddall JR: The ocular toxic findings with prolonged and high dosage chlorpromazine intake. Arch Ophthalmol *74:*460, 1965.
41. Black RL, Oglesby RD, VonSallmann L, Bunim JJ: Posterior subcapsular cataracts induced by corticosteroids in patients with rheumatoid arthritis. JAMA *174:*166, 1960.
42. Lubkin VL: Steroid cataract—a review and a conclusion. J Asthma Res *14:*55, 1977.
43. Becker B: Intraocular pressure response to topical corticosteroids. Invest Ophthalmol *4:*198, 1965.
44. Francois J: Glaucome apparement simple, secondaire a la cortisonotherapie locale. Ophthalmologica (Suppl):*142:*517, 1961.
45. Goldmann H: Cortisone glaucoma. Arch Ophthalmol *68:*621, 1962.
46. Ono S, Hirano H, Obara LO: Absorption of cortisol-4-C^{14} into rat lens. Jap J Exp Med *41:*485, 1971.
47. Ono S, Hirano H, Obara K: Presence of cortisol-binding protein in the lens. Ophthalmic Res *3:*307, 1972.
48. Ono S, Hirano H, Obara K: Study on the conjugation of cortisol in the lens. Ophthalmic Res *3:*307, 1972.
49. Hamming NA, Apple DJ, Goldberg MG: Histopathology and ultrastructure of busulfan-induced cataract. Albrecht v Graefes Arch Ophthalmol *200:*139, 1976.
50. Petursson GJ, Fraunfelder FT, Meyer SM: Oral contraceptives. Ophthalmology *88:*368, 1981.
51. Nichols CW, Lambertsen CJ: Effects of high oxygen pressures on the eye. N Engl J Med *281:*25, 1969.
52. Patz A: Retrolental fibroplasia. Surv Ophthalmol *14:*1, 1969–70.
53. Arden GB, Kolb H: Antimalarial therapy and early retinal changes in patients with rheumatoid arthritis. Br Med J *1:*270, 1966.
54. Bernstein H: The ocular toxicity of chloroquine. Surv Ophthalmol *12:*415, 1968.
55. Brinkley JR, Jr, DuBois EL, Ryan SJ: Long-term course of chloroquine retinopathy after cessation of medication. Am J Ophthalmol *88:*1, 1979.
56. Burns RP: Delayed onset of chloroquine retinopathy. N Engl J Med *275:*693, 1966.
57. Carr R, Gouras F, Gunkel R: Chloroquine retinopathy. Arch Ophthalmol *75:*171, 1966.
58. Fishman GD: Chloroquine retinopathy. *In* Hughes WF (ed): The Year Book of Ophthalmology: Chicago Year Book Medical Publishers, 1980, p 223.
59. Lawhill R, Appleton B, Altstatt L: Chloroquine accumulation in human eyes. Am J Ophthalmol *65:*530, 1968.
60. MacKenzie AH, Scherbel AL: A decade of chloroquine maintenance therapy: Rate of administration governs incidence of retinotoxicity. Arthr Rheum *11:*496, 1968.
61. Nylander V: Ocular damage in chloroquine therapy. Acta Ophthalmol *92:*1, 1967.
62. Bernstein HN: Ophthalmic considerations and test-

ing in patients receiving long-term antimalarial therapy. Am J Med *75*(Suppl):25, 1983.
63. Easterbrook M: Dose relationships in patients with early chloroquine retinopathy. J Rheumatol *14*:472, 1987.
64. Mackenzie AH: Dose refinements in long-term therapy of rheumatoid arthritis with antimalarials. Am J Med *75*(Suppl):40, 1983.
65. Hart WM, Burde RM, Johnson GP, Drews RC: Static perimetry in chloroquine retinopathy. Perifoveal patterns of visual field depression. Arch Ophthalmol *102*:377, 1984.
66. Easterbrook M: The use of Amsler grids in early chloroquine retinopathy. Ophthalmology *91*:1368, 1984.
67. Easterbrook M: The sensitivity of Amsler grid testing in early chloroquine retinopathy. Trans Ophthalmol Soc UK *104*:204, 1985.
68. Finbloom DS, Silver K, Newsome DA, et al: Comparison of hydroxychloroquine and chloroquine use and the development of retinal toxicity. J Rheumatol *12*:692, 1985.
69. Abraham R, Hendy RJ: Irreversible lysosomal damage induced by chloroquine in the retinae of pigmented albino rats. Exp Mol Pathol *12*:185, 1970.
70. Gregory MH, Rutty DA, Wood RD: Differences in retinotoxic action of chloroquine and phenothiazine derivatives. J Pathol *102*:139, 1970.
71. Ramsey MS, Fine BS: Chloroquine toxicity in the human eye. Am J Opthalmol *73*:229, 1972.
72. Rosenthal AR, Kolb H, Bergsma D, Huxsoll D, Hopkins JL: Chloroquine retinopathy in the rhesus monkey. Invest Ophthalmol Vis Sci *17*:1158, 1978.
73. Weekley R, Potts A, Reboton J, May R: Pigmentary retinopathy in patients receiving high doses of a new phenothiazine. Arch Ophthalmol *64*:65, 1960.
74. Appelbaum A: An ophthalmic study of patients under treatment with thioridazine. Arch Ophthalmol *69*:578, 1963.
75. Connell MM, Poley BJ, McFarlane JR: Chorioretinopathy associated with thioridazine therapy. Arch Ophthalmol *71*:816, 1964.
76. Meier-Ruge W, Kalberer F, Cerletti A: Microhistoautoradiographic investigations of the distribution of trituim-labeled phenothiazine derivatives in the eye. Experientia *22*:153, 1966.
77. Potts AM: The reaction of uveal pigment *in vitro* with polycyclic compounds. Invest Ophthalmol Vis Sci *3*:405, 1964.
78. Goar EF, Fletcher MC: Toxic chorioretinopathy following the use of NP 207. Trans Am Ophthalmol Soc *54*:129, 1956.
79. Cerletti A, Meier-Ruge W: Toxicological studies on phenothiazine induced retinopathy. Proc Eur Soc Study Drug Toxicity *9*:170, 1968.
80. Bard L, Gills J: Quinine amblyopia. Arch Ophthalmol *72*:328, 1964.
81. Behrman J, Mushin A: Electrodiagnostic findings in quinine amblyopia. Br J Ophthalmol *52*:925, 1968.
82. Francois J, De Rouck A, Cambie E: Retinal and optic evaluation in quinine poisoning. Ann Ophthalmol *4*:177, 1972.
83. Fong LP, Kaufman DV, Galbraith JEK: Ocular toxicity of quinine. Med J Aust *141*:528, 1984.
84. Cibis GN, Burian HM, Blod FL: Electroretinography changes in acute quinine poisoning. Arch Ophthalmol *90*:307, 1973.
85. Dickinson P, Sabto J, West RH: Management of quinine toxicity. Trans Ophthalmol Soc NZ *33*:56, 1981.
86. Karpe G: Early diagnosis of siderosis retinae by the use of electroretinography. Doc Ophthalmol *2*:227, 1948.
87. Rosenthal AR, Appelton B, Hopkins JL: Intraocular copper foreign bodies. Am J Ophthalmol *78*:671, 1974.
88. Davies SC, Marcus RE, Hungerford JL, Miller MH, Arden GB, Huehns ER: Ocular toxicity of high-dose intravenous desferrioxamine. Lancet *2*:181, 1983.
89. Lakhanpal V, Schocket SS, Jiji R: Deferoxamine (Desferal)-induced toxic retinal pigmentary degeneration and presumed optic neuropathy. Ophthalmology *91*:443, 1984.
90. Olivieri NF, Buncic JR, Chew E, Gallant T, Harrison RV, Keenan N, Logan W, Mitchell D, Ricci G, Skarf B, Taylor M, Freedman MH: Visual and auditory neurotoxicity in patients receiving subcutaneous deferoxamine infusions. N Engl J Med *314*:869, 1986.
91. Rahi AHS, Hungerford JL, Ahmed AI: Ocular toxicity of desferrioxamine: Light microscopic histochemical and ultrastructural findings. Br J Ophthalmol *70*:373, 1986.
92. Weleber RG, Shults WT: Digoxin retinal toxicity. Clinical and electrophysiologic evaluation of a cone dysfunction syndrome. Arch Ophthalmol *99*:1568, 1981.
93. Carr Rd, Henkind PL Ocular manifestations of ethambutol. Toxic amblyopia after administration of an antituberculous drug. Arch Ophthalmol *67*:566, 1962.
94. Delacoux E, Moreau Y, Godefroy A, Evstingneeff T: Prevention de la toxicite oculaire de l'ethambul: Interete de la zincemie et de l'analyse du sens chromatique. J Fr Ophthalmol *1*:191, 1978.
95. Leibold JE: Drugs having a toxic effect on the optic nerve. Int Ophthalmol Clin *11*:137, 1971.
96. Leopold IH: Drug-induced optic atrophy. *In* Fraunfelder F, Roy F (eds): Current Ocular Therapy. Philadelphia, W.B. Saunders, 1980.
97. Meadows SP: Lesions of the optic nerve. *In* Rose FC (ed): Medical Ophthalmology. London, Chapman and Hall, 1976.
98. Carrol FD: Toxicology of the optic nerve. *In* Srinvasan BD (ed): Ocular Therapeutics. New York, Masson Publishing, 1980.
99. Quere MA, Ballereau L, Baikoff G: Le traitement des nevrites optiques graves a l'ethambutol. Bull Soc Ophthalmol Fr *76*:935, 1976.
100. Kass I, Mandel W, Cohen H, Dressler SH: Isoniazid as a cause of optic neuritis and atrophy. JAMA *164*:1740, 1957.
101. Haining WM, Beveridge GW: Toxic amblyopia in a patient receiving ethchlorvynol as a hypnotic. Br J Ophthalmol *48*:598, 1964.
102. Brown E, Meyer GG: Toxic amblyopia and peripheral neuropathy with ethchlorvynol abuse. Am J Psychiatr *128*:882, 1969.
103. Cocke JG, Brown RE, Geppert LJ: Optic neuritis with prolonged use of chloramphenicol. J Pediatr *68*:27, 1966.
104. Harley RD, Huang NN, Macri CH, Green WR: Optic neuritis following chloramphenicol in cystic fibrosis patients. Trans Am Acad Ophthalmol Otolaryngol *74*:1011, 1970.
105. Joy RLT, Scalettar R, Sodee DB: Optic and periph-

eral neuritis. Probable effect of prolonged chloramphenicol therapy. JAMA *173:*1732, 1960.
106. Humblet M: Nervite retrobulbaine chronique par Antabuse. Bull Soc Belge Ophthalmol *104:*297, 1953.
107. Norton AL, Walsh FB: Disulfiram-induced optic neuritis. Trans Am Acad Ophthalmol Otolaryngol *76:*1263, 1972.
108. Nikae K, Yamamoto S-I, Igata A: Sub-acute myelo-opticoneuropathy (SMON) in Japan. Lancet *2:*520, 1971.
109. Oakley GP: The neurotoxicity of the halogenated hydroquinolines. JAMA *225:*395, 1973.
110. Standvik B, Zetterstrom R: Amaurosis after broxyquinolin. Lancet *1:*922, 1968.
111. Gittinger JW, Jr, Asdourian GK: Papillopathy caused by Amiodarone. Arch Ophthalmol *105:*349, 1987.
112. Bronte-Stewart J, Pettigrew AR, Foulds WS: Toxic optic neuropathy and its experimental production. Trans Ophthalmol Soc UK *96:*355, 1976.
113. Benton CJ Jr, Calhoun FP, Jr: The ocular effects of methyl alcohol poisoning. Report of a catastrophe involving 320 persons. Am J Ophthalmol *36:*1677, 1953.
114. Vigliani EC: Clinical observations on carbon disulfide intoxication in Italy. Industr Med Surg *19:*240, 1950.
115. Wirtschafter ZT: Toxic amblyopia and accompanying physiological disturbances in carbon tetrachloride intoxication. Am J Public Health *23:*1035, 1933.
116. Smith AR: Optic atrophy following inhalation of carbon tetrachloride. Arch Industr Hyg *1:*348, 1950.
117. Gray I: Carbon tetrachloride poisoning: Report of seven cases with two deaths. NY J Med *47:*2311, 1947.
118. Sollier P, Jousset X: Nevrites nitro-phenolees. Clin Ophthalmol *22:*78, 1917.
119. Keane JR: Toluene optic neuropathy. Ann Neurol *4:*390, 1978.
120. Feibel RM: Current concepts in retrobulbar anesthesia. Surv Ophthalmol *30:*102, 1985.
121. Kobet KA: Cerebral spinal fluid recovery of lidocaine and bupivacaine following respiratory arrest subsequent to retrobulbar block. Ophthalmic Surg *18:*11, 1987.
122. Hamilton RC: Brainstem anesthesia following retrobulbar blockade. Anesthesiology *63:*680, 1985.
123. Smith JL: Retrobulbar marcaine can cause respiratory arrest. Ann Ophthalmol *14:*1005, 1982.
124. Van Buskirk EM: Adverse reactions from timolol administration. Ophthalmology *87:*447, 1980.
125. Lawrsen SO, Bjerrum P: Timolol eyedrop-induced severe bronchospasm. Acta Med Scand *211:*505, 1982.
126. Noyes JH, Chervinsky P: Case report. Exacerbation of asthma by timolol. Ann Allergy *45:*301, 1980.
127. Altus P: Timolol-induced congestive heart failure. South Med J *74:*88, 1981.
128. Olson RJ, Bromberg BB, Zimmerman TJ: Apneic spells associated with timolol therapy in a neonate. Am J Ophthalmol *88:*120, 1979.
129. Burnstine RA, Felton JL, Ginther WH: Cardiorespiratory reaction to timolol maleate in a pediatric patient. Ann Ophthalmol *14:*905, 1982.
130. Harris L, Greenstein S, Bloom A: Respiratory difficulties with betaxolol. Am J Ophthalmol *102:*274, 1986.
131. Ronholt PC: Betaxolol and restrictive airway disease. Arch Ophthalmol *105:*1172, 1987.
132. Ball S: Congestive heart failure from betaxolol. Arch Ophthalmol *105:*320, 1987.
133. Fraunfelder FT, Scafidi AF: Possible adverse effects from topical ocular 10% phenylephrine. Am J Ophthalmol *85:*447, 1978.
134. Kim JM, Stevenson CE, Mathewson TS: Hypertensive reactions to phenylephrine eyedrops in patients with sympathetic denervation. Am J Ophthalmol *85:*862, 1978.
135. Borromeo-McGrail V, Bordiuk JM, Keitel H: Systemic hypertension following ocular administration of 10% phenylephrine in the neonate. Pediatrics *51:*1032, 1973.
136. Beswick JA: Psychosis from cyclopentolate. Am J Ophthalmol *53:*879, 1962.
137. Carpenter WT Jr: Precipitous mental deterioration following cycloplegia with 0.2% cyclopentolate HCl. Arch Ophthalmol *78:*445, 1967.

CHAPTER 18
DEVELOPMENTAL TOXICOLOGY

Celeste Martin Marx, Pharm.D.
John F. Pope, M.D.
Jeffrey L. Blumer, Ph.D., M.D.

The field of teratology is the study of birth defects, which are deviations from normal development resulting from prenatal or perinatal influences. Birth defects, comprising not only congenital malformations but also prenatal infections, chromosomal abnormalities, and genetic diseases, are the leading cause of infant mortality.[1] Chronic illness due to congenital anomalies alone accounts for one half of all hospital days.[2, 8] The medical costs of the care of children with birth defects are far in excess of $13 billion annually in the United States.[3]

The birth of an abnormal child causes much anguish and guilt. It is commonly felt in the lay community that most birth defects are preventable by avoidance of toxic exposures or better obstetric care.[4] At present, the overwhelming majority of birth defects are not preventable. Only a small fraction of defects are known to occur as a result of avoidable causes (Fig. 18–1).[5] Such toxic developmental influences include uncontrolled maternal diseases, such as diabetes mellitus and phenylketonuria; infections, including rubella; and, to a much lesser extent, environmental exposures to drugs, chemicals, radiation, and other agents.

The specter of environmental influences that adversely affect human offspring is a realistic concern. A small percentage change in the development of defects still results in a large number of babies affected. Maternal exposure to chemicals with undefined human reproductive effects occurs at unprecedented levels in occupational and home settings. Therapeutic exposure to medication is usually far more controlled, because more reproductive toxicity data are available to guide use in the gravid patient. Unfortunately, therapeutic misadventures, environmental accidents, and suicide attempts have produced a significant body of literature on drug and chemical poisonings in pregnancy. Other women, seeking sensorial pleasures, intentionally ingest substances of undefined purity, and their fetuses are subjected to all manner of uncontrolled risks.

This chapter addresses one area in particular—the role of medications, chemicals, and environmental agents as they relate to the production of such defects and disorders. It is not our goal to generate comprehensive lists of agents that produce birth defects; this information may be found elsewhere.[3, 9–14] This chapter aims to provide both the basic principles of how development may be influenced and a framework by which to look at such influences and their ability to cause abnormal development. It is, therefore, important to understand the normal pattern of prenatal development and the mechanisms by which this development may be disordered.

REVIEW OF NORMAL HUMAN DEVELOPMENT

The onset of pregnancy has been previously defined as conception, which is marked

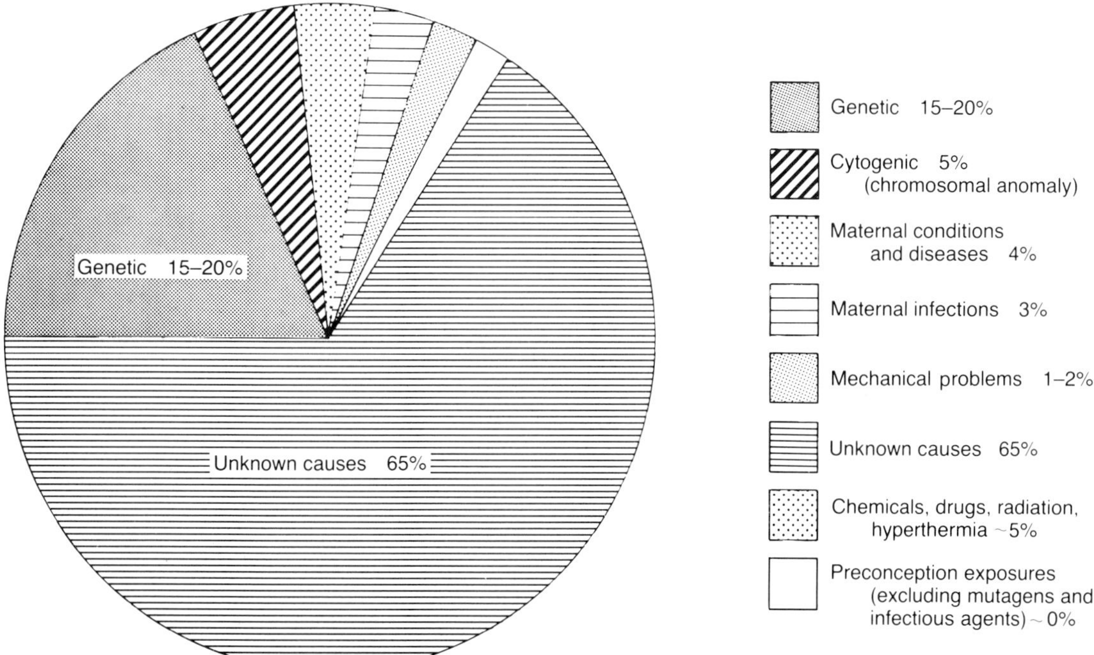

Figure 18–1. Etiologies of human malformations observed in the first year of life, using data of Wilson as adapted in Beckman DA, Brent RL: Mechanism of known environmental teratogens, drugs and chemicals. Clin Perinatol *113*:649–687, 1986.

by implantation of the fertilized egg. For reasons that will become clear as this discussion progresses, in consideration of adverse prenatal influences, it is more relevant to identify the onset of human development as the fertilization of the female's oocyte (egg) with the male's sperm. When using postfertilization conceptus age as a means of dating human pregnancy, it is critical to recognize the distinction from common practice in clinical obstetrics. Obstetricians date pregnancies from the first date of the last maternal menstrual cycle. Onset of menses is a clinically observable milestone, whereas fertilization (with rare technologic exception) is not clinically perceptible. Unfortunately, menstrual dating is notoriously unreliable, even in the minority of women who keep careful records. For the purposes of this chapter, conceptus ages are described in days or weeks postfertilization, which are generally 10 to 18 days less than the obstetric menstrual date.

Human development may be divided into three main periods: preimplantation development, the embryonic period, and the fetal period. Three other developmentally important intervals are described as the perinatal period, the neonatal period, and the nursing interval. The timing of and major activities that take place in each time period are diagrammed in Figure 18–2. *Organogenesis* is the period of embryonic differentiation, that is, the process by which cells become distinct and organs are organized. Selective activation and deactivation of genes orchestrate differential protein synthesis in various cells. Cellular movement, stimulated by selective mitosis in cell groups, begins as early as blastocyst implantation. Mitotic stimulation ultimately results in differential growth and modeling of groups of cells. This stimulation is determined by induction of protein synthesis. Any agent capable of interfering with mitotic division or protein synthesis thus has the potential to evoke a marked dysmorphogenic (malforming) action by disrupting the normal sequence of development. The limited nutritional requirements of the embryo, even to effect differentiation, imply that nutritional deficiencies in the embryonic period may permit ongoing differentiation, even as growth is impaired.

In experimental work with selectively deficient embryos, growth retardation has been observed in normal differentiation of early embryos so deprived. Organogenesis is commonly considered to be the time of highest susceptibility to malforming influences. After differentiation, adverse influences may still impair growth or organ maturation or may induce physiologic dysfunction. Such influences do not have to occur during organogenesis but may persist from prior exposure. An example of this is the possibility of malformations caused by slow release of high maternal tissue stores of etretinate (a vitamin A compound) or from polychlorinated biphenyls encountered months previously.

The *fetal period* extends from the ninth week of gestation until birth. The events of the fetal period are less dramatic than events that occur in preceding periods. Organ differentiation is continued. Organogenesis per se is not complete at the end of the embryonic period. Further growth, storage of energy substrate, and maturation of organ function are other activities that occur in this developmental period. Any adverse effect that results in delayed maturational growth during the fetal period is usually without serious consequence because the challenge of functional independence does not come until birth. Important exceptions include the birth of premature infants, for whom delayed maturation may greatly influence the chance of intact survival. Another exception is the infant born to a diabetic mother; a delay in maturation of the infant's lung function is sometimes seen to produce neonatal respiratory distress, even when the baby is full-term.

Of course, the development of an organ includes not only structural formation but also functional maturation. For example, the lung is not fully mature until the end of human gestation, and the period of its physical and functional maturity continues for more than 1 year after birth. The brain is similarly immature at birth, far more so in the human than in nearly all mammalian species. The myelinization of the brain and maturation of its function continues for years after birth. Thus, the period of organogenesis bridges the late embryonic and early fetal periods. The length of these periods varies among species. The difference in timing or organogenesis, as well as other gestational events between species, is summarized in Table 18–1. A timetable of the development of specific organs in the human is illustrated in Figure 18–3. Even after formation of an organ, injury can lead to disruption of its

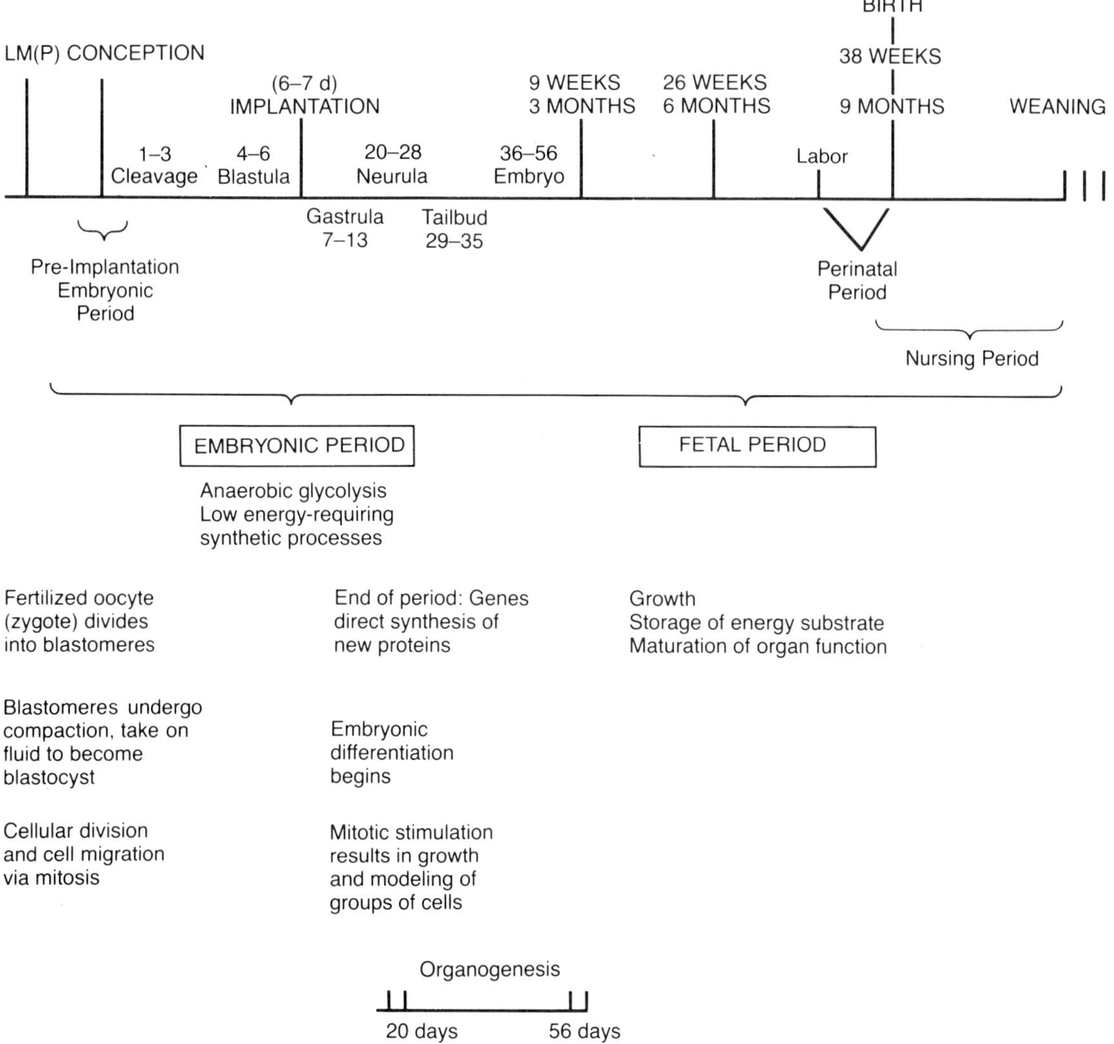

Figure 18–2. Time table of normal human development. Specified events may vary in day of timing in individual pregnancies.

structure. For example, in utero intraventricular hemorrhage may lead to formation of a cyst within the brain. The effect has been attributed to a variety of influences, including hypoxia and the oral anticoagulant warfarin.

The *perinatal period* begins with the onset of maternal labor and includes the *neonatal period*, from birth to 30 days after birth. The perinatal period comprises the baby's rigorous transition to extrauterine existence and the challenge of relatively independent survival. During and beyond the perinatal period is the once obligatory, but now optional, period of maternal-fetal exchange through breast-feeding. During the nursing period, as in all phases of prenatal development, there remains the potential for adverse influences, in addition to all the positive, growth-promoting and development-promoting influences to be passed from mother to infant.

SPONTANEOUS RISK OF ABNORMAL PREGNANCY OUTCOME

Human prenatal development is a remarkably complex yet successful process. An estimated 70 to 85 per cent of all conceptions are carried at least into the twenty-ninth week of pregnancy, and 93 per cent reach

Table 18–1. TIMING OF EARLY DEVELOPMENT IN SOME MAMMALIAN SPECIES*

	IMPLANTATION	ORGANOGENESIS PERIOD	LENGTH OF GESTATION
Mouse	4–5	6–15	19
Rat	5–6	6–15	22
Rabbit	7–8	6–18	33
Sheep	17–18	14–36	150
Monkey (rhesus)	9–11	20–45	164
Human	8–13	21–56	267

*Days from the time of ovulation.

(Adapted from Manson JM: Teratogens. *In* Klaassen CD, et al: Casarett and Doull's Toxicology; The Basic Science of Poisons. 3rd ed. New York, Macmillan, 1986.)

fetal maturity.[15] When one considers the inverse of reported incidences of various adverse pregnancy outcomes (Table 18–2), the remarkable efficiency of human reproduction is apparent. Moreover, of spontaneous abortions between 8 and 28 weeks, 30 to 40 per cent of the fetuses demonstrate chromosomal anomalies, and approximately 30 per cent have structural malformations.[5, 16] Thus, the rates of normal infants born and the apparently small risk of adverse prenatal influence may be biased by a natural process by which abnormal fetuses are lost. Recognition of avoidable adverse prenatal influences thus may be impaired as well.

The effects of a toxin which invariably results in failure of embryonic implantation may go unrecognized because the pregnancy is not identified. The investigation of adverse prenatal influences should, therefore, consider altered fertility as well. In the United States, an estimated 11 to 15 per cent of couples experience infertility, which is defined as a delay of over 1 year to achieve a successful pregnancy. Conversely, over 85 per cent of couples are able to successfully conceive within 1 year.

These positive figures and success rates are of little solace for the infertile couple or the parents of a child with a birth defect. The individual impact of these events should not be ignored. Given the present birth rate, another interpretation of the low risk of adverse pregnancy outcome is that over 200,000 children with birth defects are born in the United States yearly.[5, 8] The numbers of children with specific problems can be extrapolated from the spontaneous adverse outcome rates in Table 18–2.

DEFINITIONS

This section defines the use of terms in the study of developmental toxins. Terminology in any field of study should be clear, concise, and uniformly accepted to facilitate communication among various researchers in the field.

Teratogen. The derivation of teratogen is from the Greek "monster maker." This vividly describes the common application of the

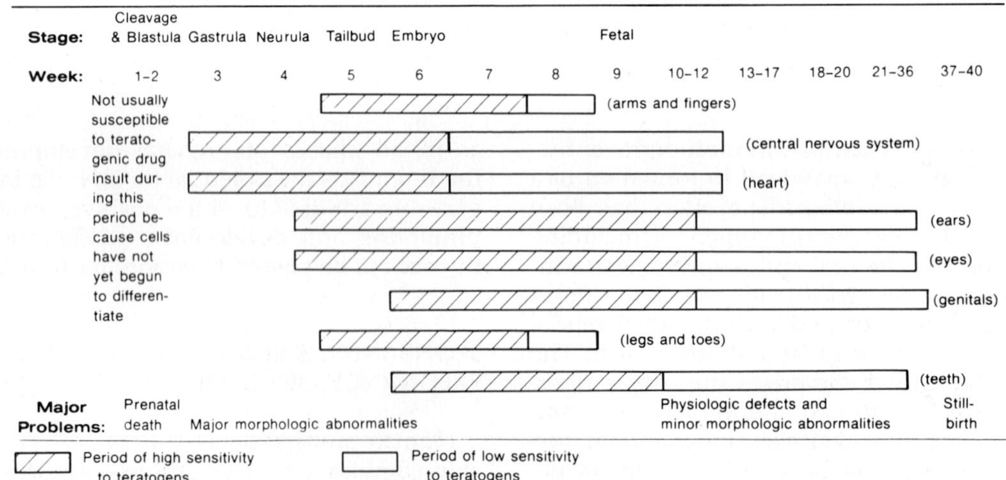

Figure 18–3. Human development with particular reference to potential teratogenic drug insults. Note: This figure is not meant to be used to exclude the possibility of adverse fetal effect. Prior exposures may produce effects prior to and during these times. (From Hays DP, Pagliaro LA: Human teratogens. *In* Pagliaro LA, Pagliaro AM (eds): Problems in Pediatric Drug Therapy. Hamilton IL, Drug Intelligence Publications, 1987.)

Table 18–2. FREQUENCY OF SELECTED HUMAN PREGNANCY OUTCOMES

EVENT	FREQUENCY OF ADVERSE OUTCOMES PER 100	STUDIED UNIT	IMPLIED "SUCCESSFUL OUTCOME" PER 100
Spontaneous abortion	10–30	Pregnancies	70–90
Chromosomal anomalies	30–40	Abortuses	60–70
Chromosomal anomalies	2	Amniocentesis specimens	98
Stillbirths	2–4	All births	96–98
Low birthweight	7	Live births	93
Major malformations	2–3	Live births	97–98
Chromosomal anomalies	0.2	Live births	99.8

(Modified from Manson JM: Teratogens. *In* Klaassen CD, et al. (eds): Casarett and Doull's Toxicology, The Basic Science of Poisons. 3rd ed. New York, Macmillan, 1986 and Wilcox AJ, Weinberg CR, O'Connor JF, et al: Incidence of early loss of pregnancy. N Engl J Med *319*:189–194, 1988.)

word to identify "teratogen," a substance that is capable of inducing gross physical malformations in the fetus. Black and Marks[17] stated that malformations should include "any disruption in organogenesis resulting in permanent, abnormal structural alteration and/or any detrimental effect on function in any fetal tissue regardless of the possible long-term effect on the animal's life." Thus, the teratogenic effects described will include not only physical disorders, but also functional and transient disorders induced by exposure. In the presence of maternal toxicity, it cannot be established that an agent directly induced the effect seen in the conceptus. The toxic effects on the mother may have caused the abnormalities in the offspring. Maternal toxicity, as defined by Black and Marks,[17] occurs when administration of substance to a pregnant animal results in any deleterious effects on maternal behavior, excretion, appearance, body weight, organ function, or incidence of gross or microscopic lesions. If any of these changes occur in the mother, the substance causing them may not be called a teratogen because any of the ill effects seen in the fetus could very well have been a result of maternal effects.

In summary, *a teratogen is a substance that causes transient or permanent physical or functional disorders in the fetus in the absence of toxic effects on the mother.*

Not all adverse effects on prenatal developmental are malforming. Some agents lead to death of the developing organism, whereas others produce only mild growth retardation. Both death and growth retardation are not considered as teratogenic events in themselves. Wilson has proposed the term *developmental toxicity* as a broader categorization of outcomes.[6] *Developmental toxicity comprises four possible manifestations of abnormal development: altered growth (growth retardation), death, malformations ("terata"), and functional deficits or impairments.* Two terms that are used frequently in teratology literature are fetotoxin and embryotoxin. Different investigators have used these terms in distinct ways.

To make reporting of research more precise and to provide uniformity to the literature in this area, the following definitions have been proposed. *Embryotoxicity* occurs when administration of a test substance to a pregnant animal results in significant embryonic loss, either by preventing implantation or by post-implantation death. This term should be used for describing significant increases in the number of in utero deaths during the period from initial test substance administration to birth or removal for examination. An embryotoxin need not produce this effect directly, as does a teratogen. *Fetotoxicity* occurs when administration of a test substance to a pregnant animal any time during gestation leads to signs of delayed development at term, compared with offspring of a control population. The offspring exposed to an agent causing fetotoxicity are usually identical in appearance to normal offspring except for reduced body weight, delayed ossification, and, sometimes, delayed development of certain organs.[18] The effect is usually transient, that is, the animal will develop normally into adulthood. Fetotoxicity is commonly caused by maternal toxicity. For example, poor maternal nutrition secondary to decreased food intake can cause fetotoxicity. By application of the more specific definitions of Black and Marks,[17] the categories as described by Wilson[6] may be adapted as in Figure 18–4.

The concept of the behavioral teratogen

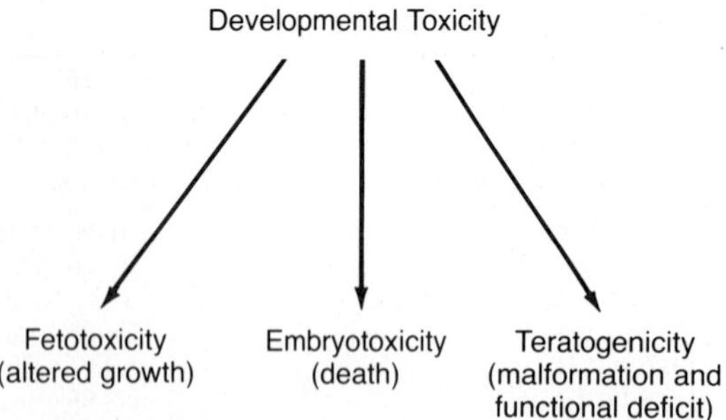

Figure 18–4. Categories of developmental toxicity.

has been described as well. This is an agent that disrupts normal behavioral development after prenatal exposure. Some authorities argue that it is a misnomer for prenatal-induced abnormal behavior. It is certainly true that the human species, with its long period of intellectual and social development, is most likely to be highly vulnerable to such effects. As some agents clearly have produced mental but not physical disturbances, it is a useful subdivision of the concept of teratogens. Because it is a term that provides more information, rather than less, it is used in this chapter independent of the direct causality implied by the term *teratogen*.

Mutagens are substances that cause permanent change in germ cell lines secondary to changes in deoxyribonucleic acid. All mutagens are teratogens, but not all teratogens are mutagens.

PRINCIPLES OF TERATOLOGY

By examining known teratogens and the factors common to their production of malformations, Wilson described the first six basic principles of teratology.[6] A seventh principle was added by Johnson.[16] These are general principles and not rules of teratology, and exceptions can be found to each maxim. Knowledge of both the concept and its limitations is critical to the application of experimental data to human risk.

In Table 18–3, vitamin A and its congeners are used to exemplify how Wilson's principles can be applied to specific agents as well as the shortcomings of these principles in characterizing all teratogens. Vitamin A has been recognized as a teratogen in animals since 1953.[19] Dietary vitamin A as carotene (beta-carotene) has not been associated with developmental toxicity in animals or humans; however, high-potency vitamin A prepared as retinol or retinyl esters has been implicated as an animal teratogen at dosages of 15 to 75 mg/kg/day and higher, producing cranial, brain, cardiovascular, limb, and genitourinary malformations. Case reports of human malformations associated with 25,000 or more international units (IU) vitamin A daily have also appeared, but no epidemiologic studies are available to verify or quantitate the risk to humans.[19, 20] Isotretinoin, an agent used for the treatment of cystic acne and an isomer of retinoic acid, has recently been implicated in the development of craniofacial, cardiac, thymic, and central nervous system (CNS) abnormalities in humans.[20–22] Etretinate, a vitamin A congener used in the treatment of psoriasis, is also a documented animal teratogen, with similar experience in humans. When a specific principle cannot be illustrated by the known experience with vitamin A congeners, other developmental toxins are used as examples.

In Table 18–3 and other illustrations in this chapter, embryologic age and teratogen susceptibility are referred to. Although embryologic timetables are helpful in studying teratogens, it is wrong to always assume that a single event occurring during the sensitive period caused the malformation seen.[23–25] Timetables may be helpful in ruling out a drug or chemical as the cause of a malformation only if it is known that the mother and conceptus were exposed to the agent at a time when the organ in question had already been fully developed and was not sensitive to chemical injury or other biochemical effects. Some of the proposed mechanisms of teratogenesis and developmental events that may be disturbed by developmental toxins are listed in Tables 18–4 and 18–5. The interaction between a developmental toxin and the organism in the production of adverse effects on its development is diagrammed in Figure 18–5.

THE MATERNAL-PLACENTAL-FETAL UNIT

The fetus is sometimes thought of as existing in a protected environment that is impervious to the world surrounding the mother. A more common opinion is that the fetus is a passive, unprotected being at the mercy of any substance that the mother may encoun-

Table 18–3. PRINCIPLES OF TERATOGENESIS

PRINCIPLE	RATIONALE	EXAMPLE
Teratogenesis depends on the genotype of the conceptus and the manner in which it reacts with environmental factors	Differences in genetic makeup lead to differences in pharmacokinetic factors or pharmacodynamic response by the mother or conceptus	Isotretinoin is highly teratogenic in humans but much less so in mice (species differences). Mice with a specific mutation ("splotch" gene) related to native spina bifida had a much higher susceptibility to isotretinoin-induced spina bifida than those without the gene. The same human mother can give birth to heteropaternal twins with very disparate fetal drug syndrome effects (phenytoin).
Susceptibility to teratogenic agents varies with the developmental stage at the time of the exposure	The conceptus passes through an orderly succession of developmental stages. Each stage represents a different susceptibility to teratogens. Prior to implantation, the conceptus is considered to be relatively resistent to harm. If too many cells are damaged, the conceptus is lost. If fewer cells are affected, there may be delayed development, but the remaining cells can take over the function of the damaged ones.	Certain agents (thalidomide, warfarin) have been shown to have organ-specific effects that are determined by the day of gestation on which exposure occurs. Other substances may effect changes by administration at the time when precursors to the organs affected were not yet present (isotretinoin in hamsters). A substance producing a persistent deficiency in a necessary substrate can act in this way.
	Organogenesis is a relatively intense period of orderly development, thus most susceptible to disruption.	Agents with long tissue storage may also induce malformations months after their actual administration (e.g., etretinate).
	Postorganogenesis anomalies may be induced by physical or biochemical alterations caused by the teratogen or by impaired maturation.	Defects may be created by in vivo exposure followed by embryo explantation or by in vitro preimplantation blastocyst exposures. Warfarin can induce damage in the already formed CNS by impaired coagulation, leading to local hemorrhage and scarring in the second or third trimester. Nonsteroidal anti-inflammatory agents (e.g., indomethacin) can close the ductus arteriosus in utero, resulting in hypertrophy of the muscular layer of the pulmonary arteries. This change may manifest as persistent pulmonary hypertension of the newborn.
	Induction of carcinogenesis is favored in the postorganogenesis period because of the high rate of cellular replication and low level of immunocompetence.	Wilms's tumor and congenital leukemia are induced in the fetal period. Phenytoin and diethylstilbestrol have been implicated as fetal carcinogens.

Table continued on following page

Table 18–3. PRINCIPLES OF TERATOGENESIS *(Continued)*

PRINCIPLE	RATIONALE	EXAMPLE
The access of adverse environmental influences on developing tissue depends on the nature of the influence (agent).	Pharmacokinetic characteristics of absorption, distribution, biotransformation, and elimination influence the ultimate amount of teratogen to reach the embryo/fetus	The relatively lesser susceptibility of mice than humans to isotretinoin teratogenicity may be related to metabolism of isotretinoin to 4-oxo-isotretinoin, a more potent teratogen that is produced more by humans than by mice.
The final manifestations of abnormal development are death, malformations, growth retardation, and functional disorders.	The type of response is determined by the individual characteristics of the exposure, particularly dosage and timing, and by the organism's susceptibility to it.	A drug such as ethanol may cause growth retardation and malformation at moderate dosage and embryotoxicity of fetal loss at near-lethal maternal exposure.
Teratogenic agents act in specific ways (mechanisms) on developing cells and tissues to initiate abnormal embryogenesis.	The same defect may be produced by agents acting via different mechanisms. Conversely, one agent may produce different developmental toxicities by the same initiating mechanism.	CNS cyst formations may occur as a result of anticoagulant-induced hemorrhage to hypoxic damage as a result of carbon monoxide poisoning. Phenytoin impairment of normal cell division can produce cleft palate and growth retardation.
The manifestations of deviant development increase in degree as dosages increase from the no-effect level to the totally lethal level.	The higher the dose, the more likely an adverse effect will be seen and the more severe it is likely to be. A threshold dose may exist below which defects are absent and above which defects are demonstrable.	Thalidomide in humans or glucocorticoids in mice can produce severe malformations in the absence of embryolethality. Cytotoxic agents that induce cell necrosis may primarily cause malformations but may be evidenced as growth retardation after repair or result in death if repair is impossible (related dose-response curves for malformations, growth retardation, or embryotoxicity). Certain agents may simultaneously cause malformations, growth retardation, and embryotoxicity in different fetuses in the same litter.
A proportional relationship exists between exposure that produced maternal toxicity and exposure that caused developmental toxicity.	Certain agents produce developmental toxicity; other substances are associated with developmental toxicity only at doses high enough to cause symptoms of toxicity in the mother.	Mercury poisoning of the fetus with irreversible CNS damage can occur in the absence of symptoms of maternal mercury toxicity. Conversely, relatively less specifically developmentally toxic substances (such as aspirin) can produce embryolethality only at doses causing severe maternal toxicity and near death although functional aspirin effects on the fetus (antiplatelet effect, constriction of the ductus arteriosus) are seen even at therapeutic dosage.

Table 18–4. MECHANISMS OF TERATOGENESIS

Cell death beyond recuperative capacity of the embryo/fetus
Mitotic delay: increase in the length of the cell cycle
Retarded differentiation: slowing or cessation in the process of differentiation
Physical constraint and vascular insufficiency
Interference with histogenesis by processes such as cell depletion, necrosis, calcification, or scarring
Inhibition of cell migration

(From Beckman DA, Brent RL: Mechanism of known environmental teratogens, drugs and chemicals. Clin Perinatol *113*:649–687, 1986.)

ter. For most developmental toxicants, the truth lies between these two extremes and effects of toxicants depend on the nature of the agent and the response of the exposed pregnancy. The reasons why the fetus is anatomically separate, but environmentally interactive, lie with the structure and function of the complex system of the maternal-placental-fetal unit.

THE MOTHER

Physiologic Changes in Pregnancy and Their Impact on Pharmacokinetic Disposition of Drugs, Chemicals, and Toxins

The changes of pregnancy are not limited to the content of the uterus. Providing for the nutritional, metabolic, and respiratory needs of the conceptus requires tremendous maternal physiologic adaptation. These changes are of great significance in the maternal therapeutic and toxic responses. They are summarized in Table 18–6.[26–28]

Table 18–5. DEVELOPMENTAL EVENTS OF EMBRYOGENESIS AND FETAL DEVELOPMENT SENSITIVE TO DISTURBANCE BY DEVELOPMENTAL TOXINS

Development and maintenance of organ fields	Formation of cell junctions and selective associations
Development and maintenance of developmental potency	Intracellular communication
Production of cell-specific organelles and products	Cellular morphogenesis
Induction	Programmed and induced cell division or death
Response to induction	Formation of intercellular material
Regulation of polarity	Tissue organization
Regulation of proportionality	Organ formation and function
Cell migration	Organ maturation
	Growth

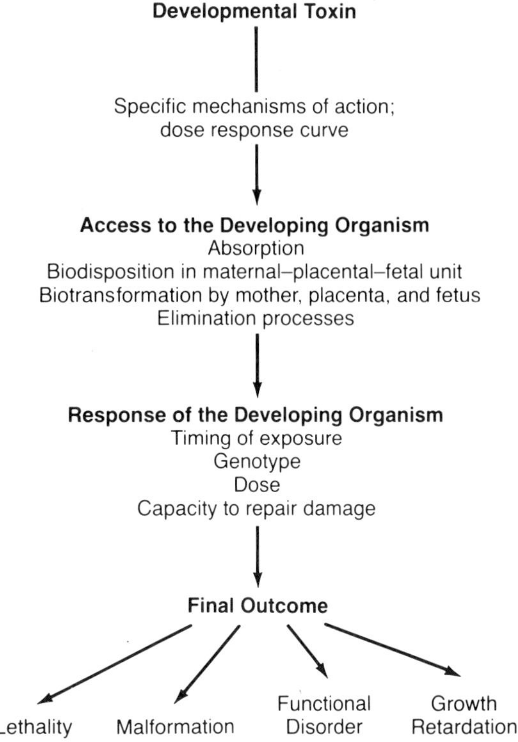

Figure 18–5. Interaction between a developmental toxin and the organism.

These physiologic changes result in differences in the pharmacokinetics and pharmacodynamics of potential developmental toxins. One of the first factors to be affected is absorption. Some substances may not even have the opportunity to be absorbed; for example, compliance with prescribed regimens may be reduced because the mother fears possible adverse effects on the fetus. Women do continue to take a remarkable number of agents during the average pregnancy. In reviews as recent as 1987, the mean number of medications ingested during pregnancy, excluding vitamins and medications for delivery, was 3.1.[29, 30]

Gastrointestinal absorption of agents may be altered by the delayed stomach emptying and decreased motility of pregnancy. Drugs that are hydrophilic and/or poorly transported across the gastrointestinal epithelium may show increased net absorption in pregnancy. Agents absorbed in the small intestine may appear in the circulation more slowly. Absorption of highly protein-bound drugs may be reduced, and secretion of substances out of the circulation may be enhanced in pregnancy.[31] This is related to the greater amount of freely diffusable compound in the

Table 18–6. PHYSIOLOGIC CHANGES OF PREGNANCY BY ORGAN SYSTEM (TIME OF DETECTED CHANGE)

OVERALL PHYSIOLOGIC CHANGES

↑ body mass 25% by term
↑ body water 7–8 L
↑ body fat 3–4 kg; 21%
↑ body temperature 0.5 C

SPECIFIC ORGAN PHYSIOLOGIC CHANGES

Renal	*Cardiovascular*	*Pulmonary*
↓ Urine concentration (5 days) Ureteral dilation due to hormonal relaxation, mechanical compression ↑ Aldosterone secretion ↑ Antidiuretic hormone secretion ↑ Plasma volume 45–50% with 70% increase in volume of extracellular fluid space ↑ Renal plasma flow 25–85% ↓ Serum creatinine; blood urea nitrogen	↑ Cardiac output (6 weeks) 35% by 10 weeks 48% by 25 weeks ↑ Heart rate 20% or 15 bpm ↑ Stroke volume 10–32% or 17 ml ↓ Peripheral vascular resistance due to low resistance placental circulatory shunt ↑ Peripheral blood flow ↑ Perfusion of skin, mucosa, epidural space ↓ Oxygen extraction ↑ Oxygen consumption 15–20%	↑ Ventilatory response to CO_2 ↑ Arterial pO_2 10 mm Hg ↓ Arterial pCO_2 10 mm Hg ↑ Minute ventilation 40–50% ↑ Alveolar ventilation ↔Vital capacity ↑ Respiratory rate 0–15% ↑ Tidal volume 40% ↓ Functional residual capacity 20% ↓ Expiratory reserve volume 20% ↓ Residual volume 20% Subjective dyspnea ↓ Airway resistance 36% Pulmonary blood flow
Gastrointestinal	***Urogenital***	***Blood***
↑ Nausea and vomiting Relaxed cardiac sphincter ↑ Gastrointestinal reflux ↓ Gastric acidity 30–50% (0–4 mo) ↓ Mucous secretion ↓ Gastric motility ↓ Small bowel motility ↑ Stomach emptying time 0–160% Hepatic metabolism ↑ or ↓ *Neurologic* ↓ Plasma cholinesterases 20%	↑ Weight of uterus 400% by 10 weeks 2000% by term	↑ Blood volume 35–40% ↑ Plasma volume 50% ↑ Red blood cell volume 18–20% 300–400 ml ↓ Hematocrit 15% ↓ Serum hemoglobin ↓ Serum iron ↑ White blood count 66% ↓ Total serum proteins 18% (3rd trimester) ↓ Serum albumin 14–30% ↑ Alpha-1, alpha-2 globulins 0–20% ↑ Serum fibrinogen 40–200% ↑ Phospholipids ↑ Cholesterol ↑ Free fatty acids

plasma with reduced albumin and total protein concentrations. This effect would not be expected for globulin-bound drugs, such as thyroid hormone, in which the increased globulin synthesis is more balanced by increased production of globulin-bound substances.

With the expanded circulating plasma and extracellular volumes in pregnancy, a resultant dampening of the effect of transport rates on compound concentrations is seen. Thus, the concentration-dependent processes, such as absorption across the gastrointestinal epithelium, take longer to complete.[31]

The increased minute ventilation in pregnancy may increase inhalant absorption of toxins or therapeutic agents. Because absorption of the same agent concentration for the same period results in approximately 30 to 50 per cent greater exposure, recommended exposure limits should be lower for pregnant women.[32] *At present, no official limits for pregnant women have been set or revisions made from standard recommendations.* Even topical absorption of agents may be enhanced. In pregnancy, the total skin surface area is increased. Circulation to the skin is enhanced, particularly to the breasts. The skin may be softer and thinner as well. All of these factors would tend to increase topical absorption of applied or contacted substances.

Distribution of Chemicals in Pregnancy

Pregnancy also results in substantial changes in body mass and fluid distribution.

The body weight increases by an average of 20 to 25 per cent. Body fat content rises by 20 per cent, from 16.5 to 20 kg on average. Much of the gain in fat weight occurs between 10 and 30 weeks' gestation (Fig. 18–6).[26]

The apparent volume of distribution (Vd) is the relationship between a dose administered and the plasma level estimated at time zero, assuming instantaneous distribution. The Vd has no physical correlate. Some substances, such as the tricyclic antidepressants, have Vd that exceeds the physical volume of the body many times (e.g., 20 to 30 L/kg).[33] This demonstrates that only a very small amount of agent is measured in plasma, relative to the much larger amount sequestered in tissue. Some substances do have a correlation between the Vd and physical volume; those that are restricted to the circulating blood volume are good examples. The Vd would be expected to increase for the pregnant woman, considering such dramatic increases in maternal aqueous and fatty tissue spaces. In fact, most substances do show increased volumes of distribution in pregnancy compared with that in the same patient prior to gestation.[34] When the total Vd is corrected for the increase in body mass, a "weight-corrected" Vd is derived. The distribution of lean and fatty tissues does not increase steadily throughout gestation; the second trimester is a relatively "fat" time, and the third trimester is relatively "leaner." It is not surprising, therefore, that the Vd is variable in the same patient at different times in pregnancy and after compared with the Vd prior to conception (Table 18–7).[34–36]

Plasma protein binding may also influence the apparent volume of distribution. More highly plasma protein-bound drugs tend to have smaller volumes of distribution. Agents such as salicylate, phenytoin, diazepam, theophylline, and dexamethasone show decreased binding to serum albumin in the pregnant woman. In all but the latter two agents, the decreased binding is accounted for by the reduced concentration of albumin.[37, 38]

The clinical significance of an increased Vd is that the same initial dose would be expected to produce lower serum concentrations in the pregnant subject. For increases in the weight-corrected Vd, the same dose per kg will result in lower plasma concentrations. A greater effect of reduced plasma albumin binding in pregnancy may be seen as levels of fetal albumin gradually rise as gestation progresses. This tends to produce a net accumulation of albumin-bound substances in the fetus as more free (nonprotein-bound) agent is available to transfer and then bind to fetal albumin. As the protein-bound drug no longer participates in the equilibrium reaction for the free drug, this encourages further transfer of free drug to the fetus to

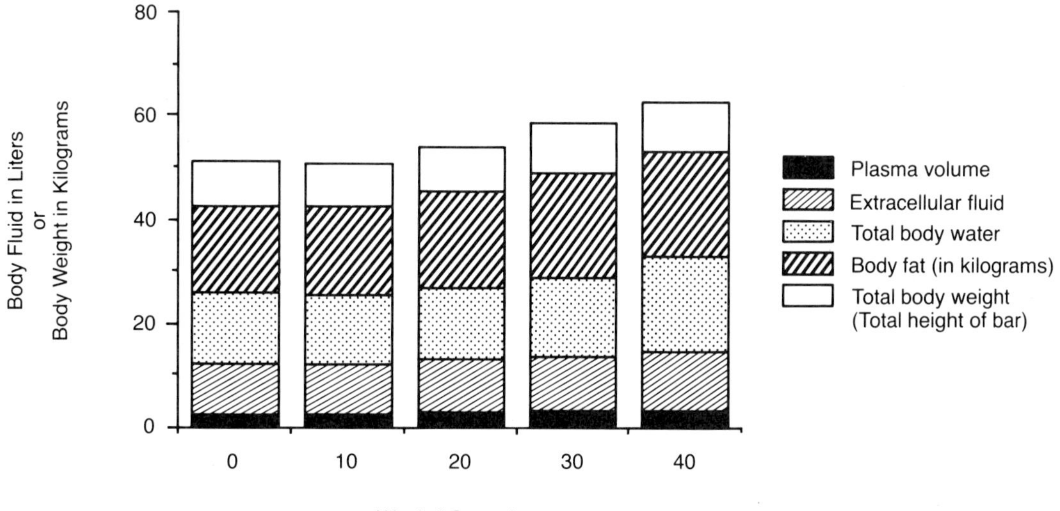

Figure 18–6. Distribution of maternal weight gain and body water distribution by duration of gestation, using data of Hytten and Leitch and Hytten and Chamberlain as tabulated by Mattison DR: Physiologic variations in pharmacokinetics during pregnancy. *In* Fabro AS, Scialli AR (eds): Drug and Chemical Action in Pregnancy. New York, Marcel Dekker, 1986.

Table 18–7. CHANGE IN APPARENT VOLUME OF DISTRIBUTION OF SELECTED AGENTS IN PREGNANCY RELATIVE TO NONPREGNANT CONTROL SUBJECTS*

	GESTATION (in Weeks) (%)				
	10	*20*	*30*	*40 (term)*	*Not Stratified*
Agent					
ampicillin	36	45	57	68	
caffeine	2	8	16	32	
cefuroxime					↔
clorazepate					33
desmethyldiazepam					72
dexamethasone					148
diazepam					49
furosemide	1	9	20	29	
meperidine	↓32	↓27	↓21	↓16	
methaqualone					↔
methimazole					20
pancuronium					↔
propranolol					↔
theophylline					20
thiopental					142
vancomycin					90

*Values are percentage increase, except as noted.
(From references 32, 34, 39, and 44.)

promote equilibrium. Of course, the maternal elimination processes concomitantly compete for the free drug, so the sum effect on fetal exchange cannot be easily predicted.[27]

The serum concentrations necessary to achieve an effect may not be the same in pregnancy. Some methods of serum level assay may be affected by endogenous substances present in the pregnant woman's circulation; digoxin serum levels can be falsely high during pregnancy because an endogenously produced digoxin-like substance (EDLS) interferes with the majority of assays. The magnitude of the falsely high digoxin values may be by as much as 0.93 ng/ml, but they vary depending on assay method.[41, 42] Additionally, there may be pharmacodynamic alterations resulting from pregnancy in which the pharmacologic response to the same plasma or tissue concentration is different. Therefore, initial dose adjustment in pregnancy should not be based on reaching a target serum concentration but rather on achieving a desired clinical effect and the absence of toxicity.

In clinical practice, the convention of obstetric drug use is to use standard dosages for nonpregnant women and adjust dosage based on effect or serum levels only when these are valid. For substances with increased pregnancy-related volumes of distribution, lower initial plasma levels would be seen. This does not, however, necessarily mean there is a lesser tissue response. For example, the lower plasma levels associated with phenytoin administration in pregnancy largely reflect reduced albumin binding.[38, 43] The larger per cent of free drug present at a given lower plasma level likely reflects a greater per cent free to act on tissue. However, that increased "free fraction" is also more available for elimination processes. The pharmacologic response to a change in serum binding in pregnancy will depend on the capacity of the gravida to eliminate the additional free drug.

Renal Elimination in Pregnancy

Consistent with the measured increase in glomerular filtration rate (GFR), the rate of elimination of some wholly renally excreted drugs is more rapid during pregnancy. Approximately 50 per cent of tested agents are more rapidly eliminated.[34] Examples of changes in renally eliminated agents in pregnancy are listed in Table 18–8.[27, 32, 34, 44]

Table 18–8. APPARENT INFLUENCE OF PREGNANCY ON THE PLASMA CLEARANCE OF DRUGS FROM LIMITED DATA

Metabolic Clearance of Drugs That Are Primarily Metabolized		
Increased	*Unchanged*	*Decreased*
acetaminophen	chlormethiazole	caffeine
betamethasone	diazepam	ketamine
carbamazepine	indomethacin	prazosin
clorazepate	labetalol	primidone
dexamethasone	meperidine	theophylline
methadone	metronidazole	
methimazole	propranolol	
metoprolol	quinine	
oxazepam		
phenytoin		
phenobarbital		
ritodrine		
terbutaline		
thiopental		
Renal Clearance of Primarily Renally Excreted Agents		
Increased	*Unchanged*	*Decreased*
amikacin	furosemide	cephalothin
ampicillin	gentamicin	methicillin
cefuroxime	vancomycin	
theophylline (but renal clearance is only a trivial part of total clearance)		

(From references 32, 34, 39, 40, 44, and 54.)

Metabolic Elimination in Pregnancy

Elimination of metabolized agents may be more rapid in pregnancy (as is seen with methimazole or phenytoin). Consistent with a reduced enzymatic activity on the basis of hepatic weight, however, many substances appear to have a slower rate of metabolic conversion (theophylline, caffeine, diazepam).[35–40] This does not necessarily mean that the dosage requirement is lessened. In the case of theophylline, the reduced intrinsic hepatic clearance caused by slower metabolic elimination is offset by reduced plasma protein binding; the sum effect is that no significant change in nonrenal clearance is seen. Concomitantly, renal theophylline clearance may be increased, particularly in the second trimester.[35, 39] The result of these changes on overall clearance and dose requirement is difficult to predict and varies among patients (see Table 18–8). Because changes in clearance cannot be readily predicted, it is even more important to titrate dosing to clinical effect and the absence of toxicity.

Measurement of Maternal-Fetal Exchange

Various methods have been used to quantify in utero drug disposition. The most common method is pooling data from various exposures (animal or human) with simultaneous maternal and fetal concentrations obtained at birth (or pregnancy termination or animal sacrifice), that is, at a known time after a known dose (Fig. 18–7). Unfortunately, although this is the most common source of data, it may not be truly reflective of normal maternal-fetal exchange. Surgery, anesthesia, and labor can markedly change maternal hemodynamic status, uteroplacental blood flow and thereby, drug transfer. Additionally, transit by the aging placenta into the mature fetus may not be a good indicator of earlier exposure. Animal models of drug transfer have traced the diffusion of substances (sometimes isotopically labeled) into fetuses serially killed at specific times after maternal exposure. This method avoids the problems of surgery or labor changing maternal-fetal exchange characteristics. However, as with all methods that pool data from a small number of pregnancies to construct maternal and fetal plasma concentration curves versus time after dosing, such curves may not give an accurate picture of the individual subject's maternal-fetal exchange, particularly where considerable interindividual variability exists.

Isolated placental preparations allow evaluation of certain placental activities, but technical limitations in collection generally restrict investigators in evaluating term placentas. In addition, the rates of perfusate flow that can be achieved in the placental preparations are low, resulting from considerable vasoconstriction that is usually present. The flow rates and transfer, therefore, may not even approximate in utero flow and transit.[45] Exteriorization and catheterization of the placenta after elective fetal animal delivery has been used to examine placental disposition of substances in somewhat earlier gestations and without the same degree of technical flow limitations.

Another common use of chronic instrumentation is that of the placenta or fetus for the collection of serial samples in utero. This is labor-intensive and risks interference with the pregnancy by catheter impedance to fetal or placental blood flow and by infection. The anesthesia used to prevent dislodgement of the equipment may also alter flow and transit. This method and sophisticated variations allow evaluation of changes in compartmental drug concentrations over time and calculation of rates of accumulation or elimination from them. The use of radionuclide-labeled microspheres as tracers to drug transfer is particularly exciting; it makes the measurement of fetal cardiac output and blood flow responses to various agents possible.[46–48]

Newer techniques combine conventional measurements with autoradiography, allowing observation of changes in the pattern of drug and metabolite disposition over time throughout the tissues of the fetus. Application of positron emission tomography (PET) methods allows investigation of the distribution and metabolism of tracer substances in the whole animal. This technique has been applied to the study of pharmacokinetics of morphine and its glucuronide metabolite in rhesus monkeys.[49] Following the administration of radiolabeled tracer substances, external detectors are used to visualize the distribution of those tracers in the maternal and fetal bodies over time.

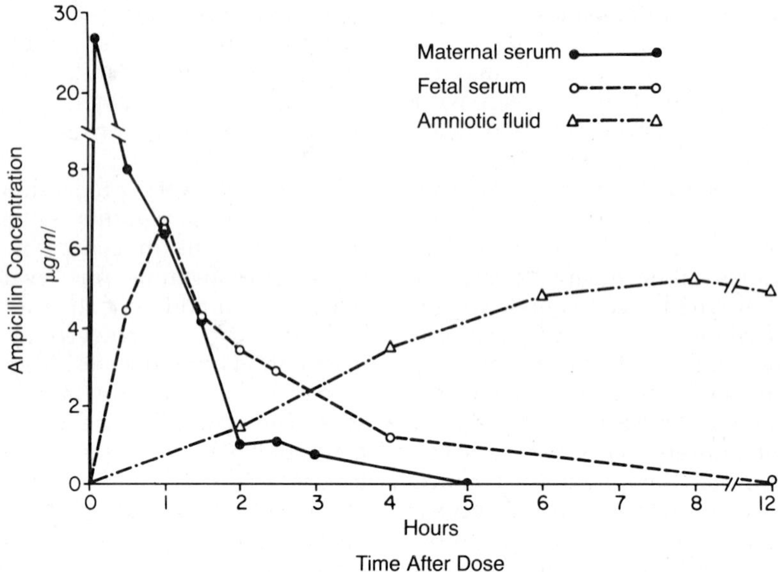

Figure 18–7. Maternal and fetal serum level curve versus time, for ampicillin. Each fetal data point is taken from the time of birth after dosing of a different baby. (From Bray RE, Boe RW, Johnson WL, et al: Transfer of ampicillin into fetus and amniotic fluid from maternal plasma in late pregnancy. Am J Obstet Gynecol 96:938–942, 1966.)

Influence of Pharmacokinetic Disposition on Teratogenicity

True (direct) teratogenic effects will depend on the toxin (or metabolite) concentrations achieved in the conceptus within a given time period. Thus, the changes in pharmacokinetic parameters and dose requirements in pregnancy may be expected to influence the risk of malformations.

There is still very limited knowledge of how to compensate for the known kinetic changes to achieve desired maternal effects or limit toxicity in humans. Most of the information in this area is derived from animal studies. Traditionally, the effect of a standard dose on the development of malformations has been evaluated. Evidence of two dose-response curves—a dose-related effect and a threshold-dose effect—has emerged from such work in the production of physical anomalies (Fig. 18–8).[16, 50] There are limitations to this approach in trying to define individual fetal-dose/teratogenic response relationships (Tables 18–9, 18–10).

It is the goal of animal experimentation in teratology to ultimately reduce the risks of unknown exposures in man. The interspecies variability in teratogenicity testing is thus a major issue. Whereas inherent species differences in susceptibility cannot be accounted for, pharmacokinetic differences in drug disposition and metabolism may be. For example, because rodents eliminate many agents much more rapidly than do humans, to produce the same kind of maternal plasma concentrations over time, it may be necessary to infuse drugs continuously or in a pulsatile fashion, using implantable pumps.

Minimization of intralitter genetic variability by selective breeding has also been accomplished to evaluate genetic influence on susceptibility to teratogens.[51] By recognizing and compensating for such controllable variables, the dose-response relationships for individual anomalies or toxic effects may become clearer. Because few agents appear to demonstrate a "threshold response" in the production of anomalies, it may be possible to establish "no obvious effect levels" (NOEL) and extrapolate such information to human exposures.[52]

Nonpharmacokinetic Maternal Influences on Teratogenicity

As noted in the foregoing discussion, environmental or therapeutic chemical exposures are only rarely known to cause birth defects. In addition to the maternal contribution to the fetus's genetic makeup and to the provision of nutrients and xenobiotics, the maternal status may influence the risk

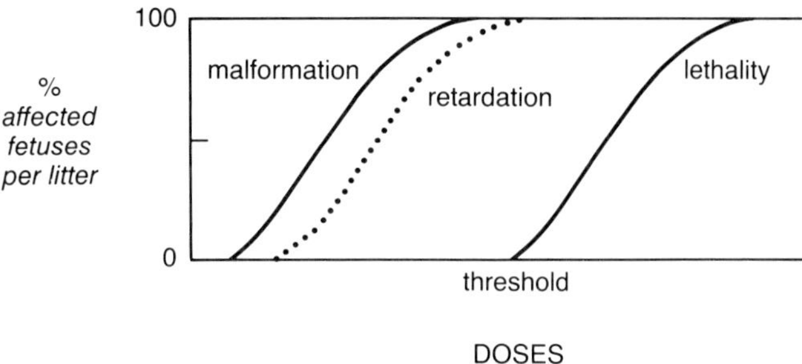

Pattern 1: Entire litter/population is malformed at exposure levels that do not cause lethality; past such exposure levels, embryotoxicity can occur, generally in conjunction with maternal toxicity (rare pattern indicative of high teratogenic potency).

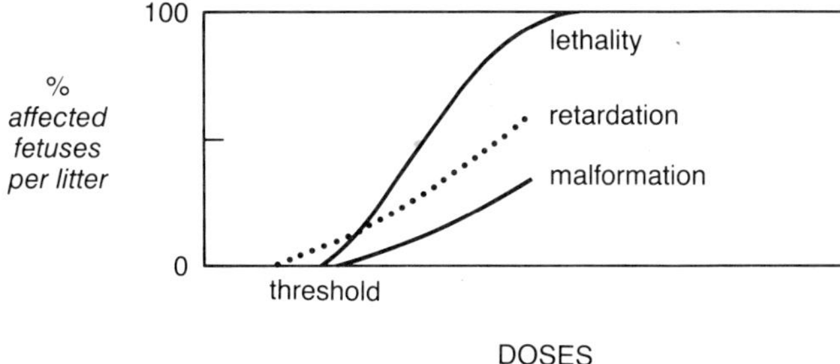

Pattern 2: Dose-related embryotoxicity with growth retardation of malformations in surviving fetuses at any given dose within the developmentally toxic range. Normal, growth-retarded, malformed, and resorbed fetuses are seen (more common pattern; indicative of primarily embryotoxic agent in this case) as lowest dose associated with embryotoxicity is close to the lowest producing teratogenic growth retardation.

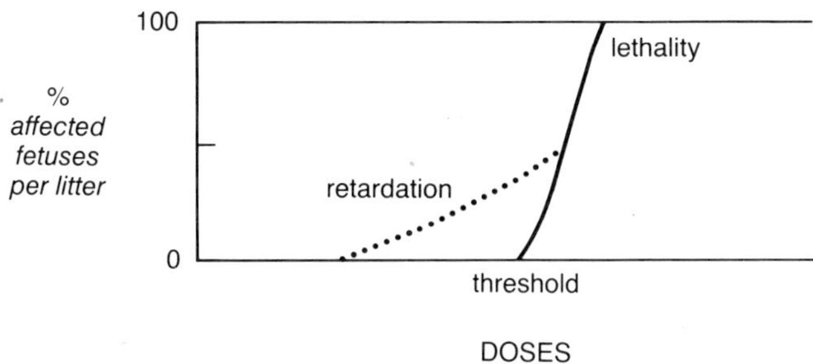

Pattern 3: Example of dose-response relationship for an agent producing growth retardation and fetal death but no increased risk of malformations (sometimes induction of embryolethality may mask production of malformations).

Figure 18–8. Dose-response patterns for different types of developmental toxicants. (Adapted from Manson JM: Teratogens. *In* Klaassen CD, Amdur MO, Doull J (eds): Casarett and Doull's Toxicology. The Basic Science of Poisons. 3rd ed. New York, Macmillan, 1986, pp 195–220.)

Table 18–9. LIMITATIONS TO INTERPRETATION OF TERATOGENICITY DATA BASED ON ADMINISTRATION OF A STANDARDIZED MATERNAL DOSE

THE SAME DOSE GIVEN TO	MAY PRODUCE	EXAMPLE
Different species	Different effects	Glucocorticoids are highly teratogenic to mice but not to humans
Different mothers of the same species	Different maternal tissue concentrations	Variability exists in maternal pharmacokinetics of many agents
The same mother in different pregnancies	Different effects	A given fetus may be more sensitive to a teratogen than its siblings or an at-risk pregnancy with uteroplacental insufficiency more sensitive to developmental toxins that restrict fetal blood flow
The same mother in a given pregnancy	Different fetal concentrations and/or effects in different fetuses	Multiple gestation animals or humans may receive different blood nutrient supply and toxin exposure, depending on site of placentation or physical constraint variables

for abnormal prenatal development, including physical malformations. Certain developmentally toxic factors specific to the mother have been determined (Tables 18–11, 18–12, and 18–13).[38, 50, 53, 55, 57, 58, 62–73]

It is clear that the uterus and placenta do not simply act as container and filter but, rather, play a dynamic role in the presence of developmental toxicity.

The Role of Maternal Toxicity in Developmental Toxicology

Not all adverse effects on the fetus depend on a toxic substance reaching the fetus. In addition to agents that poison the placenta and put the fetus at risk, other indirect developmental toxins exist. These agents disrupt the healthy balance of the fetal-placental-maternal unit. Because the fetus is biologically expendable for maternal survival, severe toxicity to the mother may initiate fetal miscarriage by release of vasoactive substances caused by maternal cardiovascular distress and local tissue damage and necrosis. One teratologist observed that any agent could produce developmental toxicity if the mother were sufficiently poisoned as to suffocate, starve, or intoxicate her.[74]

Table 18–10. LIMITATIONS TO ASSUMING A UNIFORM FETAL EXPOSURE FROM THE ADMINISTRAION OF A UNIFORM WEIGHT-ADJUSTED DOSE TO THE MOTHER IN TERATOGENICITY STUDIES

VARIATION EXISTS IN	RESULTING FROM DISPARITY IN
Interindividual disposition	Maternal absorption Maternal distribution Maternal metabolism/elimination
Placental transfer	Uterine blood flow Placental blood flow Placental thickness and surface area Placental metabolism
Fetal tissue exposure	Fetal position/site of placentation Fetal tissue distribution Fetal metabolism/elimination

Substances that produce their effect by adverse actions on maternal status are of particular interest to teratologists. Clearly, such influences should be isolated when examining direct teratogenic or embryo/fetotoxic effects. To accomplish this, changes in maternal health must be catalogued as carefully as the fetuses are examined. The Environmental Protection Agency (EPA) has identified six measurable endpoints that should be reported in experimental teratology studies using animal models. (Table 18–14). A dose-related incidence of signs of maternal toxicity in concert with adverse fetal effects is considered by some to indicate developmental toxicity occurring secondary to maternal toxicity.

The absence of fetal adverse effects in the absence of evidence of maternal drug/chemical effects is not considered to constitute an acceptable trial, except in cases in which the dose given to the mother extends over the expected range of therapeutic doses by a

Table 18–11. EXAMPLES OF MATERNAL FACTORS THAT MAY INFLUENCE THE RISK FOR ABNORMAL PRENATAL DEVELOPMENT

Factor	Effect
MATERNAL DISEASES	
Congenital Infections	
Rubella	Malformation
Cytomegalovirus	Growth retardation
AIDS	Mental retardation
Noninfectious Diseases	
Diabetes mellitus	Uteroplacental blood flow
Heart disease	Oxygen supply
Essential hypertension	Fetal survival
Renal insufficiency	Growth retardation
Severe anemia	
Autoimmune Diseases	
Systemic lupus erythematosus	Congenital heart block
Graves' disease	Neonatal thyrotoxicosis
Sensitization to exposure to fetal blood cells with rhesus antibody	Erythroblastosis fetalis
Metabolic Disorders	
Virilizing tumors producing androgens	Irreversible or reversible masculinization of female fetuses
Phenylketonuria	Risk of mental retardation; risk of malformations
MATERNAL NUTRITION	
Iodine	Fetal goiter
Nondietary vitamin A excess	Malformation
Caloric deprivation	↓ Mean birthweight: in humans: no risk for malformations; in rodents: risk for malformations
MATERNAL STRESS	
(animal): transportation, restraint, food and water restriction	
Developmental toxicity in laboratory animals	
MATERNAL AGE	
Advanced	↑ Risk chromosomal of anomalies ↑ Risk of certain malformations (Anencephaly) ↓ Capacity to maintain pregnancy
Adolescent	↑ Small for gestational age ↑ Infant mortality ↑ Certain malformations (Anencephaly)
MATERNAL SIZE	
Reduced	↓ Fetal size (animals only)
GRAVIDITY	
Increased	↑ Flaccidity of uterine blood vessels ↓ Uterine blood flow (animals)
MATERNAL TEMPERATURE REGULATION	
Fever/Hyperthermia	Retrospective analysis: ↑ risk of anencephaly (contribution of unrecognized congenital infection) Induced hyperthermia in experimental animals, dose-dependent malformations (especially neural tube defects)
Saunas/hot tub use	No evidence of increased risk of human malformations (including anencephaly)

wide margin. Therefore, the majority of animal toxicity studies are performed at very high doses relative to normal human therapeutic/occupational exposures. These studies would be expected to produce *both* dose-related direct teratogenic/toxic effects and indirect teratogenic effects caused by the same exposure.

Table 18–12. EXAMPLES OF FACTORS THAT REDUCE UTEROPLACENTAL BLOOD FLOW

DECREASED EFFECTIVE PLASMA VOLUME
Hypovolemia/dehydration
Excessive diuretic use
Peripheral vasodilation without volume expansion
Diazoxide
Nitroglycerin
Hydralazine
UTERINE VASCULAR CONSTRICTION
Hydroxyurea
Serotonin
Alpha-adrenergic vasconstrictors
Epinephrine, norepinephrine
Phenylephrine
Sympathomimetic amines in excess
Phenylpropanolamine
? Dopamine in excess
Indirect agents
Ephedrine
Cocaine
Nicotine
UTERINE CONTRACTIONS
Labor
Increased gastrointestinal motility
Substances inducing contractions (oxytocics)
Oxytocin
Prostaglandins ($F_{2\alpha}$, 15 methyl, E_2)
Ergot alkaloids
CHRONIC PLACENTAL INSUFFICIENCY
Chronic hypertension
Diabetes mellitus
SURGICAL LIGATION OF HYPOGASTRIC ARTERY
(transient decrease in uterine blood flow)

Table 18–13. FACTORS DEMONSTRATING THE INFLUENCE OF CONSTRAINT ON NORMAL PRENATAL DEVELOPMENT

Polytocal—animals that bear multiple young at one time	↓ Fetal and placental weight per fetus
Human multiple gestation	Variation in fetal size related to position and site of placentation, altered ability to compete for maternal nutritional resources or toxins
Malformed uteri Abdominal gestation Oligohydramnios	Deformed fetuses (often reversible)
Amniotic bands	Fetal deformities include disruption or approximation of the effects of chemical teratogens (i.e., limb-reduction anomalies and facial clefts)

Table 18–14. MEASURABLE END-POINTS TO BE REPORTED IN EXPERIMENTAL TERATOLOGY STUDIES AS EVIDENCE OF MATERNAL TOXICITY

Maternal mortality
Pregnancy rates
Body weight change or failure to gain weight
Consumption of food and water
Clinical signs of toxicity
Maternal organ weights

Note: The presence of two of these factors (mortality of less than 10 per cent and slight weight loss) is sufficient to define the presence of maternal toxicity in EPA regulatory documents.

It is completely reasonable that the maternal response to toxic substances may include changes in maternal heart rate, peripheral vascular resistance, uteroplacental blood flow or respiration, maternal acid-base balance, or other factors that will influence the amount of a direct teratogen or proteratogen that reaches the fetus.

Identification of substances that are relatively more teratogenic is a first step in teratogen screening. Such testing must include an assessment of the presence of maternal toxicity as above. In addition to helping to clarify whether the agent may be directly or indirectly toxic, this allows determination of the Developmental Toxicity Index (A/D ratio). In animal or in vitro embryo testing, the substance is administered at certain fractions of the maternal dose at which 50 per cent of pregnant animals die (LD_{50}). The mean embryotoxic or teratogenic dose is then compared with the adult LD_{50}. The Adult/Developmental Toxicity ratio has varied widely in tested substances (<1 to 64). Johnson has described various developmental toxicity classes based on the A/D ratio (Table 18–15).[52, 75, 76] No ratio defines an absolutely safe agent.

There are two other interesting indices of fetal toxicity commonly used in screening potential toxins. The Reproductive Toxicity Index compares the lethal dose to 1 per cent of mothers to the dose that is teratogenic (or embryotoxic) in 5 per cent of fetuses.[52] The TD_{50} is the dose that is developmentally toxic to 50 per cent of fetuses. Jusko has described two kinds of relationships between the TD_{50} and the maternal LD_{50}.[77] Class I agents appear to inflict damage independent of maternal dose. Class II agents require a minimum dose (threshold exposure) before malformations are seen. The existence of such a threshold and, by analogy, safe exposure below

Table 18–15. PROPOSED CLASSIFICATION OF DEVELOPMENTAL TOXINS FROM THE PERSPECTIVE OF DEVELOPMENTAL BIOLOGY

A/D RATIO	AGENT CLASSIFICATION		SUGGESTED NATURE OF EFFECTS
Very high (≧ 10)	A-Primary developmental hazards	Developmentally targeted	Fetal effect limited by location of sensitive developmental event. Range of effects increased by wider distribution of the event affected
Moderate (≧ 3 to < 10)		Ontogenetically targeted	Fetal effect dependent on sensitive developmental stage; range of effects broadened by persistence of toxicant; species-specific effects possible
Low (< 3)	B-Co-affective agents	Maternally associated	Fetal effects dependent on sensitive developmental stage to a degree; in general, effects are developmental delays. Occasionally, severe defects may be produced by specific agent action. Species-specific effects likely
Very low (≦ 1)		Maternally mediated	State-dependent effects present to a lesser degree. Fetal effects more dependent on maternal response

(Adapted from Johnson EM, Christian MS, Dansky L, Gabel BEG: Use of the adult developmental relationship in pre-screening for developmental hazards. Teratogenesis Carcinog Mutagen 7:273–285, 1987.)

this dose, is predicated on observed receptor interactions or enzyme interactions. Toxins that produce effects by receptor-type interactions should have a threshold dose for toxicity. Agents acting by other mechanisms, for example, modification of deoxyribonucleic acid leading to a transcription error, would be expected to produce a linear dose-response curve down to very low levels.

The relationship between maternal toxicity and malformation risk remains a matter of debate.[78] Whereas clear knowledge of such a relationship is critical to the interpretation of experimental teratogenicity studies, human clinical experience provides clear evidence of secondary developmental toxicity such as diabetes mellitus[79] and also for developmental toxicity in the apparent absence of maternal toxic response (e.g., methylmercury, thalidomide).[79–81] Various mechanisms certainly exist. We generally think of the relationship of direct and indirect prenatal toxic influences as distinct. It is conceivable that such mechanisms may not only coexist but also interact to modify severity of fetal exposure and response to potential harm. (Fig. 18–9).

THE PLACENTA

The placenta is a tissue of fetal origin. Its functions during gestation are several including protection of the conceptus, maintenance of pregnancy, prevention of maternal rejection of the pregnancy as foreign tissue, transportation of nutrients and wastes, metabolism of endogenous and xenobiotic substances, and endocrine activity.[82–85]

The protective functions of the placenta are often overrated. Nearly any drug or environmental agent that gains access to the maternal blood stream will reach the fetus by "crossing" the placenta. Much has been made of information regarding chemical characteristics of xenobiotics that reduce or limit placental transit. As discussed further in the chapter, this rarely results in a substance being completely prohibited to the fetus, and failure to be passed through the placenta does not exclude the possibility of fetal harm.

Substances do not even have to reach the fetus to harm the pregnancy. The placenta itself may be the target of an embryotoxin or teratogen. Adverse effects or anomalies may be induced in the fetus by interfering with normal placental function. Cadmium, for example, can disturb placental function and lead to fetal toxicity before reaching significant concentrations in fetal circulation.[84, 86] Trypan blue dye may produce physical disruption of fetal tissues by interfering with normal pinocytotic activity, despite being "trapped" in the placenta and not reaching the fetus.[87] The way

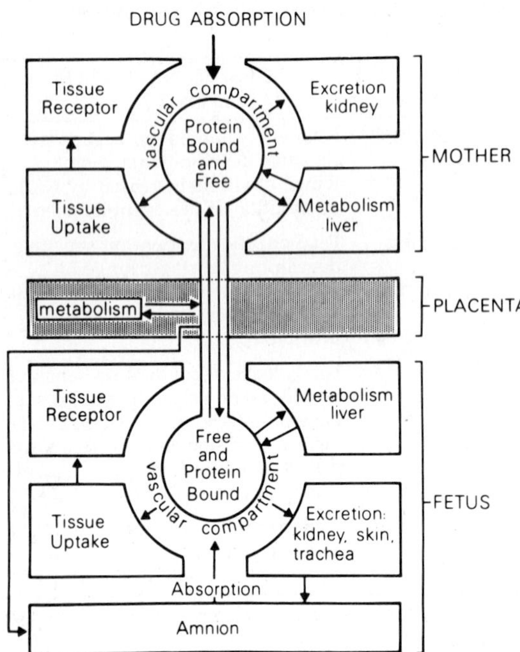

Figure 18–9. The maternal-placental-fetal unit. (From Rajchgot P, MacLeod S: Perinatal pharmacology. *In* MacLeod SM, Okey AB, Spielberg SP (eds): Developmental Pharmacology. New York, Alan R. Liss, 1983, pp 3–23.)

in which this may occur is explained by the structure and function of the placenta.

The implantation of the fertilized ovum, developed to the blastocyst stage, in the endometrial lining of the uterus is the beginning of placental development. In human development, there are actually two placentas. The first one that is formed is the yolksac placenta. It is present until its regression in the fourth month of gestation. The primary function of the yolksac is to form red blood cells, but it also participates in other embryo-maintenance activities such as absorption of maternally secreted nutrients from the exocoelomic cavity and secretory functions. It also participates in the formation of the embryonic midgut. The yolksac is thus a critically important interim structure, present during the most sensitive time of development, and yet its chemical transfer functions have not been evaluated. The classic requirements for "placental transfer," studied in late-gestation mature placentas, may not necessarily apply.

The second placenta is the chorioallantoic placenta. It also begins to form at implantation. It gradually invades maternal endometrial glands, stroma, and arterial walls to access the maternal blood supply in a villous structure that maximizes the surface area for exchange. The structure allows the high-resistance maternal arterial system to become a low-resistance system in the spiral arteries. Maternal and fetal blood circulate in proximity by the third week of gestation. Until 12 weeks' gestation, there are four tissue layers separating the maternal and fetal circulation. These are the syncytiotrophoblast (the outer layer of the trophoblast), cytotrophoblast, villus connective tissue cores, and fetal capillary endothelium. By the third trimester, the cytotrophoblast has become discontinuous and only three layers separate the circulations.[83, 84]

At term, blood comes into the spaces between the villi from over 100 spiral arteries; over 150 ml of blood may be contained in these spaces at a given time. The rate of blood flow increases during gestation from 50 ml/min at 10 weeks' gestation to 600 ml/min at term. Thus, at term, this relatively "slow" circulation replaces the blood volume in the spaces three to four times each minute.[83]

The human placenta produces a number of steroid and protein hormones for pregnancy maintenance, including human chorionic gonadotropin (the "pregnancy test" hormone), human placental lactogen (which has a role in preparation of the breasts for lactation), estrogen, and progesterone.[85]

Placental Transit

Much has been made of the role of physicochemical characteristics of toxins and drugs in determining if an agent will "cross the placental barrier." The phrase is misleading. It has been criticized in the medical literature for implying that a barrier is present that will exclude most toxic substances and that any agent that does reach the fetus is necessarily toxic. Nearly all substances tested will be found in the fetus after administration to the mother. A teleologically based efficiency of the fetus in garnering maternal nutritional resources may be in part responsible for this finding. The placenta may modify the course of transfer, but it rarely excludes a substance from the fetus. Thus, the issue is not whether a given agent will cross the placenta, but rather how rapidly, in what form, over what time course, how it will be distributed to the fetus, and what effects will accrue. The basic process by which substances access the fetus is *simple diffusion*.[88, 89] Because the placenta may be considered a series of specialized semipermeable membranes, the Fick equation should describe the transfer of substances by simple diffusion. The various transfer processes and determinants are presented in Table 18–16.

The importance of ionization and lipid solubility can be seen in the fact that mercury vapor tends to accumulate in the fetus because its volatility gives it tissue access; the fetal tissues then generate Hg^{2+}, which is trapped in tissue. Organic mercury (such as methylmercury) on the other hand, is easily distributed to the fetus, including the fetal brain, where it is highly toxic.[91, 92] It is of concern that simple complexation of substances with limited fetal distribution can so dramatically change the risk of developmental toxicity.

Table 18–16. TRANSFER PROCESSES INVOLVED IN PLACENTAL TRANSIT AND SPECIFIC FACTORS INFLUENCING THEM

SIMPLE DIFFUSION

Transfer described by Fick's law
Rate of diffusion: $K\ A\ (C_m - C_{fetal})/P$

where K = constant
A = surface area of the placenta
P = thickness of the placental layers

Net diffusion is a result of the difference in maternal and fetal concentrations ($C_m - C_{fetal}$)

Maternal concentrations are reduced by:
Limited maternal absorption,
Extensive tissue distribution, or
Rapid elimination

Uteroplacental blood flow influences transfer
Decreased flow due to uteroplacental insufficiency or shunting reduces transfer

Chemical characteristics of substance favoring rapid transfer:
Less bound to plasma proteins
Un-ionized species
pKA (ratio of un-ionized/ionized at physiologic pH)
Lower molecular weight
< 10 or < 100 MW fit through membrane pores (i.e., urea)
Greater lipid solubility (except must complete with tendency to move to maternal fat tissue)

Diffusion is the overwhelming process for transfer of exogenous substances
Application of Fick equation is limited by normal presence of shunting within the placenta
Placental "trapping" by binding or placental metabolism reduces fetal exposure

FACILITATED TRANSPORT

A saturable process for substances of specific conformation and physical structure (i.e., D-glucose but not L-glucose)

May be influenced by substances that compete for the carrier moiety in carrier-mediated transport

ACTIVE TRANSPORT

An energy-consuming process particularly vital to placental transport of nutrients: vitamins
calcium
amino acids
iron

May be limited by transport maximums

Uses specific receptor sites

PINOCYTOSIS

High molecular weight substances can reach the fetus by this membrane invagination process (animals)

Placental Metabolism

The placenta is not often thought of as an active organ that changes the substances transferred through it. In fact, enzymes capable of metabolizing drugs and other chemicals are present and active in the placenta. The human placenta contains multiple enzyme systems including those responsible for oxidation, reduction, hydrolysis, and deconjugation.[93, 94] These systems are primarily involved with endogenous steroid metabolism, and their role in the biotransformation of possible developmental toxins is not clear. The level of activity of these enzymes, although generally sensitive to induction, remains insignificant relative to that of maternal or fetal organs (including liver, kidney, and adrenal gland). When xenobiotic metabolism is considered, the presence of enzyme systems in the placenta does not contribute markedly to overall drug clearance. The significance of their presence is related to the two ways in which substances presented to the placenta may be bioconverted: detoxification and activation. In light of the present state of knowledge of its metabolic activity, the tendency to think of the placenta as fetoprotective is misapplied. The ability of the placenta to *detoxify* chemicals has not been established. The four major classes of enzyme systems involved in inactivation of reactive intermediates may be found in the placenta. They include glucuronyl transferases to create glucuronides, sulfotransferases for sulfation, epoxide hydrolases for reduction of toxic epoxides, and gluthathione-S-transferase. Lesser systems responsible for methylation, acetylation, and glycine conjugation are also present in minor amounts. Unfortunately, all of these placental systems appear to be of very low activity and refractory to induction.[93, 95] Thus, fetal exposure to bioactive forms would not be expected to be markedly decreased by the placenta.

Placental capacity to *activate* substrates to more toxic intermediates is more established.[85, 93, 96, 97] Oxidative, reducing, and hydrolytic enzymes are all present. The mono-oxygenase systems of the placenta, in particular, are highly inducible with polycyclic aromatic hydrocarbon agents and capable of producing potentially toxic metabolites. Placental metabolism usually results in metabolites that are less active, rather than more so; however, the chemical nature of the substrate appears to be the primary determinant of how much reactive intermediates will be produced. Some highly reactive intermediates that could be formed would be expected to be toxic to the placenta cell in which they were generated. Little direct fetal toxicity would be expected, but indirect harm due to placental damage could occur. It would be only the more stable intermediates that would reach maternal, as well as fetal, circulation. The effect would be expected to be more diffuse because it would be widespread, but embryo/fetal toxicity would not be impossible. It is established that toxic exposures, including cigarette smoke, polyhalogenated biphenyls, and dioxins, may induce the mono-oxygenase system.[93, 97, 98] There is substantial evidence that cigarette smoke increases the capacity of the human placenta to generate toxic metabolites.[97, 98]

Placental Toxin Sequestration

It is tempting to consider the accumulation of developmental toxins by the placenta as a protective function. In fact, the deterioration of the placenta, which is produced by agents such as cadmium, results in fetal harm by impairment of the aforementioned essential functions of the placenta.

In summary, without pharmacokinetic investigation, it is not possible to predict the fate of chemical substances during their passage from the mother to the fetus.

THE FETUS

Toxin Transport into Preimplantation Embryos

Placental passage is not critical to embryo exposure. From animal research data, it is clear that blastocysts may take on xenobiotics, even before they are implanted.[99] The chemical characteristics that favor drug transfer into blastocyst, as studied in the rabbit embryo model, are analogous to those promoting placental exchange (see Table 18–16).[99, 100] Interestingly, the degree of protein binding does not appear to be critical to drug transfer into the blastocyst. Blastocyst transfer appears to be rapid, occurring within 1 to 20 minutes after maternal dosing, depending on lipophilicity of the substance to be transferred. Some highly lipophilic agents that have been studied, such as thiopental, achieve peak blastocyst levels in 1 to 2 minutes.[99]

Some very interesting work with the mouse embryo examined the effects of cyclophosphamide. Radiolabeled cyclophosphamide achieved measurable levels in maternal tissue rapidly, but the amount of label in the embryo did not reach quantifiable limits. Indirect evidence of embryo transfer was present. Although there were no malformations, there was substantial embryotoxicity.[101]

Another indirect measure of toxic effect on the embryo was seen by examining embryonic chromosomes for evidence of sister chromatid exchange frequency in cultured embryos after maternal cyclophosphamide exposure. The frequency of this toxic effect is maternal-dose related.[102] Furthermore, exposure to a substance that is nonteratogenic in humans but teratogenic in mice such as caffeine can produce superadditive toxicity. Caffeine is believed to inhibit embryonic repair of DNA damage induced by cyclophosphamide.[103]

It is often said that the preimplantation human embryo is insensitive to adverse environmental exposures. Accumulating experimental data may question unconditional acceptance of this. The animal work demonstrates that preimplantation embryos are vulnerable to maternal exposures and may demonstrate toxicity from them. The significance of these experimental findings to early human pregnancy exposures is not known. It is, in fact, very interesting that cyclophosphamide demonstrates dose-related toxicity in embryos in culture. Although cyclophosphamide is a known developmental toxin, it must be metabolically activated to be effective or toxic. Such embryotoxicity has been taken as evidence of the ability of the embryo to bioactivate toxins.

Postimplantation Embryonic Drug Transfer

In general, most drugs pass freely to the postimplantation embryo. It has been observed that drug concentrations in animal embryonic tissue generally are lower than concomitant maternal concentrations.[104, 105] After bolus injection of the agent to the mother, whole rodent embryo drug concentrations during organogenesis are usually lower than late-gestation whole fetal concentrations.[106] A number of investigators have demonstrated that substances, such as salicyclic acid, diethylstilbestrol, and the herbicide 2,4,5-T, are present in increasing amounts in fetal tissues as the gestation advances.[107–109] Even some substances that are not well transferred to the embryo (such as phenothiazines) are found in higher concentrations in the fetus. In part, this may be related to a pH difference at the different stages of development. Experimental work with the agent dimethyloxazolidinedione (a trimethadione metabolite) has been used to calculate embryonic intracellular pH.[109] The data suggest that the early embryo is, in fact, more alkalotic than the mother and particularly more than the fetus. The corollary to this is that drug transfer to the early embryo may not favor accumulation of weak bases, but rather, favor accumulation of weak acids because it would be those agents that would be relatively trapped in embryonic tissue.

The pattern of drug distribution in prenatal tissues also shows ontogeny. Early in embryonic development, the neuroepithelium tends to accumulate substances, perhaps owing to a high metabolic activity. The blood-brain barrier to substance diffusion is not developed until the second half of pregnancy.[110] The susceptibility of the CNS to developmental toxins may be in part related to this preferential distribution. Retinoic acid, a known neuroteratogen, has been shown to accumulate in early neuroepithelium and neural crest tissue. When evaluated kinetically, the accumulation is saturable and appears to be mediated by a receptor expressed preferentially during development.[111]

In the fetus, the pattern of drug distribution is more similar to that seen in the mother. As the fetus matures, fetal tissues with storage capacity are formed and mature (Table 18–17).[27, 48, 112, 113] A rapid equilibrium between mother and fetus/embryo is expected for agents that are of low molecular weight and highly lipid-soluble, such as chloroform. Using sophisticated autoradiographic techniques, Ghantous and colleagues have shown that the embryo/fetal distribution is surprisingly low and ends very quickly after the end of maternal exposure.[114] Although the metabolites of chloroform accumulate in fetal tissue, especially in early epithelium, little accumulation is seen in late fetal brain. This may reflect a lesser lipophilicity of the metabolites than of the parent compound, which is generally true of highly lipophilic agents. When the distribution of the less lipophilic metabolite is compared with that of the parent, preferential distribution does not occur to such a degree, and appearance in the embryo/fetus is permitted.

Table 18–17. DISTRIBUTION OF XENOBIOTICS IN FETAL TISSUES

Fetal liver	Particularly able to store xenobiotics
Fetal gut	Found to contain metabolites of maternally administered agents
Fetal urine	May have either active or biotransformed substances
Fetal skeleton	Can accumulate metals and particularly substances with metal affinity (such as tetracycline and other chelating agents)
Fetal fat stores	Higher total body water content of the early fetus drops as fat is accrued
	Fat-soluble agents tend to have greater fetal distribution as the fetus ages
	Fetuses weighing less than 1 kg have very limited body fat, which may explain limited fetal concentrations of very fat-soluble substances
	Lesser fetal accumulation and retention may be related to higher maternal fat stores acting as a "bank"; equilibrium favors transfer to the large maternal "bank." Equilibrium concentration established with small quantity of fetal fat tissue is low

Fetal Metabolism

Once an agent traverses the placenta, it may be transformed by fetal tissues. Because the flow of blood to the fetus is via the umbilical vein, substances are first presented to the fetal liver. If fetal liver metabolism is active, a substantial reduction in fetal plasma concentrations may occur rapidly, as a "fetal first-pass effect." As the fetus matures, the enzyme systems of the liver develop and are capable of such biotransformation.

Generally speaking, the enzyme systems of the fetus are first detectable at 5 to 8 weeks' gestation, and their activity increases until 12 to 14 weeks, reaching only a fraction of adult levels.[93, 94, 114–123] In fact, it is not until approximately 1 year postnatal age that liver enzymatic activity is comparable to that of the adult. The first system to be developed in the fetus is the cytochrome P-450 group (or microsomal mixed-function oxidase) of enzymes, which mediates xenobiotic transformation, that is, this group affects metabolism of amino acids, ethanol, therapeutic medication, environmental pollutants, and industrial toxins. These enzymes are present as soon as the smooth endoplasmic reticulum is formed (40 to 60 days human gestation, later in most laboratory species).[93, 94] It is most active in the fetal adrenal gland and somewhat less so in the fetal liver. The fetal kidney and gut systems have even lower activity.[115]

The mono-oxygenases may comprise thousands of inducible forms; the group may be divided into two major groups—phenobarbital or polycyclic aromatic hydrocarbons (such as 3-methylcholanthrene)—based on which substance may induce their activity. The latter group includes such enzymes as the aryl hydrocarbon hydroxylases, which metabolize benzo(a)pyrene and other polycyclic aromatic hydrocarbon molecules. These hydroxylases (AHH) are present even in the blastocyst.[116] Their level of activity in the fetus is very low (2 to 4 per cent of adult activity) but may be induced by maternal smoking, as may the placental aryl hydrocarbon hydrolases.[93] It appears that fetal induction of this enzyme activity shows ontogeny, that is, a given level of maturity must be achieved before the system is inducible. There also appears to be genetic factors that govern inducibility of these hydroxylases. The phenobarbital-inducible mono-oxygenases appear early in development and gradually increase in activity until midgestation, when a low level of activity (20 to 40 per cent of adult activity) is achieved.

Hydrolytic enzymes, particularly epoxide hydrolases, which convert stable or reactive epoxides to dihydrodiols, are capable of detoxifying toxic epoxides. Epoxide formation is part of the destructive, precarcinogenic metabolism of deoxyribonucleic or ribonucleic acids. The epoxide hydrolases can repair such precancerous changes. They are also present in the fetus by 5 weeks of gestation.[117] The activity of the epoxide hydrolases is inducible and does not appear to show interindividual variability on a genetic basis, in comparison to the aforementioned mono-oxygenases.

Another group of enzymes that may have great toxicologic importance is the liver alcohol dehydrogenases. These enzymes, which are capable of catalyzing the metabolism of ethanol to aldehyde, are present at 6 weeks' gestation.[124] Multiple forms of the enzyme are present, composed of two subunits each. There is ontogenetic regulation of the enzyme produced. Separate gene loci exist for the production of three different subunits.[118, 119] Initially, the fetus produces subunits from only one of the gene loci, and the enzyme has two identical subunits. As gestation progresses, the second subunit gene begins to be expressed, and the third is not expressed until 3 to 6 months postnatally. It is not certain when the reducing enzymes for further detoxification of the formed aldehyde are active in the fetus.

The activities of conjugative pathways, including those of glycine conjugation, glucuronidation, sulfation, and glutathione formation, are very low in most laboratory animals prior to birth, even though the enzymes necessary may be present very early.[120–122] Glutathione-S-transferase is present by 6 weeks' gestation, and sulfotransferase by 10 weeks' gestation. Human fetuses generally have fairly well-developed conjugative activity for all of the systems except for glucuronidation, which remains low until shortly before term. The earlier presence of the other conjugative systems in the human fetus may indicate an endogenous role in the modulation of activity of endogenous steroids. Conjugative metabolism generally results in products that are of increased water solubility and, therefore, more excretable. For xenobiotics so transformed, they are generally less pharmacologically active. For endogenous compounds, conjugation may enhance activity. For example, certain steroid glucuronides and sulfates have greater potency than the parent steroid.[123]

In view of the limited protection provided by the placenta, the ability of the fetus to metabolize xenobiotics may appear fortuitous. In fact, it may sometimes be detrimental. Fetal metabolism (just as that of the adult and the placenta) can take agents that are nontoxic and activate them to toxic metabolites. This may indicate a role for fetal pharmacogenetics in the determination of susceptibility to developmental toxins. Fetal metabolism may ultimately result in the production of water-soluble metabolites, which are not free to back-diffuse across the placenta, becoming trapped in the fetus. If the metabolite is itself toxic, biotransformation may lead to toxin accumulation.[93]

A further effect of induction of metabolism in utero is that postnatal xenobiotic metabolism may be changed after prenatal exposures. Such exposures may enhance metabolism of the same or unrelated agents. For example, the ability of the newborn infant to metabolize bilirubin by conjugation may be induced by prenatal maternal anticonvulsants. The enzymatic capacity for phenytoin metabolism is higher in newborns whose mothers have been given phenytoin, carbamazepine, or phenobarbital. Accelerated metabolic clearance of transplacentally transferred anticonvulsants and increased labeled carbon dioxide exhalation after radiolabeled aminopyrine demethylation have been described in such infants.[124]

A further effect of fetal drug exposure is that alterations in pharmacologic response to the substance may be produced. Fetal receptors for many diverse substances have been identified. These include acetylcholine, insulin, digoxin, alpha-adrenergic agents, beta-adrenergic agents, and glucocorticoids.[124] It is conceivable that the fetus may display tolerance to or dependence on the previously administered substance or analogues, from alterations in such receptor activities or other mechanisms. Although neonatal narcotic abstinence syndrome is the best described, abstinence syndromes or persistent neonatal effects from numerous substances have been identified. These are not limited to drugs of abuse but include antihistamines and antipsychotic agents as well.[125] The relationships between pharmacokinetic and pharmacodynamic processes in the maternal-placental-fetal unit are diagrammed in Figure 18–9.

From the foregoing discussion of postfertilization development and how it may be deranged, one must not contend that these are the only mechanisms of developmental toxicity. Certainly, prefertilization influences of either parent may affect development. The best example is the potentially mutagenic effect of damage to germ cells. Abnormal spermatogenesis is better documented than abnormal oogenesis because of greater accessibility of cells for study. The effects of environmental agents on sperm production and quality have been comprehensively reviewed.[126–128] The relationship of such damage to developmental toxicity is not well defined. Sperm damage caused by toxins would appear to be a cause of infertility. Even without apparent morphologic abnormalities, heritable effects could be produced by chromosomal damage. In animal studies and human reports, such exposures may increase the risk of spontaneous abortion. The relationship to physical malformation or childhood cancer is less established. As an obvious example, there does not appear to be an increased risk of congenital malformations in those children able to be conceived after cancer chemotherapy, relative to their siblings.[129]

Counseling the Parent(s) Regarding Exposure Risks

By the time that the concerned parents are referred to a teratologist or toxicologist about the risks of a drug or toxin exposure, they generally have already spoken to any number of persons. Laypersons (primarily friends and relatives) have usually offered their advice. Often, the family physician or prescribing physician has also been consulted. The problem with having so many sources of information is the inconsistency of information. Furthermore, when laypersons or health care personnel in nonobstetric specialties are polled about whether a drug can produce birth defects, they tend to overestimate the risk. It is not unusual to consult with women for whom therapeutic abortion has been unequivocally recommended, even following exposure to agents that are not known to markedly influence the risk of an abnormal pregnancy outcome.[130] For the majority of marketed drugs, the information presented in readily available resources is not reassuring, even for agents that are not known to be developmental toxins; the most commonly used reference, the Physician's Desk Reference,[131] generally provides animal toxicity data and the manufacturer's recommendation that the drug is not to be used in pregnancy. These defensive statements are intended to discourage use when treatment of a pregnant woman is planned; they are more commonly taken to indicate that harm is inevitable through such wording as: "Safe use in pregnancy has not been established"; ". . . should not be used in pregnant women, unless in the judgment of the physician, the potential benefits outweigh the possible hazards"; and ". . . crosses the placenta and is found in fetal tissues."

For agents labeled or relabeled since November 1980, the system of Food and Drug Administration–mandated "pregnancy categories" provides a slightly more weighted picture of the relative teratogenic risks (Table 18–18).[132] It still does not guide the nonexpert in gauging what the parent wants to know: "How will this (exposure) affect my baby?" In fact, that question cannot be answered for the overwhelming majority of cases. *It is impossible to predict and, certainly, to guarantee outcome after drug or toxin exposure in pregnancy.* Even for extremely common ingestions (e.g., alcohol), data are not sufficient to give an accurate risk estimate. The question that can be evaluated is "Is this exposure known to change my chance of having a healthy baby?" Commonly, the parent(s) will ask if the exposure warrants pregnancy termination. When such information is not readily available, it has been observed that many professionals advise interruption on the basis of the labeled statement that an agent is "not proven safe for pregnant women or children."[133] This occurs even when no adverse effect could be documented. By such nonweighted advisory, the physician, and most particularly, the pregnant woman and her fetus are done a disservice.

A further problem is the delay in seeking specialized information, during which time the family is subjected to tremendous stress. Specialized information is increasingly available to prospective parents and their health care professionals in the form of reproductive toxicity information or counseling services. These services must be distinguished from simple Birth Defects Registries intended to identify changing patterns in malformations and their potential associated factors. Over twenty of the specialized information services have been established nationwide. Few of these systems have published their experience; however, from a series of presentations, a picture of the range of services provided may be drawn.[133] Activities vary from straightforward teratogen information systems/hotlines to comprehensive programs that use telephone self-referral and physician referrals[130–134] to introduce patients to integrated genetic risk consultation, advanced prenatal diagnostic programs, and teratogenicity management programs.[130–135] Ready availability of these services encourages professionals in other medical specialties to use them rather than to make a possibly incorrect or overly conservative recommendation.

It is becoming increasingly clear that it is not enough to provide information about potential drug-induced birth defects without a complete evaluation of the risks that the

Table 18–18. FOOD AND DRUG ADMINISTRATION'S PREGNANCY CATEGORIES

CATEGORY A
Controlled studies in women fail to demonstrate a risk to the fetus in the first trimester (and there is no evidence of a risk in later trimesters), and the possibility of fetal harm appears remote.
CATEGORY B
Either animal reproduction studies have not demonstrated a fetal risk, but there are no controlled studies in pregnant women, or animal-reproduction studies have shown an adverse effect (other than a decrease in fertility) that was not confirmed in controlled studies in women in the first trimester, and there is no evidence of a risk in later trimesters.
CATEGORY C
Either studies in animals have revealed adverse effects on the fetus (teratogenic or embryocidal effects or other) and there are no controlled studies in women, or studies in women and animals are not available. Drugs should be given only if the potential benefit justifies the potential risk to the fetus.
CATEGORY D
There is positive evidence of human fetal risk, but the benefits from use in pregnant women may be acceptable despite the risk (e.g., if the drug is needed in a life-threatening situation or for a serious disease for which safer drugs cannot be used or are ineffective). There will be an appropriate statement in the "warnings" section of the labeling.
CATEGORY X
Studies in animals or human beings have demonstrated fetal abnormalities, or there is evidence of fetal risk based on human experience, or both, and the risk of the use of the drug in pregnant women clearly outweighs any possible benefit. The drug is contraindicated in women who are or may become pregnant. There will be an appropriate statement in the "contraindications" section of the labeling.

(Modified from Millstein LG: FDA's pregnancy categories. N Engl J Med *303*:706, 1980.)

pregnancy bears. This includes risks on a genetic basis and in consideration of occupational exposures, alcohol or other drug use, or known health problems. Similarly, it is essential to follow the counsel given with referral for genetic counseling, obstetric care, substance abuse programs, ultrasound examination, or emergency treatment, as appropriate. The provider has a responsibility to evaluate the outcome of infants born to women so advised. This assures more consistent examination and reporting of anomalies and appropriate referral for specialized pediatric services. Teratogen hotlines and registries must guard against providing or collecting information without accurate history or follow-up. Without this, such services could miss either the outcome or the wealth of nonteratogenic exposures and collect a biased view of the harm stemming from exposures. When a center can integrate all of the needed services, there may be less time for the family to worry and more time to plan for a likely normal or recognized exceptional infant.

Counseling regarding a pregnancy exposure should be performed in a scholarly and sympathetic manner to avoid creating inappropriate alarm in the patient.[135] It is an overwhelming responsibility to translate the sometimes complex and inconsistent teratogenicity data into clear information than can be presented in terms understandable to the family. It is essential that the family is given the best opportunity to hear what is actually being said.

Additionally, consistency in counseling is important. It is useful to develop a "disclaimer statement" that clearly states the limitation of information in this area. It is helpful to guarantee that each patient counseled is patiently given the following type of information:

"All normal, healthy women have a risk of having a baby with a birth defect. This is about three to five out of every one hundred babies. When the mother has health problems, the risk may be higher . . .

"The medical information about (medications/chemicals/drugs) and birth defects is not as scientific as other medical information. We cannot do the kind of research needed to tell just how a chemical can affect the baby. So, any data we have comes from studies in animals (that may not have the same risk) or from reports of doctors who have given the medicine to women who needed it. Because doctors who see what they feel may be a problem from the use are more likely to report it than doctors whose patients had normal babies, medical reports may not tell us the real risk. For example, if one hundred pregnant women are exposed to a chemical that is not a problem, we expect at least three to five of them to have a baby with a birth defect anyway. That would be just from the normal risk of being human. So you see that many false reports may exist for any chemical.

"It is not possible to give you a precise risk of whether your pregnancy will be harmed. What we can tell you is whether there is information that says there may be a higher than usual risk. We can also refer you to services that can help tell if the pregnancy appears normal."

By providing the prospective parents with plans by which they may gain more information, they frequently become more hopeful and less anxious. In particular, information regarding the use of prenatal diagnostic aids (e.g., amniocentesis, ultrasonography, clinical laboratory testing) and their applicability or limitations for detecting a given defect is often helpful. Very frequently, the patient will ask "What would you do if you were me?" This is generally a request for an honest, informed opinion and not for a decision. It is generally wise to preface any information given in such a circumstance with an acknowledgment that what is right for one person or most women may not be the best for an individual and her family.

Use of Animal Teratogenicity Data to Evaluate Human Risk

Because scientific research cannot be conducted ethically on the human embryo/fetus, much of the information available regarding potential developmental toxicity is the result of animal teratology studies. Very little data are available regarding the most frequent environmental exposures. Despite federal mandates involving safety in the workplace and premarketing evaluation of synthetic chemicals, only 3 of over 88,700 agents in common use have been regulated, largely resulting from concern over their male reproductive toxicity. In contrast, guidelines for reproductive safety evaluation of drugs for human use, household products, pesticides, and food additives have been issued and regulatory agencies established[136, 137] (Table 18–19). Depending on their use, premarketing testing may be required to include both short-term and long-term (multigenerational) exposures. Outcome variables assessed include fertility, number of fetuses, gender ratio, fetal deaths, viability, newborn size, and presence of anomalies. Animals with short gestation, generally rodents, are used in most cases.

The use of animal data provides an inaccurate assessment of the agent's potential human toxicity. The reasons for this disparity include both pharmacokinetic and pharmacodynamic factors (Table 18–20). Although teratologists may be able to overcome the pharmacokinetic disparity by carefully managing administration of the agent, metabolites, or enzyme inhibitors, species-specific pharmacodynamic differences may not be so amenable to being minimized.

The majority of reproductive insults demonstrated in animals have not been confirmed in man. Shepard enumerates just over 900 animal teratogens in his 1986 Catalog of Teratogenic Agents; only about 18 of those substances have been classified as proven human teratogens.[8] The majority of human teratologic responses, however, can be reproduced in certain animals. No one species is clearly superior as a model of human effect. Animal studies suggest human effect, but they do not reliably underestimate or overestimate it.

Despite these limitations on human pregnancy exposures, prudence suggests that the results of available animal studies be known so that a plan for evaluating the pregnancy for such effects can be developed.

In a review of reproductive hazards in the workplace, Paul and Himmelstein have recommended a four-step approach to chemical exposure assessment and control.[139] The first step is *identification of the exposure and its potential health effects*. A complete history is taken of both parents, including occupational and nonoccupational exposures such as alcohol, smoking, home environment, and hobbies. A complete medical and reproductive history is essential. The Federal Hazards Communication Standard and some states' right-to-know legislation is making available an extensive list of chemical agents encountered in each workplace, with specific toxicity data when this is available. Material Safety Data Sheets provide much useful toxicity data but, in general, no information about reproductive risk. Additional information should be sought from published resources, including the Registry of Toxic Effects of Chemical Substances in book[140] or microfiche forms. Computerized data bases (including REPROTOX from the Reproductive Toxicology Center in Washington, DC) and local

Table 18–19. CHARGES AND REGULATORY AUTHORITY OF UNITED STATES GOVERNMENT AGENCIES REGARDING TOXIC EXPOSURES

AGENCY	LAW	COVERAGE	AUTHORITIES		
			Pre-marketing Approval	*Testing by Manufacturer*	*Reporting of Data*
Food and Drug Administration (FDA) A unit of health and human services with authority over the regulation of medical and veterinary drugs, foods and food additives, cosmetics	Food, Drug and Cosmetics Act	Drugs	X	X	X
		Food		X	
		Food Additives	X		
		Cosmetics			
Environmental Protection Agency (EPA) Independent agency (i.e., not part of a cabinet department); administers a number of diverse laws concerned with human health and the environment	Federal Insecticide, Fungicide and Rodenticide Act	Pesticides	X	X	X
	Toxic Substance Control Act	Industrial chemicals	(X)*	X	X
	Clear Air Act	Air pollutants			
	Resource Conservation and Recovery Act	Industrial waste		X	X
Occupational Safety and Health Administration (OSHA) A unit of the Department of Labor that regulates workplace conditions	Occupational Safety and Health Act	Occupational exposure			X
Consumer Product Safety Commission (CPSC) Regulates a variety of consumer products including household chemicals and fabric treatments	Federal Hazardous Substance Act	Consumer products		X	
	Consumer Product Safety Act	Consumer products			X

*Authority to test based on available data.
(Modified from Reiter LW: Neurotoxicology in regulation and risk assessment. Dev Pharmacol Ther *10*:254–358, 1987.)

Table 18–20. REASONS FOR DISPARITY BETWEEN HUMAN AND EXPERIMENTAL ANIMAL MODEL SUSCEPTIBILITY TO DEVELOPMENTAL TOXINS

Intrinsic sensitivity differences between species on a genetic basis.

Species-specific pharmacokinetic differences lead to variable exposure of the embryos of various species.
- Absorption
  - Stomach emptying times tend to vary directly with the size of the stomach and the size of the animal. Smaller animal species have faster stomach emptying.
- Presystemic drug clearance
  - First-pass effect or plasma hydrolysis may prevent appearance of xenobiotic in certain species' fetuses.
- Distribution
  - When corrected for body weight differences, variability in the volume of distribution contributes only slightly to human/animal differences.
- Plasma protein bindings
  - Animal species tend to have lower percentages of plasma protein binding. Tissue binding is very similar when humans and animals are compared. Pattern of drug distribution to tissue varies significantly between species, as a result of differences in relative body water and fat.
- Drug elimination
  - Renal elimination or metabolism tends to be much more rapid in laboratory animals used for testing. Metabolic pathways may vary in significance between species.

Pharmacokinetic diversity may be compensated for by careful management of the administration of the agent, metabolite, or enzyme inhibitors.

(From Nau H: Species differences in pharmacokinetics, drug metabolism and teratogenesis. *In* Nau H, Scott WJ (eds): Pharmacokinetics in Teratogenesis. Vol 1. Boca Raton, FL, CRC Press, 1987, pp 81–127; and Kimmel CA, Young FJ: Correlating pharmacokinetics and teratogenic endpoints. Fund Appl Toxicol *3*:250–258, 1983.)

regulatory agencies such as the Occupational Safety and Health Administration (OSHA) and National Institute for Occupational Safety and Health (NIOSH) can be highly useful in identifying information not yet available in books or medical journals.

The second step is to *characterize the extent of exposure*. This may be done by assessing the contamination of air in the worksite (industrial hygiene assessment) or by analyzing the amount of chemical an individual has absorbed (biologic monitoring). The worker and his or her physician have the right to review results of all occupational health monitoring that has been conducted. The employer must conduct specific exposure studies as requested by the practitioner; if the employer does not cooperate, federal or state agencies can conduct such inspections and measurements.

After the data are compiled, the third step is *risk assessment*. The data are examined to define the risks of a given exposure. In essence, a certain degree of risk is defined as acceptable in order to establish an acceptable exposure level. The difficulty in reproductive toxicology is in defining what an acceptable level of poor pregnancy outcomes is. Most patients feel that only no or neglible risk is acceptable. This may not be a realistic outlook, given the aforementioned frequencies of abnormal outcomes. Thus, chemical exposure limits for pregnant workers are not established. Neither NIOSH has recommended nor OSHA has mandated pregnancy-specific exposure limits, even though the pregnant woman may have increased exposure (relative to nonpregnant workers, vide infra) and altered sensitivity to certain agents.

The reproductive hazard in question should be put into perspective relative to the mother's total reproductive risk. The sufficiency of the data and the effects demonstrated in animal studies should be reviewed to formulate a plan for controlling the hazard. If the animal toxicity data indicate that the potential effects can be followed safely by, for example, ultrasonic evaluation of fetal structures, growth and development, or chromosomal analysis, it may be reasonable to have the mother continue working, with appropriate industrial hygiene measures taken to limit exposure to potential hazards. Such measures may include the use of gloves or a respirator to limit absorption, appropriate shielding, monitoring exposure with available tests (radiation badges, urine mutagenicity studies, or other laboratory tests), or a request for limited duties. Longer-term concerns may be addressed by ensuring proper ventilation or a controlled chemical handling space. Substitution of a relatively safer chemical is another option. Concomitantly, maternal habits that would complicate the risk, such as smoking or drinking alcoholic beverages, must also be controlled. If none of these is adequate, feasible, or acceptable, it may be necessary to arrange a temporary job transfer or leave of absence. Because present worker's compensation or liability policies do not address reproductive hazards, it may be necessary to work with the employee's health care providers, insurance carriers, union representatives, or attorneys to arrange alternative work assignments or disability or unemployment compensation.

In Table 18–21, selected agents with suspected or demonstrated developmental or reproductive toxicity are presented.

Table 18–21. SELECTED ENVIRONMENTAL/OCCUPATIONAL CHEMICALS WITH PURPORTED OR DOCUMENTED DEVELOPMENTAL TOXICITY

aniline
nitrobenzene
benzene
beryllium
cadmium
carbon disulfide
carbon monoxide
carbaryl
chlordane
chlordecone (Kepone)
2-chlorobutadiene
dibromochloropropane
cigarette smoking
epichlorohydrin
ethylene dibromide
ethanol
fluorides
formaldehyde
gases, anesthetic
ethylene oxide
lead
manganese
mercury
trichloroethylene
tetrachloroethylene
carbon tetrachloride
TCDD (dioxin)
polychlorinated biphenyls
polybrominated biphenyls
phthalates
radiation
styrene
toluene

The prospective parent(s) must never be given the impression that by taking such measures they will be guaranteed a normal child or even one free of the effect of developmental toxins. In human reproduction, the only alternative to taking a risk of an abnormal baby is not to have one.

Management of Environmental and Therapeutic Ingestions in the Nursing Mother

If the specter that the exposures of daily living may be hazardous is troubling, how much more so the thought that mother's milk itself may provide the infant with something less noble than nutrition and nurture. In a sense, the issue of toxic substances reaching the infant through mother's milk is one that has been more controversial than is due. However, for one aspect of the controversy, the significance of infant exposures is not yet fully recognized.

The lactating breast is an extremely proficient organ. The arrangement of alveolar cells in which milk is produced are said to resemble a bunch of grapes in the way that their tear-drop shape connects with a central lumen.[158] The lumena connect into larger ducts that feed into still larger channels. A number of channels exit at the nipple so that milk is excreted in a more spray-like manner than in a flowing manner, as from a nursing bottle.

Milk, sugar, proteins, and fat are synthesized within the alveolar cell and secreted across the membrane of the alveolar cell into the lumen. For chemical substances in the mother's blood to be secreted into milk, they generally pass across the epithelium of the capillary, through the interstitial space and the basement membrane of the alveolar cell into the alveolar cell cytoplasm. The agent then must exit the cell into the lumen. It may do so by passive diffusion, by "transcellular diffusion" of small molecules (as with membrane pores), by carrier-mediated facilitated diffusion, and perhaps by diffusion through the spaces between the alveolar cells.

The majority of substances circulating in the maternal blood stream will be found in milk.[159–168] The rate of blood flow to the breasts is less of a rate-limiting factor to simple diffusion into milk than it is for placental transit. Therefore, the chemical characteristics of water-soluble chemicals are to an extent *more* important in influencing the rate at which substances pass into milk. Molecular weight considerations associated with the placenta (vide infra) also apply to diffusion across breast tissue membranes into milk. The degree of protein binding has a balanced effect on chemical excretion into milk. Whereas agents bound to protein are not free to participate in simple diffusion, the free fraction that does diffuse may become bound to milk proteins and not diffuse back.

Human milk is slightly more acidic than maternal plasma (usually having a pH of approximately 7.0). The degree of ionization at maternal physiologic pH (pKa) is an important determinant of the tendency of substances to accumulate in mother's milk. Weak acids generally are expected to reach concentrations less than or equal to those found in plasma, by simple diffusion. Weak bases are expected to be present in milk in similar or greater amounts relative to those found in plasma. Such substances (including diazepam, cimetidine, and erythromycin) are present in plasma in a largely un-ionized form, of which a high proportion of the un-ionized species is free to diffuse. After diffusing into the more acidic milk, a relatively higher fraction becomes ionized and unable to diffuse back. This is the reason one would expect weak bases to be relatively concentrated in milk.[159]

As with passage to the fetus, there is a limitation in predicting milk concentrations from the chemical characteristics of a medication or toxin. The majority of such calculations are based on assessment of diffusion into milk ultrafiltrate, not on whole milk.[159] The differences are the most profound influences on milk excretion of xenobiotics: fat and protein. Because milk has a very high fat content, the constituents of which vary with postnatal maturity, lipid solubility is a major determinant of ultimate milk concentration. It appears at times to be even more important than the maternal milk–concentration gradient because some very lipid soluble substances are highly accumulated in milk (polychlorinated biphenyls, DDT).[160] Of course, as with fetal distribution, very highly fat-soluble substances may be distributed to maternal fat and not be found in extraordinarily large amounts in milk relative to the maternal dose. Active transport processes, as for the placenta, may also influence milk concentrations; their role is clear from the number of endogenous substances that are secreted to form milk (lactose, proteins). Because milk composition is somewhat variable, the only way to determine the potential exposure of a nursing infant is to test the milk or rely on surveys of other representative women whose milk has been tested.

At this point, human milk has been tested for over 300 substances.[161] The vast majority of these agents have been found in quantities similar to those seen in maternal plasma. It is not the concentration in milk relative to the maternal plasma level, however, (i.e., the milk/plasma ratio) that is important. The *absolute* concentration of an agent in milk and its range over the nursing interval are the determinant of the dose an infant will receive for a given milk intake. For example, cimetidine is highly concentrated in milk (M/P 7–12) relative to maternal plasma. The dose that one may predict the infant will ingest during a given feeding at the reported concentrations (4.9 to 6.0 μg/ml) would be determined by the equation:

$$\text{Dose feeding} = \frac{AUC_3}{t\beta} \cdot V_{3,t\beta}$$

where AUC_3 is the area under the milk concentration versus time curve during the feeding interval ($t\beta$), and $V_{3,t\beta}$ is the volume of milk ingested.[159, 162] Greatly simplified to provide an estimate, and by assuming a very large milk intake and that the range of reported concentrations is representative and continuously maintained, the dose would be as determined by the equation below.

By these methods, infant exposure may be calculated or estimated. It is then important to compare that exposure to recommended infant therapeutic doses or to exposure limits for toxins. For cimetidine in the foregoing example, the recommended therapeutic dose would depend on infant age and maturity. For the same calculated exposure, it would represent (a) to (e) in the next column:

(a) 12 to 50 per cent of the recommended *premature* infant therapeutic dose;
(b) 4 to 8 per cent of the recommended term infant therapeutic dose;
(c) 2.5 to 5 percent of the pediatric weight-corrected dose (mg/kg/day);
(d) 5 to 9 per cent of the maternal weight-corrected dose (800 to 1200 mg/day ÷ 60 kg); and
(e) 0.08 to 0.125 per cent of the maternal dose.

Of course, it is the last of these that is least relevant to the infant capacity to handle such exposure. Unfortunately, this is the comparison that is made in a majority of milk pharmacokinetic studies.

Milk excretion is not a major route of elimination for most agents (PCBs are a notable exception); it does not contribute significantly to overall maternal drug clearance or alter the maternal dose requirement for medications. The real limitation, considering the amount of chemical present in milk as a proportion of the maternal dose, is that it does not give information about what that signifies relative to the infant's ability to pharmacokinetically handle and pharmacodynamically respond to the exposure. It is the infant's pharmacologic ability to deal with the exposure that matters. By comparing the limited information available on excretion of xenobiotics into milk to age-appropriate infant doses, a very different and more practical view of infant exposures through breastfeeding is gleaned.[163] For example, cimetidine appears on the American Academy of Pediatrics list of drugs and chemicals that are contraindicated for mothers of nursing infants.[164] The available alternatives to this therapy do not make avoiding its use much of a hardship. The major concern usually expressed, however, is cimetidine's very high *relative* concentration (M/P ratio of 7–12) in milk. As calculated above, with every attempt made to overestimate exposures, infant exposure would not be expected to exceed the infant therapeutic dose. Toxic effects from this magnitude of exposure is unlikely

$$4.9 - 6.0\ \mu g/ml \quad \times \quad 200\ ml/kg/d \quad = \quad 1.0 - 1.2\ mg/kg/d$$

Reported range of concentrations in milk	×	High normal infant milk intake	=	Estimated infant dose

for any except an infant with impaired elimination (i.e., extreme prematurity, liver failure, kidney dysfunction, congestive heart failure). Nondose-related reactions, such as allergic or idiosyncratic effects, are not necessarily any less likely to occur with these small exposures. Infants nursing during maternal drug therapy have been reported to display a range of probable reactions, including rashes, apparent food allergy, and hemolytic anemia.[161] The exposure of a nursing baby to a drug for which there is no expected therapeutic benefit would require a very high safety assessment to constitute an acceptable risk/benefit ratio.

Certain agents are so inherently toxic and result in such severe adverse reactions that even exposure to low levels has the chance of producing adverse effects. One of the major reasons why recommendations on which drugs must be contraindicated while nursing are so disparate is that different authorities have varying *tolerance* for the risks of potential adverse effects. For some, a rare but deadly adverse effect (such as aplastic anemia from chloramphenicol) is intolerable just because it is avoidable. For others, the known benefits of breastfeeding are felt to outweigh the unlikely risk of such an occurrence. The possible effects of the exposure on the infant should be considered. The medical advantages of breastfeeding are well known.[165, 166] Many highly individual and personal considerations must be factored into the risk/benefit equation as well. Other criteria that should be weighed are included in Table 18–22.

There are only very few exposures requiring that breast-feeding be prohibited (Table 18–23). In general, these indicate a temporary cessation until the offending agent is largely eliminated from milk. Statements in the medical literature that women will not tolerate a 7- to 14-day period of expressing milk to maintain lactation underestimate the motivation of many mothers and the efficiency of electric breast pumps. The problem comes in that for many substances, the time period until infant milk exposure does not bear a significant risk is unknown. For a few agents, reports of the duration of time until a substance was below measurable levels in milk have been made (Table 18–24). Unfortunately, below-quantifiable limits does not necessarily indicate an insignificant dose. Particularly for some older data, in which sensitivity of assays was not as great, the conclusions may be misleading. For example, in an older report, atropine was noted as being present at a concentration less than 1 μg/ml.[167, 168] Using the estimated infant dose calculations, even a one half concentration of this would signify 2 1/2 times the infant therapeutic dose. Thus, nondetectable does not necessarily mean absent or insignificant.

For the majority of substances recently studied, by the time that 90 to 95 per cent of the offending agent is out of the milk, the risk to the infant would be considered insignificant. An exception is the toxic ingestion, in which it is not the remaining percentage, but the absolute amount, that matters. Another exception is for agents that are potentially carcinogenic or radioactive, in which even a minute amount may be considered unacceptable.

For substances present in milk, the time for 90 to 95 per cent of the agents to be eliminated would be expected to be 3.3 to 5 milk elimination half-lives. This value is available for only a minority of reported medications and chemicals. For substances present in milk in amounts very similar to those in plasma, it may generally be estimated to be from 3.3 to 5 plasma elimination half-lives. For agents with significant fat solubility and fat storage, the plasma half-life may grossly underestimate the time for milk concentrations to fall by this degree. For example, oxycodone, with plasma half-lives of 0.8 to 2.1 hours, may be predicted to reach 90 to 95 per cent elimination in milk within 10 hours. In fact, oxycodone may be measured in milk for more than 8 hours after a single dose but for 36 hours after multiple doses.[169] Another limitation to using such formulas is that the plasma half-life may not indicate true elimination from the body but distribution into fat tissue. In this case, excretion out of tissue storage may take much longer than the plasma half-life would indicate, and milk excretion may continue over an extended period. For this reason, maternal burden of highly toxic agent with long tissue storage for which infant risk is not dose-related (e.g., carcinogens) is considered to indicate artificial feeding (see Table 18–24).

The major difference in considering fetal exposure in utero and infant exposure through nursing is that the excreted/secreted agent must undergo the additional step of gastrointestinal absorption. Therefore, some

Table 18–22. CRITERIA FOR JUDGING THE ADVISABILITY OF BREASTFEEDING THE INFANT OF A MOTHER EXPOSED TO A DRUG OR TOXIN

THE QUANTITY OF AGENT IN MILK RELATIVE TO THE INFANT CLEARANCE CAPACITY Pharmacokinetics of agent in milk Maturity of the infant Health of the infant Quantity of milk consumed (number of feedings/day, supplemental, beikost)	The risk of dose-related effects of the agent (toxicity) will be determined by actual intake and the ability of the infant to absorb, detoxify, and eliminate it. The sensitivity of the infant to the same exposure may vary with age and health. Premature and sick infants may tolerate a given exposure differently, generally less well.
EXPERIENCE WITH USE BY NURSING MOTHERS Demonstration of idiosyncratic effects on nursing in clinical use	Clinical use can reveal unexpected or previously undocumented effects on nursing or the infant. For example, an agent that reduces milk flow may be perceived as causing infant "fussiness."
INHERENT TOXICITY AND ADVERSE EFFECTS PROFILE OF THE AGENT Adverse effect of the agent on lactation Severity of uncommon effects (i.e., bone marrow depression, carcinogenicity) Incidence of less severe adverse effects Idiosyncratic effects reported after infant exposure	These factors often require a value judgment about the risks of drug exposure at the estimated level relative to the known benefits of breastfeeding.
EXISTENCE OF THERAPEUTIC ALTERNATIVES	Most authorities agree that the safest therapeutic alternative for which there is reasonable amount of experience with use by the nursing mother should be chosen. For example, the use of insulin, rather than tolbutamide or chlorpropamide, would be preferable for the nursing diabetic mother because insulin would not be expected to be present in significant amounts in milk because of its high molecular weight and even if present would not be bioavailable through oral ingestion in milk by the infant.
ANTICIPATED DURATION OF BREASTFEEDING	Most physicians think of breastfeeding as the sole means of infant feeding until weaning and estimate risks on that basis. In many cases, breastfeeding constitutes only part of the infant diet or is planned as a short-term, emotionally meaningful experience until the mother resumes working. The acceptability of such a shorter period of exposure may be higher.
NAIVETE OF THE BABY TO EXPOSURE	If an infant has been exposed to the same substance throughout gestation, the risk of a very likely much lesser dose provided through milk is not a new risk, but a continued one. It is an avoidable risk, likely for the first time. Whether it should be avoided depends on the nature of the risk.
TOLERANCE OF THE PARENTS REGARDING UNKNOWN RISKS	Certain families have an exceptionally low tolerance for risk for their child. The importance of their concern or anxiety should not be overlooked. It often requires guidance and may be a major factor in deciding on the advisability of nursing.
RELIABILITY OF THE PARENTS FOR MONITORING AND REPORTING POTENTIAL ADVERSE EFFECTS	Methadone-treated mothers, for example, may be motivated not to report apparent oversedation or withdrawal.
AVAILABILITY OF PEDIATRIC FOLLOW-UP	If the parents prefer to avoid traditional medical care, the use of an agent that may reasonably indicate regular blood tests may be less acceptable.
OTHER FACTORS THAT MAY MAKE NURSING DETRIMENTAL TO MATERNAL HEALTH	For example, borderline nutritional status and high nutritional demands, as in a new mother with advanced cystic fibrosis. The risks of antibiotic medications present in milk to the infant may be less than the risk of nursing to the mother, unless adequate supplementation can be ensured.

Table 18–23. EXPOSURES CONSIDERED TO CONTRAINDICATE BREASTFEEDING

Antimetabolites (cancer chemotherapy drugs, including: amethopterin, cyclophosphamide, doxorubicin, methotrexate)	§Mercury, methylmercury
Androgens (e.g., testosterone)	*Methimazole
*Bromides (high dose)	Metronidazole
†Bromocriptine	Nalidixic acid
*Chloramphenicol	Nitrofurantoin
*Cimetidine	‡Phencyclidine (PCP)
*Clemastine	†Phenelzine
‡Cocaine	*Phenindione
‡Ergot alkaloid (high dose)	§Pesticides
Gold salt	§Polybrominated biphenyls
‡Heroin	§Polychlorinated biphenyls
*Indomethacin	§Polychlorinated terphenyls
Iodides	Radiopharmaceuticals
§Lead (if mother intoxicated)	§^{89}Strontium, ^{90}Strontium
‡Marijuana	Sulfonamides (for neonates)
	§Tetrachloroethylene
	*Thiouracil

*Although use of these agents during nursing should not result in excessive infant exposure (at usual doses), alternative therapeutic agents exist that do not share the same risk of serious adverse effects or case reports of adverse occurrences.

†May suppress lactation.

‡Use of these substances as drugs of abuse results in uncontrolled infant exposure because of unknown quality and purity of street drugs. Abstinence should be encouraged.

§Testing of milk indicated if mother is known to be exposed in excess to environmental chemicals for which infant sensitivity is not defined.

(Adapted from references 159–161 and 166–168.)

potent agents present in milk have very little risk for the normal nursing infant, because they are not orally absorbed or bioavailable (Table 18–25).[170] Others may still effect a local response in the gastrointestinal tract (e.g., the aforementioned antibiotics and the poorly absorbed cephalosporins and penicillins such as ticarcillin and methicillin). Some poorly absorbed cancer chemotherapeutic agents with carcinogenic potential, such as cisplatin and doxorubicin, may pose a carcinogenic risk locally in the gastrointestinal tract and may be considered unacceptable for use during nursing despite their nonabsorption.

Aside from trying to choose a rational time to resume nursing after use of the few agents that contraindicate nursing, manipulation of the breastfeeding "schedule" is to be avoided. Many authors recommend that nursing be avoided when the milk or plasma concentration is at a peak or that the mother wait until nursing is completed to take medication. Because milk is not stored in full quantity in the breast prior to feeding, even with considerable engorgement, the concen-

Table 18–24. DURATION OF TIME UNTIL SELECTED AGENTS FALL BELOW MEASURABLE MILK CONCENTRATIONS (SEE TEXT) OR CALCULATED TO EQUAL 3.3 MILK ELIMINATION HALF-LIVES

Cimetidine	12 hr
Cocaine	24 hr
Cocaine metabolite (benzyl) (ecogonine)	36 hr
Gold salts	"Many weeks"
Methimazole	16.5 hr (calculated)
Metronidazole	24 hr
Polychlorinated biphenyls	Years
Radiopharmaceuticals	
Gallium	2 weeks after 2 mCi (4 weeks after 3 mCi)
^{125}I	12 days
^{123}I	2–3 days after 10–30 mCi
^{131}I	24 hr–8 weeks
^{99}Tc Pertechnate	48 hr (after 20 mCi)
^{99}TC labeled albumin	24 hr (after 4 mCi)
Sulfisoxazole	24–30 hr

Table 18–25. SUBSTANCES WITH NEGLIGIBLE ORAL BIOAVAILABILITY WHEN FOUND IN MILK

ACTH	epinephrine
amikacin	gentamicin
amphotericin B	heparin
carbenicillin	insulin
cefamandole	kanamycin
Cefazolin	methicillin
cefonicid	moxalactam
cefoperazone	neomycin
ceftizoxime	streptomycin
cephalothin	ticarcillin
cisplatin	trimethaphan
doxorubicin	vancomycin
	vasopressin

(Adapted from Rivera-Calimlim L: The significance of drugs in breast milk; Pharmacokinetic considerations. Clin Perinatol *14*:51–70, 1987.)

trations in milk generally reflect the transfer processes acting on the maternal plasma concentrations at the time of nursing or shortly before. If one breast is continuously sampled for drug concentrations and the other is milked only at the beginning and the end of sample collection, it is commonly observed that the milk concentrations in the less-sampled breast are not significantly different than concentrations in the sampled breast. "Emptying" the breast does not significantly decrease chemical exposure of the infant by eliminating all the chemical that has "accumulated" between feedings. In fact, for fat-soluble substances, the higher concentrations seen in hind-milk—the higher fat content milk near the end of nursing—may actually increase exposure.

In general, it is a very poor idea to suggest manipulation of the times of nursing. Newborn nursing infants feed very frequently, every 1 1/2 to 3 hours; older infants may nurse less often but may desire the breast for comfort. Except for agents that are very rapidly absorbed and eliminated, the time of "peak" milk concentrations from an agent taken after nursing will often come very close to the next nursing period. For the majority of chemicals and medications, such manipulations only slightly reduce exposure. On the contrary, the potential harm that is done is considerably greater. For example, it is common practice not to medicate postpartum mothers for pain until they have nursed. Most of the narcotic and analgesic agents in common use have a "lag period" of about 30 minutes before measurable concentrations are found in milk. The mother in pain does not relax and lactate efficiently. The baby may sense the maternal tension and be frustrated by poor milk flow. It is far more reasonable to treat the mother for pain and have her nurse as soon as she is more comfortable. In general, the nursing period ends before the expected appearance of even low concentrations of the drug in milk. A further problem may be created by not allowing the baby to nurse on demand. Frequently, the result is a frustrated baby, an exhausted mother, and a compromised milk supply.

The decision to breastfeed is often made because it is in the best interest of the baby. There is growing concern about infant exposure to environmental and occupational chemicals that may be present in milk.[160, 161, 164, 171] When a question arises about contamination of milk, the issue can usually be resolved by a combination of actions.

If a specific substance is in question, it may be possible to have the milk tested. The local office of the EPA or the OSHA, as appropriate, can be helpful in identifying resources for milk and infant blood analysis and reference values. The use of reference values to compare the findings with nonnursed babies and the milk of nonexposed women is very important. Many substances are found in low amounts in milk, as they are encountered in food, water, or air. For example, the great concern about maternal exposure to gamma-benzene-hexachloride shampoo (Lindane, Kwell) during the nursing period is often put into perspective by the information that small amounts of this agent are generally found in most mothers' milk.[161]

By using the available data on milk excretion, the estimated infant dose can be compared with the set Maximum Allowable Concentrations or Allowable Daily Intake for the agent, if known.

Some substances are stored in maternal fat and would be expected to be mobilized as the maternal fat stores were lost. For women whose milk is known to have low or borderline amounts of potentially toxic substances, it may be prudent to avoid intentional fat weight loss until nursing is complete. For agents that are not stored in maternal fat, it may be possible to reduce milk excretion by a combination of industrial hygiene and common sense. Chemical exposures should be avoided or minimized. As with pregnancy exposures, appropriate shielding should help to reduce ongoing accumulation. For many agents, the time to clear maternal tissues is known or can be estimated.

As with medication exposures, a risk-benefit analysis of the estimated contaminant dose, toxicity, and factors regarding choice of breastfeeding should made (see Table 18–22). This will permit an acceptable decision to be reached in the best interest of the mother and child.

Poisoning or Overdose in Pregnant Patients

In terms of risks of drug therapy or toxin exposure, pregnant women are considered to be a vulnerable population. There is scattered information that one may draw on to identify the potential risks of an overdose or toxic ingestion by a pregnant woman. There are, however, no published reviews that summarize experience with management of various poisonings in pregnancy. A 1984 article on overdose in pregnancy, characterizing the nature of ingestions by pregnant women over a 4-year period in the Ann Arbor, Michigan area, commented only that the "treatment recommendations (by the poison control center) were essentially the same as for nonpregnant patients."[172] In fact, as the peculiar response of pregnant women to therapeutic and toxic agents becomes better understood, necessary distinctions in their poisoning management may be found and tested. Until such information is available, professionals likely to treat pregnant women must consider the potential difference in the risks of the ingestion and the risks of its treatments in this population.

The risk for toxic exposure does not appear to be lessened in pregnancy. Women continue to ingest toxins accidentally, compulsively, and/or intentionally. Despite well-publicized risks of drug and toxin exposure in pregnancy, women in the U.S. take an average of 2.1 to 11.0 drugs during pregnancy. These numbers include the most common exposures, prenatal vitamins and iron tablets.[29, 30, 173] When these are excluded, the rate of exposure falls to a mean of 3.1 agents.[29] Analgesics (now primarily acetaminophen or codeine) are also common. The routine taking of vitamin and iron prenatal tablets occasionally leads to an inadvertent ingestion of medication intended for another family member or a pet. In addition, the preparation of the home for a new family member often includes the use of solvents, varnishes, paints, and other chemicals. Maternal concern about the use of these agents is common. Pica, the enigmatic compulsion to ingest nonfood items in pregnancy, has been implicated in a number of maternal poisoning, with agents including lead and mothballs.[174, 175]

In addition, suicide attempts appear to be no less common in pregnant than in nonpregnant women. Ingestion of large amounts of tablets has been reported to be the most common method of attempted suicide by women of reproductive age, regardless of gravidity.[176] The majority of case reports of ingestions in pregnancy state that the maternal motivation was suicidal or "depression."[172, 176, 177–185] Successful suicide in pregnancy, once as high as one for every 88,000 to 400,000 live births prior to the legalization of abortion, is now believed to be much less common.[172] However, pregnancy is unique in that a mother may ingest toxins or employ weapons as an abortifacient measure, without the apparent intent to harm herself.[177] The disturbed maternal-fetal emotional relationship is made clear in such efforts. Finally, the state of knowledge about dose requirements in pregnancy is still very limited; iatrogenic overdoses and dosing errors have been reported on this basis.[178]

The gravida may be more susceptible to toxicity from chemical exposures, both therapeutic and toxic in origin. The changes in pharmacokinetic parameters during pregnancy have been stated above; some of those factors most pertinent to toxic ingestions are summarized in Table 18–26.

Pharmacodynamic responses to toxic agents may also be influenced by pregnancy, in a similarity dramatic fashion. As noted in the foregoing discussion, pregnancy produces remarkable changes in nearly every organ system. It may increase the risk of organ damage in response to toxins. The risk of hepatotoxicity from certain agents (e.g., tetracycline and erythromycin) is increased even in therapeutic doses.[186, 187] The most common effects of excessive drug dose or irritant ingestion include nausea or vomiting; the pregnant woman may be less tolerant to these effects. With the already increased cardiac output, the demands of a toxic ingestion may overwhelm the maternal ability to compensate. It is unclear whether pregnancy produces changes in the seizure threshold; some women appear to have increased susceptibility, whereas others do not.

In addition to the effects of the pregnancy on the course of the poisoning, the poisoning may put the pregnancy itself in jeopardy. Miscarriage or premature labor may occur in response to extreme maternal stress, including hypovolemia, acidosis, and hypoxia. A large number of the case reports of poisonings in midtrimester or late trimester pregnancy are complicated by such adverse outcomes.[183, 188, 189] Certain drug agents may selectively compromise uteroplacental blood flow and are to be avoided during pregnancy for that reason (see Table 18–12). Many of these have had heart rate patterns consistent with fetal distress reported in association

Table 18–26. INFLUENCE OF PREGNANCY ON TOXICOLOGIC RISK

Delayed gastrointestinal absorption	May facilitate decontamination procedures for orally ingested agents
Increased apparent volume of distribution (Vd)	May improve tolerance to toxins where effect is related to plasma concentration
Increased fat stores	May serve as a depot for toxic substances; with lysis of body fat, previously stored toxins may be released to maternal circulation
Decreased protein binding	May increase or decrease toxicity, depending on how readily the free (unbound) drug can be eliminated
Altered metabolism/elimination capacity	Challenge of the overdose will tend to reveal whether ability to detoxify is enhanced or impaired in pregnancy

with their use. Excessive diuretic therapy, particularly in the pre-eclamptic woman, may produce the same effects.[190] Agents that reduce blood flow in uterine vessels, such as cocaine or sympathomimetic amines with alpha-adrenergic activity may similarly produce fetal distress.[124, 64–67] The administration of substances that stimulate uterine contraction, such as ergot derivatives or prostaglandins of the E or F series, may also produce fetal distress or initiate labor. Any agent that can perturb the normal endocrine balance of pregnancy may also change the risk of pregnancy loss.

MANAGEMENT OF THE OVERDOSE OR TOXIC INGESTION IN THE PREGNANT PATIENT

Decontamination

The primary importance of decontamination is not different in pregnancy but the method may be. Emesis has been said to be contraindicated in "late-stage" pregnancy.[191] Certainly, the safety of vomiting itself in first- and second-trimester gestation has been documented by generations of mothers-to-be. The limits of this safety have been tested by many patients with hyperemesis gravidarum. It is important to avoid protracted vomiting, which may lead to dehydration or esophageal bleeding. The relative inefficacy and toxicity of home remedies such as sodium chloride, copper sulfate, or tartar emetic is well known, but avoidance in pregnancy is even more important because there is little benefit to outweigh any unknown risk.

The risk of fetal damage from maternal xenobiotic exposure has been reviewed above; it is a continuing concern in both ingestion and its management. The risk to the fetus should be a factor in making decisions in which therapeutic options exist. In the absence of specific experience, it is reasonable to consider that when therapeutic options exist, the treatment that avoids another fetal drug exposure may be preferred.

Ipecac (syrup of ipecacuana) is not specifically contraindicated in early pregnancy. Its use has been considered contraindicated in late pregnancy because of concern about the emesis it produces.[191] There are no data available regarding reproductive toxicity of ipecac; no animal reproductive toxicity studies have been undertaken.[192] Many people think of ipecac as a noxious substance that induces emesis locally and is eliminated as it acts. In fact, it is a systemically absorbed and centrally acting agent that is only very slowly eliminated from the body after use.[192]

When no delay will be engendered by choice of decontamination procedure, as in emergency department treatment, gastric lavage is a relatively nonsystemic alternative to ipecac. It appears to be equally efficacious for many poisonings when properly performed.[192–196]

Detoxification

The use of activated charcoal for gastrointestinal dialysis is generally considered to be a nonsystemic method of reducing total body burden of certain poisons. For serious poisoning in which charcoal therapy has been proven efficacious or may be helpful, charcoal should be instituted for the pregnant patient. Numerous case reports have noted the administration of activated charcoal in pregnancy, although they have not documented specifically continuous or repeated administration.

The routine administration of saline cathartics such as magnesium citrate or high-concentration sorbitol to hasten gastrointestinal elimination of charcoal should be recommended with caution in women in the third trimester prior to term. Catharsis may stimulate premature labor or produce electrolyte imbalance and dehydration, with resultant hypovolemia.[197]

Similarly, the risks of fetal compromise resulting from possible adverse effects of these methods of detoxification should be weighed. The institution of hemodialysis, hemofiltration, and peritoneal dialysis all carry the risk of maternal hypotension and resultant fetal hypoperfusion.[198, 199] Infectious risks caused by invasion of the body's protective tissue barriers are also increased. When heparin anticoagulation is required for such a procedure, the risks to the pregnancy, although not directly to the fetus, are of concern. Such higher-risk methods would be reserved for cases in which they are clearly indicated by the nature of the ingestion and by the maternal and fetal responses to it.

The administration of potentially life-saving antidotes or treatments should not be withheld because of fear of unknown adverse fetal effects. There are unfortunate case reports in which both mother and fetus were lost resulting from failure to administer otherwise indicated therapy.[200] In some cases, treatments may be indicated, even though they are known to be developmental toxicants. For example, it would appear to be unreasonable to withhold ethanol therapy for treatment of life-threatening ethylene glycol ingestion, despite the knowledge that high-dose or chronic ethanol is a teratogen. Certainly, it is prudent to administer the minimum effective dose as indicated by serum level monitoring. In some poisonings, it may even by reasonable to deliver a term or mature fetus so that both patients may be guaranteed specific treatment. In general, however, the cardiovascularly stable mother is a far more efficient detoxification system than those that may be offered ex utero.

The use of palliative therapies or treatments of unproven efficacy in non–life-threatening poisonings should be weighed against evidence of their safety. There are several reported poisonings that illustrate management issues peculiar to pregnancy.

Insulin Overdose. Insulin is an agent very commonly administered during pregnancy. There are few reports of insulin overadministration in pregnancy. Because of the fetal risks of hypoglycemia, glucose, which is actively transported across the placenta, should be rapidly administered. The use of glucagon will help correct maternal hypoglycemia and directly increase fetal glucose as well; no direct fetal effect of glucagon is expected because of its high molecular weight.[201]

Carbon Monoxide. There are many case reports, experimental primate studies, and at least one excellent review of the course of carbon monoxide poisoning in pregnancy.[188, 202–205] This exposure is actually more dangerous for the pregnant woman, who produces nearly twice as much carbon monoxide endogenously each day, and particularly for the pregnant smoker. The increased minute ventilation of gestation also tends to enhance the severity of exposure. Carbon monoxide diffuses readily across placental membranes or uses carrier-mediated facilitated transfer. While the mother is treated and recovers, the infant may show neurologic or behavioral effects of the prenatal exposure. Fetal CNS damage following nonfatal maternal exposures has been seen in humans and reproduced in animals.[204] From the primate model, the hemispheric destruction and microgyric and multicystic cavitary degeneration which, seen in the brain, resembles the results of other forms of perinatal hypoxic-ischemic encephalopathy.

The threshold time or carbon monoxide content for fetal damage is not known. Normal infant outcome has been reported after maternal coal furnace and smoking exposure produced carbon monoxide concentrations of at least 24.5 per cent over a number of hours prior to 8 weeks' gestation.[203] The infant was of low birth weight (1950 gm at 38 weeks' gestation), but normal development through 6 months of age at the time of the report was found.

In second- and third-trimester exposures, stillbirth has occurred shortly after exposure or has been delayed by several weeks.[202] Cerebral palsy and behavioral disturbances have been observed in surviving fetuses, in addition to normal developmental outcomes.

The prompt administration of oxygen is critical to maternal and fetal survival. In gestationally appropriate pregnancies, it is reasonable to use indicators of adequate fetal oxygenation central nervous system responsiveness (heart rate and variability), in addition to response of the mother and her laboratory findings, in adjusting or terminating oxygen therapy. To ensure adequate treatment of the fetus, it has been recommended that the mother receive oxygen therapy for five times as long as it is expected to require to return her carbon monoxide concentrations to normal; this is how long it may take for fetal levels to normalize.[202] The maternal carboxyhemoglobin elimination rate can be increased from a half-life of 2 to 3 hours to ¾ of an hour by breathing 100 per cent oxygen; fetal carboxyhemoglobin half-lives are expected to decrease from 6 to 7 hours to 2 to 4 hours by the use of maternal oxygen therapy. The fetal rate of elimination remains slower than that of the mother.

Acetaminophen. Analgesics were the most commonly overdosed substance during pregnancy, according to a recent publication (18 of 111 cases);[172] a separate summary of 59 cases has also been published.[185] Absorption of acetaminophen (APAP) is not significantly different during the 36th week of gestation than at 6 weeks' postpartum.[206] Even though the renal clearance is over twice as high during pregnancy (0.61 ± 0.64 versus 0.35 ± 0.34 ml/min), it still accounts for only a trivial part of overall clearance, and elimination half-lives are not significantly different. The volume of distribution was considerably higher, either on a total weight or weight-corrected basis. The amount of drug cleared by nontoxin generating pathways (e.g., glucuronidation) did not appear to be enhanced by gestation in this therapeutic dose study (1 gm single dose).

As noted above, there have been many case reports of APAP ingestion during pregnancy described in the medical literature (plus 11 cases in the survey by Rayburn, which are not detailed). In the majority, these occurred in the second or third trimester, but at least 12 have been first trimester overdoses.[172, 179–185] In the most detailed reports, five of the six cases were treated with acetylcysteine and the sixth with methionine (after elective delivery of the 36-week-gestation fetus).

One of the cases resulted in fetal demise prior to presentation. Nearly 30 gm of APAP had been taken over a period of less than 24 hours; at the end of this time, the last fetal movements were felt. There were very high concentrations of APAP (250 μg/gm) in the 29-week-gestation fetal liver, despite the maternal level of less than 10 μg/ml at the time of uterine evacuation 3½ days after the last dose. The back-extrapolated maternal serum APAP concentration was 300 μg/ml at 4 hours after the last dose. This woman demonstrated increased liver enzymes, peaking at 4 days after the end of ingestion. She also had elevated prothrombin times, with consumption of clotting factors V, VII, and X, attributed to impending disseminated intravascular coagulation rather than to liver dysfunction. After delivery, she recovered completely. None of the other mothers treated with acetylcysteine or S-adenosyl methionine developed signs of liver toxicity.

In two infants whose maternal ingestions occurred shortly prior to delivery (1 elective, 2 spontaneous), elimination of APAP has been evaluated. The neonate of 29 weeks' gestation eliminated APAP primarily by sulfation, with a plasma half-life of 26 hours (despite attempts at elimination by exchange transfusion); the neonate of 36 weeks' gestation eliminated APAP primarily by glucuronidation, secondarily by sulfation, and only partially by mercapturic acid conjugation (the potentially toxic metabolic pathway), with a plasma half-life of 10 hours.

The criteria of extended plasma half-life and increased toxicity of APAP in the adult does not appear to extend to the slower neonatal metabolism. The fetal liver is capable of oxidative activation of APAP to toxic acetamidoquinone, which is then normally detoxified by glutathione pathways in the adult.[184] In excess, the glutathione pathway could become substrate deficient. *N*-Acetylcysteine can donate sulfhydryl groups to replete this substrate. Infants and children appear to be much more tolerant, perhaps as a result of greater reliance on sulfation for detoxification and lesser dependence on glutathione conjugation. The capacity of the human fetus to detoxify acetamidoquinone has not been evaluated. No neonatal APAP toxicity was observed. Very interestingly, both of the infants studied died of "cot death," the British term for sudden infant death syndrome (SIDS), at 106 and 155 days, respectively.

Amitriptyline. Tricyclic antidepressant poisonings are among the most worrisome. Amitriptyline is so extensively distributed throughout the body that little of the drug is available for standard means of accessory elimination by charcoal administration of various filtration or dialysis methods.[208] Ingestion of between 1 and 1.5 gm of amitriptyline resulted in coma and unexpectedly severe ophthalmoplegia in a pregnant woman.[209] Following administration of physostigmine, the patient became agitated and combative, but the eye findings persisted. After 1 hour, lethargy returned. By the next day, the eye findings had resolved. No fetal response or outcome were noted.

Extrapyramidal reactions to drug agents may be more likely in pregnancy; metoclopramide may produce abnormal head movements (including spasmodic torticollis and oculogyric crisis).[207] Young females show a preponderant sensitivity to these disorders, which may be related to higher estrogen levels.

The life-threatening toxic effects of amitriptyline, including seizures and arrhythmias, require that treatment of the mother ensure oxygenation and circulation to the fetus. The administration of phenytoin to treat arrhythmias or seizures should not be considered contraindicated despite the fact that phenytoin is a recognized teratogen; hypoxia, due to toxic seizures, is a profound teratogen, and fetal hypoperfusion, due to maternal arrhythmias, is a developmental toxin.[210] The use of alkalinization therapy may be somewhat more controversial in pregnancy. It is possible that alkalinization will reduce the free, unionized amitriptyline, producing arrhythmias and favoring fetal transfer. There is the possibility of altered maternal respiration caused by the sedative effects of such an ingestion and of induced alkalosis; proper ventilation is essential if this mode of therapy is needed. The use of physostigmine, as in the reported case, does not appear to be of certain benefit in nongestational ingestions, thus it is less advisable than other therapies on that basis.

Iron. A very high percentage of all pregnant women take iron tablets. Only three iron poisonings, all in the second or third trimester, have appeared as case reports in the medical literature since 1970,[189, 210, 211] with another seven noted but not described by Rayburn.[172] The first poisoning was severe, with a serum iron of 1700 μg/dl despite presentation within 1 hour of ingestion and administration of ipecac.[189] Deferoxamine (DFO) was withheld because of concern over possible adverse fetal effects. The patient miscarried and subsequently succumbed with pulmonary edema, renal and hepatic dysfunction, and gastrointestinal bleeding.

In the two other case reports, slightly lesser degrees of iron ingestions were treated with DFO.[211, 212] In one, spontaneous labor began 8 hours after the ingestion at 34 weeks' gestation; an infant with normal iron and iron binding values was born. The baby subsequently required iron supplementation for low iron levels (21 μg/dl at 12 hours of life). Residual DFO from prenatal administration and loss of placental active acquisition is a likely cause of this.

In the other iron poisoning, deferoxamine was given only until it was known that the iron-binding capacity had not been exceeded. The deferoxamine was discontinued and the patient recovered uneventfully. Subsequent labor and delivery were unremarkable, as was the newborn examination. Deferoxamine has been administered to one woman for the first 16 weeks of gestation, until the pregnancy was identified.[213] The treatment had been given for chronic iron intoxication due to beta-thalassemia minor. The infant was premature but without physical anomalies.

In iron intoxication in pregnancy, the use of sodium bicarbonate solution (100 ml of 1 per cent solution) has been recommended over activated charcoal to reduce further iron absorption. Use of deferoxamine should not be withheld because of concern over adverse fetal effects. The infant should be followed for signs of iron deficiency if this treatment is used.

Lead. Pica in pregnancy may lead to congenital and maternal lead intoxication.[214, 215] Furthermore, natural calcium supplement products, such as dolomite or bonemeal, which may be used by the pregnant woman, have been found to be sometimes contaminated with lead.[216]

A woman presented at 8 months' gestation in labor with basophilic stippling on examination of the blood smear and a history of eating paint chips. The labor was halted, but amniocentesis raised concerns about congenital lead intoxication.[214] Calcium ethylenediaminetetra-acetic acid (EDTA) was given for 3 days. The infant was spontaneously delivered on the eighth day of hospitalization. The baby was appropriately sized for gestational age, but the head circumference was in the tenth percentile and length was in the twenty-fifth percentile. The cord blood lead concentration was 60 μg/dl, and a free erythrocyte protoporphyrin was 330 μg/dl. No basophilic stippling of the red blood cells was observed. Radiologic examination demonstrated metaphysitis, submetaphyseal lucencies, and sclerosis of the shafts. Red blood cell fragility tests showed increased osmotic resistance. Nearly one half of the infant's chromosomes analyzed had simple breaks, relative to 5 per cent normal. At 2 weeks of age, the infant was chelated with EDTA for 5 days. The blood lead at the end of treatment was 40 μg/dl. This rose to 48 mcg/dl by 2½ months later and the baby was chelated once more, to a post-treatment level of 21 μg/dl. By 7 months of age, the electroencephalogram and developmental examination were within normal limits, and the bony abnormalities had resolved. This case demonstrated that a short course of in utero chelation may not be sufficient to treat congenital lead poisoning.

Organophosphate Poisonings. In a published case report, a woman at 34 to 35 weeks' gestation presented in acute respiratory distress with cyanosis and tachypnea and bilateral rhonchi and crepitation.[217] Her heart rate was 78 beats per minute and her blood pressure 120/80 mm Hg, with a fetal heart rate of 140 beats per minute. The mother was salivating markedly and her pupils were reduced to "pinpoint size." An uncorrected metabolic acidosis was diagnosed. Serum and erythrocyte acetylcholinesterase determinations were near zero. Cholinesterase inhibitor poisoning was felt to be the likely cause of disorders. Administration of atropine 2.4 mg intravenous bolus with infusion of 0.02 mg/kg/hr lead to unacceptable fetal tachycardia. The woman had shown increased cooperativeness and secretion control until the atropine had to be stopped. A cesarean section was performed for delivery of a hypotonic infant with a 1-minute Apgar score of 3. The baby was mechanically ventilated for 2 days and required atropine therapy at 0.1 mg/kg/hr for 8 days. The mother required 8 days of mechanical ventilation and 11 days of atropine therapy. In this case, the infant appeared relatively less poisoned than the mother by a presumed organophosphate exposure.

This infant was delivered to accomplish specific treatment and to avoid side effects of maternal treatment. Two alternative therapies were subsequently advised that may have allowed continuation of the gestation.[218] Glycopyrrolate is a quaternary anticholinergic agent that would be expected to reduce maternal secretions without direct fetal effect because quaternary ionized compounds would not be expected to be readily diffusable across the placenta. This would not, therefore, treat the fetal poisoning. The threat to maternal and infant survival appeared to be profound lethargy and excessive secretions, which compromised ventilation. If the mother were adequately treated, the fetus should have been able to achieve sufficient oxygenation, despite ongoing fetal cholinergic toxicity. Only after the fetus was delivered did its poisoning become unmasked by the challenge of independent respiration. The other recommended alternative was the use of pralidoxime (2-PAM) to counteract the skeletal muscle weakness seen in these patients.[218] Because atropine could be readily administered after delivery of the fetus, the authors felt that there was no advantage to the use of 2-PAM over atropine therapy.[219]

Thus, there are several areas of concern when managing two poisoned patients simultaneously. It is essential to treat the mother adequately to treat the fetus. The fetus may respond adversely to management that the mother tolerates. In addition, the fetus may require specific in utero therapies, delivery, or continued postnatal treatments to overcome the effects of the exposure.

References

1. National Center of Health Statistics Advance Report, Final Mortality Statistics 1982. Monthly Vital Statistics Reports Vol 33. No 9, Suppl DHHS Publications No PHS 85–1120. Frequency of human congenital malformations. Clin Perinatol *13*:543–554, 1986.
2. Hall JH, Powers EK, McLivaine RT, Ean VH: The frequency and financial burden of genetic disease in a pediatric hospital. Am J Med *1*:417–436, 1978.
3. Schardein JL: Chemically induced birth defects. New York, Marcel Dekker, 1985.
4. Brent RL: The law and congenital malformations. Clin Perinatol *13*:505–544, 1986.
5. Beckman DA, Brent RL: Mechanism of known environmental teratogens, drugs and chemicals. Clin Perinatol *113*:649–687, 1986.
6. Wilson JF, Fraser FC (eds): Handbook of Teratology. Vols I–IV. New York, Plenum Press, 1977.
7. Roberts RJ: Fetal and infant intoxication. *In* Roberts RJ (ed): Drug Therapy in Infants—Pharmacologic

Principles and Clinical Experience. Philadelphia, WB Saunders Co, 1984.
8. Shepard TH: Catalog of Teratogenic Agents. 5th ed. Baltimore, Johns Hopkins University Press, 1986.
9. Heinonen OP, Sloane D, Shapiro S: Birth Defects and Drugs in Pregnancy. Boston, John Wright PSG Incorporated, 1982.
10. Kalter H, Warkany J: Congenital malformations; Etiologic factors and their role in prevention. (Part I) N Engl J Med *308*:424–431, 1983.
11. Kalter H, Warkany J: Congenital malformations; Etiologic factors and their role in prevention. (Part II) N Engl of Med *308*:491–497, 1983.
12. Nishimura H, Tanimura T (eds): Clinical Aspects of the Teratogenicity of Drugs. New York, Elsevier, 1976.
13. Briggs GG, Freeman RK, Yaffe SJ: Drugs in Pregnancy and Lactation. 2nd ed. Baltimore, Williams & Wilkins, 1986.
14. Hays DP, Pagliaro LA: Human teratogens. *In* Pagliaro LA, Pagliaro AM (eds): Problems in Pediatric Drug Therapy. Hamilton, IL, Drug Intelligence Publications, 1987.
15. Wilcox AJ, Weinberg CR, O'Connor JF, Baird DD, Schlatterer JP, Canfield RE, Armstrong EG, Nisula BC: Incidence of early loss of pregnancy. N Engl J Med *319*:189–194, 1988.
16. Manson JM: Teratogens. *In* Klaassen CD, Amdur MO, Doull J (eds): Casarett and Doull's Toxicology; The Basic Science of Poisons. 3rd ed. New York, Macmillan Publishing Company, 1986, pp 195–220.
17. Black DL, Marks TA: Inconsistent use of terminology in animal developmental toxicology studies; A discussion. Teratology *33*:333, 1986.
18. Shardein JL: Approaches to defining the relationship of maternal and developmental toxicity. Teratogenesis Carcinog Mutagen *7*:255–271, 1987.
19. Cohlan SQ: Excessive intake of vitamin A as a cause of congenital anomalies in the rat. Science *117*:535–536, 1953.
20. Teratology Society: Teratology Society position paper; Recommendations for vitamin A use during pregnancy. Teratology *35*:269–275, 1987.
21. Lammer EJ, Chen DT, Hoar RM: Retinoic acid embryopathy. N Engl J Med *313*:837–841, 1985.
22. Rosa FW, Wilk AL, Kelsey FO: Teratogen update; Vitamin A congeners. Teratology *33*:355–364, 1986.
23. Kapron-Bras CM, Trasler DB: Gene-teratogen interaction and its morphological basis in retinoic acid-induced mouse spina bifida. Teratology *30*:143–150, 1984.
24. Shenefelt RE: Morphogenesis of malformations in hamsters caused by retinoic acid; Relation to dose and stage at treatment. Teratology *5*:103–118, 1972.
25. Kopchnar DM, Penner JD: Developmental effects of isotretinoin and 4-oxo-isotretinoin; The role of metabolism in teratogenicity. Teratology *36*:67–75, 1987.
26. Hytten FE, Leitch I: The Physiology of Human Pregnancy. 2nd ed. Oxford, Blackwell Scientific Publications, 1971.
27. Krauer B, Krauer F, Hutten FG: Drug disposition and pharmacokinetics in the maternal-placental-fetal unit. Pharmacol Ther *10*:301–328, 1980.
28. Zuspan FP: Physiologic changes of pregnancy. *In* Fabro S, Scialli AR (eds): Drug and Chemical Action in Pregnancy. New York, Marcel Dekker Incorporated, 1986.
29. Bodendorfer TW, Briggs GG, Gunning JT: Obtaining drug exposure histories during pregnancy. Am J Obstet Gynecol *135*:490, 1979.
30. Piper JM, Baum C, Kennedy DL: Prescription drug use before and during pregnancy in a Medicaid population. Am J Obstet Gynecol *157*:148–156, 1987.
31. Jackson MF: Drug absorption. *In* Fabro AS, Scialli AR (eds): Drug and Chemical Action in Pregnancy. New York, Marcel Dekker Incorporated, 1986.
32. Mattison DR: Physiologic variations in pharmacokinetics during pregnancy. *In* Fabro AS, Scialli AR (eds): Drug and Chemical Action in Pregnancy. New York, Marcel Dekker Incorporated, 1986.
33. Hurst HE, Jarboe CE: Clinical findings, elimination pharmacokinetics and tissue drug concentrations following fatal amitriptyline intoxication. Clin Toxicol *18*:119–125, 1983.
34. Cummings AJ: A survey of pharmacokinetic data from pregnant women. Clin Pharmacokinet *8*:344–354, 1983.
35. Gardner MJ, Schatz M, Cousins L, Zeiger R, Middleton E, Jusko WJ: Longitudinal effects of pregnancy on the pharmacokinetics of theophylline. Eur J Clin Pharmacol *31*:289–295, 1987.
36. Aldridge A, Bailey J, Neims AG: The disposition of caffeine during and after pregnancy. Semin Perinatol *5*:310–314, 1981.
37. Dean M, Stock B, Patterson RJ, Levy G: Serum protein binding of drugs during and after pregnancy in humans. Clin Pharmacol Ther *28*:253–261, 1980.
38. Perucca E, Crema A: Plasma protein binding of drugs in pregnancy. Clin Pharmacokinet *7*:336–352, 1982.
39. Frederickson MC, Ruo TS, Chow MJ, Atkinson AJ: Theophylline pharmacokinetics in pregnancy. Clin Pharmacol Ther *40*:321–328, 1986.
40. Carter BL, Driscoll CE, Smith DG: Theophylline clearance during pregnancy. Obstet Gynecol *68*:555–559, 1986.
41. Phelps S, Cochlan EB, Gonzales-Ruiz A, Tolley EA, Hammond ED, Sibai BM: The influence of gestational age and pre-eclampsia on the presence and magnitude of serum endogenous digoxin-like immunoreactive substance(s). Am J Obstet Gynecol *158*:34–39, 1988.
42. Gonzales AR, Phelps S, Cochlan EB, Sibai BM: Digoxin-like immunoreactive substance in pregnancy. Am J Obstet Gynecol *157*:660–664, 1987.
43. Perucca E, Richens A, Ruprah M: Serum protein binding of phenytoin in pregnant women. J R Soc Med *74*:422–423, 1981.
44. Perucca E: Drug metabolism in pregnancy, infancy and childhood. Pharmacol Ther *34*:129–143, 1987.
45. Rudolph AM: Animal models for study for fetal drug exposure. *In* Chiang CN, Lee CC (eds): Prenatal drug exposure kinetics and dynamics. NIDA Research Monograph 60. Rockville, MD, US Department of Health and Human Services, 1986, pp 5–16.
46. Rudolph AM, Heymann MA: Methods for studying the circulation of the placenta in utero. *In* Nathanielsz PW (ed): Animal Models in Fetal Medicine. Amsterdam, North Holland Biomedical Press, 1980, pp 1–57.
47. Miller RK: Placenta transfer and function; The interface for drugs and chemicals in the conceptus. *In* Fabro S, Scialli AR (eds): Drug and Chemical

Action in Pregnancy. New York, Marcel Dekker Incorporated, 1986, pp 123–152.
48. Wang LH, Rudolph AM, Benet LZ: Pharmacokinetics of drugs and metabolites in the maternal-placental-fetal unit; General principles. *In* Chiang CN, Lee CC (eds): Prenatal Drug Exposure Kinetics and Dynamics NIDA Research Monograph No. 60. Rockville, MD, US Department of Health and Human Services, 1986, pp 25–38.
49. Lindberg BS, Hartrig P, Lilja A, Lundquist H, Langstrom B, Malmborg A, Rimland A, Svard H: Positron-emission tomography; A new approach to feto-maternal pharmacokinetics. *In* Chiang CN, Lee CC (eds): Prenatal Drug Exposure Kinetics and Dynamics NIDA Research Monograph No. 60. Rockville, MD, US Department of Health and Human Services, 1986, pp 88–97.
50. Neubert D, Barrach HJ, Merker HJ: Drug-induced damage to the embryo or fetus. Curr Top Pathol, *69*:242–324, 1980.
51. Finnell RH, Chernoff GF: Gene-teratogen interactions; An approach to understanding the metabolic basis of birth defects. *In* Nau H, Scott NJ, Jr (eds): Pharmacokinetics in Teratogenesis. Vol I. Experimental Aspects In Vivo and In Vitro. Boca Raton, CRC Press, Inc. 1987, pp 97–109.
52. Johnson EM, Christian MS, Dansky L, Gabel BEG: Use of the adult developmental relationship in prescreening for developmental hazards. Teratogenesis Carcinog Mutagen *7*:273–285, 1987.
53. DeSesso JM: Maternal factors in developmental toxicity. Teratogenesis Carcinog Mutagen *7*:225–240, 1987.
54. Gross AS, Baird-Lambert JA, Brown KF: Disposition of ritodrine in pregnancy and non-pregnant women. Br J Clin Pharmacol *25*:155P–156P, 1988.
55. Gruenwald P: Pathology of the deprived fetus and its supply line. *In* Elliot K, Knight J: Size at Birth. Ciba Foundation Symposium Number 27. New York, Associated Scientific Publishers, 1974, pp 3–26.
56. Taylor PV, Scott JS, Gerlis LM, Esscher E, Scott O: Maternal antibodies against fetal cardiac antigens in congenital complete heart block. N Engl J Med *315*:667–672, 1986.
57. Shardein JL: Congenital abnormalities and hormones during pregnancy; A clinical review. Teratology *22*:251–270, 1980.
58. Ayromlooi J: Congenital goiter due to maternal ingestion of iodides. Obstet Gynecol *39*:818–822, 1972.
59. Rosa FW, Wilk AL, Kelsey FO: Teratogen update; Vitamin A congeners. Teratology *33*:355–364, 1986.
60. Ceelen JAG: Hypervitaminosis A-induced teratogenesis. CRC Crit Rev Toxicol *6*:351–375, 1979.
61. National Center for Health Statistics. Trends in teen childbearing United States 1970–1981. US DHHS Publications 84–1919.
62. Biggers JD: Problems concerning the uterine causes of embryonic death with special reference to the effects of the aging of the uterus. J Reprod Fertil (suppl) *8*:27, 1969.
63. Taffel S: Congenital anomalies and birth injuries among live births in the United States 1973–1974. US DHEW Publication PHS 79–1909.
64. Beard RW: Response of human fetal heart and circulation to adrenaline and noradrenaline. Br Med J *1*:443–446, 1962.
65. Ugen KE, Scott WJ Jr: Acetazolamide teratogenesis in Wistar rats potentiation and antagonism by adrenergic agents. Teratology *34*:195–200, 1986.
66. Robson JM, Sullivan FM: Effect of 5-hydroxytryptamine on maintenance of pregnancy, congenital abnormalities and the development of toxemia. Adv Pharmacol *6*:187–189, 1968.
67. Chasnoff IJ, Burns WJ, Schnoll SH, Burns KA: Cocaine use in pregnancy. N Engl J Med *313*:666–669, 1985.
68. Brent RL, Franklin JB: Uterine vascular clamping; New procedure for the study of congenital malformations. Science *132*:89–91, 1960.
69. Warkany J: Teratogen update; Hyperthermia. Teratology *33*:365–371, 1986.
70. Edwards MJ: Hyperthermia as a teratogen; A review of experimental studies and their clinical significance. Teratogenesis Carcinog Mutagen *6*:563–582, 1986.
71. Saxen L, Holmberg PC, Nurminen M, Kuosma E: Sauna and congenital defects. Teratology *25*:309–313, 1982.
72. Smith DW: Recognizable Patterns of Human Deformation. Philadelphia, WB Saunders Co, 1981.
73. Graham JM Jr, Miller ME, Stephan MJ, Smith DW: Limb reduction anomalies and early in utero limb compression. J Pediatr *96*:1052–1056, 1980.
74. Fraser FC: Relation of animal studies to the problem in man. *In* Wilson JG: Handbook of Teratology. Vol I. New York, Plenum Press, 1977.
75. Shardein JL: Approaches to defining the relationship of maternal and developmental toxicity. Teratogenesis Carcinog Mutagen *7*:255–271, 1987.
76. Rogers JM: Comparison of maternal and fetal toxic dose responses in mammals. Teratogenesis Carcinog Mutagen *7*:297–301, 1987.
77. Jusko WJ: Pharmacodynamic principles in chemical teratology-dose effect relationships. J Pharmacol Exp Ther *183*:469–480, 1972.
78. Khera KS: Maternal toxicity in humans and animals; Effects on fetal development and criteria for detection. Teratogenesis Carcinog Mutagen *2*:287–295, 1987.
79. Soler NG, Walsh SH, Melius SM: Congenital malformations in infants of diabetic mothers. Q J Med *45*:303–313, 1976.
80. Murakami U: The effect of organic mercury on intrauterine life in drugs and fetal development. *In* Klingberg MA, Abramovici A, Chemke J (eds): International Symposium on the Effect of Prolonged Drug Usage on Fetal Development. (Advances in Experimental Medicine and Biology, Vol. 27.) New York, Plenum Press, 1971, 301–336.
81. Neuhaus G, Ibe K: Clinical observations on a suicide attempt with 144 tablets of Contergan Forte (N-pthalyglutarmide). Med Klin *55*:544–554, 1960.
82. Pritchard JA, MacDonald PC, Gant NF: Diseases and abnormalities of the placenta and fetal membranes. *In* Pritchard JA, et al: Williams's Obstetrics. Norwalk, CT, Appleton-Century-Crofts, 1984, pp 441–466.
83. Khong TY, Pearce JM: Development and investigation of the placenta and its blood supply in the human placenta. *In* Lavery JP (ed): The Human Placenta; Clinical Perspective. Rockville, MD, Aspen Publishers, 1986, pp 25–36.
84. Swartz WJ: Early mammalian embryonic development. Am J Ind Med *4*:51–61, 1983.
85. Miller RK: Placental transfer and function; The interface for drugs and chemicals in the conceptus.

In Fabro S, Scialli AR (eds): Principals of Drugs and Chemical Action in Pregnancy. New York, Marcel Dekker, 1986, pp 123–151.

86. Miller RK, Wier PJ, Mavlik D, DiSan'Agnese PA: Human placenta *in vitro*; Characterization during 12 hours of dual perfusion. Contrib Gynecol Obstet *13*:77–84, 1985.
87. Tuchmann-DuPlessis H, Mercier Parot L: A propos de malformations produit par le bleu trypan. Biol Med *48*:238–251, 1959.
88. Wilkening RB, Anderson S, Martensson L, Meschia G: Placenta transfer as a function of uterine blood flow. Am J Physiol *242*:429–436, 1982.
89. Tropper PJ, Petrie RH: Placental exchange. *In* Lavery JP (ed): The Human Placenta. Rockville, Aspen Publishers, 1987, pp 199–206.
90. Nau H: Species differences in pharmacokinetics, drug metabolism and teratogenesis. *In* Nau H, Scott WJ (eds): Pharmacokinetics in Teratogenesis. Vol I. Boca Raton, CRC Press Inc, 1987, pp 81–127.
91. Khayat A, Dencker L: Fetal uptake and distribution of metallic mercury vapor in the mouse; influence of ethanol and aminotriazole. Int J Biol Res Pregnancy *3*:38, 1982.
92. Weiss B, Clarksson TW: Mercury toxicity in children; In Chemical and Radiation Hazards to Children. Ross Pediatric Conferences. 1982, pp 52–58.
93. Pelkonen O: Biotransformation of xenobiotics in the fetus. Pharmacol Ther *10*:261–281, 1980.
94. Blank A, Rane A, Toftgard R, Gustafsson J: Biotransformation of benzo(a)pyrene and 7-ethoxyresorufin and heme-staining proteins in microsomes from human fetal liver and placenta. Biochem Pharmacol *32*:1547–1552, 1983.
95. Jones AH, Fantel AG, Kocan RA, Juchau MR: Bioactivation of procarcinogens to mutagens in human fetal and placenta tissues. Life Sci *21*:1831–1836, 1977.
96. Manchester DK, Jacoby EH: Resolution and reconstitution of human placental mono-oxygenase activity responsive to maternal cigarette smoking. Dev Pharmacol Ther *5*:162–172, 1982.
97. Sieber SM, Fabro S: Identifications of drugs in the preimplantation blastocyst and in the plasma, uterine secretion and urine of the pregnant rabbit. J Pharmacol Exp Ther *176*:65, 1971.
98. Juchau MR, Rettie AE: The metabolic role of the placenta. *In* Fabro SE, Scialli AR (eds): Principles of Drug and Chemical Action in Pregnancy. New York, Marcel Dekker, Inc, 1986, pp 153–169.
99. Thinthanpanda A: Characteristics of drugs that penetrate the preimplantation blastocyst. Biochem Pharmacol *29*:1663, 1980.
100. Spielmann H, Jacob-Müller U: Investigation on cyclophosphamide treatment during the preimplantation period. II. In vitro studies on the effects of cyclophosphamide and its metabolites 4-OH-cyclophosphamide, phosphoramide mustard, and acrolein on blastulation of four-cell and eight-cell mouse embryos and on their subsequent development during implantation. Teratology *23*:7–13, 1981.
101. Spielmann H, Vogel R: Transfer of drugs into the embryo before and during implantation. *In* Nau H, Scott WJ Jr (eds): Pharmacokinetics in Teratogenesis. Vol I. Boca Raton, CRC Press, Inc 1987, pp 55–69.
102. Spielmann H, Kruger C, Tenschert B, Vogel R: Studies on the embryotoxic risk of drug treatment during the preimplantation period in the mouse. Arzneim Forsch Drug Res *36*:219–223, 1986.
103. Dencker L, Danielsson BRG: Transfer of drugs to the embryo and fetus after placentation. *In* Nau H, Scott WJ Jr. (eds): Pharmacokinetics in Teratogenesis. Vol I. Boca Raton, CRC Press, 1987, pp 55–69.
104. Dencker L: Disposition of chemicals in the developing embryo and fetus. Int J Biol Res Pregnancy *3*:114, 1982.
105. Dencker L: Tissue localization of some teratogens at early and late gestation related to fetal effects. Acta Pharmacol Toxicol (Suppl) *39*:1, 1976.
106. Kimmel CA, Wilson JG, Schumacher JH: Studies on the metabolism and identification of the causative agent in aspirin teratogenesis in rats. Teratology *4*:15, 1971.
107. Shah HC, McLachlan JA: The fate of diethylstilbestrol in the pregnant mouse. J Pharmacol Exp Ther *197*:687, 1976.
108. Nau H, Bass R: Transfer of 2,3,7,8 tetrachlorodibenzo-p-dioxin (TCDD) to the mouse embryo and fetus. Toxicology *20*:299, 1981.
109. Scott WJ, Nau H: Accumulation of weak acids in the young mammalian embryo. *In* Nau H, Scott WJ Jr (eds): Pharmacokinetics in Teratogenesis. Vol I. Boca Raton, CRC Press, Inc, 1987, pp 71–77.
110. Grimm VE: Effect of teratogenic exposure on the developing brain; Research strategies and possible mechanisms. Dev Pharmacol Ther *10*:328–345, 1987.
111. Dencker L, Danielsson BRG, Ghantous H, D'Argy R, Sperber G: Saturable accumulation of retinoic acid in neural and neural crest-derived cells in early embryonic development. Dev Pharmacol Ther *10*:212–223, 1987.
112. Dencker L: Disposition of chemicals in the developing embryo and fetus. Int J Biol Res Pregnancy *3*:114, 1982.
113. Danielsson BRG, Dencker L, Lindgren A: Transplacental movement of inorganic lead in early and late gestation in the mouse. Arch Toxicol *54*:97, 1983.
114. Danielsson BRG, Ghantous H, Dencker L: Distribution of chloroform and methyl chloroform and their metabolites in pregnant mice. Biol Res Pregnancy Perinatol *7*:77, 1986.
115. Pelkonen O: Transplacental transfer of foreign compounds and their metabolism by the foetus. *In* Bridges JW, Chasseaud LF (eds): Progress in Drug Metabolism. Vol II. New York, John Wiley & Sons, Inc, 1977, pp 119–161.
116. Filler R, Lew KJ: Developmental onset of mixed function oxidase activity in pre-implantation mouse embryos. Proc Natl Acad Sci USA, *78*:6991, 1981.
117. Pelkonen O, Karki NT, Korhonen P, Koivisto M, Tuimala R, Kauppila A: Inducibility of monooxygenase activities in the human fetus and placenta. *In* Olive G (ed): Advances in Pharmacology and Therapeutics. Vol 8. Drug-Action Modification-Comparative Pharmacology. Oxford, Pergamon, 1978, pp 101–111.
118. Smith M, Hopkinson DA, Harris H: Studies on the properties of the human alcohol dehydrogenase isoenzymes determined by the different loci ADH, ADH_2, ADH_3. Ann Hum Genet *37*:49–67, 1973.
119. Smith M, Hopkinson DA, Harris H: Developmental changes and polymorphism in human alcohol dehydrogenase. Ann Hum Genet *34*:251, 1971.
120. Dutton GJ: Glucuronide synthesis in fetal liver and other tissues. Biochem J *71*:141–48, 1959.

121. Hirvonen T: Fetal and postnatal development of glucuronide formation in mammalian tissue slices. Ann Univ Turkvensis AII/*38*:1–68, 1966.
122. Irjala K: Synthesis of p-aminohippuric, hippuric and salicyluric acids in experimental animals and man. Ann Acad Sci Fenn (A) 5/*154*:1–40, 1972.
123. Ingelman-Sundberg M, Rane A, Gustafsson J: Properties of hydroxylase systems in the human fetal liver active on free and sulfoconjugated steroids. Biochemistry *14*:429–437, 1975.
124. Rajchgot P, MacLeod S: Perinatal pharmacology. *In* MacLeod SM, Okey AB, Spielberg SP (eds): Developmental Pharmacology. New York, Alan R. Liss, Inc, 1983, pp 3–23.
125. Marx CM, Cloherty JP: Drug withdrawal. *In* Cloherty JP, Stark AR: Manual of Neonatal Care. 2nd ed. Boston, Little, Brown, 1985, pp 17–28.
126. Dixon RL: Toxic responses. *In* Klaassen CD, Amdur MD, Doull J (eds): Casarett and Doull's Toxicology; The Basic Science of Poisons. 3rd ed. New York, MacMillan Publishing Co, 1986, pp 432–477.
127. Hatch M, Stein ZA: Agents in the workplace and effects on reproduction. *In* Stein ZA, Hatch MC (eds): Reproductive Problems in the Workplace. Vol I. Occupational Medicine; State of the Art Reviews. Philadelphia, Hanley and Belfus, 1986, pp 531–534.
128. Wyrobek AJ, Watchmaker G, Gordon L: An evaluation of sperm tests as indicators of germ cell damage in men exposed to chemical or physical agents. Teratogenesis Carcinog Mutagen, *4*:83, 1984.
129. Blatt J, Mulvihill JJ, Ziegler JL, Young RC, Poplack DG: Pregnancy outcome following cancer chemotherapy. Am J Med *69*:828–832, 1980.
130. Koren G, Feldman Y, Shear N: Motherrisk—A new approach to antenatal counselling of drug/chemical exposure. Vet Hum Toxicol *28*:563–565, 1986.
131. Physician's Desk Reference. 42nd ed. Oradell, NJ, Medical Economics Co, 1988.
132. Millstein LG: FDA's pregnancy categories. N Engl J Med *303*:706, 1980.
133. Program and Abstracts. Behavioral Teratology Society, Tenth Annual Meeting. Boston, July 6–8, 1986. *33*:5C–17C, 1986.
134. Rayburn W, Wilson G, Schreck J, Louwsma G, Hamman J: Prenatal counselling; A state-wide telephone service. Obstet Gynecol *60*:243–246, 1982.
135. King CR: Genetic counselling for teratogen exposure. Obstet Gynecol *67*:843–847, 1986.
136. Goldenthal EI: Guidelines for reproduction studies for safety evaluation of drugs for human use. Drug Review Branch Division of Toxicological Evaluation, Bureau of Science. US Food and Drug Administration. January 1966.
137. Reiter LW: Neurotoxicology in regulation and risk assessment. Dev Pharmacol Ther *10*:254–358, 1987.
138. Kimmel CA, Young JF: Correlating pharmacokinetics and teratogenic endpoints. Fundamen Appl Toxicol *3*:250–258, 1983.
139. Paul M, Himmelstein J: Reproductive hazards in the workplace; What the practitioner needs to know about chemical exposures. Obstet Gynecol *71*:921–938, 1988.
140. Lewis RJ, Tatker RL (eds): Registry of Toxic Effect of Chemical Substances (microfiche). US Department of Health and Human Services, Centers for Disease Control. Rockville, National Institute for Occupational Safety and Health. April 1987.
141. NIOSH Pocket Guide to Chemical Hazards. US Department of Health and Human Services, Centers for Disease Control. National Institute for Occupational Safety and Health. Publication No 85–114. February, 1987.
142. Council on Environmental Quality. Chemical Hazards to Human Reproduction. National Institute for Occupational Safety and Health. Doc. Washington, DC, US Government Printing Office. January, 1981.
143. Infante PF, Tsongas TA: Occupational reproductive hazards; Necessary steps to prevention. Am J Ind Med *4*:383–390, 1983.
144. Haas JF, Schottenfeld D: Risks to the offspring from parental occupational exposure. J Occup Med *21*:607–613, 1979.
145. Prevention of leading work-related diseases and injuries. MMWR *34*(35), 1985.
146. American College of Obstetricians and Gynecologist Guidelines on Pregnancy and Work. Contract No 210-76-0159. US Department of Health, Education and Welfare. Centers for Disease Control. Rockville, National Institute for Occupational Safety and Health, Sept 1977.
147. Brent RL: Radiation Teratogenesis. *In* Sever JL, Brent RL (eds): Teratogen Update; Environmentally-induced Birth Defect Risks. New York, Alan R. Liss, Inc, 1986, pp 145–163.
148. Heminki K, Vineis P: Extrapolation of the evidence on teratogenicity of chemicals between humans and experimental animals; Chemicals other than drugs. Teratogenesis Carcinog Mutagen *5*:251–318, 1985.
149. El Batawi MA, Fomenko V, Hemminki K, Sorsa M, Vergieva T: Effects of occupational health hazards on reproductive functions (report). Geneva, World Health Organization, Aug 4–8, 1986.
150. Barlow SM: Reproductive effects of occupation. *In* Fabro S, Scialli AR (eds): Drug and Chemical Action in Pregnancy. New York, Marcel Dekker 1986, pp 353–371.
151. Hatch MC, Stein ZA: Agent Orange and risks to reproduction; The limits of epidemiology. Teratogenesis Carcinog Mutagen *6*:185–202, 1986.
152. Kaul AF, Sooney PF, Osathanondth R: A review of possible toxicity of Di-2-ethylhexylpthalate (DEHP) in plastic intravenous containers: Effects on reproduction. Drug Intell Clin Pharm *16*:689–692, 1982.
153. Ritter EJ, Scott WJ, Randall JL, Ritter JM: Teratogenicity of di(2-ethylhexyl) pthalate, 2-ethylhexanol, 2-ethylhexanoic acid and valproic acid and potentiation by caffeine. Teratology *35*:41–46, 1987.
154. Weiss B: Environmental contaminants and behavior disorders. Dev Pharmacol Ther *10*:346–353, 1987.
155. Grimm VE: Effect of teratogenic exposure on the developing brain; Research strategies and possible mechanisms. Dev Pharmacol Ther *10*:328–345, 1987.
156. Gofmekler VA: Effect on embryonic development of benzene and formaldehyde in inhalation experiments. Gig Sanit *33*:12–16, 1968.
157. Moore JA: Problems facing the decision-maker in the risk assessment process. Teratogenesis Carcinog Mutagen *7*:205–209, 1987.
158. Berlin CM: The pharmacology of drugs and chemicals in human milk. *In* Goldfarb J, Tibbetts E (eds): Breastfeeding Handbook. 3rd ed. Hillside, NJ, Enslow Publishers, 1989, pp 46–60.
159. Wilson JT: Pharmacokinetics of drug excretion. Wilson JT (ed): Drugs in Breast Milk. Australia, ADIS Press, 1981.

160. Rogan WJ: Epidemiology of Environmental Clinical Contaminants in Breast Milk in Human Lactation. New York, Plenum Publishing Corporation, 1986.
161. Marx CM: Medications and chemicals in the nursing mother. *In* Lauwers J, Woessner C (eds): Counseling the Nursing Mother. 2nd ed. New York, Avery Publishing Group, Inc, 1989, pp 449–493.
162. Wilson JT, Brown DR, Hinson JL, Dailey JW: Pharmacokinetic pitfalls in the estimation of the breast milk/plasma ratio for drugs. Annu Rev Pharmacol Toxicol *25*:667–689, 1985.
163. Marx CM: Drug use by nursing mothers. *In* Cloherty JP, Stark AR (eds): Manual of Neonatal Care. 2nd ed. Boston, Little, Brown, 1985, pp 559–599.
164. American Academy of Pediatrics Committee on Drugs: The transfer of drugs and other chemicals into human breast milk. Pediatrics *72*:376–383, 1983.
165. Goldfarb J, Tibbetts E: Breastfeeding Handbook. 2nd ed. Hillside, NJ, Enslow Publishers, 1989, pp 9–244.
166. Lawrence RA: Breastfeeding; A Guide for the Medical Profession. 2nd ed. St. Louis, CV Mosby, 1985.
167. Knowles J: Excretion of drugs in milk; A review. J Pediatr *66*:1068–1082, 1965.
168. Anderson PO: Drugs and breastfeeding; A review. Drug Intell Clin Pharm *11*:208, 1977.
169. Marx CM, Pucino F, Carlson JD, Driscoll J, Ruddock VM: Oxycodone excretion in human milk in the puerperium (abs). Drug Intell Clin Pharm *20*:474, 1986.
170. Rivera-Calimlim L: The significance of drugs in breast milk; Pharmacokinetic considerations. Clin Perinatol *14*:51–70, 1987.
171. Wolff MS: Occupationally derived chemicals in breast milk. Am J Ind Med *4*:259–281, 1983.
172. Rayburn W, Aranow R, Delancey B, Hogan MJ: Drug overdose during pregnancy; An overview from a metropolitan Poison Control Center. Obstet Gynecol *64*:611–614, 1984.
173. Goodwin J, Harris D: Suicide in pregnancy; The Hedda Gabler syndrome. Suicide Life Threat Behav *9*:105–115, 1979.
174. Anziulewicz JA, Dick HJ, Chiarulli EE: Transplacental naphthalene poisoning. Am J Obstet Gynecol *78*:519–521, 1959.
175. Campbell DM, Davidson RL: Toxic hemolytic anemia in pregnancy due to a pica for paradichlorobenzene. Am J Med Sci *274*:139–146, 1977.
176. Whitlock RA, Edwards JE: Pregnancy and attempted suicide. Compr Psychiatry *9*:1, 1968.
177. Buchsbaum HJ, Stapeles PP: Self-inflicted gunshot wounds to the pregnant uterus; Report of two cases. Obstet Gynecol *65*:32S–35S, 1985.
178. Brandstettler RD, Gotz V: Inadvertent overdose of parenteral terbutaline. Lancet *1*:485, 1980.
179. Byer AJ, Traylor TR, Semmer JR: Acetaminophen overdose in the third trimester of pregnancy. JAMA *247*:3114–3115, 1982.
180. Robertson RG, VanCleave BL, Collins JJ Jr: Acetaminophen overdose in the second trimester of pregnancy. J Fam Pract *23*:267–268, 1986.
181. Stokes IM: Paracetamol overdose in the second trimester of pregnancy; Case report. Br J Obstet Gynecol *91*:286–288, 1984.
182. Lederman S, Fysh WJ, Tiedgerf M, Gamsu HR: Neonatal paracetamol poisoning; Treatment by exchange transfusion. Arch Dis Child *58*:631–633, 1983.
183. Hatbach H, Akhter JE, Muscato MS, Cary PL, Hoffman MI: Acetaminophen overdose with fetal demise. Am J Clin Pathol *82*:240–242, 1984.
184. Roberts I, Robinson MS, Muighal MZ, Ratcliffe JG, Prescott LF: Paracetamol metabolites in the neonate following maternal overdose. Br J Clin Pharmacol *18*:201–206, 1984.
185. Bronstein AC, Rumack BH: Acute acetaminophen overdose during pregnancy; Review of 59 cases. Vet Hum Toxicol *26*(Suppl 2):44, 1984.
186. Gwee MCE: Can tetracycline-induced fatty liver in pregnancy be attributed to choline deficiency. Med Hypotheses *9*:157–162, 1982.
187. McCormack WM, George H, Donner A, et al: Hepatotoxicity of erythromycin estolate during pregnancy. Antimicrob Agents Chemother *12*:630–635, 1977.
188. Cramer CR: Fetal death due to accidental maternal carbon monoxide poisoning. J Toxicol Clin Toxicol *19*:297–301, 1982.
189. Strom RL, Schiller P, Seeds AE, Bensel TR: Fatal iron poisoning in a pregnant female. Minn Med *7*:483–489, 1976.
190. Witter FR, King TM, Blake DS: Adverse effects of cardiovascular drug therapy on the fetus and neonate. Obstet Gynecol *58*:100S, 1981.
191. Rogers GC, Matyunas NJ: Gastrointestinal decontamination for acute poisoning. Pediatr Clin North Am *33*:261–285, 1986.
192. Ipecac (Oral-Local) in U.S.P.D.I. 7th ed. U.S. Pharmacopedial Convention, Inc, 1987, pp 1022–1023.
193. Boxer L, Anderson FP, Rowe DS: Comparison of ipecac-induced emesis with gastric lavage in the treatment of acute salicylate ingestion. J Pediatr *74*:800–803, 1969.
194. Burke M: Gastric lavage and emesis in the treatment of ingested poisons; A review and a clinical study of lavage in ten adults. Resuscitation *1*:91–105, 1972.
195. Comstock EG, Faulkner TP, Boisaubin EV, et al: Studies on the efficacy of gastric lavage as practiced in a large metropolitan hospital. Clin Toxicol *18*:581–597, 1981.
196. Matthew H, Macintosh TF, Tompsett SL, et al: Gastric aspiration and lavage in acute poisoning. Br Med J *1*:1333–1337, 1966.
197. D'Ascoli P, Gall SA: Common Poisons. *In* Gleicher N (ed): Principles of Medical Therapy in Pregnancy. New York, Plenum Press, 1985.
198. Peterson RG, Peterson LN: Cleansing the blood; Hemodialysis, peritoneal dialysis, exchange transfusion, charcoal hemoperfusion, forced diuresis. Pediatri Clin North Am *33*:675–689, 1986.
199. Colton CK, Lowrie EG: Hemodialysis; Physical principles and technical consideration. *In* Brenner BM, Rector FC (eds): The Kidney. Philadelphia, WB Saunders Co, 1981.
200. Freed CR: Treatable drug overdoses. Cleve Clin J Med *54*:255–257, 1987.
201. Rayburn W, Piehl E, Sanfield J, Compton A: Reversing severe hypoglycemia during pregnancy with glucagon therapy. Am J Perinatol *4*:259–261, 1987.
202. Longo LD: The biological effects of carbon monoxide on the pregnant woman, fetus and newborn infant. Am J Obstet Gynecol *129*:69–103, 1977.
203. Copel JA, Bowen F, Bolognese RJ: Carbon monoxide intoxication in early pregnancy. Obstet Gynecol *59*:26S–28S, 1982.
204. Ginsburg MD, Myers RE: Fetal brain injury after maternal carbon monoxide intoxication. Neurology *26*:15–23, 1976.
205. Caravati EM, Adams CJ, Joyce SM, Schafer NC:

Fetal toxicity associated with maternal carbon monoxide poisoning. Ann Emerg Med 17:714–717, 1988.
206. Rayburn W, Shukla V, Stetson P, Piehl E: Acetaminophen pharmacokinetics comparison between pregnant and nonpregnant women. Obstet Gynecol 155:1353–1356, 1986.
207. Pentel PR, Benowitz NL: Tricyclic antidepressant poisoning; Management of arrhthmias. Med Toxicol 1:101–121, 1986.
208. Spector RH, Schnapper R: Amitriptyline-induced ophthalmoplegia. Neurology 21:1188–1190, 1981.
209. Askenasy JJ, Streifler M, Felner S: The synaptic significance of metoclopramide induced dyskinetic-dystonic head and neck movements in pregnancy. J Neural Transmission 42:73–84, 1978.
210. Witter FR, King TM, Blake DS: Adverse effects of cardiovascular drug therapy on the fetus and neonate. Obstet Gynecol 58:100S, 1981.
211. Rayburn WF, Donn SM, Wulf ME: Iron overdose during pregnancy; Successful therapy with desferroxamine. Am J Obstet Gynecol 147:717–719, 1983.
212. Blanc P, Hryhorczuk D, Danel I: Deferoxamine treatment of acute iron intoxication in pregnancy. Obstet Gynecol 64:12S–14S, 1984.
213. Proudfoot AT, Simpson D, Dyson EH: Management of acute iron poisoning. Med Toxicol 1:83–100, 1986.
214. Timpo AE, Amin JS, Caslino MB, Yuceoglu AM: Congenital lead intoxication. J Pediatr 94:765–767, 1979.
215. Sensirivatana R, Supachadhiwong O, Phancharoen S, Mitrakul C: Neonatal lead poisoning. Clin Pediatr 22:582–584, 1983.
216. Roberts HJ: Potential toxicity due to dolomite and bonemeal. South Med J 76:556–559, 1983.
217. Weis OF, Muller FO, Lyell H, Badenhorst CH, Van Niekerk P: Maternal-fetal cholinesterase inhibitor poisoning. Anesth Analg 62:233–235, 1983.
218. Sosis M, Bodner A, Ahmad I: Management of cholinesterase inhibitor poisoning in obstetrics (letter). Anesth Analg 62:1135, 1983.
219. Muuler FO, Weis OF: Reply to letter to the editor. Anesth Analg 62:1136, 1983.

CHAPTER 19

TOXIC EMERGENCIES IN THE NEONATE

Michael S. Weinstock, M.D., FAAP, FACEP
Lorraine Hartnett, M.D., FAAP, A.B.M.T.

Neonatal intensive care units have had a profound effect on decreasing the morbidity and mortality of sick neonates. However, neonatal poisoning has only recently been recognized as a significant threat. Aggressive therapeutic intervention with potent pharmacologic agents and sophisticated modification of the environment have placed the newborn infant at risk for therapeutic misadventures or accidental exposure to potential environmental toxins.

Symptoms range from subtle changes in feeding and sleeping patterns to overt clinical signs and symptoms of seizures, metabolic derangement, circulatory lability, renal or hepatic failure, cardiac arrhythmias, and neurologic changes. Death may occur.

This chapter will be devoted to the early recognition, understanding, and appropriate intervention and treatment of the poisoned neonate.

NEONATAL PHARMACOKINETICS

Preterm infants born in North America can be exposed to multiple pharmacologic agents during parturition and confinement in the nursery. Four to ten medications may be given to the mother that may reach the fetus transplacentally prior to birth or may affect the infant through breast milk after birth. In the nursery, another seven drugs are routinely used and approximately seven more for specific indications.[1]

Neonatal exposure to poisons or toxic agents is a result of environmental contamination, accidental administration of toxic doses of pharmacologic agents, or therapeutic misadventures. All these can contribute to toxic emergencies. Routes of entrance may also contribute to the toxicity of the agent and should be considered. Substances enter the neonate via the respiratory tract, gastrointestinal tract, and parenteral route (IM, IV), and by direct absorption through skin and mucous membranes.

The skin of the immature infant is remarkably permeable, and percutaneous absorption of toxic compounds, resulting in illness and death, has had impressive documentation in the newborn infant.[2] Percutaneous absorption is inversely related to the thickness of the stratum corneum and directly related to skin hydration and is therefore increased in the newborn infant.[3]

There are age related differences in absorption, distribution, metabolism, and excretion of agents in preterm neonates, full-term infants, and older infants.[3] Drug absorption is quite variable from the gastrointestinal tract and depends on the maturational age of the gut. Other considerations, such as reduced plasma protein binding, distribution of the drug between body organs, and the maturity of the liver as it relates to drug biotransformation, all play a significant role in the toxicity of any exposure. The kidneys are functionally immature and may delay excretion, thereby resulting in excessive loads and toxic exposure.

ACCIDENTAL ENVIRONMENTAL EXPOSURE

Boric Acid

Boric acid has been widely used in medicine as an irrigant, antiseptic, food preservative, and treatment for dermatologic disorders. It now exists in many therapeutic forms of topical application.[4] Its use in talcum powders and ointments has been discontinued for the most part.[5] Boric acid is rapidly absorbed from the gastrointestinal tract and mucosal surfaces. The most frequent cause of intoxication in infants involves chronic topical application. Regardless of the route of absorption, the common types of manifestations are cutaneous, resembling toxic epidermal necrolysis or the "boiled lobster" appearance. Other manifestations of toxicity are irritability, seizures, and gastrointestinal effects, including nausea, vomiting, and diarrhea.[6] In moderate-to-severe poisoning, oliguria or anuria from renal tubular necrosis may occur.

Treatment consists of removal of the offending agent and supportive care. Maintenance of adequate urine output is noted to increase boric acid and borates in the urine, therefore appropriate fluid therapy is important in the treatment of boric acid poisoning. Dialysis may be indicated in the event of renal failure.

Baby Powders

Baby powders are used for the skin care of infants throughout the world. Inhalation of toxic and fatal quantities of baby powder have been reported.[7] Mortality rates greater than 20 per cent have been noted.[8] The actual incidence of morbidity and mortality secondary to aspiration of baby powders has probably been underestimated.

Commercial talcum powder is a mixture of talc (hydrous magnesium silicate) and other silicates. Some contain calcium undecylenate as an added medication.

The treatment is avoidance of exposure. Containers of talc should include a warning that the ingredients may be hazardous, and the practice of using baby powders on young infants and children should be condemned and well publicized.[9]

Heavy Metals

Neonatal accidental exposure to heavy metals is of historical interest; it is rarely seen in the neonate except as an unusual sporadic event.

Acute and chronic lead intoxication is rare. Pica is not found in the neonatal age group, and the opportunity for exposure to lead-based paints is unreported during the neonatal period. Acute and chronic lead poisoning is a disease of older children, usually greater than 6 months of age. However, the effects of lead crossing the placenta, resulting in abortion and fetal loss, are well known. Rarely have cases of fetal lead intoxication been reported. Timpo and colleagues described a case of fetal lead intoxication transplacentally in an infant who was exposed during chelation therapy of the mother with calcium-EDTA.[10]

Neonatal exposure to metallic mercury and

its salts is widely reported. Acrodynia (pink disease, dermatopolyneuritis) was described in early accounts by Bilderback.[11] Clinical manifestations include extreme irritability and restlessness alternating with periods of apathy, insomnia, anorexia, profuse perspiration with attendant thirst, pink hands and feet, rosy cheeks, and variable skin rashes with desquamation.

More than 1600 babies were poisoned by mercury-contaminated commercially laundered diapers in Argentina in 1981.[12] Mercury thermometers are no longer used in incubators because of unacceptable levels of mercury vapor exposure. In 1979 the journal *Pediatrics* noted the potential hazards of, and commented on, the levels of potential mercury vapor exposure in newborn nurseries.[13]

The management of heavy metal toxicity is similar in both neonates and adults and depends upon the form (metallic, organic, or inorganic) and whether the exposure is acute or chronic.

Immediate removal from exposure, along with supportive measures, should be initiated. Several chelating agents should be employed to treat heavy metal intoxication, depending on the type of compound. BAL (dimercaprol) 4 mg/kg/dose every 4 hours, calcium disodium edetate (calcium disodium versenate, EDTA), 50 mg/kg/24 hr divided into four doses, and penicillamine, 35 to 100 mg/kg/24 hr divided into four doses are the most commonly employed agents.

In acute mercury vapor exposure, chelation therapy with BAL, 4 mg/kg/dose every 4 hours, deep intramuscularly, should be started immediately. Tapering of the dose depends upon blood and urine mercury levels. After the initial course of BAL, oral penicillamine, 35 to 100 mg/kg/24 hr, may be administered up to 10 days.

Patients with symptomatic lead intoxication should receive combined BAL in the previously noted dosage schedule along with EDTA.[14] The dose is 50 mg/kg/24 hr in four divided doses and should not be administered until the second dose of BAL.

IATROGENIC POISONING IN THE NEONATE

Advances in neonatal medicine have brought about therapeutic exposure of premature infants and neonates to a wide variety of pharmacologic agents. With therapeutic effect comes the risk of toxicity, and in sick premature babies and neonates the risk is perhaps even greater than in the child or adult, because of several factors: altered pharmacokinetics; unfamiliarity with drug effect in this population; and inadvertent overdose because of errors in calculation.

The neonatal intensive care unit is a fast paced, dynamic, and stressful environment. Meticulous attention must be paid by physicians and nurses alike to the accuracy of written orders in order to avoid overdose. The dynamic nature of the sick neonate may mask signs and symptoms of drug toxicity; often toxicity has the same manifestations of common neonatal illness—sepsis, respiratory distress, feeding problems, fluid and electrolyte abnormalities. Because of the paucity of specific toxic syndromes in the neonate, consideration of drug reaction or overdose must be made when assessing the patient.

It is beyond the scope of the chapter to present the manifestations of toxicity of every drug used in neonatal medicine. Commonly used preparations with reported toxicity and some unusual syndromes which have been reported in the literature will be examined. Table 19–1 addresses some of the common side effects and recognized symptoms of toxicity of commonly used drugs in the neonate.[15]

Opiates

Neonates are often exposed to opiates as a result of prepartum use to relieve maternal pain during labor, or from maternal narcotic abuse. Classically, the affected neonate at delivery exhibits some degree of poor muscle tone, decreased activity, poor respiratory effort, bradycardia, and hypotension.

The severity and duration of toxic manifestations depend on several factors, including (1) the narcotic in question (meperidine has a longer half-life than does morphine or heroin); (2) the dose of narcotic; (3) the timing of the dose; (4) the size of the neonate; and (5) the individual pharmacokinetics (the sick neonate may have a decreased renal or hepatic function).

In any neonate who has been exposed to opiates and exhibits signs of toxicity in the postnatal period, naloxone, 0.01 mg/kg/dose, should be administered via the intramuscular, intravenous, sublingual, or endotracheal

Table 19–1. COMMONLY USED DRUGS AND THEIR POTENTIAL TOXICITY IN NEONATES

DRUG	TOXICITY
amikacin	Nephrotoxicity, ototoxicity
aminophylline	Tachycardia, abdominal distention, GI hemorrhage, jitteriness, or seizures
amoxicillin	Nephrotoxic, vitamin K depletion, distal renal tubular acidosis
ampicillin	Rare; increased transaminase; eosinophilia; irritability
atropine sulfate	Tachycardia, urine retention, hyperthermia
belladonna, tincture of	Hyperthermia, dry secretions, flushing
bicarbonate	Transient hyperosmolarity, alkalosis, hypernatremia
caffeine citrate	Tachycardia, seizures, abdominal distention
calcium gluconate	Bradycardia, sloughing and calcification with IV infiltration; potentiates digitalis effect
carbenicillin	Hypernatremia, sloughing with IV infiltration; transaminase elevation, platelet dysfunction
cephalothin	Nephrotoxicity, neutropenia, false-positive Coombs' test, allergic rash, poor passage through blood-brain barrier
cefazolin	Neutropenia, thrombocytopenia, false-positive Coombs' test, transient transaminase elevation
chloral hydrate	Gastric irritation, paradoxic excitement
chloramphenicol	May cause "gray baby syndrome" with toxic level; potentiates Dilantin effect, reversible bone marrow depression
chlorothiazide	Hyperglycemia, hypokalemia, hyponatremia, alkalosis
cholestyramine	Steatorrhea, GI dysfunction, malabsorption of fat-soluble vitamins; metabolic acidosis
diazepam	Sodium benzoate diluent, competes with bilirubin for albumin binding sites; respiratory depression, hypotension
diazoxide	Hypotension, hyperglycemia, sodium and water retention
digoxin	Toxicity: bradycardia, vomiting, arrhythmias, poor feeding
epinephrine	Tachycardia, arrhythmia
furosemide	Hypokalemia, hyponatremia, hypochloremia, alkalosis, dehydration, ototoxicity with aminoglycosides, renal calcifications; enchances nephrotoxicity of cephaloridine
gentamicin	Nephrotoxicity, ototoxicity
glucagon	Rebound hyperglycemia
hydralazine HCl	May cause hypotension or tachycardia
indomethacin	Transient renal and liver dysfunction, decreased platelet aggregation, hyponatremia, hypoglycemia
isoproterenol	Marked inotropic effect, hypotension, arrhythmia
kanamycin	Nephrotoxicity, ototoxicity
lidocaine HCl	Hypotension, seizures, respiratory arrest, asystole
magnesium sulfate	Hypotension, CNS depression
mannitol	Rebound edema and/or circulatory overload
moxalactam	Thrombocytopoenia, platelet dysfunction, hypothrombinemia
naloxone HCl	Tachycardia, hypertension, tremors, seizures
nitroprusside	Hypotension, tachyphylaxis, thiocyanate toxicity with long-term use
oxacillin	Penicillin sensitivity, nephrotoxicity
paraldehyde	Cardiopulmonary depression, CNS depression, pulmonary edema
phenobarbital	CNS depression with respiratory arrest with overdose
phenytoin	Bone marrow depression, nystagmus
prostigmine	Respiratory failure, cardiovascular collapse
streptomycin sulfate	Nephrotoxicity, ototoxicity, cardiovascular collapse
thorazine	Hypotension, hypothermia rare, liver disease and bone marrow depression
ticarcillin	Bleeding problems, hypernatremia
tobramycin sulfate	Nephrotoxicity, ototoxicity
vancomycin	Nephrotoxicity, ototoxicity, histamine-like response

(Adapted and modified from Harper RG, Jing JY: Handbook of Neonatology. 2nd ed. Chicago, Year Book Publishing Company, 1987.)

route. The dose will depend on the response of the infant. Repeat doses in 15 minutes or an intravenous infusion may be necessary.[16]

Antibiotics

Neonates often require treatment of sepsis with a variety of antibiotics, such as penicillins, cephalosporins, aminoglycosides, and chloramphenicol. The manifestations of toxicity must be familiar to those caring for the neonate, and careful observation for signs of toxicity must be undertaken. Adverse effects range from ototoxicity and nephrotoxicity associated with aminoglycosides to the consequences of bilirubin displacement seen with sulfa compounds. The gray baby syndrome associated with use of chloramphenicol is well documented.[17, 18] The inability of the neonate to glucuronidate chloramphenicol is responsible for the gray baby syndrome seen in some newborn infants. Attention to dosing and monitoring of drug levels (peak and trough) are paramount in preventing this potentially fatal disorder. The manifestations of gray baby syndrome are lethargy, poor feeding, abdominal distention, vomiting, tachypnea, cyanosis, hypotension, and acidosis. This symptom complex can result from toxic chloramphenicol levels (therapeutic range, 10 to 25 μg/ml). Treatment requires meticulous supportive care, exchange transfusion, and/or charcoal hemoperfusion if available.

Alcohols

Exposure of the neonate to alcohols may cause toxic manifestations. Classic methanol poisoning, with metabolic acidosis and retinal changes, is reported secondary to methanol absorption percutaneously[19] or in formula.[20] Treatment with ethanol is indicated in these cases. The usual dose to maintain a blood level of 100 mg/dl of ethanol should begin with a loading dose of 0.6 mg/kg.[21] Hemodialysis should be instituted at blood methanol concentrations greater than 50 mg/dl.

Intoxication with both ethanol and isopropyl alcohol may result following sponging an infant with these alcohols to reduce body temperature[22] or through intravenous ethanol administration.[23] Hypoglycemia with central nervous system depression and coma is frequently observed in such cases. Treatment is supportive.

The "gasping baby" syndrome was described in 1982[24] in premature infants exposed to benzyl alcohol used as an antibacterial agent in bacteriostatic saline and bacteriostatic water in parenteral solutions. The clinical syndrome observed was one of gasping progressing to apnea, metabolic acidosis, seizures, progressive central nervous system dysfunction, coma, intracranial hemorrhage, and death. The syndrome is prevented by avoidance of solutions containing benzyl alcohol.

Hexachlorophene

Hexachlorophene was once one of the most commonly used topical antiseptics in the neonatal nursery. Topical application of this substance was implicated in the deaths of 36 French babies in 1972.[25] The manifestations of poisoning included seizures and central nervous system depression. Animal studies revealed cerebral edema and vacuolization of myelin in the brain and central nervous system,[26] with similar changes found in premature infants similarly exposed to hexachlorophene.[27] Routine use of hexachlorophene-containing compounds has been discontinued.

Corticosteroids

Percutaneous absorption by the neonate of corticosteroid-containing compounds may result in Cushing's syndrome[28] (round facies, hirsutism, obesity, buffalo hump). Prolonged administration may depress the hypothalamic-pituitary-adrenal axis in these infants. Withdrawal of the offending steroid usually reverses the symptoms, but administration of corticosteroids in tapering doses may be required if adrenal suppression has occurred.

Verapamil

Supraventricular tachycardia may require treatment in the neonate. Although verapamil is often used successfully to convert such a dysrhythmia in adults and older children, its use in neonates and infants has resulted, in some cases, in life-threatening bradyarrhythmias, asystole, hypotension, and cardiac arrest,[29] even in supposedly therapeutic doses of 0.1 mg/kg over 30 seconds.[30]

Because of these potential complications, it is felt that paroxysmal supraventricular tachycardia in neonates is best treated with digoxin and, if necessary, cardioversion.

Theophylline

Theophylline preparations are used in the sick neonate as a treatment for apnea of prematurity. Accurate dosing and monitoring of theophylline levels are mandatory in caring for these infants. If these safeguards are not taken, serious overdose may occur in those neonates in whom theophylline exhibits a prolonged half-life and decreased clearance. Symptoms of overdose include tachycardia, jitteriness, tremors, seizures, hyper-reflexia, ventricular dysrhythmias, abdominal distention, and vomiting.[31] Should toxic manifestations occur, discontinuing the drug is mandatory, and symptomatic treatment of seizures or dysrhythmias is advisable. Exchange transfusion has not been effective.

Charcoal hemoperfusion is the preferred treatment for life-threatening overdose in children and adults, but, at present, insufficient documentation exists for neonates.

Ophthalmic Drops

Small term neonates who require oxygen therapy or who are at risk for cerebral hemorrhage require frequent fundoscopic examinations while in the nursery. Mydriatic and cyclopegic ophthalmic drugs are used to facilitate fundoscopic examination. These agents have the potential for adverse reaction in all age groups, including hypertension, blanching of the skin of the eyelids, subarachnoid hemorrhage, ventricular arrhythmia, and tachycardia.[32] Two cases of paralytic ileus, one fatal, followed instillation of a 1 per cent solution of cyclopentolate hydrochloride (Cyclogyl) ophthalmic drops. These cases were associated with serum concentrations of the drug to support the clinical impression of Cyclogyl intoxication.[32]

Current recommendations are to use a solution of cyclopentolate hydrochloride 0.5 per cent, tropicamide (Mydriacyl) 1 per cent, and phenylephrine 2.5 per cent in term infants.[33] Preterm infants require further dilution of the drug.

Treatment of the side effects of mydriatic agents is rarely necessary, and the approach to therapy is essentially supportive, in addition to avoidance of the offending agent.

NEONATAL CONSEQUENCES OF MATERNAL SUBSTANCE ABUSE

Pollution of the intrauterine environment by maternal use of licit and illicit drugs causes a multitude of problems in the fetus and neonate. Alcohol is the drug most abused by mothers in the United States. The impact of maternal alcohol use has been well documented in the literature, and further discussion of the fetal alcohol syndrome[34, 35] will not be pursued. Withdrawal from alcohol in the neonatal period has been described[36] but is usually short-lived and requires no treatment. Neonatal narcotic withdrawal is a serious problem in the infants of heroin, methadone, and polydrug abusers. The use of cocaine during pregnancy[37] reflects the increase in use by the general population and results in many adverse consequences to the fetus and neonate.

The long-term teratogenic effects, short-term withdrawal symptoms, and early neurodevelopmental effects of maternal drug abuse are only the beginning of a larger picture of social, psychologic, and educational turmoil for the child introduced to such an environment. The thrust of treatment for such pervasive destructive phenomena must be in prevention of drug use in our society.

Maternal Narcotic Abuse

Opiates easily cross the placenta, inducing dependency in the fetus of the narcotic-addicted mother. Abrupt discontinuation of placental opiate transfer after birth results in onset of neonatal withdrawal[38] anywhere from 72 hours to 2 weeks after birth, depending on the offending opiate. In general, heroin withdrawal symptoms will occur early in the postnatal period, reflecting its short half-life, whereas in the infant of the methadone-dependent mother the onset of withdrawal symptoms may be delayed as much as 2 weeks after birth.

The signs and symptoms of withdrawal vary in severity and affect the central nervous system, gastrointestinal tract, and respiratory tract (Table 19–2).

The clinical withdrawal syndrome has similar signs and symptoms, regardless of the

Table 19–2. SIGNS AND SYMPTOMS OF NARCOTIC WITHDRAWAL IN INFANCY

CENTRAL NERVOUS SYSTEM	GASTROINTESTINAL	RESPIRATORY	MISCELLANEOUS
Irritability	Poor suck/swallow	Tachypnea	Dehydration
Shrill cry	Vomiting	Amniotic fluid aspiration	Poor weight gain
Tremors	Colicky	Meconium aspiration	Electrolyte imbalance
Hyperreflexia	Abdominal pain		Small for gestational age
Seizures	Diarrhea		Skin excoriations
Poor sleeping			

maternal dependency on various opiates (heroin, methadone, pentazocine, propoxyphene, codeine), barbiturates,[39] or benzodiazepines,[40] although the severity and time of onset may differ. The preponderance of polydrug abuse makes delineation of distinct syndromes difficult.

Diagnosis of the withdrawal syndrome is vital for both the physical and psychosocial development of the affected neonate. Once diagnosis is made, close observation of the neonate is essential to determine the necessity for pharmacologic intervention. Observation may be undertaken in the regular newborn nursery as long as frequent vital signs, behavioral observation, and accurate recording of intake and output are achieved. Early social service intervention is necessary at this time to assure maternal counseling and proper placement of the infant after treatment.

Initial treatment of the affected neonate includes placement in a quiet environment to minimize environmental stimulation. Swaddling the infant minimizes infant movement and the risk of excoriation and promotes sleep. Frequent small feedings should be instituted to maximize caloric intake and weight gain. The infant must be examined several times daily, and the data collected should be assessed.

Indications for institution of pharmacologic therapy include severe irritability, seizures, dehydration, electrolyte abnormalities (these should not occur if the patient is closely monitored), persistent diarrhea or vomiting, and poor or no weight gain. If other medical conditions supervene, such as meconium aspiration or sepsis, the patient should not be allowed to exhibit signs of withdrawal.

If treatment is necessary, a narcotic (such as paregoric or tincture of opium) or a sedative (such as phenobarbital) may be used. Paregoric has fallen into disfavor as a treatment because of potential local mucosal irritation from its constituents—anise oil, benzoic acid, and camphor. Tincture of opium, diluted 25-fold, yields the same concentration as paregoric. The usual dose of equivalent to morphine is 0.08 mg to 0.32 mg every 3 hours. The dosing regimen must be titrated according to the patient response, with the end-point being good weight gain (in the usual patient, other signs will abate as this is achieved). Several days after good weight gain is achieved, a slow tapering of opium dosage should be commenced. The duration of treatment varies according to the offending narcotic and the severity of the maternal habit.

Phenobarbital has also had good results in treating narcotic withdrawal.[41] It is not a specific treatment for narcotic withdrawal but is the specific treatment for neonatal barbiturate withdrawal and for multidrug withdrawal. The dose must be titrated to patient response and slowly tapered once positive results are achieved. Little difference in efficacy of therapy has been noted in infants treated with either regimen.

Clonidine is a centrally acting alpha-adrenergic agonist that has been used successfully in the treatment of narcotic withdrawal in adults. Some work has been done using clonidine in the management of narcotic-addicted infants,[42] but its use remains experimental.

Maternal Cocaine Abuse

Women of childbearing age increasingly abuse cocaine, as its popularity as a recreational drug flourishes in the United States. Since it is a strong psychologically addictive drug, usage generally continues despite pregnancy, thereby exposing the fetus to the ill effects of cocaine.[43] Regardless of the route of administration (nasal, intravenous, "free base"), cocaine causes central nervous system stimulation, mood alteration, and wide-ranging physiologic changes in the user, including tachycardia, hypertension, ventricular dysrhythmias, acute myocardial infarction, CVA, pulmonary edema, and sudden death.

Cocaine readily crosses the placenta, causing profound alterations in the fetal/placental unit. Vasoconstriction of placental vessels may lead to abruptio placenta,[44] a potential disaster for both mother and fetus. Tachycardia and hypertension with resultant cerebral infarction have been noted in the fetus of a cocaine user.[45]

The question of teratogenicity secondary to maternal cocaine abuse is still debated, although anomalies of the genitourinary tract have been observed. Chasnoff and colleagues have observed significant change in interactive behavior and abnormal response to environmental stimuli in infants born to cocaine users.[43] There is no significant deviation from normal gestational age, birth weight, length, or head circumference.

Although cocaine is a highly addictive drug, physiologic dependence does not occur, hence a physiologic withdrawal state does not exist. No well-defined neonatal cocaine withdrawal state has been described.

CONCLUSION

The intensivist in the neonatal care unit, as well as the pediatrician, family practitioner, and the emergency physician, need to consider toxic emergencies when confronted with a neonate exhibiting signs and symptoms not otherwise easily explained. Neonatal sepsis can mimic poisoning, and unless the practitioner has a high index of suspicion the diagnosis will be delayed.

The actual incidence of toxic emergencies in the neonate is not known. The possibility of intoxication requires continued diligence by the physician to ensure early recognition and treatment.

References

1. Roberts RJ: Principles of Neonatal Pharmacology. *In* Avery ME, Taeusch HW Jr: Schaffer's Diseases of the Newborn. 5th ed. Philadelphia, WB Saunders, 1984.
2. Nachman RL, Esterly NB: Increased skin permeability in preterm infants. J Pediatr *79*:628–632, 1971.
3. Morselli PL, Franco-Morselli R, Bossi L: Pharmacokinetics in newborns and infants. Age-related differences and therapeutic implications. Pharmacokinetics *5*:485–527, 1980.
4. Goldbloom RB, Goldbloom A: Boric acid poisoning. Pediatrics, *43*:631, 1953.
5. Elhassani SB: Neonatal poisoning; Causes, manifestations, prevention and management. South Med *79*:12, 1986.
6. Roberts RJ: Drug Therapy in Infants: Pharmacological Principles and Clinical Experience. Philadelphia, WB Saunders, 1984.
7. Motomatsu K, Adachi H, Uno T: Two infant deaths after inhaling baby powder. Chest *75*:448, 1979.
8. Brouilette F, Weber ML: Massive aspiration of talcum powder by an infant. Can Med Assoc J *119*:354, 1978.
9. Mofenson HC, Greensher J, DiTomasso A, Okun S: Baby powder—a hazard. Pediatrics *68*:265, 1981.
10. Timpo AE, Amin JS, Casalino MB, et al: Congenital lead intoxication. Pediatrics *94*:765–767, 1979.
11. Bilderback JB: Group of cases of unknown etiology and diagnosis. Northwest Med *19*:263, 1920.
12. Banzan TM: Mercury poisoning in Argentine babies linked to diapers. Pediatrics *67*:637, 1981.
13. Mercury vapor contamination of infant incubators: A potential hazard. Pediatrics *67*:640, 1979.
14. Chisholm JJ: Management of increased lead absorption and lead poisoning in children. N Engl J Med *289*:1016, 1973.
15. Harper RG, Jing JY: Handbook of Neonatology. 2nd ed. Chicago, Year Book Publishing Company, 1987.
16. Tennenbein M: Continuous naloxone infusion for opiate poisoning in infancy. Pediatrics *105*:645, 1984.
17. Burns LE, Hodgman, JE, Cass AB: Fatal circulatory collapse in premature infants receiving chloramphenicol. N Engl J Med *261*:1318–1321, 1956.
18. Sutherland JM: Fatal cardiovascular collapse in infants receiving large amounts of chloramphenicol. Am J Dis Child *97*:7657, 1959.
19. Kahn A, Blum D: Methyl alcohol poisoning in an eight month old boy: An unusual route of intoxication. Pediatrics *94*:841, 1979.
20. Wenzl JE, Mills SD, McCall JT: Methanol poisoning in an infant: Successful treatment with peritoneal dialysis. Am J Dis Child *116*:445, 1968.
21. McCoy HG, Cipolle RJ, Ehlers SM, Sawchuck RJ, Zaske DE: Severe methanol poisoning. Am J Med *67*:804, 1979.
22. Moss MH: Alcohol-induced hypoglycemia and coma caused by alcohol sponging. Pediatrics *46*:445, 1970.
23. Peden VH, Sammon TJ, Downey DA: Intravenously induced infantile intoxication with ethanol. Pediatrics *83*:40, 1973.
24. Gershanik J, Boecler B, Ensley H, McCloskey S, George W: The gasping syndrome and benzyl alcohol poisoning. N Engl J Med *307*:1384–1388, 1982.
25. Martin-Boyer G, Lebreton R, et al: Outbreak of accidental hexachlorophene poisoning in France. Lancet *1*:91, 1982.
26. Lampert PW, Obrian JS, Garrett R: Hexachlorophene encephalopathy. Acta Neuropathol *23*:326–333, 1973.
27. Shuman RM, Leach RW, Alvord EC: Neurotoxicity of hexachlorophene in humans. Arch Neurol *32*:320, 1973.
28. Gemme G, Ruffa G, Borioli F, et al: Cushing's syndrome due to topical corticosteroids. Am J Dis Child *138*:987–988, 1984.
29. Soler-Soler J, Sagaista-Sauleda J, Cabrera A, Sauleda-Pares J: Effect of verapamil in infants with paroxysmal supraventricular tachycardia. Circulation *59*:876–879, 1979.

30. Porter CJ, Gillehe PC, Garson A Jr, Hesslein PS, Karpawich PP, McNamara DG: Effects of verapamil on supraventricular tachycardia in children. Am J Cardiol *48*:487–491, 1981.
31. Wells DH, Ferlanto JJ: Survival after massive theophylline overdose in a premature infant. Pediatrics *64*:252–253, 1979.
32. Bauer CR, Trottier MCT, Stern L: Systemic cyclopentolate (cyclogyl) toxicity in the newborn infant. J Pediatr *82*:501, 1973.
33. Caputo AR, Schnitzer RE, Linquist TD, et al: Dilation in neonates: A protocol. Pediatrics *69*:77–80, 1982.
34. Jones KL, Smith DW, Ulleland CN, et al: Pattern of malformation in offspring of alcoholic mothers. Lancet *1*:1267–1271, 1973.
35. Lemoine P, Harrousseau H, Borteylu JP, et al: Les enfants des parents alcoholiques. Ouest Med *21*:477–482, 1968.
36. Coles CD, Smith IE, Fernhoff PM, Falek A: Neonatal withdrawal: Characteristics in clinically normal nondysmorphic infants. Pediatrics *105*:445–451, 1984.
37. Chasnoff IJ, Burns WJ, Schnoll SH, Burns KA: Cocaine use in pregnancy. N Engl J Med *313*:666–669, 1985.
38. Hill R: Effects of maternal addiction on the fetus and neonate. *In* Mead Johnson Symposium on Perinatal and Developmental Medicine, Perinatal Pharmacology. Vail, Colorado, 1974.
39. Desmond MM, Schwanecke RP, Wilson GS, et al: Maternal barbiturate utilization and neonatal withdrawal symptomatology. Pediatrics *80*:190–197, 1972.
40. Rementeria JL, Bhatt K: Withdrawal symptoms in neonates from intrauterine exposure to diazepam. Pediatrics *90*:123–126, 1977.
41. Finnegan LP, Leifer MH: The use of phenobarbital in treating abstinence in newborns exposed in-utero to psychoactive drugs. Pediatr Res *17*:371, 1983.
42. Hoder EL, et al: Clonidine treatment of neonatal abstinence syndrome. Psychiat Res *13*:243–251, 1984.
43. Chasnoff IJ, Burns WJ, Schnoll SH, Burns KA: Cocaine use in pregnancy. N Engl J Med *313*:666–669, 1986.
44. Acker D, Sachs BP, Tracey KG, Wise WE: Abruptio placentae associated with cocaine use. Am J Obstet Gynecol *146*:220–221, 1983.
45. Chasnoff IJ, Bussey ME, Savich R, Stack CM: Perinatal cerebral infarction and maternal cocaine use. Pediatrics *108*:456–459, 1986.

CHAPTER 20
GERIATRIC TOXICOLOGY

James Raymond, M.D., FACEP
Timothy Mader, M.D.

Age-dependent changes in the body's physiologic functions often result in unpredictable and eccentric responses to administered drugs. In this chapter we review these consequences of aging and their effects upon drug pharmacology and toxicology. The phenomenon of acute poisoning and its treatment are discussed and strategies for the prevention of drug toxicity are outlined.

THE DIMENSIONS OF AGING

The United States, like many technologically advanced nations, consists of an aging population. Twelve per cent of our population is over 65 years of age, and this proportion is steadily growing.[1, 2] It is estimated to double by the year 2030.[3] Geriatric patients, by their very numbers and their multiple medical problems, present serious logistic challenges to the health care system. They also constitute the most medicated group in society; over 30 per cent of all prescription medicines go to the elderly and some of these drugs tend to be hazardous.[4, 5]

Many factors complicate drug therapy in the geriatric patient. The most important of these include the physiologic alterations of aging, associated disease states, and diminished patient compliance. When evaluating an older polymedicated patient with several chronic illnesses, the clinician is faced with determining whether a particular complaint represents a consequence of normal aging, a manifestation of disease, or an adverse reaction to a medication. Adding to the challenge, some symptoms occur so commonly among the elderly that their diagnostic importance is lost.

Lamy has advocated an approach to this

dilemma based on a division of the aging process into primary (physiologic), secondary (pathophysiologic), and tertiary (sociogenic) aging.[6, 7] *Primary aging* describes the normal physiologic alterations in body function and composition that occur with growing old. These age-related changes affect all organ systems to various degrees and will be discussed briefly in the following section. *Secondary aging* refers to pathophysiologic deviation from the normal process and has been termed "chronic" disease. The heterogeneity of the elderly population is largely attributable to secondary aging. *Tertiary aging*, the effect of imposed socioeconomic factors on the condition of the older patient, is often overlooked as a contributor to aging dynamics. The physician must be aware that the older individual may be living alone on a fixed income, or caring for an incapacitated spouse, with minimal or no outside support from family or friends. Tertiary aging is an important determinant of the success or failure of the elderly person's treatment plan.

AGE-RELATED PHYSIOLOGIC CHANGES AND DRUG DISPOSITION IN THE ELDERLY

Normal aging has important implications for the absorption, distribution, and elimination of drugs (see Chapter 2, Principles of Pharmacology for the Clinician). This section will discuss these age-related physiologic changes and how they affect body composition, organ function (Table 20–1), and drug disposition.

Table 20–1. AGE-RELATED PHYSIOLOGIC CHANGES

BODY COMPOSITION
1. Decreased lean body mass
2. Increased fat
3. Decreased plasma volume
4. Decreased total body water
5. Decreased total plasma albumin

CARDIOVASCULAR SYSTEM
1. Heart
   Decreased cardiac output
   Hypertrophy
   Decreased response to stress
2. Circulation
   Increased systolic blood pressure
   Decreased blood vessel resiliency
   Increased thickness of vessels
   Decreased perfusion to organs, especially kidneys, but also liver, brain, muscles, and gastrointestinal tract

KIDNEYS
1. Decreased glomerular filtration rate and renal blood flow
2. Serum creatinine same but decreased creatinine clearance
3. Decreased tubular maximum for many substances

GASTROINTESTINAL TRACT
1. Decreased gastric secretions
2. Increased gastric pH
3. Decreased active transport
4. Decreased amplitude of esophageal peristalsis
5. Decreased rate of stomach emptying

LIVER
1. Decreased size
2. Decreased number of hepatocytes
3. Altered phase I drug metabolism
4. Decreased protein synthesis

(Modified from Lamy PP: Comparative pharmacokinetic changes and drug therapy in an older population. J Am Geriatr Soc *30*:11, 1982.)

Body Composition

Significant changes occur in body composition during aging.[8] There is a decrease in lean body mass and a proportionate increase in adipose tissue.[9] This shift from lean mass to adiposity, independent of accompanying obesity, occurs in both the active and the sedentary individual. Associated with this are decreases in intracellular and extracellular water.[10] There is also a decline in plasma albumin concentration—a consequence of decreased synthesis, increased catabolism, or both.[11]

Changes in body composition have important implications for drug metabolism. The decrease in total body water results in higher concentrations. The increased ratio of fat to lean body mass alters the volume of distribution for lipophilic and hydrophilic drugs. Finally, the relative decrease in serum albumin levels influences a drug's free concentration through its protein binding affinity.

Cardiovascular System

Occult cardiovascular disease occurs frequently and makes defining normal aging difficult. The influence of diet, smoking, activity, and genetic factors further confuses the distinction. Nevertheless, certain age-related changes occur regularly, which suggests primary aging as their basis. Hypertrophy of the left ventricle develops independently of clinical cardiovascular disease, and overall it appears that cardiac output declines with age.[12–14] Blood vessels generally become thickened and less resilient. These changes may lead to decreased perfusion of the kidneys and liver, and delivery of drugs to other tissues, such as the central nervous system, may be reduced.

Kidneys

Renal plasma flow, glomerular filtration rate, creatinine clearance, and renal tubular function decline with age.[15] In spite of these, the serum creatinine level does not predictably rise because of the elderly person's diminished muscle mass. The creatinine level therefore, is an unreliable guide to renal excretory capacity.[16]

These changes in the kidney influence the clearance of drugs. Alterations in body composition and cardiac output also affect drug excretion through decreased delivery to the kidney. Secondary aging factors (heart and renal diseases) may accentuate this excretory impairment.

Gastrointestinal Tract

Gastric mucosal changes result in altered secretory function and an increased incidence of achlorhydria, which reaches 20 to 30 per cent by the eighth decade.[17, 18] There is also evidence that gastric emptying becomes progressively delayed with age.[19] These observations have important implications with respect to the rate of delivery of drugs to the small intestine, their major site of absorption. Impaired active transport of selected nutrients in the gut has also been documented. These observations may reflect a general reduction in all intestinal active transport, including drugs.[20]

Since most drugs are administered orally, these changes might be expected to impair absorption of many medications. The longer transit time may lead to food-drug interactions, further decreasing absorption. Reduced splanchnic blood flow and active transport may also retard drug absorption and thereby alter the substance's pharmacokinetic properties.

Liver

The weight of the liver decreases after age 50 years. This correlates histologically with a decrease in the number of hepatocytes.[21] Accompanying these gross and microscopic changes are ultrastructural and biochemical alterations that have implications for drug detoxification and metabolism.[22] These latter changes appear to alter phase I drug metabolism while having little effect on phase II reactions.[23] This is of minor importance, however, compared with the metabolic decrease prompted by diminished hepatic blood flow and loss of functioning hepatocytes.

SPECIAL CONSIDERATIONS IN GERIATRIC TOXICOLOGY

Adverse Drug Reactions

Adverse drug reactions (ADRs), which are noxious or unintended responses to the usual doses of drugs, are assumed to occur more frequently with increasing age. This is by no means definitive, as some investigators have found a positive correlation whereas others have not.[24] Most studies demonstrating an association have been conducted on hospital inpatients. Fewer studies have been performed in the outpatient setting where the evidence is mixed. More attention has been focused upon ADRs as a cause of hospitalization, and there appears to be a linear increase with age.[25, 26] Up to 10 per cent of elderly peoples' hospital admissions are the result of ADRs, although one cannot infer from this that the elderly are more susceptible.[27]

Factors independent of age alone appear to be more important as a cause of ADRs. These include multiple drug therapy, chronic illnesses, altered pharmacokinetics and pharmacodynamics, and the types of drugs prescribed. The increased incidence of adverse reactions with aging may be explained by the congregation of many of these factors in the older patient.

Polymedicine

The average number of prescription medications taken by the elderly outpatient is between two and three, with a smaller subset of patients taking five or more.[28] These estimates do not include the consumption of over-the-counter medications, which may be considerable. The highest incidence of polymedicine is in the chronically institutionalized patient, who receives an average of seven drugs.[29, 30]

The incidence of ADRs increases exponentially with the number of drugs taken, indicating that these adverse reactions are not merely additive.[24] A major reason for this nonlinear relationship is that patients taking large numbers of medications are often severely ill and thereby may be predisposed to adverse drug effects. Drug doses are also likely to be higher in the severely ill, thus increasing the probability of ADRs.[31] Finally, drug-drug interactions are more common as the number of medications increases. All these factors present a hazard in the elderly and elimination of even one or two drugs from their formulary may reduce this risk.

Multiplicity and Severity of Disease

The diseases necessitating drug therapy in the elderly tend to be serious and often require aggressive medical management. This may involve the use of potent drugs that have a potential for untoward effects. The low therapeutic indices of many of these (digoxin, coumadin, insulin, antiarrhythmic agents, and antihypertensive agents) create a situation conducive to toxicity and ADRs.

With aging, chronic diseases are accumulated and carried along. These illnesses, along with their escalating drug therapy, also increase the likelihood of ADRs and drug-disease interactions.

Drug-Drug Interactions

Administration of two or more drugs within a relatively short time may result in potentiation of action, accumulation of side effects, antagonism, or indifference.[32] Potentiation refers to the enhancement of one drug's action by another. Antagonism is the reduction in a drug's action by another. Accumulation of side effects occurs when drugs with similar side effects are given together. The elderly are at risk from all these possible reactions because they are usually taking multiple medications. Over-the-counter medications can possess serious side effects as well as being another source of potential drug-drug interactions.

Drug-Disease Interactions

Secondary aging effects (i.e., chronic illness) influence drug disposition in important ways. Congestive heart failure—for instance, through reduced organ perfusion—may hamper absorption and distribution of some drugs. Hepatic dysfunction, an accompaniment of some chronic illnesses, may interfere with drug metabolism and clearance. Renal impairment also has predictable effects on drug excretion.

Certain drugs used to treat one disease may exacerbate another. The use of beta-adrenergic blockers for hypertension or angina pectoris can exacerbate asthma or existing cardiac disease. Nonsteroidal anti-inflammatory drugs used in musculoskeletal disorders may worsen or precipitate renal dysfunction. It is likely that these drug-disease interactions occur with more frequency in the elderly than do drug-drug interactions.[32]

Drug-Nutrition Interactions

Malnutrition, the state of many elderly patients, increases the risk for ADRs. Inadequate intake of essential nutrients can alter the pharmacokinetics of many drugs.[33] Certain foods may reduce the bioavailability of drugs, and some medicines can influence food absorption, which then may modify the gastrointestinal uptake of ingested drugs. The elderly are at risk for many of these interactions.

ACUTE POISONING IN THE ELDERLY

Unintentional Poisoning

Most acute poisonings are unintentional. While the majority of these involve children 5 years old or younger, the most serious ones occur in adults and account for 95 per cent of reported deaths.[34] Thirteen per cent of accidental poison deaths are in patients 65 years or older, and the highest death rate for any age group occurs in those over 80 years (3 to 4 deaths per 100,000 population).[35]

Poisoning agents include a wide variety of drugs, chemicals, natural substances, and commercial products. Commonly ingested drugs include sedative-hypnotics, analgesics, cardiovascular agents, and antidepressants. Although most of these mishaps occur in the home environment, a smaller yet significant number occur in nursing homes and hospitals.

Kline-Schwartz and associates[34] have studied poisoning exposures in the elderly and have categorized the principal contributing factors: senility or confusion, improper use of a product, improper storage of an agent, or mistaking one agent for another. Prevention efforts should take these precipitants into consideration.

Intentional Poisoning

Suicide is a serious problem among geriatric patients. Persons over 65 years of age account for 25 per cent of all successful suicides.[36] Elderly white men are particularly susceptible, and they commit suicide at a rate four times that of the national average. Suicide attempts among the aged tend to be more serious than in the younger individual. An unsuccessful attempt in the older patient usually leads to a successful one within a year of the initial incident.[37]

The major predisposing factors to geriatric suicide appear to be the presence of significant underlying medical or psychiatric illness. Batchelor reported that among elderly patients who attempted suicide, 60 per cent had serious underlying medical disease and 80 per cent were suffering from depression.[38] Organic brain syndrome has been reported to correlate highly with suicide attempts in the older individual. There is some controversy about this association, however, since successful suicide involves coordination, planning, and an awareness of reality, all of which may be impaired by this disorder.[36]

Following gunshots and hanging, drug ingestion is the third most popular method of suicide in the aged; one third of these involve prescribed drugs.[39] Most individuals poison themselves with readily available substances. The elderly have more access to prescription drugs than any other segment of the population, and they may hoard these medications over a long period of time. Benson and Brodie have pointed out the decreasing use of barbiturates and the increasing role of the newer tranquilizing agents and antidepressants.[39] Flanagan and associates, reporting on their experience from the United Kingdom, note that the three most frequently ingested drugs in decreasing order were benzodiazepines, barbiturates, and tricyclic antidepressants.[40] A majority of the patients ingested two or more drugs. It is possible that the spectrum of ingested drugs will evolve as new pharmaceuticals reach the market and physicians' prescribing habits change.

As the percentage of aging individuals grows, their incidence of suicide is likely to increase. The problem of prevention will be a difficult one. Apart from the treatment of mental and physical illness, the physician must be alert for those at risk and cautious in drug-dispensing practices.

Management of Acute Ingestions in the Elderly

With two major caveats, the principles of management are identical to those for the younger patient (see Chapter 1, The Emergency Management of Poisoning). First, most elderly patients are suffering from at least one chronic disease. Treatment of the ingestion should not exacerbate these illnesses if at all possible. As a general rule, avoiding forced diuresis precludes the risk of volume overload, a hazard in older individuals. Second, many geriatric patients are taking more than one medication. The superimposed acute ingestion can give rise to ADRs and

Table 20–2. RECOMMENDATIONS FOR THE PREVENTION OF DRUG TOXICITY IN THE ELDERLY

Take a careful drug history.
Know the pharmacokinetics of the drug(s).
Individualize the dose and titrate, starting with smaller doses.
Simplify the drug regimen and review it regularly.
Avoid polymedicine at all costs.
Use medication cards, diaries, and so on.
Have the patient bring in all medication bottles.
Destroy old medicines.
Educate the patient and family concerning medications prescribed.
Educate the patient and family about over-the-counter drugs.
Maintain a high index of suspicion for drug toxicity.

(Modified from Tandberg D: How to treat and prevent drug toxicity. Geriatrics *36*:64, 1981.)

drug-drug interactions that may complicate the patient's management. After satisfactory recovery, psychiatric evaluation is imperative in cases of intentional ingestion.

Old age itself should never be a deterrent to aggressive therapy. In acute overdose, a complete medical history is often unavailable. Although the patient may have an underlying terminal illness or a severe debilitating one, these facts may not come to light until the initial resuscitation has been completed. There is time enough after the patient's admission to decide how intensive subsequent management should be.[41] The ethical issues surrounding the management of suicide in the elderly have been thoughtfully addressed by Bromberg and Cassel.[42]

DRUG TOXICITY PREVENTION IN THE ELDERLY

Prevention of drug toxicity is a major responsibility facing the physician who cares for the older patient. Unfortunately, few busy physicians take the time required to give information about the drugs they are prescribing. Patient noncompliance may further compound this situation.

As a first step, the physician needs a detailed drug history; this should not be restricted to current prescription medications and drug allergies but must include information about the use of over-the-counter drugs, the patient's reliability in taking scheduled drugs, diet, the use of alcoholic beverages, and the ability to pay for medications. The patient must then receive clear information from the physician concerning prescribed drugs. A drug's action should be explained in simple, nonscientific terms and the dosing regimen carefully detailed. Side effects should be discussed as well as the interactions of the drug with food, alcohol, and other medications. Finally, the use of generic substitutes should be explained.

Tandberg has developed a list of suggestions to help reduce the potential for adverse drug effects (Table 20–2).[43] By following these simple, logical recommendations, it may be possible to prevent some of the serious consequences of drug toxicity in the elderly.

References

1. US Department of Commerce: Statistical Abstract of the United States. Washington, DC, Bureau of Census, 1985.
2. Grundy E: Demography and old age. J Am Geriatr Soc *31*:325, 1983.
3. Pegels CC: Health care expenditures for the elderly. Prim Care *9*:249, 1982.
4. Lamy PP: New dimensions and opportunities. Drug Intell Clin Pharm *19*:399, 1985.
5. Lamy PP: Comparative pharmacokinetic changes and drug therapy in an older population. J Am Geriatr Soc *30*:11, 1982.
6. Michocki RJ, Lamy PP: A "risk" approach to adverse drug reactions. J Am Geriatr Soc *36*:79, 1988.
7. Lamy PP: Renal effects of nonsteroidal anti-inflammatory drugs. Heightened risk of the elderly? J Am Geriatr Soc *34*:586, 1986.
8. Bruce A, Anderson M, Arvidsson B: Body composition. Prediction of normal body potassium, body water and body fat in adults on the basis of body height, body weight and age. Scand J Clin Lab Invest *40*:461, 1980.
9. Forbes GB, Reina JC: Adult lean body mass declines with age: Some longitudinal observations. Metabolism *19*:653, 1970.
10. Shock NW, Watkins DM, Viengst BS: Age differences in the water content of the body as related to basal oxygen consumption in males. J Gerontol *18*:1, 1963.
11. Greenblatt DJ: Reduced serum albumin concentration in the elderly: A report from the Boston Collaborative Drug Surveillance Program. J Am Geriatr Soc *27*:20, 1979.
12. Port S, Cobb FR, Coleman E: Effect of age on the response of the left ventricular ejection fraction to exercise. N Engl J Med *303*:1133, 1980.
13. Gerstenblith G, Lakatta EG, Weisfeldt ML: Age changes in myocardial function and exercise response. Prog Cardiovasc Dis *19*:1, 1976.
14. Julius S, Antoon A, Whitlock LS, Conway J: Influence of age on the hemodynamic response to exercise. Circulation *36*:222, 1967.
15. Rowe JW, Andrew R, Robin JD: The effect of age on creatinine clearance in men: A cross-sectional and longitudinal study. J Gerontol *31*:155, 1976.
16. Cockroft DW, Gault MH: Prediction of creatinine clearance from serum creatinine. Nephron *16*:31, 1976.
17. Andrews GR, Haneman B, Arnold BJ: Atrophic gastritis in the aged. Austr Ann Med *16*:230, 1967.
18. Geokas MC, Haverback BJ: The aging gastrointestinal tract. Am J Surg *17*:881, 1969.
19. Brandt LJ: Gastrointestinal disorders in the elderly. *In* Rossman I (ed): Clinical Geriatrics. 3rd ed. Philadelphia, JB Lippincott, 1986, p 260.
20. Montgomery R, Hazney MR, Ross IN: The aging gut: A study of intestinal absorption in relation to nutrition in the elderly. Q J Med *47*:197, 1978.
21. Thomas FB, Clausen K, Greenberger NJ: Liver disease in multiple myeloma. Arch Intern Med *132*:195, 1973.
22. Tauchi H, Sato T: Some micromeasuring studies of hepatic cells in senility. J Gerontol *17*:254, 1962.
23. Schmucker DL: Drug disposition in the elderly: A review of the critical factors. J Am Geriatr Soc *32*:144, 1984.
24. Nolan L, O'Malley K: Prescribing for the elderly. Part I: Sensitivity of the elderly to adverse drug reactions. J Am Geriatr Soc *36*:142, 1988.
25. McKenney JM, Harrison WL: Drug-related hospital admissions. Am J Hosp Pharm *33*:792, 1976.
26. Levy M, Lipshitz W, Eliakim M: Hospital admissions

due to adverse drug reactions. Am J Med Sci 227:49, 1979.
27. Williamson J, Chopin JM: Adverse reactions to prescribed drugs in the elderly: A multicentre investigation. Age Ageing 9:73, 1980.
28. Nolan L, O'Malley K: Prescribing for the elderly. Part II: Prescribing patterns: Differences due to age. J Am Geriatr Soc 36:245, 1988.
29. Segal JL, Thompson JF, Floyd RA: Drug utilization and prescribing patterns in a skilled nursing facility: The need for a rational approach to therapeutics. J Am Geriatr Soc 27:117, 1979.
30. Bergman HD: Prescribing of drugs in a nursing home. Drug Intell Clin Pharm 9:365, 1975.
31. Steel K, Gertman PM, Crescenzi C, Anderson J: Iatrogenic illness on a general medical service at a university hospital. N Engl J Med 304:638, 1981.
32. Lamy PP: The elderly and drug interaction. J Am Geriatr Soc 34:586, 1986.
33. Lamy PP: The elderly, undernutrition and pharmacokinetics. J Am Geriatr Soc 30:560, 1983.
34. Klein-Schwartz W, Oderda GM, Booze L: Poisoning in the elderly. J Am Geriatr Soc 31:195, 1983.
35. Oderda GM, Klein-Schwartz W: Poison prevention in the elderly. Drug Intell Clin Pharm 18:183, 1984.
36. Sendbuehler JM, Goldstein S: Attempted suicide among the aged. J Am Geriatr Soc 25:245, 1977.
37. Gardner E, Bahn A, Mack M: Suicide and psychiatric care in the aging. Arch Gen Psychiat 10:547, 1964.
38. Batchelor IRC: Management and prognosis of suicidal attempts in old age. Geriatrics 10:291, 1955.
39. Benson RA, Brodie DC: Suicide by overdoses of medicines among the aged. J Am Geriatr Soc 23:304, 1975.
40. Flanagan RJ, Caldwell R, Lewis RR, Corless D: Toxicological investigations in the detection of drug-induced disease in elderly patients. Hum Toxicol 2:371, 1983.
41. Crome P: ABC of poisoning: The elderly. Br Med J 289:546, 1984.
42. Bromberg S, Cassel CK: Suicide in the elderly: The limits of paternalism. J Am Geriatr Soc 31:698, 1983.
43. Tandberg D: How to treat and prevent drug toxicity. Geriatrics 36:64, 1981.

CHAPTER 21
PSYCHIATRIC EVALUATION OF THE SUICIDAL PATIENT

Richard B. Warner, M.D.

SUICIDE EVALUATION AND CRISIS INTERVENTION

Two principal psychiatric tasks should be accomplished with any suicidal patient who presents to an emergency setting. These are the *evaluation of suicide potential* and the *initiation of crisis intervention.* The evaluation of suicide potential involves an assessment of the circumstances in a patient's life that have become sufficiently overwhelming to motivate a suicidal response. It also includes inquiry about the patient's plan for suicide and evaluation of several releasing factors that contribute to overcoming the patient's usual inhibition of suicide. The role of significant people in promoting or restraining the patient's suicidal activity also must be considered.

The first step of crisis intervention is helping the patient achieve a definition of the problems that are overwhelming him or her. Attempts at coping with the problems are also reviewed, and the patient should be helped to wonder how he or she selected suicide as a solution. Possible resources should be explored and alternatives to suicide promoted. At the end of the initial evaluation, it is hoped that the patient will emerge with a better understanding of the crisis and how it has affected him or her and a more adaptive plan for dealing with it. The extent to which this has happened will have an important bearing on further treatment planning.

Although the tasks of evaluation and intervention may be conceptualized separately, in practice they have much in common. Both tasks require that the interviewer attempt to form a working relationship with the patient and try to understand the meaning of the suicidal fantasy or behavior. Suicide is usually a response to some set of recent circumstances that the patient feels cannot be controlled by less drastic means. Many times the patient does not have a clear idea of the precipitant of the suicidal behavior or why an event should have such a drastic or overwhelming impact.

Taking a history of the circumstances that have led to the self-destructive behavior can help both the interviewer and the patient understand the motivation of the behavior. Taking such a history is also the first step in helping a patient put an overwhelming situation into a more definable and manageable perspective.

The Psychology of Suicide

Several psychologic phenomena characteristic of suicidal thinking have both diagnostic and therapeutic implications. The first of these is ambivalence. Every patient, no matter how hopeless or determined he or she may seem, is of two minds in the face of dying. Dying may be attractive as a method of withdrawing from a situation or assuming final control. Killing oneself may be a way of dealing with another terrifying impulse, such as killing someone else. Self-injury may be a form of self-punishment or a means of inflicting guilt on and extracting love from another. A suicidal fantasy may have any or several of these motives, and the patient should be helped to talk about them because in articulating them, some of their magical power tends to be dissipated. At the same time, the prospect of self-annihilation is usually terrifying, and it is helpful to point out some of the actions that suggest the patient wants help in resisting such impulses. This is not done in a spirit of arguing with the patient or proving to him that he does not want to die. Rather, it is important to help the patient recognize his own wish for help and to reassure him that this wish will be taken seriously.

Although suicide may often seem at first glance the act of a person in isolated despair, it is usually a dyadic event. The patient's suicidal fantasy usually involves at least one other person. This is most obvious in the case of a young person who reacts to rejection by a boyfriend or girlfriend with a sublethal overdose of medicine. In such cases a desperate attempt to force love is the primary purpose; dying is a remote consideration. In an older person reacting to loss of physical health and youthful self-image, the communicational aspect of a suicide may be harder to discern. But the act is often an indictment of persons perceived as not being sufficiently caring or responsive. This communication may be disguised in the patient's talk of being a burden on family. Clues to the communication inherent in the suicidal behavior may be found in suicide notes, good-byes, or the choice of means, e.g., a spouse's pills or a doctor's prescription. The important other person in the patient's fantasy may not be someone in the immediate surroundings but a person who has died previously and is ambivalently missed and thought of as having abandoned the patient. The patient may not be readily aware of this aspect of the suicidal behavior, and its elucidation is a part of the crisis intervention.

A person who is overwhelmed in a crisis and feels helpless typically regresses to the magical thinking characteristic of children.[1, 2] An awareness of this fact can help the interviewer use his or her imagination to appreciate the power of the suicidal patient's fantasies. In such a state of mind, the patient is more egocentric than usual, expects others to see the world just as he or she does, and has difficulty appreciating another person's range of feelings. The patient has trouble appreciating subtleties and options; rather, he or she sees matters in a black or white fashion.

Feeling powerless, the patient may ascribe great power to others, wishing them to be all-loving, all-knowing, and all nurturing, and fearing them to be all-hating and destroying. Such a psychologic position often engenders a patient's resentment toward the more powerful people who disappoint him, which may affect the budding relationship with a clinician who is trying to be helpful. Resorting to the opposite of powerlessness, the patient may magically expect to control others completely by his own actions and therefore be further disappointed when he fails. The patient may cope with his or her helplessness by infecting others with the same feeling and taking some consolation from the shared misery. Recognizing this regression in thinking is a diagnostic aid to the interviewer, and helping the patient see the unrealistic absolutes around which his thinking has become organized can be a first step toward regaining a more mature perspective, which the interviewer models.

Clinical Interactions

If the interviewer is aware of the regressed modes of thinking, he or she is likely also to be more understanding of the concomitant emotions that the patient may be experiencing. It is common to encounter feelings of embarrassment, shame, guilt, hostility, and self-depreciation. These feelings may be related not only to the crisis that has precipitated the suicidal behavior but also may be a reaction to the regression, the state of helplessness, and the behavior that has resulted.

Unfortunately, patients may find these feelings reinforced by the punitive response they may find in a hospital emergency room. Patients may encounter overt hostility in comments that are made to them by physicians and nurses, or they may find themselves the object of not so "benign neglect" as they lie unattended for several hours. These reactions to suicidal patients are usually the result of discomforting feelings they arouse in people who usually want to be helpful. An awareness of the source of these reactions is essential to the clinician who deals with such patients if a therapeutic outcome is to be achieved.[3]

Two of the more common feelings that clinicians hold toward suicidal patients are anger and disgust. If acted upon directly, these feelings can motivate sadistic behavior toward a patient. On the other hand, attempts at denying such feelings may result in other inappropriate behaviors, such as being overly solicitous toward patients or prematurely withdrawing from them. Anger and disgust in a professional who does not usually feel this way toward patients may reflect an intolerable feeling of helplessness resulting from interacting with suicidal patients.

Suicidal patients can behave in a number of ways that frustrate attempts to help and make the clinician feel helpless and inclined to an angry response. Patients may openly express hostility and denigrate the interviewer. They may express their hostility more passively by not talking with the interviewer or by saying that their problems are their own business and no one else's. In these situations it is sometimes helpful toward establishing a working relationship with patients to point out that they are acting as though their main problem is with the interviewer. In reality the problems that have brought them to desperate measures lie elsewhere in their lives, and that is what needs talking about. If the clinician can remain firm, warm, responsive, and nonjudgmental, most patients will respond with better cooperation.

ASSESSMENT OF SUICIDE POTENTIAL

In the course of the evaluation, several factors must be considered in judging the patient's lethal potential (Table 21–1).

Demographic Data

Certain demographic data relating to suicide potential are often cited.[4] It is a fact that older people are more often lethal in their suicide attempts than are younger people. Likewise, men are more often successful than women, and single people are at greater risk than married people. However, although such statistical considerations should raise the level of concern about people who are in high-risk categories, it cannot be concluded that people in the lower risk categories are not potentially lethal. The clinician should have criteria by which individualized assessment of patients can be accomplished.

Precipitating Crisis

First of all, it is important to get as clear a picture as possible of the circumstances to which the patient is reacting. Most often this will involve some elements of loss or threat of loss for the patient. Some of the more obvious and dramatic losses are interpersonal, as in death, divorce, or rejection by a loved one. Other crises include loss of phys-

Table 21–1. FACTORS IN AN EVALUATION OF SUICIDE POTENTIAL

Demographic data
Precipitating crisis
Suicide plan
History of previous attempts
Releasing factors
Hopelessness
Depression
Psychosis, organic or functional
Drugs and alcohol
Isolation and dissociation
Role of others

ical well-being, job, home, or financial status. Medical illness is often implicated in suicide among the elderly. The prospect of legal prosecution may threaten the patient's security.

Some losses are more subtle, as when a person reacts desperately to the threat of increased responsibility and loss of the familiar routine, which can attend a success such as a job promotion. In such an instance, a person may be reacting to the prospect of humiliation, an emotion that is commonly involved in suicidal behavior.

Obviously, most people sustain losses without resorting to suicide, and it is important to understand the meaning of the loss to the patient in order to understand why the person is now suicidal. Such meaning may not at first be obvious to the outside observer, but nonetheless, the losses may be devastating to the patient's self-image and sense of security and control over his or her own destiny.

Suicide Plan

The presence of a suicide plan is an ominous sign, and the patient's thoughts about such a plan should be explored in detail. How long has the patient been considering the plan, and has he or she become more obsessed with it? What means of suicide is being considered, and how lethal is that method likely to be? How available is the means to the patient? For example, if the patient is talking about using a gun to commit suicide, the interviewer would want to know if the patient has a gun or has taken any steps to acquire one. Also, has the patient settled on a particular time, place, or set of circumstances in which the plan will be enacted? Such detailed thinking bespeaks of the patient's serious intentions. In addition to a specific plan for suicide, the interviewer should also inquire about other indications of deliberate death-oriented activity such as putting business affairs in order, writing or revising a will, and instructing others about how certain matters should be handled in the patient's absence.

Although the presence of any of these indicators of suicidal intention is ominous, their absence should not be taken as a sign that the patient is not in danger. The planned suicide is characteristic of the depressed patient who has been inadequately coping with loss, actual or impending, for a period of time. Many suicides are committed impulsively in response to the patient being overwhelmed by both circumstances and dysphoric affect, often when judgment is impaired by psychosis or intoxication.

History of Previous Attempts

Previous suicide attempts in the patient's history should be thoroughly reviewed for several reasons. Previous attempts will often be evidence of an underlying psychiatric disorder, most commonly an affective disorder, which warrants diagnosis and treatment. Inquiry about specific methods attempted and how the patient happened to survive can help the interviewer gauge how lethal the patient has been in the past. Recalling circumstances in the patient's life which led to such despair may also shed light on the meaning of the current situation. The patient should also be asked about the response of other people to the prior attempts. That response may have a bearing on the communicative aspect of the current suicidal fantasy. The very fact of a previous attempt is important as an indicator of the patient having previously overcome the usual taboo or inhibition of suicide. With successive attempts and recurrent suicidal thinking, the patient may become desensitized to the horror of suicide and find it easier to enact.

A history of suicide in the patient's family or other close relationships also can be significant. Such a suicide may provide a model for the patient, or the patient may be entertaining a fantasy of reunion in the afterlife. Occasionally, a patient will become increasingly suicidal around the time of the anniversary of a parent's suicide or at the age at which the parent died. Aside from the meanings that a suicide in the family may hold, a family history of suicide may also be important in terms of a major psychiatric disorder with a genetic component, such as schizophrenia or an affective disorder.

Releasing Factors

Although many people entertain thoughts of suicide at some time in their lives, and some people think about it throughout their lives and occasionally enact such thoughts, all people maintain an inhibition of the suicidal impulse most of the time. It is important, then, to evaluate several acute phenomena that act as releasing factors, allowing the person to enter a state of mind in which the inhibition of suicide is lessened. The first of these has been mentioned, an overwhelming personal crisis, which the person cannot set into a manageable perspective with options for mastery. Constricted thinking in reaction to the crisis leads to a settling on suicide as the solution.[5] In the chronically suicidal person, the precipitating crisis usually is seen by the person as the latest in a long series of defeats. Often the particular meanings of the current crisis are quickly generalized to such global statements as "life is not worth living" or "no one cares what happens to me." In considering the patient's suicide potential, the clinician should judge the patient's ability to restore the crisis to discrete proportions, to locate it in time and place, and to deal with it as a problem on which he or she wants to work. If the crisis remains mired in a global sense of life's futility, then the patient has made no progress in gaining a more adaptive perspective.

Other factors that allow a person to enter a suicidal state of mind include hopelessness, depression, psychosis, intoxication, and dissociation.

Hopelessness

An entrenched sense of hopelessness is a particularly ominous sign and plays an important role in releasing inhibitions of suicide.[6, 7] The person who despairs of any improvement in his or her future situation usually feels isolated, is unable to think creatively, and is more likely to be motivated toward suicide by magical fantasies of withdrawal and relief or punishment and destruction. Some patients may not talk directly of feeling hopeless, and the interviewer's clue to such feelings may be personal frustration and hopelessness while listening to the patient's story. Patients should be asked directly if they see any prospect of their situation improving and what would be needed for any improvement. Hopeless people have great difficulty imagining their future in any but bleak terms. A person in true despair may have trouble remembering a time as bad as the present. However, asking the patient to compare the present with other difficult times can lead to a discussion of how the person did manage to cope with earlier crises, which may be helpful in the current crisis.

Depression

Hopelessness is often a prominent symptom of depression. Depression, considered as an illness, often fosters the suicidal state of mind and releases the inhibition against suicide. The clinician should ask about the development of the other common symptoms of depression and consider that diagnosis. Depressive symptoms can be considered in three groups.[8, 9] The first is an emotional grouping and includes persistent mood disturbances such as sadness, crying, anxiety, and irritability. The second cluster consists of cognitive manifestations that reflect a disturbance in how one views the self, the environment, and the future. Included in this group is a preoccupation with guilt, lowered self-esteem, loss of interest in usual activities and friends, and a negative outlook on the future. The third grouping consists of biologic or vegetative alterations. The most common of these are disturbed appetite with weight loss; disturbed sleep, particularly early morning awakening; and easy fatigability. Loss of libido is also a common symptom. Difficulty with concentration; slowing down of motor movements, speech, and thinking; and a diurnal variation in symptoms (the worst occurring in the morning) may also accompany depression. Finally, a persistent preoccupation with somatic complaints can be a sign of depression. When a patient has several of the symptoms just mentioned for longer than 1 month, the diagnosis of depression should be made. Further psychiatric evaluation should be arranged to discern subtypes of affective disorders and to institute any appropriate pharmacologic or somatic treatments.

Psychosis

Psychosis of any origin can aggravate a person's tendency toward suicide, often in an impulsive and unpredictable manner. Psychosis is defined as a severe mental disorder that interferes grossly with a person's ability to cope with the demands of everyday life. This interference may result from delusions and hallucinations, which compromise the person's capacity to apprehend reality. Cognitive abilities such as attention, memory, and abstract thinking may be impaired to a degree that also disturbs reality testing and judgment. In severe affective disorders, the person's mood may be so altered that appropriate reactivity to the environment is severely limited.

Discerning the presence of psychosis is a major diagnostic task in any suicide evaluation. It is accomplished by consideration of the history of the patient's recent behavior, the patient's demeanor and thought processes as evidenced through the interview, and specific features of the mental status examination. Delusional thinking usually becomes apparent in the course of the interview, but specific inquiry to determine the extent and elaboration of delusions can be helpful. Similarly, the patient should be asked about hallucinations, particularly hearing voices or seeing things; and, if the patient has experienced such phenomena, how disturbing are the hallucinations? Testing of cognitive abilities of orientation of time, place, and person; memory of three items after 5 minutes; and serial subtraction of sevens comprise a minimal screening procedure that will help to ascertain the presence of impaired thinking.

The diagnosis should lead to further differentiation of functional and organic etiologies. Delirium, or acute organic brain syndrome as it is often labeled, is a common entity in an emergency department, and delirious patients are at high risk for impulsive suicidal behavior. The diagnosis of delirium should be considered in the presence of fluctuating levels of consciousness, disorientation, and memory impairment. There are often hallucinations, most commonly visual, and the patient's speech may be incoherent. Sleep disturbances and altered psychomotor activity are also common features. Diagnosing the presence of delirium does not indicate the etiology, which can include any process that has a pathologic effect on brain tissue. Intoxication, metabolic imbalance, infection, circulatory disturbance, trauma, and mass lesions all must be considered.

The most common functional psychoses seen in emergency department settings are schizophrenia and mania. These patients have markedly disorganized thought processes and may entertain bizarre delusions. Their hallucinations are more commonly auditory. The disorganization often puts these patients at the mercy of their own dangerous impulses because the patients have less ability to tolerate the fears accompanying the delusions. Again, further psychiatric evaluation will need to be arranged to provide a more specific diagnosis and appropriate treatment.

Drugs and Alcohol

A very common factor in the release of suicide inhibition is drug intoxication. Alcohol is particularly notorious for its effects both on mood and rational judgment. The fact that alcohol alters consciousness not only puts the suicidal patient at a higher risk when intoxicated but also makes it hard for the patient to fully appreciate his own suicidal state of mind after he sobers up. Commonly, an alcoholic patient minimizes not only the extent of his drinking problem but also his lethality and likelihood of re-entering the suicidal state of mind. Clinicians are often tempted to collude with patients in regarding the episode of suicidal behavior as "just something that happened" when the patient was drunk. The likelihood of the patient's continuing to drink must be estimated.

Alcohol is a factor in suicide not only through its acute effect of intoxication but also through the deteriorating lifestyle of the chronic alcoholic. Approximately 15 per cent of alcoholics end their lives by suicide.[10] This is not hard to understand when one considers the loss of relationships, employment, and physical health that attend alcoholism. These events commonly result in intense feelings of loneliness, worthlessness, and hopelessness, which provide a setting for suicide.

In considering the lethal effects of alcohol, one should mention not only its psychologic and social effects but also its toxicologic interaction with other central nervous system depressants. People who abuse alcohol commonly have access to other medications, which may be abused as well. The combination of barbiturates and alcohol is a lethal and common example of this.

Although alcohol is the most common drug of abuse, the whole range of substances that alter mood and consciousness must be considered, both for their acute effects and their association with depression and a deteriorating lifestyle. Stimulants, depressants, and hallucinogens have all been implicated in suicide.

Isolation and Dissociation

The dyadic aspect of suicidal behavior was stressed earlier, but consideration must also be given to the extent and the ways in which the patient has become isolated. People who have attempted suicide with lethal intent often have reduced their contact with others and, perhaps more important, have reduced the significance they assign to their relationships. The movement into a suicidal state of mind is often abetted by a dissociation in which the person does not experience bonds of affection with their usual strength. This allows the person to rationalize that his or her death will have no real effect on other people. At the same time, people contemplating suicide may also be dissociated from their own feelings and may experience an emotional numbness that allows them to see their own lives as holding less value. Such a state of mind makes the act of suicide easier to commit.

Role of Others

Another dimension to assess is the role of other people in either the inhibition or aggravation of suicide.[11] In many cases, family members may overtly encourage the patient to commit suicide by making statements that leave little doubt that they would be happier with the person dead. Such statements can include sarcastic comments made after an unsuccessful suicide attempt, or there may be taunts and dares provoking the person to complete the threatened suicidal act. More often, a family's death wishes will be expressed covertly through ignoring clues to the person's intentions. The family's attitude toward the patient can be surmised from the manner in which family members mobilize at the time of the emergency department visit. The clinician should observe such reactions as a reluctance to become involved, a tendency to deny the seriousness of the person's difficulties or motivations, or oversolicitousness in a way that prevents the person from ventilating any angry feelings. Such behavior can be more important than stated intentions to be available to the patient.

Family and other intimates should be interviewed not only to assess their attitudes toward the patient but also to provide more information about events that have led up to the suicide attempt. The patient may have minimized or hidden information or may be so compromised by a mental disorder that outside information is essential. Another source of information will often be a psychotherapist or physician whom the patient has seen recently. Many suicidal patients are already in treatment, and their primary therapist should be involved in both the suicide assessment and treatment planning.

Treatment Planning

In considering the factors discussed so far, it should be apparent that there are no simple items that can reliably assure the clinician that a patient does not pose a further risk of suicide. These areas of assessment cannot be added together to give a score that indicates whether the patient should be hospitalized or sent home. Rather, they are each an aspect of a multifaceted evaluation, and any of them can be sufficiently prominent in a particular patient to lead the clinician to decide that further hospitalization is necessary to protect the patient. In general, the treatment decisions should be made conservatively, with a thorough understanding of those factors that impel the patient toward suicide and those that offer hope of resolving the crisis in a more constructive way. When there is no sense that a crisis is moving toward resolution or when releasing factors remain active, hospitalization usually will be indicated. On the other hand, in the case of a patient who has been able to engage in a discussion that moves toward hope and mastery and who has reliable support, hospitalization may be counterproductive, and outpatient treatment is indicated.

CONCLUSION

Having discussed the range of factors to be considered in evaluating suicidal potential, I will make a few suggestions about working with the patient who has made a suicide attempt. In addition to keeping in mind the psychologic characteristics discussed in the early part of this chapter, the clinician must appreciate the extent to which the patient's thinking is organically impaired by the overdose itself. The patient should be given plenty of time to achieve a sober state of mind. In addition, some attention to physical comfort will aid the development of a working relationship. A question like "How are you feeling?" should precede any discussion of "Why have you done this?"[12]

Although any emergency department setting must place a premium on efficient work, the evaluation of the suicidal person should not be rushed.[13] Premature dispositions are often not effective and may aggravate the person's dangerousness. One of the ways in which the clinician's impatience can be manifested is taking over decisions and making plans for the patient. Psychologic regression is more effectively interrupted when a clinician (1) facilitates the patient's ability to do whatever is possible for him- or herself and (2) supports whatever mature functioning is possible.

Before deciding to release a patient from the emergency department, the clinician should be able to satisfy several questions. (1) Do I have a good picture of the patient's state of mind in which suicide was attempted? (i.e., motivation, crisis, releasing factors that foster or allow suicidal thoughts). (2) What is the likelihood of the patient getting into the state of mind again in the near future? (3) Has there been any movement toward mastering the crisis? (4) Will others support or undermine that mastery? The clinician without mental health specialty training and experience will usually seek psychiatric consultation to get these questions answered. Finally, no suicidal patient should be returned to an environment of isolation but should have a clear and open line of communication to a helpful person.

References

1. Odier C: Anxiety and Magic Thinking. New York, International Universities Press, 1956.
2. Horowitz MJ: Stress Response Syndromes. New York, Jason Aronson, 1976.
3. Maltsberger JT, Buie DH: Countertransference hate in the treatment of suicidal patients. Arch Gen Psychiatr *30*:625, 1974.
4. Robins E: Suicide. *In* Kaplan HI, Sadock BJ (eds): Comprehensive Textbook of Psychiatry. 4th ed. Baltimore, Williams & Wilkins, 1985.
5. Shneidman ES: Some essentials of suicide and some implications for response. *In* Roy A (ed): Suicide. Baltimore, Williams & Wilkins, 1986.
6. Minkoff K, Bergman E, Beck AT, Beck R: Hopelessness, depression, and attempted suicide. Am J Psychiatr *130*:455, 1973.
7. Beck AT, Kovacs M, Weissman A: Hopelessness and suicidal behavior: An overview. JAMA *234*:1146, 1975.
8. Beck AT: Depression: Causes and Treatment. Philadelphia, University of Pennsylvania Press, 1967.
9. Dubovsky SL, Weissberg MP: Clinical Psychiatry in Primary Care. 3rd ed. Baltimore, Williams & Wilkins, 1986.
10. Klerman GL: Clinical Epidemiology of Suicide. J Clin Psychiatr *48*suppl:33, 1987.
11. Rosenbaum M, Richman J: Suicide: The role of hostility and death wishes from the family and significant others. Am J Psychiatr *126*:1652, 1970.
12. Spitz L: The evolution of a psychiatric emergency crisis intervention service in a medical emergency room setting. Compr Psychiatr *17*:99, 1976.
13. Weissberg MP: Emergency room medical clearance: An educational problem. Am J Psychiatr *136*:787, 1978.

CHAPTER 22
DRUG-DRUG INTERACTIONS

Michael D. Reed, Pharm.D., FCCP, FCP
Jeffrey L. Blumer, Ph.D., M.D.

Despite the introduction of drugs with increasing potency and pleiotypic effects, clinically important drug interactions are relatively infrequent. Nevertheless, the potential for drug interactions remains great and as a result, the practitioner is inundated with anecdotal reports and poorly designed studies that are often accepted with an uncritical eye. Part of the problem is that in the current definition of a drug interaction, the clinical importance of the effect is assumed rather than proved. If the definition were limited to those interactions resulting in new or unexpected effects that complicate clinical management, a better perspective might be obtained. This would limit the consideration of interactions to certain types of drugs and certain types of patients (Table 22–1). Nevertheless, the importance of such interactions cannot be overstated.

Clinically important interactions among drugs administered with therapeutic intent, as well as the effects of individual patient lifestyles, including diet, alcohol and tobacco use, and environmental exposures, on the therapeutic efficacy and safety of these agents, represent an often overlooked component of clinical practice.[1] Despite this relative complacency on the part of many health care practitioners, the potential for drug interactions to occur is limitless. In 1975, Robinson estimated that a drug formulary containing only 200 drugs theoretically possesses an astounding 19,900 pair combinations.[2] Furthermore, the increasing prevalence of polypharmacy further predisposes patients to the possibility of adverse drug interactions.[3]

Table 22–1. CHARACTERISTICS OF DRUGS AND PATIENTS AT RISK FOR DRUG INTERCTIONS

DRUGS
Potent
Widely used
Affect vital organ functions—i.e., clotting mechanisms, cardiac rhythms, glucose homeostasis
Narrow therapeutic index
Saturable hepatic metabolism
PATIENTS AT RISK
Critically ill
Receiving polypharmacy
With impaired hepatic or renal function
With hypoxemia
With metabolic disturbances
Elderly

Drugs may interact via a number of different mechanisms, which may be classified on a pharmaceutic, pharmacokinetic, and/or pharmacodynamic basis (Table 22–2). Any or all of these interactions may result in unpredictable clinical effects or toxicologic responses. Pharmaceutic interactions include those resulting in drug inactivation when compounds are physically mixed together before patient administration in syringes, infusion tubing, or parenteral fluid preparations. The inactivation of aminoglycosides by certain β-lactam antibiotics, when these drugs are mixed together in the same intravenous fluid, represents one of the more common clinically relevant examples of this type of interaction.[4] Pharmacokinetic interactions can occur when the disposition characteristics of one compound (i.e., absorption, distribution, metabolism, and/or excretion) are influenced by those of another. This type of interaction may involve one or more specific aspects of a drug's pharmacokinetic profile. For example, one drug may reduce the rate but not the overall extent of absorption; in another case, a compound may displace a drug from its protein-binding sites while concomitantly retarding its elimination from the body. Finally, drugs may interact pharmacodynamically, i.e., compete for the same receptor or physiologic system, altering a patient's response to drug therapy.

The number of known, clinically important drug interactions, combined with the ever-increasing number of available pharmacologic agents, underscores the need to understand the pharmacologic basis of drug interactions. A number of excellent texts[5, 6] and reviews[2, 7–11] have been published on the subject of drug interactions, emphasizing

Table 22–2. PRIMARY MECHANISMS OF CLINICALLY IMPORTANT DRUG INTERACTIONS

PHARMACEUTIC
Drug compatibility
Drug stability
PHARMACOKINETIC
Absorption
Distribution
Metabolism
Excretion
PHARMACODYNAMIC
Mechanism of action
Receptor binding
Receptor reactivity
Safety profile

both their importance and the clinical neglect of the issue. In this chapter, we will review and specifically evaluate the pharmacokinetic and pharmacodynamic mechanisms of drug interactions by using clinically important interactions as examples where appropriate. Furthermore, we have incorporated, where available, data obtained from reports of drug overdose and/or toxic exposure.[12, 13]

EPIDEMIOLOGY

Drug interactions are a common occurrence in medical practice and occur more frequently than clinically recognized.[1] In 1972, the Boston Collaborative Drug Surveillance Program,[14] reporting on 9900 consecutively monitored hospitalized patients who collectively had 83,200 drug exposures, found 3600 reported adverse drug reactions, of which 234 (6.9 per cent) were attributed to drug interactions. In another series, 22 per cent of the adverse drug reactions recognized on medical wards were attributed to drug interactions.[15] Durrence and coworkers[16] determined that 17 per cent of 1825 general surgical patients received potentially interacting drug combinations. Further experience has extended these observations beyond hospitalized patients to patients receiving care in both ambulatory settings and extended care facilities.

A number of epidemiologic evaluations have demonstrated clearly that the incidence of adverse drug reactions increases as the number of simultaneously prescribed drugs increases.[2, 11, 17, 18] This problem is compounded further by potential complications arising from self-medication with over-the-counter (OTC) products and alcohol and/or tobacco use. Recently, our group undertook a prospective evaluation of adverse drug reactions among 193 noninstitutionalized residents of Cuyahoga County who were 65 years of age or older.[18] A total of 1204 medications were taken by the study subjects (volunteers); 37 per cent of these agents were OTC medications. Moreover, 57 per cent of subjects reported they had experienced at least one adverse drug reaction from their medications. Not surprisingly, a significant correlation ($p < 0.005$) was observed between the number of prescription drugs taken and the incidence of adverse drug reactions.[18]

PHARMACOKINETIC MECHANISMS OF DRUG INTERACTIONS

Gastrointestinal Absorption

Absorption is defined as the translocation of drug from its site of administration into the systemic circulation. Drugs administered extravascularly, including the oral, sublingual, or intramuscular routes, must cross multiple membranes to reach the systemic circulation before distribution to their sites of action. The process of absorption can be divided, for pharmacokinetic purposes, into two distinct domains, rate and extent. Both of these domains are influenced by the physicochemical properties of the drug as well as a variety of host factors.[19] The physicochemical properties of a drug that affect absorption include molecular weight, degree of lipid solubility, extent of ionization at physiologic pH and the type of formulation administered (e.g., tablet, capsule, suspension, and so forth). Independent of the site of administration, a drug must be in solution to be available for absorption. Thus, for a drug administered orally via a solid dose form (e.g., tablet or capsule), the dissolution rate, or the rate at which a drug dissolves into solution, is the rate-limiting step in the absorption process.

Clearly, a number of potential types of interactions between two or more compounds may influence directly the rate and/or amount of drug absorbed (Table 22–3). Theoretically, foods or drugs capable of altering gastrointestinal pH could modify the absorption characteristics of a compound by changing the proportion of drug that is in the unionized (more lipid-soluble) state. Thus, the

Table 22–3. MECHANISMS INVOLVED IN INTERACTIONS THAT AFFECT DRUG ABSORPTION

Alteration of gastric emptying rate and/or gastrointestinal motility
Modification of the volume, composition, and/or viscosity of gastrointestinal secretions
Effects of pH on drug ionization and dissolution
Effects on mucosal and bacterial drug metabolism
Interactions with active transport systems
Alterations of splanchnic blood flow
Complexation and chelate formation
Toxic effects on gastrointestinal mucosa

(Adapted from Pond SM: Pharmacokinetic drug interactions. *In* Benet LZ, Massoud N, Gambertoglio JG (eds): Pharmacokinetic Basis for Drug Treatment. New York, Raven Press, 1984, pp 195–220.)

coadministration of antacids or histamine H_2-receptor blocking agents, which alter gastrointestinal pH, may substantially influence the amount of drug—particularly a weak base—absorbed from the stomach. However, in practice, this is generally not the case because the majority of drugs, independent of their pKa values, are absorbed from the small intestine.[20, 21] Conversely, these drugs, by decreasing gastric acid secretion, might promote an increase in the absorption of acid-labile drugs. Again, few data are available evaluating the clinical relevance of these potential pharmacokinetic interactions.[9, 11, 20, 21]

In contrast, drug chelates with food or other compounds resulting in decreased absorption (i.e., tetracycline plus divalent cations; ferrous sulfate plus calcium carbonate) would appear the more common and clinically relevant interactions (Table 22–4). Moreover, gastric complexation with orally administered activated charcoal, which markedly inhibits the systemic absorption of numerous compounds, remains the mainstay of clinical toxicology practice. The coadministration of cholestyramine resin also has been shown to reduce the systemic absorption of a limited number of compounds.[22]

Drugs that influence gastrointestinal motility may influence the gastrointestinal absorption of orally administered drugs by controlling the rate of drug delivery to, as well as the duration of contact time with, the major absorptive surfaces. For example, the coadministration of the anticholinergic agent propantheline has been shown to increase the rate and extent of digoxin absorption, whereas digoxin absorption was decreased following metoclopramide administration.[22]

Distribution

Drug distribution describes the movement of a pharmacologically or toxicologically active moiety from the systemic circulation into various body compartments, tissues, and cells. The pharmacokinetic parameter estimate, volume of distribution (Vd), is an apparent value that attempts to describe the relationship between the amount of drug in the body and its serum concentration. The process of distribution depends on the partition coefficient of a drug between blood and tissue, regional blood flow, and the extent of binding to plasma protein and/or tissues.

Alterations in drug distribution most commonly result from the displacement of bound drug from circulating plasma proteins. Acidic compounds bind most often to albumin, whereas basic compounds bind predominantly to α_1-acid glycoprotein.[23–25] It is assumed that the free or nonprotein-bound fraction of a compound is the pharmacologically active moiety capable of diffusing into tissues traversing cellular membranes and binding to receptors.[23] As such, changes in drug binding that result in an increase in the

Table 22–4. SELECTED CLINICALLY IMPORTANT INTERACTIONS DUE TO ALTERATION OF DRUG ABSORPTION

DRUG	COMPOUND AFFECTED	EFFECT ON ABSORPTION *(Pharmacokinetic Parameter Estimate)*
antacids	clorazepate	AUC
	tetracyclines	AUC
	warfarin	AUC
	ciprofloxacin	AUC
	isoniazid	Peak serum concentration
cholestyramine	digitalis glycosides	AUC
	thyroid hormone	AUC
kaolin	lincomycin	AUC

AUC = Area under the serum concentration time curve.

amount of free drug available may increase the amount of drug available for tissue distribution and may possibly increase the drug's concentration at the site of action.[25] The displacement of dicumarol-like oral anticoagulants (e.g., warfarin) from serum albumin–binding sites by other highly protein-bound compounds (e.g., aspirin, phenylbutazone, and so forth) represents a classic example of such an interaction. However, this more traditional view as a simple competitive displacement reaction is based on a number of assumptions, many of which defy physiologic validation (see below). Moreover, it is important to recognize that displacement interactions have been evaluated primarily in vitro and, in fact, have been very difficult to corroborate in vivo.

A number of variables may directly influence the physiologic impact of a drug-displacement interaction. In order for such reactions to be important clinically, both compounds must be ≥80 to 90 per cent bound to the same protein species. In addition, the displaced compound must exhibit capacity-limited clearance, or it must have a relatively small apparent Vd:<0.15 L/kg.[25, 26] This last factor is likely to be the most important because as the Vd increases, less of the total amount of drug in the body is present in the plasma compartment. Thus, with proportionately less compound to displace and a larger "space" in which to distribute, the effect of a displacement interaction would be, at best, only transient. Finally, it is important to recall that increasing the amount of free drug will concurrently increase the amount of compound available for metabolism and/or excretion.

Clearly, the physiologic impact of drug displacement reactions depends on the balance among a large number of variables. In the overdose situation, this is compounded further because very little is known about the impact of a single large dose of a displacing agent on the overall biodisposition of the displaced agent. The result will depend largely on whether exposure to the displacing agent occurs under single- or multiple-dose conditions. Moreover, the magnitude and duration of the interaction will be determined by the clearance rate of the displacing agent.

Despite the perception that these displacement reactions are of clinical importance, very few have actually been documented.[26] The traditionally cited interaction between oral anticoagulants and salicylates leading to an increased hypoprothrombinemic effect is most likely due to a combination of mechanisms rather than simply drug displacement.[27] First, acetylation of the platelet by salicylate and its derivatives inhibits adenosine diphosphate–induced platelet aggregation. Second, oral salicylate administration increases gastrointestinal blood losses. Finally, chronic administration of aspirin may interfere with warfarin protein-binding by actually altering the structure of the serum albumin molecule. Another example in which a combination of mechanisms rather than simply a protein displacement reaction more clearly accounts for a clinically important drug interaction involves phenylbutazone. This highly protein-bound drug may displace warfarin from albumin[28] but also inhibits the metabolism of the potent warfarin S-isomer, which leads to an accumulated hypoprothrombinemic effect. A similar interaction has been suggested for sulfonamides combined with oral sulfonylurea hypoglycemic agents.

In contrast to the interactions just discussed, changes in Vd resulting from altered tissue binding, although rare, are exemplified by the now well-known interaction between digoxin and quinidine.[29] The decrease observed in quinidine Vd and concurrent increase in serum digoxin concentrations is most likely due to digoxin tissue-binding displacement by quinidine. These changes in digoxin pharmacokinetics have been described after administration of a single dose of quinidine. In addition to tissue displacement, quinidine also decreases the renal and nonrenal clearance of digoxin. Quinine, the S-isomer of quinidine, has also been shown to interfere with the nonrenal clearance of digoxin.[30]

Metabolism

Although a number of organs, including the adrenal glands, kidney, lung, placenta, and gut, are capable of drug metabolism, the liver is the primary organ involved in the biotransformation of endogenous and exogenous substances. Most compounds are hepatically biotransformed by the mixed-function oxidase (cytochrome P-450) system. Considering the large number of endogenous and exogenously administered compounds

Table 22–5. SELECTED CLINICALLY IMPORTANT INTERACTIONS DUE TO INDUCTION OF DRUG METABOLISM

INDUCER	COMPOUND AFFECTED	PHARMACOKINETIC PARAMETER MEASURED (U)	CHANGE	
			Before	*After*
phenobarbital	alprenolol	AUC (ng/mL/hr)	706	154
	digitoxin	t½ (d)	7.8	4.5
	doxycycline	t½ (hr)	15.3	11.1
	quinidine	t½ (hr)	4	1.6
	warfarin	Css (mg/L)	0.73	0.18
	nortriptyline	Css (ng/mL)	28	18
rifampin	disopyramide	AUC (μg/mL/hr)	20	8
	metoprolol	AUC (μg/L/hr)	930	624
	warfarin	AUC (μg/mL/hr)	600	258
	digitoxin	t½ (d)	12	3.2
	tolbutamide	t½ (hr)	5.4	3.3
	oral contraceptives	t½ (hr)	7.5	3.3
tobacco smoke	lidocaine	t½ (min)	96*	88†
	propranolol	Mean Css (mg/L)	—	>200
	theophylline	t½ (hr)	11.5	7.4

AUC = area under the serum concentration time curve.
t½ = elimination half-life.
Css = steady state serum concentration.
*Nonsmoker.
†Cigarette smoker.
(Adapted from Pond SM: Pharmacokinetic drug interactions. *In* Benet LZ, Massoud N, Gambertoglio JG (eds): Pharmacokinetic Basis for Drug Treatment. New York, Raven Press, 1984, pp 195–220.)

that are partially or completely metabolized by the liver, it is easy to recognize the vulnerability of this site relative to drug interactions. A large number of drug-drug, drug-disease, and drug-nutrient interactions have been described in the literature as a result of one agent or process influencing the metabolism of another. Obviously, this influence could involve either an increase or a decrease in the metabolic clearance rate of a given compound. For drugs that are completely eliminated from the body via hepatic biotransformation, total body clearance is a function of liver blood flow and the ability of the liver to extract the drug.[31, 32] Thus, in addition to metabolic capacity, liver blood flow may be an important determinant of a drug's clearance, most notably for those drugs with high hepatic extraction ratios (e.g., lidocaine, propranolol).[32]

Drugs well known to be potent and predictable inducers of hepatic cytochrome P-450 activity[9, 11, 32–34] include the barbiturates,[35] glutethimide,[35] carbamazepine,[36] rifampin,[37] and griseofulvin.[33, 34] In addition, it is important to recognize that other drugs such as phenytoin,[38] ethanol (chronic use/abuse),[39, 40] environmental pollutants including tobacco smoke,[41] organochlorine insecticides, polychlorinated phenols,[42] foods such as Brussels sprouts and cabbage,[43] and charcoal broiling[44] all can stimulate the hepatic metabolism of drugs.[33, 34, 42, 45] Interactions of potential clinical importance with selected metabolic inducers are outlined in Table 22–5.[9]

The clinical impact of enzyme induction on drug action has been recognized for decades[33, 34, 45] and is exemplified by the now classic interaction involving the decrease in the hypoprothrombinemic effect of warfarin by the coadministration of phenobarbital.[35] Induction, or the stimulation of cytochrome P-450 activity, appears to be a result of an increase in the absolute number of cytochrome P-450 molecules.[33, 34] This increase in P-450 molecules also appears to involve the many forms of P-450.

Agents capable of inducing the hepatic cytochrome mono-oxygenase system represent a wide array of differing chemical moieties, including drugs, hormones, and environmental pollutants.[34, 42] In addition, the time course of induction varies with both the type and dose of the inducing agent.[34, 45–47] Potent inducing compounds such as phenobarbital and rifampin may begin to induce enzyme activity after only 1 to 2 days of therapy.[47, 48] Return to constitutive enzyme activity following withdrawal of the inducing agent appears quite variable but would be influenced by the inducer's body clearance rate combined with the microsomal enzyme turnover rate.[48] Dossing and associates,[48] using the antipyrine saliva test and the ami-

Table 22–6. SELECTED CLINICALLY IMPORTANT INTERACTIONS DUE TO INHIBITION OF DRUG METABOLISM

INHIBITOR	COMPOUND AFFECTED	PHARMACOKINETIC PARAMETER MEASURED (U)	CHANGE	
			Before	*After*
Chloramphenicol	dicumarol	t½ (hr)	8.7	25
	phenytoin	t½ (hr)	12	28
	tolbutamide	t½ (hr)	5.2	14.1
Phenylbutazone	phenytoin	t½ (hr)	13.7	22
	tolbutamide	t½ (hr)	8	23
	antipyrine	Cl (mL/kg/min)	37.7	26.6
Oral contraceptives	nitrazepam	Cl (mL/min)	459	323

t½ = elimination half-life.
Cl = body clearance.
(Adapted from Pond SM: Pharmacokinetic drug interactions. In Benet LZ, Massoud N, Gambertoglio JG (eds): Pharmacokinetic Basis for Drug Treatment. New York, Raven Press, 1984, pp 195–220.)

nopyrine breath test in an elaborate investigation involving four healthy subjects, described enhanced clearance occurring after 1 week and persisting for 10 days after cessation of phenobarbital administration.

As previously stated, a number of drugs are also capable of inhibiting hepatic microsomal mono-oxygenase activity, thus partially or completely inhibiting the metabolism of another compound (Table 22–6).[45] This inhibition can decrease the hepatic clearance of drugs, which consequently prolongs the total body clearance rate of a compound. Drugs commonly used in the clinical setting that are capable of inhibiting cytochrome P-450 activity include phenylbutazone,[28, 49] cimetidine,[20, 32] chloramphenicol,[50] erythromycin, ethanol (acute consumption and/or intoxication),[40, 51] and oral contraceptive steroids.[31] Interactions of potential clinical importance involving some of these agents are shown in Table 22–6; Table 22–7 shows the effects of cimetidine on various drugs.[9, 11, 20, 21, 40, 45]

The histamine H_2-receptor antagonists cimetidine, famotidine, nizatidine, and ranitidine are among the most widely prescribed drugs today. Of these four agents, cimetidine is a potent inhibitor of hepatic microsomal enzyme activity.[20, 32] Concurrent cimetidine administration has been reported to inhibit the metabolism of over 25 different compounds (see Table 22–7). Dossing and colleagues[48] found that the inhibitory effect of cimetidine on microsomal enzyme activity occurred 24 hours after drug initiation and subsided within 2 days after the last dose. In rodents, the inhibition of microsomal enzyme activity by cimetidine has been shown to decrease the hepatotoxicity of certain drugs,[32] such as acetaminophen[52, 53] and cocaine,[53] which suggests a possible therapeutic value for this metabolic interaction. However, the time course of the inhibitory effect of cimet-

Table 22–7. INFLUENCE OF CIMETIDINE ON THE DISPOSITION OF SELECTED DRUGS

DRUG AFFECTED	PHARMACOKINETIC PARAMETER MEASURED (U)	CHANGE	
		Before	*After*
diazepam	Cl (mL/min)	19.9	11.4
imipramine	t½ (hr)	10.8	22.7
lidocaine	Cl (mL/min)	766	576
meperidine	Cl (L/kg/hr)	0.6	0.47
procainamide	t½ (hr)	2.9	3.7
propranolol	AUC (µg/L/hr)	450	727
theophylline	t½ (hr)	11.5	14.1
triamterene	Renal Cl (mL/min)	71	27

t½ = elimination half-life.
Cl = body clearance.
AUC = area under the serum concentration time curve.
(Adapted from the following: Pond SM: Pharmacokinetic drug interactions. *In* Benet LZ, Massoud N, Gambertoglio JG (eds): Pharmacokinetic Basis for Drug Treatment. New York, Raven Press, 1984, pp 195–220; Somogui A, Muirhead M: Pharmacokinetic interactions of cimetidine 1987. Clin Pharmacokinet 9:493–510, 1984; and Powell JR, Donn KH: Histamine H-2 antagonist drug interactions in perspective: Mechanistic concepts and clinical implications. Am J Med 77(suppl 5B):57–84, 1984.)

idine on hepatic microsomes[48] appears to limit the drug's clinical utility as an adjunct in the treatment of acetaminophen intoxication. In addition, cimetidine, more so than other H_2-receptor antagonists, is capable of reducing hepatic blood flow, which further compromises the metabolism of high extraction ratio drugs.

Cimetidine has also been shown to decrease the renal clearance of a number of cationic drugs, including procainamide, *N*-acetyl procainamide,[54] and triamterene, by inhibition of renal proximal tubule cationic secretion.[20, 32, 55] In contrast to cimetidine, clinically significant drug interactions with ranitidine, famotidine, or nizatidine are rare[21, 32, 56, 57] and involve only a few case reports.[21] Although ranitidine has been shown to bind cytochrome P-450,[21, 58] the drug's binding affinity is approximately tenfold lower than that described for cimetidine.[21, 32, 58] Similar such observations have been reported for both famotidine and nizatidine.

More recently, viral infections and vaccines have been shown to decrease the clearance of a number of drugs, including theophylline, phenytoin, and warfarin.[59–61] In 1982, Kraemer and colleagues[60] described theophylline toxicity in 11 children who were stabilized on oral theophylline for several months during an influenza B outbreak. Two of these eleven children had seizures as the primary manifestation of theophylline toxicity. Similar observations have been described after influenza vaccine administration and respiratory tract infections due to influenza A and adenovirus. The mechanism by which certain viral infections alter drug metabolism is unknown but appears to be a result of endogenous interferon synthesis. Drugs known to induce endogenous interferon production have been shown to interfere with hepatic drug metabolism.[61] The interactions between specific viruses and/or vaccines and hepatic microsomal enzyme activity are currently the subject of aggressive evaluation.

Last, a number of compounds can interfere with or directly inhibit hepatic drug metabolism via nonmicrosomal pathways. Allopurinol, a xanthine oxidase inhibitor used to decrease endogenous uric acid production, also inhibits the metabolism of other xanthine analogues, most notably 6-mercaptopurine and its prodrug azathioprine.[62] Although this drug combination has been used for its therapeutic potential, it has also led to serious adverse drug effects, of which enhanced myelosuppression is the most notable.[62] Disulfiram (Antabuse) is a potent inhibitor of acetaldehyde dehydrogenase, the enzyme primarily responsible for the metabolism of ethanol to acetic acid. Concurrent ethanol consumption and disulfiram administration lead to acetaldehyde accumulation and the classic "Antabuse reaction," characterized by the following unpleasant symptoms: flushing, throbbing, headache, nausea, vomiting, sweating, palpitations, hypotension, and syncope. Another frequently cited reaction mediated via a nonmicrosomal pathway is the hypertensive crisis resulting from the coadministration of sympathomimetic amines and consumption of tyrosine-containing foods (cheese, red wine) by patients receiving drugs that inhibit monoamine oxidase activity.[5, 6, 9]

Elimination

The most common pathway by which drugs and/or their metabolites are eliminated from the body is via the kidney. Interactions that influence renal clearance of a compound primarily involve the physiologic processes of glomerular filtration, tubular reabsorption, or active tubular secretion. Additionally, agents that alter renal blood flow may also influence renal elimination. Consequently, alterations in renal clearance represent an important mechanism of drug interaction. Nevertheless, for such interactions to be of clinical importance, the overall elimination of active drug must depend primarily on renal mechanisms. As discussed in the Distribution section, displacement interactions (i.e., displacement from binding sites) may transiently increase the amount of free drug in the vascular compartment, resulting in an increase in the amount of drug available to be filtered by the glomerulus. However, to our knowledge this has not been reported as the sole mechanism responsible for a clinically important drug interaction.

In contrast to displacement interactions, a number of drugs can directly influence glomerular filtration through another mechanism. Recently, the nonsteroidal anti-inflammatory drugs (NSAIDs)—aspirin, fenoprofen, ibuprofen, indomethacin, naproxen, and others—have all been shown to reversibly depress renal function in certain patients.[63] This drug-induced decrease in renal function is most likely a result of NSAIDs' inhibition of renal prostaglandin synthesis[63] and has resulted in increased side effects because of accumulation of other concurrently administered drugs. The dienoic prostaglandins PGI_2, PGE_2, and PGF_2 produced by the medullary interstitial cells of the kidney are believed to be important vasodilators responsible for maintaining "vascular balance" and renal blood flow. Their synthesis and secretion appear to occur as a result of renal vascular ischemia. Individuals predisposed to NSAID-induced renal toxicity would be patients who have pre-existing renal disease, hypertension, and congestive heart failure. In intoxications involving NSAIDs, this secondary renal effect would appear to be of primary clinical importance in those patients with some degree of pre-existing renal compromise (e.g., the elderly), because it is in these patients that prostaglandins exert an important role in maintaining renal function.[63]

In clinical practice, interactions that influence renal tubular function are observed frequently and can result in serious consequences (Table 22–8). The tubular secretion of organic acids and bases is an active process that most likely involves distinct pathways.[64, 65] The classic uricosuric agents probenecid and sulfinpyrazone[66] are among the most potent inhibitors of organic acid secretion by the proximal tubule. Probenecid has been shown to inhibit the renal clearance of a number of drugs including sulfinpyrazone and indomethacin and has been used clinically to maintain serum penicillin (β-lactam) concentrations for the treatment of uncomplicated gonorrhea and other systemic infectious processes. Although interactions involving organic bases would similarly be expected, those of clinical importance primarily involve those already described after chronic cimetidine administration.[20, 54, 55]

Modification of the passive distal tubular reabsorption of weak acids and bases is another mechanism whereby drugs may interact and represents a potentially important therapeutic modality in the treatment of certain intoxications (see Table 22–8). An inverse relationship exists between the compound's degree of ionization and the overall amount of a compound reabsorbed from the urine, i.e., the greater the amount of compound present in the urine in the nonionized, more lipid-soluble state, the greater the amount reabsorbed. In general, for renal clearance to be sensitive to changes in urine pH, acidic and basic drugs must have pKa values that range between 3 to 7.5 and 7 to 11, respectively.[65] This principle of altering urinary pH has been used in the management of a number of drug intoxications, including those by the salicylates, phenobarbital, amphetamine, and phencyclidine.[9, 11] Alkalinization of urine by either intermittent or continuous intravenous infusion of sodium bicarbonate can dramatically decrease distal tubular reabsorption of salicylate and phenobarbital.

Intraluminal trapping of acids in their ionized form appears to be greatest when urine pH is ≥ 7.5.[65] Conversely, urinary acidification with either ammonium chloride administered orally or dilute hydrochloric acid administered intravenously can markedly augment the renal clearance of amphetamine and phencyclidine. Although the manipulation of urinary pH to promote "ion trapping" and augment renal clearance appears desirable, it is not without risk. Needless to say, raising or lowering urinary pH "rapidly"

Table 22–8. CLINICALLY IMPORTANT INTERACTIONS OF DRUG ELIMINATION DUE TO ALTERATION IN RENAL EXCRETION

	COMPOUND AFFECTED	EFFECT ON EXCRETION
Probenecid	β-lactam antibiotics	Secretion
	indomethacin	Secretion
	sulfinpyrazone	Secretion
Urinary alkalinization (sodium bicarbonate)	salicylate	Reabsorption
	phenobarbital	Reabsorption
Urinary acidification (ammonium chloride)	amphetamine	Reabsorption
	chloroquine	Reabsorption
	lidocaine	Reabsorption

requires alteration of the blood pH, a change which may be undesirable and possibly detrimental in certain instances. Furthermore, the clinician must carefully weigh the associated risks of pH manipulation and the time necessary to achieve effective changes in urinary pH with the effectiveness of other therapeutic modalities, and most important, with the anticipated duration of serious symptomatology.

Last, the bile represents an often overlooked but relatively important means for the elimination of a number of drugs and substrates. Parent compounds and/or their metabolites (pharmacologically active or inactive) excreted via the bile may be reabsorbed/absorbed respectively into the systemic circulation from the intestine. This process of enterohepatic circulation is an important mechanism responsible for delayed and prolonged drug absorption and elimination of a number of commonly used drugs including phenothiazines, phenobarbital, carbamazepine, spironolactone, and others. Increasing the total body clearance of many of these compounds by interfering with the enterohepatic circulation process underscores the importance of administering repeated doses of oral activated charcoal to patients who experience intoxications involving compounds that undergo substantial enterohepatic circulation.[67]

DRUG-NUTRIENT INTERACTIONS

Nutritional habits may dramatically influence the response to pharmacologic intervention. The type and quantity of food consumed as well as the overall nutritional status of a patient may directly or indirectly alter drug disposition characteristics. For decades, it has been recognized that malnutrition and starvation can suppress a number of important endogenous enzymatic processes responsible for drug biotransformation and elimination.[40, 68] These nutrient-drug effects may result from simple cofactor (e.g., vitamin, trace metal/mineral) deprivation leading to inhibition of specific enzymatic reactions[40, 69] to modifying renal function[70] and/or the quantity and functional activity of the hepatic mixed function oxidase system.[71] Obviously, the impact of these effects is difficult to predict and would appear to be at least partially responsible for interindividual variation frequently observed in many pharmacologic evaluations. Moreover, certain drugs may directly alter or impair a patient's underlying nutritional status, e.g., electrolyte and mineral depletion following chronic diuretic therapy.

The specific composition of a meal as well as one's overall diet can markedly alter drug absorption (Table 22–9). The most notable example of food-associated inhibition of drug absorption involves the complexation of tetracycline compounds when coadministered with divalent cation-containing compounds (e.g., milk, cheese, antacids, vitamins).[9, 11, 19] Such an interaction resulting in decreased systemic bioavailability is unusual. What occurs more frequently is that the rate but not the overall extent of drug absorption is decreased when the drug is administered in the presence of food. The intestinal absorption of some commonly administered drugs, such as acetaminophen, digoxin, levodopa, many penicillin and cephalosporin analogues, and phenytoin, may be delayed or reduced when these agents are given in the presence of food. Conversely, the bioavailability of some orally administered drugs including spironolactone, griseofulvin, and cefuroxime axetil can be increased when the drugs are administered in the presence of food.

Both hepatic drug metabolism and renal elimination can be influenced by the type and quantity of nutrient consumed. Cabbage, Brussels sprouts, and cauliflower have all been shown to contain certain indoles that are potent inducers of intestinal and hepatic drug-metabolizing enzymes.[43] Diets high in protein (e.g., >40 per cent total calories) have been shown to increase the metabolic capacity of the hepatic mixed-function oxidase system; this results in increased clearances of a number of drugs, including antipyrine, theo-

Table 22–9. INFLUENCE OF FOOD ON BIOAVAILABILITY OF SELECTED DRUGS

TOTAL AMOUNT OF DRUG ABSORBED	
Increased	*Decreased*
spironolactone	isoniazid
hydralazine	rifampin
hydrochlorothiazide	tetracyclines
griseofulvin (↑ fat)	erythromycin stearate
diazepam	levodopa
cefuroxime axetil, erythromycin	methyldopa
erythromycin ethylsuccinate, and estolate	

phylline, and propranolol.[43, 44, 68, 69, 72] This increase in body clearance is not observed when similar quantities of either carbohydrate or fat are substituted for protein.[69, 71, 72] In addition, diets deficient in protein are associated with altered renal hemodynamics, a condition that leads to marked decreases in glomerular filtration,[70] further influencing a drug's body clearance and pharmacodynamics.

PHARMACODYNAMIC MECHANISMS OF DRUG INTERACTIONS

In patients receiving multiple drugs, the overall effects manifested are a summation of the similar or opposing but independent actions of these multiple agents on a given cell or organ system.[11] Historically, these interactions have not been considered drug interactions; yet many are of extreme clinical importance. These interactions are properly termed pharmacodynamic drug interactions and are thought to involve drug-receptor interactions either directly or indirectly.

The types of interactions that might occur at the receptor level are varied. Moreover, the understanding of these interactions is often confounded because simple potentiation and/or antagonism are distinctly uncommon. Most of these interactions occur through an interplay of receptor mechanisms controlling the function of a given tissue or organ system. In a similar fashion, drugs may interact with physiologic or biochemical control loops, a process that leads to alterations in response to normal stimuli and input signals. Finally, one drug may prevent access of another to its site of action, thus abrogating the pharmacodynamic process.

Direct Receptor Effects

We will cite a few instances of drug interactions that occur through direct receptor-site antagonism. Consider, for example, the asthmatic patient receiving a β_2-agonist bronchodilator (e.g., albuterol, terbutaline) who develops angina and is treated with propranolol. Clearly, there is potential for the nonselective β-blocker propranolol to inhibit the bronchodilator effect of the β_2-agonist drug.[73] This risk is especially great in today's climate of medical practice in which organ system subspecialists have largely supplanted the general practitioner, and prescriptions targeted by one clinician to ameliorate symptoms in one system may unwittingly interfere with drugs prescribed by another physician who is focusing on another organ system.

Another example of direct pharmacodynamic interaction can occur during therapy with the coumarin anticoagulants. The effects of these agents may be potentiated by dextrothyroxine[74] and antimicrobial agents containing a thiomethyltetrazole ring.[75] In addition, quinidine appears to augment the cellular uptake of warfarin, thus increasing warfarin's effective concentration at the site of action. Finally, certain broad spectrum antibiotics may enhance the efficacy of warfarin through the eradication of gut bacteria responsible for vitamin K_1 synthesis.

Indirect Receptor Effects

Pharmacodynamic interactions associated with indirect receptor effects refer to those side effects of one drug that mimic the pharmacologic effects of another. The augmentation of the hypoglycemic effects of insulin and oral hypoglycemic agents by nonselective β-blocking agents is an example of agents with differing mechanisms of action producing the same clinical effect.[5, 6, 11]

The use of drugs with actions on the myocardium, cardiac conduction system, and/or capacitance and resistance vessels predisposes to a large number of pharmacodynamic interactions. Calcium channel blockers and β-receptor antagonists will often augment the myocardial depressant, bradycardic, and hypotensive effects of one another when used in concert.[76] Other effects augmented by the simultaneous administration of vasoactive drugs and β-blocking agents include exacerbation of first-dose hypotensive effects of prazosin, enhancement of the hypertensive response during clonidine withdrawal, and peripheral ischemia associated with ergotamine administration.

The importance and proliferation of NSAIDs has focused attention on a number of serious interactions that may occur with these agents.[63] The sodium and water retention that result from the chronic use of these agents may blunt the antihypertensive effects of thiazide diuretics and β-blocking agents.[77] These effects may also offset the benefits of

Table 22–10. PHARMACODYNAMIC AUGMENTATION OF DRUG EFFECTS

EFFECT	COMBINED AGENTS
Central nervous system depression	Benzodiazepines, alcohol, opioids, antidepressants, anticonvulsants, neuroleptics
Bleeding diathesis	Coumarin anticoagulants, heparin, streptokinase, NSAIDs, salicylates, antineoplastic agents, certain antibiotics (e.g., moxalactam)
Hyperglycemia	Corticosteroids with diuretics
Hypoglycemia	Sulfonylureas with salicylates, phenytoin
Hypokalemia	Corticosteroids with diuretics
Hyperkalemia	KCl with potassium-sparing diuretics or ACE inhibitors
Hypotension	Antihypertensives with tricyclic antidepressants, phenothiazines, antianginals, vasodilators

(Adapted from McInnes GT, Brodie MJ: Drug interactions that matter. A clinical reappraisal. Drugs *36*:83–110, 1988.)

diuretic therapy in mild-to-moderate congestive heart failure. Moreover, the gastrointestinal ulcerations often found in patients receiving these agents may predispose those patients receiving concomitant anticoagulant therapy to hemorrhage.

Other examples of drugs associated with indirect pharmacodynamic effects include the following: coadministration of spironolactone and potassium chloride, resulting in life-threatening hyperkalemia; various antibiotic combinations that show synergy or antagonism; and enhanced neurotoxicity of neuroleptics when coadministered with lithium.

Cellular Transport Mechanisms

A number of classic drug interactions involve the uptake and release of neurotransmitters at the nerve terminal. These include interactions between tricyclic antidepressant agents and certain antihypertensive agents.[5, 6] Fortunately, the use of newer antidepressant drugs has largely eliminated these effects as clinically important problems.

SUMMARY

Drug interactions remain an important consideration when assessing a patient's response to pharmacologic intervention. It is clear that the pharmacologic response of a drug can be markedly influenced by the concurrent administration of another therapeutic agent or food. These interactions may result in a decreased therapeutic effect or an increase in the amount and extent of untoward reactions. Despite the well-described and real clinical consequences of drug interactions,[1, 6, 9–11] this aspect of patient care continues to be too often overlooked.

Drugs can interact via a number of mechanisms but most notably on a pharmaceutic, pharmacokinetic, or pharmacodynamic basis. These interactions may occur as a result of concurrently prescribed therapeutic modalities, environmental variables, or the patients' specific habits, such as diet and alcohol and tobacco use/abuse. The unpredictable nature of drug interactions underscores how important it is for all health care practitioners to understand the mechanisms of interaction and be suspicious of their occurrence.

Generally, pharmacodynamic drug interactions result in adverse effects either through the augmentation of the effects of one drug by another having similar effects (Table 22–10) or less frequently, through the antagonism of the effects of one drug by the side effects of another. As our therapeutic armamentarium increases in size as well as potency and efficacy, the potential for these adverse reactions increases. The seriousness of this issue is compounded by the increasing subspecialization of medicine and the attendant, independent prescribing practices of these various physicians.

References

1. Faich GA, Knopp D, Dreis M, Turner W: National adverse drug reaction surveillance: 1985. JAMA *257*:2068–2070, 1987.
2. Robinson DS: The application of basic principles of drug interaction to clinical practice. J Urol *113*:101–107, 1975.
3. May FE, Stewart RB, Cluff LE: Drug interactions and multiple drug administration. Clin Pharmacol Ther *22*:322–328, 1977.
4. Pickering LK, Rutherford I: Effect of concentration and time upon inactivation of tobramycin, genta-

micin, netilmicin and amikacin by azlocillin, carbenicillin, mecillinam and piperacillin. J Pharmacol Exp Ther *217*:345–349, 1981.

5. Evaluations of Drug Interactions. 2nd ed. Washington, DC, American Pharmaceutical Association, 1976.
6. Hansten PD: Drug Interactions. 5th ed. Philadelphia, Lea & Febiger, 1985.
7. Gillette JR, Pang KS: Theoretic aspects of drug interactions. Clin Pharmacol Ther *22*:623–639, 1977.
8. Aarons L: Kinetics of drug-drug interactions. Pharmacol Ther *14*:321–344, 1981.
9. Pond SM: Pharmacokinetic drug interactions. *In* Benet LZ, Massoud N, Gambertoglio JG (eds): Pharmacokinetic Basis for Drug Treatment. New York, Raven Press, 1984, pp 195–220.
10. May JR, DiPiro JT, Sisley JF: Drug interactions in surgical patients. Am J Surg *153*:327–335, 1987.
11. McInnes GT, Brodie MJ: Drug interactions that matter. A clinical reappraisal. Drugs *36*:83–110, 1988.
12. Rosenberg J, Benowitz NL, Pond S: Pharmacokinetics of drug overdose. Clin Pharmacokinet *6*:161–192, 1981.
13. Drew RH: Applying pharmacokinetic principles to the management of drug poisoning. Pediatr Ann *16*:913–924, 1987.
14. Boston Collaborative Drug Surveillance Program: Adverse drug interactions (editorial). JAMA *220*:1238–1239, 1972.
15. Borda IT, Slone D, Jick H: Assessment of adverse reactions within a drug surveillance program. JAMA *205*:645–647, 1968.
16. Durrence CW, DiPiro JT, May JR, Nesbit RR, Jr, Sisley JF, Cooper JW: Potential drug interactions in surgical patients. Am J Hosp Pharm *42*:1553–1556, 1985.
17. Smith JW, Seidl LG, Cluff LE: Studies on the epidemiology of adverse drug reactions. V. Clinical factors influencing susceptibility. Ann Intern Med *65*:629–640, 1977.
18. Reed MD, Amer MK, Blumer JL: Drug use in the elderly. The Cleveland Foundation Report, 1985.
19. Welling PG: Effects of gastrointestinal disease on drug absorption. In Benet LZ, Massoud N, Gambertoglio JG (eds): Pharmacokinetic Basis for Drug Treatment. New York, Raven Press, 1984, pp 29–47.
20. Somogui A, Muirhead M: Pharmacokinetic interactions of cimetidine 1987. Clin Pharmacokinet *12*:321–366, 1987.
21. Kirch W, Hoensch H, Janisch HD: Interactions and non-interactions with ranitidine. Clin Pharmacokinet *9*:493–510, 1984.
22. Manninen V, Apajalahti A, Melin J, Karesoja M: Altered absorption of digoxin in patients given propantheline and metoclopramide. Lancet *1*:398–400, 1973.
23. Meyer MC, Guttman DE: The binding of drugs by plasma proteins. J Pharm Sci *57*:895–918, 1968.
24. Piafsky KM: Disease induced changes in the plasma binding of basic drugs. Clin Pharmacokinet *5*:246–262, 1980.
25. Svensson CK, Woodruff MN, Baxter JG, Lalka D: Free drug concentration monitoring in clinical practice: Rationale and current status. Clin Pharmacokinet *11*:450–469, 1986.
26. Sellers EM: Plasma protein displacement interactions are rarely of clinical significance. Pharmacology *18*:225–227, 1979.
27. O'Reilly RA: Warfarin metabolism and drug-drug interactions. Adv Exp Med Biol *214*:205–212, 1987.
28. Lewis RJ, Trager WF, Chan KK, Breckenridge A, Orme M, Rowland M, Schary W: Warfarin: Stereochemical aspects of its metabolism and the interaction with phenylbutazone. J Clin Invest *53*:1607–1617, 1974.
29. Schenck-Gustafsson K, Jogestrand T, Nordlander R, Dahlqvist R: Effect of quinidine on digoxin concentration in skeletal muscle and serum in patients with atrial fibrillation. Evidence for reduced binding of digoxin in muscle. New Engl J Med *305*:209–211, 1981.
30. Wandell M, Powell JR, Hager WD, Fenster PE, Graves PE, Conrad KA, Goldman S: Effect of quinine on digoxin kinetics. Clin Pharmacol Ther *28*:425–430, 1980.
31. MacKinnon M, Sutherland E, Simon FR: Effect of ethinyl estradiol on hepatic microsomal proteins and the turnover of cytochrome P-450. J Lab Clin Med *90*:1096–1106, 1977.
32. Powell JR, Donn KH: Histamine H-2 antagonist drug interactions in perspective: Mechanistic concepts and clinical implications. Am J Med *77*(suppl 5B):57–84, 1984.
33. Conney AH: Pharmacologic implications of microsomal enzyme induction. Pharmacol Rev *19*:317–366, 1967.
34. Gelehrter TD: Enzyme induction. New Engl J Med *294*:522–526; 589–595 and 646–651, 1976.
35. MacDonald MG, Robinson DS, Sylwester D, Jaffe JJ: The effects of phenobarbital, chloral betaine, and glutethimide administration on warfarin plasma levels and hypoprothrombinemic responses in man. Clin Pharmacol Ther *10*:80–84, 1969.
36. Rapeport WG, McInnes GT, Thompson GG, Forrest G, Park BK, Brodie MJ: Hepatic enzyme induction and leucocyte delta-aminolaevulinic acid synthase activity: Studies with carbamazepine. Br J Clin Pharmacol *16*:133–137, 1983.
37. Baciewicz AM, Self TM: Rifampin drug interactions. Arch Intern Med *144*:1667–1671, 1984.
38. Heincke RJ, Stohs SJ, Al-Turk W, Lemon HM: Chronic phenytoin administration and the hepatic mixed function oxidase system in female rats. Gen Pharmacol *15*:85–89, 1984.
39. Vessell ES, Page JG, Passananti GT: Genetic and environmental factors affecting ethanol metabolism in man. Clin Pharmacol Ther *12*:192–201, 1971.
40. Hoyumpa AM, Schenker S: Major drug interactions: Effect of liver disease, alcohol and malnutrition. Annu Rev Med *33*:113–149, 1982.
41. Jusko WJ: Role of tobacco smoking in pharmacokinetics. J Pharmacokinet Biopharm *6*:7–39, 1978.
42. Alvares AP: Interactions between environmental chemicals and drug biotransformation in man. Clin Pharmacokinet *3*:462–477, 1978.
43. Pantuck EJ, Pantuck CB, Anderson KE, Wattenberg LW, Conney AL, Kappas A: Effect of brussel sprouts and cabbage on drug conjugation. Clin Pharmacol Ther *35*:161–169, 1984.
44. Kappas A, Alvares AP, Anderson KE, Pantuck EJ, Pantuck CB, Chang R, Conney AH: Effect of charcoal-broiled beef on antipyrine and theophylline metabolism. Clin Pharmacol Ther *23*:445–450, 1978.
45. Park BK, Breckenridge AM: Clinical implications of enzyme induction and enzyme inhibition. Clin Pharmacokinet *6*:1–24, 1981.
46. Breckenridge A, Orme MLE, Davies L, Thorgeirsson SS, Davies DS: Dose-dependent enzyme induction. Clin Pharmacol Ther *14*:514–520, 1973.

47. Ohnhaus EE, Park BK: Measurement of urinary 6-β-hydroxycortisol excretion as an in vivo parameter in the clinical assessment of the microsomal enzyme-inducing capacity of antipyrine, phenobarbitone and rifampin. Eur J Clin Pharmacol *15*:139–145, 1979.
48. Dossing M, Pilsgaard H, Rasmussen B, Enghusen-Poulsen H: Time course of phenobarbital and cimetidine mediated changes in hepatic drug metabolism. Eur J Clin Pharmacol *25*:215–222, 1983.
49. Pond SM, Birkett DJ, Wade DN: Mechanisms of inhibition of tolbutamide metabolism: Phenylbutazone, oxyphenbutazone, sulfaphenazole. Clin Pharmacol Ther *22*:573–579, 1977.
50. Christensen LK, Skovsted I: Inhibition of drug metabolism by chloramphenicol. Lancet *2*:1397–1399, 1969.
51. Rubin E, Gang H, Misra PS, Lieber CS: Inhibition of metabolism by acute ethanol intoxication: A hepatic microsomal mechanism. Am J Med *49*:801–806, 1970.
52. Abernethy DR, Greenblatt DJ, Divoll M, Ameer B, Shader DI: Differential effect of cimetidine on drug oxidation (antipyrine and diazepam) vs conjugation (acetaminophen and lorazepam): Prevention of acetaminophen toxicity by cimetidine. J Pharmacol Exp Ther *224*:508–513, 1983.
53. Peterson FJ, Knodell RG, Lindemann NJ, Steele NM: Prevention of acetaminophen and cocaine hepatotoxicity in mice by cimetidine treatment. Gastroenterology *85*:122–129, 1983.
54. Somogyi A, McLean A, Heinzow B: Cimetidine-procainamide pharmacokinetic interaction in man: Evidence of competition for tubular secretion of basic drugs. Eur J Clin Pharmacol *25*:339–345, 1983.
55. van Crugten J, Bochner F, Keal J, Somogyi A: Selectivity of the cimetidine-induced alterations in the renal handling of organic substrates in humans. Studies with anionic, cationic and zwitteronic drugs. J Pharmacol Exp Ther *236*:481–487, 1986.
56. Abernethy DR, Greenblatt DJ, Eshelman FN, Shader RI: Ranitidine does not impair oxidative or conjugative metabolism: Noninteraction with antipyrine, diazepam and lorazepam. Clin Pharmacol Ther *35*:188–192, 1984.
57. Kelly HW, Powell JR, Donohue JF: Ranitidine at very large doses does not inhibit theophylline elimination. Clin Pharmacol Ther *39*:577–581, 1986.
58. Rendic S, Kajfez F, Ruf H-H: Characterization of cimetidine, ranitidine and related structures interaction with cytochrome P-450. Drug Metab Disp *11*:137–142, 1983.
59. Meredith CG, Christian CD, Johnson RF, Troxell R, Davis GL, Schenker S: Effects of influenza virus vaccine on hepatic drug metabolism. Clin Pharmacol Ther *37*:396–401, 1985.
60. Kraemer MJ, Furukawa CT, Koup JR, Shapiro GG, Pierson WE, Bierman CW: Altered theophylline clearance during an influenza B outbreak. Pediatrics *69*:476–480, 1982.
61. Azhary RE, Mannering GJ: Effects of interferon inducing agents on hepatic hemoproteins, heme metabolism and cytochrome P450-linked monooxygenase systems. Molecular Pharmacol *15*:698–707, 1979.
62. Murrell GAC, Rapeport WG: Clinical pharmacokinetics of allopurinol. Clin Pharmacokinet *11*:343–353, 1986.
63. Dunn MJ: Nonsteroidal anti-inflammatory drugs and renal function. Ann Rev Med *35*:411–428, 1984.
64. Weiner IM, Mudge GH: Renal tubular mechanisms for excretion of organic acids and bases. Am J Med *36*:743–762, 1964.
65. Peterson RG, Peterson LN: Cleansing the blood: Hemodialysis, periotoneal dialysis, exchange transfusion, charcoal hemoperfusion, forced diuresis. Pediatr Clin North Am *33*:675–689, 1986.
66. Perel JM, Dayton PG, Snell MM, Yu TF, Gutman AB: Studies of interactions among drugs in man at the renal level: Probenecid and sulfinpyrazone. Clin Pharmacol Ther *10*:834–840, 1969.
67. Park GD, Spector R, Goldberg MJ, Johnson GF: Expanded role of charcoal therapy in the poisoned and overdosed patient. Arch Intern Med *146*:969–973, 1986.
68. Krishnaswamy K: Drug metabolism and pharmacokinetics in malnutrition. Clin Pharmacokinet *3*:216–240, 1978.
69. Hathcock JW: Nutrient-drug interactions. Clin Geriatric Med *3*:297–307, 1987.
70. Fernandez-Repollet E, Tapia E, Martinez-Maldonado M: Effects of angiotensin-converting enzyme inhibition on altered renal hemodynamics induced by a low protein diet in the rat. J Clin Invest *80*:1045–1049, 1987.
71. Pantuck EJ, Pantuck CB, Weissman C, Askanazi J, Conney AH: Effect of parenteral nutritional regimens on oxidative drug metabolism. Anesthesiology *60*:534–536, 1984.
72. Fagan TC, Walle T, Oexmann MJ, Walle UK, Bai SA, Gaffney TE: Increased clearance of propranolol and theophylline by high-protein compared with high-carbohydrate diet. Clin Pharmacol Ther *41*:402–406, 1987.
73. Powels R, Shinibourne E, Hamer J: Selective cardiac sympathetic blockade as an adjunct to bronchodilator therapy. Thorax *24*:616–618, 1969.
74. Solomon HM, Shiogie JJ: Change in receptor site affinity: A proposed explanation for the potentiating effect of D-thyroxine on the anticoagulant response to warfarin. Clin Pharmacol Ther *2*:797–799, 1967.
75. Lipsky JJ: Antibiotic associated hypoprothrombinaemia. J Antimicrob Chemother *21*:281–300, 1988.
76. McInness GT, Thomson GD, Murray GD, Thompson GG, Brodie MJ: Intravenous verapamil during β-receptor blockade with propranolol. Br J Clin Pharmacol *21*:580P, 1986.
77. Webster J: Interactions of NSAID's with diuretics and β-blockers: Mechanisms and clinical implications. Drugs *30*:32–41, 1985.

CHAPTER 23

THE POISON INFORMATION TELEPHONE CALL

Anthony S. Manoguerra, Pharm.D., DABAT

For most poisoning episodes, the poisoned victim or caretaker of the victim establishes first contact with the health care system by telephone. In areas of the country served by a regional poison center, that first contact is usually with the center's staff. In other areas of the country, that first contact may be with emergency department physicians or nurses or the office staff of a primary care physician. Regardless of the location of that first contact, evaluation and assessment of the poisoning exposure requires the ability to gather appropriate information from the caller by telephone and accurately gauge the potential health risk to the victim. This is substantially different from the typical emergency department situation where the victim is physically present and an evaluation using all available senses can be performed. Nonverbal communication can occur in the emergency department setting, and the accuracy of the information can be more easily assessed. When responding by telephone, the questioning of the caller must be far more extensive, and because nonverbal communication cannot be used, the wording of the questions and instructions to the caller is vitally important.

The ability to effectively take telephone histories and effectively transmit information by telephone requires extensive training and experience. In addition, telephone evaluation requires the ability to assess the potential threat to the victim rapidly and accurately. If there exists a threat to the patient's life, emergency transport and prehospital supportive care must be started immediately. However, only approximately 5 to 10 per cent of calls to poison centers require this high level of emergency response. Most victims reported to poison centers, as many as 70 to 80 per cent, require reassurance and first aid. Therefore, the telephone evaluation is essential. If all persons exposed to chemicals or drugs arrived in emergency departments without prior telephone evaluation, the emergency departments would be overloaded by patients requiring no care or simple first aid. To be able to properly evaluate a poisoning exposure by gathering a history over the telephone and to provide a proper assessment and referral requires considerable training and experience.

The American Association of Poison Control Centers has implemented two programs that assess the capabilities of a poison center. The first program is a certification program for regional poison centers whereby a center is certified as providing comprehensive poison center services. To become certified, a center must apply to the Association and meet an established set of criteria.[1] The second program certifies staff operating in poison centers through a written examination that measures both the ability of an individual to gather correct information concerning a case and the level of toxicologic knowledge. Following successful completion of the examination, the person is allowed to use the designation Certified Specialist in Poison Information.

The types of calls that are received by regional poison centers are varied. This is best illustrated by briefly examining data from the National Data Collection System of the American Association of Poison Control Centers. The program was initiated in 1983, and in the first 4 years of operation, the system has collected data on 4,152,616 poisoning exposure cases reported to poison centers around the country. This is the largest poisoning incidence data collection ever compiled. In 1987, 1,166,940 human exposure cases were reported to the system by 63 poison centers.[2] Children under 5 years of age accounted for 62.2 per cent of the cases, whereas 26.6 per cent of cases occurred in adults. The victim's residence was the site of exposure in 91.9 per cent of cases. For pediatric exposures, there was a male predominance, but this gender distribution was reversed in teenage and adult exposures. Accidents caused 83.8 per cent of the exposures, whereas 5.8 per cent were intentional in nature.

Ingestion was the most common route of exposure (77.5 per cent), followed in descending frequency by dermal, ophthalmic, inhalation, bites and stings, and parenteral exposures. In 74.8 per cent of the cases, victims were managed in a nonhealth-care facility, typically their homes. For 23 per cent, treatment in a health-care facility was required, and 17.7 per cent required hospital admission. Three hundred ninety-seven cases ended in a fatal outcome. Twenty-two fatalities were victims under 6 years of age; 3, victims 6 to 12 years; 30, victims 13 to 17 years; and 342, adults. Children and adults most commonly ingest drug products, but exposures can involve the entire spectrum of potential toxic substances. In fatal poisoning exposures, drug products far exceed all other substances. The data just cited show that the typical call to a regional poison center involves the ingestion of a commercial product or drug by a child less than 6 years of age who can be managed at home with first aid and follow-up calls. However, the staff of poison centers are called on to manage and consult on cases involving all age groups, a wide variety of toxic exposures, and the entire spectrum of severity from no effect to fatal poisoning.

When taking a telephone call dealing with a poisoning exposure, the following is the minimum information that should be obtained from the caller:

Who was exposed? The age, sex, and weight of the victim must be obtained. Age and weight are important in determining the potential severity of an exposure. Many assessment algorithms estimate the potential severity of the exposure based on the amount ingested per kilogram of body weight. For example, acetaminophen toxicity is generally felt to occur at single acute doses greater than 140 mg/kg of body weight in healthy adults.

What was (were) the substance(s) involved in the exposure? The exact name of the product must be obtained. The caller should be instructed to provide the name and manufacturer of the product directly from the label. This is extremely important, because slight differences in the name of a product can mean substantial differences in the ingredients and therefore, potential toxicity. For example, Excedrin Extra-Strength Capsules from Bristol-Meyers contain acetaminophen 250 mg, aspirin 250 mg, and caffeine 65 mg, whereas Excedrin Extra-Strength Aspirin Free Capsules from Bristol-Meyers contain only acetaminophen 500 mg.

How much of the substance was involved in the exposure? The quantity of material involved is extremely important in assessing the potential risk from the exposure. Great care must be exercised in questioning the caller to obtain as accurate an estimate as possible. If a solid dose form of a drug is involved, the caller should be asked to determine how many tablets or capsules were present in the container before the exposure and how many are present now. If the drug is a prescription medication, the caller should be asked when it was prescribed and whether the owner has been taking the drug as prescribed. This helps to judge how many were present before the incident. If necessary, the caller should be instructed to count the remaining tablets or capsules in the container.

For liquids, the caller should be asked how much the bottle originally held. Have the caller read this directly from the container. Recent research has shown that the public has substantial difficulty in estimating fluid volumes.[3] Is any of the liquid spilled on the clothing or the floor? Does the victim's breath have the same odor as the product? All these questions will assist in estimating the amount of substance involved. Typically, adults tend to overestimate the volume of a liquid material that a child may have ingested. Many products have a pleasant taste, such as ethylene glycol or scented cleaners, and it may be reasonable to assume that the amount missing was also the amount ingested, particularly if the child was alone with the product for a long period of time. For products with a disagreeable taste, it is unlikely that large volumes will be ingested because the average volume capacity of a typical 2 year old child's mouth ranges from approximately 1.5 ml to 5 ml, depending on the size of the container.[4] In order for a child to ingest 30 ml of gasoline, for example, the child would need to ingest 6 swallows, which is highly unlikely. However, when making an assessment in a situation where the amount is unknown, it is better to make a reasonable overestimation of the potential amount involved and base the assessment accordingly. In this way, any error made in assessing the amount will be on the side of safety.

When did the exposure occur? This will

assist in determining the urgency of the situation. If the substance is expected to cause immediate symptoms and the victim has remained asymptomatic for hours, then the accuracy of the exposure history can be questioned and the patient observed. If the exposure just occurred, and the usual pattern for that particular substance may be delayed, then automobile transport to the hospital can be used. If the ingestion just occurred and the onset of symptoms is rapid, then activation of the emergency medical transport system to provide transportation to the hospital and life support may be needed.

Does the patient have any pre-existing medical problems? Existence of medical problems may complicate a poisoning exposure. For example, reactive airway disease may be triggered by irritant gases that normally would cause minimal problems in a healthy individual.

What is the condition of the victim at this time? The presence or absence of symptoms helps to confirm the history. Are the symptoms likely to have been caused by the alleged material involved in the exposure, or are they not compatible with the history? The onset or absence of symptoms can also help judge when the exposure took place. Most important, the presence or absence of symptoms assists in determining the type and rapidity of medical response the victim requires. Obviously, a victim who is exhibiting life-threatening signs such as coma or seizures requires a response by paramedics, whereas an asymptomatic victim may be observed at home or if further medical evaluation is warranted, that person can be transported by private vehicle to the hospital.

What first-aid procedures have been performed? The primary purpose in asking this question is to determine whether the procedures have been adequate or potentially harmful. For example, a child who has ingested an amount of aspirin that at most is expected to produce mild symptoms would normally be managed at home with ipecac-induced emesis. If this has already been done, then additional treatment may not be necessary. Conversely, if a child who has ingested a nontoxic material has been given salt water as an emetic, then immediate referral to an emergency department for evaluation and treatment is indicated because fatal hypernatremia may occur.[5]

In addition to the information just discussed, the name of the victim and caller should be obtained as well as the telephone number of the caller. If an ambulance is needed to transport the victim, then the address should also be obtained.

Once all of the historical information has been gathered, then an assessment of the potential risk of the exposure must be performed. In order to do this, appropriate reference materials must be readily available and in use often enough to ensure that the person doing the assessment will draw proper conclusions. Regional poison centers often supplement the reference materials with guidelines or protocols that help guide the poison information specialist in making a decision.

The assessment should determine whether the victim is in no danger, potential danger, or immediate danger from the exposure. If the victim is determined to be in no danger, then the caller can be provided with reassurance that the victim will not likely develop symptoms. Unless the material involved is totally nontoxic, e.g., silica gel ingestion or blackboard chalk ingestion, follow-up calls should be performed to the caller at appropriate times to assure that the history was accurate and that the victim is not becoming symptomatic.[6] For victims in immediate danger, the emergency medical services response system should be activated for transport to the hospital and provision with life support, if necessary. For victims in potential danger, some may be adequately managed with first-aid procedures and close observation at home, whereas others may require emergency department evaluation and treatment. If home therapy is instituted, the caller must be provided with explicit instructions in the required first-aid procedures and also about those circumstances that may develop that would indicate the necessity for additional treatment. Follow-up calls to the caller are absolutely essential in these situations. *If follow-up calls cannot be made, then home first-aid therapy should not be initiated.* If the victim is referred to a medical facility, that facility should be notified in advance of the victim's arrival so that needed preparations can be made for treatment to begin immediately. Following completion of the call, all the historical information, the basis for assessment, and the instructions to the caller need to be recorded in a written document for both legal and quality assurance purposes.

The person assessing the exposure must be able to perform some basic calculations in order to properly use the references and draw proper conclusions. For example, simple calculations such as converting pounds to kilograms may be needed to determine the dose per kilogram of body weight. Many products report their active ingredients as per cent solutions or percentages of active ingredients in a mixture. Staff responding to calls must be able to rapidly convert percentages to milligrams per milliliter in order to determine the dose to which the victim was exposed. Laboratory values are often reported in different units by different laboratories. When evaluating laboratory results, it is imperative, first of all, to know the units reported with the result and then to be able to quickly convert between units for comparison of the results with reported levels in the literature. For example, in the literature, theophylline plasma levels are most commonly reported in micrograms per milliliter (μg/ml). Many laboratories report the results in milligrams per liter (mg/L) or milligrams per deciliter (mg/dl). It is important to understand that μg/ml and mg/L are the same, whereas mg/dl is not equivalent. For example, a theophylline plasma level of 100 μg/ml is also equal to 100 mg/L and 10 mg/dl.

The history taking and assessment procedures just outlined are absolutely essential for proper handling by telephone of potential poisoning victims. To appropriately train staff to function in this capacity requires considerable resource commitment in time and funding. Regional poison centers are set up to operate in this fashion, efficiently handling large numbers of cases daily and thereby building a sizable experience base. It is not feasible to expect that the staff of most physicians' offices or emergency departments could develop the same level of expertise to function comparably with the staff of a regional poison center.[7]

It is therefore imperative that emergency departments and all physicians within a region develop a close working relationship with the regional poison center to facilitate the care of poisoned patients. Primary care providers should assist the regional poison center by informing the public that the proper entry point into the health care system in the event of a poisoning is through telephone contact with the regional poison center.

References

1. American Association of Poison Control Centers: Criteria for Certification as a Regional Poison Center. April, 1988.
2. Litovitz TL, Schmitz BF, Matyunas N, Martin TG: 1987 Annual report of the American Association of Poison Control Centers national data collection system. Am J Emerg Med *6*:479, 1988.
3. Normann SA, Manoguerra AS: Evaluation of Volume Perception of Adults. Presented at the AAPCC/AACT/ABMT/CAPCC annual meeting. San Diego, CA, October 1984.
4. Watson WA, Bradford DC, Veltri JC: The volume of a swallow: Correlation of deglutition with patient and container parametrs. Am J Emerg Med *3*:278, 1983.
5. Barer J, Hill LL, Hill RM, Martinez WM: Fatal salt poisoning from salt used as an emetic. Am J Dis Child *125*:889, 1973.
6. Litovitz TL, Elshami JE: Poison center operations: The necessity of follow-up. Ann Emerg Med *11*:348, 1982.
7. Thompson DF, Trammel HL, Robertson NJ, Reigert JR: Evaluation of regional and nonregional poison centers. N Engl J Med *308*:191, 1983.

CHAPTER 24

PREVENTION OF CHILDHOOD POISONINGS

Alan Woolf, M.D., M.P.H.
Frederick H. Lovejoy, Jr., M.D.

During the past 25 years, childhood morbidity and mortality due to poisoning have decreased as a result of new prevention strategies, along with improved triage and management techniques. Although prevention of poisonings might be broadly defined to include prevention of excessive morbidity and mortality from the injury once a poison exposure has taken place, in this chapter the definition of prevention is restricted to those measures that attempt to avert the poisoning exposure itself. Indeed, improved education, technology, and government regulations in the interests of poisoning prevention all have served as models for efforts to prevent other types of injuries as well.

PASSIVE VERSUS ACTIVE STRATEGIES

Poisoning prevention strategies can be divided conceptually into *passive* and *active* interventions. Passive interventions are those measures that do not depend on behavioral changes by the public for their success. Examples include federal regulations prohibiting the retail sales of caustic agents in household products in concentrations higher than those regarded as safe for home use. Because highly caustic agents have become less accessible to the public, the probability that they will cause poisoning is automatically reduced.

Another example of a passive safety strategy is packaging potentially dangerous medications in child-resistant containers. Such packaging limits a young child's chance of exposure to a toxic dose of the drug before being discovered by a supervising adult. Because the child-resistant cap is automatically part of the packaging, a parent does not need to make an active decision to implement this safety measure.

Active poisoning prevention strategies, on the other hand, are those that require sustained behavioral changes in the target population in order to be effective. For example, counseling parents to poison-proof their household requires continued vigilance for potential toxins entering the household and a sustained and repeated effort to store safely those household products that might be poisonous to toddlers.

THE ECOLOGY OF POISONING

Children living in families whose system of supervision has broken down are at high risk for poisoning. Some particular stress such as a recent move, family loss, or financial hardship can cause parents to relax their vigilance. Poisonings often occur when a parent is distracted—for example, around mealtime or when entertaining guests. Many poisonings occur when the parent-child interaction is not in the "business-as-usual" routine of everyday life. For example, at holiday time new hazards are introduced into a child's environment (e.g., Christmas trees and ornaments) and the parents may be distracted from their usual supervision activities by parties and family social gatherings. Previous studies have suggested that many childhood poisonings occur when a product is in use,[1] reinforcing the idea that lack of supervision is what places the child at high risk.

There is considerable evidence that complex family dynamics often underlie poisoning incidents. Families of childhood poisoning repeaters are characterized as disorganized, socially isolated, and operating under the stress of poor housing, frequent moves, or the psychiatric or physical illness of family members.[2–6] Sobel and Margolis have suggested that children who repeatedly poison themselves use such incidents as tactics in an ongoing power struggle with their parents.[7] They found that the mothers of such poisoning repeaters often came from broken homes, had alcoholic parents, and had poor parental role models; the parents were frequently sexually incompatible, and the child was the product of an unexpected and unwanted pregnancy. The children tended to be hyperactive and negativistic. The importance of such disordered family relationships in poisoning causation is reinforced by Baltimore and Meyer's findings that the poisoning recognition and storage habits of parents of 52 poisoned children were no different from those of parents of 52 control children.[8] Thus, the environmental hazards present seemed to be the same; what differed between families with and without injuries seemed to be *psychosocial* and *behavioral* factors.

Poisoning prevention strategies that fail to address important moderators such as the behavior of the child, the organization and structure of the family, and the nature of the child-parent interaction have little chance for success. Although child-proofing changes in the house may remain static, the circumstances in which the threshold to a poisoning injury is breached are dynamic (e.g., opened household products or medications, poor supervision, altered family routines). Modification of these circumstances requires patience, counseling, increased social supports, and behavioral adaptations by both children and parents. These goals are somewhat elusive and are part of the challenge in the development of new poisoning prevention strategies.

GENERAL POISONING PREVENTION STRATEGIES

Model poisoning prevention strategies have sought to combine improved technologic advances with enlightened government regulations and effective public education to reduce the risk of a poisoning injury. Baker and colleagues[9] described such general injury prevention strategies, when applied to poisonings, to include the following:

1. Banning or reducing the manufacture or sale of an injurious toxin
2. Decreasing the concentration of a poison or the total amount of a poison available to the individual to subinjurious levels
3. Preventing access to the substance
4. Creating barriers between the host and agent during the use of the toxin
5. Substituting products with less inherent toxicity but equal efficacy for more dangerous products
6. Changing the formulation of a product to make it less injurious

Each of these various principles has been successfully applied to various causes of poisoning among adults as well as children. The banning of aldrin and DDT exemplifies legislation targeted at preventing environmental toxic exposures. Limiting baby aspirin to 36 per bottle reduces the likelihood that toddlers will poison themselves. Child-resistant containers and safe storage of hazardous products prevent access. Use of particulate respirator masks during removal of paint provides a barrier to prevent toxicity due to inhalation of lead. The substitution of acetaminophen for propoxyphene gives equal analgesia while avoiding propoxyphene's considerable toxicity in the event of overdose. The reformulation of children's cough and cold preparations to exclude alcohol removes a potential source of toxicity to infants.

Although a number of excellent poisoning prevention strategies have been implemented to reduce adult injuries from exposure to occupational or environmental poisons, this chapter addresses only those specific prevention strategies effective in reducing acute home poisoning among children. The following strategies to prevent home poisonings are discussed:

1. Product packaging changes
2. Sticker trials
3. Communitywide programs
4. Clinic-based counseling
5. Creation of poison control centers

SPECIFIC POISONING PREVENTION STRATEGIES

Child-Resistant Containers

As early as 1960, the federal government began to take regulatory steps to reduce the incidence of poisoning in the United States by passing the Federal Hazardous Substance Labeling Act. This consumer-oriented legislation required proper labeling of products but did not attempt to regulate their packaging, sale, or use.[10]

During the next 15 years, better designs of

child-resistant containers were developed and field tested. The rationale for such technology was developmental — that children at highest risk for accidental poisoning (i.e., those 18 to 36 months old) lacked the ability to combine gross motor skills (the palmar exertion of sufficient straight vector force) simultaneously with fine motor skills (the finger-exerted twisting of sufficient torque force) to open easily products secured by child-resistant containers.

The technologic and design engineering advances of effective packaging, combined with enough education of the public to convince them of the potential worth of such product changes, culminated in passage of the Poison Prevention Packaging Act in 1972.[11] This legislation established standards for special packaging of household products and pharmaceuticals, defined appropriate testing procedures and those products that were subject to the regulation, and set a timetable for gradually phasing in the regulations during an 8-year period. The first products to be regulated were those containing aspirin. The list of the products covered and the dates of implementation are shown in Table 24–1. This regulation provides that if a consumer product presents a serious danger to children and special packaging is both technically feasible and practical, then a safety closure design must be submitted before the product is approved for marketing. In a 5-minute period, 85 per cent of a panel of 200 children under the age of 5 must fail to open the package. A panel of adults are also allowed a single 5-minute period, in which 90 per cent must be able to open the safety closure after reading the opening instructions on the package.

The purpose of child-resistant caps is to separate the child physically from the potential poison by providing a barrier between the two. The intent of the regulation was not to poison-proof the container but simply to delay children long enough in their attempts to get to a poison for an adult to discover and correct the hazardous situation. Follow-up studies suggest that the effectiveness of child-resistant containers has been dramatic. Accidental ingestion of aspirin by children under the age of 5 accounted for 26 per cent of all accidental ingestions in 1965, but salicylate poisonings accounted for only 4.7 per cent of all ingestions by 1974.[10] Deaths due to aspirin poisoning, approximately 400 per year in 1945, declined to 46 in 1972, and even further to 17 deaths in 1975. Other studies have shown that poisonings by safety-packaged products decreased nationally by 38 per cent from 1973 to 1976 among the age group between birth and 4 years (Table 24–2); poisonings by unregulated products increased by 20 per cent during the same period among children of the same age group.[12]

As a result of child-resistant packaging, an estimated 86,000 poisoning injuries were averted between the years 1974 and 1981.[13] Walton's study during a 6-year period (1972–1978) demonstrated a decline from 7500 to 2300 ingestions during the first 6-year period after the regulations took effect, whereas ingestions of various unregulated products either rose or stayed the same.[14]

In one public survey, more than 98 per cent of parents could describe safety packaging or safety caps.[15] An overwhelming 85 per cent of the 636 families surveyed approved of the idea of safety packaging, and 89 per cent had safety packages in the home. Only 3 per cent of respondents had discontinued use of a product because of difficulty with the package.

The Poison Prevention Packaging Act is a model example of well-crafted legislation brought about by the successful combination of physician advocacy, improved technology, and effective public education.

Other Packaging Methods

More recent product changes have included the use of unit dosing with *blister packs*. Such dispensers are expensive but accomplish the dual purposes of lowering the risk of unintentional drug overdoses because of misinterpretation of dosing instruction and decreasing the risk of an accidental overdose by children, who must spend more time unwrapping each individual pill and thus hopefully cannot ingest a harmful quantity before being discovered.

The advent of *tamper-resistant containers* with protective plastic-wrapped seals has also decreased the risk that a product might be intentionally altered without being noticed by an unwary consumer. Such an outer wrap theoretically imposes yet another barrier to children as well. The success of such tamper-proof packaging in preventing poisonings has yet to be fully evaluated. The fact that

Table 24–1. PRODUCTS COVERED BY THE POISON PREVENTION PACKAGING ACT

PPPA REGULATION	EFFECTIVE DATE	CHARACTERISTICS OF PRODUCTS REGULATED
Aspirin	8/14/72	Products containing aspirin for oral human use
Furniture polish	9/13/72	Nonemulsion liquid form, low viscosity, containing at least 10% mineral seal oil or petroleum distillates
Methyl salicylate	9/21/72	Liquid products containing more than 5% by weight
Controlled drugs	10/24/72	For oral human use
Sodium and/or potassium hydroxide	4/11/73	Dry forms at least 10% by weight; other forms at least 2% by weight
Turpentine	7/1/73	Liquid form at least 10% by weight
Kindling and/or illuminating preparations	10/29/73	Prepackaged liquid, low viscosity, containing at least 10% petroleum distillates
Methyl alcohol	7/1/73	Liquids containing at least 4% by weight
Sulfuric acid	8/14/73	Substances containing at least 10% by weight
Prescription drugs	4/16/74	For oral human use
Ethylene glycol	6/1/74	Liquids containing at least 10% by weight
Paint solvents	4/23/77	Solvents for paints that contain 10% or more by weight of benzene, toluene, xylene
Iron-containing drugs	10/17/78	Noninjectable animal and human drugs containing 250 mg or more elemental iron (total package)
Dietary supplements	10/17/78	Dietary supplements containing 250 mg or more elemental iron (total package)
Acetaminophen	2/27/80	Preparations for oral human use with 1 gram or more acetaminophen (total package)

(From Walton W: An evaluation of the poison prevention packaging act. Pediatrics *69*:364, 1982.)

most childhood poisonings occur with opened products already in use perhaps reduces the expectation that such packaging will offer substantial prevention gains.[16]

Sticker Trials

Older children can be educated to recognize hazardous agents and avoid them. Such education usually includes the use of warning stickers that parents affix to hazardous household products to alert children to the danger. These stickers, picturing a skull and crossbones, angry serpent, or frowning face (Mr. Yuk), are meant to evoke psychologically unpleasant or fearsome images in a child's mind so that she or he will be deterred from sampling the poisonous contents. Braden found that such a method of discriminating hazardous agents was necessary; preschool children incorrectly identified 40 per cent of poisonous products with which they were confronted. When children were exposed to an educational program on products labeled with warning stickers, their accuracy of recognition improved to 86 per cent.[17] Krenzelok and Garber introduced poison recognition teaching aids into a day-care center program serving 3285 children 30 to 60 months old and tested 195 randomly selected children 6 weeks later. The children showed improvements in their recognition of the warning symbol, Mr. Yuk, and in their understanding of which products were poisonous.[18]

Table 24–2. CAUSES OF FATAL POISONING AMONG CHILDREN AGES 0–4, 1960 AND 1980

AGENT	1960	1980
Aspirin	144	12
Lead	78	2
Petroleum products	48	9
Caustics/cleaning agents	23	7
All other solids and liquids	152	23
TOTAL	445	73
Death rates per 100,000 population	2.2	0.5

(From Baker S, O'Neill B, Karpf R: The Injury Fact Book. Lexington, MA, Lexington Books, 1984, p 191.)

No decrease in the incidence of poisonings has been associated with exposure to such a program, however. When Fergusson's group performed a controlled field trial that distributed labels to 583 families with 543 matched controls, no significant differences in poisoning rates could be appreciated.[19] More than 40 per cent of the parents thought Mr. Yuk labels were not useful, had misgivings about the program, or did not use the warning labels to cover all the poisons in the home. The success of an educational effort employing warning stickers probably is contingent on reinforcement of the learning; continuity of medical care (and repetition of the education) may improve the effectiveness of such a program.[20]

Other concerns have been expressed about the use of warning stickers on household products. Some researchers and parents fear that young children may be attracted instead of repulsed by the warning stickers or may not be able to understand what a poison means.[21] Furthermore, many poisons (e.g., plants) cannot be labeled with a warning. Finally, those poisoning incidents occurring outside the household—which may represent as many as 13 per cent of all poisonings in children under the age of 5[22]—cannot be effectively forestalled by a home-centered program.

Communitywide Educational Efforts

Relatively few programs have attempted to implement poisoning prevention on a communitywide basis. The health department or a poison control center has usually spearheaded such projects with the cooperation of local government officials, health professionals, community action groups, and even businesses and merchandisers. Fisher and colleagues[23] introduced one such intervention, which included community outreach seminars, school curriculum changes, point of purchase education efforts by retailers, and mass media and educational material distribution activities in Monroe County, New York. As a result, the number of poisonings requiring emergency department treatment in area hospitals dropped 66 per cent and poisoning admissions dropped 71 per cent, whereas hospitalization rates in comparable control communities remained stable. Maisel and associates[24] organized a poisoning prevention project in Charleston County, South Carolina, involving education of the public about the recognition of potential poisons and techniques for their safe storage. Activities such as programs for community groups, poster contests, mass media presentations, and group discussions were used. Results of pre- versus postintervention surveys suggested that 88 per cent of parents had been reached by the educational campaign and had implemented the recommendations. Researchers noted that the number of children hospitalized in Charleston County for poisoning declined. Both of these model programs have demonstrated that community awareness about poisoning prevention can be increased and can lower the rate of poisoning. How long such educational efforts can be sustained remains unclear; whether a more modest but self-perpetuating program of education can be as effective a deterrent needs to be tested.

Clinic-Based Educational Programs

One strategy for promoting the prevention of poisonings among young children is clinic-based education for their parents. Such education invariably includes information about the *recognition* of hazardous chemicals in the home environment; *elimination* of the hazard by not purchasing the poison, safely storing it in the home, and disposing of partially used products; *readiness* for a poisoning event by the home storage of syrup of ipecac and use of telephone stickers with emergency telephone numbers; and the appropriate first *response* (first aid) if a toxic exposure occurs in the home.

The success of such programs has been found to depend on a number of factors (Table 24–3):

1. *Content:* The educational message must be clear, readable at the fifth grade level, succinct, and targeted at the intended audience in terms of sophistication.

2. *Timeliness:* Education is most effective when the audience is addressed during a window of receptivity to such a message—that is, when they recognize its im-

Table 24–3. ATTRIBUTES OF IDEAL POISONING PREVENTION EDUCATION

Clear content
Timeliness
Relevance
Recommendations easy to implement
Repetitive intervention
Effective educator
Brief format

portance, are not distracted, and are personally motivated enough to take action.

3. *Relevance:* The message must be important to the audience and perceived as crucial to their well-being. They must be motivated by its relevance to their own health or that of their family in order to take action.

4. *Lack of barriers:* The education must give information that is practical and for which compliance is not too difficult or beset with barriers (interposed tasks the parent must complete to make the effort effective).

5. *Repetitiveness:* The most effective educational modules are repeated to reinforce the message if it is intended that the parent will routinely carry out active safety behaviors (e.g., checking labels for toxic ingredients and containers for child-resistant caps).

6. *Educator:* The professional stature of the educator has been found to relate to the success of the compliance with educational recommendations. Parents are much more likely to value their physician's personal suggestions than they are a written summary or slide show, for example. Other cultural, ethnic, and social forces may also enhance or detract from the educator's effectiveness in delivering the message.

7. *Attention span:* The educational program cannot be so abbreviated that the parent does not recognize its importance. Conversely, the education should not be preachy or tax the attention or time constraints of the audience. A program that engages parents in an active and collaborative learning experience is more effective.

Previous investigations of clinic-based educational programs have been limited by structural or research design problems. Alpert and Heagarty developed a program that used coupons that parents could redeem for poison prevention packs at their local pharmacy. However, this multistep program proved to be too complicated for parents, and the expected results were not achieved. Less than 3 per cent of the coupons were turned in; thus parents did not receive the intended ipecac or the poisoning prevention message.[25] Dershewitz and Williamson failed to show an effect when a safety counseling program to generally child-proof a home was instituted in the clinic setting.[26]

Several recent studies have shown that a more focused message directed at a specific population might be more effective. Dershewitz and colleagues, with a short poisoning prevention message delivered to mothers by a physician during the well child-care visit, demonstrated that parents would remember a simple message and would implement the suggested safety measures at home.[27] Because these mothers were attending the clinic in a health maintenance organization, the universal efficacy of such a program may be questionable. Ipecac kept in the home has been shown to be an effective part of family readiness for a poisoning, and it can prevent injury and reduce the need to seek medical assistance.[28–30] In a follow-up study of 202 families counseled in the emergency clinic setting, Woolf and colleagues showed that such counseling can increase the availability of ipecac in the home 6 months later from 37 to 68 per cent.[31] Thus, a clinic-based counseling program, combined with other prevention measures, can substantially improve family safety practices and readiness in the event of an emergency.

Poison Control Centers

The regionalization of poison control centers across the United States during the past 15 years has contributed to the remarkable progress in poisoning prevention and improvements in management. This success is derived from the leadership that poison control centers have provided in four different areas:

1. Accuracy of toxicologic information
2. Advocacy as a lead agency in poisoning prevention
3. Training for health professionals
4. Research into the ecology, management, and prevention of poisonings

There is little doubt that access to a regional poison control center improves the medical triage and management of a toxic exposure, thus preventing excessive morbidity and mortality. Studies of the use of health services in states with and without poison control centers demonstrate remarkable improvements in telephone triage patterns, avoidance of excess emergency department visits, and improved quality and quantity of pertinent information given for those poisonings in states with regional poison control centers.[32–35]

It is perhaps underappreciated that poison control centers also serve a focusing role as lead agencies in the community for poisoning prevention programs. Poison control centers are a valuable resource for public and professional information about the identification of toxic compounds, acceptable exposure levels, and safe storage and use. Poison control centers also have increasingly expanded their role to service those calls requesting information about occupational or environmental exposures and toxicology. Finally, poison control centers serve as a highly visible networking resource that can make referrals to other community facilities with more specialized knowledge about teratogenicity, public health implications of specific exposures, and plant or animal identifications.

Poison control centers also serve in poisoning prevention by improving the toxicology training of health professionals through tutorials, staff lectures, in-service programs, and regional workshops and symposia. Additionally, poison control centers can serve to alert health professionals, through surveillance of adverse drug reactions, of changes in prescribing style or precautions that must be taken. By pursuing active public education goals via newsletters, public service announcements, health fairs, and media campaigns (e.g., National Poison Prevention Week), poison control centers help to keep the public alert to the principles of poisoning prevention.

Finally, poison control centers often serve as the stimulus to develop new techniques in poisoning prevention. The centers accumulate a dynamic clinical poisoning experience from which epidemiologic trends in poisoning types and circumstances can be identified. Ideally, such an early warning surveillance system regarding a community's specific toxic exposure problems can lead to directed programs aimed at averting microepidemics of poisoning injuries. Because poison control centers are respected by the public and by health professionals for possessing a particular type of expertise, they can stimulate interest in new research and regulations for poisoning prevention.

THE PHYSICIAN'S RESPONSIBILITY

Physicians have a dual role in the prevention of poisonings, as advocates for their patients and patients' families and also as influential and respected community leaders. Physicians must recognize those circumstances that pose a higher than usual potential risk for a poisoning and must take corrective action. This action may include diverse recommendations, such as changing or simplifying a prescribed drug or recommending or advocating day-care, nursing home care, other social supports, psychiatric evaluation, or family counseling. Physicians must give adequate attention to the topic of poisoning prevention within the larger scope of preventive medicine topics that they discuss with patients as part of their routine health maintenance.

Physicians, in their capacity as community leaders, have an obligation to advocate changes necessary to decrease the risk of poisoning and to alert the community to new or previously unrecognized toxic hazards. Such advocacy includes support for the local or regional poison control service serving the community and for its programs in poisoning prevention. Physicians might also make use of public forums to change the public perceptions of poisoning prevention strategies (e.g., the need for child-resistant containers, the importance of following directions for the use of medications, and the dangers of drug abuse). Physicians can also be influential consultants to legislative bodies considering new initiatives restricting the marketing of hazardous substances or regulating their use and disposal.

Dedicated health professionals must make a concerted effort to continue the momentum and consolidate the gains that have been made in poisoning prevention and to advance new aspects of the field.

References

1. Jensen G, Wilson W: Preventive implications of a study of 100 poisonings in children. Pediatrics *65*:490–496, 1960.
2. Sibert R: Stress in families who have ingested poisons. Br Med J *3*:87–89, 1975.
3. Julyan M, Kuyenko J: Accidental poisoning in children: The "sick family." Practitioner *210*:813–815, 1973.
4. Beautrais A, Fergusson D, Shannon T: Accidental poisoning in the first three years of life. Aust Paediatr J *17*:104–109, 1981.
5. Bithoney B, Snyder J, Michalek J, Newberger E: Childhood ingestions as symptoms of family distress. Am J Dis Child *139*:456–459, 1985.

6. Rogers J: Recurrent childhood poisoning as a family problem. J Fam Pract *13*:337–340, 1981.
7. Sobel R, Margolis J: Repetitive poisoning in children: a psychosocial study. Pediatrics *35*:641–651, 1985.
8. Baltimore C, Meyer R: A study of storage, child behavioral traits, and mother's knowledge of toxicology in 52 poisoned families and 52 comparison families. Pediatrics *44*:816–820, 1969.
9. Baker S, O'Neill B, Karpf R: Poisonings. *In* The Injury Fact Book. Lexington, Mass., Lexington Books, 1984.
10. McIntire M: Safety packaging: A model for successful accident prevention. Pediatr Ann *6*:706–708, 1977.
11. Federal Register: Title 16—commercial practices. Chapter II. Consumer Product Safety Commission, Subchapter E—Poison Prevention Packaging Act of 1970 Regulations (1973). Vol 38, No. 151, pp 21247–21250. Tuesday, August 7, 1973.
12. Fisher L: An integrated model for childhood preventive programs. Vet Hum Toxicol *23*:261–264, 1981.
13. Centers for Disease Control: Update: Childhood Poisonings—United States. MMWR *34*:117, 118, 1985.
14. Walton W: An evaluation of the poison prevention packaging act. Pediatrics *69*:363–370, 1982.
15. McIntire M, Angle C, Sathees K, Lee P: Safety packaging—what does the public think? Am J Public Health *67*:169–171, 1977.
16. Jackson R, Walker J, Wynne N: Circumstances of accidental poisoning in childhood. Br Med J *4*:245–248, 1968.
17. Braden B: Validation of a poison prevention program. Am J Public Health *69*:942–944, 1979.
18. Krenzelok E, Garber R: Teaching poison prevention to preschool children, their parents, and professional educators through child care centers. Am J Public Health *71*:750–752, 1981.
19. Fergusson D, Horwood L, Beautrais A, Shannon F: A controlled field trial of a poisoning prevention method. Pediatrics *69*:515–520, 1982.
20. Phillips W, Little T: Continuity of care and poisoning prevention education. Patient Counsel Health Educ, 2:170–173, 1980.
21. Vernberg K, Culver-Dickinson P, Spyker D: The deterrent effect of poison-warning stickers. Am J Dis Child *138*:1018–1020, 1984.
22. Polakoff J, Lacouture P, Lovejoy F: The environment away from home as a source of potential poisoning. Am J Dis Child *138*:1014–1017, 1984.
23. Fisher L, Van Buren J, Nitzkin J, Lawrence R, Swackhamer R: Highlight results of the Monroe County poison prevention demonstration project. Vet Hum Toxicol *22*(Suppl. 2):15–17, 1980.
24. Maisel G, Langdoe B, Jenkins M, Aycock E: Analysis of two surveys evaluating a project to reduce accidental poisoning among children. Public Health Rep *82*:555–560, 1967.
25. Alpert J, Heagarty M: Evaluation of a program for distribution of ipecac syrup for the emergency home management of poison ingestions. J Pediatr *69*:142–146, 1960.
26. Dershewitz R, Williamson J: Prevention of childhood household injuries: a controlled clinical trial. Am J Public Health *67*:1148–1153, 1977.
27. Dershewitz R, Posner M, Paichel W: The effectiveness of health education on home use of ipecac. Clin Pediatr *22*:268–270, 1983.
28. Amitai Y, Mitchell A, Carrel J, Lucino H, Lovejoy F: Patterns of calling time and ipecac availability among poison center callers. Am J Dis Child *141*:622–625, 1987.
29. Hurst J, Dozzi A: The emergency treatment of poisoning in children. Med J Aust *2*:432–438, 1975.
30. Mofenson H, Greensher J: Controversies in the prevention and treatment of poisonings. Pediatr Ann *6*:60–74, 1977.
31. Woolf A, Lewander W, Filippone G, Lovejoy F: Prevention of childhood poisoning: Efficacy of an educational program carried out in an emergency clinic. Pediatrics *80*:359–363, 1987.
32. Sagotsky R, Gouveia W, Lovejoy F: Evaluation of the effectiveness of a poison information center. Clin Toxicol *11*:581–586, 1977.
33. Thompson D, Trammel H, Robertson N, Reigart J: Evaluation of regional and nonregional poison centers. N Engl J Med *308*:191–194, 1983.
34. Chafee-Bahamon C, Caplan D, Lovejoy F: Patterns in hospital's use of a regional poison information center. Am J Public Health *73*:396–400, 1983.
35. Chafee-Bahamon C, Lovejoy F: Effectiveness of a regional poison center in reducing excess emergency room visits for children's poisonings. Pediatrics *72*:164–169, 1983.

CHAPTER 25

DISASTER MANAGEMENT OF MASSIVE TOXIC EXPOSURE

Constance J. Doyle, M.D., FACEP
Mark J. Upfal, M.D., M.P.H.
Neal E. Little, M.D., FACEP

Exposure to hazardous materials is unfortunately as much a fact of modern life as such things as vehicular accidents and poisonings. The term hazardous material is used here to mean any substance that can be harmful to humans, animals, or the environment when released in any uncontrolled manner.[1] This chapter focuses on the management principles applicable to acute exposure to hazardous materials. Therefore, it will not address the issues surrounding chronic lower-level exposure.

One need not live near a chemical manufacturing plant, heavy industry, or a chemical dump site to be at risk for exposure to hazardous materials. A source of potential exposure is the nearest road, railroad track, or waterway. Enormous volumes of hazardous materials are transported every day. Materials for industry and agriculture are in constant movement within our transportation system. Accidents can and obviously do happen, and, as a result, people and their environment can suddenly and unexpectedly become exposed.

In 1980, several billion tons of hazardous materials were transported in the United States. Additionally, billions of tons of hazardous materials were in storage sites. Approximately 40 per cent of these materials are transported by truck.[2] Over 100,000 shippers and 40,000 motor carriers transport hazardous materials.

During 1987, CHEMTREC (a Chemical Manufacturers Association service providing assistance for hazardous materials emergencies) logged over 55,000 calls. Approximately 10 per cent of calls came from nontransportation emergencies, such as fixed sites or storage facilities. In 1984, the National Response Center received over 10,000 notifications of spills or accidents.[3] It has been estimated that approximately 80 per cent of all accidents involving the release of hazardous materials occurs on highways, with a somewhat lower percentage occurring on railroads.[2] However, railroad accidents contribute to a significant number of injuries from the transportation of hazardous chemicals.

Another consideration is the potential result from combinations of hazardous materials, such as the many new compounds generated in fires at manufacturing and storage facilities or at chemical dump sites. Furthermore, toxic injuries may be associated with other injuries as well. For example, a train derailment in a heavily populated area could encompass many problems: fire with burn injuries, explosion with physical trauma, noxious gases with respiratory injury, chemical burns, and systemic poisoning. As an isolated problem, each is difficult enough to treat. The magnitude of each problem may increase exponentially, with mass casualties, injured rescuers, and medical needs outstripping the resources to deal with them.

A brief hypothetical example of a hazardous material emergency will illustrate these facets.

A train derails near a populated suburb next to the river that is the source of the city's water supply. Multiple chemical tank cars are damaged, and the accident involves a moderate number of human casualties. Someone who has seen the wreck calls for help.

Immediately, several issues are apparent. First and foremost, what are the chemicals and how can one identify them?[4] Is it safe to approach the train to remove the wounded? Is there a fire or explosion hazard? Is the water supply to the city in danger, and, if so, what can one do about it? Do rescuers need respiratory and skin protection? Can victims be brought to the hospital emergency department without exposing the emergency department personnel and patients to chemical hazards? Should nearby residents be evacuated and how far? How does one know that the overturned tank cars are leaking? Who should be notified? Who is in charge? Who is responsible? Who will pay?

THE BHOPAL EXPERIENCE

Let us turn to an example of a real major disaster. On the night of December 3, 1984, a cloud of methyl isocyanate gas leaked from a storage tank at the Union Carbide plant in Bhopal, Mahdya Pradesh, India. Approximately 500 people in the surrounding area were killed before reaching medical treatment, and the total death count was approximately 2500.[5–7] Over 250,000 people were affected. One hospital alone treated 25,000 patients in the first 24 hours.[7] Ten thousand people were admitted to the J.P. Narayan hospital alone.[8]

Immediate respiratory symptoms consisted of severe coughing, dyspnea, pharyngitis, respiratory distress, and pulmonary edema. Severe eye irritation, lacrimation, eyelid edema, and corneal ulceration were also present. Gastrointestinal symptoms consisted of increase in salivation, nausea, vomiting, abdominal pain, and defecation; increase in urination was also noted. Central nervous system symptoms were manifested by coma, seizures, dizziness, limb weakness, and tremors.

Methyl isocyanate is used in the manufacture of carbamate insecticides. It is a liquid that has a low boiling point and is heavier than air in its gaseous form. It has a strong odor and is irritating to the eyes, skin, and respiratory tract. It may be toxic both by inhalation and cutaneous exposure. At the time of the Bhopal incident, there was a paucity of toxicologic data in the literature about exposure to this chemical.

A crowded shantytown existed immediately outside the Union Carbide plant. Residents were sleeping, and no warning was sounded at the time of the gas release. The hutlike dwellings provided little protection against the gas. Ninety to ninety-five per cent of the dead and severely injured came from this area.[7] A crowded railway station situated 1 kilometer from the plant had more than 100 dead;[7] 200 people were unconscious and 600 were lying around injured.[9]

Several studies of survivors were undertaken 3.5 months after the incident. Patients in these studies were categorized according to their distance from the plant on the night of the accident. Group I consisted of those 0.5 to 2 kilometers from the plant, and Group II was composed of those at least 8 kilometers from the plant. The groups were similar socioeconomically and demographically. One hundred per cent of the Group I sample and forty-two per cent of Group II had symptoms at the time of the incident. At the time of the study, 80 per cent of Group I and 28 per cent of Group II had continued respiratory complaints consisting of cough with or without sputum production, breathlessness, and chest pain. Fifty-seven per cent of Group I had abnormal chest radiographs, forty-nine per cent had documented restrictive defects, and twenty-one per cent had obstructive defects. Smokers numbered 11.6 per cent.[10] It is unclear whether prior pulmonary disease was present or whether some patients had both restrictive and obstructive pulmonary disease.

In a group of children categorized in the same manner, the most symptomatology occurred in the immediate area of the plant, although the more remote group was not without symptoms. Ninety-five per cent of those children from Group I had immediate cough and seventy-four per cent experienced breathlessness. Three months later, 84 per cent noted persistent cough and 48 per cent suffered from continued breathlessness. Abnormal radiographs were found in 66 per cent of Group I children, compared with 8.1 per cent of Group II children. Pulmonary testing was performed on children over the age of 7 years. Obstructive defects were found in 28 of 33 children. Persistent abdominal pain and anorexia were found in the Group I children only. Group I children experienced persistent conjunctivitis, and 10 per cent demonstrated visual abnormalities. There were no persistent eye abnormalities in those situated 8 km from the plant (Group II). Persistent neurobehavioral symptoms consisted of poor memory and weakness. Comprehensive psychologic testing was not performed. Some children who later developed obvious psychic disturbances had been classified as dead at the time of the accident and had been initially placed in morgues. Others had witnessed the deaths of parents or siblings.[11]

The local lake had measurable levels of isocyanates for 9 months after the incident. Such levels were not detectable, however, 1 year after the incident.

At the time of the incident, there were no existing plans to alert the local population in the event of disaster. Methods of protection or routes of evacuation were not publicized.

The plant was located in a densely populated area, with a shantytown around the plant. There was no widespread knowledge of the hazardous materials being used or the products manufactured. There were no standard operating practices and few engineering controls.[6] It is estimated that approximately 50,000 pounds of methyl isocyanate in liquid and vapor form were released into the atmosphere when a valve on a storage tank opened for approximately 2 hours.[7] Light winds prevented rapid dispersion of the heavier-than-air cloud. The accident happened at night when most of the residents were sleeping. Because of the rapid onset of symptoms and the large numbers affected, local hospitals were rapidly overwhelmed. Many patients were treated in the hospital garden. Local citizens helped each other in the initial rescue attempt. No local medical authority on methyl isocyanate was immediately available.

In summary, methyl isocyanate is used in the manufacture of carbamate pesticides. The major acute effects resulting from the exposures at Bhopal were related to local respiratory and eye irritation. Methyl isocyanate at higher exposure levels causes asthmatic reactions and pulmonary edema. Diisocyanates are known to be potent sensitizing agents, capable of inducing bronchospasm at minuscule exposure levels in sensitized individuals. However, this reaction to monoisocyanates such as methyl isocyanate has not yet been documented.[12] Data regarding the chronic effects of methyl isocyanate are lacking, and the long-term effects of this incident may not become apparent for many years. One might expect to see cases of chronic obstructive pulmonary disease, bronchiolitis, and restrictive lung disease resulting from pulmonary fibrosis.

DISASTER PLANNING

Planning is essential for communities at risk for chemical disasters. In the medical management of large-scale chemical exposure emergencies, numerous considerations are paramount. Individual patient care issues must be considered, as well as the overall management of the incident. As with acute trauma, one must first focus on the airway, breathing, and circulation. Then, other body systems such as the central nervous system can be addressed. In some cases, antidotes may be required. Sometimes decontamination of the victims becomes an important consideration to minimize the contamination of rescuers, medical personnel, and medical facilities.

Hospitals must plan for major chemical incidents. Large amounts of antidotes specific to the potential exposures must be available. Most hospitals in the United States do not have enough atropine (hundreds of milligrams, or even grams may be required) to treat large numbers of organophosphate-poisoned patients. Treatment locations must be planned. Twenty-five thousand patients would overwhelm even the largest hospital system. In some geographic locations, inclement weather may preclude the treatment of patients on the hospital grounds, as in India. Plans would need to include large sheltered treatment areas. Hospitals in the path of a chemical cloud may need to be evacuated unless indoor air quality could be maintained. Any emergency department could be faced with a large-scale hazardous materials emergency resulting from a transportation accident. An estimated 6000 United States facilities manufacture potentially hazardous chemicals. There are approximately 180,000 shipments by truck and rail on a daily basis.[5] There is little regulation limiting which routes and times of day may be used for hazardous materials transportation.

Most chemical substances do not fall under the regulations of the Toxic Substances Control Act of 1976 (TOSCA) which requires that *new* chemicals be reviewed. The Clean Air Act allows the Environmental Protection Agency to regulate emissions from plants under *normal* conditions, rather than emergency incidents such as Bhopal.

Multiple manufacturing facilities have located in third world countries to utilize inexpensive labor and to be closer to those markets. Technologic support is sparse and unevenly distributed. Maintenance of equipment may be poor, and manufacturing standards and controls are a far cry from those of the developed world. Regulations governing plant site planning and regulations governing manufacturing of chemicals are few. In third world countries, very dense residential areas spring up around manufacturing facilities, allowing poor workers easy and inexpensive commutes.[6]

Neither Bhopal nor a similar facility in

Institute, West Virginia, had evacuation plans at the time of the Bhopal disaster. The Institute plant had recorded 84 "escapes" of methyl isocyanate and phosgene during the 5-year period between 1980 and 1985. Some of these were not "reportable" under current regulations, since the amounts were too small.[13] Prevention issues were not even addressed.[6]

Since the Bhopal incident, many chemical industries in the United States have reviewed their safety standards. Site plans are now required for all facilities using hazardous materials and Material Safety Data Sheets must be on site. In addition, computerized site plans with maps of local areas may be available, providing such information as wind direction and other weather data to facilitate evacuation decisions. Local medical authorities should be informed of hazardous materials used in various manufacturing processes so that they can plan treatment in the event of an emergency. Sheltered off site locations for treatment should be available if a hospital is overwhelmed or must be evacuated. Warning mechanisms and a plan for early evacuation will minimize injuries. Hazardous materials training of first responders is paramount. Rescuers must be trained in the use of protective equipment and in decontamination procedures to minimize contamination of medical personnel, vehicles, medical facilities, and the environment.

Table 25–1 lists a few of the known hazardous materials tragedies the world has endured.

LEGISLATION

As required by the OSHA Hazard Communication Standard, "hazards of all chemicals produced or imported by chemical manufacturers or importers [must be] evaluated, and . . . information concerning their hazards [must be] transmitted to affected employers and employees within the manufacturing sector. This transmittal of information is to be accomplished by means of comprehensive hazard communication programs, which are to include container labeling and other forms of warning, material safety data sheets, and employee training" (29 Code of Federal Regulations 1910.1200). Workers must know the hazards of the chemicals with which they work and methods to protect themselves in the event of an accident or incident. There should also be some training in first aid and decontamination procedures at the plant. In addition to this worker "right to know" law, there is also a community "right to know" mandated by the Comprehensive Environmental Response, Compensation, and Liability Act (CERCLA) amendments of 1986, otherwise known as the Superfund Amendments and Reauthorization Act of 1986 (SARA). A balance must be achieved between worker safety, community safety, and production for profit.

Title III of SARA required that a state emergency response commission be established by April, 1987, in each state. This commission, appointed by the governor of the state, must coordinate community emergency planning committees in the development of plans for emergency response to chemical emergencies. A list of 402 extremely hazardous materials, published in the Federal Register November 17, 1986, gave threshold planning quantities. If these materials are produced, used, or stored in quantities exceeding the thresholds, they become subject to the emergency planning requirements. Additionally, requirements were set for emergency notification whenever a release of hazardous material exceeded a reportable quantity. The "community right to know" provisions of SARA require facilities to provide Material Safety Data Sheets and chemical inventories to local emergency planning committees, local fire departments, and state emergency response commissions.

DISASTER MANAGEMENT

A disaster means that needs outstrip resources to deal with the emergency in a time frame appropriate to its treatment. *The primary theme of disaster management is information management. Timely information can change the entire character of an accident.* For example, if one knew immediately that a tank car contained a particular poisonous gas and that it was leaking, then rescuers would not approach the scene without respiratory and skin protection. If one knew immediately that a certain spilled chemical could contaminate the water supply but was otherwise innocuous, then immediate containment would be in order. If the local emergency facility knew that all victims incurred carbon monoxide

Table 25–1. EXAMPLES OF SOME MAJOR HAZARDOUS MATERIALS DISASTERS

December, 1984
Bhopal, India: 2500 deaths and 250,000 injuries resulted from a leak of methyl isocyanate at a Union Carbide plant (see text).

November, 1984
Mexico City, Mexico: Over 400 deaths and 4000 injuries resulted from a liquefied gas explosion.

July, 1976
Seveso, Italy: A chemical plant explosion resulted in a massive release of dioxin (2,3,7,8-tetrachlorodibenzo-para-dioxin) in an urban area, resulting in many cases of chloracne (primarily among children and young adults), but no deaths.

July, 1975
Hopewell, Virginia: Life Science Products plant closed after 16 months' operation, having exposed approximately 150 employees to exceedingly high levels of kepone (an organochlorine pesticide), and polluted the surrounding environment, creating a major community health problem and millions of dollars in damage. Approximately 30 employees were hospitalized for acute poisoning.

June, 1974
Flixborough, Humberside, England: 28 workers killed when a chemical plant pipe ruptured and an explosion resulted. Every building on a 60-acre site was destroyed.

July, 1948
Ludwigshafen, Germany: Dimethylether explosion of a rail car, killing over 200 and injuring 4000 people.

April, 1947
Texas City, Texas: Ammonium nitrate fertilizer explosion on board a freighter in the harbor, spreading to a nearby Monsanto styrene plant, which subsequently exploded, along with another freighter also carrying nitrates. Almost 600 persons were killed, and 2000 were seriously injured.

exposure, they could arrange for auxiliary oxygen sources, as well as transportation for hyperbaric oxygen treatment if indicated. If the emergency department receives large numbers of victims who all have an indentical injury, the resources needed to treat that one injury might be depleted. However, when many of these questions cannot be answered in an appropriate time frame, a potential disaster can turn into a true disaster.

The emergency department must also have rapid access to information about the management of exposures to exotic materials that rarely present to the physician. For example, arsine, a highly toxic gas used in the semiconductor industry, requires a specific protocol for management (see Chapter 59). However, since exposures are fortunately rare, few physicians will have the opportunity to treat arsine poisoning prior to an acute incident. Thus, information about proper workup and treatment must be readily available. One excellent source of this information is the Poisindex. Another source of information about the ingredients, the toxicology, and other hazardous properties of specific chemicals and mixtures, as well as limited medical management information, is the Material Safety Data Sheet (MSDS). The MSDS is available from the manufacturer of all chemical products and is required to be present and available in all industrial plants using the product.

The second principle of proper disaster management is that of procurement of resources in a time frame appropriate to the situation. For example, a dozen people with moderate carbon monoxide poisoning could be handled by most emergency departments. A hundred victims would overwhelm the system if they arrived unannounced. But with sufficient time and planning to procure the necessary supplies, even this number could be handled in a large building such as a movie theater or a school. Few, if any, hospitals could handle a hundred serious burn victims.

The third principle of disaster management is planning. It is said that once a disaster is planned for, the disaster no longer exists. Each community should have developed and put in place an emergency contingency plan that details specific actions and responsibilities of various community services in the event of a crisis situation. There may be a specific hazardous materials annex. This contingency plan, which should be brought up to date yearly, will contain detailed instructions to follow, including emergency response operations; a roster of emergency assistance phone numbers; a description of each service's legal authority and responsibility during an emergency; a description of the structure and responsibility of the designated response organization; a section on spill clean-up techniques; a section on resource laboratories for analysis of chemical and patient data; and a clean-up and disposal equipment resource section.[14–16]

In addition to community disaster planning, industrial sites using hazardous materials must also have a disaster site plan. Plants using large quantities of hazardous materials (e.g., chemical companies), or using unusually toxic materials (e.g., semiconductor facilities) and the local hospitals should work together to plan for emergency response. Information about all significant hazards should be made available to the emergency facility. Ideally, such a plant's MSDSs should be on file in the emergency department and emergency physicians should be familiar with them. Additionally, patients should be transported from the plant to the department along with copies of the appropriate MSDSs.

In general terms, the sequence of events in a disaster is as follows: An accident occurs. Knowledge of it is transmitted to appropriate agencies; these agencies respond and gather more data. They may activate other resources. Control of the scene is secured. The scope of the problem is defined. The necessary plans for the solution of the problem are activated, and follow-up and evaluation are accomplished.

First and foremost is notification of appropriate agencies—that is, police, fire department, emergency medical system, local disaster coordinator, county and state officials, and federal agencies. It is beyond the scope of this chapter to say who must be notified in any given incident. This will vary with the incident and with local and state regulations. Various local and state agencies may have jurisdiction over a particular kind of hazard.[1] These interests may overlap, depending on the nature of a chemical, the location of a spill, and the various laws in a state. Local government sources are probably the best initial resource concerning all the possible agencies that might be involved (Table 25–2).

A police agency is responsible for securing the site: i.e., crowd control, control of access to the site, and evacuation. In general, the police agency is in charge of the overall site. A fire agency will have responsibility to respond to the chemical or fire hazard and possibly initiate extrication and initial treatment of victims. An emergency medical service (EMS) agency is responsible for medical decisions and treatment. Both fire and EMS personnel work with the police concerning their areas of responsibility. Other agencies may have greater jurisdiction and authority, such as the Centers for Disease Control (CDC), the Environmental Protection Agency (EPA), the Occupational Safety and Health Administration (OSHA), the Federal Emergency Management Agency (FEMA), the Agency for Toxic Substances and Disease Registry (within the Public Health Service), and the State Health Department.

Local municipal authorities must know how to gain access to other sources of help, including state and federal agencies. At all times, it is critical for all responders to know who is in control. The agency that assumes control may change as more information concerning the exact nature of the hazard becomes available. It is obvious that obtaining

Table 25–2. AGENCIES POTENTIALLY INVOLVED IN HAZARDOUS MATERIALS EMERGENCIES

Agency for Toxic Substances and Disease Registry (ATSDR)
Environmental Protection Agency (EPA)
State Emergency Planning Commissions (as per SARA)
Local Emergency Planning Committees (as per SARA)
Occupational Safety and Health Administration (OSHA)
Centers for Disease Control (CDC)
National Institute for Occupational Safety and Health (NIOSH)
Nuclear Regulatory Commission
Military/National Guard
Coast Guard
Department of Natural Resources
Fire Department
Police Department
Fish and Game Commission
Highways/Transportation Department
Flood Control
Harbor Commission/Port Authority
Public Health Department
Emergency Department/Emergency Medical Services
Civil Defense
Conservation
Forestry
Water Resources
Public Safety
Public Works
Federal Emergency Management Agency (FEMA)
Referral Hospital/Regional Poison Center

Table 25–3. RESOURCES AVAILABLE IN PLANNING FOR HAZARDOUS MATERIALS EMERGENCIES

Planning Guide and Checklist for Hazardous Materials by the Federal Emergency Management Agency, Washington, DC.
US Coast Guard Chemical Hazard Response Information System. Available through National Response Center. Phone : (800) 422–8802.
NIOSH/OSHA Pocket Guide to Chemical Hazards from US Government Printing Office, Washington, DC 20402. This pocket guide provides quick reference tables for chemical hazard information for a large number of common chemical substances.
NIOSH/OSHA Occupational Health Guidelines for Chemical Hazards from US Government Printing Office. This three volume reference contains specific information for a large number of chemical agents regarding toxicology, emergency procedures, leak procedures, and respiratory and other personal protective equipment.

information in an appropriate time frame is critical in all phases of response to a hazardous material emergency. Table 25–3 lists some resources available to help in the planning phase.

Plans at the local and hospital levels should include local sources of expertise that can be contacted for technical assistance. Sources may include an emergency physician, a toxicologist, a pharmacologist, an industrial hygienist, an occupational medicine specialist, testing laboratories, and chemists. Plans should include potential sources of specialized equipment that may be needed for a given hazard—e.g., equipment for extrication, decontamination showers, oxygen, chemicals for "neutralization," protective gear, and transportation vehicles.

Table 25–4 lists sources of information concerning an emergency response to a spill.

PREHOSPITAL SITE MANAGEMENT

Plan. Planning for the treatment of those exposed to chemicals involves all levels of the health care team, from emergency medical services personnel to emergency department physicians. It is essential to insure that exposure is limited to the fewest people possible.

Equipment. Equipment to handle spills and protective equipment for rescuers must be strategically located in the community, and its location must be known to all responders. An adequate supply of air tanks for self-contained breathing apparatuses (SCBAs) or equipment to refill tanks with adequate-quality breathing air must be available. Persons utilizing SCBAs must be properly trained in their use and understand the limitations of the equipment. Specifically, the time limitations of the supply tank and the reserve tank must be understood so that egress from the contaminated area can be accomplished prior to loss of supply air. The hazard, and necessary equipment, must be determined *before* first responders enter an area of chemical spill.

Many first responders (police and fire department personnel, EMS people, and even physicians and nurses) have been so thoroughly trained to aid an injured victim immediately that a hazard to their own health may be disregarded. As a result, the rescuer entering the contaminated area also may become contaminated and thus, a victim.[17–20] Although rescue of any injured or ill victims who are unable to leave the spill site is of paramount importance, rescue should be attempted only after one ascertains that any rescuers will not themselves become victims.

Identification of the Spill. Identification of the hazardous material should be attempted prior to approach to the spill. One can read the placarding on the truck or train car from afar. Binoculars are an invaluable aid. The bill of lading (cargo manifest) is located in the cab of a truck but may not be accessible without full protective gear. The diamond-shaped placard on the side of a tank or rail car with the Department of Transportation (DOT) number on it or the DOT number on the back of a truck or tank car will identify by chemical group the material being shipped. Rapid information can be obtained from the 1987 DOT Guidebook (#DOT P 5800.4), which lists chemicals by number, name, and hazard class.[4] Some states also have numbered placards with emergency information numbers to call. Similar numbers can be found on the shipping papers or package. If no number is found, then the various symbols within the diamond-shaped

Table 25–4. SOURCES OF INFORMATION AND ASSISTANCE FOR EMERGENCY RESPONSE

Chemical Transportation Emergency Center (CHEMTREC):
(800) 424–9300 (continental USA)
(202) 483–7616 (outside continental USA or Washington, DC)

Chemical Referral Center:
This is CHEMTREC's nonemergency line.
(800) 262–8200 (9 AM–6PM EST, M–F)
(202) 887–1255 (Washington, DC)

National Response Center:
(800) 424–8802 (Outside Washington, DC)
(202) 267–2675 (Washington, DC)

Coast Guard Atlantic Strike Force:
Coast Guard Pacific Strike Force:
Response teams for major spills.
(205) 694–6601 (Atlantic)
(415) 883–3311 (Pacific)

National Pesticide Telecommunications Network:
(800) 858–7378 (or 800–858–PEST)
(806) 743–3091 (Texas)

EPA RCRA/Superfund Hotline:
(800) 424–9346 (8:30 AM–4:30 PM EST, M-F)

EPA Chemical Emergency Preparedness Program:
(800) 535–0202

Toxic Substances Control Act (TOSCA) Hotline:
(202) 554–1404

Department of Transportation (DOT)
Office of Hazardous Materials Transportation:
(202) 366–4488

Centers for Disease Control (CDC):
(404) 633–5313

Department of Energy (DOE):
(301) 352–5555

National Institute for Occupational Safety and Health (NIOSH):
(404) 329–3061

Occupational Safety and Health Administration (OSHA):
(202) 523-8017

placard (Fig. 25–1)[4] should identify the general class of material being shipped. General emergency information as well as evacuation distances also can be found in this guidebook. Identification of the shipper may be possible by reading the markings on the truck from a distance. The shipper may be contacted to assist in chemical identification and provision of resources.

On a train, the waybill can be found with the conductor, who rides in either the caboose or engine. Call the nearest company trainmaster, relaying the number of the car and the location, who can get information and handling information from the tracking computer.[16] The waybill contains an STC (Standard Transport Code) number that identifies the specific chemical. Chemicals with numbers beginning with 49 are classified as hazardous.[21] The waybill contains specific chemical names and handling information as well. Additional detailed information can be obtained from the Association of American Railroads' book, Emergency Handling of Hazardous Materials in Surface Transportation (1987).[21] With train cars numbered from engine to caboose, one can thus learn what chemical the car may be carrying.[16]

Rapid emergency information can be obtained by calling CHEMTREC at 1–800–424–9300 and giving the *name* of the compound. CHEMTREC is an emergency-only communications resource. The agency will connect emergency personnel with the manufacturer's and/or shipper's personnel who can advise on emergency handling. They can then advise what sort of rescue gear may be needed and what decontamination, if any, is needed at the site.[22, 23] Most manufacturing plants have a site plan showing the location of hazardous material.

Police are needed to secure an area or initiate evacuation when danger from fumes, fire, or explosion exists. They must control crowds so that others do not become casualties. When evacuation is necessary, those downwind from the hazard should be evacuated first.

In the event that the chemical is unknown, the safest way to rescue any victim is for rescuers to enter the area in fully encapsulated suits with positive pressure, self-contained breathing apparatus.[18–20, 24] In most communities the fire department has "full turnout gear," which includes self-contained breathing apparatus. Firefighters are trained in use of the gear, whereas many EMS rescue teams are not. Some localities have access to special acid suits and other protective gear. Under medical guidance, the firefighters may begin decontamination and rescue the patient or patients. The fire department is the most qualified to assess the potential for fires and explosions and to advise medical personnel of such.

The smallest number of rescuers possible

USE ONLY IF MATERIALS CANNOT BE SPECIFICALLY IDENTIFIED
THROUGH SHIPPING PAPERS OR MARKINGS.
POISON GAS
Guide 15
POISON
Guide 55
CORROSIVE
Guide 59
DANGEROUS
Guide 11
FLAMMABLE GAS
Guide 19
FLAMMABLE SOLID
Guide 38
COMBUSTIBLE
Guide 26
FLAMMABLE
Guide 26
BLASTING AGENTS
Guide 46

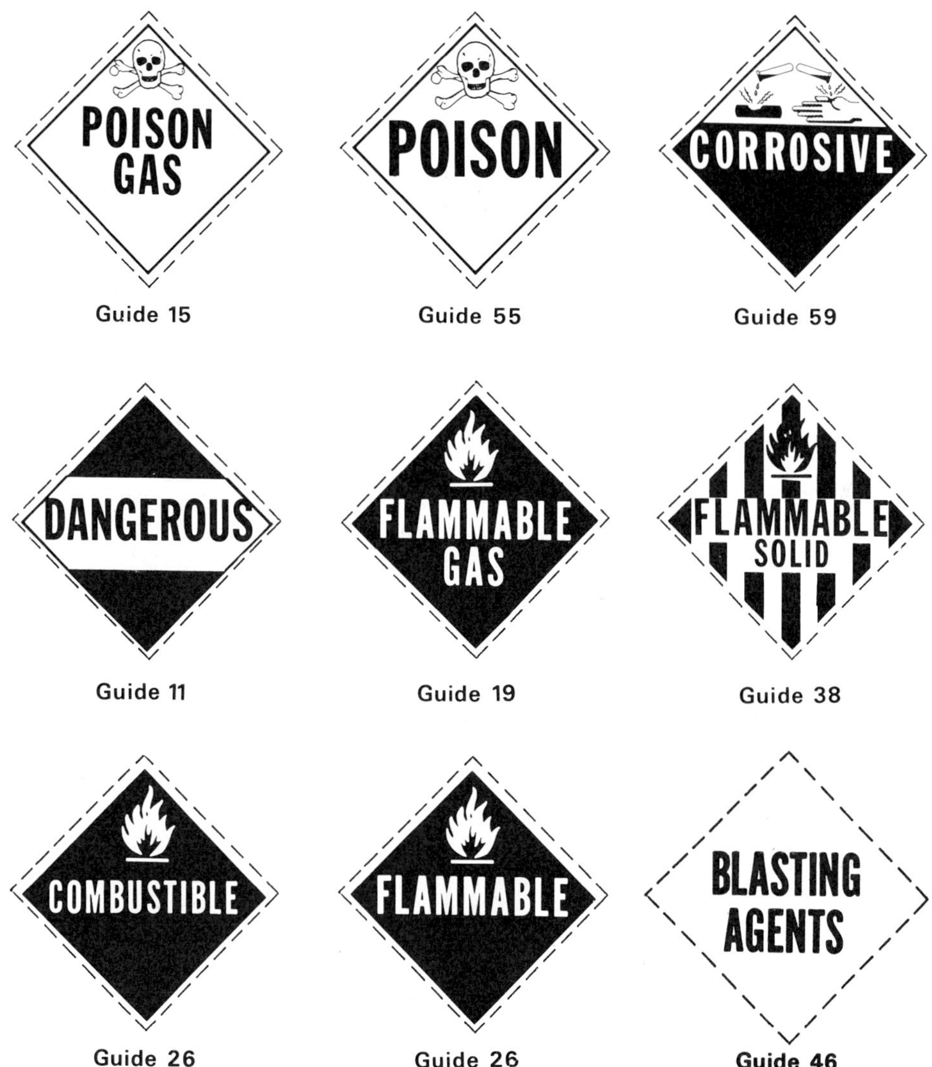

Figure 25–1. Table of placards and applicable response guide pages. (From Emergency Response Guidebook, Office of Hazardous Materials Regulation, Materials Transportation Bureau, US Department of Transportation, Washington, DC, 1980.)

Illustration continued on following page

should enter the contaminated area. At least two should go in together on a buddy system to assure each other's safety. A back-up person with suitable protective equipment should remain at the boundary to assist the rescuers in the event of an accident.[18, 19, 25]

Exposure Assessment

In general, the assessment of exposure risks in the industrial or environmental setting requires equipment and methods from the field of industrial hygiene. The industrial hygienist can perform qualitative and quantitative studies both on site and in the laboratory. Before discussing actual monitoring methods, however, it would be useful to define some terms and review some fundamental industrial hygiene concepts.

First, any chemicals can be handled safely *if* proper precautions are taken. In an uncontrolled release, this means that if there is no fire, explosion, or hazardous reaction, chem-

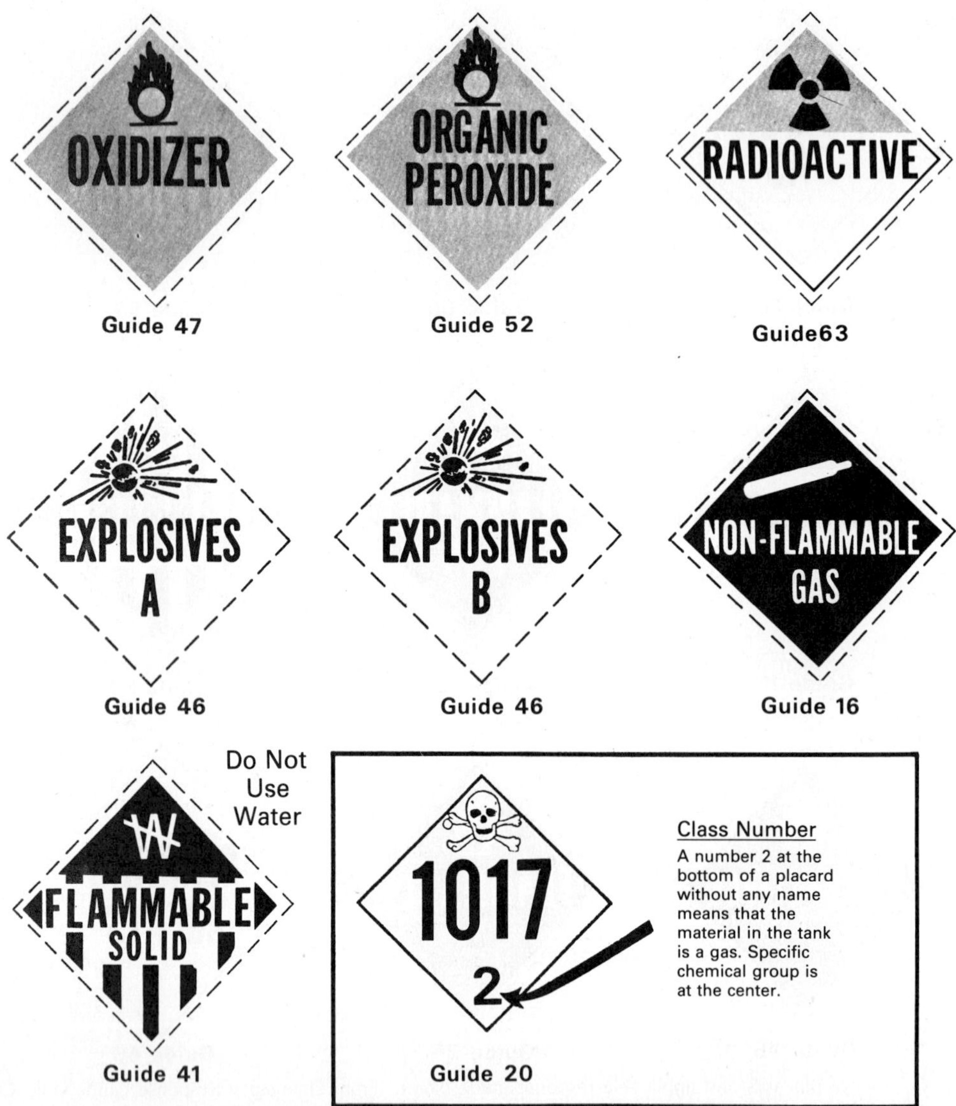

Class Numbers: 1. Explosive 2. Gases 3. Flammable and Combustible Liquids 4. Flammable Solids 5. Oxidizers and Organic Peroxides 6. Poisons 7. Radioactive Material 8. Corrosives

Figure 25–1 *Continued*

ical releases can be approached with proper personal protective equipment. In most major incidents and in some minor incidents, this will include full body suits impermeable to the hazardous material, and a positive-pressure demand style of self-contained breathing apparatus (SCBA). Personnel wearing an SCBA must be fully trained in its use, limitations, and what to do if the equipment fails. These persons must be medically cleared for SCBA use in order to be part of an emergency response team. The SCBA must have been properly inspected, maintained, and cleaned at regular intervals. A full respirator program as required by OSHA (29 CFR 1910.134) must be in place.

Secondly, any chemical, no matter how nontoxic, can be hazardous if handled inappropriately. For example, a release of methane or nitrogen in an enclosed space can cause asphyxiation. There have been numerous reports of attempted rescues in such "nontoxic" environments, in which the initial victim and the rescuers all died of simple asphyxiation.

The identity of the specific agent is only one of a number of factors affecting the actual hazard. Other factors include the air concentration, potential for skin contact, duration of exposure, temperature of the material, and individual susceptibility of the exposed persons.

Inhalation of air contaminants is the most frequent route of exposure for hazardous materials. Air contaminants may be found in a variety of forms, such as gases, vapors (the gaseous form of a substance that is primarily liquid or solid at room temperature), dusts (solid particles entrained in air), fumes (tiny solid particles often formed when a metal is heated, as in welding), mists (liquid particles entrained in air), and smoke (carbon or soot particles from incomplete combustion). Fumes, dusts, and smoke are measured in mass units of contaminant per volume unit of air (e.g., mg/m^3). Gases and vapors may be measured in either mg/m^3 or parts per million (ppm). These two units can be easily interconverted if molecular weight, temperature, and altitude are known. Because fumes are minute solid particles, respirators designed for protection against fumes will have no efficacy against vapors or gases, and vice versa.

Once an air concentration is determined, several criteria exist for assessing the risk of exposure. The IDLH (immediately dangerous to life and health) level "represents a maximum concentration from which, in the event of respirator failure, one could escape within 30 minutes without experiencing any escape-impairing or irreversible health effects."[26] The IDLH level is used to determine the unquestionable need for a reliable positive-pressure demand SCBA. Standby personnel with full protective gear and a lifeline should be available when the IDLH level is exceeded. Specific IDLH values can be found in the NIOSH Pocket Guide to Chemical Hazards.[26]

The most widely used criteria for assessing exposure levels are the Threshold Limit Values (TLVs) for hundreds of common industrial chemicals, which are updated and published annually by the American Conference of Governmental Industrial Hygienists. They "represent conditions under which it is believed that nearly all workers may be repeatedly exposed day after day without adverse effect."[27] Most TLVs are established for 8-hour time-weighted average exposures (TWAs). In general, these values protect against the effects of a lifetime of chronic exposure. However, there are also short-term exposure limits and ceiling limits for some substances included in the TLV list.

TLVs are designed to protect a population of healthy workers and are not meant to be applied to a general community population that may include infants, the elderly, and the infirm. Thus, an industrial hygienist should be consulted when interpretations based on TLVs are to be made.[27] In addition to TLVs, there are a set of legally enforceable workplace standards, known as permissible exposure limits (PELs). These have been promulgated by OSHA, based on the 1968 TLVs. PELs are not brought up to date annually and do not reflect the state of the art because of the considerable lag time in effecting changes in federal statutes.

A common fallacy is the use of odor as a measure of exposure. Information about odor may sometimes be helpful in the qualitative identification of agents, or as a *crude* guide to the exposure level. Odor thresholds for a wide variety of materials have been published. However, wide variations between reference sources and considerable individual variation in the ability to perceive specific odors may occur. For example, up to 40 per cent of the population cannot detect the almond-like odor of cyanide.[28] Thus, quantitative assessments based on odor thresholds are quite unreliable.

Some materials have excellent warning properties. For example, if the odor or irritation of ammonia is absent, one can be sure that there will be no toxic sequelae due to exposure to this agent. On the other hand, some materials, such as carbon monoxide, are odorless at lethal levels. Other agents such as hydrogen sulfide have a characteristic odor initially but induce olfactory fatigue. As a result, lethal exposures may result as exposed individuals perceive levels to be diminishing.[29]

Air concentrations can be measured at specific locations and computer models can sometimes be used to predict worst case ambient concentrations at downwind locations. Environmental monitoring can be performed with direct reading instruments providing real time measurements of levels, or it can be performed by taking air samples that can be subsequently analyzed.

Direct reading instruments include photoionization detectors, portable gas chromatographs, portable infrared spectrophotometers, portable carbon monoxide detectors, flammable gas detectors, and oxygen detectors. A simpler direct reading method for instantaneous levels is the colorimetric detector tube. In addition to monitoring the environment, it will be important to provide medical surveillance for exposed victims and rescuers. This is both to assess potential health effects and to provide information about exposure. Excellent documentation is essential because many of these incidents result in litigation. The physician's initial charting may be a deciding factor in determining whether or not someone gets their deserved compensation. It may also determine whether or not abuses of the system occur, costing public and private organizations large sums of money.

It is important to document subjective and objective findings thoroughly and document assessments carefully. One should not document that symptoms are all due to a "toxic exposure" unless this is clearly the case. Describe actual clinical findings as they present. Numerous cases of mass psychogenic illness have been reported in which victims complain of a toxic exposure and present with a variety of nonspecific symptoms mimicking a toxic exposure.[30] In any true hazardous materials incident, there is always a significant potential for considerable catecholamine release in both affected and unaffected individuals. This may exacerbate symptoms and morbidity in affected individuals and cause individuals unaffected by the toxic agent to present to the physician.

DIAGNOSTIC STUDIES

The tests indicated for symptomatic individuals will depend upon their clinical presentation and the specific agents to which they are exposed. Considerations may include chest radiographs, complete blood counts, liver function tests, urinalyses, arterial blood gases, pulmonary function tests, and biologic monitoring tests specific to the substances present in the environment. Baselines are essential for materials with potential for delayed actions (e.g., chest radiograph for materials such as oxides of nitrogen, which may cause delayed pulmonary edema or fibrosis).

Tests on asymptomatic individuals might look for subclinical effects or indices of exposure. Some emergency response team members may be involved periodically in handling a number of incidents. If proper personal protective equipment is used and if all proper precautions are taken, exposures should be well within acceptable limits. However, periodic medical surveillance of team members is necessary to ensure that unexpected exposures are not occurring.

Biologic monitoring may look for the unchanged parent substance, a metabolite, or a biochemical change as marker for exposure. Blood, urine, exhaled breath, hair, and other tissues may be analyzed. Biologic monitoring, however, may be useful only for certain substances and exposure conditions. Results of these studies must be interpreted differently in the context of an acute hazardous materials incident than in chronic exposure to workers or repeated exposure in emergency response team members.

Lead can be found in blood, urine, and other body tissues such as hair or bone. Blood is the most common specimen obtained and the best supported by the literature. Levels above 40 μg per dl may be associated with symptoms. Erythrocyte protoporphyrins (ZPP and FEP) reflect lead's inhibition of enzymes within the heme synthesis pathway. Acutely, one would see an elevated blood lead, but not an elevated ZPP or FEP. Protoporphyrins may provide a better assessment of subacute or chronic exposure. Inorganic mercury, arsenic, and most other toxic metals can be detected by atomic absorption spectrographic analysis of a 24-hour urine specimen.

Solvents or their metabolites can be detected in urine specimens. Occasionally, blood or breath (e.g., ethyl alcohol [ETOH]) analysis may be indicated. Benzene is monitored by analyzing for urinary phenols: toluene—urinary hippuric acid; xylene—urinary methyl hippuric acid; trichloroethylene and perchloroethylene—urinary trichloracetic acid; and formaldehyde—urinary formic acid.

Organophosphate pesticide exposure can

be evaluated with red blood cell acetylcholinesterase activity measurements and plasma pseudocholinesterase. These two levels should be followed for several weeks to months after acute exposure.[34] However, results must be interpreted cautiously if no baseline levels are available, since there is a wide range of normal values in the general population.

Carboxyhemoglobin levels can be determined directly in blood or can be estimated from exhaled breath analysis. In many cases, patients may have received oxygen therapy prior to having levels drawn. Thus it may be necessary to extrapolate an approximate initial carboxyhemoglobin level prior to oxygen treatment, based on a reduced half-life of carbon monoxide with treatment. Levels should be repeated at frequent (e.g., 2-hour) intervals, until they become normal. In patients with underlying coronary artery disease, levels above 15 per cent can precipitate sequelae of coronary vascular insufficiency.[31] Carboxyhemoglobin levels should be obtained whenever there is a suspicion of carbon monoxide exposure (any fire or case of incomplete hydrocarbon combustion) or methylene chloride exposure, since this substance metabolizes to form carbon monoxide.

Cyanide, as well as thiocyanate, a metabolite of cyanide, can be measured in blood. Like carbon monoxide, it may be formed from incomplete combustion and may be present in fires or cigarette smoke. Smokers normally will have elevated cyanide and carboxyhemoglobin levels.

Significant exposures to hydrofluoric acid will require monitoring of fluoride, potassium, calcium, and magnesium levels. Fatal systemic fluoride poisoning has been described with profound hypocalcemia and hypomagnesemia,[32] as well as fatal hyperkalemia following acute fluoride intoxication.[33]

In addition to using biologic monitoring to assess exposures, a variety of tests may be performed to assess functioning of the neurologic, cardiac, renal, hepatic, respiratory, and hematologic systems.

Numerous substances can cause central or peripheral nervous system effects following acute high-level exposure. An acute polyneuropathy may result from exposure to certain organic solvents such as *n*-hexane and methyl *n*-butyl ketone (MBK). Simultaneous exposure to methyl ethyl ketone (MEK) may increase the neurotoxicity of MBK.[34] Acutely, most solvents can cause narcosis and can cause respiratory depression and coma at high enough concentrations. Organophosphate pesticides cause hyperstimulation of the parasympathetic nervous system by inhibiting acetylcholinesterase. Symptoms of both muscarinic and nicotinic overstimulation are seen. Some of the older organophosphate pesticides such as triorthocresyl phosphate (TOCP) were capable of causing a severe, delayed peripheral motor neuropathy with gradual progression and slow and sometimes incomplete recovery. This syndrome, associated with a "dying back" axonopathy, is no longer seen with pesticides in current use in the United States.

Acute exposure to carbon monoxide may result in delayed neurologic deterioration weeks after exposure, which may include parkinsonian symptoms and a variety of other central and peripheral effects. Other well-described neurotoxins include heavy metals such as mercury, lead, arsenic, and manganese, and plastic components such as acrylamide, dimethylaminopropionitrile (DMAPN), and styrene.

A full neurologic examination should be performed on all patients following a toxic exposure. For known neurotoxins, or for patients with neurologic signs or symptoms, further testing may be indicated. Neurophysiologic testing may include electromyography, nerve conduction testing, and electroencephalography in certain cases. Neurobehavioral testing may include personality tests such as the Minnesota Multiphasic Personality Inventory (MMPI) and performance tests such as the Wechsler Adult Intelligence Scale (WAIS).

A number of solvents (especially the chlorinated hydrocarbons), organic amines, organic nitro compounds, and inorganic materials such as lead, arsenic, antimony, and copper may be hepatotoxic. Baseline and progressive liver function studies should be performed for toxic exposures when there is potential for hepatotoxicity.

Many heavy metals (e.g., lead, mercury, and cadmium), solvents (e.g., carbon tetrachloride and ethylene glycol), arsine, and ionizing radiation can be toxic to the kidney. Urinalysis and renal function studies (e.g., blood urea nitrogen, creatinine) are useful screens. However, these tests may be insensitive, and, for renal toxins, a 24-hour urine collection for creatinine clearance, protein, and low molecular weight proteins such as β_2-microglobulin may be indicated.[34]

Irritants and other pulmonary toxins may require evaluation with chest radiography, arterial blood gases, spirometry, and other pulmonary function testing. In some cases laryngoscopy or bronchoscopy may be indicated, particularly if there are signs of upper airway obstruction. Blood gases should also be evaluated for exposure to chemical asphyxiants such as carbon monoxide, cyanide, or hydrogen sulfide.

Acute cardiovascular effects of hazardous materials exposures should be considered in all patients at risk for cardiovascular disease. Any material that causes hypoxia (e.g., carbon monoxide, methylene chloride, cyanide) can exacerbate cardiac ischemia and precipitate angina or a myocardial infarction. Catecholamine release related to panic in a real or perceived exposure situation may result in chest pain of cardiac or noncardiac (e.g., hyperventilation syndrome) origin. Nitrates such as nitroglycerin can cause a rebound spasm of the coronary arteries within several days of exposure. Nitrates may also induce methemoglobinemia, which may exacerbate cardiac ischemia.

Dysrhythmias may be caused acutely by a variety of solvents such as benzene, chlorinated solvents, and fluorocarbons (Freons). Sudden death may occur. It is thought that the mechanism may be a sensitization of the myocardium to endogenous catecholamines. Electrocardiographic changes such as Q-T interval prolongation may also be seen acutely with arsenic and arsine exposures. Electrocardiographic changes may also be seen with materials, such as hydrofluoric acid, that cause significant electrolyte abnormalities.

To evaluate potential cardiovascular effects of toxic materials, a 12-lead electrocardiogram and rhythm strip should be obtained. Chest pain should always be evaluated to rule out ischemia as a cause.

FIELD DECONTAMINATION AND TRIAGE

Standard principles of triage apply in a chemical disaster. In very toxic substance exposures, the patient, injured or not, must be decontaminated prior to transport to the emergency department to protect EMS and emergency department staff. One possible exception to field decontamination might be an emergency department with a special decontamination room. It should be open to the outside, have showers and a collection unit for waste water, and have protective equipment for the emergency department staff. One would want to at least remove as much of the substance as quickly as possible by disrobing and washing the patient. If possible, the person should be wrapped in "clean" blankets, and a minimum of first aid that can be given with protective equipment worn should be performed. Hemorrhage control, sealing of sucking chest wounds, airway attention, and oxygen by mask should be accomplished on site and upwind from the spill. Bag-mask ventilation within a spill site would not be used for one would be bagging more toxic fumes into the victim's lungs. A self-contained demand valve could be used with the caution that if it is contaminated it may need to be left in the contaminated area and a switch made to a second device as one leaves the contaminated area.[20]

Transport of an individual who is even partially contaminated should be in a non-ALS (Advanced Life Support) vehicle if at all possible. Transport persons should wear appropriate protective gear, as should emergency department personnel at the receiving hospital. Few hospitals have such decontamination units. Those that do can treat only a limited number of individuals, usually one or two at a time.

Decontamination of specialized suits, emergency suits, and equipment is costly. If time can be taken, decontamination in the field is less costly and the hazardous material can be contained on site. Once human injuries have been cared for, environmental clean-up can be accomplished at a much more leisurely pace.[18–20] See Figure 25–2 for field decontamination procedures.

Illustrative Example

The sequence for field decontamination can be illustrated in this way: A truck transporting a concentrated liquid chemical turns over on a highway, and the tank begins to leak. A large pool of chemical is rapidly filling a low section of roadway, and a hazy cloud begins to form over the pool. The driver and companion, who are both injured, begin to

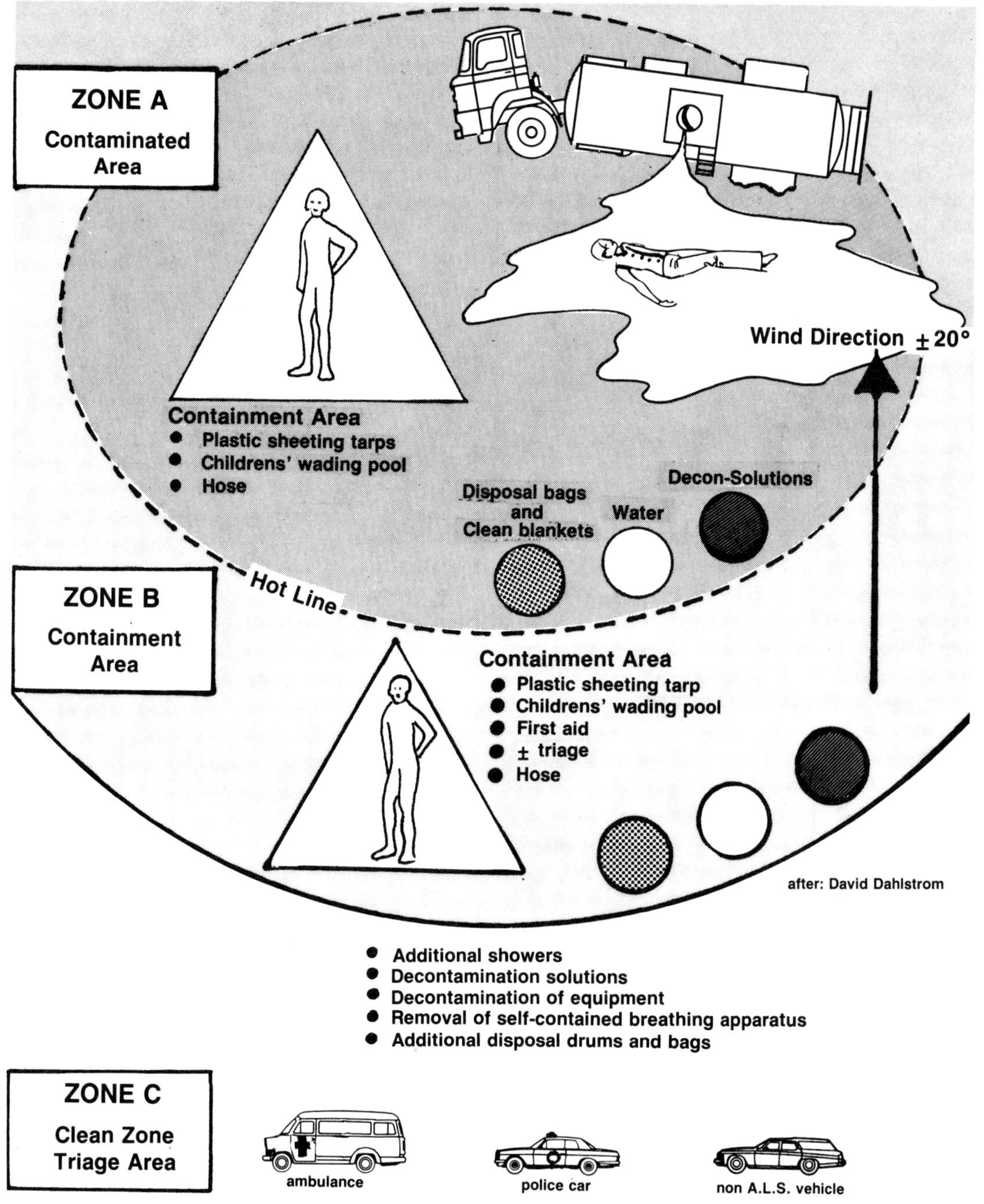

Figure 25–2. Sequence for field decontamination.

move away under their own power. Then they begin to cough and choke and pass out. Several bystanders enter to help and are overcome and lose consciousness. In the meantime, all the victims have chemical on their clothing (Fig. 25–2).[16, 18–20] Without going into specific details of particular chemicals, how might rescue be effected?

The first responders must attempt to identify the chemical from the placard on the truck. Especially note the logo ₩, which means USE NO WATER. The chemical may ignite, explode, or produce toxic fumes with water.[4] They should notify Central Dispatching for fire department, police, and EMS back-up and indicate that specialized resources or expertise may be required for a hazardous materials incident. If the placard can be read, the dispatcher can call CHEMTREC and get specific handling information. Police, fire, or EMS personnel should have access to the 1987 DOT Emergency Response Guide: Emergency Handling of Hazardous Materials in Surface Transportation. Access to other guides, Poisindex, or a poison control center for further information should be available, if possible. A triage or medical station should be set up upwind from the site at a "safe" distance. Distances are listed in the DOT Emergency Response Guidebook. An area designated as contaminated or hot should be defined (Fig. 25–2). An intermediate or containment area should be established. Rescuers can continue decontamination and emergency treatment in this area.[16, 18–20]

Rescuers should enter the contaminated area with full protective gear unless the hazard assessment indicates otherwise. Information is contained in several guides available to rescue personnel or from CHEMTREC.

Only a minimum of first aid, such as attention to the airway, cervical spine, and exsanguinating hemorrhage, should be attempted in a highly toxic environment. Move victims from the immediate area of the spill. Remove all clothing. In general, wash the entire body, including the hair, quickly with water: Exceptions to this rule include calcium oxide, chlorosulfonic acid, and titanium tetrachloride, which react violently with water (W̶). All the wash water must be contained. This can be done in a number of ways. Children's plastic wading pools or plastic sheeting may be used with an earthen dam or brick border to prevent used wash water from entering ground water. Three fire ladders may be laid sideways in a triangle and tarpaulins placed over them to form a pool. All waste water, hoses, tarpaulins, pools, and so on are left inside the hot line for the environmental clean-up team.[16, 18–20]

The victims may then move or be moved across the hot line to the containment reduction area for further decontamination. Rescuers then discard outer layers of gloves, boot covers, and suits and place these in disposal containers in the hot area before crossing the line. Self-contained breathing apparatus may need to be left on and is the last piece of equipment removed. In the containment area, more thorough washing should take place. This may be done in a similar manner by setting up a hose or some type of shower. All waste water must be contained so as not to spread contamination.[16, 20]

More thorough attention to injuries and advanced airway management can be given in this zone. With very toxic materials, rescuers still will be hampered in their efforts by protective suits and self-contained breathing apparatus.

The victims are wrapped again in clean blankets as they move from Zone B (containment area) to Zone C (clean area). Rescuers discard additional protective clothing, and the self-contained breathing apparatus is removed last, on entering the clean zone. All contaminated equipment and clothing is placed in bags and drums for later decontamination or disposal.[16, 20] Here, more extensive triage can take place, and intravenous lines and other advanced life support treatment can take place. Note that all movement is upwind from the spill.

Since one cannot be absolutely sure that decontamination is complete in the field, one should use a non-ALS vehicle if possible. Decontamination of an ALS vehicle is not only time consuming and costly, but only a limited number of ALS vehicles are available. To have one out of service for decontamination imposes a hardship on the community.

All equipment and gear in vehicles and in the emergency department should be protected from any contamination by layers of plastic and blankets, if possible.

Decisions about evacuation are based on the identification of the chemical, information from the transporter or manufacturer, chemical characteristics, explosive characteristics, and danger of fire.[4, 21, 35–40]

Additional community planning for chemical hazards involves surveying local industries for products manufactured and products imported into the community that are used in the manufacturing process. As previously mentioned, material safety data sheets should be available for all such materials from the plant using the materials. Surveying for major pipelines in one's area and knowing major rail shipping routes and train make-up areas in one's community will help. Enlisting the support of all agencies involved in a chemical disaster and instituting several mock disasters or disaster drills can point out inefficiencies in the plan and areas in which interagency communication is lacking.[16]

REGIONAL ASSESSMENT OF EXPOSURE

A major hazardous spill may raise fears in the general population of possible long-term toxic effects. Patients and workers immediately exposed to the chemical hazard, such as firefighters, EMS personnel, and police, may require on-going medical surveillance. The long-term environmental impact also needs to be assessed. If a survey of the immediate area and patient population shows no significant hazard, then the public may be reassured. In the event a persistent hazard is determined to exist, local and national authorities may need to expand testing in concentric circles from the exposure site.

The physician, however, also must be aware of the mass psychogenic component that is commonly present in perceived environmental exposures. Whether or not patients are suffering toxic effects, it is likely that they also will experience symptoms and signs of catecholamine release. Some persons may have nonspecific symptoms such as headaches, nausea, vomiting, hyperventilation, chest pain, and paresthesias. Objective signs other than tachycardia, tachypnea, mild hypertension, and respiratory alkalosis are generally lacking when symptoms are caused only by this syndrome. However, secondary cardiac ischemia, seizures, and other acute emergency conditions may present in the absence of toxic exposure, precipitated by the panic condition.

HOSPITAL MANAGEMENT

The two most common routes of injury from exposure to hazardous materials are *inhalation* and *cutaneous contact.* Decontamination for cutaneous exposure may not be adequately completed in the field. Thorough lavage must continue in the emergency facility until all hazardous materials are completely removed. Efforts to minimize contamination of the emergency facility may require using a separate decontamination area, with isolation of rinse water, and personal protective clothing for medical personnel. Medical management within the department may include trauma management, 100 per cent oxygen for inhalation injury, antidotal therapy when indicated, and general supportive therapy. Long-term follow-up care is essential to both detect and manage chronic injury.

References

1. Federal Emergency Management Agency, US Environmental Protection Agency: Planning Guide and Checklist for Hazardous Materials Contingency Plans. Washington, DC, US Government Printing Office, 1981.
2. Quarantelli EL: Transportation Accidents Involving Hazardous Chemicals Versus Those Involving Dangerous Nuclear Material. Columbus, OH, Ohio State University, Disaster Research Center, 1982.
3. Walter RA, DiGregorio RC, Kooyoomjian KJ, Eby TL: A Statistical Analysis of Hazardous Material Releases Reported to the National Response Center. Proceedings of the 1986 Hazardous Materials Spills Conference. St. Louis, 1986, pp 163–171.
4. US Department of Transportation: Hazardous Materials 1987 Emergency Response Guidebook. Washington, DC, 1987.
5. Aydelotte C: Bhopal tragedy focuses on changes in chemical industry. Occup Health Safety *54*(3):33–35, 1985.
6. Bhopal Working Group: The public health implications of the Bhopal disaster. Am J Public Health *77*(22):230–235, 1987.
7. Lorin HG, Kuling PEJ: The Bhopal tragedy—What has Swedish disaster medicine planning learned from it? J Emerg Med *4*:311–316, 1986.
8. Das JJ: The Bhopal tragedy. J Indian Med Assoc *83*(2):73–74, 1985.
9. Kamat SR, et al: Early observations on pulmonary changes and clinical morbidity due to the isocyanate gas leak at Bhopal. J Postgrad Med *31*(2):63–72, 1985.
10. Naik SR, et al: Medical survey of methyl isocyanate gas–affected population of Bhopal, Part I. J Postgrad Med *32*(4):175–184, 1986.
11. Irani SF, Mahashur AA: A survey of Bhopal children affected by methyl isocyanate gas. J Postgrad Med *32*(4):195–198, 1986.
12. Rumack BH, Hall AH: Methyl Isocyanate Management. TOMES Information System. Vol 55. Denver, Micromedex, Inc, 1988.
13. Marwick C: Bhopal tragedy's repercussions may reach American physicians. JAMA *253*(14):2001–2004, 2009–2014, 1985.
14. Jackson County Office of Emergency Measures: Hazardous Materials Response Plan. Jackson, MI, 1981.
15. Winnebago County Emergency Services and Disaster Agency: Hazardous Materials Response Plan. Rockford, IL, 1980.
16. Michigan Chapter, American College of Emergency Physicians, and Michigan State University, Institute for Community Development: Hazardous Materials Emergency Medical Treatment Symposium. East Lansing, MI, 1982.
17. Levy KD, Carr MW: US Coast Guard Site Entry Procedures for Hazardous Material Incident Response. Proceedings of the 1982 Hazardous Material Spills Conference. Milwaukee, WI, 1982.
18. Dahlstrom D: Site entry. *In* US Environmental Protection Agency and Ecology and Environment: Personnel Protection Safety Training Manual. Buffalo, NY, 1981.

19. Dahlstrom D: Personnel protection. *In* US Environmental Protection Agency and Ecology and Environment: Personnel Protection Safety Training Manual. Buffalo, NY, 1981.
20. Dahlstrom D: Decontamination. *In* US Environmental Protection Agency and Ecology and Environment: Personnel Protection Safety Training Manual. Buffalo, NY, 1981.
21. Association of American Railroads, Bureau of Explosives: Emergency Handling of Hazardous Materials in Surface Transportation. Washington, DC, 1981.
22. Zercher JC: Emergency Response—A Changing Industry Attitude. Proceedings of the 1982 Hazardous Material Spills Conference, Milwaukee, WI, 1982.
23. Taylor F: Hazardous Materials Emergency Response System. Proceedings of the 1982 Hazardous Material Spills Conference. Milwaukee, WI, 1982.
24. Dahlstrom D: Environmental disasters and medical response. *In* US Environmental Protection Agency and Ecology and Environment: Personnel Protection Safety Training Manual. Buffalo, NY, 1981.
25. US Environmental Protection Agency: Levels of Protection. Washington, DC, 1981.
26. National Institute for Occupational Safety and Health (NIOSH): Pocket Guide to Chemical Hazards. Washington, DC, US Department of Health and Human Services, Public Health Service, Centers for Disease Control, NIOSH Publication No. 85–114, Sept 1985.
27. American Conference of Governmental Industrial Hygienists: Threshold Limit Values and Biological Exposure Indices for 1987–1988. Cincinnati, 1987.
28. Kirk RL, Stenhouse NS: Ability to smell solutions of potassium cyanide. Nature *171*:698, 1953.
29. Rom WN (ed): Environmental and Occupational Medicine. Boston, Little, Brown, 1983.
30. Boxer PA: Occupational mass psychogenic illness: History, prevention, and management. J Occup Med *27*:867–872, 1985.
31. Rumack BH, Hall AH: Carbon monoxide management. TOMES Information System. Vol 58. Denver, Micromedex, Inc, 1988.
32. Tepperman PB: Fatality due to acute systemic fluoride poisoning following a hydrofluoric acid skin burn. J Occup Med *22*:691–692, 1980.
33. McIvor ME: Delayed fatal hyperkalemia in a patient with acute fluoride intoxication. Ann Emerg Med *16*:1165–1167, 1987.
34. Rosenstock L, Cullen MR: Clinical Occupational Medicine. Philadelphia, WB Saunders, 1986.
35. American Lung Association of West New York, Inc: Chemical Emergency Action Manual. 1981.
36. US Department of Transportation: Hazardous Material–Emergency Action Guide. Washington, DC, 1977.
37. National Fire Protection Association: Fire Protection Guide on Hazardous Materials. Boston, 1978.
38. National Fire Protection Association: Fire Protection Handbook. Boston, 1981.
39. Proctor NH, Hughes JP: Chemical Hazards of the Workplace. Philadelphia, JB Lippincott, 1978.
40. Hilbert GD, Berkley JH Jr, Qum FM: Mississauqua: Lessons in Large-Scale Evacuation. Proceedings of the 1982 Hazardous Material Spills Conference. Milwaukee, WI, 1981.

SPECIFIC POISONS

PART II

Natural and Environmental Toxins

CHAPTER 26

ENVIRONMENTAL TOXICOLOGY

A. Overview

Philip S. Guzelian, M.D.

Environmental toxicity has leapt to the forefront of public consciousness, as evidenced by the Time Magazine "Planet of the Year" issue on The Endangered Earth (January 2, 1989).

This section provides a brief overview of Environmental Toxicology, followed by specific sections on carcinogenesis and environmental effects on growth and hormones; then by specific examples of environmental toxins: dioxin, formaldehyde, and chronic pesticide exposure.

The public is now more aware that substances in the air, soil, and water may produce adverse effects on a variety of living systems. This has prompted increasing concern about potentially adverse health consequences for humans exposed to these potentially toxic agents and the difficulties in defining human health risks. There is growing recognition that these agents may persist in the environment for decades. Furthermore, exposure to such substances may be by inconspicuous contact through eating, breathing, or touching. Most importantly, the toxic consequences of exposure to small amounts of environmental toxins may require years or even generations to become manifest. Attention to this concept of environmental toxicity has been reinforced by frequent, dramatic incidents of area-wide ecodisasters. Examples are the radiation disaster in Chernobyl, Russia (April 26, 1986); the methyl isocyanate disaster at the Union Carbide Plant in Bhopal, India, on December 3, 1984; the recent exposure of the entire population of Michigan to polybrominated biphenyls; contamination of the Tidewater Region of Virginia with an organochlorine pesticide, Kepone; and dissemination of toxic chemicals from Love Canal and other abandoned industrial dump sites for chemicals.

The practicing physician can deal with acute, overt poisonings caused by agents discussed in other chapters of this book in a relatively straightforward manner. The diagnosis often can be made easily, and treatment can be initiated. When there is no effective therapy available, at least the prognosis can be stated with some degree of certainty. In contrast, when dealing with a patient exposed to small amounts of potentially toxic substances in the environment, the physician is confronted by an entirely different set of problems. For example, a pregnant woman who discovers she has had contact with polychlorinated biphenyls may adduce no present ill effects. However, she likely will have many questions and anxieties regarding the consequences of her exposure to the health of the unborn baby, or the consequences of breast-feeding to the health of the newborn infant. In this instance, the clinician's task is complicated by the lack of conclusive information regarding the risk of immediate or long-term adverse health effects of this chemical and the dose at which risks become significant in humans.

Given the absence of this critical information (and doubts that needed data will be available soon, if ever), I believe clinicians can best approach this problem by being acquainted with current ideas on mechanisms of pathophysiology of environmental toxicity and by using this information to formulate their own best judgment in a particular situation. Therefore, in this chapter, I have elected to present an overview of the metabolic fate of environmental chemicals in the body and the relationship of metabolism to carcinogenesis. Although cancer is perhaps the most feared and best known of the chronic pathologic effects of environmental chemicals, it should be recognized that environmental agents may cause other forms of chronic illness, including birth defects, reproductive impairment, or behavioral abnormalities.

Sources of Environmental Toxins. Natural and manufactured toxic agents are present throughout the environment—in the air, food and water, and soil. Consequently, exposure to such agents may occur at home, in the workplace, in areas of recreation, indoors, or outdoors. Most of the pollutants in air can be accounted for as carbon monoxide, sulfur oxides, hydrocarbons, particulate matter, and nitrogen oxides (although virtually any toxin can be disseminated in the air). The amounts of airborne pollutants vary according to the distance and location (upwind versus downwind) from the source of pollution. The concentration can sometimes be extremely high, as exemplified by lead or beryllium poisoning in residents located near smelters. Acute toxic manifestations of air pollution involve pulmonary irritation and respiratory compromise of patients with preexisting cardiac or pulmonary diseases. Prolonged contact with air pollutants is associated with chronic pulmonary diseases such as bronchitis, obstructive ventilatory disease, and lung cancer.

Most chemicals of human manufacture are disposed of ultimately in the soil and water. The spectacular increase in tons of chemicals produced during the last 15 years has provided a severe challenge to the soil and water to absorb and dispose of such wastes. Industrial, agricultural, and domestic users release chemicals into the environment continually, although in some dramatic instances, massive dissemination may occur from a single source, as with the explosion in a Northern Italian factory that released dioxin into the air. Not only are there increasing discharges of chemicals into the environment, but also many chemicals such as the organochlorine pesticides are extremely resistant to natural processes of decay in the environment. Consequently, they may persist in the soil and water for decades after their production. Moreover, many of these agents are poorly excreted from living systems and, hence, they progressively accumulate in plants and animals as they advance through the food chain. For example, although DDT is present in air and rain water in less than 1 part per billion (ppb), this chemical can be found in concentrations of 50 ppb in plants, in 500 ppb in aquatic animals, in 1000 ppb in herbivorous and insectivorous mammals and birds, and in greater than 5000 ppb in the body fat of humans in many parts of the world.

Food supplies represent another potential source of exposure to environmental chemicals. There are strict governmental controls on the amounts and nature of additives that can be intentionally combined with food stuffs. However, nonintentional adulterants in food may come from many sources during production of food as the animal or plant material is being raised, during processing of the food, or during its packaging and storage (Table 26–1). These unintentional additives are not exclusively manufactured substances and include naturally occurring toxins as

Table 26–1. SOURCES OF NONINTENTIONAL FOOD ADULTERANTS

DURING PRODUCTION
- Animal and insect filth (including insects and insect parts)
- Antibiotics and other agents used for prevention and control of disease
- Growth-promoting substances
- Microorganisms of toxicologic significance
- Parasitic organisms
- Pesticide residues (insecticides, fungicides, herbicides, etc)
- Toxic metals and metallic compounds
- Radioactive compounds

DURING PROCESSING
- Animal and insect filth (including insects and insect parts)
- Microorganisms and their toxic metabolites
- Processing residues and miscellaneous foreign objects
- Radionuclides

DURING PACKAGING AND STORAGE
- Animal and insect filth
- Labeling and stamping materials
- Microorganisms and their toxic metabolites
- Migrants from packaging materials
- Toxic chemicals from external sources (including vapors and solvents)

(Adapted from Cassaret LJ, Doull J [eds]: Toxicology: The Basic Science of Poisons. New York, Macmillan, 1980, p 602.)

well. Hence, as Ames and his associates have emphasized, there is no assurance that consumption of a "natural" diet offers protection from environmental toxins.

Finally, household risks for exposure to toxins other than food consumption are being increasingly recognized. One example is the syndrome of "indoor air pollution." The air indoors can become contaminated with products of combustion of gas, oil, or other fuel sources. The air also may contain chemicals used in building materials, such as formaldehyde in particle board or urethane in insulation. This problem is further aggravated by efforts to insulate homes to prevent heat loss, which at the same time decreases air exchange from the outdoors.

Toxic Manifestation of Environmental Chemicals. Table 26–2 lists some established clinical effects of exposure to environmental chemicals. Most of the chemicals listed are found in the workplace. Occupational exposures are useful for defining toxic manifestations because the offending agent is present in high concentrations and because the period of exposure can be defined. Note that no organ system is immune from the toxic effects of environmental agents; that the offending agent may be in the form of a liquid, solid, or vapor; and that there is an impressive diversity in the chemical forms such agents may display.

Although toxicity may appear as an acute poisoning, of more concern for purposes of this chapter is that there are chronic manifestations of toxicity. These include gradually debilitating diseases such as chronic bronchitis/emphysema and osteomalacia, diseases with a symptom-free period such as cancer, and possibly reproductive abnormalities. The latent period even may extend over generations as with women exposed to diethylstilbestrol whose female offspring are at elevated risk for development of vaginal adenocarcinoma. The long latent period between the contact with environmental chemicals and the appearance of pathologic effects complicates efforts to establish cause and effect relationships or to quantitatively define human health risks. The breach created by this uncertainty invites reliance on opinions and political considerations, rather than rigorous adherence to scientific information in governmental regulatory decision making.

Metabolic Fate of Environmental Chemicals. Much remains to be learned in identifying environmental toxins and elucidating the mechanisms of their toxic effects. However, progress has been made in understanding the relationship between the metabolic disposition of chemicals and their toxicity. This research has focused on the liver as the major site in the body for biotransformation of foreign substances (xenobiotics), although the hepatic enzyme systems responsible for metabolism of foreign chemicals exist in other tissues as well. Most of the chemicals in question are quite lipophilic and, therefore, are not readily excreted in aqueous media such as urine or bile. Were it not for metabolism, many of these lipophilic chemicals, including such drugs as phenobarbital, would remain in the body indefinitely.

An important group of enzymes that carry out biotransformation reactions are the monooxygenase enzymes located in the endoplasmic reticulum or "microsomes," as these membranes are called when extracted from cells. Key enzymes are the cytochromes P-450, a collective term for a group of hemoproteins that bind foreign chemicals and catalyze their oxidation by inserting one molecule of oxygen (oxygenation). Such hydroxylation reactions convert many water-insoluble foreign compounds to more polar derivatives, which are then more easily excreted (Fig. 26–1). Often associated with conversion to polar metabolites is loss of pharmacologic or toxicologic effects of drugs or other foreign substances. However, it is well recognized that many natural or manufactured chemicals capable of producing toxicity must first undergo metabolic activation ("toxification"). This occurs by oxidation through the same cytochrome P-450–dependent enzymes in the liver or in extrahepatic tissues (Fig. 26–1). Unless disposed of by detoxification systems in the cell, these oxygenated metabolites may interact chemically with important genetic (DNA, RNA) or structural (proteins, lipids) macromolecules in the cells. These interactions can initiate a chain of events ultimately leading to cell death, to mutations, or to transformation of normal cells into malignant cells.

The potential detrimental effects of metabolically activated toxins are counteracted by an array of conjugating enzymes located throughout the cell. These conjugating enzymes catalyze the conversion of oxygenated metabolites to even more water-soluble derivatives through addition of polar ligands.

Table 26–2. EXAMPLES OF TOXIC MANIFESTATIONS OF ENVIRONMENTAL SUBSTANCES

ORGAN	SYMPTOM/SIGN	EXAMPLES OF TYPICAL EXPOSURE
Eye	Corneal edema	Vapors
	Corneal inflammation	Vapors, dusts
	Cataracts	Systemic chemicals
	Lens deposits	Metals
	Papilledema	Ethylene glycol, lead
	Ptosis	Thallium
Nervous system	Headache	Lead compounds
	Drowsiness	Many organic chemicals
	Convulsions	Organochlorine pesticides
	Cerebrospinal effects	Metals
	Peripheral neuropathy	Metals, acrylamide
Head and neck	Rhinitis	Solvents
	Salivation	Organophosphates, mercury
	Cancer of sinuses	Nickel carbonyl
Pulmonary	Pneumonitis, asthma	Gases, dusts
	Fibrosis	Fibrinogen dusts
	Cancer	Asbestos, lung carcinogens
Cardiovascular	Hypotension	Nitrites, depressants
	Arrhythmias	Carbon tetrachloride, phenols
	Myocardial degeneration	Antimony, carbon disulfide
Digestive	Nausea/vomiting	Many depressants, irritants
	Colic	Metals, organophosphates
	Constipation	Metals
	Jaundice	Hepatotoxins, hemolytic agents
	Angiosarcoma	Vinyl chloride, thorium, arsenic
Genitourinary	Nephrosis	Dioxane, uranium compounds
	Bladder tumors	Azo dyes
Musculoskeletal	Osteonecrosis	Phosphorus
	Osteosclerosis	Fluorides
	Osteomalacia	Cadmium
	Osteosarcoma	Radium
Hematopoietic	Anemia	Lead, hemolytic agents
	Leukemia	Benzene, radioactive compounds
Skin	Dermatitis	Solvents, gases, irritants
	Purpura	Some hepatotoxins
	Acne	Chlorinated biphenyls, dioxins
	Photosensitization	Tars
	Keratosis/cancer	Soot, pitch, tars

(Adapted from Procter NH, Hughes JP [eds]: Chemical Hazards of the Workplace. Philadelphia, JB Lippincott, 1978, p 40.)

In most instances, the conjugated products are inactive with respect to pharmacologic or toxic effects.

Several examples of enzymes serve to detoxify the activated metabolites formed by the cytochrome P-450 enzymes. Liver cytosol contains a series of glutathione-S-transferases that catalyze the combination of oxygenated species with glutathione. The latter is a sulfur-containing tripeptide present in high concentrations in many cells, including the hepatocyte. Glutathione likely serves as an important buffer, preventing interactions between oxygenated metabolites and the sulfhydryl groups of important macromolecules. Another conjugating enzyme is microsomal epoxide hydratase, which promotes conversion of potentially reactive epoxides or arene oxides (products of cytochrome P-450 reactions) to water-soluble dialcohols.

The preceding discussion of enzymes involved in metabolism of foreign chemicals provides a basis for understanding differences among individuals in the consequences of exposure to lipophilic chemicals. The amount of the proximate toxin that accumulates in the cell will represent the net effects of enzymatic conversion of the parent compound through toxic pathways ("toxification") balanced against the capacity of the cell to convert activated substances to inactive, excretable metabolites ("detoxification"). It follows, therefore, that factors that alter the levels of activating or detoxifying

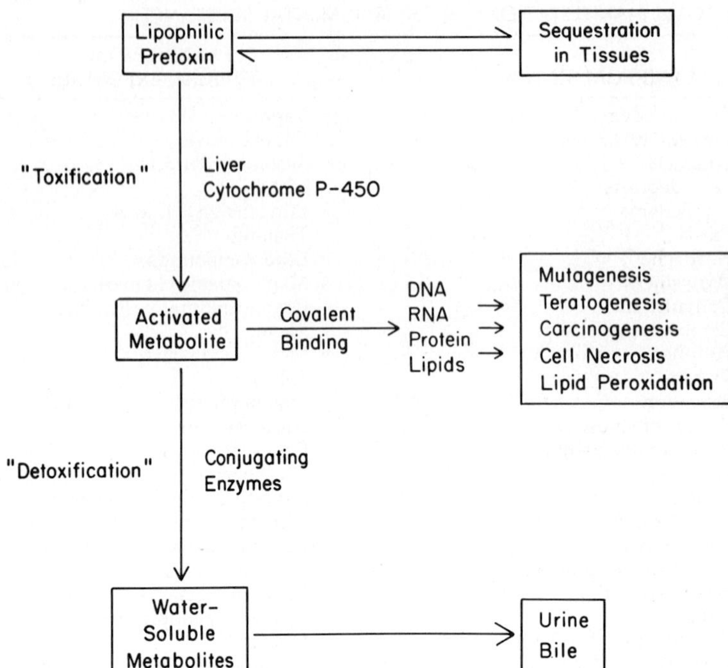

Figure 26–1. Pathways of hepatic metabolism of some environmental toxins.

enzymes in a given tissue may importantly affect the fate of a potentially toxic environmental substance. For example, we know that cytochrome P-450 is inducible by many of its own substrates, including lipophilic drugs, carcinogens, some natural substances, and numerous environmental pollutants.

One example of the latter is the organochlorine pesticide DDT. When given to rats, DDT produces proliferation of the smooth endoplasmic reticulum in the liver, accompanied by a prompt rise in the level of cytochrome P-450. If exposure to DDT ceases, the amounts of this chemical in the liver fall as a result of accelerated metabolism and excretion, plus redistribution of DDT to other tissues. Therefore, the stimulus to induce cytochrome P-450 is decreased, and the concentration of this cytochrome declines, returning to basal, steady state levels. It should be recalled that cytochrome P-450 is a collection of nonspecific enzymes capable of metabolizing a diverse array of substances with different structures. Therefore, an individual whose level of cytochrome P-450 is increased due to exposure to DDT might be either more susceptible or less susceptible to a simultaneous exposure to another potentially toxic compound, depending upon whether the cytochrome serves to activate or inactivate the toxin metabolically. Contrary effects might arise in conditions associated with reduced levels of hepatic cytochrome P-450 as in protein malnutrition, hepatitis, or cholestasis. The levels of cytochrome P-450 also may be altered depending upon gender or other genetic factors.

It may be concluded that because cytochrome P-450 is under multifactorial regulatory control, individual differences in the effects of exposure to some environmental chemicals may be expected. This same conclusion may also apply to the other side of the metabolic equation; namely, the conjugating enzymes. The amounts of the latter enzymes present, as well as the availability of their cofactors required for conjugating activity, likely are important in providing a given individual resistance to the effects of activated toxins.

Another category of chemicals, ubiquitous in the environment, does not readily fit into the presently discussed scheme for xenobiotic metabolism. These are extremely hydrophobic chemicals that are metabolized only minimally in the liver or in extrahepatic tissues. Hence, they are excreted from the body only very slowly, if at all. Examples are the organochlorine pesticides (DDT, chlordane, dieldrin, Kepone), polychlorinated biphenyls, and dioxins. Although usually humans are exposed only to low concentrations of these chemicals, the contact often occurs for many years. Because the excretion of these chemicals is minimal, they accumulate in tissue and membrane lipids throughout the body. Measurable amounts of such chemicals (DDT, polychlorinated biphenyls, dioxin) may be found in the fat of virtually all adult Americans. The health consequences of maintaining this body burden of chemicals are a subject of ongoing debate.

One concern arises from the fact that breast milk, being rich in lipids, accumulates these chemicals and, hence, infants may be exposed to markedly higher concentrations of chemicals than are present in the environment. Another concern is that sequestration of environmental chemicals in human tissues may foster malignancy, since many of these agents are known to cause tumors in the liver and other organs when administered chronically to experimental animals. A final concern is that maintaining a burden of chemicals would provide a persistent stimulus to induction of the cytochrome P-450 system. This in turn might render an individual more susceptible to subsequent exposure to other environmental procarcinogens or protoxins. Note, however, that continual induction might prove to be protective depending on the profile of enzymes induced and the particular substrates in the environment.

Based on the foregoing discussion, it might reasonably be asked whether practical tests are available to determine the status of "toxifying" and "detoxifying" enzymes in a given individual. Unfortunately, clinical tests for monitoring the human hepatic drug-metabolizing system are not in wide use and are restricted to research purposes. Such tests include assessment of the liver-dependent clearance of model drugs (e.g., theophylline, antipyrine), measured either by the rate of disappearance of the drug from blood or by the rate of appearance of metabolites in the breath. Morphologic examination of liver biopsy through the electron microscope can provide evidence for proliferation of the smooth endoplasmic reticulum, but quantification of this change is difficult. Another approach is to examine the urine for metabolites of endogenous substrates of hepatic microsomal oxidases as, for example, steroid metabolites. The urine also contains breakdown products of the hepatic endoplasmic reticulum. Glucaric acid, a derivative of glucuronic acid, has been used as an indirect means for the detection of proliferation of the smooth endoplasmic reticulum of the liver. Finally, some investigators have proposed that serum gamma-glutamyltranspeptidase activity is elevated in individuals receiving drugs that induce hepatic cytochrome P-450. However, it is important to note that this test is nonspecific and also may give false negative results for induction of the hepatic drug-metabolizing system by certain environmental chemicals.

Even though it is not practical at present to assess the metabolic fate of an environmental agent in a given patient, the physician now has available new tools to help manage individual cases in the clinical setting. Remarkable advances in analytic methods make it possible to measure the *dose* of an environmental agent directly in the patient rather than to assume dosing has occurred simply from exposure (defined as an opportunity for contact with an agent). Thus biologic monitoring (such as measuring the blood concentrations of dioxin at the parts per quadrillion level) should be substituted (where possible) for environmental monitoring (measuring dioxin levels in soil for determining whether the "exposed" patient actually received a significant dose). The modern approach offers the additional advantage of ability to evaluate the patient risk without having to account for the uncertainty in extrapolating to humans the toxic effects of an agent in animals. Thus, if the body content of the "exposed" patient is within the range of that found in the general population, then the patient may be reassured that he or she is at no unusual risk for whatever adverse health effects are attributed to the agent in question. Moreover, if the patient's level, even if evaluated, is similar to that of population groups studied epidemiologically, then this may serve as the basis of a rational risk assessment for a given patient.

In summary, comparative human toxicology relying on the dose response principle offers an important new way for the clinician to approach the patient exposed to environmental agents.

Additional Suggested Reading

1. Ames BN: Dietary carcinogens and anticarcinogens. Oxygen radicals and degenerative diseases. Science *221*:1256–1264, 1983.

2. Ashby J: Comparison of techniques for monitoring human exposure to genotoxic chemicals. Mutat Res *204*:543–551, 1988.
3. Bryant MS, Skipper PL, Tannenbaum SR, Maclure M: Hemoglobin adducts of 4-aminobiphenyl in smokers and nonsmokers. Cancer Res *47*:602–608, 1987.
4. Dean JH, Thurmond LM: Immunotoxicology: An overview. Toxicol Pathol *15*:265–271, 1987.
5. Dybing E: Predictability of human carcinogenicity from animal studies. Reg Toxicol Pharmacol *6*:399–415, 1986.
6. Ellenhorn MJ, Barceloux DG (eds): Medical Toxicology. Diagnosis and Treatment of Human Poisoning. New York, Elsevier, 1988.
7. Gosselin RE, Smith RP, Hodge HC (eds): Clinical Toxicology of Commercial Products. Baltimore, Williams & Wilkins, 1984.
8. Guzelian PS: Chlordecone poisoning: a case study in approaches for detoxification of humans exposed to environmental chemicals. Drug Metab Rev *13*:663–679, 1982.
9. Guzelian PS: Hepatic injury due to environmental agents. Clin Lab Med *4*:483–488, 1984.
10. Harris CC: Future directions in the use of DNA adducts as internal dosimeters for monitoring human exposure to environmental mutagens and carcinogens. Environ Health Perspect *62*:185–191, 1985.
11. Patterson DG Jr, Needham LL, Pirkle JL, et al: Correlation between serum and adipose tissue levels of 2,3,7,8-tetrachlorodibenzo-*p*-dioxin in 50 persons from Missouri. Arch Environ Contam Toxicol *17*:139–143, 1988.
12. Perera FP: Molecular cancer epidemiology: A new tool in cancer prevention. J Natl Cancer Inst *78*:887–898, 1987.
13. Perera FP, Weinstein IB: Molecular epidemiology and carcinogen-DNA adduct detection: New approaches to studies of human cancer causation. J Chron Dis *35*:581–600, 1982.
14. Rom WN (ed): Environmental and Occupational Medicine. Boston, Little, Brown, 1983.
15. Schulte-Hermann R: Tumor promotion in the liver. Arch Toxicol [Suppl] *57*:147–158, 1985.
16. Speizer FE: Overview of the risk of respiratory cancer from airborne contaminants. Environ Health Perspect *70*:9–15, 1986.
17. Willett WC, MacMahon B: Diet and cancer—an overview (parts one and two). N Engl J Med *310*:633–701, 1984.

B. Carcinogenesis

David J. Holbrook, Ph.D.

SCOPE OF THE PROBLEM

Environmental factors have been estimated to cause more than 85 per cent of human cancers, but in such cases the term *environmental* is all-inclusive and pertains to essentially all causative agents other than genetic factors. Environmental chemicals may be responsible for 75 per cent of human cancer, but such environmental chemicals include those manufactured, those resulting from the industrial or work environment, natural plant or fungus-produced toxins (e.g., aflatoxins), and inorganic salts (either metallic or nitrite/nitrate). Exposure to carcinogens may occur from occupational sources, diet, or lifestyle characteristics (smoking or alcohol use). Physical agents such as naturally occurring radioactive isotopes, ultraviolet radiation (e.g., sunlight), X-radiation, cosmic radiation, and viruses contribute to the "environmental" incidence of human cancers.

The occupational chemical exposure in the work environment has been estimated by most reasonable sources to cause 5 to 6 per cent of the cancers in men and approximately 2 per cent in women,[1, 2] but extreme estimates have ranged from 2 to 3 per cent to 20 to 30 per cent of human cancers. The lists of carcinogenic or probably carcinogenic chemicals vary with the source. The International Agency for Research on Cancer (IARC) compiles one representative list that includes 50 entities (chemicals, groups of chemicals, or industrial processes) that are carcinogenic to humans, and additional lists of 37 and 159 entities that are classified as "probably" and "possibly" carcinogenic to humans, respectively.[3] The IARC list is discussed at the end of this section.

PRINCIPLES OF CHEMICAL CARCINOGENESIS

Classification of Chemical Carcinogenesis: Genetic and Epigenetic Agents. Two categories of carcinogens, genotoxic and epigenetic carcinogens, are distinguished by their probable mechanism of action. *Genotoxic carcinogens* are agents that form a reactive ultimate carcinogen and are capable of reacting covalently with DNA to form various adducts with the DNA; covalent reaction may also occur with other macromolecules such as proteins and RNA. The chemicals in this category are typically studied by their ability to damage DNA or bring about DNA repair in mammalian cellular systems or to be mutagenic in model bacterial test systems. In contrast, the *epigenetic carcinogens* may act through alterations in differentiation, the effects of which include alterations in hormonal status or immunosuppression, or through support of chronic tissue injury.[4] The epigenetic carcinogens do not cause genomic damage directly. That is, they (probably) do not cause DNA damage. It has been proposed that epigenetic carcinogens may exert their effects by promotion of pre- (or "fortuitously") initiated cells.[5] The epigenetic carcinogens that do not appear to form electrophilic reactive carcinogens include asbestos, hormones, and plastics.

Metabolic Activation of Carcinogens. Most organic chemical carcinogens normally exist as relatively nonreactive parent compounds, referred to as procarcinogens (or precarcinogens). The procarcinogen requires metabolic activation to form a product, the ultimate carcinogen, capable of reacting with a target macromolecule to initiate the carcinogenic process. In some cases, one or more proximate carcinogens (or biotransformation intermediates) may exist in the pathway between the procarcinogen and the ultimate carcinogen. Although some notable exceptions exist, most of the chemical carcinogens are activated by the cytochrome P-450–dependent mixed function oxidase system. The mixed function oxidase system is a family of enzymatic activities that are markedly inducible; that is, the preexposure of mammalian cells to inducers (including certain carcinogens) brings about the increased synthesis of the enzymes capable of the metabolism of the carcinogen and other compounds. For example, the treatment of animals for several days with the carcinogens 3-methylcholanthrene or benzo(a)pyrene markedly increases the subsequent metabolism of these carcinogens to reactive species capable of covalent reaction with DNA.

The metabolism of procarcinogens typically results in a number of reactions that lead to different competing pathways: either the conversion of the procarcinogen to the ultimate carcinogen and reaction with DNA or other target macromolecule, or inactivation leading to a nonreactive metabolite. The induction of the mixed function oxidases does not always lead to the increased covalent reaction of carcinogens with DNA or to the increased formation of tumors.

A few intrinsically reactive or "direct-acting" carcinogens do not require metabolic activation to form reactive species. This group includes certain chemical intermediates and cancer chemotherapeutic agents, but the direct-acting carcinogens do not usually exist in the environment because of their chemical instability.

With either the metabolically activated or direct-acting organic carcinogens, the reactive species that is formed is an electrophilic (or relatively electron-deficient) moiety that can react covalently with a number of nucleophilic (or relatively electron-rich) sites, e.g., oxygen, nitrogen, or sulfur atoms of macromolecules. Reaction with certain low molecular weight molecules, such as glutathione, probably leads to the effective inactivation of the carcinogen.

Carcinogenesis as a Multistep Process. The development of cancer is a multistep process. The general classification distinguishes three major stages: initiation, promotion, and progression.

Initiation. Initiation is the production of a heritable change that predisposes a cell to uncontrolled growth. The initiation stage is rapid and irreversible.

In the case of the genotoxic carcinogens, with either the metabolically activated or direct-acting carcinogens the reactive species initiates the carcinogenic process by reacting with a sensitive target macromolecule. DNA, because of its role in carrying genetic information, is functionally the likely target macromolecule for reaction with ultimate carcinogens since a permanent neoplastic state may be due to alterations in the genome. Although most of the research interest is on the covalent reaction with DNA, carcinogens also form covalent adducts with RNA and proteins. Theoretically, interactions of carcinogens with proteins that regulate gene expression or that alter DNA coding of RNA synthesis (e.g., alteration of enzymatic methylation of DNA which, in turn, alters the rate of RNA transcription) may also permanently alter cellular replication and function.[6]

The initiation is a relatively rare event. Although most cells in a tissue may undergo damage by a chemical carcinogen, most cells die, undergo repair, or survive damage to noncritical sites and, thus, do not develop into preneoplastic nodules or tumors. The estimates are that the initiation occurs in only one per hundred thousand cells or one per million cells.[7] Tumor-initiating substances react with DNA, but the reaction alone does not lead to a tumor. Most covalent reaction of a carcinogen with DNA is repaired (or the damage may exist in a noncritical region) with no development of tumors. A few cells that have been damaged by a carcinogen will develop into preneoplastic nodules, and a few of the preneoplastic nodules will develop into tumors. There are active processes for the repair of damage to DNA; damage to other macromolecules (e.g., RNA or protein) is corrected by the degradation of the damaged macromolecule and its resynthesis.[6]

Although most DNA damage is repaired, cell division may occur before the repair if the cells are rapidly dividing; the damaged DNA is used as a template for DNA replication (i.e., in postreplication repair). In such a case, use of the damaged DNA during replication may result in the permanent alterations in the genome and a fixation of a mutagenic event. Abnormal cells may undergo proliferation to form preneoplastic nodules.

Certain human diseases characterized by deficiencies in DNA repair or metabolism predispose the individuals to the development of cancers. *Xeroderma pigmentosum* is accompanied by a deficiency in the DNA incision stage of repair and is associated with an extremely high incidence of skin cancers initiated by ultraviolet radiation. Patients with ataxia telangiectasia, Fanconi's anemia, and Bloom's syndrome also are characteristically deficient in DNA metabolism and are susceptible to high rates of cancer development.[8]

Promotion. Cells may undergo initiation to yield dormant or suppressed preneoplastic cells without the progressive growth to form neoplasms. Subsequent exposure (usually repeated exposures) to promoters releases the cells from the normal regulatory control and leads to uncontrolled growth and development of neoplasms.[6]

The classic experiments of initiation and promotion were conducted by painting carcinogens on mouse skin with subsequent prolonged treatment with various promoters. In the often-cited pattern of such experiments, the following principles were established:

(a) The animals could be treated with a single low dose of initiator without initiation of cancer; therefore, there exists a subcarcinogenic dose. It is critical in such an analysis that this applies only within the statistical limitations of the experiment, because there is a valid question whether such a threshold actually does exist for a genotoxic carcinogen.

(b) Repeated treatment of animals with the low, subcarcinogenic dose of the carcinogen results in tumor formation; therefore, the effects of the (initiator) carcinogen treatments are cumulative.

(c) Repeated treatments with a promoter alone do not result in tumor formation; therefore, many promoters are not carcinogenic by themselves.

(d) A single or a few treatments with a subcarcinogenic dose of initiator, followed even weeks or months later by repeated treatments with a promoter, result in tumor formation; this is the classic initiation-promotion experiment. One interpretation is that the initiator produced a damaged DNA, and the subsequent treatment with the promoter caused the replication of cells before the full repair of the damaged DNA and the fixation of a somatic mutation. Some promoters cause increased cellular proliferation and their action would be consistent with such a proposal; however, not all promoters cause cellular proliferation.

(e) Repeated treatment with a promoter followed some time later by a single treatment with an initiator does not cause tumor formation; i.e., reversing the sequence of the treatments in (d) does not result in tumor formation.

The original studies on initiation and promotion were conducted on mouse skin. The initiation-promotion stages also have been demonstrated in a number of other tissues such as liver, lung, bladder, colon, esophagus, mammary gland, stomach, and pancreas in experimental animals.[9]

The studies in mouse skin have typically used the phorbol esters, the active ingredient in croton oil, as tumor promoters. The active promoting agents represent a wide variety of chemicals, both in terms of structure and biochemical activity, and include bile acids, saccharin, hormones, phenobarbital, polychlorinated or polybrominated biphenyls, and butylated hydroxytoluene.[9] In liver carcinogenesis studies, experimental animals are treated with an *N*-nitroso compound and subsequently treated with the promoter phenobarbital in the drinking water. Although phenobarbital is a promoter in rat liver carcinogenesis, a committee of the International Agency for Research on Cancer (IARC) concluded that phenobarbital is not a carcinogenic risk in humans after a review of epidemiologic studies in humans, e.g., in epileptic patients who are treated for long intervals with high dosages. The absence of human carcinogenicity upon high-level exposure has been noted for several agents, such as phenobarbital and saccharin, which are epigenetic carcinogens in experimental animals.[10]

Progression. Tumor progression is characterized by increases in growth rate, invasiveness, and metastases.[5] Neoplasms undergo qualitative changes in their phenotypic properties, which in some cases include the transition from benign to malignant growth characteristics. Biochemically, there are changes in the molecular structure (arrangement) of the genes, increases in the number of copies of certain genes (gene amplification), instability in the chromosomal structures (leading to changes in the karyotypes within malignant cells) and loss of copies of other genes (deletion).[5]

Chemical Carcinogenesis and Oncogenes. Certain normal cellular genes (proto-oncogenes) are homologous with certain oncogenic RNA retroviruses that replicate via a DNA provirus integrated into cellular DNA. Proto-oncogenes are cellular genes that are expressed during normal growth and developmental processes, and they normally function as genes for growth factors, growth factor receptors, and regulatory proteins or as kinases. The abnormal activation of the proto-oncogenes to activated oncogenes capable of cellular transformation includes point mutations, gene amplification (an increased number of copies of a specific gene per cell), chromosomal rearrangement, and promoter insertion (insertion of a new regulatory sequence for gene use).[11] The activation of the proto-oncogenes may result in increased levels of normal proteins involved in cellular growth or in normal or altered levels of expression of an abnormal protein.[11] The activated oncogenes can transform cells in culture to grow in a pattern consistent with uncontrolled growth and induce neoplasia when the transformed cells are injected into immunocompromised mice. The activation and expression of more than one proto-oncogene may be necessary to cause the transformation of a normal cell into a tumorigenic cell.[11]

Several oncogenes have been detected in human tumors by the transfer ("transfection") in vitro of tumor DNA into mouse fibroblasts and, upon injection into mice, the subsequent in vivo tumor development in immunocompromised mice. Activated *ras* genes have been detected in 27 per cent of cases of acute myeloid leukemia examined in humans, and the Ha-*ras* gene was detected in four of the six examined human squamous cell carcinomas.[11] Likewise, oncogenes are detected in spontaneous and carcinogen-induced tumors in experimental animals.[11]

It is suggested that "conversion of proto-oncogenes to oncogenes by genetic alterations contributes to the neoplastic transformation of cells. . . . Investigations in several rodent models for chemical carcinogenesis imply that oncogenes are activated by carcinogen treatment and that this activation process is causally involved in tumor induction."[12] Chemicals and radiation can cause activation of oncogenes by production of point mutations in animal tumor studies. However, oncogene activation may not always be a result of chemical interaction with DNA.[11, 13] Alternatively, in animal carcinogenesis studies the chemical may increase "the background tumor incidence by a mechanism such as cytotoxicity or receptor-mediated promotion."[11]

NITROSAMINES AND OTHER *N*-NITROSO CARCINOGENS

The discussion of specific carcinogens will be limited to agents that reflect high levels of exposure or exposure to a large fraction of the general population.

Biochemistry. The carcinogenic *N*-nitroso compounds may be characterized chemically in two groups: (1) the nitrosamines, which are not intrinsically reactive and require metabolic activation by the cytochrome P-450–dependent mixed function oxidase system to form the electrophilic ultimate carcinogens, and (2) the *N*-nitrosoamides, including nitroso(alkyl)ureas, nitroso(alkyl)guanidines, and nitrosourethanes or nitrosoalkylcarbamates. The latter group are intrinsically reactive (with DNA and other macromolecules) and thus are direct-acting carcinogens that do not require metabolic activation.[14, 15]

Exposure and Occurrence—Preformed. Human exposure to nitrosamines may occur either through exposure to preformed nitrosamines (in food, water, or air) or through exposure to nitrosamines potentially formed in vivo.[15] Nonoccupational exposure to preformed nitrosamines may occur from food (e.g., nitrite-cured meat products or fish, or malt-beverages),[16] household goods (e.g., rubber), tobacco and tobacco smoke, cosmetics, drugs, pesticides, and indoor air (e.g., frying of nitrite-cured meat with release of volatile nitrosamines).[15] The greatest exposure of humans to nitrosamines occurs from dietary sources.[14]

Nitrosamine formation occurs during the heating of nitrite-cured meat products, such as bacon;[15] the nitrite or nitrate is added during the curing process to prevent the germination of spores and thereby prevent botulism.[17] Current technology has led to markedly reduced concentrations of nitrosamines; the amounts of nitrite salts added have been reduced and the addition of nitrosation inhibitors, such as ascorbic acid, has reduced the preformed nitrosamine concentrations and the amounts formed during frying.[15, 17]

Very low levels of nitrosamine contamination of fish or cheese have occasionally been reported, but such levels are very low, typically less than 1 part per billion (ppb) (1 μg/kg).[15, 17] Early findings of preformed nitrosamines in beer and other malt beverages have brought about changes in the methods of preparation and a marked decrease in the contamination by nitrosamines.[14, 15] However, even with new preparative technology, beer and other malt beverages typically contain low levels (usually less than 1 μg/kg) of nitrosamines.[15]

In smokers, the greatest nonoccupational source of exposure to preformed nitrosamines is tobacco and tobacco smoke.[15] The nitrosamine formation in tobacco smoke from tobacco amines and nitrous gases is suggested as a contributor to the known carcinogenicity of tobacco smoke,[15] although tobacco smoke also contains other chemical carcinogens such as polycyclic aromatic hydrocarbons and metallic cations.[17] Harvested tobacco is practically free of nitrosamines,[16] but both curing and combustion result in the formation of nitrosamines.[15] The concentrations of formed nitrosamines are a function of the nitrate concentration of the tobacco[15] and of the nitrosatable constituents derived from pesticides (amines, amides, and carbamates) and other compounds such as alkaloids and amino acids.[17]

Other sources of exposure to nitrosamines are cosmetics (ointments, creams, shampoos, and lipsticks) and the preformed nitrosamines in drugs and pesticides.[15] In addition, nitrosatable amines are used as accelerators and stabilizers in rubber production, and the nitrogen oxides in the ambient air may act as nitrosating agents during production or storage.[15]

Indoor air may result in the exposure to substantial quantities of volatile nitrosamines (especially from tobacco use but also from the frying of cured meats).[15] In contrast, outdoor air in urban areas or in automobile exhausts does not contain detectable levels of nitrosamines.[15]

Occupational exposure to preformed nitrosamines may occur in the rubber industry from use of nitrosamines during the production, in leather tanning that uses reactive amines in the tanning process, in chemical industries using amines, and in metal-working industries that use nitrosamine-containing grinding fluids.[15]

Exposure and Occurrence—In Vivo Formation. Nitrosamines can be formed from amines (especially secondary and tertiary amines) and amides by the reaction of nitrosating agents. The chemistry of the reaction varies with the nature of the nitrosatable compound.[15] Nitrite, under acidic conditions, yields an active nitrosating medium for secondary amines,[15] and the nitrosation reaction occurs more rapidly with secondary amines than with tertiary amines.[14] In vivo formation of nitrosamines occurs from nitrosatable amino compounds present in foods, drugs, or cosmetics and from nitrosating agents such as nitrite or nitrogen oxides.[15] The nature of the reaction in an acidic medium implies that the reaction can occur in the acidic medium of the stomach from ingested nitrosatable compounds. This is supported by experiments in vitro and in vivo. A number of studies have demonstrated that the combined oral administration of nitrosatable amino compounds and nitrite to experimental animals results in tumor development,[18] but tumors are not observed when nitrite or the amino compounds are given alone.[18]

Nitrite and nitrogen oxides are effective nitrosating agents. Nitrate is ubiquitous, and high concentrations are present in vegetables and in drinking water. The salivary glands secrete nitrate with saliva, and the oral microflora rapidly reduce nitrate to nitrite. In the acidic medium of the stomach, the conditions are favorable for the in vivo nitrosation of ingested nitrosatable compounds (especially secondary amines). Although the potential for the formation of carcinogenic nitrosamines in humans exists, the conditions of pH and the concentrations of nitrite and the nitrosatable amines may not be conducive to such formation.

The average American diet contains approximately 75 mg of nitrate and 0.8 mg of nitrite daily, and vegetables contribute most of the nitrate ingested.[19] Nitrite ingestion is due predominantly to cured meats (more than 33 per cent), to baked goods and cereals (approximately 33 per cent), and to vegetables (less than 20 per cent).[19] It is estimated that approximately 25 per cent of the ingested nitrate is secreted into the saliva, and approximately 20 per cent of the salivary nitrate is reduced to nitrite.[19]

A number of naturally occurring inhibitors of nitrosation exist. Ascorbic acid (vitamin C) reacts with nitrite (or nitrous acid) and yields nitric oxide (nitrogen monoxide, NO) which is not a nitrosating agent.[15, 20] Alpha-tocopherol (vitamin E) is another effective inhibitor of nitrosation.[15, 19]

Carcinogenesis. A majority of, but not all, *N*-nitroso compounds are carcinogens in *experimental animals;* in one compilation, 90 per cent of the 300 *N*-nitroso compounds studied are carcinogenic.[14, 18] All animal species are susceptible to carcinogenesis induced by *N*-nitroso compounds, including nitrosamines.[14, 17] In the evaluation of the potential of human carcinogenesis of *N*-nitroso compounds, both preformed compounds and those that may be formed in vivo, i.e., through the participation of nitrite or nitrate conversion to nitrite, must be considered.

Although great potential exists for the role of *N*-nitroso compounds as human carcinogens, there is a general lack of acceptance that current data firmly support such a role. Preussmann and Eisenbrand "do not think that sufficient data exist for meaningful evaluation," and, "therefore, estimation of nitrosamine contribution to human cancer risk is largely speculative."[15]

Since nitrates are reduced to nitrites by the bacteria in saliva, the possible carcinogenicity of nitrate has been studied. The quantities of *N*-nitroso compounds formed in vivo depend on the availability of nitrite (either present as such or formed from nitrate by the bacterial nitrite reductase) and conditions (pH, temperature, absence of antioxidants) favorable to chemical nitrosation. In animals, nitrite is "probably not carcinogenic" and nitrate has not been shown to be carcinogenic.[19] If the *N*-nitroso compounds formed in vivo are important in human cancer, populations with higher dietary consumption of nitrate (or nitrite) would be expected to have a higher incidence of cancer in the appropriate target organs.[21] It has been concluded that there is insufficient evidence that nitrates (or nitrites formed in vivo) cause cancer in humans, and that "the epidemiological evidence currently available is qualitatively inadequate to justify any useful conclusions on the role of *N*-nitroso compounds or nitrates in human carcinogenesis."[22] Although it is acknowledged that endogenous formation of *N*-nitroso compounds has been associated with increased risk of certain cancers, e.g., stomach and esophagus, it was concluded that "no convincing epidemiological evidence has been presented concerning the etiological role of these compounds in human cancer."[20] Likewise, in spite of several epidemiological studies "consistent with the hypothesis that exposure of humans to high levels of nitrate and/or nitrite may be associated with an increased incidence of cancers of the stomach and esophagus," the overall "epidemiological evidence suggesting that nitrate, nitrite, and *N*-nitroso compounds play a role in the development of cancer in humans is largely circumstantial."[19]

AFLATOXINS

Role and Exposure. Aflatoxins are only one of the groups of the carcinogenic compounds derived from soil-based microorganisms.[17, 19] Aflatoxins are produced by *Aspergillus flavus*, other *Aspergillus* species, and perhaps by some *Penicillium* and *Rhizopus*.[16, 23] These fungal-produced toxins exist as heterogeneous mixtures and occur as food contaminants. Aflatoxin B1 is the carcinogenic natural product with the most significant impact,[17] is the most potent hepatocarcinogen known,[19] and is carcinogenic in a number of animal species (with varying sensitivities in different species),[10, 19] with development of liver neoplasms predominantly.

Human exposure to aflatoxins may occur by the consumption of foods that have been contaminated by certain strains of *Aspergillus flavus* or *Aspergillus parasiticus* during growth, harvest, or storage.[23] Nearly all agricultural products are potentially subject to contamination with aflatoxins. Common sources include grains (e.g., corn, rice, sorghum), peanuts, oilseeds (e.g., cottonseed oil, copra), legumes (soybeans, other beans), and tree nuts (e.g., almonds, pecans, walnuts).[23, 24] The use of aflatoxin-contaminated feed for domestic animals may result in secondary exposure to humans by the consumption of products such as meat, milk and cheese, and eggs that contain residues of the aflatoxins or their toxic metabolites.[23]

The FDA established enforcement levels of 0.5 part per billion in milk and 20 parts per billion for other food products.[25] In the United States, concentrations of up to 20 ppb are permitted in human foods.[10, 19] Levels of up to 200 ppb are permitted in animal feeds,[10] although there may be a concern for secondary exposure to aflatoxins from the use of animal products.

Carcinogenesis—Animal Studies. Aflatoxin B1 is a potent hepatocarcinogen in experimental animals, but tumors may also occur in the colon and kidneys.[25] In rats, tumors develop after the administration of 0.2 μg per day or a single dose of 0.5 mg of aflatoxin B1; the tumor incidence is 50 per cent at 26 months after the latter treatment.[16] There are marked differences in the susceptibility of various species to carcinogenesis by aflatoxin B1; rats are much more susceptible than mice.

Carcinogenesis—Human Studies. The National Toxicology Program[25] includes the aflatoxins in the list of substances or groups of substances that may reasonably be anticipated to be carcinogens.

Very high levels of aflatoxins occur in foods in certain regions of Africa and Asia, and people in these regions suffer a high incidence of liver cancer. Within Swaziland, Kenya, Uganda, and Thailand, where epidemiologic studies have been conducted, in certain areas the climatic conditions (i.e., high temperatures and high humidity)[25] are favorable for fungal growth; the food supply shows a relatively high aflatoxin contamination, and the average aflatoxin consumption exceeds 10 μg per kg of body weight per day.[16] In other areas of the same countries where lower temperatures and lower humidity prevail, the food supply shows a relatively lower aflatoxin contamination and the average human aflatoxin consumption is less. Within each country, there is a direct relationship between the incidence of liver tumors (cases/100,000 people/year) and the average daily dietary intake of aflatoxins in contaminated agricultural products.[10, 16]

Although aflatoxin B1 is a potent liver carcinogen in animals, in the epidemiologic studies in Africa and Asia it is difficult to ascribe the incidence of human liver cancers solely to aflatoxin B1 because of the concurrent exposure to other potentially causative agents (hepatitis B virus, other carcinogenic mycotoxins, and liver parasitism) that may be enhancing factors due to liver cell damage and replication.[10, 19]

In the United States, it is estimated that 0.15 to 0.50 μg of aflatoxins is consumed daily,[25] equivalent to 0.002 to 0.007 μg per kg per day for the hypothetical 70-kg adult. The contamination of foods, greater in the southeastern United States, results in the greatest dietary exposure from corn and peanuts. The exposure from other dietary sources such as tree nuts (almonds, walnuts, pecans, and pistachios) is probably of minor significance because of the small quantities consumed or infrequent contamination.[19] Secondary exposure potentially may occur by the consumption of products (e.g., meat, milk, other dairy products, and eggs) derived from animals that have consumed aflatoxin-contaminated feeds.[23] However, a National Academy of Sciences committee concluded that it is unlikely that significant secondary exposure, or at least negligible exposure compared to other sources, results from the consumption of animal tissues or milk;[19] although large amounts of milk are consumed, there is generally an absence of detectable levels of aflatoxin B1 metabolite in milk samples in the United States.[24]

A National Academy of Sciences committee has concluded that "there is no epidemiological evidence that aflatoxin contamination of foodstuffs is related to cancer risk in the United States."[19] Unlike the epidemiologic studies in Africa and Asia, in the United States neither of the states with the highest average consumption of aflatoxins is among the states with the highest incidence of liver cancer, and thus other carcinogens are apparently more important in the development of liver cancers.

Biochemistry. Among the toxic aflatoxins, aflatoxins B1 and G1 are the most biologically active, but other derivatives also exhibit carcinogenicity.[23] Aflatoxin B1 requires metabolic activation by the cytochrome P-450–dependent mixed-function oxidase to be converted to the reactive 2,3-epoxide, the ultimate carcinogen. The aflatoxins, e.g., aflatoxin B1, are genotoxic carcinogens and the reactive metabolites react with DNA. The major adduct formed with DNA in intracellular reactions is formed from the 2-position of aflatoxin B1 and the N-7 position of guanine in DNA.

POLYCYCLIC AROMATIC HYDROCARBONS

Polycyclic aromatic hydrocarbons (PAH) are widespread contaminants in the environment, and they occur primarily as a result of incomplete combustion and pyrolysis of organic materials, for example, fossil fuels. In many cases, benzo(a)pyrene, a carcinogenic PAH, is used as the model compound to assess exposure to PAH.

The greater exposure of the general population to ambient air PAH is derived from heat and power generation, refuse burning, and coke production.[26] The greatest occupational exposure occurs in workers engaged in tarring (road surfaces and roofs) and coke oven operations.[26]

Motor vehicle exhausts contribute only a small percentage (approximately 1 per cent) of the total environmental presence to PAH, and benzo(a)pyrene constitutes approximately 3 to 5 per cent of the identified PAH emitted from motor vehicles.[26] The newer statutory standards for hydrocarbon emissions have resulted in reductions in the total contribution of motor vehicles to environmental contamination by PAH.

In addition to ambient air, exposure to PAH also occurs in the indoor environment, in part from cigarette smoke. Except in certain occupational groups, generally cigarette use is the most important overall source of exposure to PAH, or benzo(a)pyrene, among smokers.[26] The one-pack-per-day smoker is estimated to inhale approximately 0.7 μg per day or 0.4 μg per day of benzo(a)pyrene from unfiltered cigarettes or filtered cigarettes, respectively,[26] in comparison to the estimate of 0.02 μg per 8-hr day due to the ambient air exposure.[26] Sidestream cigarette smoke, i.e., the passive inhalation of smoke by a nonsmoker in the presence of smokers, also results in appreciable exposure in the indoor environment. PAH are not the only carcinogens present in smoke; other carcinogens include volatile nitrosamines and heavy metals.[27] Certain methods of cooking (in homes, or in restaurants along with cigarette smoke) also increase the level of PAH in the indoor environment.

Biochemistry. A number of PAH are carcinogenic in laboratory animals. The parent compounds are nonreactive but are metabolized by the cytochrome P-450 to form proximate carcinogens (metabolic intermediates) and ultimate carcinogens (reactive electrophilic moieties that covalently react with DNA and other macromolecules).

The most commonly used model compound of the PAH is benzo(a)pyrene. As is characteristic of most PAH, a large number of metabolites are produced but only a few react with DNA. The most reactive site on the benzo(a)pyrene is the K region and the formation of the corresponding K region epoxide. Structural studies of the adducts formed between benzo(a)pyrene and DNA demonstrate that the K-region epoxides are not common adducts with cellular DNA. Although the K-region epoxide is formed, the compound appears to be rapidly inactivated in cellular systems by either epoxide hydrolase (an enzyme which hydrolyzes the epoxide ring to form a dihydrodiol) or by glutathione sulfotransferase (which forms a nonreactive conjugate of the epoxide). The metabolic pathway leading to the ultimate carcinogen of benzo(a)pyrene consists of a cytochrome P-450–dependent mixed-function oxidase activity to yield an epoxide, the epoxide hydrolysis by epoxide hydrolase to form a dihydrodiol, and a second reaction catalyzed by the cytochrome P-450–dependent mixed-function oxidase to form the ultimate carcinogen, 7,8-dihydro-7,8-diol-9,10-epoxide.

The ultimate carcinogen is a "bay region" epoxide, i.e., an epoxide which is on a ring joined to the remainder of the condensed ring system by only two carbons. The reactivity of this bay region epoxide is increased by the ability to form an intramolecular hydrogen bond between one of the hydroxyl groups and the epoxide oxygen. In addition, the dihydrodiol epoxides are poor substrates for the inactivation reactions normally catalyzed by epoxide hydrolase or glutathione sulfotransferase. Thus, increased reactivity due to intramolecular hydrogen bonding and decreased breakdown of the reactive epoxide are conducive to covalent reaction of the ultimate carcinogen with DNA and other macromolecules.

The formation of a carcinogenic bay region epoxide is not limited to benzo(a)pyrene; a large number of other PAH also are metabolized to carcinogenic bay region epoxides. The formation of a bay region epoxide is not an absolute requirement for the formation of ultimate carcinogens. A few PAH-related compounds structurally cannot form bay region epoxides, but these compounds are carcinogenic.

Exposure of an animal to PAH results in an induced synthesis of the types of cytochrome P-450 (specifically cytochrome P[1]-450 or P-448) that metabolize the PAH to reactive metabolites that are capable of covalent attachment to DNA. Consequently, the repeated exposures to PAH increase the metabolism of the PAH to ultimate carcinogens and other metabolites. Thus, repeated exposure not only increases the likelihood of initiation but also increases the metabolism of the procarcinogen to an ultimate carcinogen.

OTHER CHEMICAL CARCINOGENS

Vinyl Chloride. Vinyl chloride (monomer) is a synthetic halogenated unsaturated hydrocarbon used in the production of polyvinyl chloride. Vinyl chloride is a genotoxic carcinogen—that is, it reacts covalently with DNA and produces liver angiosarcomas in experimental animals.[10] The most definitive activity of vinyl chloride in humans is the development of hepatic angiosarcoma. The incidence caused by occupational exposure is highest in "reactor cleaners."[10]

Benzidine. Benzidine (or 4,4′-diaminobiphenyl) is an intermediate in the synthesis of dyes. It has also been used in clinical laboratories for the detection of blood. Benzidine is a genotoxic carcinogen in laboratory animals. Although the target site of carcinogenesis in laboratory animals varies in different species, benzidine induces urinary bladder cancer in humans.[10]

Diethylstilbestrol. Diethylstilbestrol (or DES) is a synthetic estrogen that was at one time used in treatments to maintain pregnancy. Diethylstilbestrol is carcinogenic in various experimental animals. Although the theory is not uniformly accepted, DES does not appear to react with DNA and therefore appears to be an epigenetic carcinogen that exerts its carcinogenicity through its hormonal activity. It is one of the few epigenetic carcinogens that is an established causative agent for cancer in humans.[10] The daughters of women treated with diethylstilbestrol during pregnancy have a markedly increased risk of clear cell adenocarcinoma of the vagina and the cervix during puberty and there may be an increased risk of vaginal adenosis and squamous carcinoma of the cervix later in life.[10]

RADIATION: RADON

Nature. Radon, or ^{222}radon, is a radioactive and nonreactive gas derived from the isotopic decay of naturally occurring ^{226}radium and itself decays into other alpha-particle–emitting isotopes.

The exposure of humans to radon includes occupational exposure in miners. However, the appearances of the radon gas and radon decay products in a small fraction of homes[28] and other exposures are major concerns. The exposures depend on a number of factors.

(1) The geology of the region around the residences—the radium content in the soil around foundations[28]—is the major source of radon and its radioactive decay products.

(2) The radium content in earth-derived building materials such as cinder block and building stone contributes to the exposure by the radon gas effusion from the materials.[29] The construction of the residence markedly affects the concentrations of radon. The radon gas from the underlying soil or the building materials may be concentrated and trapped in the residence. In well-ventilated homes with higher levels of air movement in living areas, the indoor concentration of radon is nearly the same as the outdoor con-

centration and is estimated to be approximately 0.2 to 0.3 picocurie per liter (pCi/L) of air in the continental United States.[29] In some homes with less ventilation, like some energy-efficient homes, the radon concentrations in the living areas may be approximately three times the external concentrations and the concentrations in basements twice the concentrations in upper floors, but the concentrations are markedly altered by the underlying construction of the residence.[29] By one estimate, the exposure to radon and radon decay products in one million residences in the United States may exceed the exposure received by current uranium miners.[30] In geographic regions where the radium content in the soil is high, the hazard from radon may be decreased by remedial modifications or alterations in new construction practices.[28] In principle, radon-associated cancers may be preventable by identification of potentially hazardous residences and construction modification to minimize radon contamination.[30]

(3) The radon content in water supplies also contributes to exposure and to indoor contamination. In one compilation of data from 39 states in which 50 or more groundwater supplies were sampled, the radon concentration in public groundwater was 500 (or more) pCi/L of water in four states (Rhode Island, New Hampshire, Vermont, and Massachusetts) and 35 (or less) pCi/L in nine states.[31]

Estimates of the role of radon as the causative agent in human lung cancer usually have been made on the basis of cancer incidence in radon-exposed miners.[32] One estimate is that approximately 10 per cent of the lung cancer in the United States is tentatively attributable to pollution by radon and its radioactive decay products in residences.[30] In more detailed estimates, radioactive decay products of radon may cause 25 per cent of the lung cancers in nonsmokers over age 60 years and a somewhat higher percentage at older ages, and about 5 per cent in smokers (a smaller percentage because of the other causative agents of lung cancer to which the smoker is exposed).[28]

^{222}Radon itself is chemically inert, has a low solubility in biologic fluids, and does not constitute a major hazard in pulmonary exposures.[28] However, the carcinogenic radon decay products,[28, 30] especially when absorbed to dust particles, are deposited in the respiratory tract, and the emitted alpha-particles irradiate the human bronchial epithelium.[32]

MECHANISM OF CARCINOGENESIS IN RELATION TO HUMAN EXPOSURE AND RISK ASSESSMENT

The genotoxic or epigenetic mechanisms of action of chemical carcinogens are important factors to be considered in the estimation of risk of carcinogens. Genotoxic carcinogens that are reactive with DNA are effective after single or limited exposure or a low-dose exposure. Thus, it is proposed that the genotoxic carcinogen is a "qualitative" hazard to humans.[6] In addition to these carcinogens being active after a single exposure or after very limited exposures, the effects of repeated exposures are cumulative, and there may be additive interactions with other genotoxic carcinogens acting in the same target tissue.[6] It is debated whether a "no adverse observed effect level" or threshold exists for genotoxic carcinogens. It is desirable to attain the lowest possible human exposure although zero exposure to genotoxic carcinogens is usually impractical.

In contrast, epigenetic carcinogens have carcinogenic effects at much higher exposures, and carcinogenic treatment dosages in experimental animals usually greatly exceed any reasonable corresponding exposure level to humans. The examples most often cited are estrogens, which are epigenetic carcinogens at nonphysiologically high dosages and after prolonged treatment, whereas exposure at physiologic levels presumably does not result in carcinogenesis. Thus, it is proposed that the risk from exposure to an epigenetic carcinogen is of a "quantitative" nature.[6] In that context, one would anticipate that there is a threshold exposure level below which there is no or minimal hazard.[4, 6] Only a few epigenetic carcinogens have been clearly established as carcinogenic in humans; diethylstilbestrol is a major example.[10]

Chemicals that are carcinogenic in experimental animals are potential cancer hazards to humans. Unlike carcinogenesis studies in experimental animals that are genetically uniform and live in controlled environments, estimations of human risk are much more difficult because humans differ in exposure to factors that alter the sensitivity to carcinogenesis: genetics, hormonal factors, dietary components that may change the abilities to activate or detoxify carcinogens, and smoking. Interactions between substances alter the susceptibility to carcinogenesis; one of the better-established examples is that smokers are much more susceptible to asbestos-induced lung carcinogenesis than nonsmokers.[10]

The generally long latent period between exposure to carcinogens and the observation of cancers in humans has made the epidemiologic studies difficult and imprecise. However, a few instances of extremely high exposures have permitted estimates of a minimum latent period to certain human carcinogens. In an analysis by Williams and colleagues, exposures were sufficient to incriminate causative agents, and the minimum latent periods for various carcinogens were as short as 2 years (e.g., benzidine) or 4 years (e.g., vinyl chloride monomer).[10]

DESIGNATIONS AND CLASSIFICATION OF CARCINOGENS BY SCIENTIFIC AND REGULATORY AGENCIES

The evaluation of potential carcinogenic agents in humans and experimental animals is a very active and somewhat changing area. Three major, commonly recognized organizations classify various substances as carcinogens for scientific or regulatory purposes.

National Toxicology Program. To June, 1987, more than 300 carcinogenicity studies in rats or mice on 308 different chemicals have been designed and evaluated by the National Toxicology Program or, in earlier studies, by the National Cancer Institute.[33] Since June, 1983, the carcinogenicity studies in experimental animals are classified by the National Toxicology Program as: (a) "clear evidence" of a chemically related increased incidence of malignant neoplasms, benign neoplasms, or combination of malignant and benign neoplasms; (b) "some evidence" of an increased incidence of benign neoplasms, marginal increases in neoplasms of several organs/tissues, or a slight increase in uncommon malignant or benign neoplasms; (c) "equivocal evidence" of a marginal increase in neoplasms; (d) "no evidence" of chemically related increases in malignant or benign neoplasms; or (e) "indequate study," a category for studies that (perhaps for major experimental flaws) cannot be evaluated for showing either the presence or absence of an increased incidence of neoplasms.[3]

The findings of 202 studies by the National Cancer Institute and 125 studies by the National Toxicology Program in rats and mice have been compiled by Haseman and associates.[33] Of the 327 reported studies (which may have involved experiments in male and female rats and mice), 49 per cent demonstrated a carcinogenic effect in at least one sex and/or species, 13 per cent gave equivocal evidence of carcinogenicity, 37 per cent showed no evidence of carcinogenicity, and 2 per cent of the studies were considered inadequate for evaluation.

The National Toxicology Program report lists 24 substances or groups of substances and 5 occupational exposures (with unknown etiologic agents) as "known carcinogens" (defined as "those substances for which the evidence from human studies indicates that there is a causal relationship between exposure to the substance and human cancer") and 119 other substances or groups of substances that may reasonably be anticipated to be carcinogenic (defined as "those for which there is a limited evidence of carcinogenicity in humans or sufficient evidence of carcinogenicity in experimental animals").[25]

United States Environmental Protection Agency, Carcinogen Assessment Group (CAG). The Carcinogen Assessment Group has prepared a list of chemical substances for which "substantial or strong evidence exists showing that exposure to these chemicals, under certain conditions, causes cancer in humans, or can cause cancer in animal species which, in turn, makes them potentially carcinogenic in humans." Substances are placed on the CAG list "only if they have been demonstrated to induce malignant tumors in one or more animal species or to induce benign tumors that are generally recognized as early stages of malignancies, and/or if positive epidemiologic studies indicated they were carcinogenic."[34]

International Agency for Research on Cancer (IARC). In a series of monographs, the IARC assesses (a) the evidence for carcinogenicity from studies in humans, (b) the evidence for carcinogenicity from studies in experimental animals, and (c) data from short-term tests (e.g., mutagenesis, DNA damage, or transformation). The latter studies are contributing and useful indicators because initiation of carcinogenesis involves (or is thought to involve) damage to DNA and a somatic cell mutation. A list of the known or suspected human carcinogenic agents, as evaluated by the IARC, is presented in Table 26–3.

The evidence of carcinogencity from *human studies* is derived from case reports and descriptive or analytic epidemiologic studies, and the degrees of evidence for carcinogenicity are categorized as (a) "sufficient evidence," a causal relationship between the agent and human cancer; (b) "limited evidence," a causal relationship is creditable but alternative explanations could not be ex-

Table 26–3. LIST OF AGENTS WHICH ARE CARCINOGENIC OR PROBABLY CARCINOGENIC TO HUMANS

CARCINOGENIC*	PROBABLY CARCINOGENIC†
Aflatoxins	Acrylonitrile
4-Aminobiphenyl	Adriamycin
Arsenic and arsenic compounds‡	Androgenic (anabolic) steroids
Asbestos	Benz[a]anthracene
Azathioprine	Benzidine-based dyes
Benzene	Benzo[a]pyrene
Benzidine	Beryllium and beryllium compounds
N,N-Bis(2-chloroethyl)-2-naphthylamine (Chlornaphazine)	*Bis*chloroethyl nitrosourea (BCNU)
Bis(chloromethyl) ether and chloromethyl methyl ether (technical grade)	Cadmium and cadmium compounds
1,4-Butanediol dimethanesulfonate (Myleran)	1-(2-Chloroethyl)-3-cyclohexyl-1-nitrosourea (CCNU)
Chlorambucil	Cisplatin
1-(2-Chloroethyl)-3-(4-methylcyclohexyl)-1-nitrosourea (methyl-CCNU)	Creosotes
Chromium (hexavalent) compounds‡	Dibenz[a,h]anthracene
Cyclophosphamide	Diethyl sulfate
Diethylstilbestrol	Dimethylcarbamoyl chloride
Erionite	Dimethyl sulfate
Melphalan	Epichlorohydrin
8-Methoxypsoralen (methoxsalen) plus ultraviolet radiation	Ethylene dibromide
2-Naphthylamine	Ethylene oxide
Nickel and nickel compounds‡	*N*-Ethyl-*N*-nitrosourea (ENU)
Sulfur mustard (mustard gas)	Formaldehyde
Treosulfan	5-Methoxypsoralen
Vinyl chloride	4,4′-Methylene *bis*(2-chloroaniline)
	N-Methyl-*N*-nitro-*N*-nitrosoguanidine (MNNG)
	N-Methyl-*N*-nitrosourea (MNU)
	Nitrogen mustard
	N-Nitrosodiethylamine
	N-Nitrosodimethylamine
	Phenacetin
	Polychlorinated biphenyls
	Procarbazine hydrochloride
	Propylene oxide
	Silica (crystalline)
	Styrene oxide
	Tris(1-aziridinyl)phosphine sulfide (thiotepa)
	Tris(2,3-dibromopropyl) phosphate
	Vinyl bromide

*Sufficient evidence of carcinogenicity in humans.

In addition to the defined chemicals concluded to be carcinogenic in humans, various mixtures are classified as carcinogenic: analgesic mixtures containing phenacetin (although phenacetin is classified as probably carcinogenic), betel quid with tobacco, coal tars and coal tar pitches, combined therapy with a number of antitumor compounds, estrogens (as replacement therapy, or nonsteroidal or steroidal), oral contraceptives (combined or sequential), mineral oils (untreated and mildly treated), shale oils, soots, talc containing asbestiform fibers, and tobacco smoke and smokeless tobacco products. Also, a number of occupations or processes containing mixtures of substances have been concluded to be carcinogenic. These activities and occupations include aluminum production, auramine manufacture, coal gasification, coke production, furniture and cabinet making, underground hematite mining with exposure to radon, iron and steel founding, isopropyl alcohol manufacture (by the strong acid process), magenta manufacture, the rubber industry, and shoe and boot manufacture and repair.

†Generally, limited evidence of carcinogenicity in humans and sufficient evidence in experimental animals.

An additional 159 entities have been classified as possibly carcinogenic in humans.

‡Evaluation of the group but not necessarily to all compounds within the group.

(Adapted from the International Agency for Research on Cancer: IARC Monographs on the Evaluation of the Carcinogenic Risk of Chemicals to Humans, Suppl 7. IARC, World Health Organization, Lyon, 1987.)

cluded; or (c) "indequate evidence" because of few pertinent data, the available data were positive but did not exclude chance, or available studies do not show evidence of carcinogenicity.[3]

Four categories are used to evaluate the studies in *experimental animals*: (a) "sufficient evidence," which indicates that there is an increased incidence of malignant tumors in multiple species or strains, in multiple experiments with various routes or dosage levels (especially with dose-response effects), or to an unusual degree in incidence, site, or type of tumor, or age at onset; (b) "limited evidence," when the data suggest a carcinogenic effect but are limited because of a single experiment; the use of a single species or strain; an inadequate dosage, duration, or number of animals; or the neoplasms produced often occur spontaneously and are difficult to classify as malignant during the histopathology; (c) "inadequate evidence," when the studies cannot be interpreted as showing either the presence or absence of a carcinogenic effect or that the chemical is not carcinogenic within the limits of the tests used; and (d) "no data" available to the review group.[3]

The demonstration of a positive carcinogenic effect by a chemical in rodents indicates that it has the *potential* for carcinogenesis in humans. To satisfy statistical considerations, the experimental studies in animals are conducted at high dosages that exceed the levels of reasonably expected exposures to humans. The high dosages used in experimental studies with rodents may not reflect the corresponding risk to humans exposed to lower levels. The higher dosages may exceed certain protective cellular systems (e.g., concentrations of intracellular glutathione or DNA repair systems), or alter the predominant metabolic pathways (e.g., cytochrome P-450–dependent mixed-function oxidase or epoxide hydrolase) when one metabolic system is saturated and a second may produce more toxic or more carcinogenic metabolites. The *risk assessment* to humans must include the level of exposure, the differences that may exist in the toxicokinetics at high versus low levels of exposure, and possible differences in metabolism or kinetics in rodents versus humans.

In spite of the difficulties encountered, the chemicals that have been demonstrated to cause cancer in humans also produce cancer in animal models and, conversely, the chemicals that are carcinogenic in rodent studies are potential carcinogenic hazards to humans.[10] "Although test animals may respond differently from humans, experience has shown that most known human carcinogens also cause cancer in experimental animals if adequately tested."[25] Vinyl chloride and *bis*(chloromethyl)ether were shown to be carcinogenic in animals before subsequent identification of cancer causation in humans.[10]

References

1. Thomas DB: Cancer epidemiology and prevention. *In* Moossa AR, Robson MC, Schimpff SC (eds): Comprehensive Textbook of Oncology. Baltimore, Williams and Wilkins, 1986, p 3.
2. Searle CE: Preface. *In* Searle CE (ed): Chemical Carcinogens. Washington, DC, American Chemical Society, 1984, p xv.
3. International Agency for Research on Cancer: IARC Monographs on the Evaluation of the Carcinogenic Risk of Chemicals to Humans, Suppl. 7. IARC, World Health Organization, Lyon, 1987.
4. Greim H, Wolff T: Carcinogenicity of organic halogenated compounds. *In* Searle CE (ed): Chemical Carcinogens. Washington, DC, American Chemical Society, 1984, p 525.
5. Pitot HC, Grosso LE, Goldsworthy T: Genetics and epigenetics of neoplasia: Facts and theories. *In* Huberman E, Barr SH (eds): Carcinogenesis. Vol 10: The Role of Chemicals and Radiation in the Etiology of Cancer. New York, Raven Press, 1985, p 65.
6. Williams GM, Weisburger JH: Chemical carcinogens. *In* Klaassen CD, Amdur MO, Doull J (eds): Toxicology: The Basic Science of Poisons. New York, Macmillan, 1986, p 99.
7. Farber E: Possible etiologic mechanisms in chemical carcinogenesis. Environ Health Perspect *75*:65, 1987.
8. Ruddon RW: Cancer Biology. New York, Oxford University Press, 1987, p 530.
9. Slaga TJ: Overview of tumor promotion in animals. Environ Health Perspect *50*:3, 1983.
10. Williams GM, Reiss B, Weisburger JH: A comparison of the animal and human carcinogenicity of environmental, occupational and therapeutic chemicals. *In* Flamm WG, Lorentzen RJ (eds): Mechanism and Toxicity of Chemical Carcinogens and Mutagens. Princeton, NJ, Princeton Scientific Publishing, 1985, p 207.
11. Stowers SJ, Maronpot RR, Reynolds SH, Anderson MW: The role of oncogenes in chemical carcinogenesis. Environ Health Perspect *75*:81, 1987.
12. Reynolds SH, Stowers SJ, Patterson RM, Maronpot RR, Aaronson SA, Anderson MW: Activated oncogenes in B6C3F1 mouse liver tumors: Implications for risk assessment. Science *237*:1309, 1987.
13. Crawford BD: Perspectives on the somatic mutation model of carcinogenesis. *In* Flamm WG, Lorentzen RJ (eds): Mechanism and Toxicity of Chemical Carcinogens and Mutagens. Princeton, NJ, Princeton Scientific Publishing, 1985, p 13.
14. Lijinsky W: Structural relations and dose response

studies in nitrosamine carcinogenesis. *In* Mehlman MA (ed): Safety Evaluation: Toxicology, Methods, Concepts and Risk Assessment. Princeton, NJ, Princeton Scientific Publishing, 1987, p 215.

15. Preussmann R, Eisenbrand G: *N*-Nitroso carcinogens in the environment. *In* Searle CE (ed): Chemical Carcinogens. Washington, DC, American Chemical Society, 1984, p 829.
16. Grasso P: Carcinogens in food. *In* Searle CE (ed): Chemical Carcinogens. Washington, DC, American Chemical Society, 1984, p 1205.
17. Weisburger EK: Carcinogenic natural products in the environment. *In* Mehlman MA (ed): Safety Evaluation: Toxicology, Methods, Concepts and Risk Assessment. Princeton, NJ, Princeton Scientific Publishing, 1987, p 243.
18. Preussmann R, Stewart BW: *N*-Nitroso carcinogens. *In* Searle CE (ed): Chemical Carcinogens. Washington, DC, American Chemical Society, 1984, p 643.
19. National Academy of Sciences, Assembly of Life Sciences, Committee on Diet, Nutrition, and Cancer: Diet, Nutrition, and Cancer. Washington, DC, National Academy of Sciences, 1982, p 234.
20. Ohshima H, Bartsch H: A new approach to quantitate endogenous nitrosation in humans. *In* Stich HF (ed): Carcinogens and Mutagens in the Environment. Vol 2: Naturally Occurring Compounds: Endogenous Formation and Modulation. Boca Raton, FL, CRC Press, 1983, p 3.
21. Fraser P: Nitrates: Epidemiological evidence. *In* Wald NJ, Doll R (eds): Intrepretation of Negative Epidemiological Evidence for Carcinogenicity. IARC Scientific Publication No. 65. Lyon, International Agency for Research on Cancer, 1985, p 183.
22. Armstrong BK: Nitrates: Conclusion. *In* Wald NJ, Doll R (eds): Intrepretation of Negative Epidemiological Evidence for Carcinogenicity. IARC Scientific Publication No. 65. Lyon, International Agency for Research on Cancer, 1985, p 195.
23. Busby WF Jr, Wogan GN: Aflatoxins. *In* Searle CE (ed): Chemical Carcinogens. Washington, DC, American Chemical Society, 1984, p 946.
24. Stoloff L: Mycotoxins as potential environment carcinogens. *In* Stich HF (ed): Carcinogens and Mutagens in the Environment. Vol 1: Food Products. Boca Raton, FL, CRC Press, 1982, p 97.
25. US Department of Health and Human Services, Public Health Service: Fourth Annual Report on Carcinogens, Summary 1985, NTP 85-002.
26. Bridbord K, Finklea JF, Wagoner JK, Moran JB, Caplan P: Human exposure to polynuclear aromatic hydrocarbons. *In* Freudenthal RI, Jones PW (eds): Carcinogenesis. Vol 1: Polynuclear Aromatic Hydrocarbons: Chemistry, Metabolism, and Carcinogenesis. New York, Raven Press, 1976, p 319.
27. Hoffmann D, Wynder EL, Hecht SS, Brunnemann KD, LaVoie EJ, Haley NJ: Chemical carcinogens in tobacco. *In* Bannasch P (ed): Cancer Risks: Strategies for Elimination. Berlin, Springer-Verlag, 1987, p 101.
28. Radford EP: Potential health effects of indoor radon exposure. Environ Health Perspect *62*:281, 1985.
29. Esmen NA: The status of indoor air pollution. Environ Health Perspect *62*:259, 1985.
30. Ames BN, Magaw R, Gold LS: Ranking possible carcinogenic hazards. Science *236*:271, 1987.
31. Andrews RNL, Turner AG: Controlling toxic chemicals in the environment. *In* Lave LB, Upton AC (eds): Toxic Chemicals, Health, and the Environment. Baltimore, Johns Hopkins University Press, 1987, p 5.
32. Jacobi W: Cancer risk from environmental radioactivity. *In* Bannasch P (ed): Cancer Risks: Strategies for Elimination. Berlin, Springer-Verlag, 1987, p 154.
33. Haseman JK, Huff JE, Zeiger E, McConnell EE: Comparative results of 327 chemical carcinogenicity studies. Environ Health Perspect *74*:229, 1987.

33a. Fishbein L: Critical elements in priority selections and ranking systems for risk assessments of chemicals. *In* Mehlman MA (ed): Safety Evaluation: Toxicology, Methods, Concepts and Risk Assessment. Princeton, NJ, Princeton Scientific Publishing, 1987, p 1.

34. National Library of Medicine, Hazardous Substance Data Bank. Bethesda, MD.

Recommended Readings

Bannasch P (ed): Cancer Risks: Strategies for Elimination. Berlin, Springer-Verlag, 1987, p 199.

Flamm WG, Lorentzen RJ (eds): Mechanism and Toxicity of Chemical Carcinogens and Mutagens. Princeton, NJ, Princeton Scientific Publishing, 1985.

Iversen OH (ed): Theories of Carcinogenesis. Cambridge, Hemisphere Publishing, 1988, p 327.

Mehlman MA (ed): Safety Evaluation: Toxicology, Methods, Concepts and Risk Assessment. Princeton, NJ, Princeton Scientific Publishing, 1987.

Ruddon RW: Cancer Biology. New York, Oxford University Press, 1987, p 530.

Searle CE (ed): Chemical Carcinogens. Vols 1 and 2. Washington, DC, American Chemical Society, 1984, p 1373.

Williams GM, Weisburger JH: Chemical carcinogens. *In* Klaassen CD, Amdur MO, Doull J (eds): Toxicology: The Basic Science of Poisons. New York, Macmillan, 1986, p 99.

C. Hormonal, Growth, and Other Effects

Alice Stark, Dr.P.H.

Human physiologic processes occur in an environment contaminated by a diverse group of xenobiotics reflecting the chemical environment in which we live. Commercial production of chemicals results in environmental distribution of the original compound or of its byproducts. Despite this, few of the approximately 3000 new compounds introduced each year have been screened for most potential health effects. Usually, adverse effects attributable to commercial chemicals have been detected only after extensive human exposure, usually in the work place where concentrations are high.

Exposure to chemical pollutants can result in alteration of complex biologic systems. These alterations may result because the pollutant mimics the action of a naturally occurring substance such as a hormone, injures a tissue or organ, or changes the balance between components or activity of elements of a system. This section examines effects on the endocrine system of widely distributed xenobiotics. Unfortunately, compounds that have been extensively studied for their effects on humans are limited in number. By pointing out what is known, it is hoped that the clinician will gain increased awareness of the potential effects of chemical exposures.

TOXIC INSULT

The endocrine system is highly susceptible to toxic insult. The toxicity can be manifested on the endocrine organs directly by altering their natural secretions, or through toxic agents acting on endocrine-responsive target tissues, producing a varied physiologic response. Understanding the mechanisms producing these effects can be complicated. Often hormonal homeostasis is maintained by multiple substances, all of which act on a specific organ to regulate its function. For example, the mammary gland will grow and differentiate under the influence of steroid hormones, but it also requires stimulation from polypeptide hormones to become a lactogenic organ. Chemicals that inhibit or decrease lactation may induce this effect indirectly by inhibiting prolactin secretion from the pituitary.

Alteration of Natural Secretions. The first major mechanism by which xenobiotics may influence the endocrine system is by alteration of natural secretions. Good examples illustrating the multiplicity of sites of toxicity are found in studies of infertility. Some chemicals have been shown to have toxicologic actions on the gonads and germ cells directly, but the toxic insult is actually mediated at other sites such as neuroendocrine centers influencing gonadotropic hormone levels. With other chemicals, toxicologic actions are on one biologic process of a gland, such as the gonad (e.g., steroidogenesis), with little effect on another (e.g., oogenesis). Although alteration of either of these processes can result in infertility, completely different mechanisms are involved.

Mimicry of Natural Hormones. The other major mechanism by which xenobiotics may influence the endocrine system is through biologic activities similar to those of natural hormones. Therefore, toxicologic effects may not be due to the adverse action of the chemical on an endocrine organ itself but rather to the chemical exerting a hormonal stimulation on a target tissue that results in a lesion. Many such effects have been seen with chemicals possessing estrogenic activity, which influence the liver, immune system, and reproductive tract. Such activities result in a hormonal imbalance that can produce a variety of endocrine disorders at different target sites.

Effects of Toxic Agents on the Ovary

The purpose of cyclic ovarian function is to provide viable oocytes for fertilization by sperm ascending through the female genital tract. Destruction of oocytes by toxins is of paramount importance, but even without loss of oocytes, subtle functional alterations in ovarian physiology can have a profound influence on reproductive efficiency. It is estimated that in approximately 40 per cent of couples with infertility, ovulatory problems are etiologic.[1] Currently, only a limited number of instances of ovulatory problems induced by known toxicants have been recognized, emphasizing the need for much more work in this area.

Few reliable data exist regarding infertility or adverse reproductive outcomes in the general population. Data are even more scanty respecting geographic or occupational distributions.[2] Among the many reasons for this are (a) the widespread use of contraception, (b) the high rate of elective abortion prior to determination of the reproductive outcome or in some cases even before clear-cut documentation of pregnancy, (c) the mobility of the United States population, and (d) the lack of an appropriate reporting system for adequate epidemiologic surveillance. As a consequence, no widely accepted "normal" or expected rates of ovulatory failure, infertility, ectopic pregnancy, and spontaneous abortion are available.

Given this medical and cultural environment, our ability to understand the effects of xenobiotics on reproduction is limited. When an effect is unique, such as the phocomelia induced by thalidomide,[3] there will be a high rate of detection. Similarly, if the frequency of the clinical problem is dramatically higher than the background rate, detection is probable. For example, farm workers exposed to dibromochloropropane (DBCP), a soil fumigant that directly inhibits spermatogenesis,[4] experienced a substantial and apparent decline in the ability to father children. It is unlikely that similar effects, if markedly less profound or striking, would be discerned through epidemiologic surveillance alone.

Ovarian toxicity can occur either as a direct action of the toxicant or indirectly if the agent requires metabolic activation to exert its effect. Direct-acting toxicants include compounds that mimic the structure of naturally occurring hormones, i.e., estrogens, or that injure cells because of general chemical reactivity, i.e., alkylating agents. Indirect-acting toxicants exert their effects usually by metabolic activation of a nontoxic compound to an active metabolite. Ovaries possess the enzymes necessary for processing many toxic chemicals,[5–7] making this mechanism possible.

Environmental and Occupational Ovarian Toxicants

Marijuana. The major psychoactive component of marijuana, Δ-9-tetrahydrocannabinol (THC) may interfere with reproduction by several mechanisms. There is evidence that secretion of gonadotropins in primates is inhibited by THC at the hypothalamic level.[8–10] Depression of gonadotropic hormone release occurs for a substantial interval of time after THC exposure and is dose-related. Administration of THC during the luteal phase of normal ovulatory cycles in monkeys did not affect progesterone production or luteal length, but altered the subsequent menstrual cycle.[8]

Alcohol. The use of alcohol in our culture is widespread, and there has been great interest in the effects of alcohol drinking on reproduction. Excessive use of alcohol during pregnancy can injure the fetus irreparably, producing the fetal alcohol syndrome.[11] Other reproductive problems have been less convincingly demonstrated. Menstrual disorders,[12, 13] frequent abortion,[14] and infertility[14, 15] have been observed without more specific mechanistic studies. Since a direct action of alcohol on the gonad can produce sterility in animals[16] and studies of female alcoholics demonstrate higher rates of infertility, more work is needed to determine the effects of alcohol, particularly at levels consistent with social consumption.

Polycyclic Aromatic Hydrocarbons. Polycyclic aromatic hydrocarbons represent a major environmental contaminant, originating from fossil fuel combustion, petroleum product synthesis, and cigarette smoking. A reasonable database is available to address the issue of reproduction only with cigarette smoking. Increased rates of infertility have been observed in smokers,[17–20] but the mechanism is unclear. Data from one study[21] suggest a toxic effect of cigarette smoking on the ovary, resulting in an earlier age at menopause. In rats, nicotine delays the rise in serum progesterone coincident with early pregnancy by approximately 12 hours, consistent with a direct effect on the gonad.[22] This may be analogous to the situation in men in whom smoking depresses not only serum testosterone levels[23] but sperm counts as well.[24] It is not known whether this is related to direct action on the testes, or is mediated through the hypothalamic-pituitary axis. With over 3000 identifiable compounds in cigarette smoke, the specific agent(s) responsible is not known.

Halogenated Polycyclic Hydrocarbons. Halogenated polycyclic hydrocarbons are widely used in agriculture and the agricultural industry. These compounds are of particular concern because they persist in the environment for extended periods of time and bio-accumulate as they move up the food chain. They are highly soluble in fats. The potential human hazard is illustrated by an episode of rice oil contamination in Japan that resulted in menstrual cycle abnormalities; however, no specific endocrinologic data are available.[25]

The prototype compound in the halogenated polycyclic hydrocarbon class is DDT. A large body of evidence suggests that DDT and many of its metabolites display estrogenic properties.[26–31] DDT is believed to act as an estrogen in a classic estrogen receptor–mediated fashion. Methoxychlor, a chemically related pesticide, also has estrogenic properties[31–34] but acts indirectly, requiring *O*-methylation to an estrogenic metabolite.[35, 36] Kepone (chlordecone) is a chlorinated polycyclic ketone that also has an estrogen-like action.[37, 38] The Kepone analogue Mirex was initially felt not to be uterotropic, but subsequent studies have demonstrated a degradation to Kepone and estrogen-like action.[39]

All the polycyclic hydrocarbons are relatively weak estrogens, but with significant exposure an estrogenic response can potentially be elicited, analogous to the effect of oral contraceptives. An infertility effect of DDT and its estrogenic derivatives has been difficult to demonstrate. However, based on the frequency of ovulatory dysfunction and season of birth,[40] it has been proposed that disorders of ovulation are related to the seasonal use of pesticides.

Effects of Toxic Agents on the Testes

Testicular function can be divided into two major components, spermatogenesis and steroidogenesis. These two functions are anatomically segregated, with spermatogenesis occurring in the seminiferous tubules and androgen biosynthesis taking place in the Leydig cells. The anterior pituitary acts in the regulation of both these functions through secretion of the gonadotropins, luteinizing hormone (LH), and follicle-stimulating-hormone (FSH). The LH acts in the control of androgen production, and FSH influences spermatogenesis.

Chemicals can affect spermatogenesis either during sperm production in the seminiferous tubules or during sperm maturation in the epididymis. Transport time through the epididymis is short (1 to 2 weeks), and damage to resident sperm would most likely result in short-term effects. Damage to the stem cells of the seminiferous tubules is more likely to be the basis of long-term effects on spermatogenesis. The potential for effect is related to the ability of the substance to enter the milieu of the seminiferous tubules or the epididymis.

The complex interactions of testicular and anterior pituitary hormones and their respective target cells produce several pathways through which chemical exposure could affect gonadal function. By determining blood levels of pituitary and testicular hormones, insight can be gained into possible damage to the testes.

The effects of a toxin on male reproduction can be manifested in several ways. These include symptoms like impotence or reduced libido, reduced fertility, alterations in sperm, changes in hormonal production, and adverse reproductive outcomes, such as spontaneous abortions or birth defects. In many instances the pathways leading from chemical exposure to these manifestations are unknown.

Occupational and environmental chemicals shown to have an effect on male reproductive function are limited in number. There are even fewer in cases of specific changes in testicular function or spermatogenesis. Table 26–4 shows the substances for which toxic effects on male reproduction have been found.[41]

Dibromochloropropane. Commercially produced since 1956, DBCP is a highly persistent, lipophilic, brominated organochlorine that has been used as a fumigant against nematodes for a wide variety of plants. In California, DBCP was used mainly on grapes, peaches, citrus fruits, and tomatoes; in the Carolinas it was used on peaches and soybeans; in Central America and Israel on bananas; and in Hawaii on pineapples. Its use in the United States has been suspended with the exception of use on pineapple fields in Hawaii.[42]

DBCP is a potent reproductive toxin presumably by a direct effect on the spermatogonia and on the seminiferous tubules. Sperm analysis of patients presenting clinically with infertility reveals a consistent pattern of azoospermia or oligospermia with a dose-response relationship to duration and degree of exposure. Following cessation of exposure there is some tendency for a resumption of normal spermatogenesis, particularly in cases of oligospermia.[43] The hormonal patterns in individuals with DBCP exposure and reduced sperm production are characterized by elevated levels of FSH, representative of tubular damage and of reduction in spermatogonia. The testicular biopsies performed show a deficit of spermatogenic cells.

Chlordecone (Kepone). This is a highly stable, chlorinated hydrocarbon pesticide introduced in 1958 as an insecticide and fungicide. Its manufacture and use were terminated in the United States in 1977 because of its acute toxicity.

Table 26–4. OCCUPATIONAL AND ENVIRONMENTAL CHEMICALS ASSOCIATED WITH ADVERSE EFFECTS ON MALE REPRODUCTIVE FUNCTION[41]

	METHOD OF EXAMINATION OF REPRODUCTIVE FUNCTION			
	Reproductive History	*Sperm Analysis*	*Hormonal Evaluation*	*Testicular Histology*
DBCP	+	+	+	+
Chlordecone (Kepone)	+	+		+
Lead	+	+	+ −	+
Carbon disulfide (CS)	+	+ −	+	

Male workers with high levels of exposure to Kepone frequently had abnormalities in sperm count, morphology, and motility. There is also evidence for histologic alterations of spermatogenesis.[44] It is believed that Kepone exerts a direct effect on testes and that the majority of patients recover.[45]

Lead. There is historical evidence that lead may decrease the fertility of exposed male workers and may affect the reproductive performance of their wives.[46] Both a reduction in the number of offspring in families of workers occupationally exposed to lead and an increase in the miscarriage rate among women whose husbands were exposed was shown.[47] Exposure resulting in blood lead levels over 50 μg per dl frequently results in disorders of sexual dynamics and decreased libido. There appears to be a direct effect on the seminiferous tubules and on spermatogenesis, producing depressed sperm counts. It is unclear whether or not there is an effect on gonadotropin or androgen production.

Carbon Disulfide (CS). This substance is used primarily in the production of viscose rayon; exposure to CS occurs not only in the preparation process but also during the spinning and washing of the viscose. CS exposure at high levels is toxic to the male reproductive system. Semen analysis indicated hypospermia, asthenospermia, and teratospermia indicating effects on the testes. Also, lowered levels of FSH and LH indicate that the pituitary/hypothalamus also may be involved.[48]

Effects of Toxic Agents on the Adrenal

As the sole site of production of glucocorticords and mineralocorticords, the adrenal cortex has far-reaching and important effects on intermediary metabolism and electrolyte balance in the body. Glucocorticords such as cortisol play a major role in the regulation of carbohydrate, protein, and lipid metabolism and also modulate the actions of other hormones on these same processes. Major sites of action of cortisol include the liver, muscles, and adipose tissue. Aldosterone, the most potent mineralocorticoid produced by the adrenal cortex, participates in the regulation of renal sodium and potassium reabsorption and excretion. The adrenal cortex also produces various androgenic and estrogenic steroids, but they are of lesser biologic importance under normal circumstances.

The adrenal cortex is very vulnerable to chemical-induced injury.[49] Although many chemicals have been shown to affect adrenocortical function adversely, for most the mechanisms involved have not been determined. The lipophilic nature of the adrenal cortex probably contributes to its vulnerability by promoting the deposition and accumulation of various hydrophobic compounds, including potentially toxic agents. Once present in the adrenal cortex, chemical toxins may exert direct effects on the gland or be metabolized by adrenal enzymes, resulting in detoxification or activation.

Among the foreign compounds metabolized by adrenal mono-oxygenases are the carcinogens benzo(a)pyrene and 7,12-dimethylbenz(a)anthracene (DMBA).[50] The latter causes adrenal necrosis, but the relationship between DMBA metabolism and the necrosis has yet to be fully resolved. However, adrenal activation of several other chemicals that results in local toxicity has been definitely established. For example, adrenal metabolism of the mineralocorticoid antagonist spironolactone,[51] or of the insecticide analogue 1-(*O*-chlorophenyl)-1-(*p*-chlorophenyl)-2,2-dichloroethane (*O*, *p*-DDD),[52] results in the formation of reactive metabolites and inhibition of steroidogenesis. For compounds such as carbon tetrachloride and chloroform, local activation is probably also involved in the adrenal necrosis produced by each.[53] The role of local metabolism in the actions of most other adrenal toxins has not been determined.[54]

Effects of Toxic Agents on the Thyroid

The thyroid gland plays a critical role in growth, development, and normal body metabolism. The thyroid gland has been shown to be a target of insult by many physical and chemical environmental factors. These factors include ionizing radiation,[55, 56] temperature,[57] and chemical agents.[58]

Follicular Cells. The follicular cells that secrete the iodothyronines are responsible for maintaining the basal metabolic rate in tissues essential for their normal function.

Agents that alter the release of thyroid-stimulating hormone (TSH) by the anterior pituitary, or thyrotropin-releasing hormone (TRH) by the hypothalamus, could significantly affect follicular cell function. It has been shown[59] that methylparathion exerts an anticholinesterase effect at the hypothalamic-pituitary axis; therefore, TRH release could be affected by exposure. It has been suggested[57] that cold stimulates release of TRH whereas warmth and trauma inhibit release of TRH from the hypothalamus.

Iodide uptake has been shown to be influenced by a number of xenobiotics. Inorganic ions such as thiocyanate and perchlorate,[60] and several dithiocarbamate fungicides—nabam, zineb, and ziram—that break down to ethylene thiourea, all inhibit iodide uptake. DDT behaves similarly.[61] However, the herbicide 2,4-D enhanced iodide uptake.[62]

Parafollicular or C Cells. The functions of the C cell are the synthesis, storage, and release of calcitonin in response to an appropriate physiologic stimulus. There is not a significant amount of evidence that xenobiotics affect the storage or release of calcitonin.

CLINICAL IMPLICATIONS

This discussion is not meant to be an exhaustive review of the effects of xenobiotics on the endocrine glands. It is meant to illustrate the wide range of chemicals that can affect the endocrine glands through a variety of mechanisms. These mechanisms include direct destruction of cells, mimicry of endocrine secretions, and alteration of balance between elements of the system.

When endocrine dysfunction is identified, the clinician needs to be aware that xenobiotics may be partially or in some case solely responsible for that dysfunction.

Few definitive tests are available to identify chemical contaminants in bodily fluids. What is more, population standards for exogenous chemicals in humans are even more scanty. Consequently, the patient's history is the most important tool for identifying a possible toxic insult. In addition to a medical and familial history, the history should include a thorough exploration of the person's occupational history, hobbies (e.g., stained-glass making, gardening), neighborhood/residential exposures (e.g., cleaners, pesticides, furnishings), use of medications, health foods, and other lifestyle factors (e.g., smoking, alcohol and drug use). It may be necessary to examine the activities of other household members as well. Generally, removal from exposure is the most important and efficacious form of treatment, although specific therapeutic measures may be available in some instances. Specialized references should be consulted once the toxic agent has been identified.

References

1. Speroff L, Glass RH, Kase NG: Investigation of the infertile couple. *In* Speroff L, et al (eds): Clinical Gynecologic Endocrinology and Infertility. 3rd ed. Baltimore, Williams and Wilkins, 1983, pp 467–492.
2. Wilcox AJ: Surveillance of pregnancy loss in human populations. Am J Ind Med *4*:285–291, 1983.
3. Shepard TH: Catalog of Teratogenic Agents. 2nd ed. Baltimore, Johns Hopkins University Press, 1976.
4. Whorton D, Krauss RM, Marshall S, Milby TH: Infertility in male pesticide workers. Lancet *2*:1259–1261, 1977.
5. Heinrichs WL, Juchau MR: Extrahepatic drug metabolism: The gonads. *In* Gram TE (ed): Extrahepatic Metabolism of Drugs and Other Foreign Compounds. New York, SP Medical and Scientific Books, 1980, pp 313–332.
6. Mattison DR, Shorgeirsson SS: Gonadal aryl hydrocarbon hydroxylene in rats and mice. Cancer Res *38*:1368–1373, 1978.
7. Sims P, Grover PL: Epoxides in polycyclic aromatic hydrocarbon metabolism and carcinogenesis. Adv Cancer Res *20*:165–274, 1974.
8. Asch RH, Smith CG, Silver-Khodr TM, Pauerstein CJ: Effects of 9-tetrahydrocannabinol administration on gonadal steroidogenesis activity *in vivo*. Fertil Steril *32*:576–582, 1979.
9. Smith CG, Besch NF, Asch RH: Effects of marijuana on the reproductive system. *In* Thomas JA, Singhal

R (eds): Advances in Sex Hormone Research. Baltimore, Urban and Schwarzenberg, 1980, pp 273–294.
10. Smith CG, Besch NF, Smith RG, Besch PK: Effect of tetrahydrocannabimol on the hypothalamic pituitary axis in the ovariectomized rhesus monkey. Fertil Steril *31*:335–339, 1979.
11. Ulleland CN: The offspring of alcoholic mothers. Ann NY Acad Sci *197*:167–169, 1972.
12. Belfer M, Shader RI, Carroll M, Harnatz JS: Alcoholism in women. Arch Gen Psychiatr *25*:540–544, 1971.
13. Podolsky E: The alcoholic woman and premenstrual tension. J Am Med Womens Assoc *18*:816–818, 1963.
14. Wilsnack SC: Sex role identity in female alcoholism. J Abnorm Psychol *82*:253–261, 1973.
15. Kinsey BA: Psychological factors in alcoholic women from a state hospital sample. Am J Psychiatr *124*:1463–1466, 1968.
16. Van Shiel DH, Gavoler JS, Lester R: Alcohol-induced ovarian failure in the rat. J Clin Invest *61*:624–632, 1978.
17. Hammond EC: Smoking in relation to physical complaints. Arch Environ Health *3*:146–164, 1961.
18. Pettersson F, Fries H, Millus SJ: Epidemiology of secondary amenorrhea. I. Incidence and prevalence rates. Am J Obstet Gynecol *117*:80–86, 1973.
19. Tokuhata G: Smoking in relation to infertility and fetal loss. Arch Environ Health *17*:353–359, 1968.
20. Vessey MP, Wright NH, McPherson K, Wiggens P: Fertility after stopping different methods of contraception. Br Med J *1*:265–267, 1978.
21. Jick H, Porter J, Morrison SA: Relation between smoking and age of natural menopause. Lancet *1*:1354–1355, 1971.
22. Yoshinaga K, Rice C, Krenn J, Pilot RL: Effects of nicotine on early pregnancy in the rat. Biol Reprod *20*:294–331, 1979.
23. Briggs WJ: Cigarette smoking and infertility in men. Med J Aust *1*:616–617, 1973.
24. Campbell JM, Harrison KL: Smoking and infertility. Med J Aust *1*:342–343, 1979.
25. Kimbrough RD: The toxicity of polychlorinated polycylic compounds and related chemicals. Crit Rev Toxicol *2*:445–498, 1974.
26. Bitman J, Cecil HC, Harris SJ, Fries GF: Estrogenic activity of *O,p'*-DDT in mammalian uterus and avian oviduct. Science *162*:371–372, 1968.
27. Burlington H, Lindeman VF: Effect of DDT on testes and secondary sex characteristics of white leghorn cockerels. Proc Soc Exp Biol Med *74*:48–51, 1950.
28. Gellert RJ, Heinricks WL, Severdloff RS: DDT homologues: Estrogen-like effects on the vagina, uterus and pituitary of the rat. Endocrinology *91*:1095–1100, 1972.
29. Heinricks WL, Gellert RJ: DDT administered to neonatal rats induces persistent estrus syndrome. Science *173*:642–643, 1971.
30. Levin W, Welch RM, Conney AH: Estrogenic action of DDT and its analogs. Fed Proc *27*:649, 1968.
31. Welch RM, Levin W, Conney AH: Estrogenic action of DDT and its analogs. Toxicol Appl Pharmacol *14*:358–367, 1969.
32. Bitman J, Cecil HC: Estrogenic activity of DDT analogs and polychlorinated biphenyls. J Agric Food Chem *18*:1108–1112, 1970.
33. Bulger WH, Muccitelli RM, Kupber D: Interactions of methoxychlor, methoxychlor base-soluble contaminant and 2,2-bis (*p*-hydroxyphenyl)-1,1,1-trichloroethane with rat uterine estrogen receptor. J Toxicol Environ Health *4*:881–893, 1978.
34. Nelson JA: Effects of dichlorodiphenyltrichloroethane (DDT) analogs and polychlorinated biphenyl (PCB) mixtures on 17β-[^{3}H]estradiol binding to rat uterine receptor. Biochem Pharmacol *23*:447–451, 1974.
35. Bulger WH, Muccitelli RM, Kupfer D: Studies on the *in vivo* and *in vitro* estrogenic activities of methoxychlor and its metabolites; Role of hepatic monooxygenase in methoxychlor activation. Biochem Pharmacol *27*:2417–2423, 1978.
36. Kapoor IP, Metcalf RL, Nystrom RF, Sangha GK: Comparative metabolism of methoxychlor, methiochlor and DDT in mouse, insects and in a model ecosystem. J Agric Food Chem *18*:1145–1152, 1970.
37. Bulger WH, Muccitelli RM, Kupfer D: Studies on the estrogenic activity of chlordecone (Kepone) in the rat: Effects on uterine estrogen receptor. Molec Pharmacol *15*:515–524, 1979.
38. Huber JJ: Some physiological effects of the insecticide Kepone in the laboratory mouse. Toxicol Appl Pharmacol *7*:516–524, 1965.
39. Carlson DA, Konyha KD, Wheeler WB, Marshall GP, Zaylskie RG: Mirex in the environment: Its degradation to Kepone and related compounds. Science *194*:939–941, 1976.
40. Bourne JP: A zodiac study of infertility: Is person of birth associated with dysfunctions in ovulation? Baltimore, Department of Maternal and Child Health, The Johns Hopkins University School of Hygiene and Public Health, 1974.
41. Sever LE, Hessol NA: Toxic effects of occupational and environmental chemicals on the testes. *In* Thomas JA, Korach KS, McLachlan JA: Endocrine Toxicology. New York, Raven Press, 1985.
42. Babich H, Davis DL, Stotsky G: Dibromochloropropane (DBCP): A review. Sci Total Environ *17*:207–221, 1981.
43. Whorton MD, Milby TH: Recovery of testicular function among DBCP workers. J Occup Med *22*:177–179, 1980.
44. Taylor JR, Selhorst JB, Houff SA, Marting AJ: Chlordecone intoxication in man. I. Clinical observations. Neurology *28*:626–630, 1978.
45. Barlow SM, Sullivan FM: *Reproductive Hazards of Industrial Chemicals.* New York, Academic Press, 1982.
46. Rom WH: Effects of lead on reproduction. *In* Infante PF, Legator MS (eds): Proceedings of a Workshop on Methodology for Assessing Reproductive Hazards in the Workplace. Cincinnati, NIOSH, 1980, pp 33–43.
47. Lancranjan I, Popescu HI, Gavanescu O, Klepsch I, Serbanesca M: Reproductive ability of workmen occupationally exposed to lead. Arch Environ Health *30*:396–401, 1975.
48. Lancranjan I: Alterations of spermatic fluid in patients chronically poisoned by carbon disulfide. Med Lav *63*:29–33, 1972.
49. Ribelin WE: Effects of drugs and chemicals upon the structure of the adrenal gland. Fund Appl Toxicol *4*:105, 1984.
50. Sims P: Studies on the metabolism of 7-methylbenz(a)anthracene and 7,12-dimethylbenz(a)anthracene and its hydroxymethyl derivatives in rat liver and adrenal homogenates. Biochem Pharmacol *19*:2761, 1970.
51. Kon H, Gillette JR: Studies on the destruction of adrenal and testicular cytochrome P-450 by spironolactone. J Biol Chem *254*:1726, 1979.

52. Martz F, Straw JA: Metabolism and covalent binding of op-DDD: Correlation between adrenocorticalytic activity and metabolic activation by adrenocortical mitochondria. Drug Metab Dispos *8*:127, 1980.
53. Colby HD, Brogan WC, Miles PR: Carbon tetrachloride–induced changes in adrenal microsomal mixed function oxidase and lipid peroxidation. Toxicol Appl Pharmacol *60*:492, 1981.
54. Colby HD, Rumbaugh RC: Adrenal drug metabolism. *In* Gram TE (ed): Extrahepatic Metabolism of Drugs and Other Foreign Compounds. Jamaica, NY, Spectrum Publications, 1980, p 239.
55. Conrad RA, Dobyns BM, Sutow WW: Thyroid neoplasia as a late effect of exposure to radioactive iodine in fallout. JAMA *214*:316–324, 1970.
56. Hempelmann LH: Risk of thyroid neoplasms after irradiation in childhood. Science *160*:159–163, 1968.
57. Ganong WF: The thyroid gland. *In* Review of Medical Physiology. Los Altos, CA, Lange Medical Publications, 1965, pp 248–265.
58. Kingsbury JM: Phytotoxicity. *In* Casarett LJ, Doull J (eds): Toxicology: The Basic Sciences of Poisons. New York, Macmillan, 1975, pp 591–604.
59. Lybeck H, Leppaluoto J, Auto H: The influence of an anticholinesterene, methylparathion on the radioiodine uptake of the rat thyroid *in vivo* and *in vitro*. Ann Med Biol Fenn, 1067: *45*:76–79, 1966.
60. Netter FH: Endocrine system and selected metabolic diseases. *In* Forsham PH (ed): The CIBA Collection of Medical Illustrations. Vol 4. New York, RR Donnelley and Sons, 1974.
61. Graham SL, Hansen WH: Effects of short-term administration of ethylenethiourea upon the thyroid function of the rat. Bull Environ Contam Toxicol *7*:19–25, 1972.
62. Florsheim WH, Velcoff SM: Some effects of 2,4-dichlorophenoxyacetic acid on thyroid function in the rat: Effects on iodine accumulation. Endocrinology *71*:1–6, 1962.

D. Polychlorinated Dibenzo-*P*-Dioxins

Donald G. Patterson, Jr., Ph.D., Larry L. Needham, Ph.D., and John S. Andrews, Jr., M.D.

Worldwide public concern about the toxicity of polychlorinated dibenzo-*p*-dioxins (PCDDs) and polychlorinated dibenzofurans (PCDFs) has spurred extensive research in toxicology; new findings are reported yearly at scientific meetings, including one international meeting devoted entirely to the subject of PCDDs and PCDFs. One of these compounds, 2,3,7,8-tetrachlorodibenzo-*p*-dioxin (2,3,7,8-TCDD), has been called the most toxic compound synthesized by human beings. However, 2,3,7,8-TCDD is only one of 22 tetrachlorodibenzo-*p*-dioxins and only one of 75 chlorinated (mono-octa) dibenzo-*p*-dioxins; there are 135 PCDFs.

None of these chemicals are produced for commercial purposes, but chlorinated PCDDs and PCDFs are produced as trace contaminants in several chemical processes, primarily the synthesis of chlorinated phenols. For example, 2,3,7,8-TCDD is a byproduct in the synthesis of 2,4,5-trichlorophenol and an intermediate in the production of 2,4,5-trichlorophenoxyacetic acid and hexachlorophene. Trace levels of these compounds are also produced during the incineration of waste materials, combustion of leaded gasoline, and bleaching of wood pulp.

Thus, these compounds can enter the environment by a variety of means. Once there, they are remarkably stable. Many of these compounds, especially highly toxic ones that are substituted with chlorine at the 2,3,7, and 8 positions, bioaccumulate in the human food chain. These compounds generally can be found at the parts per trillion (ppt) levels in the lipid stores of humans, especially those living in an industrialized society. For example, 2,3,7,8-TCDD is normally found in the adipose tissue and serum of adults at levels below 20 ppt.[1] The half-life of 2,3,7,8-TCDD in humans has been estimated to be about 7 years.[2]

As mentioned, 2,3,7,8-TCDD has been shown to be very toxic, although its toxicity varies in the animal species tested. The hamster has been shown to be the least sensitive, with a median lethal dose (LD_{50}) in the low mg/kg range, and the guinea pig is the most sensitive, with a LD_{50} in the low μg/kg range. The most common symptoms of animals after lethal exposure are loss of body weight, "wasting away" syndrome, and thymic atrophy.[3] Researchers have shown that 2,3,7,8-TCDD is carcinogenic in rats and mice and that it causes teratogenic effects.[4, 5] Also, 2,3,7,8-TCDD has been shown to be a potent inducer of microsomal enzymes and to be acutely immunotoxic.[6] Using 2,3,7,8-TCDD as the reference, the toxicity of chlorinated dibenzo-*p*-dioxins and dibenzofurans decreases with a decreasing or an increasing number of chlorines. Congeners with chlorine substitution at the 2,3,7,8 positions are the most toxic.

Toxic effects of chlorinated dibenzo-*p*-dioxins and dibenzofurans in humans are not so apparent. To detect any such adverse effects, populations unduly exposed via unintentional releases or occupation have been examined. Several of these populations are described.

VIETNAM VETERANS

From 1962 to 1970, the herbicide Agent Orange [a 1:1 mixture of 2,4-dichlorophenoxyacetic acid (2,4-D) and 2,4,5-trichlorophenoxyacetic acid (2,4,5-T) in diesel oil] was used as a defoliant in Vietnam. The herbicide was contaminated with 2,3,7,8-TCDD to an extent ranging from less than 1 part per million (ppm) to greater than 20 ppm.[7, 8] 2,3,7,8-TCDD was formed as an unintentional byproduct during the manufacture of 2,4,5-T. Many Vietnam veterans have expressed concern that their health may have been adversely affected by exposure to Agent Orange and its 2,3,7,8-TCDD contaminant. In response to these concerns, the United States Congress in 1979 passed Public Law 96-151 (House Resolution 3892), mandating epidemiologic studies of possible health effects in Vietnam veterans due to exposure to herbicides.

New Jersey,[9] Massachusetts,[10] the Centers for Disease Control (CDC),[11–15] the United States Air Force,[2, 16, 17] and the Veterans Administration (VA)[18] have all conducted studies on Vietnam veterans. Gross and associates, in a VA-sponsored study, were the first to measure 2,3,7,8-TCDD levels in the adipose tissue of Vietnam veterans some 10 years after their exposure had ceased.[18] The results of this study showed that several veterans classified as "heavily exposed" had higher 2,3,7,8-TCDD levels than did a group of veterans classified as "nonexposed." This finding, along with the study by Rappe and colleagues showing detectable levels of PCDFs in the blood of survivors of the Yusho incident in Japan about 11 years after their exposure ceased, suggested that elevated levels of 2,3,7,8-TCDD might still be measured in veterans many years after their exposure ceased.[19] The veterans in studies that actually measured 2,3,7,8-TCDD body burden levels can be subdivided into two groups: (1) those veterans who handled Agent Orange as part of their military duties (Operation Ranch Hand), and (2) those veterans who served in a combat role but did not directly handle Agent Orange (ground troops). The largest such studies have been conducted by the CDC and the Air Force in collaboration with the CDC.

Ground Troops. A large-scale study of United States Army veterans was conducted by the CDC to determine whether military records could be used to identify veterans exposed to Agent Orange.[11] The CDC compared current serum 2,3,7,8-TCDD levels of Vietnam veterans with exposure estimates based on military records and with 2,3,7,8-TCDD levels of veterans not serving in Vietnam. The indirect exposure measures were: (1) weighted number of days within 2 km of an Agent Orange spray within 6 days after the spray; (2) weighted number of days within 2 km of a previous Agent Orange spray; (3) the same scores for sprays with unknown herbicide agents; (4) the number of days in five heavily sprayed areas; and (5) two self-reported measures of exposure. None of the indirect measures of exposure and neither type of self-reported exposure identified Vietnam veterans who had currently elevated serum 2,3,7,8-TCDD levels. The distributions of current 2,3,7,8-TCDD levels were nearly identical (Fig. 26–2) in Vietnam (mean: 4.2 ± 2.6 ppt, N = 646) and non-Vietnam (mean: 4.1 ± 2.3 ppt, N = 97) veterans. Two Vietnam veterans had levels above 20 ppt, as shown in Figure 26–2 (2,3,7,8-TCDD levels in individuals from the general population generally are below 20 ppt).[1] These two men each reported their health status as "excellent" and did not attribute any health problems to Agent Orange exposure.

Because no significant differences were seen in the TCDD levels between cases and controls, further studies of adverse health effects caused by TCDD exposure in these ground troop veterans were deemed unwarranted.

Agent Orange Handlers. In 1978, the Air Force responded to the Congressional mandate with the Air Force Health Study, which involved all 1267 members of the Ranch Hand unit and a series of matched controls. The two groups were given detailed physical examinations in 1982,[20] 1985,[21] and 1987–1988. These same veterans will be examined

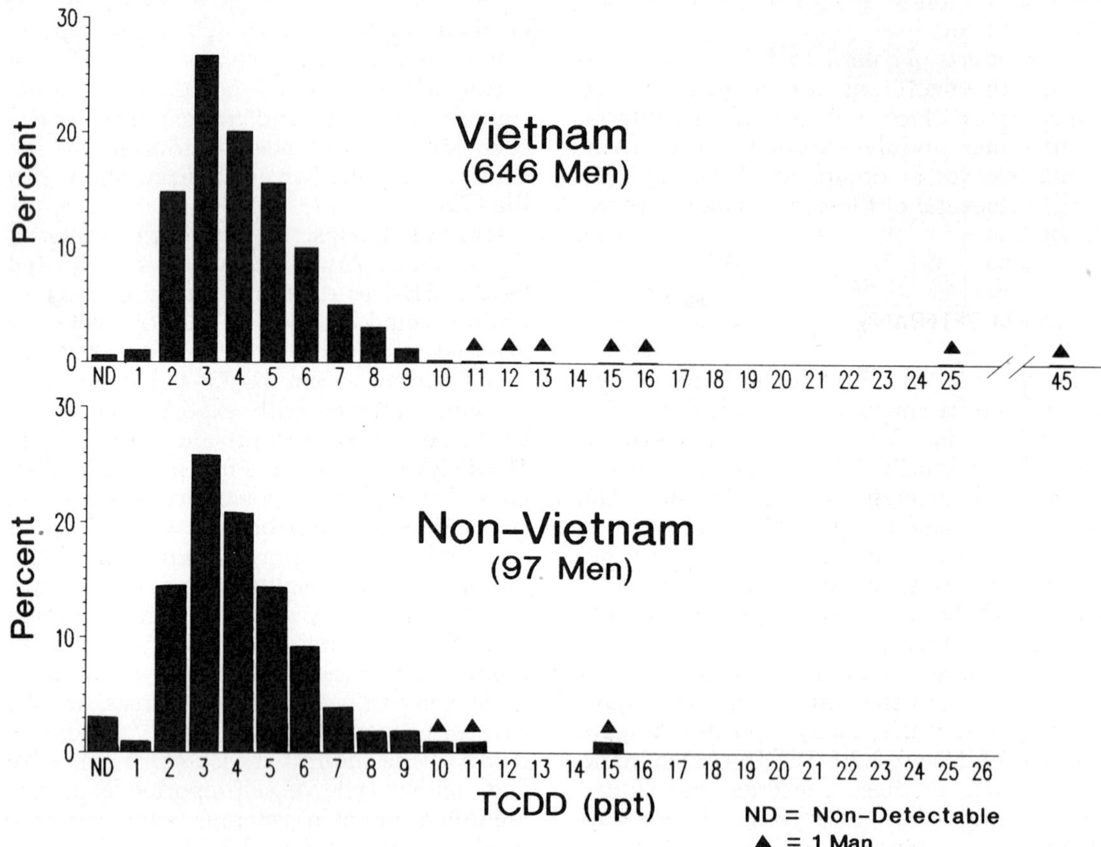

Figure 26–2. Serum 2,3,7,8-TCDD levels of Vietnam and non-Vietnam veterans in the Agent Orange Validation Study.

again in 1992, 1997, and 2002. In 1987, the Air Force in collaboration with the CDC conducted a pilot study to evaluate the Air Force exposure index for Ranch Hand veterans. The pilot study measured 2,3,7,8-TCDD levels in 150 Ranch Hand veterans and in 50 controls. The results from this study showed a large difference between the mean level in the Ranch Hand veterans (49 ppt, $N = 147$) and the controls (5 ppt, $N = 49$). Additionally, the distribution of levels in the two groups differed markedly (Fig. 26–3), indicating that some Ranch Hand personnel have had unusually heavy 2,3,7,8-TCDD exposure. However, as can be seen from the data plotted in Figure 26–3, approximately 38 per cent of the Ranch Hand veterans had levels of less than 20 ppt, which is within the range normally found in unexposed populations.[1] Because of potentially large misclassification of exposure using an exposure index, the Air Force decided to analyze the serum from nearly all members of the Ranch Hand unit for 2,3,7,8-TCDD. These analyses will be completed in 1990, at which time the relationship between 2,3,7,8-TCDD levels and the many results of the medical examinations will be determined.

Two other studies, funded by New Jersey[9] and Massachusetts,[10] have determined PCDD and PCDF levels in small cohorts of Vietnam veterans (ground troops and Agent Orange handlers). Both studies found that Agent Orange handlers had elevated 2,3,7,8-TCDD levels in blood and adipose tissue whereas ground troops were within the normal background range. These results are consistent with the CDC and Air Force studies.

2,3,7,8-TCDD Half-Life in Humans. The half-life of 2,3,7,8-TCDD in animals is less than 1 year, with some variability among species. Several studies indicate that the half-life in humans may be longer than 1 year. The finding of elevated 2,3,7,8-TCDD levels in occupationally exposed workers many years after their exposure ceased suggested that 5 to 8 years was a more reasonable estimate of 2,3,7,8-TCDD half-life in hu-

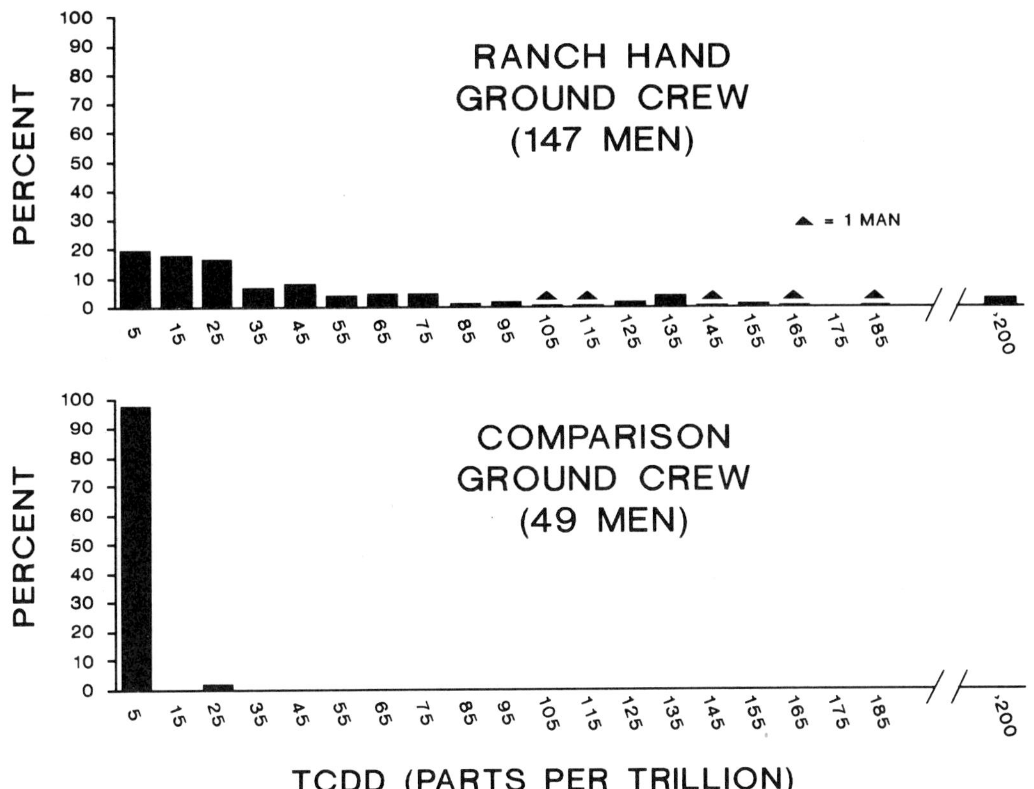

Figure 26–3. Serum 2,3,7,8-TCDD levels of Ranch Hand and control veterans in the 1987 Air Force Health Study.

mans.[22] A researcher who had ingested radiolabeled 2,3,7,8-TCDD estimated a half-life of 5.8 years based on his urinary and fecal excretions.[23] Because of the very limited half-life data available, the CDC collaborated with the Air Force in a study of Vietnam veterans to better estimate the half-life of 2,3,7,8-TCDD in humans.[2] In this study, 2,3,7,8-TCDD levels for 36 Ranch Hand veterans were determined in serum collected in 1987, as well as in serum from the same individuals that had been collected and stored since 1982. The median half-life for these 36 Ranch Hand veterans was 7.1 years (95 per cent confidence interval about the median of 5.8 to 9.6 years).

A half-life of 7 years in humans suggests that about two to four 2,3,7,8-TCDD half-lives have elapsed since the potential exposure of Vietnam veterans to Agent Orange and that 2,3,7,8-TCDD can serve as a biologic marker for previous 2,3,7,8-TCDD exposure in Vietnam veterans.

SEVESO, ITALY

In July, 1976, an explosion at a factory in Meda, Italy, that produced 2,4,5-trichlorophenol contaminated parts of the towns of Seveso, Meda, Cesano Maderno, and Desio with 2,3,7,8-TCDD. Within 20 days of the explosion, Italian authorities had evacuated all families from the area immediately surrounding the explosion site (Zone A) and had taken measures to minimize exposure of nearby residents (Zone B). The blood and adipose tissue of one person, a resident within Zone A who died from pancreatic adenocarcinoma 7 months after the explosion, were measured for 2,3,7,8-TCDD. Her 2,3,7,8-TCDD levels (whole-weight bases) were 1840 ppt in adipose tissue and 6 ppt in blood.[24]

In April, 1988, Italian scientists and the CDC agreed to analyze 14 of the more than 30,000 serum samples (1 to 3 ml) that had been collected from residents of four zones during July, 1976, through 1985. The purpose of this pilot study[25] was to assess whether serum methodology developed at the CDC[26] could be used to measure 2,3,7,8-TCDD in these low-volume samples. The pilot study analyzed serum samples from five Zone A residents who had the most severe types (III or IV) of chloracne; four Zone A residents

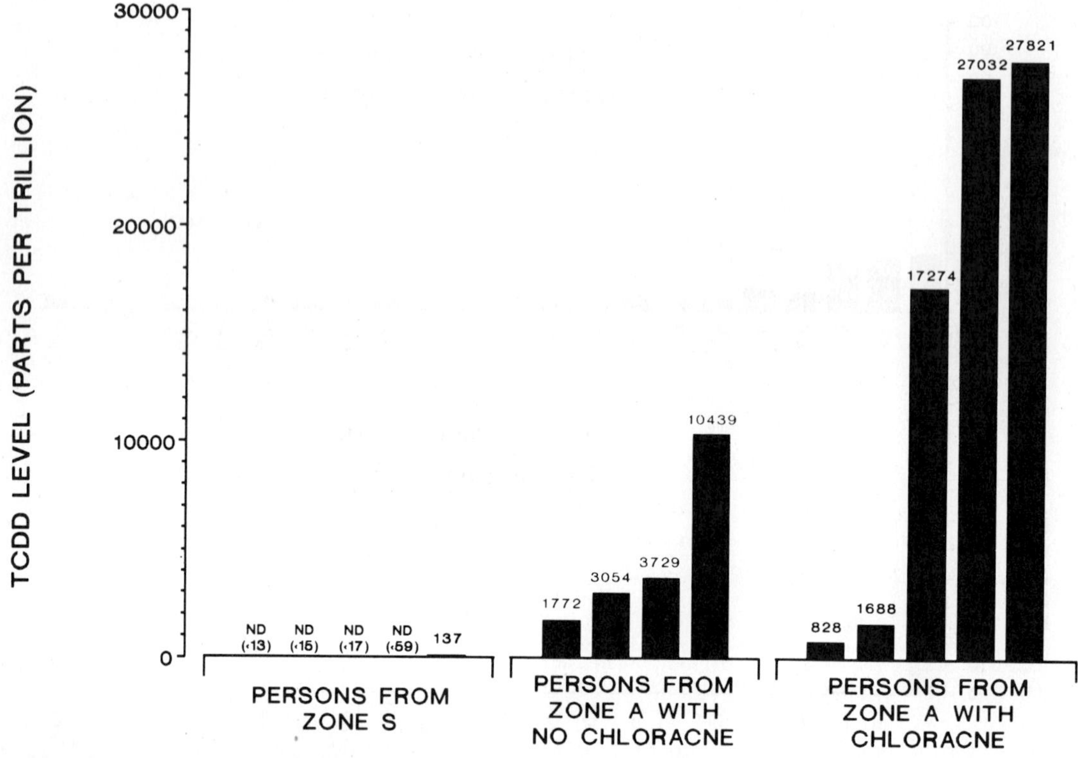

Figure 26–4. Serum 2,3,7,8-TCDD levels of Zone A residents (with and without chloracne) and controls (Zone S), Seveso, Italy.

who did not develop chloracne; and five persons from Zone S (a control zone outside the contaminated area). All these samples, collected in 1976 and stored since then at −30°C, were analyzed at the CDC without any sample identification. The 2,3,7,8-TCDD levels detected in some of these samples are the highest ever reported in humans (Fig. 26–4). The three highest levels (more than 17,000 ppt) are from children who developed the most severe types of chloracne. However, as can be seen in Figure 26–4, no apparent threshold level for chloracne is obvious.

The potentially exposed populations and selected controls underwent physical examinations from 1976 to 1985. Although some liver function tests in several of the populations were higher than those in other groups, no groups had levels outside the normal concentration range.[27] The only abnormal clinical finding has been chloracne. Because some of the adverse health effects may have a longer latency period, approximately 250 more of these stored serum samples will be analyzed for 2,3,7,8-TCDD. These data will contribute to our knowledge of the half-life of 2,3,7,8-TCDD in men, women, boys, and girls. These results also will be forthcoming in 1990.

MISSOURI, UNITED STATES

A chemical plant in Verona, Missouri, produced 2,4,5-T from 1968 to 1969 and, after

Table 26–5. ADIPOSE TISSUE 2,3,7,8-TCDD LEVELS IN PPT IN EXPOSED AND CONTROL PARTICIPANTS, MISSOURI, 1986

EXPOSURE STATUS	*N*	Range	Mean	SD	Median
TCP production	9	41.9–750	245	287	122
Horse arena	16	5.0–577	145	202	24.1
Residential	16	5.2–59.1	26.8	18.9	19.5
Waste hauling	10	3.7–25.8	12.4	8.3	9.0
Controls	128	ND–20.2	7.0	4.0	6.1

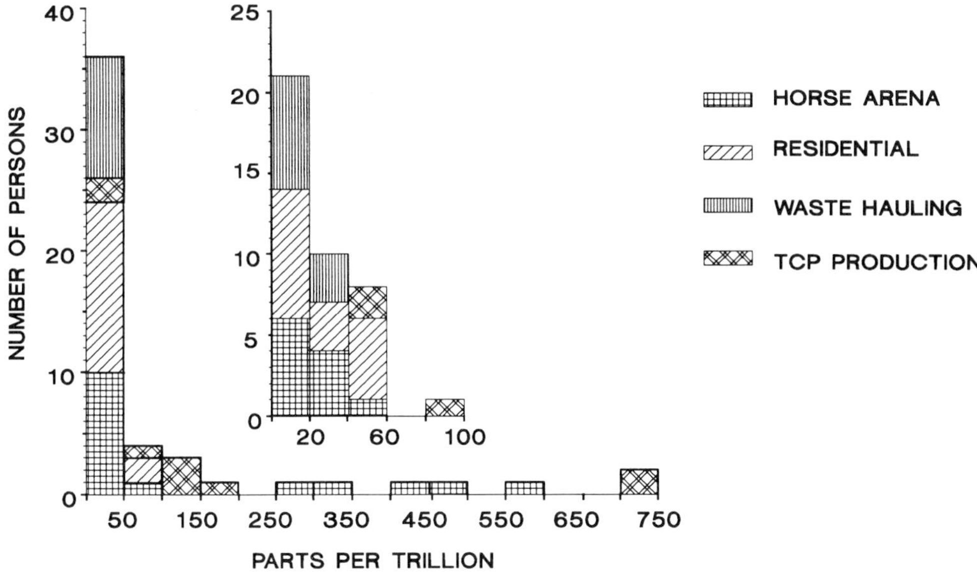

Figure 26–5. Adipose tissue 2,3,7,8-TCDD levels in exposed and unexposed persons in Missouri, 1986.

sitting idle for a year, produced hexachlorophene until it was closed in December, 1971. Approximately 29 kilograms of 2,3,7,8-TCDD–contaminated sludge wastes produced at the Verona plant were mixed with waste oils and sprayed in 1971 for dust control on areas of eastern Missouri (horse arenas, parking lots, and residential roads). More than 250 sites in Missouri are suspected of having been contaminated, and 45 have been documented to have had greater than 1 part per billion of 2,3,7,8-TCDD in the soil (two thirds of these sites are residential). The Missouri Department of Health compiled between 1983 and 1985 a central listing of more than 2000 persons who believed they had been exposed to TCDD.

From 1985 to 1986, a study of adipose tissue levels of 2,3,7,8-TCDD in Missouri residents was conducted under a cooperative agreement between the Missouri Department of Health and the CDC (funded by an interagency agreement with the Agency for Toxic Substances and Disease Registry).[22, 28] The group consisted of 51 individuals who were classified into one of four exposure categories: (1) produced 2,4,5-trichlorophenol (TCP); (2) transported contaminated wastes, performed truck maintenance, or worked for a trucking company where contaminated oil

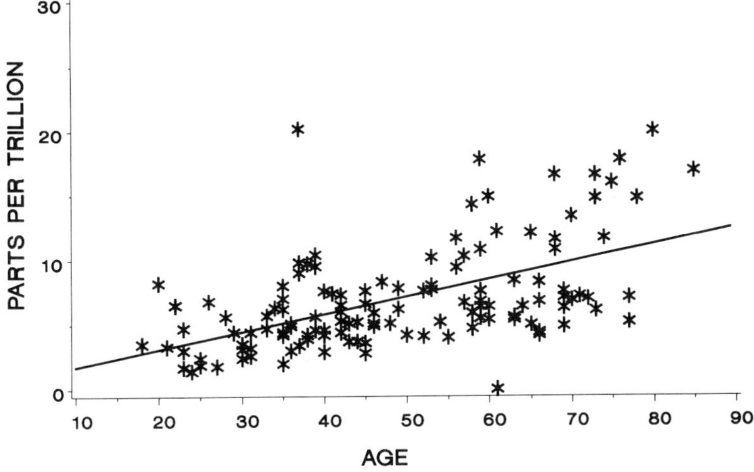

Figure 26–6. Correlation of adipose tissue 2,3,7,8-TCDD levels with age from 128 general Missouri residents, 1986.

Table 26–6. CONCENTRATION OF 2,3,7,8-TCDD IN HUMAN ADIPOSE TISSUE AND SERUM FROM INDIVIDUALS WITH NO KNOWN EXPOSURE TO 2,3,7,8-TCDD

SOURCE OF ADIPOSE TISSUE	N	WHOLE WEIGHT BASIS Mean (ppt)	Range (ppt)	MEAN AGE (Range)	Reference
Adipose tissue from elective surgical patients in Missouri, 1985	128	7.0(6.1[a])	ND[b],1.4–20.2	49.0 (18–85)	22 28
Adipose tissue from (autopsy) Georgia and Utah, 1984	35	7.1[a]	2.7–19	55.8 (16–85)	29
Adipose tissue from (autopsy) sudden deaths in St. Louis, Missouri	35	7.2[a]	2.2–20.5	41.5 (15–88)	30
Adipose tissue from (autopsy) the general Canadian adult population, 1976	46	6.4[c]	ND,2.0–13	39.7	39
Adipose tissue from (adult controls) Binghamton, New York	8	7.2	1.4–17.7	—	39
Adipose tissue from hospital patients, Umea, Sweden	31	3.0	0–9	—	40
Adipose tissue composites[d] from the EPA FY'82 NHATS Repository, 1982	46	5.0[e]	ND–10	—	41
Adipose tissue from cancer patients in Japan, 1985	12	9.0	6–18	—	42
Adipose tissue from general surgical patients in Shanghai, China, 1984	7	ND	Detection limit 2 ppt	54	43
Adipose tissue from (autopsy) general adult population in southern Japan, 1984	6	6.6[e,f]	ND–9.7	59 (46–70)	44
Adipose tissue from (autopsy) accidental death or illness in Japan	17	13.2	2.6–33	49.5 (27–74)	45
Serum from New Jersey controls, 1987	19	8.2[g]	3.7–17.1	54	46
Serum from elective surgical patients in Missouri, 1985	21	7.6[g]	1.9–26.0	42.5 (19–70)	26
Serum from U.S. Army veterans (non-Vietnam), 1987	97	4.1[g]	ND–15	39 (33–46)	11
Serum from U.S. Air Force (non-Vietnam) controls, 1987	49	4.8[g,h]	2–9.7	49	16
Blood from general population in Hamburg, FRG	10	4.0[i]	ND(<1.5)–9.1	37.1 (24–48)	47
Adipose tissue from (autopsy) general adult population in Munich, FRG	44	5.9[e,j]	ND(<1)–18.2	60.5 (15–85)	48,49
Adipose tissue from general adult population in Hamburg, FRG, 1986	21	—	1.5–18	—	50
Adipose tissue from U.S. Army controls (non-Vietnam)	7	3.2	1–5	—	9
Adipose tissue from veteran controls, 1978	4	5.1	3–8	—	18

[a]Geometric mean.
[b]Not detected.
[c]Mean is of 25 positive samples, 21 samples were NDs.
[d]Composites from over 900 specimens.
[e]Lipid-adjusted basis.
[f]Mean is of 4 positives, 2-NDs.
[g]Serum on a lipid-adjusted basis.
[h]Excludes one person (21.3 ppt) documented to have had exposure to industrial chemicals.
[i]Whole blood on lipid-adjusted basis.
[j]Mean is of 22 positive samples, 22 samples were NDs.

had been used for dust control; (3) cared for or rode horses in contaminated arenas; and (4) resided in areas sprayed with contaminated oil. The control group consisted of 128 persons who donated 20 gm of omental adipose tissue during elective abdominal surgery at one of three hospitals in Kansas City, St. Louis, or Springfield. All but one of the participants had detectable adipose tissue levels of 2,3,7,8-TCDD, as shown in Table 26–5. The distributions of the 2,3,7,8-TCDD level are shown in Figure 26–5. The adipose tissue 2,3,7,8-TCDD levels for persons with no known exposure was below 20.2 ppt.

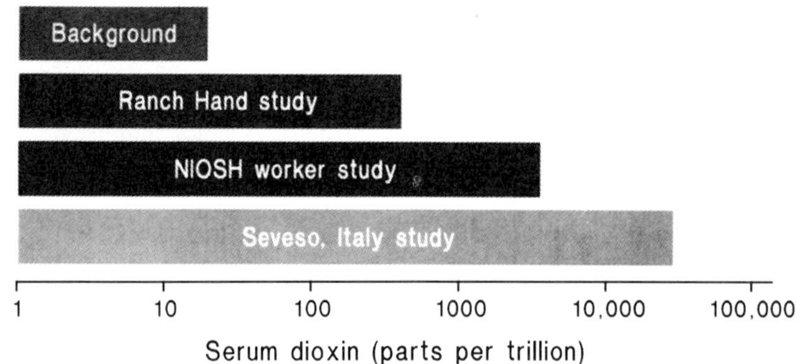

Figure 26–7. Ranges of measured serum 2,3,7,8-TCDD levels in selected studies.

Ninty-five per cent of the levels were 16.6 ppt or less. There were no significant differences by sex, race, or city of residence or by rural, suburban, or urban status. In the control group, the mean and median adipose tissue 2,3,7,8-TCDD levels increased about 20 per cent per decade of age for both men and women (Fig. 26–6). This is consistent with the findings of other studies.[29, 30]

Significant differences were evident in levels for the persons with no known exposure versus all 51 exposed persons, and for three of the four exposure categories (TCP production, horse arena, and residential exposure). Twenty-two (43 per cent) of the 51 exposed participants had levels less than the highest level of the control participants. Significant is the fact that these 22 individuals were thought to have been exposed to 2,3,7,8-TCDD on the basis of epidemiologic evidence but did not show evidence of exposure on the basis of objective laboratory data. Therefore, we must have an objective measure of exposure to minimize misclassification before looking at outcomes such as health effects.

Various populations potentially exposed to 2,3,7,8-TCDD in Missouri have been examined for adverse health outcomes, including abnormal serum enzyme levels[31] and immunotoxicity.[32, 33] No adverse health outcomes in these populations have been confirmed.

SUMMARY OF HUMAN LEVELS AND TOXIC EFFECTS

In general, the background levels of 2,3,7,8-TCDD reported in the literature are less than 20 ppt (Table 26–6). Levels reported in Vietnam veterans who handled Agent Orange; residents of Seveso, Italy; and occupationally exposed workers in the United States have been substantially above this background level (Fig. 26–7). Many large epidemiologic studies (Air Force Ranch Hand, National Institute of Occupational Safety and Health [NIOSH] workers, Seveso), which have detailed medical information as well as a laboratory measurement of 2,3,7,8-TCDD serum levels, are still ongoing. These studies offer the best opportunity to find any possible correlation between health effects and 2,3,7,8-TCDD exposure.

Thus far, the only effect clearly demonstrated in humans is chloracne. Several epidemiologic studies of humans exposed to herbicides contaminated with 2,3,7,8-TCDD have been conducted to determine whether an association exists between exposure and cancer. The evidence from these studies is difficult to assess because the exposure to TCDD is not documented by analytic measurements, and potential exposure to other active materials was evident. Some of the studies found an association between potential exposure and lymphomas and soft tissue sarcomas (in various body sites)[34, 35] and stomach cancer.[36] Other studies did not show any associations.[37, 38] Existing data are insufficient to evaluate reliably a causal association between exposure to 2,3,7,8-TCDD and cancer in humans. Again, we must have an objective measure of exposure on at least a representative segment of the population in order to decrease misclassification in these studies.

References

1. Patterson DG Jr, Fingerhut MA, Roberts DR, et al: Levels of PCDDs and PCDFs in workers exposed to 2,3,7,8-TCDD. Am J Indust Med, *16*:135, 1989.
2. Pirkle JL, Wolfe WH, Patterson DG Jr, Needham LL, Michalek JE, Miner JC, Peterson MR: Estimates

of the half-life of 2,3,7,8-TCDD in Ranch Hand veterans. J Toxicol Environ Health, *27*:165, 1989.
3. Courtney KD, Putnam JP, Andrews JE: Arch Environ Contam Toxicol *7*:395–396, 1978.
4. Kociba RJ, Keyes DG, Beyer JE, et al: Results of a two-year chronic toxicity and oncogenicity study of 2,3,7,8-tetrachlorodibenzo-*p*-dioxin in rats. Toxicol Appl Pharmacol *46*:279–303, 1978.
5. Courtney KD, Moore JA: Teratology studies with 2,4,5-trichlorophenoxy-acetic acid and 2,3,7,8-tetrachlorodibenzo-*p*-dioxin. Toxicol Appl Pharmacol *20*:396–403, 1971.
6. Vos JG, Moore JA, Zindl JG: Effect of 2,3,7,8-tetrachlorodibenzo-*p*-dioxin in the immune system of laboratory animals. Environ Health Perspect *5*:149–162, 1973.
7. Young AL, Calcagnic JA, Tremblay JW: The Toxicology, Environmental Fate, and Human Risk of Herbicide Orange and Its Associated Dioxin. United States Air Force Occupational and Environmental Health Laboratory Technical Report TR-78-92. San Antonio, TX, Brooks Air Force Base, 1978.
8. Hagenmeier H: Determination of 2,3,7,8-tetrachlorodibenzo-*p*-dioxin in commercial chlorophenols and related products. Fresenius Z Anal Chem *325*:603–606, 1986.
9. Kahn PC, Gochfeld M, Nygren M, et al: Dioxins and dibenzofurans in blood and adipose tissue of Agent Orange–exposed Vietnam veterans and matched controls. JAMA *259*:1661–1667, 1988.
10. Schecter A, Constable JD, Bargest JV, et al: Isomer specific measurement of PCDD and PCDF isomers in human blood from American Vietnam veterans two decades after exposure to Agent Orange. Chemosphere *18*:531, 1989.
11. Centers for Disease Control Veterans Health Studies Group: Serum 2,3,7,8-TCDD levels in U.S. Army Vietnam-era veterans. JAMA *260*:1249–1254, 1988.
12. Centers for Disease Control Vietnam Experience Study: Health status of Vietnam veterans: I. Psychosocial characteristics. JAMA *259*:2701–2707, 1988.
13. Centers for Disease Control Vietnam Experience Study: Health status of Vietnam veterans: II. Physical health. JAMA *259*:2708–2714, 1988.
14. Centers for Disease Control Vietnam Experience Study: Health status of Vietnam veterans: III. Reproductive outcomes. JAMA *259*:2715–2719, 1988.
15. Centers for Disease Control Vietnam Experience Study: Postservice mortality among Vietnam veterans. JAMA *257*:790–795, 1987.
16. Centers for Disease Control: Serum levels of 2,3,7,8-TCDD in Vietnam veterans of Operation Ranch Hand. MMWR *37*:309–311, 1988.
17. Lathrop GD, Wolfe WH, Albanese RA, Moynahan PM: Epidemiologic Investigation of Health Effects in Air Force Personnel Following Exposure to Herbicides: Study Protocol. National Technical Information Service Document No. AD A 122 250. Brooks Air Force Base, Texas: United States Air Force School of Aerospace Medicine, 1982.
18. Gross ML, Lay JO, Lyon PA: 2,3,7,8-TCDD levels in adipose tissue of Vietnam veterans. Environ Res *33*:261–268, 1984.
19. Rappe C, Nygren M, Buser HR, et al: Identification of PCDDs and PCDFs in human samples: Occupational exposures and Yusho patients. *In* Tucker RE, Young AL, Gray AP (eds): Human and Environmental Risks of Chlorinated Dioxins and Related Compounds. New York, Plenum Press, 1983, pp 241–253.
20. Lathrop GD, Wolfe WH, Albanese RA, Moynahan PM: An Epidemiologic Investigation of Health Effects in Air Force Personnel Following Exposure to Herbicides: Baseline Morbidity Study Results. National Technical Information Service Document No. AD A 138 340. Brooks Air Force Base, San Antonio, TX: United States Air Force School of Aerospace Medicine, 1984.
21. Lathrop GD, Machado SG, Karrison TG, et al: Air Force Health Study: An Epidemiologic Investigation of Health Effects in Air Force Personnel Following Exposure to Herbicides: Final Report. National Technical Information Services Document No. AD A 188 262. Brooks Air Force Base, San Antonio, TX: United States Air Force School of Aerospace Medicine, 1987.
22. Patterson DG Jr, Hoffman RE, Needham LL, et al: Levels of 2,3,7,8-TCDD in adipose tissue of exposed and control persons in Missouri–An interim report. JAMA *256*:2683–2686, 1986.
23. Poiger H, Schlatter C: Pharmacokinetics of 2,3,7,8-TCDD in man. Chemosphere *15*:1489–1494, 1986.
24. Facchetti S, Fornari A, Montagna M: Distribution of 2,3,7,8-TCDD in the tissues of a person exposed to the toxic cloud at Seveso. Forensic Environ Appl *1*:1406–1444, 1981.
25. Centers for Disease Control: Preliminary Report: 2,3,7,8-TCDD exposure to humans—Seveso, Italy. MMWR *37*:733–736, 1988.
26. Patterson DG Jr, Hampton L, Lapeza CR Jr, et al: High-resolution gas chromatographic/high-resolution mass spectrometric analysis of human serum on a whole-weight and lipid basis for 2,3,7,8-TCDD. Anal Chem *59*:2000–2005, 1987.
27. Mocarelli P, Marocchi A, Brambilla P, et al: Clinical laboratory manifestations of exposure to dioxin in children: A six-year study of the effects of an environmental disaster near Seveso, Italy. JAMA *256*:2687–2695, 1986.
28. Andrews JS, Garrett WA, Patterson DG Jr, et al: 2,3,7,8-TCDD levels in adipose tissue of persons with no known exposure and in exposed persons. Chemosphere *18*:499–506, 1989.
29. Patterson DG Jr, Holler JS, Smith SJ, et al: Human adipose data for 2,3,7,8-TCDD in certain U.S. samples. Chemosphere *15*:2055–2060, 1986.
30. Graham M, Hileman FD, Orth RG, et al: Chlorocarbons in adipose tissue from a Missouri population. Chemosphere *15*:1595–1600, 1986.
31. Stehr PA, Stein G, Falk H, et al: A pilot epidemiologic study of possible health effects associated with 2,3,7,8-tetrachlorodibenzo-*p*-dioxin contamination in Missouri. Arch Environ Health *41*:18–22, 1986.
32. Hoffman RE, Stehr-Green PA, Webb KB, et al: Health effects of long-term exposure to 2,3,7,8-TCDD. JAMA *255*:2031–2038, 1986.
33. Evans RG, Webb KB, Knutsen AP, et al: A medical follow-up of the health effects of long-term exposure to 2,3,7,8-TCDD. Arch Environ Health *43*:273, 1988.
34. Hardell L, Standstrom A: Case-control study: Soft-tissue sarcomas and exposure to phenoxyacetic acids or chlorophenols. Br J Cancer *39*:711–717, 1979.
35. Eriksson M, Hardell L, O'Berg N, Moller T, Axelson O: Soft-tissue sarcomas and exposure to chemical substances: A case-referent study. Br J Indust Med *38*:27–33, 1981.
36. Axelson O, Sundell L, Anderson K, Edling C, Hogstedt C, Kling H: Herbicide exposure and tumor mortality: An updated epidemiologic investigation on Swedish railroad workers. Scand J Work Environ Health *6*:73–79, 1980.

37. Cook RR, Bond GG, Olsen RA, Ott MG: Evaluation of the mortality experience of workers exposed to the chlorinated dioxins. Chemosphere *15*:1769, 1986.
38. Smith AH, Fisher DO, Giles HJ, Pearce N: The New Zealand Soft Tissue Sarcoma Case-Control Study: Interview findings concerning phenoxyacetic acid exposure. Chemosphere *12*(4/5):565–571, 1983.
39. Schecter A, Ryan JJ, Gitlitz G: Chlorinated dioxin and dibenzofuran levels in human adipose tissues from exposed and control populations. *In* Rappe C, Choudhary G, Keith LH (eds): Chlorinated Dioxins and Dibenzofurans in Perspective. Chelsea, MI, Lewis Publishers, 1986, pp 51–65.
40. Rappe C, Nygren M, Lindstrom G, Hansson M: Dioxins and dibenzofurans in biological samples of European origin. Chemosphere *15*:1635–1639, 1986.
41. Stanley JS, Boggess KE, Onstot J, Sack TM: PCDDs and PCDFs in human adipose tissue from the EPA FY'82 NHATS Repository. Chemosphere *15*:1605–1612, 1986.
42. Ono M, Wakimoto T, Tatsukawa R, Masuda Y: Polychlorinated dibenzo-*p*-dioxins and dibenzofurans in human adipose tissues of Japan. Chemosphere *15*:1629–1634, 1986.
43. Ryan JJ, Schecter A, Masuda Y, Kikuchi M: Comparison of PCDDs and PCDFs in the tissue of Yusho patients with those from the general population in Japan and China. Chemosphere *16*:2017–2025, 1987.
44. Ryan JJ: Variation of dioxins and furans in human tissues. Chemosphere *15*:1585–1593, 1986.
45. Ogaki J, Takayama K, Miyata H, Kashimoto T: Levels of PCDDs and PCDFs in human tissues and various foodstuffs in Japan. Chemosphere *16*:2047–2056, 1987.
46. Fingerhut MA, Sweeney MH, Patterson DG Jr, et al: Levels of 2,3,7,8-TCDD in the serum of U.S. chemical workers exposed to dioxin-contaminated products; Interim results. Chemosphere, in press.
47. Päpke O, Ball M, Lis ZA, Scheunert K: PCDD/PCDF in whole blood samples of unexposed person. Chemosphere, in press.
48. Thoma H, Mücke W, Kretschmer E: Untersuchung von Humanfettproben auf PCDD/F. VDI-Berichte *634*:383–387, 1987.
49. Thoma H, Mücke W, Kretschmer E: Concentrations of PCDD and PCDF in human fat and liver samples. Chemosphere *18*:491–498, 1989.
50. Beck H, Eckart K, Mathar W, Wittkowski R: Levels of PCDDs and PCDFs in adipose tissue of occupationally exposed workers. Chemosphere *18*:507–516, 1989.

E. Formaldehyde

Alice Stark, Dr.P.H.

Formaldehyde is a colorless gas with a pungent odor. It reacts readily with compounds that have active hydrogen atoms such as alcohols, phenols, ammonia, amines, and amides; such reactivity is of particular concern because of the ubiquity of nitrogen compounds (DNA, RNA, proteins, amino acids) in biologic systems. Formaldehyde is very soluble in water; in aqueous solution at body temperature, it is relatively stable and exists in an equilibrium state with the hydrated form. Formaldehyde polymerizes readily in both the liquid and solid states. This polymerization process is delayed by the presence of water. Commercial formaldehyde preparations, known as formalin or formol, are aqueous solutions containing 37 to 50 per cent formaldehyde by weight; 10 to 15 per cent methyl alcohol is also added to these aqueous solutions as a polymerization inhibitor.

Potential Sources of Exposure

American manufacturers produce about 7 billion pounds of formaldehyde each year. It is used primarily in the production of urea-, phenol-, acetal-, and melamine-formaldehyde resins. The remainder is used to make other industrial chemicals, leather products, and agricultural products, and to prepare vaccines, drugs, disinfectants, and fumigants. Formaldehyde-based resins are used as adhesives in making plywood, veneers, and particleboard and in the production of plastics, textiles, insulating materials, paper, and rubber products.[1] Formaldehyde exposure in these manufacturing processes is a risk to those employed in the plants and possibly to residents in their immediate vicinity.

The potential for exposure to formaldehyde outside the workplace is widespread. It has been estimated that about 11 million people live in homes containing urea-formaldehyde foam insulation (UFFI) or particleboard made with urea-formaldehyde resins.[2] Concentrations ranging from 0.01 to 10.6 parts per million (ppm) in air have been measured in homes, with most residential exposure being below 0.5 ppm. Formaldehyde is also used in permanent press clothing and in many cosmetics, causing exposure through direct contact. The greatest overall cause of formaldehyde sensitization appears to be clothing.[3] Other potential sources of formaldehyde include combustion in gas stoves and heaters, the breakdown of cooking oils, cigarette smoke, and automobile exhausts.

Metabolism

Formaldehyde is a normal metabolite in the human body, resulting from the metabolism of food. As a normal intermediary metabolite, formaldehyde occupies a central role in the one-carbon pool as methylene tetrahydro-folate.[4] Human beings are capable of handling normal levels of formaldehyde and some excess.[5] The free compound usually is not found in body tissues and fluids. Endogenous formaldehyde is rapidly metabolized to formate or it enters the one-carbon pool. Exogenous exposure, which can occur by the respiratory, oral, or dermal routes, also results in rapid oxidation of formaldehyde to formate and carbon dioxide or incorporation into other molecules.[6]

Physiologic End-points

Acute ingestion of formalin by humans has resulted in loss of consciousness, vascular collapse, pneumonia, hemorrhagic nephritis, and abortion. Formaldehyde has occasionally injured the larynx and trachea, but damage to the gastrointestinal tract occurs primarily in the stomach and lower esophagus. Fatalities have resulted from ingestion of as little as 30 ml of formalin.[7,8] The use of formaldehyde to devitalize dental pulp has produced paresthesia, soft tissue necrosis, and sequestration of bone.[9–11] Filters impregnated with melamine-formaldehyde resin were associated with an outbreak of hemolytic anemia among hemodialysis patients.[12]

HEALTH EFFECTS IN HUMANS

Acute

Ear, Nose and Throat Injury. Even at low doses, formaldehyde is a strong irritant, producing symptoms in the eyes and nose and other parts of the upper respiratory system. Complaints include headaches, fatigue, sore throat, inability to concentrate, and thirst. The most sensitive person experiences slight eye irritation at 0.01 ppm and some can perceive the odor at concentrations as low as 0.05 ppm. At 0.1 to 3.0 ppm most people experience eye, nose, and throat irritation. The number of symptoms, their severity, and the number of people affected increases with dose. Formaldehyde splashed in the eyes is capable of causing blindness.[2]

Airway Injury. Formaldehyde is a direct airway irritant that causes bronchoconstriction and aggravates pre-existing asthmatic conditions and allergic rhinitis. Reactions may be immediate or delayed, suggesting different mechanisms. Currently, there is insufficient evidence to determine whether or not formaldehyde is capable of actually causing asthma.[2] But in nonsmoking asthmatics subjected to 3 hours of exposure to 3 ppm of formaldehyde, there were no significant changes in pulmonary function (FVC, FEV, FEF 25–27 per cent, SGaw, or FRC) or airway reactivity.[13] The concentration ranges at which effects have been reported in the literature are shown in Table 26–7.

Direct Tissue Injury. Substantial information exists to indicate that at levels as low as 0.12 ppm of formaldehyde many people develop irritant effects from exposure. The irritation that results is from stimulation of the trigeminal nerve endings, evoking a burning sensation of the nasal passages and burning and tearing of the eyes. The effect is readily reversible once exposure ceases. Formaldehyde not only stimulates nerves, it also

Table 26–7. REPORTED HUMAN HEALTH EFFECTS OF FORMALDEHYDE AT VARIOUS AIRBORNE CONCENTRATIONS

HEALTH EFFECTS	APPROXIMATE FORMALDEHYDE CONCENTRATION (PPM)
Neurophysiologic effects	0.05–1.50
Odor threshold	0.05–1.0
Eye irritation	0.01–2.0*
Upper airway irritation	0.10–25
Lower airway and pulmonary effects	5–30
Pulmonary edema, inflammation, pneumonia	50–100
Death	100+

*The low concentration (0.01 ppm) was observed in the presence of other pollutants that may have been acting synergistically.

(Data from CIR Expert Panel: Final report on the safety assessment of formaldehyde. J Am Coll Toxicol 3:157–184, 1984.)

causes tissue damage at the site of contact. At low levels of exposure, recovery occurs during periods of nonexposure. Even more advanced pathologic changes possess a degree of reversibility. At some point, however, the process becomes irreversible and a carcinoma is produced. Irritation, therefore, should be viewed as an early warning stage in a process that can lead to progressively more severe health effects.[1, 5]

Dermal Injury. Formaldehyde is both a dermal irritant and a sensitizer.[16, 17] About 5 per cent of the general population in the United States reacts to 1 per cent formalin administered by occluded patch testing.[3] The threshold for induction of allergic contact dermatitis in previously unsensitized individuals may be less than 1 per cent formalin. Once sensitized, an individual's threshold reduces to about 0.006 per cent formalin. There is also evidence that exposure through inhalation can result in dermatitis in sensitized people; both dermal and respiratory symptoms can be evoked simultaneously.

Dermal responses, like respiratory effects, can be of two types, immediate or delayed. Urticaria, the immediate and less prevalent response, could be of immunologic origin or a skin response directly triggered by release of histamine and other vasoactive substances. Delayed allergic contact dermatitis is clearly hypersensitivity.

Other Effects. Embryotoxicity, teratogenicity, and reproductive effects of formaldehyde do not appear to be important at the low concentrations that cause irritation or sensitization in a substantial number of individuals.[18]

Chronic

The United States Environmental Protection Agency (EPA) has classified formaldehyde as a "probable human carcinogen." Based on a review of epidemiologic studies, the EPA has concluded that there is limited evidence to indicate that formaldehyde may be a carcinogen in humans. Nine studies reported statistically significant associations between site-specific respiratory neoplasms and exposure to formaldehyde or formaldehyde-containing products.[19]

An examination of studies in animals has indicated that there is sufficient evidence of carcinogenicity of formaldehyde in animals by the inhalation route. This is based on the induction by formaldehyde of an increased incidence of a rare type of malignant tumor, nasal squamous cell carcinoma. The effect was produced in both sexes of rats, in multiple inhalation experiments, and in multiple species (i.e., rats and mice). In these long-term laboratory studies, tumors were not observed beyond the initial site of nasal contact. Because humans breathe through both the nose and mouth, it is biologically feasible that an increased risk of cancer of the buccal cavity and pharynx also exists.[19, 20]

The mechanisms of action leading to formaldehyde's expression of a carcinogenic effect are at least partially understood. As concentration increases, a series of reactions in the exposed tissues occur, starting with irritation, dysplasia, hyperplasia, metaplasia, and carcinoma in situ and ending finally in frank squamous cell carcinoma. This ability to cause tissue damage and subsequent cell proliferation depends highly on concentration and is not well correlated with length of exposure. At low concentrations, tissue recovery after only short rest periods appears to occur. As concentration increases, repair becomes more and more difficult and the damage is ultimately irreversible.

An increased risk of nasal cancer appears to be associated with histories of nasal polyps, recurrent nose bleeds, and sinus disorders. This points out the importance of noncarcinogenic effects in the prediction of risk of development of cancer.

Clinical Recommendations

The focus of this section has been on health effects resulting from formaldehyde exposure in the home and workplace. The levels may range from less than 0.1 ppm to well above the Occupational Safety and Health Administration—Permissible Exposure Level (OSHA—PEL) of 3 ppm, an 8-hour time-weighted average. Generally, outside the occupational setting ambient levels will tend to be at the lower end of the range. The signs and symptoms produced by formaldehyde also can result from exposure to numerous other chemical, biologic, or physical agents. Therefore, the essential and difficult task of the clinician is to identify the specific causative agent so that appropriate treatment can be instituted.

History

A most valuable tool is a detailed patient history that includes, in addition to the standard items, questions relating to the person's work and lifestyle. These questions should be specific and focus on the past as well as the present. Questions regarding the type of housing (e.g., mobile home), furnishings, insulation, use of various consumer products (e.g., cosmetics, shampoos, and so on), type of home heating, and presence of industrial sites in the residential area can provide useful leads. The presence of similar complaints in household members or coworkers can point to common exposures.

Many states have worker right-to-know laws in addition to the OSHA hazard communication standard. These laws and regulations require that employers provide workers with health and safety information about the chemicals they come in contact with at the workplace. The patient, therefore, may already know about workplace exposures and if not can request the information. This source may prove valuable to the physician. Table 26–8 lists occupations that have a potential for formaldehyde exposure.[21]

Based on the history, it may be possible to conclude that formaldehyde is the causative agent or that it is likely to be. If the exposure is occurring at home, air measurements can be suggested as a means of verification.

Table 26–8. POTENTIAL OCCUPATIONAL EXPOSURES TO FORMALDEHYDE

Anatomists	Glue and adhesive makers
Agricultural workers	Hexamethylenetetraamine makers
Bakers	Hide preservers
Beauticians	Histology technicians (assumed to include necropsy and autopsy technicians)
Biologists	Ink makers
Bookbinders	Lacquerers and lacquer makers
Botanists	Medical personnel (assumed to include pathologists)
Crease-resistant textile finishers	Mirror workers
Deodorant makers	Oil well workers
Disinfectant makers	Paper makers
Disinfectors	Particleboard makers
Dress goods shop personnel	Pentaerythritol makers
Dressmakers	Photographic film makers
Drugmakers	Plastic workers
Dyemakers	Resin makers
Electrical insulation makers	Rubber makers
Embalmers	Soil sterilizers and greenhouse workers
Embalming fluid makers	Surgeons
Ethylene glycol makers	Tannery workers
Fertilizer makers	Taxidermists
Fireproofers	Textile mordanters and printers
Formaldehyde resin makers	Textile waterproofers
Formaldehyde employees	Varnish workers
Foundry employees	Wood preservers
Fumigators	
Fungicide workers	
Furniture dippers and sprayers	
Fur processors	
Glass etchers	

Diagnostic Tests

Changes in pulmonary function tests have not been consistently present, have been small, and have not shown a regular association with exposure. Even individuals with pre-existing asthma have not been shown to experience significant bronchoconstriction when exposed to 3 ppm of formaldehyde for 3 hours. Therefore, pulmonary function tests and provocative inhalation tests are not useful for assessing formaldehyde exposure or sensitivity.[13, 22]

The incidence of sensitivity to formaldehyde in the general population is not insignificant. Formaldehyde is the tenth leading cause of skin reactions among patients with dermatitis. An occluded patch test of 2 per cent formalin is suggested as a diagnostic aid.[23] Because it seems likely that patch testing itself can induce sensitivity, it is not recommended for pre-employment or routine medical surveillance.[15]

Examination of formic acid levels in urine as a biologic indicator of formaldehyde exposure revealed extreme variability both among individuals and in repeat tests of individuals. Thus, formic acid in urine is not a good index of exposure.[24]

Treatment

Persons who have ingested formaldehyde should be made to swallow milk or water containing ammonium acetate, and vomiting should be induced. This should be followed by gastric lavage with a weak (0.1 per cent) ammonia solution that will convert the formaldehyde to relatively inert pentamethylenetetramine (10 liters of 0.1 per cent ammonia converts 4 grams of formaldehyde). Gastric lavage is warranted only in the first 15 minutes following ingestion.[25] Circulatory and respiratory function should be adequately managed.

Removal from formaldehyde exposure is of prime importance for the alleviation of all symptoms. If dermatitis is present, additional treatment as appropriate may be required.[23]

Contaminated skin should be washed with soap and water; splashes in the eye should be treated by irrigation for 15 minutes.[25]

Hemodialysis is effective for the removal of formic and lactic acids and for the correction of metabolic acidosis.[5] However, hemodialysis should be used only if the acidosis is uncorrectable with sodium bicarbonate or sodium lactate solutions. It should be considered in the early management of severe formaldehyde ingestion.

References

1. Sheldrich JE, Stadman TR: Final report on product/industry profile and related analysis on formaldehyde and formaldehyde-containing products. Part II, CSPC-C-78-0091. Unpublished data. Columbus, OH, Batelle, Feb, 1979.
2. National Research Council, Committee on Aldehydes, Board on Toxicology and Environmental Health Hazards: Health effects of formaldehyde. *In* Formaldehyde and Other Aldehydes. Washington, DC, National Academy Press, 1981, Chapter 7.
3. Feinman SE: Formaldehyde Sensitization. Draft report prepared by the Consumer Product Safety Commission, 1984.
4. McGilvery RW: Biochemistry, A Functional Approach. 2nd ed. Philadelphia, WB Saunders, 1979, p 605.
5. Ells JT, McMartin KE, Black K, Virayotha V, Tisdell RH, Tephly JTR: Formaldehyde poisoning: Rapid metabolism to formic acid. JAMA *246*:1237–1278, 1981.
6. Gescher A, Heckman JA, Stevens MFG: Oxidative metabolism of some *N*-methyl-containing xenobiotics can lead to stable progenitors of formaldehyde. Biochem Pharmacol *28*:3235–3238, 1979.
7. Bohmer K: Formalin poisoning. Dtsche Z Ges Gerichtl Med 1934:*23*:7–18, 1934; Chem Abs *28*:5884, 1934.
8. Kline BS: Formaldehyde poisoning; With report of a fatal case. Arch Intern Med *36*:220–228, 1925.
9. Grossman LI: Paresthesia from N2 or N2 substitute; Report of a case. Oral Surg Oral Med Oral Pathol *45*:114–115, 1978.
10. Heling B, Ram Z, Heling I: The root treatment of teeth with Toxavit; Report of a case. Oral Surg Oral Med Oral Pathol *43*:306–309, 1977.
11. Montgomery S: Paresthesia following endodontic treatment. J Endodont *2*:345–347, 1976.
12. Orringer EP, Mattern WD: Formaldehyde-induced hemolysis during chronic hemodialysis. N Engl J Med *294*:1416–1420, 1976.
13. Sauder LR, Green DJ, Chatham MD, Kulle TJ: Acute pulmonary response of asthmatics to 3.0 ppm formaldehyde. Toxicol Ind Health *3*:569–578, 1987.
14. CIR Expert Panel: Final report on the safety assessment of formaldehyde. J Am Coll Toxicol *3*:157–184, 1984.
15. Preliminary Assessment of the Health Effects of Formaldehyde. Office of Risk Assessment, Directorate of Health Standards Programs, OSHA, 1984.
16. Fisher AA: Contact Dermatitis. Philadelphia, Lea and Febiger, 1967.
17. Cronin E: New allergens of clinical importance. Semin Clin Dermatol *1*:33–41, 1982.
18. Consensus Workshop Group: Deliberations of the Consensus Workshop on Formaldehyde. Little Rock, Arkansas, Oct, 1983.
19. Assessment of Health Risks to Garment Workers and Certain Home Residents from Exposure to Formaldehyde. Environmental Protection Agency, Office of Pesticides and Toxic Substances, Apr, 1987.
20. Stayner L, Smith AB, Reeve G, Blade L, Elliott L, Keenlyside R, Halperin W: Proportionate mortality study of workers exposed to formaldehyde in the garment industry. Am J Epidemiol *120*:458–459, 1984.
21. IARC Monographs on the Evaluation of the Carcinogenic Risk of Chemicals to Humans. Vol 29: Some Industrial Chemicals and Dyestuffs. Lyon, 1982, p 352.
22. Harving H, Korsgaard J, Dahl R, Pedersen OF, Molhave L: Low concentrations of formaldehyde in bronchial asthma: A study of exposure under controlled conditions. Br Med J *293*:310, 1986.
23. Proctor NH, Hughes JP (eds): Chemical Hazards of the Workplace. Philadelphia, JB Lippincott, 1978.
24. Gottschling LM, Beaulieu HJ, Melvin WW: Monitoring of formic acid in urine of humans exposed to low levels of formaldehyde. Am Ind Hyg Assoc J *45*:19–23, 1984.
25. Zurlo N: Formaldehyde and derivatives. *In* Encyclopedia of Occupational Health and Safety. Vol 1, 3rd ed. Geneva, International Labor Office, 1983, pp 914–915.

F. Chronic Pesticide Poisoning

Wayne R. Snodgrass, M.D., Ph.D.

Estimates of acute pesticide poisoning place the number of cases at 1 million,[1–3] but the incidence and severity of chronic pesticide poisoning are unknown. One reason for this is the difficulty of defining chronic pesticide toxicity in human beings. Is it the incidence of neuropsychologic deficits caused by chronic pesticide toxicity? If so, how do we measure such adverse effects objectively and quantitatively? Is it the incidence of chemically induced cancer caused by chronic pesticide exposure and long-term body burdens of certain long-lasting pesticides? Quantification of the risk for chemically induced human cancer is difficult in part because of the long (often 5 to 20 years or more) but unknown lag time period for the tumor to appear clinically, and the widely variable genetic susceptibility in different individuals. Despite these difficulties, certain principles and guidelines are available to clinicians to assist in the evaluation of patients claiming to be or suspected to be chronically exposed to pesticides. This chapter focuses on the diagnosis and management of chronic pesticide poisoning.

TYPES OF CHRONIC PESTICIDE TOXICITY

The types of chronic pesticide toxicity may be categorized by chemical class, e.g., organophosphate or organochlorine; by the presence or absence of current ongoing exposure; or by the extent of the long-term body burden, i.e., a chemical with a very long total body elimination half-time measured in months to years.

Organophosphate poisoning usually is considered to be relatively acute and it is considered that, following termination of exposure, clinical toxicity resolves. However clinical data clearly document persistent adverse effects of organophosphates persisting long beyond the last period of exposure. There are two general types of persistent organophosphat[illegible] neurotoxicity an[illegible]

The so-called [illegible] organophosphor[illegible] toxicity poisoning is distinct from inhibition of plasma pseudocholinesterase or inhibition of erythrocyte cholinesterase.[4, 5] In the classic presentation of NTE-type toxicity, ataxic signs occur 1 to 3 weeks after an acute exposure. Painful, transient paresthesias develop in a stocking-glove distribution over the lower extremities and rapidly extend to motor weakness and ataxia, with later involvement of the upper extremities.[4, 5] Evidence in laboratory animals points toward greater symptoms from multiple subchronic doses compared with a large single dose. Subchronic dermal exposure appears to be the most potent route of dosing.[4, 5] Structure-activity relationships of organic phosphonates versus phosphenates versus phosphates and the ability to have a chemical leaving group correlate with ability to inhibit the NTE enzyme. Thus, not all organophosphates pose a risk for NTE inhibition, and only a few have been documented to cause clinical delayed neurotoxicity. In the future, a lymphocyte NTE test may be available to help assess exposure of an individual patient.[6]

The second type of delayed organophosphate toxicity consists of neuropsychologic deficits.[7] Abnormalities of memory, abstraction, mood, intellectual functioning, and flexibility of thinking can be demonstrated in subjects with a last prior organophosphate poisoning of 7 years or more.[7] These individuals may have neuropsychologic test results similar to those of subjects with cerebral damage or dysfunction. These sequelae are sufficiently subtle that clinical neurologic examination, clinical electroencephalography, and audiometric, ophthalmic, and blood chemistry testing cannot discriminate poisoned subjects from controls.[7] The physician cannot rely solely on the standard neurologic examination or on clinical intuition in evaluating a patient who has been poisoned by organophosphates. The usual clinical neurologic examination does not thoroughly assess higher-level cognitive skills but rather focuses on sensory and motor functioning. The major deficits in these patients are cognitive and appear on neuropsychologic tests of abilities that receive limited emphasis in the usual neurologic examination. Thus, the two methods, *clinical neurologic examination and neuropsychologic testing, provide a more thorough evaluation of such patients with chronic cognitive deficits following organophosphate poisoning.*[7] Nerve conduction studies in acute organophosphate poisoning usually have been reported as normal.[8] The muscle response to single stimulation shows a repetitive response. This repetitive response disappears on repeated stimulation, and this finding is thought by some to be characteristic.[8]

Organochlorine chronic pesticide poisoning presents equally difficult challenges to the physician. Halogenated hydrocarbons include those used as pesticides, as well as many fumigants and solvents. The fumigants and solvents, usually with molecular weights of less than approximately 236 daltons, are generally considered to have shorter half-lives, in part resulting from their greater vapor pressures. The halogenated hydrocarbon insecticides, usually with molecular weights of approximately 291 to 545, have lower vapor pressures and include lindane (gamma-BHC or gamma-benzene hexachloride), chlordane, heptachlor, methoxychlor, aldrin, Mirex, toxaphene, and many others.[9] Other halogenated hydrocarbon environmental contaminants also pose a toxicity risk for humans and include TCDD (dioxin or 2,3,7,8-tetrachlorodibenzo-*p*-dioxin), PBBs (polybrominated biphenyls), and PCBs (polychlorinated biphenyls). Many of these less volatile halogenated hydrocarbons share the properties of high lipid solubility and extensive distribution and storage into body fat; they are poorly metabolized with a resulting long total body half-life.

An especially important factor in chronic pesticide poisoning is the potential for chronic persistent accumulation in the body. This accumulation occurs in *all* individuals because of nonoccupational exposure through food (even though the absolute amount may be low), inhalation, or skin absorption. Thus, in the general population a background concentration, e.g., in body fat, of certain halogenated hydrocarbons is detectable, including PCBs, DDT, DDE (metabolite of DDT), hexachlorobenzene, dieldrin, lindane and its isomers, and sometimes TCDD (dioxin), pentachlorophenol, and BHT (butylhydroxytoluene). In lower concentrations in body fat in non-occupationally exposed individuals are detected (sometimes less consistently) chemicals such as aldrin, heptachlor, oxychlordane, Mirex, Kepone, DDD, PBBs, chlorinated benzenes, polychlorinated terphenyls, tetrachlorophenol, toxaphene, phthalate esters (e.g., DEHP, used as a plasticizer in plastics), and a variety of more volatile chlorinated aliphatic hydrocarbons.[10] Thus, a definite body burden of halogenated hydrocarbons exists, a priori, in every patient. Subtle neuropsychologic testing of absolutely unexposed individuals (controls), including infants and children, does not exist; all individuals have some exposure to halogenated hydrocarbons.

One may assess the potential for accumulation by use of *a calculated bioconcentration factor (BCF).*[10] The BCF is the ratio between the concentration of a chemical in tissue (e.g., fat) (mg/kg) and the concentration of the same chemical in the diet (mg/kg). A BCF of 1 or less means that no accumulation has occurred. Table 26–9 lists the BCFs for several chemicals and pesticides. Some of these numbers are rather sobering. Such data are valuable in assessing relative risk for body accumulation. Another conceptually useful method for assessment of chronic toxicity, particularly in occupational exposure, is the Chronic Exposure Index (CED).[11]

$$\text{CED} = \log_{10} \frac{[y \times D - 1]}{(\text{age} - 18)},$$

where Y is the number of years of exposure to a pesticide and D is the most recent estimate of number of days of usage of pesticides per year. Index values from the median value to the highest value for a particular group of subjects are defined as high chronic exposure; those from the lowest to the median value are called low chronic exposure.[11] In addition, knowledge of relative chronic toxicity data also is useful in assessing overall risk,[12] as is information on specific mecha-

Table 26–9. BIOCONCENTRATION FACTORS OF CHEMICALS IN HUMANS (FAT)

CHEMICAL	BCF
PCBs (polychlorinated biphenyls)	251
Dioxin (2,3,7,8-TCDD)	170
DDT (DDT + DDE + DDD)	1279
Hexachlorobenzene (HCB)	674
beta-Hexachlorocyclohexane (beta-HCH)	527
gamma-Hexachlorocyclohexane (lindane)	18.6
Pentachlorophenol	3.7
BHT (butylated hydroxytoluene)	0.55

(Modified from Regulat Toxicol Pharmacol 6:313, 1986.)

nisms, such as metabolite-related tissue binding of halogenated hydrocarbons that result in more selective tissue toxicity.[13]

Symptoms and signs of chronic organochlorine/halogenated hydrocarbon pesticide poisoning are illustrated by the cyclodiene pesticides. These include chlordane, heptachlor, aldrin, and dieldrin. Two types of chronic exposure syndromes occur.[14] In one, the exposure is continuous and leads to a slow accumulation of insecticide along with progressive symptoms. In the second type of chronic syndrome, insecticide exposure remains below that needed to cause symptoms; however, the individual becomes very sensitive to further intake.[14] In 10 to 20 per cent of sprayers applying dieldrin who became poisoned, the earliest clinical signs developed in 3 months of exposure, but most workers required 8 or more months of exposure.[14] Mild illness consisted of headache (that often was unresponsive to drugs and was persistent), dizziness, general malaise, insomnia, nausea, increased sweating, nystagmus, diplopia, tinnitus, slight involuntary movements, and blurred vision. Severe illness included progression to myoclonic jerking involving one or more limbs, sometimes accompanied by brief loss of consciousness. Approximately half of the 10 to 20 per cent of cases progressed to convulsions.[14]

Persistent neurologic sequelae from cyclodiene chronic poisoning include EEG abnormalities lasting long after objective signs of toxicity have resolved. Normalization of the EEG after exposure has stopped may require up to 3 months for endrin, a year for dieldrin and more than a year for telodrin.[14] During continued chronic exposure to a mixture of chlorinated hydrocarbons, organophosphates, and carbamates in asymptomatic, occupationally exposed workers, chronic elevation of serum epinephrine and of serum glucose (77 versus 127 mg/dl, controls vs. exposed) was reported.[11] Thus, neurologic effects of chronic pesticide exposure apparently include sympathetic stimulation of the adrenal glands. Similar data for altered neurologic and altered dopamine and pituitary function are reported for exposure to the hydrocarbon styrene.[15]

Chronic poisoning from halogenated hydrocarbons results in measurable neurophysiologic and neuropsychologic abnormalities. Chronic toxic encephalopathy, once established, improves only slightly or not at all with time. Older individuals are more severely affected and less likely to recover. In one study, psychometric retesting 4 years later (4 years' exposure free) showed significant deterioration in verbal memory with improvement in visual memory.[16] Computed tomography of the brain may or may not demonstrate loss of brain substance.[17]

Similarly, persistent long-term neurophysiologic effects of TCDD (dioxin) have been studied.[18] No clinically evident neurotoxicity was noted in an unreported study cited by Young[19] of prison volunteers in the mid-1960s who were exposed dermally to 2,3,7,8-TCDD (dioxin). The experiment was done to determine the dose of TCDD required to induce chloracne. A suspension of 1 per cent TCDD in chloroform/alcohol was applied to the backs of 10 subjects on alternate days for 1 month. The cumulative applied dose was 7500 μg of TCDD. Eight of the ten subjects developed chloracne, which lasted 4 to 7 months. Blood chemistry determinations, including hematologic, liver, and kidney function, remained within normal limits.[19] TCDD is highly persistent, with a whole body half-life of approximately 5 years. Poiger dosed himself orally with 105 ng of 3H-TCDD in corn oil.[20] The dose of 1.14 ng per kg contained only 13 microcuries of tritium. Approximately 88.5 per cent of the dose was absorbed. Radioactivity was detected only in the feces and was excreted at a rate of 0.03 per cent of the body burden per day; the whole body half-life was estimated to be 5.8 years.[20] Pharmacokinetic approaches to such long half-life chemicals are still being developed.[21]

The Bhopal incident of massive methyl isocyanate exposure is an example of chronic chemical exposure. Although often considered a relatively short-term exposure, increasing evidence exists that the methyl isocyanate exposure at Bhopal has resulted in persistent long-term sequelae in survivors.[22] The primary sequela is chronic pulmonary damage, a combined obstructive and restrictive type. Methyl isocyanate–specific antibodies have been detected in the serum of some of the victims upon follow-up, and the antibody titer seems to correlate with the severity of the lung injury.[22] Of over 200,000 people exposed to methyl isocyanate, most probably about 5,000 died within 2 days, and about 60,000 individuals require long-term medical management.[22]

ASSESSMENT OF EXPOSURE HISTORY

One of the most difficult aspects in evaluating a patient claiming to have or presenting with chronic pesticide poisoning is obtaining a meaningful medical history. Those individuals who already decided that they will pursue legal redress for their exposure often have attributed (sometimes unknowingly) many minor and nonspecific complaints to the alleged exposure. Other individuals with legitimate medical toxicologic events may be unable to reconstruct a completely useful history despite skillful questioning.

In an attempt to obtain a more consistent and thorough history, many medical toxicologists have constructed patient history and physical examination forms. One example of such a form is shown in Figure 26–8. The primary purpose of such a form is to assist in the completeness of the evaluation and secondarily to expedite the process. Such a form is particularly useful in the setting of an environmental-occupational toxicology clinic.

For the physician evaluating an individual patient, an exposure history as complete as possible and general knowledge of the toxicity effects on humans of the individual chemical(s) are usually the best information available for making a diagnosis and patient management recommendations. Equally important in regard to chemical exposure is information regarding the patient's general medical status, past medical history, and specific susceptibilities, e.g., known history of allergies or family history of cancer.

Knowledge of the individual chemical(s)' bioconcentration factor (BCF) may be of use for selected chemicals. For infants, it is useful to know that breast-fed neonates potentially may be subjected to much higher halogenated hydrocarbon pesticide intake per kilogram of body weight than are adults because of the much higher concentration of these chemicals in human milk.[23] Indeed, milk is the major route of excretion of body burdens of highly fat-soluble chemicals such as dioxin (TCDD). Matsamura writes, "If a 5-kg infant consumed 0.7 liter of human milk daily containing DDT at an average concentration of 0.08 ppm, the resulting dosage would be 0.0112 mg/kg/day. This value may be compared with the average adult daily intake of 0.0005 mg/kg/day. Assuming a 2- to 3-fold increased sensitivity to the toxic effects of DDT in infants compared to adults, this amounts to eight times more than the FAO-WHO–recommended maximum acceptable dose!"[23] Similar considerations for lindane isomers (total benzene hexachloride) reveal that up to 1000 times more than the daily adult per kg intake may be "dosed" to infants![23] Subcutaneous fat concentrations of chlorinated hydrocarbons from infants and children sampled in 1982 reflected a highly significant association with the quantity of mother's milk consumed.[24] Some individual fat concentrations were higher than the mean values for adults from other areas.[24] Because hydrocarbons have been documented to alter biochemically the developing brain in young laboratory animals,[25] these human infant data have to be viewed with concern.

Increasing data are available on quantification of pesticide exposure in various situations. Home gardening exposure to the carbamate carbaryl is approximately 8.5 mg per 10 grams of pesticide applied to garden plants.[26] Protective clothing reduced exposure by 20-fold. Since 92.5 per cent of suburban residents are reported to use pesticides around the home, such exposure has considerable significance.[26] Similarly, the risk of aerial pesticide spraying is unknown and requires further evaluation.[27]

Assessment of Symptoms

Assessment of symptoms is a subjective evaluation. This is particularly difficult in chronic pesticide poisoning for at least two reasons: (1) many symptoms are nonspecific (e.g., headache, intermittent dizziness) or vague (e.g., general malaise), and (2) in the United States the patient may be planning legal action or be seeking workmen's compensation relating to the pesticide exposure and thus may perceive his or her symptoms differently. It is important for the physician to exercise skillful judgment and, if possible, rely on prior experience. In the end, a judgment of the relevance of the complaints to the chemical exposure has to be made.

Assessment of Signs

Assessment of signs is generally an objective evaluation. In chronic pesticide poisoning, the physical examination should be done

TOXICOLOGY CLINIC

HISTORY

1. Name: (Last) (First) (Middle) 2. Date:

3. Age: 4. Birthdate: 5. Personal Physician:

6. Employer's Name and Address:

PAST HISTORY

A. Have you ever had a serious illness? yes no

B. Have you had any illness requiring a physician in the past two years? yes no

C. Have you any trouble or disability at present? yes no

D. Where do you work? ________________

E. What type of product is made or what is the nature of business where your work?
____

F. What is your job title? ________________

G. What exactly do you do in your job? ________________
____

H. What is (are) the name(s) of chemical(s) or products manufactured in your area of work? ________________
____

I. Are you exposed to fumes, dust, chemicals, or radiation? ________________
If so, list any medication you are taking now:________________
____

J. Are you on any medication? ________________
If so, list any medication your are taking now:________________
____

Have you ever been a patient in a hospital? yes no
If yes, for what reason?
____

Have you ever received x-ray or radiation therapy? yes no
____

Are you in an area or profession where special health hazards are present or tested for? yes no
____

Are you subject to hives? yes no
____

Are you allergic to anything? yes no
____

Are you allergic to or have you had any ill effect from any drugs or medications? yes no
If yes, list:
____

Have you had a skin disorder or rash within the last two years? yes no
____

Have you gained or lost weight in the last year? yes no
gain: loss:
____

Do you use tobacco? yes no
To what extent?
____

Have you had or have you now any of the following?

	yes	no		yes	no		yes	no
Cancer	[ ]	[ ]	Drowsiness	[ ]	[ ]	Sore throat	[ ]	[ ]
Epilepsy	[ ]	[ ]	Nausea/vomiting	[ ]	[ ]	Difficulty swallowing	[ ]	[ ]
Heart disease	[ ]	[ ]	Gout	[ ]	[ ]	Hoarseness	[ ]	[ ]
Kidney trouble	[ ]	[ ]	Tremors	[ ]	[ ]	Twitching muscles	[ ]	[ ]
Asthma	[ ]	[ ]	Headaches	[ ]	[ ]	Chest pain	[ ]	[ ]
Jaundice	[ ]	[ ]	Fainting	[ ]	[ ]	Shortness of breath	[ ]	[ ]
Pleurisy	[ ]	[ ]	Dizziness	[ ]	[ ]	High blood pressure	[ ]	[ ]
Tuberculosis	[ ]	[ ]	Convulsions	[ ]	[ ]	Palpitations/pounding of the heart	[ ]	[ ]
Pneumonia	[ ]	[ ]	Rheumatism	[ ]	[ ]	Asthma	[ ]	[ ]
Arthritis	[ ]	[ ]	Easy fatigability	[ ]	[ ]	Persistent cough	[ ]	[ ]
Migraine	[ ]	[ ]	Memory difficulty	[ ]	[ ]	Persistent/frequent diarrhea	[ ]	[ ]
Stomach ulcer	[ ]	[ ]	Ringing in ears	[ ]	[ ]	Excessive fat/cholesterol in blood	[ ]	[ ]
Blood in urine	[ ]	[ ]	Loss of hearing	[ ]	[ ]	Large amounts of sputum	[ ]	[ ]
Diabetes	[ ]	[ ]	Difficulty breathing	[ ]	[ ]	Indigestion or nervous stomach	[ ]	[ ]
Goiter	[ ]	[ ]	Irritability	[ ]	[ ]			

Figure 26–8. Personal history form.

with particular attention toward target organs for toxicity of a particular chemical, if known. The neurologic examination and close scrutiny for signs compatible with cancer, when there is a long history of exposure, are important.

Biologic monitoring is becoming increasingly sophisticated and helpful in the initial assessment of chronic pesticide exposure and for follow-up. Biologic monitoring includes a variety of approaches—measurement of air levels of a specific chemical; direct measurement of blood, urine, or fat levels of a specific chemical; measurement of a metabolite in urine or of a toxicologically relevant (e.g., thioether compounds) metabolite in urine; or measurement of a biochemical effect relevant to toxicity risk (e.g., DNA-adducts in urine; urine porphyrins). Unlike environmental monitoring, biologic monitoring can assess exposure by all routes, not just by the inhalation route. Biologic monitoring potentially may assess the actual uptake of a chemical by an individual. Also, biologic monitoring, depending on the specific parameter, may take into account, at least in part, individual variability for risk from a given level of exposure. A biologic exposure index (BEI) theoretically can be developed for many specific chemicals.[28] For trichloroethylene, the BEI is 100 mg of TCA (trichloroacetic acid) per liter of urine, with the specimen collected at the end of the work week; this is the acceptable upper limit of exposure. Greater concentrations indicate excessive exposure requiring further investigation.

One useful approach to biologic monitoring, especially for low-level exposure, has been the repeated sequential measurement of plasma pseudocholinesterase to monitor organophosphate exposure of agricultural field workers and those exposed to pesticide spray drift.[29] Small but definite intra-individual plasma pseudocholinesterase differences over time were found in individuals intermittently exposed to organophosphate spray drift compared with those not exposed.[29] Measurement of urinary alkylphosphates may be a more sensitive method for biologic monitoring of low-level organophosphate exposure.[29, 30] Sequential monitoring for specific pesticides also appears indicated for indoor work areas such as greenhouses.[31, 32]

Biologic monitoring for risk of developing organophosphate-induced polyneuropathy (NTE inhibition) appears possible with the development of a lymphocyte or platelet NTE assay.[6] Validation by careful clinical studies is needed prior to more widespread use of this test.

The porphyrin excretion pattern in urine may become a useful biologic monitor for certain pesticides and chemicals. Chemicals considered porphyrinogenic include PCBs, PBBs, TCCD, vinyl chloride, chlorinated naphthalenes, and some organophosphorus and organochlorine pesticides.[33] Chemically induced porphyria occurs owing to inhibition of uroporphyrinogen decarboxylase, an enzyme that is part of heme synthesis. Inhibition of this enzyme results in accumulation and increased excretion of uroporphyrin and heptacarboxylic porphyrin.[33] Only small elevations in urinary porphyrins have been seen generally in individuals exposed to chemicals such as PCBs. In one study, a few individuals had a urinary uroporphyrin excretion of 66 to 106 μg per 24 hours following exposure to PCBs, compared with a nonexposed group whose values measured less than 60 μg per 24 hours.[34] Other studies have suggested that a total porphyrin (not uroporphyrin) excretion in adults of up to 200 μg per liter of urine is normal.[33] The pattern of porphyrins excreted rather than the total amount appears more significant for biologic monitoring purposes.[33, 34] An increase in uroporphyrin and heptacarboxylic porphyrin may be an early finding in chemically induced porphyria.[33] An increase in uroporphyrin and a decrease in coproporphyrin was seen following PCB exposure.[34]

Another potentially useful and rational approach to biologic monitoring for selected pesticides and chemicals is the measurement of urinary thioethers.[35, 36] A usual but not necessary requirement is that the chemical be metabolically activated to an electrophilic (positively charged), short-lived toxic metabolite by the cytochrome P-450 microsomal mixed-function oxidase drug-metabolizing enzymes. Besides electrophilic intermediates, such chemicals as aliphatic and aromatic halides and alpha-beta unsaturated ketones may undergo direct (nonglutathione transferase) conjugation with glutathione. The technique exploits the fact that conjugation with glutathione, followed by urinary elimination as mercapturic acid metabolites, is a significant metabolic pathway, especially for putative toxic metabolites. Urinary thioethers potentially may indicate the extent of internal contamination of an exposed individual. Gasoline station attendants who dispensed gasoline directly at full-serve pumps versus those attendants who did not (self-serve pumps) had urinary thioether concentrations (median value, 7 to 8 pm per urine void) of approximately 8 μmol-SH/mmol of creatinine versus approximately 2 μmol-SH/mmol of creatinine, respectively.[35] Although urinary thioether output detects dose-related increases in chemical exposure in animal models,[37] this has not yet been demonstrated conclusively in clinical studies. Inhibition of red blood cell glutathione-S-transferase potentially may be another useful marker of toxic chemical body burden.[38] Some organochlorine and halogenated hydrocarbon pesticides (many of which are no longer marketed in the United States) are known to be metabolically activated and also known, upon chronic high-dose exposure, to be carcinogenic in laboratory animals.[39, 40] Assessment of chronic exposure to these or similar pesticides by urinary thioether measurement in the future may become a useful biologic monitor. Certainly this approach deserves further careful, well-designed, prospective clinical studies.

An exciting and potentially highly significant biologic monitor is DNA-adduct formation. DNA-adduct formation represents a direct chemical covalent bond between one of the bases of DNA and a chemical. The combination may be measured as a DNA-adduct. Such adduct formation may be one of the initial steps necessary for chemically induced carcinogenesis. However, one has to be very cautious in attempting to apply such information clinically unless solid data validate a correlation between a given monitoring technique and the risk of human cancer.

DNA-adduct measurement in the white blood cells of iron foundry workers correlated quantitatively with air concentrations of polycyclic aromatic hydrocarbons, such as benzpyrene.[41] The mean adduct levels (femtomoles of adduct per microgram of DNA) ranged from 0.24 to 1.5 fmol/μg (or, expressed differently, 0.80 to 5.0 mean adducts/10^7 nucleotides) and correlated with air concentrations of less than 0.05 to over 0.2 μg of benzpyrene per cubic meter of air in the workplace. Similarly, vinyl chloride, known to cause angiosarcoma of the liver in humans, reacts to form DNA-adducts.[42] One has to be cautious in interpreting data. For example, although styrene, used in the manufacture of plastics, produces chromosome aberrations in cultured blood lymphocytes in vitro, workers exposed to low levels of styrene show no measurable chromosome abnormalities.[43] Hemoglobin adducts of certain chemicals represent another biologic monitoring endpoint and are described for ethylene oxide, benzene, benzpyrene, and dimethylnitrosamine.[44]

In summary, many techniques exist or are being developed for biologic monitoring. Some will prove more predictive than others. Biologic monitoring of chronic pesticide exposure will expand as mechanisms of toxicity and new techniques advance.[45, 46]

WORK-UP OF NEUROTOXICITY

The work-up of neurotoxicity in individual patients can be divided into the assessment of the peripheral nervous system (PNS) and the central nervous system (CNS). In general, somewhat more objective measurements (neurophysiologic testing) can be made in examination of the PNS compared with the CNS (neuropsychologic testing), with the exception of evoked potential measurements.

For PNS function, it is important to remember that axonal neuropathies are associated often with deficits of both sensory and motor function.[47] Motor function testing includes inspection for muscle atrophy and unusual movements; analysis of coordination; testing muscle tone and resistance to passive stretch of an extremity; the Babinski reflex; and analysis of strength of individual muscles. Sensory function testing includes evoking the sensations produced by warmth and cold, pinprick, joint movement, tuning fork vibration, and shapes of complex objects. Cranial nerve examination, especially optic (II) and trigeminal (V) nerve function, is important in evaluation of toxic exposures.[47] Similarly, evaluating the autonomic nervous system for bladder, bowel, and sexual function, pupil response, lacrimation, salivation, sweating, and supine-upright blood pressure is important.

Knowledge of the specific toxin is helpful in planning and analyzing PNS evaluation. For example, in acrylamide neuropathy, sensory symptoms and signs are prominent.[48] By contrast, neurotoxic esterase (NTE) neuropathy from organophosphates may show retention of sensory function in the face of significant distal wasting and weakness.[48] Nerve conduction velocity may not be altered in organophosphate NTE neuropathy, but a large drop in muscle action potential amplitude (EMG testing) may be observed. Acrylamide toxicity can be detected earlier by monitoring vibration sensation in fingers, e.g., using a portable Optacon device.[47] In hexacarbon solvents, e.g., *n*-hexane or methylbutyl ketone toxic neuropathy, use of nerve motor conduction velocity measurements is valuable because these solvents affect conduction.[48] Blue-yellow color vision loss from solvent exposure is well documented.[49] The Lanthony D-15 desaturated panel test for color vision loss has been validated for use at the workplace as an initial screening tool.[49]

For CNS function, evaluation of mental status includes assessment of the level of consciousness, orientation, concentration, memory, cognitive functions, behavior, mood, and affect. The most frequently reported behavioral effect of chemicals is a disturbance in psychomotor functioning. Usually, this is characterized by a delay or slowness in response time, clumsy or awkward eye-hand coordination or dexterity, or a combination of these. Diminished attention also has been found.[50] For a thorough evaluation of suspected neuropsychologic deficits, use of a standard battery of psychologic tests is the best available procedure.[47] Such testing is time consuming and usually is done by psychologists trained in the use of such tests. There is a need for standardized neuropsychologic tests of a sufficient degree of simplicity and speed of administration such that they can be administered more readily to blue collar industrial workers as well as individuals with non-occupational environmental exposures. Furthermore, such test results must be adjusted for age and education level.

One example of a neuropsychologic test battery with published normative data from a control population with no known previous history of occupational exposure to industrial chemicals is the POET (Pittsburgh Occupational Exposure Test) battery.[51] Other descriptions of neuropsychologic testing results support the use of computed tomography (CT) head x-ray scans and targeting specific neuropsychologic tests for specific exposure situations.[17, 52, 53] A few specific examples of chemicals for which formal neuropsychologic testing for exposure effects has been done include organophosphates, inorganic lead, carbon disulfide, mercury, styrene, perchloroethylene and trichloroethylene,[50] chlorinated solvent mixtures such as that of methylene chloride plus Freon 113 plus trichloroethylene,[54] and the fumigants methyl bromide and sulfuryl fluoride.[55]

TREATMENT

Treatment of chronic pesticide poisoning or exposure requires careful medical evaluation and a thorough assessment of the exposure situation. Recommendation that the patient be removed from further exposure may be more easily followed for nonoccupational exposures. For occupational exposures, removal of the worker to another area of the work site where lower exposure occurs may, on occasion, be acceptable medically. Alternatively, temporary removal while clean-up measures are begun also, on occasion, may be acceptable medically. Monitoring exposure at the work site by a medically suitable means should be a part of all recommendations and follow-up evaluations of workers with chronic pesticide toxicity.

Treatment of symptoms, other than removal from further exposure, often may be symptomatic only. Protective clothing can be recommended and should be worn for certain chemical exposure situations. More published data are becoming available to identify improved protective clothing materials,[56, 57] e.g., polyvinyl alcohol polymer material to resist permeation of methylene chloride.[58]

Gastrointestinal dialysis may offer the possibility of enhancing the rate of removal of the body burden of certain chemicals that have long residence times (measured in months to years) and are sequestered in kinetically deep storage sites (usually body fat). A well-documented example was the use of repeated oral cholestyramine therapy to increase the removal of chlordecone (Kepone), a highly neurotoxic chemical.[59] Other examples include the use of repeated oral mineral oil to enhance excretion of chlordane and lindane.[60–62]

In summary, diagnosis and management of chronic pesticide poisoning presents a significant challenge to current medical toxicology capabilities. With careful attention to the details of exposure history and clinical findings in each individual patient, coupled with knowledge of the chemical involved, an individualized management plan can be formulated that should be beneficial for most patients.

References

1. WHO: Safe use of pesticides. Tech Report Series 513. Geneva, 1973.
2. Editorial: Health problems of pesticide usage in the third world. Br J Indust Med *42*:505, 1985.
3. Maugh TH: Chemicals: How many are there? Science *199*:162, 1978.
4. Cherniack MG: Organophosphorus esters and polyneuropathy. Ann Intern Med *104*:264, 1986.
5. Hollingshaus JG, Fukuto TR: Effect of chronic exposure to pesticides on delayed neurotoxicity. *In* Chambers JE, Yarbrough JD (eds): Effect of Chronic Exposures to Pesticides on Animal Systems. New York, Raven Press, 1982, p 85.
6. Lotti M: Biological monitoring for organophosphate-induced delayed polyneuropathy. Toxicol Lett *33*:167, 1986.
7. Savage EP, Keefe TJ, Mounce LM, Heaton RK, Lewis JA, Burcar PJ: Chronic neurological sequelae of acute organophosphate pesticide poisoning. Arch Environ Health *43*:38, 1988.
8. Wadia RS, Chitra S, Amin RB, Kiwalkar RS, Sardesai HV: Electrophysiological studies in acute organophosphate poisoning. J Neurol Neurosurg Psychiatr *50*:1442, 1987.
9. Hayes WJ: Pesticides Studied in Man. Baltimore, Williams and Wilkins, 1982, p 172.
10. Geyer H, Scheunert I, Korte F: Bioconcentration potential of organic environmental chemicals in humans. Regulatory Toxicol Pharmacol *6*:313, 1986.
11. Berberian IG, Evan EE: Neurotoxic studies in humans occupationally exposed to pesticides. J Soc Occup Med *37*:126, 1987.
12. De Rosa CT, Stara JF, Durkin PR: Ranking chemicals based on chronic toxicity data. Toxicol Indust Health *1*:177, 1985.
13. Brandt I: Metabolism-related tissue binding of halogenated hydrocarbons. Ups J Med Sci *91*:289, 1986.
14. Eicobichon DJ, Joy RM: Pesticides and Neurological Diseases. Boca Raton, FL, CRC Press, 1982, p 134.
15. Arfini G, et al: Impaired dopaminergic modulation of pituitary secretion in workers occupationally exposed to styrene: Further evidence from PRL (prolactin) response to TRH stimulation. J Occup Med *29*:826–830, 1987.
16. Orbaek P, Lindgren M: Prospective clinical and psychometric investigation of patients with chronic toxic encephalopathy induced by solvents. Scand J Work Environ Health *14*:37, 1988.
17. Orbaek P, Lindgren M, Olivecrona H, Haeger-Aronsen B: Computed tomography and psychometric test performances in patients with solvent-induced chronic toxic encephalopathy and healthy controls. Br J Indust Med *44*:175, 1987.
18. Barbieri S, et al: Long-term effects of 2,3,7,8-tetrachlorodibenzo-*p*-dioxin on the peripheral nervous system. Clinical and neurophysiological controlled study on subjects with chloracne from the Seveso area. Neuroepidemiology *7*:29, 1988.
19. Young AL: Determination and measurement of human exposure to the dibenzo-*p*-dioxins. Bull Environ Contam Toxicol *33*:702, 1984.
20. Poiger H, Schlatter C: Pharmacokinetics of 2,3,7,8-TCCD in man. Chemosphere *15*:1489, 1986.
21. McNamara PJ, Fleishaker JC, Hayden TL: Mean residence time in peripheral tissue. J Pharmacokinet Biopharm *15*:439, 1987.
22. Varma DR: Anatomy of the methyl isocyanate leak in Bhopal. *In* Saxena J (ed): Hazard Assessment of Chemicals. Washington, DC, Hemisphere Publishing Corporation. 1987, p 233.
23. Matsumura F: Hazards to man and domestic animals. *In* Matsumura F (ed): Toxicology of Insecticides. 2nd ed. New York, Plenum Press, 1985, p 566.
24. Niessen KH, Ramolla J, Binder M, Brugmann G, Hoffmann U: Chlorinated hydrocarbons in adipose tissue of infants and toddlers: Inventory and studies on their association with intake of mothers' milk. Eur J Pediatr *142*:238, 1984.
25. Bhatt A, Kahn S, Pandya KP, Sabri MI: Effect of hexacarbons on selected lipids in developing rat brain and peripheral nerves. J Appl Toxicol *8*:53–57, 1988.
26. Kurtz DA, Bode WM: Application exposure to the home gardener. *In* Honeycutt RC, Zweig G, Ragsdale NN (eds): Dermal Exposure Related to Pesticide Use. Washington, DC, American Chemical Society, 1985, p 139.
27. Ratner D, Eshel E: Aerial pesticide spraying: An environmental hazard. JAMA *256*:2516, 1986.
28. Lowry LK: The biological exposure index: Its use in assessing chemical exposures in the workplace. Toxicology *47*:55–69, 1987.
29. Richter ED, Rosenvald Z, Kaspi L, Levy S, Gruener N: Sequential cholinesterase tests and symptoms for monitoring organophosphate absorption in field workers and in persons exposed to pesticide spray drift. Toxicol Lett *33*:25, 1986.
30. Franklin CA, Muir NI, Moody RP: The use of biological monitoring in the estimation of exposure during the application of pesticides. Toxicol Lett *33*:127, 1986.
31. Kundiev YI, Krasnyuk EP, Viter VP: Specific features of the changes in the health status of female workers exposed to pesticides in greenhouses. Toxicol Lett *33*:85, 1986.
32. Desi I, Palotas M, Vetro G, Csolle I, Nehez N, Zimanyi M, Ferke A, Huszta E, Nagymajtenyi L: Biological monitoring and health surveillance of a group of greenhouse pesticide sprayers. Toxicol Lett *33*:91, 1986.
33. Strik JJT: Porphyrins in urine as an indication of exposure to chlorinated hydrocarbons. Ann NY Acad Sci *514*:219, 1987.
34. Osterloh J, Cone J, Harrison R, Wade R, Becker C: Pilot survey of urinary porphyrins from persons transiently exposed to a PCB transformer fire. J Toxicol Clin Toxicol *24*:533, 1987.
35. Stock JK, Priestly BG: Urinary thioether output as an index of occupational chemical exposure in petroleum retailers. Br J Indust Med *43*:718, 1986.
36. Lafuente A, Cobos A, Mallol J: A pilot study of urinary thioethers as biological indicators of the urban contamination. Public Health *101*:267, 1987.
37. Rozman K, Summer KH, Rozman T, Greim H: Elimination of thioethers following administration of naphthalene and diethylmaleate to the rhesus monkey. Drug Chem Toxicol *5*:265, 1982.

38. Ansari GAS, Singh SV, Gan JC, Awasthi YC: Human erythrocyte glutathione-S-transferase: A possible marker of chemical exposure. Toxicol Lett *37*:57, 1987.
39. Epstein SS: The carcinogenicity of heptachlor and chlordane. Sci Total Environ *6*:103, 1976.
40. Infante PF, Epstein SS, Newton WA: Blood dyscrasias and childhood tumors and exposure to chlordane and heptachlor. Scand J Work Environ Health *4*:137, 1978.
41. Perera FP, Hemminki K, Young TL, Brenner D, Kelly G, Santella RM: Detection of polycyclic aromatic hydrocarbon DNA adducts in white blood cells of foundry workers. Cancer Res *48*:2288, 1988.
42. Bolt HM, Laib RJ, Peter H, Ottenwalder H: DNA adducts of halogenated hydrocarbons. J Cancer Res Clin Oncol *112*:92, 1986.
43. Maki-Paakkanen J: Chromosome aberrations, micronuclei and sister-chromatid exchanges in blood lymphocytes after occupational exposure to low levels of styrene. Mutat Res *189*:399, 1987.
44. Farmer PB, Neumann HG, Henschler D: Estimation of exposure of man to substances reacting covalently with macromolecules. Arch Toxicol *60*:251, 1987.
45. Ashby J: Comparison of techniques for monitoring human exposure to genotoxic chemicals. Mutat Res *204*:543–551, 1988.
46. Symposia: Biological monitoring of workers manufacturing, formulating and applying pesticides. Proceedings of the Seventh International Workshop of the Scientific Committee on Pesticides of the International Commission on Occupational Health. Toxicol Lett *33*:1, 1986.
47. Spencer PS, Arezzo J, Schaumburg H: Chemicals causing disease of neurons and their processes. *In* O'Donoghue JL (ed): Neurotoxicity of Industrial and Commercial Chemicals. Vol I. Boca Raton, FL, CRC Press, 1985, pp 1–14.
48. LeQuesne PM: Neurophysiological investigation of subclinical and minimal toxic neuropathies. Muscle Nerve *1*:392–395, 1978.
49. Mergler D, Blain L: Assessing color vision loss among solvent exposed workers. Am J Indust Med *12*:195–203, 1987.
50. Feldman RG, Ricks NL, Baker EL: Neuropsychological effects of industrial toxins: A review. Am J Indust Med *1*:211–227, 1980.
51. Ryan CM, Morrow LA, Bromet EJ, Parkinson DK: Assessment of neuropsychological dysfunction in the workplace: Normative data from the Pittsburgh Occupational Exposures Test battery. J Clin Exper Neuropsychol *9*:665–679, 1987.
52. Anger WK: Neurobehavioral tests used in NIOSH-supported worksite studies, 1973–1983. Neurobehav Toxicol Teratol *7*:359–368, 1985.
53. Maurissen JPJ: Psychophysical testing in human populations exposed to neurotoxicants. Neurobehav Toxicol Teratol *7*:309–317, 1985.
54. Rasmussen K, Sabroe S: Neuropsychological symptoms among metal workers exposed to halogenated hydrocarbons. Scand J Soc Med *14*:161–168, 1986.
55. Anger WK, Moody L, Burg J, Brightwell WS, Taylor BJ, Russo JM, Dickerson N, Setzer JV, Johnson BL, Hicks K: Neurobehavioral evaluation of soil and structural fumigators using methyl bromide and sulfuryl fluoride. Neurotoxicology *3*:137–156, 1986.
56. Brown DP: Mortality of workers exposed to polychlorinated biphenyls—an update. Arch Environ Health *42*:333–339, 1987.
57. Stampfer JF, McLeod MJ, Betts MR, Martinez AM, Berardinelli SP: Permeation of eleven protective garment materials by four organic solvents. Am Indust Hyg Assoc J *45*:642–654, 1984.
58. Berardinelli SP, Hall R: Site-specific whole glove chemical permeation. Am Indust Hyg Assoc J *46*:60–64, 1985.
59. Vahdat N: Permeation of protective clothing materials by methylene chloride and perchloroethylene. Am Indust Hyg Assoc J *48*:646–651, 1987.
60. Cohn WJ, Boylan JJ, Blanke RV, Fariss MW, Howell JR, Guzelian PS: Treatment of chlordecone (Kepone) toxicity with cholestyramine. N Engl J Med *298*:243–248, 1978.
61. Snodgrass WR, Kisker S, Rozman K: Enhanced elimination of an environmental chlorinated hydrocarbon in man: Use of oral mineral oil and cholestyramine. Vet Human Toxicol *25*(Suppl 1):59, 1983.
62. Snodgrass WR, Morgan DP, Winsett O, Roy D, Hadrzynski CL: Mobilization of a halogenated hydrocarbon pesticide from body fat in man: Lindane. Vet Human Toxicol *28*:471, 1986.

CHAPTER 27
POISONOUS SNAKEBITE

Lester Haddad, M.D.
George Podgorny, M.D.

Even as we approach the year 2000, the treatment of snakebite remains controversial. The purpose of this chapter is to review the present thinking on snakebite therapy and to develop a rational approach to the subject.

Mention will also be made of the other venomous reptile, the lizard *Heloderma suspectum,* or the Gila monster. Venomous arthropods and marine life are each discussed in separate chapters. The only venomous mammal in the United States is the short-tailed shrew, *Blarina brevicauda,* which rarely, if ever, has inflicted envenomation on humans.[1] No bird species has ever been known to be poisonous.

CLASSIFICATION OF SNAKES

The major snake families are the Colubridae, the Elapidae, the Hydrophidae, and the Viperidae (Table 27–1).

Colubridae

The principal snake family is the Colubridae, an enormous group of approximately 1400 species that includes roughly two thirds of the world's snakes, most of which are harmless. This group includes rat snakes, bull snakes, and garter snakes; there are 38 genera in the United States alone. King snakes are also nonpoisonous.

Bites of harmless snakes are significant only as contaminated puncture wounds. Harmless snakes have rows of teeth and frequently the imprints of the teeth are seen on the skin. Cleansing, debridement, and administration of tetanus prophylaxis as indicated usually suffice. The use of broad-spectrum antibiotics may be indicated because the mouth of the snake is a veritable pool of microorganisms. Infrequently, the bite of a harmless snake will produce swelling, itching, and erythema. This is an allergic reaction to the snake's saliva, and an antihistamine will quickly relieve the symptoms.

Recent reports indicate that perhaps 10 per cent of the colubrid snakes possess rear fangs and may occasionally cause an envenomization, which is usually very low-grade, producing only mild symptoms. Usually, treatment of the local symptoms will be sufficient. Such snakes include the hog-nosed snake, the corn snake, and the so-called lyre snakes of the genus *Trimorphodon*. These snakes inhabit areas of Arizona, California, Texas, and Mexico.

Fibrinolysis from these "harmless" colubrids has occasionally been reported, such as that from the bite of a red neck keelback, *Rhabdophis subminatus,* a supposedly harmless snake bought in the pet store.[2] Fibrinolysis from colubrid bites in Japan has also been reported.[3–5]

Africa has the only colubrid that is dangerous, the boomslang *(Dispholidus typus).*

Elapidae

The elapid family includes the highly poisonous coral snakes; the cobras; the African mambas; the kraits; and the Australian/Pacific elapids, which as a group represent nearly all of the poisonous snakes of Australia.

Coral

The only species of Elapidae native to the United States are coral snakes (see Figs. 27–5 and 27–6*). Coral snakes are small, slender, and shy reptiles. The eastern coral snake is *Micrurus fulvius*, and the Arizona or Sonoran coral snake is *Micruroides euryxanthus*. It is fortunate that both species possess a unique coloration that easily provides identification. Wide red and black bands are separated by narrow yellow rings; in the Sonoran coral snake, there is less disparity in the width of the yellow rings versus the black and red bands. This scheme is true of the main trunk

*On Color Plate I at the front of this book.

Table 27–1. CLASSIFICATION OF IMPORTANT POISONOUS SNAKES

FAMILY	COMMON NAME	SCIENTIFIC NAME
Colubridae	Boomslang	*Dispholidus typus*
Elapidae	Coral	
	Eastern coral	*Micrurus fulvius fulvius*
	Arizona or Sonoran coral	*Micrurus euryxanthus*
	Cobra	
	Egyptian	*Naja haje*
	Indian	*Naja naja naja*
	King	*Ophiophagus hannah*
	Mamba	
	African green	*Dendroaspis angusticeps*
	African black	*Dendroaspis polyepis*
	Krait	
	Malayan	*Bungarus candidus*
	Australian/Pacific	
	Common death adder	*Acanthophis antarctica*
	Tiger snake	*Notechis scutatus*
	Taipan snake	*Oxyuranus scutellatus*
Hydrophidae (Sea Snakes)		
Viperidae		
Subfamily: Old World "True" Viper		
	Russell's viper	*Vipera russelli*
	Common puff adder	*Bitis arietans*
	African gaboon viper	*Bitis gabonica*
	Carpet or "saw-scaled" viper	*Echis carinatus*
Subfamily: Crotalidae, the Pit Vipers		
	Agkistrodon (see Table 27–2)	
	Mamushi	*Agkistrodon halys*
	Bothrops	
	Barba amarilla	*Bothrops atrox*
	New World pit viper, or true fer-de-lance	*Bothrops lanceolatus*
	Crotalus (see Table 27–2)	
	Rattlesnakes	
	Lachesis	
	Bushmaster	*Lachesis mutus mutus*
	Sistrurus (see Table 27–2)	
	Trimeresurus	
	Okinawan habu	*Trimeresurus flavorviridis*
	Chinese habu	*Trimeresurus mucrosquamatus*

of the snake and does not hold constant on the head and tail. The snout of the coral snake is black.

A useful jingle for identification is

"Red on yellow—kill a fellow,
Red on black—venom lack."

Coral snakes have small heads and jaws and also possess small, nonmovable posterior fangs. The injection apparatus is not as efficient as that of vipers, and envenomation requires a longer period of the snake holding on to the prey. Because of this, the bites of coral snakes may present clinically as only scratch marks or as a minuscule puncture with little swelling.

Mamba

A most deadly group of elapids are the mambas of Africa: the black mamba, *Dendroaspis polyepis*, and the green mamba, *Dendroaspis angusticeps*.

Although mambas usually choose to flee rather than strike, they can kill a human in 15 minutes. They usually live in trees, although they have the ability to raise their bodies almost 2 feet above the ground as they scoot along on their tails at up to 7 miles an hour.

Kraits

Kraits are found throughout most of South Asia. They are characterized by a medium to large size, ranging from 3 to 4 feet and frequently are 6 or 7 feet in length. Furthermore, they often have colorful patterns of light and dark bands. Their fangs are short, and the venom is fairly toxic. Kraits belong to the genus *Bungarus*, and the two most common ones are *B. fasciatus*, the banded krait, and *B. coeruleus*. The major components of *Bungarus* venom are hemolysins, cholinesterase, and neurotoxins.

There is a minimal local reaction to the krait bite. However, within an hour or two, neurotoxic symptomatology similar to the bite of the coral snake appears.

Treatment of the krait bite is immediate administration of specific antivenin. In southern Asia, many antivenins are available to treat the krait bite. In Sri Lanka, India, and Bangladesh, an antivenin produced in India is used. Additional antivenins are produced in Bangkok, including a monovalent antivenin for the bite of the banded krait.

Viperidae

This family includes 2 major groups or subfamilies: the "true vipers" (vipers without a pit) of the Old World, and the Crotalidae, the pit vipers of America (and Asia).

Three "true" vipers of major importance include *Bitis arietans*, the common puff adder, which is the number one cause of death from snakebite in Morocco and North Africa; *Vipera russelli*, or Russell's viper, a major cause of death from snakebite in Thailand, Burma, and India; and *Echis carinatus*, the carpet or saw-scaled viper found from West Africa through the Middle East to Sri Lanka.

The Crotalidae (Table 27–2) is a major subfamily that includes the pit vipers. This group includes the rattlesnakes, the water moccasin (cottonmouth), and the copperhead, which account for over 90 per cent of poisonous snakebites in the United States.

The Crotalidae includes the genus *Bothrops* or American lancehead. Barba amarilla *(B. atrox)* is the number one snake to cause death in Central America. *B. atrox* is often mistakenly called the fer-de-lance; the true fer-de-lance, *B. lanceolatus*, is found only in Martinique. One of the most common snakes causing death in South America is the cascabel, the South American rattlesnake *(Crotalus durissus terrificus)*.

Although most pit vipers are in the Americas, the Agkistrodon has relatives in Japan and the Far East: *A. halys*, the mamushi, and *A. rhodostoma*, the Malayan pit viper. A relative of Bothrops is the genus *Trimeresurus*, or Asian lancehead, represented by the Chinese habu, *T. mucrosquamatus*, and the Okinawan habu, *T. flavorviridis*.

Pit vipers are distinguished by a facial pit on each side of the head situated a little below midway between eye and nostril. The pit is a heat-sensing organ that helps the snake to aim when striking at warm-blooded prey. *Any snake with such a pit is poisonous*. Pit vipers are further characterized by (1) an elliptical pupil, as opposed to round pupils in harmless snakes; (2) single caudal plates, as opposed to double caudal plates in harmless snakes; (3) well-developed fangs that protrude from the anterior aspect of the mouth; (4) a triangular-shaped head, and (5) rattles, on rattlesnakes only. A rattle is added each time a rattlesnake sheds its skin, which may occur up to 3 to 4 times a year. Although most rattlesnakes usually live 10 years, some have lived up to 20 years.[1]

Hydrophidae

Sea snakes have evolved from Elapidae and belong to the family Hydrophidae. Some of them are actually sea kraits. Sea snakes are totally aquatic and helpless on land. Their anatomy has been highly adapted for marine life; the body and particularly the tail are vertically compressed to provide swimming ability; the nostrils are on the top of the head rather than on the side, and specialized glands excrete salt in order to permit life in a saline environment.

Sea snakes inhabit the Pacific Ocean, and various species are found anywhere from South America to Southeast Asia to Australia and New Zealand.[6, 7] There are some sea snakes in the Indian Ocean as well. At this time, no venomous sea snake is known to inhabit the Atlantic Ocean. However, plans to create a sea level canal to replace or supplement the Panama Canal likely will result in the appearance of venomous sea snakes in the Atlantic Ocean.

Sea snake bites are said to be often almost painless. The fangs are extremely small, frequently only 2 to 3 millimeters in length. A major component of the venom of the sea snake is neurotoxin. Sea snake venoms are poor antigens, therefore interfering in the preparation of satisfactory antivenins. However, some antivenins are available. Symptomatology is similar to that of elapid snakes

Table 27–2. VENOMOUS PIT VIPER SNAKES (SUBFAMILY CROTALIDAE) OF AMERICA

COMMON NAME	SCIENTIFIC NAME	GEOGRAPHIC DISTRIBUTION
Rattlesnakes	***Genus:*** *Crotalus*	
Eastern diamondback	*Crotalus adamanteus*	Eastern seaboard; tidal and adjoining areas from North Carolina to Florida; Gulf Coast areas of Alabama, and Mississippi
Timber rattlesnake	*C. horridus*	North and northeast, except Maine and immediate area of Great Lakes; west of Mississippi into Central States and eastern Texas
Prairie rattlesnake	*C. viridis viridis*	Great Plains, including midwestern and prairie states
Western diamondback rattlesnake	*C. atrox*	Texas, Oklahoma, and west into southeastern California
Great Basin rattlesnake	*C. viridis lutosus*	Basin between Rocky and Sierra Nevada Mountains; Idaho, Utah, Arizona, Nevada, California, and Oregon
Northern Pacific rattlesnake	*C. viridis oreganus*	Pacific slope from British Columbia to California, including Washington, Oregon, and western Idaho
Southern Pacific rattlesnake	*C. viridis helleri*	Southern California and northern Baja California
Mojave	*C. scutulatus*	Southwestern Texas, Arizona, and southern Nevada to California
Mojave Desert sidewinder	*C. cerastes*	Utah, Arizona, and California
Central American	*C. durissus durissus*	Central America
South American	*C. durissus terrificus*	South America
Massasauga/pigmy	***Genus:*** *Sistrurus*	
Massasauga	*Sistrurus catenatus*	Florida to Tennessee, Arkansas, and Oklahoma; into Nebraska, Iowa, Colorado, Texas, and Arizona
Pigmy	*S. milliarius*	North Carolina to Florida and west to Oklahoma and Texas
Copperhead/cottonmouth	***Genus:*** *Agkistrodon*	
Southern copperhead	*Agkistrodon contortix*	Central Massachusetts to northern Florida and west to Illinois and eastern Texas
Eastern/Western cottonmouth	*A. piscivorus*	Southernmost Virginia to Florida and west from Florida to eastern Texas, Mississippi Valley, Illinois, and Indiana

and mostly represents neurotoxic findings similar to the bite of the coral snake.

Sea snakes have been reported to be aggressive. Bite victims are mainly fishermen. Very few sea snakes are in captivity in the United States.

The most common sea snake is *Pelamis platurus* or the yellow-bellied sea snake.[8]

CHARACTERISTICS OF SNAKES

Probably no other animal has been so scrutinized, maligned, and talked about as the snake. From time immemorial—in the Old Testament and Greek mythology to the folklore of the Middle Ages and that of the western United States—the snake has been a subject of attention and fascination.

It is estimated that nearly 50,000 people die yearly of snakebite; 75 per cent of these deaths occur in India.[1]

Snakes are unique animals because of their elongated, cylindrical body construction with an egg-shaped or occasionally triangular head. In most snakes, the body tapers caudad, ending sharply, except in rattlesnakes (Color Plate I, Figs. 27–1 and 27–2*). Snakes are limbless, although occasionally a few species exhibit limbal skeletal remnants.

Two other animals resemble the general configuration of the snake, namely eels and legless lizards. The former are fish, and the latter (only a few species) can be distinguished by having eyelids. Snakes possess an endoskeleton, and their surface is covered with hard and dry articulating scales.

The habitat of the snakes of North America ranges all over the continent, from the east-

*On Color Plate I at the front of this book.

ern Pennsylvania woods to the swamps of Florida, to the bayous of Louisiana, through the prairie, and into the Mojave Desert and to the West Coast. Rattlesnakes are the most adaptive in regard to their habitat and ecology, whereas moccasins prefer moisture and proximity to bodies of water.

The moccasin (Color Plate I, Fig. 27–3*) is also called the cottonmouth because of its white buccal mucosa. This snake prefers an almost amphibious habitat. It tends to be somewhat smaller than a rattlesnake, but its venom's potency characteristics parallel those of the rattlesnake. Another species is called the copperhead (Color Plate I, Fig. 27–4*) because of the copper-like coloration of many mature specimens. This snake is the predominant venomous snake in the United States, but fortunately it possesses the least potent venom. Copperheads predominate in wooded areas and open fields. Coral snakes have the smallest range and are somewhat shy and secretive.

Most of the snakes in North America basically withdraw in the face of danger. Attacks on humans and other animals occur as a part of self-defense. Because of the predominance of copperheads east of the Mississippi, most of the poisonous snakebites in this region are caused by them. West of the Mississippi, most of the poisonous bites are caused by rattlesnakes. A few coral snakebites occur in Florida, Georgia, the southern portions of South Carolina, and occasionally Arizona (Color Plate I, Figs. 27–5 and 27–6*). East of the Mississippi, bites mostly involve the extremities of humans; west of the Mississippi, bites frequently are found on the trunk.

The venom apparatus of snakes consists of venomous glands (anlage of the parotid glands) that produce and store the venom, venom canals that connect the glands to the fangs, and the palatine muscles that squeeze the glands and inject the venom. The fangs in pit viters are specialized hollow teeth, located anteriorly in the maxilla, whereas in coral snakes they are located posteriorly and are small and nonmovable; thus the coral snake must bite and chew to inject venom. In vipers, the fangs are normally folded underneath the premaxilla to swing out and be ready for injection before strike. The length of fangs ranges between 5 and 20 millimeters, and the distance between them ranges between 5 and 20 millimeters. *The size of the snake and, therefore, its potential envenomization ability, can be judged by the distance between the fangs, as exhibited by fang marks. A distance of 10 or fewer millimeters signifies a small snake, 10 to 15 millimeters represents a medium-sized snake, and over 15 millimeters is evidence of a large, venomous snake.*

So-called defanged snakes can ultimately be dangerous because all snakes periodically grow new fangs. When manipulated, a dying or dead snake may exhibit a reflex of palatine muscles and effect a bite.

Venom

Snake venoms are highly complex substances containing a mixture made primarily of proteins, many of which have enzymatic activities, such as proteinases, phospholipases, cholinesterases, and hyaluronidases.[9] The action of the venom as a whole is now known to be quite different than its separate components, because isolated peptides may be 3 to 25 times more toxic than the crude venom. The practice of dividing snake venoms into neurotoxins, fibrinolysins, cardiotoxins, and the like is clinically misleading. For example, coagulant, anticoagulant, and fibrinolytic activities may vary with each species of snake and even among different-aged snakes of the same species,[10, 11] possibly producing a variable and unpredictable coagulopathy in any particular patient. Thus, it is best to realize that snake envenomization may produce an entire spectrum of clinical illness with each individual patient.

The severity of poisoning is usually related to the location and severity of bite; the species and size of snake; the amount of injected venom; the age and size of the victim; and the sensitivity of the victim to the injected venom.

The size of the victim is important; therefore, children and infants are more vulnerable. The condition of the victim will seriously affect the outcome. Such conditions as hypertension, diabetes, advanced age, debility, or coagulation disorders are aggravated by venomous snakebite. Individuals who have bleeding tendencies, such as hemophiliacs or those receiving anticoagulant therapy; patients with active peptic ulcers; and patients with open wounds are more susceptible to

*On Color Plate I at the front of this book.

bleeding secondary to envenomation. Menstruating women may bleed excessively after pit viper bite. Women who have endometriosis may bleed excessively and develop severe pain. Cases have been reported of abortion in pregnant women who have been bitten by pit vipers.

The location of the bite is of great significance. Venomous snakebites on the head and trunk are two to three times more serious than those on the extremities. Bites on the upper extremities carry a worse prognosis than those on the lower extremities. Incidental penetration of the fangs into a blood vessel and the consequent injection of venom is usually catastrophic.

CLINICAL PRESENTATION

All snakebites fall within two broad categories: *asymptomatic*, inflicted by nonvenomous snakes or caused by venomous snakes without evidence of envenomation and therefore without bite-related symptomatology; and *symptomatic*, inflicted by venomous snakes causing identifiable and potentially significant envenomation. (Specifics of the recognition and treatment of this second category will follow.)

Clinical observation is the only means of distinguishing between these two all-important categories, and the decision resulting from this observation is one of the most important judgments a physician must face in the management of snakebites. If the offending snake has been specifically identified as a nonvenomous one and no symptoms appear after 4 hours, the patient may be sent home from the emergency department. If 4 to 6 hours have elapsed without symptoms since the bite of a snake known or presumed to be poisonous, it can be assumed that venom was not introduced. *Occasionally, a delayed reaction may occur and should be anticipated*, and the patient's family should be so advised and instructed as to pertinent signs and symptoms.

Evaluation of the Bite

The initial effort should be an efficient and comprehensive evaluation of the patient, with particular attention to the local area of the bite. The following items should be noted and described where appropriate, preferably on an hourly basis for the first 12 hours:

Fang marks, if present. If there are two punctures, measure the distance between the two. Although uncommon, bleeding fang marks are a poor prognostic sign.

Pain, if present.

Swelling and its extent. One method is to circle the margin of edema every hour and to chart the time for each margin. Measure and record the circumference of the swollen limb in comparison to the other.

Color. Is erythema present?

Local reaction. Are blebs present? Although muscle fasciculations, petechiae, and/or ecchymoses are not specifically local reactions, inspection of the wound is an opportunity to watch for these phenomena.

Systemic symptoms, if present.

Clinical Signs and Symptoms

The presence and severity of signs are paramount guidelines in proper assessment of the snakebite victim. Repeated, often hourly evaluations in the early hours of management are necessary to properly treat these patients.

Symptoms seen with pit viper snakebite include varying degrees of pain, nausea and vomiting, diaphoresis, dizziness, chills, and paresthesias. Because snakebite is such a frightening event, several of the symptoms just mentioned may simply be due to emotional stress. For example, nausea, vomiting, and diaphoresis just after the event may well be due to emotional fright. However, nausea and vomiting that develop 4 hours after the actual event in a patient who had previously been calm may well represent a systemic manifestation and indicate a worsening of the patient's condition.

Physical findings from pit viper snakebite primarily include erythema and edema at the site of the fang marks. Fever, rapid respiratory rate, or sinus tachycardia may be seen. The development of any of the following should be considered systemic manifestations and should indicate significant envenomation—petechiae, ecchymoses, or frank bleeding from single or multiple sites; oliguria or anuria; nystagmus, muscle fasciculations, muscle weakness, paralysis, coma, or convulsions; respiratory distress; shock; or cardiac dysrhythmia or cardiac arrest.

Laboratory Data

Elevations of the white blood cell count are commonly seen in snakebite victims. The following laboratory findings herald significant envenomation: the development of anemia; coagulation abnormalities such as hypofibrinogenemia, thrombocytopenia, prolongation of either the prothrombin time or the partial thromboplastin time; elevation of the blood urea nitrogen (BUN) or creatinine levels, or metabolic abnormalities; or cardiac dysrhythmia.

Although enzyme-linked immunosorbent assay and radioimmunoassay tests for detection of snake venom have been developed,[12] until they become more specific and practical with respect to availability and running time, they are presently of limited usefulness.

CONTROVERSIES IN THERAPY

Throughout the ages, various therapies have been proposed for the treatment of venomous snakebites. After widespread clinical use and study, just as many therapies have fallen into disfavor and have been summarily dismissed. Recent casualties include en bloc excision (poor cosmetic outcome); ice immersion (high incidence of amputations); and EDTA chelation therapy.

Although their applications have been significantly modified, the oldest methods to survive are the limited use of a tourniquet and early use of incision and suction. Once touted for routine use, fasciotomy still plays a limited role in the management of compartmental syndrome. Clearly, the latest and most sensational controversy involves electric shock therapy of snakebite with a modified "stun gun." Before we recommend our preferred method of treatment, a brief discussion of these treatment entities will be presented.

Tourniquet

Obviously, ligature should be venous in order not to occlude the flow of arterial blood to the area. In fact, such a ligature should be lymphatic, because the uptake of the venom and its transport occurs via the lymphatics. In moderate to severe envenomations, one can clinically observe the gradual proximal advance of the edema. Application of a ligature does not prevent the spread of edema, even though the generally held belief is that ligature does slow the advance of the edema. Experience indicates that if an appropriate venous-type ligature is applied immediately or within minutes after venomous snakebite, it may prove beneficial in slowing the uptake of the venom.

Once edema has progressed beyond the location of the tourniquet, the tourniquet will be of no value. Also, application of a tourniquet an hour or later following the bite will be of no particular value.[13]

Incision

Theoretically, incision into the so-called venom pool is an attractive treatment mode. In practice, three major problems emerge:

Location. The appropriate location is believed to be an incision through the fang mark. Fangs of most of the pit vipers are curved and, depending on the relative position of the portion of the human anatomy and of the head of the snake, as well as on the length of the fang and the degree of penetration, the deposit of the venom may occur at any point on a periphery of a circle equivalent to the length and direction of the fangs through the skin.

Direction. Direction of the incision is also problematic, particularly on the limbs. Incisions made perpendicular or tangential to skinlines and to the long axis of the limb do not heal as well and produce a more noticeable scar than those made parallel to the long axis. Additionally, if carried to adequate depth, an incision may damage vessels, nerves, and tendons. It is therefore imperative that if an incision is made, it be *parallel* to the long axis of the limb. It is also important to consider the combination of the location and direction of the incisions. An incision made parallel to the long axis of the limb through the fang mark will potentially lead to the venom pool only if the fangs were directed, so to say, at the 12 o'clock and 6 o'clock positions.

Depth. The depth of the incision is of great significance. Most serious envenomations occur secondary to bites of sizable snakes whose fangs penetrate well into the subcutaneous tissues and, indeed, into muscles. In order to contact the venom pool, it would therefore be necessary to carry the depth of the incision to at least the subcutaneous or areolar tissues and on to the muscles.

Suction

Parenthetically, it should be mentioned that suction could be achieved either by utilizing a suction apparatus (such as a cup) or by the mouth. The snake venom is a protein that will be digested in the stomach, and no ill effects will result to the person performing suction unless there are fresh cuts or abrasions in the buccal mucosa or on the tongue. Fresh postextraction dental sockets will also permit absorption of the venom. Snake venom has mild topical anesthetic properties that might be felt in the mouth of the individual providing the suction. Increased tissue damage to the wound may result from suction.

Fasciotomy

In the past, fasciotomy had been proposed as the sole means of treatment of serious venomous snakebite, mostly through the efforts of Glass, who recommended routine fasciotomies and debriding of the necrotic muscle.[14, 15] Others have used the procedure when it was specifically indicated. Presently, fasciotomy may be a useful surgical adjunct to therapy only when specifically indicated, such as for relief of compartmental syndrome. The routine procedure of fasciotomy requires incision through the thickness of the skin and subcutaneous areolar tissue into the fascia of the muscles. Such incisions permit bulging of the edematous and frequently necrotic muscle through the incision, therefore relieving the tightness that frequently leads to the embarrassment of arterial circulation.

Fasciotomies are typically performed for a compartmental syndrome on the limbs, particularly the forearm and the leg. Usual indications for fasciotomy, whether a venomous snakebite or secondary to mechanical trauma or other causes of hemorrhage and/or necrosis in the muscles, depend on the physical condition, laboratory findings, and particularly on the weakening of the arterial pulse distal to the area of swelling.

In our experience and that of others,[9] fasciotomy is infrequently needed. There is no evidence that debriding the involved muscle mass somehow precludes the systemic spread of the venom. Fasciotomy should be performed only when specifically indicated and only after measurement of compartment pressure has documented compartmental syndrome.

Electric Shock Therapy

In 1986, Guderian and coworkers[16] presented successful management of 34 cases of snakebite by electroshock therapy alone within 30 minutes of the bite. The authors used a "modified" stun gun with a 9-volt battery to deliver a direct pulsating current of approximately 25,000 volts (25kV) and less than 1 milliampere. In this procedure, one probe acts as the ground terminal, whereas the other applies the current to the site of the bite. A lead attached to the spark plug of an outboard motor at half-throttle has also been used. This type of current supposedly does not stimulate cardiac muscle. Usually, 4 to 5 shocks at 10-second intervals are applied. The authors stated, "We have records on 34 cases of bites on limbs where there was evidence of penetration of the skin. The current was applied within 30 minutes, and 10 to 15 minutes later all pain had gone and the usual sequelae of an untreated bite (swelling, serosanguineous bullae, bleeding, shock, and renal failure) did not develop. No patient died. After an hour the patient was usually able to go home. At follow-up there was no necrosis of tissue around the bite due either to the bite or the treatment. Seven people who refused the shock treatment experienced the classic complications and 2 needed life-saving amputations."[16]

This proposed treatment has been greeted with sensationalism, skepticism, and even outright cynicism.[17, 18] However, it is important to keep an open mind to any new idea. Electroshock treatment of snakebite should be studied in an objective and scientific fashion before any final recommendation is made.

TREATMENT OF SNAKEBITE ENVENOMATION

The key to proper management of snakebite envenomation includes repeated hourly assessment with thorough documentation of any progression of signs and/or symptoms; clinical judgment tempered by pragmatic common sense; antivenin therapy when appropriate; and observation and supportive therapy.

First Aid

The best first aid is to get to a hospital emergency department as soon as possible. Although helpful, having the patient, police, or emergency medical squad try to identify or capture the snake may be time-consuming and even fraught with danger.

The following first-aid measures may be used in the field during transport of the patient and immediately on arrival at the emergency department. The patient must be kept at rest and preferably supine; the bitten part of the body, particularly if it is a limb, should be immobilized and kept in a dependent position to decrease the spread of venom. Reassurance is very useful.

A tourniquet carefully applied by experienced personnel in such a manner to occlude venous and lymphatic return is appropriate. A palpable pulse must be present distal to the tourniquet. The tourniquet should be applied a few inches above the bite, loosened every 15 to 30 minutes, and reapplied above the level of progressive edema.

Emergency Department Assessment

On the arrival of a snakebite patient to the emergency department, the emergency physician must first do a quick history and physical to determine if there was definitely a snakebite (often the history is not clear); if possible, the type of snake should be determined, and a thorough evaluation of the bite itself (as described) should be made to determine the presence of fang marks, erythema, pain, or swelling. *Time your findings.* Circle and time the margin of edema—this is most helpful in your decision to render antivenin. Timed measurement of limb circumference is also most helpful. When indicated, incision and suction of the bite may be done in the first 15 minutes by experienced personnel. Incisions should be placed parallel to each other and somewhat above the fang marks along the long axis of the limb. The depth of the incision should extend through the subcutaneous fat and to the fascia of the muscle. Incisions should be 2 centimeters apart. Incisions should not be cruciate because the benefit is not greater, and scarring is excessive. Although there is no evidence that irrigation of the incision with saline alters the course of the condition, the wound should be thoroughly scrubbed with soap and water or cleansing solution such as povidone-iodine (Betadine). The complications of improper incision include neurovascular or tendon injury and infection.

An intravenous line in an uninvolved extremity should be begun, and blood should be immediately sent for complete blood count, type and crossmatch, prothrombin time, partial thromboplastin time, fibrinogen, blood urea nitrogen, creatinine, and electrolyte studies; also, extra blood should be obtained for coagulation or other studies. Urinalysis is essential as well as a 12-lead electrocardiogram and cardiac monitoring.

A more thorough history and physical should then be obtained, and any early systemic manifestations should be timed and documented. A moment for reassurance and emotional support early on is important in establishing long-term rapport with the patient.

Tetanus prophylaxis for the contaminated puncture wound and a broad-spectrum antibiotic are both indicated. Relief of pain early on may obscure assessment and is usually, if possible, reserved until after a decision concerning antivenin therapy is made.

Hourly assessment with properly timed documentation will clearly indicate significant envenomation and determine the mode of therapy.

Table 27–3 lists guidelines for treatment of pit viper bites, which account for over 90 per cent of snakebites in the United States. Rapid progression of swelling within 4 hours, especially involving the trunk; the presence of systemic symptoms such as altered mental status, coma, or convulsions; petechiae, ecchymoses, or frank bleeding; shock, pulmonary edema, or other major complications indicate major (Stage III or IV) envenomation and the probable if not definite need for antivenin therapy.

Antivenin

The major consideration today in symptomatic snakebite therapy is whether or not to give the patient antivenin.

Table 27–3. GUIDELINES FOR TREATMENT OF PIT VIPER (RATTLESNAKE, COTTONMOUTH, AND COPPERHEAD) BITES*

GRADES OF POISONING	SYMPTOMS AND SIGNS WITHIN 4 HR	SURGICAL MEASURES	MEDICAL MEASURES	ANTIVENIN DOSAGE WHEN INDICATED
0	Fang marks No local or systemic signs	—	—	—
I–Minimal	Moderate pain and erythema Local swelling No progression of signs No systemic symptoms	Incision and suction may be indicated within the first 30 min by trained personnel	Tetanus prophylaxis Antibiotic Antihistamine Observation	—
II–Moderate	Progressive pain, erythema and edema extending 10–15″ from site of bite. Minor constitutional symptoms such as fever, vomiting, or dizziness	As above Immobilization of the injured part	Observation Above supportive ℞. IV† antivenin therapy on occasion may be indicated in rapidly progressive situations, especially with rattlesnake or cottonmouth bites‡	0–5 vials of Wyeth's crotalid polyvalent antivenin
III–Severe	Rapidly progressive pain, erythema 15–20″ from site of bite by 12 hr. Ecchymosis, petechiae, and systemic signs such as vertigo, tachycardia	As above	Observation Above supportive ℞. IV† antivenin therapy is probably indicated, especially with rattlesnake or cottonmouth bites	5–10 vials may be necessary, depending on patient response
IV–Very severe	Rapidly progressive swelling and erythema extending to trunk within 4 hr; shock, coma, convulsions, renal failure, muscle fasciculations, and cardiac arrest may ensue	Fasciotomy is usually indicated only for compartmental syndrome and/or vascular compromise	IV† antivenin therapy Blood transfusions, steroids, and critical care in an intensive care unit will probably be indicated	Up to 10–20 vials may be indicated, depending on patient response

*These are guidelines only. The management of snakebite poisoning remains controversial, demands considerable clinical judgment, and varies with the type of snake, the extent of bite and envenomation, and the geographic region. Children generally require more antivenin than adults.

†IV = intravenous.

‡Copperhead bites in general do not require antivenin therapy.

Physicians are perhaps more conservative today about administering antivenin. Indeed, a recent report[19] from Texas noted that 81 patients who had crotalid envenomation were successfully treated with intravenous fluids, antibiotics, tetanus prophylaxis, immobilization of the injured part, and supportive therapy. None of these patients received antivenin, and there were no deaths or amputations. However, this series included only 4 patients who had Stage IV rattlesnake bites. Generally, antivenin therapy is not indicated for the most common snakebite in the United States, that of the copperhead.[1, 20]

The use of antivenin has been further challenged because it is potentially hazardous when allergic complications occur.[21, 22] Immediate hypersensitivity (anaphylaxis) and delayed-type hypersensitivity (serum sickness) are definite concerns. In a recent study[23] of 40 patients who received antivenin, 60 per cent developed allergic reactions; however, treatment of these antivenin allergic reactions was uniformly effective, with no mortality, minimal morbidity, and no chronic sequelae. *Antivenin remains the mainstay of treatment of serious snakebite envenomation.*[1, 9, 20, 23]

Types of Antivenin. Wyeth's Crotalidae polyvalent antivenin, equine origin, is the most frequently administered antivenin in the Americas today. The antivenin is a purified (by ammonium sulfate precipitation) serum from horses hyperimmunized against 4 species of pit vipers found in the Americas—*Crotalus atrox*, the western diamondback rattlesnake; *Crotalus adamanteus*, the eastern diamondback rattlesnake; *Bothrops atrox*; and *Crotalus durissus terrificus*, the South American rattlesnake. The venom of these four snakes contains antigens basic to most of the pit vipers throughout the world. Thus, in addition to being effective against the rattlesnakes (*Crotalus* and *Sistrurus*) and the copperhead and water moccasins *(Agkistrodon)*, this antivenin is also effective against the Central American snakes, the bushmaster *(Lachesis)*, *Bothrops*, the South American pit vipers *(C. durissus terrificus)*, and even Old World Eastern snakes, the mamushi *(Agkistrodon halys)*, and the true viper *Trimeresurus* species, the habu vipers.

Wyeth coral snake antivenin is monovalent and specific for the Eastern coral snake, *Micrurus fulvius*, although it may also be used for the Texas coral snake. Currently, no antivenin is available for the Arizona or Sonoran coral snake. Unlike the pit vipers, coral snakes throughout the world are antigenically distinct, and a universal antiserum is an impossibility.[24]

Snakebite by exotic snakes is becoming more commonplace. The source, location, and availability of exotic antivenins can be obtained from the Arizona Poison Control Center in Tucson, Arizona (telephone [602] 626-6016).

Skin Testing for Sensitivity to Antivenin. Practically all snake antivenins currently available in the world are prepared from the serum of horses. Thus, any patient who is to receive antivenin should be questioned concerning allergy to horses or horse serum, history of urticaria, multiple allergies, or history of reactions to horse serum injections.

Skin testing is preferable to conjunctival sac testing and should only be performed once a physician decides antivenin is indicated.[24] The Wyeth preparation contains a small vial of normal horse serum that can be used as prepared 1:10. The appearance of any of the following phenomena within 30 minutes indicates a positive skin reaction: wheal, with or without pseudopods; erythema; or itching. *A negative skin test does not preclude a serious allergic reaction when antivenin is administered.*[1, 23, 24]

A positive skin test, a history of horse serum allergy, or severe allergic reaction to antivenin administration may weigh against administration of antivenin. In a critically ill patient who may die without antivenin administration, it may be necessary to go ahead and give antivenin with concomitant use of diphenhydramine (Benadryl) 50 to 100 mg IV and an epinephrine (1 mg in 100 mL saline) intravenous drip.[23, 24] Although controversial, corticosteriods are probably a useful adjunct in both prevention and treatment of allergic response to antivenin. Corticosteroids are definitely indicated in the management of serum sickness, an almost universal occurrence in patients receiving 7 to 8 vials or more of antivenin.

Administration of Antivenin. Antivenin should always be given intravenously. One 10-ml vial is diluted in 100 ml of normal saline, and up to 5 vials in 500 ml may be administered over 1 to 2 hours (e.g., to a patient with a Stage IV rattlesnake bite). Antivenin should be administered as soon as possible, preferably within 4 hours of the bite; it is usually ineffective 12 to 24 hours after the bite. Patients begun on antivenin therapy should be admitted to the intensive care unit. Children usually require more antivenin than adults.

Table 27–3 relates the number of vials that may be indicated for treatment to the stages of envenomation in pit viper bites. When a decision to administer antivenin has been made, it has been our experience that at least 5 vials are necessary to be effective. Some parameters indicating an end-point for administration of antivenin include a halt in the rapid advance of swelling; an increase in blood pressure in a patient in shock; a stop in the fall of platelet or fibrinogen levels with a subsequent rise; improvement in a sense of well-being, or a general improvement in the patient's clinical condition.[1, 9, 10, 19, 20, 23, 24]

Bites of the coral snake are managed differently. Systemic signs usually occur late with the bite of the coral snake. Earlier systemic signs relate to the paralysis of cranial nerves, causing mydriasis, strabismus, ptosis, slurring of speech, dysphagia, and nonspecific muscle weakness. The respiratory muscles are affected last, resulting in respiratory muscle paralysis, which is the leading cause of death due to the bite of the coral snake. Once neurotoxic signs develop following coral snake envenomation, it may well be too late to administer the antivenin. Thus, 3 or 4 vials are administered to the asymptomatic patient following a bite from a coral snake, and up to 10 vials are administered to the symptomatic patient.[1, 24]

Supportive Therapy

Fasciotomy may be indicated in the event of compartmental syndrome and/or vascular compromise. Platelet and/or blood transfusions or fresh frozen plasma may be necessary in the patient who has coagulation abnormalities and frank bleeding. Ventilator therapy with positive end-expiratory pressure may be indicated in the patient who has adult respiratory distress syndrome. Dialysis may be necessary in patients who develop renal shutdown. Critical care with multispecialty consultation in an intensive care unit may be necessary for the gravely ill patient.

LONG-TERM COMPLICATIONS

Tissue necrosis and slough may be the result of inadequate treatment of the pit viper bite. In the absence of or with delay of administration of specific antivenin, extensive vasculitis, necrosis, and sloughing of the skin and subcutaneous tissues may occur.

Later, fibrosis frequently occurs, particularly after rattlesnake and water moccasin bites. Bites on the hand, both on the dorsum and on the palm, are particularly susceptible to late fibrosis and contractures. As the result of these changes, limitation of motion in flexion and extension frequently results. In anticipation of this, major snakebites should be photographed early and continuously in treatment for documentation purposes.

Acute and chronic pituitary failure resembling Sheehan's syndrome has been described following snakebite by Russell's viper *(Vipera russelli)* in Burma.[25]

THE FUTURE

Present antivenin is a mixture of antibody and foreign protein source. The need for a purified antivenin devoid of adverse human effect is clearly recognized. IgG(T) is a highly purified antibody that has been isolated from commercial antivenin.[26] Research to develop F(ab) fragments is presently under way. It is hoped that the future will give us an affordable, allergy-free method for the management of snakebite victims.

GILA MONSTER

The Gila monster *(Heloderma suspectum)* is a venomous lizard that inhabits the southwestern United States. The venom apparatus consists of eight glands in the floor of the mouth, which are an adaptation of the sublingual salivary glands. Venom is secreted into the oral cavity and then flows along through the grooves in the teeth. Because of this rather primitive and inefficient injection apparatus, lizards have to hang on tenaciously and chew on the soft tissues of their prey to introduce a sufficient amount of venom to immobilize the prey. To detach the Gila monster from the victim, introduce a hemostat, stick, or spoon between the jaws posteriorly and pry them apart.

The venom is primarily neurotoxic and produces pain, edema, and mostly local reaction. A recent case report[27] of life-threatening anaphylaxis following Gila monster bite, characterized by hypotension and severe angioedema of the upper airway, was treated successfully with intravenous fluids, epinephrine, and corticosteroids.

There are no documented deaths from the Gila monster. There is no known antivenin. Supportive measures, tetanus prophylaxis, and relief of pain are indicated for treatment.

References

1. Podgorny G: Venomous reptiles of the United States and Canada. In Haddad LM, Winchester JF (eds): *Clinical Management of Poisoning and Drug Overdose.* Philadelphia, WB Saunders, 1983, pp 275–294.
2. Cable D, McGehee W, Wingert WA, Russell FE: Prolonged defibrination after a bite from a "nonvenomous" snake. JAMA *251*:925, 1984.
3. Mather HM, Mayne S, McMonagle TM: Severe envenomation from a 'harmless' pet snake. Br Med J *1*:1324, 1978.
4. Minton SA: Beware: Nonpoisonous snakes. Clin Toxicol *15*:259, 1979.
5. Mandell F, Bates J, Mittleman B, Loy J: Major coagulopathy and 'nonpoisonous' snake bites. Pediatrics *65*:314, 1980.

6. Reid HA: Sea-snake bites. Br Med J *2*:73, 1956.
7. Reid HA: Diagnosis, prognosis, and treatment of sea-snake bite. Lancet *1*:399, 1961.
8. Halstead BW: Poisonous and Venomous Marine Animals of the World. Rev ed. Princeton, NJ, Darwin Science Press, 1978.
9. Russell FE: Snake Venom Poisoning. Philadelphia, JB Lippincott, 1980.
10. Curry SC, Kunkel DB: Death from a rattlesnake bite. Am J Emerg Med *3*:227, 1985.
11. Simon TL, Grace TG: Envenomation coagulopathy in wounds from pit vipers. N Engl J Med *305*:443, 1981.
12. Minton SA: Present tests for detection of snake venom: Clinical applications. Ann Emerg Med *16*:932, 1987.
13. Gennaro JF, McCullough NC: Comments on the contemporary treatment of poisonous snakebite in North America. Med Rec Ann *46*:224, 1961.
14. Glass TG: Early debridement in pit viper bite. Surg Gynecol Obstet *136*:774, 1974.
15. Glass TG: Early debridement in pit viper bites. JAMA *235*:2513, 1976.
16. Guderian RH, MacKenzie CD, Williams JF: High voltage shock treatment for snake bite. Lancet *2*:229, 1986.
17. Russell FE: Another warning about electric shock for snakebite. Postgrad Med *82*:32, 1987.
18. Pearson CA: High-voltage shock treatment for snakebite (letter). Lancet *2*:461, 1986.
19. Burch JM, Agarwal R, Mattox KL, Feliciano DV, Jordan GL: The treatment of crotalid envenomation without antivenin. J Trauma *28*:35, 1988.
20. Pennell TC, Babu SS, Meredith JW: The management of snake and spider bites in the southeastern United States. Am Surgeon *53*:198, 1987.
21. Buerk CA: The treatment of crotalid envenomation without antivenin. J Trauma *26*:669, 1986.
22. Lindsay D: Controversy in snake bite—time for a controlled appraisal. J Trauma *25*:462, 1985.
23. Jurkovich GJ, Luterman A, McCullar K, Ramenofsky ML, Curreri PW: Complications of Crotalidae antivenin therapy. J Trauma *28*:1032, 1988.
24. Otten EJ: Antivenin therapy in the emergency department. Am J Emerg Med *1*:83, 1983.
25. Tun-Pe, Phillips RE, Warrell DA, Moore RA, Tin-Nu-Swe, Myint-Lwin, Burke CW: Acute and chronic pituitary failure resembling Sheehan's syndrome following bites by Russell's viper in Burma. Lancet *2*:763, 1987.
26. Sullivan JB: Past, present, and future immunotherapy of snake venom poisoning. Ann Emerg Med *16*:938, 1987.
27. Piacentine J, Curry SC, Ryan PJ: Life-threatening anaphylaxis following Gila monster bite. Ann Emerg Med *15*:959, 1986.

CHAPTER 28
POISONOUS ARTHROPODS

Table 28–1 lists the poisonous arthropods that will be discussed in this chapter.

A. Spiders and Scorpions

George Podgorny, M.D.
Brad S. Selden, M.D.
Donald B. Kunkel, M.D.

SPIDERS

Practically all spiders are venomous; however, only two of them in the United States can be considered dangerous to humans. The minuscule size of the body and therefore of the venom quantity is the reason that most spider bites hardly ever cause symptoms in humans. An allergic reaction occasionally may be misinterpreted as envenomation. Most but not all spiders spin webs to intercept their prey. Spiders basically feed on insects and each other and are, in general, beneficial. Most of the spider venoms contain neurotoxins and tissue lysins. This combination, when injected into the prey, paralyzes it while aiding in the digestion of the victim's body; the victim's contents are sucked out later. It is precisely because of these characteristics that the two dangerous American spiders present medical problems.[1]

Black Widow *(Latrodectus mactans, Latrodectus hesperus)*

Only the female of this species is of any significance. She frequently devours her mate and thus is aptly named. The black widow possesses one of the most potent animal venoms known, far more potent than that of a poisonous snake. Primarily a neurotoxin, it binds to neuromuscular synaptic membranes.[2, 3] Fortunately, the amount of venom present in a given spider is so minuscule that human envenomations present only moderate clinical symptomatology.

The black widow spider is small and shiny black. *The female exhibits a very constant, discernible, hourglass-shaped, bright red marking on the ventral side of the abdomen.* The male of the species is much smaller and displays only a small, reddish dot. Occasionally, a younger specimen may lack the hourglass marking or may even appear to be mottled brown.

This spider is ubiquitous in most of the United States, particularly in the Southeast. The habitat is usually outdoors, and the most common encounter classically occurs in an outhouse[4] and involves the male genitalia. The victim is usually a camper. Frequently, people who are bitten, particularly children, are aware of a bite by virtue of an initial, sudden, burning pain, which frequently is the extent of the initial symptomatology. Despite various "classic" descriptions of the appearance of the black widow bite, most of them cannot be distinguished from a flea bite.

Systemic symptoms usually develop anywhere between 1 and 12 hours after the bite but generally within the first 4 hours. Symptoms primarily include the initial burning

Table 28–1. THE POISONOUS ARTHROPODS

PHYLUM: ARTHROPODA
Characteristics: Exoskeleton, made of chitin, shed at intervals; segmented body; jointed appendages

- Subphylum: Chelicerata
  - Class Arachnida: Six pairs of appendages, four pairs of legs
    - Araneae: Spiders, tarantulas
    - Scorpionida
    - Acarina: Ticks, mites
- Subphylum: Mandibulata
  - Class Crustaceae: Lobster, shrimp
    - Insecta:
      - Hymenoptera: Bees, wasps, ants
      - Lepidoptera: Butterflies and moths (and their caterpillars)
    - Myriapoda
      - Diplopoda: Millipedes
      - Chilopoda: Centipedes

pain at the site of the bite; abdominal pain and severe, cramping spasms that bring the patient to the emergency department; and weakness of the lower extremities.

The abdominal pain and associated spasm are intense; on examination, the patient may also exhibit muscular guarding and often a boardlike abdomen. *The lack of fever and leukocytosis and the history of a bite distinguishes this condition from an acute abdomen,* the major diagnostic pitfall. Other signs include the development of erythema at the site of the bite, muscular spasm in the lower extremities, restlessness, and sinus tachycardia. Bites of the upper extremities result in chest pain and spasm of the pectoralis and intercostal muscles.

Treatment of the severely symptomatic patient includes hospital admission for intravenous fluids, tetanus prophylaxis, pain relief with judicious use of intravenous morphine, and intravenous calcium gluconate. Calcium gluconate, 10 ml of a 10 per cent solution, is quite effective in relieving the pain, muscular spasm, and boardlike rigidity of the abdomen and will prove most comforting to the patient. Repeated doses may be necessary.

Muscle relaxants such as diazepam (Valium) and methocarbamol (Robaxin) have been used with some success, especially as an adjunct to calcium gluconate therapy. In our experience, the use of intravenous diazepam or methocarbamol reduces the frequency of use of calcium gluconate.

A commercially prepared antivenin for black widow spider bite is available. It is an equine serum product and therefore should be used with caution and only after appropriate sensitivity testing. In our experience, the need for this antivenin is rare, because most cases are self-limiting or respond well to calcium gluconate or a muscle relaxant or both. Antivenin (Merck) is available in vials of 6000 units. The lyophilized material is diluted in 2.5 ml of sterile water. A single vial constitutes a dose for intramuscular injection.

Brown Recluse "Fiddle-Back" Spider *(Loxosceles reclusa)*

The brown recluse spider has become a significant cause of cutaneous necrosis and delayed wound healing, particularly in the southeastern United States.

The brown recluse may have been imported from its basic habitat in Central and South America. Such importation most likely occurred in shipments of food and vegetables. During the past 50 years, the range of this spider has extended steadily from its epicenter in Louisiana toward Texas and Arkansas as well as northeast and north; cases of bites have also been reported as far east as Virginia and West Virginia. Once reclusive and found in abandoned buildings, the brown recluse has begun to adapt its natural habitat to include homes, garages, and barns. Brown recluse spider bites are becoming more common.

The spider is somewhat nondescript, brownish to tan, small, and frequently indistinguishable from other spiders. A fiddle-shaped design is discernible on the dorsum of the thorax, but this design sometimes may be vague, requiring the use of a magnifying glass to be seen. The brown recluse is probably the only spider in North America that has only three pairs of eyes. The usual number is four pairs.

The brown recluse venom has a high content of lysins that cause tissue necrosis and vasculitis. The bites of the brown recluse vary in their severity from being almost asymptomatic to displaying a major systemic reaction. Fortunately, the latter reaction and even the more common local necrotic reaction are infrequent.

Typically, initial symptomatology may be none or limited to mild pain. Within 24 to 48 hours, erythema and some swelling occur at the site of the bite. The lesion may not progress further and follow a benign course. Or there may be a rapid increase in swelling, tenderness, and the development of a central zone of purplish discoloration with surrounding erythema. A central blood-filled vesicle may occur. In 3 to 5 days, the vesicle disappears and is replaced by necrotic crust. When the crust is removed, a deep ulcer becomes evident. This ulcer, which frequently becomes secondarily infected, heals in an extremely variable fashion.

A systemic reaction may also infrequently occur, manifested by fever, chills, nausea, and myalgia 12 to 24 hours after the bite. Thrombocytopenia, hemolytic anemia,[5] and disseminated intravascular coagulation[6] have all been reported to occur, with subsequent shock, renal failure, and, rarely, death.

Treatment of the progressive cutaneous reaction has been revolutionized through the work of Rees and coworkers,[7–10] who have administered the leukocyte inhibitor Dapsone, 4–4′-diaminodiphenylsulfone (DDS). A course of Dapsone, from 50 to 100 mg a day for 14 days, has proved most effective if begun *before* cutaneous necrosis appears, i.e., during the period of purplish discoloration but before vesicle or eschar formation. A test documenting the presence of G6PD before commencing Dapsone therapy is desirable, if the test is available. A CBC (complete blood count) should be performed prior to the institution of Dapsone and repeated during therapy. The recommended starting dose for Dapsone is 25 mg twice a day.

Unfortunately, many patients do not present to the emergency department until actual necrosis or ulceration has set in. Once frank necrosis occurs and a clear area of demarcation exists, it is time to undertake debridement. Warm saline soaks will result in the earlier separation of devitalized tissue. Debridement can be accomplished surgically or by the use of proteolytic enzymes such as Elase (fibrinolysin and deoxyribonuclease, combined [bovine]).

Smaller ulcers can be attended to by debridement, cleansing, use of antibiotics such as cephalexin (Keflex), and can be given an opportunity to heal by secondary intention. Whenever the ulcer crater is larger than the size of a quarter or is present on the exposed skin of a female patient, surgical excision and full-thickness skin grafting are indicated.

Tarantula (Dugesiella)

The tarantula is a large, frequently hairy, jumping spider present in many areas of the United States, particularly in the Southwest. Its size, appearance, and undeserved reputation create an aura of fatal danger. Tarantulas possess venoms that are so mild that they rarely, if ever, cause a medical problem in humans. Occasional allergic reactions to the venom can occur. Lately, these spiders have become popular as pets and therefore can frequently be seen in homes. Occasionally, they are used by jewelry stores to prevent unauthorized attempts to reach into the window displays.

SCORPIONS

Scorpions are land cousins of the invertebrate crustaceans (shrimp and lobster). Having eight legs makes the scorpion a member of Class Arachnida along with spiders. The scorpion has an elongated, segmented body similar to that of the shrimp and a relatively long, segmented, and highly mobile "tail," which is actually a continuation of the segmented body. The last segment of the tail is equipped with a stinger called a telson. In the front of the body are a pair of large pincers called pedipalps. Between the bases of the pedipalps, the scorpion has a small mouth with a pair of mouth pincers called chelicerae.

In comparison with other groups of animals, scorpion species are somewhat limited; less than 700 are known. In some tropical and arid areas of the world, scorpions approach a length of 20 centimeters. About 40 species of scorpion have been identified in the continental United States and Canada. Apparently, scorpions do not exist or are extremely scarce in the Great Lakes area, but stowaway scorpions have caused stings as far north as Michigan.[12] Most of the species of scorpions range in the southern states[11] and along the sunbelt to the west coast. The only American species of clinical consequence, *Centruroides sculpturatus* Ewing, is indigenous to Arizona, with a range into Mexico and colonies in California, Texas, New Mexico, and southern Nevada.[13] This scorpion is relatively small and usually tan.

Scorpions are nocturnal predators and seek cover in the daytime. Because they are attracted to moisture and dampness, they may crawl into a moist shoe overnight. In areas of heavy infestation, an old method of control has been to spread out a large, wet burlap sack overnight. Scorpions will seek out the sack and crawl underneath, where they can be located in the morning and destroyed.

Scorpion Venom and Its Clinical Effects

Essentially all non-American scorpions of medical significance are of the family Buthidae. The venoms are low molecular weight proteins with a variety of actions, depending on the species.[14] A hyperadrenergic state with high levels of circulating catecholamines, hypertension, cholinergic signs, pulmonary edema, myocardial injury, cardiac dysrhythmia, cardiovascular collapse, and death can occur with stings by the yellow scorpion *Leirus quinquestriatus* (range: Turkey, Lebanon, Syria, Jordan, and northern Africa).[15] Similar effects are seen from stings of the common North African *Adroctonus* spp.[15] Hypertension, cholinergic symptoms, convulsions, coma, and death can be seen following stings by the South American *Tityus* spp.[15] Hemolysis, renal failure, bleeding disorders (including disseminated intravascular coagulation), tissue necrosis, pancreatitis, and neurotoxicity also have been described as a result of stings from non-American scorpions.[13, 15, 16] Effective antivenins are produced in Mexico, Brazil, Turkey, Algeria, and Egypt for the aforementioned species[15] and adrenergic receptor blocking agents, such as propranolol and phentolamine, have been used effectively in animal models to treat hyperadrenergic effects of *Leirus* spp venom.[16]

The effects of *Centruroides* venom seem to be entirely neurotoxic. There are no enzymes that cause tissue destruction, which explains the usual lack of inflammatory findings at the sting site. A first group of protein neurotoxins bind neuronal sodium channels to cause incomplete sodium channel activation; then a second type causes or enhances repetitive firing of axons.[14] Clinical findings are consistent with this increased presynaptic activity at the neuromuscular junction, parasympathetic nerves, and possibly adrenergic nerve endings and adrenal medulla (see Table 28–2).

The stings of other American species, including *Vejovis* spp (striped-tail scorpion) and *Hadrurus* spp (giant hairy scorpion), may produce local swelling, edema, and pain. Although envenomations by the aforementioned non-American scorpions still cause fatalities,[15] no deaths have been reported in the United States in recent years.

Table 28–2. GRADES OF *CENTRUROIDES SCULPTURATUS* ENVENOMATION[13]

GRADE I	Local pain and/or paresthesias at the site of envenomation
GRADE II	Pain and/or paresthesias remote from the site of envenomation, in addition to local findings
GRADE III	*Either* cranial nerve *or* somatic skeletal neuromuscular dysfunction: (1) cranial nerve dysfunction: blurred vision, wandering eye movements, hypersalivation, trouble swallowing, tongue fasciculations, problems with upper airway, slurred speech (2) somatic skeletal neuromuscular dysfunction: jerking of extremities, restlessness, severe involuntary shaking and jerking which may be mistaken for (but is not) seizure activity
GRADE IV	*Both* cranial nerve *and* somatic skeletal neuromuscular dysfunction

Evaluation and Management of *Centruroides* Envenomations

The Samaritan Regional Poison Center in Phoenix, Arizona, was consulted in over 1300 cases of scorpion envenomation in 1988 and manages significant envenomations directly in the emergency department. In an extensive 1984 review of experiences there, Curry and associates devised a grading system of severity of *Centruroides sculpturatus* envenomation, based on clinical signs and symptoms, that is used to guide therapy (Table 28–2).[13] Patients with Grade I and Grade II envenomations are usually treated at home with cautious application of ice to the sting site for pain relief and with oral analgesics, although the efficacy of antivenin for severe Grade II symptoms is currently being evaluated. Antivenin therapy may be recommended in those patients with Grade III envenomations and is usually necessary in those with Grade IV.

Specific *Centruroides* antivenin derived from goat serum is available from Antivenom Production Laboratories, Arizona State University, Tempe, Arizona. It is not approved for general use by the Food and Drug Administration but is available within the state of Arizona by special action of the Arizona State Board of Pharmacy.

In cases requiring antivenin, advanced life support measures are first implemented (reversal of neuromuscular impairment by antivenin may take 15 to 30 minutes or longer). Special attention is given to airway management, as this may be compromised in severe cases with increased secretions and impaired cranial nerve function. A skin test for hypersensitivity to the goat antiserum is then performed. One vial of reconstituted antivenin is then diluted in 50 ml of crystalloid and given intravenously over 15 to 30 minutes. Even in the presence of a negative skin test, the infusion should be initiated at just a few microdrops per minute, and the intravenous drip rate rapidly increased while the patient is closely monitored for signs of anaphylactic/anaphylactoid response. If severe envenomation symptoms persist 1 hour after the end of the first infusion, a second vial is given.

Complications of antivenin therapy include rare anaphylactic/anaphylactoid reactions and delayed hypersensitivity (serum sickness) in some patients.

ARTHROPODS

Centipedes and Millipedes

Centipedes and millipedes together form the group Myriapoda. American millipedes (Diplopoda) are virtually harmless to human beings. The centipedes (Chilopoda) are frequently venomous and will bite. Allergic reactions to the bites have been reported occasionally. The American centipedes rarely produce medical problems, short of some local pain. They possess a posterior "claw"; however, the claw has no stinger; instead, centipedes bite.

Occasionally, a giant centipede produces an intensely itching path of red dots over the skin where it has walked, embedding its legs partially into the skin. Such allergic reactions should be treated under general principles and do not require any specific measures.

Lepidoptera

Lepidoptera (butterflies and moths) and certain larvae (caterpillars) are capable of injury by so-called passive stinging, that is, using toxin contained in spines found over most of their body. When such a caterpillar is picked up, some of the hairlike spines break off into the skin, causing intense pain and occasionally rash. Analgesics and antihistamines are useful. A most common offender is the so-called puss caterpillar *(Megalopyge opercularis)*.

References

1. Podgorny G: Venomous Reptiles and Arthropods of the United States and Canada. In Haddad LM, Winchester JF (eds): Clinical Management of Poisoning and Drug Overdose, Philadelphia, WB Saunders, 1983, pp 275–294.
2. Moss HS, Binder LS: A retrospective review of black widow spider envenomation. Ann Emerg Med *16*:188, 1987.
3. Baba A, Cooper JR: The action of black widow spider venom in synaptosomes. J Neurochem *34*:1369, 1980.
4. Parrish HM: Analysis of 460 fatalities from venomous animals in the United States. Am J Med Sci *24*:35, 1963.
5. Chu JY: Hemolytic anemia following brown recluse spider bite. Clin Toxicol *12*:531, 1978.
6. Vorse M: Disseminated intravascular coagulation following fatal brown spider bite. J Pediatr *80*:1035, 1972.
7. Rees RS, Schak R, Withers E: Management of the brown recluse spider bite. Plast Reconstr Surg *68*:768, 1981.
8. King LE, Rees RS: Dapsone treatment of brown recluse spider bite. JAMA *250*:648, 1983.
9. Rees RS, Altenbern DP, Lynch JB, King LE: Brown recluse spider bites: A comparison of early surgical excision versus dapsone and delayed surgical excision. Ann Surg *202*:659, 1985.
10. Rees RS, Campbell D, Reiger E, King LE: The diagnosis and treatment of brown recluse spider bites. Ann Emerg Med *16*:945, 1987.
11. Stahnke HL: Arizona's lethal scorpion. Ariz Med *29*:490, 1972.
12. Trestrail JH: Scorpion envenomation in Michigan. Vet H Toxicol *23*:8, 1971.
13. Curry SC, Vance MV, Ryan PJ, et al: Envenomation by the scorpion *Centruroides sculpturatus*. J Toxicol Clin Toxicol *21*:417–449, 1983–84.
14. Wang GK, Strichartz GR: Purification and physiological characterization of neurotoxins from venoms of the scorpions *Centruroides sculpturatus* and *Leiurus quinquestriatus*. Molec Pharmacol *23*:519–533, 1983.
15. Keegan HL: Scorpions of Medical Importance. Jackson, Miss, University Press of Mississippi, 1985.
16. Geuron M, Adolph R, Grupp IL, Gabel M, Grupp G, Fowler NO: Hemodynamic and myocardial consequences of scorpion venom. Am J Card *45*:979, 1980.

B. Stinging Insects

L. Reed Shirley, M.D.

Man and nature have established what at times appears to be a precarious relationship. Mankind's food chain is partially dependent on insects and their function in cross-pollination. Mankind also relies on their assistance in the processes of natural decay. In contrast, insects have been implicated in the transmission of particular infectious illnesses. In the case of certain protozoan infections (e.g., malaria), insects are an integral part of the infectious organism's life cycle. Perhaps through the process of natural selection, some insects have developed stingers. These modified ovipositors may assist insects in their food gathering and in other instances may serve as defense mechanisms.

The universal human response to a Hymenoptera insect sting is local pain and irritation. In over 90 per cent of Hymenoptera sting victims, the resulting swelling and erythema are less than 2 inches in diameter, and the process resolves within 24 hours. Although a nuisance, this response cannot be interpreted as a health hazard. However, a few victims will have more serious effects of envenomation. For the most part, these serious reactions constitute immediate hypersensitivity reactions.

Von Pirquet coined the term allergy after a Greek word for "changed activity." He used this to designate states of altered reactivity distinct from the general population. Only a subset of susceptible and previously sensitized victims will have these responses when challenged. This is in contrast to toxins and poisons that bear expected consequences of exposure. The health hazards of plant toxins and poisonous reptile and arthropod bites are related to the "dose" of toxin/poison and to the victim's size. Manifestations are not dependent on the host's prior exposure or on his ability to mount an allergic antibody response.

The human consequences of an insect sting range from pain and local irritation to anaphylaxis. A fatal reaction to either a hornet or wasp sting was first recorded in Egyptian hieroglyphics (ca. 2600 BC). Waterhouse reported the anaphylactic potential of an insect sting in 1914.[1] Over the past 75 years, clinical observations and experimental evidence have allowed dissection of the allergic response into a specific immunologic process. The allergic antibody has been purified, IgE receptor and target cells identified, and mediators described. This chapter addresses the health hazards of the stinging insects. The pathophysiology and clinical expression of allergic reactions to stinging insects and treatment will be stressed.

CLINICAL FEATURES

Prevalence

The United States vital statistics registries estimate 40 to 50 fatal insect stings per year. Most authorities believe that this understates the true prevalence of the problem.[2] They suggest that unreported insect stings probably account for at least some of the cases that otherwise appear to be unexplained sudden death or idiopathic anaphylaxis.

Surveys have recorded that 0.4 to 0.8 per cent of Boy Scouts have a history of systemic reaction following an insect sting.[3, 4] This is compared with a survey of adults reporting a 4 per cent prevalence of systemic reactions following insect stings.[5] Differences between these reports include not only the age but also the geographic distribution of the study populations and the methods of data acquisition. The relevance of these differences to an estimate of the true prevalence of allergic reactions to stinging insects remains speculative.

Demographics

Systemic reactions appear more likely to occur in young adult males. In a three-year collaborative study[6] including 3236 Hymenoptera allergic subjects, the mean age was 30.5 years (62 per cent men). This male predominance, greater than that observed for some other hypersensitivity states, suggests that either males are more likely to be stung or that their immunologic response to venom allergens is particularly intense.

Thirty-two per cent of the subjects in this collaborative study had concomitant asthma, allergic rhinitis, or allergic skin disease. This is contrasted to the estimated frequency of 10 to 20 per cent of the general population who have atopic illness. Considering that all respondents were practicing allergists/immunologists, this difference may reflect their referral patterns and subject selection. Other studies have noted that the frequency of personal or family history of allergy in insect allergic subjects is no greater than that in the general population.[7–9]

The Insect

Members of the class Insecta responsible for insect allergic reactions belong to the phylum Arthropoda. Arthropods are characterized as invertebrates with hard, jointed exoskeletons and paired, jointed appendages. The order Hymenoptera is one of the largest and most highly developed orders of the class Insecta. Characteristically, these insects live in large colonies with a complex social organization. They undergo a complete metamorphosis that usually includes a footless grub in the larval stage. Other identifying features include two pairs of well-developed, membranous wings.

As depicted in Table 28–3, Hymenoptera of medical importance include the Apidae, Vespidae, and Formicidae families. The genus *Apis* includes the common honeybee *(A. mellifera)* and the bumblebees. In contrast to the other stinging insects, bees are docile and tend to sting only when provoked. Honeybees live in hives and during winter months remain dormant. As a result of its barbed tip, the bee's stinger is left in the victim, and the bee self-eviscerates. According to conventional wisdom, a bee is the culprit when a stinger is found at the sting site. However, recent evidence indicates that on occasion, the yellow jacket may also leave its stinger.

The yellow jacket is a member of the family Vespidae. In contrast to bees, Vespidae feed on various vegetable and animal matter, and because their colonies are destroyed by cold weather, they usually don't store food. Their nests generally consist of one or more combs of papery material that is usually horizontally placed so that the cells are vertical, with the open end down. Several species of yellow jacket are included in the subgenus *vespula.* This aggressive insect nests in the ground and in decaying wood. It is the insect most commonly cited as responsible for stinging allergic reactions.

The New World hornets *Vespula maculata* (bald-faced hornet) and *Vespula arenaria* (yellow hornet) are closely related to the yellow jacket. They comprise the subgenus *dolichovespula* of the genus *Vespula thomson*. In contrast to yellow jackets (genus *Vespula thomson,* subgenus *vespula*), New World hornets build papier-mâché nests in trees and bushes. Hornets common to Europe *(Vespa crabro* and *Vespa orientalis)* are included in a separate genus *(Vespa).*

Wasps are included in the genus *Polistes.*

Table 28–3. HYMENOPTERA OF MEDICAL SIGNIFICANCE

ORDER	FAMILY	GENUS	SUBGENUS	SPECIES
Hymenoptera	Apidae	*Apis*		*A. mellifera*
		Bombus		
	Vespidae	*Vespa*		*V. crabro*
				V. orientalis
		Vespula thomson	*Dolichovespula*	*D. maculata*
				D. arenaria
			Vespula sensu strictu	*V. vulgaria*
				V. maculifrons
				V. germanica
				V. squamosa
		Polistes		*P. exclamans*
				P. fuscatus
				P. annularis
	Formicidae	*Solenopsis*		*S. invicta*
				S. richteri

These insects tend to live in mud or open-comb nests in protected places such as building eaves.

The imported fire ants present within the United States belong to the species *Solenopsis invicta* and *Solenopsis richteri*. This aggressive insect entered the United States during the first part of this century. *S. invicta*, the dominant species, has since spread from the lower Gulf Coast throughout the entire Gulf Coast and the Southeast, whereas *S. richteri* remains confined to a small region bordering Alabama and Mississippi.[10] In contrast, bees, yellow jackets, wasps, and hornets are present in all regions of the United States and represent a potential for anaphylaxis in any given area.

Fire ants live in large colonies and form mounds which, on occasion, are of sufficient size to damage farm machinery and crops. The fire ant first bites and then rotates around a pivot point, inflicting multiple stings with its modified ovipositor. These stings result in a 2- to 3-millimeter diameter sterile pustule. This universal response clearly indicates that the fire ant was responsible for envenomation, and in the case of an allergic response, the appearance of the pustule removes other insects from consideration. As members of the order Hymenoptera, fire ants are winged insects. However, these wings are vestigial structures; therefore the fire ant crawls to its victim. In this manner, stings are more likely on the extremities. Furthermore, in contrast to the victims of the other Hymenoptera members, young children are more commonly stung.

The use of whole body extract in the treatment of insect-allergic patients was first reported in 1930.[11] An intrinsic bee protein present in all bee body parts and responsible for insect-allergic reactions was hypothesized in an effort to justify whole body extract therapy. However, access to relatively pure insect venoms has convincingly established the therapeutic benefit of venom immunotherapy and demonstrated that the clinical effects of whole body extract injections are indistinguishable from those of placebo injections.[12] Because there are no detectable venom proteins in the commercially prepared whole body extracts, this mode of therapy and the concept of an intrinsic bee protein have fallen by the wayside.[13] We herein present the current approach.

The Antigen

Each species has a unique, complex mixture of enzymes, peptides, and biologically active amines (Table 28–4). Honeybee venom has been the most intensively studied. Enzymes common to all the stinging insects include hyaluronidase and phospholipase. Through degradation of extracellular ground substance (hyaluronic acid), hyaluronidase acts as a spreading factor, potentiating the effects of other venom constituents. Phosphoglycerides, the substrate for phospholipase, are an integral part of biologic membranes. Therefore, in contrast to hyaluronidase, phospholipase has direct biologic effects. It may induce smooth muscle contraction, hypotension, altered vascular permeability, and mast cell histamine release.

From a biochemical and immunologic perspective, the stinging insects vary in their phospholipase activity. Honeybee venom has only phospholipase A_2 activity, with a molecular weight of 15,800.[14] In contrast, yellow jacket, hornet, and wasp venoms have both phospholipase A_1 and B activities, with a molecular weight of 37,000. Phospholipase A_1 specifically hydrolyses the ester bond at the C1 position of the phosphoglyceride. Phospholipase A_2 removes the fatty acid from the C2 position. Phospholipase B removes fatty acids from both the C1 and C2 carbons. These differences in biochemical function and molecular weights imply distinct enzymes with potentially distinct antigenic determinants.

Other venom proteins with enzymatic activity include acid phosphatase, histidine decarboxylase, cholinesterase, and protease. Acid phosphatase is present in honeybee venom, but authorities differ as to this enzyme's activity in vespid venoms. Yellow jacket venom is the only Hymenoptera venom in which histidine decarboxylase and cholinesterase enzyme activities have been demonstrated, whereas protease activity has been isolated in both yellow jacket and hornet venoms.

Peptides without enzymatic activity contained in honeybee venom include melittin, apamine, mast cell degranulating peptide, and minimine. Melittin constitutes 50 per cent of honeybee venom. When injected into human volunteers, this substance produces pain and local inflammation. It will also stimulate contraction of smooth muscle, augment

Table 28–4. HYMENOPTERA VENOM

	Venom Antigen	*Honeybee*	*Yellow Jacket*	*Hornet*	*Wasp*	*Fire Ant*	*Allergen*
ENZYMES	Hyaluronidase	x	x	x	x	x	x
	Phospholipase	A_2	A_1/B	A_1/B	A_1/B	x	x
	Acid phosphatase	x	(?)	(?)	(?)		x
	Histidine decarboxylase		x				
	Cholinesterase		x				
	Protease		x		x		
NONENZYMATIC PEPTIDES	Melittin	x					
	Apamine	x					
	MCDP*	x	x	x	x		
	Minimine	x					
	Antigen 5		x	x	x		x
	Kinins		x		x		
	Hornet kinin			x			
AMINES	Histamine	x	x	x	x		
	Dopamine	x	x	x			
	Norepinephrine	x	x	x			
	Epinephrine		x	x			
	Acetylcholine			x			
	Serotonin		x	x	x		

*MCDP = Mast cell degranulating peptide; activity in honeybee venom has 2600 MW and that in vespid venoms has MW 1600.

capillary permeability, lower systemic blood pressure, and may induce histamine release. The effects of apamine are primarily restricted to the central nervous system. It will induce long-lasting stimulation in mice and modify reflex action potentials in cats. Mast cell degranulating peptide, as its name implies, promotes the noncytolytic release of histamine from mast cell preparations. However, it also has anti-inflammatory properties through reduction in vascular permeability.[15] Minimine, when given in the larval stages of *Drosophila melanogaster* development, results in miniature, adult flies.

Antigen 5 is apparently absent in honeybee venom but is a major allergen contained in yellow jacket, hornet, and wasp venoms. In a similar manner, kinins have been identified in yellow jacket and wasp venoms but not in honeybee venom. A specific kinin, designated "hornet kinin," has also been recognized. Another peptide with mast cell degranulating properties has been identified in vespid venoms. In contrast to the protein seen in honeybees with a molecular weight of 2600 daltons, the mast cell degranulating peptide in vespid venoms has a molecular weight of 1600 daltons.

Histamine is detectable in all vespid (yellow jacket, hornet, and wasp) and honeybee venoms. Honeybee, yellow jacket, and hornet venoms contain both dopamine and norepinephrine, and yellow jacket and hornet venoms contain epinephrine. Acetylcholine has been isolated from hornet venom, and serotonin is included in yellow jacket, hornet, and wasp venoms.

Before emphasizing these apparent differences in the composition of insect venoms, it is important to stress that the number of studies of wasp venoms is relatively limited. Less is known about fire ant venoms. The majority of fire ant venom is water-insoluble piperidine alkaloids, but small quantities of phospholipase and hyaluronidase activity have been identified. Furthermore, there may be seasonal variation in the fire ant's venom content.[16]

The biologic activities of the various compounds contained in Hymenoptera species venom likely contribute to the universal, responses to a sting challenge. However, the response of major clinical significance and with which this chapter is concerned is the allergic response. Allergenic components of venom have been limited to phospholipase A_1 and A_2, hyaluronidase, acid phosphatase, melittin, and antigen 5.

The taxonomy and venom analysis as just outlined help in understanding potential cross-sensitivity. In a study of 99 insect-allergic patients, only 46 per cent had IgE class antibodies to a single insect venom.[17] Most had antibody that cross-reacted with at least one other venom, and in almost one fourth, antibody reacted to all three venoms tested.

Hypothetically, individuals who were sensitized to only one insect mounted an IgE class antibody response to venom component unique to that particular insect. In cases of sensitivity to multiple venoms, there may be multiple sensitization or more likely, sensitization to antigens common to the insect venoms in which sensitization was documented. In theory, an allergic antibody with specificity for an epitope unique to phospholipase A_2 may be dominant in one insect-allergic subject, whereas in another subject, the IgE antibody may be specific for an epitope common to both phospholipase A_1 and phospholipase A_2. This immunologic possibility further complicates interpretation of studies noting cross-sensitivity.

Clinical Manifestations of Insect Allergy

The universal response to Hymenoptera envenomation is local erythema and pain. In the case of fire ants, a sterile pustule develops at the sting site. The extent and duration of these local reactions is variable, but most are less than 2 inches in diameter and resolve within 24 hours. This variability may, in part, be due to differences in skin texture and blood vascular supply at the site of the insect sting. However, host factors may also contribute to this individual variability. Among individuals who experience extensive, local reactions, approximately 50 per cent will have allergic antibody to the appropriate venom. This suggests that the immunologic response may contribute to the differences seen in local responses.

Acute, systemic reactions also differ in their clinical expression. Fortunately, these anaphylactic events account for only a small fraction of Hymenoptera species insect stings. Expressions of anaphylaxis include generalized urticaria and/or angioedema, laryngeal edema, bronchospasm, hypotension, and uterine and bowel smooth muscle contractions. In most instances, symptoms develop within minutes of exposure, and the likelihood of severity seems related to this time of onset.[6] Of 3236 subjects enrolled in the collaborative Hymenoptera venom study,[6] 51 per cent of systemic reactions developed within 10 minutes of the insect sting and 72 per cent were considered moderate to severe in nature. This is contrasted to subjects with reactions developing between 11 and 21 minutes after the sting; 63 per cent of this group had moderate-to-severe reactions. Of those reactions appearing between 301 minutes and 2880 minutes following insect envenomation, 58 per cent were mild. However, there were 4 cases of severe anaphylaxis among the 38 patients whose symptoms developed 300 minutes after the insect sting.

In a retrospective analysis of 400 stinging insect–associated fatalities, 69 per cent of the cases available for analysis had documented respiratory tract findings at autopsy.[18] In almost half of these cases, pathology leading to upper airway obstruction was evident. Unfortunately, the initial clinical signs and symptoms suggesting anaphylaxis were not described. However, in analysis of 43 fatal cases of drug-induced anaphylaxis, only 37 per cent of the cases presented with respiratory distress.[19] Pathologic findings indicative of pulmonary congestion were present in 90 per cent of the 40 cases available for review. Furthermore, in 50 per cent of cases, evidence of pulmonary edema existed, and 45 per cent had increased tracheobronchial secretions. Laryngeal edema was evident in 15 of the 40 cases. Other presenting manifestations of fatal drug-induced anaphylaxis included circulatory collapse (14/43), seizures (11/43), cyanosis (11/43), nausea and vomiting (10/43), dizziness and weakness (6/43), skin eruptions (3/42), numbness and tingling sensations (3/42), and facial swelling (1/43).

The allergic response is notable for its longevity and specificity. Unless symptoms are pharmacologically modified, recurrence is expected on antigen rechallenge. However, for stinging insect allergy, the exact expression of insect sting–associated anaphylaxis (e.g., laryngeal edema or hypotension) may vary when the susceptible individual is rechallenged with the appropriate venom. Furthermore, not all challenges will result in a systemic reaction. In a study of 3236 stinging insect–allergic subjects, 31 per cent of subjects had no significant reaction following field challenges.[6] Although field stings and voluntary case reports may include challenges with irrelevant antigens, this rate of no response is similar to that noted with experimental challenges where the stinging insect is carefully controlled.[12] With the exception of variable expression, both the clinical features of anaphylaxis and the observation that almost all subjects who have these systemic reactions have positive immediate skin test reactions to venom preparations support an allergic pathophysiology for most, if not all, adverse reactions following Hymenoptera sting challenge.

Pathogenesis of the Allergic Response

The allergic antibody, like other antibody classes, is a complex polypeptide composed of two heavy chains (epsilon) and two light chains (kappa or lambda). Disulfide bonds within each chain identify specific antibody regions or domains, and the covalent bonds between the heavy chains and between the light and heavy chains establish a stable complex. The intact molecule has a molecular weight of 190,000 daltons. Amino acid sequencing has identified constant and hypervariable regions within both heavy and light chains. The hypervariable regions presumably confer antigen specificity and are located toward the N-terminal region of both light and heavy chains. The C-terminal half of the epsilon chain contains determinants unique for its biologic function, including the ligand for the IgE receptor.

IgE receptors are contained on the surface of human mast cells and basophils. Cultured human basophils have, on the average, 270,000 IgE receptors per cell.[20] Their high affinity helps explain the observations that minute quantities of IgE antibody may induce homologous tissue sensitization. Although there is a noncovalent bond between the IgE molecule and its receptor, the remarkably low dissociation constant explains the persistence of sensitization in passive transfer experiments. IgE receptors are also present on neutrophils, eosinophils, macrophages, and platelets. However, in contrast to mast cells and basophils, the number of these receptors per cell varies from 1000 to 60,000. IgE receptors on nonmetachromatic cells are structurally distinct from those on mast cells and basophils and have a much lower affinity.

IgE antibody bound to the IgE receptor forms complexes that migrate in the surface membrane of mast cells and basophils. Antigen binding to adjacent IgE antibodies modifies membrane function and promotes calcium influx (Fig. 28–1). This event signals the noncytolytic release of biogenic amines, neutral proteases, proteoglycans, acid hydrolases, and chemotactic factors. In addition to the release of these preformed mediators, activated mast cells and basophils begin to synthesize and later release products of arachidonic acid metabolism (eicosanoids) and an alkylglycerylетherphosphorylcholine designated PAF-acether.

Biogenic amines of human mast cells are limited to histamine; the rat mast cell contains both histamine and serotonin. The biologic properties of histamine are mediated through binding and activation of H_1 and H_2 cell surface receptors. In general, histamine promotes airway and gastrointestinal smooth muscle contraction and arteriolar vasodilation. Histamine also stimulates afferent nonmyelinated nerve endings. Antidromic neural conduction results in the release of neuropeptides, including substance P. In addition to vasodilation, neuropeptides also promote mast cell activation. Contraction of endothelial cells within the postcapillary venules follows. This process results in the exudation of plasma fluid and the production of edema.

Heterogeneity of the human mast cell population has recently been discovered.[21] Among other distinguishing characteristics, mucosal mast cells and cutaneous mast cells differ in some of their mediators. Both cell populations contain the neutral protease tryptase, whereas only cutaneous mast cells contain chymase. Proteoglycan content also helps distinguish these two cell populations. Chondroitin sulfate is the major proteoglycan in mucosal mast cells, whereas heparin predominates in cutaneous mast cells. Apparently, both cell populations contain the acid hydrolases β-hexosaminidase, β-glucuronidase, β-D-galactosidase, and arylsulfatase. Chemotactic factors include an oligopeptide (ECF-A) that preferentially attracts and activates eosinophils. Neutrophil chemotactic factor of anaphylaxis (NCF-A) is a high molecular weight glycoprotein which, as its name implies, preferentially attracts and activates neutrophils.

Mast cell activation augments phospholipase activity, which in turn promotes hydrolysis of membrane associated phosphoglycerides. Products of hydrolysis include diacyl glycerol and arachidonic acid.[22] Diacyl glycerol promotes membrane fusion and presumably assists the mast cell in release of the preformed mediators contained within the cytoplasmic granules. Arachidonic acid acts

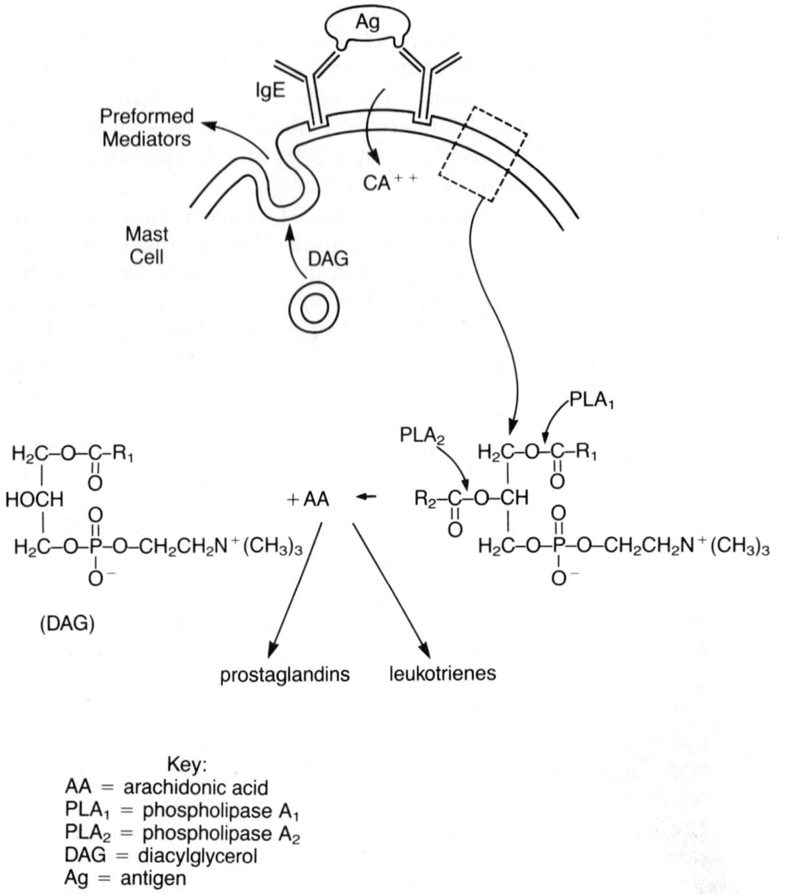

Key:
AA = arachidonic acid
PLA_1 = phospholipase A_1
PLA_2 = phospholipase A_2
DAG = diacylglycerol
Ag = antigen

Figure 28–1. Mast cell activation.

as the substrate for the newly synthesized mast cell mediators. The predominant metabolite of the cyclooxygenase pathway in human mast cells is the prostanoid PGD_2. Prostaglandin PGE_2, $PGF_2\alpha$, 6-keto-$PGF_1\alpha$, and thromboxane are minor components of arachidonic metabolism in human pulmonary mast cells.[23] Lipoxygenase pathway enzymes yield unstable acyclic hydroperoxyeicosantetraenoic acids (HPETEs), which undergo enzymatic and nonenzymatic conversion to hydroxyeisocatetraenoic acids (HETEs). In particular, 5-HPETE forms the 5,6-epoxide LTA_4. This is converted to LTC_4, LTD_4, and LTE_4, which, in combination, comprise slow-reacting substance of anaphylaxis (SRS-A).[24] LTA_4 is also the substrate for a 5,12-diHETE called LTB_4.

Biologic properties of PGD_2 include bronchoconstriction, peripheral vasodilatation, coronary and pulmonary vasoconstriction, inhibition of platelet aggregation, enhanced neutrophil chemokinesis, and basophil histamine release. LTB_4 promotes neutrophil chemotaxis and adherence and modifies vascular permeability. LTC_4, LTD_4, and LTE_4 also augment vascular permeability, and both LTC_4 and LTD_4 are potent stimuli for bronchoconstriction. LTC_4 also constricts arterioles.

Platelet activating factor is another newly synthesized mast cell mediator. Phospholipase A_2 promotes hydrolysis of 1-*O*-alkyl-2-acyl-glyceryl-3-phosphorylcholine to lyso-PAF. This substrate is acetylated to PAF-acether. In addition to stimulation of platelet aggregation and degranulation, PAF-acether promotes neutrophil chemotaxis and activation, pulmonary vasoconstriction and edema, systemic hypotension, and bronchoconstriction.

In combination, preformed and newly synthesized mast cell and basophil mediators are proinflammatory. A case can be made for most of the mast cell/basophil mediators in the pathogenesis of stinging insect anaphylaxis. However, histamine is the only mediator identified with certainty as influential.[25]

Histamine, when injected into humans, may result in urticaria, angioedema, hypotension, altered coronary blood flow, an increase or a decrease in respiratory rate, vomiting, and tenesmus.

Unusual Reactions

Most adverse reactions following stinging insect challenge are anaphylactic in nature. However, occasionally there are reactions involving the neurologic or vascular systems without associated findings of anaphylaxis. Vasculitis, nephrosis, serum sickness, neuritis, and encephalopathy have followed Hymenoptera species stings. These reactions may be noted several days to a week following the insect challenge, and fatalities have been reported. Although the pathogenesis remains to be defined, these unusual reactions do not seem to be related to allergic antibody and mast cells/basophils.

DIAGNOSIS

Signs and symptoms of acute anaphylaxis occurring shortly after a painful insect sting should suggest Hymenoptera species hypersensitivity. The essential features necessary for this diagnosis are:

1. Signs and symptoms of acute anaphylaxis
2. History or clinical evidence of Hymenoptera species envenomation
3. Demonstration of allergic antibody with specificity for a stinging insect venom.

The presenting manifestations must be compatible with anaphylaxis. Although the history of an antecedent sting is necessary, there may be problems in recognition when a toddler or unconscious patient cannot relate this information. On occasion, a careful examination may uncover signs of insect envenomation. The fire ant leaves its hallmark of a sterile pustule. The remnants of the barbed honeybee stinger would suggest a honeybee sting, but as mentioned previously, on a rare occasion the yellow jacket may also leave its stinger.

The events surrounding the patient's episode of anaphylaxis may also prove helpful in clarification of the precipitating event. Outdoor activities during summer months would enhance the chances of insect anaphylaxis. In contrast, in most locations of the Northern Hemisphere, stinging insect allergic reactions are unlikely during winter months. In a like manner, fire ant allergy is unlikely in regions where this insect has not been seen. A history of previous insect anaphylaxis would prove helpful in making the diagnosis. However, in a substantial number of cases, there is no prior evidence of Hymenoptera species venom hypersensitivity. Family history of atopy in general or insect allergy in particular offers no particular assistance to the diagnosis.

Patient identification of the particular Hymenoptera species responsible for envenomation is generally considered unreliable. With the exception of fire ants and honeybees, there are no reliable clues on physical examination. Identification and differentiation between the wasp, yellow jacket, and hornet is extremely difficult in the brief moments before a sting. On occasion, the nest or dead insect may be retrieved.

Confirmation of anaphylaxis due to Hymenoptera species envenomation hinges on demonstration of allergic sensitization. Reliable methods include skin tests with appropriate insect venoms and radioallergosorbent (RAST) tests. In the case of fire ants, venom is not yet commercially available. Practicing allergists confronted with potentially fire ant allergic subjects therefore rely on whole body fire ant extracts for diagnosis. Comparative studies suggest that the purified fire ant venoms are more potent than whole body extracts.[26, 27] However, the whole body fire ant extracts appear sufficiently potent to reliably identify allergic subjects.[28, 29]

At concentrations of up to 1 μg/ml, apid and vespid venoms are reliable skin test antigens. At 1 μg/ml, most sensitive patients will have flare and wheal responses by 15 minutes. With concentrations greater than this, nonspecific reactions are seen in a respectable number of nonallergic subjects. In contrast, defining sensitivity as a positive immediate skin test reaction to an intradermal injection of venom at concentrations up to and including 1 mg/ml, the false-positive reaction rate is quite small.[30] Insect skin tests are associated with a small chance of anaphylaxis. For this reason, intradermal skin tests are preceded by epicutaneous skin testing. The response dictates the initial dose selected for intradermal skin test injections. RAST analysis provides a convenient alternative, but variability between laboratories provides a complicating factor in analysis of results.

As implied, the presence of signs or symptoms of an allergic reaction are critical in the diagnosis of Hymenoptera species venom allergy. Patients without manifestations of an allergic response who present for emergency care following an insect sting generally do not need specific venom testing. Patients with large, local reactions following stinging insect envenomation are one possible exception. Case reports of insect anaphylaxis preceded by large local reactions have been used as justification for testing this patient population for insect hypersensitivity. However, considering that approximately 50 per cent of subjects with large local reactions may have venom specific IgE antibodies, this practice is debatable.

THERAPY

Therapy for allergic illness includes the classic triad of avoidance, medications, and modification of host immunity using antigen injections (Table 28–5). This remains true for stinging insect allergy. There are no studies regarding the efficacy of avoidance measures, but logically these guidelines should reduce risk of exposure for the insect-allergic patient. When nests are identified, an exterminator (or individual without insect hypersensitivity) should be asked to remove and destroy them. In the case of fire ant hypersensitivity, ant mounds can be treated with an insecticide. The insect-allergic patient should avoid sandals and bare feet when outside and should wear a hat, long sleeves, and pants when flying insects are anticipated. When gardening or handling piled trash, lumber, or stone, one should wear gloves. The allergic individual should avoid trimming hedges, bushes, and trees and should have others mow the lawn. In particular, caution should be taken in picnic areas, around garbage cans, and near fruit trees or roadside fruit stands where food may attract insects. In addition, the insect-allergic patient should not attract insects by wearing brightly colored clothes or scented cosmetics. When an insect begins to swarm, the person should stay calm and slowly move away and should not provoke the insect by swatting.

Table 28–5. THERAPY FOR INSECT STING ANAPHYLAXIS

Avoidance
Nests
Nonprotective clothing
Perfumed cosmetics
Medication
Epinephrine HCl, 0.01 ml/kg up to 0.3–0.5 ml of 1:1000 concentration given subcutaneously
Volume expansion with normal saline, Ringer's lactate or colloid; vasopressors for unresponsive hypotension
Inhaled adrenergics for respiratory distress unresponsive to epinephrine; may need airway stabilization
Steroids
Patient identification
Immunotherapy

Although histamine is one of the mast cell mediators contributing to the pathophysiology of the patient's symptoms (elevated levels of the substance have been documented during episodes of insect anaphylaxis), clinical experience clearly demonstrates that antihistamines are of little benefit in treating hypotension, laryngeal edema, or bronchospasm. This experience suggests that the doses of antihistamines customarily used may be insufficient. It also illustrates the fact that for maximal effect, antihistamines should be given prior to histamine release. However, this clinical experience is also used to support the concept that mast cell mediators other than histamine have major significance in the pathophysiology of anaphylaxis.

In contrast, *epinephrine* may prove life-saving in cases of anaphylaxis. In 50 fatal episodes of Hymenoptera envenomation, only 6 per cent of patients received therapy within the first hour after being stung.[18] This outcome is contrasted to 100 nonfatal outcomes in which 87 per cent of cases received treatment within the same time period. In most cases, the clinician needs to use both the α- and β-adrenergic effects of epinephrine; therefore, this agent is preferable to the more selective β_2-adrenergics such as terbutaline sulfate.

When a patient who has insect anaphylaxis presents with findings of systemic hypotension, *volume expansion* is indicated. This can be accomplished with either normal saline, Ringer's lactate, or colloid. Vasopressors may be added if, after correction of the intravascular depletion induced by vasodilatation and increased capillary permeability, hypotension persists. With severe respiratory distress that is insufficiently responsive to epinephrine, inhaled bronchodilators may prove helpful. As noted, respiratory distress may be due to bronchospasm or airway edema. Ultimately, stabilization of the airway may become necessary. In cases of hypotension or respiratory distress, parenteral steroids are usually added to the treatment regimen.

The insect-allergic patient should have ready access to epinephrine. Prepackaged needles and devices that automatically inject standard doses of epinephrine are readily available. Just as for the patient with diabetes mellitus or epilepsy, the insect-allergic patient should also be advised to wear some form of identification indicating the medical condition.

Venom injections represent the third aspect of therapy. Graded doses of venom, given by injection on a regular basis, modify the insect-allergic patient's clinical sensitivity. A study of 59 insect-allergic patients given either placebo, whole body extract, or specific venom and then challenged by an insect sting in a controlled setting clearly demonstrated efficacy of venom injections.[12] Only one of twenty subjects with a history of stinging insect anaphylaxis and venom specific IgE who received venom injections had any clinical evidence of allergic sensitization when rechallenged. This was statistically different from the 40 per cent to 60 per cent who, despite administration of whole body extract injections or placebo, had clinical manifestations of insect anaphylaxis on rechallenge.

Immunologic effects of venom injections include both the generation of venom specific IgG class antibodies and augmentation of subsequent venom specific IgE synthesis. With initial injections, the concentration of IgE specific for the venom proteins increases. However, with continued injections, the concentration then falls. In some cases, the venom specific IgE becomes nondetectable.

Venom injection therapy is not indicated for patients with adverse reactions (such as nephrosis) following an insect sting that are not mediated by an allergic response. Prevention of fatal anaphylaxis has been used as justification for these costly and potentially dangerous injections. Some have argued that relatively infrequent fatal reactions in children should influence the decision regarding this mode of therapy. They would limit therapy to those individuals with a previous life-threatening reaction and would withhold such therapy from children whose previous manifestations were limited to generalized urticaria.

Unresolved issues regarding insect venom immunotherapy include clarification of the immunologic events that confer protection, duration of therapy, antigen cross-reactivity (and venoms selection criteria), and efficacy of fire ant whole body extract injections. As with other allergens, efforts at chemical modifications of venom that could maintain immunogenicity while reducing allergenicity, if effective, should prove rewarding.

NONVENOMOUS INSECT ALLERGY

A few insects have been associated with inhalant allergy. The caddis fly, mayfly, aphid, and cockroach are generally recognized as carriers of potent inhalant allergens. Symptoms exhibited on exposure to the sensitive subject include those of allergic rhinitis, allergic conjunctivitis, and asthma. In unusually heavy exposures to moths, butterflies, bees, beetles, and screwworms, inhalant allergy has also been suggested, and positive skin test reactions have been identified.

Some of the biting insects have been associated with anaphylaxis. Although the fire ant first bites and thereby anchors its position on the victim, as previously described, this process is followed by envenomation with the modified ovipositor. In contrast, the kissing bug, bedbug, and deerfly lack a stinging apparatus and only bite. Each has been associated with systemic anaphylaxis. In the case of deerflies, immediately positive intradermal skin tests suggest an allergic pathogenesis.[31] The rather common experience of immediate and delayed local reactions following mosquito and flea bites has prompted studies investigating an immunologic response. Although an immediate skin test response has been documented with appropriate extracts, an allergic pathogenesis remains speculative because of the apparent difficulty in conferring this response in passive transfer experiments.

References

1. Waterhouse AT: Bee sting and anaphylaxis. Lancet 2:946, 1914.

2. Barnard JH: Studies of 400 Hymenoptera sting deaths in the United States. J Allergy Clin Immunol *52*:259, 1973.
3. Settipane GA, Boyd GK: Prevalence of bee sting allergy in 4,992 Boy Scouts. Acta Allergol *25*:286, 1970.
4. Settipane GA, Newstead GJ, Boyd GK: Frequency of Hymenoptera allergy in an atopic and normal population. J Allergy Clin Immunol *50*:146, 1972.
5. Golden DBK, Valentine MD, Kagey-Sobotka A, et al: Prevalence of Hymenoptera venom allergy. J Allergy Clin Immunol *69*(suppl):124, 1982.
6. Lockey RF, Turkeltaub PC, Baird-Warren IA: The Hymenoptera venom study I, 1979–1982: Demographics and history-sting data. J Allergy Clin Immunol *82*:370, 1988.
7. Settipane GA, Klein DE, Boyd GK: Relationship of atopy and anaphylactic sensitization: A bee sting allergy model. Clin Allergy *8*:259, 1978.
8. Huber P, Hoigne R, Schmid P, Dozzi M, et al: Atopy and generalized allergic reactions to Hymenoptera stings. Monogr Allergy *18*:147, 1983.
9. Grant JA, Rahr R, Rhueson D, et al: Diagnosis of Polistes wasp hypersensitivity. J Allergy Clin Immunol *72*:399, 1983.
10. Rhoades RB, Schafer WL, Schmid WH, et al: Hypersensitivity to the imported fire ant: A report of 49 cases. J Allergy Clin Immunol *56*:85, 1975.
11. Benson RL, Semenov H: Allergy in its relation to bee sting. J Allergy *1*:105, 1930.
12. Hunt KJ, Valentine MD, Sobotka AK, et al: A controlled trial of immunotherapy in insect hypersensitivity. N Engl J Med *299*:157, 1978.
13. Wypych JI, Reisman RE, Elliott WB, et al: Immunologic and biochemical evaluation of the potency of whole insect body extracts. J Allergy Clin Immunol *63*:267, 1979.
14. Valentine MD: Insect venom allergy: Diagnosis and treatment. J Allergy Clin Immunol *73*:299, 1984.
15. Cavagnol RM: The pharmacological effects of Hymenoptera venoms. Annu Rev Pharmacol Toxicol *17*:479, 1977.
16. Hannan CJ, Stafford CT, Rhoades RB, et al: Seasonal variation in antigens of the imported fire ant *Solenopsis invicta*. J Allergy Clin Immunol *78*:331, 1986.
17. Light WC, Reisman RE: Stinging insect allergy: Changing concepts. Postgrad Med *59*:153, 1976.
18. Barnard JH: Studies of 400 Hymenoptera sting deaths in the United States. J Allergy Clin Immunol *52*:259, 1973.
19. Delage C, Irey NS: Anaphylactic deaths: A clinicopathologic study of 43 cases. J Forensic Sci *17*:525, 1972.
20. Ogawa M, Nakahata T, Leary AG, et al: Suspension culture of human mast cells/basophils from umbilical cord blood mononuclear cells. Proc Natl Acad Sci USA *80*:4494, 1983.
21. Enerback L: Mast cell heterogeneity: The evoluation of the concept of a specific mucosal mast cell. *In* Befus AD, Bienenstock J, Denburg JA (eds): Mast Cell Differentiation and Heterogeneity. New York, Raven Press, 1986, p 1.
22. Warner JA, Peters SP, Lichtenstein LM, et al: ^{3}H arachidonic acid incorporation and metabolism in purified human basophils (abst). Fed Proc *45*:735, 1986.
23. Lewis RA, Soter NA, Diamond PT, et al: Prostaglandin D_2 generation after activation of rat and human mast cells with anti-IgE. J Immunol *129*:1627, 1982.
24. Hammarstrom S: Leukotrienes. Annu Rev Biochem *52*:355, 1983.
25. Wasserman SI, Marquardt DL: Anaphylaxis. *In* Middleton E, Reed CE, Ellis EF, Adkinson NF, Yunginger JW (eds): Allergy: Principles and Practice. St. Louis, CV Mosby, 1988.
26. Paull BR, Coghlan RH, Vinson SB: Fire ant venom hypersensitivity. J Allergy Clin Immunol *71*:101, 1983.
27. Reed MA, deShazo RD, Ortiz AA, et al: Comparison between RAST with imported fire ant (IFA), whole body extracts (IFAWBE), and venom (IFAV). J Allergy Clin Immunol *79*:217, 1987.
28. Strom GB, Boswell RN, Jacobs RL: In vivo and *in vitro* comparison of fire ant venom and fire ant whole body extract. J Allergy Clin Immunol *72*:46, 1983.
29. Triplett RF: Sensitivity to the imported fire ant: Successful treatment with immunotherapy. South Med J *66*:477, 1973.
30. Hunt KJ, Valentine MD, Sobotka AK, et al: Diagnosis of allergy to stinging insects by skin testing with Hymenoptera venoms. Ann Intern Med *85*:56, 1976.
31. Wilber RD, Evans RE: An immunologic evaluation of deer fly hypersensitivity. J Allergy Clin Immunol *55*:72, 1975.

CHAPTER 29
MUSHROOMS

Jeffrey Brent, M.D., Ph.D.
Ken Kulig, M.D.
Barry H. Rumack, M.D.

It is probably easiest to understand mushroom toxicology by categorizing mushrooms into groups based on the toxins they contain and the symptoms and signs they may cause. Given a history of mushroom ingestion, it should be possible for one to determine to which groups the mushroom may belong based on the clinical picture, pending definitive identification of the mushroom in question. The possible mushroom-associated syndromes and the typical causative species are listed in Table 29–1. This determination of the types of mushrooms ingested based on the presenting syndrome is quite similar to what is encountered daily in the emergency department, where patients are seen after overdosing on unknown medications.

GENERAL MANAGEMENT

As with all poisonings, supportive care is of primary importance. Airway management and cardiopulmonary resuscitation, along with maintenance of vital signs, should take priority over identification of the toxin and concern about antidotes.

Guidelines for initial management are listed in Table 29–2. Most patients who have symptoms after mushroom ingestion will have prominent gastrointestinal complaints: vomiting, diarrhea (often bloody), and abdominal pain. It is important to determine the time course of the development of symptoms after ingestion. If they developed later than 6 hours after ingestion it can be assumed that the mushrooms belonged either to the cyclopeptide (the deadly *Amanitas*), monomethylhydrazine, or orelline group. With mushrooms from the orelline group, symptoms may develop later than 24 hours after ingestion. It is emphasized, however, that gastrointestinal symptoms occurring within a few hours of ingestion do not rule out poisoning by these mushrooms; the patient also may have ingested a number of different mushrooms that cause early symptoms.

Activated charcoal may be of benefit in absorbing any toxin remaining in the gut. If the patient presents within 1 hour of the time of ingestion and has not spontaneously vomited, it may be useful to lavage the stomach with a large-bore tube. Activated charcoal may be administered via the tube after the lavage. Any gastric contents obtained either by spontaneous emesis or lavage should be saved and examined for spores.

To examine for spores, the gastric aspirate or emesis sample should be filtered through cheesecloth, centrifuged for 10 minutes, and the heavier layer at the bottom of the test tube containing the spores removed carefully with a pipette. Add a drop of water and a cover slip and place under the oil-immersion lens. Mushroom spores, in general, are essentially the same size as red blood cells (8 to 20 μm). Spores found in either the gastric contents or lamellae should be examined under the microscope for (1) general appearance, (2) shape, (3) color, (4) thick or thin walls; and (5) the presence of pores.

A spore print can be helpful in identifying the mushroom in question. This is formed by placing the cap of the mushroom on a white piece of paper (Fig. 29–1) and allowing the spores to fall on the paper, imparting a characteristic color. An example of a spore print is shown in Figure 29–2. Because it generally takes several hours for an adequate spore print to develop, one should be started as soon as possible. It is usually helpful to cover the cap with a glass or bowl while the spore print is being formed to prevent the dispersion of spores by drafts.

Because even veteran mushroom hunters occasionally make an error, many have adopted the practice of only eating one kind of mushroom at a time and saving a sample in case unanticipated effects occur.

If you are fortunate enough to have a professional mycologist in your area, he or she should be able to tell you the principal types of mushrooms in your region and assist you in mushroom identification. Local or

Table 29–1. SUMMARY OF COMMON MUSHROOM-ASSOCIATED SYNDROMES

SYNDROME	CLINICAL COURSE	TOXINS	TYPICAL CAUSATIVE MUSHROOMS*
Delayed gastroenteritis followed by hepatorenal syndrome	Stage I: 6–24 hr post ingestion: onset of nausea, vomiting, profuse cholera-like diarrhea, abdominal pain, hematuria Stage II: 12–48 hr post ingestion: apparent recovery; hepatic enzymes are rising during this stage Stage III: 24–72 hr post ingestion: progressive hepatic and renal failure, coagulopathy, cardiomyopathy, encephalopathy, convulsions, coma, death	Cyclopeptides principally amatoxins	"Deadly *Amanitas*," *Galerina* sp.
Anticholinergic syndrome	30 min–2 hr post ingestion: delirium and hallucinations typically associated with anticholinergic findings	Muscimol, ibotenic acid	*Amanita muscaria*, *A. pantherina*
Delayed gastroenteritis with central nervous system abnormalities	6–24 hr post ingestion: nausea, vomiting, diarrhea, abdominal pain, muscle cramps, delirium, convulsions, coma; hemolysis and methemoglobinemia may occur	Monomethyl-hydrazine	*Gyromitra esculenta* ("false morel")
Cholinergic syndrome	30 min–2 hr post ingestion: bradycardia, bronchorrhea, bronchospasm, salivation, perspiration, lacrimation, convulsions, coma	Muscarine	*Boletus* sp., *Clitocybe* sp., *Inocybe* sp., *Amanita* sp.
Disulfuram-like reaction with ethanol	30 min after drinking ethanol (may occur up to 1 wk after eating coprine-containing mushrooms): flushing of skin of face and trunk, hypotension, tachycardia, chest pain, dyspnea, nausea, vomiting, extreme apprehension	Coprine	*Coprinus atramentarius*
Hallucinations	30 min–3 hr post ingestion: hallucinations, euphoria, drowsiness, compulsive behavior, agitation	Indoles, psilocybin, and psilocin	*Psilocybe* sp.
Delayed gastritis and renal failure	Abdominal pain, anorexia, vomiting starting over 30 hr post ingestion followed by progressive renal failure 3–14 days later	Orelline, orellanine	*Cortinarius* sp.
General gastrointestinal irritants	30 min–2 hr post ingestion: nausea, vomiting, abdominal cramping, diarrhea; may recover without treatment	Unidentified, probably multiple	*Chlorophyllum molybdites*, backyard mushrooms ("little brown mushrooms"), many others

*See Table 29–3 for an extensive list of mushrooms causing these syndromes.

regional poison centers should know how to reach mycologists in their region. When a patient is seen following a mushroom ingestion, ask a family member or friend to bring in a similar mushroom (if possible) for identification purposes. Keep the specimen under refrigeration wrapped in wax paper and stored in a paper bag. (A thorough discussion of mushroom identification may be found in the literature.[1])

The greatest concern is for the ingestion of deadly *Amanitas*. There have been many antidotes and treatments suggested for this kind of poisoning, most of them unproven. If vomiting and diarrhea are severe enough to result in significant fluid loss, intravenous replacement of volume and electrolytes is important. The intravenous solution should contain glucose.

By consulting Table 29–1, it should be apparent to which group the ingested mushrooms may belong. For ease of discussion, further management recommendations are described under the specific toxins. Common mushroom species containing the toxins discussed appear in Table 29–3.

CYCLOPEPTIDES

(Color Plate II, Figs. 29–3, 29–4, and 29–5)*

The cyclopeptide-containing mushrooms are responsible for over 90 per cent of all

*On Color Plates II and III at the front of the book.

Table 29–2. GENERAL MANAGEMENT OF MUSHROOM INGESTION

1. Determine history of ingestion: how many types of mushrooms ingested, what time, if anyone else ate them, and what symptoms are present.
2. History of symptom presentation with emphasis on chronology. Attempt to determine which of the possible syndromes (see Table 29–1) the patient may have. For example, gastrointestinal symptoms occurring more than 6 hours post ingestion strongly suggest cyclopeptide, monomethylhydrazine, or *Cortinarius* poisoning.
3. Administer activated charcoal. If the patient has diarrhea, do not give a cathartic. Repeat the activated charcoal every 4 hours until charcoal-laden stools are passed. If a cathartic is used, give it only with the first dose of activated charcoal.
4. If feasible, and when indicated, send gastric aspirate or emesis, along with any remaining mushrooms, to a mycologist for identification.
5. Try to perform a preliminary identification of mushroom and spores. Start to develop a spore print as soon as possible.
6. Maintain supportive measures, including airway support, intravenous fluids, and vasopressors (if needed).
7. If the ingested mushroom is of the cyclopeptide or orelline group, admit patient and follow hepatic and renal function until recovery.
8. Avoid antispasmodics for gastrointestinal symptoms.

deaths from mushroom poisonings. Although there are a variety of mushrooms in this group (see Table 29–3), almost all fatalities and serious poisonings are caused by the deadly *Amanitas*, particularly *Amanita phalloides.* The cyclopeptides consist primarily of amatoxins, which contain eight amino acids in their structure, and phallotoxins, which contain seven. Over 15 cyclopeptides have been isolated from the genus *Amanita.* Note, however, that not all mushrooms of the

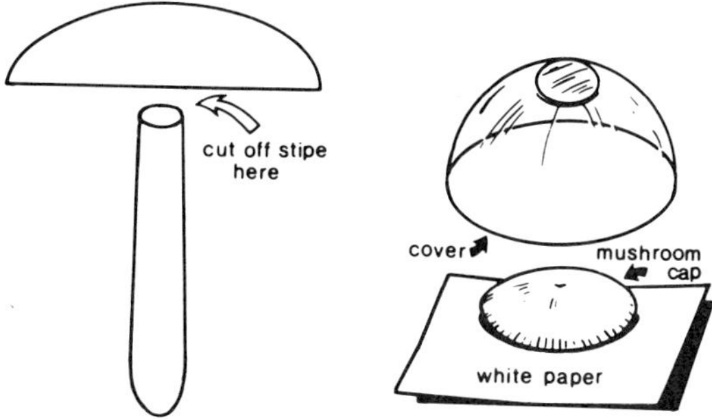

Figure 29–1. Technique of developing a spore print. (Reprinted with permission from Rumack BH, Salzman E (eds): Mushroom Poisoning: Diagnosis and Treatment. West Palm Beach, FL, CRC Press, 1978. Copyright The Chemical Rubber Company, CRC Press, Inc.)

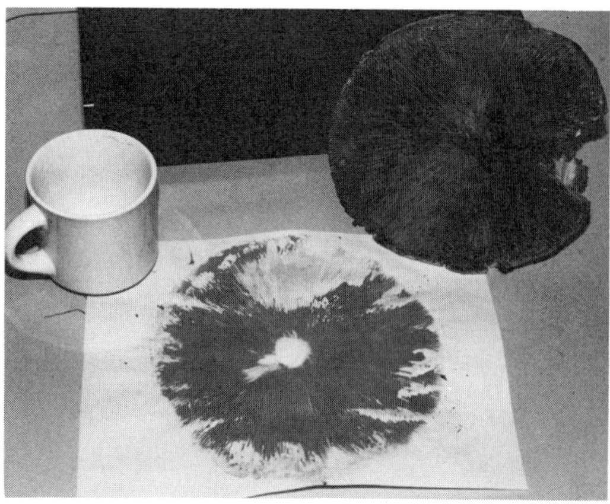

Figure 29–2. Spore print of *Chlorophyllum molybdites.* Courtesy of Lynn Augenstein, M.D., and the Rocky Mountain Poison Center, Denver.

Amanita species contain significant quantities of amatoxin. *Amanita muscaria* and *A. pantherina,* for example, contain no amatoxin.

The phallotoxins are extremely potent hepatotoxins but are not well absorbed from the gastrointestinal tract and therefore contribute little to *Amanita* toxicity. They may contribute to the initial gastroenteritis-like picture, however. Laboratory animals cannot be poisoned by oral administration of phalloidin, whereas they die within hours after intravenous injection.

Amatoxins have been demonstrated to be actively absorbed and potent hepatotoxins. Alpha-amanitin is the principal toxin in this group. The nucleoli of liver cells disintegrate soon after exposure to alpha-amanitin, which interferes with transcription of deoxyribonucleic acid (DNA) by inhibiting ribonucleic acid (RNA) polymerase II. For this reason alpha-amanitin is used as a research tool in molecular biology.

Circulating amatoxins can be detected for approximately 24 hours after ingestion. Most of the ingested alpha-amanitin is excreted renally, and urine levels tend to be higher than serum levels. Although amatoxins can be detected by very sensitive radioimmunoassay or high pressure liquid chromatographic methods, these are not usually clinically available. The Meixner test is a bedside assay that can detect amatoxins. In this test, gastric material or pulverized mushroom juice is spotted on pulp paper (e.g., newspaper) and allowed to dry. A blue color developing within ½ hour of applying several drops of concentrated hydrochloric acid to the spot constitutes a positive test.

Table 29–3. SOME MUSHROOM SPECIES, BY CLINICAL GROUPING OF TOXINS

CYCLOPEPTIDES (AMATOXINS, PHALLOTOXINS)
Amanita phalloides ("death cap")
A. verna ("death angel") (see Fig. 29–3)
A. virosa ("destroying angel") (see Fig. 29–4)
A. bisporigera
A. ocreata
A. suballiacae
A. tenuifolia
Galerina autumnaluis (see Fig. 29–5)
G. marginata
G. venerata
Lepiota helveola
L. vosserandii
Conocybe filaris

MUSCIMOL, IBOTENIC ACID
Amanita muscaria ("fly agaric") (see Fig. 29–6)
A. pantherina (see Fig. 29–7)
A. gemmata
A. cokeri
A. cothurnata

MONOMETHYLHYDRAZINE
Gyromitra esculenta ("false morel") (see Fig. 29–8)
G. gigas
G. ambigua
G. infula (see Fig. 29–9)
G. caroliniana
G. brunnea
G. fastigiata
Paxina sp.
Sarcosphaera coronaria

MUSCARINE
Boletus calopus
B. luridus
B. pulcherrimus
B. satanas
Clitocybe cerrusata (see Fig. 29–10)
C. dealbata
C. illudens
C. riuulosa
Inocybe fastigiata (see Fig. 29–11)
I. geophylla
I. lilacina
I. patuoillardi
I. purica
I. rimosus
*Amanita muscaria**
*A. pantherina**

COPRINE
Coprinus atramentarius ("inky cap") (see Fig. 29–12)
Clitocybe clavipes

INDOLES
Psilocybe cubensis (see Fig. 29–13)
P. caerulescens
P. cyanescens
P. baeocystis
P. fimentaria
P. mexicana
P. pelluculosa
P. semilanceata
P. silvatica
Conocybe cyanopus
Gymnopilus aeruginosa
G. spectabilis
G. validipes
Panaeolus foenisecii ("mowers mushroom")
P. subbalteatus
Stropharis coronilla

ORELLINE/ORELLANINE
Cortinarius orellanus
C. speciosissinus (see Fig. 29–15)
C. splendoma
C. gentilis

GENERAL GASTROINTESTINAL IRRITANTS
Many species from diverse genera
"Little brown mushrooms" (backyard mushrooms)
Chlorophyllum molybdites (see Fig. 29–14)
Orphalates illudens ("jack-o'-lantern")

*Although *A. muscarina* and *A. pantherina* contain muscarine in small quantities, anticholinergic symptoms usually predominate.
All figures are in Color Plates II and III.

The cyclopeptides are not denatured by boiling, and hence cooking the deadly *Amanita* mushrooms does not render them nontoxic. It has been estimated that one *A. phalloides* cap may be lethal to an adult.

The identification of the deadly *Amanitas* in the field should not be difficult, yet for a variety of reasons even those who have picked and consumed mushrooms for many years with impunity are not immune to making that fatal mistake. Figure 29–16 demonstrates the maturation of a typical *Amanita* mushroom and how the classic annulus and "death cup" develop. These structures are not always obvious, however, and may be obliterated in the act of picking the mushroom out of the ground. The immature "buttons" in many ways resemble edible puff-

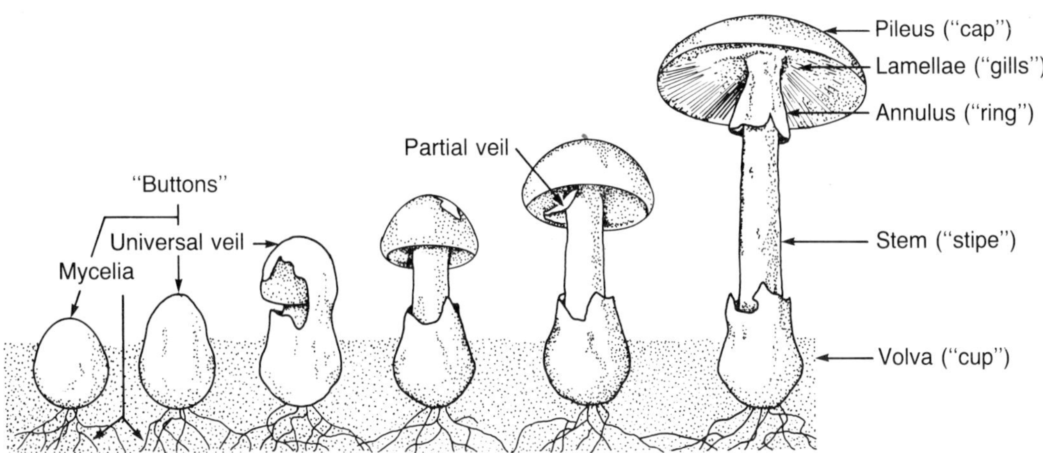

Figure 29–16. Maturation of *Amanita* species. The early stages ("buttons") may resemble nontoxic "puffballs." The lamellae and spores are white in all *Amanita* species, whereas the pileus may be white, as in *A. phalloides, A. verna,* or *A. virosa,* or bright orange-red, as in *A. muscaria.* The distinguishing features of all amanitas include the annulus and volva ("death cup"); however, these are frequently destroyed in the process of picking and preparing the mushroom. The amanitas are toxic during all stages of development. (Adapted from Litten W: The most poisonous mushrooms. Sci Am *232*:90, 1975.)

balls. It is useful to remember that all species of deadly *Amanitas* have white gills and spore prints.

The classic clinical presentation of *Amanita* poisoning consists of three stages. Patients do not have gastrointestinal symptoms for at least 6 hours after ingestion and then suddenly develop colicky abdominal pain, vomiting, and severe diarrhea (stage I). The diarrhea may contain blood and mucus and may be so severe that it has been termed cholera-like.

Even without treatment, patients may go on to apparent recovery (stage II), although during the next day hepatic enzymes may be rising. Two to 4 days after ingestion, the patient may then progress to fulminant hepatic, cardiac, and renal failure; pancreatitis; diffuse intravascular coagulation; convulsions; and death (stage III).

The pathologic picture of hepatic necrosis tends to be most marked in the centrilobular areas. In a series of aggressively treated patients the death rate from *Amanita phalloides* poisoning is in the range of 9 to 11 per cent. Although most patients with cyclopeptide-induced hepatotoxicity will have a full recovery, a small percentage will develop immune complex–mediated chronic active hepatitis.

A wide variety of antidotes to *Amanita* poisoning have been touted to be beneficial, but for the most part clinical reports have been anecdotal. The use of thioctic acid has been lauded in the European literature based on anecdotal reports. Being a dithiol compound, it has been postulated to function as a free radical scavenger. However, there is no convincing human evidence of its efficacy.

Intravenous penicillin has also been recommended on the theory that it inhibits the uptake of amatoxin by hepatocytes. A variety of other protective mechanisms for penicillin have also been proposed. Animal data and retrospective human data suggest that benzylpenicillin (penicillin G) in the dose range of 300,000 to 1,000,000 units/kg/day was hepatoprotective; however, this could not be demonstrated in a prospective study.

Silibinin, a component of silymarin, an abstract of thistle, has been shown to be effective in animals in reducing hepatotoxicity by inhibiting amatoxin uptake by hepatocytes. It has also been postulated to act as a free radical scavenger. However, there are no convincing data that it is useful in humans, and its routine use therefore cannot be recommended.

There have been anecdotal reports and preliminary animal data on a number of additional antidotes including hyperbaric oxygen, cimetidine, ascorbic acid, cephalosporins, corticosteroids, cytochrome C, bile salts, heavy metal salts, *D*-penicillamine, and diethyldithiocarbamate. However, there are no firm clinical data indicating that any of them are useful.

Although it is unclear if any of these antidotes are of value in the management of amatoxin poisoning, there is little doubt that aggressive optimization of the patient's fluid status is of paramount importance.

Charcoal hemoperfusion or hemodialysis may be theoretically useful in enhancing elimination early after ingestion. However, this has never been known to be beneficial and may be impractical since most patients present late.

Liver transplantation has been successfully performed on several patients with severe cyclopeptide-induced hepatotoxicity. Since most patients with amatoxin poisoning will recover with aggressive supportive care, transplantation should not be considered to be standard treatment for hepatotoxicity. However, if a patient shows signs of severe hepatotoxicity, transfer to a transplantation center may be beneficial to facilitate the procedure should it become necessary.

Because amatoxins have been reported to undergo enterohepatic recirculation, it may be useful to administer activated charcoal for at least 24 hours post ingestion.

Although several other genera of mushrooms contain the toxic cyclopeptides (see Table 29–3), the *Amanitas* (Figs. 29–3 and 29–4) are by far the most commonly ingested that result in significant clinical toxicity. Several species of *Galerina* (Fig. 29–5) contain amatoxin, but these mushrooms are quite small; approximately 15 to 20 *Galerina* mushrooms contain the same amount of toxin as 1 mature *Amanita phalloides.*

One of the common errors made in identification of mushrooms of the *Amanita* species is confusing them with *Chlorophyllum molybdites* mushrooms (see Color Plate III, Fig. 29–14), which also possess an annulus and a swelling at the base resembling a cup. Patients ingesting *C. molybdites* mushrooms, however, usually develop severe vomiting and diarrhea within 2 hours, although many people are able to consume these mushrooms without becoming symptomatic. Differentiating between *C. molybdites* and *Amanitas* should not be difficult. *Chlorophyllum* sp. are the only mushrooms with greenish gills and spores, and the spores are thick walled and contain pores. The mushroom itself will stain a reddish-orange color where it is injured, and the annulus is moveable, as opposed to *Amanita,* in which the annulus is fixed.

MUSCIMOL, IBOTENIC ACID
(Color Plate II, Figs. 29–6 and 29–7)*

Muscarine was first extracted from *Amanita muscaria* in 1869, and its use as a pharmacologic research tool has enhanced our knowledge of the "muscarinic" receptors of the parasympathetic nervous system. Paradoxically, most patients poisoned by *A. muscaria* have anticholinergic findings, as the mushroom contains more potent toxins that have a physiologic effect opposite that of muscarine.

Mushroom species of this group contain the closely related substances muscimol, a hallucinogen, and ibotenic acid, a potent insecticide. *A. muscaria* is commonly known as the "fly agaric" because it attracts and kills flies that land on it. These mushrooms have been utilized for at least 3000 years in the rituals of many Asian and Indian tribes. Within 30 minutes of ingestion, intoxication with ataxia, euphoria, visual perceptual changes, and hallucinations occurs. If the amount is not carefully titrated, however, frank psychosis, convulsions, and coma can develop.

Both *A. muscaria* and *A. pantherina* are very common mushrooms with wide geographic distribution.

Because these mushrooms contain muscarine, a cholinergic agent, atropine has been advocated for years as a specific antidote. Although this may be true in some cases, in the experience of most investigators serious poisoning by *A. muscaria* is associated with anticholinergic-like signs. Delirium and coma have been reversed by physostigmine in many cases. However, because of the dangers inherent in the use of physostigmine, its administration should be restricted to patients with either a severe anticholinergic syndrome or a serious diagnostic dilemma. Usually the diagnosis of an anticholinergic syndrome can be made by careful examination and attention to vital signs.

The identification of *A. muscaria* should be relatively easy. The cap is bright orange or red and is covered with "warts," which are remnants of the universal veil (see Fig. 29–16). As in all *Amanita* species, the annulus and vulva are prominent, and the spores are hyaline, thin walled, and without pores.

---

*On Color Plates II and III at the front of the book.

Many cases of *A. muscaria* poisoning are seen in individuals who deliberately seek and ingest the mushroom for its hallucinogenic properties, and so the history is very important. The purposeful ingestion of urine from people who have eaten these mushrooms has been reported as a way to elicit the psychoactive effects of the excreted muscimol. The treatment consists of supportive care and the use of physostigmine (only if the poisoning is life-threatening or if the patient is psychotic and a danger to himself or herself) or atropine, depending on whether anticholinergic or cholinergic signs predominate.

MONOMETHYLHYDRAZINE

(Color Plate II, Fig. 29–8, and Color Plate III, Fig. 29–9)*

The *Gyromitra* spp., or false morels, are an extremely interesting genus toxicologically. Many species of *Gyromitra* contain monomethylhydrazine (CH_3NHNH_2) or its precursor gyromitrin. Monomethylhydrazine is also used in a variety of industrial processes and as rocket fuel.

Monomethylhydrazine poisoning causes symptoms and signs similar to those seen after isoniazid overdose, and both agents are felt to inhibit the formation of gamma-aminobutyric acid (GABA) in the brain by inducing a state of pyridoxine deficiency. GABA is the primary inhibitory neurotransmitter of the central nervous system.

Six to 24 hours after ingestion of mushrooms from the *Gyromitra* spp., patients develop vomiting, diarrhea, dizziness, fatigue, and muscle cramps. Usually these symptoms are mild, but delirium, coma, and convulsions may occur. Methemoglobinemia and hemolysis may be life-threatening, and in parts of Eastern Europe fatalities from *G. esculenta* are common. Hepatic and renal failures occur with fatal ingestions.

The treatment consists of supportive care, administration of methylene blue for methemoglobin levels greater than 30 per cent, blood transfusions if required, and intravenous pyridoxine for monomethylhydrazine-induced seizures. Pyridoxine (vitamin B_6), which is depleted in poisoning by hydrazines, is a cofactor in the synthesis of GABA. Pyridoxine also forms a chemical complex with hydrazines, and this may play a role in its antidotal effect in treating monomethylhydrazine poisoning.

High doses of pyridoxine are known to cause peripheral neuropathy, so its excessive use should be avoided. If the patient is seizing, a dose of 5 gm should be administered intravenously. This should be repeated only for recurrent seizures.

The *Gyromitra* spp. are nongilled fungi, the spores of which develop in asci, or microscopic sacs, on the surfaces of the fruiting bodies. The bodies of *Gyromitra* spp. are extremely convoluted, hence the nickname "brain fungi." Many species of *Gyromitra* are edible, but determining which ones is best left only to experts.

MUSCARINE

(Color Plate III, Figs. 29–10 and 29–11)*

Unlike the anticholinergic *Amanitas*, mushrooms in this group predictably cause symptoms and signs of muscarine poisoning. Thirty minutes to 1 hour after ingestion, patients may develop the classic syndrome called cholinergic crisis, consisting of bradycardia, bronchospasm, profuse bronchorrhea, miosis, seizures, salivation, lacrimation, involuntary loss of urine and stool, and vomiting. Unlike the cholinergic crisis seen after poisoning by organophosphate insecticides, the syndrome in these cases is usually mild and seldom life-threatening. This may be at least partially due to the poor gastrointestinal absorption of muscarine. Muscarine is heat labile, so vigorous cooking of these mushrooms may prevent their cholinergic effects.

Treatment consists of supportive care and administration of atropine. The antidote should be given as frequently as necessary to dry pulmonary secretions.

More than 30 species of *Inocybe* and 6 species of *Clitocybe* contain muscarine. These inconspicuous mushrooms commonly grow in lawns and public parks.

Amanita pantherina and *A. muscaria* contain muscarine (hence the name) but usually in quantities that are insufficient to cause a cholinergic syndrome. Muscarine was initially isolated from *A. muscaria*.

*On Color Plates II and III at the front of the book.

COPRINE
(Color Plate III, Fig. 29–12)*

Coprine poisoning is most commonly associated with ingestion of *Coprinus atramentarius,* or the "inky cap." It is so called because the mature specimens have lamellae that deliquesce into an inky black fluid that is obvious on examination of the mushroom. The mushrooms themselves are quite edible. However, they contain coprine, which is a glutamic acid derivative that induces hyperacetaldehydemia in the presence of ethanol. Its mechanism of action is unknown, but it has been speculated that the coprine, like disulfiram (Antabuse), inhibits the metabolism of ethanol at the acetaldehyde dehydrogenase step, resulting in clinical symptoms.

The Antabuse-like reaction may occur after the ingestion of alcohol as long as 1 week after consumption of *C. atramentarius.* Symptoms include flushing of the face and trunk, palpitations, dyspnea, chest pain, and diaphoresis. Hypotension may occur secondary to peripheral vasodilatation.

Treatment of this syndrome consists primarily of the administration of intravenous fluids. There is no specific antidote. The syndrome usually abates within several hours.

INDOLES
(Color Plate III, Fig. 29–13)*

The psilocin-psilocybin–containing mushrooms have been used by American Indians in religious ceremonies for thousands of years. The *Psilocybe* genus contains more than 100 species of small, brown, slender-stalked mushrooms. They are commonly but not exclusively found growing in piles of dung and fertilized grasses, especially after a spring rain. They are found in moist areas all over the United States, most commonly in the South. The spores are purple and smooth and contain pores. A classic feature is the blue-green color of the *Psilocybe* mushroom in areas where it is injured or handled.

Thirty to 60 minutes after ingesting the psychotropic *Psilocybe,* a feeling of euphoria develops, followed by perceptual distortions and hallucinations that are usually, but not always, considered pleasant. These effects are caused by the indoles psilocybin and psilocin, which are chemically related to serotonin. Because of the small amounts of psychoactive indoles in these mushrooms, the ingestion of many "caps" is usually required to elicit a hallucinogenic effect. Tachycardia, mydriasis, and paresthesias are common. Seizures have been reported. The experience generally lasts 4 to 6 hours. Flashbacks may occur.

Patients who come to the emergency department usually need reassurance only, but sedation may be required. Benzodiazepines are probably the drugs of choice in this case.

ORELLINE AND ORELLANINE
(Color Plate III, Fig. 29–15)*

Some mushrooms of the genus *Cortinarius* contain the bipyridyl toxins orrelline and orellanine. Ingestion of these mushrooms may result in the development, after a 1-day delay, of gastritis, chills, headaches, and myalgias. A small percentage of these cases will progress to renal failure, evident days later. Few cases of *Cortinarius* poisoning have been reported in the United States, but there have been many documented occurrences in Europe and Japan. Some species of *Cortinarius* are edible, creating a dangerous temptation to the seasoned yet adventurous mushroom hunter. Mushrooms of this genus are distinguished by their rusty-brown spores. *Cortinarius* is the largest genus of mush-

Table 29–4. POSSIBLE PITFALLS IN THE TREATMENT OF MUSHROOM POISONING

1. Forgetting that "mushroom poisoning" may actually be an allergic reaction or food poisoning secondary to bacteria.
2. Forgetting that "mushroom poisoning" may actually be secondary to pesticides sprayed on the mushroom or edible mushrooms being laced with drugs (e.g., phencyclidine) or from a concomitant medical or surgical disease.
3. Assuming that all persons ingesting the same mushroom must become ill.
4. Assuming that if symptoms occur before 6 hours post ingestion, deadly *Amanitas* could not have been eaten.
5. Discharging patients without follow-up when they appear to have recovered from their gastrointestinal symptoms when those symptoms developed more than 6 hours post ingestion.
6. Forgetting the principles of supportive care while concentrating on toxin identification and antidotes.

*On Color Plates II and III at the front of the book.

rooms, containing over 800 species, making the differentiation between the edible and poisonous varieties extremely difficult.

Orelline and orellanine are heat-stable toxins that are chemically closely related to the herbicide diquat. Poisoning by these compounds results in tubulo interstitial nephritis and fibrosis. There are no antidotes for poisoning by these mushrooms. Since the patients tend to become symptomatic more than 24 hours post ingestion, it is unlikely that activated charcoal would be of much benefit. Treatment therefore consists of aggressive fluid management and close monitoring of renal function.

GASTROINTESTINAL IRRITANTS

This group has traditionally been a catchall for mushrooms that (1) usually produce vomiting and diarrhea shortly after ingestion; (2) do not produce systemic symptoms or signs; and (3) usually result in a benign clinical course not requiring treatment.

The number of species that fall under this classification is so great that to list them would be unproductive. Not all species of this group of mushrooms will cause symptoms in all people who ingest them. The same species may cause symptoms in one person at one time and not at another time. The toxins responsible for the gastrointestinal symptoms are, for the most part, unidentified.

Among the most common species causing acute gastroenteritis is *Chlorophyllum molybdites* (Color Plate III, Fig. 29–14). In its juvenile form it resembles the "shaggy mane," and it is quite often mistaken for this edible mushroom. It is, however, easily distinguished from virtually all other mushrooms by its green gills and spore print (see Fig. 29–2).

Many of the common "backyard mushrooms" or "little brown mushrooms" can be considered to be in this group. When these mushrooms are ingested by children, however, or in large quantities by adults, it is still safest to presume them to be toxic and have them identified.

CONCLUSION

The toxicology of mushrooms has been discussed in only modest detail. The management of mushroom poisoning is best thought of by dividing mushrooms into clinical syndromes based on the toxins they contain. The treatment of mushroom poisoning is not significantly different from that for drug overdose; supportive care must take highest priority pending identification of the toxin.

Common pitfalls in the management of mushroom poisoning are listed in Table 29–4. By avoiding these common errors and emphasizing supportive care and continued monitoring, the outcome in most cases of mushroom poisoning should be favorable.

General References

1. Rumack BH, Salzman E (eds): Mushroom Poisoning: Diagnosis and Treatment. West Palm Beach, FL, CRC Press, 1978, p 263.
2. Aboul-Enen HY: Psilocybin: A pharmacological profile. Am J Pharmacol *146*:91, 1974.
3. Alleva FR, Balazs T, Sager AO, et al: Failure of thioctic acid to cure mushroom-poisoned mice and dogs. Toxicol Appl Pharmacol *33*:122, 1975.
4. Bartter F: Thioctic acid and mushroom poisoning. Science *187*:216, 1975.
5. Becker CE, Tong TG, Boerner UDO, et al: Diagnosis and treatment of *Amanita phalloides*–type mushroom poisoning. West J Med *125*:100, 1976.
6. Blayney D, Rosenkranz E, Zettner A: Mushroom poisoning from *Chlorophyllum molybdites*. West J Med *132*:74, 1980.
7. Finestone AJ, Berman R, Widmer B, et al: Thioctic acid treatment of acute mushroom poisoning. Penna Med *75*:49, 1972.
8. Fiume L: Mechanism of action of amanitins. Curr Probl Clin Biochem *7*:20, 1977.
9. Faulstich H: Structure of poisonous components of *Amanita phalloides*. Curr Probl Clin Biochem 71, 1977.
10. Floersheim GL: Antagonistic effects against single lethal doses of *Amanita phalloides*. Arch Pharmacol *293*:171, 1976.
11. Floersheim GL: Treatment of human amatoxin mushroom poisoning. Myths and advances in therapy. Med Toxicol *2*:1, 1987.
12. French AL, Garrettson LK: Poisoning with the North American Jack O'Lantern mushroom, *Omphalotus illudens*. Clin Toxicol *26*:81, 1988.
13. Kisilevsky R: Hepatic nuclear and nucleolar changes in *Amanita* poisoning. Arch Pathol *97*:253, 1974.
14. Klein AS, Hart J, Brems JJ, et al: *Amanita* poisoning: Treatment and the role of liver transplantation. Am J Med *86*:187, 1989.
15. Lampe KF, McCann MA: Differential diagnosis of poisoning by North American mushrooms, with particular emphasis on *Amanita phalloides*–like intoxication. Ann Emerg Med *16*:956, 1987.
16. Lincoff G, Mitchel DH: Toxic and Hallucinogenic Mushroom Poisoning. New York, Van Nostrand-Reinhold, 1977, p 263.
17. Litten W: The most poisonous mushrooms. Sci Am *232*:90, 1975.

18. McCormick DJ, Avbel AJ, Gibbons RB: Nonlethal mushroom poisoning. Ann Intern Med *90*:332, 1979.
19. McDonald A: Mushrooms and madness. Hallucinogenic mushrooms and some psychopharmacological implications. Can J Psychiatr *25*:586, 1980.
20. Mitchel DH: *Amanita* mushroom poisoning. An Rev Med *31*:51, 1980.
21. Mitchel DH: Mushrooms—cyclopeptides (management/treatment protocol). *In* Rumack BH (ed): Poisindex Information System. Denver, CO, Micromedex, Inc. (edition expires 5/31/89).
22. Mitchel DH: Mushrooms—orellanine/orelline (management/treatment protocol). *In* Rumack BH (ed): Poisindex Information System. Denver, CO, Micromedex, Inc. (edition expires 5/31/89).
23. Paaso B, Harrison DC: A new look at an old problem: Mushroom poisoning. Am J Med *58*:505, 1975.
24. Peden NR, Bissett AF, Macaulay KEC, et al: Clinical toxicology of "magic mushroom" ingestion. Postgrad Med J *57*:543, 1981.
25. Richard JM, Louis J, Cantin D: Nephrotoxicity of orellanin, a toxin from the mushroom *Cortinarius orellanus*. Arch Toxicol *62*:242, 1988.
26. Rumack BH: Diagnosis and treatment of mushroom poisoning. Topics Emerg Med *1*:85, 1979.
27. Scheider SM, Borochovitz D, Krenzelok E: Cimetidine protection against alpha-amanitan hepatotoxicity in mice: A potential model for the treatment of *Amanita phalloides* poisoning. Ann Emerg Med *16*:1136, 1987.
28. Simmons DM: The Meixner test for amatoxins in mushrooms. Clin Toxicol *16*:401, 1980.
29. Teutsch C, Brennan RW: *Amanita* mushroom poisoning with recovery from coma. Ann Neurol *3*:177, 1978.
30. Vesconi S, Langer M, Gaetano I, et al: Therapy of cytotoxic mushroom intoxication. Crit Care Med *13*:402, 1985.
31. Wieland T, Faulstich H: Amatoxins, phallotoxins, phallolysin, and antamanide: The biologically active components of poisonous *Amanita* mushrooms. CRC Crit Rev Biochem *5*:185, 1978.

CHAPTER 30
POISONOUS PLANTS

Donald B. Kunkel, M.D.

The toxic properties of some plants are well known, but those of many are relatively obscure and difficult to ascertain. The list of plants known to cause adverse effects in human beings and other animals is overwhelming and constantly being expanded. It is of interest to the practitioner that so few cases of human death occur following exposure to poisonous plants, for the exposures are many and result in a great number of inquiries to poison control centers. It is estimated that 5 to 10 per cent of all such calls concern plants, yet hospitalizations are rare. It seems there might be "much ado about nothing" in this virtual jungle of toxins, yet the concerns are real, and the offending plants may be capable of producing serious intoxication.

PLANT IDENTIFICATION

A significant problem in dealing with a plant exposure inquiry is proper identification of the plant itself, especially over the telephone. Surprisingly few of us are aware of even the common local names, let alone botanic names, of many plants regularly encountered. Attempting to ascertain the identity of the ubiquitous "little red berry" on the telephone with a distraught mother whose child has just feasted on one can be a frustrating experience.

The problem of absolute lack of knowledge of the plant is compounded by difficulties in the nomenclature of plants, which exist at several levels. Names for plants tend to vary geographically, and one plant may have several common names depending on locality. For example, yellow oleander *(Thevetia peruviana)* is also known as "lucky nut" and "be-still tree." Botanists have not made the identification of plants easier for the practitioner, as botanic names tend to change occasionally, sometimes for obscure reasons.

It is best to become an amateur botanist if one is dealing often with plant inquiries. A general knowledge of poisonous and nonpoisonous plants in a particular locale can be time saving and realistically can provide better patient care, since more than a few children and adults are given an emetic to cause vomiting "to be on the safe side" because the plant was not identified. Local experts are usually quite happy to become involved in the medical system as informal consultants, and even nursery people can be quite helpful.

It is best to have relatives or friends of the patient bring in plant specimens when any question exists on the identity of the plant. Specimens of vomitus containing plant material should be saved for possible use in determining the type of plant ingested.

The references at the end of this chapter are those I have found especially helpful in plant identification and in the treatment of exposures.

PROBLEMS IN CLINICAL EVALUATION

To treat or not to treat, that is the question. Once the plant is properly identified, and identified as a "poisonous plant," can one with consistency predict toxicity? Many factors enter into an evaluation of potential toxicity; some are listed here.

Human Versus Animal Data. Much of the literature concerning poisonous plants is abstracted from veterinary experience, especially livestock studies. This information is of undoubted interest to the clinician, but must be interpreted with care. What is relevant to a herd of sheep may not indicate treatment of a child.

Geographic and Seasonal Variables. Plants known to be toxic in one part of the world may not be so very toxic in other areas. An example of this phenomenon is the chinaberry tree, which is known to cause central nervous system stimulation and death in its native Africa but seems to cause only gastroenteritis in the United States. Most likely, soil conditions and climate account for these variances.

Plant Part Ingested. A plant may be listed as poisonous, but certainly all parts of the plant are not consistently toxic in each case. The common garden tomato, a solanine alkaloid-containing plant, has perfectly edible fruit, but stems and leaves are known to be toxic. Likewise, peaches and apricots contain a cyanide-producing principle, amygdalin glycoside, within the fruit kernel and leafy portions of the tree, but the fruits are common staples.

Absorbability of Toxins. Some plant products listed as extremely toxic, such as castor beans, many times are limited in toxicity because of factors that impede absorption across the gut wall. Castor beans have a very tough seed coating that inhibits release of the active principles unless the bean is chewed. Dieffenbachia usually presents no problem with systemic absorption of oxalates because of the violent oropharyngeal reaction following chewing of the leaf.

Controversies. The available literature is uneven in regard to the potential toxicity of some plants. Evolving evidence is constantly changing the toxic or nontoxic status of some plants. Controversies rage in respect to the true poison potential of some plants. Pyracantha is listed in some texts as a poisonous plant, yet delicious jellies made of pyracantha berries are commercially available. Because of a 1919 report of a child's death following ingestion of wild poinsettia, hybrid poinsettias have been labeled as very poisonous until recently and are now thought to cause only mild gastroenteritis following ingestion, if any symptoms occur at all.

The physician must take the above factors and, above all, the patient's presenting and continuing clinical picture into consideration when formulating a treatment plan. The sage warning, "Just don't do something, stand there!" is probably cogent in many cases of plant ingestions.

MECHANISMS OF EXPOSURE

In my experience, poisonous plant contacts are generated in the following ways in declining frequency:

"Accidental" Childhood Exposures. Usually no "accident," actually. Children are attracted to bright berries and shiny leaves and will ingest plant parts as an expression of their own innate inquisitiveness and "texturing" of a new product as a form of learning. Most childhood ingestions (usually in the 2 to 3 year old age group) are nontoxic or relatively benign episodes, and simple reassurance of the parent is indicated after the plant is reasonably well identified. On occasion, home emesis or other measures, such as milk administration for dieffenbachia ingestions, may be advised, with careful home management protocols established by the physician or poison control center. On rare occasions, referral to a physician or hospital emergency department may be necessary.

Accidental Dermal Exposures. Fairly frequent calls are received concerning skin rashes (some with systemic sequelae) and punctures caused by plants. Some rashes may be due to applied pesticides, but most can be managed safely at home. On occasion I have seen severe neurologic and shocklike clinical presentations following punctures by palm fronds and century plant blades.

Use of Plants as Drugs of Abuse. A number of plants containing psychoactive principles are rather commonly abused, some with treacherous sequelae. Jimson weed is used fairly commonly in my experience but usually not more than once because of the severe hallucinations and peripheral anticholinergic effects, which usually prompt an evaluation in an emergency department. Many of the common street drugs are plant derivatives (heroin) or intact plant products (marijuana), and the entire area of poisonous plants begins to meld into the arena of drug abuse.

Foraging Incidents. Serious plant intoxications occur through experimenting, for food-gathering purposes, in tasting and ingesting unknown plants or plants morphologically similar to known edible wild plants. This sometimes fatal mistake seems to occur repeatedly with umbellifers, plants which are represented by not only the common carrot but also the water hemlock. Similarly, toxic mushrooms can be mistaken for edible ones (see Chapter 29).

Use of Herbs as Medication and Food Supplements. The utilization of a wide variety of plants as home remedies, beverages, and food supplements is certainly not new. Indeed, many modern drugs are either derivatives of plants or modifications of known plant chemical products. Twenty-five per cent of today's pharmacopeia is estimated still to be of natural origin. Various ethnic groups have contributed herbal lore that is spread by word of mouth and popular publications. Commercialization of herbal products has resulted in therapeutic alternatives to traditional medicine. Unfortunately, perhaps largely due to misidentification of plants and their overzealous use, illness and death have occurred. Striking recent examples have been tragic results from the use of amygdalin (Laetrile), pennyroyal, and gordolobo yerba.

ADVICE FOR THERAPY

Reassurance. Most plant exposures require only well-informed explanations after the plant is identified. The reassurance must be firmly given and reasonably stated, for the fixation on "poisonous plants" is strong.

Decontamination. General principles of any poisoning episode are to be followed with some minor exceptions:

(1) *Ingestion:* It is very difficult to remove leafy material, twigs, large berries, and so on from the gut with a tube, even a large-bore orogastric hose. Likewise, it may be somewhat hazardous to induce emesis in a situation of ingestion of *large* amounts of leafy plant product (possible glottic obstruction). If ingestions of large amounts of plant material are known, it is probably safer and more efficacious to induce emesis in a medical facility where resuscitative equipment is immediately available. This is particularly true in persons who may be prone to impairment of protective airway reflexes (for example, retarded or intoxicated individuals). If emesis is contraindicated, as in a comatose patient, the task of removing material may be formidable. The use of activated charcoal is recommended. Cathartics may be of benefit to hasten elimination.

(2) *Injection (puncture wounds):* Penetrating wounds by thorns, cactus spikes, palm fronds, and so on are notoriously prone to early inflammatory reaction and secondary infection. Careful removal of imbedded foreign material with meticulous cleansing is important. Tetanus prophylaxis is recommended, and antibiotics may be necessary for infectious complications. Deep punctures into joint spaces may be especially troublesome.

Elimination of Absorbed Toxin. Most plants contain complex mixtures of organic and inorganic (e.g., selenium) compounds. Attempts at speeding renal elimination by forced diuresis or the use of extracorporeal devices seem to be futile and potentially harmful in most cases of intoxication by plant material. The use of *repeated* doses of activated charcoal orally has not been studied sufficiently in plant ingestions.

Antidotes. Physiologic antagonists do exist

for the effective treatment of physiologic effects of some plant intoxications. These will be discussed. Emphasis always should be on basic resuscitation and accurate diagnosis before use of potentially harmful drugs as "antidotes."

Supportive Care. As in any intoxication, general supportive care is paramount. Careful attention to airway, ventilation, cardiovascular status, control of seizures, management of body core temperature, and so on is essential. Remember that plant poisonings may be complex and not well delineated in existing literature, and multisystem problems may be anticipated, even though the plant may be in a specific toxin category.

SYMPTOM COMPLEXES AND APPROACHES TO SPECIFIC THERAPY

As noted, most plant poisonings are complex in clinical presentation. Numerous structural variants of the same general class of toxins may be present within a plant (for example, the various alkaloids of jimson weed) or totally different toxins may be present in the same plant (for example, castor oil and ricin in castor beans). Gastrointestinal symptoms are almost universally found, but other organ system involvement may occur. As more experience with plant poisonings is documented, these syndromes undoubtedly will become better defined, but many plant intoxications remain confusing. An excellent chart of symptomatic responses to common poisonings, as modified from Barreuther, Pichioni, and Arena is presented at the end of this chapter.

An attempt follows to organize the toxicity and basic management of ingestion of some of the better-recognized poisonous plants into a "target organ" scheme. It is recognized that such a delineation may be misleading in that many toxic plants affect more than one organ system, as any single drug might do.

Gastrointestinal/Mucous Membrane. Probably the organ system most often affected by plant ingestion, the gastrointestinal system, including here the buccal cavity and the liver, may be solely affected or may be only an early precursor of other organ toxicity.

Buccal/Pharyngeal Irritation. Many of the oxalate-containing plants, such as dieffenbachia, contain spicule-like crystals of oxalic acid, which probably act in concert with plant enzymes to produce severe irritation that may cause upper airway compromise. (Thus the common name, *dumb* cane, as a result of aphonia.) Chewing of the rosary pea (jequirity bean) may cause a reaction described as caustic in nature. Milk may be advised for limited topical irritation. Watch for upper airway obstruction.

Gastroenteritis. Nausea, vomiting, or diarrhea may be the only clinical findings in a particular plant poisoning, or they may be premonitory signs of systemic involvement. The numbers of plants known to cause gastrointestinal disturbance are overwhelming, but examples of potential local irritation follow the ingestion of wisteria seeds or pods and the pods of the Mexican bird of paradise (poinciana). Gastrointestinal symptoms that may be an early indication of systemic toxicity are observed in the ingestion of oleander parts and castor bean seeds. Management is by replacement of intravascular fluid and electrolytes, with symptomatic treatment of bowel cramping and hypermotility in severe cases. Of course, if absorbable toxins affecting other organ systems potentially are present, attention must be paid to progressive findings and specific treatment anticipated, if available.

Hepatic Involvement. Direct hepatic involvement by plant materials is rare and is largely confined to the pyrrolizidine alkaloid-containing plants, such as the herb gordolobo *(Senecio longilobus)*, which may cause veno-occlusive disease. The herb pennyroyal has been associated with centrilobular hepatic necrosis. Various bulb plants (iris, daffodil, narcissus) have been implicated in hepatic complications following ingestion. Hepatic failure may occur following prolonged shock and renal failure as a secondary effect of poisoning. Care is largely supportive.

Renal. Deposition of products of intravascular hemolysis, as in castor bean intoxication from absorption of toxalbumins, or oxalate crystals, reported with the cooking and eating of rhubarb leaves, may result in renal failure. In the former, urinary alkalinization may be of benefit. In the latter, attention must be turned to correction of hypocalcemia and to maintenance of urine output. Hemodialysis as supportive care may be necessary. Ingestion of the autumn crocus (colchicine poisoning) may cause primary renal failure.

Hematopoietic. As noted, certain plants

contain phytotoxins (toxalbumins), which may cause hemagglutination, hemolysis, and renal failure. Included in this group are such plants as castor bean or jequirity bean. If hemolysis should occur (apparently a very rare event), exchange transfusion may be considered, along with renal care as just noted above. Favism in glucose-6-phosphate dehydrogenase-deficient individuals is well known as a cause of hemolysis.

Some plants contain excessive amounts of nitrates, depending on types of agricultural fertilizers used. Infant methemoglobinemia has been traced to the feeding of vegetables with high nitrate content and subsequent intraluminal conversion to absorbable nitrite. Treatment is supportive, with consideration of methylene blue infusion in a severe situation.

Cardiovascular. A number of plants can cause variable effects on the heart and peripheral vascular system, as a result of direct or indirect causes. Plants and fungi are the sources of some commercial cardiac/vascular preparations (for example, digitalis, ergot). The group of plants containing the cardiac glycosides (digitalis-like compounds) deserves special attention. Foxglove, oleander, yellow oleander, lily of the valley, and others contain glycosides capable of causing intoxication associated with gastrointestinal symptoms, followed by progressive A-V block. Treatment should be aimed at gut decontamination, correction of electrolyte imbalance (usually *hyper*kalemia in acute poisoning) with ion-exchange resins or hemodialysis, and correction of severe bradycardia (atropine) and conduction block (phenytoin). In an extremely severe situation, electrical pacing might be indicated. Digoxin-specific Fab antibodies *should* reverse foxglove toxicity and *may* reverse oleander toxicity, although reports are few.

Ergot alkaloids are discussed in Chapter 99.

Respiratory. Plant pollens account for the seasonal miseries of a significant portion of the population. Although not considered a true "poisoning" problem in the context of this book, nonetheless more human morbidity undoubtedly results from hypersensitivity reactions than from classic plant intoxications.

Cellular respiration may be impaired by cyanide intoxication secondary to gut hydrolysis of ingested plant parts containing amygdalin glycoside. Treatment is supportive, with use of the Lilly cyanide kit necessary in severe poisoning. (For antidotal therapy with amyl nitrite, sodium nitrite, and sodium thiosulfate, see Chapter 70.)

Central Nervous System. Many sources refer to a plant as causing central nervous system "stimulation" or "depression." This differentiation may be somewhat artificial, as a person who is agitated initially may progress to coma. Likewise, seizure activity may not be a primary result of central nervous system stimulation but may reflect cerebral hypoxia secondary to depressive effects. Plants have been used therapeutically primarily for sedation and analgesia but have been used selectively for religious and recreational purposes for many effects, including arousal (coca leaf), hallucinations (peyote cactus), and sedation (opium poppy). Therapy, of course, varies widely depending on clinical presentation and knowledge of the pharmacologic action of the plant used or abused.

Autonomic Nervous System. Many naturally occurring substances, particularly those affecting the central nervous system, also affect the autonomic nervous system. One outstanding group of plants in this regard is those that produce atropine-like alkaloids. The prime plant of current concern is jimson weed. The clinical presentation of intoxication by this plant is that of central and peripheral anticholinergic effect: hallucinations, tachyarrhythmias, hypertension, elevated body temperature, dilated pupils, dry and flushed skin, decreased bowel activity, and urinary retention. Treatment is largely supportive, although physostigmine may be used cautiously for life-threatening conditions, as a diagnostic tool, and for hallucination and hyperactivity control in select situations.

Skin and Eye. Topical irritation of exposed skin or mucous membranes may be caused by contact with the sap of some plants. I have recently seen several persons with severe, hemorrhagic rash that developed immediately after exposure to the sap of the century plant (an agave). Most dermatitis following plant exposure seems to be based on a hypersensitivity reaction, with poison

Text continued on page 600

SOME TOXIC PLANTS FOUND IN THE UNITED STATES

COMMON NAME	SCIENTIFIC NAME	TOXIC PARTS	POISONOUS PRINCIPLES	SYMPTOMS
Akee	*Blighia sapida*	Fruit, except ripe aril, which is edible	Hypoglycins A and B	Vomiting ("Jamaican vomiting sickness"), convulsions, coma; may be lethal. Severe hypoglycemia may be found
Apricot (also applies to parts of other fruits whose kernels or seeds contain amygdalin glycoside, e.g., peach, apple, pear)	*Prunus* spp.	Fruit kernels, foliage	Amygdalin glycoside (cyanogenic—produces free cyanide ion following hydrolysis in the gut)	Symptoms and findings of cyanide poisoning, such as shock, hyperpnea, and coma. Breath may have "bitter almond" odor. Metabolic acidosis usually marked. Deaths have been reported from ingestion of these natural products or the purified amygdalin glycoside (Laetrile)
Autumn crocus or meadow saffron	*Colchicum autumnale*	All parts	Colchicine alkaloid	Burning pain and rawness in mouth and throat. Vomiting, diarrhea, shock, renal failure. Symptoms usually appear 2–6 hr after ingestion. Death may occur during relapse after period free of symptoms
Azalea—see Rhododendron				
Bird of paradise (Mexican bird of paradise or poinciana)	*Casesalpinia gilliesii*	Pods	Unknown	Vertigo, severe vomiting and diarrhea, dehydration (symptoms may persist for 24 hr)
Black locust (Color Plate IV, Fig. 30–1)*	*Robinia pseudoacacia*	Inner bark, young leaves, and seeds	Robin (phytotoxin) and robitin (glycoside)	Vomiting, diarrhea, shocklike picture, CNS depression
Bleeding-heart	*Dicentra formosa*, other species	Foliage, roots	Several isoquinoline-type alkaloids, including apomorphine, protoberberine, and protopine	Tremors, staggering gait, labored breathing, salivation, convulsions. Death may be due to paralysis
Buckeye (Color Plate IV, Fig. 30–2)*	*Aesculus* spp.	Leaves, flowers, and seeds	Esculin (glycoside)	Vomiting, diarrhea, pupillary dilation, muscle twitching, weakness, ataxia, CNS depression, and paralysis
Burn bean—see Texas mountain laurel				
Caladium—see Philodendron				
Castor bean (Color Plate IV, Fig. 30–3)*	*Ricinus communis*	All parts, mainly seeds	The phytotoxins—ricin and ricinine (toxalbumins)	Nausea, vomiting, violent purging, burning sensation in mouth and throat, hemolysis of red blood cells, kidney failure, death. 2–4 seeds produce serious poisoning in adults. 1–3 seeds in a child could be lethal if chewed. Hard seed coating is protective
Century plant (Color Plate IV, Figs. 30–4 and 30–5)*	*Agave americana*	Sap	Unknown	Skin exposure to sap may cause severe dermatitis, sometimes hemorrhagic. Rash may be associated with fever and leucocytosis
Chinaberry (Color Plate IV, Fig. 30–6)*	*Melia azedarach*	Fruit	Probably a resinoid	Has caused serious poisoning in certain animals (hogs and sheep), including dyspnea, sluggish movements, weak and fast pulse, vomiting. 6–8 fruit may be lethal to a child, but human exposures in USA seem limited to severe gastroenteritis
Christmas holly—see Holly				
Christmas rose	*Helleborus niger*	Rootstocks and leaves	Two very toxic glycosides, helleborin and belleborein	Juice produces inflammation and numbing sensations in mouth. Vomiting, diarrhea, and possible convulsions; affects central nervous system

*On Color Plates IV, V, and VI at the front of this book.

Table continued on next page

SOME TOXIC PLANTS FOUND IN THE UNITED STATES *Continued*

COMMON NAME	SCIENTIFIC NAME	TOXIC PARTS	POISONOUS PRINCIPLES	SYMPTOMS
Daffodil—see Narcissus				
Daphne	*Daphne mezereum* and other species	Berries, bark, leaves	Daphnin and vesicant resin, mezerenic acid anhydride	Plant intensely acrid, producing vesication when rubbed on skin; ingestion produces burning sensation in mouth. Vomiting, diarrhea with blood and mucus, stupor, kidney failure, weakness, convulsions and death. Mortality is about 30%.
Desert potato	*Jatropha macrorhiza*	Plant root	Phytotoxins	Nausea, vomiting abdominal cramps, profuse watery diarrhea that may lead to dehydration
Dieffenbachia, dumb cane (Color Plate IV, Fig. 30–7)*	*Dieffenbachia seguine* or *picta*	All parts, including sap	Calcium oxalate crystals, toxic protein	Burning of mouth, tongue, lips; inflammation of larynx, may affect breathing. Juice in the eye causes marked burning and inflammation; direct eye contact may cause corneal opacity
Digitalis—see Foxglove				
Dutchman's-breeches	*Dicentra cucullaria*	See Bleeding-heart		
Elephant ear—see Philodendron				
Fava bean	*Vicia faba*	Bean or plant pollen	Sensitivity to beans or inhaled pollen noted in individuals deficient in glucose-6-phosphate dehydrogenase	Sensitive persons may experience headache, nausea, vomiting, abdominal pain, and hyperthermia. More severe reactors may develop sudden hemolytic anemia with secondary hemoglobinuria and icterus. Occurs in persons of Mediterranean extraction
Four-o'clock	*Mirabilis jalapa*	Root, seed	The alkaloid trigonelline	Irritant to skin, mouth, and throat. Causes purgation
Foxglove (Color Plate IV, Fig. 30–8)*	*Digitalis purpurea*	Leaves and seeds	Several glycosides, mainly digitoxin, digitalin, digitonin	One of the sources of the drug digitalis, used to stimulate the heart. In large amounts the active principles cause A-V block and slow pulse and other cardiac arrhythmias. See Chapter 88 on digitalis
Golden chain	*Laburnum anagyroides*	Beanlike capsules in which the seeds are suspended	The quinolizidine alkaloid cytisine	Dysphagia, possible pupil dilation, excitement, incoordination, vomiting, renal failure, convulsions, coma, and death through asphyxiation. Considered very poisonous shrub or tree in Britain. Action similar to that of nicotine
Gordolobo—see Threadleaf				
Groundsel—see Threadleaf				
Holly	*Ilex* spp.	Berries	Ilicin	Nausea, abdominal pain, severe vomiting, and diarrhea
Hyacinth	*Hyacinthus orientalis*	Bulb	Probably narcissine-like alkaloids	Intense digestive upset, vomiting, diarrhea; severe purgation
Hydrangea (Color Plate V, Fig. 30–9)*	*Hydrangea* spp.	Entire plant	A cyanogenic glycoside (hydrangin)	See Apricot
Indian licorice—see Rosary pea				
Indian tobacco	*Lobelia inflata*	Entire plant	Alkaloids of lobeline, lobelamine, etc	Nausea, vomiting, weakness, tremors, convulsions, coma, and death
Iris (blue flag)	*Iris versicolor*	Leaves and root stalks	Acrid resinous substances irisin, irigenin, iridin	Acts on GI tract, liver, and pancreas causing purging and congestion of the intestinal tract. Can also cause dermatitis
Jack-in-the-pulpit (Indian turnip)	*Arisaema triphyllum*	Rhizome	Calcium oxalate crystals	Intense irritation of mouth and throat; burning pain; inflammation of larynx (resembles dumb cane)
Jasmine—see Yellow jessamine				
Jequirity bean—see Rosary pea				
Jerusalem cherry	*Solanum pseudocapsicum*	Berries	Solanine and related alkaloids	Headache, abdominal pain, vomiting, diarrhea, circulatory collapse, convulsions, CNS and respiratory depression

*On Color Plates IV, V, and VI at the front of this book.

SOME TOXIC PLANTS FOUND IN THE UNITED STATES *Continued*

COMMON NAME	SCIENTIFIC NAME	TOXIC PARTS	POISONOUS PRINCIPLES	SYMPTOMS
Jimson weed (thorn apple) (Color Plate V, Fig. 30–10)*	*Datura stramonium, D. metel, D. inoxia, D. suaveolens,* and other species	All parts, especially seeds	The solanaceous alkaloids atropine, hyoscyamine, and scopolamine	Symptoms include intense thirst, urinary retention, dryness of mouth, rapid pulse, delirium, incoherence; later, slow respiration, high temperature, convulsions or coma preceding death. Handling leaves or seeds followed by rubbing eyes can cause dilation of pupils
Laburnum—see Golden chain				
Lantana (Color Plate V, Fig. 30–11)*	*Lantana camara*	Berries (unripe)	A polycyclic triterpenoid named lantadene A	Extreme muscular weakness, GI irritation, lethargy, cyanosis, and circulatory collapse. Syndrome resembles atropine poisoning in some respects.
Larkspur	*Delphinium ajacis* and other species	Young plant, seeds	Poisonous alkaloids, mainly delphinine	Ingestion produces digestive upset, respiratory depression, paresthesias, salivation, headache, hypotension, and cardiac arrhythmias
Laurel—see Texas mountain laurel *or* Mountain laurel. (Caveat: Many "laurels" are nontoxic)				
Lily of the valley	*Convallaria majalis*	Leaves, flowers, roots	The cardiac glycosides convallarin, convallamarin, and convallatoxin	Cardiac effects similar to digitalis glycosides. Dizziness and vomiting may occur in 1–2 hours, if large quantities are eaten
Locust—see Black locust				
Mescal—see Peyote				
Mescal bean (Color Plate V, Fig. 30–12)*—see Texas mountain laurel				
Mistletoe (Color Plate V, Fig. 30–13)*	*Phoradendron* spp.	Berries	Beta-phenylethylamine and tyramine, choline	Several deaths among children have been attributed to eating the berries. Tea brewed from berries has caused fatality. Death occurred about 10 hr after symptoms of acute gastroenteritis and cardiovascular collapse. Acute GI symptoms of nausea, vomiting, diarrhea; respiratory difficulties, bradycardia, delirium, hallucinations, cardiovascular collapse, and coma
Monkshood	*Aconitum napellus* and other species	Roots, seeds, leaves	Poisonous alkaloids, mainly aconitine, a polycyclic diterpene	Alkaloids cause vagal stimulation and bradycardia. Also, tingling and numbing sensation of the lips and tongue; irregular pulse; dimness of vision; GI upset with nausea, vomiting and diarrhea; respiratory failure
Morning-glory (Heavenly blue, pearly gates, flying saucer varieties)	*Ipomoea violacea*	Seeds	The olavine alkaloids ergine, isoergine, elymoclavine and others; all chemically related to LSD	From 50–200 ingested powdered seeds are capable of inducing psychotomimetic effects for several hours (hallucinations). Used by thrill-seekers because of LSD-like effects. Produce nausea, uterine stimulation, euphoria
Mountain laurel	*Kalmia latifolia* and *angustifolia*	All parts	Andromedotoxin, a resinoid substance	Curare-like effect on skeletal muscles. Stimulation of skeletal muscle followed by paralysis. Inhibitory action on heart tissues. Depresses the CNS, causing respiratory failure and ultimately death
Narcissus or daffodil	*Narcissus* species	Bulb	Narcissine, lycorine, and other alkaloids	Severe gastroenteritis, vomiting, purging, trembling, convulsions, hypotension, possible hepatic degeneration
Nightshade family (includes many wild and cultivated plants, such as black nightshade, potato, tomato, eggplant, and some "jessamines") (Color Plate V, Fig. 30–14)*	*Solanum* spp.	Variable with species; some have edible fruit (tomato, eggplant) or tubers (potato)	Solanine alkaloids (see Jerusalem cherry)	See Jerusalem cherry

*On Color Plates IV, V, and VI at the front of this book.

Table continued on next page

SOME TOXIC PLANTS FOUND IN THE UNITED STATES *Continued*

COMMON NAME	SCIENTIFIC NAME	TOXIC PARTS	POISONOUS PRINCIPLES	SYMPTOMS
Oleander (Color Plate V, Figs. 30–15 and 30–16)*	*Nerium oleander*	All parts, green or dry. Single leaf, well-chewed, reportedly lethal	Cardiac glycosides; oleandroside, oleandrin, nerioside	Local irritation of mucous membranes, mouth, and stomach. Nausea, vomiting, diarrhea, slow and irregular pulse changing to rapid and thready pulse, and ventricular fibrillation and death
Pencil tree	*Euphorbia tirucalli*	Leaves, stems, milky sap	Irritant in sap	Irritation to lips, tongue, and mouth. Sap may blister skin and irritate eyes
Peyote (Color Plate VI, Fig. 30–17)*	*Lophophora williamsii* and *L. diffusa*	All parts, usually cactus "button" used	Various alkaloids, of which mescaline is only one	Sensory distortion, hallucinations (primarily visual)
Philodendron Caladium Elephant ear	*Philodendron* spp. *Caladium bicolor* *Colocasia antiquorum*	Entire plant Entire plant Entire plant	Calcium oxalate Calcium oxalate Calcium oxalate	Local irritation to mucous membranes, swelling of lips and tongue, along with excessive salivation, may lead to difficulty in swallowing. Excessive swelling of tongue and pharyngeal edema may inhibit respiration. No systemic effects have been reported
Poison hemlock (Color Plate VI, Fig. 30–18)*	*Conium maculatum*	All parts	Coniine (alkaloid)	Nausea, vomiting, early CNS stimulation, followed by severe CNS depression, associated muscle paralysis, and respiratory failure
Poison ivy (erroneously called poison oak)	*Toxicodendron radicans* or *Rhus toxicodendron*	All parts, even the smoke from burning it	An oily resin called urushiol which is made up of phenolic substances like 3-*N*-pentadecylcatechol	Produces a severe allergenic response causing dermatitis upon contact, resulting in inflammation, blistering, and vesicles. As skin breaks, a liquid exudes and scabs of crusts form
Pokeweed (pigeonberry, inkberry)	*Phytolacca americana, P. decandra*	Roots and leaves; fruit is least toxic, but has also caused poisoning	A resinous material and a water-soluble saponin, glycoprotein, and possibly two other alkaloids—phytolaccine and phytolaccotoxin	Produces burning sensation in mouth, gastrointestinal cramps, vomiting, diarrhea (also amblyopia and tremors). Later, visual disturbance, perspiration, salivation, lassitude, prostration, and weakened respiration and pulse may be seen. If recovery does not occur in 24 hr, may be fatal
Privet	*Ligustrum japonicum*	All parts	Perhaps andromedotoxin. Most sources state the principle is unknown	Poisoning seems to be rare in USA, but in Europe children have died from eating fruit. In animals it causes severe vomiting, colic, and diarrhea
Red squill	*Urginea maritima*	Bulb	Cardiac glycosides	Similar to Oleander
Rhododendron (also azalea)	*Rhododendron* spp.	All parts	Andromedotoxin	Salivation, nasal discharge, nausea, vomiting, diarrhea, muscle weakness, labored breathing, coma (based on animal studies), dullness of vision, paralysis, hypotension, lacrimation, anorexia
Rhubarb (Color Plate VI, Fig. 30–19)*	*Rheum rhaponticum*	Leaf *blade* (not the petiole, which is edible)	Oxalic acid	Severe intermittent abdominal pains, vomiting, diarrhea, headache, weakness and hemorrhages. Muscular cramps and tetany due to hypocalcemia may occur. Large amounts of raw and cooked leaves can cause convulsions and coma, followed rapidly by death associated with renal failure
Rosary pea (crabseye, precatory bean, jequirity bean, Indian licorice)	*Abrus precatorius*	Seeds	The phytotoxin abrin and the tetanic glycoside abric acid	Seed is caustic. Causes burns to mouth and esophagus. Less than one seed, if chewed, may be fatal. Symptoms resemble those of castor bean poisoning. Nausea, vomiting, severe diarrhea, weakness, shock, trembling of hands, oliguria, hemolytic anemia, hallucinations in children and fatal uremia

*On Color Plates IV, V, and VI at the front of this book.

SOME TOXIC PLANTS FOUND IN THE UNITED STATES *Continued*

COMMON NAME	SCIENTIFIC NAME	TOXIC PARTS	POISONOUS PRINCIPLES	SYMPTOMS
Star-of-Bethlehem (snowdrop)	*Ornithogalum umbellatum*	All parts	Alkaloids (related to colchicine)	Nausea, nervous symptoms, and general disturbances of the intestinal tract
Sweet pea	*Lathyrus odoratus*	Seeds	Aminopropionitrile	Skeletal deformity and growth suppression; muscle paralysis (from animal studies)
Texas mountain laurel (Color Plate V, Fig. 30–12)*	*Sophora secundiflora*	Entire plant	Cytisine	Increased salivation, nausea, vomiting, headache, vertigo, confusion, hallucinations, excessive thirst, muscle fasciculation, convulsion, and respiratory stimulation followed by failure.
Thorn apple—see Jimson weed				
Threadleaf groundsel (Senecio)	*Senecio longilobus*	Entire plant	Pyrrolizidine alkaloids	Chronic ingestion may cause enlarged liver, ascites, abdominal pain, nausea, vomiting, diarrhea, headache, apathy, and emaciation. Poisoning usually occurs in drinking certain herbal teas. Senecio is a major cause of hepatic veno-occlusive disease (see Chapter 13)
Tobacco (and wild tobacco, tree tobacco) (Color Plate VI, Fig. 30–20)*	*Nicotiana* spp.	Probably all parts	Nicotine and related alkaloids	Nausea, vomiting, muscular fasciculation; early CNS stimulation followed by severe CNS depression in association with muscle paralysis and respiratory failure
Water hemlock (cowbane) (Color Plate VI, Fig. 30–21)*	*Cicuta maculata* and other species	All parts, mostly the roots	Resin-like substance called cicutoxin	Symptoms appear in 15 min and include severe stomach pain, great mental excitation and frenzy, vomiting, salivation, and violent spasmodic convulsions alternating with periods of relaxation. Pupils dilate and delirium is common. Death may occur within 15 min after ingestion of lethal amount
Wisteria (Color Plate VI, Fig. 30–22)*	*Wisteria floribunda* (Japanese) and *W. sinensis* (Chinese)	Seeds or pods	Poisonous resin and a glucoside, wisterin	Mild to severe gastroenteritis with repeated vomiting, abdominal pain, and diarrhea
Yellow jessamine (Carolina jessamine)	*Gelsemium sempervirens*	Whole plant, berries	Toxic alkaloids gelsemine and gelseminine	The alkaloids chiefly depress and paralyze motor nerve endings. Depression of the motor neurons of the brain and spinal cord results in respiratory arrest
Yellow oleander (be-still tree) (Color Plate VI, Fig. 30–23)*	*Thevetia peruviana*	All parts; fruit ("lucky nut") most attractive to children	Cardiac glycosides (thevetin A and B, thevetoxin)	See Oleander
Yew (Color Plate VI, Fig. 30–24)*	*Taxus baccata and T. canadensis*	All parts, especially *seed* if chewed; fleshy red pulp of fruit least harmful	Taxine, an alkaloid	Nausea, vomiting, diarrhea, abdominal pain, circulatory failure, and difficulty in breathing. The alkaloid depresses heart function. Can cause dermatitis

Gratitude is extended to Alan Barreuther, Phar. D., and Albert L. Picchioni, Ph.D., for allowing abstraction from Toxic Plants, a compendium released by the Arizona Poison and Drug Information Center of the Arizona Poison Control System. Special recognition to Jay M. Arena, M.D., of Duke University, whose compendia appear in many publications and whose foresight has brought us to the present state of the art.

Michael D. Ellis, M.S., Texas State Poison Center, University of Texas Medical Branch, Galveston, graciously permitted use of Figures 30–8, 30–9, 30–13, 30–16, 30–21, and 30–22 from his private collection. All other figures are from the private collection of the chapter author, Donald B. Kunkel, M.D.

*On Color Plates IV, V, and VI at the front of this book.

ivy and poison oak being prime offenders. Treatment is usually symptomatic, although severe reactions may require antihistaminics and corticosteroid therapy.

Conjunctival irritation following direct contact with dieffenbachia sap is a known phenomenon. Allergic conjunctivitis and corneal abrasions following contact with many plants are more common manifestations of plant exposure.

TOXIC PLANT CHART

This chapter outlines a general approach to toxic plant exposure. The preceding chart lists the major toxic plants in the United States, with their toxic parts, chemistry, and symptomatology. The reader is referred to the following reference material for a more detailed description of a specific plant.

References

STANDARD MEDICAL TEXTS

1. Lampe KF, McCann MA: A.M.A. Handbook of Poisonous and Injurious Plants. Chicago, American Medical Association, 1985. (State-of-the-art reference; highly recommended)
2. Hardin JW, Arena JM: Human Poisoning from Native and Cultivated Plants. Duke University Press, Durham, NC, 1974. (Medically oriented)
3. Kingsbury JM: Poisonous Plants of the United States and Canada. Prentice-Hall, Englewood Cliffs, NJ, 1964. (Excellent coverage of plant toxins and nomenclature; oriented toward the veterinarian)

BOTANIC REFERENCES

1. Muenscher WC: Poisonous Plants of the United States. Collier Books (Macmillan), New York, 1975. (Good line drawings)
2. Perry F (ed): Complete Guide to Plants and Flowers. Simon and Schuster, New York, 1974. (Good color plates)
3. Clark DE (ed): New Western Garden Book. Lane Publishing Company, Menlo Park, CA, 1979. (Good cross-referencing to common and botanic names; primarily for use in western USA, but useful elsewhere)

CHAPTER 31
TOXIC MARINE LIFE

Lester M. Haddad, M.D.
Richard F. Lee, Ph.D.

Herman Melville wrote of the mystery of the sea. Long a source of inspiration and of fear, the sea has also proved to be a cause of human morbidity and mortality.

Reference to poisonous and venomous marine animals dates back to ancient Greek and Roman times.[1] In the Bible (Deuteronomy 14:9–10), Moses cautions the Israelites: "Of all that are in the waters you may eat whatever has fins and scales. And whatever does not have fins and scales you shall not eat; it is unclean." Moses gave his people sound medical advice: The poisonous puffer fish and venomous marine animals such as the sea snake (Color Plate VII,* Fig. 31–1), sea wasp, moray eel, stingray, sea urchin (Color Plate VII,* Fig. 31–2), Portuguese man-of-war, and blue-ringed octopus (Color Plate VII,* Fig. 31–3) all lack fins and scales.

Some of the substances known to be most toxic to human beings are found in marine organisms (Table 31–1). Toxins injected by an animal into its prey are usually high-molecular-weight proteinaceous substances known as *venoms*. Toxins that produce clinical symptoms after consumption are called *poisons;* they are generally low-molecular-weight molecules.

Marine life is toxic to humans by stinging (jellyfish, corals, and sea anemones), by ingestion (ciguatera, puffer fish poisoning,

*On Color Plate VII at the front of this book.

Table 31–1. REACTIVE TOXICITIES OF A SELECTED GROUP OF TOXIC SUBSTANCES

TOXIN	MINIMUM LETHAL DOSE (μg/kg)*	SOURCE
Botulinus toxin A	0.00003	Bacterium: *Clostridium botulinum*
Tetanus toxin	0.00010	Bacterium: *Clostridium tetani*
Ricin	0.02000	Plant: castor bean, *Ricinus communis*
Palytoxin	0.15000	Zoanthid: *Palythoa* spp.
Crotalus toxin	0.20000	Snake: The rattlesnake, *Crotalus atrox*
Diphtheria toxin	0.30000	Bacterium: *Corynebacterium diphtheriae*
Cobra neurotoxin	0.30000	Snake: *Naja naja*
Kokoi venom	2.7	Frog: *Phyllobates bicolor*
Tarichatoxin	8	Newt: *Taricha torosa*
Tetrodotoxin	8	Fish: *Sphoeroides rubripes*
Saxitoxin	3.4–9	Produced by the dinoflagellate *Gonyaulax catenella* transvected by shellfish
Bufotoxin	390	Toad: *Bufo vulgaris*
Curare	500	Plant: *Chondodendron tomentosum*
Strychnine	500	Plant: *Strychnos nux-vomica*
Muscarin	1100	Mushroom: *Amanita muscaria*
Samandarin	1500	Salamander: *Salamandra maculosa*
Disopropyl fluorophospate	3000	Synthetic nerve gas
Sodium cyanide	10,000	Inorganic poison

*Minimal lethal dose refers to mouse, except for ricin, in which it refers to guinea pig, and for bufotoxin and muscarin, in which it refers to cat.

(Reprinted with permission from Mosher HS, Fuhrman FA, Buckwald HD, Fisher HG: Tarichatoxin-tetrodotoxin: A potent neurotoxin. Science *144*:1103, 1964. Copyright 1964 by The American Association for the Advancement of Science.)

paralytic shellfish poisoning), by spinous puncture injury (stingray, catfish, scorpion fish, cone shell, sea urchin, and sponges), and by bites by the sea snake and the neurotoxic Australian blue-ringed octopus, *Octopus maculosa*. Shark bite is the most obvious example of marine trauma. This chapter reviews the more common marine toxins that have clinical significance.

The three most common marine organisms causing emergency department visits in the mainland United States are stingrays, catfish, and jellyfish,[2] whereas coral injuries, coelenterate stings, and sea urchin toxicity are the three most common in Hawaii.[3, 4]

JELLYFISH AND THE COELENTERATES

The phylum Coelenterata is composed of invertebrates that have the dominant characteristic of tentacles equipped with nematocysts. The phylum[1] is divided into three classes:

1. **Hydrozoa.** This group includes *Physalia physalis*, or the Portuguese man-of-war (bluebottle) and its Pacific relative, *Physalia utriculus*, found off Hawaii and in the Indo-Pacific; and the hydroid corals, which are commonly found growing in tufts on rocks, seaweed, and dock pilings. Examples include *Millepora alcicornus*, the stinging fire coral; and *Lytocarpus philippinus*, the feather hydroid, usually attached to the sea floor.[1]
2. **Scyphozoa.** This group includes the jellyfish, such as the Chesapeake sea nettle, *Chrysaora quinquecirrha*; the deadly sea wasp or boxjelly of Australian waters, *Chironex fleckeri* Southcott; the deadly sea wasp of Philippine waters, *Chiropsalmus quadrigatus* Haeckel; and *Carukia barnesi* Southcott, the cause of "Irukandji stings" to swimmers around Queensland, Australia.[1]
3. **Anthozoa.** This group includes the sea anemones and the corals. Venomous sea anemones of the anthozoan class include the *Anemonia sulcata*, *Actinodendron plumosum* Haddon, *Rhodactis howesi*, *Triactis producta*, the rosy anemone *Sagartia elegans*, *Radianthus paumotensis*, and others.[1]

The coelenterates produce human injury by firing off their *nematocysts* on contact. Nematocysts, or stinging cells, are actually cell organoids in specialized epithelial cells. At least 17 types of nematocysts are found in coelenterates. In general, they consist of a capsule wall enclosing a tightly coiled hollow tube that bursts forth like a dart on contact with a human being or animal (Fig. 31–10). The fluid in the capsules is the venom. Nematocysts range from 5 μm to 1.12 mm in length.

When activated, the nematocysts discharge forcibly. During discharge, the coiled internal tubule everts progressively, bringing its armament of chitinous spikes and spines to the external surface. Actual penetration of the prey is facilitated by the continuously renewed crest of spines created at the tip of the everting tubule when spines that were previously internal reach the tip and become superficial.[5] The venom in the capsule is conveyed to the victim through the thread. Robson described the process in these terms: "The tip of the shaft is formed by a constantly renewed spearhead of opposed barbs. These flick out sharply and take their positions in each of the spiral rows."[6] Although all coelenterates have nematocysts, most are not injurious to people.

The severity of stinging to human beings depends on the type of nematocysts, their penetrating power, the area of the victim's skin exposed, and the sensitivity of the victim to the venom. Injurious effects resulting from an encounter with coelenterate nematocysts range from mild dermatitis to instant death.

Portuguese Man-of-War

The Portuguese man-of-war (Color Plate VII,* Fig. 31–4) is characterized by a floating stem with several tentacles dangling from the underside of the float. One or more of the tentacles are markedly elongated and are called fishing tentacles. *Physalia* is pelagic or inhabits the surface of the sea and is found worldwide in warmer waters. One fishing tentacle may contain almost a million nematocysts. The sting from a Portuguese man-of-war is far more severe than that from the common jellyfish and often produces intense local pain extending up the extremity, similar to an electric shock. Generalized symptoms such as headache, urticaria, shock, muscle cramps, nausea, and vomiting all may occur. Death from *Physalia* has been reported but is unsubstantiated.

*On Color Plate VII at the front of this book.

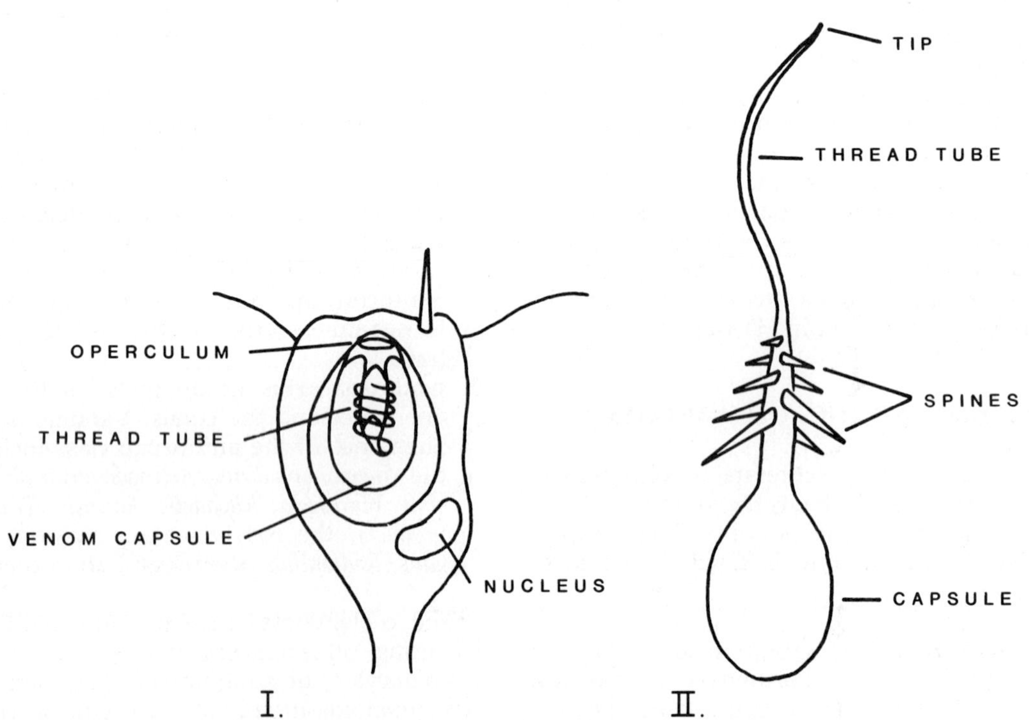

Figure 31–10. Generalized coelenterate nematocyst. I. Undischarged. II. Discharged. (Modified from Halstead BW: Poisonous and Venomous Marine Animals of the World. Rev ed. Princeton, NJ, Darwin Press, 1980.)

Hydroid Coral

Hydroid corals are upright, clavate, bladelike, or branching calcareous growths or encrustations that are important in the development of reefs. The stinging coral is not a true coral but a hydroid characterized by an exoskeleton of calcium carbonate, the surface of which is covered with numerous minute pores. Hydroid corals vary in color from white to yellow-green and are widely distributed throughout tropical seas in shallow water. *Millipora* is the best-known genus. The hydroid corals are a nuisance to divers off the Florida Keys and in the Caribbean.

Jellyfish

Jellyfish are the most common of the coelenterates that produce clinical injury and account for a significant number of emergency department visits in United States coastal areas during the summer.

Jellyfish are marine, and most are pelagic. They display a wide variety of sizes, shapes, and colors. Many appear semitransparent or glassy, and they often have brilliantly colored gonads, tentacles, or radial canals. They may vary in size from a few millimeters to more than 2 meters across the bell (top), with tentacles up to 36 meters in length. Because the tentacles in some species are long, it is possible to encounter them without seeing the bell. After a storm during which jellyfish have been broken up and washed ashore, one can be stung while walking along a beach by stepping on tentacles containing undischarged nematocysts. Even when dry, the nematocysts retain the capacity to discharge and produce typical symptoms.

Sea Wasp

Sea wasps (Color Plate VII,* Fig. 31–5) are the lethal cubomedusans, *C. fleckeri* of Australia and *C. quadrigatus* Haeckel of the Philippines. In Australian waters, the Cubomedusae were responsible for more than 50 deaths from 1950 to 1970. Death in less than 3 minutes has been caused by *C. fleckeri* stings. Another cubomedusan from the family Carybdeidae, *C. barnesi*, has been described by Southcott[7] as the causative agent of the Irukandji syndrome, or Type A stinging, as described by Flecker[8, 9] in swimmers in northern Queensland, Australia. Type A stinging is said to occur in swimmers who suffered severe generalized symptoms but no wheals after a sting. Type B stinging refers to urticaria but no generalized symptoms.

Stings from *Chironex* and *Chiropsalmus* are dangerous. The effects usually consist of extremely painful localized areas of wheal, edema, and vesiculation, which later result in necrosis involving the full thickness of the skin. The initial lesions, caused by the structural pattern of the tentacles, are multiple linear wheals with transverse barring. The purple or brown tentacle marks form a whiplike skin lesion. Painful muscle spasms, respiratory distress, a rapid and weak pulse, prostration, pulmonary edema, shock and respiratory failure, or death may result. The pain is said to be excruciating, with the victim frequently screaming and becoming irrational. Death may take place within 30 seconds to 2 or 3 hours, but the usual time is less than 15 minutes. The cough and mucoid expectoration that result from some of the other forms of jellyfish attacks are generally absent in patients with *Chironex* and *Chiropsalmus* stings.

Sea Anemones and Corals

Sea anemones are some of the most abundant seashore animals. Most are sessile, ranging in size from a few millimeters to a half meter in diameter. Anemones have a flower-like appearance under water when their tentacles are extended. When irritated or when the water recedes, the tentacles invaginate and the body contracts rapidly. In addition to having stinging nematocysts, some sea anemones are poisonous if eaten.

Corals are the major constituent of living reefs, such as the Great Barrier Reef off the northeastern shore of Queensland, Australia. They are composed of an external calcium carbonate skeleton that houses small, anemone-like polyps. The actual stinging ability of true corals is exaggerated. More dangerous are the cuts and lacerations one can suffer from handling coral or brushing against it.

Coral stings have been described as a distinct stinging sensation, followed by weeping of the lesion, wheal formation, and itching.

*On Color Plate VII at the front of this book.

If coral cuts or stings are left untreated, a superficial scratch may within a few days become an ulcer, with a septic sloughing base surrounded by a painful zone of erythema. Cellulitis, lymphangitis, enlargement of the local lymph glands, fever, and malaise are commonly present. The ulcer may be quite disabling, and the pain is usually out of proportion to the physical signs. If the ulcer occurs in a lower extremity, the patient may be unable to walk for weeks or months after the injury. Relapses, which occur without warning, are common.

Diagnosis

Diagnosis of jellyfish sting can be aided by the patient or a companion. When a patient experiences an unknown sting, the diagnosis is usually made by observing a row of urticarial lesions or the presence of a tentacle adherent to the patient's skin. Stingrays leave a penetrating wound, and snakes leave fang marks. Catfish leave a barb, and this occurs only on handling the catfish.

A differential diagnosis with respect to the type of coelenterate is not so important in the United States, but where lethal coelenterates exist, as in Australia, identification of nematocysts on the patient by examining the skin wheals of the victim is important. Halstead suggests that the wheal should be scraped with the edge of a microscope slide or scalpel and the material microscopically examined for the presence of nematocysts. Nematocysts may also be obtained by microscopic examination of a strip of transparent tape that has been pressed against the surface of the wheal. The nematocysts will adhere to the sticky side of the tape. Identification of nematocysts from the skin of the victim will yield positive identification of a coelenterate sting, but it will not provide positive information regarding species identification.

Treatment

Treatment of coelenterate stings is symptomatic and supportive. Advanced cardiac life support may be necessary in patients who sustain cardiac arrest, either from toxic effects of the venom (e.g., *C. fleckeri*) or from anaphylaxis. Unfortunately, it is not uncommon for patients with sea wasp stings to be beyond resuscitation by the time they reach the hospital (personal communication, Peter Bastable, MD, Second International Conference of Emergency Medicine, Brisbane, Australia, October, 1988). For those who are fortunate enough to arrive alive at the hospital after a *Chironex* sting, rapid IV administration of sea wasp antivenin (Commonwealth Serum Laboratories, Australia) may be lifesaving. Tentacle removal should also be safely accomplished using a surgical hemostat.

For anaphylactic shock, epinephrine IV, oxygen, IV fluids, dopamine, diphenhydramine, and a glucocorticoid such as Solu-Medrol may be indicated.

For asthma-like attacks, epinephrine, oxygen, normal saline, IV fluids, a bronchodilator, and perhaps a steroid may be considered, generally depending on the patient's presentation and response to treatment.

For paresthesia, and as reported for muscle spasms,[10–12] intravenous calcium chloride (e.g., 10 ml of 10 per cent for adults, administered slowly) has proved useful, but should be performed with cardiac monitoring.

Antitetanus immunization updating and treatment should be provided as indicated.

Considerable success has been achieved by using the following steps in management of jellyfish and Portuguese man-of-war stings.[2]

1. At the scene, advise the emergency medical service personnel or available family member or companion to remove any jellyfish tentacles that may be adhering to the skin, using sand held by a bath towel. Do not rub off the tentacles, rather pull them off. Care must be taken not to expose the treating individual, who also might be stung. As long as the tentacles are on the skin, they will continue to discharge their nematocysts.
2. The wound should be washed with alcohol to fix the remaining nematocysts, thus preventing them from discharging.
3. A paste of baking soda (sodium bicarbonate) should be applied to the wound, affording considerable local relief. After an hour, moisten the baking soda with water and scrape it off with a dull object, like a spoon, to remove any remaining nematocysts.
4. Jellyfish often cause allergic reactions, and generalized urticaria and intense pruritus are common. Parenteral Benadryl, 50 mg IV in an adult, or a steroid, such as Solu-Medrol, 125 mg IV, or both may be indi-

cated. Patients should be discharged with a prescription for an antihistamine or a steroid or both, to use as an outpatient. For as long as 1 to 2 weeks after the initial sting, it is not uncommon for patients to return for recurrence of urticarial lesions at the site of the sting.[2] These should be treated symptomatically with antihistamines. For this reason, follow-up is recommended to all patients with jellyfish stings.

5. Patients who incur Portuguese man-of-war stings may have severe radiating pain and generalized symptoms. Morphine may be necessary to relieve pain. Generalized symptoms, including hypotension, may be present, and IV fluid therapy with normal saline and general supportive measures may be indicated.

STINGRAYS

Stingrays are a common cause of emergency department visits; approximately 750 people are stung yearly along United States coasts. Three common stingrays are the round stingray, *Urolophus halleri,* the larger stingrays, *Dasyatis sayi* (found primarily in the Atlantic), and *Aetobatus narinari* (found primarily in the Pacific). The electric ray, *Torpedo marmorata,* is able to generate an electrical discharge capable of temporarily disabling an adult man.[1] Some stingrays display an interesting characteristic: They have a sense of territory and usually do not stray too far from their claimed "turf."

The *Dasyatis* stingrays (Color Plate VII,* Fig. 31–6) are difficult to detect because of their habit of lying buried in the mud or sand with only a portion of the body exposed.

Accidents usually occur when bathers step on a buried ray. The ray then whips its tail up and forward, driving the stinger into the foot or leg. Shuffling the feet in murky water causes stingrays to swim away from the immediate area. Commercial fishermen are sometimes stung in the hand or arms when emptying nets. Divers may be stung on the chest or abdomen.

The tail is armed with one or more venomous spines. The spine has a sharp, arrow-like tip and backward-pointing serrations along the sides so that after penetration the barb is difficult to remove and lacerates the tissues as it is withdrawn. The venom apparatus consists of a spine, integumentary sheath, and associated venom glands. When the spine penetrates the flesh, the sheath is torn, the venom is released, and a violent tissue reaction is produced. Russell has carried out research on the pharmacology, clinical aspects, and treatment of stingray envenomation.[13–15]

Pharmacology

The venom is primarily protein, and extracts contain serotonin and enzymes such as 5′-nucleotidase and phosphodiesterase.

Stingray venom is one of the most powerful vasoconstrictors found among animal toxins. Coronary vessel spasm, with resultant ST changes on the electrocardiogram and actual myocardial injury with subsequent decrease in cardiac output and hypotension, and arrhythmias, including cardiac standstill, have been observed experimentally in cats.[15] The venom is highly unstable and is markedly heat labile.

Clinical Aspects

Most stings occur on the ankle or foot. The stingray spine is very sharp, and by virtue of the mechanism of injury, it is common for a patient to receive a laceration rather than a puncture wound. The three patients who presented to our emergency department in two recent weeks all described walking in the ocean and feeling a "fluttering" under their foot and then a sudden "stabbing" pain. The usual presenting symptom is severe shooting pain that increases in intensity over the first hour.

Systemic symptoms, such as chest pain, syncope, and other neurologic sequelae, have been described. Death has been reported but is uncommon.

Treatment

The key to therapy involves care of the wound, relief of pain, observation, and even hospitalization in severe cases.

Therapy should be begun immediately, with irrigation of the wound with saltwater. The wound should then be immersed continuously in hot water for at least 60 minutes; this deactivates the heat-labile venom and

*On Color Plate VII at the front of this book.

also relieves pain. The use of hot water immersion is based on extensive clinical evidence[1, 2, 14, 15] and is a standard of care.

In the emergency department, hot water immersion should be continued. Often hot water immersion alone will provide pain relief, and pain medication is not necessary. After an hour of continuous hot water immersion, have the patient take the foot or affected part out of the water: if he or she suffers no pain, then one can stop treatment. Extremity wounds should then be irrigated, cleansed, debrided, and explored if necessary to remove any foreign body. An x-ray to rule out foreign body may be useful. Lacerations may then be surgically closed.

Patients with systemic symptoms should be observed, and patients with chest pain, irregular pulse, or hypotension should have an electrocardiogram and should be placed on a cardiac monitor. Hospitalization may be necessary when symptoms persist. Supportive therapy may be indicated.

Patients who suffer a sting on the chest or abdomen may require surgical exploration.

Most cases will respond to treatment in the emergency department. Tetanus prophylaxis is necessary. Antibiotics are usually required. Serious wounds may require outpatient follow-up.

CATFISH

Marine catfish are abundant silvery fishes with a smooth, scaleless skin. They have four to five barbels or "whiskers" around the mouth, giving them their name. The dorsal and pectoral spines of many species, especially juvenile catfish, are venomous and capable of inflicting very painful wounds. Stinging usually results from handling the fish, such as when removing the fish from the net or taking a hook out of its mouth. The venom of one species, the Indo-Pacific catfish *Plotosus lineatus,* has been reported to be lethal.[1]

Catfish stings are common and painful and often become secondarily infected. Irrigation to remove venom, cleansing, debridement, and removal of the catfish barb are essential to management. A patient will often have a painful, swollen, and infected wound days after the initial result. The typical history is that the person was stung while handling a catfish but thought that the barb had been removed. X-ray films are indicated, as catfish barbs are radiopaque. If the foreign body is seen on the radiograph, the wound should then be opened and explored and the catfish spine removed.

Both tetanus and antibiotic coverage are indicated; in the authors' experience, cephalexin (Keflex) is the preferred antibiotic.

SEA URCHINS

The invertebrate phylum Echinodermata includes the venomous sea urchins (see Color Plate VII,* Fig. 31–2), such as *Diadema setosum, Toxopneustes pileolus lamarck, Toxopneustes gratilla linnaeus,* and *Echinothrix calamaris;* starfish, such as *Acanthaster planci,* or the crown-of-thorns starfish, and sea cucumbers.[1] Both venomous sea urchins and the venomous starfish have venomous spines.

Sea urchin (and starfish) toxin is remarkably heat labile, and hot water immersion therapy is indicated,[3, 4] taking care not to burn the patient. Surgical removal especially of the thick calcium-containing spines may be indicated,[4] as well as tetanus prophylaxis.

SCORPION FISH AND STONEFISH

The stonefish (*Synanceja* sp.) (Color Plate VII,* Fig. 31–9) and scorpion fish (*Notesthes* sp.) belong to the family Scorpaenidae. Other examples of venomous fish in this family include the butterfly fish *(Pterois lunulata),* zebra fish (Color Plate VII,* Fig. 31–8), sculpin (*Scorpaena* sp.), and rockfish (*Sebastes* spp.). Most venomous Scorpaenidae are found in tropical water, but a somewhat less venomous species of scorpion fish occurs along the coast of California and the southeastern coast of the United States. Most scorpion fish stings occur during handling of the fish. Venomous dorsal spines, which cause the injury, are characteristic of these fish.

Inoculation of infectious material as well as a pain-producing venom can complicate the spine-puncture wound.[16] Some venomous fish spine puncture wounds may be "dry," indicating that a puncture wound has occurred without the injection of venom. Unless an antivenin is available (e.g., for

*On Color Plate VII at the front of this book.

stonefish, the stonefish antivenin from Commonwealth Serum Laboratories in Australia), treatment is similar to that for stingray injury (hot water immersion, wound debridement as indicated, and supportive therapy for systemic reactions, if present). Several deaths have been attributed to stonefish injury, dating back to antiquity.[1]

TOXIC MARINE INGESTION

In addition to the forms of marine life that cause bacterial, allergic, and other human illnesses after their ingestion, some species contain one or more toxins and can cause illness, such as ciguatera, puffer fish "fugu" poisoning, and paralytic shellfish poisoning.

On initial consideration of the treatment for ingestion of toxic marine organisms, the patient history, physical examination, actual seafood consumed, available laboratory test results, emergency status, clinical manifestations, and course of the illness should be evaluated.[17] For some illnesses, the emergency and the nature of the poisoning may require aggressive emergency and critical care until the patient is able to metabolize the toxin.[17] For puffer fish poisoning and paralytic shellfish poisoning (red tide), only supportive treatment may be available.[1, 2] Severe, prolonged, life-threatening illnesses may occur in remote areas where advanced cardiac life support, mechanical ventilation, IV fluids, and other supportive therapy may be required until the patient can be evacuated to a suitable medical facility for definitive care.[4] In divers, toxic marine ingestion may need to be considered as well as air embolism, decompression sickness (e.g., the "bends"), and other diving emergencies.[4, 17]

Paralytic Shellfish Poisoning

More than 1000 cases of paralytic shellfish poisoning have been reported, with fatalities in approximately 20 per cent of cases. Paralytic shellfish poisoning results from consumption of mollusks (e.g., mussels, clams, scallops, and oysters) that have fed on certain toxic *Gonyaulax* species. These unicellular algae or phytoplankton from red tides concentrate the toxins in their digestive glands ("hepatopancreas," "liver") or siphon. Mollusks feed by filtering seawater that contains phytoplankton. The shellfish are not adversely affected by the algal toxins.[18–24]

There is no known antidote to the most potent toxins, which include saxitoxin and analogues.[25, 29] Oral ingestion of 0.5 to 1.0 mg of poisonous shellfish can be fatal.[25, 27] These toxins block action potentials by preventing the flow of sodium, thus impeding nerve conduction. Immunity is not engendered through antibody production after exposure to sublethal doses. Poisonous shellfish cannot be recognized by appearance, odor, or any method other than chemical analysis and (mouse toxicity) bioassay. Cooking, frying, and baking only partially ameliorate toxicity.[18, 26] A victim's prognosis depends on the quantity ingested.[29]

The best prevention of paralytic shellfish poisoning in humans is strict adherence to public health agency guidelines on harvesting, processing, and consumption of shellfish.[18, 26] The sporadic and unpredictable nature of red tides and paralytic shellfish poisoning further argues for stringent compliance with quarantine regulations.

"Red tides" result from excessive growth (bloom) of particular unicellular algae (phytoplankton), giving the water a red-brown appearance due to the pigments contained in the algae.[28] Factors involved in the initiation, subsequent development, and continuation of a red tide are not totally understood. Red tides occur sporadically and are usually of short duration. In general, the abundance and seasonal distribution of dinoflagellates are intimately related to temperature, salinity, light, nutrients, and hydrographic conditions, including currents and water column stability in the sea.[23] However, toxic red tides are essentially a coastal phenomenon.

Poisonings related to ingestion of shellfish were described in the time of Moses, about 1491 B.C.[25] Blooms or red tides of oceans are mentioned in the Bible in Exodus 7:20–21: "And all the waters that were in the river were turned to blood. And the fish that was in the river died; and the river stank, and the Egyptians could not drink the water of the river." Because of the red tide in 208 B.C., the name Red Sea was applied by the ancient Greeks to all coasts of Arabia. The red tides were mentioned in the Iliad as well as in the writings of Tacitus. As early as 1689, the first case of paralytic shellfish poisoning was described.

Medical history gives accounts of incidents

of shellfish poisoning in many parts of the world between 1827 and 1909. The great Wilhelmshaven outbreak that took place in Germany in 1885 attracted scientists' attention to the red tide as a health hazard.[18]

The first large epidemic recorded in the United States was in San Francisco in 1927; 102 persons became ill, and 6 died.[32]

The work of Somner and his associates in the 1930s proved that the California mussel *Mytilus californianus* lost its toxicity in filtered water but regained it in seawater taken from a red tide area. These same scientists correlated the increase of toxicity of mussels with the number of *Gonyaulax catanella* present in their environment.[18] This finding was confirmed several years later by other investigators.

In the 1940s, Woodcock first demonstrated that the toxin of *Gymnodinium breve,* which causes the red tide off the Florida coast, could act as an upper respiratory tract irritant. Death of large numbers of fish became associated with blooms of this microorganism, as did seabird fatalities and shellfish poisoning.[18]

From this research, paralytic shellfish poisoning was clearly shown to originate from red tides, with filter-feeding bivalve mollusks as transvectors, especially mussels and clams—for example, *Mytilus edulis* (mussel), *M. californianus* (mussel), and *Saxidomus gigantus* (Alaskan butter clam) in northeastern Pacific Ocean coastal waters; and *Mya arenaria* (soft-shell clam), *Placopecten magellanicus* (sea scallop), and *Mytilus edulis* in northwestern Atlantic Ocean coastal waters.[20, 22, 33]

Although shellfish include mollusks such as clams, oysters, and scallops, and crustaceans such as shrimp, lobsters, and crabs, mollusks that have a hard shell are particularly prone to cause paralytic shellfish poisoning. Crustaceans can have softer shells; however, where there is an outbreak of paralytic shellfish poisoning, much of the marine life can be involved, and fish, shellfish, and other seafoods may be poisonous or restricted.

Rates of accumulation and loss of toxin and anatomic distribution of toxin differ among species.[26] In mussels, for example *Mytilus* spp., the toxins are concentrated in the digestive glands ("hepatopancreas," "liver," or "dark glands"). Toxicity is usually lost within weeks from mussels in seawater that does not contain toxic dinoflagellates. In the Alaskan butter clam *(S. gigantus),* for example, the principal storage sites of the toxin after the initial accumulation in the digestive glands are the gills and siphons. Butter clams can maintain toxicity for as long as 2 years after initial accumulation of toxin from a red tide.

Fortunately, the muscular tissues (white meat) of mollusks (mantle muscle, adductor muscles, foot, and body—exclusive of digestive glands) tend to store relatively small amounts of poison. These are the tissues most commonly eaten by people.[26]

Crustacean shellfish such as lobsters are only very rarely transvectors of paralytic shellfish poisoning.[34]

The toxic principals of *Gonyaulax* species, of which mollusks are transvectors, are substituted tetrahydropurine structures that include saxitoxin 1, neosaxitoxin 2, gonyautoxin 3 (II), gonyautoxin 4 (III), and gonyautoxin 5 (VII).[31]

The chemical and physiologic characteristics of saxitoxin 1 and analogues are very similar. The toxicity of each compound is approximately 5000 mouse units (MU)/mg (1 MU is the amount of poison that kills a 20-gm laboratory white mouse within 15 minutes after intraperitoneal injection). One mouse unit of saxitoxin by intraperitoneal injection is approximately 0.18 mg.[25] Saxitoxin is among the most potent human poisons known. A dose of purified saxitoxin or analogues lethal to humans is 0.1 mg.[26]

If a patient is overwhelmed by paralytic shellfish poisoning, apnea, respiratory paralysis, and motor paralysis resembling curarization[32, 35] can occur. The initial manifestations of poisoning may consist of numbness and tingling around the lips, mouth, upper airway, and fingers, which may be apparent within a few minutes after eating poisonous shellfish.[1, 35] These sensations are followed by a feeling of numbness in other parts of the body. Nausea, vomiting, and diarrhea can occur. Floating sensations may be reported by the patient. Until proven otherwise, paralytic shellfish poisoning is a life-threatening emergency. As the illness progresses, respiratory distress and muscle paralysis become more severe. Death results from respiratory paralysis within 2 to 12 hours, depending on the magnitude of the dose. If a patient survives for 24 hours, the prognosis is good, and there appears to be no lasting effect.[27]

Diagnosis

Without an adequate history, diagnosis can be, and often is, most puzzling. A complete history is essential for proper diagnosis—a presumptive diagnosis of paralytic shellfish poisoning should be made in a patient who develops neurologic symptoms after ingestion of mussels during seasons of risk in areas where paralytic shellfish poisoning occurs. Other causes of neurologic illness may appropriately have to be ruled out. Obtaining saxitoxin from the implicated shellfish, identifying the toxin in the patient, and identifying the toxin in an algal organism such as *G. catenella*[36] may be helpful. Analyses of toxic shellfish and toxic dinoflagellate algal organisms for toxins have helped establish a diagnosis in patients involved in certain outbreaks of shellfish poisonings, particularly because the seawater is not always abnormally pigmented or may not manifest a pigmented tide until late in the outbreak.[35] It is preferable that all the toxins be rapidly identified from the patient's blood or urine.

Management

The treatment of paralytic shellfish poisoning is symptomatic and supportive. Although there is no proven antidote, antisaxitoxin-antibody treatment has experimentally been effective in animals[37] and may not only be useful in treating patients who have sustained a poisoning by saxitoxin (with or without other toxins) but may also serve as a model for treating poisoning caused by saxitoxin-like purines and similar compounds. Gastric lavage and activated charcoal are indicated, as saxitoxin is readily absorbed on charcoal. An alkaline diuresis with sodium bicarbonate may be of value, as the toxins are reportedly unstable in an alkaline medium. Steroids[25] such as hydrocortisone may be indicated. Respiratory support, cardiac monitoring, and maintenance of blood pressure are often necessary, as these patients are usually in critical condition.

Puffer Fish Poisoning

Puffer fish poisoning[1, 40] can be a highly lethal form of fish poisoning. The puffer fish toxin tetrodotoxin can produce a prolonged state of suspended animation resembling death.[1, 39, 40] Fugu in Japan and the tambore puffer in Cuba are popular fish eaten by some persons in some cultures. In Japan,[1] a 59 per cent mortality was reported in 6386 cases of puffer fish poisoning during a period of 78 years. Although selected outbreaks of marine poisonings may cause greater mortality, puffer fish poisoning overall appears to cause the greatest mortality on a consistent basis. At least three deaths from eating puffers have been reported in Florida.

Puffer fish are named for their ability to inflate themselves to a nearly spherical shape when disturbed (Color Plate VII,* Fig. 31–7). Some common names for tetrodotoxic puffers in various areas of the world are tambores (Cuba), fugu (Japan), West Indian swellfish, blowfish, globefish, Sphaeroides, balloon fish, tetraodon, porcupine fish, toadfish, tiger puffer, jug fish, rabbit fish, and botete.[1]

Toxicology

The toxin that causes puffer fish poisoning is tetrodotoxin.[1, 10] Tetrodotoxin is a basic compound that is readily soluble in water. It is *not* heat labile, and boiling or heating the fish will not deactivate the poison. Tetrodotoxin is a specific inhibitor of sodium conductance by nerve cells.[1, 10]

Social Aspects

In Japan, fugu is considered a delicacy, and all cooks and restaurants handling fugu must be specially licensed to prepare fugu. The muscle of the fish is the part that is eaten, usually during the winter months (during the nonreproductive season for puffers). Even with extensive regulations, fugu is still the major cause of death from food poisoning in Japan.

Clinical Presentation

The clinical manifestations of puffer poisoning include paresthesia about the lips, fingertips, and elsewhere; diaphoresis, hyperemesis, dysphonia, floating sensations, progressive muscle paralysis, cyanosis, and many other manifestations may be present.[1, 10, 38]

A most unusual phenomenon has been described: Patients may be completely para-

*On Color Plate VII at the front of this book.

lyzed, have absent corneal reflexes, and have dilated, fixed pupils but on recovery are found to have had complete retention of consciousness while in such a state.[1, 40]

Treatment

Management is symptomatic and supportive. Airway management, endotracheal intubation, and mechanical ventilation may be required in apneic patients, who may have extensive respiratory and muscle paralysis.[38] Atropine and/or a cardiac pacemaker may be useful in managing symptomatic bradycardia.[38] Cardiac arrhythmias should be managed appropriately. Normal saline IV infusion and perhaps dopamine may be helpful in managing symptomatic hypotension. Gastric lavage may be performed, with deposition of activated charcoal into the stomach after lavaging with a 2 per cent sodium bicarbonate solution (IV).[38]

Considerable caution is urged when pronouncing death due to puffer poisoning, because the toxin may produce a deceptive state of suspended animation.[1, 40]

Ciguatera

Numerous species of predominantly reef fish have been linked to ciguatera.[1, 41, 42] Apparently, toxins including those from the benthic dinoflagellate algal organism *Gambierdiscus toxicus* pass up the food chain of fishes and poison individuals consuming sufficient amounts of toxic fish.[42–44] Sensitized persons, who are susceptible to small amounts of toxic fish, can become quite ill and may require aggressive treatment.

Barracuda, amberjack, kingfish, dolphin fish, wrasses, triggerfish, the moray eel, surgeon fish, filefish, and even such delicacies as grouper, red snapper, herring, and pompano are among the approximately 300 species that have at various times been implicated in causing ciguatera. Sixty per cent of the cases reported in the Miami study[43] followed ingestion of grouper. So many reports of ciguatera followed the ingestion of barracuda that its sale is prohibited in Miami.

The characteristic clinical syndrome of ciguatera occurs after eating a ciguatoxic fish and includes both gastrointestinal and neurologic symptoms. The characteristic features of ciguatera include paresthesia of the perioral region and distal extremities and a cold-to-hot sensory reversal dysesthesia—the patient usually describes a burning hot sensation while picking up a cold drink. The presence of these two unique symptoms in conjunction with gastroenteritis permit the clinical diagnosis of ciguatera.[1, 2, 42–44]

Bagnis and associates[42] reviewed 3009 cases of ciguatera in the South Pacific and noted paresis involving the extraocular muscles or the lower extremities in 10.5 per cent of patients, paralysis of the lower extremities in 0.6 per cent of patients, and only three deaths, or 0.1 per cent of the total group.

Ataxia, headache, arthralgias, and vertigo are also common complaints. Pruritus is present. Another unusual feature is that patients may complain that their teeth feel loose and are painful.[41–44] Oropharyngeal paresthesia, acral paresthesia, and even total-body paresthesia can develop. Nausea, vomiting, and diarrhea may be severe. Hypotension that is symptomatic and symptomatic bradycardia (including heart blocks) can develop.

Paresthesia and prolonged weakness after the acute phase may persist for several weeks.[41–44] It has also been noted that repeated episodes of ciguatera may be more severe in character.[42–44]

Treatment

A promising new treatment of acute and chronic ciguatera in appropriate patients is IV mannitol.[45] After establishing an IV infusion of normal saline or lactated Ringer's solution, 20 per cent mannitol is given as a piggyback (IV) solution. The dose of mannitol is calculated to a maximum of 1 gm/kg of body weight and given at a rate of 500 ml/hour. Thus, a 70-kg man would receive 70 gm of 20 per cent mannitol, or 350 ml over 42 minutes. Symptomatic and supportive therapy may also be indicated.[41–50]

Some patients feel well before the infusion is completed.[45] However, patients should still be placed on a ciguatera diet[44] avoiding fish, shellfish, alcoholic beverages, nuts or nut products, and seeds or seed products for 6 to 12 months.

Acute and chronic ciguatera has been managed using amitriptyline.[49, 50] Remissions and exacerbations may occur.[44, 45, 47, 48]

References

1. Halstead BW: Poisonous and Venomous Marine Animals of the World. Revised ed. Princeton, NJ, Darwin Press, 1978.
2. Haddad LM, Lee RF, McConnell OJ, Targett NK: Toxic marine life. *In* Haddad LM, Winchester JF (eds): Clinical Management of Poisoning and Drug Overdose. Philadelphia, WB Saunders, 1983, pp 303–317.
3. Sims JK: Dangerous marine life. *In* Shilling CW, Carlston CB, Mathias RA: The Physician's Guide to Diving Medicine. New York, Plenum Press, 1984, p 427.
4. Sims JK: Emergencies related to marine fauna. *In* Tintinalli JE, Rothstein RJ, Krome RL (eds): Emergency Medicine: A Comprehensive Study Guide. New York, McGraw-Hill, 1985, pp 364–366.
5. Lane CE: Nematocyst toxins of coelenterates. *In* Humm HJ, Lane CE (eds): Bioactive Compounds from the Sea. New York, Marcel Dekker, 1974, p 123.
6. Robson EA: Nematocysts of *Corynactis*: The activity of the filament during discharge. Q J Microsc Sci *94*:229, 1953.
7. Southcott RV: Revision of the Irukandji syndrome. Aust J Zool *15*:651, 1967.
8. Flecker H: Fatal stings to N. Queensland bathers. Med J Aust *1*:35, 1952.
9. Flecker H: Irukandji sting to N. Queensland bathers. Med J Aust *2*:89, 1952.
10. Halstead BW: Poisonous and Venomous Marine Animals of the World. Vol. 1. Washington, DC, United States Government Printing Office, 1965.
11. Ellis MD: Dangerous Plants, Snakes, Arthropods and Marine Life. Hamilton, Ill. Drug Intelligence Publications, 1978, p 214.
12. Halstead BW: Hazardous marine life. *In* Strauss RH (ed): Diving Medicine. New York, Grune & Stratton, 1976, p 227.
13. Russell FE: Injuries by venomous animals in the U.S. JAMA *177*:85, 1961.
14. Russell FE: Stingray injuries: Discussion of treatment. Am J Med Sci *226*:611, 1953.
15. Russell FE: Report of 2 fatal case studies on mechanism of death from stingray venom. Am J Med Sci *235*:566, 1958.
16. Sims JK, Enomoto PI, Frankel RI, Wong LMF: Marine bacteria complicating seawater near-drowning and marine wounds: A hypothesis. Ann Emerg Med *12*:212, 1983.
17. Sims JK: A theoretical discourse on the pharmacology of toxic marine ingestions. Ann Emerg Med *16*:1006, 1987.
18. Ahles MD: Red tide: A recurrent health hazard. Am J Public Health *64*:807, 1974.
19. Bates HA, Kostriken R, Rapoport H: A chemical assay for saxitoxin: Improvements and modifications. J Agric Food Chem *26*:252, 1978.
20. Bond RM, Medcof JC: Epidemic shellfish poisoning in New Brunswick, 1957. Can Med Assoc J *19*:19, 1978.
21. Collins M: Algal toxins. Microbiol Rev *42*:725, 1978.
22. Hsu CP, Marchand A, Shimizu Y, Sims GG: Paralytic shellfish toxins in the sea scallop, *Placopecten magellanicus*, in the Bay of Fundy. J Fish Res Board Can *36*:32, 1979.
23. LoCicero VR (ed): Proceedings of The First International Conference on Toxic Dinoflagellate Blooms. The Massachusetts Science and Technology Foundation, Wakefield, Mass., 1975.
24. Meyer KF: Food poisoning. N Engl J Med *249*:765, 804, 843, 1953.
25. Morse EV: Paralytic shellfish poisoning: A review. J Am Vet Med Assoc *171*:1178, 1977.
26. Ray SM: Current status of paralytic shellfish poisoning. *In* Proceedings of Third International Congress of Food Science and Technology, 1971, p 717.
27. Schantz EJ: The dinoflagellate poisons. *In* Kadis S, Aegler A, Ajl S (eds): Microbial Toxins. Vol 7. New York, Academic Press, 1971, p 3.
28. Schantz EJ: Poisonous red tide organisms. Environ Lett *9*:225, 1975.
29. Schantz EJ: Immunological aspects of fish and shellfish poisons. *In* Catsimpoolas N (ed): Immunological Aspects of Food. AVI Publishing Company, Westport, Conn., 1977, p 260.
30. Schmidt RJ, Loeblich AR III: Distribution of paralytic shellfish poison amoung pyrrhophyta. J Mar Biol Assoc UK *59*:479, 1979.
31. Shimizu Y, Hus CP, Fallon WF, Oshima Y, Miura I, Nakanishi K: Structure of neosaxitoxin. J Am Chem Soc *100*:6791, 1978.
32. Sommer H, Meyer KF: Paralytic shellfish poisoning. Arch Pathol *24*:560, 1937.
33. Tennant AD, Naubert J, Corbeil HE: An outbreak of paralytic shellfish poisons. Can Med Assoc J *72*:436, 1955.
34. Yentsch CM, Balch W: Lack of secondary intoxification by red tide poison in the American lobster *Homanus americanus*. Environ Lett *9*:249, 1975.
35. Hughes JM, Merson MH: Current concepts—fish and shellfish poisoning. N Engl J Med *295*:1117, 1976.
36. Bates HA, Kostriken R, Rapoport H: The occurrence of saxitoxin and other toxins in various dinoflagellates. Toxicon *16*:595, 1978.
37. Davio SR: Neutralization of saxitoxin by antisaxitoxin rabbit serum. Toxicon *23*:669, 1985.
38. Sims JK, Ostman DC: Pufferfish poisoning: Emergency diagnosis and management of mild human tetrodotoxication. Ann Emerg Med *15*:1094, 1986.
39. Russell FE: Marine toxins and venomous and poisonous marine plants and animals (invertebrates). Adv Mar Biol *21*:59, 1984.
40. Torda TA: Pufferfish (tetrodotoxin) poisoning: Clinical record and suggested management. Med J Aust *1*:599, 1973.
41. Bagnis R, Berglund F, Elias PS, van Esch GJ, Halstead BW, Kojima K: Problems of toxicants in marine food products. I: Marine biotoxins. Bull WHO *42*:69, 1970.
42. Bagnis R, Kuberski T, Laugier S: Clinical observations on 3009 cases of ciguatera in the South Pacific. Am J Trop Med Hyg *28*:1067, 1979.
43. Lawrence DN, Enriquez MB, Lumish RM, Maceo A: Ciguatera fish poisoning in Miami. JAMA *244*:254, 1980.
44. Gillespie NC, Lewis RJ, Pearn JH, Bourke ATC, Holmes MJ, Bourke JB, Shields WJ: Ciguatera in Australia—occurrence, clinical features, pathophysiology and management. Med J Aust *145*:584, 1986.
45. Palafox NA, Jain LG, Pinano AZ, Gulick TM, Williams RK, Schatz IJ: Successful treatment of ciguatera fish poisoning with intravenous mannitol. JAMA *259*:2740, 1988.

46. Chretien JH, Fermaglich J, Garagusi VF: Ciguatera poisoning—presentation as a neurologic disorder. Arch Neurol *38*:783, 1981.
47. Engleberg NC, Morris JG, Lewis J, McMillan JP, Pollard RA, Blake PA: Ciguatera fish poisoning: a major common source outbreak in the U.S. Virgin Islands. Ann Intern Med *98*:336, 1983.
48. Morris JG, Lewin P, Hargrett N, Smith CW, Blake PA, Schneider R: Clinical features of ciguatera fish poisoning. A study of the disease in the Virgin Islands. Arch Intern Med *142*:1090, 1982.
49. Bowman PB: Amitriptyline and ciguatera. Med J Aust *140*:802, 1984.
50. Davis RT, Villar LA: Symptomatic improvement with amitriptyline in ciguatera fish poisoning (letter). N Engl J Med *315*:65, 1986.

CHAPTER 32
FOOD POISONING

Corey M. Slovis, M.D., FACP, FACEP

Many different organisms and toxins are capable of causing food poisoning. This chapter is primarily devoted to food-borne botulism, the most deadly food-related toxicologic disease known. In addition to a review of the various forms of botulism, the chapter contains information on the food-borne, toxin-related diseases of *Staphylococcus aureus*, *Clostridium perfringens*, cholera and noncholera vibrios, *Bacillus cereus*, and Jamaican vomiting sickness.

BOTULISM

Botulism is probably the best known rare disease in the United States and Canada.[1, 2] Botulism is the clinical syndrome that results from the actions of the botulinal toxin–a neurotoxin produced by the anaerobic, spore-forming, gram-positive rod *Clostridium botulinum*.[3, 4] There are four relatively distinct forms of botulism: (1) food-borne botulism; (2) infant botulism; (3) wound botulism; and (4) botulism, classification undetermined.[3]

Food-borne botulism is the best-known form of botulism. It occurs when an individual consumes food contaminated with preformed toxin.[1, 3] Infant botulism is now the most common form of botulism and occurs in infants who have ingested foods contaminated by spores of *C. botulinum*. Disease occurs if the spores germinate in the infant's intestine and produce toxin.[5] Wound botulism, a rare form of the disease, occurs when wounds become colonized by *C. botulinum*, and toxin is absorbed systemically.[3, 6] The newest category of botulism is "classification undetermined." This category is used for cases of botulism that occur in patients older than 1 year of age in whom no obvious food or wound source can be identified.[1, 3]

Bacteriology

The *C. botulinum* species is subdivided based on the immunologically distinct toxin type that each subspecies produces. There are eight different serologic types: A, B, C_1, C_2, D, E, F, and G, and all but the C_2 type produce disease in humans or animals.[3, 4, 7] The botulinal toxin is produced after the botulinum spore germinates and begins cell growth. Release of the toxin usually results when the mature cell's wall lyses.[7, 8]

The dormant spores of *C. botulinum* are highly resistant to heating, freezing, aerobic and anaerobic conditions, ionizing radiation, and exposure to various chemical agents.[3, 4, 9] Spores can survive boiling, and temperatures above 120° C for at least 30 minutes are required to destroy the spores.[7, 10] Although spores may remain potentially viable despite markedly adverse conditions, their germination requires the presence of a number of factors. Germination requires the following: the organic acids alanine or cysteine, lactate or bicarbonate, a pH of 4.6–7.0, and a temperature between 4° and 70° C.[2, 7, 11] An alkaline medium prevents spore germination.[9] Once germination occurs, continued organism growth requires even more specific conditions, which include the presence of nine amino acids, three vitamins, an anaerobic environment, a low redox state, a neutral pH, and a temperature in the range of 15 to 45° C.[3, 11] Not all types of botulism are so fastidious; growth of type E organisms has been reported in temperatures as low as 3° C and in nonanaerobic environments.[3]

The Botulinal Toxin

The botulinal toxin, botulin, is the most powerful and dangerous toxin known, with the lethal dose as small as 0.5 μg.[12] Although botulinum spores are relatively heat resistant, botulin is heat sensitive.[3] Heating at 80° C for 30 minutes or 100° C for 10 minutes will destroy any active toxin.[9, 13] Boiling under pressure is required at higher altitudes.[10] If the organism is allowed to mature in a food substance, it will synthesize a protoxin that can be released before and during cell lysis. Ingestion allows the stomach's proteases to cleave portions of the protoxin into the active form, which is then rapidly absorbed in the small bowel.[4, 14] Once the toxin has been absorbed, it spreads via blood and the lymphatic system to nerve terminals and neuronal tissue throughout the body.[4, 14] The toxin binds to extracellular cholinergic nerve membranes and enters the nerve cell by endocytosis.[4] After the toxin enters the cell, a process called the "lytic" or "paralytic step" occurs.[3, 7, 8] This step results in the blockade of subsequent acetylcholine release from nerve terminals.[4, 7, 8]

The exact mechanism by which botulinal toxin blocks acetylcholine release is not presently known nor is the toxin's exact site of action.[4] However, multiple studies have suggested that the toxin's actions are mediated by decreasing or blocking the calcium-dependent exocytosis of acetylcholine.[4, 7, 8] The toxin's blockade of acetylcholine release occurs at four separate sites: (1) the neuromuscular junction; (2) ganglionic nerve endings; (3) postganglionic parasympathetic nerve endings; and (4) postganglionic sympathetic nerve endings that use acetylcholine.[7] The toxin only affects the release of acetylcholine and does not affect acetylcholine's synthesis, storage, or metabolism.[7, 8] Botulinal toxin does not affect impulse conduction down nerves or impulse conduction at nerve terminals.[4, 8, 15]

Food-Borne Botulism

Clinical Presentation

Food-borne botulism usually presents within 12 to 48 hours of ingestion of infected foods.[3, 16–21] Symptoms may be delayed, however, as long as 8 days post ingestion.[20, 22] The usual initial symptoms are gastrointestinal (GI) with nausea, vomiting, diarrhea, and abdominal distention being the most common early symptoms.[17–19, 22] Abdominal distention in association with abdominal pain and increasing patient anxiety may falsely suggest the diagnosis of an acute abdomen.[30] Up to 70 per cent of patients will develop constipation as the illness evolves.[17] Although gastrointestinal symptoms are seen in most patients, they are not present in approximately one third of patients.[37, 38]

Patients may also present with neurologic symptoms due to cholinergic blockade. Visual disturbances, dysarthria, dysphagia, and a dry mouth are the four most common specific neurologic symptoms.[3, 17, 18, 20, 21] Various other nonspecific neurologic complaints seen in patients suffering from botulism include malaise, generalized weakness, headache, dizziness, and paresthesias.[3, 17, 20, 21, 33] Symmetric weakness and decreasing respiratory strength are seen as the disease progresses.

Ocular changes are an especially common cranial nerve finding in botulism.[3, 22] Lateral rectus weakness, ptosis, and pupillary abnormalities are seen in almost every patient who develops neurologic symptoms.[17, 20, 21] Fixed or dilated pupils are seen in almost half the patients who present in botulism epidemics.[6] Because botulism is so rare and associated with numerous nonspecific symptoms, the Centers for Disease Control[3] and others[20, 21, 23] have suggested various constellations of signs and symptoms to help clinicians consider the diagnosis of botulism early in its presentation (Table 32–1).

Most patients in whom the disease is suspected do not turn out to have botulism, and up to half of these patients with suspected cases either have no illness or receive no final

Table 32–1. MOST COMMON PRESENTATIONS OF FOOD-BORNE BOTULISM

Presenting complaints	Dry mouth and/or dysphagia Abdominal symptoms
Initial appearance	Anxious Normal mental status Weak
Medical history	Previously well
Vital signs	Afebrile Slow or normal pulse
Physical examination	Dysphonia Dysarthria Symmetric ocular weakness Symmetric neurologic abnormalities

diagnosis.[3] The disease most commonly confused with botulism is Guillain-Barré syndrome. Approximately 10.5 per cent of persons with suspected cases of botulism reported to the Centers for Disease Control eventually are diagnosed as having Guillain-Barré syndrome. Other diseases commonly confused with botulism include carbon monoxide poisoning (3.4 per cent of reported cases of botulism), food poisoning—etiology unknown (3.2 per cent), and food poisoning due to staphylococcal organisms (3.0 per cent).[3] Table 32–2 presents a comprehensive list of the diseases cited in the differential diagnosis of botulism.[1, 2, 3, 10, 19, 24] Physicians should always consider botulism whenever a patient presents with weakness of any kind (ie, generalized, ocular, laryngeal, and so forth).

Diagnosis

A definite diagnosis of botulism is best made by confirming the presence of botulinal toxin in the patient's serum.[3] Unfortunately, only one third of patients with botulism will have the toxin detected in their serum.[25] False-negative results are especially common when the patient's serum is examined late in the course of the illness.[3] Stool examination for preformed toxin and botulinum organisms is very helpful in the early diagnosis of botulism. When both stool and serum testing are used, the diagnosis of botulism may be confirmed by the laboratory in approximately 75 per cent of cases.[25] Stool should be obtained for analysis without the use of enemas and before antibiotic therapy.[3, 25] Without stool and/or serum confirmation, botulism may be difficult to diagnose. The finding of preformed toxin or the organism in food ingested by an affected patient is supportive evidence for the diagnosis.[3] The electromyogram (EMG) may be very useful in correctly differentiating botulism from myasthenia gravis, Guillain-Barré syndrome, and the Eaton-Lambert syndrome. The EMG in a patient suffering from botulism shows a decrease in the evoked action potential at slow frequency stimulation (2 Hz/sec), whereas at rapid stimulation (50 Hz/sec), there is an increase in the evoked action potential.[10, 26] Post-tetanic potentiation may also be seen with repetitive high frequency stimulation.[10, 12] The EMG findings in myasthenia gravis show decreased evoked muscle responses at both slow and fast stimulation, and these EMG findings improve with tension.[10] There is usually a decrease in evoked potential as the muscle is repetitively stimulated, the opposite of what is found in botulism.[10, 12] The EMG findings in a patient who has the Eaton-Lambert syndrome are very similar to those in a patient suffering from botulism.[10, 16, 26] EMG findings for botulism, however, are very dissimilar between different muscle groups and evolve over time, whereas EMG findings between different muscles for the Eaton-Lambert syndrome are very similar and stay relatively stable over time. EMG findings for the Guillain-Barré syndrome usually show patchy slowing, which is indicative of demyelinization.[12] EMG findings alone should never be used to differentiate any disease from botulism, because (1) up to 15 per cent of cases of botulism may have normal EMGs;[16, 17] (2) improvement with edrophonium may be seen in up to one quarter of patients with proven cases of botulism;[10, 17] and low-frequency findings supportive of myasthenia gravis may be seen in almost 20 per cent of patients who suffer from botulism.[19]

In summary, the diagnosis of botulism may be difficult to make on initial patient presentation. The common presenting symptoms (see Table 32–1), the keys for differential diagnosis (see Table 32–2), and the patient's EMG results should be helpful. Until absolutely certain of another diagnosis, the physician should always consider botulism in the differential diagnosis of any patient who has a suspected case of food poisoning and in any patient who presents with a neurologic or neuromuscular complaint.

Table 32–2. DIFFERENTIAL DIAGNOSIS IN BOTULISM

Disease or Condition	Differential Manifestations
Neurologic Diseases	
Guillain-Barré syndrome	Usually ascending paralysis Elevated CSF protein Paresthesias Preceding viral illness common Absent deep tendon reflexes
Myasthenia gravis	Lack of autonomic findings Increased fatiguability Improvement with edrophonium EMG findings
Eaton-Lambert syndrome	Underlying malignancy, especially oat cell Progression much slower Predominant thigh and pelvic muscle involvement Extraocular muscle involvement rare Pupillary findings almost never present EMG findings
Cerebrovascular accident	Asymmetric Unilateral Vascular distribution Asymmetric deep tendon reflexes
Biologic Infections and Toxins	
Bacterial food poisons (staphylococcal, clostridial, and so forth)	Rapid onset Gastrointestinal complaints predominate No paralysis No cranial nerve involvement
Diphtheria	Pseudomembrane Pharyngitis Schick test Limb paralysis occurs weeks after cranial nerve involvement
Poliomyelitis	Fever Meningeal signs Crampy muscle pain Asymmetric distribution CSF may show encephalitis pattern
Tick paralysis	More common in children Tick(s) found on physical examination Paralysis usually ascending Deep tendon reflexes may be absent
Encephalitis	Altered mental status Fever Meningeal signs Abnormal CSF
Saxitoxin	Symptoms within 1 hour of fish ingestion Paresthesias of face predominate Tachycardia Vertigo
Trichinosis	Fever Myositis Periorbital edema Eosinophilia
Amanita	Coma Violent vomiting Hepatic failure
Tetanus	Trismus Risus sardonicus Neck and jaw stiffness Muscle spasms
Poison and Overdose	
Phenothiazine reaction	Spastic muscle contractures Resolution with antihistamines
Carbon monoxide poisoning	Headache Altered mental status Elevated CO level
Organophosphate overdose	Fasciculations Cholinergic symptoms Resolution with atropine
Anticholinergic poisoning	Fever Altered mental status Tachycardia and vasodilation No cranial nerve involvement
Aminoglycoside-induced paralysis	Medication history Post anesthesia History of renal impairment Serum levels
Heavy metal exposure	Exposure history Rapidity of onset Serum or urine levels
Hypermagnesemia	Medication history Renal impairment Serum magnesium level
Medical Conditions and Emergencies	
Acute myocardial infarction Appendicitis Bowel obstruction Bowel infarction	Classic signs and symptoms should evolve over time
Acute intermittent porphyria	History or family history Cranial nerve involvement rare Prior psychiatric or CNS complaints Urinary test abnormalities
Carcinomatous invasion of the base of the skull	Cranial nerves V and VIII involvement only Meningeal signs and symptoms
Hysteria	Variable, inconsistent findings No objective findings
Sepsis	Fever Leukocytosis Localized sites of infection Abnormal CSF findings Positive blood cultures

Compiled in part from information contained in references 1, 2, 3, 10, 12, 24, and 37.

Epidemiology and Types of Botulism

Geographic Distribution

Toxin types A, B, and E account for almost all cases of human botulism.[3, 9] Types F and G are very rare in humans, although type G toxin was recently implicated in the sudden deaths in a cluster of five patients.[9] Toxin types C and D are associated with botulism in mammalian animals and birds.[9]

Approximately one half of the recent outbreaks of food-borne botulism have been due to type A, 21 per cent to type B, and 12 per cent to type E; in 16 per cent of recent outbreaks, the toxin type was never determined.[3, 9, 17] In the United States, the majority of type A outbreaks have occurred west of the Rocky Mountains whereas type B outbreaks almost always have occurred east of the Mississippi.[3, 9, 11] Type B is the predominant toxin type in Europe.[9] This geographic distribution correlates highly with the frequency of occurrence of botulism spores in soil samples from these regions.[12] Spores of *C. botulinum*, type E are commonly found in silt from the waters of Alaska, Canada, and the Great Lakes; these same regions are the areas where type E botulism occurs.[3, 27]

Food Types

The name "botulism" originally comes from the Latin word "*botulus*," meaning sausage. Blood sausage was the first known food to be associated with causing botulism.[16] Although in the past poorly preserved meat was the cause of most cases, at present improper home canning techniques for vegetables are by far the most common cause of types A and B botulism. In the past 20 years, approximately 90 per cent of botulism outbreaks have involved only 1 to 2 people.[3, 13] Although restaurant-acquired botulism accounts for only 4 per cent of the total number of outbreaks, restaurant-associated outbreaks account for 40 per cent of the total number of patients seen with botulism.[13]

The largest outbreak in the United States involved 59 people and occurred because of improper home canning of jalapeno peppers for a restaurant hot sauce.[22] Before making the hot sauce, many of the home-canned jars of peppers had exploded on the restaurant's shelves. Unfortunately, the contaminated but as yet unexploded portions were used in the hot sauce.

Although poor home canning or preparation techniques cause most cases, some recent large outbreaks have been caused by onions and potatoes that were left at warm temperatures for more than 12 hours in incubator-like conditions.[13, 20, 28] The onions, which were immersed in butter, were used in patty melt sandwiches; this resulted in 28 cases.[13, 20] The potatoes were wrapped in aluminum foil and later used in potato salad, which resulted in 34 cases.[28] A similar incubation process has occurred in recent outbreaks involving beef and chicken pot pies and turkey loaf, all of which were left to stand in warm ovens at least overnight and then eaten without reheating.[13, 29]

Cases of type E botulinum food poisoning result from either poor vacuum packing or improper home preparation/preservation techniques.[23, 27] It is a common practice in the Inuit Eskimo communities to prepare urraq (uncooked seal flipper in seal oil); muktuk (chunks of white whale skin, blubber, and meat); and fermented salmon eggs; these foods allow growth of the botulinum organism when left to ferment at room temperature because the foods are low in carbohydrates and thus do not become acidic.[27]

Treatment

The treatment of botulism requires early and aggressive stabilization with meticulous attention to airway and ventilatory status. Most early deaths are due to respiratory failure before the patient has presented for health care or to the failure of health care workers to recognize early signs of respiratory impairment once the patient has presented.[30–33]

If the diagnosis of botulism is suspected, patients should have their "ABCs secured," that is, their airway patency, ability to breathe, and cardiovascular status assessed and stabilized. They should be placed in a well-observed treatment room on an electrocardiogram monitor, and an intravenous line should be established. Patients suspected of having botulism should be carefully and calmly interviewed. They should be asked if any of their family or friends have similar symptoms. Although any food ingested during the past 8 days could possibly cause botulism, food consumption during the past 2 to 3 days is of most importance. Patients should be asked if they have had any home canned foods, eaten in a restaurant, or eaten unusually prepared meats (especially in Alaska and Canada).

Pulmonary function tests are required in all patients with suspected botulism.[34] Although arterial blood gas measurements may be helpful in the complete assessment of any patient, they are not helpful in predicting a declining respiratory reserve.[30, 31] Hypercarbia due to respiratory muscle weakness is usually seen very late in the course of botulism, immediately before the patient's respiratory arrest.[30] In an effort to predict those patients who will experience a declining ventilatory status, values for baseline vital capacity and forced inspiratory volume should be obtained regularly at 2 to 4 hour intervals. In one study, all adult patients with vital capacities less than one third of that predicted eventually required mechanical ventilation.[30] Elective intubation before respiratory arrest dramatically decreases the mortality in botulism.[17]

After the patient's ventilatory status has been assessed (assuming mechanical ventilation is not required), the next step is to call the state health department consultant.[34] The Centers for Disease Control maintains a 24-hour telephone number to provide callers with their state's on-call consultant (404–639–2888). This telephone number provides 24-hour access to consultation regarding suspected cases of botulism. Information will also be provided concerning the nearest location for obtaining the antitoxin, which is usually at or near regional airports and quarantine stations.

After notifying the state health officer, serum and stool samples should be obtained for processing by the Centers for Disease Control.[34] These samples should be kept refrigerated but not frozen.[3] It is preferable to obtain serum before antibiotic administration and to obtain the stool sample spontaneously rather than post enema.[3] If this cannot be accomplished, it should be appropriately noted on the specimen label.

Because botulism has anticholinergic effects, unabsorbed toxin-containing food may still be present in the patient's stomach or lower GI tract. Upper and lower gastric decontamination with an orogastric tube and high enemas should be performed. The efficacy of an oral gut lavage solution in suspected cases of botulism is yet to be evaluated. After gastric decontamination has been performed, the patient should be admitted to a monitored area where close observation is possible.

In all but asymptomatic patients, the use of a trivalent (A,B,E) antitoxin should be administered. There have been very few studies that have critically evaluated the efficacy of antitoxin.[3, 13, 30, 32] Hypersensitivity reactions are seen in approximately one in ten patients treated with the horse serum–prepared antitoxin.[33, 35] More than half of these reactions are nonfatal acute hypersensitivity reactions (urticaria and anaphylaxis), whereas the remainder are delayed serum sickness type hypersensitivity reactions.[33, 35] Skin testing before treatment does not reliably separate those patients who will or will not have immediate or delayed allergic reaction.[35] Serum sickness is more likely to occur in patients treated with more than four vials (40 mL) of the trivalent antitoxin.[35] Because of the incidence of side effects and the fact that not all patients who have eaten the same foods develop botulism, physicians must use their judgment in administering the antitoxin to asymptomatic patients. It is probably most prudent to closely follow up patients and only give the toxin if some GI symptoms, neurologic complaints, or cranial nerve findings develop.

Once the patient has been stabilized in an intensive care unit, numerous telephone calls should be made to alert all neighboring emergency departments.[18] Similarly, local and state health departments should be mobilized, and in proven cases or epidemics, the media should be utilized to alert any potential victims.

The mortality for botulism has fallen dramatically from over 60 per cent to between 5 and 15 per cent during the past 30 years.[3, 13, 17, 30] There are multiple reasons for this, including more widespread media coverage, more aggressive early care, availability of an antitoxin, and the emergence of intensive care expertise by physicians. Botulism patients should be cared for by experts in ventilator management and intensive care medicine. In recent reports, almost all in-hospital deaths have been due to pulmonary- and/or ventilator-related complications.[17, 30, 31]

Patients who develop botulism from toxin type A are more likely to have a more severe and protracted clinical course than those patients who develop botulism from types B or

E.[11, 17] Although patients with type A may see a physician sooner after onset of symptoms, they are more likely to require mechanical ventilation than patients with types B and E.[13, 17] This is probably due to both the greater potency of type A and its increased affinity for nerve tissue.[15]

Recovery from botulism may be delayed for months.[10] Patients often describe weakness and easy fatiguability up to a year after their acute disease.[36, 37] Guanidine has been used to increase nonrespiratory muscle strength but has many side effects.[1, 36] This agent may be helpful for selected patients but is not believed to be curative.[3, 5, 30]

Infant Botulism

Infant botulism is a newly recognized disease. It was first described in 1976, and since that time increasing numbers of cases have been reported.[3, 38, 39] It has recently been identified as one of the occult causes of the sudden infant death syndrome.[5, 40] Two nonbotulinum *Clostridium* organisms, *Clostridium butyricum* and *Clostridia barati*, have been shown to cause infant botulism by elaboration of botulism toxins type E and F, respectively.[5, 41] At present, more than 400 cases of infant botulism have been reported to the Centers for Disease Control, making the disease the most common form of botulism.[42]

Unlike adult botulism, which results from ingestion of preformed toxin, infant botulism is due to in vivo germination of botulism spores. Symptoms occur when the bacteria colonize the infant's intestine and begin to produce toxin.[43] The relative uniqueness of spore germination in infants is due to the differences between infant and noninfant GI tracts. Botulism spores will not germinate in the presence of high acidity, a complex mix of aerobic and anaerobic bacteria, or a mature gastrointestinal immune system.[40, 44] Infants are at risk until the age of about 4 to 6 months because their GI tracts have a relative paucity of bacterial types and number; are more alkaline; and lack a mature mucosal immune system of lysozymes, complement, and secretory IgA.[40, 42, 44]

Breast feeding compared with formula feeding provides some immunity from infant botulism, but breast fed infants become at increased risk within 4 weeks from the initiation of solid foods.[5, 40, 42] In one outbreak involving 44 infants, all had been breast fed, but most had been recently introduced to new foods.[42] Other risk factors for infant botulism include residence in regions that have high soil counts of botulinum spores, alkaline soil, nearby construction or soil disruption, high dust counts, and the ingestion of honey, which may harbor botulinum spores.[45, 46] More than 50 per cent of reported cases have come from three states: California, Utah, and Pennsylvania.[47]

The symptoms of infant botulism are well described.[42, 45, 47, 48] The syndrome usually begins with constipation in infants 6 weeks to 6 months of age.[3] Numerous nonspecific symptoms then develop including decreased feeding, poor sucking reflex, decreased spontaneous activity, a weakened cry, and increased fatigue.[42, 45, 48] Parents often complain that the baby has been "floppy."[42, 45] Infants may not present, however, until the more severe signs and symptoms of ptosis, decreased gag reflex, generalized hypotonia, absent deep tendon reflexes, and respiratory distress are present.[42, 45, 48] On average, some symptoms have been present for approximately 4 to 5 days.[3, 42, 45]

The diagnosis of infant botulism should initially be made based on the presence of some of the symptomatology just mentioned. Assays for toxin are rarely positive in infant serum samples, but the diagnosis may be confirmed by the finding of botulinum toxin or the organism in stool.[3] The EMG, if performed, may reveal brief small abundant motor-unit action potentials.[38, 48]

The mortality for infant botulism is very low as long as health care is obtained and the diagnosis is made before the development of respiratory insufficiency.[42, 45, 47] In one large study, there was a 2 per cent mortality rate.[42] Care is mainly supportive, with careful feeding, close monitoring of ventilatory status, and observation for secondary complications such as otitis media, pneumonia, ARDS, and the syndrome of inappropriate antidiuretic hormone.[3, 42] Penicillin use, in an attempt to eradicate intestinal botulinum organisms, is theoretically contraindicated because toxin is released when cell wall lysis occurs.[3, 7] Aminoglycosides should not be used to treat secondary infections because they potentiate botulinum-induced neuromuscular blockade.[45, 47]

Wound Botulism

Wound botulism is a very rare form of botulism, with only 30 cases reported in the United States between 1950 and 1985.[3, 6, 49, 52] It presents exactly like classic food-borne botulism, with only a few exceptions: there are no early GI complaints; fever may be present; the incubation period is longer (4 to 14 days); and it does not occur in epidemics.[6, 50] The diagnosis is confirmed by the finding of botulinal toxin in the patient's blood, the wound, or both.[6]

Although it was previously thought that dirty wounds predisposed to wound botulism, in one recent report of 13 cases, 8 individuals had clean wounds at the time of diagnosis.[49] Most patients who develop wound botulism are young to middle-aged adults, although the disease has been seen in a 6 year old child a few days after a compound lower arm fracture.[49, 51]

Wound botulism should be suspected in any postoperative or wounded patient who develops the signs and symptoms of botulism.[49] It should also be considered in patients who develop unexplained weakness or declining respiratory effort, especially if they have received treatment with aminoglycosides.[49–51]

The care of patients who have wound botulism centers on debridement and drainage of the infected wounds.[49] Close monitoring of respiratory status, along with early intubation for respiratory compromise, is indicated. Trivalent antitoxin should be administered as soon as possible.[3, 49]

Wound botulism is now being reported with an increasing frequency in intravenous drug abusers.[52, 53] Most of these patients have not had prominent skin infections but presented due to cranial nerve dysfunction.[52, 53] Because intravenous drug abuse has again become an epidemic in this country, physicians should be actively aware of this new clinical setting for wound botulism. Patients suspected of having wound botulism should undergo careful skin examinations, their serum and wounds should be cultured, and they should be given intravenously administered antibiotics and antitoxin.

Botulism, Classification Undetermined

A fourth form of botulism, classification undetermined, was established by the Centers for Disease Control in 1978.[3] By definition, patients in this group must be older than 1 year of age and cannot have any foodstuff or wound as their source of disease. It is possible that many of the patients in this group represent an adult variant of infant botulism.[54, 55] These patients usually have some abnormalities of their GI tracts that could potentially allow spore germination such as achlorhydria, a relatively sterile intestinal lumen due to pretreatment with broad-spectrum antibiotics, or abnormal gut physiology resulting from recent surgery or inflammatory bowel disease.[3, 54, 55]

ADDITIONAL SELECTED FOOD-RELATED TOXINS
(Table 32–3)

Staphylococcus aureus

Staphylococcal food poisoning is one of the most common causes of food poisoning in the United States.[56] During one 5-year period, over 7000 cases were reported to the Centers for Disease Control.[56] Disease is caused by one or more of the six heat-stable enterotoxins produced by the staphylococcus organism.[57] Any proteinaceous food that is stored between 3° C (40° F) and 60° C (140° F) can allow staphylococcal growth and toxin elaboration.[56, 58]

The classic symptoms of staphylococcal food poisoning are the triad of abdominal pain or nausea, followed by vomiting or diarrhea.[56, 59] Although staphylococcal food poisoning is thought not to be associated with fever, patients often feel febrile, and in one large outbreak almost half the patients had temperatures over 38° C.[60] The disease is usually mild and self-limited, although patients may develop mild to moderate hypotension, dehydration, and bloody diarrhea.[56, 59, 60] Death is rare but has been reported in up to 4.4 per cent of the population of one series.[56, 61]

The most common foodstuffs associated with staphylococcal food poisoning are ham and other pork products, meats, poultry, baked goods with cream fillings, and potato or egg salads.[57, 58] Milk and dairy products are rarely the sole cause of staphylococcal outbreak.[56] All of the foods just mentioned are high in protein and will permit staphylococcal growth when they are allowed to sit

Table 32–3. MOST COMMON SOURCES AND INCUBATION PERIODS OF SELECTED FOOD TOXINS

Disease	Incubation Period	Source of Toxins
Botulism		
Types A and B	1–2 d	Home-canned, low acidity vegetables (potatoes, onions, garlic, beans)
Type E	1–2 d	Fermented fish and fish products (seal meat, whale meat, salmon eggs)
Bacillus Cereus		
Emetic type	1–6 h	Fried rice
Diarrheal type	12–16 h	Reheated meats
Cholera and other vibrios	12–14 h	Raw shellfish (especially raw oysters and crabs)
Clostridia perfringens	12–24 h	Meats and poultry, meat stew
Staphylococcus aureus	1–6 h	Foods stored at room temperature (especially ham, meats, potato and egg salads, and baked goods with cream fillings)
Jamaican vomiting sickness	1–3 h	Unripe akee fruit

at room temperature for even a few hours.[56] Because of the relatively ubiquitous nature of staphylococcus, foods can become tainted during normal preparation as a result of staphylococcus-contaminated equipment or when unsanitary preparation techniques are used by food handlers.[56, 58]

Clostridium perfringens

Clostridium perfringens food poisoning is another very common type of food poisoning that occurs in the United States.[62, 63] It typically occurs when heat-stable spores germinate in meat or meat-contaminated gravy that is left at room temperature after being cooked.[64–66] Outbreaks are usually associated with institutional settings where the incriminated food has been cooked the previous day and left to slowly cool rather than being promptly refrigerated.[63, 64] Reheating the food to 75° C or greater will inactivate the heat-labile toxin, and retrospective reviews of large outbreaks show lack of reheating to be a common omission.[63, 64, 66]

Symptoms from clostridial food poisoning are due to an enterotoxin;[64, 65] although *C. perfringens* is capable of producing 12 toxin types, all food-borne disease in the United States has been due to type A strains.[67] The enterotoxin causes fluid, sodium, and chloride secretion into the lumen of the small intestine.[62, 63]

Symptoms of *C. perfringens* food poisoning occur within 12 to 24 hours of onset.[62–64] Diarrhea and abdominal cramps are usually the only symptoms, although patients occasionally complain of nausea. Vomiting and fever or chills occur infrequently, and serious illness is almost never seen.[62–64] Deaths reported from this usually mild disease have either been in elderly, debilitated patients or in rare outbreaks from type C strains in Germany and New Guinea.[62, 63] Treatment is supportive only.

Vibrio

Vibrios are motile gram-negative rods that are endemic to the waters of many southern coastal areas of the United States. At present, ten species of vibrios have been identified that have the potential to cause human disease.[67, 68]

Illness due to cholera is mediated by an enterotoxin called the cholera toxin, which blocks sodium absorption and enhances secretion of chloride by directly stimulating adenyl cyclase in gut epithelial cells.[69] Large cholera epidemics are not seen in the United States, but small periodic outbreaks due to the El Tor strain of vibrio cholera do occur.[69, 70]

Vibrio cholera causes an intense watery diarrhea that may result in fluid losses of up to 1 liter per hour.[67, 68] In severe cases (cholera gravis), volume losses may result in dehydration and death if not aggressively treated.[68] Patients have noncrampy "rice water"–like grayish stools and may in some cases develop vomiting.[67–69]

Most vibrio infections in the United States are due to disease from vibrio organisms that produce enterotoxin without cholera-like activity.[67, 71] The most important of these are non-01 serotype *V. cholerae, V. parahaemolyticus, V. fluvialis,* and *V. mimicus.*[71, 72] These organisms, which are also endemic to coastal areas, produce diarrhea, abdominal pain and cramping, nausea and vomiting, and in up to one third of patients, fever and chills. Bloody diarrhea may be seen in noncholera vibrio infections.[67, 71, 72]

Patients usually develop gastroenteritis from both chlorea and noncholera vibrioses within 24 hours of raw seafood ingestion. Raw oysters and incompletely cooked crabs are the two most common sources of cholera and noncholera vibrio infection in the United States.[67, 71] Treatment of these diseases is generally supportive. Aggressive oral or intravenous volume glucose and electrolyte replacement is required.[67, 68] Drugs that interfere with adenyl cyclase or electrolyte fluxes across gut epithelial cells may significantly decrease volume losses.[69] Chlorpromazine, aspirin, indomethacin, and nicotinic acid have all been shown to be effective in treating cholera.[67, 69]

Bacillus cereus

Bacillus cereus is a relatively common, underreported form of food poisoning that may mimic staphylococcal, clostridial, or vibrio food-borne illness.[73, 74] *B. cereus* is an aerobic, spore-forming, gram-positive rod.[74] Illness due to *B. cereus* is via elaboration of either of two different enterotoxins. One of the enterotoxins is a heat-labile enterotoxin that causes a diarrheal type illness.[73, 75] The other enterotoxin is heat stable and causes a disease that predominantly affects the upper GI tract.[73, 75] Spores of *B. cereus* are commonly found in cereals, rice, vegetables, spices, and pasteurized fresh and powdered milk.[76, 77]

The upper gastrointestinal form of the disease, also called the emetic form, has a more rapid onset and shorter clinical course than the diarrheal form. Patients usually become ill within 1 to 6 hours of ingestion and recover within 24 hours.[73, 75] This form of the disease closely resembles staphylococcal food poisoning.[74, 75] Diarrhea and abdominal cramps may occur but are not the prominent feature of the emetic form.[75]

Fried rice is the usual foodstuff associated with the emetic form of *B. cereus* infection.[75, 76] The heat-resistant spores germinate when already cooked rice is left to cool and is unrefrigerated for 2 or more hours.[74, 77]

The diarrheal form of the disease is caused by a toxin that stimulates adenyl cyclase in intestinal epithelial cells.[73] The resultant watery diarrhea and abdominal cramps are quite similar to but milder than the symptoms of cholera.[73, 75] Upper gastrointestinal complaints such as nausea and vomiting are seen in less than 25 per cent of affected individuals, and fever is rare.[73, 75] Illness usually occurs within 12 hours of the ingestion of contaminated foods, and symptoms usually last for 24 to 36 hours.[73–76] The usual mode of transmission of this disease is via inadequate refrigeration of already cooked foods.[74]

Stool examination is not generally useful to diagnose *B. cereus.* The diagnosis can best be made by detecting 10^5 or more organisms per gram of food.[73] Treatment of this usually mild, self-limited disease is supportive only.

Akee Fruit Poisoning (Jamaican Vomiting Sickness)

Jamaican vomiting sickness is a relatively rare disease characterized by the acute onset of vomiting within 2 to 3 hours of eating a meal. The disease is caused by the ingestion of the unripe akee fruit, a fruit that is not usually available or eaten outside of Jamaica.[78] Seizures, coma, and death occur in severe cases.[78, 79]

The arillus and seeds of the unripe akee fruit contain the amino acids hypoglycin A and B (L-alpha-amino-methylene cyclopropionic acid and its gamma-glutamyl conjugate, respectively).[78] Hypoglycin A, which is also called hypoglycin, is more potent than hypoglycin B. The amino acids in hypoglycin A and B cause their toxicity by blocking long chain fatty acid metabolism and subsequent gluconeogenesis at the mitochondrial level.[78, 80] Blockade is via inhibition of several cofactors, including different acyl coenzyme A and carnitine.[78] The result is profound hypoglycemia to levels as low as 3 mg per dl.[78, 79] Hypoglycin may also cause vomiting and central nervous system depression in the absence of significant hypoglycemia.[81] Hepatotoxicity, similar to that of Reye's syndrome, has been found at postmortem study.[78, 81]

Intravenous glucose infusion and supportive care are the mainstays of therapy in treating Jamaican vomiting sickness. In untreated persons who develop hypoglycemic coma, the mortality rate may be as high as 80 per cent.[79]

Acknowledgments

The author acknowledges Linda Markwell, M.L.S., for her tireless reference assistance and Pamela Rye, C.D.A., for her secretarial and administrative support.

References

1. Sellin LC: Botulism—An update. Milit Med *149*:12–16, 1984.
2. Henderson DK, Tillman DB, Webb HH, et al: Infectious disease emergencies: The clostridial syndromes (specialty conference). West J Med *129*:101–120, 1978.
3. Centers for Disease Control: Botulism in the United States, 1899–1977: Handbook for Epidemiologists, Clinicians, and Laboratory Workers. Washington, DC, 1979, pp 1–41.
4. Simpson LL: The action of botulinal toxin. Rev Infect Dis *1*:656–662, 1979.
5. Arnon, SS: Infant botulism: Anticipating the second decade. J Infect Dis *154*:201–206, 1986.
6. Merson MH, Dowell VR Jr: Epidemiologic, clinical and laboratory aspects of wound botulism. N Engl J Med *289*:1105–1110, 1973.
7. Simpson LL: The orgin, structure, and pharmacological activity of botulinum toxin. Pharmacol Rev *33*:155–188, 1981.
8. Sugiyama H: Clostridium botulinum neurotoxin. Microbiol Rev *44*:419–448, 1980.
9. Dowell VR Jr: Botulism and tetanus: Selected epidemiologic and microbiologic aspects. Rev Infect Dis *6*(suppl 1):202–207, 1984.
10. Cherington M: Botulism: Ten-year experience. Arch Neurol *30*:432–437, 1974.
11. Smith LDS: Clostridium botulinum: Characteristics and occurrence. Rev Infect Dis *1*:637–641, 1979.
12. Case records of the Massachusetts General Hospital. Weekly clinicopathological exercises. Case 48–1980. N Engl J Med *303*(23):1347–1355, 1980.
13. MacDonald KL, Cohen ML, Blake PA: The changing epidemiology of adult botulism in the United States. Am J Epidemiol *124*:794–799, 1986.
14. Bonventre PF: Absorption of botulinal toxin from the gastrointestinal tract. Rev Infect Dis *1*:663–667, 1979.
15. Sellin LC, Thesleff S, Dasgupta BR: Different effects of types A and B botulinum toxin on transmitter release at the rat neuromuscular junction. Acta Physiol Scand *119*:127–133, 1983.
16. Sanders AB, Seifert S, Kobernick, M: Botulism: Clinical review. J Fam Pract *16*:987–1000, 1983.
17. Hughes JM, Blumenthal JR, Merson MH, et al: Clinical features of types A and B food-borne botulism. Ann Intern Med *95*:442–445, 1981.
18. Ruthman JC, Hendricksen DK, Bonefeld R: Emergency department presentation of type A botulism. Am J Emerg Med *3*:203–205, 1985.
19. St. Louis ME, Peck SHS, Bowering D, Morgan GB, et al: Botulism from chopped garlic: Delayed recognition of a major outbreak. Ann Intern Med *108*:363–368, 1988.
20. MacDonald KL, Spengler RF, Hatheway CL, et al: Type A botulism from sauteed onions: Clinical and epidemiologic observations. JAMA *253*:1275–1278, 1985.
21. Terranova W, Breman JG, Palumbo JN: Ocular findings in botulism type B. JAMA *241*:475–477, 1979.
22. Terranova W, Breman JG, Locey RP, Speck S: Botulism type B: Epidemiologic aspects of an extensive outbreak. Am J Epidemiol *108*:150–156, 1978.
23. Whittaker RL, Gilbertson RB, Garrett AS: Botulism, type E: Report of eight simultaneous cases. Ann Intern Med *61*:448–454, 1964.
24. Goldfrank LR, Flomenbaum NE, Weisman RS: Hysteria or botulism: A fatal misdiagnosis. *In* Goldfrank's Toxicologic Emergencies. 3rd ed. Norwalk, CT, Appleton-Century-Crofts, 1986, pp 527–537.
25. Dowell VR Jr, McCroskey LM, Hatheway CL, et al: Coproexamination for botulinal toxin and *Clostridium botulinum*: A new procedure for laboratory diagnosis of botulism. JAMA *238*:1829–1837, 1977.
26. Gutmann L, Pratt L: Pathophysiologic aspects of human botulism. Arch Neurol *33*:175–179, 1976.
27. Hauschild AHW, Gauvreau L: Food-borne botulism in Canada, 1971–84. Can Med Assoc J *133*:1141–1146, 1985.
28. Mann JM, Martin S, Hoffman R, et al: Patient recovery from type A botulism: Morbidity assessment following a large outbreak. Am J Public Health *71*:266–269, 1981.
29. Centers for Disease Control. Botulism and commercial pot pie—California. MMWR *32*:39–40, 45, 1983.
30. Schmidt-Nowara WW, Samet JM, Rosario PA: Early and late pulmonary complications of botulism. Arch Intern Med *143*:451–456, 1983.
31. Hughes JM, Tacket CO: 'Sausage poisoning' revisited (editorial). Arch Intern Med *143*:425–427, 1983.
32. Tacket CO, Shandera WX, Mann JM, Hargrett NT, Blake PA: Equine antitoxin use and other factors that predict outcome in type A foodborne botulism. Am J Med *76*:794–798, 1984.
33. Merson MH, Hughes JM, Dowell VR, et al: Current trends in botulism in the United States. JAMA *229*:1305–1308, 1974.
34. Centers for Disease Control. Release of botulism antitoxin. MMWR *35*:490–491, 1986.
35. Black RE, Gunn RA: Hypersensitivity reactions associated with botulinal antitoxin. Am J Med *69*:567–570, 1980.
36. Puggiari M, Cherington M: Botulism and guanidine: Ten years later. JAMA *240*:2276–2277, 1978.
37. Mann J: Prolonged recovery from type A botulism (letter). N Engl J Med *309*:1522–1523, 1983.
38. Pickett J, Berg B, Chaplin E, Brunstetter-Shafer MA: Syndrome of botulism in infancy: Clinical and electrophysiologic study. N Engl J Med *295*:770–772, 1976.
39. Midura TF, Arnon SS: Infant botulism: Identification of Clostridium botulinum and its toxins in faeces. Lancet *2*:934–936, 1976.
40. Arnon SS: Breast feeding and toxigenic intestinal infections: Missing links in crib death? Rev Infect Dis *6*(suppl 1):193–201, 1984.
41. Aureli P, Fenicia L, Pasolini B, et al: Two cases of type E infant botulism caused by neurotoxigenic *Clostridium butyricum* in Italy. J Infect Dis *154*:207–211, 1986.

42. Long SS, Gajewski JL, Brown LW, Gilligan PH: Clinical, laboratory, and environmental features of infant botulism in Southeastern Pennsylvania. Pediatrics *75*:935–941, 1985.
43. Wilcke, BW Jr, Midura TF, Arnon SS: Quantitative evidence of intestinal colonization by Clostridium botulinum in four cases of infant botulism. J Infect Dis *141*:419–423, 1980.
44. Sugiyama H: Animal models for the study of infant botulism. Rev Infect Dis *1*:683–688, 1979.
45. Thompson JA, Glasgow LA, Warpinski JR, Olson C: Infant botulism: Clinical spectrum and epidemiology. Pediatrics *66*:936–947, 1980.
46. Istre GR, Compton R, Novotny T, et al: Infant botulism: Three cases in a small town. Am J Dis Child *140*:1013–1014, 1986.
47. Gay CT, Marks WA, Riley HD Jr, et al: Infantile botulism. South Med J *81*:457–460, 1988.
48. Arnon SS, Midura TF, Clay SA, et al: Infant botulism: Epidemiological, clinical and laboratory aspects. JAMA *237*:1946–1951, 1977.
49. Hikes DC, Manoli A II: Wound botulism. J Trauma *21*:68–71, 1981.
50. Thorne FL, Kropp RJ: Wound botulism: A life-threatening complication of hand injuries. Plast Reconstr Surg *71*:548–550, 1983.
51. Keller MA, Miller VH, Berkowitz CD, Yoshimori, RN: Wound botulism in pediatrics. Am J Dis Child *136*:320–322, 1982.
52. MacDonald KL, Rutherford GW, Friedman SM, Dietz FR, et al: Botulism and botulism-like illness in chronic drug abusers. Ann Intern Med *102*:616–618, 1985.
53. Rapoport S, Watkins PB: Descending paralysis resulting from occult wound botulism. Ann Neurol *16*:359–361, 1984.
54. Case 48–1980: Botulism (letter). N Engl J Med *304*(13):789–791, 1981.
55. Chia JK, Clark JB, Ryan CA, Pollack M: Botulism in an adult associated with food-borne intestinal infection with Clostridium botulinum. N Engl J Med *315*:239–241, 1986.
56. Holmberg SD, Blake PA: Staphylococcal food poisoning in the United States: New facts and old misconceptions. JAMA *251*:487–489, 1984.
57. Todd JK: Staphylococcal toxin syndromes. Annu Rev Med *36*:337–347, 1985.
58. Staphylococcal food poisoning from turkey at a country club buffet—New Mexico. MMWR *35*(46):715–716, 721–722, 1986.
59. Eisenberg MS, Gaarslev K, Brown W, et al: Staphylococcal food poisoning aboard a commercial aircraft. Lancet *1*:595–599, 1975.
60. Effersoe P, Kjerulf K: Clinical aspects of outbreak of staphylococcal food poisoning during air travel. Lancet *2*:599–600, 1975.
61. Currier RW 2d, Taylor A Jr, Wolf S, et al: Fatal staphylococcal food poisoning. South Med J *66*:703–705, 1973.
62. Shandera WX, Tacket CO, Blacke PA: Food poisoning due to *Clostridium perfringens* in the United States. J Infect Dis *147*:167–170, 1983.
63. Loewenstein MS: Epidemiology of *Clostridium perfringens* food poisoning. N Engl J Med *286*:1026–1028, 1972.
64. Petersen LR, Mshar R, Cooper GH Jr, et al: A large *Clostridium perfringens* foodborne outbreak with an unusual attack rate pattern. Am J Epidemiol *127*:605–611, 1988.
65. McDonel JL: The molecular mode of action of *Clostridium perfringens* enterotoxin. Am J Clin Nutr *32*:210–218, 1979.
66. Bartholomew BA, Stringer MF: *Clostridium perfringens* enterotoxin: A brief review. Biochem Soc Trans *12*:195–197, 1984.
67. Morris JG Jr, Black RE: Cholera and other vibrios in the United States. N Engl J Med *312*:343–350, 1985.
68. Gangarosa EJ, Barker WH: Cholera: Implications for the United States. JAMA *227*:170–171, 1974.
69. Holmgren J: Actions of cholera toxin and the prevention and treatment of cholera. Nature *292*:413–417, 1981.
70. Blake PA, Allegra DT, Snyder JD, et al: Cholera—A possible endemic focus in the United States. N Engl J Med *302*:305–309, 1980.
71. Hughes JM, Hollis DG, Gangarosa EJ, et al: Non-cholera vibrio infections in the United States. Ann Intern Med *88*:602–606, 1978.
72. Shandera WX, Johnston JM, Davis BR, et al: Disease from infection with *Vibrio mimicus*, a newly recognized Vibrio species. Ann Intern Med *99*:169–171, 1983.
73. Terranova W, Blake PA: *Bacillus cereus* food poisoning. N Engl J Med *298*:143–144, 1978.
74. Giannella RA, Brasile L: A hospital food-borne outbreak of diarrhea caused by *Bacillus cereus*: Clinical, epidemiologic, and microbiologic studies. J Infect Dis *139*:366–370, 1979.
75. Bandhaya MS: Food poisoning and other clinical diseases caused by *Bacillus cereus*. J Med Assoc Thail *68*:427–431, 1985.
76. Centers for Disease Control: *Bacillus cereus*—Maine. MMWR *35*:408–410, 1986.
77. Blakey LJ, Priest FG: The occurrence of *Bacillus cereus* in some dried foods including pulses and cereals. J Appl Bacteriol *48*:297–302, 1980.
78. Tanaka K, Kean EA, Johnson B: Jamaican vomiting sickness. N Engl J Med *295*:461–467, 1976.
79. Bressler R: The unripe akee—forbidden fruit. N Engl J Med *295*:500–501, 1976.
80. Billington D, Osmundsen H, Sherratt HSA: The biochemical basis of Jamaican akee poisoning. N Engl J Med *295*:1482, 1976.
81. Tanaka K, Isselbacher KJ: Isovaleric and -methylbutyric acidemias induced by hypoglycin A: Mechanism of Jamaican vomiting sickness. Science *175*:69–71, 1972.

CHAPTER 33
RADIATION POISONING

Richard B. Yow, M.D.

In the early morning hours of April 26, 1986, an improbable event occurred: there was an explosion and subsequent "core meltdown" at reactor #4 in the Chernobyl nuclear plant in the Soviet Union. A plume of radioactive particulate matter and gases was released before any containment could be established. Fortunately, the prevailing winds initially drove the radioactive cloud over relatively sparsely populated areas. Nevertheless, in the aftermath of the incident, countries around the world recorded increased radiation levels as a result of the atmospheric and "fall-out" radioactivity. Over 50 million curies were released into the environment.[1–10]

All that is visible now of the reactor #4 complex is a 28-story concrete and steel containment—the "Sarcophagus," as it has become known. Appropriately named, this structure is a memorial to the event, while the place name "Chernobyl" has become a symbol for the global interdependence that must be realized in this era of nuclear technology.

The experience of the Chernobyl incident has taught many lessons, from disaster preparedness to medical assessment and intervention in the care of radiation accident victims.[11, 12] More importantly, however, it has spawned a reassessment of the very necessity and the safety of nuclear technology. In the wake of the Three Mile Island incident of 1979, public concern in the United States grew as an increased awareness of the potential hazards of nuclear technology was heightened by mass media coverage.[7] The Chernobyl incident had an even greater effect on a worldwide scale. There has been an international response by regulatory agencies, as well as from the nuclear industry itself. The National Academy of Science, in 1987, revealed numerous unreported serious accidents that have occurred at the Savannah River plant, an American nuclear weapons facility.[13] This report stimulated several other investigations that have revealed safety hazards at other nuclear weapons facilities.[14]

It is apparent that the increased use of radioactive materials in industry, medicine, and weaponry mandates the most rigorous safety standards applied to all levels of production, transport, and waste disposal. A breach of safety at any level could result in harmful exposure of an individual or the public.

As health care professionals, we have a responsibility for the health and welfare of the public. We must, therefore, become involved in the technical, political, and social reform of the nuclear industry to insure that a preventive approach is emphasized. Then, when the highly "improbable" event of a radiation accident occurs, we must be prepared to deal with the complex illness known as radiation poisoning in a competent fashion.[15, 16]

PHYSICAL PRINCIPLES OF RADIATION

All atoms of a given chemical element are designated by an atomic number, *z*. This number designates the quantity of protons in the nucleus and also determines the number of orbital electrons in the electrically neutral atom and therefore the chemical characteristics of that atom.

The Nucleus

The nucleus of an atom is characterized by the number of neutrons and protons it contains. The total quantity or sum of protons and neutrons is the *mass number*, or *A*. The term used for nuclear particles collectively is *nucleons*. A *nuclide* is a nuclear species characterized by an exact nuclear composition, including the mass number, *A*, and the *atomic number*, or *z*.

The notation for a nuclide is an abbreviation of its chemical name, *X*, along with its mass number, *A*, and atomic number, *z*: for example $^{A}_{z}X$. Nuclides with differing mass numbers but the same atomic number (number of protons) are called *isotopes*. A good example is the element iodine, which has 53 protons. Iodine has several isotopes that are important to this chapter. ^{131}I, or iodine-131, is a radioactive isotope used in nuclear medicine for evaluating thyroid function. In greater quantities, it is used for ablating hyperfunctioning thyroid tissue or thyroid cancer, and it is also an important isotope released in nuclear accidents, such as that at Chernobyl.[1, 17] It is a major byproduct of nuclear fission and therefore is in great quantity within the core materials of nuclear power plants.[7] Other isotopes of iodine are iodine-123 (^{123}I), iodine-125 (^{125}I), and iodine-131 (^{131}I). (Notice that the z number has been omitted since the "I" indicates that the element is iodine, which by definition has 53 protons.)

The simplest example of isotopes is hydrogen, which has one proton. There are three isotopes of hydrogen: H, ^{2}H, and ^{3}H, or hydrogen, deuterium, and tritium. Tritium is of particular interest because it is a byproduct of the weapons facility type of nuclear reactor processing.[13] When released into the environment, tritium is easily oxidized to tritiated water. Therefore, contamination of water sources is a hazard.

Some isotopes are stable; that is, there is no significant tendency to transform the nuclear configuration. Others have an unstable nuclear configuration and, therefore, transform to a more stable state. Nuclear transformations involve discrete and exact amounts of energy released as emitted particles or *photons* (electromagnetic waves), thus the production of radiation.

Radiation means the transfer of energy. This transfer may be accomplished by energetic particles (alpha particles, beta particles, neutrons, or protons) or by electromagnetic waves (gamma rays, x-rays, ultraviolet, visible light, infrared, microwaves, radiowaves—in order of decreasing energy). The term *ionizing radiation* refers to either particles or waves that are energetic enough to cause *ionization* in the cells of the body. Ionization refers to the creation of an electrical imbalance in atoms or molecules and is the underlying mechanism responsible for the biologic effects of radiation. It is also the mechanism by which most radiation detectors work.

Radioactivity is the property of a substance to emit radiation while transforming from one nuclide to another, the process known as *radioactive decay*. Radioactive decay is a spontaneous event that is described by mathematical probability. The average decay rate is defined by a decay constant that is characteristic for each radionuclide.[17] Since the decay constant is predictable for a given radionuclide, we can predict the amount of isotope in a sample that will be remaining after a given time, if we know the original amount, by the formula

$$N(t) = N(0)\, e^{-\lambda T}$$

where:

N(t) = number of atoms remaining after time
N(0) = number of atoms at time 0
λ = decay constant
T = time interval
e = base of natural logarithm

The amount of radioactivity (A) is proportional to the number of radioactive atoms, and this (A) activity may be substituted for N in the equation.

Half-Life

A much more practical physical property of a radioactive substance is its *half-life*, which is derived from the equation just discussed and is inversely proportional to the decay constant: $T\frac{1}{2} = .693/\lambda$. The half-life is the time required for a radionuclide to decay to 50 per cent of its initial activity. Isotopes with long half-lives, such as cesium-137, which has a half-life of 30 years, pose a long-term threat to the public when released into the environment. After the Chernobyl release, elevated levels of Cs-137 and Cs-134 were found throughout Europe in food products and even in breast milk.[4, 8, 9]

The *effective half-life* is also an important factor. This takes into account the excretion of a substance from the body, or the biologic half-life. Therefore, effective half-life is shorter than the physical half-life; for example, the effective half-life of Cs-137 is about 110 days.

Radiation Dose and Dose Rate

The *roentgen* (R) is a unit of measure of energy deposited in air. It is of no clinical value.

In order to define the absorbed dose in a tissue, the rad is used. One rad is that dose that deposits 100 ergs of energy in 1 gram of tissue. A newer system, the International System, or SI unit, for tissue dose is the *gray*

(Gy), equivalent to 1 joule deposited in 1 kilogram of tissue. One hundred rads equal 1 gray (100 rads = 1 Gy).

To account for differences in the biologic damage caused by various ionizing radiation, the rem (roentgen equivalent man) was developed. This dose-equivalent unit is calculated by multiplying the absorbed dose (rad) by a quality factor (QF) that is applied for each type of radiation. For gamma and x-rays and beta particles, the quality factor is, for all practical purposes, 1. Alpha particles and neutrons have a QF of greater than 1. The newer SI unit for rem is the *sievert* (Sv). One hundred rem equal one sievert. *Dose rate* is simply the dose in rad or rem (Gy or Sv) expressed in terms of time interval of exposure: for example, rem/hr. Lower doses/rates are expressed as millirem (mrem) or one thousandth of a rem.

The background radiation we are subjected to as the result of cosmic rays, naturally occurring radioactivity in the soil, building materials, and substances in our bodies is in the 100 mrem/year range.[18]

Activity

Historically, the *curie* was the unit used to describe the amount of a radioactive substance. It was originally defined as the rate at which 1 gram of radium decayed. Currently, the curie is defined as 37 billion (3.7×10^{10}) disintegrations per second. The newer unit becquerel (Bq) is a simpler system to use. One becquerel is defined as one disintegration per second. One curie equals 3.7×10^{10} Bq.

A typical nucl306 medicine examination uses approximately 10 millicuries of activity or 10 one thousandths of a curie. Compare that with the release of over 50 million curies from Chernobyl—a factor of 10 to the 8th power.

EXPOSURE TO RADIATION

Background Radiation. The world population is constantly bombarded by radiation. Natural background radiation from the earth and cosmic rays accounts for approximately 100 mrem per year per person. It may be as much as 100 times that per year in areas of Brazil and India. Medical exposures are in the range of 100 mrem per year when averaged over the entire population. A small amount, 1 to 5 mrem per year from atomic weapons testing fall-out and other lower level sources, also contributes. Combined, these exposures total approximately 200 mrem per year averaged over the entire population.[18]

Some unusual exposures that have occurred are from luminous wrist watches, television sets, dental porcelain material, and smoke detectors. Cigarette smoking, both active and passive, causes significant radiation doses to the lung epithelium as a result of radioactive substances that are concentrated in the tobacco leaf from the soil and are deposited along the epithelial lining when the smoke is inhaled.[19–21]

Radon. A recent concern is the presence of radon in homes.[22] Radon is virtually ubiquitous. It is the decay product of radium-226, which is the fifth daughter of the decay of uranium-238. U-238 and therefore radium-226 are present in varying concentrations in all soil and rock. Many houses that have been surveyed show very high levels of radon, which apparently concentrates particularly in those dwellings that have an easy flow of air from the soil into the house but poor ventilation of the air mass within the house.[23] A causal relationship between radon exposure and lung cancer has been established in uranium miners, and the Environmental Protection Agency (EPA) characterizes radon as the second leading contributor to lung cancer.[22, 24] Radon is a chemically inert gas with a half-life of approximately 4 days. Two of the decay products of radon are alpha emitters, and it is suspected that the tissue damage in the lungs is due to these high-energy alpha particles.

No clear understanding exists of the threshold concentration for risk exposure to radon. A national standard for risk assessment and the establishment of a strategy for policy concerning radon in the United States and elsewhere are needed. The effects of radon are cumulative over a long period. The only treatment is identification of the problem and a preventive approach.

RADIATION POISONING

Any dose of radiation that exceeds the background dose is *radiation poisoning*. Radiotherapy is an intentional radiation poisoning of a focal area in the body.

Radiation poisoning may be due to an external radiation source, to an internal source, or to surface contamination of the skin. Any combination of these is possible. *Irradiation* is a general term to describe exposure to radiation from any type of source and is used interchangeably with radiation exposure, dose, or radiation poisoning.

EXTERNAL RADIATION

External radiation is a specific term that refers to a source with no direct contact with the person exposed. A very important implication of this type of exposure is that the irradiation is usually due to a gamma, x-ray, or possibly a highly energetic beta particle source. (Neutron exposure also would be an external radiation but is very unlikely, unless a patient were exposed through a break in the shielding of a reactor or to a neutron source such as those used for calibration of detectors at nuclear power plants.) *The patients are not radioactive and therefore pose no threat to the attendant medical personnel.*

The exposure may be whole body or confined to a more localized region of the body. The dose from an external source depends on three factors: time, distance, and shielding. The time spent in a radiation field is critical. Obviously, the longer someone is exposed to a given dose rate, the higher the total dose. The dose rate is inversely proportional to the square of the distance from the source. For example, if the dose rate is 8 Gy/hour at a distance of 4 feet, at 8 feet the dose rate would be only 2 Gy/hour [$(4\text{ ft}/8\text{ ft})^2 \times 8$ Gy/hr or $\frac{1}{4}(8) = 2$ Gy/hr]. Shielding between the source and the person reduces the dose rate in a complex fashion dependent on (1) the type of radiation and its energy, (2) the type of shielding material, and (3) the thickness of the shielding material. A partially shielded body may have a dramatic effect on prognosis, since portions of the bone marrow may be shielded. Effective hematopoiesis then might be maintained. In general, a dense, thick shielding, such as concrete, steel, or lead, is required for x-rays and gamma rays. Beta particle doses are not usually considered as whole body, since they do not penetrate deeper than the subcutaneous tissue. Two to three centimeters of almost any material denser than air are adequate to attenuate most beta particle exposures.

Local Exposures to External Radiation

Assessment. Chronic exposures to radiation are most likely in individuals whose occupation may subject them to radiation sources. Industrial radiographers may present with signs or symptoms of chronic exposure to extremities or the hands. Usually the history alone will be diagnostic, but other sources of chronic injury must be ruled out as well.

Hospital radiology workers and nuclear technology workers must be carefully evaluated when presenting with skin or extremity symptoms. Chronic ill health, malaise, and possible anemia also may be clues to chronic irradiation, either whole body or local exposures.

Acute local exposures are most likely in radiation workers, but in the case of nuclear accidents, such as weaponry or power plant accidents, the public also may be exposed. An associated whole body dose must be considered whenever a local exposure is found, even if the history seems clear. Assessment for whole body penetrating exposure is covered later in this chapter.

Skin. Radiation burns and subcutaneous tissue injuries, to varying degrees, are common following radiation therapy, nuclear power plant accidents, or industrial radiation accidents. Skin damage is inversely proportional to the energy of gamma rays or x-rays. The less energetic x-rays are more likely to deposit their energy in the skin and subcutaneous tissues than is the more energetic gamma radiation. Beta particles rapidly give up their energy in skin and subcutaneous tissues, therefore, skin and subcutaneous damage is very likely when beta exposure is present. Whatever the type of radiation, if the dose is high, skin effects are to be expected.[25, 26]

Erythema is the hallmark of a radiation exposure involving the skin. The rapidity of onset from the time of the exposure correlates with the dose. At very high doses—for example, in excess of 5000 rad (50 Gy)—the erythema, severe pain, and sensation of heat appear very rapidly, within minutes to a half-hour. For doses in the moderate range, 2 to

6 Gy, the onset of the initial erythema is more likely to be 2 to 3 hours after exposure.

After the initial transient erythema has cleared, a latency period may appear, followed by a second period of erythema known as *fixed erythema*. This has an appearance similar to that of thermal burns. The latency period depends on the dose: the greater the dose, the shorter the latency period. For moderate doses, in the 2 to 6 Gy range, the latency period is 2 to 3 weeks. No significant latency period is seen with doses greater than 50 Gy (5000 rad), and blistering and desquamation may occur very rapidly.[27]

Subcutaneous Tissue. The amount of subcutaneous tissue damage is usually underestimated when first evaluated. Unlike the case with thermal burns, the energy from radiation is deposited in the deeper tissues as well as the upper layers. Nerve endings, sweat glands, and hair follicles are affected. Most important is the process of *obliterating endarteritis* that may progress for months and cause a progressive tissue necrosis. Epilation may occur at doses greater than 2 to 4 Gy (200 to 400 rad). The hair loss usually occurs 2 to 3 weeks after exposure. Up to the dose range of 7 Gy (700 rad), hair follicles probably will regenerate. Doses above 7 Gy probably will kill the hair follicle, and therefore epilation will be permanent.[27]

Management of Radiation Burns

The care of radiation burns is similar to that for thermal burns. Irritating lotions and coverings should be avoided. Use only bland lotions. Cortisone creams may be used, with the usual precautions. If the damage progresses to dry desquamation, an aqueous solution of 1 per cent gentian violet may be applied. Adequate pain relief is important. It must be remembered that the pain may be severe and prolonged due to underlying subcutaneous injury. The choice of an analgesic should be selected with the longevity of the use in mind. Drugs that may cause bone marrow suppression should be avoided, since an associated irradiation of bone marrow may cause suppression of hematopoiesis.

Standard care for desquamation and tissue necrosis will be necessary for higher-dose exposures. Superinfection must be treated promptly with appropriate antibiotics. Due to the difficulty of estimating the extent of the injury in deep tissues, decisions concerning skin grafting, amputation, or excisions should be made cautiously. Tissue viability is difficult to assess because of the progressive endarteritis that may be present in deep tissues without concomitant overlying superficial damage.[28] Radionuclide scanning may be used to assess microcirculation and tissue viability when surgical intervention is contemplated.

Since concomitant whole body penetrating exposures are possible, appropriate laboratory tests for dosimetric evaluation should be obtained from the onset. This is discussed in the section on management of *acute radiation syndrome*. Superficial contamination by radioactive dust or liquid and potential *internal contamination* should be managed as discussed later.

External Contamination by Radioactive Materials[35]

Radioactive particles or liquids can cause external contamination of the skin and clothing. Concomitant ingestion, inhalation, or absorption through the skin may occur. External contamination most likely would occur at a nuclear installation, hospital, or industrial laboratory where radioisotopes are used. The fall-out from a nuclear weapon explosion or accident such as that at Chernobyl is a potential source of light or heavy contamination. All installations that handle radioisotopes have monitoring devices to detect surface contaminations. If an incident or contamination occurs at a nuclear facility, it is expected that the appropriate immediate actions would be taken by trained personnel at the installation. In the event of a nuclear accident, or if concomitant nonradiation injuries are present, physicians outside of an installation may be required to manage patients who are contaminated.

It is unlikely that the level of contamination would be sufficient to be harmful to attendant personnel, but radiation monitoring should be done as soon as possible. The total dose to any attendant should not exceed 1 Gy (100 rad). Skin and subcutaneous tissue damage is expected from contamination by beta and low energy gamma emitters. Alpha particles are not a threat unless ingested or inhaled, since they cannot penetrate the outer layer of skin because of their large size and electrical charge. Most radioisotopes emit more than one type of radiation. Gamma and beta emitters are common among the most likely sources of external contamination. The monitors used in installations where radioisotopes are found will usually detect both gamma and beta radiation. Such monitors are required in hospital nuclear medicine laboratories and therefore would be available for the assessment of a potentially contaminated patient.

Physicians, nurses, and other trained medical personnel are well equipped to handle external contamination. If contaminated patients are treated as though they were infected and adequate barrier precautions are established, the potential spread or cross-contamination of radioactive dust will be minimized.

Whole Body Penetrating External Radiation and the Acute Radiation Syndrome

This section deals with exposures to penetrating ionizing radiation, primarily gamma and x-ray. Neutron exposures are very unlikely, as previously mentioned. Accidental exposures to harmful amounts of x-rays and gamma rays have occurred in the past owing to failure of safety devices, but most data concerning the radiobiology of high doses of external radiation come from the studies of the Japanese victims of the A-bomb.[29, 30] If wartime casualties are excluded, the 31 deaths associated with acute radiation poisoning at Chernobyl nearly equal the total number of deaths occurring until that time throughout the entire nuclear industry.[30] Until the medical reports from the Chernobyl incident were published, modern medical literature included few experiences with radiation accidents or the medical management of persons exposed to high levels of radiation. A private physician or hospital staff is unlikely to encounter victims of accidental radiation exposure from other than industrial accidents or nuclear weapons detonation. Although radiation protection personnel from nuclear installations and disaster team personnel will probably be available for help with management of victims, the private physician or emergency room staff may be called upon to triage victims, initiate supportive therapy, deal with associated nonradiation injuries, and perform an inclusive evaluation of each patient.

The Acute Radiation Syndrome

Acute radiation syndrome (ARS)[29, 30] results from multiorgan damage by penetrating external radiation distributed throughout the whole body. It represents the most dramatic manifestation of external radiation exposure. As previously noted, the acute radiation syndrome may be associated with other radiation poisoning, radiation burns, local radiation injury, surface contamination, or internal contamination. Acute penetrating radiation exposures produce a constellation of nonstochastic injuries, that is, injuries that are dose dependent and that result from a threshold effect.

Many factors influence the biologic effects of a penetrating radiation exposure. The most important is the dose and dose rate (Table 33–1). If the dose rate is low and the exposure is spread out in time, there is more chance for cellular repair. Thus, if a given dose is received at a low dose rate, its biologic effect is expected to be less than from one received at a high dose rate. In radiation therapy, *fractionation* refers to giving a fraction of the total dose at intervals over several weeks.

The type and energy level of radiation are also a factor. This has been discussed previously.

The distribution of the exposure is critical. The whole body dose will yield the most effect. As the volume percentage of the body exposed is decreased, the effects dramatically diminish. For example, the dose that causes death is four times greater when only half the body is exposed compared with a whole body exposure.

Significant individual variation in radiosensitivity exists, as evidenced by dose-effect curves for lethality. The variation is approximately a factor of three from the less to more sensitive individuals. Age is also a factor; children and infants have a greater sensitivity to radiation than do adults.

Diagnostic medical exposures are not whole body doses but are relatively confined to the area of interest. A direct comparison between diagnostic x-ray doses and whole body doses, therefore, cannot be made. However, the relative values may be helpful in conceptualizing the magnitude of the doses stated herein. For a posterior-anterior

Table 33–1. DOSE-EFFECT RELATIONSHIPS FOLLOWING ACUTE WHOLE BODY IRRADIATION (X = OR GAMMA)

WHOLE BODY* DOSE (RAD)	CLINICAL AND LABORATORY FINDINGS
5–25	Asymptomatic. Conventional blood studies are normal. Chromosome aberrations detectable.
50–75	Asymptomatic. Minor depressions of white cells and platelets detectable in a few persons, especially if baseline values established.
75–125	Minimal acute doses that produce prodromal symptoms (anorexia, nausea, vomiting, fatigue) in about 10–20% of persons within 2 days. Mild depressions of white cells and platelets in some persons.
125–200	Symptomatic course with transient disability and clear hematologic changes in a majority of exposed persons. Lymphocyte depression of about 50% within 48 hours.
240–340	Serious, disabling illness in most persons with about 50% mortality if untreated. Lymphocyte depression of about 75+% within 48 hours.
500+	Accelerated version of acute radiation syndrome with GI complications within two weeks, bleeding, and death in most exposed persons.
5000+	Fulminating course with cardiovascular, GI, and CNS complications resulting in death within 24–72 hours.

*Conversion of rad (midline) dose to radiation measurement in R can be made roughly by multiplying rad times 1.5. For example, 200 rad (midline) is equal to about 300 R (200 × 1.5).

(From Mettler FD: Emergency management of radiation accidents. J Am Coll Emerg Phys 7:302, 1978. Used by permission.)

chest radiograph, the dose to the chest is around 20 to 50 mrad (1/1000 rad) for thin chests and 200 to 400 mrad for thick chests. An air contrast barium enema may range from 100 to 1500 or more mrad.

An acute whole body radiation dose greater than 1 Gy (100 rad) is likely to cause clinically apparent signs and symptoms. Below 1 Gy, minor symptoms may occur, but no therapy is necessary beyond psychologic care. With increasing doses, above 1 Gy, the clinical manifestations become more evident and dramatic. The LD-50/60 (estimated median radiation dose leading to death in 60 days) ranges from approximately 3 Gy (300 rad) to 6 Gy (600 rad). The value primarily depends on the level of medical care given. The LD-50/60 value of 6 Gy is feasible only when the most sophisticated medical management is available.

It is apparent from the LD-50/60 data that doses from 1 Gy (100 rad) to 10 Gy (1000 rad) will manifest a spectrum of clinical findings from mild changes to death. Acute radiation syndrome (ARS)[30] will be present in this dose range. The ARS may be divided into hematologic, gastroenteric, and central nervous system/cardiovascular phases. An estimate of the actual dose received can be made from the temporal sequence and severity of the clinical findings as seen in Table 33–1. These groupings on clinical bases are helpful for management and treatment strategies.

Clinical Features of ARS. A prodromal illness, similar to motion sickness, may have its onset rapidly or several hours after exposure. The higher the dose, the sooner the onset and the more severe the prodromal symptoms. Malaise, anorexia, vomiting, nausea, and rarely diarrhea characterize the prodromal phase. These symptoms may be caused by a psychoneurotic reaction to an accident or viral syndrome, and therefore only subsequent medical evaluations may clarify the diagnosis. These symptoms are due to parasympathetic reactions to radiation, not gastrointestinal damage.

Latent Period. Following the prodromal phase, a latent period of relative well-being usually is present. This latent period is shortened as the dose increases. Above 6 Gy, the latency may be nonexistent. With lesser doses it may last a few weeks.

Third Phase. Gastrointestinal symptoms and hematologic changes become manifest as this phase develops. The third phase may last for weeks to months and is followed by either slow recovery or death, depending on the severity of the dose and the injury to the gastrointestinal system and bone marrow, or on concomitant nonradiation injury. Vomiting, diarrhea, fluid and electrolyte loss, intestinal ulcerations, and hemorrhage characterize the gastrointestinal symptoms. The bone marrow depression will overlap and dominate if the patient survives the gastrointestinal-associated symptoms. Bacterial infections, leukopenia, and anemia may be severe.

At exposure levels greater than 6 Gy (600 rad), the gastrointestinal symptoms probably will become manifest quite early and will dominate the clinical picture.

What used to be referred to as the central nervous system (CNS) syndrome, the immediate onset of severe neurologic symptoms, has been produced in animals with doses in the range of 1000 Gy but has not been observed in humans. The CNS syndrome is now subdivided into the cardiovascular phase and the CNS phase. At levels of exposure greater than 20 Gy (2000 rad), no prodromal or latency is expected. Cardiovascular collapse and hypotensive shock, followed by convulsions, coma, and death, are expected.

Management of Acute Radiation Syndrome. The accident history should be obtained from the appropriate people, and each patient's potential for exposure is evaluated. A thorough clinical evaluation of all systems should be done immediately after lifesaving supportive therapy is instituted.

The degree of biologic damage may not be clinically evident on the initial physical examination of the patient. Laboratory tests are essential to the assessment of estimated exposure, management planning, and prognosis.[31]

Leukocyte, platelet, absolute lymphocyte, and neutrophil counts should be obtained initially and every 6 hours for the first 48 hours. Complete blood counts and blood chemistry determinations should be obtained for baselines.

The absolute lymphocyte count is the most valuable triage test during the initial 2 days. If the count drops rapidly in the first 48 hours, a significant exposure has occurred. A drop to an absolute value of less than 1000 cells/mm^3 in that time frame indicates a severe injury and a grave prognosis. If no early initial drop occurs, the dose is probably less than 1 Gy (100 rad).

The granulocyte count becomes an important indicator of injury only after the first few days. There is usually a rise in the granulocyte count for 3 to 10 days, which cannot be used as an indicator. If a subsequent rapid drop in the count occurs over the next 10 to 20 days, a moderate-to-severe dose was received. In the mid-dose range (200 to 500 rad), a paradoxic rise in count may occur. This rise may be of value for dosimetric estimates, since its presence suggests a dose of less than 5 Gy (500 rad).

The nadir of the granulocyte count appears at about day 25 to 30. A subsequent slow rise in the granulocyte count is expected. If levels drop to 100 to 200 cells/mm^3 in less than 20 days, the prognosis is guarded.

Platelet counts have changes similar to those of granulocytes but lag those counts by 2 to 3 days.

Other tests that require more sophisticated equipment and procedures include cytogenetic examination of lymphocytes[32] and blood typing for transfusions and possible bone marrow transplantation. Early consultation with a specialty unit should be obtained for details of blood collection and handling requirements.

The cytogenetic examination takes advantage of changes that occur in the chromosomes as a result of radiation injury. Dicentric chromosomes and fragments are increased because of radiation injury, and the number of dicentrics can be correlated with good estimates of whole body doses. When it has been established that a significant dose has been received [greater than 1 Gy (100 rad)], appropriate infection control procedures should be instituted. The subsequent clinical course will dictate the need for sophisticated isolation procedures.

All patients will probably need some treatment for anxiety and the cardinal symptoms of the prodromal illness. Tranquilizers and antiemetics are appropriate, but standard antiemetics such as the neuroleptics (chlorpromazine, promethazine) may have undesirable secondary effects. Depression of gastric emptying is a feature of the prodromal syndrome and may be worsened by these antiemetics. Newer antiemetics without gastrokinetic suppression are being evaluated, but currently none are available.[33] Treatment of the gastroenteric injury will require fluid and electrolyte replacements and nonabsorbed antibiotic therapy to counteract the intestinal immune suppression and subsequent bacterial overgrowth.

The treatment of the hematologic derangements will be dictated by the specific changes in the patient's status over the course of the illness. Transfusions of platelets and red blood cells should be given as necessary. If a severe prodromal period and no latent period are observed, death is inevitable and only symptomatic therapy is needed. Patients with doses in the 200 to 600 rad range will require hematologic support.

Bone marrow transplantation has potential in ARS patients.[34] The recent experience with transplantation of 13 patients from the Chernobyl incident suggests potential benefit in selected cases. Adverse consequences of transplantation also must be considered. These include drug toxicity, graft versus host disease, and iatrogenic immune suppression. The data analysis is confounded by the complexity of radiation-induced injuries and the associated nonradiation injuries. Therefore, bone marrow transplantation in ARS patients remains investigational and should be instituted only by experienced specialists.

GENERAL MANAGEMENT OF EXTERNAL CONTAMINATION

Concomitant life-threatening conditions should be dealt with as necessary, while maintaining nursing barrier procedures similar to standard operating room protocols and infectious disease control procedures. Attendant personnel should wear protective radiation aprons, gowns, gloves, and masks, doubled when possible. The patient should be treated in a room separated from other patients and free from traffic. If a hospital does not have a specific room set aside for radiation emergencies, a room such as an autopsy room that is not essential to routine patient care should be used.

Detailed monitoring for surface contamination should be a first priority after lifesaving measures are instituted. Attendant personnel should be minimized to restrict potential spread of contamination. Contaminated clothing should be removed carefully and slowly to minimize spread to the patient and the environment. All potentially contaminated materials should be placed in plastic bags and sealed carefully. Any fluids used for decontamination should be collected in appropriately annotated containers.

The patient should be assessed for concomitant whole body irradiation when such an exposure is a possibility. Appropriate laboratory tests should be obtained. (See section on Acute Radiation Syndrome.) Urine, feces, and sputum of patients should be collected and saved in sealed containers for future monitoring to evaluate potential internal contamination. These samples can be screened for radioactivity with the same monitoring devices as are used for surface contamination; however, a negative screen does not exclude internal contamination. Any wounds or abrasions should be covered with waterproof protection to avoid contamination from other areas of the body during decontamination.

Decontamination Guidelines

A complete body survey for contaminated areas should be made. If a monitoring device is not available, the patient should be transferred to a facility with such capabilities; if the patient's condition prevents transfer, survey devices and experienced personnel should be brought to the patient.

Most contamination can be removed with soap and water or mild detergents, since radioactive substances usually adhere to or rest on the oily film of the skin. Dry skin and breaches in the integrity of the integument are much harder to decontaminate due to adsorption, adherence, and absorption. When decontamination progresses to the need for stronger agents to remove the outer horny skin layer, the possibility of absorption is enhanced. Some radionuclides (for example, tritium) can be absorbed through intact skin if the contact time is prolonged.

Initial decontamination can be carried out by physicians and staff without special training if the guidelines stated here are followed. When feasible, any decontamination beyond soap and water should be done by experienced personnel at a dedicated site. The physician should realize that "complete decontamination of the skin does not have to be performed within the shortest period of time." The initial gentle decontamination with soap and water will reduce the levels of residual contamination sufficiently to eradicate almost completely any further potential tissue damage. When possible, any persistent contamination may be handled by experienced personnel.

Decontamination of radioactive substances should be carried out by starting at the periphery of the contaminated area and working toward the center. (Note that this is opposite to the general procedure for "prepping" an area for a surgical incision.) It is imperative that no washings be allowed to contaminate wounds, body orifices, or adjacent areas of the body that are not contaminated. Contamination near the nose and other orifices should be removed first. The skin should not be rubbed during washing. Undue pressure or irritation could push contaminated material deeper into the interstices of the skin. Contaminated wounds should be washed by irrigating generously with sterile saline or water. Free bleeding may help decontaminate. A wound may need to be enlarged to irrigate adequately. The level of contamination and type of radiation must be established accurately. When it is apparent that further irrigation is ineffective in lowering contamination levels, the risk of further intervention such as debridement must be assessed and compared with the long-term risks of the remaining contamination. This will require decision-making by a team of experienced personnel.

A contaminated wound may be the portal of entry for internal contamination. It is especially important to collect feces and urine for monitoring under these circumstances.

Further decontamination after soap and water washing by experienced personnel at an appropriate facility might include the use of a saturated solution of potassium permanganate, followed by 10 per cent solution of sodium metabisulfite. (The potassium permanganate will discolor the skin while the sodium metabisulfite will remove the discoloration.)

INTERNAL CONTAMINATION

A radioactive substance may enter the body by ingestion, inhalation, or breaks in the integument. Direct absorption through intact skin is unusual, but tritium is a notable exception.

The risks associated with internal contamination are primarily the late effects of radiation, such as cancer induction, rather than an immediate threat to the patient's life. It would take an exceptionally large intake by ingestion or inhalation to result in doses capable of the acute radiation syndrome.

Unlike external radiation poisoning in which the exposure was completed prior to the patient's being seen by medical personnel, the internally contaminated patient will continue to be exposed until the substance is eliminated from the body or it decays naturally to negligible levels. This type of radiation poisoning affords the physician an opportunity to decrease the patient's exposure and thus decrease the morbidity.

The types of radionuclides potentially encountered in patients internally contaminated are numerous. Those radioisotopes potentially encountered in nuclear accidents associated with weaponry or power plants will be discussed. Internal contamination of exposed persons at Chernobyl included over 20 different radionuclides, but iodine and cesium accounted for most of the doses received internally.[34]

Detection devices for internal contamination, termed whole body scintillation counters, are very sophisticated units unlikely to be available except at very highly specialized facilities. Treatment may have to be instituted based on a high probability of contamination as indicated in the history. In the case of fallout from accidents, such as Chernobyl, prevention of ingestion by avoiding contaminated food supplies is paramount.

Management of the patient will depend on the type of radionuclide, the route of entry, and the time interval between the intake and the institution of treatment.

General Treatment

Gastrointestinal Tract. Material may enter the gastrointestinal tract either by direct ingestion or by inhalation and subsequent clearance into the pharynx by ciliary action of the respiratory system. Whether or not the ingested substance is absorbed from the intestine, immediate general treatment should be instituted.

Gastric lavage or emesis with syrup of ipecac should be performed if ingestion has been recent. Appropriate precautions for aspiration should be maintained. A cathartic should be given to limit the time the substance is present within the intestine.

If a specific radioisotope is known, isotopic dilution may be used: a nonradioactive ion that will compete with the radioactive material for absorption is given in large quantities.

Respiratory Tract. The lungs are the most probable portal of entry for radioactive materials, because airborne particulate material and radioactive gases pose the greatest hazard when released into the environment during a nuclear accident.

Large particles, greater than 5 microns, will deposit in the large bronchi, be transported by ciliary action, and swallowed. The treatment for orally ingested materials, described earlier, would be efficacious. For smaller particles of less than 5 microns, deposition will occur in the lung parenchyma. If the material is insoluble, the lung itself becomes the target organ. If soluble, the material will translocate to the blood stream and then on to the target organ. Treatment in this case is directed toward enhancing natural excretion. When insoluble materials are retained in the lung parenchyma, expectorants may be helpful, but treatment is largely ineffective.

Treatment for Specific Radionuclides

Radioiodine.[36] Iodine-131 is a major contributor to radioactivity released as a result of a core meltdown or nuclear bomb explosion. An estimated 20 million curies or more were released from Chernobyl into the environment.[1] Although external radiation to the thyroid can induce thyroid neoplasia (both benign and malignant), available data suggest that radioiodine *may* induce cancer in the human thyroid but to a much lesser extent than does external radiation.

Intake may be either by ingestion or inhalation. Iodine-131 is absorbed in the gastrointestinal tract and the lungs within 30 minutes of intake. It is then rapidly concentrated by the thyroid, with maximum uptake at 48 hours. Nearly instantaneous incorporation into thyroxine takes place, with a subsequent slow release from the thyroid (biologic half-life, 8 days). Six hours after a single oral dose, about 25 per cent of the activity is found in the thyroid.

Potassium Iodide Administration. Nonradioactive iodine, given orally in the form of potassium iodide (KI), will rapidly block accumulation of radioiodine in the thyroid by saturating the transport mechanism of iodide, inhibiting organification of iodide, and diluting the radioactive iodide atoms. Increased urinary excretion of I-131 is also accomplished, which reduces the whole body dose.

If 100 mg of KI is given at the same time as exposure to I-131, thyroid blockade is nearly 97 per cent effective. Given after the exposure, the protection rapidly declines to near ineffectiveness after 6 hours.

Adverse reactions to KI administration are rare but must be considered when mass distribution of KI to potentially exposed persons is contemplated. These reactions include hypothyroidism, dermatitis, and the more potentially serious iodide sensitivity reactions, which can be life threatening. Thus, KI must be given conscientiously only after a risk assessment shows the thyroidal dose is likely to exceed that of the Food and Drug Administration's protective action guideline dose.

Treatment consists of oral administration of 100 to 170 mg per day of KI, depending on the KI commercially available. The FDA has approved KI for use in radiation emergencies. The adult dose recommended by the FDA is 130 mg of KI; for children aged under 1 year, it is 50 mg of KI.[37] The guidelines for a distribution policy are set forth by the Federal Emergency Management Agency. For maximum effectiveness, KI must be given immediately before or during the exposure and continued as long as a significant exposure continues. Obviously, if persons can be evacuated from the area, that would be optimal. This should be strongly encouraged for pregnant women, since KI can induce hypothyroidism goiter in the neonate.

Cesium. Cs-137 and Cs-134 are also major radionuclides released from accidents such as that at Chernobyl. They are concentrated in muscle and other soft tissues but are continually secreted into the gut and reabsorbed. Treatment with Prussian blue, 1 gram dissolved in water, taken three times daily, will help prevent the reabsorption and therefore will increase excretion in feces. Treatment should be continued until excretion of cesium ceases.

Tritium. As discussed earlier, tritium is absorbed through skin, or it may be ingested or inhaled. Its distribution in the body is that of water. Treatment therefore is directed toward excretion in urine. Forced fluid intake and use of diuretics until no further significant excretion is obtained are recommended.

Plutonium and Other Radionuclides. Plutonium and other radionuclides that may be responsible for internal contamination are less likely to be encountered. The treatment can be very complex, depending on the type of material and route of intake. The management of these patients should be referred to experienced personnel, as should all cases of internal contamination after initial therapy is instituted as outlined in this chapter.

LONG-TERM EFFECTS OF RADIATION

It is important to put into perspective the acuteness of the injuries described. There are also long-term effects of radiation that must be dealt with in the survivors of the higher doses and also in the patients who receive doses below the thresholds for signs and symptoms. The absolute risks of low level radiation are still controversial. The association of radiation and the induction of cancer is based primarily on data for acute high doses (greater than 1 Gy). Epidemiologic data indicate that cancer of the bone marrow, breast, thyroid, bone, and lung can be associated with high radiation doses. The absolute threshold dose for induction of carcinogenesis is not known. Common sense dictates that radiation exposures should be kept as low as possible.

Cataracts, chronic dermatitis, and possible genetic effects are all potential late effects of radiation exposure.

Concluding Remarks

Radiation injury is complex, owing to the potential for multiorgan insult and the variety of types of exposures. The practicing physician is unlikely to encounter such injury, but the ever-increasing peacetime use of radionuclides and the wide distribution of nuclear weaponry make it more probable that the emergency physician might become involved in the care of radiation-injured patients.

The recent Chernobyl incident enlightened us all to the potential risks of the nuclear industry. It also has given us much data and new experience in the management of nuclear disasters and radiation-injured persons.

It is unfortunate that the price of knowledge is so high. Humanity has paid a significant debt for the knowledge gained from the catastrophes of Nagasaki, Hiroshima, and Chernobyl. It is hoped that future advances in the care and treatment of radiation injuries can be developed with the aid of computer models rather than requiring animal research and human tragedy.

References

1. International Atomic Energy Agency: Summary Report on the Post-Accident Review Meeting on the Chernobyl Accident. Safety Series Report No. 75-INJAG-1. Vienna, 1986.
2. Goldman M, Catlin RJ, Anspaugh L, et al: Health and environmental consequences of Chernobyl nuclear power plant accident. Department of Energy publication No. DOE/ER-0332. Springfield, VA, National Technical Information Service, 1987.
3. Ahearne JF: Nuclear power after Chernobyl. Science *236*:673–679, 1987.
4. Fry FA: The Chernobyl reactor accident: The impact on the United Kingdom. Br J Radiol *60*:1147, 1987.
5. USSR State Committee on the Utilization of Atomic Energy: The accident at Chernobyl nuclear power plant and its consequences. IAEA (International Atomic Energy Agency) Bulletin, Vienna, 1986.
6. Watson WS: Human Cs^{137}/Cs^{134} levels in Scotland after Chernobyl. Nature *323*:723, 1986.
7. International Conference on Non-military Radiation Emergencies Proceedings. November 1986.
8. Haschke F, Pietschnig B, Karg V, Vanura H, Schuster E: Radioactivity in Austrian milk after the Chernobyl accident. N Engl J Med *316*:409, 1987.
9. Gori G, Carna G, Guerreri E, Corchi G, Dalla Cera P, Guttavecchia E, Ghini S, Tonelli D: Radioactivity in breast milk and placenta during the year after Chernobyl. Am J Obstet Gynecol *159*:1232, 1988.
10. US Nuclear Regulatory Commission: Report on the Accident at the Chernobyl Nuclear Power Station. Publication No. NUREG-1250. Washington, DC, US Nuclear Regulatory Commission, 1987.
11. Paretzke HG: The impact of the Chernobyl accident on radiation protection. Health Physics *55*:139, 1988.
12. Coesel CK: Political and medical lessons of Chernobyl. JAMA *256*:630, 1986.
13. National Research Council: Safety Issues at Defense Production Reactors: Report to the US Department of Energy Commission to Assess Safety and Technology at DOE Reactors. Washington, DC, National Academy Press, 1987.
14. Crawford M: Watkins takes the helm at DOE Science *243*:1136, 1989.
15. Cassel C, Jameton A: Medical responsibility and thermonuclear war. Ann Intern Med *97*:426–432, 1982.
16. Health Policy Committee: The medical consequences of radiation accidents and nuclear war. Ann Intern Med *97*:447, 1982.
17. Sorenson J, Phelps ME: Physics in Nuclear Medicine. New York, Grune and Stratton, 1980.
18. Facts about Low Level Radiation. Printed by American Nuclear Society, with permission from International Atomic Energy Agency. American Nuclear Society, LaGrange Park, IL, 1982.
19. Martell EA: Radioactivity of tobacco trichomes and insoluble cigarette smoke particles. Nature *249*:215–217, 1974.
20. Radford EP Jr, Hunt VR: Polonium-210: A volatile radioelement in cigarettes. Science *143*:247–249, 1964.
21. Little JB, Radford EP Jr, McCombs HL, Hunt VR: Distribution of polonium in pulmonary tissues of cigarette smokers. N Engl J Med *273*:1343–1351, 1965.
22. Samet JM, Nero AV: Indoor radon and lung cancer. N Engl J Med *320*:591, 1989.
23. Council on Scientific Affairs, American Medical Association: Radon in homes. JAMA *258*:668, 1987.
24. Committee on Biological Effects of Ionizing Radiation, National Research Council: Health risks of radon and other internally deposited alpha-emitters. Washington, DC, National Academy Press, 1988.

25. Knowlton NP, Leifer E, Higness JR, et al: Beta ray burns of human skin. JAMA *141*:239, 1949.
26. Thomas GE, Wald N: The diagnosis and management of accidental radiation injury. J Occup Med *1*:421, 1959.
27. Jamnet H, Daburon F, Gerber GB, Hopewell JW, Haybrittle JL, Whitfield L: Radiation damage to the skin: Fundamental and practical aspects. Proceedings of a workshop held in Saclay, France. Br J Radiol (Suppl) *19*:1, 1986.
28. Stern PJ: Surgical Approaches to Radiation Injuries of the Hand. The Medical Basis of Nuclear Accident Preparedness. Amsterdam, Elsevier North Holland, 1980, p 257.
29. Keller PD: A clinical syndrome following exposure to atomic bomb explosions. JAMA *131*:504, 1946.
30. Finch SC: Acute radiation syndrome. JAMA *258*:664, 1987.
31. Saenger EL: Acute effects of external radiation. *In* Proceedings of International Conference on Nonmilitary Radiation Emergencies, Washington, DC. Chicago, AMA, 1986, p 146.
32. International Atomic Energy Agency: Biological dosimetry: Chromosomal aberration analysis for dose assessment. IAEA Technical Report No. 260. Vienna, 1986.
33. Dubois A, Walker RI: Prospects for management of gastrointestinal injury associated with the acute radiation syndrome. Gastroenterology *95*:500, 1988.
34. Baranov A, Gale RP, et al: Bone marrow transplantation after the Chernobyl nuclear accident. N Engl J Med *321*:205, 1989.
35. Management of Persons Accidentally Contaminated with Radionuclides. NCRP Report No. 65. Bethesda, MD, National Council on Radiation Protection and Measurements, 1980.
36. Becker DV: Reactor accidents: Public health strategies and their medical implications. JAMA *258*:649, 1987.
37. Potassium Iodide as a Thyroid-Blocking Agent in a Radiation Emergency: Final Recommendations on Use. Washington, DC, Bureau of Radiological Health and Bureau of Drugs, Food and Drug Administration, 1982.

SECTION B

Centrally Active Agents

CHAPTER 34

TRICYCLIC AND NEWER ANTIDEPRESSANTS

Paul R. Pentel, M.D.
Daniel E. Keyler, Pharm.D.
Lester M. Haddad, M.D.

Tricyclic antidepressant (TCA) toxicity is a leading cause of hospitalization and death due to intentional drug overdose. TCA toxicity was first noted in 1966, when Fréjaville and associates[1] described 100 cases of TCA overdose with a 20 per cent mortality rate. Despite the introduction of specific therapies and improved methods of supportive care, mortality from TCA overdose remains appreciable and a leading cause of toxic death.

TCAs remain the most commonly prescribed drugs for the treatment of depression, despite the recent introduction of nontricyclic antidepressants (trazodone, fluoxetine, and many others outside the United States) and a resurgence of interest

Table 34–1. COMMERCIAL PREPARATIONS OF TRICYCLIC ANTIDEPRESSANTS (AVAILABLE AS THE HYDROCHLORIDE) IN THE UNITED STATES[1]

Imipramine	**Desipramine**
Tofranil[5]	Norpramin
Janimine	Pertofrane[5]
Imipramine	**Nortriptyline**
Berkomine[4]	Pamelor
Amitriptyline	Allegron[4]
Elavil[5]	**Doxepin**
Endep	Sinequan
Amitriptyline	Adapin
Triavil[2]	**Protriptyline**
Etrafon[2]	Vivactil
Limbitrol[3]	Concordin[4]
Domical[4]	**Maprotiline**
Lentizol[4]	Ludiomil[5]
Saroten[4]	**Amoxapine**
Tryptizol[4]	Asendin

[1]This table includes the TCA-related compounds maprotiline and amoxapine.
[2]In combination with a phenothiazine, perphenazine.
[3]In combination with a benzodiazepine, chlordiazepoxide.
[4]Commercial trade name in England (British National Formulary).
[5]Same name in England and U.S.A.

in the monoamine oxidase inhibitors (Table 34–1).

Factors contributing to the large number of serious TCA overdoses include (1) the widespread availability of TCAs to depressed patients at high risk for suicide by drug ingestion, (2) the severity of cardiovascular and central nervous system effects associated with overdose, and (3) the limited efficacy of available treatments for overdose.

Quality of the Available Information

Data regarding TCA overdose in humans are derived from case reports and patient series. The commonly prescribed TCAs are well represented in these reports, but information regarding trimipramine, protriptyline, butriptyline, and clomipramine is limited. Many controlled animal studies of TCA toxicity are available, but no controlled trials of therapy for TCA overdose in humans have been reported.

CLASSIFICATION

TCAs may be classified as secondary or tertiary amines (Fig. 34–1). The tertiary amines are demethylated in vivo to their corresponding secondary amines, and several of these metabolites (desipramine, nortriptyline) are also available for clinical use. At therapeutic doses, the clinically available TCAs may be distinguished from one another by their relative abilities to inhibit the reuptake of neurotransmitters (norepinephrine, dopamine, serotonin), their anticholinergic and antihistaminic potencies, and their tendency to sedate.[2, 3] At toxic doses, these differences are unimportant, and the toxicities of most TCAs are qualitatively and quantitatively similar. One possible exception is the tertiary amine lofepramine, which is slowly metabolized to desipramine, and because of the limited rate at which desipramine is formed, may be less toxic than other TCAs, although specific clinical data are lacking.

Amoxapine is structurally related to the TCAs and has similar therapeutic actions. Amoxapine overdose, however, is characterized by a higher incidence of seizures, and cardiovascular toxicity is rare[4–6] (Table 34–2). The tetracyclic antidepressant maprotiline is also more likely than TCAs to produce seizures but is associated with cardiovascular toxicity typical of the TCAs at sufficient doses.[7, 8] Trazodone and fluoxetine represent a growing number of structurally diverse atypical or nontricyclic antidepressants whose toxicity is quite distinct from that of the TCAs. These drugs do not produce cardiac conduction delays, hypotension, or arrhythmias; even massive overdoses are generally well tolerated.[9, 10] A variety of other atypical antidepressants are available outside the United States or are undergoing clinical trials, and these also lack the serious toxic effects of the TCAs.[11, 12] The monoamine oxidase inhibitors are discussed in Chapter 44B.

PHARMACOKINETICS

Peak serum TCA concentrations occur 2 to 8 hours after administration of a therapeutic dose.[13, 14] After overdose, the anticholinergic properties of the TCAs may slow gastric emptying and further delay drug absorption. Nevertheless, the onset of toxicity after overdose is typically rapid, and most deaths occur within several hours of presentation. This time course probably reflects the potencies of the TCAs such that absorption of even a

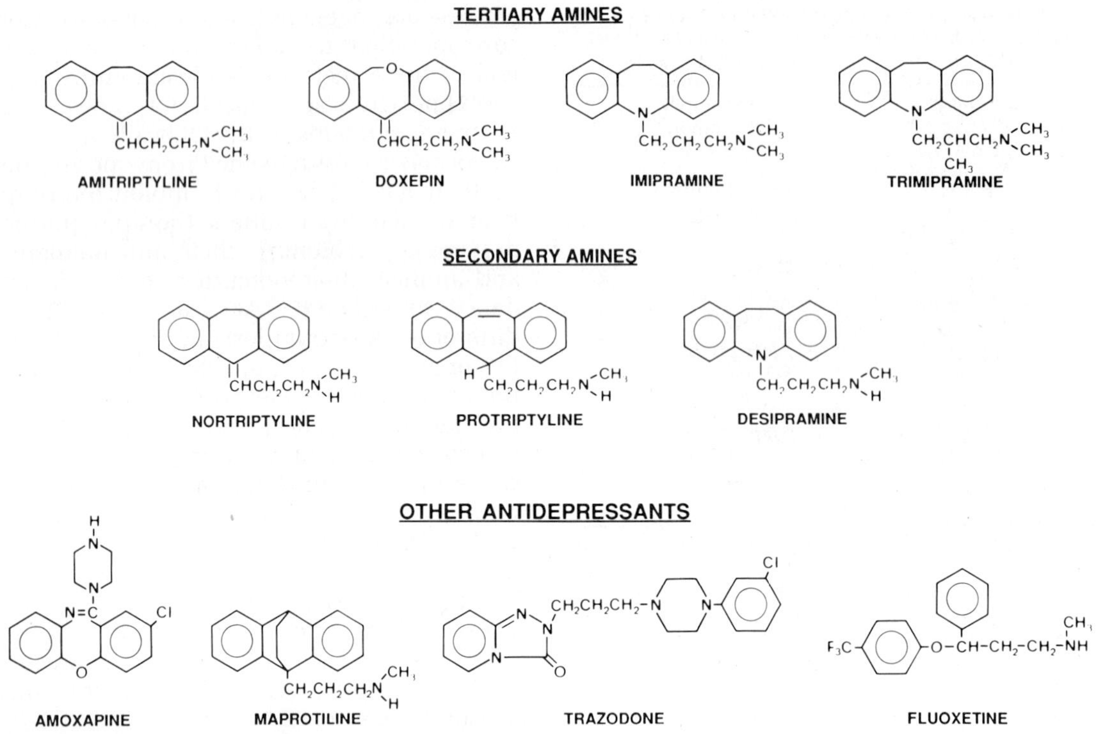

TERTIARY AMINES

AMITRIPTYLINE DOXEPIN IMIPRAMINE TRIMIPRAMINE

SECONDARY AMINES

NORTRIPTYLINE PROTRIPTYLINE DESIPRAMINE

OTHER ANTIDEPRESSANTS

AMOXAPINE MAPROTILINE TRAZODONE FLUOXETINE

Figure 34–1. Structures of some antidepressants. (From Richardson JW, Richelson E: Antidepressants: A clinical update for medical practitioners. Mayo Clin Proc *59*:330, 1984.)

fraction of the ingested dose may prove toxic or fatal. First-pass hepatic metabolism of therapeutic doses of TCAs is extensive (23 to 73 per cent for imipramine) but may become saturated with overdose, resulting in increased bioavailability.[15]

All TCAs have a large volume of distribution (10 to 20 L/kg), and in some tissues drug concentrations are 10 to 100 times that of blood.[16, 17] Distribution of TCAs to tissue is rapid, and less than 1 to 2 per cent of the ingested dose is present in the blood even in the early hours following overdose.[18] Both mono- and biexponential kinetics have been described for the disappearance of TCAs from serum.[19, 20] Elimination half-lives for therapeutic doses of TCAs average 8 to 30 hours (55 to 127 hours for protriptyline), with longer half-lives in the elderly[19, 21, 22] (Table 34–3). The elimination half-life after overdose may be somewhat longer owing to saturable metabolism[20, 23, 24] but is still generally within the range reported for therapeutic doses.

Elimination of TCAs is almost entirely due to hepatic metabolism; renal excretion of these drugs, which are weak bases, is negligible even when urine is acidified.[25] The TCAs are first converted to demethylated and hydroxylated metabolites[26–28] that are quantitatively and qualitatively similar in toxicity to their parent compounds.[29] The serum concentration of active metabolites in the first few hours after overdose is generally low, but metabolites may contribute to toxicity after the first 12 to 24 hours.[20, 30] Active metabolites undergo further demethylation or conjugation to inactive compounds that are excreted in urine. There is little biliary excretion of TCAs as parent drug or active metabolite.[31, 32]

Hydroxylation of some TCAs by hepatic microsomes displays genetic polymorphism that is linked to debrisoquin hydroxylation. In the United States, 90 to 95 per cent of patients are rapid hydroxylators and have a much shorter desipramine half-life (13 to 23 hours) than slow hydroxylators (81 to 131 hours).[33] Slow recovery from desipramine overdose has been reported in one patient owing to slow hydroxylation.[24]

The TCAs (as well as amoxapine and maprotiline) are extensively bound to serum proteins, primarily alpha-1 acid glycoprotein (AAG).[34] Changes in the serum AAG concentration[35, 36] or pH[37] may markedly affect the bound fraction of TCAs, but it is

Table 34–2. TYPES OF ANTIDEPRESSANTS AND THEIR OVERDOSE TOXICITY

TYPE	PRINCIPAL TOXIC EFFECTS
Tricyclic Antidepressants	
Tertiary amines	
imipramine	
amitriptyline	
doxepin	
trimipramine	
clomipramine*	
butriptyline*	Hypotension, arrhythmia, coma, seizure, hyperthermia
Secondary amines	
desipramine	
nortriptyline	
protriptyline	
Tetracyclic Antidepressant	
maprotiline	Like other TCAs, but seizures more likely
Dibenzoxazepine	
amoxapine†	Seizures, coma; little cardiovascular toxicity
Benzodiazepine	
alprazolam	Sedation
Atypical Antidepressants	
trazodone	
fluoxetine	
fluvoxamine*	Sedation
mianserin*	
zimelidine*	
buproprion*	
Monamine Oxidase Inhibitor‡	
tranylcypromine	Coma, seizure, hyper- or hypotension, hyperthermia
phenelzine	

*Not marketed in the United States as of 1/89.
†Sometimes classified as a TCA.
‡Discussed in Chapter 44.

unlikely that changes in binding affect overdose toxicity (see discussion of $NaHCO_3$).

MECHANISMS OF TCA TOXICITY

Overview

The most important toxic effects of TCA overdose are hypotension, arrhythmias, coma, seizures, and hyperthermia. Cardiotoxicity results from multiple effects on the cardiac cell action potential, direct effects on vascular tone, and indirect effects mediated by the autonomic nervous system (Table 34–4). Hyperthermia is due to excessive muscular activity in the presence of high anticholinergic tone. Central nervous system toxicity is less well understood; anticholinergic and antihistaminic effects may contribute.

Cardiac Cell Action Potential

The normal features of the action potential in cardiac cells are shown in Figure 34–2. The most prominent electrophysiologic action of the TCAs is inhibition of the fast sodium channel and the slowing of phase 0 depolarization in His-Purkinje tissue and ventricular myocardium. In this respect, the TCAs resemble Class I antiarrhythmic agents (e.g., quinidine, procainamide, encainide, flecainide).[38, 39] Impaired depolarization of cells within the His-Purkinje system slows ventricular depolarization and appears on the electrocardiogram as prolongation of the QRS interval, the hallmark of TCA overdose (Fig. 34–3).

Slowed conduction may contribute to the development of ventricular arrhythmias. Nonuniform slowing of conduction could lead to unidirectional block and re-entry, a well-recognized mechanism of ventricular tachycardia.[40] In support of this possibility, ventricular tachycardia is a general feature of toxicity due to other drugs that slow ventricular depolarization, such as Class I antiarrhythmic agents.

Impaired phase 0 depolarization may also contribute to hypotension after TCA over-

Table 34–3. PHARMACOKINETICS AND CLINICAL PARAMETERS OF SOME ANTIDEPRESSANTS

DRUG	VOLUME OF DISTRIBUTION (L/kg)	ELIMINATION HALF-LIFE (hr)	USUAL DAILY DOSE—YOUNG HEALTHY ADULT (mg)	THERAPEUTIC SERUM CONCENTRATION (ng/ml)	ACTIVE METABOLITES
amitriptyline	10–19	10–25	50–300	125–250*	Nortriptyline 10-OH-amitriptyline 10-OH-nortriptyline
imipramine	20–40	18–34†	50–300	150–300*	Desipramine 2-OH-imipramine 2-OH-desipramine
doxepin	9–33	8–24 (doxepin) 33–81 (desmethyldoxepin)	50–300	75–200*§	Desmethyldoxepin
trimipramine	NA	NA	50–300	50–300*‖	Desmethyltrimipramine
nortriptyline	21–57	16–36	30–100	50–150	10-OH nortriptyline
desipramine	22–59	12–30†	50–300	150–300	2-OH desipramine
protriptyline	19–26	55–127	15–60	50–150	
amoxapine	NA	8 (amoxapine) 30 (8-hydroxyamoxapine)	50–300	160–800‡	8-OH amoxapine 7-OH amoxapine
maprotiline	15–28	47	50–300	200–300	Desmethylmaprotiline
trazodone	NA	3–6	50–600	500–2000‖	m-Chlorophenyl piperazin
fluoxetine	12–43	26–220 (fluoxetine) 77–235 (norfluoxetine)	20–30	20–250‡	Norfluoxetine

Adapted from references 2, 150 through 155.
*Parent compound plus demethylated metabolite.
†Longer for slow hydroxylators.
‡Parent compound plus metabolite.
§Not well established.
‖Numbers refer to usage serum concentrations; optimal therapeutic concentrations not established.
NA = not available.

dose. The intracellular movement of sodium during phase 0 is closely coupled to the release of intracellular calcium stores and cellular contraction.[41] Impaired entry of sodium into cardiac cells may therefore impair cellular contractility. This action is, like ventricular tachycardia, also a general feature of toxicity due to Class I antiarrhythmic agents.

Sodium channel inhibition in vitro is sensitive to pH, and increasing the extracellular pH minimizes TCA-induced slowing of phase 0 depolarization. Elevating the blood pH has been shown to have a beneficial effect in a variety of animal models of TCA overdose, resulting in improvements in intraventricular conduction delays, hypotension, and ventricular arrhythmias.[18, 42, 43] Conversely, acidosis may aggravate TCA cardiotoxicity.[18] Increasing the extracellular sodium concentration also minimizes the effects of TCAs on phase 0 depolarization. Together with increasing blood pH, increasing the serum sodium concentration probably contributes to the therapeutic effect of hypertonic [1 molar

Table 34–4. MECHANISMS OF TCA CARDIOTOXICITY

TOXIC EFFECT	MECHANISM
Conduction Delays	
QRS prolongation Atrioventricular block	Sodium channel inhibition producing slowed conduction
Arrhythmias	
Sinus tachycardia	Cholinergic blockade, inhibition of catecholamine reuptake
Ventricular tachycardia	? Re-entry due to slowed conduction
Torsades de pointes	Prolonged repolarization
Ventricular bradyarrhythmias	Impaired automaticity
Hypotension	
Decreased cardiac contractility	Sodium channel inhibition
Vasodilation	Alpha-adrenergic blockade with decreased cardiac filling pressure or peripheral vascular resistance
Tachy- or bradyarrhythmia	Rate-related decrease in cardiac output

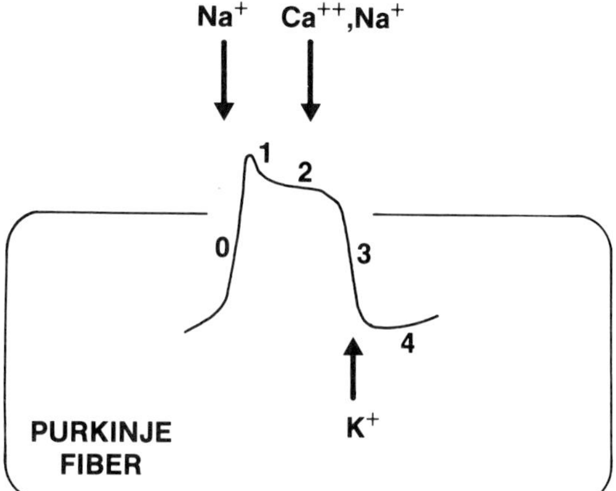

Figure 34–2. Normal Purkinje fiber action potential. Phase 0 depolarization is due to activation of the fast sodium channel and the resulting inward sodium current. Depolarization is maintained during phase 2 by an inward current caused by calcium and sodium. Repolarization (phase 3) is due in part to an outward potassium current. In cells with intrinsic automaticity, spontaneous depolarization during phase 4 initiates phase 0 depolarization when the threshold voltage is reached. (From Pentel PR, Benowitz NL: Tricyclic antidepressant poisoning: Management of arrhythmias. Med Toxicol *1*:101, 1986.)

(1M)] sodium bicarbonate on TCA cardiotoxicity.

Other effects of the TCAs on the cardiac cell action potential include slowing of repolarization and phase 4 (spontaneous) depolarization and calcium channel inhibition.[44] Prolongation of repolarization, as well as the QT interval, is a feature of both therapeutic and toxic doses of TCAs. QT prolongation predisposes to the development of torsades de pointes, which has been reported in patients taking therapeutic doses of TCAs.[45] Torsades de pointes typically occurs when the ventricular rate is slow. Because the underlying rhythm in patients with TCA overdose is most often sinus tachycardia, torsades de pointes is an uncommon feature of overdose. Slowing of phase 4 depolarization inhibits ventricular automaticity. At toxic doses, impaired automaticity may suppress ventricular escape rhythms and lead to marked bradycardia. The importance of calcium channel inhibition in TCA overdose is unclear; in massive TCA overdose it could contribute to the occurrence of high-grade atrioventricular block or sinus node arrest.

Neurotransmitter Reuptake

The inhibition of neuronal neurotransmitter reuptake (norepinephrine, dopamine, serotonin) and the resulting increase in synaptic neurotransmitter levels are thought to be important in mediating the antidepressant effect of TCAs.[3] With overdose, increases in the cardiac concentration of catecholamines may contribute to sinus tachycardia.[46, 47] Increases in vascular catecholamines may contribute to the transient hypertension occasionally observed early in the course of TCA overdose.[48, 49] Increased concentrations of catecholamines might also contribute to ventricular arrhythmias, but data on this question are limited.

It has also been suggested that profound or prolonged inhibition of norepinephrine reuptake could cause hypotension by depleting neuronal reserves of the neurotransmitter. The limited efficacy of high doses of catecholamines in correcting severe TCA-induced hypotension argues against this being the predominant mechanism for hypotension.

Cholinergic Blockade

The anticholinergic actions of TCAs contribute to the development of sinus tachycardia, hyperthermia, ileus, urinary retention, pupillary dilatation, and probably coma.[50] Of these, the most important is hyperthermia, which is caused by impaired sweating and is most often observed in patients who are generating excessive heat due to repetitive seizures, myoclonus, or agitation.[51] It has been suggested that seizures are also anticholinergic in origin, but this question has not been adequately investigated. Preliminary in vitro data suggest that the ability of TCAs to produce seizures may be related to inhibition of GABA receptor–mediated neuronal chloride uptake.[52]

Alpha Blockade

At therapeutic doses of TCAs, alpha-adrenergic blockade causes vasodilation and postural hypotension. At toxic doses, both venodilation and arteriolar dilation are important contributors to hypotension.[53, 54]

Protein Binding

The serum protein binding of TCAs is enhanced in vitro by increasing pH.[55] It has

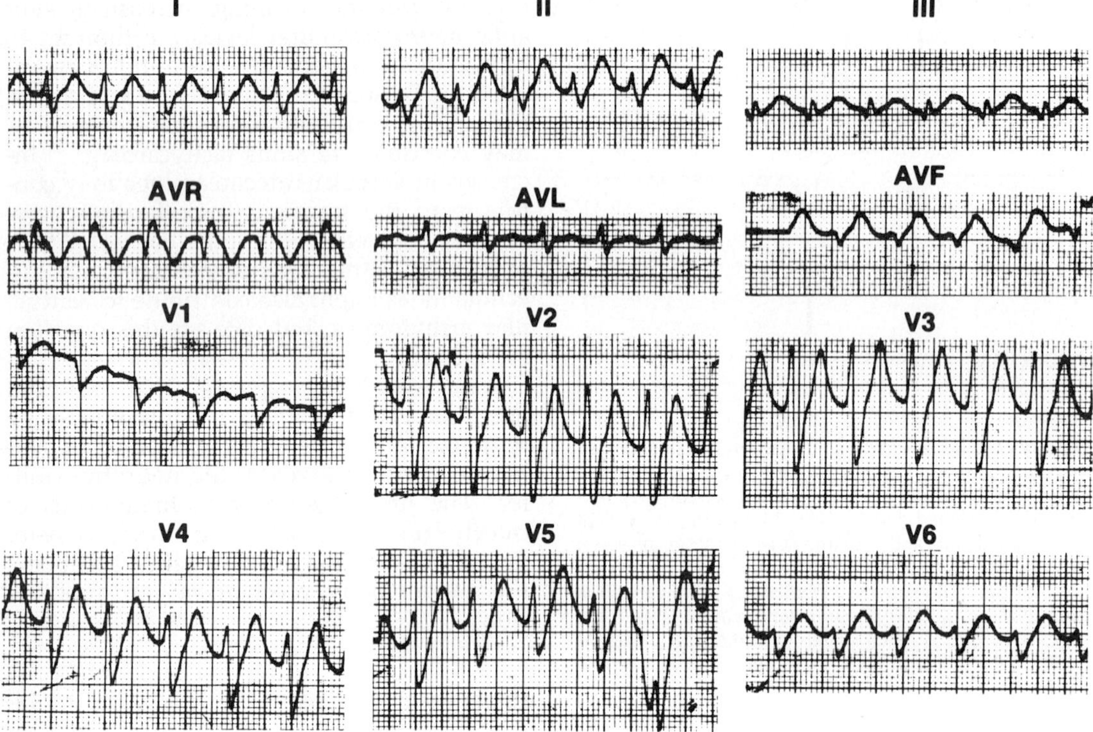

Figure 34–3. Typical 12-lead electrocardiogram of a patient with tricyclic antidepressant toxicity. Note the rapid rhythm with markedly prolonged QRS duration. P waves are not clearly visible. (From Pentel PR, Benowitz NL: Tricyclic antidepressant poisoning: Management of arrhythmias. Med Toxicol *1*:101, 1986.)

therefore been postulated that the beneficial effect of $NaHCO_3$ on TCA cardiotoxicity might be due to increasing blood pH, enhancing protein binding, and reducing the concentration of unbound (pharmacologically active) drug. The failure of exogenously administered alpha-1-acid glycoprotein to ameliorate TCA toxicity in rats, despite markedly increasing its binding in serum, argues against this hypothesis.[36]

PRESENTATION

General

Life-threatening overdose is usually associated with ingestion of more than 1 gm of TCA. Of patients who reach the hospital, many deaths occur within several hours of presentation, and most occur within the first 24 hours.[56–59] It is not uncommon for a patient's clinical condition to deteriorate rapidly in the first few hours after drug ingestion, with the patient progressing from an asymptomatic state to life-threatening cardiotoxicity or seizures in less than 1 hour.[57, 60]

Cardiovascular

QRS Morphology. *QRS interval prolongation is the most distinctive feature of serious TCA overdose*[61, 62] (see Fig. 34–3). QRS morphology is usually that of a nonspecific intraventricular conduction delay; discrete bundle branch block is less common.[58] TCA-induced conduction delay is rate dependent, and tachycardia exaggerates QRS prolongation.[42] *The QRS axis is typically shifted to the right.*[63]

QRS prolongation is not in itself harmful, but it serves to identify patients at risk of developing further complications.[56, 64] In one study, a QRS duration of greater than 0.16 second identified patients at greatest risk of ventricular arrhythmias, and a QRS duration of greater than 0.10 second identified patients at greatest risk of seizures. However, these and other complications may occur with a lesser degree of QRS prolongation, and patients with any degree of QRS prolongation are generally considered at risk for developing life-threatening TCA toxicity. In contrast to the seizures induced by TCAs and maprotiline, seizures due to amoxapine usually occur in the absence of cardiovascular toxicity.[4]

Atrioventricular Block. The PR interval in TCA overdose is prolonged, but second- or third-degree atrioventricular block is rare.[58, 61]

QT Interval. The QT interval is mildly prolonged with therapeutic doses of TCAs and is more prolonged with overdose. However, the degree of QT prolongation is not a useful predictor of complications.

Sinus Tachycardia. The most common rhythm associated with TCA overdose is sinus tachycardia, which is present in more than 50 per cent of patients.[65] The sinus rate is usually modest (less than 160 beats/per/min) and does not cause hemodynamic compromise. The severity of sinus tachycardia is not a useful predictor of other complications.[66] Sinus tachycardia may be aggravated by concurrent hypoxia, hypotension, hyperthermia, or the use of beta-1 adrenergic agonists.

Ventricular Arrhythmias. Ventricular tachycardia is probably the most common ventricular arrhythmia in patients with TCA overdose. However, it may be quite difficult to distinguish from sinus tachycardia when QRS prolongation is marked and P waves are not visible (see discussion of wide-complex tachycardia without P waves hereafter). It is likely that some reports of ventricular tachycardia (and its treatment) in the literature are actually cases of supraventricular rhythms. The present discussion of ventricular tachycardia should be interpreted with this limitation in mind.

Ventricular tachycardia most often occurs in patients with marked QRS prolongation and/or hypotension[64, 67] and may be precipitated by seizures.[68] Other predisposing factors include hypoxia, hypothermia, acidosis, and the use of beta-1 adrenergic agonists. Mortality in patients with ventricular tachycardia is high.

Premature ventricular beats are uncommon in patients with TCA overdose. Ventricular fibrillation is usually a terminal rhythm that occurs as a complication of ventricular tachycardia and/or hypotension. Torsades de pointes has been reported with TCA overdose[69, 70] but is rare and more often complicates therapeutic use of TCAs.[71] Slow ventricular rhythms may occur with massive TCA overdose.

Wide-complex Tachycardia Without P Waves. One of the most difficult diagnostic problems in patients with TCA overdose is classifying the cardiac rhythm when P waves are not visible. A common underlying rhythm in this situation is sinus tachycardia with QRS prolongation. P waves may be obscured by the preceding T wave because of prolonged PR and QT intervals and the rapid heart rate. When QRS duration is markedly prolonged, this rhythm may be indistinguishable from ventricular tachycardia. A 12-lead electrocardiogram may reveal P waves not visible on a rhythm strip. If time allows, an electrocardiogram obtained using an esophageal electrode or an intra-atrial pacemaker as a sensing lead may help by revealing P waves that the standard 12-lead electrocardiogram does not. When patients present soon after overdose, serial observation of the electrocardiogram is often helpful. A gradual evolution of QRS morphology prior to the loss of P waves suggests that the wide-complex rhythm is supraventricular. The observation of atrioventricular dissociation or fusion beats would, as in other settings, suggest that the rhythm is ventricular in origin. Other criteria commonly used to differentiate ventricular and supraventricular rhythms, such as QRS morphology and duration, have not been tested in patients with TCA overdose and may not be applicable in this setting.

Late Arrhythmias. TCA toxicity usually resolves in 24 to 48 hours,[56] although slower recovery has been reported in slow hydroxylators.[24] Maximal toxicity and almost all deaths occur within 24 hours of presentation.[57–59] However, a few cases of arrhythmias or sudden death 2 to 5 days after TCA ingestion have been described. Most of these cases involve patients with residual TCA toxicity or coexisting disease,[72–74] although one report describes a patient with apparently full resolution of cardiac toxicity 24 hours prior to a bradycardic arrest.[75] Several retrospective reviews specifically addressing this question have failed to find any cases of late, unexpected deterioration or death.[58, 66, 76, 77] Moreover, the pharmacokinetics of the TCAs offer no theoretical basis for the late reappearance of toxicity. If late arrhythmias are in fact a feature of TCA overdose, their incidence must be quite low.

Hypotension. Hypotension in TCA overdose is due to both impaired cardiac contractility and/or vasodilation.[53, 54] The presence of hypotension correlates poorly with QRS duration.[67] Other factors contributing to hypotension include very fast or very slow heart rates, intravascular volume depletion, hypoxia, hyperthermia, acidosis, seizures, and the coingestion (or therapeutic use) of other cardiodepressant or vasodilating drugs.

Central Nervous System

Coma. Central nervous system depression is usually present in patients with QRS prolongation. Coma may also occur when QRS duration is normal, particularly when other central nervous system depressant drugs are coingested.

Delirium. Delirium may occur with the ingestion of modest doses of TCAs or early in the course of more massive TCA overdose. It is characterized by agitation, disorientation, or psychotic behavior. The presumed mechanism is cholinergic blockade in the central nervous system, and other anticholinergic signs (such as hyperthermia, dry skin, mydriasis, sinus tachycardia, ileus, and urinary retention) may be present.

Seizures and Myoclonus. Seizures are most common in patients with QRS prolongation[64] but may also occur in those with a normal QRS duration.[68] Maprotiline and amoxapine are more likely than other cyclic antidepressants to cause seizures.[4, 7] One retrospective study also found a higher incidence of seizures with desipramine, but the number of patients studied was small.[8] Seizures due to TCAs most often occur within 1.5 hours of presentation. They are usually generalized, brief, and single and subside before an anticonvulsant can be administered.[68] Seizures may result in acidosis, hyperthermia, or rhabdomyolysis but are usually well tolerated.[68, 78] In one series, however, 4 of 30 patients with seizures due to TCA overdose developed marked cardiovascular deterioration (hypotension, ventricular arrhythmias) during seizures or within minutes of their cessation.[68] It was speculated that cardiovascular deterioration may have been due to seizure-induced acidosis.

A further illustration of the potential consequences of seizures is provided by amoxapine overdose. Although this drug has little cardiovascular toxicity, one study found amoxapine overdose to have a substantially higher incidence of seizures and higher mortality than the TCAs.[4]

Myoclonus is less common than seizures, although the reported incidence varies. Potential complications are the same as for seizures but are less likely to occur.[79]

Hyperthermia

Hyperthermia in TCA overdose results from excessive heat generation (seizures, myoclonus, or agitation) in the presence of impaired heat dissipation (decreased sweating). Death or permanent neurologic sequelae have been reported in patients with drug overdose (including TCA overdose) when core temperature exceeds 105°F for periods as brief as several hours.[51] The unusually high morbidity and mortality associated with overdose-induced hyperthermia may be due to the coexistence of multiple cerebral insults, such as hyperthermia, hypotension, and hypoxia.

Other

Urinary retention and ileus are common in TCA overdose. Pupil size is variable owing to the opposing influence of cholinergic and alpha-adrenergic blockade. Pupils nonreactive to light have been reported but are rare.[79, 80] Pulmonary complications include aspiration pneumonitis and the adult respiratory distress syndrome.[81] These complications are most likely secondary to coma, hypotension, pulmonary infection, or excessive fluid administration rather than primary toxic effects of the TCAs.

DIFFERENTIAL DIAGNOSIS

Overdoses most likely to be confused with TCA toxicity are those that produce QRS prolongation. TCA cardiotoxicity may be indistinguishable from overdose with Class IA (quinidine, procainamide, disopyramide) or Class IC (flecainide, encainide, propafenone) antiarrhythmic agents (see Chapter 97). Other potential causes of QRS prolongation include massive propranolol overdose,[82] quinine overdose,[83] antipsychotic drug overdose,[84] chloroquine overdose,[85] hyperkalemia, cardiac ischemia, and disease of the cardiac conduction system. Carbamazepine (Tegretol) has been described as having toxicity similar to that of the TCAs. Although carbamazepine may produce or aggravate atrioventricular block,[86] it does not prolong QRS duration with overdose.[87] The muscle relaxant cyclobenzaprine (Flexeril) has also been described as having TCA-like toxicity,[88] but there is no evidence of QRS prolongation or important cardiac toxicity with overdose.[89]

MANAGEMENT

Treatment of TCA overdose must be aggressive from the start. All patients with known TCA overdose in the prehospital phase are placed on electrocardiographic telemetry. Depending on the clinical situation, the emergency physician may consider it appropriate to initiate oral activated charcoal and, in a life-threatening emergency, intravenous bicarbonate therapy. Intravenous access is established, generally with D5W at a "keep open" rate, and oxygen is begun.

In the emergency department,[90] airway management is secured, and blood for baseline studies, including arterial blood gases, is drawn. Adequate oxygenation and ventilation are essential. Maintenance intravenous fluids only are generally indicated throughout the hospital stay, as the goal is to keep the patient in a normovolemic state. Intravenous expansion with normal saline may be appropriate for the hypotensive patient requiring volume expansion. Cardiac monitoring and a 12-lead electrocardiogram are obtained.

A general assessment of the patient is indicated. Is there evidence of concomitant trauma? Are there other underlying medical conditions requiring management? Are there indications of other drugs involved in overdose? Has the patient aspirated? In summary, a general history, physical, and overall assessment as outlined in Chapter 1 are essential to proper management.

Recommendations on admission criteria, cardiac monitoring, activated charcoal administration, and sodium bicarbonate therapy (as well as other modalities) are herein described.

Admission Criteria. Patients who have ingested TCAs but show no signs of toxicity during 6 hours of observation (and have received oral activated charcoal) require no further medical monitoring.[57, 91, 92] Psychiatric evaluation should be obtained. Patients with sinus tachycardia alone have a low incidence of other complications but are generally admitted for observation.[65, 66]

Monitoring. Because of the possibility of rapid deterioration, early initiation of cardiac monitoring and intravenous access are useful in patients who have ingested TCAs. Monitoring of vital signs should include frequent measurement of temperature, particularly in patients with agitation or seizures. If respiratory depression or hypotension is present, arterial blood gases should be monitored.

Duration of Monitoring. Cardiac monitoring of patients after TCA overdose is generally recommended until all signs of toxicity are absent for 24 hours.[77] QRS duration may be considered normal if it is less than 0.10 second or similar to the duration prior to overdose. When QRS duration is marginally prolonged (0.10 to 0.12 second) and no baseline electrocardiogram is available, it may be unclear whether the observed QRS duration is normal for that patient or prolonged owing to TCA ingestion. In this situation, measurement of the serum TCA concentration may be helpful. A clearly elevated TCA concentration would suggest that the QRS prolongation is drug induced and that continued cardiac monitoring is indicated.

Reducing Absorption. Gastric emptying and administration of activated charcoal (50 gm with a cathartic) are generally recommended.[93] Whether this regimen is superior to activated charcoal alone is not known. Although ileus is common with TCA overdose, decreased or absent bowel sounds are not contraindications to administration of activated charcoal unless there is reason to suspect additional gastrointestinal pathology. Gastric lavage is preferred for gastric emptying because ipecac-induced emesis may promote aspiration in patients who cannot protect their airway owing to seizures or an impaired level of consciousness.

$NaHCO_3$. *Aside from gastric decontamination, intravenous sodium bicarbonate ($NaHCO_3$) is the most useful single intervention for the management of TCA toxicity.* 1M $NaHCO_3$ is effective in treating each of the most important manifestations of TCA cardiotoxicity: QRS prolongation, ventricular arrhythmias, and hypotension (Fig. 34–4). It is also one of the

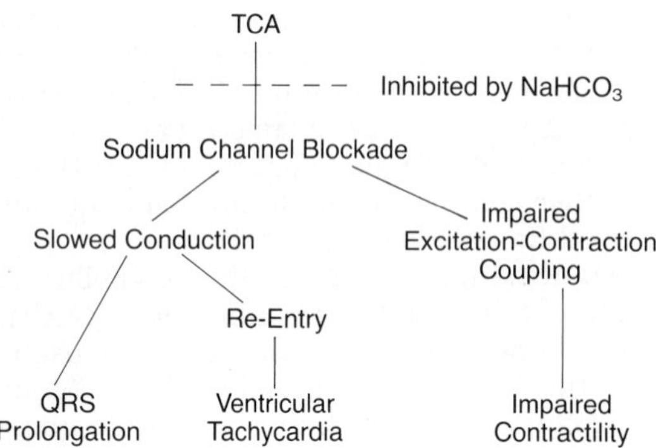

Figure 34–4. Role of cardiac sodium channel inhibition in mediating TCA toxicity.

safest therapies available for TCA toxicity. The usual commercial preparation of intravenous sodium bicarbonate is a hypertonic solution of 1 molar (1M, or 1 molar, or 1 mEq/ml) sodium bicarbonate, 50 mEq/50 ml of sodium bicarbonate.

When TCAs were introduced into clinical use, TCA overdose was noted to share many of the features of quinidine toxicity.[94] 1M sodium lactate (which is rapidly metabolized to bicarbonate) had been reported to be beneficial in treating quinidine toxicity,[94–96] and this therapy was therefore suggested for patients with TCA overdose as well. In uncontrolled studies, 1M sodium lactate and 1M $NaHCO_3$ appeared to be of benefit for TCA cardiotoxicity.[97–101] Subsequent controlled studies in animals clearly established that $NaHCO_3$ is effective in reducing QRS prolongation, increasing blood pressure, and suppressing ventricular ectopy due to TCA toxicity.[18, 43, 48, 102, 103] Controlled studies in patients have not been reported, but a large body of anecdotal data suggests that $NaHCO_3$ is effective in humans as well.

Because acidosis aggravates TCA cardiotoxicity, the beneficial effect of $NaHCO_3$ lies partly in the correction of acidosis. It is clear, however, that $NaHCO_3$ is effective even when blood pH is normal. This beneficial effect appears to be mediated by increases in both blood pH and sodium concentration,[104] although the relative contribution of each differs in various animal models.[18, 43]

There are few data commenting on the optimal dose of 1M $NaHCO_3$ in TCA overdose. It is common practice to administer 50 mEq of $NaHCO_3$ (1 mEq/ml) as an initial IV bolus, with repeat doses as needed for cardiotoxicity or until the arterial blood pH is 7.45 to 7.55. Because marked alkalosis can precipitate ventricular arrhythmias even in the absence of TCAs, the safety of increasing blood pH further is not known. If increasing the serum sodium concentration is important in humans, then administering $NaHCO_3$ as a bolus may be preferable to diluting it in IV fluids prior to administration.

There is no evidence that $NaHCO_3$ is effective for treating TCA-induced seizures.

Hyperventilation. Hyperventilation has been reported to benefit patients with TCA-induced cardiotoxicity,[105, 106] but clinical data are less abundant than data on the use of $NaHCO_3$. The efficacy of hyperventilation for ventricular ectopy has been demonstrated in dogs.[43] Hyperventilation, however, is less effective than $NaHCO_3$ for cardiotoxicity in rats,[18] possibly because $NaHCO_3$ increases the serum sodium concentration, whereas hyperventilation does not. Because hyperventilation in other clinical settings may provoke seizures, the possibility that it might aggravate TCA-induced seizures has been raised.[107] $NaHCO_3$ is therefore generally preferred to hyperventilation for TCA cardiotoxicity. Nevertheless, hyperventilation may be useful if $NaHCO_3$ is relatively contraindicated, such as in a patient with pulmonary edema.

Phenytoin. Phenytoin enhances intracardiac conduction in some experimental settings and has therefore been studied and suggested[108] as a treatment for TCA cardiotoxicity. Phenytoin has been reported to improve QRS duration in patients,[109, 110] including one preliminary report that noted more rapid improvement of cardiovascular toxicity in patients randomized to phenytoin,[109] but these studies lacked controls and are difficult to interpret. Animal studies have not demonstrated a beneficial effect,[111–113] and possible aggravation of ventricular ectopy was noted in one report.[113]

Phenytoin has also been used in TCA overdose as an anticonvulsant, although its efficacy for this purpose is not established. When administered as a pretreatment, phenytoin has been reported to reduce the incidence of amoxapine-induced seizures in dogs.[114] However, phenytoin was not effective for imipramine-induced seizures in rats;[115] in the same study, diazepam and phenobarbital were effective.[115] (See further discussion on management of seizures.)

Physostigmine. The cholinesterase inhibitor physostigmine may antagonize some anticholinergic features of TCA overdose, such as sinus tachycardia and coma,[116] but these complications can generally be treated supportively. Physostigmine is otherwise ineffective for, and may even exacerbate, TCA cardiotoxicity. Severe bradycardia and asystole have been reported with its use in TCA overdose.[117] Physostigmine has also been used to terminate TCA-induced seizures and myoclonus. Although efficacy has been reported anecdotally, physostigmine may also, paradoxically, precipitate seizures.[7] In view of this toxicity, there is no role for physostigmine in the management of TCA overdose.

Beta Blockers. Beta blockers have been reported to reduce QRS prolongation in patients with TCA overdose.[118] Because QRS prolongation is rate dependent, this effect may be secondary to slowing of the heart rate.[42] The possibility of hemodynamic deterioration with beta blockers argues against their use.

Enhancing Elimination. Enhancing elimination of the TCAs is difficult owing to their large volume of distribution and the small fraction of the absorbed dose that is present in blood. Repeated oral doses of activated charcoal have been reported to have no effect on the clearance of therapeutic doses of imipramine[119] and to shorten the elimination half-life of amitriptyline by 20 per cent.[25] Because most deaths from TCA overdose occur within hours of drug ingestion, a small increase in clearance is not likely to alter outcome. It is possible, however, that repeated doses of charcoal might shorten the duration of toxicity in slow hydroxylators who have very long TCA half-lives. Little active TCA is excreted in urine, and measures to enhance urinary TCA excretion have a negligible effect on total clearance.[25]

Hemodialysis is ineffective in enhancing the elimination of TCAs because of their extensive protein binding and lipid solubility.[120] Hemoperfusion overcomes these limitations but is relatively ineffective because of the large volume of drug distribution. One study reported removal of less than 2 per cent of the ingested dose of imipramine as parent drug or active metabolite during 6 hours of hemoperfusion.[30] Nevertheless, rapid improvement in cardiotoxicity after TCA overdose has been anecdotally reported during hemoperfusion.[121–123] Because these reports are based on uncontrolled observations, it is possible that improvement was coincidental with, rather than a consequence of, hemoperfusion. In support of this possibility, serum TCA levels often decreased rapidly in the first few hours after admission even without hemoperfusion, presumably because of drug distribution.[60] Animal data are not available. There is, therefore, little support for the use of hemoperfusion in the management of TCA overdose.

Mechanical Support of the Circulation. Because TCA toxicity is reversible, temporary mechanical support of the circulation might be useful in hypotensive patients who are unresponsive to other measures. Serum TCA levels often decline rapidly after overdose owing to distribution of drug to tissues.[60] A temporary period of mechanically assisted circulation might therefore allow time for spontaneous improvement. There is one report of a child who survived 2.5 hours of closed-chest cardiac massage during nonperfusing ventricular tachycardia due to imipramine overdose.[124] Preliminary data in dogs suggest that cardiopulmonary bypass may allow survival after a fatal dose of TCA.[125] Although further study is needed, cardiopulmonary bypass or intra-aortic balloon counterpulsation (for patients with a spontaneous rhythm) should be considered for viable patients who cannot be otherwise supported.

Use of Drug Levels. TCAs can be detected qualitatively in urine by thin-layer chromatography or quantitatively in serum by liquid or gas chromatography. Active demethylated metabolites are usually measured by these methods, but hydroxylated metabolites are not. Therapeutic TCA concentrations (parent compound) are generally in the range of 50 to 300 ng/ml[126] (see Table 34–3).

The correlation of serum TCA concentrations with toxicity is imprecise,[64, 127–129] and their measurement adds little to the management of TCA overdose. Serum concentrations of less than 1 μg/ml are usually associated with minimal toxicity, although even these concentrations may prove toxic with mixed drug ingestions.[58, 130] Life-threatening toxicity is usually accompanied by a serum concentration of greater than 1 μg/ml, and concentrations of greater than 3 to 5 μg/ml are often fatal.[62] The serum TCA concentration may increase up to fivefold post mortem. When using TCA levels to determine cause of death, the measurement of liver drug concentrations[131] or parent/metabolite drug ratios[132] is preferable. Some side effects associated with therapeutic dosing of TCAs are listed in Table 34–5.

Specific Complications

See Table 34–6 for an overview of toxic effects and the treatment of these effects.

QRS Prolongation. QRS prolongation identifies patients at risk for developing arrhythmias, hypotension, or seizures. In the absence of these complications, it is not known whether there is any benefit to treating the QRS duration per se. The potential adverse effects of prophylactic therapy include pulmonary edema from large doses of $NaHCO_3$ (50 mEq sodium/50-ml ampule) and possible aggravation of seizures by hyperventilation. A reasonable approach to patients with QRS prolongation is to correct any factor that might aggravate toxicity (acidosis, hypoxia, dehydration) and institute further therapy only as needed for specific complications.

Sinus Tachycardia. Treatment for sinus tachycardia is not generally needed. Beta blockers may slow the sinus rate but can also impair cardiac output and cause hypotension. Physostigmine can also slow the sinus rate but may precipitate seizures, bradycardia, or asystole.

Atrioventricular Block. First-degree atrioventricular block requires no treatment. Second- (type II) or third-degree atrioventricular block may be managed with a pacemaker or isoproterenol. Owing to the rarity of these complications, data regarding the efficacy of these interventions are lacking.

Table 34–5. ADVERSE EFFECTS OF THERAPEUTIC DOSES OF TCAs

COMMON[156–158]
Postural hypotension
Anticholinergic
Constipation
Urinary retention
Blurred vision
Dry mouth
Sedation
Diaphoresis
UNCOMMON
Agitation[159]
Seizures
Aggravation of seizure disorder[160–162]
New onset of seizures (maprotiline)[163]
Neonatal withdrawal with maternal use of clomipramine[164]
Aggravation of cardiac conduction delay[165–167]
Tardive dyskinesia (amoxapine)[168]
Syndrome of inappropriate antidiuretic hormone[169, 170]
Neuroleptic malignant syndrome (amoxapine)[171]

Ventricular Tachycardia. Predisposing factors such as acidosis, hypotension, and hyperthermia should be corrected. If a beta-1 agonist is being used for inotropic support, the lowest effective dose should be used. The only measures that have been experimentally demonstrated as beneficial for ventricular arrhythmias are $NaHCO_3$, hyperventilation, and lidocaine. $NaHCO_3$ may be administered until the arrhythmia subsides or arterial blood pH is 7.5 to 7.55. Lidocaine may be used if $NaHCO_3$ is ineffective but should be administered slowly to avoid precipitating seizures. The use of other antiarrhythmic agents is limited because Class IA or IC drugs may worsen sodium channel inhibition and aggravate cardiotoxicity.[133] DC countershock may be useful if hypotension is present. Overdrive pacing has been suggested for refractory ventricular arrhythmias,[107] but its efficacy is not known.

Wide-complex Tachycardia. Diagnostic strategies for differentiating ventricular tachycardia from sinus tachycardia with QRS prolongation have been discussed previously (see section on wide-complex tachycardia without P waves). When diagnosis of the rhythm is not possible, it is reasonable to correct potential aggravating factors and administer $NaHCO_3$ as described previously for ventricular tachycardia. These maneuvers may correct ventricular tachycardia and are not likely to compromise the patient if the rhythm is supraventricular. It has been suggested that further measures be withheld if blood pressure is stable and that the rhythm be considered ventricular tachycardia (and treated as such) if the patient is hypotensive.[107]

Ventricular Bradycardia. This rhythm is often agonal, and there are no data regarding its management in TCA overdose. The usual therapy in other situations is a pacemaker or isoproterenol.

Hypotension. Acidosis and hyperthermia should be corrected. A fluid challenge often corrects mild hypotension[53] and may facilitate the management of more severe hypotension. For hypotension unresponsive to fluids, both $NaHCO_3$ and sympathomimetic agents have been shown useful. $NaHCO_3$ is generally used first because of its safety.

Table 34–6. TREATMENT OF TCA TOXICITY

TOXIC EFFECT	TREATMENT
Cardiovascular	
QRS prolongation	$NaHCO_3$ (not clear if treatment indicated in the absence of arrhythmias or hypotension)
Atrioventricular block —type II 2° or 3°	Pacemaker Isoproterenol
Severe hypertension	Nitroprusside
Hypotension	Correct: acidosis, hyperthermia, seizures Intravascular volume expansion $NaHCO_3$ Vasopressors (norepinephrine) Inotropes (dopamine, dobutamine) Mechanical support: intra-aortic balloon pump, cardiopulmonary bypass
Sinus tachycardia	Rarely needed
Ventricular tachycardia	Correct: acidosis, hyperthermia, hypotension, seizures $NaHCO_3$ Lidocaine DC cardioversion Overdrive pacing Avoid Class IA or IC antiarrhythmic agents
Torsades de pointes	Pacemaker Isoproterenol
Premature ventricular beats	$NaHCO_3$ Lidocaine
Ventricular bradycardia	Correct hypoxia Pacemaker Isoproterenol
Other	
Delirium	Restraints usually sufficient Benzodiazepine Neuromuscular blockade for severe hyperthermia
Seizures	Diazepam Phenytoin Neuromuscular blockade for severe acidosis, hyperthermia
Hyperthermia	Control: seizures, myoclonus, agitation Cooling: external or ice gastric lavage

In animals, a variety of inotropic and vasopressor agents have been reported to be useful for TCA-induced hypotension; these include dopamine, norepinephrine, isoproterenol, and prenalterol.[120, 134, 135] It is not clear which agent is most effective, and no comparisons of these drugs are available in patients. Because both vasodilation and impaired cardiac contractility may contribute to hypotension, the requirements of individual patients for inotropic or vasopressor drugs may differ. A pulmonary artery catheter is often helpful in tailoring therapy, but treatment must generally be initiated before such a catheter can be placed. One approach is to start with a vasopressor such as norepinephrine[54] and, if necessary, add an inotrope such as dopamine or dobutamine. The theoretical advantage of this sequence is that norepinephrine, with less beta-1 agonist activity, is less likely to aggravate or precipitate ventricular tachycardia. Alternatively, the initial use of a drug such as dopamine would provide inotropic as well as vasopressor actions.

Hypertension. Hypertension is generally mild, of short duration, and requires no treatment. If severe (blood pressure > 170 mmHg systolic or 110 mmHg diastolic), a rapidly titratable drug such as nitroprusside should be used because TCA-induced hypotension may develop later.

Seizures. Because seizures may aggravate cardiotoxicity, their early termination is important. Controlled studies of seizure management in patients are not available. However, anecdotal observations in patients suggest that diazepam is effective for terminating seizures and does not worsen hypotension or arrhythmias, even with repeated doses.[68, 134] Intravenous phenytoin at a dose of 15 mg/kg is subsequently administered at a rate of 20 to 40 mg/min for control of TCA-induced seizures.[108] (See Chapter 1 for further discussion of seizure management.)

In addition to anticonvulsant therapy, the consequences of seizures should be managed supportively. Acidosis may be minimized by ensuring adequate ventilation during seizures (using manual bag ventilation if mechanical ventilation is ineffective). Prolonged seizures, and the resulting lactic acidosis, may also require administration of $NaHCO_3$. Core temperature should be obtained and hyperthermia treated. In patients with frequent seizures or status epilepticus, conservative measures may fail to prevent acidosis or hyperthermia. Such patients may benefit from a brief period of neuromuscular blockade.[51] Prolonged paralysis should be avoided so that seizures are not obscured. As in other clinical situations, prolonged seizures (> 2 hours) carry the risk of permanent brain injury.

Delirium. Mechanical restraint is usually sufficient, but other measures may be needed in agitated patients to allow tracheal intubation or control of hyperthermia. Sedation may precipitate respiratory depression. If sedation is required, a benzodiazepine is least likely to aggravate cardiotoxicity.[68, 134] Neuromuscular blockade has been useful in patients with severe agitation and hyperthermia.[51]

Coma. Management of a decreased level of consciousness may require tracheal intubation and mechanical ventilation. Physostigmine may improve the level of consciousness but is contraindicated because it may precipitate seizures or asystole.

Hyperthermia. Patients at highest risk for hyperthermia (those with agitation, myoclonus, seizures) should have their core temperature measured at least every 30 minutes because of the rapidity with which hyperthermia may develop.[51] A core temperature of more than 105°F may cause neurologic damage.[51] Cooling should be initiated well before this temperature is reached. Cooling may be accomplished by standard measures, including external application of ice, evaporative cooling, or ice-water gastric lavage.[51] If seizures or agitation cannot be adequately controlled, paralysis may be needed to facilitate cooling.

DRUG INTERACTIONS

Some TCA drug interactions are listed in Table 34–7. Concurrent overdose with monoamine oxidase inhibitors and TCAs has been reported to produce seizures, coma, and hyperpyrexia. Because these toxic effects may also occur with either drug alone, the extent to which this represents an interaction is unclear. Similar toxicity has been reported with therapeutic doses of TCAs and monoamine oxidase inhibitors together, particularly clomipramine or TCAs that inhibit serotonin reuptake.[136, 137] Recent reports suggest that other TCAs may be safely combined with monoamine oxidase inhibitors for the treatment of refractory depression. Some authors recommend that treatment be initiated with the TCA alone and that the monoamine oxidase inhibitor be added several days later.[3]

Recent data suggest that administration of

Table 34–7. DRUG INTERACTIONS WITH TCAs

DRUG	INTERACTION
	Therapeutic Dose
ethanol (chronic)	Increased TCA clearance[13]
disulfiram	Decreased TCA clearance[172]
cimetidine	Decreased TCA clearance[173, 174]
halothane	Arrhythmias[175]
sympathomimetics phenylephrine norepinephrine epinephrine	Increased pressor response to sympathomimetic[176]
monoamine oxidase inhibitors	Seizures, coma, hyperthermia[136, 137, 177]
clonidine	Loss of clonidine's antihypertensive effect[178]
guanethidine	TCAs antagonize antihypertensive effect[179]
cocaine	Exaggerate increase in heart rate and blood pressure (desipramine)[139]
anticholinergics	Additive effects[146, 157]
vasodilators	Additive effects[146, 157]
	Overdose
beta blockers	Additive negative inotropic effect
Class Ia or Ic antiarrhythmic agents	Additive conduction delay
physostigimine	Bradycardia, asystole, seizures[7, 58]

desipramine to cocaine abusers may reduce their craving for cocaine and may have a role in the treatment of cocaine addiction.[138] However, desipramine inhibits neuronal norepinephrine reuptake and may exaggerate the increases in heart rate and blood pressure associated with cocaine abuse.[139] The safety of administering desipramine to cocaine abusers therefore requires further study.

Pharmacodynamic interactions of importance in the setting of TCA overdose may be seen with drugs that have similar toxic effects, such as impairment of cardiac contractility (beta blockers) or conduction (Class IA and IC antiarrhythmic agents). Cholinergic agonists such as physostigmine may cause severe bradyarrhythmias or asystole in patients with TCA overdose.[117]

ATYPICAL ANTIDEPRESSANTS

Trazodone

Trazodone (Desyrel) is a selective inhibitor of neuronal serotonin uptake. It lacks the quinidine-like toxicity (sodium channel inhibition) of the TCAs[140] and has little anticholinergic activity. Overdose toxicity (of an ingested dose up to 9.2 gm) is largely limited to nausea, vomiting, and a decreased level of consciousness.[9, 141, 142] Although trazodone is an alpha-adrenergic blocker, hypotension has not been a feature of overdose. Reported deaths have generally involved other sedating drugs in addition to trazodone. Priapism, usually a complication of therapeutic dosing, may also occur after overdose.[143] Single case reports have implicated trazodone in aggravating pre-existing ventricular tachycardia[144] and contributing to sinus arrest following electroconvulsive therapy,[145] but a causal role for trazodone in these instances is not established.

Fluoxetine

Like trazodone, fluoxetine (Prozac) selectively inhibits neuronal serotonin uptake. There is little binding to histaminic, cholinergic, or alpha-adrenergic receptors.[146] Fluoxetine does not inhibit the fast sodium channel of myocardial cells and is devoid of the cardiac toxicity of TCAs.[147] In mice and rats, the principal toxic effect of very high doses (25 to 56 mg/kg) is seizures.[148] Experience with overdose in humans is limited. One patient had two brief seizures after ingesting 3 gm fluoxetine. Eight additional patients tolerated overdose of fluoxetine with minimal or no symptoms. The only reported death involved multiple additional drugs.[148] An interaction between therapeutic doses of fluoxetine and monoamine oxidase inhibitors has been reported, consisting of shivering, nausea, confusion, and anxiety.[149]

References

1. Fréjaville JP, Nicaise AM, Christoforov B, Sraer JD, Pebay-Payroula F, Gaultier M: Étude statistique d'une seconde centaine d'intoxications aiguës par les dérivés de l'iminodibenzyle (tofranil, pertofan, G 34, surmontil) et ceux du dihydrobenzocyclohepadiène (laroxyl, elavil). Bul Soc Med Hop Paris *117*:1151, 1966.
2. Richardson JW, Richelson E: Antidepressants: A clinical update for medical practitioners. Mayo Clin Proc *59*:330, 1984.
3. Brotman AW, Falk WE, Gelenberg AJ: Pharmacologic treatment of acute depressive subtypes. *In* Meltzer HY (ed): Psychopharmacology: The Third Generation of Progress. New York, Raven Press, 1987, p 1031.
4. Litovitz TL, Troutman WH: Amoxapine overdose—seizures and fatalities. JAMA *250*:1069, 1983.
5. Kulig K, Rumack B, Sullivan JB: Amoxapine overdose: Coma and seizures without cardiotoxic effects. JAMA *248*:1092, 1982.
6. Munger MA, Effron BA: Amoxapine cardiotoxicity. Ann Emerg Med *17*:274, 1988.
7. Knudsen K, Heath A: Effects of self-poisoning with maprotiline. Br Med J *288*:601, 1984.
8. Wedin GP, Odera GM, Klein-Schwartz W, Gorman R: Relative toxicity of cyclic antidepressants. Ann Emerg Med *15*:797, 1986.
9. Gamble ED, Peterson LG: Trazodone overdose: Four years of experience from voluntary reports. J Clin Psychiatry *47*:544, 1986.
10. Chand S, Crome P, Dawling S: One hundred cases of acute intoxication with mianserin hydrochloride. Pharmakopsychiatr Neuropsychopharmacol *14*:15, 1981.
11. Crome P: Overdose of selective antidepressants. *In* Costa E, Radagni G (eds): Typical and Atypical Antidepressants: Clinical Practice. New York, Raven Press, 1982.
12. Cassidy S, Henry J: Fatal toxicity of antidepressant drugs in overdose. Br Med J *295*:1021, 1987.
13. Ciraulo DA, Barnhill JG, Jaffe JH: Clinical pharmacokinetics of imipramine and desipramine in alcoholics and normal volunteers. Clin Pharmacol Ther *43*:509, 1988.
14. Alexanderson B, Borga O, Alvan G: The availability of orally administered nortriptyline. Eur J Clin Pharmacol *5*:181, 1973.
15. Brosen K, Gram LF: First-pass metabolism of imipramine and desipramine: Impact of the sparteine

oxidation phenotype. Clin Pharmacol Ther *43*:400, 1988.
16. DeVane CL, Simpkins JW, Stout SA: Cerebral and blood pharmacokinetics of imipramine and its active metabolites in the pregnant rat. Psychopharmacol Bull *84*:225, 1984.
17. Della Corte L, Sgaragli GP: Tissue distribution of chlorimipramine and its demethylated metabolite after a single dose in the rat. Pharmacol Res Commun *16*:207, 1984.
18. Pentel P, Benowitz N: Efficacy and mechanism of action of sodium bicarbonate in the treatment of desipramine toxicity in rats. J Pharmacol Exp Ther *230*:12, 1984.
19. Schultz P, Turner-Tamiyasy K, Smith G, Giacomini KM, Blaschke TF: Amitriptyline disposition in young and elderly normal men. Clin Pharmacol Ther *33*:360, 1983.
20. Gram LF, Bjerre M, Kragh-Sorenson P, Kvinesdal B, Molin J, Pedersen OL, Reisby N: Imipramine metabolites in blood of patients during therapy and after overdose. Clin Pharmacol Ther *33*:335, 1983.
21. Abernathy DR, Greenblatt DJ, Shader RI: Imipramine disposition in users of oral contraceptive steroids. Clin Pharmacol Ther *35*:792, 1984.
22. Dawling S, Crome P, Graithwaite R: Pharmacokinetics of single oral doses of nortriptyline in depressed elderly hospital patients and young healthy volunteers. Clin Pharmacokinet *5*:394, 1980.
23. Nelson JC, Jatlow PI: Nonlinear desipramine kinetics: Prevalence and importance. Clin Pharmacol Ther *41*:666, 1987.
24. Spina E, Henthorn TK, Eleborg L, Nordin C, Sawe J: Desmethylimipramine overdose: Nonlinear kinetics in a slow hydroxylator. Ther Drug Mon *7*:239, 1985.
25. Karkkainen S, Neuvonen PJ: Pharmacokinetics of amitriptyline influenced by oral charcoal and urine pH. Clin Pharmacol Toxicol *24*:326, 1986.
26. Hucker HB, Balletto AJ, Demetriades J, Arison BH, Zacchei AG: Urinary metabolites of amitriptyline in the dog. Drug Metab Disp *5*:132, 1977.
27. Tasset JJ, Pesce AJ: Amoxapine in human overdose. J Anal Toxicol *8*:124, 1984.
28. Bickel MH, Baggiolini M: The metabolism of imipramine and its metabolites by rat liver microsomes. Biochem Pharmacol *15*:1155, 1966.
29. Jandhyala BS, Steenberg JM, Perel JM, Manian AA, Buckley JP: Effects of several tricyclic antidepressants on the hemodynamics and myocardial contractility of the anesthetized dog. Eur J Pharmacol *42*:403, 1977.
30. Pentel PR, Bullock ML, DeVane CL: Hemoperfusion for imipramine overdose: Elimination of active metabolites. J Toxicol—Clin Toxicol *19*:239, 1982.
31. Breyer-Pfaff U, Prox A, Wachsmith H, Yao P: Phenolic metabolites of amitriptyline and nortriptyline in rat bile. Drug Metab Disp *15*:882, 1987.
32. Gard H, Knapp D, Walle T, Gaffney: Qualitative and quantitative studies on the disposition of amitriptyline and other tricyclic antidepressant drugs in man as it relates to the management of the overdosed patient. Clin Toxicol *6*:571, 1973.
33. Brosen KD, Otton V, Gram LF: Imipramine demethylation and hydroxylation: Impact of the sparteine oxidation phenotype. Clin Pharmacol Ther *40*:543, 1986.
34. Javaid JI, Hendricks K, Davis JM: Alpha-1-acid glycoprotein involvement in high affinity binding of tricyclic antidepressants to human plasma. Biochem Pharmacol *32*:1149, 1983.
35. Freilich DI, Giardina EV: Imipramine binding to alpha-1-acid glycoprotein in normal subjects and cardiac patients. Clin Pharmacol Ther *35*:670, 1984.
36. Pentel PR, Keyler DE: Effects of high dose alpha-1-acid glycoprotein on desipramine toxicity in rats. J Pharmacol Exp Ther *246*:1061, 1988.
37. Levitt MA, Sullivan JB Jr, Owens SM, Burnham L, Finley PR: Amitriptyline plasma protein binding: Effect of plasma pH and relevance to clinical overdose. Am J Emerg Med *4*:121, 1986.
38. Connolly SJ, Mitchell LB, Swerdlow CD, Mason JW, Winkle RA: Clinical efficacy and electrophysiology of imipramine for ventricular tachycardia. Am J Cardiol *53*:516, 1984.
39. Weld FM, Bigger JT Jr: Electrophysiological effects of imipramine on ovine cardiac Purkinje and ventricular muscle fibers. Circ Res *46*:167, 1980.
40. Wit AL, Cranefield PF, Hoffman BF: Slow conduction and re-entry in the ventricular conducting system. Circ Res *30*:11, 1972.
41. Reiter M: Calcium mobilization and cardiac inotropic mechanisms. Pharmacol Rev *40*:189, 1988.
42. Nattel S: Frequency-dependent effects of amitriptyline on ventricular conduction and cardiac rhythm in dogs. Circulation *72*:898, 1985.
43. Nattel S, Mittleman M: Treatment of ventricular tachyarrhythmias resulting from amitriptyline toxicity in dogs. J Pharmacol Exp Ther *231*:430, 1984.
44. Tamargo J, Rodriguez S, Garcia De Jalon P: Electrophysiological effects of desipramine on guinea pig papillary muscles. Eur J Pharmacol *55*:171, 1979.
45. Krikler DM, Curry PVL: Torsade de pointes, an atypical ventricular tachycardia. Br Heart J *38*:117, 1976.
46. Schwartz R, Esler M: Catecholamine levels in tricyclic antidepressant self-poisoning. Aust NZ J Med *4*:479, 1974.
47. Harvengt C, Desager JP, Vanderbrist M, Bogaert M, Moerman E: Sympathetic nervous system response in acute cardiovascular toxicity induced by amitriptyline in conscious rabbits. Toxicol Appl Pharmacol *44*:115, 1978.
48. Jackson JE, Banner W: Tricyclic antidepressant intoxication: Effects of physostigmine and bicarbonate. Vet Hum Toxicol *24*:39, 1982.
49. Sigg EB, Osborne M, Kobol B: Cardiovascular effects of imipramine. J Pharmacol Exp Ther *141*:237, 1963.
50. Richelson E: Antimuscarinic and other receptor-blocking properties of antidepressants. Mayo Clin Proc *58*:40, 1983.
51. Rosenberg J, Pentel PR, Pond S, Benowitz N: Hyperthermia associated with drug intoxication. Vet Hum Toxicol *26*:413, 1984.
52. Malatynska E, Knapp RJ, Masaaki I, Yamamura HI: Antidepressants and seizure-interactions at the GABA-receptor chloride-ionophore complex. Life Sci *43*:303, 1988.
53. Langou RA, Van Dyke C, Tahan SR, Cohen LS: Cardiovascular manifestations of tricyclic antidepressant overdose. Am Heart J *100*:458, 1980.
54. Teba L, Schiebel F, Dedhia HV, Lazzell VA: Beneficial effect of norepinephrine in the treatment of circulatory shock caused by tricyclic antidepressant overdose. Am J Emerg Med *6*:566, 1988.
55. Levitt A, Sullivan J, Owens M, Finley F, Burnham L: Change in amitriptyline plasma protein binding

with increase in plasma pH over 7.4. Vet Hum Toxicol *26*:399, 1984.
56. Hulten BA, Heath A: Clinical aspects of tricyclic antidepressant poisoning. Acta Med Scand *213*:275, 1982.
57. Callaham M, Kassel D: Epidemiology of fatal tricyclic antidepressant ingestion: Implications for management. Ann Emerg Med *14*:1, 1985.
58. Pentel P, Sioris L: Incidence of late arrhythmias following tricyclic antidepressant overdose. Clin Toxicol *18*:543, 1981.
59. Crome P, Newman B: Fatal tricyclic antidepressant poisoning. J Royal Soc Med *72*:649, 1979.
60. Bramble MG, Lishman AH, Purdon J, Diffey BL, Hall RJC: An analysis of plasma levels and 24-hour ECG recordings in tricyclic antidepressant poisoning: Implications for management. Q J Med *56*:357, 1985.
61. Thorstrand C: Clinical features in poisonings by tricyclic antidepressants with special reference to ECG. Acta Med Scand *199*:337, 1976.
62. Biggs JT, Spiker DG, Petit JM, Ziegler VE: Tricyclic antidepressant overdose: Incidence of symptoms. JAMA *238*:135, 1977.
63. Niemann JT, Bessen HA, Rothstein RJ, Laks MM: Electrocardiographic criteria for tricyclic antidepressant cardiotoxicity. Am J Cardiol *57*:1154, 1986.
64. Boehnert MT, Lovejoy FH: Value of the QRS duration versus the serum drug level in predicting seizures and ventricular arrhythmias after an acute overdose of tricyclic antidepressants. N Engl J Med *313*:474, 1985.
65. Frommer DA, Kulig K, Marx JA, Rumack B: Tricyclic antidepressant overdose. JAMA *257*:521, 1987.
66. Foulke GE, Albertson TE, Walby WF: Tricyclic antidepressant overdose: Emergency department findings as predictors of clinical course. Am J Emerg Med *4*:496, 1986.
67. Shannon M, Merola J, Lovejoy FH: Hypotension in severe tricyclic antidepressant overdose. Am J Emerg Med *6*:439, 1988.
68. Ellison DW, Pentel PR: Clinical features and consequences of seizures due to cyclic antidepressant overdose. Am J Emerg Med *7*:5, 1989.
69. Davison ET: Amitriptyline-induced torsade de pointes: Successful therapy with atrial pacing. J Electrocardiol *18*:299, 1985.
70. Curtis RA, Giacona N, Burrows D, Baumann JL, Schaffer M: Fatal maprotiline intoxication. Drug Intell Clin Pharmacol *18*:716, 1984.
71. Hermann HC, Kaplan LM, Bierer BE: Q-T prolongation and torsades de pointes ventricular tachycardia produced by the tetracyclic antidepressant agent maprotiline. Am J Cardiol *51*:904, 1983.
72. Barnes RJ, Kong SM, Wu RWY: Electrocardiographic changes in amitriptyline poisoning. Br Med J *3*:222, 1968.
73. Freeman JW, Mundy GR, Beattie RR, Ryan C: Cardiac abnormalities in poisoning with tricyclic antidepressant. Br Med J *2*:610, 1969.
74. Sedal L, Korman MG, Williams PO, Mushin G: Overdosage of tricyclic antidepressants: A report of two deaths and a prospective study of 24 patients. Med J Aust 2:74, 1972.
75. McAlpine SB, Calabro JJ, Robinson MD, Burkle FM: Late death in tricyclic antidepressant overdose revisited. Ann Emerg Med *15*:1349, 1986.
76. Greenland P, Howe TA: Cardiac monitoring in tricyclic antidepressant overdose. Heart Lung *10*:856, 1981.
77. Goldberg RJ, Capone RJ, Hunt JD: Cardiac complications following tricyclic antidepressant overdose. JAMA *254*:1772, 1985.
78. Jennings AE, Levey AS, Harrington JT: Amoxapine-associated acute renal failure. Arch Intern Med *143*:1525, 1983.
79. Burks JS, Walker JE, Rumack BH, Ott JE: Tricyclic antidepressant poisoning: Reversal of coma, choreoathetosis, and myoclonus by physostigmine. JAMA *230*:1405, 1974.
80. Nosko MG, McLean DR, Chin WDN: Loss of brain stem and pupillary reflexes in amoxapine overdose: A case report. Clin Toxicol *26*:117, 1988.
81. Shannon M, Lovejoy FH: Pulmonary consequences of severe tricyclic antidepressant ingestion. Clin Toxicol *25*:443, 1987.
82. Buinsohn A, Eisenberg ES, Jacob H, Rosen J, Bock J, Frishman WH: Seizures and intraventricular conduction defect in propranolol poisoning. Ann Intern Med *91*:860, 1979.
83. Boland ME, Roper SM, Henry JA: Complications of quinine poisoning. Lancet *1*:384, 1985.
84. Baker PB, Merigan KS, Roberts JR, Pesce AJ, Kaplan LA, Rashkin MC: Hypothermia, hypertension, hypertonia and coma in a massive thioridazine overdose. Am J Emerg Med *6*:346, 1988.
85. Riou B, Barriot P, Rimailho A, Baud FJ: Treatment of severe choroquine poisoning. N Engl J Med *318*:1, 1988.
86. Beermann B, Edhag O, Vallin H: Advanced heart block aggravated by carbamazepine. Br Heart J *37*:668, 1975.
87. Weaver DF, Camfield P, Fraser A: Massive carbamazepine overdose: Clinical and pharmacologic observations in five episodes. Neurology *38*:755, 1988.
88. O'Riordan W, Gilette P, Calderon J, Stennes RL: Overdose of cyclobenzaprine, the tricyclic muscle relaxant. Ann Emerg Med *15*:592, 1986.
89. Linden CH, Mitchiner JC, Lindzon RD, Rumack BH: Cyclobenzaprine overdosage. J Toxicol Clin Toxicol *20*:281, 1983.
90. Haddad LM: Tricyclic antidepressant overdose. *In* Haddad LM, Winchester JF (eds): Clinical Management of Poisoning and Drug Overdose. Philadelphia, WB Saunders, 1983, pp 359–371.
91. Stern TA, O'Gara PT, Mulley AG, Singer DE, Thibault GE: Complications after overdose with tricyclic antidepressants. Crit Care Med *13*:672, 1985.
92. Tokarski GF, Young MJ: Criteria for admitting patients with tricyclic antidepressant overdose. J Emerg Med *6*:121, 1988.
93. Crome P, Dawling S, Graithwaite RA, Masters J, Walkey R: Effect of activated charcoal on absorption of nortriptyline. Lancet *2*:1203, 1977.
94. Wasserman F, Brodsky L, Dick MM, Kathe JH, Rodensky PL: Successful treatment of quinidine and procainamide intoxication: Report of three cases. N Engl J Med *259*:797, 1958.
95. Bellet S, Hamdan G, Somylo A: The reversal of cardiotoxic effects of quinidine by molar sodium lactate. Clin Res *6*:226, 1958.
96. Bellet S, Hamdan G, Somylo A, Lara R: The reversal of cardiotoxic effects of quinidine by molar sodium lactate: An experimental study. Am J Med Sci *237*:165, 1959.
97. Bismuth C, Peray-Peyroula F, Frejaville J-P, Efthy-

miou M-L, Fournier E: Nouveaux cas d'intoxication aigue par les derives tricycliques: Traitement par les sels de sodium. J Eur Toxicol *6*:285, 1969.
98. Brown TCK: Sodium bicarbonate treatment for tricyclic antidepressant arrhythmias in children. Med J Aust *2*:380, 1976.
99. Brown TCK, Barker GA, Dunlop ME, Loughnan PM: The use of sodium bicarbonate in the treatment of tricyclic antidepressant-induced arrhythmias. Anaesth Intensive Care *1*:203, 1973.
100. Gaultier M, Pebay-Peyroula F: Intoxication aigue par antidepresseurs tricycliques. La Revue du Praticien *21*:2259, 1971.
101. Hoffman JR, McElroy CR: Bicarbonate therapy for dysrhythmia and hypotension in tricyclic antidepressant overdose. West J Med *134*:60, 1981.
102. Nattel S, Keable H, Sasyniuk BI: Experimental amitriptyline intoxication: Electrophysiologic manifestations and management. J Cardiovasc Pharmacol *6*:83, 1984.
103. Hedges JR, Baker B, Tasset JJ, Otten EJ, Dalsey WC, Sverud SA: Bicarbonate therapy for the cardiovascular toxicity of amitriptyline in an animal model. J Emerg Med *3*:253, 1985.
104. Sasyniuk BI, Jhamandas V: Mechanism of reversal of toxic effects of amitriptyline on cardiac Purkinje fibers by sodium bicarbonate. J Pharmacol Exp Ther *231*:387, 1984.
105. Bessen HA, Niemann JT, Haskell RJ, Rothstein RJ: Effect of respiratory alkalosis in tricyclic antidepressant overdose. West J Med *139*:373, 1983.
106. Kingston ME: Hyperventilation in tricyclic antidepressant poisoning. Crit Care Med *7*:550, 1979.
107. Pentel PR, Benowitz NL: Tricyclic antidepressant poisoning: Management of arrhythmias. Med Toxicol *1*:101, 1986.
108. Frommer DA, Kulig KW, Marx JA, Rumack BH: Tricyclic antidepressant overdose. A review. JAMA *257*:521–526, 1987.
109. Boehnert M, Lovejoy FH Jr: The effect of phenytoin on cardiac conduction and ventricular arrhythmias in acute tricyclic antidepressant (TCA) overdose. Vet Hum Toxicol *27*:297, 1985.
110. Hagerman GA, Hanashiro PK: Reversal of tricyclic-antidepressant-induced cardiac conduction abnormalities by phenytoin. Ann Emerg Med *10*:82, 1981.
111. Kulig K, Bar-or D, Marx J, Wythe E, Rumack BH: Phenytoin as treatment for tricyclic antidepressant cardiotoxicity in a canine model. Vet Hum Toxicol *26*:399, 1984.
112. Mayron R, Ruiz E: Phenytoin: Does it reverse tricyclic antidepressant induced cardiac conduction abnormalities? Ann Emerg Medicine *14*:505, 1985.
113. Callaham M, Schumaker H, Pentel P: Phenytoin prophylaxis of cardiotoxicity in experimental amitriptyline poisoning. J Pharmacol Exp Ther *245*:216, 1988.
114. Gerdes DA, Krenzelok EP: Seizure prophylaxis in amoxapine overdose (abs). Vet Hum Toxicol *26*:399, 1984.
115. Beaubien AR, Carpenter DC, Mathieu LF, MacConaill M, Hrdina PD: Antagonism of imipramine poisoning by anticonvulsants in the rat. Tox Appl Pharmacol *38*:1, 1976.
116. Slovis TL, Ott JE, Teitelbaum DT, Lipscomb W: Physostigmine therapy in acute tricyclic antidepressant poisoning. Clin Toxicol *4*:451, 1971.
117. Pentel P, Peterson CD: Asystole complicating physostigmine treatment of tricyclic antidepressant overdose. Ann Emerg Med *9*:588, 1980.
118. Freeman JW, Loughhead MG: Beta blockade in the treatment of tricyclic antidepressant overdosage. Med J Aust *1*:1233, 1973.
119. Goldberg MJ, Park GD, Spector R, Fischer LJ, Feldman RD: Lack of effect of oral activated charcoal on imipramine clearance. Clin Pharmacol Exp Ther *38*:350, 1985.
120. Heath A, Wickstrom I, Martensson E, Ahlmen J: Treatment of antidepressant poisoning with resin hemoperfusion. Hum Toxicol *1*:361, 1982.
121. Diaz-Buxo JA, Farmer CD, Chandler JT: Hemoperfusion in the treatment of amitriptyline intoxication. Trans Am Soc Artif Intern Organs *24*:699, 1978.
122. Marbury T, Mahoney J, Foller T, Juncos L, Cade R: Treatment of amitriptyline overdosage with charcoal hemoperfusion. Kidney Int *12*:485, 1978.
123. Pedersen RS, Jorgensen KA, Olesen AS, Christensen KN: Charcoal haemoperfusion and antidepressant overdose. Lancet *1*:719, 1978.
124. Southall DP, Kilpatrick SM: Imipramine poisoning: Survival of a child after prolonged cardiac massage. Br Med J *4*:508, 1974.
125. Martin TG, O'Connell JJ, Pentel PR, Miller DL, Keyler DE: Resuscitation from severe cyclic antidepressant toxicity using cardiopulmonary bypass (abs). Vet Hum Toxicol *30*:354, 1988.
126. Perry PJ, Pfohl BM, Holstad SG: The relationship between antidepressant response and tricyclic antidepressant plasma concentrations. Clin Pharmacokinet *13*:381, 1987.
127. Rudorfer MV: Cardiovascular changes and plasma drug levels after amitriptyline overdose. J Toxicol Clin Toxicol *19*:67, 1982.
128. Nicotra MB, Rivera M, Pool JL, Matthew WN: Tricyclic antidepressant overdose: Clinical and pharmacologic observations. Clin Toxicol *18*:599, 1981.
129. Salzman C: Clinical use of antidepressant blood levels and the electrocardiogram. N Engl J Med *313*:512, 1985.
130. Crome P, Braithwaite RA: Relationship between clinical features of tricyclic antidepressant poisoning and plasma concentrations in children. Arch Dis Child *53*:902, 1978.
131. Apple FS, Bandt CM: Liver and blood postmortem tricyclic antidepressant concentrations. J Clin Pathol *89*:794, 1988.
132. Bailey DN, Shaw RF: Interpretation of blood and tissue concentrations in fatal self-ingested overdose involving amitriptyline: An update (1978–1979). J Anal Toxicol *4*:232, 1980.
133. Schwartz JB, Keefe D, Harrison DC: Adverse effects of antiarrhythmic drugs. Drugs *21*:23, 1981.
134. Follmer CH, Lum BK: Protective action of diazepam and of sympathomimetic amines against amitriptyline-induced toxicity. J Pharmacol Exp Ther *222*:424, 1982.
135. Sangster B, de Groot G, Borst C, de Wildt D: Dopamine and isoproterenol in imipramine intoxication in the dog. Clin Toxicol *23*:407, 1985.
136. Marley E, Wozniack KM: Clinical and experimental aspects of interactions between amine oxidase inhibitors and amine re-uptake inhibitors. Psychol Med *13*:735, 1983.
137. Beaumont G: Clomipramine (anafranil) in the treatment of pain, enuresis and anorexia nervosa. J Int Med Res *1*:435, 1973.
138. Kosten TR, Schumann B, Wright D, Carney MK,

Gawin FH: A preliminary study of desipramine in the treatment of cocaine abuse in methadone maintenance patients. J Clin Psychiatry *48*:442, 1987.
139. Fishman MW, Folton RW: Effects of desipramine maintenance on cocaine self-administration in humans. Psychopharmacol Bull *96*:520, 1988.
140. Byrne JE, Gomoll AW: Differential effects of trazodone and imipramine on intracardiac conduction in the anesthetized dog. Arch Int Pharmacodyn Ther *259*:259, 1982.
141. Lesar T, Kingston R, Dahns R, Saxena K: Trazodone overdose. Ann Emerg Med *12*:221, 1983.
142. Hassan E, Miller DD: Toxicity and elimination of trazodone after overdose. Clin Pharmacol *4*:97, 1985.
143. Scher M, Krieger JN, Sjergens JN, Juergens S: Trazodone and priapism. Am J Psychiatr *140*:1362, 1983.
144. Vlay SC, Friedling S: Trazodone exacerbation of ventricular tachycardia. Am Heart J *106*:604, 1983.
145. McCracken J, Radoslav K: Trazodone administration during ECT associated with cardiac conduction abnormality. Am J Psychiatr *141*:1488, 1984.
146. Stark P, Fuller RX, Wong DT: The pharmacologic profile of fluoxetine. J Clin Psychiatry *46*:7, 1985.
147. Steinberg MI, Smallwood JK, Holland DR, Bymaster FP, Bemis KG: Hemodynamic and electrocardiographic effects of fluoxetine and its major metabolite, norfluoxetine, in anesthetized dogs. Toxicol Appl Pharmacol *82*:70, 1986.
148. Wernicke JF: The side effect profile and safety of fluoxetine. J Clin Psychiatry *46*:59, 1985.
149. Sternbach H: Danger of MAOI therapy after fluoxetine withdrawal. Lancet 2:850, 1988.
150. Lemberger LD, Bergstrom RF, Wolen RL, Farid NA, Enas GG, Aranoff GR: Fluoxetine: Clinical pharmacology and physiologic disposition. J Clin Psychiatry *46*:14, 1985.
151. Hollister LE: Current antidepressants. Ann Rev Pharmacol Toxicol *26*:23, 1986.
152. Ziegler VE, Biggs JT, Wylie LT, Rosen SH, Hawf DJ, Coryell WH: Doxepin kinetics. Clin Pharmacol Ther *23*:573, 1978.
153. Ziegler VE, Biggs JT, Wylie LT, Coryell WH, Hanifl KM, Hawf DJ, Rosen SH: Protriptyline kinetics. Clin Pharmacol Ther *23*:580, 1978.
154. Ankier SI, Martin BK, Rogers MS, Carpenter PK, Graham C: Trazodone: A new assay procedure and some pharmacokinetic parameters. Br J Clin Pharmacol *11*:505, 1981.
155. Alexanderson B: Pharmacokinetics in desmethylimipramine and nortriptyline in man after single and multiple oral doses: A cross-over study. Eur J Clin Pharmacol *5*:1, 1972.
156. Henry JA, Martin AJ: The risk-benefit assessment of antidepressant drugs. Med Toxicol 2:445, 1987.
157. Stark P, Hardison CD: A review of multicenter controlled studies of fluoxetine vs. imipramine and placebo in outpatients with major depressive disorder. J Clin Psychiatry *46*:53, 1985.
158. Glassman AH, Bigger JT, Giardina EV, Kantor SJ, Davies M: Clinical characteristics of imipramine-induced orthostatic hypotension. Lancet *1*:468, 1979.
159. Weiss RD: Relapse to cocaine abuse after initiating desipramine treatment. JAMA *260*:2545, 1988.
160. Jimenez MD, Guharoy S: Tricyclic-induced seizures activity. Drug Intell Clin Pharm *17*:644, 1983.
161. Dallos V, Heathfield K: Iatrogenic epilepsy due to antidepressant drugs. Br Med J *4*:80, 1969.
162. Petti RA, Campbell M: Imipramine and seizures. Am J Psychiatry *132*:538, 1975.
163. Bernard PG, Levine MS: Maprotiline-induced seizures. South Med J *79*:1179, 1986.
164. Cowe L, Lloyd DJ, Dawling S: Neonatal convulsions caused by withdrawal from maternal clomipramine. Br Med J *284*:1837, 1982.
165. Glassman AH: Cardiovascular effects of tricyclic antidepressants. Ann Rev Med *35*:503, 1984.
166. Smith RB, Rusbatch BJ: Amitriptyline and heart block. Br Med J *2*:514, 1967.
167. Kantor SJ, Bigger JT, Glassman AH, Macken DL, Perel JM: Imipramine-induced heart block: A longitudinal case study. JAMA *231*:1364, 1975.
168. Tao GK, Harada DT, Koosikas ME, Dordon MN, Brinkman JH: Amoxapine-induced tardive dyskinesia. Drug Intell Clin Pharm *19*:548, 1985.
169. Lydiard RB: Desipramine-associated SIADH in an elderly woman: Case report. J Clin Psychiatry *44*:153, 1983.
170. Abbott R: Hyponatremia due to antidepressant medications. Ann Emerg Med *12*:708, 1983.
171. Taylor NE, Schwartz HI: Neuroleptic malignant syndrome following amoxapine overdose. J Nerv Ment Dis *176*:249, 1988.
172. Ciraulo DA, Barnhill J, Boxembaum H: Pharmacokinetic interaction of disulfiram and antidepressants. Am J Psychiatry *142*:1373, 1985.
173. Curry SH, DeVane CL, Wolfe MM: Cimetidine interaction with amitriptyline. Eur J Clin Pharmacol *29*:429, 1985.
174. Wells BG, Pieper JA, Stewart CF, Waldon SL, Bobo L, Warner C: The effect of ranitidine and cimetidine on imipramine disposition. Eur J Clin Pharmacol *31*:285, 1986.
175. Edwards RP, Miller RD, Roizen MF, Ham J, Way WL, Lake DR, Roderick L: Cardiac response to imipramine and pancuronium during anesthesia with halothane or enflurane. Anesthesiology *50*:421, 1979.
176. Boakes AJ, Laurence DR, Teoh PC, Barar FSK, Benedikter LT, Prichard BNC: Interactions between sympathomimetic amines and antidepressant agents in man. Br Med J *1*:311, 1973.
177. Rom WN, Benner EJ: Toxicity by interaction of tricyclic antidepressant and monoamine oxidase inhibitor. Calif Med *117*:65, 1972.
178. Briant RH, Reid JL, Dollery CT: Interaction between clonidine and desipramine in man. Br Med J *1*:522, 1973.
179. Mitchell JR: Antagonism of the antihypertensive action of quanethidine sulfate by desipramine hydrochloride. JAMA *202*:973, 1973.

CHAPTER 35
LITHIUM

James F. Winchester, M.D.

Lithium carbonate has revolutionized psychiatric treatment. It has become an indispensable psychiatric tool, responsible for changing many patients with manic-depressive illness from custodial care to almost total rehabilitation. In the United States alone the saving in health care dollars has been estimated to be around 4 billion dollars in the first 10 years (1972–1982) that lithium was approved for restricted use by the Food and Drug Administration. These costs include savings in psychiatric care as well as increased economic production.

Despite the suggestion in 1897 by Lange[1] that lithium might have an effect on depression, not until 1949 did Cade[2] report an effect on mania. Since then, largely from the work of Schou and coworkers,[3, 4] lithium has found its way into standard psychiatric treatment.[5] It is difficult to determine the incidence of lithium intoxication, but approximately 200 cases have been reported, most of them since 1963.[6] As will be outlined, lithium has a narrow therapeutic index, therefore elevations of serum levels above well-defined ranges will result in toxicity. A gradual onset of intoxication is far more common than acute overdose. After cessation of lithium in an intoxicated patient, the symptoms may persist for some time, reflecting the pharmacokinetic and pharmacodynamic handling of lithium. In many cases of lithium intoxication, predisposing factors and drug interaction play major roles.

Acute overdosage results in a mortality rate of 25 per cent, whereas the mortality rate in patients intoxicated during maintenance treatment with lithium is around 9 per cent; in addition, persistent central nervous system or renal damage or both occur in approximately 10 per cent of patients.[6]

Prior to 1950, lithium had been used as a "salt substitute" and had been the major constituent of "7-Up," a well-known American soft drink. The increasing use of lithium in nonpsychiatric disorders (see Table 35–2) will result in an even larger number of patients being exposed to the potential toxicity of lithium in the future.

PHARMACOLOGY AND PHARMACOKINETICS

In the United States, lithium carbonate is the principal formulation used, but lithium citrate is also available in syrup form. In other countries different salts of lithium are available, but the predominant formulation in Canada, the United Kingdom, and Scandinavia is lithium carbonate. In the United Kingdom, 400-mg tablets are available; in Scandinavia, the United Kingdom, and the United States, sustained release formulations may also be obtained. The available lithium preparations are shown in Table 35–1. Lithium is the lightest of all the known metals and exists in nature in various ionized forms and salts. Lithium bromide was used in the past as a hypnotic sedative agent, and lithium chloride at one time was used as a table salt substitute. Its molecular weight is approximately 74 daltons, its atomic number is 3, and atomic weight is 6.94. It is handled by the body very similarly to sodium, but it shows a different emission line than sodium on the flame photometer at around 671 nm. Although lithium chloride was introduced for treatment of manic-depressive psychosis, lithium carbonate was found to be a more stable compound, and accordingly it has come into widespread use.

Lithium produces many metabolic and neuroendocrine changes, but no conclusive evidence favors one particular mode of action. In terms of mineral metabolism, lithium competes for sodium, potassium, magnesium, and calcium, in that order, and displaces them from intracellular and bone sites in this progression. Lithium ions affect neurotransmitter impulses by several methods:[7–9] (1) inhibition of release and augmentation of reuptake of norepinephrine at nerve endings; (2) inhibition of the hydro-osmotic effect of arginine vasopressin[10] via reduction of receptor-mediated synthesis of cyclic AMP from inhibition of the enzyme adenylate cyclase (a mechanism probably responsible for the nephrogenic diabetes insipidus and alterations in thyroid function seen in some pa-

Table 35–1. AVAILABLE LITHIUM (Li) PREPARATIONS*

TRADE NAME	CHEMICAL FORMULATION	DOSAGE FORMS
United States		
Lithane (Miles Pharmaceutical)	lithium carbonate	Tablets, 300 mg
lithium carbonate USP	lithium carbonate	Capsules, 150 mg, 300 mg, 600 mg, and tablets, 300 mg
lithium citrate syrup USP (Roxane)	lithium citrate	Syrup, 8 mEq/5 ml—equivalent to 300 mg of lithium carbonate
Cibalith-S (CIBA)	lithium citrate	Syrup, 8 mEq/5 ml—equivalent to 300 mg of lithium carbonate
Lithobid (CIBA)	lithium carbonate	Tablets, 300 mg (sustained release)
Eskalith (SmithKline)	lithium carbonate	Capsules and tablets, 300 mg
Eskalith CR (SmithKline)	lithium carbonate	Tablets, 300 mg, 450 mg, and capsules, 300 mg (sustained release)
Canada		
Carbolith (ICN)	lithium carbonate	Capsules and tablets, 300 mg
Lithane (Pfizer)	lithium carbonate	As above
Lithizine (Maney)	lithium carbonate	As above
United Kingdom	lithium carbonate	400 mg tablets also available
Scandinavia	lithium carbonate	Sustained release formulation
Litarex		

*Molecular weight = 73.89 daltons; atomic number, 3; atomic weight, 6.94; emission line on flame photometer, 671 nm.

tients). In addition, long-term lithium administration has been shown to stimulate the release of endogenous serotonin from the hippocampus but not from the cortex in animal brains[11]—data which are consistent with the concept that lithium stabilizes serotoninergic neurotransmission. Regardless of its biochemical mechanisms, it is clear that lithium is able to affect receptor sensitivity and bring about changes in neurotransmission. Because of its chemical similarity to sodium, potassium, calcium, and magnesium, lithium may interact or interfere with biochemical pathways for these substances at the cell membrane level and also within the cell.[12]

Gastrointestinal absorption of lithium is rapid and complete following oral administration of tablets or the liquid form of lithium. Peak serum levels are reached within 1 to 2 hours (with the exception of sustained-release formulations), and the drug is freely distributed in whole body water but with a slow uptake by, and release from, central nervous system tissue. In fact, it may take 24 hours for lithium to cross the blood-brain barrier effectively. Lithium is neither protein-bound nor tissue-bound, and with the usual oral doses of 1200 to 1800 mg daily, steady state plasma levels are reached within 5 to 6 days.[4] Conventionally, blood levels for monitoring serum lithium are taken 12 hours after the last dose.

Excretion is predominantly by the kidney, with trace amounts being found in the stools. Approximately 80 per cent of lithium is reabsorbed at the proximal renal tubule, and 20 per cent is excreted in the urine.[13] The avid proximal tubular reabsorption explains the fact that distal tubular diuretics (thiazides, and so on) may cause compensatory increases in proximal tubular reabsorption of both sodium and lithium,[14] while loop diuretics (furosemide and ethacrynic acid) cause continued sodium and lithium excretion.[15] It is of interest that the serum half-life of lithium is shorter in a young person compared with an older person; values of 18 hours in the former and 36 hours in the latter have been reported.[16] On average, the half-life of elimination ($\tau_{1/2}$) is approximately 29 hours for an adult; thus serum levels normally would fall by about 20 per cent within 6 hours of stopping lithium therapy.[17] It is important that the $\tau_{1/2}$ correlates with the glomerular filtration rate, since renal lithium clearance is estimated to be approximately a quarter of that of creatinine clearance.[15] In view of the pharmacokinetic handling of lithium in elderly patients and in those with diminished renal capacity, it is essential that levels in patients receiving lithium be monitored almost continuously. Lithium renal clearance (C_{Li}) is normally 10 to 40 ml per min, and the fractional excretion of lithium ($FE_{Li} = C_{Li}/C_{creatinine}$) is approximately 17 to 30 per cent. The apparent volume of distribution of lithium is slightly greater than whole body water—around 0.79 liter per kg of body weight.

The renal elimination of lithium is influenced by several factors, including sodium and water balance, the presence of drugs that affect renal tubular reabsorption of sodium, and other phenomena. As will be discussed, any condition leading to sodium and water imbalance may seriously affect the handling of lithium by the kidney and consequently may predispose to toxicity. Another interesting phenomenon not fully explained is that manic patients may tolerate high levels of lithium during the initial control of their manic state, but after control it has been observed that patients become less tolerant to high serum levels of lithium.[18] On the other hand, lithium toxicity may appear in the elderly patient at lower serum levels than usual, and, in the elderly, therapeutic levels may be around 0.2 mEq per liter.[7]

THERAPEUTIC USES

Table 35–2 outlines the therapeutic uses of lithium. In the United States, lithium is approved only for the treatment of manic-depressive (bipolar) illness, but as can be seen from Table 35–2, it has been used experimentally in a wide variety of psychiatric and nonpsychiatric disorders. Because of the observation that lithium induces leukocytosis as a side effect of treatment,[19] lithium carbonate has been used to reduce infection and leukopenia in patients receiving systemic chemotherapy.[20]

Table 35–2. THERAPEUTIC USES OF LITHIUM

PSYCHIATRIC DISORDERS	NONPSYCHIATRIC DISORDERS
Manic-depressive (bipolar) illness*	Pain
Unipolar depressive illness	Premenstrual tension
Behavior disorders	Leukopenia/chemotherapy
Character disorders	Felty's syndrome
Pain	Thyrotoxicosis
Alcoholism/drug abuse	Tardive dyskinesia
Premenstrual tension	Huntington's chorea
Organic brain syndrome	? Pancreatic cholera syndrome
Cycloid psychosis	? Syndrome of inappropriate antidiuretic hormone secretion
Anorexia nervosa	
Schizoaffective disorders	
Steroid-induced psychosis	

*Only approved use for lithium in the USA; other uses are experimental.

Table 35–3. SERUM LITHIUM AND TOXIC MANIFESTATIONS*

SEVERITY OF SYMPTOMS	TOXIC STAGE†	SERUM LITHIUM CONCENTRATION *(mEq/L)*
No toxicity (therapeutic)	0	0.4–1.3
Mild toxicity	I	1.5–2.5
Serious toxicity	II	2.5–3.5
Life-threatening toxicity	III	>3.5

*N.B.: Lithium toxicity may become manifest even at therapeutic levels, especially in the elderly when the therapeutic level may be 0.2 mEq/L.

†Classification of Hansen and Amdisen.[6] (Stages I and II: apathy, tremor, weakness, ataxia, motor agitation, rigidity, fascicular twitching, nausea, vomiting, and diarrhea. Stage III: Latent convulsive movements, stupor, and coma.)

LITHIUM INTOXICATION

As noted, most cases of lithium intoxication arise during prolonged therapy,[6, 21] although acute ingestion is recognized.[22] Small adjustments in dosage or frequency of administration commonly give rise to toxic manifestations, and only in a minority of cases is self-poisoning responsible for the intoxication. In general, therefore, it follows that lithium toxicity may not present dramatic symptomatology, and the psychiatrist or other physician managing patients may be unaware of the subtle changes occurring in the prodromal phase of lithium poisoning.

The *prodromal phase* lasts for several days to weeks and may be manifested by a combination of the following symptoms: vomiting, diarrhea, drowsiness, coarse muscle tremor, muscle twitching, lethargy, tinnitus, nystagmus, slurred speech, and, in severe cases, polyuria and polydipsia. It is not surprising that the symptoms can be mistaken for those of the primary depressive illness. Good correlation exists between the symptomatology of lithium poisoning and the serum lithium concentration.[6] In the full-blown syndrome, the toxic manifestations can be graded on a scale of I to III, as shown in Table 35–3. The full syndrome of lithium toxicity may take many days to dissipate following cessation of lithium. As noted, the central nervous system manifestations may never completely regress,[23-28] even up to 5 years following intoxication,[27] and in certain situations lithium toxicity has an appreciable mortality rate.

Systemic Manifestations[6, 7]

Central Nervous System

After a fine hand tremor is observed, the patient may develop muscular and reflex hyperirritability; spastic, dystonic[29] or choreiform movements; cogwheel rigidity; parkinsonism; confusion; mental lapses with prolonged memory impairment (the latter for 2 months in a patient acutely poisoned and treated with hemodialysis[30]); neurologic asymmetry; cutaneous hyperalgesia; and polyneuropathy.[31] Other manifestations are anxiety, delirium, hyperpyrexia, and stupor progressing to coma. The electroencephalogram may well be abnormal, with some patients showing 2 to 5 Hz patterns with spikes and sharp waves. Cerebellar signs may predominate.[32] Paradoxically, in otherwise well-controlled patients mania is the principal manifestation of toxicity.[33, 34]

Gastrointestinal System

Severe gastroenteritis often occurs initially following acute overdose of lithium.

Cardiovascular System

Arrhythmias, hypotension, circulatory failure, and interstitial myocarditis have been reported. The electrocardiogram may show depressed S-T waves or T inversion in chest leads V4 to V6,[6] premature atrial contractions,[35] or complete heart block.[36] Myocytic degeneration and lymphocyte, histiocyte, and plasma cell infiltration, exacerbated by uremia, with severity closely correlated with plasma lithium levels, have been observed in rats chronically intoxicated with lithium.[37]

Miscellaneous

As mentioned, leukocytosis occurs with predominant neutrophilia in the peripheral blood and in bone marrow, with accompanying lymphocytopenia. Isolated cases of leukopenia also have been reported.[38] Increased calcium, magnesium, and parathyroid hormone levels may be observed in blood samples. Increases in serum calcium and parathyroid hormone within the normal range occur in 80 per cent of patients in the early weeks of lithium therapy and exceed the normal range in 10 per cent on long-term therapy.[39] In chronically treated patients, osteoporosis has been reported and disturbed iodine metabolism is common; 4 per cent of patients develop a goiter, but rarely hypothyroidism. Rare cases of exophthalmos have occurred during lithium treatment, as has thyrotoxicosis.[40] Weight gain is also reported, but the mechanism is unknown. Lithium also affects glucose metabolism by enhancing uptake and utilization of glucose in muscle and stimulating the release of insulin from the pancreas. Other miscellaneous side effects are acne, exacerbation of psoriasis, production of other rashes, and hair loss. Reduction in body temperature also has been observed.[41] Adult respiratory distress syndrome also has been observed in severe poisoning that is being treated.[42]

Teratogenicity[6]

Chronic lithium treatment of pregnant women has been associated with fetal cardiac abnormalities, particularly of the tricuspid valve, in 11 of 13 offspring of patients exposed to lithium. In addition, congenital goiter has been reported. During pregnancy, lithium clearance increases by approximately 100 per cent and decreases abruptly after delivery to prepregnancy levels. Breast milk contains lithium in concentrations of approximately half the maternal serum concentration. In view of this, bottle feeding is recommended, since lithium intoxication can occur in infants. The babies are described as hypotonic, floppy, and listless, but revert to normal over time.

The Kidney[43]

Since the body's handling of lithium is so closely related to renal function, it follows that even subtle alterations of renal function may seriously affect lithium excretion and lead to toxicity. Lithium competes with sodium and potassium at the renal tubular level, therefore sodium and water balance control not only the serum level of lithium but also its toxicity. Conditions that enhance proximal tubular reabsorption of lithium constitute a very significant hazard since they occur episodically and may go undetected. These conditions include hyponatremia, administration of diuretics that act on the distal tubules, low salt or weight-reducing diets, and administration of nonsteroidal anti-inflammatory agents such as indomethacin, phenylbutazone,[44] mefenamic acid,[45] and piroxicam.[46] Loop diuretics have no direct effect on lithium reabsorption, but if they precipitate sodium depletion, a reduction in the fractional excretion of lithium (FE_{Li}), with retention of lithium by the kidney, may occur. Lithium itself may affect the thirst center, turn off the normal response to hyperosmolality, and promote dehydration.

The predominant effect that lithium has on the kidney, however, is the production of nephrogenic diabetes insipidus, with polyuria and polydipsia. This syndrome does not respond to exogenous antidiuretic hormone (ADH) and is due to a vasopressin-insensitive defect in urine concentration at the tubular level, manifested by the fact that most patients have high endogenous vasopressin during the polyuric phase. Polyuria and polydipsia are present in about 30 per cent of patients receiving lithium, but in only 10 per cent of all lithium patients is the effect serious enough to lead to dehydration.[47] Urinary incontinence developed in 17 per cent of women taking lithium and was ascribed to lithium-induced changes in bladder cholinergic-adrenergic balance.[48] As shown in Figure 35–1, sodium and water deficiency or renal impairment leads to a reduction of the fractional excretion of lithium and lithium clearance, which, in turn, may promote sodium loss by the kidney, leading to a vicious cycle and further complicating the lithium toxicity. Lithium itself may produce a urinary acidification defect, probably as a result of a distal renal tubular acidosis.[49] Lithium-induced urinary concentration defects are most often reversible when the drug is discontinued, although in some patients the concentration defect may persist for some time.[50, 51]

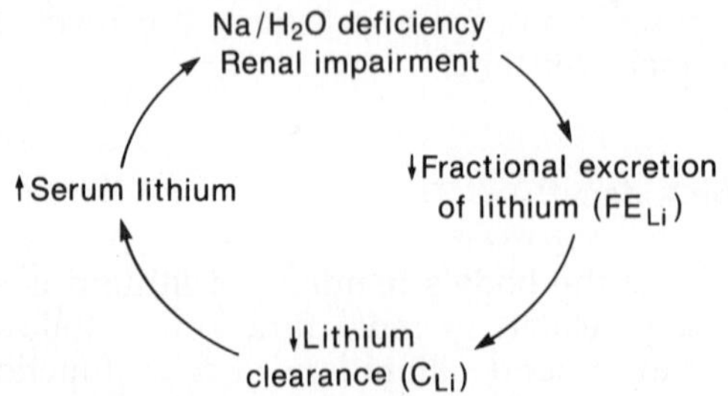

Figure 35–1. The vicious cycle of sodium depletion and lithium toxicity.

Several other renal effects of lithium have been observed. In patients with lithium intoxication, renal biopsy has revealed changes consistent with acute tubular necrosis; whether this is due to lithium or to the accompanying circulatory collapse of lithium poisoning has not yet been determined.[52, 53] Acute renal failure, presumably from acute tubular necrosis, has been described.[53, 54] Nephrotic syndrome due to minimal change disease ("lipoid nephrosis")[55] or focal segmental glomerular sclerosis[56] also has been reported in patients receiving lithium; variable degrees of proteinuria (not in the nephrotic range) commonly are observed in lithium-treated patients. At present, the literature presents conflicting reports on the incidence of chronic interstitial nephropathy in patients receiving lithium, with or without accompanying changes in renal function, albuminuria, and urinary enzyme abnormalities.[43, 57, 58] However, the incidence of chronic interstitial nephritis and renal insufficiency in patients receiving lithium therapy apparently is fairly low, and the etiologic role of lithium is in doubt.[43] It is of interest that patients with severe psychiatric illness may well be at greater risk for developing renal disease than normal individuals, further complicating the etiologic role of lithium in induction of interstitial nephritis.[59] Moreover, a prospective study of the glomerular filtration rate in patients before and after lithium treatment, with an average of 6 years of treatment, has shown no differences in renal function before and after therapy.[60, 61] On the other hand, rats ingesting lithium over a prolonged period do develop renal interstitial fibrosis.[62, 63]

Pathophysiology of Lithium Intoxication

As noted, lithium excretion depends on sodium and water balance and the glomerular filtration rate. Any increase in serum lithium leads to toxicity, to a reduction of lithium clearance, and to a protracted elimination half-time owing to a reduced fractional excretion of lithium by the kidney (Fig. 35–1). In addition, increases in serum lithium also promote natriuresis with further obligatory water loss and lead to the vicious cycle seen in Figure 35–1. Diabetes insipidus also may promote sodium and water loss, particularly if the polyuria leads to water loss in excess of water intake—a particular condition of patients whose manic-depressive illness is exacerbated.

Lithium toxicity may arise from several predisposing factors. The most important of these are dehydration, dietary restriction of sodium, anorexia, vomiting, diarrhea, and extreme exercise—all of which will produce sodium and water imbalance. Additionally, following parturition the glomerular filtration rate, and consequently lithium clearance by the kidney, drop precipitously to half the level during pregnancy. Certain drugs may affect the handling of lithium by the kidney, whereas other drugs may interact with lithium in the central nervous system to produce toxic effects. These drugs are outlined in Table 35–4. Finally, primary renal disease from any cause predisposes to lithium intoxication. Note that primary renal disease seems to be more common in manic-depressive patients and may arise from other drug toxicity, such as excessive analgesic intake, and in particular nonsteroidal anti-inflammatory agents.

Table 35–4. KNOWN DRUG INTERACTIONS WITH LITHIUM

	EFFECTS OF INTERACTION
Haloperidol	Rigidity, ataxia, oral tardive dyskinesia, ↑ depression, ↑ haloperidol toxicity
Tricyclic antidepressants (TCA)	Additive antidepressant effect, hypotension, delirium, seizures, increase in blood pressure if hypotension secondary to TCA
Phenothiazines	↑ Lithium and phenothiazine toxicity, ↑ depression along with toxicity
Benzodiazepines	↑ Depression
Neuromuscular blockers	↑ Neuromuscular blockade
Methyldopa	↑ Parkinsonian-like syndrome
Nonsteroidal anti-inflammatory drugs: indomethacin piroxicam mefenamic acid phenylbutazone	Partial reversal of nephrogenic diabetes insipidus and ↑ serum lithium, ↓ renal lithium clearance
Phenytoin	Polyuria, polydipsia, tremor
Calcium channel blockers: verapamil nifedipine diltiazem	Additive or synergistic action with lithium
Diuretics	
Thiazides	↑ Serum lithium
Osmotics, acetazolamide, sodium bicarbonate	↑ Urinary lithium excretion
Furosemide	No change in serum lithium, unless induces significant sodium loss
Potassium-sparing diuretics and K supplements	Abolishes distal renal tubular acidosis and may prevent renal lithium toxicity

Laboratory Manifestations

In general, the serum levels of sodium are within the normal (or low normal) range, whereas lower sodium concentrations may be encountered in the cerebrospinal fluid (CSF). A *low anion gap* may serve as a useful diagnostic aid when a history of lithium ingestion cannot be obtained; such an observation was made in two severely intoxicated patients (serum Li > 4 mEq/L), which was corrected with dialysis, and was not observed in patients with therapeutic lithium levels.[64] No changes are seen in potassium concentrations in blood or CSF. Serum calcium and magnesium occasionally may be found in increased concentration in the blood, but the most important abnormality is a serum lithium concentration usually in excessive range, as shown in Table 35–3. Of research interest rather than practical use are the findings of increased plasma concentrations of antidiuretic hormone (vasopressin), parathyroid hormone, thyroid-stimulating hormone, aldosterone, and renin.

The glomerular filtration rate may be reduced during the acute illness, but this should respond to adequate fluid replacement. During the acute phase of the illness, the renal lithium clearance and fractional excretion of lithium are reduced. Clinically, the most impressive renal manifestation is polyuria; in one series of patients, polyuria exceeding 3 liters per day was observed in approximately 30 per cent of the patients.[65] Other abnormalities are defects in renal concentration ability in about 80 per cent of the patients, a low urinary sodium concentration, and a distal tubular acidosis.[43]

Treatment

By far the most important aspect of treatment of lithium poisoning is its anticipation *before* serious intoxication occurs. Regular serum lithium measurements should be taken in patients who are undergoing long-term management, and dosage adjustment should be made on the basis of the measurements. Five to seven days may be required after dosage adjustment for serum lithium levels to fall within the desired range. It is most important that patients be cautioned to avoid sodium and water restriction, particularly in the early stages of treatment with lithium. Patients should promptly report any intercurrent illness with pyrexia in which sweating may become excessive, leading to sodium and water loss.

In certain situations the urinary concentration defect resulting in severe polyuria may benefit from modest doses of a thiazide diuretic, which may allow continued treatment with lithium.[66] In addition, nonsteroidal anti-inflammatory agents such as indomethacin and phenylbutazone may help reduce lithium-induced polyuria.[67] It is of interest that potassium supplementation or potassium-sparing diuretics such as triamterene and amiloride may reverse the lithium-induced inhibition of water transport and may also restore urinary acidification, but in general these drugs have no effect on the lithium clearance.[68] It follows, therefore, that serum potassium also must be monitored during lithium treatment.

Definitive Steps to Be Taken

1. Whenever lithium toxicity is suspected, the patient should be *admitted to hospital*. Although symptomatology in general progresses slowly, seizure activity may arise unexpectedly and may become life-threatening.

2. In all cases, *lithium carbonate should be withdrawn* and any concomitant diuretic therapy such as thiazide diuretics should be withheld. If self-poisoning is the reason for the intoxication, *gastric lavage* should be performed. It is worth reiterating that symptoms may progress despite cessation of lithium or thiazide in view of the prolonged elimination half-time of lithium.

3. *Restore sodium and water balance.* In infected or dehydrated patients, appropriate attention to fluid balance and control of pyrexia must be maintained. In patients with nephrogenic diabetes insipidus, infusion of standard (normal) saline infusions may induce a hypertonic state,[69] which itself raises the appreciable morbidity and mortality. In the latter situation, half-normal saline or other hypotonic fluid may be required, or thiazide diuretics may be reintroduced to control the diabetes insipidus. Amiloride, by inhibiting water transport in the collecting tubule, has been shown to reduce the mean urine volume from 4.7 to 3.1 liters and induce a rise in mean urinary osmolality from 575 to 699 mOsm per kg in a series of 9 patients, also avoiding the necessity for potassium supplementation.[70] Amiloride also has been used successfully in other reports.[71]

4. Forced diuresis/sodium infusion. *Forced diuresis has no role*[6, 21] in the management of lithium intoxication unless the glomerular filtration rate is below normal, on restoration of which the serum lithium should fall to around 1 mEq per liter within 30 hours of stopping diuretic treatment. Sodium chloride had long been proposed as useful in enhancing excretion of lithium by the kidney, but current evidence does not favor an effect of sodium chloride on lithium excretion, and the fractional excretion of lithium did not change consistently during sodium infusion.[6, 21] Only in the presence of reduction in glomerular filtration rate due to hypovolemia would sodium chloride infusions have any effect on increasing the fractional excretion of lithium, being accompanied also by an increase in creatinine clearance due to volume expansion. It is recommended that fluid therapy or forced diuresis be used only when the serum lithium level has been elevated for a few days and not above 2.5 mEq per liter; in this situation, measurements of serum lithium should be determined frequently. If serum lithium fails to fall to 1 mEq per liter within 30 to 36 hours of treatment, then dialysis should be considered (see paragraph 6).

5. Antidotes. Direct adenylate cyclase stimulators, such as forskolin, have met with no success in a mouse model of lithium

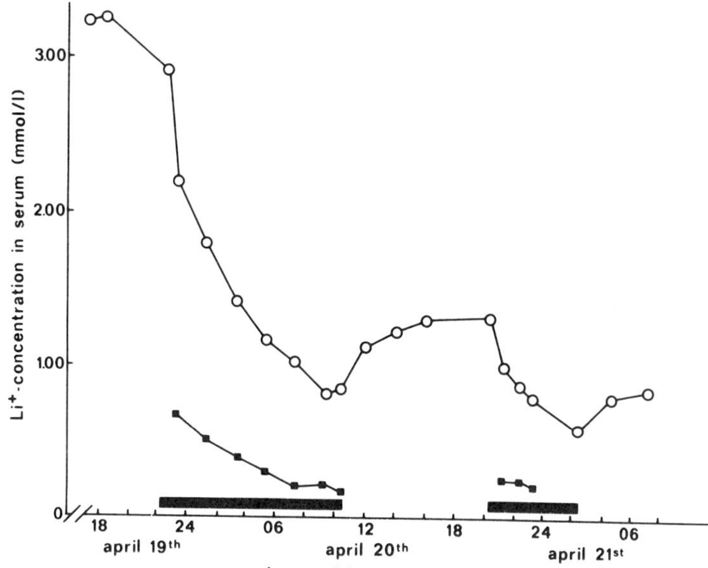

Figure 35–2. Serum lithium response to hemodialysis in a 66 year old man.
○, Dialyzer inlet lithium concentration; ■, dialyzer outlet lithium concentration; ▬, hemodialysis periods. (From Hansen HE, Amdisen A: Lithium intoxication. Q J Med *47*:123, 1978, with permission.)

toxicity[72] and are not recommended until definitive studies are performed to demonstrate their efficacy.

6. *Hemodialysis.* This is the *treatment of choice* for severe lithium intoxication.[6, 21, 73–76] When hemodialysis is not immediately available, peritoneal dialysis may be instituted initially. Lithium is the most dialyzable toxin known, in view of its small molecular weight, negligible protein-binding, and behavior similar to that of sodium. Extraction of lithium by hemodialysis, therefore, is greater than 90 per cent. Hemodialysis has been shown to reduce the elimination half-time substantially

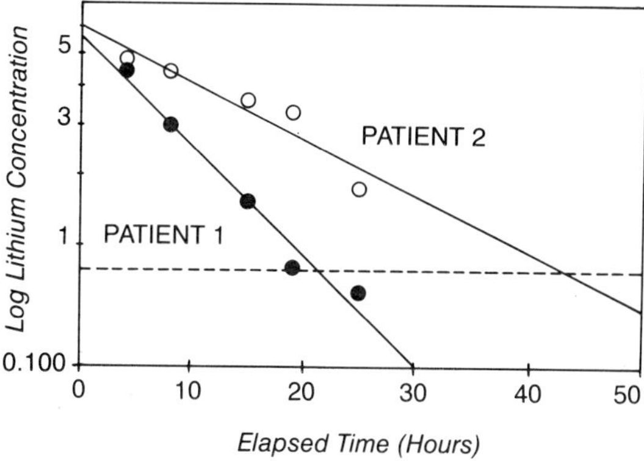

Figure 35–3. Log plasma lithium levels plotted against time in two patients. In patient 1 (●), the predicted level of 0.6 mEq/L occurs at 24 hours, while in patient 2 (○), the predicted level of 0.6 mEq/L occurs at 45 hours. Dialysis would be recommended in patient 2.

and also to reduce serum lithium levels rapidly[6] (Fig. 35–2). Several investigators recommend a protracted hemodialysis (10 to 12 hours), to be repeated as necessary until the serum lithium level remains at less than 1 mEq per liter 6 to 8 hours after dialysis.[6, 21, 22] As with any drug intoxication, "rebound" in plasma levels occurs owing to lithium redistribution or continued gastrointestinal absorption. In my experience, however, a 6-hour hemodialysis with modern high surface area hemodialyzers substantially reduces serum lithium, and only rarely have I had to repeat hemodialysis to maintain a low serum lithium level.

A guide to the necessity for initial hemodialysis, arising from the known first-order elimination of lithium and suggested by several investigators[6, 77] is depicted in Figure 35–3. Hemodialysis should be performed in unstable patients or if three or more serum lithium concentrations plotted on a log-linear scale against time predict that the lithium concentration will not fall below 0.6 mEq per liter within 36 hours or longer.

7. *Maintenance of water balance.* It must be appreciated that persistent sodium and water loss may occur for days to weeks after lithium intoxication,[50, 51] and patients require careful monitoring of fluid balance during this stage.

8. Finally, one of the most distressing features of lithium intoxication may be the persistent neurologic/renal defects that occur in

approximately 10 per cent of patients.[6, 23–26] Consequently, neurology/nephrology follow-up is advised.

References

1. Lange: 1897. Cited in Hansen and Amdisen.[6]
2. Cade J: Lithium salts in the treatment of psychotic excitement. Med J Aust *36*:349, 1949.
3. Schou M, Juel-Nielsen N, Stromgren E, Volby H: The treatment of manic psychosis by the administration of lithium salts. J Neurol Neurosurg Psychiatr *17*:25, 1954.
4. Schou M: Lithium studies. 3. Distribution between serum and tissues. Acta Pharmacol Toxicol (Kbh) *15*:115, 1958.
5. Schou M: Lithium treatment of manic-depressive illness. Past, present and perspective. JAMA *259*:1834, 1988.
6. Hansen HE, Amdisen A: Lithium intoxication. Q J Med (New Series) *47*:123, 1978.
7. Rosenbaum AH, Maruta T, Richelson E: Drugs that alter mood. II. Lithium. Mayo Clin Proc *54*:401, 1979.
8. Coyle JT: Psychiatric drugs in medical practice. Med Clin North Am *61*:891, 1977.
9. Schou M: Pharmacology and toxicology of lithium. Annu Rev Pharmacol Toxicol *16*:231, 1976.
10. Christensen S, Kusano E, Yusufi AN, Murayama N, Dousa TP: Pathogenesis of nephrogenic diabetes insipidus due to chronic administration of lithium in rats. J Clin Invest *75*:1869, 1985.
11. Treiser SL, Cascia CS, O'Donohue TL, Thoa NB, Jacobowitz DM, Kellar KJ: Lithium increases serotonin release and decreases serotonin receptors in the hippocampus. Science *213*:1529, 1981.
12. Ehrlich BE, Diamond JM: Lithium, membranes and manic-depressive illness. J Membrane Biol *52*:187, 1980.
13. Thomsen K, Schou M: Renal lithium excretion in man. Am J Physiol *215*:823, 1968.
14. Petersen V, Hvidt S, Thomsen K, Schou M: Effect of prolonged thiazide treatment on renal lithium clearance. Br Med J *3*:143, 1974.
15. Jefferson JW, Kalin NH: Serum lithium levels and long-term diuretic use. JAMA *241*:1134, 1979.
16. Prien PF: Lithium in the treatment of affective disorders. Clin Neuropharmacol *3*:113, 1978.
17. Mason RW, McQueen EG, Keary PJ, James N: Pharmacokinetics of lithium: Elimination half-time, renal clearance and afferent volume of distribution in schizophrenia. Clin Pharmacokinet *3*:241, 1978.
18. Fyro B, Sedvall G: The excretion of lithium. *In* Johnson FN (ed): Lithium Research and Therapy. Academic Press, New York, 1975, p 287.
19. Shopsin B, Friedmann R, Gershon S: Lithium and leukocytosis. Clin Pharmacol Ther *12*:923, 1971.
20. Lyman GH, Williams CC, Preston D: The use of lithium carbonate to reduce infection and leukopenia during systemic chemotherapy. N Engl J Med *302*:257, 1980.
21. Amdisen A: Clinical features and management of lithium poisoning. Med Toxicol Adverse Drug Exp *3*:18, 1988.
22. Jacobsen D, Aasen G, Fredericksen P, Eisenga B: Lithium intoxication: Pharmacokinetics during and after terminated hemodialysis in acute intoxication. J Toxicol Clin Toxicol *25*:81, 1987.
23. Von Hartitszch B, Hoenich NA, Leigh RS, Wilkinson R, Frost TH, Weddel A, Posen GA: Permanent neurological sequelae despite haemodialysis for lithium intoxication. Br Med J *4*:757, 1972.
24. Juel-Jensen P, Schou M: Permanent brain damage after lithium intoxication. Br Med J *4*:673, 1973.
25. Nagaraja D, Taly AB, Sahu RN, Channabasavanna SM, Nayaranan HS: Permanent neurological sequelae due to lithium toxicity. Clin Neurol Neurosurg *89*:31, 1987.
26. Modestin J, Foglia A: Lithium poisoning with persistent neurological sequelae. Schweiz Med Wochenschr *118*:173, 1988.
27. Izzo KL, Brody R: Rehabilitation in lithium toxicity: Case report. Arch Phys Med Rehabil *66*:779, 1985.
28. Adityanjee A: The syndrome of lithium effectuated neurotoxicity. J Neurol Neurosurg Psychiatr *51*:1246, 1987.
29. Goetting MG: Acute lithium poisoning in a child with dystonia. Pediatrics *76*:978, 1985.
30. Saxena S, Mallikarjuna P: Severe memory impairment with acute overdose lithium toxicity. Br J Psychiatr *152*:853, 1988.
31. Chang YC, Yip PK, Chiu YN, Lin HN: Severe generalized polyneuropathy in lithium intoxication. Eur Neurol *28*:39, 1988.
32. Tesio L, Porta GL, Messa E: Cerebellar syndrome in lithium poisoning: A case of partial recovery. J Neurol Neurosurg Psychiatr *50*:235, 1987.
33. El Mallakah RS, Kantesaria AN, Chaikovsky LI: Lithium toxicity presenting as mania. Drug Intell Clin Pharm *21*:979, 1987.
34. Nurnberger JI Jr: Diuretic-induced lithium toxicity presenting as mania. J Nerv Ment Dis *173*:316, 1985.
35. Dhillon AS, Adams JS: Lithium-related premature atrial contractions. J Clin Psychiatr *48*:305, 1987.
36. Salama AA: Complete heart block associated with mesoridazine and lithium combination. J Clin Psychiatr *48*:123, 1987.
37. Baandrup U, Bagger JP, Christensen B: Myocardial changes in rats with lithium-induced uremia. Acta Pathol Microbiol Immunol Scand [A] *93*:317, 1985.
38. Green ST, Dunn FG: Severe leucopenia in fatal lithium poisoning. Br Med J *290*:517, 1985.
39. Mallette LE, Eichhorn E: Effects of lithium carbonate on human calcium metabolism. Arch Intern Med *146*:770, 1986.
40. McDermott MT, Burman KD, Hofeldt DT, Kidd GS: Lithium-associated thyrotoxicosis. Am J Med *80*:1245, 1986.
41. Follézou JY, Bleibel JM: Reduction of temperature and lithium poisoning. N Engl J Med *313*:1609, 1985.
42. Lawler PG, Cove-Smith JR: Acute respiratory failure following lithium intoxication. A report of two cases. Anaesthesia *41*:623, 1986.
43. Singer I: Lithium and the kidney. Kidney Int *19*:374, 1981.
44. Frolich JC, Leftwich R, Ragheb M, Oates JA, Reimann I, Buchanan D: Indomethacin increases plasma lithium. Br Med J *1*:1115, 1979.
45. Shelley RK: Lithium toxicity and mefenamic acid. A possible interaction and the role of prostaglandin inhibition. Br J Psychiatr *151*:847, 1987.
46. Walbridge DG, Bazire SR: An interaction between lithium and piroxicam presenting as lithium toxicity. Br J Psychiatr *147*:206, 1985.
47. Forrest JN, Cohen AD, Torretti J, Himmelhoch JM,

Epstein FH: On the mechanism of lithium-induced diabetes insipidus in man. J Clin Invest *53*:1115, 1974.
48. Rosenbaum JF, Pollack MH: Treatment-emergent incontinence with lithium. J Clin Psychiatr *46*:444, 1985.
49. Perez GO, Oster JR, Vaamonde CA: Incomplete syndrome of renal tubular acidosis induced by lithium carbonate. J Lab Clin Med *86*:386, 1975.
50. Mann J, Branton LJ, Larkins RG: Hyperosmolality complicating recovery from lithium toxicity. Br Med J *2*:1522, 1978.
51. Cairns SR, Wolman R, Lewis JG, Thakker R: Persistent nephrogenic diabetes insipidus, hyperparathyroidism, and hypothyroidism after lithium treatment. Br Med J *290*:516, 1985.
52. Lavender S, Brown JN, Berrill WT: Acute renal failure and lithium intoxication. Postgrad Med J *49*:277, 1973.
53. Dias N, Hocken AG: Oliguric renal failure complicating lithium carbonate therapy. Nephron *10*:246, 1972.
54. Fenves AZ, Emmett M, White MG: Lithium intoxication associated with acute renal failure. South Med J *77*:666, 1985.
55. Richman AV, Masco HL, Rifkin SL, Acharya MK: Minimal change disease and nephrotic syndrome associated with lithium therapy. Ann Intern Med *92*:70, 1980.
56. Santella RN, Rimmer JM, MacPherson BR: Focal segmental glomerulosclerosis in patients receiving lithium carbonate. Am J Med *84*:951, 1988.
57. Hestbech J, Hansen HE, Amdisen A, Olsen S: Chronic renal lesions following long-term treatment with lithium. Kidney Int *12*:205, 1977.
58. Hansen HE, Hestbech J, Sorensen JC, Norgard K, Heilskov J, Amdisen A: Chronic interstitial nephropathy in patients on long-term lithium therapy. Q J Med *48*:577, 1979.
59. Kincaid-Smith P, Burrows GD, Davies BM, Holwill B, Walter M, Walker RG: Renal biopsy findings in lithium and prelithium patients. Lancet *2*:700, 1979.
60. DePaulo JR, Correa EL, Sapir DG: Renal toxicity of lithium and its complications. Johns Hopkins Med J *149*:15, 1981.
61. DePaulo JR Jr, Correa EI, Sapir DG: Renal function and lithium: A longitudinal study. Am J Psychiatr *143*:892, 1986.
62. Ottosen PD, Nyengard JR, Olsen TS, Christensen S: Interstitial focal fibrosis and reduction in proximal tubular length in adult rats after lithium treatment. Acta Pathol Microbiol Immunol Scand [A] *94*:401, 1986.
63. Samiy AH, Rosnick PB: Early identification of renal problems in patients receiving chronic lithium treatment. Am J Psychiatr *144*:670, 1987.
64. Keleher SP, Raciti A, Arbeit LA: Reduced or absent serum anion gap as a marker of severe lithium intoxication. Arch Intern Med *146*:1839, 1986.
65. DePaulo JR, Correa EL, Sapir DG: Lithium and renal tubular and glomerular function. Abstract. American Psychiatry Association, 1981, p 254.
66. Levy ST, Forrest JN, Heninger GR: Lithium-induced diabetes insipidus, manic symptoms, brain and electrolyte correlates and chlorothiazide treatment. Am J Psychiatr *130*:1014, 1973.
67. Rapoport J, Chiamovitz C, Alroy GG, Better OS: Lithium-induced nephrogenic diabetes insipidus: Studies of tubular function and pathogenesis. Israel J Med Sci *15*:765, 1979.
68. Mehta PK, Sodhi B, Arruda JAL, Kurtzman NA: Interaction of amiloride and lithium on distal urinary acidification. J Lab Clin Med *93*:983, 1979.
69. Verbov JL, Phillips JD, Fife DG: A case of lithium intoxication. Postgrad Med J *41*:190, 1965.
70. Batlle DC, von Riotte AB, Gaviria M, et al: Amelioration of polyuria by amiloride in patients receiving long-term lithium. N Engl J Med *312*:408, 1985.
71. Kosten TR, Forrest JN: Treatment of severe lithium-induced polyuria with amiloride. Am J Psychiatr *143*:1563, 1986.
72. Kaplan Z, Schreiber G, Belmaker RH: Lack of effectiveness of forskolin or inositol as antidote in lithium toxicity. Short note. J Neurol Trans *72*:167, 1988.
73. Amdisen A, Skjoldborg H: Haemodialysis for lithium poisoning. Lancet *2*:213, 1969.
74. Winchester JF, Gelfand MC, Knepshield JH, Schreiner GE: Dialysis and hemoperfusion of poisons and drugs—update. Trans Am Soc Artif Intern Organs *23*:762, 1977.
75. Bismuth C, Baud FJ, Buneaux F, Du Fretay X: Spontaneous toxicokinetics of lithium during a therapeutic overdose with renal failure. J Toxicol Clin Toxicol *24*:261, 1986.
76. Jaeger A, Sauder P, Kopferschmitt J, Jaegle ML: Toxicokinetics of lithium intoxication treated by hemodialysis. J Toxicol Clin Toxicol *23*:501, 1985–86.
77. Simard M, Gumbiner B, Lee A, Lewis H, Norman D: Lithium carbonate intoxication. A case report and review of the literature. Arch Intern Med *149*:36, 1989.

CHAPTER 36
TOXICOLOGY OF DEPENDENCY

A. The Alcoholic Patient

Charles E. Becker, M.D.

Emergency physicians and toxicologists are paying increasing attention to the acute and chronic effects of alcohol, alone or in conjunction with other toxins. The purpose of this chapter is to review the settings in which an alcoholic patient is likely to be seen as a toxicologic emergency. Special emphasis will be placed on key physical findings, laboratory analysis, important alcohol-drug interactions, and the unique management of intoxicated patients.

Alcohol is the most common single drug taken by patients. Alcohol (ethanol—C_2H_5OH) is a sedative-hypnotic drug, which, in acute overdose, may result in respiratory depression, cardiovascular collapse, and death. Chronic ingestion of large amounts of alcohol causes damage to many organ systems. Alcohol is commonly taken along with other drugs in overdose cases. It is recognized that chronic alcoholism is associated with important psychologic problems, including a high incidence of depression and suicide.[1] The alcoholic patient's psychologic problems are often treated with psychopharmacologic agents that may provide a means for carrying out a suicide intent.

When alcoholic patients are no longer able to obtain alcohol, they may try to produce their own beverage or purchase congeners, thus creating toxic hazards of alcohol substitutes and illicit alcoholic spirits. These alcohol substitutes are of great interest because they provide examples of lethal synthesis—that is, the metabolic products of a given toxin are even more toxic than the parent agent, such as formic acid from methanol. Because of the acute and chronic central nervous system (CNS) effects of alcohol, the history given by an alcoholic individual in a toxic emergency may be unreliable. The physician, therefore, must depend on physical examination and laboratory tests to identify and treat the acute problem.

The gastrointestinal tract may be injured by alcohol or alcohol substitutes. Gastritis, pancreatitis, and liver disease are common events in alcoholic patients and must be managed appropriately. Other complicating medical conditions, such as associated burns, injuries to extremities, or alcohol withdrawal, may complicate the picture. Finally, a special type of toxic emergency in an alcoholic patient involves injury to the fetus of a pregnant alcoholic woman.

IMPORTANT PHYSICAL FINDINGS

Obviously, everyone who has alcohol on his or her breath does not need a work-up for alcohol toxicology emergencies and their complications. As a general rule, intoxicated patients who are comatose or unable to walk should have an evaluation of their alcoholic status.

An acute brain syndrome in an alcoholic patient is one of the most difficult differential diagnoses for a physician. Table 36–1 lists some of the key physical findings in this setting. Special attention must be paid to physical findings that give clues to the diagnosis of altered mental status. The physical examination may often be limited by hostility of the patient or associated severe trauma.

Once the airway is protected, vital signs must be carefully assessed. Special attention should be given to recording the body temperature. Alcoholic individuals are very susceptible to hypothermia, as alcohol causes vasodilatation that contributes to heat loss. Because of alcohol-induced vasodilatation, the patient may not feel cold and yet have a

Table 36–1. IMPORTANT PHYSICAL FINDINGS IN ALCOHOLIC PATIENTS

Careful vital signs: special emphasis on temperature and blood pressure
Careful mental status examination
Neurologic examination with special attention to eye movements, pupil size, and evidence of head trauma
Blood behind the tympanic membrane
Odor on the breath
Signs of chronic liver disease and check for occult blood
Size of thyroid

low body temperature. Arrhythmias may be caused by hypothermia. Hypothermic alcoholic patients should be suspected of having hypoglycemia. There is an approximately linear relationship between the degree of hypoglycemia and body temperature. If the thermometer is only shaken down to a normal level and the temperature recorded, hypothermia may be completely missed. It is imperative to record the patient's true temperature on admission to the emergency department. Overzealous use of room temperature fluids may further lower the temperature.

It is also imperative to monitor the blood pressure carefully and relate this to the pulse. Alcoholic individuals frequently have postural hypotension or may have autonomic insufficiency that may complicate the diagnosis and management of the overdose.

An alcoholic patient must always be suspected of having head trauma. Conjunctival hemorrhages, blood behind the tympanic membranes, spinal fluid rhinorrhea, nystagmus, and inequality of the pupils must be noted. In view of the complexity of the clinical setting, it is usually best to avoid giving additional medications to an already confused patient so that the natural history of the confusional state can be observed. From clinical experience in dealing with alcoholic patients with altered mental states and potential head trauma, one must always suspect a subdural hematoma or other CNS injury.

Breath odors in an alcoholic patient may give important clues to the cause of the confusional state. The breath may suggest alcohol or its congeners, specific solvents, hydrocarbons, cyanide, liver failure, or metabolic disturbances. While the vital signs, neurologic examination, and odors are being detected, the clothes of the patients should be completely removed and the skin observed carefully. Needle marks may suggest parenteral drug abuse. Skin disease (e.g., scabies and pediculosis) under treatment may suggest Kwell (gamma benzene hexachloride) therapy leading to convulsions. Easy bruising suggests vitamin C or vitamin K deficiency.

The thyroid should be palpated, as an alcoholic patient with thyroid storm may mimic severe withdrawal or toxic emergency. The size of the liver and physical findings for hepatic coma or severe liver disease should be sought. Obvious asterixis, ascites, jaundice, signs of portal hypertension, or hemorrhage into the abdominal flanks may strongly suggest associated pathologies that will complicate the toxic emergency. A rectal examination and a stool sample for occult blood are required. Because the history will likely be unreliable in this setting, the physical findings may provide the clue to the suspected toxin, and laboratory analysis will give further confirmation of the initial impression.

Patients who are markedly vitamin deficient may exhibit symptom complexes such as Wernicke's encephalopathy and Korsakoff's psychosis. Wernicke's encephalopathy is characterized by paralysis of eye movements, ataxia, and mental disturbance. Impairment of eye movements consists of paralysis or weakness of the external recti, nystagmus both vertical and horizontal, and various palsies of conjugate gaze. Sixth-nerve palsy is most often bilateral, but not always symmetric, and results in diplopia and internal strabismus. Korsakoff's psychosis is characterized by retrograde and anterograde amnesia. Patients exhibit large gaps in memory and are unable to remember recent events in their proper temporal sequence, usually resulting in a tendency to confabulate.

Both Wernicke's encephalopathy and Korsakoff's psychosis are indicators of severe thiamine deficiency and often indicate a poor prognosis. Thiamine replacement along with replacement of all water-soluble vitamins must be rapidly instituted.

KEY LABORATORY FINDINGS

Table 36–2 lists key laboratory determinations in alcoholic patients with toxic emergencies.

Blood Alcohol Level

The mental state of an intoxicated patient may not always correlate with the blood alcohol level. The blood level of alcohol is related to its volume of distribution and closely approximates total body water, which is 60 to 70 per cent of body weight. The lethal dose of alcohol and its relationship to the effects are in part determined by tissue tolerance. The estimated oral dose that would cause the death of 50 per cent of patients is

Table 36–2. KEY LABORATORY TESTS IN ALCOHOLIC PATIENTS

Blood alcohol determination
Osmolality:

$$2\ \text{Na} + \frac{\text{Blood glucose}}{18}(\text{mg/dl}) + \frac{\text{BUN}}{3}(\text{mg/dl}) = 285 \pm 5\ \text{mOsm/kg}\ H_2O$$

Electrolytes with special attention to potassium
Determination of anion gap:

$$(\text{Na} + \text{K}) - (\text{Cl} + HCO_3) = 8 \text{ to } 12 \pm 3\ \text{mEq/liter}$$

Arterial blood gases
Blood glucose
Urinalysis for crystals—BUN and creatinine, myoglobin
Blood and urine ketone tests
Calcium, phosphorus, magnesium
Amylase
Electrocardiogram
Flat plate radiograph of abdomen

that quantity producing a blood level in the range of 450 to 500 mg/dl (0.50 per cent). Thus the measurement of the blood alcohol level is essential to compare the degree of neurologic impairment with the blood level. It is important in toxicology emergencies to be able to anticipate the meaning of a blood alcohol level as well as to back-calculate estimated blood alcohol levels. Because alcohol distributes in body water and a blood alcohol level can usually be obtained, it is possible to estimate the dose of alcohol that has been ingested and to predict the blood alcohol level at a given time if there is complete alcohol absorption.

The term *usual dose of alcohol* describes a 1-ounce drink of approximately 80 to 86 proof. The word *proof* in the United States is defined as 50 per cent by volume. Because alcohol is usually administered as a "shot," one shot is 1 ounce or 30 ml. If alcohol is 80 proof, the concentration would be 40 per cent by volume. Thus, a 1-ounce shot of 80 proof contains 12 ml of pure alcohol. The specific gravity of alcohol is .79. Thus, 1 ounce of alcohol contains only approximately 10 ml of 100 per cent alcohol. The volume of distribution of alcohol is approximately 70 per cent of body weight. Therefore, in a standard 70-kg patient, 70 per cent by volume would be approximately 50 liters. If 10 gm of alcohol (10 ml of 100 per cent alcohol) in a typical drink are placed in 50 liters, the blood alcohol concentration will be 20 mg/dl or 0.020 per cent. In many states, the legal definition for "under the influence of alcohol" is 100 mg/dl, or 0.1 per cent.

At the usual "clinical" doses, the metabolism of alcohol is at a fixed rate over time known as zero-order kinetics. For most patients with normal liver function, the elimination rate of alcohol is approximately 15 to 20 mg/dl/hour. Thus, if alcohol is completely absorbed, one can back-calculate the estimated alcohol at a given time. In the presence of liver disease, this rate may be somewhat slower. When liver function is normal, there is an increase to a maximum of 30 mg/dl/hour with chronic alcohol use. One must be always cautious about estimating effects from a given alcohol level because of tissue tolerance for a given alcohol level. For example, it is quite possible for an individual to appear normal by routine examination at 100 mg/dl alcohol because his or her nervous system is tolerant to this level.

Once alcohol is absorbed, equilibration is rapid, and it is distributed throughout total body water. The simplest method to estimate total body water is 60 to 70 per cent of the lean body mass. After the blood alcohol level peaks, it declines at a relatively fixed rate as determined by metabolism, in which 95 per cent of ethanol is removed by oxidation and approximately 5 per cent removed by the lungs and the kidneys. Most of the metabolism takes place in the liver, with extrahepatic metabolism accounting for a relatively small percentage. It is generally accepted that the zinc-containing NAD-dependent enzyme alcohol dehydrogenase, located in the cytosol of the liver cell, is the major enzyme responsible for alcohol metabolism. The first metabolite of alcohol, acetaldehyde, has been a subject of intense study during the past 5 years. Questions now are being asked about the toxicology of acetaldehyde and its effects on intoxication. Although alcohol metabolism previously was thought to occur at a constant rate independent of concentration, more recent studies have suggested much more complicated elimination kinetics for alcohol.

Serum Osmolality and Osmolar Gaps

Serum osmolality is an important parameter to assess. Solutes that may contribute to osmolalities are ethanol, isopropanol, ethylene glycol, and methanol. Table 36–3 lists the molecular weight and approximate effects on osmolality at dangerous levels. It is important to recognize, however, that most drugs that would be taken by intoxicated

Table 36–3. ALCOHOL AND ALCOHOL SUBSTITUTES

	MOLECULAR WEIGHT	APPROXIMATE LETHAL DOSE	APPROXIMATE LETHAL LEVEL	mOsm/L	ACIDOSIS	KETOSIS	CLINICAL MANIFESTATIONS
Ethanol	46	4 gm/kg	500 mg/dl	100	+/−	+/−	Acidosis uncommon.
Methanol	32	1 gm/kg	100 mg/dl	30	4 +	None	Metabolized to formate; no odor; visual signs common, ⊕ CT; ↑ mean corpuscular volume.
Ethylene glycol	62	2 gm/kg	200 mg/dl	35	3 +	None	Metabolized to oxalic acid; no odor; CNS excitation; no visual signs; oxalate crystals in urine; delayed renal failure.
Isopropanol	60	2 gm/kg	200 mg/dl	35	None	4 +	Metabolized to acetone; typical odors; gastritis common; ketonemia without acidosis and normal sugar.
Paraldehyde	132	1–2 gm/kg	50 mg/dl	4	None	+/−	Typical pungent odor; severe gastritis.

alcoholic patients cannot be screened by osmolalities, because the serum levels are so low and the molecular weights so high that they do not become a significant osmolar force.[2] One of the values of performing serum osmolality is as a quick indication of the cause of intoxication; the osmolality determination does not destroy the sample, and the serum can be saved for later toxicologic analysis.

To detect various alcohols by osmolality, the laboratory must perform the test by the freezing point method; the blood must not be drawn in oxalate or EDTA, which would falsely elevate the osmolality. Table 36–3 illustrates the molecular weight, the approximate lethal dose, osmolality, and clinical manifestations of common alcohol and alcohol substitutes. It is clinically useful to estimate the expected osmolality by doubling the sodium, adding the blood sugar divided by 18 and the blood urea nitrogen (BUN) divided by three. This will usually create a normal osmolality of approximately 285 ± 5 mOsm. One can thereby estimate what the osmolality should be and confirm this with a blood alcohol test. If there is a difference between what is observed and what is expected, then there are extra osmolar forces that are not explained. By determining blood alcohol level and osmolality, one can thereby infer that extra osmolar forces are present, possibly suggesting methanol, ethylene glycol, or isopropyl alcohol. To estimate quickly the cause of excess osmolar forces, one can estimate alcohol by multiplying the osmolar difference by 4.6, with methanol by 3.2, and ethylene glycol by 6.2. These figures provide rough estimates for the expected levels for these individual alcohols.

Serum Electrolytes and Anion Gap

In addition to the osmolality, serum electrolyte determinations should be performed on all acute alcoholic patients. The anion gap is usually defined as the sodium and potassium concentration minus the chloride and the bicarbonate. This normal value is 8 to 12 mEq/liter. In the absence of renal failure or diabetic ketoacidosis, the identification of an anion gap greater than 15 mEq/liter requires further explanation. Ethylene glycol and methanol increase the anion gap as a result of production of unique acids and lactate. In alcohol-intoxicated patients without other toxins, the increased anion gap may suggest alcoholic ketoacidosis. In alcoholic ketoacidosis, the increase in the anion gap is probably due to hydroxybutyrate metabolites that may not be detected by Acetest tablets (used to measure ketones); thus, it is important to measure the serum ketones. Gabow and associates[3] suggested that the increased anion gaps in patients without uremia, chemical or drug intoxication, or evidence of ketoacidosis are not due to lactate but to other unidentified or "idiogenic" anions.

Urinalysis

Urinalysis must also be included in the metabolic profile of an alcoholic patient. Urinalysis is especially important if ethylene glycol ingestion is considered likely, because oxalate crystals may be identified. In addition, very dark urine in an alcoholic patient may indicate rhabdomyolysis.

Additional Studies

Calcium, magnesium, and phosphate levels also may be useful in the metabolic profile. Alcoholic patients who do not have renal insufficiency frequently will have a low phosphate level. The phosphate is decreased even more by the intravenous infusion of glucose, insulin, or bicarbonate. Low serum phosphate levels may mimic CNS, muscle, hematopoietic, and liver dysfunction, which may further confuse the toxic emergency. Arterial blood gas determinations may be necessary to define the severity of the metabolic derangements in alcoholic patients. However, the blood pH is not nearly as important a factor as is the osmolality in such patients. Alcohol itself and low levels of blood urea are not osmotically active in that they have free access to cells. However, hyperglycemia may create an altered mental status, by causing marked disturbances in osmolality. It is critical to detect a high blood glucose level and to measure the osmolality, as this is a key factor in determining the outcome of the patient.

It is clear that all these metabolic abnormalities must be interpreted in the light of renal function as measured by the BUN and creatinine levels. With acute muscle destruction caused by alcohol, phencyclidine, or solvents, there may be alterations in creatinine, potassium, and phosphate levels; all may be elevated while the BUN determination is relatively normal. It may be useful to monitor the metabolic milieu of the heart and cardiovascular system by reviewing the electrocardiogram in toxic emergencies. A prolonged Q-T interval may suggest quinidine-like medications, or a widened QRS may suggest overdose with tricyclic antidepressants. T-wave changes also may be noted with electrolyte abnormalities of calcium, potassium, and magnesium. If chemical asphyxiants are present, such as hydrogen sulfide, carbon monoxide, or cyanide, then acute ST segment elevations may be identified in all leads of the electrocardiogram, suggesting diffuse cardiac injury. Hypothermia changes may also be diagnosed with J wave phenomena on the electrocardiogram. Some alcoholic patients with ethylene glycol poisoning may show evidence of hypocalcemia, suggested by a prolonged Q-T interval.

Abdominal pain is a frequent occurrence in acute alcoholic patients. Serum amylase and serum lipase determinations are essential to rule out pancreatitis. The amylase clearance may be helpful in the diagnosis of acute pancreatitis in patients who already have experienced normalization of the serum amylase level. Some substances are radiopaque and can be observed on a flat plate of the abdomen. These include heavy metals (iron, lead, arsenic), some psychotropic agents, and enteric coated tablets. A radiograph of the abdomen also may show pancreatic calcification, suggesting chronic pancreatitis. Blood ammonia or CNS glutamate determinations may help diagnose hepatic coma.

The use of a blood or urine toxicology screen in all alcoholic patients with an altered mental state is not worthwhile. The toxicology laboratory tests should be selected according to the clinical presentation of the patient, the physical findings, and other laboratory tests. The blood alcohol level and the osmolality are very useful, as are acetaminophen and aspirin determinations. If an alcoholic patient is found in a closed space or is involved in a fire, a carboxyhemoglobin determination is useful. Unusual circumstances, such as home brew created in battery casings or fermented grain that has been contaminated with pesticides, may indicate the need for lead or arsenic determinations. If an alcoholic patient is receiving therapy for tuberculosis, it may be necessary to determine an isoniazid level if the patient has seizures or profound metabolic acidosis. Even if these are unlikely, it is a wise practice to save a sample of serum in all alcoholic patients with altered mental state should the need arise for subsequent toxicologic analysis.

ALCOHOL-DRUG INTERACTIONS

Perhaps the reason that alcohol is so often involved in toxic emergencies is because alcohol is commonly taken by patients and interacts with almost all other medications.[1] Drug interactions may be *direct*—that is, the specific chemical effect of the alcohol itself—or *indirect*—that is, a pharmacologic effect of alcohol interacting with another pharmacologic agent. Sometimes it is also useful to consider alcohol-drug interactions as *pharmacokinetic*, in which alcohol itself alters the kinetics or metabolism of another medication, or *pharmacodynamic*, in which the pharmacologic effects interact. *Table 36–4* lists common anticipated alcohol-drug interactions.

As more has been learned about alcohol-drug interactions, their complexity has become evident.[4] Much of the complexity is related to whether alcohol is acutely or chronically administered. When alcohol is simultaneously administered with other medications, such as sedative-hypnotic drugs, synergistic or potentiating pharmacologic effects at least occur. Alcohol also may acutely block the metabolism of other medications. Alcohol ingested chronically creates metabolic as well as tissue tolerance. The balance of these acute and chronic effects is complicated and probably depends in part on genetic susceptibility of rates of metabolism as well as adaptive effects at primary tissue sites.

Table 36–4. ANTICIPATED ALCOHOL-DRUG INTERACTIONS

Direct (pharmacokinetic)
Direct effect on metabolism—acute and chronic
Enhanced liver toxicity
Fructose
Monoamine oxidase (MAO) inhibitors
Disulfiram-like reactions
Methanol, ethylene glycol
Indirect (pharmacodynamic)
Sedative-hypnotic
Minor and major tranquilizers
Gastric irritants (aspirin)
Antihistamines
Hypoglycemic agents
Narcotics
Anticonvulsants
Vasodilators
Diuretics
Alcohol effects on common laboratory tests
Increases uric acid
Glucose intolerance
Mild anemia with increased mean corpuscular volume
Hypokalemia, hypophosphatemia, hypomagnesemia

By far the most common problem in a toxic emergency is the simultaneous ingestion of alcohol with other drugs. It has been shown that acute alcohol administration inhibits the metabolism of various medications.[4] This fact has special importance in fatal and nonfatal traffic accidents in which a relatively small amount of alcohol may be present along with perhaps marijuana, other sedative-hypnotic drugs, or tranquilizers. Because alcohol acutely competes for metabolic pathways with other drugs, a marked decrease in drug metabolism may occur, with subsequent high levels of a parent drug leading to markedly altered levels of consciousness.

It is important to anticipate alcohol-drug interactions. Highly protein-bound drugs with low intrinsic hepatic clearances are among those that exhibit kinetic alterations with alcohol (e.g., benzodiazepines, phenytoin, and warfarin). Less highly bound drugs are less consistently affected (e.g., glutethimide). Acute intake of alcohol inhibits mixed-function oxidase activity and prolongs the elimination of sedative drugs, whereas chronic intake of alcohol with a normally functioning liver causes proliferation of hepatic smooth endoplasmic reticulum, resulting in an increase in drug-metabolizing ability. Alcohol also may affect drug distribution as well as the tissue binding and alter the first-pass phenomenon for those drugs with high intrinsic clearance.

Acute alcohol intoxication affects not only drugs acting on the nervous system, but may also enhance the hypotensive effect of phenothiazines or narcotics because alcohol has vasodilating properties. Alcohol also may alter anticoagulant metabolism, with the attendant risk of bleeding; mixed with aspirin it may enhance the likelihood of gastrointestinal bleeding.

Of special importance are drug interactions with alcohol in which enhanced toxin production caused by the stimulation of microsomal enzyme activity may occur. Carbon tetrachloride probably exerts its toxicity after conversion to active metabolites. The hepatotoxicity of acetaminophen is caused by a toxic metabolite excess after glutathione depletion. Thus, chronic alcohol ingestion may enhance the hepatotoxicity of both these agents. It is emphasized that the chronic effects of alcohol occur after only 2 to 3 weeks of continued alcohol use and may persist for as long as 4 to 9 weeks.[5]

On occasion, toxicity is created by the constituents of alcoholic beverages. Common nonalcoholic components of alcoholic beverages may include tyramine in wines, and some types of beer contain dihydroxyphenylalanine. Both these compounds can precipitate a hypertensive crisis in patients being treated with monoamine oxidase inhibitors. By injuring the liver, alcohol may alter plasma protein binding of drugs and toxins. Therapy directed at enhancing metabolism of alcohol with fructose may lead to hyperuricemia, lactic acidosis, and enhanced risk of seizure.

If alcohol is administered simultaneously with disulfiram or other drugs with disulfiram-like activity, nausea, vomiting, headache, and convulsions may occur. Some antibiotics, oral hypoglycemics, and cancer chemotherapeutic agents have been suggested to cause disulfiram-like reactions, although these are usually mild.[6] If alcohol is ingested simultaneously with a compound possessing toxic metabolites (such as methanol or ethylene glycol), then the apparent toxicity of these noxious agents may be delayed until alcohol has been metabolized, because the enzyme degradation of alcohol is preferential. This action forms the basis of a component of therapy for these intoxications (see Chapter 37) but also may delay the full presentation of a toxic event.

One also must recognize that alcohol itself commonly affects laboratory tests that may suggest other disease processes. Hyperuricemia, glucose intolerance, hypokalemia, mild anemia with an increased mean corpuscular volume, and abnormal liver function test results may be associated with chronic alcohol ingestion; these findings may mislead the physician to prescribe nonindicated medications.

CLINICAL PRESENTATION—INTOXICATION

The acute alcoholic patients may present in one of three ways: intoxicated, undergoing withdrawal, or in the postwithdrawal period.[7] A nontolerant individual may suffer an acute, sedative-hypnotic-like overdose if he or she consumes a large amount of alcohol and has no tissue or metabolic tolerance. An individual who is tolerant to alcohol still may become severely intoxicated by consuming large quantities of alcohol. The degree of intoxication depends on three factors: the blood alcohol concentration, the rapidity of the blood alcohol rise, and the period during which the alcohol level is maintained. The pattern of the drinking, the state of the absorptive surface of the stomach and the gastrointestinal tract, and the presence of other medications also contribute to the degree of intoxication. Although alcohol may cause various degrees of intoxication, it uncommonly causes coma by itself.[1]

TREATMENT OF ACUTE ETHANOL INTOXICATION

The most important single factor in the treatment of the acutely alcohol-intoxicated patient is to provide cardiopulmonary support. The lethal dose of alcohol varies by a factor of two or three depending on tolerance. Severe hepatic insufficiency may further complicate alcohol metabolism. Because alcohol is responsible for so many metabolic alterations, an intoxicated patient may have disturbances that can influence the level of consciousness. These include fluid and electrolyte imbalance, hypoglycemia, and nutritional deficiencies. Alcoholic cardiomyopathy with its attendant complications may ensue. Death, if it results from alcohol alone, is usually caused by respiratory depression. Other metabolic disturbances leading to circulatory collapse can complicate the condition.

During the acute phase of intoxication with alcohol alone, one must be certain to measure blood glucose. Hypoglycemia is common, easily diagnosed, and easily treated. Children ingesting even small amounts of alcohol are quite susceptible to hypoglycemia. Alcoholic adults who are malnourished and have little liver glycogen also may be unable to elevate blood glucose by glycogenolysis.

Because alcohol is readily absorbed from the gastrointestinal tract, gastric lavage, induction of emesis, and activated charcoal are not indicated in cases of alcohol intoxication alone; they may be indicated when concomitant drug ingestion is suspected.[8] There is rarely a good substitute for supportive care. Administration of stimulants, forced exercise, cold showers, or unusual remedies for curtailing alcoholic intoxication should be avoided.

Intravenous infusions of fructose increase the rate of alcohol metabolism.[9] However, oral administration of fructose causes gastrointestinal upset, and parenteral administration of large doses may result in hyperuricemia, lactic acidosis, alterations of the liver, and osmotic diuresis.[9] Valid scientific studies have failed to provide convincing evidence for the usefulness of other medications (amantadine and fenmetozole) in altering alcohol intoxications.

Alcohol-intoxicated individuals may become belligerent and require special precautions and attention. An acute toxic psychiatric emergency due exclusively to alcohol ingestion requires that patients be protected from themselves and others. This is much easier said than done. Practical experience indicates that some physicians are not always skilled in managing acutely belligerent patients. The presence of many trained individuals makes the patient realize that it is pointless to resist judicious restraints, whereas token attempts at restraints using insufficient force exacerbate belligerence.[7] Sharp objects, eyeglasses, and dangling clothing must be removed from staff members until such a patient can be controlled. An intoxicated patient should be restrained on the side or face down in a quiet and comfortable environment and observed frequently. Use of physical restraint devices without monitoring the patient can be hazardous because the patient may vomit, aspirate, or suffer musculoskeletal injury. Because patients are usually deficient in thiamine, folate, and magnesium, empiric replacement may be indicated.

ALCOHOL WITHDRAWAL

When alcohol ingestion is discontinued abruptly, a characteristic syndrome of motor agitation, anxiety, insomnia, and reduction of seizure threshold occurs and may be confused with other toxic emergencies. The severity of the withdrawal syndrome is usually proportional to the dose and the duration of the preceding alcohol intake.[10] However, administration of other sedative medications and concomitant medical or surgical complications can markedly alter the severity of the alcohol withdrawal syndrome. In its mildest form, the alcohol withdrawal syndrome presents as tremor, anxiety, and insomnia, which usually occur 6 to 8 hours after cessation of alcohol. Seizures during the early phase of alcohol withdrawal are typically grand mal and occur in bursts of two or three beginning 12 hours after cessation of drinking. Some alcoholic patients with major medical or surgical complications may suffer more severe reactions, with hallucinations, total disorientation, and marked abnormalities of vital signs.

The later, severe withdrawal syndrome occurring usually 48 to 72 hours after cessation of drinking is known as delirium tremens. Delirium tremens is characterized by tremulousness, visual hallucinations, agitation, confusion, disorientation, and autonomic overactivity. Estimates of the mortality rate of severe alcohol withdrawal have probably been overstated in the past, and the prognosis is most probably related to the underlying precipitating medical or surgical complication.[1] It is important to rule out head trauma, rib fractures, lung infections, hypoglycemia, pancreatitis, and gastritis in these patients. Thyroid storm may be difficult to differentiate from delirium tremens; an enlarged thyroid gland may suggest the diagnosis of thyroid storm.

The major objective of any pharmacologic assistance in the alcohol withdrawal syndrome must be based on ruling out other toxic emergencies and attempting to prevent seizures, delirium, and arrhythmias. If other intoxications are suspected, most patients undergoing mild alcohol withdrawal do not need pharmacologic therapy and should be carefully observed. Maintenance of fluid and electrolyte balance is critical, and losses caused by increased temperature, diaphoresis, and vomiting should be replaced. Total body magnesium may be decreased in alcoholic patients unless they have been taking magnesium-containing antacids. Replacement of potassium and phosphate is indicated, especially when large amounts of glucose are given. Vitamins (especially thiamine and other water-soluble vitamins) are essential. It has been alleged that acute carbohydrate administration to a starved alcoholic patient may precipitate acute thiamine deficiency and worsen encephalopathy. It is probably safe to give 100 mg of thiamine to all alcoholic patients in withdrawal.

Most alcoholic patients treat their own alcohol withdrawal symptoms by continuation of alcohol intake, although the alcohol dose can be slowly tapered. Not only is it psychologically undesirable to maintain a patient on alcohol, but also the metabolic abnormalities created by chronic alcohol use persist. Paraldehyde was used to treat alcohol withdrawal for many years, but its adverse reactions occur at higher frequency than in diazepam-treated patients with delirium tremens. Paraldehyde may also worsen metabolic abnormalities, has a disagreeable odor, and is dangerous as an intramuscular injection. Phenothiazines have potentially serious side effects that probably outweigh their benefit in treating alcohol withdrawal. These effects include postural hypotension, extrapyramidal syndromes, alteration of temperature regulation, lowering of the seizure threshold, and many dermatologic and hematologic abnormalities.[7] Antihistamines also have been used to treat alcoholic withdrawal but are probably less effective in preventing seizures than other medications. In older alcoholic patients, the anticholinergic effects of the antihistamines may lead to complications of urinary retention, constipation, and confusion.

Based on clinical experience and some studies, the drugs of choice in the alcohol withdrawal syndrome are the benzodiazepine derivatives.[10] Current evidence does not show clear-cut superiority for any of these drugs. They all are more effective than placebo in preventing seizures and in treating the symptoms of alcohol withdrawal. Because both chlordiazepoxide (Librium) and diazepam (Valium) are long-acting compounds with active metabolites, they must be given with caution, especially if other toxins have been ingested. Many benzodiazepines also are absorbed erratically from intramuscular sites and have active metabolites that accumulate, thereby enhancing the likelihood of delayed sedation, prolonged hospitalization, and increased risk of respiratory embarrassment. Oxazepam (Serax) is converted rapidly to inactive water-soluble metabolites and will probably not accumulate even in patients with liver disease. Unfortunately, oxazepam is not available for parenteral administration. When rapid clinical action is required to manage the withdrawal syndrome, the intravenous route for the benzodiazepines is preferred. This is especially important if the patient is having life-threatening seizures.

In general, administering low doses of intravenous diazepam and loading the seizing patients with phenytoin in order to prevent continued seizure activity is preferred. It is important to emphasize that most of the benzodiazepines will accumulate and also lead to a withdrawal syndrome; therefore, the dose of these medications must be tapered gradually over 4 to 7 days.

Because alcohol withdrawal is so easily confused with other toxic emergencies and is extremely variable in character, the dose of medication required to manage the withdrawal varies widely. It is unwise to have routine standing orders for medications or for fluid balance in patients undergoing alcohol withdrawal. It is not necessary to suppress all the symptoms of the alcohol withdrawal syndrome, especially the tremor, as this will lead to excessive sedation. Routine use of phenytoin in the treatment of the alcohol withdrawal syndrome is controversial. When treated with phenytoin and varying doses of benzodiazepines, alcoholic patients with previous histories of seizures had better results with the combination of phenytoin and benzodiazepines than with benzodiazepines alone.[11] If phenytoin is used, it should not be maintained past the withdrawal period except in patients with underlying epilepsy. The development or presence of ataxia in an alcoholic patient taking phenytoin suggests phenytoin toxicity, and the phenytoin blood level should be measured. Use of β-blocking drugs to alter adrenergic activity may be effective and shorten hospitalization but is probably too dangerous for routine use.

ALCOHOL TOXIDROMES

When faced with a toxic alcoholic patient, it is useful to have in mind the typical syndrome or toxidromes that may be involved (Table 36–5). Alcoholic patients often have metabolic acidosis that may suggest paraldehyde ingestion, alcoholic ketoacidosis, lactic acidosis occurring spontaneously or with fructose therapy, isoniazid or aspirin poisoning, carbon monoxide poisoning, or the ingestion of alcohol substitutes.

Alcohol Metabolic Acidosis

Alcoholic ketoacidosis is an especially common problem. The patient usually vomits

Table 36–5. ALCOHOL TOXIDROMES

Metabolic acidosis

Paraldehyde: unique odor, increased anion gap, gastritis, no increase in serum osmolality

Ethanol: depressed sensorium, odor, metabolic acidosis, mild ketosis

Fructose therapy: metabolic acidosis, no increase in serum osmolality, hyperuricemia

Isoniazid: coma, persistent seizures, metabolic acidosis

Salicylate: hyperventilation, vomiting, fever, bleeding, tinnitus, increased anion gap

Carbon monoxide: presence or absence of coal gas odor, bullae on the skin, metabolic acidosis, relatively normal oxygen tension

Methanol: normal breath, no ketosis, normal Q-T on electrocardiogram, high white blood cell count, abnormal eye examination, increased osmolality, visual disturbance, increased mean corpuscular volume

Ethylene glycol: renal failure, crystals in the urine, anion gap, increased osmolality

Isopropanol: severe gastritis, acetonemia with normal glucose, increased serum osmolality, coma, pancreatitis

Other

Gamma benzene hexachloride: skin rash, application of medication, seizures

Lithium: tremor, seizure, polyuria, delayed CNS toxicity, narrow anion gap

Solvents: acetone, unique odor, CNS depression

Arsenic: garlicky breath, profuse diarrhea, hair loss, Mees' lines on the fingernails, increased skin pigmentation, neuropathy

Lead: abdominal pain, convulsions, metallic taste, motor neuropathy, hypertension and gout

and has moderate acidosis and mild glucose intolerance. It is essential to rule out pancreatitis in this setting. Only moderate ketosis is often encountered in the early phases of the illness, as most of the acidosis is caused by hydroxylated derivatives that do not induce a color change to blue with the nitroprusside tablet test. With adequate supportive care the acidosis is reversible, especially with appropriate hydration. Paraldehyde overdose also may present metabolic acidosis and an anion gap. In this circumstance paraldehyde is excreted in the breath and has a unique odor. When paraldehyde is taken orally, gastritis is frequent. Lethal doses of paraldehyde cause only slight abnormalities of serum osmolality. In alcoholic patients who are treated with fructose in an attempt to enhance alcoholic metabolism, lactic acidosis may result. In general it is unwise to use fructose in this setting because severe acidosis can be caused by the therapy.

Alcoholic patients may have tuberculosis or may have a conversion of a negative tuberculin test. Large amounts of isoniazid will cause prolonged seizures and metabolic acidosis.[12] This topic is discussed in Chapter 54.

Aspirin also may be ingested by alcoholics to treat a hangover or for other associated medical conditions. In excess, it may cause metabolic acidosis and a wide anion gap. A salicylate level determination is required to rule out this intoxication. Urine screening tests cannot be relied on for salicylate, as urinary clearance of salicylate depends on urine pH. Patients who are severely toxic from salicylate may have an acid urine that will contain very little salicylate.

Alcoholic individuals often fall asleep with a lighted cigarette or are involved inadvertently in a fire. Inebriated and impoverished persons also may attempt to keep themselves warm during the winter with poorly ventilated heating devices. Severe metabolic acidosis in an alcoholic patient found in a closed environment or in a fire requires carboxyhemoglobin determinations to rule out carbon monoxide poisoning.

In any alcoholic patient with metabolic acidosis, an increased anion gap, and an increased serum osmolality, one must consider the ingestion of alcohol substitutes. These are discussed in detail elsewhere. Methanol, ethylene glycol, and isopropyl alcohol all may cause metabolic acidosis, increased anion gap, and increased osmolality.

Alcoholic patients may inhale various organic solvents in a deliberate attempt to induce intoxication and euphoria. Solvent inhalation may induce a syndrome of muscle destruction, renal tubular acidosis, or gastrointestinal toxicities. The key factor in detecting an alcoholic patient with solvent inhalation is the identification of paint on the face or a unique odor. Some alcoholic individuals die suddenly while inhaling solvents, sometimes because of direct pulmonary injury or fatal arrhythmias. As alcoholic beverages become more expensive, it is anticipated that alcoholic patients will seek cheap substitutes, especially inexpensive organic solvents. The importance of solvent inhalation in alcoholic patients is emphasized in a report by Ramu and associates.[27]

DISULFIRAM

Disulfiram (Antabuse) is commonly used by many recovering alcoholic patients.[7] Any alcoholic patient ingesting disulfiram may potentially have a series of toxicologic problems. Disulfiram was discovered by accident during an investigation of its use as an anthelmintic agent, when, after ingestion, an investigator became ill when drinking alcohol. Disulfiram's potential value in treating alcoholism and its pharmacology were studied; it was used initially as an aversive method of treatment. The major pharmacologic and toxicologic action of disulfiram is thought to be a result of its capacity to form complex chelates with many heavy metals. Alcoholic patients were initially treated with many grams of disulfiram a day. Much toxicity occurred when the drug was first used, because patients were challenged with alcohol.

When disulfiram is taken with alcohol, severe, sometimes fatal reactions occur. Recent studies have found that disulfiram is excreted rapidly in the urine and breath, with 90 per cent of the oral dose excreted in 3 days.[28] Absorption of labeled disulfiram is almost complete but may be altered by simultaneous administration of antacids or iron. The onset of a disulfiram reaction after the first dose occurs 6 hours after the drug is first taken and usually persists for at least 24 hours after the drug is discontinued, except in patients who have abnormal liver function, in whom the reaction may continue for as long as 96 hours.

The metabolites of disulfiram may be detected in the breath and urine and used as markers of compliance.

A most interesting new area concerning the toxicology of disulfiram has been its effect on the adrenergic nervous system. The conversion of dopamine to norepinephrine is the final step in catecholamine biosynthesis and is catalyzed by the enzyme dopamine beta-hydroxylase. This enzyme is inhibited by a variety of chelating agents and disulfiram. Disulfiram itself is not a potent chelating agent, but its metabolic products are potent copper chelators. The in vivo conversion of exogenous dopamine to norepinephrine appears to be dose dependent and may be associated with some alteration in blood pressure.[30] It is possible that some of the potential therapeutic benefit of disulfiram is related to alterations in catecholamine pathways.

Clinical Presentation of the Alcohol-Disulfiram Reaction

Within a few minutes after the ingestion of even minute quantities of alcohol in disulfiram-treated patients, toxic reaction occurs. The patient first notes a feeling of warmth in the face. The skin, especially in the upper chest and face, becomes bright red, and a pounding sensation occurs in the head. Respiratory difficulties, nausea, vomiting, sweating, weakness, dizziness, blurred vision, and confusion all may be part of the reaction. With large doses of alcohol and disulfiram, the reaction may be extremely severe and even life threatening. Reactions are usually proportional to the amount of alcohol ingested and the dose of disulfiram. Reactions may last a few minutes in mild cases to several hours in severe ones. The mechanism of the phenomenon has been studied but is not completely clear. Study of reactions is limited by the difficulty of measuring disulfiram and acetaldehyde, as well as by problems in interpreting animal studies and the dangers of human experimentation.

Disulfiram and its metabolites are thought to block the oxidation of acetaldehyde. Acetaldehyde then causes vasodilation and decreases the blood pressure. In some studies, disulfiram significantly increases the acetaldehyde level in normal nondrinking subjects and dramatically increases acetaldehyde after ingestion of alcohol. Disulfiram-alcohol reactions themselves are not totally explicable on the basis of high acetaldehyde concentrations. In animals it is not possible to relate the acute disulfiram reaction to acetaldehyde, disulfiram, or the metabolites of disulfiram. It has been suggested that other compounds may cause the severe reactions. In animals it is also evident that disulfiram prevents the stimulant effect of alcohol and acetaldehyde on heart rate, arterial pressure, and myocardial contractility.[7] It is difficult to study disulfiram in anesthetized animals because the disulfiram may interact with the anesthetic agents, causing altered cardiovascular effects.

Because of the difficulty in measuring blood levels of disulfiram and acetaldehyde, better studies are required. Studies by Iber and Chowdhury found highly variable acetaldehyde levels in reactors and nonreactors on disulfiram who were tested with alcohol.[29] Because disulfiram inhibits dopamine beta-hydroxylase, it is possible that the drug produces a catecholamine deficiency state.[29] The best current explanation for the disulfiram reaction is a combination of a direct blood vessel-relaxing effect of acetaldehyde and an adrenergic insufficiency state produced by disulfiram.

Some patients taking disulfiram accidentally ingest alcohol or deliberately take alcohol in an attempt to verify the efficacy of the drugs or to commit suicide. Some patients with mild reactions never seek medical attention. However, occasional cases may require immediate medical attention. Even though the disulfiram-alcohol reaction is usually short lived and without sequelae, severe reactions can occur. Intracranial hemorrhages or acute myocardial infarction may occasionally occur.

Treatment

Fluid administration, oxygen, and supportive therapy are presently the mainstay of therapy in these patients.

There is little definitive information concerning the appropriate treatment of disulfiram-alcohol reactions. Information supplied by the manufacturer about disulfiram refers primarily to unreferenced sources and recommends administration of oxygen and carbon dioxide (95 per cent oxygen, 5 per cent carbon dioxide), ephedrine sulfate, and intravenous ascorbic acid or antihistamines. It is difficult to document the therapeutic efficacy of any of these procedures. Strict guidelines on human experimentation make it difficult to carefully study these therapeutic maneuvers. It is suggested on the basis of uncontrolled studies that intravenous administration of iron salts might be capable of reversing the alcohol-disulfiram reaction, but this has not been uniformly substantiated.

Administration of antihistamines is often recommended to treat the alcohol-disulfiram reaction, but there is no evidence that histamine plays a part in these reactions, even in laboratory animals. Phenothiazines are also occasionally administered for gastrointestinal distress, nausea, and vomiting. These drugs seem to be contraindicated because of the likelihood of precipitating hypotension. The administration of carbon dioxide seems contraindicated because a patient undergoing this reaction is apparently already maximally vasodilated.

Complications

Side effects of disulfiram may occasionally be difficult to distinguish from other toxic emergencies. Neuropsychiatric and cardiovascular side effects have been of great concern.[31–34] Carbon disulfide, a metabolite of disulfiram, may have important cardiovascular and psychiatric complications.[30] Workers who are exposed to carbon disulfide in the manufacture of viscose rayon and also in the vulcanization of rubber have been noted to experience irritability, memory defects, altered sexual function, and accelerated cardiovascular disease. Acute brain syndromes also may result from exposure to carbon disulfide.[30] It is possible that neuropsychiatric changes could be related to alteration of biogenic amines associated with disulfiram and its metabolites. It may be difficult to distinguish disulfiram-induced encephalopathy from psychogenic disorders induced by the drug or as a primary component of alcoholism. Hotson and Langston reported two patients who had disulfiram-induced encephalopathy and who exhibited paranoid ideation, disorientation, impaired memory, ataxia, dysarthria, and abnormal electroencephalograms.[33] Grand mal seizures also may be part of this syndrome.

It may be difficult to distinguish disulfiram-induced psychosis from a toxic reaction to carbon disulfide or the abstinence from alcohol. Peripheral and optic neuritis occurring in alcoholic patients also has been associated with disulfiram rather than alcohol. Any neuropathic toxicity of disulfiram would be difficult to distinguish from toxicity of chronic alcohol alone. Rainey reviewed the neurotoxic effects of disulfiram and compared them with those of carbon disulfide. He concluded that there appears to be "at least a superficial" relationship between the behavioral and neurologic effects of disulfiram and carbon disulfide. He also suggested that thiamine supplementation might prevent disulfiram-induced neuropathy.[34]

Because of the possibility of neuropsychiatric and cardiovascular complications of disulfiram, psychosis and active cardiovascular diseases thus may become relative contraindications to the use of the medication. Complicated medical conditions requiring drug treatment in which disulfiram may precipitate drug interactions or worsen those medical conditions should make physicians wary of prescribing the drug. In light of these hazards, mandatory treatment with the drug is inadvisable and questionable. Patients also must know the alcohol content of common

Table 36–6. ALCOHOL CONTENT (%) OF SOME COMMON NONPRESCRIPTION AND PRESCRIPTION PREPARATIONS

Cough preparations		Tonics	
Vicks Formula 44	10	Geritol	12
Romilar CV	10	Bronchodilators	
Pertussin Plus	25	Elixophyllin	20
Nyquil	25	Brondecon	20
Robitussin	3	Other	
Mouthwashes		Paregoric tincture	45
Listerine	25	Terpin hydrate elixir	42
Scope	18		
Colgate 100	17		
Tincture	50		
Elixirs	25		

nonprescription and prescription medications (Table 36–6).

Drug Interactions with Disulfiram

Many drugs have been noted to shorten the duration of action of other drugs by accelerating the rate of biotransformation. The number of drugs causing much more serious reactions by inhibiting drug metabolism is relatively small. Disulfiram may prolong the half-life of some drugs by inhibiting hepatic microsomal mixed-function oxidases.

The clinical effects of disulfiram on other drugs are quite variable, possibly because of individual differences in gastrointestinal absorption or genetic differences in the capacity of disulfiram to inhibit drug-metabolizing enzymes. A marked decrease in the metabolism of aminopyrine with disulfiram is reported, whereas phenobarbital enhanced the metabolism of aminopyrine.[7] It was also found that disulfiram increases the anticoagulant effect of warfarin in most but not all subjects by inhibiting the metabolism of warfarin in the liver. Administration of disulfiram plus phenytoin results in a 100 to 500 per cent increase in serum concentrations of phenytoin in some patients. Disulfiram also may inhibit the metabolism of isoniazid, causing coordination difficulties and changes of behavior.

Disulfiram has been administered with methadone to alcoholic heroin addicts, and no major demonstrable clinically apparent interaction occurs. Rifampin and disulfiram have been administered to a few patients without major observable reactions. Levodopa and disulfiram have caused no observable toxicity. Although severe clinical drug interactions seem to be relatively uncommon with disulfiram, it seems wise to monitor blood levels of drugs simultaneously administered with disulfiram.

References

1. Becker CE, Roe RL, Scott RA: Alcohol as a Drug. Huntington, NY, Robert E. Krieger Publishing Company, 1979.
2. Glasser L, Sternglanz PD, Combie J, Robinson A: Serum osmolality and its applicability to drug overdose. Am J Clin Pathol *60*:695, 1973.
3. Gabow PA, Kaehny WD, Fenessey PV, Goodman SI, Gross TA, Schrier RW: Diagnostic importance of increased serum anion gap. N Engl J Med *303*:854, 1980.
4. Lieber CS: Interactions to ethanol and drug metabolism. J Adv Alcohol *1*:1, 1980.
5. Iber FL: Drug metabolism in heavy consumers of ethanol. Clin Pharmacol Ther *22*(art 2):735, 1978.
6. Linnolla M: Alcohol withdrawal and noradrenergic function. Ann Intern Med *107*:875, 1987.
7. Becker CE: Pharmacotherapy in the treatment of alcoholism. *In* Mendelson JH, Mell NK (eds): Diagnosis and Treatment of Alcoholism. New York, McGraw-Hill Book Company, 1979.
8. David DJ, Spyker DA: The acute toxicity of ethanol: Dosage and kinetic nomograms. Vet Hum Toxicol *21*:2726, 1980.
9. Levy R, Eco T, Hanenson IB: Intravenous fructose treatment of acute alcohol intoxication. Arch Intern Med *137*:1176, 1977.
10. Sellers EM, Kalant H: Alcohol intoxication withdrawal. N Engl J Med *294*:757, 1976.
11. Sampliner R, Iber FL: Diphenylhydantoin control of alcohol withdrawal seizures. JAMA *230*:1430, 1974.
12. Coyer N: Isoniazid-induced convulsions. South Med J *138*:294, 1976.
13. Becker CE: Acute methanol poisoning—"The blind drunk"—Medical Staff Conference, University of California, San Francisco. West J Med *135*:122–128, 1981.
14. Becker CE: Methanol poisoning. J Emerg Med *1*:51–58, 1983.
15. Osterloh JD, Pond SM, Grady S, Becker CE: Serum formate concentrations in methanol intoxication as a criterion for hemodialysis. Ann Intern Med *104*:200–203, 1986.
16. Jacobsen D, McMartin KE: Methanol and ethylene glycol poisonings: Mechanism of toxicity, clinical course, diagnosis and treatment. Med Toxicol *1*:309–334, 1986.
17. Jacobsen D, Jansen H, Wiik-Larsen E, Bredesen JE, Halvorsen S: Studies on methanol poisoning. Acta Med Scand *212*:5–10, 1982.
18. Jacobsen D, Bredesen JE, Eide I, Ostborg J: Anion and osmolal gaps in the diagnosis of methanol and ethylene glycol poisoning. Acta Med Scand *212*:17–20, 1982.
19. Methanol poisoning (editorial). Lancet, 1:910–912, 1983.
20. Wu AHB, Stout R, McComb RB: Case Report—falsely high serum creatinine concentration associated with severe methanol intoxication. Clin Chem *29*:205–208, 1983.

21. Swartz RD, Millman RP, Billi JE, et al: Epidemic methanol poisoning: Clinical and biochemical analysis of a recent episode. Medicine *60*:373–382, 1981.
22. Ekins BR, Rollins DE, Duffy DP, Gregory MC: Standardized treatment of severe methanol poisoning with ethanol and hemodialysis. West J Med *142*:337–340, 1985.
23. Ley CO, Gali FG: Parkinsonian syndrome after methanol intoxication. Eur Neurol *22*:405–409, 1983.
24. Andrews LS, Clary JJ, Terrill JB, Bolte HF: Subchronic inhalation toxicity of methanol. J Toxicol Environ Health *20*:117–124, 1987.
25. Starr HG, Clifford NJ: Acute lindane intoxication. Arch Environ Health *25*:374, 1972.
26. Wheeler M: Gamma benzene hexachloride poisoning in children. West J Med *127*:518, 1977.
27. Ramu A, Rosenbaum J, Blaschke TF: Disposition of acetone found in the acute acetone intoxication. West J Med *129*:429, 1978.
28. Iber FL, Dutta S, Shamszad M, Krause S: Excretion of radioactivity following administration of ^{35}sulfur-labeled disulfiram in man. Alcohol Clin Exp Res *1*:359, 1977.
29. Iber FL, Chowdhury B: The persistence of the alcohol-disulfiram reaction after dissemination of drug in patients with and without liver disease. Alcohol Clin Exp Res *1*:365, 1977.
30. Rogers WK, Benowitz NL, Wilson KM, Abbott JA: Effect of disulfiram on adrenergic function. Clin Pharmacol Ther *25*:469, 1979.
31. Davidson M, Feinle BM: Carbon disulfide poisoning: A review. Am Heart J *83*:100, 1972.
32. Gardner-Thorpe C, Benjamin S: Peripheral neuropathy after disulfiram administration. J Neurol Neurosurg Psychiatry *34*:253, 1971.
33. Hotson JR, Langston JW: Disulfiram-induced encephalopathy. Arch Neurol *33*:141, 1976.
34. Rainey JM: Disulfiram toxicity and carbon disulfide poisoning. Am J Psychiatry *134*:371, 1977.

B. Evaluation of Drug Use in the Adolescent

Richard L. Jones, M.D.

The pervasive availability of psychotrophic chemicals, such as alcohol, marijuana, tobacco, cocaine, heroin, LSD, PCP, and many others, has profoundly altered the cultural environment in which we live, work, and attempt to rear our children. In the last half of the twentieth century, drug experimentation, use, and abuse have so invaded our society that millions of vulnerable youth and adults must decide *daily* whether they should or when they will use drugs. Clinicians caring for patients of any age must have the skills and knowledge to educate in prevention those patients whose background suggests an increased vulnerability to abuse or addiction. Clinicians also must have the resources to identify, intervene with, and appropriately refer those patients whose abuse of chemicals has affected their physical, emotional, or social health.

For adolescents in our culture, deciding what role the various available chemicals will play in their lives is a task they must confront from an early age. Macdonald and Newton have characterized the continuum of chemical use-abuse-addiction, which, if kept in mind by clinicians, can serve as a framework for judging the extent of patient disability and, thus, the appropriate intervention strategy (Table 36–7).

A substantial minority of patients have an increased likelihood of developing drug and alcohol dependency. The studies of Goodwin, Schuckit, Cloninger, and others strongly suggest a genetic risk for alcoholism (and presumably for drug dependency). Essentially, two types of inheritable predispositions to alcoholism exist: milieu-limited and male-limited. In the milieu-limited type, environmental factors may help reduce the actual risk of alcoholism, whereas in the male-limited type, environmental factors will not alter the chances of alcoholism developing but may reduce its severity.

Risk factors that may identify patients at increased risk for the development of chemical abuse problems are listed in Table 36–8. Of particular importance is the concept of *heightened vulnerability* to the psychotropic effects of chemicals. Adolescents, especially those who are socially immature, who are genetically vulnerable to alcoholism or mental illness, or who have impulse control problems, are probably at such increased risk that, when they are seen for any kind of medical problem, repeated preventive education is warranted. Efforts should be made to get them to postpone experimentation with alcohol and drugs as long as possible in order to permit neurologic and social maturation.

Longitudinal studies by Kandel and Logan have defined a period of "transitional" heavy alcohol (and presumptively drug) use during the late teens and early twenties. It is encouraging that in Jessor and Jessor's studies, 53 per cent of men and 70 per cent of women

Table 36–7. STAGES OF DRUG ABUSE

STAGE	MOOD ALTERATION	FEELING	DRUGS	SOURCES	BEHAVIOR	FREQUENCY
1. Learning the mood swing	Euphoria Normal Pain	Feel good; few consequences	Tobacco Marijuana Alcohol	"Friends"	Little detectable change; moderate "after the fact" lying	Progresses to weekend usage
2. Seeking the mood swing	Euphoria Normal Pain	Excitement; early guilt	All of the above plus inhalants, hash oil, hashish, "uppers," "downers," prescriptions	Buying	Dropping extracurricular activities and hobbies; mixed friends (straight and druggie); dress changing; erratic school performance and "skipping"; unpredictable mood and attitude swings; "conning" behavior	Weekend use progressing to four to five times per week; some solo use
3. Preoccupation with the mood swing	Euphoria Normal Pain	Euphoric highs; doubts, including severe shame and guilt; depression; suicidal thoughts	All of the above plus "mushrooms," PCP, LSD, cocaine	Selling	"Cool" appearance; straight friends dropped; family fights (verbal and physical); stealing (police incidents); pathologic lying; school failure, skipping, expulsion; jobs lost	Daily Frequent solo use
4. Using drugs to feel normal	Euphoria Normal Pain	Chronic guilt, shame, remorse, depression	Whatever is available	Any way possible	Physical deterioration (weight loss, chronic cough); severe mental deterioration (memory loss and flashbacks); paranoia, volcanic anger, and aggression; school dropout; frequent overdosing	All day, everyday

(From Macdonald DI, Newton M: Drugs, Drinking, and Adolescents. Chicago, Year Book Medical Publishers, Inc., 1984.)

who were diagnosed as problem drinkers as teenagers "matured" into socially acceptable drinkers by their early twenties. Likewise, the period of peak drug use (alcohol, tobacco, marijuana, and cocaine) in Kandel's studies was between 16 and 22 years of age, followed by a marked reduction in both the frequency and variety of drugs used thereafter by most individuals.

This period of "transitional" drug and alcohol abuse from mid-adolescence to young adulthood increases the difficulty of diagnosing correctly those adolescents and young adults who have chemical abuse problems. Table 36–9 lists the behavioral problems adolescents and young adults manifest when Stages 2 and 3 of chemical abuse (see Table 36–7) have developed. In general, any adolescent with depression, runaway behavior, school problems, or family problems should be evaluated for possible chemical abuse. In contrast, adolescents with court-related alcohol or drug problems or any delinquency, those with histories of any type of recurrent accidents, and those with depressive-suicidal behavior should be *assumed* to have chemical abuse problems *until proved otherwise.* This diagnostic approach will identify as chemical abusers some patients who will "mature into social users." It is better to err in overdiagnosing this population of patients, however, even though clinicians may lose some patients by an aggressive intervention strategy.

When the clinician decides that a chemical abuse assessment is warranted, a medical-counseling evaluation (Table 36–10) should be activated, utilizing all resources available to the clinician. It is important that the clinician remain an active participant in the eval-

Table 36–8. RISK FACTOR CHECKLIST FOR SUBSTANCE/ALCOHOL ABUSE

Family history of alcoholism on either side of the family, including all relatives
Availability of alcohol and/or drugs
Early use of any mind-altering drugs—especially alcohol, tobacco, marijuana, cocaine
Family history of teetotalism
Use of cross-dependent drugs (marijuana, sedatives, tranquilizers)
Preference for drug-using peer group
Ethnic background with an increased reported incidence of alcoholism
Attentional deficit disorder and/or learning disabilities (especially if exposure to drugs/alcohol occurs early and if associated with academic underachievement)
Family problems, including divorce, abuse, and inconsistent and impulsive parenting and supervision
Male sex

(Adapted from Jones RL: Identification and management of the toxic adolescent. Semin Adolesc Med *1*:239, 1985, with permission.)

uation process and in rendering a diagnosis to the patient and family, as well as in discussing the referral options. Unquestionably, this evaluation process will be somewhat confrontational for everyone, may expose heretofore unknown family problems, may not be as cost-effective as other clinical activities, and frequently may not be completed because of patient or family noncompliance.

Adolescents with evidence of gastritis, peptic ulcer disease, hepatitis, chronic nonasthmatic/allergic bronchitis, hypertension, sexually transmitted diseases (especially recurrent), and blackouts should be closely scrutinized. Laboratory evaluation is rarely conclusive by itself (even urine screening). A systematic plan for evaluation and treatment

Table 36–9. BEHAVIORAL PARAMETERS SEEN IN SUBSTANCE/ALCOHOL ABUSERS

A worsening in school performance
School truancy
Symptoms of acute and/or chronic depression
Unexplained or recurrent accidents or fights
Repeated overt intoxications
Preoccupation with social activities in which alcohol/drugs might be present
Decreased communication with other family members
Drug-using peer group
Changes in dress and personal habits of hygiene
Runaway behavior
Court involvement regarding charges such as drunk and disorderly conduct, driving while intoxicated, and so on

(From Jones RL: Identification and management of the toxic adolescent. Semin Adolesc Med *1*:239, 1985, with permission.)

should be formulated (Table 36–10). Psychologic/chemical abuse profiles like the Michigan Alcohol Screening Test (MAST), the WASP Test (Table 36–11), the CAGE Test (Table 36–12), the symptom checklist for substance abuse (Table 36–13), and the adolescent failure syndrome test (Table 36–14) can provide nonconfrontational approaches to evaluating personality function and mood. The WASP and CAGE questions are easily learned and can be incorporated into history taking as a means of assessing chemical abuse risk. Professional colleagues such as psychologists, psychiatrists, and psychiatric social workers are especially helpful in providing some or all of the behavioral portion of the evaluation.

The evaluation will necessarily require several visits, during which time the behaviors that prompted the assessment may worsen, necessitating therapeutically short-term solutions, emergency interventions, or shortening of the evaluation schedule. Invariably, related problems such as parental alcohol or drug abuse, family difficulties, evidence of physical or sexual abuse, financial woes, or related problems will complicate the evaluation and narrow the referral and treatment options. Parents may need referral for treatment themselves or to support groups like Tough Love and Adult Children of Alcoholics.

At the end of the evaluation process (which it is hoped is *not* the last session with the family), a summary session should be held to discuss referral options, which include the following:

Stage 1 Experimentation (see Table 36–7)

The problem behaviors do not include any biopsychosocial evidence of chemical abuse. These patients will need ambulatory individual or family therapy or both and not hospitalization. Printed reminders regarding the inappropriate and (probable) illegal use of chemicals should be given along with preventive education, especially if alcoholism, drug abuse, or mental illness exists within the family.

Stage 2 Chemical Use (see Table 36–7)

All patients with substantial chemical use will benefit from a period of required abstinence and therapeutic intervention in a facility providing both alcohol and drug withdrawal education and behavior modification (a dual diagnosis facility). This is especially warranted when a family history of chemical abuse or mental illness or both exists.

Table 36–10. MEDICAL-COUNSELING EVALUATION

Appropriately done by clinicians who are
- familiar with the patient/family
- familiar with the risk factors and behavioral toxicities common to adolescent/young adult drug abusers (Stage 2–Stage 4)
- have some interest or experience in counseling-assessment

Evaluation process should involve 1–5 visits, including a physical examination and appropriate laboratory evaluation, which should be done during the initial visit

The visits after the initial interview/physical examination/mental status assessment may number 2–4, depending upon the clinician's ongoing assessment. The clinician, however, should, estimate for the family the total number of expected visits at the first visit

Patients should be seen for 30–60 minutes for each visit. Counseling-assessment is best done before or at the end of office hours (noontime or prior to afternoon hours is appropriate as well)

The limits of confidentiality should be defined during the first visit. Although a complex issue, continued confidentiality with the patient should be judged by the dictum, "If the patient is going to hurt himself/herself or someone else or run away, then the clinician must bargain/plead to convince the patient how—to whom—what—when the information will be shared with the family"

Additional counseling-assessment sessions are used to
- obtain the patient's/family's confidence so that more extensive and reliable history can be obtained
- explore relevant family issues (i.e., divorce, parenting, emotional issues, potential/existing parental alcohol or substance abuse)
- obtain additional history through use of questionnaires like The Michigan Alcoholic Screening Test (MAST), Symptom Checklist for Substance Abuse (Table 36–13), Adolescent Failure Syndrome Test (Table 36–14), and the CAGE and WASP Screening Questions (Tables 36–11 and 36–12)
- provide the patient and family with drug/alcohol education
- encourage and educate parent(s) to use appropriate community support groups (e.g., AA, Alanon, Tough Love, etc.) and to monitor more closely the patient's behavior (e.g., phone calls, friends, curfew, etc.) and search for drugs/drug paraphernalia (in the patient's room, car, etc.)
- provide ongoing urine monitoring for drugs(s)—if appropriate and requested by the parent(s) or patient
- reach agreement with the patient about what information needs to be shared (in the clinician's judgment) at the summary session

The summary visit should be spent simultaneously reviewing with the patient and parent(s) pertinent risk factors, behavioral parameters, and physical examination and laboratory results, including urine results

Recommendations. The interpretative report should provide the patient and family with several treatment options that may or may not continue to involve the clinician:
- If the problem(s) prompting evaluation do not seem alcohol- and drug-related, appropriate referral to other counseling, therapy, or school resources is indicated. Experimental drug use should warrant guidance with regard to risk factors and dysfunctional behaviors
- If alcohol and drug use is occurring but only as a covariable in the adolescent's life, referral as above should occur along with the option to provide further management and, one would hope, abstinence from the alcohol/drug use through random urine screening or referral to an ambulatory drug treatment program
- If the adolescent's alcohol/drug use is abusive and the clinician believes it is a primary cause of the dysfunctional behavior and physical abnormalities, either a comprehensive ambulatory or inpatient substance abuse program should be recommended
- If the patient's evaluation suggests a primary psychiatric etiology, referral to a psychiatrist or therapist may be warranted. If the patient has concomitant alcohol/drug experimentation and has any risk factors, referral should be to a psychiatrist, who can continue to monitor for the development of abusive alcohol/drug use. Offering to screen the patient's urine for drugs as he or she continues to work with the parents and therapist may be valuable

Most frequently, however, these patients are referred to community-based day treatment or chemical abuse programs in which intervention and education are attempted. Many of the patients worsen with ambulatory attempts to alter chemical use behavior or are held in limbo until their behavior(s) either improve or worsen, prompting hospitalization, which their insurance will then cover partially or fully.

Stage 3 and 4 Abuse/Addiction (see Table 36–7)

All these patients will need *prompt* hospitalization, either in a chemical dependency (CD) program (if most or all of the biopsychosocial problems are thought to be secondary to the chemical abuse) or a psychiatric chemical dependency (dual diagnosis) program that provides a behavioral-psychiatric treatment modality as well as CD education. *These patients invariably are unsuccessfully treated in ambulatory programs.* Most of them, in fact, will need long-term residential treatment (following the 4- to 8-week dual diagnosis hospitalization) to cope with the abnormal behaviors and strategies learned during their period of chemical abuse.

Stages 1 and 2 Chemical Use with Sub-

Table 36–11. WASP TEST FOR SYMPTOMS AND SIGNS OF ALCOHOL ABUSE

W	*W*ithdrawal symptoms—adolescents usually do not have classic alcohol withdrawal symptoms
A	*A*lcohol tolerance—commonly seen in adolescent drinkers
S	*S*pite drinking—adolescents who spite drink do so despite the usually adverse psychosocial consequences that occur to them. Uncommonly, physical problems like gastritis or postbinge seizures or, commonly, physical trauma may occur
P	*P*athology—evidence for target organ pathology, especially the brain, is common in adolescent drinkers

(From Gitlow SE, Peyser HS (eds): Alcoholism: A Practical Treatment Guide. New York, Grune and Stratton, 1980, with permission.)

stantial Psychiatric Dysfunction (see Table 36–7)

These patients' biopsychosocial abnormalities result from psychiatric dysfunction induced by the neurochemical effects of alcohol and drug use. Psychiatric referral and possible hospitalization should be recommended.

In completing the medical-counseling evaluation for suspected chemical abuse, clinicians should remember the following points:

1. These evaluations virtually always trigger emotional turmoil in family and patient. Empathy, patience, and flexibility in scheduling the visits, and completing the evaluation are crucial to its success.
2. To refer the patient and family appropriately, counseling skills and correctly staging the severity of the adolescent's chemical use/abuse (see Table 36–7) are more important than knowing either the specific DSM-III-R* diagnosis or the specific kinds or amounts of chemicals being consumed.
3. Providing the most appropriate medical or psychiatric diagnoses will be crucial in qualifying the patient and family for an insurance-covered therapeutic program

Table 36–12. CAGE QUESTIONNAIRE FOR ALCOHOLISM

- Have you ever felt you ought to Cut down on your drinking?
- Have people Annoyed you by criticizing your drinking?
- Have you ever felt bad or Guilty about your drinking?
- Have you ever had a drink first thing in the morning to steady your nerves or get rid of a hangover (Eye-opener)?

One positive response calls for further inquiry.
Two or more positive answers strongly suggest alcoholism.

(From Ewing JA: Detecting alcoholism; The CAGE Questionnaire. JAMA 252:14, 1985. Reprinted with permission.)

Table 36–13. A SYMPTOM CHECKLIST FOR SUBSTANCE ABUSE*

	Yes	No
I. PSYCHOLOGIC COMPLICATIONS		
Has family member expressed concern about person's drug use?	____	____
Does person drink or use other drugs at home and in front of parents?	____	____
Does person's drug use cause family fights or arguments?	____	____
Has person's drug use caused problems with parents or friends?	____	____
Has person every been in drug treatment?	____	____
Has person ever been arrested for drug use?	____	____
II. BIOMEDICAL COMPLICATIONS		
Has person ever shown behavioral changes as a result of drug use?	____	____
Has person every had memory blackouts caused by drug use?	____	____
Has person ever used drugs in the morning?	____	____
Has person every had hallucinations secondary to drug use?	____	____
Has person ever had "shakes" due to drug use?	____	____
III. SCHOOL PROBLEMS		
Has person ever been using drugs while truant from school?	____	____
Has person ever used illicit drugs or alcohol on school grounds?	____	____
Has person ever missed school as a result of drug use or its effects?	____	____
Has person ever used drugs while in school building?	____	____
Has person kept or carried alcohol or drugs in school?	____	____
Has person needed to use drugs before going to school?	____	____
Has person seen school social worker or counselor because of drug use?	____	____

*Substance or drug abuse represents alcohol or illicit substances or both.

(Adapted from Halikas J, Lyttle M, Morse C, et al: Proposed criteria for the diagnosis of alcohol abuse in adolescence. Comp Psychiatry *25*(6):581–585, 1984, with permission.)

*Diagnostic and Statistical Manual of Psychiatric Diagnosis-Revised.

Table 36–14. ADOLESCENT FAILURE SYNDROME TEST* (AN AID TO PARENTS CONCERNED THAT ADOLESCENTS MAY BE HARMFULLY INVOLVED WITH DRUGS)

	DOES NOT APPLY	POSSIBLY APPLIES	DEFINITELY APPLIES
1. A change in the family's communication with adolescent. Refusal to take part in discussions concerning unacceptable behavior. Previous closeness may dissipate, and disciplinary talk may be interrupted either by "tuning out" or angry outbursts.	0	1	2
2. Refusal of the adolescent to recognize the impact on the family of unacceptable behavior, e.g., arguments, intoxicated events, or delinquent acts.	0	2	4
3. Concern expressed by others, e.g., siblings, classmates, teachers, other family members, or authority figures, concerning personality changes, suspected drug usage, or traveling with the "wrong crowd."	0	2	4
4. Expressed concern for oneself, e.g., "I'm worried I might get involved with drugs or alcohol," or "My life is meaningless, and I want to die."	0	2	4
5. Involvement in hard rock music, preoccupation with rock stars, attendance at rock concerts.	0	1	2
6. "Rebellious" dress style, e.g., rock or beer commercial T-shirts, army jackets, worn jeans, long hair.	0	1	2
7. Poor choice of friends, choosing to be with kids known or suspected of being delinquent and/or involved with drugs and alcohol.	0	2	4
8. Mysterious comings and goings, frequent telephone calls and visits by unfamiliar youth.	0	2	4
9. Change in social group, grade school friends left behind for a more "down and out group."	0	2	4
10. Incidents of untrustworthiness, particularly incorrect explanations of absence from school or lies about location of parties or parental chaperoning.	0	2	4
11. Unexcused absences from school or missed classes.	0	1	2
12. Minor or major delinquent involvement, especially where participants were intoxicated or drugs were involved.	0	2	4
13. Any violence or threat of violence toward parents or siblings.	0	2	4
14. Any violent episode away from home, including injury to self or others.	0	1	2
15. Minor or major automobile accidents.	0	1	2
16. Vocal disrespect for parents, teachers, or other authorities.	0	1	2
17. Unhealthy relationships. This includes a variety of unfortunate social styles, e.g., isolation from any close friends, or choice of a single friend to the exclusion of all others. No healthy involvement or interest in the opposite sex.	0	1	2
18. Premature adult behaviors, e.g., seductive dress or behavior, pseudosophisticated "existential" concerns, unreasonable questioning or rejection of family values, especially regarding "recreational" drug usage.	0	1	2
19. Early sexual involvement, e.g., concerns of pregnancy or discovery of birth control materials.	0	2	4
20. Mood swings, such as depression, irritability, or unexplained euphoria and talkativeness.	0	2	4
21. Sleep disturbances, particularly staying awake for long periods at night or going to bed.	0	2	4
22. A drop in grade averages, perhaps accompanied by a stated loss of interest in school.	0	1	2
23. Money problems: missing money from purses or coin collections at home or at babysitting jobs or homes of grandparents, or holds a steady job but does not show money in savings.	0	2	4

Table 36–14. ADOLESCENT FAILURE SYNDROME TEST* (AN AID TO PARENTS CONCERNED THAT ADOLESCENTS MAY BE HARMFULLY INVOLVED WITH DRUGS) *Continued*

	DOES NOT APPLY	POSSIBLY APPLIES	DEFINITELY APPLIES
24. Annoyance or tantrums occur when questioned, e.g., about possible drug involvement.	0	2	4
25. Cigarette smoking.	0	2	4
26. Discovery of marijuana, pills, or alcohol. Missing bottles of liquor or diluted liquor in the family supply.	0	2	4
27. Discovery of a diary recounting drug experiences or involvement with the drug scene or finding notes stating usage or drug exchange.	0	2	4
28. Episodes of intoxication, either marijuana or alcohol.	0	2	4

Parents should score their children on each item: 0 for not at all, the intermediate column for possible or single occurrence; and the "Definitely Applies" column where it applies without question or if there has been more than one instance. The entire score on all statements should then be added. A total of 8 should be viewed as suggestive, that is, worthy of gathering further information; a score of 12 or more is probable for harmful involvement with drugs worthy of further data gathering and evaluation by a knowledgeable person. A score of 16 or more should be viewed as nearly diagnostic; a full evaluation should be carried out, and serious consideration should be given to seeking treatment.

*Copyright by David G. Logan, MD, and Ronald E. Harrison, 2217 Packard Road, Suite 13, Ann Arbor, MI 48104. Used with permission.

that makes the clinician's efforts worthwhile.

4. Issues of confidentiality with the patient must involve consideration of the degree of biopsychosocial dysfunction induced by chemical use or abuse. *Clinicians must be advocates for the patient's health, whatever they perceive it should be.* This principle should guide the clinician's approach in dealing with information during the evaluation.
5. These families are universally in turmoil. Clinicians shouldn't expect much, if any, appreciation from the patients or families. *Interventions can be successful in dramatically altering the course of a patient's life.*

Evaluation of adults with suspected chemical abuse differs substantially from that of adolescents. Frequently, work and family problems or the development of a disabling medical symptom may trigger a patient's self-referral or force a family or company referral. Risk factor assessment (see Table 36–8) is useful, as are the incorporation of questions from the WASP (Table 36–11) and CAGE (Table 36–12) tests in eliciting historical clues suggesting substantial alcohol or drug use. Abuse of "gateway" drugs (alcohol, tobacco, marijuana, and cocaine) occurs in adults along with use of drugs such as narcotics, barbiturates, and tranquilizers that adolescents rarely use.

Unlike adolescents in whom dysfunctional behaviors are the predominant abnormalities that prompt an evaluation, adults may have medical symptoms of alcohol withdrawal that initiate a visit to the clinician's office. Underestimation of use and conscious lying regarding chemical use always should be suspected when symptoms or physical findings suggest otherwise. Laboratory testing should be used aggressively to substantiate suspected abuse. Requests for pain medications (narcotics especially) or for drugs cross-addictive with alcohol (sedatives, tranquilizers, and most sleeping pills) should prompt at least a historical review of risk and chemical abuse symptoms as listed previously. Multiple drug and alcohol abuse by adults is not unusual.

Unlike adolescents, adults must, except in rare instances, agree to participate in a treatment program. The negotiations for treatment with patients may be easier if court-related offenses prompted the evaluation, if the patient's employer has a dependency referral option, or if the patient's physical symptoms are clearly related to chemical abuse. The details of treatment of adults are beyond the scope of this chapter.

SUMMARY

Regardless of the age of the patient, clinicians are more apt to consider the diagnosis of chemical abuse in their patients if they:

- have a high index of suspicion,
- are familiar with the symptoms and signs of chemical abuse,
- have a systematic plan for evaluation of such patients,
- understand the community-based referral options available to them, and
- have an interest and proclivity in treating patients with these kinds of problems.

Bibliography

AMA Council on Scientific Affairs: Marijuana: Its health hazards and therapeutic potentials. JAMA 246:1823–1827, 1981.

Cloninger CR, Bohman M, Sigvardsson S: Inheritance of alcohol abuse. Arch Gen Psychiatry *38*:861–868, 1981.

Copeland KC, Underwood LE, Van Wyk JJ: Marijuana smoking and pubertal arrest. N Eng J Med *96*:1079–1080, 1980.

DuPont RL: Getting Tough on Gateway Drugs: A Guide for the Family. Washington, D.C., American Psychiatric Press, Washington, DC, 1984.

Ewing JA, Rouse BA, Pellizar ED. Alcohol sensitivity and ethnic background. Am J Psychiatry *131*:206, 1974.

Gitlow SE, Hennecke L (eds): Etiology of alcoholism: A new theoretic mosaic. Semin Adoles Med *1*:235, 1985.

Gitlow SE, Peyser HS (eds): Alcoholism: A practical Treatment Guide. New York, Grune and Stratton, 1980.

Gold MS, Dackis GA: Role of the laboratory in the evaluation of suspected drug abuse. J Clin Psychiatry *48*(Suppl):17–23, 1986.

Goodwin DW: Alcoholism and heredity: A review hypothesis. Arch Gen Psychiat *36*:57, 1979.

Goodwin DW: Studies of familial alcoholism: A review. J Clin Psychiatry *45*:14–17, 1984.

Halikas JA, Weller WA, Morse CL, et al: A longitudinal study of marijuana effects. Int J Addictions *20*:701–711, 1985.

Jaffe JH: Drug addiction and drug abuse. *In* Gilman AG, Goodman LS, Goodman A (eds): The Pharmacologic Basis of Therapeutics. 6th ed. New York, Macmillan, 1980, pp 535–584.

Jessor R, Jessor SL: Adolescent development and the onset of drinking. J Stud Alcohol *36*:27–51, 1975.

Jones RL (ed): The toxic adolescent. Semin Adoles Med *1*:4, 1984.

Jones RL: Identification and management of the toxic adolescent. Semin Adoles Med *1*:239, 1985.

Kandel DB, Logan JA: Patterns of drug use from adolescence to young adulthood. I. Periods of risk for initiation, continued use and discontinuation. Am J Public Health *74*:660–666, 1984.

Macdonald DI, Newton M: The clinical syndrome of adolescent drug abuse. Adv Pediatr *25*:1–25, 1981.

Rogers PP (ed): Chemical dependency. Pediatr Clin North Am *34*:2, 1987.

Schuckit MA, Goodwin DW, Windkur G: A half-sibling study of alcoholism. Am J Psychiatry *128*:1132–1136, 1972.

Wesson DR, Smith DE: Cocaine: Treatment perspectives. Natl Inst Drug Abuse Res Monogr Ser *61*:1983–203, 1985.

Wilford BB: Drug Abuse. A Guide for the Primary Care Physician. Chicago, American Medical Association, 1981.

References

1. Austin GA: Perspectives on the History of Psychoactive Substance Abuse, Rockville, MD, National Institute of Drug Abuse, 1978.
2. Bissell LB, Haberman P: Alcoholism in the Profession, New York, Oxford University Press, 1984.
3. Blaskinsky M, Russell GK: Urine Testing for Marijuana use: Implications for a Variety of Settings, American Council for Drug Education, 1981.
4. Braude MC, Szara S (eds): Pharmacology of Marijuana, New York, Raven Press, 1976.
5. Criteria Committee National Council on Alcoholism: Criteria for the diagnosis of alcoholism. Ann Intern Med 77:249, 1972.
6. DeLuca JR (ed): Fourth Annual Report to the U.S. Congress on Alcohol and Health, Rockville, MD, U.S. Government Printing Office, 1981.
7. Dependency and Age, A World Survey. World Health Organization, 1980.
8. Donegan NH, Rodin J, O'Brien CP, Solomon RL: A learning-theory approach to commonalities. *In* Levinson PK, Gerstein DR, Maloff DR (eds): Commonalities in Substance Abuse and Habitual Behavior. Lexington, MA, Lexington Books, 1983.
9. DuPont RL: Marijuana, alcohol, and adolescence: A malignant synergism. Seminars in Adolescent Medicine, 1:4, 311, 1985.
10. Eckardt MJ, et al.: Health hazards associated with alcohol consumption. JAMA 246:648, 1981.
11. Ellinwood EG, Kilbey MD (eds): Cocaine and Other Stimulants, New York, Plenum Press, 1979.
12. Fishman HC: A family approach to marijuana use. *In* Marijuana and Youth: Clinical Observations on Motivation and Learning, Rockville, MD, National Institute on Drug Abuse, 1982.
13. Gay GR, Way EI: Pharmacology of the opiate narcotics. *In* Smith DE, Gay GR (eds): It's So Good, Don't Even Try It Once, Englewood Cliffs, NJ, Prentice-Hall, Inc. 1972.
14. Gitlow SE, Peuser HS: Alcoholism: A Practical Treatment Guide, New York, Grune and Stratton, 1980.
15. Gold MS: 800-Cocaine, New York, Bantam Books, 1984.
16. Gold MS, Dackis CA: New insights and treatments: Narcotics and cocaine addiction. Clin Therapeut 7:6, 1985.
17. Gold MS, Semlitz L, Dackis CA, Extein I: The adolescent cocaine epidemic. Semin Adoles Med 1:4, 303, 1985.
18. Gritz ER: Smoking behavior and tobacco abuse. *In* Mello NK (ed): Advances in Substance Abuse. Greenwich, CN, JAI Press, 1980.
19. Haddad LM: Cocaine in perspective. JACEP 8:374, 1979.
20. Haddad LM, Winchester JF: Clinical Management of Poisoning and Drug Overdose. Philadelphia, W.B. Saunders Co., 1983.
21. Johnson L, Bachman J, O'Malley P: Student Drug Use, Attitudes and Beliefs: National Trends 1975–1982. Rockville, MD, National Institute on Drug Abuse, 1984.

22. Jones RL: Drug Use and Abuse. *In* Shearin RB, Wientzen RL: Clinical Adolescent Medicine. Boston, GK Hall, 1983.
23. Kandel D: Stages in adolescent involvement in drug use. Science 190:921, 1975.
24. Kulberg A: Substance abuse: Clinical identification and management. *In* Blumer JL, Reed MD (eds): Pediatric Toxicology. Ped Clin N Am 33:2, 325, 1986.
25. Macdonald DI, Newton M: Drugs, Drinking and Adolescents. Chicago, Year Book Medical Publishers, 1984.

CHAPTER 37

METHANOL, ISOPROPYL ALCOHOL, HIGHER ALCOHOLS, ETHYLENE GLYCOL, CELLOSOLVES, ACETONE, AND OXALATE

James F. Winchester, M.D.

This chapter deals with substances that produce metabolic complications, particularly the production of an acidosis. Poisoning by several of these substances requires early intervention, in the case of methanol to prevent ocular and central nervous system toxicity and in the case of ethylene glycol to prevent renal failure.

METHANOL

Methanol (methyl alcohol, wood spirits) is a widely used commercial, industrial, and marine solvent and paint remover as well as a solvent in paints, varnishes, shellacs, and photocopying fluid. It may be used alone as an antifreeze fluid (starting concentration 95 per cent) and is commonly used in windshield washing fluids (starting concentration 35 to 95 per cent). In addition, it can be formulated as a solid canned fuel (4 per cent), along with ethanol and soap, or as a liquid fuel for heating small engines used in various hobbies.[1] In the United Kingdom, methanol is adulterated with a purple dye to distinguish it from ethanol; for use in small quantities, it is available only through the pharmacist as "methylated spirits," for which the user must sign a register. However, its widespread industrial use in laboratories, schools, and industrial processes accounts for the fact that large volumes may be obtained, commonly resulting in epidemic outbreaks of methanol poisoning. (See Chapter 76 for a table of selected products containing methanol.)

Methanol is widely used in industry as a solvent and an adulterant to make ethyl alcohol unfit to drink when the latter is used for cleaning purposes. Since methanol can be purchased tax free and is considerably less expensive than normal alcoholic beverages, it is not surprising that the alcoholic derelict may consume such compounds. Methanol has no therapeutic properties and is considered only as a toxicant. It has been reported that 6 per cent of all cases of blindness in the US Armed Forces in World War II were caused by methanol.[2] The fatal dose is said to be between 60 and 240 ml,[1] or 15 to 30 ml of a 40 per cent solution. However, with aggressive treatment, survival may be achieved at much higher intake.

Toxicology and Pharmacology

Although toxicity has been reported after inhalation or skin absorption,[3] the main route of toxicity is ingestion. Methyl alcohol is readily absorbed from the gastrointestinal tract after ingestion to give peak blood levels in 30 to 90 minutes, to be widely distributed in body tissues with a distribution of 0.6 to 0.7 L/kg.[4–7] A small amount of methanol is found in the expired breath of normal subjects,[4] possibly by endogenous metabolic production.[6] In animals most infused methanol is excreted by the respiratory tract (30 per cent of the ingested dose),[5] but this is not the prime mode of excretion in man.[7] The kidney in untreated patients excretes less than 5 per cent of unchanged methanol, and the remaining methanol (90 to 95 per cent) is excreted by hepatic biotransformation to other compounds. The majority of methanol, therefore, is converted to breakdown products, principally in the liver, by the metalloenzyme alcohol dehydrogenase to produce formaldehyde. Thereafter, formaldehyde is converted to formate by such enzyme systems as aldehyde dehydrogenase, xanthine oxidase, glyceraldehyde-3-phosphate hydrogenase, catalases, peroxidase, aldehyde oxidase, and a glutathione-dependent formaldehyde dehydrogenase.[8] The elimination half-life of methanol varies between 14 and 20 hours (mild intoxication) and 24 and 30 hours (severe intoxication) in untreated patients, and this is prolonged to 30 to 35 hours by the administration of ethanol.

Unlike poisoning by ingestion of formaldehyde, which does not produce retinal damage (see Chapter 26), local production of formaldehyde from methanol in the retina is felt to be principally responsible for optic papillitis and retinal edema with subsequent blindness,[8, 9] although *continuous* infusion of formate may produce optic nerve edema.[10] The ability to oxidize methanol to formic acid and to oxidize formic acid varies considerably with different animal species. For instance, the rabbit excretes only 1 per cent of methanol as urinary formic acid compared with 20 per cent in the dog; the oxidation capabilities of humans are intermediate.[11] Oxidation of methanol, like that of ethanol, proceeds independently of the blood concentration, but at a rate only one-seventh that of ethanol, accounting for the fact that complete oxidation and excretion of methanol require several days. Although oxidation is ostensibly achieved within the liver, it also occurs within the kidney.[11] The enzyme alcohol dehydrogenase, the principal enzyme involved in oxidation of ethanol, is also utilized in the oxidation of methanol. However, ethanol is preferentially metabolized by this enzyme, and administration of ethanol delays its clinical and biochemical effects. It is for this reason that ethyl alcohol is used clinically to slow down the metabolic transformation of methanol to the toxic product (formic acid), itself the product of oxidation. The metabolic pathways for the breakdown of methanol are shown in Figure 37–1.

Clinical Manifestations of Methanol Intoxication

Symptoms of methanol poisoning may be delayed for 12 to 18 hours, and this latent period is thought to be due to the delayed metabolism of methanol to the principal toxic product, formic acid.[12] The manifestations are as follows: a minor central nervous system intoxication similar to that seen with ethyl alcohol intoxication, a major acidosis due to the production of formic acid[12] and lactic acidosis,[13–15] and the most serious toxicity to the retinal cells by the local production of formaldehyde in the retina and optic disc,[9, 16] enhanced by acidosis.[17] In animals (monkeys and rats), it has been demonstrated that folate deficiency seems to promote the acidosis, and there is some evidence in animals that folic or folinic acid enhances the breakdown of formic acid to carbon dioxide and water and may prevent ocular toxicity.[10, 18–20]

The fatal human dose lies between 60 and 240 ml, although survivors have been reported toward the upper end of this range. As little as 10 ml has been considered toxic; although death may be prompt, it is usually delayed for several days. Even before hemodialysis was used as specific therapy for this intoxication, *institution of therapy before visual disturbances occurred appeared to promote an improved prognosis.*[5] As mentioned, methanol may be consumed along with ethyl alcohol, but, even when consumed alone, inebriation and subsequent drowsiness are noticed to be mild and somewhat transient.

Characteristically, the period of inebriation is followed by an asymptomatic period; then within 6 to 30 hours (which may be protracted if ethanol was also ingested) the characteristic symptoms and signs occur (Table 37–1). The major symptoms and signs of methanol poisoning consist of vertigo, vomiting, severe abdominal pain, diarrhea, back pain, dyspnea, motor restlessness, cold and

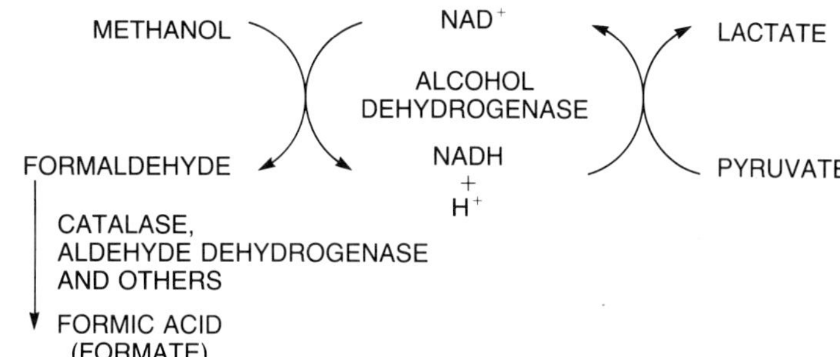

Figure 37–1. Metabolic degradation of methanol.

clammy extremities, blurring vision, and hyperemia of the optic disc with occasional blindness. Blood pressure is usually well maintained, but in the severely ill patient the pulse may be slow; this confers a grave prognostic sign. Since the visual disturbance can proceed to blindness, pupillary light reactions may be absent. In very severe cases, restlessness and delirium may be marked features, and in the presence of severe acidosis, Kussmaul respiration may or may not be seen. Death may be rapid or may occur many hours after the onset of coma. A curious feature of the modus of death is the occurrence of inspiratory apnea and terminal opisthotonos and convulsions.[5] Another clinical feature is the finding of pancreatitis on autopsy of severe cases of methanol poisoning, a feature that might explain the severe abdominal pains accompanying acute methanol poisoning.[21–23] Hyperamylasemia[7] (salivary[24]) has been observed, as has myoglobinuric acute renal failure.[25] In the latter regard, a diagnosis of renal failure based on serum creatinine alone may be false, since methanol interferes with creatinine determination.[26] Becker, in a review of methanol poisoning, points out that permanent optic nerve damage occurs in 25 per cent of poisoned subjects.[7] Other permanent neurologic features include parkinsonism and necrosis of the putamen observed either at autopsy or on computed axial tomography (CT) of the brain.[27, 28]

Factors in the Production of Acidosis

It has long been felt that formic acid was the prime metabolite responsible for the profound metabolic acidosis seen in methanol poisoning. However, for a long time it has been known that formic acid production accounts for only half the anion gap seen in this condition.

Early evidence[14, 15] favored the production of lactic acidosis, as shown in Figure 37–1. It appears that lactic acid[29] accumulates as a result of reversal of normal oxidation of lactate to pyruvate because of the trapping of NAD+ as NADH in the liver as a consequence of the oxidation of methanol to formic acid. This is still controversial because McMartin and associates found that the increase of blood formate in their study corre-

Table 37–1. METHANOL INTOXICATION

MAJOR SYMPTOMS/SIGNS	LABORATORY FEATURES
Early	May have detectable serum ethanol and methanol levels
Inebriation	
Drowsiness	
Delayed (6–30 hr)	
Vomiting, vertigo	Systemic acidosis with low bicarbonate*
Upper abdominal pain	Formic acidemia
Dyspnea	Lactic acidemia*
Acidosis (± Kussmaul respiration)	↑ Hematocrit*
Blurred vision	↑ Anion gap
Hyperemia of optic disc	↑ Mean corpuscular volume*
Blindness	↑ Blood glucose
Dilated pupils → absent light reflex	↑ Serum amylase
	↑ Osmolal gap
Urinary formaldehyde smell	Methanol > 30 mg/dl†

*More severe abnormalities correlate with poor outcome.
†Hemodialysis should be instituted at blood methanol concentrations > 50 mg/dl.

lated best with the anion gap increase.[30] On the other hand, Smith and coworkers found no such correlation in a single patient intoxicated with methanol.[14] Occasionally mild ketonuria may be observed. Swartz and colleagues showed that acidosis (and particularly the low serum bicarbonate concentration) correlated better with the blood methanol level as well as with the gastrointestinal and central nervous system symptomatology.[31] In addition, they showed that the red blood cell mean corpuscular volume (MCV) in severely intoxicated patients was higher than in those patients with mild intoxication and that it correlated well with the degree of acidosis and symptomatology. The changes in MCV were not related to hemodilution nor hemoconcentration, nor was it felt that they were related to abnormalities in folic acid metabolism, but rather they were produced by the direct toxic effect of formaldehyde on cellular ion transport. Incubation of red blood cells with formic acid did not produce toxic swelling of the red blood cells.[32]

More recently, because of the introduction of a rapid assay for blood formate,[33] it has been shown that formate accounts for over 50 per cent of the bicarbonate deficit and that mortality correlates better with the degree of acidosis than with the blood methanol concentration.[34] It also appears that serum formate concentration may be a better guide to hemodialysis.[34]

Treatment of Methanol Intoxication

As can be seen from Table 37–2, in the era before hemodialysis was demonstrated to be effective[5, 35] in removing methanol, formic acid, and formaldehyde,[32] outbreaks of methanol intoxication were associated with a very high mortality and morbidity from permanent optic atrophy following a period of papilledema.[36] Dialysis methods have largely centered on the more efficient method of hemodialysis;[30, 32, 34, 37–46] however, in certain situations peritoneal dialysis,[41, 43–46] although less efficient than hemodialysis, may be of some benefit in the treatment of this disease. Not every patient requires hemodialysis for a successful outcome,[31, 32, 35, 37–42] and this will be discussed more fully in the section on management of an epidemic of methanol poisoning. Certain forms of dialysate regeneration for hemodialysis markedly decrease the efficiency of methanol and formate removal.[47]

The following guidelines, however, are suggested for the routine management of methanol intoxication:

1. If the patient is seen early, gastric lavage for the removal of residual gastric methanol should be instituted as rapidly as possible.
2. Following this, ethanol (ethyl alcohol) should be administered to all patients while awaiting methanol determination. The usual dose to maintain a blood level of 100 mg/dl of ethanol should begin with a loading dose of 0.6 gm/kg,[40] and this can be maintained with an ethanol infusion of 66 mg/kg/hr for nondrinkers (154 mg/kg/hr for chronic ethanol drinkers) in view of the increased hepatobiliary transformation of ethanol in the latter group. Ethanol alone may be all that is required for a blood concentration less than 20 mg/dl.[48] Ethanol should be given as an intravenous infusion of 10 per cent ethanol diluted in D5W.
3. Initial correction of the acidosis with bicarbonate is imperative, particularly if the serum bicarbonate concentration is below 15 mEq/L and the plasma pH is below 7.35[31] (see also Chapter 7). (Large quantities may be required.)
4. Extracorporeal hemodialysis that achieves a methanol clearance of approximately 150 ml/min using a blood flow of between 200 and 300 ml/min through a dialyzer of surface area 1.0 m^2 is associated with a more rapid fall in blood methanol levels compared with conservative management alone.[31] It is imperative that ethanol be replaced for that removed during dialysis, and this can be achieved by increasing the ethanol infusion rate to 7.0 gm/hr[40] or by adding ethanol to the hemodialysate.[31] Hemodialysis should be instituted if the blood methanol concentration is greater than 50 mg/dl and should be continued until the serum methanol level is reduced to the range of 20 mg/dl. Ethanol removal is very similar to methanol removal in terms of clearance, and values are reported to lie between 100 and 150 ml/min of ethanol clearance.

In one patient reported by Swartz and associates, the addition of ethanol to the

Table 37–2. METHANOL POISONING AND OUTCOME

	NUMBER OF PATIENTS	SURVIVED	DIED	OUTCOME UNKNOWN	NORMAL VISION	PERMANENT IMPAIRED VISION	DIALYSIS USED
Bennett et al.[5]	323	282	41	—	7	7	no
Tonning et al.[42]	49	49	—	—	49	—	no
Anonymous[35]	11	8	3	—	7	1	no*
Kane et al.[41]	18	24	8	—	7	—	yes
Gonda et al.‡[37]	35	2	7	4	15	8	yes
McCoy et al.[40]	2	?	—	—	2	—	yes
Tobin and Lianos[39]	1	1	?	?	?	?	yes
McMartin et al.[30]†	2	2	1	—	1	—	yes
Lins et al.[15]	4	24	2	—	2	—	yes§
Swartz et al.[31]	46	19‖	—	—	22	2	no
			—	—	13	6	yes

*One patient had peritoneal dialysis.
†Only one death in hospitalized patients.
‡Includes all reports of hemodialysis up to 1978 and 9 patients treated by the authors.
§Combined hemodialysis/charcoal hemoperfusion was used.
‖22 patients referred for tertiary care; group above not referred for tertiary care.

dialysate decreased the clearance of ethanol by approximately 30 per cent, and the patient did not require more vigorous ethanol replacement during hemodialysis. Another interesting feature these workers observed was that in seven of nine patients who underwent hemodialysis, the blood methanol level increased by as much as 20 mg/dl, even up to 36 hours after hemodialysis was terminated.[31] Such "rebound" rises in methanol levels were previously reported[30] and are consistent with observations of other drug removals with hemodialysis, reflecting the movement of methanol from tissues to the plasma compartment (see Chapter 8). It must be remembered, however, that dialysis must be continued, along with ethanol administration, until the methanol levels are below 30 mg/dl. Since profound acidosis is a common feature, it is prudent to use bicarbonate-based dialysate for methanol poisoning.

5. Experimental evidence shows that administration of pyrazole, which inhibits alcohol dehydrogenase, may be used with some success for the treatment of methanol poisoning in monkeys.[49] In humans it has been used to inhibit the oxidation of ethanol for experimental purposes. Folinic or folic acid to promote catalase-mediated metabolism of formate has also been administered to monkeys to enhance the metabolism of formate to carbon dioxide and water.[50, 51] However, there is incomplete evidence on which to base clinical recommendations on the use of these experimental compounds.

Management of an Epidemic

As has been pointed out, sporadic cases of methanol poisoning are fairly rare, and the largest experiences are generally gained from managing methanol intoxication epidemics. Swartz and colleagues experienced an epidemic at a Michigan state prison, and their observations allow a few statements to be made on the triage management of such epidemics.[31] Management of methanol intoxication can be divided into those patients who were referred for tertiary care in hospitals and those who were not. This division was based predominantly on manifestations in the central nervous, ocular, and gastrointestinal systems. Those who exhibited major symptoms in each of these systems were referred for further treatment. However, Swartz and colleagues pointed out that hemodialysis, although useful for enhancing elimination of methanol—especially when blood levels were greater than 100 mg/dl or the acidosis was refractory to standard management—was not always necessary.[31] When hemodialysis might be associated with a high risk, such as upper gastrointestinal hemorrhage or hemodynamic instability, conservative treatment or peritoneal dialysis might suffice to stabilize the patient during the phase of slow but efficient pulmonary elimination of residual methanol. They also pointed out that in certain cases the initial severe central nervous system complications might prove irreversible, even with aggressive treatment. This accounts for some of the deaths associated with methanol poisoning as reported in Table 37–2 and the permanent central nervous system manifestations.[27, 28]

ISOPROPYL ALCOHOL

Isopropyl alcohol (2-propanol, isopropanol) is an important aliphatic alcohol widely used in industry and the home as a solvent and in medicine as a rubbing alcohol or sterilizing agent. In the home, isopropyl alcohol may be found in rubbing alcohol, skin lotion, hair tonics, aftershave lotions, and window cleaning fluids.[52] Like methanol, isopropyl alcohol is ingested by the debilitated or misguided alcoholic because it is cheaper than standard ethanol. Isopropanol intoxication is second to ethanol ingestion in this category as reported to the American Association of Poison Control Centers.[53] However, certain features differentiate the ingestion of isopropyl alcohol from that of ethanol and methanol, principally the production of ketonuria, because approximately 15 per cent of an ingested dose of isopropyl alcohol is metabolized to acetone.

Pharmacology and Toxicology

Isopropyl alcohol appears to be more toxic than ethyl alcohol but less toxic than methanol. It is about twice as potent as ethanol and is metabolized at a much slower rate than ethanol. The reported lethal dose in adults is 240 ml; intoxicating doses as low as 20 ml have been reported.[52] It is interesting that in alcoholics tolerant to ethanol there seems to be some cross tolerance to isopropyl alcohol,[54, 55] although this is not invariable.[56] Within 30 minutes 80 per cent of an oral dose is absorbed, with complete absorption within 2 hours.[57] The apparent volume of distribution is 0.6 to 0.7 L/kg, and the compound is excreted by first-order kinetics,[57] with a T½ of 2.5 to 3.2 hours[58] and a pulmonary alveolar clearance of 8 L/min.[59] The kidney accounts for 20 to 50 per cent of unchanged isopropanol excretion.[58] The oxidation of isopropanol to *acetone*[60] probably involves the enzyme alcohol dehydrogenase;[61] however, ethanol administration has not been used clinically in this condition, although it has been demonstrated that the metabolic rate of isopropanol cannot be accelerated by insulin or glucose.[61] Although ingestion of isopropanol is the major route for intoxication, accidental inhalation of isopropanol vapor during massage or alcohol sponging of pyrexial patients in poorly ventilated areas has been reported to produce deep coma.[52] One disturbed individual administered isopropyl alcohol as an enema and became toxic, since the alcohol is readily absorbed from the bowel.[62] The clinical signs of isopropyl alcohol persist for two to four times the usual duration of those seen with ethanol, again reflecting the slower metabolism of the drug.[60, 63]

The signs and symptoms of isopropyl alcohol poisoning are similar to those of ethanol. Characteristically, the patient may be in deep coma after an acute ingestion, with the coma preceding a respiratory arrest—all taking place within a few hours of ingestion. Isopropyl alcohol, like ethanol, also leads to cardiomyopathy, which may manifest as an arrhythmia or severe hypotension, a bad prognostic sign.[56] Dehydration and hemorrhagic gastritis (a striking feature of isopropyl alcohol ingestion) may contribute to hypotension.[64, 65] As with all central nervous system depressants, aspiration of stomach contents into the lungs is a definite risk. Severe hypotension is a bad prognostic sign; it may result in renal shutdown. Hepatic cellular damage also has been described as a result of isopropyl alcohol intoxication;[55] in animals, the fatty (triglyceride) content of the liver is increased significantly, as with ethanol. Since other ingredients, such as menthol, camphor, methylsalicylate, and naphthalene, may be ingested concomitantly, the central nervous system signs normally associated with isopropyl alcohol alone may be superseded by the central stimulatory effects of these ingredients. Other rare symptoms of isopropyl intoxication are hemolysis and myopathy (including myoglobinuria[66]); the mechanism for production of these symptoms is unknown. In coingestions with hydrocarbons, there is good evidence that isopropanol enhances the toxicity of hydrocarbons.[67, 68]

Diagnosis of Isopropyl Alcohol Poisoning

The principal features outlined previously should suggest the diagnosis. In the alcoholic patient, the characteristic smell of rubbing alcohol on the breath combined with acidosis should alert the physician to the possibility of isopropanol ingestion; however, the symptoms and signs are similar to those of methanol and ethylene glycol intoxication and alcoholic ketoacidosis although they lack the retinal toxicity of formaldehyde in methanol poisoning and the oxalate crystals in urine in ethylene glycol poisoning. Usually there is evidence of an osmolal gap (0.17 mOsm/kg for every 1 mg/dl isopropanol), as in ethanol intoxication itself. Clues to the diagnosis of acidosis in alcoholic patients are given in Chapter 7. The patient poisoned with isopropanol will show ketones in the urine and blood and an osmolal gap, but without glycosuria. Renal dysfunction may occur if coma and hypotension have been prolonged, and there may be evidence of mild hepatic dysfunction. Increased cerebrospinal fluid protein has been recorded, but the etiology of this is unknown. Although tachycardia is common,[69] bradycardia and other arrhythmias may be detected on clinical and electrocardiographic examinations. Hypoglycemia may also be a prominent feature.[69]

The presence of isopropanol can be detected in both blood and gastric contents; serum levels around 50 mg/dl indicate mild intoxication, whereas serum levels of 150 mg/dl have been associated with deep coma.[70] However, a pediatric patient recovered after treatment despite an isopropanol blood level of 520 mg/dl,[71] whereas adult recovery with blood levels of 346 to 560 mg/dl have been recorded.[72]

Treatment

As with most other ingested poisons, gastric lavage is one of the most important methods of treatment. Most isopropanol recovery from the stomach is within 2 hours of ingestion, but even when the gastric lavage is delayed a large amount of isopropyl alcohol can still be removed. Activated carbon adsorbs isopropanol at a rate of only 500 mg/gm carbon. As with other poisons, attention must be paid to the preservation of a patent airway during gastric lavage. If there is evidence of alveolar hypoventilation, oxygen administration and artificial respiration may be required. The two main methods of treatment for isopropyl alcohol poisoning are (1) preservation of fluid balance and blood pressure, which may require the use of intravenous fluids and pressor drugs, and (2) hemodialysis to reduce blood levels of isopropanol.

Several investigators have now reported beneficial clinical outcomes with the institution of early hemodialysis in this rare but serious condition.[73] Freireich and associates demonstrated that isopropanol and its metabolite acetone were removed with hemodialysis,[74] whereas King and colleagues reported a fall in blood isopropanol from 440 to 100 mg/dl after 5 hours of hemodialysis.[75] In the latter report, the clinical response was dramatic; the patient was in stage 4 coma at the start of hemodialysis and became normotensive and responsive after a 5-hour hemodialysis. Another patient dialyzed for isopropyl alcohol poisoning along with a severe disulfiram reaction also showed a dramatic clinical response to hemodialysis.[76] If hemodialysis is not available for treatment of isopropanol poisoning, peritoneal dialysis is the second choice. Dua has reported a successful clinical outcome after 20 hours of peritoneal dialysis despite the fact that the acetone level was 1878 mg/dl at the initiation of therapy.[77] However, in this patient no isopropyl alcohol removal was noted. A further report of successful recovery from "near fatal" isopropanol poisoning in a child treated with peritoneal dialysis has been published.[78]

As mentioned, although it is expected that isopropanol is metabolized through alcohol dehydrogenase, differences in the kinetics of elimination between isopropanol and ethanol or methanol elimination in dogs and rats exist. Alcohol administration has not been used in humans to inhibit the formation of the toxic metabolite to the same degree as it is used clinically in methanol or ethylene glycol poisoning.

NORMAL PROPYL ALCOHOL

Normal propyl alcohol (propanol-1, *N*-propanol) is related to isopropyl alcohol but may be more toxic, although it appears to induce the same metabolic effects.[52] A human fatality has been recorded.[79]

THE HIGHER ALCOHOLS

A full discussion of this group of alcohols is included to point out that the higher saturated aliphatic alcohols have some toxicity. The higher liquid alcohols are butyl, amyl, ethyl, hexyl, and so on, and the solid fatty alcohols include lauryl, myristyl, cetyl, and stearyl. The liquid alcohols are used as solvents, and the solid fatty alcohols are used in cosmetics.[80] The butyl alcohols are generally less toxic than the amyl alcohols to the central nervous system, but they are two to five times more toxic than ethanol in the rat.[81] However, in general, the order of increasing toxicity by single oral doses is as follows: ethyl, isopropyl, sec-butyl, *N*-butyl, ter-butyl, iso-butyl, and amyl alcohol. *N*-Butyl alcohol vapors have produced conjunctivitis and keratitis, and, although skin irritation is common with the liquid alcohols, percutaneous absorption does not seem to occur. However, vapor inhalation may produce pulmonary injury. *N*-Butyl alcohol does not appear to produce ill effects after intravenous infusion.[82] However, extrapolation of animal data to humans gives a calculated mean oral lethal dose of *N*-butyl alcohol of 90 to 210 ml.[80]

The amyl alcohols are more toxic, and the ingestion or rectal instillation of about 30 ml has proved lethal in human adults.[61] In addition, glycosuria and methemoglobinemia may result from the ingestion of isoamyl alcohol in the fermentative fusel alcohol.[81]

Animal data have established that the alcohols in this group are indeed toxic, but very few cases of human toxicity have been described. In general, the major clinical effects are in the central nervous system, particularly with vaporizing compounds, and include headache, muscle weakness, giddiness, ataxia, confusion, delirium, and coma. If ingested, gastrointestinal effects are principally vomiting and diarrhea, with the odor of the alcohol being present. Death is mainly due to respiratory failure, but it may also occur from cardiac arrhythmias.

Treatment of Higher Alcohol Poisoning

The main method of treatment after ingestion is gastric lavage until all the alcohol is removed. Some have suggested mineral oil instillation into the stomach, although there is no clinical evidence to support its use.[80] Since the primary alcohols—the group containing ethyl, isopropyl, butyl, and amyl alcohols—are oxidized to the aldehydes and acids, significant metabolic acidosis may result. The secondary alcohols are converted to ketone, which may also cause central nervous system depression, and should be managed appropriately. Fortunately, the tertiary alcohols are metabolized slowly and incompletely and excreted in the urine as glucuronides.[80]

BENZYL ALCOHOL

Although not reported to be an adult human toxic agent, there had been some concern over the presence of benzyl alcohol concentrations in a stable dialysis population at levels significantly higher than those in normal controls.[84] Benzyl alcohol is administered along with heparin to preserve the heparin solution necessary for anticoagulation during dialysis. Although levels of benzyl alcohol are lowest at the end of dialysis, indicating that the substance was dialyzable, substantial rises in benzyl alcohol concentrations in the interdialytic period occur, suggesting that tissue uptake of benzyl alcohol occurs early after administration, with subsequent transfer from tissues into the plasma compartment. The normal detoxification of benzyl alcohol is by way of oxidation to benzoic and hippuric acids, following which these compounds are excreted rapidly in the urine. However, in dialysis patients hippuric and benzoic acids can be removed in the absence of renal function.

Benzyl alcohol–preserved intravenous solutions have been associated with deaths in premature infants, given in an average dosage of 130 to 405 mg/kg/day, in whom high urine and serum benzoate levels were detected as well as high urinary hippurate levels.[85] It has since been confirmed that a specific syndrome, the "gasping syndrome," is seen in premature infants with progressive central nervous system depression[86] and intraventricular hemorrhage[87] given large quantities of benzyl alcohol–preserved intravenous solutions. The syndrome is one of metabolic acidosis, bradycardia, skin breakdown, respiratory depression with "gasping," hypotonia, hepatorenal failure, hypotension, and central nervous system depression.[86] Benzyl alcohol–containing solutions should be avoided in premature infants.

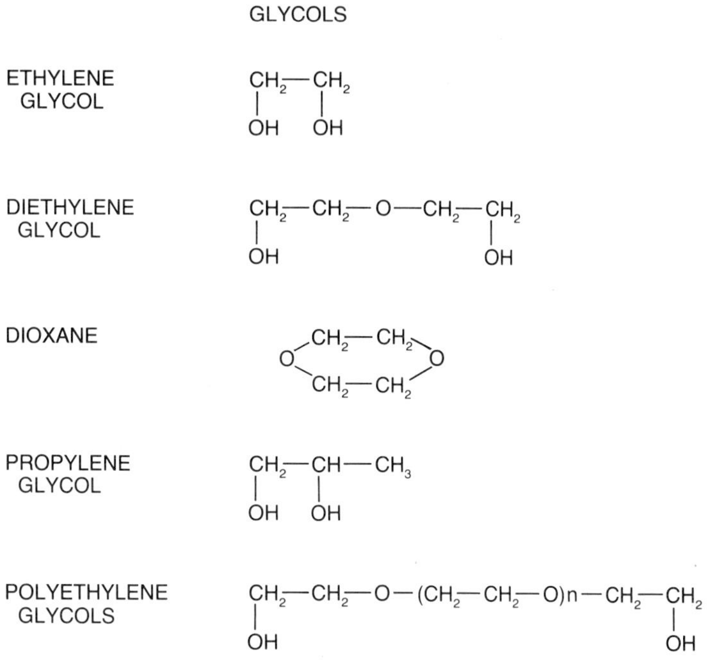

GLYCOLS

ETHYLENE GLYCOL	$CH_2(OH)—CH_2(OH)$
DIETHYLENE GLYCOL	$CH_2(OH)—CH_2—O—CH_2—CH_2(OH)$
DIOXANE	$O(CH_2—CH_2)_2O$ (ring: $CH_2—CH_2$ / O / O / $CH_2—CH_2$)
PROPYLENE GLYCOL	$CH_2(OH)—CH(OH)—CH_3$
POLYETHYLENE GLYCOLS	$CH_2(OH)—CH_2—O—(CH_2—CH_2—O)n—CH_2—CH_2(OH)$

Figure 37–2. Glycols.

ETHYLENE GLYCOL

Ethylene glycol intoxication is one of the most serious and dramatic poisonings encountered in clinical toxicology. As with methanol and isopropanol, ethylene glycol is commonly ingested by the debilitated or misguided alcoholic patient, but, unlike methanol poisoning, which usually occurs in epidemics, ethylene glycol ingestion is sporadic.

Ethylene glycol is a simple but important starting material for many chemical manufacturing processes. In addition, it is a widely used solvent and is found in cosmetic preparations and antifreeze solutions for internal combustion engines. A large group of glycols exists, and they vary in their toxicity, chemical structure, and metabolism (Fig. 37–2).[88] Since ethylene glycol is the more common clinical entity, it will be discussed in some detail and reference to the others will follow. Although epidemics of ethylene glycol poisoning are unusual, the first clinical report of poisoning did involve an epidemic in which 76 people succumbed after using an elixir of an antibiotic (sulfanilamide) that contained 72 per cent of a related compound, diethylene glycol.[89] More than 50 human fatalities from ethylene glycol ingestion have been reported in the United States; in Europe several deaths have been reported, although the ingestion appears to be less common.

Pharmacology and Toxicology

Ethylene glycol itself appears to be nontoxic, although skin irritation and skin penetration have been described as well as acute iridocyclitis following accidental eye contact.[90] After ingestion, peak blood levels occur at 1 to 4 hours, and the unchanged compound undergoes glomerular filtration and passive reabsorption.[83] The compound is highly toxic owing to its breakdown products and the induction of acidosis. Inhalation is not generally associated with toxicity, although cases of chronic poisoning with nystagmus and recurrent attacks of unconsciousness have been reported in factory workers exposed to vapors of ethylene glycol.[91] Although the accepted lethal dose of ethylene glycol ingestion in adults is 100 ml, recovery has been reported following ingestions ranging from 240 to 970 ml.[89]

The major toxicity of ethylene glycol results from accumulation of its four major breakdown products (Fig. 37–3). Ethylene glycol is an odorless solution, and the patient can appear to be inebriated as with methanol, although the absence of an alcoholic breath helps in the differential diagnosis. Ingestion is usually concomitant with ethyl alcohol, although the compound has been taken alone in many cases. In the severest form of intoxication, accumulation of the four breakdown

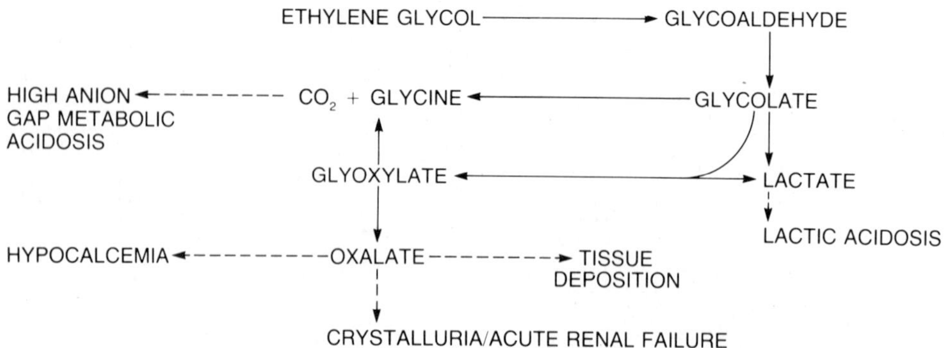

Figure 37–3. Metabolic degradation of ethylene glycol.

products (aldehydes, glycolate, oxalate, and lactate) accounts for all the symptomatology. In the more fulminant form, the patient is in a profound coma with seizure activity, which in turn may be complicated by respiratory failure, cardiovascular collapse, pulmonary edema, and an increase in the existing severe metabolic acidosis.[88, 92] Death may follow in 8 to 24 hours if not treated. Survivors of the acute phase experience renal failure. On renal biopsy or autopsy, extensive destruction of the renal substance is seen, caused by deposition of birefringent oxalate crystals in the renal tubules, with evidence of interstitial nephritis and focal hemorrhagic necrosis in the cortex as well as acute tubular necrosis.[93–95]

The underlying basis for the toxicity can be divided into two major categories: tissue destruction due to deposition of calcium oxalate crystals, and production of severe acidosis due to aldehyde, glycolate, and lactate production. The changes just outlined in the renal substance are not limited to the kidney but have been shown in the meninges of the brain,[93, 96] blood vessels,[97] liver,[97, 98] and pericardium.[96] The tissue destruction is due to the deposition of calcium oxalate crystals, as a consequence of which calcium ions are chelated and hypocalcemia may follow.[98] Tissue destruction generally will improve following the removal of ethylene glycol to remove or prevent the formation of calcium oxalate crystals. Although renal failure usually reverses, permanent renal and central nervous system damage frequently have been reported. It is felt that the initial central nervous system depression is from glycol itself or the production of aldehydes, which follows 6 to 12 hours after ingestion of ethylene glycol during the height of aldehyde production.[99, 100]

The metabolic acidosis is produced by the combination of lactic acidosis (resulting from trapping of nicotinamide adenine dinucleotide during the breakdown of ethylene glycol) and the byproducts of glyoxalate metabolism, which inhibit the citric acid cycle; both increase lactic acid production (see Fig. 37–3). In addition, glycolate (and to a lesser extent glyoxalate) recondense under the activity of pyridoxal phosphate and glyoxalate transaminase enzymes to form glycine and carbon dioxide; glycine production is associated with the consumption of bicarbonate and accounts for the profound metabolic acidosis seen in this condition (see Chapter 7).

The metabolism of ethylene glycol (spontaneous half-life, 3 hours) depends on alcohol dehydrogenase contained in the hepatocytes. Only a small amount of glycol is excreted in the urine after an oral dose; rather, the production of the metabolites in the sequence outlined in Figure 37–3 accounts for the major toxicity,[101, 102] and it appears that tissue damage occurs predominantly in those species that preferentially metabolize ethylene glycol to oxalate (including man).[101, 102]

Urinary hippurate crystals have been mentioned in several case reports of ethylene glycol poisoning. Evidence, however, does not favor glycine conjugation with benzoic acid to form hippurate; the crystals that appear to be hippurate have been analyzed by x-ray diffraction and seem to be calcium oxalate monohydrate, which appears as a monoclinic crystal (see Fig. 37–4*B*).[103, 104]

Clinical Presentation

The clinical presentation of ethylene glycol toxicity occurs in three fairly well defined phases:[105] the first phase occurs within 30 minutes to 12 hours after ingestion of ethylene glycol. The patient appears to be drunk, but without the alcohol smell on the breath, and may experience nausea, vomiting, and hematemesis. However, the major effects are on the central nervous system. The patient may be in coma with seizure activity that is often focal in nature. Other central nervous system effects are nystagmus, paralysis of external muscles of the gait and eyes, depressed reflexes, myoclonic seizures, and tetany due to hypocalcemia.

In phase 2 of intoxication, which begins 12 to 14 hours later, the patient may experience tachycardia, mild hypertension, pulmonary edema, and congestive cardiac failure, all of which are felt to be due to the deposition of calcium oxalate crystals within the vascular tree, the myocardium, and the lung parenchyma.

Phase 3 of ethylene glycol poisoning, which comes on between 24 and 72 hours following ingestion, is marked by the predominance of flank pain, with costovertebral angle tenderness and evidence of acute tubular necrosis, usually in the form of oliguric acute renal failure.

Diagnosis of Ethylene Glycol Poisoning

Ethylene glycol poisoning should be strongly suspected in patients who appear to be inebriated but have no alcohol smell on the breath. Other diagnostic features of ethylene glycol poisoning include the presence of calcium oxalate crystals in the urine, either as dihydrate or monohydrate crystals (Fig. 37–4). In addition, microscopic hematuria may occur during the third phase of the poisoning, and oliguria, proteinuria, and urine with a low specific gravity may be observed. Any evidence of renal failure will be manifested by a rise in serum creatinine and blood urea nitrogen. The more profound features, however, are those associated with metabolic acidosis: the patient may have Kussmaul respiration, with a large anion gap and evidence, also, of an osmolal gap (0.2 mOsm/kg for every 1 mg/dl ethylene glycol) (see Chapter 7). A persistent high osmolal gap with low ethylene glycol levels may be due to persistence of glycolate in plasma.[106] In addition to these features, lactic acidosis complicates the picture. During the initial phase of toxicity, hypocalcemia may be observed in addition to the profound acidosis, and, if renal failure supervenes, hyperkalemia may develop. Additionally, a raised white cell count is commonly found, and lumbar puncture may reveal high protein values. Ethylene glycol may be detected in gastric fluid as well as in urine and blood. Oxalic acid (oxalate) levels also may be extremely high.

Treatment

At one time it was felt that ethylene glycol poisoning should be managed in the same way as systemic oxalate poisoning (see hereafter), with soluble calcium salts. However, evidence to support the use of this treatment is not forthcoming, since hypocalcemia is not an invariable complication of glycol poisoning. Aggressive treatment of the acidosis and institution of hemodialysis[73, 95] form the mainstay of therapy.

Treatment should include gastric lavage for removal of residual ethylene glycol, correction of dehydration and shock, and management of fluid balance in the presence of pulmonary edema, which might be due to the toxic effects of ethylene glycol metabolites or the sodium overload. In addition, hypocalcemia should be corrected with calcium chloride, depending on serum calcium levels. The mainstay of treatment, however, is correction of the metabolic acidosis, which often requires massive doses of sodium bicarbonate administration (as much as 1000 to 2000 ml); such obligatory sodium administration requires early institution of hemodialysis.

As in methanol poisoning, ethyl alcohol[107] is administered to act as a preferential substrate for the enzyme hepatic alcohol dehydrogenase; as in methanol poisoning, administration of ethyl alcohol should be gauged to maintain a plasma ethanol level of 100 to 200 mg/dl. Also as in methanol poisoning, hepatic enzyme induction may be present in a habitual alcoholic, so more ethanol may be required than in a patient who has been abstinent from alcohol. Ethanol should be given as an intravenous infusion of 10 per cent ethanol diluted in D5W.

Peterson and colleagues examined the pharmacokinetics of ethanol and ethylene glycol before and during hemodialysis for the treatment of ethylene glycol poisoning.[108] Blood ethylene glycol levels before dialysis

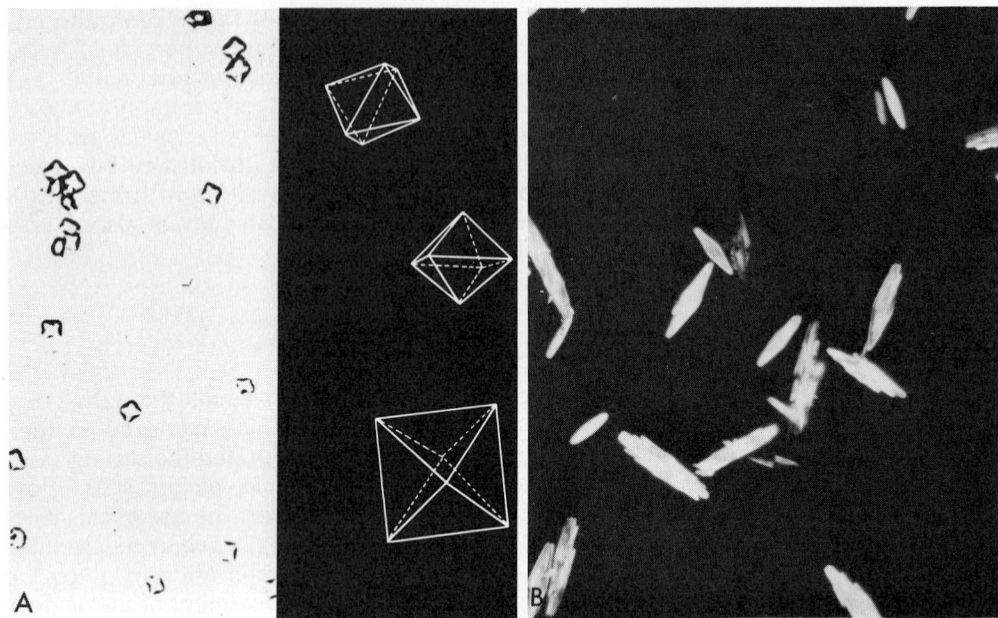

Figure 37–4. *A,* Calcium oxalate dihydrate crystals in urinary sediment and drawing of octahedral crystals (courtesy of Dr. G. E. Schreiner). *B,* Calcium oxalate monohydrate crystals in urinary sediment (courtesy of Dr. A. Terlinsky). These crystals are monoclinic in shape and were previously thought to be "hippurate" crystals.

were 50 mg/dl; the measured osmolality was 422 mOsm/kg and the calculated osmolality was 312 mOsm/kg. They demonstrated that the spontaneous elimination half-time of ethylene glycol during administration of 5 per cent ethanol intravenously was 3 hours; during the oral administration of ethanol the elimination half-time was prolonged to 17 hours, when the blood levels of ethanol ranged between 130 and 200 mg/dl. During dialysis and continued oral ethanol therapy, the half-life of ethylene glycol was reduced to 2.5 hours. Ethylene glycol removal (clearance) was demonstrated to be 210 ± 3.0 ml/min with a blood flow rate through the dialyzer of 227 ml/min, a result that correlates closely with urea clearance. In this single patient, 111 gm of ethylene glycol were removed with dialysis, compared with 10 gm of ethylene glycol excretion in the urine over the same 6-hour hemodialysis period. The investigators, therefore, recommended that in the management of ethylene glycol poisoning an oral loading dose of 0.6 gm of 50 per cent ethanol/kg body weight be given, followed by oral maintenance doses of 109 mg of 20 per cent ethanol/kg/hr, and that dialysis be initiated rapidly. During hemodialysis, 230 mg of ethanol/kg/hr should be administered to maintain blood ethanol levels of 100 to 200 mg/dl. These measures should be continued until ethylene glycol has been eliminated from the blood (< 10 mg/dl).

Subsequent correspondence, however, highlighted the fact that oral ethanol administration would be hazardous in an unconscious patient and that higher concentrations of intravenous ethanol would be required.[109] In addition, Freed and associates[109] pointed out that the enzyme alcohol dehydrogenase is 50 per cent inhibited at an ethanol concentration of 2 mg/dl and more than 90 per cent saturated at 50 mg/dl;[110] however, ethylene glycol requirements to saturate the enzyme by 50 per cent are reported to be much higher at 326 mg/dl.[111]

Peterson and associates also pointed out that alcohol can be added to the dialysate bath to give a dialysate level of 100 mg/dl using 95 per cent ethanol[108]; stabilization of blood ethanol levels was easier than with intravenous or oral ethanol therapy. Bicarbonate dialysis is most appropriate. Aggressive therapy has been associated with survival with blood concentrations of 145 mg/dl at 8 hours and 560 mg/dl at 1 hour in two patients, the authors suggesting that dialysis be recommended at levels above 50 mg/dl.[112] Others have reported aggressively treated survivors with concentrations up to 650 mg/dl and deaths in patients with ethylene glycol levels between 98 and 775 mg/dl.[103, 108, 112, 113] Recently Gabow and colleagues have demonstrated in a small series of patients that glycolic acid concentrations are invariably elevated, lactic acidosis may be present, and glycolic acid is well dialyzed (105 ml/min at a blood flow rate of 200 ml/min measured in one of three patients).[114] Glycolic acid is the major contributor to the profound acidosis[114, 115] and has an elimination half-life of 7 hours (ethylene glycol itself had a half-life of 8.4 hours, which was prolonged more than tenfold by ethanol).[115] Clearance of ethylene glycol by the kidney was at a rate of 27.5 ± 4.5 ml/min and a fractional renal clearance of 19.8 ± 1.5 per cent (both lower than respective urea clearances), whereas hemodialyzer clearance was 156 ml/min.[115] It is well recognized that coingestion of ethyl alcohol may reduce symptomatology from ethylene glycol,[116] but what is less well recognized is that the anion gap acidosis may be normalized with ingestion of exogenous anions, e.g., bromide.[117]

Hemoperfusion has been attempted in a single patient with ethylene glycol poisoning.[118] During the first 2 hours of charcoal hemoperfusion, plasma ethylene glycol clearance was 72 mg/min at a blood flow rate of 300 ml/min. This compared with only 39 mg/min eliminated by the kidney. At about 2 hours the column became saturated, and removal of ethylene glycol fell to negligible limits. This demonstrates that charcoal hemoperfusion should probably not be used unless the columns are changed regularly at 1.5- to 2-hour intervals. In addition, correction of acid base changes is not possible with hemoperfusion, as has been pointed out in Chapter 8.

Pyridoxine (500 mg IM four times daily, which stimulates the metabolism of glyoxalate to glycine) and thiamine (100 mg IM four times daily, which stimulates glyoxalate to alpha-OH-beta-ketoadipate) are cofactors for the metabolism of ethylene glycol and have been suggested as antidotes.[119]

Other experimental therapies for the treatment of ethylene glycol poisoning include the use of pyrazole and 4-methyl pyrazole (4-MP).[120, 121] Blomstrand and Theorell had shown that, in monkeys, methanol poisoning can be successfully treated with 4-MP, which is a potent inhibitor of alcohol dehydrogenase.[122] Pyrazole, however, has been found to be toxic in doses sufficient to inhibit alcohol dehydrogenase. 4-MP has been used in rats and monkeys with some benefit in the treatment of ethylene glycol poisoning.[121, 122] Arising from studies of 4-MP in humans,[120] Baud and associates treated three patients with oral 4-MP (20 mg/kg/day[123] or intermittent intravenous 4-MP 9.5 mg/kg at 9 hours after glycol ingestion, decreasing to 0.6 mg/kg at 57 hours after glycol ingestion)[124] until plasma ethylene glycol determinations were negative. No patient was treated with hemodialysis. A mild metabolic acidosis in two patients, a skin rash in one, and possible eosinophilia in the others were the only associations with treatment with 4-MP.

As with methanol poisoning, the primary ingested substance is not directly responsible for the toxicity; it is the metabolites that produce the serious consequences of both methanol and ethylene glycol poisoning. Therefore, it is mandatory not only to remove the intoxicating substance but to prevent the formation of the metabolites or remove them by hemodialysis. This is easily accomplished clinically and has been demonstrated in animals and humans[113] to prevent both morbidity and mortality in ethylene glycol poisoning. Not only correction of acidosis but also diversion of the alcohol dehydrogenase enzyme activity to another substrate (ethanol) is extremely important in this regard.

DIETHYLENE GLYCOL

Many of the derivatives of ethylene glycol are available in commercial and industrial settings.[88] However, in the 1920s 105 deaths were reported from renal failure owing to diethylene glycol,[125] which was used as a vehicle (73 per cent) for the preparation of 10 per cent sulfanilamide, which itself had the potential for producing renal damage. Although no oxalate crystals have been demonstrated in the kidney,[126] the renal pathology closely resembles ethylene glycol toxicity, as do the pathologic findings in the liver, lungs, heart, and meninges.[97, 126] The structure of diethylene glycol (see Fig. 37–2) and the simple esters of diethylene glycol contain a stable ether linkage that is resistant to metabolism to oxalate or formate. This explains the fact that metabolic acidosis is encountered rarely and has only been reported in childhood diethylene glycol poisoning.[127] However, the ether linkage in diethylene glycol, dipropylene glycol, dioxane, and monomethyl- and butyl-ethers of diethylene glycol is associated with a far higher degree of renal damage.[128]

The simple ethers of ethylene glycol and diethylene glycol appear to be more toxic than the parent alcohol and produce severe nephrotoxicity partly compounded by the intravascular hemolysis that occurs with several of these compounds in addition to the production of central nervous system depression, mild liver damage, and pulmonary edema.[88]

Management of the ethers of ethylene glycol poisoning is similar to management of intoxication with the parent compound. The use of ethanol in treatment has not been studied.

CELLOSOLVES

Cellosolves, used as solvents for resins, paints, inks, and industrial coatings and cleaners, are the monoalkyl ethers of ethylene glycol and principally consist of methyl cellosolves and butyl cellosolves.[88] Toxicity arises from these compounds by inhalation of their vapors to produce toxic encephalopathy and bone marrow depression without hemolysis. However, in rats but not in canine species, hemoglobinuria has been observed, particularly with butyl cellosolves rather than ethyl or methyl cellosolves. As with the simple ethers of ethylene glycol, pulmonary, renal, and hepatic changes that resemble toxicity from diethylene glycol have been observed. Severe metabolic acidosis also has been reported after ingestion of the monomethyl ether of ethylene glycol.[129] Management of cellosolve poisoning is essentially similar to that of diethylene glycol, but particular attention must be paid to the correction of the acidosis and the occasional renal failure.

POLYGLYCOLS AND PROPYLENE GLYCOL

Triethylene glycol, the lowest molecular weight polymer to be derived from the series of ethylene and diethylene glycols, has a molecular weight of around 200 daltons and is a liquid; such polymers remain liquid up to a molecular weight of 1000 daltons, after which they become solid and are termed carbowaxes.[88] The toxicity decreases with ascending molecular weight, but as a class this group of compounds is in general of very low toxicity.[130] Reported deaths appear to occur from renal injuries rather than central nervous system depression. Chronic toxicity may arise from chronic ingestion of the polyethylene glycols ranging in molecular weight from 200 to 6000 daltons, but there is good evidence that compounds with a molecular weight greater than 6000 daltons have less toxicity. Polyethylene glycol of a molecular weight of 400 daltons is recovered in the urine in about 80 per cent of the ingested dose. However, these remarks apply to experiments in rats and dogs; it appears that even compounds with a molecular weight of 6000 daltons are excreted to a high degree in human urine after intravenous administration.

Propylene glycol, however, has been reported to be completely innocuous and as such has been allowed by the Food and Drug Administration for use in cosmetics and foods and as a solvent for certain drugs. Recently, however, in a patient with renal failure who was unable to excrete propylene glycol in the urine, such retention caused severe central nervous system depression.[131] In addition, lactic acidosis was a prominent feature in this patient, with a large anion gap and a lactic acid level of 80 mEq/L. The patient responded rapidly to intravenous fluids and sodium bicarbonate and on recovery volunteered a history of "gas" exposure. Propylene glycol levels of 70 and 60 mg/dl were found in blood and urine, respectively.[131] Two previous cases of childhood poisoning with propylene glycol have been recorded: stupor and seizures developed, and the symptoms regressed on cessation of propylene glycol exposure.[132, 133] One horse that received 2.84 L of propylene glycol also became stuporous.[134] Propylene glycol contamination of intravenous nitroglycerine preparations has been associated with hyperosmolar coma and a high osmolal gap without acidosis; the patient responded to hemodialysis.[135]

It appears that propylene glycol is metabolized to lactic acid, which subsequently enters the glycolytic pathway.[136] Cate and Hedrick felt that propylene glycol probably accumulated in blood because of impaired renal clearance, with resultant lactic acidosis and stupor.[131] Management of such toxicity is fairly simple with the use of sodium bicarbonate and intravenous fluids.

In lithograph workers myeloid hypoplasia has been observed as well as birth defects and testicular damage with glycol ether and methyl cellosolves,[137, 138] and it has been suggested that ethoxyacetic acid, the major urinary breakdown product, be measured as a means of following industrial exposure.[137]

ACETONE

Acetone is included in this chapter because of its relationship to isopropyl alcohol metabolism and its important toxicity. Although not commonly reported, acetone ingestion does produce certain clinical effects.[139–142] Acetone (dimethylketone, beta-ketopropane, propanone, and pyroacetic ether) is a component of a large number of industrial and household cleaners, glues, and solvents and is commonly found in the household as nail polish remover. Other ketone derivatives, such as ethyl-butyl-ketone, isobutyl-ketone, and methyl-ethyl-ketone in addition to such solvents as chloroform, carbon tetrachloride, and so on, are found in paint and varnish removers, industrial metal cleaners, carburetor cleaners, and shoe polish. Acetone is relatively nontoxic, and ingestions of 200 to 400 ml may not be serious.[142, 143] The odor of acetone is characteristic, and it has narcotic properties.

Apart from ingestion, the compound may be inhaled, and the recommended threshold limit for industrial hygiene is 1000 ppm for workers exposed 8 hours a day. With inhalation, recent reports suggest that acetone also may be a solvent abused for recreational purposes by young people,[144] although it appeared at one time that industrial exposure was more prevalent.[145] Ingested acetone, which produces significant blood levels equal to those of toxic ethanol concentrations, is said to produce similar symptomatology, although its anesthetic potency is greater.[146] The pharmacokinetics of acetone indicate that the half-life in plasma lies between 19 and 31 hours, with a mean half-life of 28 hours.[139] The major excretory route is through the lungs, and the fruity odor of the breath is characteristic of acetone poisoning. The kinetics of elimination indicate that since the volume of distribution is 0.82 L/kg body weight, with an average minute ventilation, several days are required for complete elimination of acetone in the breath.

Clinical symptomatology from acetone inhalation includes cough, bronchial irritation, headache, and fatigue; after oral ingestion, gastrointestinal symptoms of vomiting and nausea occur. In severe cases, central nervous system depression similar to that seen with alcohol occurs. The patient may appear drunk,[139] but the progression to coma appears to be more rapid than with ethanol. Other reported symptoms are a red and swollen pharynx with erosions of the soft plate, lethargy, stupor, and coma. In addition, acidosis has been reported,[139] although it is not clear whether this was due to central nervous system depression or the toxicity of acetone itself.

Treatment

After inhalation, the patient should be removed into an area of fresh air and oxygen administered as required. If the patient has ingested acetone, gastric lavage should be performed or an emetic given. Attention to correction of acidosis and maintenance of respiration is extremely important, and it should not be expected that the patient will recover rapidly. As Ramu and associates have pointed out, 2 to 3 days will be required for a progressive but slow improvement in consciousness.[139] A concentration of acetone in blood (measured by gas chromatography) at the height of toxicity in the patient described by Ramu and associates was 0.25 gm/dl,[139] and at levels greater than 1 gm/dl the elimination of acetone is determined by the respiratory route; no acidosis was observed even with such concentrations. At lower levels, saturable metabolism of acetone also has been documented, with conversion of acetone into glucose.[146]

OXALATE

Oxalic acid is included in this chapter because of its relationship to ethylene glycol poisoning; however, it is a dangerous poison in its own right. Oxalic acid is found in bleaches and metal cleaners and also in many plants, such as rhubarb leaves, *Dieffenbachia* leaves (dumb cane), citrus fruit, beet, mangold, halogeton, sorrel, purslane, dock, greasewood, and Russian thistle.[147] Oxalate formation may also occur spontaneously in vivo in primary oxalosis. Ascorbic acid ingestion in high doses is associated with oxalate deposition in tissue in dialysis patients.[148]

The poisoning mainly relates to the oxalic acid and its soluble salts, which have corrosive activity on the alimentary tract with production of severe gastroenteritis and hypotension, the former of which may last for 1 week.[149, 150] Prolonged inhalation of fumes produced by boiling oxalic acid solutions also may lead to oxalic acid poisoning with renal impairment. Gangrene of the hands has been reported following immersion of the hands in cases of oxalate solutions.[151] Absorption in less severe cases of oxalate poisoning produces chelation of calcium to produce symptoms related to hypocalcemia, such as muscle twitching, cramps, and central nervous system depression,[152] the severity of which may produce cardiac arrhythmias.[153] As with ethylene glycol poisoning, oxalate deposition in blood vessels, kidney, liver, heart, and lungs occurs.[98, 153] The mean lethal dose is between 15 and 30 gm, with death usually following within a few hours.[149] If the patient survives, the picture is almost identical to that of corrosive acid poisoning, with the almost invariable occurrence of acute renal failure. Urinalysis may reveal oxalate crystals as well as hematuria and albuminuria (see Fig. 37–4).

Symptoms include pain in the throat, esophagus, and stomach, with the mucous membranes taking on a whitish opaque appearance. Hematemesis is a possibility, and extreme diarrhea also has been reported, often leading to shock. Tetany, convulsions, stupor, coma, and death also may result from hypocalcemia, and renal failure is seen.

Treatment

Treatment should be rapidly instituted by giving a dilute solution of calcium lactate, lime water, finely pulverized chalk, plaster, and/or milk to supply large amounts of calcium to inactivate oxalate by forming an insoluble calcium salt in the stomach. Gastric lavage is controversial, since this may compound an already severe corrosive lesion in the esophagus or stomach. However, if used, gastric lavage should be done with limewater (calcium hydroxide). Intravenous gluconate or calcium chloride solutions should be given to prevent hypocalcemic tetany; in severe cases parathyroid extract also has been given. Strictures may develop in the survivors, as well as other gastrointestinal lesions that should be managed as outlined in Chapter 65. Additionally, acute renal failure should be anticipated, and careful fluid management is necessary.

Removal of oxalate (in primary oxalosis) with hemodialysis is of the order of 650 mg/4.5 hr, whereas long-dwelling peritoneal dialysis using four 2-L exchanges in 24 hours approximates 300 mg/day of oxalate removal. For this reason, although hemodialysis or peritoneal dialysis has never been suggested in the past for oxalate poisoning, it is possible that oxalate removal with these techniques might prevent acute renal failure and certainly will help correct the hypocalcemia since dialysate calcium concentrations are around 6.4 mg/dl (Winchester, 1982, personal observations). Hemoperfusion with activated charcoal has been attempted in primary oxalosis for the removal of oxalate. Maggiore and associates demonstrated 44 per cent decrease in plasma oxalate levels during a 2-hour hemoperfusion.[154] The total quantity of oxalate removed, however, is around 150 mg with a 4-hour charcoal hemoperfusion, but with saturation of the charcoal observed at 2 hours (Winchester, 1982, personal observation).

References

1. Gosselin RE, Smith RP, Hodge HC (eds): Methyl alcohol. *In* Clinical Toxicology of Commercial Products. 5th ed. Baltimore, Williams & Wilkins, 1984, p III-275.
2. Greer JN: The cause of blindness. *In* Zahl PA (ed): Blindness: Modern Approach to the Unseen Environment. Princeton, Princeton University Press, 1950, p 100.
3. Kahn A, Blum D: Methyl alcohol poisoning in an 8 month old boy. An unusual route of intoxication. J Pediatr *94*:841, 1979.
4. Eriksen SP, Kulkarni AB: Methanol in normal human breath. Science *141*:639, 1963.
5. Bennett IL, Carey FH, Mitchell GL, Cooper MN: Acute methyl alcohol poisoning: A review based on experiences in an outbreak of 323 cases. Medicine *32*:431, 1953.
6. Axelrod J, Daly J: Pituitary gland: Enzymic formation of methanol from 5-methyl adenosine. Science *150*:892, 1965.
7. Becker CE: Methanol poisoning. J Emerg Med *1*:51, 1983.

8. Cooper JR, Kini MM: Editorial. Biochemical aspects of methanol poisoning. Biochem Pharmacol *11*:405, 1962.
9. Potts AM, Johnson LV: Studies on the visual toxicity of methanol. I. The effect of methanol and its degradation products on retinal metabolism. Am J Ophthalmol *35*:107, 1952.
10. Martin-Amat G, Tephly TR, McMartin KE, Makar AB, Hayreh MD, Hayreh SS, Baumabach G, Cancilla P: Methyl poisoning. II. Development of a model for ocular toxicity in methanol poisoning using the rhesus monkey. Arch Ophthalmol *95*:1847, 1977.
11. Ritchie JM: The aliphatic alcohols. *In* Gilman AG, Goodman LS, Gilman A (eds): The Pharmacological Basis of Therapeutics. 6th ed. New York, Macmillan, 1980, p 376.
12. Clay KL, Murphy RC, Watkins WD: Experimental methanol toxicity in the primate: Analysis of metabolic acidosis. Toxicol Appl Pharmacol *34*:49, 1975.
13. Harrop GA, Benedict EM: Acute methyl alcohol poisoning associated with acidosis. Report of a case. JAMA *74*:25, 1920.
14. Smith SR, Smith SJM, Buckley BM: Combined formate and lactic acidosis in methanol poisoning. Lancet *2*:1295, 1981.
15. Lins RL, Zachee P, Christiaens M, Van De Vivjer F, De Waele L, Sandra P, DeBroe ME: Prognosis and treatment of methanol intoxication. *In* Holmstedt B, Lauwerys R, Mercier M, Roberfroid M (eds): Mechanisms of Toxicity and Hazard Evaluation. New York, Elsevier/North Holland Biomedical Press, 1980, p 415.
16. Kini MM, Wing DW, Cooper JR: Biochemistry of methanol poisoning. V. Histological and biochemical correlates of effects of methanol and its metabolites on the rabbit. J Neurochem *9*:119, 1962.
17. Mardones J: The alcoholic. *In* Root WS, Hofmann FG (eds): Physiologic Pharmacology. New York, Academic Press, 1963.
18. McMartin KE, Makar AB, Martin-Amat G, Palese M, Tephly TR: Methanol poisoning. I. The role of formic acid in the development of metabolic acidosis in the monkey and the reversal by 4-methylpyrazole. Biochem Med *13*:319, 1975.
19. Hayreh MD, Hayreh SS, Baumbach G, Cancilla P, Martin-Amat G, Tephly TR, McMartin KE, Makar AB: Methyl alcohol poisoning. III. Ocular toxicity. Arch Ophthalmol *95*:1851, 1977.
20. Baumbach GL, Cancilla PA, Martin-Amat G, Tephly TR, McMartin KE, Makar AB, Hayreh MD, Hayreh SS: Methyl alcohol poisoning. IV. Alterations of the morphological findings of the retina and optic nerve. Arch Ophthalmol *95*:859, 1977.
21. Bennett IL, Nation TC, Olley JR: Pancreatitis in methyl alcohol poisoning. J Lab Clin Med *40*:405, 1952.
22. Kaplan K: Methyl alcohol poisoning. Am J Med Sci *244*:170, 1982.
23. Yant WP, Shrenk HH: Distribution of methanol in dogs after inhalation, and administration by stomach tube and subcutaneously. J Ind Hyg Toxicol *19*:337, 1937.
24. Eckfeldt JH, Kershaw MJ: Hyperamylasemia following methanol intoxication. Source and significance. Arch Intern Med *146*:193, 1986.
25. Grufferman S, Morris D, Alvarez J: Methanol poisoning complicated by myoglobinuric acute renal failure. Am J Emerg Med *3*:24, 1985.
26. Wu AH, Short R, McComb RB: Falsely high serum creatinine concentration associated with severe methanol intoxication. Clin Chem *29*:205, 1983.
27. Guggenheim MA, Couch JR, Weinberg W: Motor dysfunction as a permanent complication of methanol ingestion. Arch Neurol *24*:550, 1971.
28. McLean DR, Jacobs H, Mielke BW: Methanol poisoning: A clinical and pathological study. Arch Neurol *8*:161, 1980.
29. Shahangian S, Ash KO: Formic and lactic acidosis in a fatal case of methanol intoxication. Clin Chem *32*:395, 1986.
30. McMartin KE, Ambre JJ, Tephly TR: Methanol poisoning in human subjects. Am J Med *68*:414, 1980.
31. Swartz RD, Millman RP, Billi JE, Bondar NP, Migdal SD, Simonian SK, Monforte JR, McDonald FD, Harness JK, Cole KL: Epidemic methanol poisoning: Clinical and biochemical analysis of a recent episode. Medicine *60*:373, 1981.
32. Marc-Aurele J, Schreiner GE: The dialysance of ethanol and methanol: A proposed method for the treatment of massive intoxication by ethyl or methyl alcohol. J Clin Invest *39*:802, 1960.
33. Grady S, Osterloh JD: Improved enzymatic assay for formate with colorimetric end point. J Anal Toxicol *10*:1, 1986.
34. Osterloh JD, Pond SM, Grady S, Becker CE: Serum formate concentrations in methanol intoxication as a criterion for hemodialysis. Ann Intern Med *104*:200, 1986.
35. Editorial: Methanol poisoning. Med J Aust *1*:818, 1974.
36. Wood CA: Poisoning by wood, or methyl alcohol and its preparations as a cause of death and blindness; a supplementary report. NY Med J *81*:5, 1905.
37. Gonda A, Gault H, Churchill D, Hollomby D: Hemodialysis for methanol intoxication. Am J Med *64*:749, 1978.
38. Felts JH, Templeton TB, Wolff WA, Meredith JH, Hines J: Methanol poisoning treated by hemodialysis. South Med J *55*:46, 1962.
39. Tobin M, Lianos E: Hemodialysis for methanol poisoning. J Dial *3*:97, 1979.
40. McCoy HG, Cipolle RJ, Ehlers SM, Sawchuk RJ, Zaske DE: Severe methanol poisoning. Am J Med *67*:804, 1979.
41. Kane RL, Talbert W, Harlan J, Sizemore G, Cataland S: A methanol poisoning outbreak in Kentucky. Arch Environ Health *17*:119, 1968.
42. Tonning DJ, Brooks DW, Harlow CM: Acute methyl alcohol poisonings in 49 naval ratings. Can Med Assoc J *74*:20, 1956.
43. Keyvan-Larijarni H, Tannenberg AM: Methanol intoxication. Comparison of peritoneal dialysis and hemodialysis treatment. Arch Intern Med *134*:293, 1974.
44. Wenzl JE, Mills SD, McCall JT: Methanol poisoning in an infant. Successful treatment with peritoneal dialysis. Am J Dis Child *116*:445, 1968.
45. Humphrey J: Methanol poisoning: Management of acidosis with combined haemodialysis and peritoneal dialysis. Med J Aust *1*:833, 1974.
46. Gjessing J: Peritoneal dialys med tham von Methanolintoxikation. Opusc Med Bd *10*:40, 1965.
47. Whalen JE, Richard CJ, Ambre JJ: Inadequate removal of methanol and formate using the sorbent based regeneration hemodialysis delivery system. Clin Nephrol *11*:318, 1979.

48. Ekins BR, Rollins DE, Duffy DP, et al: Standardized treatment of severe methanol poisoning with ethanol and hemodialysis. West J Med *142*:337, 1985.
49. Blomstrand R, Ostling-Wintzell H, Lof A, McMartin K, Tolf BR, Hedstrom KG: Pyrazoles as inhibitors of alcohol oxidation and as important tools in alcohol research: An approach to therapy against methanol poisoning. Proc Natl Acad Sci *76*:3499, 1979.
50. Editorial: Use of folate analogues in treatment of methyl alcohol toxic reactions is studied. JAMA *242*:1961, 1979.
51. Billings RE, Tephly TR: Studies on methanol toxicity and formate metabolism in isolated hepatocytes. Biochem Pharmacol *28*:2985, 1979.
52. Gosselin RE, Smith RP, Hodge HC (eds): Isopropyl alcohol. *In* Clinical Toxicology of Commercial Products. 5th ed. Baltimore, Williams & Wilkins, 1984, p III-217.
53. Litovitz TL, Schmitz BF, Matyunas N, Martin TG: 1987 Annual report of the American Association of Poison Control Centers Data Collection System. Am J Emerg Med *6*:479, 1988.
54. Mendelson J, Wexler D, Leiderman PH, Solomon P: A study of addiction to non-ethyl alcohols and other poisonous compounds. Q J Stud Alcohol *18*:561, 1957.
55. Chapin MA: Isopropyl alcohol poisoning with acute renal insufficiency. J Maine Med Assoc *40*:288, 1949.
56. Adelson L: Fatal intoxication with isopropyl alcohol (rubbing alcohol). Am J Clin Pathol *38*:144, 1962.
57. Lacouture PG: Isopropyl alcohol. Clin Toxicol Rev *3*:3, 1980.
58. Daniel DR, McAnally BH, Garriott JC: Isopropyl alcohol metabolism after acute intoxication in humans. J Anal Toxicol *5*:110, 1981.
59. Brugnone F, Perbellini L, Apostoli P, Belloni M, Caretta D: Isopropanol exposure. Environmental and biological monitoring in a print works. Br J Ind Med *40*:160, 1983.
60. Williams RT: Detoxication Mechanisms. 2nd ed. New York, John Wiley & Sons, 1959.
61. Lehman AJ: Effect of insulin, insulin-dextrose and water diuresis on metabolism of isopropyl alcohol. Proc Soc Exp Biol Med *62*:232, 1946.
62. Corbett J, Meier G: Suicide attempted by rectal administration of drug. JAMA *206*:2320, 1968.
63. Morris HJ, Lightbody HD: The toxicity of isopropanol. J Ind Hyg Toxicol *20*:428, 1938.
64. Fuller HC, Hunter OB: Isopropyl alcohol—an investigation of its physiologic properties. J Lab Clin Med *12*:326, 1927.
65. Lehman AJ, Chase HF: The acute and chronic toxicity of isopropyl alcohol. J Lab Clin Med *29*:561, 1944.
66. Kulig K, Duffy JP, Linden CH, et al: Toxic effects of methanol, ethylene glycol and isopropyl alcohol. Top Emerg Med *6*:14, 1986.
67. Cornish HH, Adefuin J: Potentiation of carbon tetrachloride toxicity by aliphatic alcohols. Arch Environ Health *14*:447, 1967.
68. Traiger GJ, Plaa GC: Chlorinated hydrocarbon toxicity: potentiation by isopropyl alcohol and acetone. Arch Environ Health *28*:276, 1976.
69. Kelner M, Bailey DN: Isopropyl ingestion: Intrepretation of blood concentrations and clinical findings. J Toxicol Clin Toxicol *20*:497, 1983.
70. McCord WM, Switzer PK, Brill HH: Isopropyl alcohol intoxication. South Med J *41*:639, 1948.
71. Visudhiphan P, Kaufman H: Increased cerebrospinal fluid protein following isopropyl alcohol intoxication. NY State J Med *71*:887, 1971.
72. Alexander CB, McBay AJ, Hudson RP: Ispopropanol and isopropanol deaths—ten years experience. J Forensic Sci *27*:541, 1982.
73. Winchester JF, Gelfand MC, Knepshield JH, Schreiner GE: Dialysis and hemoperfusion of poisons and drugs—update. Trans Am Soc Artif Intern Organs *23*:762, 1977.
74. Freireich AW, Cinque TJ, Xanthaky G, Landau D: Hemodialysis for isopropanol poisoning. N Engl J Med *277*:699, 1967.
75. King LH, Bradley KP, Shires DL: Hemodialysis for isopropyl alcohol. JAMA *211*:1855, 1970.
76. Morris AJ: Personal communication. Cited in reference 73.
77. Dua SL: Peritoneal dialysis for isopropyl alcohol poisoning. JAMA *230*:35, 1974.
78. Depner TA, Mecckalsic MD: Peritoneal dialysis for isopropanol poisoning. West J Med *137*:322, 1981.
79. Durwald W, Degen W: Eine todliche Vergiftung mit N-Propyl-Alkohol. Arch Toxikol *16*:85, 1956.
80. Gosselin RE, Hodge HC, Smith RP, Gleason MH (eds): Higher alcohols. *In* Clinical Toxicology of Commercial Products. 4th ed. Baltimore, Williams & Wilkins, 1976, p 6.
81. Treon JF: Alcohols. *In* Irish DD, Fassett DW (eds): Patty's Industrial Hygiene and Toxicology. 2nd ed. New York, Interscience Publishers, 1963, p 1409.
82. Welt B: N-Butanol: Its use in control of post operative pain in otorhinollaryngolgical surgery. Arch Otolaryngol *52*:549, 1950.
83. Von Oettingen WF: The aliphatic alcohols, their toxicity and potential dangers in relation to their chemical constitution and their fate in metabolism. Washington, DC, US Public Health Service, Public Health Bulletin 281, 1943.
84. Bowen D, Cowburn D, Renekamp M, Sullivan J: Benzyl alcohol: High levels found in plasma of uremic patients on hemodialysis. Clin Chim Acta *61*:399, 1975.
85. Brown WJ, Buist NRM, Gipson HTC, Huston RK, Kennaway NG: Fatal benzyl alcohol poisoning in a neonatal intensive care unit. Lancet *1*:1250, 1982.
86. Gershanik J, Boecker B, Ensley H, McLoskey S, George W: The gasping syndrome and benzyl alcohol poisoning. N Engl J Med *307*:1384, 1982.
87. Hiller JC, Benda GI, Rahatzad M, Allen JR, Culner DH, Carlson CV, Reynolds JW: Impact on mortality and intraventricular hemorrhage among very low birth weight infants. Pediatrics *77*:500, 1986.
88. Gosselin RE, Smith RP, Hodge HC (eds): Ethylene glycol. *In* Clinical Toxicology of Commercial Products. 5th ed. Baltimore, Williams & Wilkins, 1984, p III-172.
89. Vale JA, Meredith TJ: Ethylene glycol poisoning. *In* Poisoning: Diagnosis and Treatment. Boston, Update Books, 1981, p 131.
90. Sykowski P: Ethylene glycol toxicity. Am J Ophthalmol *34*:1599, 1951.
91. Troisi FM: Chronic intoxication with ethylene glycol vapour. Br J Ind Med *1*:65, 1950.
92. Friedman EA, Greenberg JB, Merrill JP, Dammin GJ: Consequences of ethylene glycol poisoning: Report of four cases and review of the literature. Am J Med *32*:891, 1962.

93. Pons CA, Custer RP: Acute ethylene glycol poisoning: A clinicopathologic report of eighteen fatal cases. Am J Med Sci *211*:544, 1946.
94. Berman LB, Schreiner GE, Feys J: The nephrotoxic lesion of ethylene glycol. Ann Intern Med *46*:611, 1957.
95. Schreiner GE, Maher JF, Marc-Aurele J, Knowlan D, Alvo M: Ethylene glycol—two indications for hemodialysis. Trans Am Soc Artif Intern Organs *5*:81, 1959.
96. Hagemann PO, Chiffelle TR: Ethylene glycol poisoning. A clinical and pathologic study of three cases. J Lab Clin Med *33*:573, 1948.
97. Smith DE: Morphologic lesions due to acute and subacute poisoning with antifreeze. Arch Pathol *51*:423, 1951.
98. Zarembski PM, Hodgkinson A: Plasma oxalic acid and calcium levels in oxalate poisoning. J Clin Pathol *20*:283, 1967.
99. Hagstam KE, Ingvar DH, Paatela M, Tallqvist H: Ethylene glycol poisoning treated by haemodialysis. Acta Med Scand *178*:599, 1965.
100. Ross IP: Ethylene glycol poisoning with meningoencephalitis and anuria. Br Med J *1*:1340, 1956.
101. McChesney EW, Goldberg L, Parekh CK, Russell JC, Min BH: Reappraisal of the toxicology of ethylene glycol. II. Metabolic studies in laboratory animals. Food Cosmet Toxicol *9*:21, 1971.
102. Hodgkinson A, Zarembski PM: Oxalic acid metabolism in man. Calcif Tissue Res *2*:115, 1968.
103. Godolphin W, Meagher EP, Sanders HD, Frohllich J: Unusual calcium oxalate crystals in ethylene glycol poisoning. Clin Toxicol *16*:479, 1980.
104. Terlinsky AS, Grochowski J, Geoly KL, Strauch BS, Hefter L: Identification of atypical calcium oxalate crystalluria following ethylene glycol ingestion. Am J Clin Pathol *76*:223, 1981.
105. Schreiner GE, Maher JF: Toxic nephropathy. Am J Med *38*:409, 1965.
106. Hewlett TP, McMartin RE: Ethylene glycol intoxication: The value of glycolic acid determination for diagnosis and treatment. Clin Toxicol *24*:389, 1986.
107. Wacker WEC, Haynes H, Druyan R, Fisher W, Coleman JE: Treatment of ethylene glycol poisoning with ethyl alcohol. JAMA *194*:1231, 1965.
108. Peterson CD, Collins A, Himes JM, Bullock ML, Keane WF: Ethylene glycol poisoning. Pharmacokinetics during therapy with ethanol and hemodialysis. N Engl J Med *304*:21, 1981.
109. Freed CR, Bobbitt WH, Williams RM, Shoemaker S, Nies AS: Ethanol for ethylene glycol poisoning. N Engl J Med *304*:976, 1981.
110. Pietruszko R, Crawford K, Lester D: Comparison of substrate specificity of alcohol dehydrogenase from human liver, horse liver and yeast towards saturated and 2-enoic alcohols and aldehydes. Arch Biochem Biophys *159*:50, 1973.
111. Pietruszko R, Voigtlander K, Lester D: Alcohol dehydrogenase from human and horse liver: Substrate specificity with diols. Biochem Pharmacol *27*:1296, 1978.
112. Stokes JB, Averon F: Prevention of organ damage in massive ethylene glycol ingestion. JAMA *243*:2065, 1980.
113. Underwood F, Bennett WM: Ethylene glycol intoxication. Prevention of renal failure by aggressive management. JAMA *226*:1453, 1973.
114. Gabow PA, Clay K, Sullivan LB, Lepoff R: Organic acids in ethylene glycol intoxication. Ann Intern Med *105*:16, 1986.
115. Cheng JT, Beysolow TD, Kaul B, Weisman R, Feinfeld DA: Clearance of ethylene glycol by kidneys and hemodialysis. J Toxicol Clin Toxicol *25*:95, 1987.
116. Egbert AM, Reed JS, Powell BJ, Liskow BI, Liese BS: Alcoholics who drink mouthwash: the spectrum of nonbeverage alcohol use. J Stud Alcohol *46*:473, 1985.
117. Heckerling PS: Ethylene glycol poisoning with a normal anion gap due to occult bromide intoxication. Ann Emerg Med *16*:1384, 1987.
118. Sangster B, Prenen JAC, DeGroot G: Ethylene glycol poisoning. N Engl J Med *302*:465, 1980.
119. Beasley VR, Back WB: Acute ethylene glycol toxicoses: a review. Vet Hum Toxicol *22*:255, 1980.
120. Chou JY, Richardson KE: The effect of pyrazole in ethylene glycol toxicity and metabolism in the rat. Toxicol Appl Pharmacol *43*:33, 1978.
121. Clay KL, Murphy RC: On the metabolic acidosis of ethylene glycol intoxication. Toxicol Appl Pharmacol *39*:39, 1977.
122. Blomstrand R, Theorell H: Inhibitory effect on ethanol oxidation in man after administration of 4-methyl-pyrazole. Life Sci *9*:631, 1970.
123. Baud FJ, Bismuth C, Garnier R, Galliot M, Astier A, Maistre G, Soffer M: 4-Methylpyrazole may be an alternative to ethanol therapy for ethylene glycol intoxication in man. J Toxicol Clin Toxicol *24*:463, 1986–87.
124. Baud FJ, Galliot M, Astier A, Bien DV, Likforman J, Bismuth C: Treatment of ethylene glycol poisoning with intravenous 4-methylpyrazole. N Engl J Med *319*:97, 1988.
125. Geiling EMK, Cannon PR: Pathologic effects of elixir sulfanilamide (diethylene glycol) poisoning; clinical and experimental correlations: Final report. JAMA *111*:919, 1938.
126. Leech PN: Elixir of sulfanilamide-Massengill. Chemical, pharmacologic, pathologic and necropsy reports; preliminary toxicity reports on diethylene glycol and sulfanilamide. JAMA *109*:1531, 1937.
127. Bowie MD, McKenzie D: Diethylene glycol poisoning in children. S Afr Med J *46*:931, 1972.
128. Kesten HD, Mullinos MC, Pomerantz L: Pathologic effects of certain glycol and related compounds. Arch Pathol *27*:447, 1939.
129. Nitter-Hauge S: Poisoning with ethylene glycol monomethyl ether. Acta Med Scand *188*:277, 1970.
130. Smyth HF, Seaton J, Fischer L: Single dose toxicity of some glycols and derivatives. J Pharm Sci *39*:349, 1950.
131. Cate JC, Hedrick R: Propylene glycol intoxication and lactic acidosis. N Engl J Med *303*:1237, 1980.
132. Martin G, Finberg L: Propylene glycol: A potentially toxic vehicle in liquid dosage form. J Pediatr *77*:877, 1970.
133. Arulanantham K, Genel M: Central nervous system toxicity associated with ingestion of propylene glycol. J Pediatr *93*:515, 1978.
134. Myers VS, Vsenik EA: Propylene glycol intoxication of horses. J Am Med Vet Assoc *155*:1841, 1969.
135. Demey H, Daelemans R, De Broe ME, Bossaert L: Propyleneglycol intoxication due to intravenous nitroglycerin. Lancet *1*:1361, 1984.
136. Miller ON, Bazzano G: Propanediol metabolism and its relation to lactic acid metabolism. Ann NY Acad Sci *119*:957, 1965.
137. Hardin BD, Lyon JP: Summary and overview of NIOSH symposium on toxic effects of glycol ethers. Environ Health Perspect *57*:273, 1984.

138. Cullen MR, Rado T, Waldrin JA, et al: Bone marrow injury in lithographers exposed to glycol ethers and organic solvents used in multicolor offset and ultraviolet curing printing processes. Arch Environ Health *38*:347, 1983.
139. Ramu A, Rosenbaum J, Blaschke TF: Disposition of acetone following acute acetone intoxication. West J Med *129*:429, 1978.
140. Browning EC: Ketones. *In* Toxicity and Metabolism of Industrial Solvents. New York, Elsevier Publishing Company, 1965, p 412.
141. Ross DS: Acute acetone intoxication involving eight male workers. Ann Occup Hyg *16*:73, 1973.
142. Gitelson S, Werczberger A, Herman JB: Coma and hyperglycemia following drinking of acetone. Diabetes *15*:810, 1966.
143. Rooth G, Ostenson S: Acetone in alveolar air and the control of diabetes. Lancet *2*:1102, 1962.
144. Oliver JS, Watson JM: Abuse of solvents "for kicks." A review of 50 cases. Lancet *1*:84, 1977.
145. Divicenzo GD, Yanno FJ, Astill BD: Exposure of man and dog to low concentrations of acetone vapor. Am Ind Hyg Assoc J *34*:329, 1973.
146. Haggard HW, Greenberg LA, McCullough-Turner J: The physiologic principles governing the action of acetone together with determination of toxicity. J Ind Hyg Toxicol *26*:133, 1944.
147. Gosselin RE, Smith RP, Hodge HC (eds): Oxalate. *In* Clinical Toxicology of Commercial Products. 5th ed. Baltimore, Williams & Wilkins, 1984, p III-326.
148. Balcke P, Schmidt P, Zaggornik J, Kopsa H, Haulenstock A: Ascorbic acid aggravates secondary hyperoxalemia in patients on chronic hemodialysis. Ann Intern Med *101*:344, 1984.
149. Webster RW: Legal Medicine and Toxicology. Philadelphia, WB Saunders, 1930.
150. Witthaus RA: Manual of Toxicology. New York, William Wood and Company, 1911.
151. Klander JV, Shelanski L, Gabriel K: Industrial uses of compounds of fluorine and oxalic acid; Cutaneous reaction and calcium therapy. Arch Ind Health *12*:412, 1965.
152. Brown SA, Gettler AO: A study of oxalic acid poisoning. Proc Soc Exp Biol Med *19*:204, 1922.
153. Polson CJ, Tattersall RN: Clinical Toxicology. Philadelphia, JB Lippincott, 1959.
154. Maggiore W, Poggi A, Parlongo S, Cerrai T: Oxalate removal by dialysis and hemoperfusion. Proc Eur Dial Transplant Assoc *16*:717, 1979.

CHAPTER 38
OPIATES AND NARCOTICS

Kathleen C. Hubbell, M.D., FACEP

HISTORY

The opiate class of drugs includes the natural alkaloids of the opium poppy and their synthetic derivatives, which share some or all of the original properties. Although some of the pharmacologic actions of the opiates mimic natural sleep, the term *narcotic* is misleading, as the major use of opiates in modern medicine is for analgesia whereas other classes of drugs are far more useful for inducing sleep. Physicians, the lay public, and regulatory agencies generally use the term *narcotic* to describe those drugs that produce dependence.

The properties of opium have been known for thousands of years. Early Egyptians used it to calm children, and other cultures used it to relieve pain and treat mental disorders. It was also eaten or smoked for recreational purposes.

Opium became a resource for modern medicine in the early 19th century when its major alkaloid was isolated and given the name morphine, after Morpheus, the god of sleep. The other principal constituents, codeine, thebaine, and papaverine, were isolated several years later. Physicians found the potent analgesia produced by morphine to be valuable in their practices. However, as medical experience with morphine grew, they became familiar with its undesirable side effects, including the development of tolerance and the production of physical and psychologic dependence. Because of the desirability of retaining a drug with morphine's potent analgesic effect in the medical armamentarium, ways were sought to modify morphine chemically to produce a drug without addiction potential. One of the earliest products of this research was heroin, the 3,6-diacetate ester of morphine. Although initially lauded as nonaddicting and potent, heroin was later found to have the same disadvantages as morphine, to which it is converted in the body.

The exact molecular structures of morphine, codeine, and thebaine were defined in the 1920s. Once they were known, a systematic program was undertaken to synthesize new and, it was hoped, potent and nonaddictive compounds by transforming the natural opiates. Many valuable drugs such as dihydromorphinone (Dilaudid), hydrocodone (Anexsia), metopon, and oxycodone (Percodan) were created in this manner, although none fulfilled the criteria of the ideal compound. Totally synthetic opiates were also developed by using only certain rings and bridges from the morphine skeleton and modifying these. Levorphanol (Levo-Dromoran), dextromethorphan, phenazocine (Narphen), meperidine (Demerol), fentanyl (Sublimaze), methadone, propoxyphene (Darvon), and diphenoxylate (of Lomotil) are just a few of the thousands of synthetic opiates that have been invented.

During the efforts to modify the natural opiates and synthesize new ones, it was noted as early as 1915 that some of the resultant compounds blocked the pharmacologic effects of the known opiate analgesics. In 1951 the relatively new drug nalorphine (Nalline) was used to reverse the symptoms of morphine poisoning in humans. In 1954 nalorphine was also found to possess potent analgesic properties in humans. This discovery spurred attempts to find new agonist-antagonist compounds that presumably would be nonaddicting. Levallorphan (Lorfan), pentazocine (Talwin), and buprenorphine (Buprenex) were among those developed. In 1961 the pure antagonist naloxone (Narcan) was synthesized.

The discovery and classification in the 1970s of the opiate receptor sites in the body provided new direction to researchers in their efforts to find the perfect opiate.[1]

PHARMACOLOGY OF THE OPIATES

Opiate Receptors

Four types of opiate receptors are thought to exist in human brain and spinal cord tissues.[2, 3] They were named according to the drug that activated them during experimental studies: *mu* receptor for morphine; *kappa* for ketocyclazocine; *sigma* for SKF 10,047; and *delta*. After discovery of the receptor sites, scientists postulated the existence of endogenous opioid substances that would interact with the sites. This led to the isolation of methionine (met−) enkephalin and leucine (leu−) enkephalin, β-endorphin, and dynorphin. These endogenous peptides are thought to act as neurotransmitters in a system similar to the adrenergic and dopaminergic systems and to be involved in the modulation of pain and possibly in the development of tolerance and addiction to exogenous opiates.[4–6]

Mu receptors are most highly concentrated in areas of the brain involved in pain sensation. They have a high affinity for the morphine-like pure agonist drugs and produce analgesia, respiratory depression, miosis, and euphoria when stimulated by these drugs. These receptors are blocked by the agonist-antagonist class.

Kappa receptors are found in the spinal cord and brain and likewise cause analgesia, respiratory depression, miosis, and sedation when binding by the agonist-antagonist-type drugs such as pentazocine (Talwin), nalorphine (Nalline), and butorphanol (Stadol) occurs.

The location of the sigma receptors is not certain. Stimulation of these receptors produces the dysphoria and hallucinations that are the side effects of certain opiates of the agonist-antagonist class.

The role of the delta receptor has not been elucidated.

The pure antagonist naloxone blocks the mu, kappa, and sigma receptors. Its ability to block the delta receptor is unknown.

Administration, Absorption, Distribution, and Excretion

Opiates (Table 38–1) may be administered orally and parenterally and may be inhaled ("snorted") or smoked. Although there are variations among the large number of available opiates, maximal toxic and therapeutic effects are generally reached in 10 minutes after IV injection, in 30 minutes after intramuscular injection, and in 90 minutes after subcutaneous or oral administration. Opiates are metabolized rapidly by the liver, minimizing their duration of action, even in over-

Table 38–1. PHARMACOLOGY OF COMMON OPIATES

TYPE	RECEPTOR
Agonist Drugs	
Apomorphine	
Codeine	
Diphenoxylate (in Lomotil)	
Fentanyl (Sublimaze)	
Heroin	
Hydromorphone (Dilaudid)	
Levorphanol (Levo-Dromoran)	
Loperamide (Imodium)	mu
Meperidine (Demerol)	?delta
Methadone (Dolophine)	
Metopon	
Morphine	
Opium powder or tincture	
Oxycodone (in Percodan)	
Paregoric	
Propoxyphene	
Agonist-Antagonist Drugs	
Buprenorphine (Buprenex)	mu kappa
Butorphanol (Stadol)	
Nalbuphine (Nubain)	kappa
Pentazocine (Talwin)	sigma
Antagonist Drugs	mu
Naloxone (Narcan)	kappa
Naltrexone	sigma
Nalmefene	?delta

dose. They are then excreted in the urine. Most opiates are not stored in body tissues, but propoxyphene and buprenorphine are fat soluble and have a prolonged duration of action in overdose.

Some of the most commonly abused opiates undergo unusual methods of preparation by addicts for their administration. These methods often contribute to the pathology suffered by the users. Other drugs differ markedly from the typical absorption and metabolism described above. These drugs are discussed below.

Heroin

Heroin (diacetylmorphine) is purchased on the street from dealers who have diluted it with various substances such as quinine, mannitol, lactose, talc, sodium bicarbonate, and occasionally antihistamines or phencyclidine. The final concentration of heroin is usually 3 to 5 per cent. Mexican brown heroin is cheaper, less potent, and contains more vegetable impurities. White Asian heroin is purer. Heroin is often sterile but may be contaminated with *Bacillus* species and diphtheroids. The heroin mixture is heated in a spoon or bottle cap over a match to dissolve the powder. It is then aspirated through cotton or a cigarette filter into a syringe, often made by the addict by attaching a needle to an eyedropper. It is then injected IV or "skin-popped" subcutaneously. When heroin supplies are low, addicts attempt to extract the drug from their homemade filters by boiling. Injection of this liquid produces "cotton fever" of unknown etiology. Alternatively, heroin can be inhaled or liquefied on aluminum foil over a candle and the fumes inhaled ("chasing the dragon"). Because of first-pass inactivation in the liver, oral doses of heroin have little euphoric or analgesic effect. The half-life of IV heroin is 3 to 20 minutes.[7, 8]

Methadone

Methadone has become the most widely used opiate for addict maintenance programs because, unlike most other opiates, it has a slow onset of action and an unusually long duration of action of almost 24 hours. It also undergoes little first-pass metabolism, making it an effective drug for oral administration. Oral overdose requires a prolonged treatment and observation period. Methadone is packaged as a diskette that contains cellulose, which forms a sludge when mixed with water to discourage parenteral use. It is also supplied as tablets, syrup, and solution. When illegally diverted to IV use, methadone is slightly more potent than morphine and can cause serious overdose in nontolerant persons.[7, 9]

LAAM (L-alpha-acetylmethadol)

LAAM is a long-acting methadone derivative with a half-life of 2 days. It enables addicts to participate in maintenance programs in which they receive their medication three times a week rather than every day. Prolonged observation is needed in case of overdose.[10, 14]

Percodan and Percocet

Oxycodone has a parenteral effect equivalent to morphine. Abusers crush and "cold shake" the tablets for IV injection. Other addicts take 30 to 40 tablets per day orally and suffer the toxic effects of the large doses of aspirin and acetominophen contained in these compounds.

Talwin

Talwin has only one-fourth the parenteral potency of morphine. However, in some parts of the United States Talwin tablets are crushed, combined with the antihistamine tripelennamine, and injected IV by heroin addicts when supplies of their preferred drug are low or of poor quality. This combination is known as "Ts and blues."[11] Talwin is now available combined with naloxone as Talwin NX. The naloxone is inactive when the combination is taken orally but will block the effect of Talwin diverted to IV use.

Because Talwin is of the agonist-antagonist class, it precipitates withdrawal in persons addicted to pure agonists. For this reason, addicts often complain of "allergy" to Talwin.

Diphenoxylate (with atropine in Lomotil)

This opiate is an effective antidiarrheal agent with very little respiratory depression, even in large doses (e.g., 75 mg) when used in adults. However, many deaths due to respiratory arrest have been reported in children under the age of 2 years who have received single doses of 7.5 mg. This is presumably because the immature blood-brain barrier of the infant allows greater penetration of the drug into the central nervous system. Use of diphenoxylate in children under the age of 2 years is contraindicated, but prescribed or accidental ingestion still occurs.

In Lomotil intoxication, the earliest signs are anticholinergic because of the atropine that is included in the preparation to discourage abuse. The onset of respiratory depression may be delayed from 6 to 14 hours after ingestion, and toxic symptoms are prolonged with cyclical waxing and waning for as long as 72 hours. Delayed gastric emptying and release from tissue storage may explain these effects. A prolonged observation period is required.[12, 13]

Naloxone (Narcan)

Naloxone was the first pure opiate antagonist to be synthesized. It can be given IV, IM, sublingually or into the endotracheal tube[14] but is ineffective orally. It blocks all opiate receptors and has no agonist activity at any opiate receptor.[15] Tolerance does not develop, and there is no abstinence syndrome after withdrawal of naloxone. There have been virtually no reports of adverse effects from naloxone, except in the anesthesiology literature in which can be found a number of case reports linking the administration of small doses of naloxone to reverse narcotic anesthesia with the onset of atrial and ventricular dysrhythmias, hypertension, pulmonary edema, and sudden death in both young and old patients who had undergone a wide variety of procedures. These effects were poorly understood, but it was postulated that opiate reversal led to an outpouring of catecholamines that were responsible for the dramatic and life-threatening complications in this patient subgroup.[60–66]

Naloxone blocks the activity of endogenous as well as exogenous opiates.[6] This property suggests that naloxone may have a role in pathologic conditions that involve the endorphins, such as shock and brain and spinal ischemia.[16, 17]

Naltrexone, a congener of naloxone, is an opiate antagonist that is effective when given orally. It should be very useful in detoxification programs when it becomes more widely available.[18]

Buprenorphine (Buprenex)

Although originally classed as a drug of the agonist-antagonist type, clinical experience has shown that buprenorphine usually behaves like a mu-agonist such as morphine. It has a high affinity for and a slow rate of dissociation from the mu receptor site, which may account for its relatively long duration of action and unpredictable reversal by naloxone.

However, buprenorphine can antagonize large doses of previously administered mu and kappa receptor agonists, while having additive effects, especially on respiratory depression, with small doses of both types of agonists.[67]

CLINICAL MANIFESTATIONS OF OPIATE USE

Clinical effects of opiates are produced through the stimulation of the opiate receptors discussed earlier. Differences between therapeutic and toxic effects are largely a matter of degree. Clinical signs are dose related, although opiate addicts develop tolerance to all effects except miosis of the pupil and reduced intestinal motility.

Opiates produce major pharmacologic and toxic effects on the central nervous system, the cardiovascular system, and the gastrointestinal system.[19] In brief, the effects on the central nervous system include increased tolerance to pain, altered psychologic response to pain, suppression of anxiety, and sedation. Opiates produce respiratory depression by a direct effect on pontine and medullary respiratory centers. Suppression of the cough reflex, nausea and vomiting from stimulation of the chemoreceptor trigger zone, and euphoria are also noted. Cardiovascular effects include orthostatic hypotension and syncope. Gastrointestinal effects include decrease in peristalsis with an increase in anal sphincter tone and ileocecal valve tone, thus explaining the antidiarrheal effects of the opiates.[19]

Patients receiving therapeutic doses of opiates develop reduced pupil size, analgesia, some respiratory depression, no significant change in other vital signs when in the supine position, possible nausea and vomiting, mild euphoria, or dysphoria if receiving one of the agonist-antagonist class, and little change in the level of consciousness.

ACUTE OPIATE OVERDOSE

Overdose produces more severe, but similar, symptoms. Miosis is caused by an effect on the Edinger-Westphal nucleus, producing an exaggerated response to light. Dilated pupils might be caused by hypoxia or other ingested nonopiate drugs. Meperidine (Demerol) may cause dilated pupils.

Opiates depress the rate but not the depth of respiration by decreasing the sensitivity of the respiratory center to the level of arterial carbon dioxide. Hypoxia develops and is the cause of death in almost all fatal opiate intoxications.[19, 24] Noncardiac pulmonary edema is present in these cases as well. Noncardiac pulmonary edema is common in heroin overdose and has occurred after oral intoxication with methadone and propoxyphene. It never occurs after therapeutic doses of opiates. Its cause is controversial but is probably related to hypoxia-induced pulmonary vasoconstriction, which causes elevated pulmonary capillary pressures and leakage of protein-rich fluid into the interstitium and alveoli.[19–23] Clinical findings of noncardiac pulmonary edema include rales, rhonchi, wheezes, and pink, frothy sputum.

Changes in blood pressure or heart rate secondary to opiate intoxication are rare in a supine patient. Peripheral vasodilatation does occur and causes orthostatic hypotension. Significant supine hypotension in a patient suffering from overdose should lead the physician to consider other drugs, severe uncorrected hypoxia, or hypovolemia.

Opiate intoxication causes contrasting signs and symptoms in the central nervous system. Heroin and potent opiates produce a euphoric "rush" for several seconds after intravenous injection. It is intensely pleasurable, even though it may be accompanied by nausea and vomiting. The nausea is produced by stimulation of the chemoreceptor trigger zone, which after the initial stimulation becomes unresponsive to further stimulus from additional doses of opiate or from an emetic such as ipecac.[19] A short period of central nervous system excitation follows. In children, seizures may result after an overdose of any opiate. In adults, seizures are usually limited to cases of meperidine or propoxyphene intoxication. Meperidine can also cause twitching and hyperreflexia. Drowsiness proceeding to unconsciousness follows the excitatory phase. Users of pentazocine or other of the agonist-antagonist opiates may experience dysphoria and hallucinations rather than euphoria.

Decreased peristalsis and urinary retention are encountered in both chronic use and overdose of opiates. Direct effects on nerve plexuses in the gastrointestinal and genitourinary tracts produce increased smooth muscle tone, causing tightening of sphincters and decreased contractions in the longitudinal muscles and resulting in slower transit times. These effects complicate management of oral ingestions involving opiates.

In addition to the physiologic responses to opiate overdose described earlier, other physical findings in chronic opiate users may provide clues to the cause of the patient's condition. "Track marks," sclerotic veins, atrophic depressed scars of "skin-popping," puffy hands and feet caused by venous insufficiency and lymphatic obliteration, and a fresh injection site are suggestive of chronic IV opiate abuse. The finding of multiple fresh injection sites is more compatible with cocaine use, which requires more frequent injections. Flushed skin, urticaria, and scratches as evidence of pruritus are seen after opiate ingestion or injection secondary to histamine release.[19] Cyanosis is, of course, a universal skin finding in severe opiate overdose.

The dose of opiate received by the patient and that patient's tolerance for opiates generally determine whether the respiratory depression produced will be profound enough to cause death. Heroin addicts die of overdose only if they mistakenly inject a purer form of heroin than that to which they are accustomed. Much lower doses may be lethal for nontolerant individuals.

A very small number of apparent opiate overdose deaths may result from causes other than opiate-induced respiratory depression. Some heroin addicts have been reported to die within minutes of injection, before significant respiratory depression had developed, and after use of nonlethal amounts of heroin. Simultaneous ingestion of alcohol and sudden arrhythmia have been postulated as causes.

Contributing somewhat to overdose morbidity and mortality are procedures performed on unconscious addicts by their friends in an attempt to revive them. Pouring milk into the mouth, injecting milk intravenously, placing an unconscious addict in a cold shower or tub, and placing paper wadding in the pharynx to prevent swallowing the tongue are some of these misguided interventions.

TREATMENT OF OPIATE OVERDOSE

As described in the previous section, respiratory depression with resultant hypoxia is the cause of death in opiate overdose. Therefore, initial patient management must be directed toward assessment of the patient's respiratory status and the provision of a patent and protected airway and adequate ventilation. In the prehospital phase of care, emergency medical technicians (EMTs) should ventilate depressed patients with a bag-valve mask with 100 per cent oxygen or endotracheally intubate and ventilate with 100 per cent oxygen, according to the EMT's training level. A finger-stick determination of blood glucose should be performed and D50W and thiamine administered if needed. However, undue time should not be spent at the scene attempting to start an IV line in a patient with sclerotic veins. Naloxone (Narcan) should only rarely be administered in the prehospital setting because of the possibility of vomiting and aspiration during treatment and the potential difficulty in controlling patients as they regain consciousness.

In the emergency department, a similar sequence should be followed. Immediate assessment and control of airway and ventilation should be accomplished by endotracheal intubation in patients with respiratory depression. An IV line should be started, blood drawn for laboratory tests, bedside determination of blood glucose performed, and D50W and thiamine given if indicated. Adequacy of circulation should be assessed, but is usually not adversely affected by opiate overdose.

Pupil size, respiratory rate, and level of consciousness should be measured, and then naloxone should be administered in an initial dose of 0.4 to 2.0 mg IV. If IV access will be delayed, naloxone is effective when instilled into the endotracheal tube in the same doses.[14] The recommended dose in children is 0.01 mg/kg; a dose of 0.1 mg/kg should be administered if the initial dose is ineffective.[25] The effects of naloxone will be seen in 1 to 3 minutes, peaking in 5 to 10 minutes. Naloxone's high affinity for the mu receptor enables it to reverse the effects of opiates that act at this receptor at the relatively low doses described. However, its affinity for the kappa and sigma receptors is less, and larger doses are required to reverse overdoses of pentazocine and the other drugs that bind these receptors. Therefore, if no response is noted to the initial dose of naloxone, an additional dose of 2 mg should be given and repeated every 5 minutes until response occurs or a maximum dose of 10 mg has been administered. If there has been no improvement after 10 mg, it is unlikely that opiates are responsible for the patient's condition. Experience has shown that large doses of naloxone are required to reverse overdoses of codeine, propoxyphene, and methadone in addition to drugs in the agonist-antagonist class. Partial response to naloxone suggests a mixed overdose, postictal state, or cerebral anoxia.[26, 27] Sublingual naloxone is also effective.

Administration of naloxone will reverse all of the pharmacologic effects of opiates, including analgesia, miosis, respiratory depression, sedation, and decreased peristalsis. In addition, emesis may occur immediately after injection and a period of hyperventilation follows as the respiratory center responds to the stimulus of the accumulated carbon dioxide. It is controversial whether naloxone protects against the seizure activity caused by meperidine and propoxyphene. Seizures occurring after naloxone may be due to cerebral anoxia, infection, trauma, or other cause.[28]

Naloxone cannot immediately reverse the noncardiac pulmonary edema encountered in many heroin overdoses because it is a result of hypoxia and not a direct pharmacologic effect of the opiate. Treatment of opiate-induced noncardiac pulmonary edema consists of reversing respiratory depression with naloxone and providing adequate oxygenation. Mild cases may be treated with high-flow oxygen by face mask, but most cases require intubation and positive-pressure ventilation with 100 per cent oxygen. Positive end-expiratory pressure may be necessary. Diuretics, digitalis, and afterload reducers have no role in treating this disorder. Noncardiac pulmonary edema generally clears within 24 to 48 hours with this treatment. Persistent clinical and radiographic abnormalities should prompt consideration of aspiration pneumonia as the cause.[29]

The half-life of naloxone is 30 to 80 minutes. Only minimal effects of a 0.4-mg dose persist 45 minutes after IV injection. Because the effects of most opiates last longer than 30 minutes, respiratory depression and sedation will recur unless repeat doses of naloxone are given. This is particularly true with long-acting or fat-soluble compounds such as methadone, propoxyphene, diphenoxylate, and buprenorphine. To prevent patient deterioration due to unnoticed recurrence of opiate effects, a naloxone infusion at 0.4 to 0.8 mg/hour can be started and titrated according to patient signs and symptoms. The infusion can be prepared by mixing 4 mg of naloxone in a liter of D5W or normal saline and running at 100 ml/hour.

A new, pure opiate antagonist, nalmefene, may prove to be useful for reversing opiate effects for much longer periods than naloxone. Nalmefene's half-life is 10.3 to 12.9 hours. A 1-mg IV dose reverses opiate effects for 4 hours, a 2-mg dose for 8 hours. A 50-mg oral dose has been shown to be effective for 48 hours. Although experience with nalmefene is limited at this time, it so far appears to be a potent and safe compound with many potential areas of application.[30]

Once the patient's condition is stabilized, a complete history and physical examination must be performed to identify any concurrent medical or traumatic conditions. Certain illnesses are common in addicts, and the septic complications of chronic IV opiate use in particular can be immediately life threatening. About 5 per cent of opiate-related deaths each year are due to infection. Table 38–2 lists a summary of medical complications.

The disposition of patients who have presented with an IV opiate overdose depends on their response to treatment. A patient whose symptoms can be fully reversed by naloxone should be observed to be asymptomatic for a minimum of 12 hours after weaning from the naloxone drip. This period is adequate to detect recurrence of opiate-induced symptoms and the delayed onset of noncardiac pulmonary edema. Patients who have injected a long-acting opiate such as methadone, LAAM, propoxyphene, or diphenoxylate must be symptom free for at least 24 hours before discharge. Patients with only partial response to naloxone, noncardiac pulmonary edema, or concurrent serious medical problems require admission.

The management of patients who have taken an oral opiate overdose is slightly different from the above. If a patient presents with a history of oral ingestion of an opiate but is asymptomatic, an observation period of 4 to 6 hours after gastric emptying is usually sufficient to determine if the ingestion is a serious one. Patients who have manifested symptoms of opiate intoxication should be observed for 12 to 24 hours. Exceptions to these guidelines occur in the case of oral opiates that possess delayed onset or prolonged duration of action, and these will be discussed later.

In the case of oral ingestion, decontamination of the gastrointestinal tract must be added to the specific recommendations for management of opiate overdose that were given above. Gastric emptying should always be undertaken, no matter how long after the ingestion. Delayed gastric emptying is characteristic of opiate overdose because of decreased peristaltic activity. Tablets have been found in the stomach more than 20 hours after ingestion. Lavage is preferred over ipecac-induced emesis, even in a conscious pa-

Table 38–2. MEDICAL COMPLICATIONS OF OPIATE USE

INFECTION
Acquired immunodeficiency syndrome (AIDS)
Endocarditis: Suspected in any user with fever of undetermined origin, murmur, pneumonia, embolic phenomena, or positive blood cultures
Bacterial: Characteristically right-sided; most commonly *Staphylococcus aureus*, generally penicillin- and possibly methicillin-resistant; *Escherichia coli, Pseudomonas*, and enterococci less frequent; prior cardiac disease is rare; slowly progressive; septic emboli to lungs
Fungal: Most frequent in users with prior cardiac disease; *Candida* most common; mycotic aneurysm
Soft tissue infections
Abscess, nodules, ulcers: Fever and leukocytosis with no source of infection are common; infections due to pathogenic contaminants and nonsterile injection technique
Tetanus: Opportunistic infection at compromised lesion site
Malaria, tuberculosis: Sharing of contaminated paraphernalia
Bacteremia, sepsis: Staphylococci most common; streptococci; pneumococci; *Salmonella*
Hepatitis: Hepatitis B most common; assumed to be present in any hospitalized addict; subclinical to lethal disease

PULMONARY
Pneumonia: Patients treated for pneumonia should be observed for 7–10 days after antibiotic therapy is completed to avoid overlooking signs of endocarditis
Bacterial: Generally staphylococci
Fungal: *Candida* predominates
Aspiration: Must be differentiated from pulmonary edema; typically produces increased respiratory rate as opposed to the slowed respiratory rate observed in pulmonary edema with respiratory center depression
Pulmonary edema: "Heroin lung." Most commonly observed in heroin, propoxyphene, and methadone poisoning; presents in combination with respiratory center depression
Embolism: May result as complication of endocarditis, especially of tricuspid and pulmonic valves, and may result in abscess formation or emboli from injected material such as talc, starch, quinine
Atelectasis
Fibrosis, granulomas: Cause not established; perhaps due to opiate diluent deposition; decreased vital capacity, mild-to-moderate decrease in oxygen diffusion capacity across alveolar capillary membrane; may result in pulmonary hypertension and precipitate heart failure; chest x-ray film may be normal or reveal bilateral reticular basilar infiltrates, pulmonary artery enlargement, or hilar adenopathy

DERMATOLOGIC "Tracks" and scars are cutaneous evidence of drug abuse; caused by nonsterile injection technique and injection of fibrogenic particulate matter
Abscess, ulcerative: Usually multiple, hyperpigmented, and linear
Cellulitis: Strong or wood-hard tenseness
Lymphangitis
Phlebitis
Sphaceloderma: Gangrene of the skin

NEUROLOGIC
Cerebral edema
Transverse myelitis: Acute paraplegia, occasionally persistent; thoracic sensory levels are characteristic; caused by adulterants, transient ischemia, hypersensitivity reaction, or direct opiate effect
Horner's syndrome: from supraclavicular injection
Postanoxia encephalopathy
Polyneuritis
Crush injury

HEPATIC
Cirrhosis: Abnormal liver function likely due to infection sequelae, toxic adulterants, and concomitant chronic alcohol ingestion
Alcoholic hepatic disease

RENAL
Nephropathy: Glomerulonephritis
Immune complex nephritis

MUSCULOSKELETAL
Infectious spondylitis, sacroiliitis: Hematogenous spread from nonsterile injection
Lumbar vertebral osteomyelitis: *Staphylococcus aureus, Pseudomonas aeruginosa, Klebsiella, Enterobacter, Mycobacterium, Serratia marcescens, Candida*
Myositis ossificans: "Drug abuser's elbow"—extraosseous metaplasia injury to brachialis muscle due to poor injection technique with calcification developing
Camptodactylia: Irreducible finger flexion and hand edema from injections into fingers and hand veins

HEMATOLOGIC
Thrombocytopenia: Immunologic mechanisms, quinine-induced
Leukopenia: Bone marrow depression
Anemia: Repetitive blood donations

LABORATORY
Hypergammaglobulinemia: Elevated IgM, IgG in 90% of addicts; may lead to false positive on many serologic tests; elevated immunoglobulins return to normal levels when street drug use is discontinued
False-positive VDRL
$\downarrow C_3$ and total complement

(Modified from Easom JM and Lovejoy FH. Opiates. *In* Haddad LM, Winchester JF (eds): Clinical Management of Poisoning and Drug Overdose. Philadelphia, WB Saunders, 1983, p 428.)

tient, because depression of the chemoreceptor trigger zone is an effect of opiates. The possibility of seizures and relatively rapid onset of sedation also favors lavage over ipecac. Unconscious patients should be lavaged only after endotracheal intubation to protect the airway. When lavage is complete, 0.4 mg of naloxone should be given IV to reverse the typical slowing of intestinal transit that occurs with opiates, even if the patient shows few other signs of intoxication. Activated charcoal and cathartic should also be administered.[31]

Three opiates—propoxyphene, methadone, and diphenoxylate—deserve special mention because their atypical time course of action requires a change in the usual handling of patients. Propoxyphene is rapidly absorbed, and most deaths due to this drug have occurred within the first 2 hours after ingestion, many within 15 minutes. This fact emphasizes the need for prompt intervention to empty the stomach with lavage, rather than induction of emesis, and for the use of the larger than usual doses of naloxone known to be needed. Despite the rapid absorption, the clinical course is prolonged in nonfatal overdoses because of the storage of propoxyphene in the body fat and its later release, causing sedation and respiratory depression. A minimum observation period of 24 hours is recommended in symptomatic patients.[32, 33]

Major symptoms of methadone overdose may not become apparent for 6 to 12 hours after ingestion and often last 24 to 48 hours. Therefore, patients must be observed for a longer period than usual after gastric emptying to identify significant overdoses (24 hours) and must be maintained on naloxone infusions for 24 to 48 hours if symptomatic to prevent late respiratory depression. If LAAM, the even longer-acting methadone derivative, was ingested, observation and treatment periods must be further lengthened.

Diphenoxylate, although safe even in large doses in adults, is extremely toxic to children under 2 years of age, presumably because it crosses the immature blood-brain barrier more easily. Death due to respiratory arrest has occurred many times in children who have been given the drug "therapeutically," as well as in those who have accidentally ingested it. Onset of respiratory depression is delayed 6 to 14 hours after ingestion, and it may last 72 hours. Consequently, it is recommended that asymptomatic children under the age of 5 years be observed for 24 hours after gastric emptying, with the caveat that early gastric decontamination does not necessarily prevent subsequent respiratory depression. Symptomatic children should receive at least 12 hours of a naloxone infusion followed by observation of at least 12 hours of symptom-free time. Asymptomatic adults may be discharged after 6 hours of observation.[12, 13, 34, 35]

ABSTINENCE SYNDROMES

It is one of the characteristic properties of opiates that their chronic use produces tolerance to their effects and that their abrupt withdrawal produces an abstinence syndrome. It is generally agreed that an opiate user must take relatively high doses of potent compounds regularly for 2 to 4 weeks before experiencing withdrawal on cessation of therapy. However, animal and human studies have shown some evidence of acute opiate dependence, with naloxone precipitating hormonal and physiologic changes after a single dose of opiate similar to those noted in withdrawal from chronic use. Acute and chronic opiate use may represent opposite ends of the spectrum of the development of dependence.[36–39]

The clinical manifestations of withdrawal from all of the different opiates are similar. The time course varies according to the potency and duration of action of the drugs. Symptoms of abstinence appear in 3 to 4 hours and subside in 4 to 5 days after cessation of short-acting opiates such as meperidine, whereas their appearance may be delayed as long as 2 days and their resolution for 2 weeks or more in the case of long-acting drugs such as methadone. The intensity of symptoms is greatest in withdrawal from potent and short-acting opiates and least in withdrawal from less potent or longer-acting drugs. Withdrawal from the agonist-antagonist class is very mild.

The initial stage of the abstinence syndrome is one of drug craving and anxiety, without objective signs. This lasts about 12 hours in morphine addicts. In the next stage, the withdrawing patient goes in and out of a restless "yen sleep" and exhibits yawning, mydriasis, lacrimation, rhinorrhea, diaphoresis, and elevated heart rate and blood pressure. Piloerection is seen, and the appearance of the skin may have given rise to the expression "going cold turkey." Nausea, vomiting, diarrhea, and abdominal pain follow in the next stage. Also common are myalgias, muscle spasms, and twitching, which may have originated the saying "kicking the habit."

Further progression of the previous symptoms and the development of fever occur next. The intensity of these symptoms peak and then resolve according to the time courses described earlier. The most severe stage with dehydration, hyperglycemia, spontaneous ejaculation or orgasm, leukocytosis, and fever is almost never encountered in the United States because of the low potency of street drugs. The abstinence syndrome is extremely distressing and uncomfortable for addicts and is accompanied by an intense craving for opiates. Addicts will feign illness and allow invasive procedures in an attempt to obtain drugs. It is important for physicians to realize, however, that opiate withdrawal, unlike alcohol withdrawal, carries no risk of death or serious morbidity. Seizures and delirium are not an element of opiate withdrawal.

Withdrawal may also be precipitated by the administration of naloxone to an addict in the course of treating an opiate overdose. Symptoms begin about 5 minutes after injection, peak in 30 minutes, and are over in 1 to 2 hours. It is not necessary to treat them.[19, 40–42]

In order to understand current therapy of opiate abstinence, it is necessary to return to the consideration of the effects of opiates on their receptors in the central nervous system. The nucleus locus ceruleus seems to be the control center responsible for producing the symptoms of withdrawal. This nucleus is richly provided with receptor sites of the opioid, α-adrenergic, and other types. Each neuron has on its surface all of the different types of receptors. It is known that stimulation of at least two types, the opioid and the α-adrenergic, produces the same response intracellularly in the neuron—that is, modification of adenyl cyclase activity. Stimulation of either of these receptors by their agonists, e.g., morphine for the opioid receptor and clonidine for the α-adrenergic receptor, produces a depression of adenyl cyclase activity and a resultant decrease in cyclic AMP. If the stimulation is continuous, however, as with opiate abuse, physiologic adaptation occurs within the neuron, producing normal levels of adenyl cyclase, despite the constant opiate binding. Should the opiate binding be abruptly terminated by discontinuation of the drug or by replacement of the drug at the receptor by an antagonist drug such as naloxone, then the depressant opioid effect will be lifted and there will be an acute rise in the level of cyclic AMP. This increased metabolic activity in the neuron correlates with the clinical hyperactivity of the withdrawing patient. However, if either the opioid or the α-adrenergic receptor is again stimulated by an agonist such as methadone at the opioid site or clonidine at the adrenergic site, adenyl cyclase activity will decrease to the normal level for the adapted cell and the patient will no longer suffer abstinence symptoms. The use of methadone to treat and to prevent withdrawal is easy to understand. The dual receptor system described earlier explains how a nonopioid drug like clonidine can be used to decrease the symptoms and discomfort of withdrawal. Lofexidine, a structural analogue of clonidine, has also been shown to reduce signs and symptoms of abstinence. Clonidine is not a perfect replacement for opioids. In the doses necessary to prevent abstinence, it produces sedation and hypotension that limit its usefulness, particularly in the outpatient setting. Lofexidine may be somewhat less potent, but has fewer side effects. Even with their disadvantages, these drugs are a resource for emergency physicians who must often deal with withdrawing patients who have, for various reasons, been separated from their maintenance supply of their chosen drug of abuse or from their methadone. One suggested dosing regimen is to give 0.1 mg of clonidine every 30 to 60 minutes until symptoms are controlled or disabling side effects prevent further administration. Experience in maintenance programs suggests that 0.7 mg/day is the average required dose. The effects of clonidine and opiates are additive, and the combination can produce severe orthostatic hypotension and sedation. This is a hazard of outpatient use of clonidine in addicts, who may succumb to the desire for opiates while on clonidine,[14, 43–55] and careful monitoring during follow-up care is necessary.

Clonidine has also been useful in the treatment of the neonatal narcotic abstinence syndrome in infants born to addicted mothers. It controls the symptoms of this disorder at doses of 3 μg/kg/day or more without serious side effects.[56]

One other interaction between clonidine and opiates is receiving much attention. It has been noted that the antihypertensive effect of clonidine can be reversed by naloxone in some individuals. It has been shown in human and animal studies that clonidine administration is associated with the release of the endogenous opiate β-endorphin from the brain stem and pituitary. It has been postulated that blocking of the actions of the endorphins by naloxone is responsible for the increase in blood pressure of clonidine-treated subjects who receive naloxone. Many reports contradict the existence of this effect. One study identified a naloxone-responsive group of patients who had higher plasma renin and adrenalin levels than the group that did not respond to naloxone with an elevation of blood pressure. Although the existence of a clonidine "antagonist" would be very desirable for clinicians, a much better understanding of this interaction is needed before it will be clinically useful.[57–59]

References

1. Fishman J, Hahn E: The opiates. *In* Richter RW: Medical Aspects of Drug Abuse. Hagerstown, Md., Harper and Row, 1975, pp 37–49.
2. Martin WR, Eades CG, Thompson JA, et al: The effect of morphine- and nalorphine-like drugs in the non-dependent and morphine-dependent chronic spinal dog. J Pharmacol Exp Ther *197*:517, 1976.
3. Snyder SH: Opiate receptors in the brain. N Engl J Med *296*:266, 1977.
4. Terenius L: Endogenous peptides and analgesia. Ann Rev Pharmacol Toxicol *18*:189, 1978.
5. Bunney WE, Pert CB, Klee W, Costa E, Pert A, Davis G: Basic and clinical studies of endorphins. Ann Intern Med *91*:239, 1979.
6. Simon EJ: Opiate receptors and their implications for drug addiction. *In* Lettieri DJ, Sayers M, Pearson HW: Theories on Drug Abuse: Selected Contemporary Perspectives. NIDA Research Monograph 30. Washington, DC, US Government Printing Office, March 1980.
7. Baden MM: Pathology of the addicted states. *In* Richter RW: Medical Aspects of Drug Abuse. Hagerstown, Md., Harper and Row, 1975, pp 189–208.
8. O'Neil P, Baker P, Gough T: Illicitly imported heroin products: Some physical and chemical features indicative of their origin. J Forensic Sci *29*:888, 1984.
9. Beaver W, Wallenstein S, Houde R, et al: A clinical comparison of the analgesic effects of methadone and morphine administered intramuscularly, and of orally and parenterally administered methadone. Clin Pharmacol Ther *8*:415, 1967.
10. Fraser H, Isbell H: Actions and addiction liabilities of alpha-acetyl methadols in man. J Pharmacol Exp Ther *105*:458, 1952.
11. Caplan LR, Thomas C, Banks G: Central nervous system complications of addiction to "T's and Blues." Neurology *32*:623, 1982.
12. Rosenstein G, Freeman M, Standard A, Weston N: Warning: The use of Lomotil in children. Pediatrics *51*:132, 1973.
13. Ginsberg CM: Lomotil intoxication: 10 cases. Am J Dis Child *125*:241, 1973.
14. Preston KL, Bigelow GE: Pharmacological advances in addiction treatment. Int J Addict *20*:845, 1985.
15. Tandberg D, Abercrombie D: Treatment of heroin overdose with endotracheal naloxone. Ann Emerg Med *11*:443, 1982.
16. Jasinski J, Martin W, Haertzen C: The human pharmacology and abuse potential of *N*-allylnoroxymorphone (naloxone). J Pharmacol Exp Ther *157*:420, 1967.
17. McNicholas LE, Martin WR: New and experimental therapeutic roles for naloxone and related opioid antagonists. Drugs *27*:81, 1984.
18. Milne B, Jhamandas K: Naloxone: New therapeutic roles. Can Anaesth Soc J *31*:272, 1984.
19. Jaffe JH, Martin WR: Opioid analgesics and antagonists. *In* Gilman AG, Goodman LS, Rall TW, et al: Goodman and Gillman's The Pharmacologic Basis of Therapeutics, 7th ed. New York, MacMillan, 1985, pp 491–531.
20. Benowitz NK, Rosenberg J, Becker CE: Cardiopulmonary catastrophes in drug-overdosed patients. Med Clin North Am *63*:278, 1979.
21. Duberstein JL, Kaufman DM: A clinical study of an epidemic of heroin intoxication and heroin-induced pulmonary edema. Am J Med *51*:704, 1971.
22. Frand UI, Shim CS: Methadone-induced pulmonary edema. Ann Intern Med *76*:975, 1972.
23. Bogartz LJ, Miller WC: Pulmonary edema associated with propoxyphene intoxication. JAMA *215*:259, 1971.
24. Greene M, Luke J, Dupont R: Acute opiate overdose: A preliminary report on mechanism of death. *In* Proceedings of the Fifth National Conference on Methadone Therapy. New York, National Association for the Prevention of Addiction to Narcotics, 1973.
25. Moore RA, Rumack B, Conner CS, Peterson RG: Underdosage after narcotic poisoning. Am J Dis Child *134*:156, 1980.
26. Martin WR: Naloxone. Ann Intern Med *85*:765, 1976.
27. Zaks A, Jones T, Fink M, Freedman AM: Treatment of opiate dependence with high dose oral naloxone. JAMA *215*:2108, 1971.
28. Gilbert PE, Martin WR: Antagonism of the convulsant effects of heroin, *D*-propoxyphene, meperidine, normeperidine, and thebaine by naloxone in mice. J Pharmacol Exp Ther *192*:538, 1975.
29. Stern WZ, Subbarao K: Pulmonary complications of drug addiction. Semin Roentgenol *18*:183, 1983.
30. Barsan WG, Seger D, Danzl D, et al: Duration of antagonistic effects of nalmefene and naloxone in opiate-induced sedation for emergency department procedures. Am J Emerg Med *7*:155, 1989.
31. Nimmo WS, Heading RC, Prescott LF: Reversal of narcotic-induced delay in gastric emptying and paracetamol absorption by naloxone. Br Med J *10*:1189, 1979.
32. Hudson P, Barringer M, McBay AJ: Fatal poisoning with propoxyphene: Report of 100 consecutive cases. South Med J *70*:938, 1977.
33. Lovejoy FH, Mitchell AA, Goldman P: The management of propoxyphene poisoning. J Pediatr *85*:98, 1974.
34. Lovejoy FH: Indications for naloxone in Lomotil poisoning. Pediatrics *54*:658, 1974.
35. Wasserman GS, Green VA, Wise GW: Lomotil ingestions in children. Am Fam Physician *11*:93, 1975.
36. Ream NW, Robinson MG, Richter RW, et al: Opiate dependence and acute abstinence. *In* Richter RW:

Medical Aspects of Drug Abuse. Hagerstown, Md., Harper and Row, 1975, pp 81–123.

37. Schulz R, Herz A: Opioid tolerance and dependence in light of the multiplicity of opioid receptors. *In* Sharp CW: Mechanisms of Tolerance and Dependence. NIDA Research Monograph 54. Washington, DC, US Government Printing Office, 1984, pp 70–80.
38. Bickel WK, Stitzer ML, Wazlavek BE, Liebson IA: Naloxone-precipitated withdrawal in humans after acute morphine administration. NIDA Research Monograph 67. Washington, DC, US Government Printing Office, 1986, pp 349–54.
39. Eisenberg RM: Further studies on the acute dependence produced by morphine in opiate naive rats. Life Sci *31*:1531, 1982.
40. Isbell H, White WM: Clinical characteristics of addictions. Am J Med *14*:558, 1953.
41. Himmelsbach C: The morphine abstinence syndrome, its nature and treatment. Ann Intern Med *15*:829, 1941.
42. Jaffe JH: Drug addiction and abuse. *In* Gilman AG, Goodman LS, Rall TW, et al: Goodman and Gilman's The Pharmacologic Basis of Therapeutics, 7th ed. New York, Macmillan, 1985, pp 541–545.
43. Bakris GL: Clonidine for opiate withdrawal in the chronic pain patient. Postgrad Med *71*:240, 1982.
44. Bakris GL, Cross PD, Hammarsten JE: The use of clonidine for management of opiate abstinence in a chronic pain patient. Mayo Clin Proc *57*:657, 1982.
45. Cuthbert NG, Francis DL, Collier HO: Adaptation of a neuron to normorphine and clonidine. Biochem Soc Trans *11*:64, 1983.
46. Eisenberg RM: Influence of clonidine on the acute dependence response elicited in naive rats by naloxone. Life Sci *32*:1547, 1983.
47. Fantozzi R, Luciani G, Masini E, et al: Clonidine and naloxone-induced opiate withdrawal: A comparison between clonidine and morphine in man. Subst Alcohol Actions-Misuse *1*:369, 1980.
48. Fink M: Narcotic antagonist therapy of opiate dependence. *In* Richter RW: Medical Aspects of Drug Abuse. Hagerstown, Md., Harper and Row, 1975, pp 160–166.
49. Gold MS, Redmond DE, Kleber HD: Clonidine blocks acute opiate-withdrawal symptoms. Lancet 2:599, 1978.
50. Gold MS, Pottash AC, Sweeney DR, et al: Lofexidine blocks acute opiate withdrawal. NIDA Research Monograph *41*:264, 1982.
51. Kleber HD, Riordan CE, Rounsaville B, et al: Clonidine in outpatient detoxification from methadone maintenance. Arch Gen Psychiatry *42*:391, 1985.
52. Kreek MJ: Methadone maintenance treatment for chronic opiate addiction. *In* Richter RW: Medical Aspects of Drug Abuse. Hagerstown, Md., Harper and Row, 1975, pp 167–185.
53. Robson LE, Mucha RF, Kosterlitz HW: The role of interaction between opiate receptors and alpha-adrenergic receptors in tolerance and dependence. Biochem Soc Trans *11*:64, 1983.
54. Strode SW: Propoxyphene dependence and withdrawal. Am Fam Physician *32*:105, 1985.
55. Preston KL, Bigelow GE, Liebson IA: Self-administration of clonidine and oxazepam by methadone detoxification patients. *In* Harris LS: Problems of Drug Dependence, 1983. Proceedings of the 45th Annual Scientific Meeting. The Committee on Problems of Drug Dependence, Inc., NIDA Research Monograph 49, 1984, pp 192–198.
56. Hoder EL, Leckman JF, Ehrenkranz R, et al: Clonidine in neonatal narcotic-abstinence syndrome. N Engl J Med *305*:1284, 1981.
57. Farsang C, Kapocsi J, Varga K, et al: Beta-endorphin and essential hypertension: Importance of the clonidine-naloxone interaction. Acta Physiol Hung *65*:217, 1985.
58. Niemann JT, Getzug T, Murphy W: Reversal of clonidine toxicity by naloxone. Ann Emerg Med *15*:1229, 1986.
59. Ramirez-Gonzalez MD, Tchakarov L, Garcia RM, et al: Beta-endorphin acting on the brainstem is involved in the antihypertensive action of clonidine and alpha-methlyldopa in rats. Circ Res *53*:150, 1983.
60. Michaelis LL, Hickey PR, Clark TA, Dixon WM: Ventricular irritability associated with the use of naloxone. Ann Thorac Surg *18*:608, 1974.
61. Kripke BJ, Finck AJ, Shah NK, Snow JC: Naloxone antagonism after narcotic-supplemented anesthesia. Anesth Analg *55*:800, 1976.
62. Flacke JW, Flacke WE, Williams GD: Acute pulmonary edema following naloxone reversal of high-dose morphine anesthesia. Anesthesiology *47*:376, 1977.
63. Azar I, Turndorf H: Severe hypertension and multiple atrial premature contractions following naloxone administration. Anesth Analg *58*:524, 1979.
64. Andree R: Sudden death following naloxone administration. Anesth Analg *59*:782, 1980.
65. Estilo AE, Cottrell JE: Naloxone, hypertension, and ruptured cerebral aneurysm. Anesthesiology *54*:352, 1981.
66. Prough DS, Roy R, Bumgarner J, Shannon G: Acute pulmonary edema in healthy teenagers following conservative doses of intravenous naloxone. Anesthesiology *60*:485, 1984.
67. Opioid (Narcotic) Analgesics (Systemic). *In* USP Dispensing Information: Drug Information for the Health Care Professional, Vol IB, 9th ed. Harrisonburg, VA, Banta Company, 1989, pp 1783–1811.

CHAPTER 39

BARBITURATES, METHAQUALONE, AND PRIMIDONE

James F. Winchester, M.D.

The epidemiology of agents responsible for poisoning is changing, throughout the world.[1–3] Over the last 15 years, an increasing number of patients have died from poisoning by analgesics, tranquilizers, and antidepressants, while the deaths from barbiturates and methaqualone have fallen considerably. Barbiturate prescription by physicians has decreased considerably, either on a voluntary basis,[4] by change in prescribing laws,[2] or by withdrawal of the agent, as with methaqualone in the United States and the United Kingdom. This has resulted in an increasing use of benzodiazepine for the induction of sleep.[5] Over a 10-year period in the United Kingdom, 6090 deaths occurred from barbiturates;[13] the American Association of Poison Control Centers (which cover approximately half the American population) in 1987 reported 4637 exposures (14 deaths) to barbiturates, and 116 exposures (no deaths) to methaqualone.[6] In the United States and in the United Kingdom, barbiturates are available legally only by prescription, and the street use of these "downers" has waned in popularity.

BARBITURATES

Barbituric acid (2,4,6-trioxo-hexa-hydropyrimidine) is the parent compound, of which the diethyl derivative (barbital) was introduced as a hypnotic sedative agent in 1903. Barbituric acid is used in vast quantities by the chemical industry in the manufacture of plastics, while the medicinal consumption of barbiturates in the United States used to exceed 400 tons annually.[7]

Pharmacology and Pharmacokinetics

A general formula with the substituted radicals for the various derivatives of barbituric acid is shown in Table 39–1. In general, any change in the molecule that increases lipid solubility decreases the duration of action and accelerates metabolic degradation, with an accompanying increase in potency for hypnosis. This is particularly seen in compounds such as thiopental, which is used as an intravenous anesthetic with onset of activity within 20 to 30 seconds. Methyl substitution at R_3 increases the lipid solubility of the drug and shortens its duration of action, although demethylation to a longer-acting metabolite may occur.[8]

Most barbiturates used clinically are given orally; after transit through the stomach, absorption takes place in the small intestine, despite the favorable pH partition occurring in the stomach. Sodium salts are more rapidly absorbed than are free acids. Absorption is more rapid when barbiturates are diluted with water and slower when the stomach contains food. In general, the more lipid-soluble the drug is, the more highly protein-bound it is. Approximately 80 per cent of thiopental, but only 5 per cent of phenobarbital, is protein bound, and both these drugs differ markedly in their lipid solubility. The unbound (free) concentration of barbiturates in plasma and cerebrospinal fluid (CSF) is equal. Barbiturates are highly lipid soluble and are distributed into the vascular areas of brain (gray matter), where maximal uptake occurs within 30 seconds, inducing sleep within a few minutes. Thirty minutes after intravenous administration, redistribution into the less vascular areas of the brain occurs, and plasma levels of barbiturate may fall to 10 per cent of peak levels. Thus no correlation exists between duration of action and elimination half-life of these drugs, since their activity depends on the rapid (vascular) distribution phase. With the less lipid-soluble barbiturates, cerebral uptake is slower, and sleep may not occur until as long as 20 minutes after intravenous administration of barbital or phenobarbital. Equilibration of barbiturates is different in different tissues and is slowest in the poorly vascular fat tissue. When steady state is reached, the highest concentrations of drug in nonadipose

Table 39–1. BARBITURATE CLASSIFICATION

GENERAL FORMULA AND SUBSTITUTED DERIVATIVES

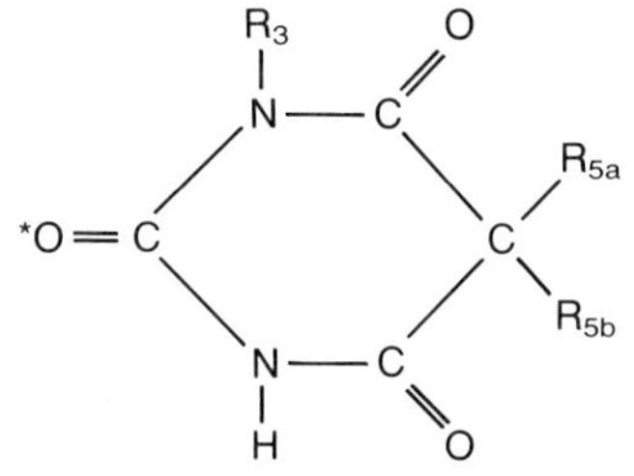

Barbiturate	*Duration of Action (Hrs)*	R_{5a}‡	R_{5b}§	R_3
Ultrashort-Acting				
thiopental*	0.3	ethyl	1-methyl butyl	—H
thiamylal*	0.3	allyl	1-methyl butyl	—H
methohexital	0.3	allyl	1-methyl-2-pentynyl	—CH_3
Short-Acting				
hexobarbital	3	methyl	1-cyclohexen-1-yl	—CH_3
pentobarbital	3	ethyl	1-methyl butyl	—H
secobarbital	3	allyl	1-methyl butyl	—H
Intermediate-Acting				
amobarbital	3–6	ethyl	isopentyl	—H
aprobarbital	3–6	allyl	isopropyl	—H
butabarbital	3–6	ethyl	sec-butyl	—H
Long-Acting				
barbital†	6–12	ethyl	ethyl	—H
mephobarbital†	6–12	ethyl	phenyl	—CH_3
phenobarbital†	6–12	ethyl	phenyl	—H
primidone*	6–12	ethyl	phenyl	—H

*Has S = substitution for O = in thiopental and thiamylal, and H_2 substitution for O = in primidone.
†Only drugs responsive to alkaline diuresis.
‡Previous notation: R_1.
§Previous notation: R_2.

tissue, although less than in fat, occur in the liver and the kidney.

Barbiturates are filtered by the renal glomerulus in quantities equivalent to the fraction unbound in plasma. Highly lipid-soluble barbiturates are not only highly protein bound but also are poorly filtered; however, they also are readily reabsorbed from the renal tubular lumen. Barbiturates with low lipid-to-water partition coefficients (for example, barbital, aprobarbital, and phenobarbital) are excreted largely unchanged in the urine, with approximately 20 per cent of an oral hypnotic dose of barbital being eliminated within 24 hours, although traces of barbital may be found up to 8 to 12 days after administration. As previously noted in Chapter 8, alkalinization of the urine tends to promote ionization of barbiturates and leads to their enhanced excretion, particularly with phenobarbital.

The bulk of barbiturate, therefore, is metabolized in the liver, although small quantities of the thiobarbiturates (thiopental and thiamylal) are biotransformed in kidney, brain, and other tissues. Although most of the biotransformation products are inactive, demethylation yields active products with certain barbiturates; for example, mephobarbital and methabarbital, respectively, give rise to phenobarbital and barbital. Barbiturates are transformed by oxidation of the radicals —R_{5a} and —R_{5b} to alcohols, ketones, phenols, or carboxylic acids, which appear in the urine as these compounds or as glucuronized conjugates. *N*— Hydroxylation, *N*— dealkylation of *N*— alkylbarbiturates, desulfuration of thiobarbiturates, and opening of the barbituric acid ring also are known to occur.[8] The biotransformation process responsible for termination of biologic activity is side-chain oxidation.

The duration of action of barbiturates has for a long time been classified as long, intermediate, short, and ultrashort (see Table 39–1). However, this classification is somewhat artificial, since the elimination half-lives of the drugs do not conform to their apparent duration of action. For instance, with drugs that are metabolized by cytochrome P-450 enzymes in the liver, repeated administration may shorten the metabolic elimination half-life. Similarly, in children, the half-life of phenobarbital is half that in adults, but in infants the elimination half-life is two to five times that of an adult. Elimination half-life is increased during pregnancy, in elderly people, in patients with impaired renal function, and, most importantly, in patients with impaired liver function.

When given in sedative or hypnotic dosage, barbiturates have little effect on skeletal, cardiac, or smooth muscle. However, in acute barbiturate intoxication, muscle inhibitory effects produce serious problems with cardiovascular stability. The desired central nervous system effects of barbiturates range from mild sedation to general anesthesia. In addition, phenobarbital and mephobarbital have selective anticonvulsant activity; some evidence indicates that barbiturates may have euphoriant activity, while there is equivocal evidence that they have an effect on anxiety. Barbiturates have no effect on pain; in small doses they are thought to increase the reaction to painful stimuli and, in certain experimental models, may antagonize the effect of analgesics. In patients with somatic pain, barbiturates may cause paradoxic excitement.

Barbiturates decrease the low-frequency electrical activity of the electroencephalogram and increase the low-voltage fast activity (15 Hz to 35 Hz), suggesting electrical arousal of the reticular activating substance, although this arousal response is incomplete due to nonstimulation of the hippocampal component. The barbiturates decrease sleep latency, increase delta activity and fast EEG activity during sleep, decrease the number of state shifts to stages 0 and 1, and decrease body movement. The pharmacologic basis for activity in the central nervous system most likely is due to the fact that low-dose barbiturates have a GABA-like action or enhance the effects of GABA (gamma-aminobutyric acid) activity within the central nervous system. However, barbiturates also may selectively abolish noradrenergic excitation (but not inhibition) in various synapses, as well as having a minor role with activity against acetylcholine. During barbiturate-induced anesthesia, there is an approximate 50 per cent fall in oxygen utilization by brain tissue. This observation has led to the clinical use of high-dose barbiturates for protection against cerebral infarction during cerebral ischemia and head injury.[9–12]

Barbiturate interaction with GABA explains the nonselective inhibition of synaptic responses, such that the neurogenic drive for respiration is eliminated by a barbiturate dose about three times greater than that normally used to induce sleep. Similarly, suppression of hypoxic and chemoreceptor drives to respiration is achieved with high doses of barbiturates; the dominant respiratory drive shifts to the carotid and aortic bodies and eventually fails. It is of interest that, unlike the opiates and opioids, barbiturates suppress the cough reflex only in doses sufficient to embarrass the respiration seriously. Apart from central depression of respiration, however, barbiturates can inhibit smooth muscle activity directly (producing laryngospasm after intravenous administration). The smooth muscle effects, however, are seen particularly in the cardiovascular system, when cardiovascular depression accompanies acute barbiturate poisoning, as does depression of vascular smooth muscle, both of which can be overcome by digitalis and beta-adrenergic agonists. The smooth muscle inhibitory effect is also observed in the gastrointestinal tract, where reduction in bowel motility is observed, which reverses on recovery from barbiturate poisoning.

Tolerance, Abuse, and Dependence[8, 13]

Tolerance to barbiturates is a well-recognized phenomenon. For example, the plasma concentration during which sleep ensues may be lower than that upon awakening, after a single dose; accordingly, this phenomenon cannot be explained on the induction of hepatic microsomal enzymes. Similarly with chronic administration, tolerance to increasing doses of barbiturates occurs to the extent that the effective dosage of barbiturate may be increased by as much as six times—a phenomenon two to three times greater than can be accounted for by enhanced hepatic metabolism. This tolerance to barbiturates is also conferred upon other central nervous system depressant drugs, such as meprobamate, glutethimide, methaqualone, and general anesthetics. In addition, cross-tolerance develops to drugs such as phenycyclidine and benzodiazepines, although there is no tolerance for the muscle-relaxant properties of benzodiazepines.

The effects of the abrupt withdrawal of barbiturates in patients who have been taking them for prolonged periods vary considerably, depending upon the degree of tolerance and the duration of abuse prior to withdrawal. However, discontinuation of barbiturates may result in progressive seizures, delirium, insomnia, tremor, anorexia, and abnormal sleep patterns. In addition, abdominal cramps, nausea, vomiting, and orthostatic hypotension are characteristic, and patients may exhibit purposive behavior patterns. Seizure activity is the most important of all the withdrawal symptoms, and the number of seizures varies from a single one to status epilepticus. Neither phenytoin nor chlorpromazine will prevent seizures, and in this case barbiturates themselves are indicated for suppression.

Drug Interactions[8] (See also Chapter 22)

An increased sedative effect is observed with other central nervous system active drugs, particularly alcohol, but also with antihistamines and other central nervous system depressants. An increased effect of barbiturates is seen during coadministration of isoniazid, methylphenidate, and monoamine oxidase inhibitors. The principal drug interactions observed, however, are through the induction of hepatic microsomal enzymes; this causes significant elimination of the following drugs: dicoumarin, digoxin, tetracycline, corticosteroids, oral contraceptives, phenytoin, sulfa drugs, tricyclic antidepressants, hormones such as testosterone, and vitamins D and K. It also has been observed that toxic metabolite formation may occur more significantly in patients who have been receiving barbiturates and coingesting other compounds, particularly the hydrocarbon anesthetics, carbon tetrachloride, and acetaminophen (see Chapter 13). As mentioned, aspirin displaces phenobarbital from its albumin-binding sites, while thyroxine is displaced by barbiturates from thyroxine-binding proteins. Barbiturates also decrease the absorption of certain drugs, such as dicoumarol and griseofulvin.

Not only is microsomal biotransformation of drugs affected, but other enzyme systems also are increased in activity; for example, delta-amino levulinic acid synthetase is increased, which is particularly important in the production of exacerbations of porphyria.

Therapeutic Uses of Barbiturates

The use of barbiturates has largely been superseded by the safer and more efficacious benzodiazepines; however, barbiturates are available as single or combined therapy for many disease states, such as functional gastrointestinal disorders, hypertension, asthma, coronary artery disease, and analgesic combinations, and for restlessness and surgical preparation for minor medical and dental procedures. Barbiturates are still used for their rapid action in the emergency treatment of convulsions from any cause, but even in this respect benzodiazepines may be superior. It must be remembered that some time is required before the anticonvulsant effect of phenobarbital develops, during which time restraint of the patient may be required. The ultrashort-acting barbiturates are still used for anesthesia and commonly as adjuncts to other agents for obstetric anesthesia. Other uses for barbiturates are in narcoanalysis and narcotherapy. Barbiturates are also used for reducing brain edema/metabolism after surgery, head injury, near-drowning, or cerebral ischemia.[9–12]

From its observed effect on hepatic microsomal enzymes, phenobarbital has been used successfully to treat hyperbilirubinemia and kernicterus and to increase bile salt metabolism and excretion in selected cases of cholestasis.

Manifestations of Barbiturate Toxicity

Most cases of barbiturate poisoning are secondary to suicide attempts, but in children or in drug abusers, accidental barbiturate poisoning is rather common. Little evidence supports "automatism" in the etiology of poisoning with barbiturates;[14] this refers to the patient who, after falling asleep from barbiturate-induced hypnosis, wakens during the night and takes more barbiturates in the mistaken belief that the original dose was not taken. Although initially it was believed this contributed to a quarter of 488 cases of intoxication,[15] subsequent studies have not confirmed the observation.[16]

It appears that the short-acting barbiturates, particularly those with short half-lives and high lipid solubility, are more potent and more toxic than the more polar, long-acting compounds, such as phenobarbital and barbital. Many patients with barbiturate poisoning are found dead at home, and in these patients the short-acting barbiturates are found at autopsy in blood specimens. Mortality rates from barbiturate poisoning range from less than 1 per cent[17] to as high as 10 per cent.[18, 19] Such studies include not only patients who have ingested small quantities of barbiturates but also patients who have been severely intoxicated. Goodman and associates demonstrated a 3 per cent mortality rate in long-acting barbiturate poisoning with blood levels exceeding 8 mg/dl, whereas there was a 5 per cent mortality rate in patients intoxicated with short-acting barbiturates in whom blood levels exceeded 3 mg/dl.[20] Mortality in these patients was confined principally to those in grade 3 or grade 4 coma,[21] in whom corresponding mortality rates were 12 per cent for long-acting barbiturate poisoning and 13 per cent for short-acting barbiturate poisoning. There was a direct correlation between the necessity for endotracheal intubation, depth of coma, presence of pneumonia, and the eventual outcome; patients with pneumonia, prolonged endotracheal intubation, pyrexia, and cardiovascular instability had the highest mortality rates.

A study from the Massachusetts General Hospital related depth of coma quite precisely to the initial plasma level of secobarbital or pentobarbital; using multiple regression and discriminate function analyses, the plasma level of barbiturate correlated most strongly with the eventual outcome and the seriousness of poisoning.[22] Other studies from the United States had reported a very high mortality (approximately 34 per cent) in patients poisoned largely with barbiturates (or glutethimide) who presented in grade 4 coma.[23] Shubin and Weil had shown that the major morbidity and mortality in patients with barbiturate poisoning was consequent on depression of autonomic central control of respiratory and circulatory function, with the eventual development of pneumonia and cardiovascular instability, the latter of which may be further impaired by the injudicious use of forced diuresis.[24]

It is difficult to state with any conviction the lethal doses of barbiturates, since widely varying ingestions with survival have been reported. However, the potentially fatal dose of phenobarbital is 6 to 10 gm and of amobarbital, secobarbital, or pentobarbital, 2 to 3 gm.[25] The highest recorded blood levels from which recovery of patients has been reported is 58 mg/dl for phenobarbital,[26] 120 mg/dl for barbital,[27] and 16 mg/dl for butethal and cyclobarbital.[28]

Ingestion of other intoxicants, such as alcohol,[29] along with barbiturates may contribute particularly to the central nervous system depression. It is interesting that Greenblatt and associates were unable to confirm any additive effect of ethanol on the degree of seriousness of intoxication, despite the fact that 40 per cent of the patients in this study had coingested other central nervous system depressants, particularly alcohol.[22]

The characteristic signs and symptoms of barbiturate poisoning are depression of the central nervous and cardiovascular systems. Mild-to-moderate intoxication resembles that seen with alcohol; with severe intoxication, the patient is comatose to a varying degree and may progress from stupor to coma, with depression and eventual loss of deep tendon reflexes. The pupils initially are constricted and react to light, but, late in the course of barbiturate poisoning, hypoxic paralytic pupillary dilatation may occur. As noted, respiration is affected early. Breathing initially may be slow, or rapid and shallow, with development of Cheyne-Stokes respiration. Eventually, depression of respiration and concomitant depression of minute volume and vital capacity occur, with accompanying evidence of hypoxemia and hypercapnia. Blood pressure may fall precipitously; this is felt initially to be due to loss of central control of blood pressure at the mid-brain level, but cardiac instability and inhibition of vascular smooth muscle tone may contribute.[24, 30] The patient in shock exhibits the classic signs of sweating, rapid weak pulse, cold and clammy skin, hemoconcentration, and oliguria. Hypothermia is common, and it must be remembered that the temperature should be taken with a rectal thermometer.

Bullous skin lesions are reported to occur

with an incidence of 6.5 per cent;[31] they occur principally over pressure areas but also between the toes and fingers. At one point they were thought to be sufficiently characteristic for acute barbiturate intoxication as to be diagnostic. However, these lesions have also been observed in overdosage with methaqualone, meprobamate, glutethimide, opiates, and tricyclic drugs.[14]

Early deaths from barbiturate intoxication are due to cardiorespiratory arrest. Delayed fatalities may arise from circulatory collapse, acute renal failure, bronchopneumonia, atelectasis, lung abscess, pulmonary edema, and cerebral edema.[20, 22, 32] In addition, in patients who have suffered prolonged hypoxia before getting to treatment centers, there may well be acute brain death; in these cases, all measures should be used to eliminate barbiturates from the body before a final diagnosis of brain death is made. Partial recovery of hypoxic neurologic lesions has been reported in patients surviving severe barbiturate overdose with prolonged coma.[33]

Management of the Poisoned Patient

The principles of management of barbiturate intoxication are like those for many other drugs and are divided into three separate subsections: prevention of drug absorption; support of circulatory and respiratory function; and expedition of barbiturate excretion.

Prevention of Drug Absorption, Emesis, and Gastric Lavage

Certainly emesis and gastric lavage should be employed in patients who are seen within 4 hours of ingestion of barbiturates and in whom there is no impairment of consciousness, since most barbiturates are rapidly absorbed from the gastrointestinal tract. It has been reported, however, that the average time between ingestion and admission to hospital is around 7 hours in barbiturate-intoxicated patients, which renders the efficacy of emesis or gastric lavage somewhat questionable.[30] In addition, Matthew and colleagues had shown that gastric lavage was of little value unless performed within 4 hours of ingestion.[34] However, there are reports of delayed gastric emptying in patients after barbiturate poisoning[35, 36] and also reports of drug mass formation (phenobarbital)[37] and gastrointestinal hypomotility, all of which suggest that gastric lavage should be attempted within 4 to 8 hours after ingestion, with caution being taken to protect the airway.

Activated charcoal has a definite role in management of barbiturate poisoning. After the initial report by Holt and Holz in 1963 of reduction of morbidity and mortality in children with barbiturate poisoning given activated charcoal,[38] other reports have attested to its efficacy.[39] In animal models, administration of activated charcoal within 30 minutes[40] to 4 hours[41] following oral overdosage of barbiturates reduces plasma drug concentrations in both the fed and unfed animal, demonstrating that activated charcoal prevents absorption of drugs passing through the stomach into the intestine. Routinely, therefore, activated charcoal slurries should be given by nasogastric tube or by mouth in the semiconscious patient. Relapse into coma during the recovery phase of barbiturate poisoning after return of gastrointestinal motility has been reported on several occasions;[42] administration of activated charcoal may prevent or retard this relapse by strongly adsorbing drugs within the gastrointestinal tract.

In view of the fact that phenobarbital may cause gastric mass formation,[37] as do carbromal, glutethimide, meprobamate, and ethchlorvynol, the practicing physician must be aware that endoscopic gastric lavage to remove such a mass may be necessary.

Support of Respiratory and Circulatory Function

Because of the dangers of sudden cardiorespiratory arrest in barbiturate-intoxicated patients, a rapid assessment of the neurologic as well as cardiorespiratory status must be obtained soon after the patient is seen either in the emergency department or in the intensive care unit. It is often necessary to place an endotracheal tube for respiration in patients who are in stage 4 coma (unconscious with little response to pain, peripheral cyanosis, depressed respiration, hypothermia, and hypotension, as well as sluggish-to-absent pupillary and deep tendon reflexes).[24] This also has the advantage of preventing aspiration pneumonia during gastric lavage.

It is well recognized that circulatory shock is common in those with severe barbiturate poisoning. The patients exhibit arterial hypotension, a low cardiac output, an absolute decrease in plasma volume, or an expansion of the vascular capacity to the extent that relative hypovolemia is seen, even with a normal or a low central venous pressure.[24, 30] The treatment of choice, therefore, is volume expansion with crystalloids and albumin, which may be aided by the use of vasoactive compounds like dopamine or dobutamine. In severely intoxicated patients, therefore, it may be necessary to place a Swan-Ganz catheter for measurement of pulmonary capillary wedge pressure, or a central venous pressure line. It also has been demonstrated that left ventricular ejection fraction is reduced in severely intoxicated animals,[43] to the extent that cardiopulmonary bypass was utilized for circulatory support during removal of barbiturates by dialysis in severely poisoned dogs.

Although the mortality rate in early reports of treatment of barbiturate poisoning with analeptic agents such as nikethimide was around 40 per cent and was less than 1 per cent with standard conservative management without the use of these agents,[17] recent reports suggest that doxapram, another central stimulant, may be used with some benefit in severe hypnotic drug overdosage.[14] In some reports, digoxin has been used to support the circulation, particularly when central venous pressure is elevated after intravenous fluid administration without accompanying diuresis.[8]

Assiduous attention must be paid to management of respiratory status. This includes standard measures for insuring a patent airway, blood gas measurements for adjustments of administered oxygen concentrations, control of acidosis, and adjustments of ventilation, all of which may be required on an ongoing basis. Only when x-ray or clinical evidence of pneumonia is observed should antibiotics be instituted.

Hypothermia requires the use of "space blankets." In certain situations, direct rewarming of cardiopulmonary bypass blood[44] or the mediastinum itself[45] or "core" warming with peritoneal dialysate[46] may be useful, since the most significant outcome of profound hypothermia in barbiturate-intoxicated patients is the induction of ventricular fibrillation and cardiac arrest. Hyperthermia may be observed rarely in barbiturate-intoxicated patients, and it is felt that sweat gland necrosis and the other skin lesions may play a role in increasing body temperatures in this regard.[47] Constant monitoring of renal function is necessary, since in the past renal function was responsible for approximately one sixth of shock and hypoxia, but, in patients who have been in prolonged coma, myoglobinuria also may contribute (this is tested for by measuring myoglobin in urine and also may be accompanied by rises in serum enzymes, creatinine phosphokinase, SGOT, or SGPT[48]). Renal failure also may be present even after recovery of consciousness following barbiturate poisoning. Here, recovery from acute renal failure (acute tubular necrosis) should be eminently possible with intermittent hemodialysis for maintenance of the uremic state, until renal function recovers.

Enhancement of Barbiturate Elimination

Forced Alkaline Diuresis. It is likely that forced alkaline diuresis has been misused frequently in the treatment of acute barbiturate overdose. Although cardiovascular and respiratory monitoring and prevention of drug absorption apply equally to short- and long-acting barbiturates, at this point the treatment becomes quite separate for both classes of barbiturates. The short-acting and intermediate-acting barbiturates have high lipid partition coefficients, high protein binding, and high dissociation constants (pK_a), the latter of which is not amenable to alteration in the renal tubule under physiologic circumstances; as a result, these drugs passively diffuse through cell membranes, with forced alkaline diuresis being of little benefit. For short-acting barbiturates, renal clearance of these drugs can be increased to only 5 ml/min with forced diuresis.[42] For a fuller discussion of this phenomenon, see Chapter 8.

Briefly, phenobarbital (pK_a, 7.24) is totally nonionized at pH 7.45, 50 per cent nonionized at pH 7.2, but less than 4 per cent nonionized at pH 7.5.[49] It follows, therefore, that attaining an alkaline urinary pH greater than 7.5 allows the excretion of predominantly ionized phenobarbital (phenobarbital diffuses across renal tubular cell membranes when nonionized, but not when ionized). On the other hand, the drug secobarbital is 99 per cent nonionized at pH 7.2 and 98 per cent nonionized at pH 7.5; therefore, with this short-acting barbiturate forced alkaline diuresis is not of any benefit.[49] For forced diuresis to be effective, there must be adequate renal and circulatory function, and precautions must be taken to anticipate the development of cardiac or pulmonary complications.

It has been observed that forced alkaline diuresis is of considerable benefit in the management of barbital, phenobarbital, and mephobarbital poisoning, with excretion of considerable quantities of drug in urine and improvement in consciousness and other manifestations of barbiturate poisoning. Renal clearance values for barbiturates may reach as high as 17 ml/min.[42] Comments have been made that the vascular volume expansion occurring during administration of fluids for forced diuresis may provide additional benefit by increasing renal blood flow.[50]

Peritoneal Dialysis. Peritoneal dialysis only achieves clearances of barbiturates up to 10 ml/min, even with pharmacologic manipulation of the dialysate.[42] Therefore, relatively low removal rates of barbiturates have been reported, again reflecting their pharmacokinetic handling, particularly of the short-acting barbiturates.

Hemodialysis. Hemodialysis has been used on many occasions with much success in the management of barbiturate poisoning. Again, the long-acting barbiturates are more readily dialyzable due to lower protein binding, and several dramatic cases of recovery from extremely severe barbiturate poisoning have been reported. In studies of simultaneous hemodialysis and forced diuresis, hemodialysis has been found to be nine times more efficient for long-acting drugs and six times more efficient for the short-acting drugs than forced diuresis.[26] In general, all the barbiturates mentioned in Table 39–1 have been reported to be removed by hemodialysis.[42] In certain situations of very severe barbiturate poisoning, hemodialysis has removed 744 mg/hr of phenobarbital, 262 mg/hr of butabarbital, and 323 mg/hr of cyclobarbital,[26] again reflecting the fact that short-acting barbiturates have greater protein binding and sequestration in adipose tissue. There is no significant advantage to adding activated charcoal or lipid to the dialysate to achieve further partitioning of barbiturates across hemodialysis membranes.

Hemoperfusion.[42, 51] Many animal studies have demonstrated that activated charcoal hemoperfusion for barbiturate poisoning is effective.[42, 51] Charcoal hemoperfusion can reduce mortality and morbidity in animals with pentobarbital and phenobarbital poisoning, with mortality of 59 per cent in the controls and 14 per cent in treated animals.[52] A study of hemodialysis, charcoal hemoperfusion, and XAD-2 resin hemoperfusion in experimental barbiturate poisoning showed a progressive increase in drug clearances in that same order.[53] Yatzidis and associates were first to report in two patients a reduction of phenobarbital and barbital blood levels with uncoated activated charcoal hemoperfusion, and eventual recovery of both patients.[54] Following this, Chang used albumin collodion-coated activated charcoal with rapid removal of phenobarbital in a poisoned patient.[55] Using charcoal particles coated with an acrylic hydrogel polymer, we achieved a phenobarbital removal rate of 640 mg/hr in one severely intoxicated patient (Fig. 39–1), with complete recovery; in the same series, a patient poisoned with secobarbital and pentobarbital responded rapidly to hemoperfusion.[56] Several other investigators have confirmed the utility of activated charcoal hemoperfusion in severe barbiturate poisoning.[57, 58] Resin hemoperfusion with the no longer available XAD-4 resin hemoperfusion device is more efficient than activated charcoal devices[59, 60] (see Chapter 8).

The indications for hemodialysis or hemoperfusion in barbiturate poisoning have been outlined in Chapter 8. Briefly, however, severely intoxicated patients in stage 4 coma with high plasma levels of phenobarbital (greater than 10 mg/dl) or short-acting barbiturates (greater than 5 mg/dl), who have not responded to intensive supportive care, should be considered for hemodialysis or hemoperfusion.[42, 51, 56, 57] However, it is worthwhile reiterating that the clinical condition of the patient is more important than the drug levels; there may be tolerance and consequently high blood levels in some patients; low blood levels may be seen in patients poisoned with multiple agents, including alcohol; and if brain death is suspected, then this diagnosis cannot be made until there is no barbiturate present within blood or cerebrospinal fluid. All these conditions suggest the use of hemodialysis or hemoperfusion. An isoelectric encephalogram should not be considered a contraindication to dialysis or hemoperfusion in patients with barbiturate poisoning, since recovery of three patients with isoelectric encephalograms has been reported following either hemodialysis

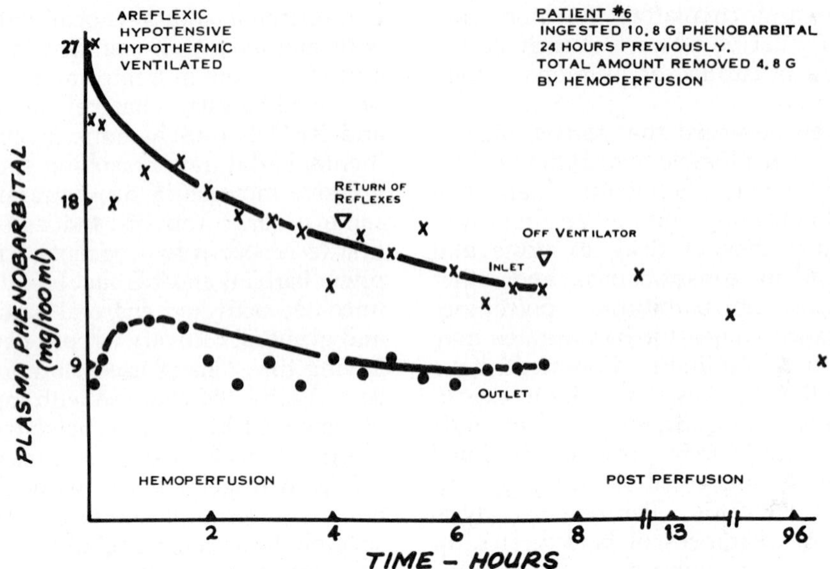

Figure 39–1. Response to charcoal hemoperfusion of a patient severely intoxicated with phenobarbital. X, Concentration (mg/dl) entering: ●, concentration leaving charcoal hemoperfusion device. (From Gelfand MC, Winchester JF, Knepshield JH, Hanson KM, Cohan SL, Strauch BS, Geoly KL, Kennedy AC, Schreiner GE: Treatment of severe drug overdosage with charcoal hemoperfusion. Trans Am Soc Artif Intern Organs *23*:599, 1977, with permission.)

alone or hemodialysis combined with forced diuresis.[42]

Conclusions

It cannot be overstated that conservative medical management of patients with barbiturate poisoning is associated with a low mortality, especially if patients are treated within a poison treatment center or medical intensive care unit. In the most severely intoxicated patients, falling into stage 3 or stage 4 coma, mortality rates are higher despite expert intensive care management. In these situations, forced alkaline diuresis, hemodialysis, or hemoperfusion should be considered in addition to intensive supportive management. This group of patients, fortunately, is a minority, and most patients can be adequately managed with a conservative approach.

METHAQUALONE

Methaqualone is included here, although it has been withdrawn from the prescription market in both the United Kingdom and the United States, because of its street availability, abuse potential, and drug dependence. Introduced in 1965 as a nonaddicting, nonbarbiturate sedative-hypnotic, it soon proved to cause physical dependence and became a major drug of abuse in the 1970s, under various street and official names (Table 39–2).[61] In 1987, the American Association of Poison Control Centers report included only 136 exposures to methaqualone with no deaths in a population base of approximately half that of the United States.[6] This contrasts to a (legal) 3.4 million dollar market in 1970,[61] and over three times that value in 1972, at the height of its use. It was mainly used orally but was also smoked in a small pipe or on a marijuana cigarette. Its addicting potential was not realized until late in its use, and it was not put on the United States Controlled Substances Act until 1973. It was withdrawn in the United Kingdom in 1981 and later in the United States.

Pharmacology

Methaqualone (2-methyl-3-*o*-tolyl-4-(3H)-quinazolinone) is highly lipid soluble, with a

Table 39–2. SYNONYMS FOR METHAQUALONE

LEGAL	STREET
Quaalude, Sopor, Mandrax, Optimil, Parest, Somnafac	sopors, sopes, ludes, heroin for lovers, love drug

pK_a of 2.4. It is a sedative-hypnotic, anticonvulsant, antitussive, and weak antihistamine. It is not an analgesic, but it may potentiate analgesic properties of opioids (e.g., codeine). It is rapidly absorbed (greater than 99 per cent) from the gastrointestinal tract, reaching peak levels in 1 to 2 hours after ingestion. In plasma, it is 70 to 90 per cent bound to serum albumin, and it is distributed to adipose and other tissues. It is metabolized in the liver (99 per cent) to eight major monohydroxylated metabolites and the *N*-oxide, which are predominantly excreted in the urine.[8] Less than 1 per cent of unchanged drug is excreted in the urine, and only 1 to 4 per cent in the bile. The pharmacokinetics follow a two-pool kinetic model with an elimination half-life of 10 to 40 hours.[8] Continuous use of methaqualone induces hepatic microsomal enzymes (mostly cytochrome P-450, but also uridine diphosphate (UDP) glucuronyl transferase). It also has an anticonvulsant effect related to inhibition of gamma-aminobutyric acid transmission.[8]

Toxicology

Drug Abuse. As Table 39–2 indicates, the drug was originally hailed as an aphrodisiac although this is not in the least true. Most drug users feel a "rush," or "buzz," and a calm, peaceful, contented feeling. If ingested in combination with diphenhydramine and methaqualone (Mandrax), users experience tingling around the lips before falling asleep with a therapeutic dose. The same feeling has also been described in street users. Inasmuch as the drug has been withdrawn from therapeutic use, its adverse effects in therapeutic dosage will not be described in any detail. It was associated with minor hemorrhagic problems such as epistaxis, dry mouth, agranulocytosis, and aplastic anemia. Teratogenic effects were not observed in humans but were observed in rats receiving high doses. Central nervous system effects were mainly presleep paresthesias, as just described, and also paresthesias of the distal extremities with rare cases of peripheral neuropathy.[62] Occasionally gross hematuria (due to the *O*-tolidine contaminant of improperly synthesized methaqualone) was observed. The overriding problem with methaqualone was the development of tolerance with chronic use, addiction, and a clear abstinence syndrome, characterized by headache, anorexia, nausea, abdominal cramps, tremor, nervousness, and insomnia, beginning 3 to 5 days after discontinuation of the drug. The syndrome may resemble that of barbiturate withdrawal or withdrawal of any other addictive substance.

Overdose. Methaqualone, as would be expected, was used in many self-poisoning incidents, particularly in the United Kingdom. In 1966, ingestion of Mandrax accounted for 5 per cent of all admissions to the Regional Poisoning Treatment Centre in Edinburgh. This figure was close to 10 per cent in 1967 and has steadily declined since that period.[63] The syndrome of methaqualone overdose differs markedly from that of other sedative-hypnotic ingestion. Toxicity is manifested by hypertonicity, exhibited in increased deep tendon reflexes and muscular hypertonicity, myoclonus, generalized muscle twitching, shivering, and occasionally seizures. The hypertonicity may require the use of pancuronium paralysis and mechanical ventilation. Salivation and excessive bronchial secretions may compromise the respiratory status, and occasionally pulmonary edema may be observed.[64] It is interesting that as the syndrome progresses the degree of hypotension or respiratory depression is much less than that observed in coma caused by other hypnotic agents. In a review of 246 fatalities from methaqualone abuse, 72 per cent of fatalities were due to somnolence, and so on, and subsequent accidental death.[65]

Treatment

As with other hypnotic agents, immediate attention is directed to preservation of the airway, the respiration, and the cardiovascular status. Tracheal intubation in a comatose patient should be followed by gastric lavage with a large-bore tube, activated charcoal, and a cathartic. There is no role for forced diuresis in the elimination of methaqualone, and in light of the earlier remarks on increased salivation and tracheobronchial secretion, this may further compromise the respiratory status. In very severe methaqualone overdose unresponsive to conservative therapy, with plasma levels exceeding 4 mg/dl, hemodialysis,[66] or more preferably sorbent hemoperfusion,[50, 51] has been shown to be effective in reversing coma, reducing plasma levels, and effecting a complete recovery.

PRIMIDONE

Primidone is considered under barbiturate poisoning, since it may be viewed as a congener of phenobarbital (a deoxybarbiturate).[67] Primidone resembles phenobarbital but appears to be more selective in modifying electric shock seizure patterns in animals and human beings. Its anticonvulsant effect is due both to the parent drug and its active metabolites phenobarbital and phenylethylmalonamide.

Pharmacology and Toxicity[67]

Primidone is rapidly and completely absorbed after oral administration, with peak levels being achieved after 3 hours. The plasma elimination half-life is approximately 7 to 14 hours, whereas the half-life of phenylethylmalonamide is 16 hours and phenobarbital, 48 to 120 hours. Approximately 40 per cent of the drug is excreted unchanged in the urine within 24 hours. Phenobarbital accumulation in plasma may be delayed several days after starting treatment with primidone.

The toxicity of primidone is very similar to that of phenobarbital, with a similar duration of action (Table 39–1). Common complaints are of sedation, vertigo, nystagmus, and an acute feeling of intoxication. In addition, acute psychotic reactions have been observed in patients with temporal lobe epilepsy. Hemorrhagic diathesis, megaloblastic anemia, and osteomalacia similarly have been reported for primidone as with prolonged use of phenytoin and phenobarbital. Large crystals have been observed in urine from intoxicated patients.[68] It is interesting that a high primidone:phenobarbital concentration ratio during chronic medication implies that the medication has not been taken regularly; concentrations of primidone alone of greater than 10 mg/dl are usually associated with ataxia and lethargy.

Treatment of Primidone Intoxication

Treatment of primidone intoxication should follow the previous recommendations for barbiturate poisoning. A handful of case reports of peritoneal dialysis, hemodialysis, and hemoperfusion is available.[51] None of these reports present primidone clearance data, although blood levels of primidone fell steadily during each of the procedures and the patients recovered.

References

1. Ekeberg O, Jacobsen D, Flaaten B, Mack A: Effect of regulatory withdrawal of drugs and prescription recommendations on the pattern of self-poisonings in Oslo. Acta Med Scand *221*:483, 1987.
2. Henry JA, Cassidy SL: Membrane stabilising activity: A major cause of fatal poisoning. Lancet *1*:1414, 1986.
3. Hardwicke C, Holt L, James R, Smith AJ: Trends in self-poisoning in Newcastle, New South Wales, 1980–1982. Med J Aust *144*:453, 1986.
4. Vale JA, Meredith TJ (eds): Poisoning—Diagnosis and Treatment. Boston, Update Books, 1981.
5. Litovitz TL: Benzodiazepines. *In* Haddad LM, Winchester JF (eds): Clinical Management of Poisoning and Drug Overdose. Philadelphia, W.B. Saunders, 1983, p 475.
6. Litovitz TL, Schmitz BF, Matyunas N, Martin TG: 1987 Annual report of the American Association of Poison Control Centers Data Collection System. Am J Emerg Med *6*:479, 1988.
7. Gosselin RE, Hodge HC, Smith RP, Gleason MN (eds): Clinical Toxicology of Commercial Products. 4th ed. Baltimore, Williams & Wilkins, 1976.
8. Harvey SC: Hypnotics and sedatives. *In* Gilman AG, Goodman LS, Gilman A (eds): The Pharmacological Basis of Therapeutics. 6th ed. New York, Macmillan, 1980, p 339.
9. Eisenberg HM, Frankowski RF, Contant CF, Marshall LF, Walker MD: High-dose barbiturate control of elevated intracranial pressure in patients with severe head injury. J Neurosurg *69*:15, 1988.
10. Bohn DJ, Biggar WD, Smith CR, Conn AW, Barker GA: Influence of hypothermia, barbiturate therapy, and intracranial pressure monitoring on morbidity and mortality after near-drowning. Crit Care Med *14*:529, 1986.
11. Smith A: Barbiturate protection in cerebral hypoxia. Anesthesiology *47*:285, 1977.
12. Miller SM, Cottrell JE, Turndorf H, Ransohoff J: Cerebral protection by barbiturates and loop diuretics in head trauma: Possible modes of action. Bull NY Acad Med *56*:305, 1980.
13. Jaffe JH: Drug addiction and drug abuse. *In* Gilman AG, Goodman LS, Gilman A (eds): The Pharmacological Basis of Therapeutics. 6th ed. New York, Macmillan, 1980, p 535.
14. Matthew H: Drug overdose. Medicine (Medical Education International Ltd) *4*:273, 1972.
15. Aitken RCB, Proudfoot AT: Barbiturate automatism—myth or malady? Postgrad Med J *45*:612, 1969.
16. Jansson B: Drug automatism as a cause of pseudosuicide. Postgrad Med J *30*:A34, 1961.
17. Clemmesen C, Nilsson E: Therapeutic trends in the treatment of barbiturate poisoning: The Scandinavian method. Clin Pharmacol Ther *2*:220, 1961.
18. Matthew H, Lawson AAH: Acute barbiturate poi-

soning—a review of two years' experience. Q J Med *35:*539, 1966.
19. Setter JG, Maher JF, Schreiner GE: Barbiturate intoxication. Evaluation of therapy including dialysis in a large series selectively referred because of severity. Arch Intern Med *117:*224, 1966.
20. Goodman JM, Bischel MD, Wagers PW, Barbour BM: Barbiturate intoxication. Morbidity and mortality. West J Med *124:*179, 1976.
21. Reed CE, Driggs MF, Foote CC: Acute barbiturate intoxication: A study of 300 cases based on a physiologic system of classification of severity of the intoxication. Ann Intern Med *37:*290, 1952.
22. Greenblatt DJ, Allen MD, Harmatz JS, Noll BJ, Shader RI: Overdosage with pentobarbital and secobarbital: Assessment of factors related to outcome. J Clin Pharmacol *19:*758, 1979.
23. Arieff AI, Friedman EA: Coma following non-narcotic drug overdosage: Management of 206 adult patients. Am J Med Sci *266:*405, 1973.
24. Shubin H, Weil MH: The mechanism of shock following suicidal doses of barbiturates, narcotics, and tranquilizer drugs, with observations on the effects of treatment. Am J Med *38:*853, 1965.
25. Berman LB, Jeghers HJ, Schreiner GE, Pallotta AJ: Hemodialysis: An effective therapy for acute barbiturate poisoning. JAMA *161:*820, 1956.
26. Kennedy AC, Lindsay RM, Briggs JD, Luke RA, Young N, Campbell D: Successful treatment of three cases of very severe barbiturate poisoning. Lancet *1:*955, 1969.
27. Bailey DN, Jatlow PI: Barbital overdose and abuse. A new problem. Am J Clin Pathol *64:*291, 1975.
28. Raeburn JA, Cameron JC, Matthew H: Severe barbiturate poisoning: Contrasts in management. Clin Toxicol *2:*133, 1969.
29. Ritchie JM: The aliphatic alcohols. *In* Gilman AG, Goodman LS, Gilman A (eds): The Pharmacological Basis of Therapeutics. 6th ed. New York, Macmillan, 1980, p 376.
30. Hadden JK, Johnson K, Smith S, Price L, Giardina E: Acute barbiturate intoxication. JAMA *209:*893, 1969.
31. Beveridge AW, Lawson AAH: Occurrence of bullous lesions in acute barbiturate intoxication. Br Med J *1:*835, 1965.
32. Afifi AA, Sacks ST, Liu VY, Weil MH, Shubin H: Accumulative prognostic index for patients with barbiturate, glutethimide, and meprobamate intoxication. N Engl J Med *285:*1447, 1971.
33. Slager UT, Reilly EB, Brandt RA: The neuropathology of barbiturate intoxication. J Neuropathol Exp Neurol *25:*237, 1966.
34. Matthew H, Mackintosh TF, Tompsett SL, Cameron JC: Gastric aspiration and lavage in acute poisoning. Br Med J *1:*1333, 1966.
35. Schreiner GE, Berman LB, Kovach R, Bloomer HA: Acute glutethimide (Doriden) poisoning: The use of bemigride (megimide) and hemodialysis. Arch Intern Med *101:*899, 1958.
36. Victor LB, Gordon EL, Greendyke RM: Therapeutic implications of autopsy findings in acute barbiturate intoxication. NY State J Med *68:*2090, 1968.
37. Johanson WG Jr: Massive phenobarbital ingestion with survival. JAMA *202:*1106, 1967.
38. Holt E Jr, Holz PH: The black bottle. J Pediatr *63:*306, 1963.
39. Hayden JW, Comstock EG: Use of activated charcoal in acute poisoning. Clin Toxicol *8:*515, 1975.
40. Corby DC, Fiser RH, Decker WJ: Re-evaluation of the use of activated charcoal in the treatment of acute poisoning. Pediatr Clin North Am *17:*545, 1970.
41. Lipscomb DJ, Widdop B: Studies with activated charcoal in the treatment of drug overdose using the pig as an animal model. Arch Toxicol *34:*37, 1975.
42. Winchester JF, Gelfand MC, Knepshield JH, Schreiner GE: Dialysis and hemoperfusion of poisons and drugs—update. Trans Am Soc Artif Intern Organs *23:*762, 1977.
43. Kennedy JH, Barnette J, Flasterstein A, Higgs W: Experimental barbiturate intoxication: Treatment by partial cardiopulmonary bypass and hemodialysis. Cardiovasc Res Center Bull *14:*61, 1976.
44. Fell RH, Gunning AJ, Bardhan KD, Triger DR: Severe hypothermia as a result of barbiturate overdose complicated by cardiac arrest. Lancet *1:*392, 1968.
45. Linton AL, Ledingham IM: Severe hypothermia with barbiturate intoxication. Lancet *1:*24, 1966.
46. Lash RF, Burdette JA, Ozdil T: Accidental profound hypothermia and barbiturate intoxication. A report of rapid "core" rewarming by peritoneal dialysis. JAMA *201:*269, 1967.
47. Leavell VW: Sweat gland necrosis in barbiturate poisoning. Arch Dermatol *100:*218, 1969.
48. Wright N, Clarkson AR, Brown SS, Fuster V: Effects of poisoning on serum enzyme activities, coagulation, and fibrinolysis. Br Med J *3:*347, 1971.
49. Robinson RR, Gunnells JC Jr, Clapp JR: Treatment of acute barbiturate intoxication. Mod Treat *8:*562, 1971.
50. Freeman JW, Beattie RR, Ryan CA: Management of patients unconscious from drug overdose. Med J Aust *2:*1165, 1970.
51. Winchester JF, Gelfand MC, Tilstone WJ: Hemoperfusion in drug intoxication: Clinical and laboratory aspects. Drug Metab Rev *8:*69, 1978.
52. Hill JB, Palaia FL, McAdams JL, Palmer PJ, Maret SM: Efficacy of activated charcoal hemoperfusion in removing lethal doses of barbiturates and salicylate from the blood of rats and dogs. Clin Chem *22:*754, 1976.
53. Medd RK, Widdop B, Braithwaite RA, Rees AJ, Goulding R: Comparison of hemoperfusion and hemodialysis in the therapy of barbiturate intoxication in dogs. Arch Toxicol *31:*163, 1973.
54. Yatzidis H, Oreopoulos D, Triantaphyllidis D, Voudiclari S, Tsaparas N, Gavras C, Stavroulaki A: Treatment of severe barbiturate poisoning. Lancet *2:*216, 1965.
55. Chang TMS: Hemoperfusion alone and in series with hemofiltration or dialysis for uremia, poisoning, and liver failure. Kidney Int *10:*S305, 1976.
56. Gelfand MC, Winchester JF, Knepshield JH, Hanson KM, Cohan SL, Strauch BS, Geoly KL, Kennedy AC, Schreiner GE: Treatment of severe drug overdosage with charcoal hemoperfusion. Trans Am Soc Artif Intern Organs *23:*599, 1977.
57. Vale JA, Rees AJ, Widdop B, Goulding R: Use of charcoal haemoperfusion in the management of severely poisoned patients. Br Med J *1:*5, 1979.
58. Barbour BJ, LaSette AM, Koffler A: Fixed bed charcoal hemoperfusion for the treatment of drug overdose. Kidney Int *7:*S333, 1976.
59. Rosenbaum JL, Kramer MS, Raja R: Resin hemoperfusion for acute drug intoxication. Arch Intern Med *136:*263, 1976.

60. Rosenbaum JL: Poisonings. *In* Giordano C (ed): Sorbents and Their Clinical Applications. New York, Academic Press, 1980, p 451.
61. Inaba DS, Gay GR, Newmeyer JA, Whitehead C: Methaqualone abuse. JAMA *224*:1505, 1973.
62. Marks P, Sloggem J: Peripheral neuropathy caused by methaqualone. Am J Med Sci *272*:323, 1976.
63. Matthew H, Proudfoot AT, Brown SS, Smith ACA: Mandrax poisoning: Conservative management of 116 patients. Br Med J *2*:101, 1968.
64. Oh TE, Gordon TP, Burden PW: Unilateral pulmonary edema and "mandrax" poisoning. Anaesthesia *33*:719, 1978.
65. Wetli D: Changing patterns of methaqualone abuse: A survey of 246 fatalities. JAMA *249*:621, 1983.
66. Proudfoot AT, Noble J, Nimmo J, Brown SS, Cameron JC: Peritoneal dialysis and haemodialysis in methaqualone poisoning. Scot Med J *13*:232, 1968.
67. Rall TW, Schleifer LS: Drugs effective in the therapy of the epilepsies. *In* Gilman AG, Goodman LS, Gilman A (eds): The Pharmacologic Basis of Therapeutics. 6th ed. New York, Macmillan, 1980, p 448.
68. Lane GP, Lewis CJ, Zail SC: Macroscopic crystalluria after primidone overdosage. Med J Aust *147*:624, 1987.

CHAPTER 40
COCAINE

Lester M. Haddad, M.D.

Cocaine is the recreational drug of choice in America today.[1] The late 1970s found cocaine, expensive and scarce, a status symbol, its use largely confined to the wealthy and socially prominent.[1, 2] Abundant in the 1980s, the abuse of cocaine has become almost commonplace. With the introduction of the inexpensive "crack," cocaine use has grown at an alarming rate. In 1986, the National Institute of Drug Abuse estimated that 3 million Americans used cocaine regularly, and at least 30 million Americans had tried cocaine at least once.[3, 4]

Cocaine is also lethal. Cocaine as a cause of cardiac arrest presenting to an emergency department was described in 1979.[1] In the 10-year period from 1976 to 1986, there was more than a 15-fold increase in emergency department visits attributed to cocaine abuse, in cocaine deaths (more than 5 per 1000 deaths), and in admissions to cocaine treatment programs.[5, 6] One hundred and thirty-five confirmed murders during cocaine-related deals and 60 cocaine overdose deaths were reported in Dade County (Florida) alone.[7]

Reports on the medical complications of cocaine have mushroomed in the medical literature during the past 5 years: today the aura of and attraction to cocaine are finally beginning to erode in the public eye.

HISTORY

Cocaine, an alkaloid of the plant *Erythoxylon coca*, grows extensively in the Andes mountains. Coca leaves mixed with lime were chewed by Peruvian Indians as early as the sixth century and were an essential part of the Incan religion.

Although explorers introduced the leaves to Europe, it was not until 1860 that Niemann isolated the alkaloid cocaine.[8] In 1883, Aschenbrandt, a German army physician, gave cocaine to Bavarian soldiers and noticed that it alleviated fatigue.[8] Sigmund Freud, the Viennese neurologist, began experimenting with cocaine in 1884 to relieve his own depression and became ecstatic about its curative abilities. He proposed in July of 1884 that cocaine be used (1) as a stimulant, (2) for digestive disorders of the stomach, (3) for cachexia, (4) for alcohol and drug addiction, (5) for asthma, (6) as an aphrodisiac, and (7) as a local anesthetic.[9] Only the last mentioned use of cocaine, that of use as a local anesthetic, has persisted in modern medicine. In 1884, Freud's close friend Karl Koller was the first to use cocaine as a local anesthetic in eye surgery and thus forever legitimized the use of cocaine in medicine. It was not until Freud had used cocaine extensively for years that he wrote his great psychiatric works.

The author Sir Arthur Conan Doyle had his famous literary detective Sherlock Holmes inject cocaine to pass the time between cases.

The history of cocaine in America is also a vivid one. William Steward Halsted, the father of modern surgery, reported in 1884 the use of cocaine in regional nerve blocks. Unfortunately, Halsted himself became heavily cocaine dependent.[10]

Cocaine was thought at one time to be a possible cure for tuberculosis. Indeed, in 1895, Robert Louis Stevenson, while undergoing cocaine therapy in a sanitarium, wrote the novel Dr. Jekyll and Mr. Hyde in only 3 days.

In 1886, John Styth Pemberton of Atlanta marketed an elixir containing cocaine from the coca leaf and caffeine from the African kola nut and appropriately named it "Coca-cola." Coca-cola rapidly became one of the most popular elixirs in the country. Not until 1906 did the Coca-Cola Company agree to use decocainized coca leaves.

Cocaine came under the strict control of the Harrison Narcotic Act and is listed as a narcotic and dangerous drug. Its illicit use is subject to the same penalties as those applied to opium, morphine, and heroin.

PHARMACOLOGY

The alkaloid cocaine (benzoylmethylecgonine, $C_{17}H_{21}NO_4$) represents roughly 1 per cent of the coca leaf. Cocaine reaches the United States primarily as cocaine hydrochloride, which is prepared by dissolving the alkaloid in hydrochloric acid to form a water-soluble salt and is marketed as crystals, granules, or white powder. Cocaine hydrochloride decomposes on heating.

It has become common in the United States today to convert cocaine hydrochloride back to its original alkaloid form, or "free-base." Free-base cocaine melts at 98°C, vaporizes at higher temperatures, and is not destroyed by heating; these properties allow it to be smoked. Cocaine hydrochloride is converted to free-base by mixing the cocaine with an alkaline solution such as ammonia and then adding a solvent such as ether. The mixture separates into two layers: The top layer contains cocaine dissolved in the solvent. The solvent can then be evaporated, leaving relatively pure cocaine crystals.[11]

"Crack" is an inexpensive form of free-base, prepared by using baking soda and water.

Intranasal use of cocaine is the most common route of administration, followed by smoking, and then by parenteral use. The effects of intranasal "snorting" begin after about 20 minutes, peak at 60 minutes, and then gradually decline for at least 3 hours after inhalation.

Smoking cocaine, either from crack cigarettes or free-base from a water-pipe, results in nearly immediate respiratory absorption and a rapid rise in blood level concentrations, producing an intense euphoria, which users often describe as the same "rush" experienced following intravenous abuse. The euphoric effects of smoking cocaine usually last only 20 minutes.

Cocaine is metabolized by plasma and liver cholinesterase to water-soluble metabolites, benzoylecgonine, and ecgonine methyl ester, and is excreted in the urine. Less than 20 per cent of cocaine is excreted unchanged in the urine. Cocaine is present in the urine of an adult for 24 to 36 hours following administration.[12–14]

Cocaine blocks the presynaptic re-uptake of the neurotransmitters norepinephrine and dopamine, producing an excess of transmitter at the postsynaptic receptor sites.[15] Thus cocaine is a powerful central nervous system stimulant and owes its popularity to this effect. It increases both heart rate and blood pressure, is a powerful sympathomimetic, and also increases body temperature.[7] Amphetamines produce effects similar to those of cocaine.[16, 17]

Although the oral lethal dose of cocaine is usually given as 1200 mg, death has been reported to follow as little as 20 mg of parenterally administered cocaine.[18, 19]

CLINICAL USE

In modern medicine, cocaine is used primarily by otolaryngologists, plastic surgeons, and emergency physicians. Cocaine is an excellent local anesthetic and vasoconstrictor of mucous membranes and as such enjoys wide use in nasal surgery, rhinoplasty, and emergency nasotracheal intubation. It is no longer used in ophthalmic surgery.

Johns and Henderson[20] concluded from clinical experience that a safe limit for nasal topical application is higher than 200 mg and that reactions to cocaine are not necessarily dose related.

The usual topical therapeutic dose is given as 2 ml of a 5 or 10 per cent solution (100 or 200 mg). We have found that 200 mg (2 ml of a 10 per cent solution) given intranasally is useful during emergency nasotracheal intubation.

RECREATIONAL ABUSE

The present epidemic of cocaine abuse is considered to be the third and most extensive occurring in the United States, the first occurring in the 1890s and the second in the 1920s.[21] Present purity levels of street cocaine may range from 20 to 90 per cent or greater, in contrast to average purity levels of 3 per cent during the 1970s. Some street names for cocaine include coke, snow, C, girl, white girl, leaf, blow, nose candy, her, and white lady.

Cocaine is variously cut into grams or "spoons" (half grams) and is usually adulterated with mannitol, sucrose, or lactose.[2] Caffeine, amphetamines, ephedrine, phenylpropanolamine, procaine, lidocaine, and other local anesthetics all have been substituted for cocaine.[22] The cocaine is chopped with a razor blade into lines or columns on a piece of glass, and the line is inhaled, usually through a rolled dollar bill.

Crack is so-called from the cracking sound made by the crystals when they are heated.[23]

CLINICAL PRESENTATION

Cocaine initially produces an excitable state, with elevation of both heart rate and blood pressure, dilated pupils, and rapid respirations. The patient may or may not have hallucinations[24] or vomiting. Such patients usually are not seen in the emergency department unless the hypertension (with concomitant headache), hallucinations, or vomiting is severe or unless they present with a secondary complication such as trauma.

In 1979 the emergency medicine literature identified cocaine as a cause of increased emergency department visits for sudden cardiac arrest, cardiac arrhythmias, and status epilepticus.[1] The list of medical complications resulting from cocaine has considerably expanded, with cardiac, neurologic, pulmonary and obstetric effects and sequelae from intravenous drug abuse primarily identified in the medical literature.

In a recent 1-year retrospective review of 137 patients presenting to an emergency department with cocaine intoxication, a wide variety of chief complaints was noted, including altered mental status (40 patients), chest pain (21 patients), syncope (19 patients), suicide attempt (13 patients), palpitations (12 patients), and seizures (12 patients), as well as one patient with cardiac arrest.[25]

Cardiac Effects

Chest Pain. Ever since Coleman, Ross, and Naughton in 1982 described a previously healthy 38 year old who sustained an acute myocardial infarction shortly after snorting cocaine (intranasally),[26] 35 additional cases[27–39] to date have been reported in the medical literature. Acute myocardial infarction has occurred in patients aged 20 to 44 years within 6 hours of cocaine use. The route of administration was primarily intranasal[26] but also intravenous,[8] free-base inhalation, and by smoking crack. All patients presented with chest pain, and most had classic electrocardiographic findings of acute myocardial infarction, with subsequent elevations in the creatine-phosphokinase–MB isoenzyme fraction.

Schachne et al, in the second modern case report (1984),[27] documented a 21 year old patient with structurally normal coronary arteries who had acute myocardial infarction following recreational abuse of cocaine; cardiac catheterization was performed 1 week following admission. It was then postulated that cocaine produced acute myocardial infarction by coronary artery spasm.

Subsequent case reports suggested that the mechanism of acute myocardial infarction following cocaine abuse might include coronary artery spasm alone, coronary artery spasm with resulting thrombus, or perhaps primary coronary thrombosis.

Smith et al,[39] in reviewing 30 cases of patients who underwent coronary angiography, noted that 19 showed either totally occluded or partially thrombosed vessels. These investigators proposed that this number may have been higher if earlier angiography—within 4 hours of presentation—had been performed, and further proposed that thrombolytic therapy may be indicated in such patients: Three of nine patients in their series were treated in such fashion.

Contraction band necrosis may be the pathologic finding in patients with acute myocardial infarction following recreational abuse of cocaine.[40] Myocardial contraction bands are probably related to elevated circulating levels of norepinephrine.[40] Cocaine abusers who presented with cardiac symptoms to an emergency department in Las Vegas were found to have dramatically elevated norepinephrine blood levels (400 to 600 ng/L) and epinephrine levels that were twice normal.[41] Within minutes of achieving elevated local concentrations of catecholamines, myofilaments actually "ratchet"[40] past each other and end up as an amorphous mass incapable of contracting again; they ultimately are replaced by fibrous tissue.[40]

All patients who present to the emergency department with chest pain should be questioned about recent recreational abuse of cocaine and should be rapidly evaluated to either document or exclude myocardial ischemia or infarction.

Palpitation. Palpitation following cocaine use is a common cause of emergency department visits. Sinus tachycardia is the most common cause, and observation and sedation are all that are usually necessary. If frequent or multifocal premature ventricular contractions are present, beta-blocker therapy with propranolol or labetalol may be indicated, as well as subsequent admission to the coronary care unit for observation. Ventricular tachycardia and other life-threatening arrhythmias are discussed later in this chapter under Emergency Management.

Neurologic Effects

Altered mental status is the most common effect of cocaine abuse; seizures, status epilepticus, headache, syncope, focal neurologic signs and symptoms, ischemic stroke, and subarachnoid and intracerebral hemorrhage have all been reported as neurologic complications following the recreational abuse of cocaine or crack.[42–46]

Grand mal seizures are the most common neurologic complication, accounting in one series[42] for 29 of 55 cases with neurologic sequelae of cocaine abuse. Grand mal seizures have been personally observed in consultation following clinical use of cocaine, during an ENT (ear, nose, and throat) procedure, and after emergency nasotracheal intubation. Seizures may be seen in either first-time or habitual abusers of cocaine. Status epilepticus is not unusual and may be accompanied by a high anion-gap metabolic acidosis.[45]

Focal neurologic signs and symptoms include transient sensory abnormalities, or transient motor and sensory complaints, and blurriness or loss of vision.[42]

Ischemic stroke in four patients ranging from age 20 to 35 have been reported following smoking crack, inhaling free-base, and intranasal use.[43–44] Subsequent angiography in one patient[43] indicated that vasospasm was the probable cause of the cocaine-induced stroke.

Chasnoff and colleagues[46] reported a mother who smoked about 1 gram of cocaine on the day of delivery of her infant, approximately 15 hours prior to delivery. Her baby was noted to have persistent tachycardia, decreased muscle tone in the right arm, and subsequent apnea, cyanosis, and seizures shortly after birth. The baby was noted to have, by noncontrast computed tomography, an acute cerebral infarction in the distribution of the left middle cerebral artery.

The "kindling phenomenon," or reverse tolerance to cocaine, has been described.[47] This is the phenomenon "in which repetitive sub-threshold electrical stimulation of the limbic system produces increasing effects on electrical activity and behavior, eventually resulting in major convulsions or reaction to a stimulation that previously produced no effect."

Young patients who present with headache or other neurologic signs or symptoms should be carefully questioned about the possible association of recent cocaine abuse and appropriately evaluated.

Psychophysiologic Effects

Occasional use of cocaine is initially associated with "positive" effects. In general, subjects experience euphoria, stimulation, reduced fatigue, sexual stimulation, increased mental ability, alertness, and increased social tendencies.[48–50] Subsequently, users discover that higher doses intensify the pharmacologic euphoria.

When does controlled or occasional use become compulsive abuse requiring treatment? Although not known at present, this line is thought to be related to the actual frequency of experience—when access to the drug increases or when the user switches to a more rapid rate of administration.[16]

Euphoria becomes so extreme that it is often compared to orgasm.[16] The memory of the euphoria begins to dominate one's life, so that the successes and joys of daily life seem commonplace and boring. Craving for such euphoria begins to preoccupy the user. The pattern of abuse progresses to prolonged periods or "binges" of abuse lasting up to 1 or 2 days. These periods are followed by periods of extreme exhaustion and depression, or "crash." A period of withdrawal follows, then craving begins anew. Once begun, this "binge-crash cycle" is extremely destructive to one's personality and lifestyle.[16] Suicide is a not uncommon event during the depressive aftermath of a binge. This behavior pattern is reached much sooner in crack and free-base abusers.[16]

Chronic use of cocaine is also associated with paranoid psychosis, severe anxiety and panic states, and depression.[16, 48–50] Perceptual changes, such as seeing halo lights around objects and extreme itching as if in response to crawling bugs—"cocaine bugs"—can occur. Hallucinations have also been described.

Cocaine has been said to cause a psychologic addiction, although it is presently thought that "a true neurophysiologic addiction occurs, whose clinical expression is psychologic."[16] The very concepts of habituation and addiction are presently in evolution.

Intravenous Cocaine and AIDS

Intravenous drug abuse is the second leading cause of the acquired immunodeficiency syndrome (AIDS) in the United States today, primarily via intravenous cocaine or heroin abuse and largely among young black males. Intravenous drug abuse of cocaine has the usual complications attendant on any drug given intravenously without proper sterile technique, such as hepatitis, AIDS, cellulitis, abscess formation, bacterial endocarditis, thrombophlebitis, polyneuropathies, myopathies, and renal failure with or without rhabdomyolysis and myoglobinuria.

Other Complications

Cardiovascular complications include renal infarction,[51] mesenteric insufficiency,[52] acute rupture of the ascending aorta,[53] and diffuse muscle and skin infarction after inhaling crack.[54] A recent report[55] has described the association of cocaine intoxication, rhabdomyolysis, acute renal failure, liver dysfunction, and disseminated intravascular coagulation in 39 patients. The presence of acute renal failure was particularly lethal.[55]

Since smoking crack and inhaling free-base are becoming more common, pulmonary effects are now being reported. Abnormally low carbon monoxide diffusion capacities were noted in 10 of 19 free-base cocaine abusers.[56] Pneumomediastinum and pneumothorax after inhaling alkaloidal cocaine has been noted.[57] A recent report described a patient who experienced three separate episodes of pulmonary infiltrates and bronchospasm after smoking crack.[58]

Nasal septal necrosis and perforation, loss of the sense of smell, and atrophy of the nasal mucosa are seen following chronic nasal administration of cocaine.

Obstetric complications include abruptio placentae,[59] higher rates of spontaneous abortion,[60] and placental vasoconstriction leading to uterine contraction and fetal hypoxemia.[61] Cocaine during pregnancy is associated with impaired fetal growth,[62] an increase in perinatal complications and mortality,[23] and perhaps an increase in congenital malformation.[63]

EMERGENCY MANAGEMENT

Cocaine toxicity should be suspected in all young patients who present to the emergency department with chest pain, palpitation, cardiac arrhythmias, or cardiac arrest; headache, seizures, or other neurologic complications; or any bizarre illness inappropriate for the patient's age.

In the emergency department, ensure that all patients with suspected cocaine overdose have a patent airway, an intravenous line, and frequent monitoring of vital signs. All suspected cocaine overdose patients should be placed on a cardiac monitor and undergo a 12-lead electrocardiogram.

Patients with chest pain should be rapidly evaluated and referred for possible admission to the hospital. Patients with electrocardiographic changes indicative of acute myocardial infarction may or may not be candidates for thrombolytic therapy at this time. Cardiology consultation should be considered to evaluate this possibility, as well as the indications for (or against) coronary angiography.

Sudden cardiac arrest may be the presenting picture of cocaine overdose.[1, 45] In 1978, a sensational case of death occurred in Atlanta: when drug inspectors boarded an airplane at the airport, a passenger ingested six cocaine-filled condoms and one burst; the victim rapidly sustained a cardiac arrest and subsequently died in spite of aggressive resuscitation attempts.[1] Intoxication from cocaine-filled condom ingestion is not a rare event. Surgery rather than endoscopy is recommended for removal of intact condoms because endoscopic manipulation has caused their rupture.[64] Whole bowel irrigation is useful for removal of cocaine packets and crack vials.

Cocaine should be considered a possible cause in all young patients who are brought to the emergency department in cardiac arrest. At least two infants who suffered cardiac arrest and death were found to have cocaine toxicity (personal communication, Boyd Stephens, MD, 1988).

For life-threatening cardiac dysrhythmia such as ventricular tachycardia when cocaine is the probable cause, intravenous propranolol may be indicated.[1, 45, 65, 66] It is given in 1-mg increments by IV push every 5 to 15 minutes, for up to five doses, by the emergency physician attending at the bedside.

Although others[65] may be more liberal, we reserve management of hypertension secondary to cocaine for severely hypertensive patients, patients who may exhibit altered sensorium, or patients who may develop possible neurologic sequelae. Antihypertensive therapy with either propranolol, labetalol, or metoprolol may be indicated.

Patients with seizures may be difficult to manage because their seizures are often prolonged and recurrent. Status epilepticus is not unusual. Diazepam is the drug of choice for management of status epilepticus secondary to cocaine overdose. In patients with seizures that are unresponsive to high doses of diazepam, or those with associated opisthotonos, pancuronium bromide paralysis and mechanical ventilation may be necessary. Patients with recurrent seizures may develop a high anion gap metabolic acidosis, usually a lactic acidosis,[45] which may require treatment with sodium bicarbonate. The patient should also be assessed for other neurologic sequelae as already described.

Dialysis has no role in the treatment of cocaine overdose because cocaine is rapidly metabolized, and only small amounts produce symptomatology.

Any patient with significant manifestations of cocaine overdose may well require admission and supportive care. Laboratory confirmation of cocaine overdose and observation is important because hyperthermia, hypertension, seizures, cardiac, neurologic, and other complications are constant concerns in these patients. Patients with intravenous cocaine abuse must be evaluated, observed, and managed for those sequelae attendant to intravenous administration. And finally, psychiatric consultation and referral is indicated when medically appropriate.

References

1. Haddad LM: 1978: Cocaine in perspective. J Am Coll Emerg Phys *8*:374, 1979.
2. Gay GR, Inaba DS, Sheppard CW, Newmeyer JA: Cocaine: History, epidemiology, human pharmacology and treatment. A perspective on a new debut for an old girl. Clin Toxicol *8*:149–178, 1975.
3. Abelson HI, Miller JD: A decade of trends in cocaine use in the household population. Natl Inst Drug Abuse, Res Monograph Ser *61*:35–49, 1985.
4. Adams EH, Gfoerer JC, Rouse BA, Kozel NJ: Trends in prevalence and consequences of cocaine use. Adv Alcohol Subst Abuse *6*:49–71, 1986.
5. Colliver J: A Decade of DAWN: Cocaine-Related Cases, 1976–1985. Washington, D.C., National Institute on Drug Abuse, Division of Epidemiological and Statistical Publication, 1987.
6. National Institute on Drug Abuse, Division of Epidemiological and Statistical Publication. Cocaine Client Admissions 1976–1985. Washington, D.C., U.S. Government Printing Office, 1987.
7. Mittleman RE, Wetli CV: Death caused by recreational cocaine use: An update. JAMA *252*:1889–1893, 1984.
8. Byck R: Cocaine Papers: Sigmund Freud. New York, Stonehill Publishing Company, 1975.
9. Musto D: The American Disease—Origins of Narcotic Control. New Haven, CT, Yale University Press, 1973.
10. Petersen RC, Stillman RE (eds): Cocaine, 1977. NIDA Research Monograph 13. National Institute on Drug

Abuse. Washington, D.C., U.S. Government Printing Office, 1977.
11. Allred RJ, Ewer S: Case Report: Fatal pulmonary edema following intravenous cocaine use. Ann Emerg Med *10*:441, 1981.
12. Baselt RC, Chang R: Urinary excretion of cocaine and benzoylecgonine following oral ingestion in a single subject. J Anal Toxicol *11*:27, 1987.
13. Van Dyke C, Byck R, Barash PG, Jatlow P: Urinary excretion of immunologically reactive metabolites after intranasal administration of cocaine, as followed by enzyme immunoassay. Clin Chem *23/2*:241, 1977.
14. AMA Council on Scientific Affairs: Scientific issues in drug testing. JAMA *257*:3110–3114, 1987.
15. Ritchie JM, Greene NM: Cocaine. *In* Gilman AG, Goodman LS (eds): The Pharmacologic Basis of Therapeutics. 7th ed. New York, Macmillan, 1985, p 309.
16. Gawin FH, Ellinwood EH: Cocaine and other stimulants. N Engl J Med *318*:1173, 1988.
17. Caldwell J, Sever PS: The biochemical pharmacology of abused drugs. Clin Pharmacol Ther *16*:625, 1974.
18. Price KR: Fatal cocaine poisoning. J Forensic Sci Soc *14*:329, 1974.
19. Miller SH, Dvorchik B, Davis TS: Cocaine concentration in the blood during rhinoplasty. Plast Reconstruct Surg *60*:566, 1977.
20. Johns ME, Henderson RL: Cocaine use by the otolaryngologist: A survey. Trans Am Acad Ophthalmol Otolaryngol *84*:969, 1977.
21. Byck R: Cocaine use and research: Three histories. *In* Fisher S, Raskin A, Uhlenhuth EH (eds): Cocaine: Clinical and Behavioral Aspects. New York: Oxford University Press, 1986.
22. Siegel RK: Cocaine substitutes. N Engl J Med *302*:817, 1980.
23. Cregler LL, Mark H: Medical complications of cocaine abuse. N Engl J Med *315*:1495–1500, 1986.
24. Siegel RK: Cocaine hallucinations. Am J Psychiatr *135*:309, 1978.
25. Deriet RW, Albertson TE: Emergency department presentation of cocaine intoxication. Ann Emerg Med *18*:182, 1989.
26. Coleman DL, Ross TF, Naughton JL: Myocardial ischemia and infarction related to recreational cocaine use. West J Med *136*:444, 1982.
27. Schachne JS, Roberts BH, Thompson PD: Coronary artery spasm and myocardial infarction associated with cocaine use. N Engl J Med *310*:1665, 1984.
28. Kossowsky WA, Lyon AF: Cocaine and acute myocardial infarction: A probable connection. Chest *86*:729, 1984.
29. Pasternack PF, Colvin SB, Baumann FG: Cocaine-induced angina pectoris and acute myocardial infarction in patients younger than 40 years. Am J Cardiol *1*:55:847, 1985.
30. Gould L, Gopalaswamy C, Patel C, Betzu R: Cocaine-induced myocardial infarction. NY State Med J *85*:660, 1985.
31. Cregler LL, Mark H: Relation of acute myocardial infarction to cocaine abuse. Am J Cardiol *56*:794, 1985.
32. Howard RE, Hueter DC, Davis GJ: Acute myocardial infarction following cocaine abuse in a young woman with normal coronary arteries. JAMA *254*:95, 1985.
33. Wilkins CE, Mathor VS, Ty RC, Hall RJ: Myocardial infarction associated with cocaine abuse. Texas Heart Inst J *12*:385, 1985.
34. Weiss RJ: Recurrent myocardial infarction caused by cocaine abuse. Am Heart J *111*:793, 1986.
35. Isner JM, Estes NAM, Thompson PD, Costanzo-Nordin MR, Subramanian R, Miller G, Katsas G, Sweeney K, Sturner WQ: Acute cardiac events temporally related to cocaine abuse. N Engl J Med *315*:1438–1443, 1986.
36. Rollinger IM, Belzberg AS, MacDonald IL: Cocaine-induced myocardial infarction. Can Med Assoc J *135*:45, 1986.
37. Chiu YC, Brecht K, DasGupta DS, Mhoon E: Myocardial infarction with topical cocaine anesthesia for nasal surgery. Arch Otolaryngol Head Neck Surg *112*:988–990, 1986.
38. Rod JL, Zucker RP: Acute myocardial infarction shortly after cocaine inhalation. Am J Cardiol *59*:161, 1986.
39. Smith HWB, Liberman HA, Brody SL, Battey LL, Donohue BC, Morris DC: Acute myocardial infarction temporally related to cocaine use. Ann Intern Med *107*:13–18, 1987.
40. Karch SB, Billingham ME: Pathology and etiology of cocaine-induced heart disease. Arch Pathol Lab Med *112*:225, 1988.
41. Karch SB: Serum catecholamine levels in cocaine-intoxicated patients with cardiac symptoms—abstract. Ann Emerg Med *16*:481, 1987.
42. Lowenstein DH, Massa SM, Rowbotham MC, Collins SD, McKinney HE, Simon RP: Acute neurologic and psychiatric complications associated with cocaine abuse. Am J Med *83*:841–846, 1987.
43. Golbe LI, Merkin MD: Cerebral infarction in a user of free-base cocaine ("crack"). Neurology *36*:1602, 1986.
44. Levine SR, Washington JM, Jefferson MF, Kieran SN, Moen M, Feit H, Welch KMA: "Crack" cocaine-associated stroke. Neurology *37*:1849, 1987.
45. Haddad LM: Cocaine. *In* Haddad LM, Winchester JF (eds): Clinical Management of Poisoning and Drug Overdose. Philadelphia, W. B. Saunders, 1983, pp 443–447.
46. Chasnoff IJ, Bussey ME, Savich R, Stack CM: Perinatal cerebral infarction and maternal cocaine use. J Pediatr *108*:456, 1986.
47. Post RM, Kopanda RT: Cocaine, kindling, and psychosis. Am J Psychiatr *133*:627, 1976.
48. Fischman MW, Schuster ER, Krasnegor NA: Physiological and behavioral effects of intravenous cocaine in man. *In* Ellinwood EH, Kilbey MD (eds): Cocaine and Other Stimulants. New York, Plenum Press, 1977.
49. Byck R, Jatlow P, Barash P, Van Dyke C: Cocaine: Blood concentration and physiological effects after intranasal application in man. *In* Ellinwood EH, Kilbey MD (eds): Cocaine and Other Stimulants. New York, Plenum Press, 1977.
50. Resnick RB, Schwartz LK: Acute systemic effects of cocaine in man: A controlled study by intranasal and intravenous routes. Science *195*:696, 1977.
51. Scharff JA: Renal infarction associated with intravenous cocaine use. Ann Emerg Med *13*:1145, 1984.
52. Nalbandian H, Sheth N, Dietrich R, Georgiou J: Intestinal ischemia caused by cocaine ingestion: Report of two cases. Surgery *97*:374, 1985.
53. Barth CW, Bray M, Roberts WC: Rupture of the ascending aorta during cocaine intoxication. Am J Cardiol *57*:496, 1986.
54. Zamora-Quesada JC, Dinerman H, Stadecker MJ, Kelly JJ: Muscle and skin infarction after free-basing cocaine (crack). Ann Intern Med *108*:564, 1988.

55. Roth D, Alarcon FJ, Fernandez JA, Preston RA, Bourgoiguie JJ: Acute rhabdomyolysis associated with cocaine intoxication. N Engl J Med *319*:673–677, 1988.
56. Itkonen J, Schnoll S, Glassroth J: Pulmonary dysfunction in "free-base" cocaine users. Arch Intern Med *144*:2195, 1984.
57. Shesser R, Davis C, Edelstein S: Pneumomediastinum and pneumothorax after inhaling alkaloidal cocaine. Ann Emerg Med *10*:213, 1985.
58. Kissner DG, Lawrence WD, Selis JE, Flint A: Crack lung: Pulmonary disease caused by cocaine abuse. Am Rev Respir Dis *136*:1250, 1987.
59. Acker D, Sachs BP, Tracey KJ, Wise WE: Abruptio placentae associated with cocaine use. Am J Obstet Gynecol *146*:220, 1983.
60. Chasnoff IJ, Burns WJ, Schnoll SH, Burns KA: Cocaine use in pregnancy. N Engl J Med *313*:666, 1985.
61. Woods JR, Plessinger MA, Clark KE: Effect of cocaine on uterine blood flow and fetal oxygenation. JAMA *257*:957, 1987.
62. Zuckerman B, Frank DA, Hingson R, Amaro H, Levenson SM, Kayne H, Parker S, Vinci R, Aboagye K, Fried LE, Cabral H, Timperi R, Bauchner H: Effects of maternal marijuana and cocaine use on fetal growth. N Engl J Med *320*:762, 1989.
63. Bingol N, Fuchs M, Diaz V, Stone RK, Gromisch DS: Teratogenicity of cocaine in humans. J Pediatr *110*:93, 1987.
64. Suarez CA, Arango A, Lester JL: Cocaine-condom ingestion—surgical treatment. JAMA *238*:1391, 1977.
65. Rappolt RT, Gay GR, Inaba DS: Propranolol in the treatment of cardiopressor effects of cocaine (letter). N Engl J Med *295*:448, 1976.
66. Fennell WH, Fischman MW, Schuster CR, Resnekov L: Cardiovascular effects of cocaine (letter). N Engl J Med *295*:960, 1976.

CHAPTER 41
MARIJUANA

Stephen Szara, M.D., D.Sc.

Marijuana continues to be by far the most extensively used illicit drug in the United States. Much of what we know today about the health hazards associated with acute and chronic use comes from clinical case reports and from results of scientific research. The modern era of scientific research began about 20 years ago when the major psychoactive component of marijuana was isolated and identified chemically as Δ_1-tetrahydrocannabinol or by the more commonly used nomenclature, Δ^9-tetrahydrocannabinol (THC for short).[1] A few years later[2] a practical synthesis of this substance was produced, and in 1968 the National Institute of Mental Health (NIMH) contracted for larger scale production of THC for distribution to the research community. With the availability of a chemically well defined active principle and the infusion of federal monies in the early 1970s, scientific research began in earnest.

Some of this research was conducted in controlled clinical settings in which acute dose-response studies of a variety of physiologic and mental effects clearly demonstrated that marijuana is indeed a drug and THC is its major active ingredient.[3] The effects of chronic drug exposure and its potential health hazards, however, are difficult to study in a laboratory setting on humans, and thus much of what we know about this aspect of marijuana use comes from clinical case studies and from experimental studies in animals. It is no wonder these findings remain controversial and ambiguous.

The ambiguity of this knowledge may be attributed to a number of factors.[4] First, it has been difficult to either prove or disprove health hazards in man by extrapolation of data from animal studies. The doses used in animals are often much larger than the average amount of drug consumed by humans, and species differences make the extrapolation difficult. Second, marijuana is still used by young persons in the best of health, frequently on an intermittent rather than a regular basis, which may lead to an underestimation of the potential impact of cannabis use on health. Third, cannabis is often used in combination with tobacco and alcohol, among licit drugs, as well as a variety of illicit drugs. This fact makes any conclusion drawn from uncontrolled clinical observation less than conclusive.

In recognition of these difficulties, more recent research is being conducted with more appropriate doses of the drug in animal studies and more careful selection of the patient population in clinical studies, utilizing appropriate control groups whenever feasible so that more confidence can be placed in the conclusions drawn from these data. The purpose of this chapter is to present the best and most recent data available on the potential health problems of marijuana use so that clinicians can recognize and treat the medical and psychologic difficulties arising from this widely used drug.

The extent of drug use and abuse in our society is estimated by periodic epidemiologic surveys[5] of three selected subject populations:

1. High school seniors from a representative sample of public and private high schools from throughout the United States are annually surveyed.
2. A periodic National Household Survey on Drug Abuse is conducted on a sample of subjects over 12 years old, living in households in the continental United States.
3. In 1985 approximately 25,000 members of the armed forces stationed at home and abroad were asked about their use of alcohol and drugs.

Without going into extensive detail on these findings,[5] marijuana is still by far the most widely used illicit drug. Some of the highlights in the report by the Secretary of the Department of Health and Human Services include the following:

- Over half (54.2 per cent) of high school seniors in the 1985 class had used marijuana, slightly down from the peak of 60.3 per cent in 1980.
- Over one quarter (25.7 per cent) of 1985 seniors were using marijuana currently, compared with 25.2 per cent the year before and the high point of 37.1 per cent in the class of 1978.
- Daily use of marijuana (20+ days per month), which peaked at 10.7 per cent among 1978 high school seniors, was down to 4.9 per cent in the 1985 senior class, about the same level as the year before (5.0 per cent).
- The 1985 National Household Survey noted a decline in marijuana use compared with the 1982 survey: 23.7 per cent of 12 to 17 year olds had used marijuana compared to 26.7 per cent in 1982; among young adults 18 to 25, a decline from 64.1 per cent to 60.5 per cent was found.
- In the military population the 1985 Survey found that nearly 20 per cent of persons in the lower three enlisted grades (E1 to E3) had used marijuana within the previous 12 months; 11 per cent reported use during the preceding month. In the higher enlisted grades (E4 to E6), 12 per cent had used marijuana in the prior year; 7 per cent during the preceding month. Rates of marijuana, cocaine, and other illicit drug use are considerably lower in the grades above E6. However, alcohol use rates seem to be consistently high across all grades. Overall, there is reason to be encouraged by the results of the 1985 Survey. In 1980, 27 per cent of military personnel reported using an illicit drug during the previous month. This figure dropped to 19 per cent in the 1982 Survey and by 1985 was down to 9 per cent.

As these statistics suggest, the use of this substance is so prevalent that clinicians should have at least a basic understanding of marijuana's effects and probably should include careful questioning about drug use in their history taking of patients in the youth and young adult age brackets.

Smoking the "joint," as the marijuana cigarette is usually called, is the most common pattern of usage in the United States. Generally, smoke from the joint (or "bong" or water-pipe) is inhaled deeply and held in the lungs for a period of 15 to 30 seconds. This is a very efficient and rapid way to "get high," and smokers can easily control their level of intoxication because effective brain levels of the active ingredients are rapidly achieved.

Oral dosage is the second most common means of intoxication. Generally, the marijuana is baked inside cookies or brownies and ingested. In this mode, the effects after ingestion do not start immediately, as with inhalation. Peak brain levels are reached approximately 120 minutes after ingestion; the effects, however, last longer. The user, in this mode of administration, cannot control the level of intoxication, and for some this is rather disconcerting. For example, oral users have periods of being "too high" and feeling anxious, interspersed with periods of not being high enough and feeling depressed or tired.

The intravenous route has been reported in the literature, although primarily in research subjects. However, some illicit intravenous use has been reported, with subjects "shooting" crude marijuana plant extracts, but this remains an extremely unusual practice.

BOTANY AND CHEMISTRY

Cannabis sativa is a hemp plant that has been used for centuries not only for its psychoactive resin but also for hemp fiber and rope. The cannabinoid Δ^9-tetrahydrocannabinol (THC) is the principal active ingredient in the *Cannabis sativa* plant. Depending on its cultivation, it can contain anywhere between 0.4 and 6 per cent of THC. There are more than 400 other chemicals, including several other cannabinoids, that have little, if any, psychoactive effect. THC is primarily found in the leaves and flowering tops of the plant.

Marijuana, in common parlance, generally refers to tobacco-like preparations of the leaves and flowers. Hashish, the resin extracted from the tops of the flowering plants, sometimes has a THC concentration of more than 10 per cent. Hash oil is a specially prepared extraction from *Cannabis* that can provide a THC concentration of 20 per cent or higher. An average marijuana cigarette has from 500 to 1000 mg of plant material with a THC concentration of approximately 1 to 3 per cent, or 5 to 30 mg. Continued monitoring of the potency of street marijuana has revealed a steady increase in average potency from 1.5 per cent of THC in the late 1970s to about 3.0 per cent in recent years.[5]

Once absorbed, THC is rapidly metabolized by the lung and liver into a host of metabolites. THC is highly lipophilic and rapidly leaves the blood stream for deposit into lipoid tissues. The peak blood level of THC is reached within minutes of inhalation and then declines rapidly. It is important to note that blood levels of THC do not correlate well with psychoactive effects, since users maintain their intoxication levels after smoking for 2 to 3 hours, and blood levels of THC were shown to have peaked long before this period. Some cannabinoid metabolites, however, such as 11-nor-Δ-9-carboxylic acid, can be detected in the blood for several days after consumption through the use of sensitive radioimmunoassay methods. The lingering presence of these metabolites thus can present significant problems for the clinician, who may not always be able to determine through blood levels alone whether the patient is acutely intoxicated or has simply used the drug several days beforehand.[4]

ACUTE EFFECTS OF MARIJUANA

Almost all the physiologic and psychologic effects of a single use of marijuana can be predicted by dose. As noted, an average street dose or marijuana joint can contain anywhere from 5 to 30 mg of THC, thus making accurate dose determination in the intoxicated patient more difficult than in the experimental setting. However, though the terms *low* dose and *high* dose are difficult to define, most effects can be reproduced in normal healthy volunteers if they are given the same low or high dose by the same route of administration.

Acute Cardiovascular Effects

It has been well established that sinus tachycardia occurs after administration of THC. This tachycardia is very reproducible and is clearly related to the dose of the drug. Marijuana may produce orthostatic hypotension at higher dosages. Electrocardiographic changes in intoxicated individuals have shown nonspecific ST-T changes as well as occasional premature ventricular contractions. The electrocardiographic changes, however, have not been easily reproduced and seem to be subject dependent. The effects on patients who have pre-existing angina pectoris can be harmful, since exercise performance in these individuals was reported to be significantly decreased following administration of marijuana. Clearly, the increased heart rate, blood pressure changes, and apparent increase in myocardial oxygen demand certainly can add to a patient's already compromised cardiovascular system. The mechanism of action for the cardiovascular effects has been shown to be primarily stimulation of the autonomic nervous system with involvement of both the parasympathetic and sympathetic pathways. No long-term cardiovascular effects have been described to date.

Respiratory Effects

Since inhalation of marijuana is the prevalent mode of administration in the United States today, the effects of the drug on the respiratory tract are of major concern. Marijuana smoke, like tobacco smoke, has a high content of particulate matter, or tar. When this matter is inhaled deeply into the lungs, it appears to produce effects at both the anatomic and cellular levels. Although these effects may occur after a single use, the primary effects are seen following subacute or chronic administration. Following acute inhalation of marijuana, bronchodilatation has been demonstrated in both normal and asthmatic patients. Additionally, following one-time administration by inhalation, the clinician may see rhinitis, pharyngitis, and hoarseness. These symptoms, however, generally occur along with an acute bronchitis-laryngitis following chronic or subacute usage.

Psychologic and Neurologic Effects

Certainly marijuana's effects on central nervous system functions such as behavior, cognition, perception, and performance have been extremely important issues for research over the years. It is important to understand the mind-altering qualities of this drug that have made it such a popular recreational drug in our society. Additionally, it is important to recognize and understand the drug's effects on cognition and performance in intoxicated individuals, particularly in social settings or situations requiring accurate psychomotor functioning, that is, on the job, in the classroom, driving on the highway. It is also extremely important to know whether or not the use of this drug over a long period of time could lead to long-term mental disabilities that might have far-reaching effects on our sociomedical system.

In the acute state, it appears that the mood-altering effects of marijuana are in fact dose dependent. Intoxicated individuals who consume low to moderate dosages of the drug generally report a feeling of well-being or euphoria, a dreamlike state, a state of pleasant relaxation, an alteration of time and space perception, and a heightening of the senses; for example, better olfaction and clearer perception of music. In addition, they may experience a loss of short-term memory and an inability to perform complex psychologic or motor tasks. In some users, or in users who inadvertently take too large a dose, symptoms may range from mild anxiety to paranoid behavior to acute psychosis, with problems in dealing with reality and obsessional thought content characterized by delusions, hallucinations, illusions, and bizarre behavior.

Cognitive functioning such as speaking and problem-solving also seem to be affected by marijuana use. These cognitive changes are apparently related not only to the dosage of the drug but also to the complexity of the task or the problem to be solved as well as the individual's familiarity with the given task. Marijuana users, while intoxicated, frequently have problems with fluency of speech and organization of thought. Marijuana has been shown to interfere with short-term memory, and this dysfunction is thought to be a major cause of poor cognitive performance while under marijuana intoxication. In addition, it appears that material and facts learned while intoxicated are less well recalled than the same material learned in a nondrug state. This finding, of course, may have a significant impact on the performance of students or individuals in work or job-training situations.

Complex Motor Functions

Complex motor functions are also impaired while individuals are in the intoxicated state. There may be far-reaching consequences for society as well as for the practicing clinician in marijuana's effect on the important tasks of driving automobiles and flying airplanes. These two activities are clearly impaired during acute intoxication with the drug. Of most importance is the fact that some performance parameters continue to be impaired even several hours after the subject no longer feels high. Motor performance impairment is additionally affected by the common combination of marijuana with alcohol. This combination is a tremendous challenge for the practicing clinician, who may see individuals with altered behavior involved in motor vehicle accidents. The behavior may be secondary to the trauma itself or to alcohol use, but, given the prevalence of marijuana use in our society today, the clinician should consider marijuana intoxication as another potential factor in the patient's altered state.

CHRONIC EFFECTS

As noted, the effects of marijuana on human subjects after subacute or chronic usage are most controversial. When one examines the difficulties of a research design investigating the drug's effects on human subjects, it is not difficult to see why so much controversy and contradiction exist. The majority of the chronic studies done with marijuana first identified chronic users and then measured physiologic and psychologic parameters compared with nonmarijuana-smoking control subjects. Obviously, unless gross physiologic or psychologic changes occurred, more subtle changes would not be noted nor be subject to researcher interpretation.

In the late 1970s several studies were conducted with chronic smokers who were maintained in a controlled setting for a period of weeks. These studies seem to have demonstrated less controversial and more reproducible data than do the epidemiologic cross-sectional medical studies on chronic users of the drug. In the early 1970s, when serious concerns about the health consequences of chronic heavy use of marijuana were first raised, there were no suitable user populations in the United States, so populations in other countries such as Jamaica, Greece, and Costa Rica, where chronic heavy use of cannabis has a much longer history, were selected for cross-sectional studies. The research from these three studies has been extensively discussed in Marijuana and Health Reports[6a] and subsequently published.[7–9] The following summary of chronic effects provides a critical overview of the potential health consequences as currently known, based on these and other, more recent clinical studies.

Chronic Pulmonary Effects

Because marijuana is typically smoked, its possible adverse effects on the lung and pulmonary function have long been of concern. If the public health experience with tobacco smoking can be considered a precedent for the pulmonary consequences of chronic inhalation of tar-containing material, we could expect the development of pathology, such as emphysema or cancer of the lung, in the cannabis user population. Thus far there is no direct evidence that smoking marijuana correlates with lung cancer. The American experience has been too brief for this to be a likely outcome. Nevertheless, there is good reason for concern about the possibility of pulmonary cancer resulting from extended use over several decades. Like tobacco smoke residuals, so-called tar cannabis residuals, when applied to the skin of experimental animals, have been shown to be tumor producing. Analysis of marijuana smoke also has revealed large amounts of cancer-producing hydrocarbons. For example, benzopyrene, a known cancer-producing chemical found in tobacco smoke, has been reported to be 70 per cent more abundant in marijuana smoke than in tobacco.[6]

Several clinical studies of human users have reported such symptoms as laryngitis, cough, hoarseness, bronchitis, and cellular change in chronic marijuana smokers, which resemble symptoms found in heavy tobacco smokers. In one study, of American soldiers stationed in Europe, these symptoms were serious enough to cause the chronic hashish user to seek medical treatment.[10] Although studies of small numbers of chronic cannabis users in Jamaica,[7] Greece,[8] and Costa Rica[9] found no evidence of lung pathology, this result may have been due to the fact that traditional users in those countries do not deeply inhale cannabis smoke and retain it in their lungs as do American users.

Very recently a research group at the University of California in Los Angeles has published a number of reports on the current results of their longitudinal studies of lung function in demographically comparable groups selected from a sample of 279 heavy, habitual marijuana smokers and a group of control nonsmokers of marijuana (including subgroups of tobacco smokers).[11–13] Results of the initial testing of participants indicated that daily smoking of marijuana was associated with physiologic and symptomatic evidence of large airways disease, whereas regular tobacco smoking affects mainly the smaller airways and the alveolated regions of the lung.[11] In follow-up testing, after a 2- to 3-year hiatus, the group succeeded in re-examining approximately half of their original cohort. Most of the re-examined participants remained in their original smoking category. Considering only those participants who did not change their smoking status, chronic respiratory symptoms remained significantly more prevalent among continuing smokers of marijuana and/or tobacco than among nonsmokers. Although the frequency of reported symptoms tended to decline slightly among the smokers of marijuana or tobacco alone, respiratory symptom prevalence tended to increase among the dual smokers of both marijuana and tobacco.

Analysis of lung function data in the retested subjects who retained their original smoking status indicated a continuing or worsening abnormality in measures of small airways function and diffusing capacity in tobacco smokers, including those who also smoked marijuana, and an increasingly high frequency of abnormalities in tests of large airways function among smokers of marijuana alone or with tobacco. These results support previous findings from an analysis of cross-sectional data[12] of a negative impact of tobacco (but not marijuana alone) mainly on small airways and alveolar function, and of marijuana (but not tobacco) predominantly on large airways function. Thus, the longitudinal data suggest an additive effect of marijuana plus tobacco, at least with respect to symptom prevalence, that was not apparent from the cross-sectional findings alone.

Fiberoptic bronchoscopy, performed in a subsample of 32 subjects, revealed airway hyperemia and other visible abnormalities in 29 subjects (91 per cent) in the three smoking groups, unlike the unremarkable findings in the nonsmoking control group.[13] Light microscopy showed two or more histopathologic changes in the bronchial epithelium of all smokers regardless of the substance smoked. Squamous metaplasia was observed in all subjects smoking both marijuana and tobacco, a prevalence that was significantly different from that in any of the other groups of subjects. Hyperplasia of basal and goblet cells and cellular disorganization were more prevalent in the marijuana users than in the respective control subjects. A direct relationship between cumulative marijuana use and bronchoscopic and histopathologic changes was not apparent in this relatively small study sample.

In summary, the total body of clinical and experimental evidence accumulated to date appears to indicate that relatively young, habitual, heavy marijuana smokers have a high prevalence of pulmonary symptoms associated with abnormal airway appearance and histologic alterations, regardless of concomitant tobacco smoking. Since marijuana users often also smoke tobacco, and the combination appears to place an additive burden on the pulmonary system, the long-term consequences of this practice may be more ominous than previously thought. These long-term consequences, however, remain to be established by additional studies.

Hormonal and Reproductive Effects

Effects on reproduction have been attributed to marijuana as far back as the earliest cannabis commission's scientific report, that of the Indian Hemp Drugs Commission of 1894.[47] In recent years, in a few experiments researchers have attempted to study marijuana's effects on the endocrine system and on reproductive functions. Some have found a decrease in male levels of serum testosterone correlated with heavy marijuana use, although several others have not. One explanation for this discrepancy in experimental findings is that, after one smokes marijuana, the temporarily depressed levels of testosterone may rapidly return to more usual levels. Depending on the time schedule in which sampling is done, the effects may be missed. Even when testosterone decreases have been found, the levels have been within normal limits. Whether more persistent, chronic use of marijuana might result in permanently depressed levels of serum testosterone is not known at this time.

Two studies of the semen of male chronic users of marijuana have found abnormalities in count, motility, and structural characteristics of the sperm examined.[14, 15] In one of these experiments, the semen of 16 healthy young men smoking marijuana under controlled conditions was studied. The levels of use, while high—8 to 20 joints per day—were comparable to those of other very heavy users in the general population. Decreases in sperm count and motility were found, together with evidence of structural spermatozoal abnormalities. A second study, of Greek chronic users, also found structural abnormalities in sperm that were associated with heavy use.[15] Although the clinical implications of these findings are by no means certain, decreased fertility might well result, especially in those of already marginal fertility. In the more controlled laboratory study, there was an apparent gradual return to normal function when marijuana use was discontinued.[14] To date, there have been no published reports relating abnormal offspring to the father's marijuana use. Whether or not alterations in reproductive function might have greater significance for the developing child or adolescent who uses marijuana is not known at this time, although this is a concern, since the younger user is probably more vulnerable during his physiologic development.

It is now generally believed that the effects of cannabinoids on the hormones that modulate the female reproductive process originate within the brain as a result of changes in such neurotransmitters as dopamine, norepinephrine, and serotonin. In animals there is good evidence that THC can suppress production of gonadotropin-releasing hormone in the hypothalamus with consequent decrease in pituitary and ovarian sex hormones. These changes, again, seem to be transitory: Tolerance was shown to develop to these hormonal changes on continuing administration of THC, and the effects also seem to be reversible when cannabis use is discontinued.[5] Data on the effects of cannabis use in human females are sparse. What data have been published are inconclusive, possibly for reasons of reversibility and tolerance as mentioned above. Still, many questions remain regarding the long-term consequences of use, especially during sensitive developmental phases such as adolescence.

Pregnancy and Fetal Development

The effects of maternal marijuana use on fetal development and the outcome of pregnancy are difficult to study because these effects are complicated by such variables as nutrition, alcohol, tobacco, other drug use, socioeconomic status, and so on, which also affect fetal health. In order to determine marijuana's effect, these variables must be equalized or controlled. Large numbers of mother/child pairs are necessary if disorders that are infrequent are to be studied.

Three studies have examined samples of sufficient size to control adequately for confounding effects. Hingston et al[16, 17] studied 1690 mother/child pairs, Gibson et al[18] sampled 7301 births, and the largest study to date, by Linn et al[19] involved 12,716 mothers and their newborn babies. The general conclusions from these studies were that marijuana users were more likely than nonusers to have had an unplanned pregnancy, premature labor, and abruptio placentae, and their children were more likely to have lower birth weight, congenital features compatible with fetal alcohol syndrome (FAS), or some other major malformation. Marijuana use was a better predictor for FAS than alcohol use in these studies. The investigators noted that tobacco and marijuana smoking frequently occur with alcohol and other drug abuse in the same women. Therefore, some of the adverse effects on fetal development attributed to maternal drinking or smoking may be due to an interaction with marijuana and other psychoactive substances. When a number of these toxic substances are consumed together, their toxic effects on the fetus may be additive.

An interesting and important question is what happens to these babies as they grow up. One study[20] found that newborn nervous system alterations, measured by standardized techniques to indicate subtle qualitative and quantitative differences in behavior in babies born to regular maternal marijuana users, apparently are not manifested by poorer performance on cognitive and motor tests after 1½ and 2 years of age. Whether this means that neurologic disturbances present at birth are transient or whether the tests used at 1½ to 2 years of age are less sensitive to marijuana-related effects is unknown.

Marijuana and the Immune System

The effect of marijuana on the immune system is another controversial area in which clinical evidence that users have decreased resistance to infection remains inconclusive. The question is of particular importance for two reasons. First, since THC is now approved by the FDA for the treatment of nausea resulting from cancer chemotherapy, and since cancer chemotherapeutic chemicals are themselves severely immunosuppressive, any additional THC-induced immunosuppression would be very undesirable. Second, in view of the prevalence of AIDS infection in the drug-abusing population, a question can be raised about the potential contribution of an immunosuppressive effect of marijuana on the spread of this virus, especially in multidrug users. These considerations have spurred renewed interest in exploring the effects of THC on various components of the immune system using various animal models.

Friedman and his group reported on the in vitro and in vivo suppressive effects of THC on interferon production of murine spleen cells.[21, 22] They also demonstrated suppression of human natural killer (NK) cell activity by THC.[23] The importance of NK cells in host defenses against tumor cells and microbial infections is recognized. Another study, using guinea pigs, has found that THC decreases host resistance to herpes simplex virus type 2. This decrease occurs in a dose-dependent fashion using amounts of THC equivalent to human consumption levels.[24] Still another group, utilizing cell culture studies, found that THC as well as some of the other cannabinoids stimulate the maturation of key immune system cells called monocytes but that this maturation is defective.[25] Cannabinoids seem to induce the expression of certain maturation-marker proteins, but the cells do not exhibit a mature monocytic morphology and produce aberrant proteins that seem to block transition of the cells from an intermediate to a more advanced state of maturation. The possible role of these effects in alteration of the normal immune response in humans remains to be explored.

Psychopathology

The most common adverse psychologic reaction of marijuana use is an exaggeration of the more usual marijuana response in which the individual loses perspective (i.e., the realization that what she or he is experiencing is a transient drug-induced distortion of reality) and becomes acutely anxious. This reaction appears to be more common in relatively inexperienced users, although unexpectedly higher doses of the drug (e.g., as with a more potent variety of marijuana) can cause such a response even in more experienced users. The symptoms generally respond to authoritative assurance and diminish in a few hours as the immediate effects of acute intoxication recede. An acute brain syndrome associated with cannabis intoxication, including such features as clouding of mental processes, disorientation, confusion, and marked memory impairment, has been reported.[26] Other cannabinoid-induced symptoms may include severe panic and anxiety states, paranoia, depression, personality changes, confusional states, and psychoses, which are indistinguishable from classic psychiatric syndromes unless the drug-induced etiology is known. The correct diagnosis often cannot and will not be made by physicians and psychiatrists unless they keep in mind this possibility and actively pursue verification by asking direct questions and following up with accurate blood and urine testing.[27]

Marijuana "flashbacks"—spontaneous recurrences of feelings and perceptions similar to those produced by the drug itself—have been reported.[28] A survey of United States Army users of marijuana found that flashbacks occurred in both frequent and infrequent users and were not necessarily related to a history of lysergic acid diethylamide (LSD) use. Such experiences may range from the quite vivid recreation of a drug-related experience to a mild evocation of a previous experience. The origin of such experiences is uncertain, but those who have had them typically require little or no treatment. Although some patients reporting flashbacks had their initial "bad trip" on drugs other than marijuana, the flashback reaction of the disturbing aspects of the original experience occurred following alcohol or marijuana use. Although there is no specific antidote for the treatment of these experiences, benzodiazepines have been useful to calm patients' anxiety.[29]

Tolerance and Dependence

Tolerance to cannabis, that is, a diminished physiologic and psychologic response to a given repeated drug dose, is now well substantiated. Tolerance development originally was suspected because experienced overseas users were able to use large quantities of the drug that would have been toxic to United States users, who were accustomed to smaller amounts. Carefully conducted studies with known doses of marijuana or THC leave little question that tolerance develops with prolonged use.[30]

The term *cannabis dependence* has often been used in an imprecise way, with meanings ranging from a vague desire to continue use of the substance if it is available, to the manifestation of physical withdrawal symptoms following discontinuance. Defining *dependence* as the experiencing of definite physical symptoms (such as irritability, restlessness, sleep disturbance, nausea, and diarrhea) following withdrawal of the drug, experimental evidence indicates that such symptoms can occur under conditions of extremely heavy administration on a research ward. At first, this evidence appeared as a theoretical curiosity, but in recent years, with the increasing potency of street marijuana and hashish, clinical reports indicate that it can also happen in real life.[31, 32]

EFFECTS OF MARIJUANA IN COMBINATION WITH ALCOHOL AND OTHER DRUGS

Since marijuana is so commonly used with alcohol and other drugs, the combined effects of these drugs have potentially important implications. Given the extremely wide range of possible doses and interactions, it is not surprising that our present knowledge is still quite limited, even of the most common combination, alcohol and marijuana. Some of the potential dangers to the outcome of pregnancy by the mother's use of both marijuana and alcohol have been alluded to earlier. In another study of 97 regular users of both drugs it was found that alcohol use preceded marijuana use by 3 years.[33] Both drugs were used in social situations, with about 10 per cent of users meeting criteria for alcoholism and the same proportion for severe marijuana abuse. Significant problems associated with alcohol included blackouts (20 per cent) and self reports of overuse (27 per cent). The significant complaints about marijuana were panic reactions (22 per cent) and feeling addicted (14 per cent). Six per cent of those interviewed reported traffic arrests while drinking compared to 15 per cent who were arrested for driving offenses while using marijuana.

A related issue is the extent to which marijuana use might displace alcohol use were both drugs equally available. Although some marijuana users in the 1960s were ideologically opposed to alcohol, it now appears that the overall as well as simultaneous use of both drugs has generally increased. Although it is not possible to be certain what would occur under conditions of equal availability, no indications exist that increased marijuana use among teenagers and young adults has resulted in decreased alcohol use; in fact, a positive correlation was observed: Those using marijuana heavily were more likely to use alcohol than those who either did not use it or used it less frequently. One large-scale longitudinal study of children from elementary to high school age has found that the early use of alcohol (and tobacco) is commoner in those who also begin marijuana use early or use it more regularly and heavily.[34] In one study of marijuana use in young men conducted in a closed experimental ward setting, marijuana smoking increased regardless of the availability of alcohol, although, conversely, alcohol use decreased when marijuana was available.[35] Thus the larger question of what would happen in American culture were marijuana more freely available cannot readily be answered. It might well depend on the kinds of informal social attitudes and controls that develop among users.

There have been few human studies of the interactive effects of marijuana with drugs other than alcohol. However, limited evidence suggests that such interactions may be significant. A study in which high doses of THC were given to young adult men indicates that chronic marijuana use may affect the persistence of barbiturates in the body as well as their rate of absorption.[36] Only limited studies have been done thus far on the combined use of amphetamines and marijuana in humans. One study found that simultaneous use resulted in an increase in the intensity and duration of the subjective high greater than that produced by the use of either alone.[37] Street marijuana is frequently adulterated (sprinkled or sprayed) with phencyclidine (PCP) and sometimes sold without special warnings. Severe toxic reactions may result from the use of such material, and attending physicians should be aware of this possibility.[29] In a report from the emergency department of a metropolitan teaching hospital in Australia toxicologic analysis of biologic specimens from patients admitted for self-poisoning revealed a prevalence of multidrug use.[38] Although barbiturates and benzodiazepines were found in about half of the cases, alcohol with other drugs (44 per cent) and cannabinoids with other drugs (32 per cent) were the next most frequent findings. Importantly, discrepancies between the purported drug consumption and the toxicologic results were frequent; complete agreement occurred in only 35 per cent of cases. Marijuana contaminated with paraquat is discussed in Chapter 69.

DIAGNOSIS AND TREATMENT

The clinical features of acute intoxication with marijuana, either administered orally or after smoking, are very nondescript. The signs of hyperemia of the conjunctivae, irritation of mucous membranes of the throat and nose (see Chapter 1), and sinus tachycardia, coupled with seeming trouble with short-term memory and its effects on continuity of conversation, fluency of speech, and performance of complex tasks, may be the only clues to marijuana use. As stated, acute panic and anxiety reactions as well as an acute toxic psychosis with hallucinations, delusions, illusions, and agitation are seen primarily in inexperienced users or in individuals who take too high a dose. These adverse reactions can generally be managed with a quiet, supportive, and protective environment, reassurance, and, if needed, mild sedation with drugs such as the benzodiazepines. The symptoms from these episodes generally subside within hours. In patients who have a genotype for schizophrenia, even a modest dose of marijuana sometimes can produce a schizophrenic type of psychosis that may be difficult to distinguish from acute toxic psychosis. In these individuals, the usual drug and support therapies for schizophrenia are needed.

In general, since the clinical presentation of acute marijuana intoxication is so subtle and its use so prevalent, clinicians should suspect use of this drug when confronted with individuals who seem to have problems with cognitive functions such as thinking, speaking, and attention span and have difficulty with complex tasks such as driving. Although assay techniques are available to determine marijuana use, these tests are not practical in the acute clinical situation of intoxication because interpretation is hampered by poor correlation between blood levels and clinical effects and continued prolonged elimination of the drug, making determination of the exact time of use difficult.

These assays, however, can be useful in identifying a user population even if they are not helpful in determining effects from acute intoxication. Early detection through urine testing has a role in identifying a potential source of problems in adolescents, such as diminished school performance, memory or concentration impairment, or the frequent "amotivational state" that develops in chronic users. It may also help to address the multitude of family problems related to drug abuse, thereby avoiding the gross family collapse that may otherwise develop. Until marijuana is clearly viewed as a potentially dangerous drug and early detection strategies are developed, including urine testing and parental awareness, treatment will occur only after a major crisis.[39]

Under the best circumstances, treatment is a difficult process, and prevention should be the treatment of first choice. Psychotherapy for this problem is often characterized by premature termination of attendance and relapse. A 12-step Alcoholics Anonymous model is often quite helpful for adolescent marijuana users and alcoholics. Positive behavior is reinforced while negative behaviors and attitudes are discouraged in a peer-oriented treatment milieu.[39]

THERAPEUTIC ASPECTS

In many parts of the world, cannabis has been and is still used as a folk medicine. The modern phase of therapeutic use of cannabis began about 140 years ago when O'Shaughnessy reported on its effectiveness as an analgesic and anticonvulsant.[46] At about the same time, others described marijuana's use in the treatment of psychiatric illnesses and some favorable results in producing sleep and enhancing appetite without causing physical addiction. It was also tried as a treatment for opium addiction, chronic alcholism, delirium tremens, and a large variety of painful disorders. The drawbacks that historically accompanied therapeutic trials of cannabis centered on the highly variable content of THC, its loss of potency while standing on pharmacy shelves, and its variable gastrointestinal absorption. Therefore, when aspirin, barbiturates, and other synthetic analgesics and sedatives became available, the medical use of extracted *Cannabis indica* faded. The Marijuana Tax Act of 1937 was the final blow that eliminated it from medical practice.

In past decades, however, not only has THC been synthesized but also researchers now have available standardized cigarettes and capsules with specific concentrations of the drug. These advances, plus public and scientific interest in the nature of marijuana's effects on human beings, have generated renewed activity in the therapeutic potential of this substance. In the past 15 years, preclinical and clinical trials have been used to investigate marijuana's efficacy as a potential analgesic and sedative-hypnotic, among other uses.[3, 40] However, the variability of the therapeutic response in limited studies evaluating the efficacy of this drug combined with the undesirable side effects and the adequacy of already marketed drugs for these purposes do not support enthusiasm for future trials.[41] Attempts to utilize the demonstrated bronchodilatory effects for the treatment of asthma and the ocular hypotensive effects for the treatment of glaucoma have largely been abandoned because of psychotomimetic side effects and because of the availability of equally effective alternative drugs for these indications.

Antiemetic Effect

THC and some of its synthetic analogues such as nabilone, Levonantradol, and Nabitan have been tested in mostly open clinical trials for antiemetic potency on cancer patients receiving chemotherapy and found to be effective in alleviating the invariable side effects of nausea and vomiting.[42] In more than 14 controlled studies THC was found to be at least as useful or superior to certain marketed drugs (such as prochlorperazine) in standard use for controlling these symptoms in cancer patients. Side effects of THC itself may still be a problem, but evidence for its efficacy for this treatment indication, especially in patients who are not responding to other drugs, has convinced the Food and Drug Administration (FDA) to make THC capsules legally available for prescription under the trade name Marinol (trademark of Unimed).[41] However, because of its high liability for abuse, prescription of THC capsules is controlled as a Schedule II drug under the Controlled Substances Act and is limited to the amount necessary for a single cycle of chemotherapy (i.e., a few days).

Anticonvulsant Effect

Marijuana's therapeutic potential as an anticonvulsant has sparked interest since a study in the 1940s showed that five retarded children, poorly controlled on conventional anticonvulsant medication, were improved after the use of cannabis.[43] Relatively recently, cannabidiol, a natural component of marijuana that has practically no marijuana-like psychoactivity, has proved to have anticonvulsant activity in animals.[44] In a clinical trial in 15 patients, cannabidiol was reported to be effective in controlling seizures.[45] Further confirmation of these results and more clinical studies will no doubt be required before cannabidiol's place in the treatment of epilepsy can be judged. Because this cannabinoid has little psychoactivity and low toxicity, its use for therapeutic purposes appears to be very promising.

References

1. Gaoni Y, Mechoulam R: Isolation, structure, and partial synthesis of an active constituent of hashish. J Am Chem Soc *86*:1646–1647, 1964.
2. Petrzilka T, Sikemeier C: Über Inhaltsstoffe des Haschisch. Helv Chim Acta *50*:1416–1419, 2111–2113, 1967.
3. Braude MC, Szara S (eds): Pharmacology of Marihuana. New York, Raven Press, 1976.
4. Hollister LE: Health aspects of cannabis. Pharmacol Rev *38*:1–20, 1986.
5. Secretary, Department of Health and Human Services: Drug Abuse and Drug Abuse Research. Second Triennial Report to Congress. DHHS Publ. No. (ADM)87–1486, Rockville, MD, 1987.
6. Peterson RC (ed): Marijuana Research Findings: 1980. NIDA Research Monograph 31. National Institute on Drug Abuse. Washington, DC, US Government Printing Office, 1980.

6a. Marijuana and Health; Fourth Report to the U.S. Congress. From the Secretary of Health, Education, and Welfare 1974. DHEW Publication No. (ADM) 75–181. Washington, DC, 1974.

7. Rubin V, Comitas L: Ganja in Jamaica. The Effects of Marihuana. New York, Anchor/Doubleday, 1976.
8. Stefanis C, Dornbush R, Fink M: Hashish: Studies of Long-term Use. New York, Raven Press, 1977.
9. Carter WE (ed): Cannabis in Costa Rica: A Study of Chronic Marihuana Use. Philadelphia, Institute for the Study of Human Issues, 1980.
10. Tennant FS: Histopathologic and clinical abnormalities of the respiratory system in chronic hashish smokers. Substance Alcohol Actions/Misuse *1*:93–99, 1980.
11. Tashkin DP, Coulson AH, Clark VA, Simmons M, Bourque LB, Duann S, Gong H: Respiratory symptoms and lung function in habitual heavy smokers of marijuana alone, smokers of marijuana and to-

bacco, smokers of tobacco alone, and nonsmokers. Am Rev Respir Dis *135:*209–216, 1987.
12. Tashkin DP, Calvarese BM, Simmons MS, Shapiro BJ: Respiratory status of seventy-four habitual marijuana smokers. Chest *78:*699–706, 1980.
13. Gong H, Fligiel S, Tashkin DP, Barbers RG: Tracheobronchial changes in habitual, heavy smokers of marijuana with and without tobacco. Am Rev Respir Dis *136:*142–149, 1987.
14. Hembree WC, Nahas GG, Zeidenberg P, Huang HFS: Changes in human spermatozoa associated with high dose marihuana smoking. *In* Nahas GG, Paton WDM (eds): Marihuana: Biological Effects. New York, Pergamon Press, 1979, pp 429–439.
15. Issidorides MR: Observations in chronic hashish users: Nuclear aberrations in blood and sperm and abnormal acrosomes in spermatozoa. *In* Nahas GG, Paton WDM (eds): Marihuana: Biological Effects. New York, Pergamon Press, 1979, pp 377–388.
16. Hingston R, Alpert J, Day N, Darling E, Kaynes H, Morelock S, Oppenheimer E, Zuckerman B: Effects of maternal drinking and marijuana use on fetal growth and development. Pediatrics *70:*539, 1982.
17. Hingston R, Zuckerman B, Frank DS, Kaynes H, Sorenson JR, Mitchell J: Effects on fetal development of maternal marijuana use during pregnancy. *In* Harvey DJ (ed): Marijuana '84; Proceedings of the Oxford Symposium on Marijuana. Oxford, IRL Press, 1984.
18. Gibson GT, Bayhurst PA, Colley DP: Maternal alcohol, tobacco and cannabis consumption on the outcome of pregnancy. Aust NZ Obstet Gynecol *23:*16–19, 1983.
19. Linn S, Schoenbaum SC, Monson RR, Rosner R, Stubblefield PC, Ryan KJ: The association of marijuana use with outcome of pregnancy. Am J Public Health *73:*1161–1164, 1983.
20. Fried PA, Makin JE: Neonatal behavioural correlates of prenatal exposure to marihuana, cigarettes and alcohol in a low risk population. Neurotoxicol Teratol *9:*1–7, 1987.
21. Friedman M, Cepero ML, Klein T, Friedman H: Suppressive effect of delta-9-tetrahydrocannabinol in vitro on phagocytosis by murine macrophages. Proc Soc Exp Biol Med *182:*225–228, 1986.
22. Blanchard DK, Newton C, Klein TW, Stewart WE 2d, Friedman H: In vitro and in vivo suppressive effects of delta-9-tetrahydrocannabinol on interferon production by murine spleen cells. Int J Immunopharmacol *8:*819–824, 1986.
23. Specter SC, Klein TW, Newton C, Mondragon M, Widen R, Friedman J: Marijuana effects on immunity: Suppression of human natural killer cell activity of delta-9-tetrahydrocannabinol. Int J Immunopharmacol *8:*741–745, 1986.
24. Cabral GA, Mishkin EM, Marciano-Cabral F, Coleman P, Harris L, Munson JH: Effect of delta-9-tetrahydrocannabinol on herpes simplex virus type 2 vaginal infection in the guinea pig. Proc Soc Exp Biol Med *182:*181–186, 1986.
25. Murison G, Chubb CBH, Maeda S, Gemmell A, Huberman E: Cannabinoids induce incomplete maturation of cultured human leukemia cells. Proc Natl Acad Sci USA *84:*5414–5418, 1987.
26. Meyer RE: Psychiatric consequences of marihuana use: The state of evidence. *In* Tinklenberg JR (ed): Marihuana and Health Hazards: Methodological Issues in Current Research. New York, Academic Press, 1975, pp 133–152.
27. Estroff TW, Gold MS: Psychiatric presentations of marijuana abuse. Psychiatr Anns *16:*221–224, 1986.
28. Stanton MD, Mintz J, Franklin RM: Drug flashbacks, II. Some additional findings. Int J Addict *11:*53–69, 1976.
29. McCabe OL: Psychedelic drug crises: Toxicity and therapeutics. J Psychedelic Drugs *9:*107–114, 1977.
30. Jones RT, Benowitz N: The 30-day trip—Clinical studies of cannabis tolerance and dependence. *In* Braude MC, Szara S (eds): Pharmacology of Marihuana. New York, Raven Press, 1976, pp 627–642.
31. Weller RA, Halikas JA: Objective criteria for the diagnosis of marijuana abuse. J Nerv Ment Dis *168:*98–103, 1980.
32. Tennant FS: The clinical syndrome of marijuana dependence. Psychiatr Anns *16:*225–234, 1986.
33. Weller RA, Halikas JA, Moorse C: Alcohol and marijuana: Comparison of use and abuse in regular marijuana users. J Clin Psychiatry *45:*377–379, 1984.
34. Smith GM, Fogg CP: High school performance and behavior before and after initiation of illicit drug use. Fed Proc *36:*564, 1976.
35. Mello NK, Mendelson JH, Kuehnle JC, Sellers ML: Human polydrug use: Marijuana and alcohol. J Pharmacol Exp Ther *207:*922–935, 1978.
36. Benowitz NL, Jones RT: Effects of delta-9-tetrahydro-cannabinol on drug distribution and metabolism. Clin Pharmacol Ther *22:*259–268, 1977.
37. Evans MA, Martz R, Rodda BE, Lemberger L, Forney RB: Effects of marijuana-dextroamphetamine combination. Clin Pharmacol Ther *20:*350–358, 1976.
38. Ray JE, Reilly DK, Day RO: Drugs involved in self-poisoning: verification by toxicological analysis. Med J Aust *144:*455–457, 1986.
39. Gold MS, Washton AM, Dackis CA, Chatlos JC: New treatments for opiate and cocaine users: But what about marijuana? Psychiatr Anns *16:*206–213, 1986.
40. Hollister LE: Cannabis: Finally a therapeutic agent? Drug Alc Depend *11:*135–145, 1983.
41. Ungerleider JT, Andrysiak T: Therapeutic issues of marijuana and THC (tetrahydrocannabinol). Int J Addict *20:*691–699, 1985.
42. Razdan RK: Structure-activity relationships in cannabinoids. Pharmacol Rev *38:*75–149, 1986.
43. Davis JA, Ramsey HD: Antiepileptic action of marihuana active substance. Fed Proc *8:*284, 1949.
44. Karler R, Turkanis SA: The cannabinoids as potential antiepileptics. J Clin Pharmacol *21:*437S–448S, 1981.
45. Carlini EA, Cunha JM: Hypnotic and antiepileptic effects of cannabidiol. J Clin Pharmacol *21:*417S–427S, 1981.
46. O'Shaughnessy WB: On the preparation of Indian hemp and gunjah. Trans Med Phys Soc Bombay *8:*421–461, 1842.
47. Kalant OJ: Report of the Indian Hemp Drug Commission, 1839–94: A critical review. Int J Addict *7*(1):77–96, 1972.

CHAPTER 42

PHENCYCLIDINE AND THE HALLUCINOGENS

Suzanne M. Shepherd, M.D.
Andy S. Jagoda, M.D.

The man who comes back through the door in the wall will never be quite the same as the man who went out.

ALDOUS HUXLEY
DOORS OF PERCEPTION, 1954

The hallucinogens are a heterogeneous group of compounds that primarily cause altered cognitive and perceptual states that cannot otherwise be experienced. These drugs have been variously referred to as hallucinogens, psychotomimetics, psychedelics, pseudohallucinogens, dysleptics, and mind expanders. The lack of agreement in terminology results from the subjective nature of the experience caused by these agents.

Hallucinogens characteristically cause illusions or alterations in perception rather than true hallucinations or perceptions with no basis in reality. True hallucinogens are quite unusual. Table 42–1 lists the eight classes of hallucinogenic agents.

HISTORICAL AND EPIDEMIOLOGIC PERSPECTIVES

The earliest documented use of hallucinogenic agents dates back to 3500 BC. They were used primarily in medicine and in religious rituals. Twentieth century use of hallucinogens originated in 1938 when Albert Hofmann, working for Sandoz Laboratories in Basel, Switzerland, first synthesized lysergic acid diethylamide (LSD, so-called LSD-25 because it was the 25th compound in the lysergic amide series). The drug was initially studied for its oxytocic and hemostatic activity. Then on April 16, 1943, Dr. Hofmann accidentally ingested a minute but unknown quantity of D-LSD. He records, ". . . there surged upon me an uninterrupted stream of fantastic images of extraordinary plasticity and vividness and accompanied by an intense, kaleidoscope-like play of colors."[1] For the next 20 years LSD was used almost exclusively to study and treat diverse "mental illnesses." It was initially hoped that it would provide a model to study schizophrenia, but it soon became apparent that LSD did not alter ego function or reality testing or produce the characteristic auditory hallucinations.

In psychotherapeutics, LSD was touted as being useful in treating everything from neurosis to alcoholism to homosexuality. It was claimed to speed the process of bringing repressed material to the surface, to increase insight, and to help the subject experience difficult affects, conflicts, and impulse strivings. Indeed, in controlled therapeutic settings with select patient populations (i.e., those with well-developed, stable egos), LSD appeared to be a safe adjunct to psychotherapy. Despite numerous subjective claims, substantial evidence that hallucinogen use resulted in any measurable lasting personality, belief, value, attitude, or behavioral changes did not emerge.

Illicit use of LSD and other hallucinogens greatly accelerated in the 1960s, as segments of society began searching for pharmacologic means of gaining inner peace and experiencing "cosmic oneness." Use was spurred on by the writings of Carlos Castaneda, Aldous Huxley, and Timothy Leary. Leary wrote in 1964 ". . . A psychedelic experience is a journey to new realms of consciousness . . . [LSD] opens the mind, frees the nervous system of its ordinary patterns and structures . . . you must remember, too, that the experience is safe."[2] By January 1967, there were enough people involved in the psychedelic culture to bring together 40,000 in San Francisco for a "tribal be-in," which then evolved into the famous "Summer of Love."

Table 42–1. HALLUCINOGENS

COMPOUND	COMMON NAME OR ABBREVIATION	ESTIMATED HUMAN HALLUCINOGENIC DOSE
I. Lysergamides		
Lysergic acid amide	Morning glory seeds	200–300 seeds
Lysergic acid diethylamide	LSD	35 μg
II. Phenylalkylamines (PAA)		
A. Phenylisopropylamines		
2,5-dimethoxy-4-methyl amphetamine	DOM, STP	1–5 mg
2,5-dimethoxy-4-ethyl amphetamine	DOET	1–4 mg
2,5-dimethoxy-4-propyl amphetamine	DOPR	1–2 mg
3,4-methylenedioxymethamphetamine	MDMA, Ecstasy	75 mg
5-methoxy-3,4-methylenedioxyamphetamine	mmDA	30–50 mg
4-bromo-2,5-dimethoxyamphetamine	bromoDMA	0.7 mg
3,4-methylenedioxyamphetamine	mDA	70–225 mg
B. Phenethylamines		
3,4,5-trimethoxyphenethylamine	mescaline	300–500 mg
3,5-dimethoxy-4-ethoxyphenethylamine	escaline	40–80 mg
3,5-dimethoxy-4-propoxyphenethylamine	proscaline	40–80 mg
III. Indolealkylamines (IAA)		
A. Methyltryptamines		
methyltryptamine		30 mg
5-methoxy methyltryptamine		5 mg
B. *N,N*-Dimethyltryptamines		
5-methyldimethyltryptamine		
N,N-dimethyltryptamine	DMT	75–100 mg
4-hydroxydimethyltryptamine	psilocin	20 mg
4-phosphorodimethyltryptamine	psilocybin	12 mg
5 hydroxydimethyltryptamine	bufotenine	
C. *N*-Alkylated tryptamines		
N,N-diethyltryptamine	DET	
dipropyltryptamine	DPT	50–75 mg
diisopropyltryptamine	DiPT	50–100 mg
4-hydroxydiethyltryptamine		15 mg
5-methoxydiisopropyltryptamine		6–10 mg
IV. Cholinergic Antagonists		
Atropine		
JB 329	Ditran	
Scopolamine		
V. Arylcyclohexylamines		
1-(1-phenylcyclohexyl)piperidine	PCP	1–10 mg
2-(O-chlorophenyl)-2-(methylamino)cyclohexanone	Ketamine	
1-(1-phenylcyclohexyl)pyrrolidine	PHP	
1-piperidinocyclohexanecarbonitrile	PCC	
N-ethyl-1-phenylcyclohexylamine	PCE	
1-(1-[2-thienyl]cyclohexyl)piperidine	TCP	
VI. Cannabinoids		
delta-9-tetrahydrocannabinol	9-THC	5–20 mg
VII. Carbolines		
harmoline		
harmine		
VIII. Nutmeg		5–15 gm
myristicin		
elemicin		
eugenol		
geraniol		
safrol		

It was during the Summer of Love that phencyclidine, the PeaCe Pill (PCP), first arrived on the illicit drug scene. Its illicit use was initially short lived owing to the unpredictable and often negative experiences that occurred. Phencyclidine re-emerged as a drug of abuse in the early 1970s. Its cheap and easy synthesis made it affordable for large numbers of recreational users, who learned to titrate its effects by smoking. By the mid 1970s an estimated 7 million people had used PCP occasionally, and 1 million people used it at least once a week. In 1975 and 1976, phencyclidine-induced psychosis was the leading cause of new admissions to St. Elizabeth's mental health facility in Washington, DC.

Demand for variety in the hallucinogenic experience resulted in the emergence of a number of other hallucinogenic agents such as dimethyltryptamine (DMT) and 2,5-dimethoxy 4-methyl amphetamine (DOM). As the number of people using unknown amounts of substances marketed as hallucinogens increased, the number of reported adverse and occasionally catastrophic effects increased. Use of most hallucinogens peaked in the late 1960s, except for PCP, which peaked in the mid 1970s.

In 1970 the Comprehensive Drug Abuse Prevention and Control Act designated LSD, mescaline, peyote, DOM, and 3,4-methylenedioxyamphetamine (mDA) as Schedule I drugs. Under the law, manufacture, production, creation, or distribution of these drugs became punishable by imprisonment or fine. In 1978 phencyclidine was classified as a Schedule II drug; this ended legal production of the drug and imposed criminal penalties for its production and sale. In 1975, 11 per cent of high school seniors claimed to have used LSD at least once. In 1979, 10 per cent claimed such use. In 1986 only 7 per cent had tried LSD. These numbers must be viewed cautiously, however, because there are no accurate means of verifying actual drug consumption.

It was almost inevitable that with the continued use of illicit drugs there would be a resurgence of interest in hallucinogen use and abuse. A number of newer "designer drugs" in the phenylalkylamine (PAA) and indolealkylamine (IAA) categories have emerged that have not been scheduled, and illegal manufacture of hallucinogens that are already scheduled continues. The physician must understand the pharmacology and clinical presentation of the hallucinogen groups in order to recognize and manage exposures appropriately.

PHENCYCLIDINE (PCP)

The arylcyclohexylamines are atypical of the other hallucinogens because of their complicated stimulant, depressant, and analgesic properties. Phencyclidine (PCP, 1-(1-phenylcyclohexyl)piperidine) is the most studied and used arylcyclohexylamine and remains today one of the most common drugs of abuse (Fig. 42–1). Street names for phencyclidine include PCP, PeaCe Pill, angel dust, elephant or horse tranquilizer, rocket fuel, and crystal (Table 42–2).

Phencyclidine was discovered in 1926. In the late 1950s Parke Davis developed phencyclidine as a general anesthetic agent, marketed under the name Sernyl. Sernyl was promoted as a non-narcotic, nonbarbiturate anesthetic that did not produce respiratory depression. In 1958 Greifenstein described profound anesthesia in patients who maintained a wide awake appearance and partial orientation and termed this a "dissociative" agent.[3] In 1965 human use of Sernyl for anesthesia was discontinued owing to dysphoria, hallucinosis, and extreme agitation after anesthesia that developed in 15 to 20 per cent of patients and lasted up to 18 hours. Phencyclidine was reintroduced as Sernylan for veterinary anesthesia in 1967, at which time it also emerged as a drug of abuse in Haight-Ashbury.

PCP is cheaply and easily synthesized in clandestine drug kitchens from locally available chemicals. Synthesis involves the addition of piperidinocyclohexane carbonitrile to phenyl magnesium bromide. An initial investment of 75 dollars yields a pound of PCP, which has a potential street value of 20,000 dollars. Phencyclidine is illicitly substituted for many desirable but often unavailable drugs including Δq-tetrahydrocannabinol (THC), LSD, mescaline, psilocybin, mDA, Hawaiian woodrose, cocaine, and other psychedelic agents.[4, 5]

Phencyclidine is available on the street in a variety of forms, including powder, tablets, leaf mixture, rock crystal forms, and liquid. The actual PCP content varies considerably among those forms, powder being the most

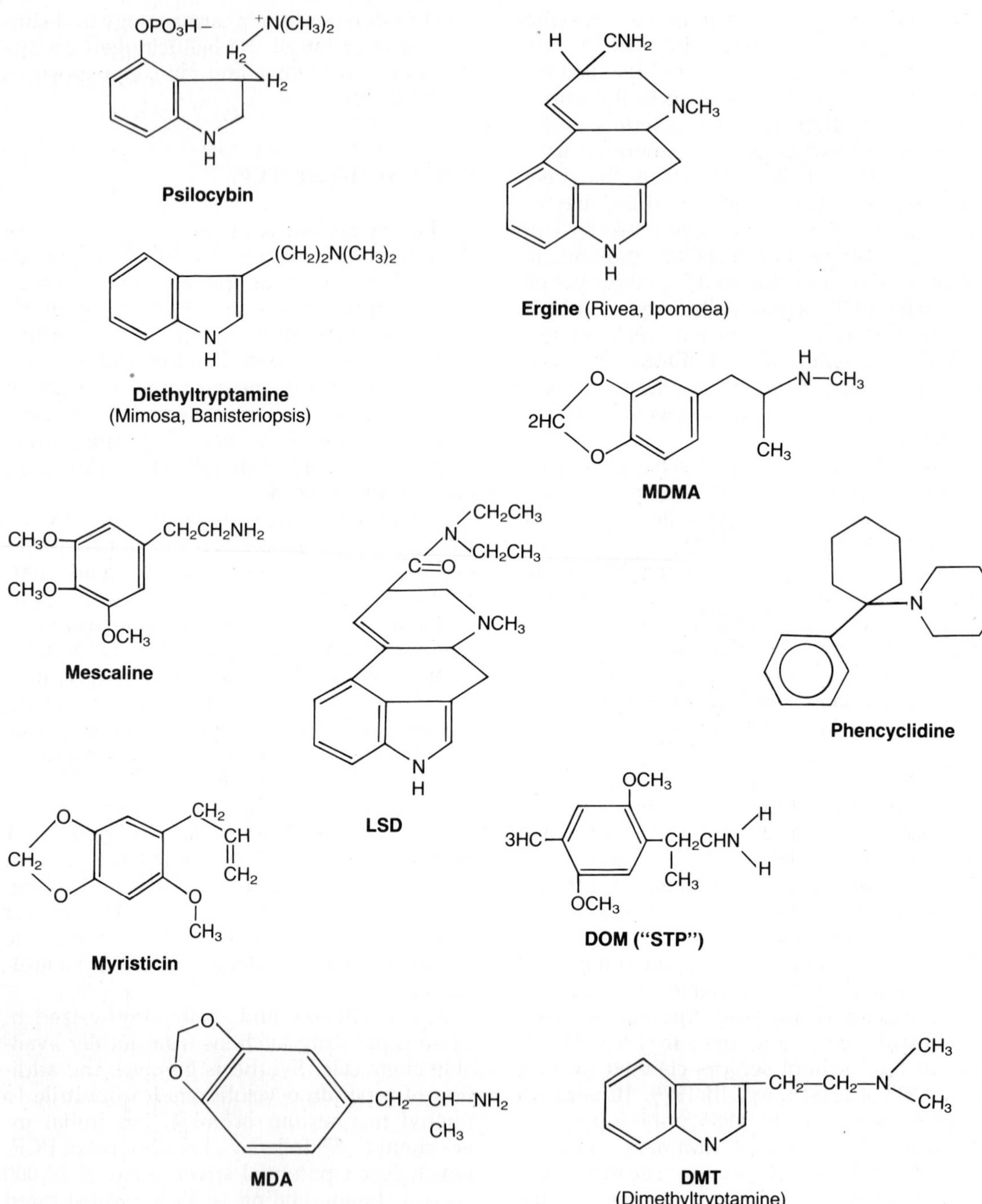

Figure 42–1. Chemical structures of hallucinogens and phencyclidine.

pure. The average dose in tablet form is 5 mg (range, 1 to 6 mg). Phencyclidine is sold sprinkled onto a variety of leafy mixtures (parsley, mint, oregano, tobacco) or rolled into a joint ("crystal joint" or "KJ") containing an average of 1 to 10 mg of PCP per joint. Chronic users may "dust" their joints with an additional 50 mg of powder. Although PCP is frequently reported to be smoked using marijuana as the leaf material ("supergrass"), this mixture is rarely sold on the street. Phencyclidine is also sold as mentholated cigarettes dipped into liquid PCP ("supercools").

Table 42–2. STREET NAMES FOR PHENCYCLIDINE

angel dust	embalming fluid	mint weed	soma
angel hair	goon	mist	stardust
angel mist	gorilla biscuits	monkey dust	supergrass
animal tranquilizer	hog	PCP	superkools
busy bee	hog dust	peace	superweed
Cadillac	horse tranquilizer	PeaCe Pill	surfer
CJ	jet fuel	peace weed	T
crystal	Kay Jay (or KJ)	pits	TAC
crystal joints	killer weed	rocket fuel	TIC
cyclones	kristal joint	scuffle	tranks
DOA	KW	Selma	whack
dust	magic mist	sheets	whacky weed
elephant tranquilizer	mint dew	Sherman	wobble weed
		snorts	zombie dust

(From Litovitz TL: Phencyclidine (PCP). *In* Haddad LM, Winchester JF (eds): Clinical Management of Poisoning and Drug Overdose. 1st ed. Philadelphia, WB Saunders, 1983, p 449.)

Phencyclidine is now most commonly smoked (by 72 per cent of users) or snorted (13 per cent). This behavior has greatly reduced the incidence of overdose. Smokers can self-titrate their exposure; higher exposures will incapacitate the user before a potentially lethal level of anesthesia is reached. In one study, 13 per cent of 1000 patients took phencyclidine pills, whereas intravenous use of phencyclidine occurred in only 1.6 per cent.[6] "Side smoke" is an interesting phenomenon described in pediatric intoxications, among law enforcement officials, and also in at least one reported accidental exposure in which a patient was intoxicated unintentionally when exposed to PCP-containing smoke vapors.[6, 7, 8]

Phencyclidine has more than 60 other psychoactive analogues. The five analogues most frequently used are ketamine, PCC (1-piperidinocyclohexanecarbonitrile), PCE (*N*-ethyl-1-phenylcyclohexylamine), TCP (1-(1-[2-thieny]cyclohexylpiperidine), and PHP (phenylcyclohexylpyrrolidine) (Fig. 42–2). *Ketamine* is the only analogue legally manufactured for human use. It is used clinically as a dissociative anesthetic in pediatrics. Ketamine is less potent, has a shorter duration of action, and produces seizures less frequently than phencyclidine. Ketamine is sold on the street as "green." *PCC* appears as a byproduct in badly synthesized batches of PCP. It is an unstable compound that degrades to piperidine; contaminated batches may be recognized by the fishy odor of piperidines. PCC in combination with PCP has been shown to potentiate its toxic and lethal effects, probably through generation of cyanide.[9] *PCE* is much more potent than PCP. It was available as a street drug for 10 years before its 1978 classification as a Schedule I drug. *TCP,* the thiophene analogue of PCP, produces similar but more intense effects than PCP. The effects of TCP are of shorter duration. TCP appeared on the street in 1972 and was classified as a Schedule I drug in 1975. *PHP,* the pyrrolidine analogue is as potent as PCP, is easily manufactured, but is only weakly reactive on radioimmunoassay (RIA) and is not detected by many commonly used drug screening systems. These factors contribute to its popularity and frequent substitution for PCP. PHP was classified as a Schedule I drug in 1978.[4, 5]

PHARMACOLOGY

Phencyclidine is a stable, water- and alcohol-soluble, white crystalline solid. It is a tertiary amine with a molecular weight of 243. The three-ring structure appears to be essential for reactivity on RIA analysis. Phencyclidine has a high lipid water partition coefficient and a pK_a of 8.5; it acts as a weak base with pH-dependent urinary excretion.

The onset of effect occurs in 30 to 60 minutes when ingested and in 2 to 5 minutes when smoked. In smokers, peak effect is noted in 15 to 30 minutes, and significant effects are noted for 4 to 6 hours. Effects resolve in 24 to 48 hours. Up to half the phencyclidine present in a burning cigarette may be converted to the relatively inactive pyrrolysis product phenylcyclohexene.

Phencyclidine is highly tissue distributed. Misra et al[11] estimated brain levels to be six to nine times higher and adipose tissue levels to be 31 to 113 times higher than those of plasma. Phencyclidine dissociates in the

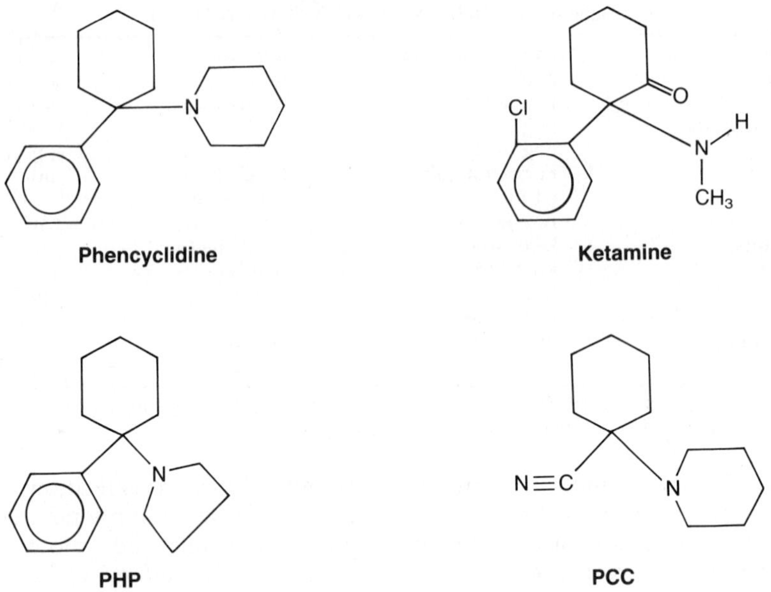

Phencyclidine

Ketamine

PHP

PCC

Figure 42–2. Phencyclidine and several of its psychoactive analogues.

physiologically slightly acidic spinal fluid (pH 7.3). It remains in the central nervous system for up to 48 hours in rat studies. This high degree of tissue distribution at least partially explains the extended duration of observed clinical effects despite often undetectable serum drug levels.[3] This large volume of distribution also partially explains the prolonged urinary excretion of metabolites. In one study,[12] only 4 per cent of urines became negative in the first week, 50 per cent became negative at the end of 2 weeks, and 1 per cent remained positive more than 30 days. Food deprivation, weight loss, exercise, and stress may act to release stored or accumulated phencyclidine from body tissues. The extent of phencyclidine protein binding is unclear, but plasma albumin and glyceroprotein binding have been demonstrated.

Phencyclidine is 90 per cent metabolized in the liver. Oxidative hydroxylation is the major mode of hepatic metabolism of PCP. The metabolites produced are inactive. These monohydrate metabolites appear as glucuronyl conjugates in the urine. Approximately 10 per cent of the drug is excreted unchanged in the urine. Pulmonary PCP metabolism has been demonstrated. PCP and metabolites are also excreted in perspiration. Phencyclidine is significantly secreted into the stomach and ionized in the acidic gastric lumen; gastric drug concentration may reach 20 to 50 times serum level, independent of the method of drug use. The drug is later resorbed from the alkaline duodenum. Intrinsic (p.o.) clearance of phencyclidine is approximately four times that of systemic clearance, supporting significant enterohepatic recirculation and a significant first-pass effect. This gastroenteric recirculation also helps to explain the waxing and waning course noted with phencyclidine.[13]

The mechanism of action of phencyclidine is complex. PCP interacts with all neurotransmitter systems studied to date. PCP has been shown to inhibit the GABA system. GABA is found in the descending pathway between the neostriatum and the substantia nigra, and acts as an inhibitory influence on nigrostriatal neurons. GABA agonists show a dose-dependent inhibition of the locomotor stimulatory effects of PCP. Benzodiazepines, which work at GABA coreceptors, are effective in treating anxiety symptoms and muscle rigidity produced by PCP.[3] Phencyclidine inhibition of GABA, with subsequent deregulation of dopaminergic activity, may partially explain PCP-induced dopaminergic symptoms.

Phencyclidine has been demonstrated to produce both an anticholinergic effect through acetylcholine receptor blockade and a sympathomimetic effect. Phencyclidine is also thought to inhibit acetyl and butyryl cholinesterase.[3] Drugs with anticholinergic activity (i.e., atropine and phenothiazines) have been shown to aggravate symptoms of

PCP intoxication. Physostigmine treatment has been shown to reverse neurologic (tremor and nystagmus) and psychiatric symptoms (agitation, hostility, and panic).[14] The sympathomimetic effect of PCP occurs through a cocaine-like potentiation of the pressor response to epinephrine, norepinephrine, and serotonin. There is also direct α-adrenergic receptor stimulation. Phencyclidine has also been shown to have opiate receptor action.[15]

In addition to all of the above effects, phencyclidine has been found to act directly on blood vessels, causing vasospasm. Phencyclidine-induced vasospasm has been prevented and reversed in vitro with verapamil.[16] The in vivo implications of this action have not been defined, but phencyclidine interaction with calcium and potassium channels is being investigated.

THE CLINICAL PICTURE

Phencyclidine is infamous for its wide spectrum of unpredictable effects. Similar doses may not produce similar effects in different users, and the symptoms may wax and wane as a result of the drug's enterohepatic circulation and large volume of distribution.

To get an overview of the clinical picture, it may help to divide intoxications into arbitrary dose-dependent categories. Lower dose exposures usually result from smoking or snorting and produce a subjective sense of intoxication with associated ataxia, slurred speech, and extremity hypesthesia. There may be sweating, muscle rigidity, and various degrees of mental status change ranging from a blank stare to aggressive hostility. As the dose increases, often because of oral ingestions, the user shows increasing degrees of anesthesia or even coma. Hypertension, tachycardia, diaphoresis, and muscle rigidity may be present. *Hallucinations, nystagmus, violent behavior, and sensory anesthesia are characteristic signs of phencyclidine intoxication.* Convulsions and death may ultimately occur.

Tolerance develops to the behavioral and toxic effects, and thus there is no absolute relationship between the serum level to clinical effect. Chronic users may be ambulatory at blood levels that would be lethal to the novice. There is also evidence that dependence on phencyclidine occurs. Unlike LSD, monkeys will self-administer phencyclidine. Abrupt withdrawal after prolonged use results in fearfulness, tremors, and facial twitches. In humans, cessation of chronic use results in anxiety, nervousness, and antisocial behavior.[17]

PSYCHOACTIVE MANIFESTATIONS

Luby first described the psychoactive manifestations of phencyclidine in 1959. Patients exposed to small amounts of PCP note distortions in body image (micropsia and macropsia, detachment of extremities), loss of body boundaries, and sensory blockade. Disorientation is common, and amnesia may be noted. Speech may be pressured or blocked, sparse, and purposeless. Thinking is disorganized and blocked and is stimulus bound. Users feel and may act inebriated. This dissociation and anesthesia are frequently described by users in terms of isolation and numbness; these effects may also result in the common delusions of superhuman strength and invulnerability. These last two delusions are perhaps the hallmark of phencyclidine intoxication. Users may also have feelings of anxiety and hostility. These delusions, illusions, and thought disturbances all contribute to the unpredictable and bizarre behavioral disturbances seen in these patients.

Hallucinations with this drug are relatively uncommon compared to those seen with the hallucinogens.[18] Patients are often described as gentle, loving, and nonviolent individuals by family and friends prior to their PCP-affected actions.[19] McCarron et al (1981), analyzing a series of 1000 patients, found an incidence of 29 per cent and 35 per cent for bizarre behavior and violence respectively.[6] With higher doses, increasing stereotypy of behavior, total disorientation, and finally mutism and catatonia occur. Mental status and behavioral aberrations may rapidly change. With chronic use, fatigue, irritability, severe depression, and memory loss occur. Users withdraw from and alienate friends and family.

PHYSICAL MANIFESTATIONS

Physical manifestations of PCP intoxication vary considerably. In milder intoxications nystagmus, hyperactive deep tendon reflexes, repetitive movements, ataxia, myoclonus, bizarre posturing, dystonia, and, more rarely, athetosis have been noted. At moderate to higher doses "lead pipe" rigidity, opisthotonos, and generalized seizures are seen. Status epilepticus producing anoxic encephalopathy, progressive renal failure, hepatic failure, and death have been described.

Patients with moderate to high dose intoxications are initially stuporous or comatose. Coma may last several hours to several days. The mechanism of production of coma is unclear. Electroencephalic changes in the comatose patient show a widespread sinusoidal theta rhythm interrupted by periodic slow delta complexes—changes that are similar to those produced by deep ketamine anesthesia.[20]

Phencyclidine intoxications have been found to cause myoglobinuric renal failure by two mechanisms. Excessive isometric muscle activity has been shown to lead to rhabdomyolysis and increased plasma creatine kinase (CPK) concentrations, which are associated with acute tubular necrosis. Malignant hyperthermia is a second mechanism.[21] McCarron[6] noted a 2.6 per cent incidence of hyperthermia in 1000 patients, but it is unclear in what percentage of these cases the condition could be attributed to malignant hyperthermia or to autonomic hyperactivity.

Sensory anesthesia and dissociation contribute to the behavioral aberrations seen with phencyclidine and also to a fairly high incidence of associated trauma. Loss of response to pain is dose related and progressive. Trauma may be self-mutilatory or accidental. Trauma may vary from minor abrasions, contusions, and lacerations to fractures and major intra-abdominal, intrathoracic, and intracranial injuries.

Signs of cholinergic stimulation are common. In low-dose ingestions flushing and diaphoresis are noted. In higher doses hypersalivation, drooling, bronchorrhea, vomiting, and urinary retention may occur. Bronchospasm is less common. These symptoms would of course be exacerbated by the use of physostigmine to treat the psychoactive symptoms.

McCarron et al noted a 57 per cent incidence of hypertension in their study.[6] Blood pressure elevation is usually mild. Studies show that the mean systolic increase is 26 mm Hg and the mean diastolic increase is 19 mm Hg.[3] In both the acute intoxication and recovery phases (72 to 96 hours) a small risk of dopaminergic hypertensive and hyperthermic crisis has been noted. One fatal case of hypertension with intracerebral hemorrhage found at autopsy has been reported.[6] Tachycardia may be present. Tachypnea occurs with low-dose intoxications. Airway patency may be effectively maintained by strap muscle and masseter spasm. Laryngeal and pharyngeal reflexes may be hyperactive; suctioning and intubation should be done with care to avoid precipitating airway spasm. At high doses ventilatory drive decreases. Apnea occurs infrequently (2.8 per cent) but is a major cause of death in cases of significant PCP intoxication. Apnea may also occur in the patient with grand mal seizures. Cardiac arrest occurs quite infrequently (0.3 per cent). Phencyclidine has been demonstrated to have a direct myocardial depressant effect, decreasing both the force of contractions and the rate of conduction.[21, 22]

LABORATORY STUDIES

Serum and urine testing for PCP do not correlate well with symptom severity. Urine levels of the drug may be undetectable in alkaline urine. A number of tests are used to test the urine qualitatively. Paper and silica gel thin-layer chromatography are good in experienced hands as a quick and cheap general screen. High performance liquid chromatography, and gas chromatography with either nitrogen phosphorus or flame ionization detection offer greater resolution and can be used to quantitate the drug. An 80 per cent false negative rate has been attributed to them.[23] Radioimmunoassay and the easier, faster, and less expensive enzyme multilinked immunoassay (EMIT) provide better specificity and accuracy. Quantitative blood levels can be obtained by enzyme immunoassay and gas chromatography–mass spectrophotometry.

Abnormal laboratory tests in the phencyclidine-intoxicated patient may include metabolic acidosis, hypoxemia, hypoglycemia, elevated serum SGOT, SGPT, uric acid, and creatine phosphokinase (CPK) levels and urine myoglobin. Twenty-two per cent of patients in McCarron's study[6] were found to have a serum glucose level of less than 70 mg per dl, with an average of 58 mg per dl.

Mild to moderate elevations of CPK (over 300), SGOT, and SGPT are not uncommon. Uric acid elevations were seen in approximately one-fourth of patients tested. Although not common, it is important to note uric acid elevation because acidification of the urine to increase phencyclidine excretion will reduce uric acid solubility and may precipitate uric acid nephropathy.

PEDIATRIC INTOXICATIONS

Phencyclidine intoxication has been reported in infants and children. They can become intoxicated in a number of ways: (1) rarely by deliberate poisoning, more likely for sedation or amusement, (2) by passive inhalation of side stream smoke, (3) by accepting and swallowing PCP tablets offered by another child—commonly seen in older infants and children, and (4) by chewing on PCP-containing cigarettes.[24] The youngest intoxicated child reported to date was 11 days old.

Children appear to be quite sensitive to phencyclidine. They present more commonly with neurologic symptoms than do adults. Lethargy is the most common symptom and may alternate with periods of agitation. Children have been noted to have decreased responses to verbal and tactile stimuli, decreased feeding, ataxia, nystagmus, and staring spells. Less commonly noted are seizures, obtundation, coma, hypertension, and opisthotonos, and these symptoms tend to occur with exposures to higher doses. Hyperreflexia, hypertonia, and rigidity are noted much less frequently than in adults. Notably absent is aggressive behavior. The differential diagnosis in these children may include seizure, Reye's syndrome, meningitis, hypoglycemia, hyponatremia, head trauma, brain tumor, and other drug intoxications.[7, 24]

Phencyclidine crosses the placenta. In humans, exposed neonates may have tremulousness, hypertonicity or opisthotonos, nystagmus, and diarrhea. The picture may be very similar to that of narcotic withdrawal, and both conditions have been successfully treated with phenobarbital. Teratogenic effects described include decreased fertility, increased fetal demise, chromosomal breaks, and an increased incidence of spinal defects.[25]

EMERGENCE

As patients recover from intoxication, physiologic changes tend to arise and disappear in a waxing and waning fashion in the reverse order of their initial appearance. The recovery phase is quite variable. Patients with mild symptoms usually recover in several hours, except for irritability and depression, which may last 24 hours. A small number of patients develop prolonged psychosis and depression that may last several months. This psychosis responds poorly to drugs but may closely resemble schizophrenic psychosis clinically. Clinical experience at one hospital with patients with prolonged phencyclidine psychosis suggests that a quarter of these patients may return within a year with acute schizophrenic psychosis.[17] Further support for a correlation between prolonged phencyclidine psychosis and the later development of schizophrenia is provided by the prolonged schizophreniform "thought disorders" and aberrant behavior produced by PCP in schizophrenic patients compared to normal volunteers. Depression in PCP-intoxicated patients during the emergence process frequently stimulates further drug abuse.[18]

MORTALITY

Budd and Lindstrom (1983)[26] reviewed 104 PCP-related deaths in Los Angeles county. Eighty-one per cent of patients were males, 73 per cent were black, 58 per cent were in their 20s, and 52 per cent were homicide victims. Fourteen per cent of patients had taken a fatal dose of phencyclidine alone or in combination with other drugs or alcohol. Fifty-one per cent of deaths occurred in May to December. Many deaths were accidental. In accidental deaths, several patients were noted to have pathologic changes in the lungs including pneumonia, pulmonary edema, and aspiration pneumonitis. As one might expect, the mean serum PCP level of patients dying from trauma or drowning (0.6 μg/ml) was considerably lower than the level in those with fatal drug ingestions (2.9 μg/ml). Drug levels of 2.0 to 2.5 μg/ml are considered uniformly fatal, with deaths occurring primarily from seizures or apnea.

TREATMENT

Phencyclidine ingestions produce unpredictable behavior, mandating an individualized therapeutic approach. Therapy is directed toward four areas as necessary: (1) life support, (2) behavior, (3) motor reactions, and (4) drug clearance.

Mildly intoxicated patients should be treated with sensory isolation in a nonthreatening environment. A room should be chosen where the patient can be watched and from which objects that the patient could use to harm himself or others have been removed. "Talking down" is ineffective and may actually agitate the patient. Physical restraints should be avoided to prevent exacerbation of rhabdomyolysis. Pharmacologic restraint is best provided with diazepam (5 to 10 mg p.o. or IV) or haloperidol (5 to 10 mg PO or IM). Phenothiazines are contraindicated because they may lower the seizure threshold, potentiate anticholinergic effects of PCP, and cause hypotension. Dystonia may be treated with diphenhydramine (50 to 100 mg).

Stuporous and comatose patients are diagnostic challenges. Naloxone should always be administered to cover cointoxication with narcotics; it may also be effective in reversing some of phencyclidine's CNS effects. A quick glucose measurement (Glucoscan, Dextrostik) should be performed or a dextrose solution administered because hypoglycemia is frequently noted. Physostigmine is currently not indicated because it may exacerbate cholinergic effects of phencyclidine and interact with other coingested drugs.

Airway management is imperative but can be difficult owing to hypersecretions, laryngospasm, and dystonia. Frequent suctioning may be necessary. Patients unable to protect their airway should be intubated. Atropine should be avoided in management of secretions because it may have a central interaction with phencyclidine, will decrease sweating, and may interact with other coingested drugs (i.e., anticholinergic agents).

Seizures can usually be controlled by intravenous administration of diazepam. Occasionally, phenobarbital, dilantin, or even general anesthesia may become necessary. Hypertension usually does not require treatment, but diazoxide, nitroprusside, propranolol, and hydralazine have been used successfully. The patient's temperature must be closely monitored. Hyperthermia should be managed with mechanical cooling methods rather than drugs. Bicarbonate administration should be considered for management of significant metabolic acidosis.

Drug clearance can be assisted in several ways. Gastric lavage and suction coupled with multidose charcoal administration are theoretically excellent adjuncts due to ion-trapping of phencyclidine and the effective adsorption of phencyclidine by charcoal. Practically, placement of a nasogastric tube is often impossible, and instrumentation in general is to be avoided in the awake patient. Urinary excretion of phencyclidine can be increased as much as 100-fold by acidification of the urine. The addition of forced diuresis, mannitol, and furosemide can further increase the rate of urinary clearance of phencyclidine. Vigorous acidification with ascorbic acid or ammonium chloride was recommended in the past. Acidification is not currently recommended, however, because it will decrease urinary myoglobin excretion, decrease uric acid solubility, and exacerbate metabolic acidosis. Acidification may also be a problem in the concomitantly head-injured patient and may further aggravate underlying hepatic damage in chronic substance abusers. Clearance data using ion-trapping, however excellent, must also be considered in relation to the relatively small role of urinary excretion in PCP clearance. Hepatic metabolism accounts for approximately 90 per cent of phencyclidine inactivation, and therefore the most active acidification may only increase excreted phencyclidine by 13 per cent.[23, 26]

Haloperidol is preferred to treat persistent phencyclidine psychosis. Giannini et al[13, 27] found that haloperidol was more effective than chlorpromazine in reducing anxiety, thought disorganization and abnormal thought content, and visual hallucinations in these patients.

LYSERGIC ACID DIETHYLAMIDE (LSD)

LSD is the "gold standard" to which all hallucinogens are compared in terms of potency, clinical effects, pharmacology, and treatment. Very little new data have accumulated since 1970, when LSD became a Schedule I drug. All information reported since then has been the result of illicit use or animal experimentation.

LSD is a water-soluble compound that has no color, taste, or odor. It is a racemic mixture of four stereoisomers: D-, L-, D-iso, and L-isoLSD. D-LSD is the only stereoisomer with hallucinogenic activity. It is usually taken orally in capsules or applied to a variety of ingestible substances. Colorful street names often reflect the form in which it is marketed—hence such names as blue and yellow dots, pink and purple wedges, animal crackers, window panes (gelatin impregnated squares), acid blotters, stamps, and many more! It produces psychoactive effects at a dose of 35 μg. Street doses usually average 150 to 300 μg (often advertised as seven to nine times the actual dose). The psychophysiologic effects are dose related between 1 and 16 μg/kg. LSD may also be insufflated or injected intravenously or subcutaneously, which produces a faster onset of effect. LSD may be impregnated on tobacco and smoked; users claim that the "high" produced is unsatisfactory. LSD equilibrates in the serum at 30 to 60 minutes. The half-life is 103 to 175 minutes, depending on the tissue compartment model used.[28] LSD is concentrated in the bile and excreted in the stool. It can be detected with spectrophotofluoroscopy; however, its rapid metabolism makes it quite difficult to detect on toxicology screening.

Tolerance to the behavioral effects of LSD develops rapidly after three to four consecutive daily doses. Sensitivity returns to baseline after 3 to 4 days of abstinence. Interestingly, there is less tolerance to the sympathomimetic effects of LSD. There is cross tolerance between LSD and the hallucinogenic PAA and IAA, possibly due to a common site of action. Cross tolerance does not develop to phencyclidine, cannabis, or amphetamines. There is no evidence of physical dependence, nor is a withdrawal syndrome produced after abrupt discontinuation of use.

The clinical syndrome, or "trip," produced by LSD can be arbitrarily divided into three overlapping phases (Table 42–3). The first manifestations of drug effect are usually somatic. There is invariably mydriasis. Other somatic effects are not consistent findings and when present are usually inconsequential. These effects include increases in heart rate, blood pressure, and reflexes, paresthesias, twitches, incoordination, and cutaneous flushing. Increases in leukocyte count, glucose, and free fatty acids have been reported and are ascribed to stress-induced release of catecholamines.

Perceptual distortions usually begin 30 to 60 minutes after oral ingestion. There is a magnified sense of color with increased vividness and contrast. Perception of distance and shape is altered, and objects appear to melt, vibrate, and flow. Sound becomes intensified, and users have difficulty locating the source of the sound. It is important to emphasize again that users do not fabricate sounds or images de novo but distort existing sensory clues. Two rather unique perceptual alterations are observed with LSD use. One is synesthesias, in which one sensory modality is translated into another, i.e., smelling colors. The other is a failure to suppress a prior image, causing an overlay of images like a photographic double exposure.

The psychic manifestations of a hallucinogenic experience consist of depersonalization, derealization, and loss of body image. Rarely, visual hallucinations occur in this phase. Emotions can rapidly change from ecstasy to despair, often triggered by sensory clues. Thoughts and memories flow incessantly, often breaking the boundaries of repression. Four to six hours into a "trip" the user often turns inward to transcendental

Table 42–3. LSD INTOXICATION

PHASE	TIME FROM INGESTION	SYMPTOMS
Somatic	0–60 minutes	Tension, lightheadedness, mydriasis, twitching, flushing tachycardia, hypertension, hyperreflexia
Perceptual	30–60 minutes	Visual, auditory, and sensory alterations; distortions of color, distance, shape, and time; synesthesias
Psychic	2–12 hours	Euphoria, mood swings, depression, feelings of depersonalization, derealization, loss of body image

or contemplative thoughts. Users often perceive themselves as communicating in great philosophical depth, while in reality their conversations make no sense to the observer.

Intellectual function during LSD use shows variable objective impairment. Tests involving attention, concentration, and motivation demonstrate decreased performance. There is no improvement in creative tasks performed under the influence of LSD, nor is there objective evidence that past use improves overall intellectual or creative abilities.

It is unfortunate, but those individuals who are most vulnerable to the adverse effects of LSD are often the ones most attracted to its use. Six factors have been identified as contributing to an adverse psychological outcome (i.e., a "bad trip"). An individual's preexisting character structure is a major predictor. It is well documented that users with poor premorbid adjustment or a personal or family history of psychiatric illness, especially schizophrenia, have an increased incidence of adverse psychiatric reactions. The setting in which the drug is taken is extremely influential on the outcome. Stressful environments can precipitate unpleasant and disruptive perceptions. "Set" refers to the user's frame of mind and expectations; if there is insufficient mental preparation the drug effect can be overwhelming. Because LSD lowers defense mechanisms, insecurity can lead to panic attacks and psychotic breaks. It is stressed that LSD should be taken with an empathetic companion who is not taking the drug. A negative experience during a trip is more likely to result in a prolonged psychiatric problem. Finally, higher doses result in more intense and longer lasting effects, including subsequent increased dissociative problems.[29] Despite these factors, there are no predictors to suggest which users will experience a bad trip. Adverse effects have been reported in all types of individuals in all kinds of sets and settings.

The most commonly observed adverse effect is the panic attack. LSD interferes with the ability to filter and integrate sensory input. As the user is bombarded by stimuli, he may lose his control and reference points to reality and become overwhelmed with the fear of impending insanity. It is during a panic attack that a user can do the most harm to himself and others. LSD does not produce aggressive or violent behavior. In fact, there is no good correlation between LSD use and true homicidal or suicidal behavior. Instead, during a panic attack an individual may jump from a building in an attempt to fly or strike out in fear. Panic attacks usually last less than 24 hours, but they can degenerate into prolonged psychotic states.

LSD toxic psychosis can last from days to months. It is controversial but generally accepted that prolonged psychosis is not actually caused by the drug. Prolonged psychosis is felt instead to be a psychotic condition that is accelerated or exacerbated by the experience.[30] Symptoms of the psychotic state therefore depend on the patient's premorbid personality and may include thought disorders, hallucinations, depression, regression, or depersonalizations.

LSD "flashbacks" also are characteristic. Studies investigating the effects of chronic LSD use are generally impaired by the lack of premorbid data. Chronic users, so-called acid or pot heads, are stereotyped as "counter cultural," artistic, mystic, and eccentric. There is no evidence that these personality traits are due to the drug. In fact, chronic use may represent an attempt on the part of the user to abolish social inhibitions and develop character insight.[31] Nor is there any evidence that chronic use is associated with brain damage. Flashbacks refer to spontaneous recurrences of the somatic, perceptual, or psychic phases of an LSD experience that occur after cessation of drug use. They may occur under benign conditions or may be triggered by stress or other drug use (i.e., barbiturates or cannabis). Flashbacks have been reported to occur up to 10 times a day and up to 18 months after LSD use. They have been reported after a single LSD ingestion; however, the incidence of occurrences increases with increased LSD use.[32]

Reports of organic side effects of LSD use have centered on chromosomal and teratogenic effects. At this time these issues are not considered significant. Early studies showed chromosomal breakage in leukocyte cultures. Similar damage has been shown to occur in numerous other drug and nondrug situations. In addition, there is neither good evidence that these chromosomal abnormalities have any clinical relevancy nor good evidence of increased incidence of birth defects or abortion related to LSD use.[33, 34]

There are no confirmed fatalities due directly to LSD toxicity. Death in animals results from respiratory failure. The LD_{50} varies widely from one species to another (i.e., in mice it is 46 μg/kg and in rabbits it is 0.3 μg/kg). Humans have ingested up to 1 mg per kg safely. There is one interesting report of eight people who "snorted" an unknown amount of pure LSD mistakenly instead of cocaine.[35] Within 5 minutes they developed anxiety, restlessness, generalized paresthesias, and vomiting. All had auditory and visual hallucinations. All had sinus tachycardia, widely dilated pupils, flushing, and sweating. Three had hypertension, and four became febrile (one to 41° C). Five became comatose. All eight had some degree of coagulopathy, and four had evidence of mild generalized bleeding. All patients recovered within 12 hours with supportive treatment.

Mechanism of Action

Albert Hofmann's discovery that microgram amounts of LSD could have profound central nervous system effects was instrumental in stimulating research into chemical mediators of brain function. It became evident early that LSD acted in the 5-HT (serotonin) pathway, which was known to act as an inhibitor or modulator in the cortex, raphe, and limbic systems. It was initially postulated that hallucinogens worked by blocking the 5-HT system, thus decreasing the filtering of cognitive perceptions that resulted in sensory overload. This was supported by the observation that serotonin depletion potentiated the effects of LSD.

It is now known that there are at least two 5-HT receptors. 5-HT1 receptors are presynaptic, and activation of these sites inhibits the release of serotonin. 5-HT2 receptors are postsynaptic and are excitatory when stimulated. There is possibly a third receptor, an autoreceptor on the raphe cell bodies, that when stimulated inhibits cell firing. There is excellent evidence that LSD acts primarily on the 5-HT2 receptor and not on the 5-HT1 receptor. Potentiation of the LSD effect by pretreatment with serotonin depleters is then explained, because presynaptic inhibition is decreased.[36] Supporting the 5-HT2 receptor theory, pipenperone (a specific 5-HT2 antagonist) blocks the ability of rats to distinguish LSD from saline.[37] In addition, compounds that are the most behaviorally active in man possess the highest 5-HT receptor affinity. There also appears to be a decrease in 5-HT binding sites with repeated hallucinogen exposure, possibly explaining the rapid tolerance (4 to 5 days) that develops to these agents.

Treatment

LSD ingestions are usually benign and self-limited and require no intervention. The most common adverse effect is the acute panic reaction, which is best managed by "talking down" the patient in an unobtrusive, reassuring manner. The patient should be placed in a quiet, comfortable room, never left alone, oriented as necessary, and reminded that the experience is drug related and will eventually end. Efforts should be made to introduce pleasant thoughts, emphasize positive aspects, and divert the patient from frightening thoughts. The talk-down process should be devoid of condemnation, judgments, or sudden movements that might be misinterpreted as threatening. The patient should be allowed to move around, although suggestions to lie down and relax can be made. Gastrointestinal decontamination and venipuncture may agitate and exacerbate the panic attack and should not be performed unless other drug ingestion is suspected. Acute panic reactions refractory to supportive care can be treated with benzodiazepines, preferably administered orally. Both diazepam (10 to 20 mg) and chlordiazepoxide (25 to 50 mg) have been used successfully. Acute psychotic reactions may need pharmacologic intervention; haloperidol (2 to 5 mg IM) is the drug of choice for this treatment. Chlorpromazine should be avoided because there have been reports of cardiovascular collapse in patients who have taken drugs mixed with belladonna alkaloids.

Flashbacks are usually self-limited and thus can be treated with the same supportive care used in acute panic attacks. Recurrent episodes that are debilitating to the patient have been treated with psychotherapy, haloperidol, phenothiazines, and benzodiazepines with varying degrees of success. Patients should be cautioned that persistent drug use of any kind can stimulate flashbacks and should be avoided.

Hospitalization is rarely needed for LSD-related events. Patients should always be discharged in the company of a responsible friend or family member.

INDOLEALKYLAMINES (IAA)

Dimethyltryptamine (DMT) is the most studied of the synthetic indolealkylamines. Dipropyltryptamine (DPT), diethyltryptamine (DET), and diisopropyltryptamine (DiPT) will also be discussed here because they are psychotomimetic, are used in psychotherapy, and are abused. Psilocin and psilocybin are the best known indolealkylamines and will be discussed later.

DMT and its 5-methoxy derivative were the active ingredients in the hallucinogenic snuff used in the pre-Columbian Americas. These snuffs were made from the leaves, seeds, and pods of *Mimosa hostilis, Pipladinia peregrina,* and *Prestolia* species. DMT was first isolated and studied in humans in 1956. At doses of 35 to 80 μg, DMT produces effects similar to those of LSD. More vivid color distortions are described with use of this drug. The effect lasts less than 1 hour and DMT has therefore been labeled the "businessman's LSD." It is not active orally. DMT is usually insufflated or smoked and more rarely is injected intravenously. Adverse effects are the same as those seen with LSD use. Panic attacks are particularly noticeable owing to the rapid onset of action. As with LSD, tolerance develops to DMT, and cross tolerance develops to the other hallucinogens.[38]

The *N-N*-diethyl and diisopropyl derivatives of tryptamine, DET and DPT respectively, are only effective when taken parenterally. They are less potent than DMT and are longer acting. At low doses, 15 to 30 μg, they are reported to cause an intensification of emotion, heightened fantasy activity, confrontation of repressed or denied aspects of self, increased recall of the past, and enhanced insight. Due to these properties, low doses of DET and DPT have been successfully used in psychotherapy.[66] At higher doses patients have been reported to lose ego boundaries and experience psychological regression.

The *N*-isopropyl homologues of DMT and 5-MeO-DMT, DiPT and 5MeO-DiPT respectively, are active orally in humans. In human volunteer studies, Shulgin and Carter[39] have shown that DiPT administration causes a passive psychotomimetic state that is characterized by auditory distortion. Administration of 5 MeO-DiPT results in a talkative and disinhibited state with easy emotional expression. It has been concluded that 5 MeO-DiPT is the better of the two for psychotherapy owing to the absence of intense sensory disturbances. The effective dose of DiPT is 20 to 50 μg and for 5-MeO-DiPT, 6 to 10 μg. Onset of effect averaged 20 to 30 minutes, with a peak effect of about 90 minutes for both.

Treatment of adverse effects resulting from the indolealkylamines is the same as that used for LSD. The patient is talked down in a supportive environment.

PHENYLALKYLAMINES (PAA)

The phenylalkylamines are divided into two groups, the phenylethylamines and the phenylisopropylamines. Mescaline is the best known of the phenylethylamines and will be discussed in the ensuing section on hallucinogens of plant origin. The phenylisopropylamines are related to both mescaline and amphetamines, and as such they are often referred to as the psychotomimetic amphetamines. 2,5-Dimethoxy-4-methyl amphetamine (DOM) and 3,4 methylene-dioxyamphetamine (mDA) were formerly the most popular agents in this group as drugs of abuse and are the best studied. In recent years newer phenylisopropylamines such as 4-bromo-2,5-dimethoxyamphetamine (bromo DMA) and 3,4-methylenedioxymethamphetamine (mDMA) have emerged with increasing notoriety.

DOM was first synthesized in 1964 and found its way into the illicit drug scene in Haight-Ashbury in 1967. It was frequently combined with anticholinergic drugs and marketed as STP. Initially named after the motor oil, STP later came to stand for "Serenity, Tranquility and Peace." Anticholinergic agents were dropped from the mixture after several years, and the two drugs became synonymous. Ironically, trips with these agents did not live up to the acronym. DOM has a longer half-life than LSD, and the trip has been reported to last up to 24 hours. The long duration of action combined with sympathomimetic side effects resulted in numerous bad trips and gradual disillusionment with the drug. By the late 1960s drug dealers were marketing their stocks of DOM as LSD. The most infamous marketing scam was the "pink wedge incident" in 1967, in which 270 μg of LSD was combined with 0.9 mg of STP and sold as 1000 μg of LSD. Eighteen patients with "death trips" were treated at the Haight-Ashbury Free Clinic in a 5-hour period.

DOM is 100 times more potent than mescaline and one-fiftieth to one-hundredth as potent as LSD. Its effects are dose related. Less than 3 mg causes mild euphoria and increased self-awareness, but there are no perceptual changes. Doses greater than 5 mg are hallucinogenic. Street doses tend to be in the 10-mg range. DOM is usually taken orally. Effects start in 1 to 2 hours and peak in 3 to 5 hours. Physical effects include mild tachycardia, hypertension, hyperthermia, diaphoresis, mydriasis, paresthesias, nausea, and dysphasia. Tolerance to DOM develops after only 2 to 3 days of use, and there is cross tolerance to other hallucinogens.

2,5-Dimethoxy-4-ethylamphetamine (DOET) is the ethyl homologue of DOM. In doses of 0.75 to 4 mg it causes mild euphoria, increased self-awareness, and mild anxiety. It is not associated with psychotomimetic activity or perceptual changes; thus it is controversial whether to classify it with the hallucinogens. Subjects in therapeutic settings tend to feel relaxed and are more accepting of new ideas and more aware of feelings and body image under the influence of this agent.[40]

MDA possesses both sympathomimetic and hallucinogenic properties at doses between 60 and 150 mg. Onset of action occurs 40 to 60 minutes after oral ingestion. Peak effect occurs at 90 minutes, and the effect terminates at approximately 8 hours. MDA causes an intensification of feeling, increased self-insight and empathy, and increased perceptual ability. Users claim that it is "more sensual than cerebral," and it therefore has been referred to as the love drug. There is no evidence of an aphrodisiac effect. The only consistently noted physical effect is mydriasis. In overdose (6 mg/kg), however, MDA has been reported to cause hyperpyrexia, hypertension, tachycardia, rigidity, seizures, rhabdomyolysis, disseminated intravascular coagulation, adult respiratory distress syndrome, and refractory shock.[70] In addition to the possibility of lethality in overdose, there is some disturbing evidence in animals that MDA is a neurotoxin that causes selective serotonergic terminal degeneration.[41] The implications of this finding have not yet been delineated.

BromoDMA is not a pharmacologic preparation but has been appearing on the illicit drug scene in the past several years. It has been referred to as 100 x, implying that it is a hundred times as strong as MDA. It is also called tiles and golden eagle, referring to the shape of the blotters it is often sold on. The street doses are extremely variable owing to the unpredictable diffusion of the liquid bromoDMA as it is absorbed onto the blotters. Doses have ranged from 0.7 mg to 4.6 mg in the same batch. Onset of action is 45 to 60 minutes, and the trip lasts from 12 to 24 hours. As with MDA, it possesses both hallucinogenic and sympathomimetic activity. Overdose can result in disorientation, panic, and violent and aggressive behavior. Grand mal seizures and death have been reported with bromoDMA use.

The last psychotomimetic amphetamine to be mentioned is mDMA. Street names for this drug include ecstasy, XTC, MDM, Adam, E, Doctor, and M and Ms. mDMA has received considerable publicity owing to its emergency Schedule I classification in 1985, based primarily on its structural similarity to MDA. Very little information has been published in the literature on this drug. It has been used as a psychotherapeutic agent based on claims that it improves mood, ability to communicate, and introspection. Illicit use of mDMA has been increasing on college campuses in recent years. Three hundred and sixty-nine undergraduates at a major college campus in California were anonymously polled, and 143 (39 per cent) reported at least one use of the drug. The median number of times of use was four, with a range of 1 to 38 times.[42] It has not been reported to cause disorientation, perceptual distortion, or psychotic states. Sympathomimetic side effects are reported to be minimal at usual doses. At higher doses one may see amphetamine-like cardiovascular and stimulatory effects and hallucinations. Psychotherapeutic doses range from 75 to 150 mg. The psychotomimetic effect lasts from 4 to 6 hours. An interesting recent report in the literature describes a patient with Nardil and mDMA interaction, and notes that the chemical structure of mDMA with its methyl-substituted alpha carbon and unsubstituted beta carbon (see Fig. 42–1) makes this compound a potent indirect sympathomimetic agent, thus placing the patient at high risk for significant MAOI-sympathomimetic toxicity.[43] In laboratory animals, mDMA has been shown to be neurotoxic. A preliminary report of mDMA-induced depletion of serotonin receptors in the brain, with a 75 per cent return of receptor sites by 6 months, was recently reported in humans.[44]

Treatment of phenylalkylamine adverse effects is largely supportive, as for LSD. For acute psychotic reactions, haloperidol is the drug of choice. Phenothiazines are contraindicated owing to reports of cardiovascular collapse in patients who have taken STP containing belladonna alkaloids.

HALLUCINOGENS OF PLANT ORIGIN

Hallucinogens occur throughout the plant kingdom. Approximately 20 species of the 800,000 plant species are hallucinogenic, with an interesting and unexplained concentration of these species on plants native to the New World. These hallucinogenic species have been used by primitive tribes in religious ceremonies and by herbalists and witch doctors for centuries. A question has been raised about whether the concept of deity arose from their use.[1] Northern Aryan peoples invaded India 3500 years ago, bringing with them the cult of a plant called soma. The plant was deified and used as a holy inebriant; some 1000 hymns to soma are included in the Rig Veda. During the ensuing 2000 years use of the original plant was abandoned. The identity of soma is uncertain but may be *Amanita.* In Central America, archaeologic excavations have found mushroom stones, indicating the existence of a sophisticated mushroom cult in Guatemala more than 3500 years ago that included the use of *Psilocybe, Stropharia, Conocybe,* and *Paneolus* in their ceremonies. Datura (Jimson weed) was used by the Chibcha Indians of South America to sedate victims of human sacrifices. In medieval Europe, many of the fantastic visions attributed to witchcraft have been hypothesized to have been caused by *Datura stramonium* and *Hyoscamine niger* (henbane) use. Modern religous use of hallucinogens is exemplified by the ritual use of peyote and mescaline in the Native American Church.

Mescaline and Peyote

Peyote and mescaline have been used in Mexican and South American religious ceremonies for centuries. Juan Cardenas, a Spanish physician in the New World, described the effects of mescaline intoxication in 1591 in his Primera Parte de los Secretos Marvilloses de las Indias. Mescaline use became so prevalent among the Spanish in the New World that an edict banning its use except by "pagan Indians" was passed in 1620. Many Spanish writings attributed diabolic properties to the Peyote cactus. In the United States, Peyote cults were established by the Kiowa and Comanche in the 1800s based on raids into Mexico. Use in native American religious ceremonies rapidly became widespread. In 1906 a loose tribal confederation, the Mescal Bean Eaters, was established. In 1918, the Native American Church was established as a defense against anti-Peyote drug legislation. Peyote and mescaline use is a sacramental rite in the Native American Church, and members are therefore exempt from prosecution under the Controlled Substances Act. In 1922, 13,300 followers were registered. More recently, the Church numbers over 200,000 followers. Medicinal use of Peyote was suggested in an 1889 Parke Davis catalog as a tincture for use in patients with angina or pneumothorax and as a respiratory stimulant.

Mescaline, the active phenethylamine alkaloid in Peyote, was isolated by Hefter in 1896. In 1918, mescaline was successfully synthesized. Its chemical structure was identified as 3,4,5-trimethoxybetaphenethylamine. Levin was one of the first to systematically describe the physiologic, pharmacologic, and psychologic properties.[45] In 1940, Stockings used mescaline as a model for psychosis.[45] Mescaline is available today synthetically or as a variety of peyote extracts. Dried peyote buttons contain 6 per cent mescaline (45 mg). Mescaline is also available as a tincture of peyote (70 per cent alcohol extract), basic panpeyote (chloroform extract of ground peyote), and soluble peyote (hydrochloride extract of basic panpeyote used for injection). Synthetic mescaline is available as the hydrochloride or sulfate salt; 375 mg of the hydrochloride salt is equivalent to 500 mg of the sulfate salt. Synthetic mescaline has been administered intravenously, orally, subcutaneously, and intramuscularly. Intravenous administration provides the most rapid onset of effect. Similar dose-response effects are provided by all routes of administration.

Peyote, the North American dumpling cactus, is a small, fleshy, spineless cactus that grows along the Rio Grande River valley and other arid areas of the southwestern United States and Mexico. Peyote is found as two variants, *Lophophora williamsii* and *L. diffusa*. Although these two are morphologically indistinct, their alkaloid compositions vary considerably. Mescaline is the major active alkaloid in *L. williamsii*. Pellotine is the major alkaloid in *L. diffusa* and possesses essentially no hallucinogenic activity. Mescaline is present in *L. diffusa* in only trace amounts.

Peyote refers to the unmodified cactus. It is used fresh or dried to increase potency. Peyote buttons are round tubercles, each with yellow-white tufts at the apex instead of spines. The buttons are sliced off. The hard brown discs produced by drying these buttons maintain hallucinogenic activity even after prolonged storage. Peyote may be swallowed intact after softening in the mouth or as a salad or tea, or it may be ground into a powder. The powder is placed in capsules or tablets to avoid the bitter taste. The drug user may buy substances labeled mesc or Big Chief; however, mescaline is rarely available on the street. Analysis of these substances has revealed the presence of LSD, PCP, amphetamines, STP, strychnine, and aspirin.[43]

A dose of 5 mg per kg of mescaline will usually produce visual hallucinations and psychic effects. Four to twelve peyote buttons must be ingested to produce an equivalent effect. Mescaline is rapidly absorbed. Nausea and vomiting are noted within 30 to 60 minutes. The user then commonly exhibits diaphoresis, mild tachycardia, hypertension, mydriasis, and hyperreflexia. Photophobia secondary to mydriasis, ataxia, nystagmus, tremors, and muscle fasciculations may also occur. Sensory changes, primarily characterized by visual hallucinations, follow, peaking at 4 to 6 hours and persisting up to 14 hours. Shimmering and intensification of the visual field and of color and texture perception are noted. Geometric imagery may be complex. The sensorium usually remains clear. This phase is vividly described by Huxley in The Doors of Perception. The user frequently experiences anxiety, paranoia, and emotional lability. Auditory hallucinations are infrequent. Tolerance, but not physical dependence, occurs. Cross tolerance with LSD and psilocybin is described. Mescaline has been found to inhibit neurons of the ventral portion of the dorsal raphe system.

Doses of 20 to 60 mg per kg have produced respiratory depression, vasodilation, and hypotension. Bradycardia is described with higher doses. Mortality is rare, but massive ingestions have produced profound central nervous system and respiratory depression. Other deaths have resulted from accidents due to the hallucinatory effects.

Treatment is supportive. Patients should be placed in a nonthreatening environment and reassured. Gastric decontamination is indicated only if the patient presents early, because mescaline is rapidly absorbed, or if more toxic drugs have been coincidentally ingested. Sedation, if necessary, should not be provided by phenothiazines. Phenothiazines may interact adversely with other ingested drugs (PCP, DOM, anticholinergics). Patients with massive mescaline ingestion may require ventilatory support.

Morning Glory Seeds

Convolvulaceae is the scientific name for this family of plants. Many of the plants in this family have been used for centuries for their hallucinogenic effects. The morning glory is illustrated and described in a voluminous study of medicinal plants, animals, and rocks of "New Spain" by Hernandez (personal physician to the King of Spain in Mexico, 1570–1575). The seeds were used for divination. Hernandez wrote, ". . . when the priests wanted to commune with their gods . . ., they ate ololiuqui seeds, and . . . a thousand visions and . . . hallucinations appeared to them."[1] Seeds were also ground into a flour, which was soaked in alcohol or cold water and then strained. The filtrate was used as a drug for divination, healing, and religious ceremonies by the Aztecs and later by the American Indians.

In the past several decades *Ipomoea* species have become a source of abused seeds. Abuse has been fueled by suggestive advertising in "new generation" magazines listing these seeds as hallucinogens. Garden catalogs list such interesting names as Flying Saucers, Summer Skies, Pearly Gates, and Heavenly Blue. The Hawaiian woodrose *(Merremia tuberosa)* and the Hawaiian baby woodrose *(Argyreia nervosa)* are other, more potent hallucinogens in this family.

In 1960, chemical analysis showed that the active components of these seeds were indole alkaloids. These alkaloids include chanoclavin, elymoclavine, penniclavine, ergine, ergometrine, isoergine, and lysergol. The principal active components of these alkaloids are D-lysergic acid, D-isolysergic acid amide, and D-lysergic acid methylcarbinolamide. The seeds are only one-tenth as potent as LSD. Three hundred Heavenly Blue seeds produce effects equivalent to 200 to 300 μg of LSD. Seeds must be ground or made into an extract prior to use.

The psychic effects of seed ingestion are similar to those of LSD. Visual deceptions and feelings of depersonalization are prominent. Periods of apathy may alternate with excitement. Recent and remote memory may be impaired. Acute psychosis has been described. One suicide resulting from persistent flashbacks was described by Cohen in 1964.[46] Flushing, hypotension, tachycardia, and mydriasis are seen. Nausea is a frequently reported symptom, which may be related to intentional fungicide-coating of these seeds by manufacturers to discourage abuse. Reassurance and supportive therapy are the mainstay of treatment.[31, 47]

Psilocybin

Spanish conquistadors described century-old Aztec rituals utilizing the sacred mushroom (Teonanacatl or "God's flesh"), ololiuqui seeds, and peyote in their chronicles. Archaeologists date a sophisticated mushroom cult to 3500 BC in Central America. This "food of the gods" was eaten ritually for worship, prophecy, and divination. At least 20 species of hallucinogenic mushrooms were utilized, including those of four genera: *Psilocybe, Conocybe, Paneolus,* and *Stropharia.* These were first identified by Wassan and Heim in the 1950s. Chemical analysis was performed by Hofman, who identified the two psychoactive components as psilocybin (4-phosphoryloxyl-*N*, *N*-dimethyl tryptamine) and psilocin (4-hydroxyl-*N*,*N*-dimethyltryptamine). Psilocybin is 1.5 times more potent than psilocin. In vivo, psilocin may actually be the active agent, because dephosphorylation is rapid by alkaline phosphatase. In 1978, psilocybin was also isolated from *Gymnopilus* species. Psilocybin is quite stable, and both dried plants and boiled extracts retain potency.

Psilocybin produces a clinical picture that is almost identical to that of LSD use. Duration of action is shorter, only 5 to 6 hours. Psilocybin effect is initially noted at 15 minutes and peaks at 90 minutes. Physical effects include tachycardia, tachypnea, mild hypertension, hyperthermia, mydriasis and blurred vision, nausea, dizziness, hyperactive deep tendon reflexes, and impaired coordination. Psychic effects include visual deceptions, time-space perception impairment, feelings of depersonalization, and often a dreamlike state. LSD is 100 to 200 times more potent than psilocybin. (One hundred micrograms of LSD is equivalent to 20 mg of fresh psilocybin or 10 mg of the dried or boiled plant). Tolerance and cross tolerance to LSD and mescaline develop.[42, 48]

Treatment is supportive. Emesis or lavage and charcoal are effective but impractical. Quiet surroundings should be provided where the patient can be reassured. A companion may be helpful. Toxic psychosis may be treated with Haldol (5 to 10 mg IM). Mortality is rare (less than 1 per cent); when reported it occurred in children. Accidental poisoning in children has been associated with hyperthermia and seizures. Seizures respond well to diazepam (0.1 to 0.3 mg/kg IV). Hyperthermia responds well to mechanical cooling methods, and aspirin is contraindicated.[30, 33]

Although serious toxicity related to psilocybin has not been reported in adults, many adults have been severely poisoned by eating other toxic species while in search of hallucinogenic mushrooms. Eighteen species of psilocybin-containing mushrooms grow in the Pacific northwest, Florida, and Hawaii. Mushrooms of the genus *Psilocybe* are small and many have conical caps, very thin stipes, attached gills, and purple to chocolate brown spore prints. The presence of hallucinogenic compounds correlates with a blue or purple stain on bruised stipes. *Paneolus* species have conical caps, thin stalks, and purple-brown to black spore prints. *Gymnopilus* species have broad yellow to orange caps, thick stalks, and rusty orange spore prints. Several "new generation" magazines offer mail order *Psilocybe* spores to grow at home.[40, 48]

Nutmeg

Nutmeg has been used as a spice for many centuries. It was introduced into Europe by the Arabs in the twelfth century. It was used as an aphrodisiac and a narcotic in India and Yemen. Nutmeg has been used unsuccessfully medicinally to treat a wide variety of illnesses including cholera, rheumatism, digestive disorders, madness, musculoskeletal disorders, skin eruptions, and menorrhagia. The first documented incident of nutmeg poisoning occurred in 1576. Many cases have been reported more recently. In the early 1900s poisonings often occurred because of the high doses of nutmeg used as an abortifacient. More recently, most poisonings reported occur in experimenting students and prison inmates deprived of other psychoactive drugs. Accidental poisonings also occur when too much nutmeg is used to top various beverages and foods. An anonymous author in Legal Highs noted "beneficial as spice or in small amounts; not recommended as hallucinogen."[1, 34, 49]

Nutmeg is obtained from the fruit of the evergreen tree *Myristica fragrans,* which grows indigenously in the Molucca Islands of the South Pacific. Nutmeg is now cultivated in Trinidad and Grenada. The *Myristica* fruit is similar to a peach or an apricot and contains a single glossy brown nut. Nutmeg is derived from the seed, whereas mace is derived from the dried scarlet aril or seed coat. The aromatic fraction of 20 gm of nutmeg produces 210 mg myristicin, 2 mg elemicin, 5 mg eugenol, 6 mg isoeugenol, 18 mg methyleugenol, 11 mg methylisoeugenol, 8 mg methoxyeugenol, and smaller fractions of geraniol, safrol, borneal, and linalol.

Each nutmeg is composed of 5 to 15 per cent volatile oil. Myristicin was initially thought to be the psychoactive agent; however, ingestion of pure myristicin does not produce the same results obtained from ingestion of the entire nutmeg. The other volatile oils may be responsible for the psychoactive effect noted. Myristicin is metabolized in vivo to the psychotomimetic compound 3-methoxy-4,5 methylenedioxyamphetamine (MMDA). Elemicin is metabolized to 3,4,5-trimethoxyamphetamine (TMA).[1, 34, 48, 50]

The toxic dose of nutmeg is 5 to 30 gm (obtained from one to three nutmegs or 0.4 to 4.5 gm of volatile oil). Symptoms begin in 3 to 6 hours and may last 60 hours. Patients may present in a detached dreamlike state. Predominantly visual hallucinations are noted. The only reported death occurred in an 8 year old boy who ate two nutmegs, became comatose, and died within 24 hours. Management is symptomatic and supportive.[51]

DIFFERENTIAL DIAGNOSIS

This chapter has dealt with phencyclidine and a number of the commonly abused hallucinogens. There may be a tremendous amount of overlap in symptoms between the drugs discussed, making drug identification difficult at best. Historical and clinical clues can help the clinician make this differentiation. Unfortunately, toxicologic screening, while invaluable in many situations of drug ingestion, plays very little role in identifying any of the hallucinogens other than phencyclidine.

Rarely, a hallucinating patient may offer historical information that helps in identifying the abused substance. Information such as ingestion of a peyote button, mushroom, or ground seeds is of obvious help. Ingestion of a carrying substance such as blotting paper or a stamp may suggest LSD ingestion. Hallucinogens and PCP are rarely administered intravenously. Histories may be unreliable, however, due to a number of factors: Drugs are often sold under false names and are often contaminated with adulterants, the patient may be amnestic, hallucinating, agitated, or withdrawn, or may not admit to illicit drug use.

Mental status testing may sometimes be of help if it is used cautiously. Users of LSD, PAAs, and IAAs usually retain intact egos and show positive results on reality testing. They are usually aware that the sensory distortions they are experiencing are drug induced and are often receptive to suggestions and help. Conversely, patients on PCP often lose the sense of body boundaries and are disorganized and disoriented. PCP-intoxicated patients tend to be delusional, and their extremely bizarre actions with violent outbursts are completely uncharacteristic of the other hallucinogens. Of note, schizophrenics, who must be differentiated from drug abusers, tend to have past mental illness histories, absent intact egos, and auditory hallucinations (not illusions!).

Clinically, the picture seen with most hallucinogens is psychoactive rather than physical. Tachycardia, hypertension, and hyperreflexia are nonspecific and are not always present. Dry mouth, blurred vision, and cycloplegia suggest atropine or *Datura* intoxication. Phencyclidine produces the most characteristic physical findings and should be suspected in any patient presenting with acute confusion or agitation with bizarre or violent behavior, ataxia, hypertension, or nystagmus. Evidence of trauma is often present. Of note, PCP users, unlike patients abusing hallucinogens, do not have mydriasis.

Phencyclidine is the only hallucinogenic agent that frequently causes stupor and coma and thus should be suspected in all such patients. Comatose PCP users show nonfocal results on neuroexamination. The presence of hypertension and hyperreflexia helps to distinguish them from patients with sedative-hypnotic and narcotic overdoses.

The therapeutic approach to the hallucinogen-intoxicated patient should always begin with the basics. Reassurance, sensory isolation, and protection of the patient and others are the cornerstones of therapy. If sedation is necessary, diazepam and haloperidol are the agents of choice; phenothiazines are relatively contraindicated. Gastric decontamination and charcoal instillation recommendations vary according to the agent taken. One should always monitor for and manage severe manifestations of intoxication early.

References

1. Hofmann A: The discovery of LSD and subsequent investigations on naturally occurring hallucinogens. *In* Ayd FS, Blackwell B (eds): Discoveries in Biological Psychiatry. Philadelphia, JB Lippincott, 1970, pp 91–106.
2. Leary T, Metzner R, Alpert R: The Psychedelic Experience: A Manual Based on the Tibetan Book of the Dead. New Hyde Park, NY, University Books, 1964.
3. Aniline O, Pitts FN: Phencyclidine (PCP): A review and perspectives. CRC Crit Rev Toxicol *10:*145–177, 1982.
4. Lundberg GD, Gupta RC, Montgomery SH: Phencyclidine: Patterns seen in street drug analysis. Clin Toxicol *9:*503–510, 1976.
5. Rainey JM, Crowder MK: Prevalence of phencyclidine in street drug preparations. N Engl J Med *290*(8):466–467, 1974.
6. McCarron MM, Schulze BW, Thompson GA, et al: Acute phencyclidine intoxication: Incidence of clinical findings in 1000 cases. Ann Emerg Med *10*(5):237–242, 1981.
7. Welch MJ, Correa GA: PCP intoxication in young children and infants. Clin Pediatr *19*(8):510–514, 1980.
8. Aniline O, Pitts FN, Allen RE, Burgoyne R: Incidental intoxication with phencyclidine. J Clin Psychiatry *41*(11):393–394, 1980.
9. Davis WM, Borne RF, Hackett RB: Piperidinocyclohexanecarbonitrile (PCC): Acute toxicity alone and potentiation of the lethality of phencyclidine (PCP). Fed Proc *38:*435–439, 1979.
10. Giannini AJ, Price WA, Loiselle RH, Malone DW: Treatment of phencyclohexylpyrrolidine (PHP) psychosis with haloperidol. Clin Toxicol *23*(2–3):185–189, 1985.
11. Misra AL, Pontani RB, Bartolomeo J: Persistence of phencyclidine (PCP) and metabolites in brain and adipose tissue and implications for long-lasting behavioral effects. Res Commun Chem Pathol Pharmacol *24*(3):431–435, 1979.
12. Patel P, Connor G: A review of thirty cases of rhabdomyolysis-associated acute renal failure among phencyclidine users. Clin Toxicol *23*(7–8):547–556, 1986.
13. Giannini AJ, Nageotte C, Loiselle RH, et al: Comparison of chlorpromazine, haloperidol and pimozide in the treatment of phencyclidine psychosis: DA-2 receptor specificity. Clin Toxicol *22*(6):573–579, 1985.
14. Castellani S, Adams PM, Giannini AJ: Physostigmine treatment of acute phencyclidine intoxication. J Clin Psychiatry *43*(1):10–11, 1982.
15. Castellani S, Giannini AJ, Boering JA, Adams PM: Phencyclidine intoxication: Assessment of possible antidotes. J Toxicol Clin Toxicol *19*(3):313–319, 1982.
16. Altura BT, Altura BM: Phencyclidine, lysergic acid diethylamide and mescaline: Cerebral artery spasm and hallucinogenic activity. Science *212:*1051–1052, 1981.
17. Petersen RC, Stillman RC (eds): Phencyclidine (PCP) abuse: An appraisal. NIDA Research Monograph, 1978, pp 1–8.
18. Luisada PV: The phencyclidine psychosis: Phenomenology and treatment. *In* Petersen RC, Stillman RC (eds): Phencyclidine (PCP) Abuse: An Appraisal. NIDA Research Monograph, 1978, pp 241–247.
19. Fauman MA, Fauman BJ: Violence associated with phencyclidine abuse. Am J Psychiatry *136*(12):1584–1586, 1979.
20. Stockard JJ, Werner SS, Aalvers JA, Chiappa KH: Electroencephalographic findings in phencyclidine intoxication. Arch Neurol *33:*200–203, 1976.
21. Goode DJ, Meltzer HY: The role of isometric muscle tension in the production of muscle toxicity by phencyclidine and restraint stress. Psychopharmacology *42:*105–108, 1975.
22. Albuquerque EX, Aguayo LG, Warnick JE: Interaction of phencyclidine with ion channels of nerve and muscle: Behavioral implications. Fed Proc *42:*2584–2589, 1983.
23. Phencyclidine. Englewood, CO, Poisindex, Micromedex, 1990.
24. Schwartz RH, Einhorn A: PCP intoxication in seven young children. Pediatr Emerg Care *2*(4):238–241, 1986.
25. Strauss AA, Modanlou HD, Bosu SK: Neonatal

manifestations of maternal phencyclidine (PCP) abuse. Pediatrics *68*(4):550–552, 1981.

26. Corales R, Maull K, Becker D: Phencyclidine abuse mimicking head injury. JAMA *243*(22):2323–2324, 1980.
27. Giannini AJ, Eighan MS, Loiselle RH, Giannini MC: Comparison of haloperidol and chlorpromazine in the treatment of phencyclidine psychosis. J Clin Pharmacol *24*:202–204, 1984.
28. Wagner J, Aghajanian G, Bing O: Correlation of performance test scores with "tissue concentration" of lysergic acid diethylamide in human subjects. Clin Pharmacol Ther *9*:635–638, 1968.
29. Cohen S: The varieties of psychotic experience. J Psychoact Drugs *17*(4):291–296, 1985.
30. Vardy M, Kay S: LSD psychosis or LSD-induced schizophrenia? Arch Gen Psychiatr *40*:877–883, 1983.
31. Strassman R: Adverse reactions to psychedelic drugs: A review of the literature. J Nerv Ment Dis *172*(10):577–595, 1984.
32. Roy A: LSD and onset of schizophrenia. Can J Psychiatry *26*:64–65, 1981.
33. Cohen M, Marinello M, Bark N: Chromosomal damage in human leukocytes induced by lysergic acid diethylamide. Science *155*:1417–1419, 1967.
34. Gilmour D, Bloom A, Lele K, et al: Chromosomal aberration in users of psychoactive drugs. Arch Gen Psychiatr *24*:268–272, 1971.
35. Klock J, Boermer V, Berher C: Coma, hyperthermia and bleeding associated with massive LSD overdose: A report of eight cases. Clin Toxicol *8*(2):191–203, 1975.
36. Glennon R, Titeler M, McKenney J: Evidence for 5HT2 involvement in the mechanism of action of hallucinogenic agents. Life Sci *35*:2505–2511, 1984.
37. Mokler D, Stoudt K, Rech R: The 5HT2 antagonist pirenperone reverses disruption of FR-40 by hallucinogenic drugs. Pharmacol Biochem Behav *22*:677–682, 1985.
38. Martin W, Swan J: Relationships of CNS tryptaminergic processes and the action of LSD-like hallucinogens. Pharmacol Biochem Behav *24*:393–399, 1986.
39. Shulgin A, Carter M: *N,N*-Diisopropyltryptamine (DiPT) and 5-methoxy-*N,N*-diisopropyltryptamine (5-MeO-DiPT): Two orally active tryptamine analogs with CNS activity. Commun Psychopharm *4*:363–369, 1980.
40. Snyder S, Weingartner H, Faillace L: DOET (2,5-Dimethoxy-4-ethylamphetamine: Effects of varying doses in man. Arch Gen Psychiatr *24*:50–55, 1971.
41. Ricuarte G, Bryan G, Strauss L, et al: Hallucinogenic amphetamine selectively destroys brain serotonin nerve terminals. Science *229*:986–988, 1985.
42. Peroutka S: Incidence of recreational use of 3,4-methylenedimethoxymethamphetamine (MDMA, "Ecstasy") on an undergraduate campus. N Engl J Med *317*(24):1542–1543, 1987.
43. Smilkstein MJ, Smolinske SC, Rumack BH: A case of MAO inhibitor/MDMA interaction: Agony after ecstasy. Clin Toxicol *25*(1,2):149–159, 1987.
44. MDMA; Preliminary reports. JAMA *258*(23):3362, 1987.
45. McCall R: Neurophysiological effects of hallucinogens on serotonergic neuronal systems. Neurosci Behav Rev *6*:509–514, 1982.
46. Schultes RE: Hallucinogens of plant origin. Science *163*:245–249, 1969.
47. Hollister L: Effects of hallucinogens in humans. *In* Jacobs BL (ed): Hallucinogens: Neurochemical, Behavioral and Clinical Perspectives. New York, Raven Press, 1984, p 19.
48. Glennon R, Titeler M, Young R: Structure-activity relationships and mechanism of action of hallucinogenic agents based on drug discrimination and radiologic binding studies. Psychopharm Bull *22*(3):953–957, 1986.
49. Shulgin AT: Chemistry of phenethylamines related to mescaline. J Psychedel Drugs *11*(1–2):41–52, 1979.
50. Geehr EC: Toxic plant ingestions. *In* Auerbach PS, Geehr EC (eds): Management of Wilderness and Environmental Emergencies. New York, Macmillan, 1983, pp 379–425.
51. Payne RB: Nutmeg intoxication. N Engl J Med *269*:36–38, 1963.

CHAPTER 43
DESIGNER DRUGS AND AMPHETAMINES

A. Designer Drugs

Patrice Barish, M.D.
Judith Tintinalli, M.D.

"Designer drugs" is the name given to a general group of synthetic controlled substance analogues, usually opioid or psychedelic derivatives, produced for the purpose of illicit distribution.[1] Underground chemists create new designer drugs by varying the chemical structure of an existing illicit or controlled substance. Producers of designer drugs can evade the law by creating new chemicals that do not fall under the jurisdiction of the United States Drug Enforcement Administration. These synthetic counterparts can be stronger and cheaper than the original drug, and in some localities, the demand for designer drugs has severely undercut the demand for traditional narcotics.

Designer drugs are not a new phenomenon.[2] In the late 1960s, a number of hallucinogenic amphetamine analogues of mescaline were produced. In the early 1970s, black market chemists produced chemical variants of methaqualone, phencyclidine, and amphetamines. An increase in designer drug use was noted in the early 1980s when several unexplained deaths, suspected to be drug-associated, occurred in Orange County, California. No evidence of narcotics was found in blood and urine specimens. Later, it was determined that these deaths were due to overdose of alpha-methyl fentanyl, which is a synthetic analogue of the legitimate anesthetic fentanyl citrate.[3]

Examples of modern designer drugs include analogues of fentanyl, such as alpha-methyl fentanyl, para-fluoro fentanyl, alpha-methyl acetylfentanyl, benzyl fentanyl, and 3-methyl fentanyl; meperidine, particularly MPPP (1-methyl-4-phenyl-propionoxypiperidine) and MPTP (*N*-methyl-4-phenyl-1,2, 3,6-tetrahydropyridine); phencyclidine; and phenylpropanolamine methylenedioxyamphetamine (MDA), and MDA's *N*-methyl analogue, MDMA.

Fentanyl Analogues

Fentanyl is a synthetic phenylpiperidine opioid, which acts as an agonist of the opiate receptor. It is commercially available as fentanyl citrate (Sublimaze), a potent, short-acting anesthetic, and its respiratory depressant and muscular rigidity effects can be reversed with naloxone. Three-methyl and alpha-methylfentanyl are synthetic analogues sold on the street as "China White" or "Synthetic," a yellow-white powder said to be about 100 times more potent than morphine.[3, 4] The sedative dose is thought to be as low as 0.05 mg. The onset of action of these analogues is extremely rapid; very small doses can cause sudden death from respiratory arrest; and they are not detected on routine drug screens. Opioid analogue overdose should be suspected as a cause of death or respiratory depression in young adults, even in the absence of overt signs of drug abuse, such as needle tracks.

Meperidine Analogues

In the illicit production of the meperidine analogue MPPP (1-methyl-4-phenyl-propionoxypiperidine), a dangerous byproduct, MPTP (N-methyl-4-phenyl-1,2,3,6-tetrahydropyridine) has been demonstrated. MPTP is a neurotoxin that appears to selectively destroy dopaminergic neurons, resulting in the development of extrapyramidal or choreiform movement disorders.[1, 5, 6] The disorder is not dose related, and, once symptoms appear, they are generally irreversible, although clinical improvement can result during treatment with l-dopa. Abuse of MPTP should be considered in any young patient presenting with parkinsonian or choreiform movement disorders. Substances similar to

MPTP may be industrial chemical byproducts and are suspected etiologic agents in the development of Parkinson's disease by people in industrial settings.

Psychedelics

The psychedelic drugs include a large group of compounds characterized by the ability to produce hallucinations, heightened awareness of sensory input, and a diminished capacity to delineate the boundaries between self and the environment. Most hallucinogenic drugs are indolealkylamines (LSD, psilocybin, dimethyltryptamine), or phenylethylamines (mescaline), or phenylisopropylamines (dimethoxyamphetamine, DMT). Countless derivations of these compounds can be synthesized and sold illicitly for their mood-altering properties.[6] Two popular street hallucinogens are MDA (3,4-methylenedioxyamphetamine) and MMDA (5-methoxy-3,4-methylenedioxyamphetamine). Besides the mood- and perception-altering effects, sympathomimetic effects such as pupil dilation, hypertension, tachycardia, hyperthermia, and hyperreflexia can occur. The general duration of action is up to 12 hours, although more prolonged panic states can occur. In some individuals, the use of psychedelic agents can produce severe depression, paranoid behavior, or psychosis.[7]

Phencyclidine is an arylcyclohexylamine that was developed as an anesthetic, but its use was abandoned because it caused delirium. Although its use has diminished, it is still manufactured and sold illicitly, often misrepresented as LSD or mescaline. The major clinical effects are nystagmus, ataxia, and dissociative anesthesia. Impressive aggressive behavior, paranoia, and agitation are also commonly evident. Hypertension, tachycardia, hyperthermia, dystonia, and rhabdomyolysis can also occur.[7]

Summary

Designer drugs can be chemically manipulated continually so that drug analysis may be negative despite the presence of an obvious toxic drug syndrome. Treatment is supportive: naloxone and supportive care for consumers of the opioid derivatives; sedation, generally with a benzodiazepine derivative, and symptomatic treatment of sympathomimetic effects, for those with the effects of the psychedelics.

References

1. Shafer J: Designer drugs. Science, March 1985, 60–67.
2. Medical News and Perspectives: A growing industry and menace: Makeshift laboratory's designer drugs. JAMA *256*:3061–3063, 1986.
3. Brittain JL: China White: The bogus drug. J Toxicol Clin Toxicol *19*:1123–1126, 1982–83.
4. Ayres WA, Starsiak MJ, Sokolay P: The bogus drug: Three-methyl and alpha-methyl fentanyl sold as "China White." J Psychoactive Drugs *13*:91–93, 1981.
5. Burns RS: The clinical syndrome of striatal dopamine deficiency. N Engl J Med *312*:1418–1421, 1985.
6. Appler WD: View from the nation's Capital. J Clin Psychopharmacol 5:350–352, 1985.
7. Jaffe JH: Drug addiction and drug abuse. *In* Gilman AG, Goodman LS, Rall TW, Murad F (eds): The Pharmacological Basis of Therapeutics. 7th ed. New York, Macmillan, 1985, pp 532–566.

B. Amphetamines

Richard O. Shields, M.D.

History

The term *amphetamines* refers to a family of structurally related compounds with limited legitimate clinical uses but vast potential for abuse, addiction, and toxicity. Racemic betaphenylisopropylamine is the prototype member of the family, first synthesized in 1887 and called "amphetamine." Manipulation of the basic amphetamine molecule in an attempt to reduce unwanted side effects and abuse potential and to enhance desired effects has led to the development of compounds with varying clinical effects and similar toxicities.

"Ice" is crystallized methamphetamine; it has gained popularity in Hawaii and on the West Coast of the United States because it is easily made, it can be smoked, and its action lasts for hours (as opposd to minutes for crack). It has a high addictive potential.

The first medical use of amphetamine was in 1932, when Smith, Kline, and French, the pharmaceutical company, introduced a new weapon in the fight against the common cold: the Benzedrine nasal inhaler. Each inhaler contained 250 mg of amphetamine base. When inhaled, Benzedrine produced relief of nasal congestion through potent local vasoconstriction.[1]

One side effect of Benzedrine inhalation was sleeplessness, an observation that soon led to the use of amphetamine in the treatment of narcolepsy. Over the next few years, amphetamines were recommended for use in the treatment of a wide variety of disorders, including obesity, drug and alcohol addiction, childhood hyperactivity, urinary incontinence, schizophrenia, and many others.[2]

Amphetamines, which were readily available without prescription, were touted as "pep" pills for the relief of fatigue and to fight off unwanted sleep. When reports of the medical complications of amphetamine abuse began appearing in the medical literature, the United States Food and Drug Administration intervened and in 1938 designated amphetamines as prescription-only drugs.

The demand and enthusiasm for amphetamines remained high, however, and the widespread use of pep pills by the combatants in World War II created a worldwide market for both prescription and black market amphetamines. Postwar epidemics of oral and intravenous abuse of readily available amphetamines occurred in Japan, Sweden, Australia, and the United Kingdom.

In the United States, the epidemic began in the early 1950s with the use of amphetamine tablets by students, long-distance truck drivers, and others seeking to avoid sleep. By the early 1960s, the intravenous injection of amphetamines became popular among the drug subculture as a means of getting "high." By the early 1970s, pharmaceutical companies were producing vast amounts of amphetamines (12 billion tablets in 1971 alone), an estimated 90 per cent of which were diverted to illicit use.[3]

In 1971, the Food and Drug Administration placed the most commonly abused amphetamines among Schedule II drugs (drugs that have some medical uses but high abuse potential) and restricted their legitimate use to the treatment of narcolepsy, hyperkinetic behavior in children, and short-term adjunctive therapy for weight reduction. Quotas on the production of amphetamines were also imposed. These measures reduced the amount of amphetamines available, but some physicians continued to write amphetamine prescriptions freely. Many abusers were able to get amphetamines from "script doctors"; physicians from whom controlled substance prescriptions could be obtained for a price. A study done by the Wisconsin Controlled Substances Board in 1976 revealed that only 26 of that states 9500 licensed practitioners had prescribed Biphetamine 20 (a combination of dextroamphetamine and amphetamine widely available on the illicit market) during 1975. Over 70 per cent of the 118,300 doses were prescribed by only five practitioners and appeared to represent diversion of the drug for illicit purposes under the guise of treating obesity.[4]

As the supply of pharmaceutical amphetamines began to decrease, amateur chemists began producing amphetamines in clandestine laboratories. Amphetamines are easy to synthesize, do not require expensive equipment, and reward the producer with large profit margins. During 1987, federal and state police agencies discovered nearly 650 clandestine laboratories, most of them in California, and many of them producing so-called "crystal meth"—a popular street amphetamine.[5]

Specific Agents

Methamphetamine and amphetamine are the most commonly abused drugs in this group, with local geographic variations based on availability, habit, price, and user sophistication. Methylphenidate is popular in some areas for intravenous use. Phentermine, phenmetrazine, phendimetrazine, diethylpropion, and fenfluramine have been used extensively as anorectic agents and are involved in accidental and intentional overdoses as well as in recreational drug use.

Hallucinogenic Amphetamines. Synthetic drugs with methoxy substitutions on the phenyl ring of the amphetamine molecule are referred to as hallucinogenic amphetamines. These drugs are also structurally sim-

Table 43–1. Amphetamines and Related Substances

Chemical or Common Names	Trade Names	Street Names
amphetamine		Speed, bennies, dex, dexies, uppers
racemic	Benzedrine	
D-isomer	Dexedrine	
methamphetamine	Desoxyn	Meth, speed, crystal meth
phentermine	Ionamin, Fastin	
phenmetrazine	Preludin	
methylphenidate	Ritalin	
diethylpropion	Tepanil, Tenuate	
methylenedioxyamphetamine		Love drug, MDA, Ecstasy, speed for lovers
3,4-methylenedioxymethamphetamine		MDMA, Ecstasy, XTC, Adam, MDM
3,4-methylenedioxyethamphetamine		MDEA, EVE
4-methyl-2,5-dimethoxyamphetamine		STP, DOM, Serenity-tranquility-peace
epinephrine	Adrenalin	
dopamine	Intropin	

ilar to mescaline and exhibit both central nervous system stimulation and hallucinogenic activity. The first of these drugs, methylenedioxyamphetamine, or MDA, was synthesized in 1910. It was patented later as an antitussive and an anorectic agent. It was rediscovered in the United States in the 1960s with the increasing popularity of "psychedelic" drugs and was widely abused. It was classified by the United States Drug Enforcement Administration as a Schedule I drug (no legitimate use, high abuse potential) in 1973, but its use in the drug subculture continued.[6] Although classified as a hallucinogen, MDA at doses of 100 to 200 mg has the purported ability to heighten self-awareness, increase esthetic sense, increase spirituality, decrease defensiveness and anxiety, and increase desire for interpersonal contact. The street names for MDA reflect this reputation: "love drug," "speed for lovers," and "harmony." The use of MDA in this dosage range has been suggested as an adjunct in psychotherapy to enhance access to feelings and emotions.[6]

At higher doses, MDA produces both stimulant and mescaline-like effects, with visual hallucinations, panic, paranoia, hypertension, tachycardia, seizures, coma, hyperthermia, rhabdomyolysis, and adult respiratory distress syndrome (ARDS). A number of deaths related to MDA usage have been reported.[7]

Methylenedioxymethamphetamine (MDMA) differs from MDA by only a single methyl group on the amino nitrogen. It was first synthesized in 1914 as an anorectic agent. In the early 1970s, some psychiatrists began using MDMA in psychotherapy, and by the early 1980s it had become a popular drug of abuse with a reputation similar to that of MDA. It was classified as Schedule I by the DEA in July, 1985, on an emergency basis because of its similarity to MDA, its widespread recreational use, and its potential toxicity. Sufficient data do not exist at this time to determine whether MDMA has legitimate medical uses.[8] Deaths have been reported related to MDMA use.[9]

In an attempt to circumvent federal restrictions, more than 50 MDA analogues have been synthesized, some of which are now available on the illicit drug market. The more popular appear in Table 43–1.

PHARMACOLOGY

Structure

Amphetamine is the name given to the racemic mixture of the optically active compound phenylisopropylamine. Its trade name is Benzedrine. The D-isomer is called D-amphetamine, dextroamphetamine, dexamphetamine, or its trade name, Dexedrine. The L-isomer is known as L-amphetamine, or levoamphetamine. This is the structure of this parent compound:

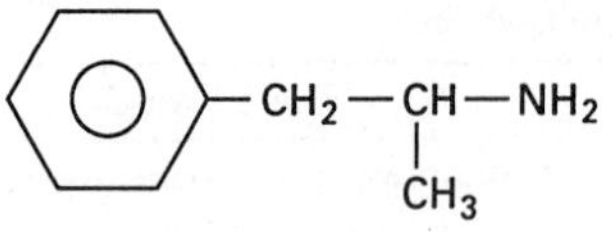

$$C_6H_5-CH_2-\underset{\displaystyle CH_3}{\underset{|}{CH}}-NH_2$$

The substitution of a methyl-group for a hydrogen on the amino-group results in methamphetamine, a drug with enhanced central CNS stimulation and high abuse potential.

Amphetamine analogues are produced by altering either the phenyl ring or the ethylamine side-chain. Adding a further methyl-group to the alpha-carbon produces phentermine, which has enhanced anorectic activity. Converting the side-chain to a cyclic structure, such as in methylphenidate, enhances the CNS stimulant effects while reducing the cardiovascular effects. Placing one or more methoxy-groups on the phenyl ring produces drugs with hallucinogenic effects similar to those of mescaline. Other modifications have produced potent monoamine oxidase inhibitors, such as tranylcypromine.

The amphetamines are indirectly acting sympathomimetic compounds with prominent central as well as peripheral activity. They are structurally very similar to the endogenous catecholamines epinephrine, norepinephrine, and dopamine. The alpha- and beta-adrenergic effects appear to result from the release of neurotransmitters from presynaptic vesicles rather than from direct stimulation of receptors. Amphetamines are also thought to block re-uptake of catecholamines by presynaptic neurons and to inhibit monoamine oxidase activity. These actions all tend to increase the concentration of neurotransmitter in the synapse and are felt to represent the mechanism of action producing the behavioral effects of amphetamines.[10]

The prominent CNS activity of amphetamines compared with other sympathomimetics accounts for their popularity as drugs of abuse. The CNS activity is mediated by both dopaminergic and adrenergic pathways in the brain that account for stereotyped behavior and locomotor activity, respectively. Stimulation of the reward center in the medial forebrain bundle may result from increased synaptic norepinephrine and produce euphoria and increased libido. Similar stimulation of the reticular activating system may result in the increased motor activity and decrease in fatigue produced by amphetamines. Stimulation of the dopaminergic system in the brain by amphetamines produces stereotypical behavior in humans and in animals and is thought to produce the schizophrenic-like symptoms of amphetamine psychosis.[11]

The so-called hallucinogenic amphetamines such as MDA and MDMA may produce perceptual and emotional alterations mediated via serotoninergic central pathways, although their exact mechanism of action remains unclear.[8]

Metabolism

Amphetamines are well absorbed across the mucosal surfaces of the GI tract, nasopharynx, tracheobronchial tree and vagina. Peak plasma levels after oral ingestion occur within 1 to 3 hours, varying somewhat with the degree of physical activity and the amount of food in the stomach. Amphetamines are highly lipid soluble and readily cross the blood-brain barrier. Protein binding and volume of distribution vary widely.

Amphetamines undergo extensive hepatic degradation with the production of numerous metabolites, some of which possess pharmacologic activity. Unchanged drug and metabolites are then excreted into the urine.

Amphetamine undergoes deamination and aromatic hydroxylation with benzoic acid and para-hydroxyamphetamine, the major metabolites that appear in the urine. *Renal excretion of unchanged amphetamine is highly variable and dependent on urinary pH. When the urine is acidic, as much as 60 per cent of a therapeutic dose of amphetamine is excreted unchanged within 48 hours. This percentage drops to about 5 per cent in alkaline urine.* The elimination half-life of about 10 hours in acid urine is prolonged two to three times when the urine pH is above 7.5.[10]

Methamphetamine undergoes *N*-dealkylation to amphetamine and aromatic hydroxylation to para-hydroxymethamphetamine. These two metabolites, along with unchanged drug, appear in the urine along with smaller amounts of other metabolites. As with amphetamine, urinary pH strongly affects the excretion of unchanged drug.[10]

Methylphenidate is metabolized almost exclusively by ester hydrolysis to the inactive metabolite ritalinic acid. Practically no unchanged drug is excreted.[10]

MEDICAL INDICATIONS

Soon after the discovery of their potent pharmacologic effects, amphetamines were being used to treat a wide variety of medical conditions. In 1946, only 14 years after the introduction of the Benzedrine inhaler, W. R. Bett listed 39 clinical uses of amphetamines. Conditions allegedly benefited by the use of amphetamines included cerebral palsy, colic, Parkinson's disease, opiate addiction, alcoholism, childhood behavior problems, epilepsy, schizophrenia, myasthenia gravis, migraine, urticaria, and dysmenorrhea.[2]

Currently, there are only three accepted medical indications for the therapeutic use of amphetamines: narcolepsy, attention deficit disorder in children, and obesity. Narcolepsy is a debilitating neurologic disorder characterized by irresistible attacks of the desire to sleep, which occur at inappropriate times and despite adequate hours of sleep. These attacks of sleep usually last only a few minutes and may occur many times a day. Amphetamine, dextroamphetamine, and methylphenidate in doses ranging from 20 to 60 mg per day have been shown to either reduce the frequency or eliminate the attacks.

Children with attention deficit disorder (ADD) exhibit impulsive behavior, inattention, and easy distractibility and may show motor hyperactivity. Methylphenidate in doses of 2.5 to 40 mg per day improves impulse control and attention in many of these children. Other amphetamines have also been used successfully in treating ADD.

Amphetamines continue to be used as an adjunct to the treatment of obesity, even though any long-term benefits are overshadowed by the very real risk of abuse and addiction. Amphetamines clearly do cause short-term suppression of appetite, but with continued use, tolerance to the anorectic effect develops. Obesity is a multifactorial behavioral and medical problem that requires emotional and lifestyle changes to combat. "Quick-fix" treatments may produce weight loss, but unless more permanent changes are made, weight is almost always regained.

PATTERNS OF ABUSE

Inhalers

Abuse of amphetamines began soon after the introduction of the Benzedrine nasal inhaler in 1932. It was soon discovered that the inhaler could be easily opened and the paper filler removed. The paper, impregnated with 250 mg of racemic amphetamine, could then be chewed and swallowed, or soaked in a variety of liquids and the liquid swallowed. Both methods extracted a significant portion of the amphetamine, making it available for absorption.[1] The manufacturer of Benzedrine attempted to reduce the misapplication of its product by making the inhaler more difficult to open and by adding picric acid to the filler, but abusers were not deterred. In 1949, with federal legislative action pending to strictly control amphetamine inhalers, Benzedrine was withdrawn from the market and a new product, Benzedrex, was introduced to replace it. The Benzedrex inhaler contained the nonamphetamine ingredient propylhexedrine, which was an effective vasoconstrictor yet had only 9 per cent of the CNS stimulation of amphetamine. Inhaler abusers had alternatives to Benzedrine, however, since other pharmaceutical companies were marketing their own amphetamine inhalers under the trade names Wyamine, Valo, and Nasal-ator. Not until 1959 did the FDA ban over-the-counter sales of amphetamine inhalers, 21 years after other forms of amphetamines were made available by prescription only.

By the early 1970s, both oral and IV abuse of the Benzedrex inhaler with some associated fatalities was being reported, especially among polydrug abusers. Propylhexedrine by the intravenous route appears to be toxic to the myocardium and pulmonary vasculature. Benzedrex inhalers remain available.

Occasional Abuse

The majority of those who use amphetamines without medical supervision do so sporadically, using small oral doses, and do not consider themselves drug abusers. Amphetamines are used to combat fatigue, enhance athletic performance, prevent drowsiness and sleep, suppress appetite during attempted weight loss, or for a temporary euphoric "high." As many as 20 per cent of American adolescents have used amphetamines, but only a small percentage of those will go on to chronic abuse.[12] Occasional use is not without its dangers, however. Small doses of amphetamines have been associated with serious toxicity in some individuals, and in some, occasional use leads to dependence, tolerance, and chronic abuse.

Chronic Oral Abuse

Tolerance to the euphoric effects of amphetamines develops rapidly, leading abusers to use larger and larger amounts of drug to attain and sustain the desired effect. Any attempt to halt or reduce drug intake produces debilitating depression and lack of energy that may last for many days. Amphetamines taken to alleviate the depression only continue the cycle. Often other drugs are used in an attempt to balance out the highs and lows. Many of these abusers were initiated to amphetamines by prescription anorectics and are sustained by obtaining prescriptions from one or more well-meaning physicians.

Intravenous Abuse

The intravenous (IV) injection of amphetamines, especially methamphetamine, produces an intense "rush" that is described as being an extremely pleasurable and powerful sensation. An intense craving for this short-lived euphoria develops, causing the IV abuser to inject repeatedly to sustain the sensation. Tolerance to IV amphetamines develops rapidly, forcing the IV abuser to use larger doses to obtain the same effect. The IV abuser's life revolves around obtaining and injecting the drug, which leads to social isolation, poor personal hygiene, criminal acts to obtain money or drugs, and other antisocial behavior. When exhaustion ensues or the drug supply is depleted, the "crash" follows. These periods are longer and more intense than those experienced by the oral abuser. Prolonged sleeping, occasionally filled with nightmares, is followed by binge eating. Profound depression occurs, sometimes precipitating suicide attempts. The abuser believes that the only way out is to inject more drug, and the cycle of "rush" and "crash" begins again.[13]

This type of amphetamine abuse is the least common but has a devastating impact on the abuser. It is difficult to treat, and relapses after apparent "cures" are common. The frequent occurrence of amphetamine psychosis further hampers treatment.

CLINICAL EFFECTS AND TOXICITY

The clinical effects of amphetamines on physiology and behavior can be predicted from their pharmacologic actions on the sympathetic and central nervous systems. Toxicity likewise can be predicted when clinical effects are excessive (acute toxicity) or prolonged (chronic toxicity).

Clinical Effects

Amphetamines became drugs of abuse because of their potent CNS stimulation. Amphetamines produce mood elevation, a feeling of self-confidence, a feeling of increased energy and decreased fatigue, anorexia, and euphoria. Intravenous abusers report a "rush" of intensely pleasurable feelings that some have described as similar to that of sexual orgasm.

The peripheral effects of amphetamines are mediated via alpha- and beta-adrenergic receptors. Stimulation of alpha-receptors produces mydriasis, increased metabolic rate, diaphoresis, increased sphincter tone, peripheral vasoconstriction, and decreased gastrointestinal motility. Stimulation of beta-receptors (both 1 and 2) produces increased heart rate and contractility, increased automaticity, and dilatation of bronchioles.[14]

Acute Toxicity

Mild toxicity usually presents with anxiety, restlessness, headache, palpitations, nausea, vomiting, insomnia, talkativeness, and irritability. Symptoms and signs that indicate more severe toxicity include confusion, agitation, stereotyped behavior, panic, hypertension, chest and abdominal pain, cardiac dysrhythmias, fever, and dilated pupils. The presence of the following symptoms indicates severe toxicity and demands immediate intervention: delirium, marked hypertension, hypotension, hyperpyrexia, coma, focal neurologic deficits, and hemodynamically significant cardiac dysrhythmias.[11]

Death from amphetamine toxicity is usually caused by acute cerebrovascular or cardiac events, including myocardial infarction and intracerebral hemorrhage.[15–21] A significant number of deaths, however, result from accidental or self-inflicted injuries. Deaths have also been reported from hyperthermia.[15] Other complications of amphetamine abuse that have been reported include cerebral vasculitis,[22] myoglobinuric renal failure,[23] cardiomyopathy with congestive cardiac failure,[24] hyperthyroxinemia,[25] hepatocellular injury,[26] and acute lead poisoning (from methamphetamine synthesized in a clandestine laboratory).[27]

The range of toxicity of amphetamines varies widely, based on individual variations and the development of tolerance. Children appear to develop toxicity at lower doses than do adults. Death has been reported with a dose as low as 1.5 mg per kg of methamphetamine in an adult male,[28] but some tolerant individuals have ingested as much as 15 gm in a 24-hour period without acute toxicity. Treatment clearly must be based on clinical findings and symptomatology rather than on estimates of the amount of drug ingested.

Chronic Toxicity

The hallmark of chronic amphetamine toxicity is the development of a paranoid psychosis resembling paranoid schizophrenia.[29] Hallucinations are usually tactile, visual, or olfactory, and repetitive stereotyped behavior is common. The psychosis usually remits upon withdrawal from amphetamines but may be reactivated by re-exposure to the drug or even by physical or psychologic stress.[10] This implies that chronic exposure to amphetamines produces long-term, if not permanent, changes in the brain. Amphetamines have also been shown to intensify psychotic symptoms or even induce psychotic episodes in some schizophrenics. This psychotomimetic effect of amphetamines is not well understood but may result from damage to nigrostriatal dopaminergic systems.

The chronic "speed freak" usually is poorly groomed, poorly fed to the point of malnutrition, paranoid, and with few close interpersonal relationships.[30]

Related Effects

Intravenous abusers of amphetamines are at risk for all the same medical complications faced by IV users of other drugs. Infectious complications include abscesses at injection sites, viral hepatitis (both beta and delta), acquired immunodeficiency syndrome, bacterial or fungal endocarditis, septic thrombophlebitis, tetanus, and pneumonia from septic pulmonary emboli. Inadvertent intra-arterial injection can lead to vasospasm, ischemia, or gangrene of the affected digit or limb. Injection of fillers or adulterants can produce toxicity related to the adulterant, or multiple microemboli to the lung, which can lead to restrictive lung disease.

TREATMENT

The treatment of amphetamine toxicity involves stabilization of vital functions, measures to prevent further absorption of ingested drug, attempts to enhance elimination of drug already absorbed, treatment of specific toxic symptoms, and disposition.

History

A brief but detailed history should be obtained from the patient or from those who brought the patient to medical attention. An accurate history may be difficult to obtain because of the fear of legal or family entanglements. The history should answer the following questions: What was taken? Was it a pharmaceutically produced drug, in which case amount and type of drug is known? Or was it a street drug, the type and potency of which may be quite variable with various adulterants present. Of 549 samples of alleged amphetamine and methamphetamine purchased "on the street" and analyzed by the Los Angeles Street Drug Identification Program from 1971 to 1980, 284 samples contained none of the alleged drug. A total of 15 substitutes were identified, including caffeine, lidocaine, ephedrine, procainamide, and benzocaine.[31] Other samplings of "street speed" have discovered more dangerous adulterants, including strychnine, barbiturates, and synthetic opiates.[32]

How was it taken? When taken intravenously, onset of action is quicker and gastrointestinal decontamination is unnecessary.

When was the drug taken? Onset of action of ingested amphetamine is 1 to 3 hours. Someone symptomatic 30 minutes after ingestion can be expected to have increased symptomatology and is a candidate for close monitoring and aggressive decontamination. Sustained release preparations are slower in onset but remain longer in the gastrointestinal tract and thus are available to decontamination measures longer.

Why was it taken? Drug-taking with self-destructive intent requires psychiatric evaluation when the patient is medically stable. Drug-taking that precipitates an emergency department visit may warrant counseling or detoxification for the patient.

Physical Examination

The examination of someone with suspected amphetamine toxicity begins with an assessment of the airway, vital signs, and neurologic status. Maintaining adequate ventilation and perfusion is the crucial first step in the management of the acutely poisoned patient.

Mild fever should be treated with cool compresses or sponging; core temperatures over 40°C or rapidly rising temperatures should be treated more aggressively with hypothermia blankets or ice baths. Dantrolene has been successfully used to treat drug-induced hyperthermia and should be considered if other methods of cooling fail.[11]

Mild hypertension with either a reflex bradycardia or a tachycardia usually requires no treatment. Severe hypertension (diastolic pressure greater than 120 mm Hg) should be treated, especially if symptoms of end-organ damage (especially CNS) are present. The treatment of choice is an IV infusion of nitroprusside, although other drugs have been suggested, including propranolol, diazoxide, chlorpromazine, nifedipine, and phentolamine. Nitroprusside is a vasodilator that opposes amphetamine-induced vasoconstriction and is rapidly effective, easily titrated, and very short-acting.

Hypotension may result from volume-depletion caused by poor intake, fever, hyperventilation, and increased metabolic rate. This volume depletion is easily correctable with IV infusions of crystalloid solutions. A more ominous cause of hypotension is left ventricular failure resulting from myocardial infarction, acute cardiomyopathy, or dysrhythmias. Ventricular dysrhythmias should be treated with IV lidocaine. Symptomatic supraventricular dysrhythmias should be treated with IV verapamil. Hypotension from infarction or cardiomyopathy may require invasive hemodynamic monitoring and the use of vasopressors such as dopamine.

Tachypnea is a frequent finding caused by increased metabolic rate, fever, and agitation. It requires no treatment, but tachypnea out of proportion to other findings requires a consideration of other reasons, such as metabolic acidosis, pulmonary edema, and pneumonia (especially in the IV abuser).

Mild agitation may be controlled by a supportive friend in a quiet setting. If agitation continues, the use of repeated small doses of IV diazepam may be needed. Agitation uncontrolled by diazepam may require IV haloperidol, droperidol, or chlorpromazine. These drugs have potential side effects of hypotension, respiratory depression, and dystonic reactions and should be used judiciously.

Seizures should be treated with aggressive airway management, ventilatory support, and IV diazepam. Seizures unresponsive to diazepam may require IV phenytoin (10 to 15 mg/kg) infused at 25 to 50 mg per min. Paralysis with pancuronium may be necessary in refractory seizures, especially those complicated by acidosis and/or rhabdomyolysis.

Acute psychotic symptoms may benefit from a supportive environment and rapid psychiatric evaluation. Suicidal ideation is common and precautions are advisable. More severe symptoms may require sedation with chlorpromazine or haloperidol.

Intracranial hemorrhage is a well-documented complication of both oral and IV amphetamine abuse.[17–20] Frequent presenting findings are severe headache, nausea, vomiting, confusion, disorientation, and focal neurologic deficits. Hypertension may be present, but a typical hypertensive hemorrhage may develop in the face of a normal blood pressure. Treatment involves rapid diagnosis by computed tomography, reduction of elevated intracranial pressure as indicated with hyperventilation and diuresis, and neurosurgical consultation for possible operative intervention.

Decontamination

The decision on how and if to decontaminate the gastrointestinal tract after oral amphetamine ingestion depends on the type of substance ingested (elixir vs. tablets vs. sustained release preparations), the time since ingestion, the amount ingested, and the level of patient agitation.

As with other drugs that may induce hypertension and seizures, syrup of ipecac–induced vomiting should probably be avoided. In the symptomatic but awake patient, activated charcoal, 30 to 100 gm in adults and 1 to 2 gm per kg in children, followed or accompanied by a cathartic such as sorbitol, may be a safer and equally efficacious choice.

If the patient is comatose, has lost the gag reflex, or has required heavy sedation, gastric lavage with a large-bore naso- or orogastric tube is preferred, followed by instillation of activated charcoal into the stomach via the tube. Protection of the airway with a cuffed endotracheal tube may be necessary.

Enhancing Elimination

Since amphetamines are basic compounds with high pKas, forced acid diuresis should enhance excretion via ion-trapping mechanisms in the renal tubule. Although there is question whether this is clinically efficacious, and although there are potential risks, including precipitating acute renal failure in the presence of myoglobinuria, acidification remains a significant therapeutic modality in amphetamine overdose. This technique should be used only with close monitoring of hemodynamic parameters, pH of blood and urine, and presence of myoglobin in the urine. Acidification can be attained using IV ascorbic acid or ammonium chloride, 1 to 2 gm every 4 to 6 hours. A urine pH of 5 is adequate with a urine output of about 5 ml per kg per hr. Arterial pH should be checked every 2 hours and acidification halted if it begins to fall from the normal range.

The use of hemodialysis, charcoal hemoperfusion, or peritoneal dialysis is indicated only if renal or hepatic failure is present, blocking normal pathways of metabolism and elimination.

SUMMARY

Amphetamines remain recreational drugs for many people and are readily available in many formulations. The medical, psychiatric, and sociologic complications of the use of amphetamines may cause the abuser to seek help from health care workers, emergency departments, poison control centers, or other resources. Treatment is directed at maintaining vital functions, treating toxic symptoms, and promoting an acid diuresis with monitoring as indicated.

References

1. Anderson RJ, Reed WG, Hillis LD: History, epidemiology, and medical complications of nasal inhaler abuse. J Toxicol Clin Toxicol *19*:95–107, 1982.
2. Bett WR: Benzedrine sulfate in clinical medicine: Survey of the literature. Postgrad Med J *22*:205–218, 1946.
3. Grinspoon L, Hedblom P: The Speed Culture—Amphetamine Use and Abuse in America. Cambridge, MA, Harvard University Press, 1975.
4. Treffert DA, Joranson D: Restricting amphetamines—Wisconsin's success story. JAMA *245*:1336–1338, 1981.
5. Lerner MA: An explosion of drug labs. Newsweek, April 25, 1988, p 25.
6. Climko RP, et al: Ecstasy: A review of MDMA and MDA. Intl J Psychiatr Med *16*:359–372, 1986–87.
7. Simpson DL, Rumack BH: Methylenedioxyamphetamine—clinical description of overdose, death, and review of pharmacology. Arch Intern Med *141*:1507–1509, 1981.
8. Seymour RB, Wesson DR, Smith DE, Zerkin EL, Novey JH (eds): MDMA: Proceedings of the conference. J Psychoact Drugs *18*:291–313, 319–327, 349–354, 1986.
9. Dowling GP, McDonough ET, Bost RO: "Eve" and "Ecstasy"—A report of five deaths associated with the use of MDEA and MDMA. JAMA *257*:1615–1617, 1987.
10. Caldwell J (ed): Amphetamines and Related Stimulants: Chemical, Biological, Clinical, and Sociological Aspects. Boca Raton, FL, CRC Press, 1980.
11. Linden CH, Kulig KW, Rumack BH: Amphetamines. Trends Emerg Med *7*:18–32, 1985.
12. Nicholi AM: The nontherapeutic use of psychoactive drugs. N Engl J Med *308*:928, 1983.
13. Smith DE, Fischer CM: An analysis of 310 cases of acute high-dose methamphetamine toxicity in Haight-Ashbury. Clin Toxicol *3*:117–124, 1970.
14. Gilman AG, Goodman LS, Rall TW, Murad F: The Pharmacologic Basis of Therapeutics. 7th ed. New York, Macmillan, 1985, pp 166–180.
15. Kalant H, Kalant OJ: Death in amphetamine users: Causes and rates. Can Med Assoc J *112*:299–304, 1975.
16. Carson P, Oldroyd K, Phadke K: Myocardial infarction due to amphetamine. Br Med J *294*:1525–1526, 1987.
17. Harrington H, Heller HA, Dawson D, Caplan L, Rumbaugh C: Intracerebral hemorrhage and oral amphetamine. Arch Neurol *40*:503–507, 1983.
18. Lukes SA: Intracranial hemorrhage from an arteriovenous malformation after amphetamine injection. Arch Neurol *40*:60–61, 1983.

19. Salanova V, Taubner R: Intracerebral haemorrhage and vasculitis secondary to amphetamine use. Postgrad Med J *60*:429–430, 1984.
20. Shukla D: Intracranial hemorrhage associated with amphetamine use. Neurology *32*:917–918, 1982.
21. Lucas PB, Gardner DL, et al: Methylphenidate-induced cardiac arrhythmias. N Engl J Med *315*:1485, 1986.
22. Matick H, Anderson D, Brumlik J: Cerebral vasculitis associated with oral amphetamine overdose. Arch Neurol *40*:253–254, 1983.
23. Scandling J, Spital A: Amphetamine-associated myoglobinuric renal failure. South Med J *75*:237–240, 1982.
24. O'Neill MB, Arnolda LF, et al: Acute amphetamine cardiomyopathy in a drug addict. Clin Cardiol *6*:189–191, 1983.
25. Morley JE, Shafer RB: Amphetamine-induced hyperthyroxinemia. Ann Intern Med *93*:707–709, 1980.
26. Stecyk O, Loludice TA: Multiple organ failure resulting from intravenous abuse of methylphenidate hydrochloride. *14*:597–599, 1985.
27. Alcott JV III, Barnhart RA, Mooney LA: Acute lead poisoning in two users of illicit methamphetamine. JAMA *258*:510–511, 1987.
28. Zalis EG, Parmley LF: Fatal amphetamine poisoning. Arch Intern Med *112*:60–64, 1963.
29. Robinson TE, Becker JB: Enduring changes in brain and behavior produced by chronic amphetamine administration: A review and evaluation of animal models of amphetamine psychosis. Brain Res Rev *11*:157–198, 1986.
30. Kramer JC, Fischman VS, Littlefield DC: Amphetamine abuse—patterns and effects of high doses taken intravenously. JAMA *201*:89–93, 1967.
31. Klatt EC, Montgomery S, et al: Misrepresentation of stimulant street drugs: A decade of experience in an analysis program. Clin Toxicol *24*:441–450, 1986.
32. Renfroe CL, Messinger TA: Street drug analysis: An eleven year perspective on illicit drug alteration. Semin Adolesc Med *1*:247–257, 1985.

CHAPTER 44
THE ANTIPSYCHOTIC DRUGS

Robert R. Bass, M.D., FACEP
Jonathan Vargas, M.D., FACEP

A. Phenothiazines and Other Psychotropics

The use of neuroleptic medications, also referred to as antipsychotic drugs or major tranquilizers, is widespread in the United States. Such drugs have remained the mainstay of treatment of psychoses since their introduction in the mid-1950s. Current indications for their use include a variety of clinical situations far beyond the realm of psychiatry. Neuroleptic drugs are used to control nausea, vomiting,[1] and intractable hiccups,[2] as well as for potentiation of analgesics and general anesthetics. Their sedative properties make them useful for sedation prior to invasive procedures and in the emergency chemical restraint of agitated patients.[3] In addition, neuroleptic agents are used in many neurologic disorders, and recently they have also been utilized as antiarrhythmics.[4]

Although five different classes of neuroleptic drugs are available, the phenothiazines and the butyrophenone haloperidol are the most commonly employed. Fatalities with the therapeutic use or abuse of neuroleptic agents are uncommon, and toxicity is less severe than that of the chemically related tricyclic antidepressants. Adverse reactions, however, are common and are usually manifested by either central nervous system (CNS) effects, such as extrapyramidal reactions or sedation, or cardiovascular effects, principally orthostatic hypotension or arrhythmias. The clinical presentation of neuroleptic toxicity can be difficult to recognize if it is not suspected. The frequent use of neuroleptics as antiemetics and for sedation in a wide range of clinical settings demands that clinicians in virtually every specialty understand the indications, actions, and adverse effects of these so-called "antipsychotic" medications.

PHARMACOLOGY OF NEUROLEPTIC DRUGS

The antipsychotic activity of neuroleptic drugs is closely associated with their propensity to block D-2 dopamine (DA) receptors in the brain.[5-7] All neuroleptic agents appear to be equally efficacious, but those with higher dopaminergic receptor affinity require a lower average daily dose to produce desired clinical effects (Fig. 44–1 and Table 44–1). Extrapyramidal symptoms occur when there is a decrease in dopaminergic activity relative to cholinergic activity in the basal ganglia.[8-10]

Neuroleptic drugs block other receptors, such as histamine (H_1 and H_2), alpha-adrenergic (alpha$_1$ and alpha$_2$), muscarinic, and serotonin receptors.[8, 11] The relative degree to which each neuroleptic agent binds these receptors determines its unique pharmacologic properties and side effects (Tables 44–2 and 44–3).

Classification

Currently available neuroleptic drugs may be divided into five major categories: phenothiazines, thioxanthines, butyrophenones, indoles, and diphenzoxapines (Fig. 44–2).

Rather than using the traditional classification of neuroleptic drugs by chemical structure, a more clinically useful classification is obtained through grouping based on relative receptor activity. For example, agents with

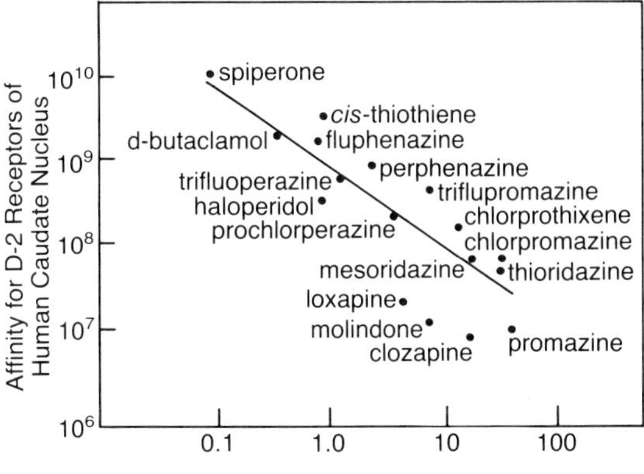

Figure 44–1. Relationship between neuroleptic affinities for the dopamine (D-2) receptor of human brain caudate nucleus and average daily dose for treating schizophrenia. (From Richelson E: Neuroleptic affinities for human brain receptors and their use in predicting adverse outcomes. J Clin Psychiatr 45:331–336, 1984. Used with permission.)

high muscarinic receptor affinity (such as thioridazine or chlorpromazine) are likely to produce sinus tachycardia or urinary retention, both of which may be a problem in elderly patients. These same agents would be less likely to produce extrapyramidal side effects, since a decrease in cholinergic activity in the basal ganglia would balance the reduction of dopaminergic blockade. In contrast, haloperidol, which has low muscarinic receptor affinity, has a high incidence of acute dystonic and extrapyramidal side effects. This classification provides a guide for selecting the most appropriate neuroleptic agent for a given patient and a better understanding of the adverse side effects and toxicity of these agents.[12]

Pharmacokinetics

The pharmacokinetics of neuroleptic drugs are variable and complex. While there may be some common elements with respect to metabolism, the kinetics have not been well studied overall, except for chlorpromazine, and little useful information is available. Chlorpromazine has been extensively studied and is a useful model, but may not be generalizable for all neuroleptic agents because of its complex metabolism.

The oral absorption of chlorpromazine tends to be erratic and unpredictable; in general, the best bioavailability is achieved through parenteral administration. In one study, chlorpromazine given as a single oral dose was shown to be only 32 per cent biologically available (range, 10 to 69 per cent) when compared with a single intramuscular injection. The reduced bioavailability of orally administered chlorpromazine appears to occur as the result of metabolism either within the gastrointestinal lumen or during absorption through the bowel wall. After one month of oral therapy, levels were even lower (by 37 per cent) than what would have been predicted from a single oral dose of chlorpromazine. This suggests that the bioavailability of orally administered chlorpromazine is further reduced in patients on chronic therapy.[13]

After absorption, peak chlorpromazine plasma levels are normally seen within 2 to 3 hours of a single oral dose, with a rapid fall-off in plasma concentration during the following 3 to 6 hours.[13]

Neuroleptic drugs are largely lipophilic

Table 44–1. NEUROLEPTIC POTENCY AND RANGE OF DAILY ORAL DOSING

NEUROLEPTIC AGENT	EQUIVALENT DOSE TO 100 MG OF CHLORPROMAZINE	RANGE OF DAILY ORAL DOSAGE
Alipathic		
chlorpromazine (Thorazine)	100	25–2000
Piperazine		
fluphenazine (Permitil, Prolixin)	2	1–25
perphenazine (Trilafon)	10	4–64
prochlorperazine (Compazine)	15	15–150
trifluoperazine (Stelazine)	5	2–64
Piperidine		
mesoridazine (Serentil)	50	75–400
thioridazine (Mellaril)	100	50–800
Butyrophenone		
haloperidol (Haldol)	2	1–30
Thioxanthene		
chlorprothixene (Taractan)	100	30–600
thiothixene (Navane)	4	6–60
Dihydroindolone		
molindone (Moban)	10	15–225
Dibenzoxazepine		
loxapine (Loxitane)	10	10–300

(Adapted from Black JL, Richelson E, Richardon JW: Antipsychotic agents: A clinical update. Mayo Clin Proc *60*:777–789, 1985.)

and are distributed throughout the body with a theoretical volume of distribution of 20 liters per kg.[13] They are extensively bound to tissues (particularly in the brain) and plasma protein (mostly albumin) and do not demonstrate simple single compartment pharmacokinetics. Neuroleptic drugs readily cross the placenta and enter the fetal circulation.[14–16] Because of its multicompartment distribution and extensive tissue binding, urinary metabolites of chlorpromazine may be seen up to several months after cessation of chronic therapy.

Neuroleptic metabolism occurs primarily in the liver. Metabolites are conjugated with glucuronic acid to produce hydrophilic compounds that can be excreted primarily in the urine and to a lesser extent in bile. Fetuses, infants, and elderly people have slower metabolic and elimination rates. Children, on the other hand, metabolize neuroleptic drugs more rapidly than do adults.[17, 18]

Table 44–2. AFFINITY OF NEUROLEPTIC AGENTS FOR SEVERAL NEUROTRANSMITTER RECEPTORS

	RECEPTOR					
		Histamine		*Adrenergic*		
ANTIPSYCHOTIC AGENT	*Dopamine D-2*	H_1	H_2	α_1	α_2	*Muscarinic*
chlorpromazine (Thorazine)	5.3	11	0.033	38	0.13	1.4
chlorprothixene (Taractan)	13	—	—	—	—	—
fluphenazine (Permitil, Prolixin)	125	4.8	—	11	0.064	0.053
haloperidol (Haldol)	25	0.053	0.0034	16	0.026	0.0042
loxapine (Loxitane)	1.4	20	—	3.6	0.042	0.22
mesoridazine (Serentil)	5.3	55	—	50	0.062	1.4
molindone (Moban)	0.83	0.00081	0.00142	0.040	0.16	0.00026
perphenazine (Trilafon)	71	12	—	10	0.20	0.067
prochlorperazine (Compazine)	14	5.3	—	4.2	0.059	0.18
thioridazine (Mellaril)	3.8	6.2	—	20	0.12	5.6
cis-thiothixene (Navane)	222	17	0.0213	9.1	0.50	0.034
trifluoperazine (Stelazine)	38	1.6	—	4.2	0.038	0.15

A higher numerical value indicates greater binding and greater antagonism of a given receptor.

(From Black JL, Richelson E, Richardson JW: Antipsychotic agents: A clinical update. Mayo Clin Proc *60*:777–789, 1985. Used with permission.)

Table 44–3. SIDE EFFECTS OF NEUROLEPTICS CAUSED BY RECEPTOR BLOCKADE

Antidopaminergic
Extrapyramidal movement disorders
Dystonia, parkinsonism, akathisia, tardive dyskinesia, rabbit syndrome
Endocrine effects
Prolactin elevation (galactorrhea, gynecomastia, menstrual changes, sexual dysfunction)
Antimuscarinic
Blurred vision
Attack or exacerbation of narrow angle glaucoma
Dry mouth
Sinus tachycardia
Constipation
Urinary retention
Speech blockage
Memory dysfunction
Decreased sweating
Antihistamine H_1
Sedation
Drowsiness
Hypotension
Weight gain
Anti-α_1-Adrenergic
Postural hypotension, lightheadedness
Reflex tachycardia

(From Richelson E: Neuroleptic affinities for human brain receptors and their use in predicting adverse effects. J Clin Psychiatry 45:331–336, 1984. Used with permission.)

Studies of chlorpromazine metabolism have demonstrated a number of oxidized metabolites that are biologically active.[17, 19] To a certain extent, the wide variation in observed therapeutic phenothiazine plasma concentrations can be explained by the presence of unmeasured metabolites with varying degrees of biologic activity. Thus, while the mean half-life for chlorpromazine is 18 hours (range, 6 to 119 hours), the biologic effects typically last much longer.[20]

TOXICOLOGY OF NEUROLEPTIC DRUGS

CNS Toxicity

The therapeutic as well as the adverse central nervous system effects of neuroleptic drugs stem from their dopamine receptor antagonism within the CNS.[8] Blockade of dopamine receptors in the nigroneostriatal neural pathways within the basal ganglia results in extrapyramidal reactions. Blockade of dopaminergic (DA) neurons by neuroleptic agents causes a loss of the normal DA inhibitory effect on cholinergic neurons with the consequent development of hypokinetic side effects (parkinsonism).[21] A similar mechanism probably explains the development of acute dystonic reactions, akathisia, and may also contribute to the malignant neuroleptic syndrome. On the other hand, chronic dopamine receptor blockade from long-term neuroleptic drug therapy may result in denervation hypersensitivity and subsequent increase in dopamine levels within the CNS, leading to hyperkinesia (tardive dyskinesia). The extrapyramidal symptoms described later occur with usual doses of neuroleptic drugs and are not dose related.

Acute Dystonic Reactions (Dyskinesia). Acute dystonic reactions usually occur within the first 4 days of therapy with a neuroleptic drug but may seen within hours of a single dose. Dystonic reactions occur in about 12 per cent of patients receiving neuroleptic agents and occur twice as often in male patients as in female patients.[22] Children are especially prone to develop severe generalized dystonic reactions.[23, 24]

Often considered benign or not recognized by inexperienced clinicians, dystonic reactions are quite distressing and occasionally may be life threatening. Spasmodic, intermittent contractions of facial, neck, or back muscles are characteristic, resulting in bizarre grimaces, tongue protrusion, trismus, torticollis, opisthotonos, or respiratory difficulty. Less commonly, spasms of the pharyngeal and laryngeal muscles can lead to choking, respiratory distress, and asphyxia. Oculogyric crisis with painful lateral or vertical deviation of the eyes and blepharospasm can also occur. The patients are often considered hysterical because of the unusual appearance of the dystonias. The focal nature of the symptoms has resulted in the misdiagnosis of seizures in some instances. The differential diagnosis includes other causes of dystonia, such as dystonic cerebral palsy, tetanus, Sydenham's chorea, and Wilson's disease. Meningitis must be considered in patients with dystonic reactions and fever.[25]

Clinicians should consider neuroleptic toxicity in patients with an appropriate clinical presentation even when no clear history of neuroleptic ingestion is apparent, since many patients are often unaware of the medication they are taking, especially elderly people.[26] Many individuals who abuse neuroleptic drugs recreationally will deny any history of drug ingestion. In these cases treatment for

PHENOTHIAZINES

Aliphatic Group	Piperidine Group	Piperazine Group
S; N; R; $CH_2CH_2CH_2—N(CH_3)_2$	S; N; R_1; R_2	S; N; R_1; $CH_2CH_2CH_2—N$ (piperazine) $N—R_2$
promazine (Sparane) chlorpromazine (Thorazine) triflupromazine (Uesprin)	prochlorpromazine (Compazine) trifluoperazine (Stelazine) fluphenazine (Prolixin) perphenazine (Trilafon)	thioridazine (Mellaril) mesoridazine (Serentil)

THIOXANTHENES

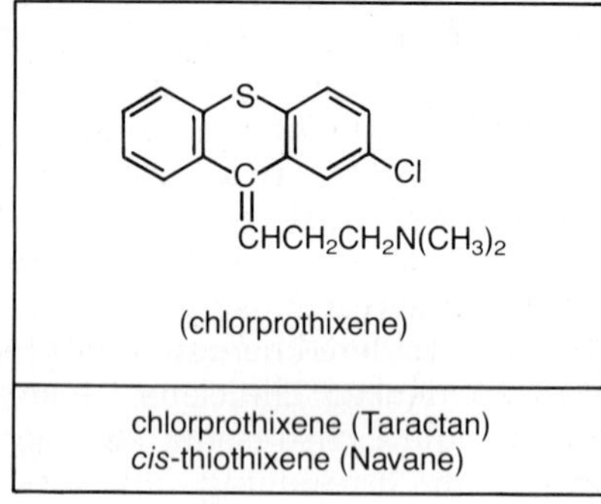

chlorprothixene (Taractan)
cis-thiothixene (Navane)

BUTYROPHENONES

O
N
OH
F
Cl
(haloperidol)

haloperidol (Haldol)
spiperone

INDOLES

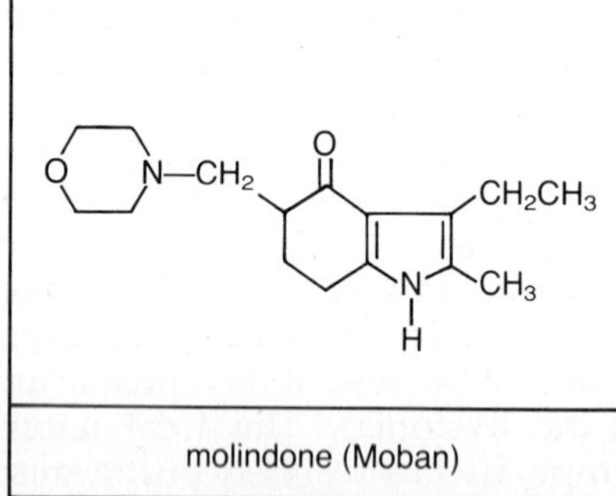

molindone (Moban)

DIBENZOXAZEPINES

NCH_3
N
N
Cl
O

loxapine (Loxitane)

Figure 44–2. Classification of neuroleptic agents by chemical structure.

possible neuroleptic-associated dystonic reactions is often diagnostic as well as therapeutic.

Parkinsonism (Akinesia). Parkinsonism is characterized by a generalized slowing of volitional movement (bradykinesia). The classic pill-rolling tremor may not be present. Parkinsonism may at first be mistaken for depression.[21] The shuffling gait may also be simply attributed to "old age." Although Parkinson's disease is found in elderly people, parkinsonism from neuroleptic drugs occurs in all age groups.[22]

Akathisia. Akathisia is characterized by motor restlessness and a subjective feeling of discomfort and unease. In severe cases the patient literally may run about constantly in a state of distress.[27] Often akathisia is mistaken for an exacerbation of psychosis, but increased doses of neuroleptic drugs in these instances only results in a worsening of the akathisia.

Tardive Dyskinesia. Tardive dyskinesia (TD) consists of involuntary choreiform movements of the lips, mouth, and tongue.[35] As opposed to the early onset of the aforementioned disorders, TD can occur within months of beginning neuroleptic drugs but the average is over 3 years. This disorder mandates careful selection of the neuroleptic agent for treatment of chronic disease states.[36]

Rabbit Syndrome. Rabbit syndrome is a focal tremor of the perioral muscles that is similar to that seen in patients with Parkinson's disease.[30]

Sleep Apnea. A possible link exists between the use of phenothiazines and sudden infant death. Sleep apnea has been demonstrated in normal infants with 1 mg per kg per day of promethazine and may explain the mechanism of sudden death associated with phenothiazine use in infants.[31] The use of neuroleptic drugs as antiemetics and antitussives in infants less than a year old, therefore, is not recommended.

Lowered Seizure Threshold. Patients with a prior history of seizures or of having a predisposing CNS lesion are at risk of developing seizures while taking phenothiazines. Status epilepticus has been reported to occur with overdoses of loxapine.[32]

Disordered Thermal Regulation. Hyperthermia can occur with therapeutic doses, either in the malignant neuroleptic syndrome or with anticholinergic impairment of sweating in elevated ambient temperatures, especially in elderly people. Hypothermia is unusual and is mild and not life threatening.

Neuroleptic Malignant Syndrome

The neuroleptic malignant syndrome (NMS) consists of hyperpyrexia up to 42.2° C, altered mental status manifested by delirium or coma, and "lead pipe" muscular rigidity. Autonomic dysfunction leads to labile blood pressure, tachycardia, diaphoresis, and urinary incontinence.[33–36] It is estimated that the NMS may occur in up to 1 per cent of patients exposed to neuroleptic drugs. The majority of affected individuals are less than 40 years of age.[30, 36] Eighty-four per cent of the reported reactions have involved the use of haloperidol, depot fluphenazine, or chlorpromazine, although other psychotropic agents have been implicated.[37] The syndrome typically develops over a period of 24 to 72 hours. The mortality rate is estimated at 20 per cent. Death is secondary to the complications of rhabdomyolysis, renal failure, cardiovascular collapse, respiratory failure, arrhythmias, or thromboembolism. Myocardial infarction has also been reported to complicate NMS.[38] The differential diagnosis includes heat stroke, lethal catatonia, central anticholinergic syndrome, intracranial hemorrhage, thyrotoxicosis, strychnine poisoning, malignant hyperthermia, meningitis, and adverse drug interaction with MAO inhibitors.[39]

Cardiovascular Toxicity

Serious cardiovascular events or deaths related to neuroleptic therapy are generally considered to be infrequent,[40] although some believe that the incidence may be underreported.[41, 42] Cardiovascular toxicity has been observed in patients on therapeutic doses of neuroleptic drugs, as well as in patients who have overdosed (Fig. 44–3).[40, 43] Certain neuroleptic agents demonstrate more cardiovascular toxicity than others, in particular thioridazine, mesoridazine, and chlorpromazine, whereas cardiac toxicity is rarely seen with the diphenzoxapines or haloperidol. Cardiovascular toxicity is usually manifested by either electrophysiologic changes or hypotension.

Electrophysiologic Changes. In therapeutic doses, neuroleptic drugs demonstrate a quinidine-like antiarrhythmic effect.[44] Electrocardiographic changes characteristically include increased PR or QT intervals, as well as nonspecific T wave widening, notching, or inversion.[45] Although cases have been reported of sudden death in patients on therapeutic doses of neuroleptic drugs, the association of these deaths and the electrocardiographic changes has not been fully established.[46]

Animal studies have suggested that antiarrhythmic and proarrhythmic effects may be dose related, with the former occurring with lower and the latter with higher or toxic doses of neuroleptic drugs.[47] At toxic levels, thioridazine has been noted experimentally to increase the likelihood of ventricular arrhythmias, which have been implicated as the most likely cause of sudden death associated with chronic phenothiazine therapy,[43] as well as with phenothiazine overdose.[40] Combined overdose of both a tricyclic anti-

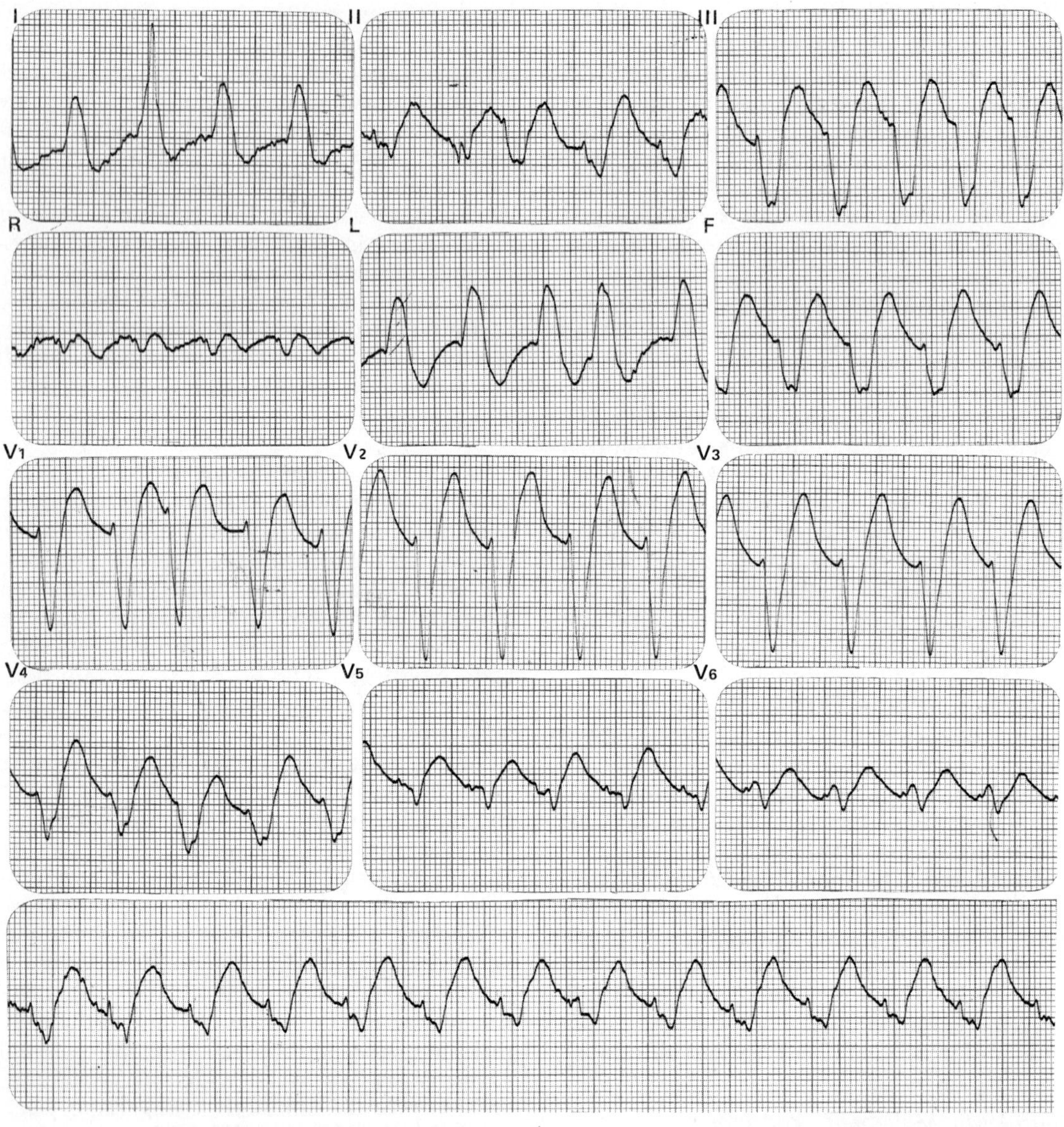

Figure 44–3. A 25 year old woman, blind since birth from retrolental fibroplasia, took an overdose of her medications: approximately 60 Serentil (mesoridazine), 100 mg per tablet, and approximately 60 Trilafon (perphenazine), 8 mg per tablet. One hour postingestion she arrived in the emergency department awake, alert, and walking, with an admission blood pressure of 142/70. Gastric lavage and instillation of activated charcoal and sodium sulfate were performed. Three hours postingestion the patient became comatose, and her blood pressure dropped to 84/60; an electrocardiogram (A) was immediately obtained, which revealed bizarre intraventricular conduction delay with a widened QRS (0.20 sec) and marked left axis deviation; P waves were not identified.

Because the patient's blood pressure improved on intravenous fluid therapy and her condition did not deteriorate further, she was managed conservatively with close observation but no drug therapy.

depressant and a phenothiazine is more likely to produce malignant arrhythmias. A particularly malignant ventricular arrhythmia, torsades de pointes, has been associated with chronic phenothiazine therapy.[48] A number of atrial arrhythmias and atrioventricular blocks have been reported in cases of neuroleptic overdose and may be of varying clinical significance.

Hypotension. A well-known side effect of neuroleptic therapy is orthostatic hypotension. Drugs with high alpha$_1$-receptor af-

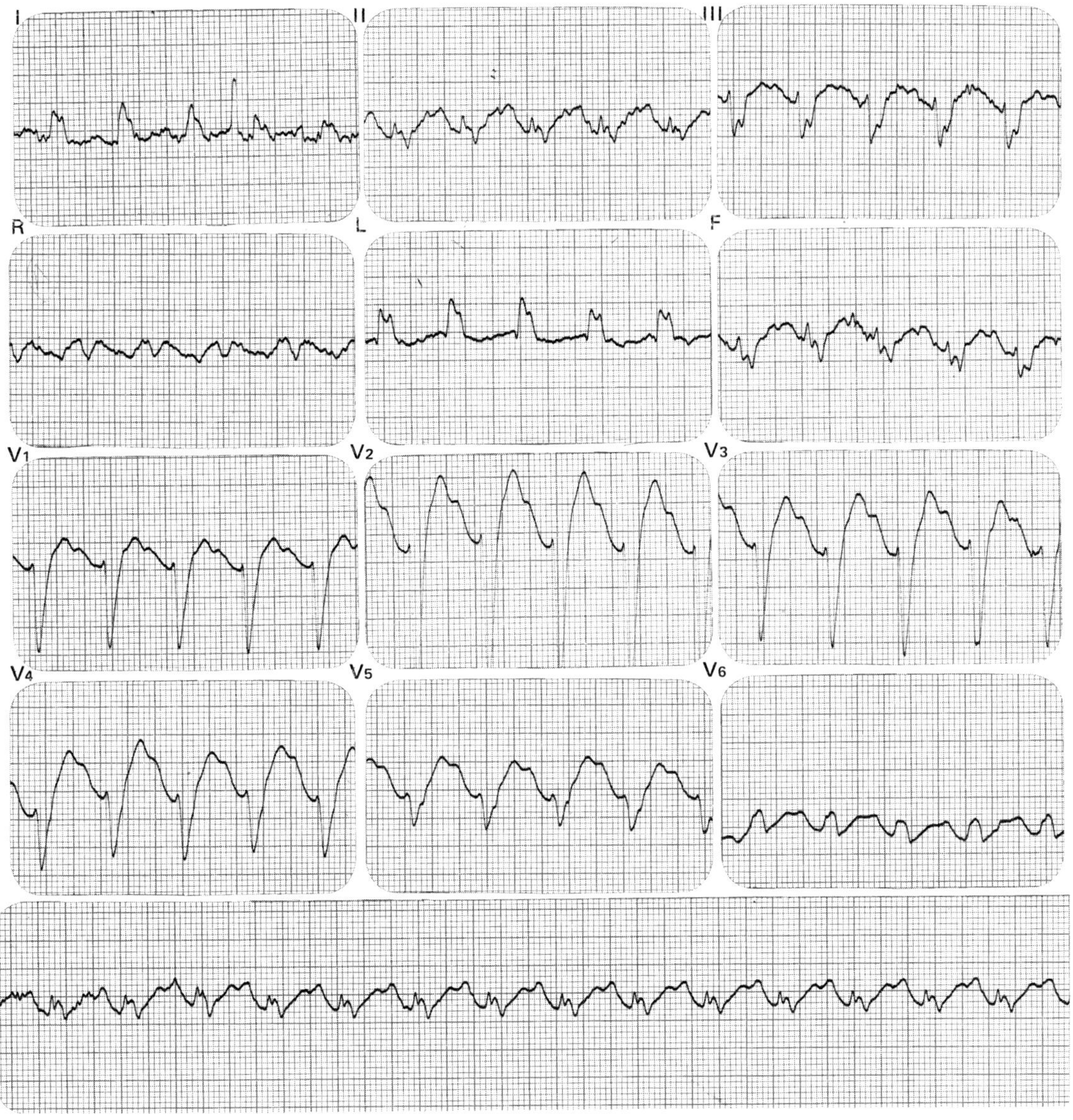

B

Figure 44–3 *Continued B,* Six hours after her hypotensive episode, a repeat ECG showed persistence of the intraventricular conduction defect, but there was perceptible narrowing of the QRS complex, and P waves were now evident.

Illustration continued on following page

tinity more commonly are associated with this problem. Frank hypotension from phenothiazine overdose may occur and most likely results from a combination of alpha$_1$-blockade as well as direct myocardial depression. Patients on antihypertensive therapy, in particular alpha$_1$-blocking agents, may experience an enhanced hypotensive effect. Paradoxic hypotension from unopposed beta-adrenergic stimulation may result if epinephrine is administered to individuals on neuroleptic therapy. Several cases of hypertension in children caused by haloperidol poisoning have been reported.[49, 50] The mechanism for this is unclear. It is recommended that children with a toxic ingestion of haloperidol be monitored for at least 48 hours for the development of hypertension.[49]

Other Cardiovascular Effects. A case of sudden death due to pulmonary edema has been reported in a patient on haloperidol.[51]

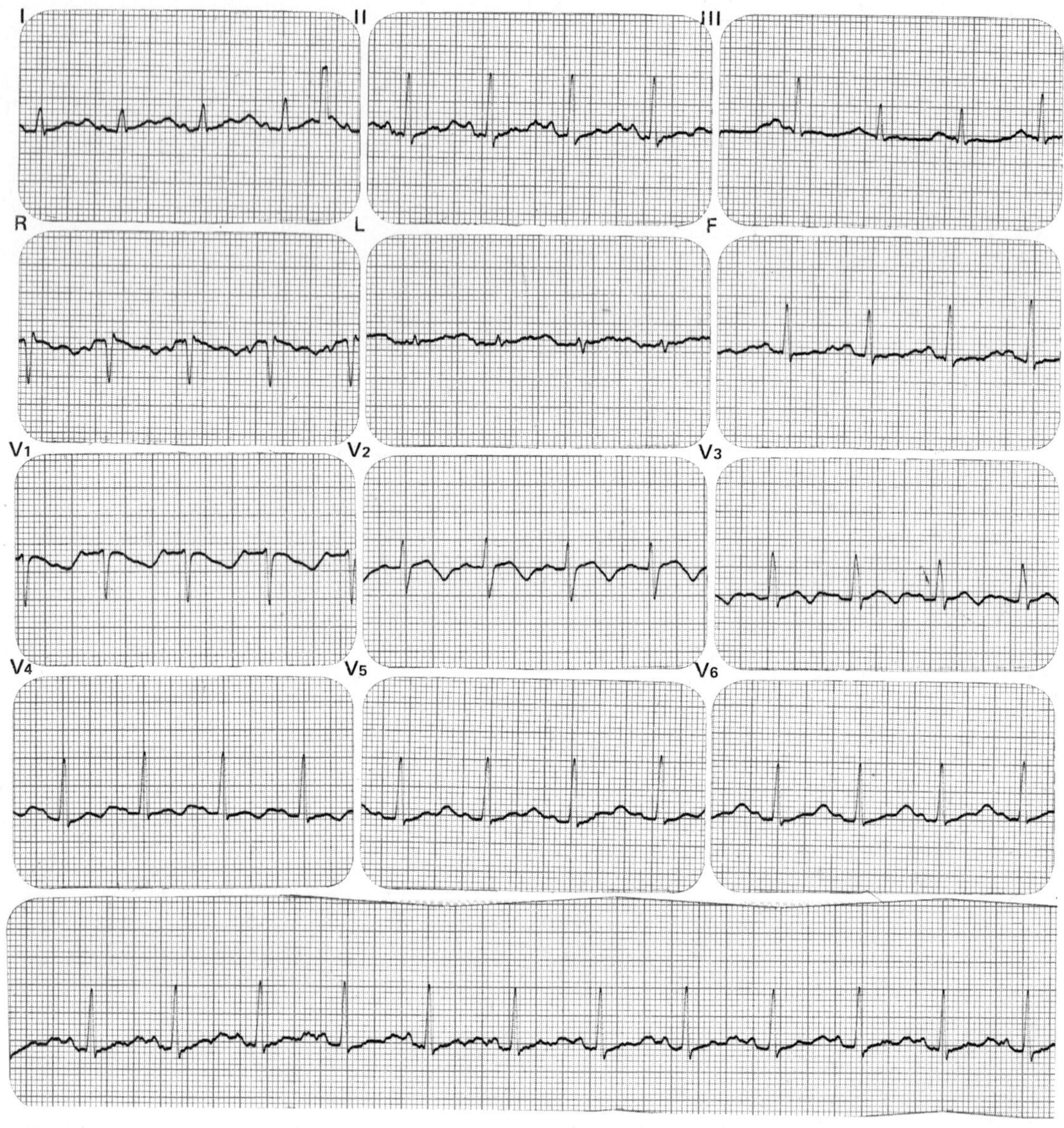

Figure 44–3 *Continued* C, The patient continued to improve, and the following day a third ECG showed resolution of the intraventricular conduction defect; the prolonged Q-T interval of 0.48 is compatible with phenothiazine effect. Following admission to the psychiatric unit after she was medically stable, the result of the admission gas chromatography drug screen confirmed the presence of phenothiazines. (Courtesy of Memorial Medical Center, Savannah, Georgia.)

The pathophysiology is unclear. Autopsies of patients who have died suddenly while on chronic phenothiazine therapy have disclosed myocardial deposits of an acid mucopolysaccharide.[52] The significance of these deposits is not known at this time.

Miscellaneous Adverse Effects

Priapism. Priapism has occurred with the use of neuroleptic drugs. It is unclear whether this is from peripheral alpha-adrenergic antagonism, central cholinergic excess, histamine receptor stimulation, or a combination of these mechanisms.[53–56]

Ocular Toxicity. Initially, many patients may complain of blurred vision secondary to the anticholinergic effects of neuroleptics on accommodation. This is usually well tolerated or may require only the wearing of reading glasses. Chlorpromazine and thioridazine have been implicated in serious ocular toxicity as well, which appears to be dose related.[57–60]

Dermatologic Reactions. Urticaria and dermatitis are common with neuroleptic use, occurring in about 5 per cent of patients on chlorpromazine. A hypersensitivity reaction may develop during the first 8 weeks of therapy and resolves with discontinuance of the neuroleptic drug. People who handle neuroleptic drugs frequently may develop a contact dermatitis.[61] Photosensitivity reactions may develop in some patients taking neuroleptic drugs; it resembles a severe sunburn.[59, 62] An effective sunscreen and the wearing of adequate covering when patients are in sunlight will help prevent this.[21]

An abnormal blue-gray pigmentation has been reported in patients receiving high-dose long-term phenothiazines. It is rarely seen with current prescribing practices.[21]

Hepatotoxicity. Cholestatic jaundice may also develop and is thought to be a hypersensitivity reaction. When neuroleptic therapy is imperative, switching to a low-potency dissimilar type of neuroleptic drug is advisable. When therapy can be discontinued, stopping the offending drug is sufficient to resolve any hepatic toxicity.[62] Cirrhosis is a late complication and fortunately is rare.[21]

Hematologic Disorders. Agranulocytosis is a rare (less than 1 in 10,000 cases) complication of neuroleptic use.[21] However, any patient who develops a sore throat or apparent upper respiratory infection, especially during the first 8 to 12 weeks of neuroleptic therapy,[63] should have a complete blood count performed to rule out a serious drug-induced blood dyscrasia.

Drug Interactions

A number of other pharmocologic agents that may interact with neuroleptics are listed in Table 44–4. Many of these interactions have already been discussed.

A few cases have been reported of an irreversible neurotoxic syndrome with symptomatology similar to the neuroleptic malignant syndrome resulting from the interaction of lithium and neuroleptic drugs. This occurs most commonly when patients are on high doses of both lithium and the neuroleptic drug, although it has been reported in patients with therapeutic serum levels of both agents.

Table 44–4. INTERACTION OF NEUROLEPTICS AND OTHER AGENTS

AGENT	ADVERSE EFFECTS
Depressants Sedatives Hypnotics Opiates Ethanol	Enhanced CNS and respiratory depression
Tricyclic antidepressants	Cardiac arrhythmias
Antiparkinsonism drugs	Enhanced anticholinergic effect
Antihypertensives MAO inhibitors	Enhanced hypotensive effect
Epinephrine	Hypotension
Antacids H_2 blocking agents	Decreased neuroleptic absorption
Warfarin	Reduced warfarin levels
Phenytoin	Increased levels of phenytoin
Tricyclic antidepressants	Increase in TCA and neuroleptic levels
Lithium	Neurotoxic syndrome

OVERDOSE

Massive overdose of a neuroleptic drug alone may cause coma, miosis, hypotension, hypothermia, dysrhythmias, or respiratory depression.[64, 65] However, the majority of overdoses involving only neuroleptic drugs are either asymptomatic or are manifested solely by antihistamine (H_1)–induced sedation.

Respiratory depression requiring endotracheal intubation is uncommon with neuroleptic overdose, but children appear to be at increased risk for developing apnea (even with therapeutic doses).[66] There is an increased risk of respiratory depression with the combined overdose of neuroleptic drugs and narcotics. In addition, combination drug therapy should not be routinely used for sedation of young children undergoing minor ambulatory care procedures.

In neuroleptic overdoses, dopamine receptor blockade within the hypothalamus may result in loss of thermoregulatory control. Hypothermia is more frequently seen than hyperthermia.[64]

Screening Tests

The Phenistix urine dipstick test is positive for phenothiazines if a violet color occurs initially and persists when 50 per cent H_2SO_4 is dropped onto the strip. A negative color reaction does not rule out phenothiazine ingestion.

An alternate approach is to add 10 to 15

drops of a 10 per cent ferric chloride solution to 1 ml of urine. Phenothiazines produce a burgundy wine and salicylates a dark purple color. A more complicated and quasi-quantitative method has also been reported, which may be helpful.[68] None of these screening tests are useful for detecting the nonphenothiazine neuroleptic drugs.

TREATMENT

Overdose

General Considerations

The initial approach to the treatment of neuroleptic toxicity should be based on the clinical scenario and presenting symptomatology. Patients with an acute overdose should be managed with attention to airway ventilation and cardiovascular support. As soon as possible, gastric contents should be evacuated, regardless of the time that has elapsed from ingestion, since gastric emptying may be delayed by the agent. Gastric lavage with a large-bore tube may be more desirable in many clinical situations. Ipecac, which is effective, should be used with caution because of the propensity for neuroleptic drugs to induce rapid sedation or seizures. When any question as to the status of the airway exists, endotracheal intubation should be accomplished prior to gastric lavage.

Hemodialysis and forced diuresis do not appear to enhance elimination because of extensive tissue- and protein-binding by neuroleptic drugs.

The majority of patients presenting with neuroleptic toxicity will be on therapeutic doses and will manifest a particular reaction to the agent, usually CNS- or cardiovascular-related. These reactions are usually not life threatening, and intervention can be directed toward reducing or eliminating the symptomatology.

Seizures

Seizures are treated initially with diazepam and then a loading dose of phenytoin. Particular attention should be paid to ruling out treatable hypoglycemia secondary to other ingested or injected substances. Patients with neuroleptic toxicity are already prone to developing hyperthermia, and this is doubly true for patients with generalized seizures. Myoglobinuria may complicate seizures leading to renal failure. Therefore, attention to maintaining optimal hydration and ensuring adequate urine output is critical.

Cardiovascular

Orthostatic hypotension or, less commonly, frank hypotension results from an alpha-adrenergic receptor blockade that reduces peripheral vascular resistance.[46, 68] Reduced myocardial contractility may play a role as well. Patients with frank hypotension should be placed supine; if there are no signs of congestive failure, a fluid challenge with an appropriate crystalloid should be initiated. If there is no response to the fluid challenge, an alpha-adrenergic agent such as norepinephrine, methoxamine, or phenylephrine may be useful. Adrenergic agents with high beta-adrenergic activity, such as epinephrine or dopamine, in theory may exacerbate the hypotension by enhancing relatively unopposed beta-adrenergic stimulation. Careful and appropriate hemodynamic monitoring should be done to ensure optimal therapy.

Patients on alpha-adrenergic blocking antihypertensive agents may experience an exaggerated antihypertensive effect when treated with neuroleptic drugs. Such patients can be managed by switching to a nonalpha-blocking antihypertensive agent or to a neuroleptic drug with less alpha-receptor affinity.

Both atrial and ventricular arrhythmias may occur as the result of neuroleptic toxicity. Underlying factors such as hypoxia, acidosis and electrolyte abnormalities should be addressed and corrected if necessary. Ventricular arrhythmias, such as premature ventricular contractions or ventricular tachycardia that is hemodynamically stable, may be treated with lidocaine or phenytoin. Agents that reduce conductivity, such as quinidine or procainamide, should be avoided. Overdrive pacing may prove useful in some cases.[69] Empiric treatment with sodium bicarbonate has been proposed but is not a proven modality. Torsades de pointes, a particularly malignant form of ventricular tachycardia, is refractory to treatment with conventional therapy and should be managed with an infusion of isoproterenol.[70] The initial infusion of isoproterenol should be 0.2 μg per minute and titrated to a heart rate of between 80 and 100 beats per minute.

Other arrhythmias, such as asystole, ventricular fibrillation, or atrioventricular blocks, should be managed with currently accepted treatment guidelines. Physostigmine, once proposed for the treatment of atrial tachycardias associated with mixed tricyclic and phenothiazine overdose, should be avoided because of its potential for inducing severe bradycardia or asystole.[71]

Dystonic Reactions

Acute dystonic reactions brought on by dopamine blockade within the central nervous system, with resultant cholinergic stimulation in the nigrostriatal system, are effectively treated with drugs that have anticholinergic actions. Benztropine, 2 mg, or diphenhydramine, 1 to 2 μg per kg (up to 50 mg) IV or IM, is recommended.[72, 73] Benztropine has the advantage of a longer duration of action. Both can cause sedation as a bothersome side effect. The initial parenteral treatment should be followed by oral benztropine or diphenhydramine for 3 to 4 days. Another oral agent, trihexyphenidyl, is also useful in controlling extrapyramidal reactions. The usual dosage is 2 to 5 mg tid with meals. Anticholinergic side effects occur in 30 to 50 per cent of patients on trihexyphenidyl. Diazepam also has been successful. Benztropine prophylaxis during the initial 7 days of neuroleptic therapy has been shown to decrease markedly the incidence of dystonic reactions.[74]

Akathisia may be seen early during treatment with neuroleptic drugs or soon after a dose increase. Most patients respond to a decrease of their medication. Propranolol and other beta-blockers with good CNS penetration, such as metoprolol and betaxolol, have been reported to be effective in about 50 per cent of cases.[75, 76] Diazepam and diphenhydramine are not as effective but may be of use. Clonidine also may offer some benefit.[77]

Tardive dyskinesia (TD) is a syndrome associated with long-term neuroleptic use. There is no effective treatment for TD currently. The best hope for minimizing it is by prevention.[36, 75] Using the lowest effective neuroleptic dose and frequently reassessing patients as to medication needs are necessary. Drug-free intervals or "holidays" have been advocated but are not proved to decrease the incidence of TD.[78] The use of neuroleptic drugs in any disorder other than schizophrenia for more than 6 months needs very careful scrutiny. Once TD develops, discontinuance of the neuroleptic agent is recommended if the patient can tolerate this. No known medication is entirely effective in treating TD, although many have been tried. Approaches have focused on influencing CNS dopamine, acetylcholine, GABA, serotonin, and neuropeptides with varying success. At present, no drug can be recommended for the treatment of TD.

Neuroleptic Malignant Syndrome

The neuroleptic malignant syndrome (NMS) is a life-threatening disorder that requires early recognition. First, the neuroleptic drug must be stopped and general measures to cool patients with severe hyperthermia should be instituted. The patients' fluid and electrolyte status should be brought to optimal function and urine output maintained to prevent myoglobin-induced renal failure.[79] Two anecdotal approaches to NMS have been reported as being successful.[80–83] Bromocriptine, a dopamine agonist, has also been successfully employed and theoretically corrects the dopamine depletion within the CNS. The oral dose of bromocriptine is 2.5 mg bid initially, gradually increasing to 5 mg tid. Doses up to 60 mg per day have been used.[80] Dantrolene, a muscle relaxant effective in malignant hyperthermia, can be given in a dose of 0.8 to 1.0 mg per kg every 6 hours orally or intravenously.[81, 82] Treatment for up to 2 weeks may be necessary. Relapses may occur, especially when the NMS is associated with depot fluphenazine, which is still effective after several weeks. Amantidine has also been successfully used to treat the NMS.[83] Levodopa, carbidopa, pancuronium bromide,[84] and sodium nitroprusside[85] have been used with some success, but little evidence supports their routine use at this time for NMS. The antimuscarinic drugs are not effective in treating NMS even though they are effective in the treatment of the neuroleptic-induced dystonias.

References

1. Ordog G, Vann PW, Owashi ND, Wassergerger J, Herman L: Intravenous prochlorperazine for the

rapid control of vomiting in the emergency department. Ann Emerg Med *13*:253, 1984.
2. Ives T, Pharm D, Fleming MF, Wert CW, Bloch J: Treatment of intractable hiccups with intramuscular haloperidol. Am J Psychiatr *142*:1368, 1985.
3. Clinton J, Sterner S, Steimachers Z, Ruiz E: Haloperidol for sedation of disruptive emergency patients. Ann Emerg Med *16*:319, 1987.
4. Pratt CM, Young JB, Wierman AM, Borland RM, Seals AA, Leon C, Raizner A, Quinones MM, Roberts R: Complex ventricular arrhythmias associated with the mitral valve prolapse syndrome. Am J Med *80*:626, 1986.
5. Creese I, Burt IR, Snyder SH: Dopamine receptor binding predicts clinical and pharmacological potencies of antischizophrenic drugs. Science *192*:481, 1976.
6. Seeman P, Lee T, Chau-Wong M, Wong K: Antipsychotic drug doses and neuroleptic/dopamine receptors. Nature *261*:717, 1976.
7. Snyder SH, Banerjee SP, Yamamura HI, Greenburg D: Drugs, neurotransmitters, and schizophrenia. Science *184*:1243, 1974.
8. Richelson E: Neuroleptic affinities for human brain receptors and their use in predicting adverse effects. J Clin Psychiatr *45*:331, 1984.
9. Delay J, Keniker P, Green A, Mororet M: Le syndrome excito moteur provoques par les medicaments neuroleptiques. Presse Med *65*:1771, 1957.
10. Ayd FJ: A survey of drug-induced extrapyramidal reactions. JAMA *175*:1054, 1961.
11. Kanba S, Richelson E: Antidepressants are weak competitive antagonists of histamine H_2 receptors in dissociated brain tissue. Eur J Pharmacol *94*:313, 1983.
12. Rifkin A, Rieder E, Sarantakos S, Saraf K, Kane J: Is loxapine more effective than chlorpromazine in paranoid schizophrenia? Am J Psychiatr *141*:1411, 1984.
13. Dahl SG, Strandjord RE: Pharmacokinetics of chlorpromazine after single and chronic dosage. Clin Pharmacol Ther *21*:437, 1976.
14. Lipton MA, Dimascio A, Killam KP: Psychotropic drugs in pregnancy. *In* Goldberg HL, DiMascio A: Psychopharmacology: A Generation of Progress. New York, Raven Press, 1978, pp 1047–1055.
15. Edlund MJ, Craig TJ: Antipsychotic drug use and birth defects: An epidemiologic reassessment. Comp Psychiatr *25*:32, 1984.
16. Tamer AK, Arias D, Fogel J: Phenothiazine-induced extrapyramidal dysfunction in the neonate. Pediatrics *75*:479, 1969.
17. Morselli PL: Psychotropic drugs. *In* Morselli PL: Drug Disposition During Development. New York, Spectrum Publications, 1977, pp 431–474.
18. Popper CW: Child and adolescent psychopharmacology. *In* Cavenar JO: Psychiatry, Philadelphia, JB Lippincott, 1985.
19. Creese I, Burt D, Snyder SH: Biochemical actions of neuroleptic drugs: Focus on dopamine receptor. *In* Iverson LL, et al: Handbook of Psychopharmacology. New York, Plenum Press, 1978, pp 37–89.
20. Whitfield LR, Kaul PN, Clark ML: Chlorpromazine metabolism. Pharmacokinetics of chlorpromazine following oral administration in men. J Pharmacokinet Biopharm *6*:187, 1979.
21. Baldessarini RJ: Drugs and treatment of psychiatric disorders. *In* Gilman AG, Goodman LS, Rall TW, Murad F: The Pharmalogic Basis of Therapeutics. New York, Macmillan, 1985, pp 387–445.
22. Black JL, Richelson E, Richardson JW: Antipsychotic agents: A clinical update. Mayo Clin Proc *60*:777, 1985.
23. Gupta JM, Lovjoy FH: Acute phenothiazine toxicity in childhood: A five year survey. Pediatrics *39*:771, 1967.
24. Knight ME, Roberts RJ: Phenothiazine and butyrophenone intoxication in children. Pediatr Clin North Am *33*:299, 1986.
25. Levinson DF, Simpson GM: Neuroleptic-induced extrapyramidal symptoms with fever. Arch Gen Psychiatr *43*:839, 1986.
26. Pall HS, Williams AC: Extrapyramidal disturbances caused by inappropriate prescribing. Br Med J *29*:30, 1987.
27. Ball R: Drug-induced akathisia: A review. J R Soc Med *78*:748, 1985.
28. Weiden J, Mann JJ, Haas G, Mattson M, Frances A: Clinical nonrecognition of neuroleptic-induced movement disorders: Cautionary study. Am J Psychiatr *144*:1148, 1987.
29. Burke RE: Tardive dyskinesia: Current clinical issues. Neurology *34*:1348, 1984.
30. Jus K, Jus A, Gautier J, Villeneuve A, Pires P, Pineau R, Villeneuve R: Studies of the actions of certain pharmacological agents on tardive dyskinesia and on the rabbit syndrome. Int J Clin Pharmacol *9*:138, 1984.
31. Kahn A, Hasaerts D, Blum D: Phenothiazine-induced sleep apneas in normal infants. Pediatrics *75*:844, 1985.
32. Peterson CD: Seizures induced by acute loxapine overdose. Am J Psychiatr *138*:1089, 1981.
33. Caroff SN: The neuroleptic malignant syndrome. J Clin Psychiatr *41*:79, 1980.
34. Guze BH, Baxter LR: Current concepts: Neuroleptic malignant syndrome. Med Intell *313*:163, 1985.
35. Rampertaap MP: Neuroleptic malignant syndrome. South Med J *79*:331, 1986.
36. Allsop P, Twigley AJ: The neuroleptic malignant syndrome. Anaesthesia *42*:49, 1987.
37. Taylor NE, Schwartz HI: Neuroleptic malignant syndrome following amoxapine overdose. J Nerv Ment Dis *176*:377, 1988.
38. Becker D, Birger M, Samuel E, Floru S: Myocardial infarction: An unusual complication of neuroleptic malignant syndrome. Nerv Ment Dis *176*:377, 1988.
39. Peebles-Brown AE: Hyperpyrexia following psychotropic drug overdose. Anaesthesia *40*:1097, 1985.
40. Davis JN, Bartlett E, Termini BA: Overdosage of psychotropic drugs: A review. Dis Nerv Syst *29*:157, 1968.
41. Neimann J, Stapczynski J, Rothstein R, Laks M: Cardiac conduction and rhythm disturbances following suicidal ingestion of mesoridazine. Ann Emerg Med *10*:253, 1981.
42. Donlon PT, Tupin JP: Successful suicides with thioridazine and mesoridazine. Arch Gen Psychiatr *34*:955, 1977.
43. Hollister LE, Kosek J: Sudden death during treatment with phenothiazine derivatives. JAMA *192*:93, 1965.
44. Fowler NO, McCall P, Chou TC, et al: Electrocardiographic changes and cardiac arrhythmias in patients receiving psychotropic drugs. Am J Cardiol *37*:223, 1976.
45. Burda AD: Electrocardiographic abnormalities induced by thioridazine (Mellaril). Am Heart J *76*:153, 1968.

46. Leetsma JE, Koenig KL: Sudden death and phenothiazines: A current controversy. Arch Gen Psychiatr *18*:137, 1968.
47. Yoon MS, Han J, Dersham GH, Jones SA: Effects of thioridazine (Mellaril) on ventricular electrophysiologic properties. Am J Cardiol *43*:1155, 1979.
48. Kemper AJ, Dunlap R, Pietro DA: Thioridazine-induced torsades de pointes. Successful therapy with isoproterenol. JAMA *249*:2931, 1983.
49. Cummingham DG, Challapalli M: Hypertension in acute haloperidol poisoning. J Pediatr *95*:489, 1979.
50. Scialli JVK, Thornton WE: Toxic reactions from a haloperidol overdose in two children. JAMA *239*:48, 1978.
51. Mahutte CK, Nakasato SK, Light R: Haloperidol and sudden death due to pulmonary edema. Arch Intern Med *142*:1951, 1982.
52. Richardson HL, Graupner KI, Richardson ME: Intramyocardial lesions in patients dying suddenly and unexpected. JAMA *195*:254, 1966.
53. Velek M, Stanford GK, Marco L: Priapism associated with concurrent use of thioridazine and metoclopramine. Am J Psychiatr *144*:827, 1987.
54. Fishbain DA: Priapism resulting from fluphenazine hydrochloride treatment reversed by diphenhydramine. Ann Emerg Med *14*:600, 1985.
55. Greenburg WM: Mechanism of neuroleptic-associated priapism. Am J Psychiatr *145*:393, 1988.
56. Greenburg WM, Lee KK: Priapism treated with benztropine. Am J Psychiatr *144*:384, 1987.
57. Prien RF, Delong SL, Cole JO, Levine J: Ocular changes with high-dose chlorpromazine therapy. Arch Gen Psychiatr *23*:464, 1970.
58. McClanahan WS, Harris JE, Knoblock WH, Treoici LM, Vadsco RL: Ocular manifestations of chronic phenothiazine derivative administration. Arch Ophthalmol *75*:319, 1966.
59. Hollister LE: Clinical Pharmacology of Psychotherapeutic Drugs. New York, Churchill-Livingstone, 1983, pp 110–171.
60. Miller FS, Bunt-Milam AH, Kalina RE: Clinical-ultrastructural study of thioridazine retinopathy. Ophthalmology *89*:1478, 1982.
61. Fisher AA: Contact Dermatitis. Philadelphia, Lea and Febiger, 1967, pp 60–61.
62. Hollister LE: Complications from psychotherapeutic drugs—1964. Clin Pharmacol Ther *5*:322, 1964.
63. DuComb L, Baldessarini RJ: Timing and risk of bone marrow depression by psychotropic drugs. Am J Psychiatr *134*:1294, 1977.
64. Allen MD, Greenblatt DJ, Noel BJ: Overdosage with antipsychotic agents. Am J Psychiatr *137*:234, 1980.
65. Chandavasu O, Chatkupt S: Central nervous system depression from chlorpromazine poisoning: Successful treatment with nalozone. J Pediatr *106*:214, 1976.
66. Whyman A: Phenothiazine death: An unusual case report. J Nerv Ment Dis *161*:214, 1976.
67. Forrest FM, Forrest IS, Mason AS: Review of rapid urine tests for phenothiazine and related drugs. Am J Psychiatr *118*:300, 1961.
68. Tri TB, Combs DT: Phenothiazine-induced ventricular tachycardia. West J Med *123*:412, 1975.
69. Tranum BL, Murphy ML: Case report: Successful treatment of ventricular tachycardia associated with thioridazine (Mellaril). South Med J *62*:357, 1969.
70. Wilson W, Weile SJ: Case report of phenothiazine-induced torsades de pointes. Am J Psychiatr *141*:1265, 1984.
71. Weisdorf D, Kramer J, Goldberg A: Physostigmine for cardiac and neurologic manifestations of phenothiazine poisoning. Clin Pharmacol Ther *24*:663, 1978.
72. Lee A: Treatment of drug-induced dystonic reactions. J Am Coll Emerg Phys *8*:453, 1979.
73. Ott D, Goeden SR: Treatment of acute phenothiazine reaction. J Am Coll Emerg Phys *8*:471, 1979.
74. Winslow RS, Sillner V, Coon DJ, Robinson MW: Prevention of acute dystonic reactions in patients beginning high-potency neuroleptics. Am J Psychiatr *143*:706, 1986.
75. Dupuis B, Catteau J, Dumon J, Lebert C, Petit H: Comparison of propranolol, sotalol, and betaxolol in the treatment of neuroleptic-induced akathisia. Am J Psychiatr *144*:802, 1987.
76. Reiters S, Adler L, Erle S, Duncan E: Neuroleptic-induced akathasia treated with pindolol. Am J Psychiatr *144*:383, 1987.
77. Alder LA, Angrist B, Peselow E, Reitano J, Totrosen J: Clonidine in neuroleptic-induced akathisia. Am J Psychiatr *144*:235, 1987.
78. Sant WW III, Ellison G: Drug holidays alter onset of oral movements in rats following chronic haloperidol. Biol Psychiatr *19*:95, 1984.
79. Eiser H, Neff MS, Slifkin RF: Acute myoglobinuric renal failure. Arch Intern Med *142*:601, 1982.
80. Meuller P, Vester JW, Fermaglich J: Neuroleptic malignant syndrome. JAMA *249*:386, 1983.
81. Coons D, Hillman FJ, Marshall RW: Treatment of neuroleptic malignant syndrome with dantrolene sodium: A case report. Am J Psychiatr *139*:94, 1982.
82. May DC, Morris SW, Stewart RM, Fenton BJ, Gaffney FA: Neuroleptic malignant syndrome: Response to dantrolene sodium. Ann Intern Med *98*:183, 1983.
83. McCarron MM, Boettger ML, Peck JJ: A case of neuroleptic malignant syndrome successfully treated with amantadine. J Clin Psychiatr *43*:381, 1982.
84. Sangal R, Dimitrievic R: Neuroleptic malignant syndrome. JAMA *254*:2795, 1985.
85. Blue MG, Schneider SM, Noro RN, Fraley DS: Successful treatment of neuroleptic malignant syndrome with sodium nitroprusside. Ann Intern Med *104*:56, 1986.

B. Monoamine Oxidase Inhibitors

Clinical interest in monoamine oxidase inhibitors (MAOI) began in 1952 when iproniazid, an isoniazid derivative studied as a possible antituberculin agent, was recognized as having mood-elevating properties.[1, 2] Later in the mid-1950s, several hydrazine-type MAO inhibitors were produced. These were effective antidepressants, but their use was limited by hepatotoxicity, though phenelzine, a member of this group, is still in use today.[3] In 1962 tranylcypromine was introduced. This nonhydrazine MAO inhibitor was more rapid acting, and liver toxicity was negligible.

MAO inhibitors were popular antidepressants from 1957 to 1962, but enthusiasm for them waned after life-threatening hypertensive crises following ingestion of tyramine-containing foods was reported.[3] It is estimated that 21 deaths occurred in about 1.5 million patients treated with tranylcypromine.[4] By the mid-1960s the tricyclic antidepressants emerged as the drugs of choice for the treatment of depression, and MAO inhibitors fell into disfavor.[5]

Renewed interest in the MAO inhibitors has occurred over the past several years because of their efficacy in the treatment of atypical depression, panic attacks, and depression refractory to other antidepressants, and with patients intolerant to tricyclic antidepressants.[6, 7] Their low therapeutic-to-toxic index and potential for serious adverse drug and food interactions, however, limits them to carefully selected compliant patients by clinicians well-versed in their use.

The three MAO inhibitors presently in use in the United States today are tranylcypromine (Parnate), phenelzine (Nardil), and isocarboxazid (Marplan).

PHARMACOLOGY

Monoamine oxidase (MAO) and catechol-*O*-methyl transferase (COMT) are enzymes that provide the principal pathways for the degradation and inactivation of nonmethylated biogenic amine neurotransmitters, such as norepinephrine, dopamine, and serotonin. MAO inhibitors, structurally similar to MAO substrates, block MAO by binding to the enzyme.[8] Most currently available MAO inhibitors bind irreversibly, and only synthesis of new MAO can restore enzyme activity.[9, 10] This process takes several weeks and accounts for the prolonged effect of MAO inhibitors.[11]

Inhibition of MAO activity alters catecholamine neurotransmitter levels in a variety of tissues. Norepinephrine accumulates in the central nervous system, which is believed to account for the mood-enhancing effect of MAO inhibitors.[7, 12] In postganglionic sympathetic nerve endings, norepinephrine stores accumulate in both stable and mobile pools.[13]

Two types of MAO enzymes have been described. MAO-A preferentially deaminates norepinephrine and serotonin, whereas MAO-B metabolizes phenylethylamine.[14] Conventional MAO inhibitors are nonselective and bind to either subtype.[7]

Only a few MAO inhibitors are approved by the US Food and Drug Administration. Phenelzine, isocarboxazid, and tranylcypromine are used in a variety of psychiatric disorders.[7, 15–17] They are not considered drugs of choice for classic depression but may be used either when other therapies have failed[7] or in combination with certain tricyclic antidepressants or lithium.[18] Pargyline[19] is a seldom-used MAO inhibitor employed in the treatment of moderate-to-severe hypertension refractory to other pharmacologic agents.[20]

MAO inhibitors are classified structurally into three groups: hydrazines (R-NH-NH-R), hydrazides (R-NH-NH-CO-R) and nonhydrazines (amine or ammonia derivatives) (Fig. 44–4).

PHARMACOKINETICS

MAO inhibitors are oral agents that are rapidly absorbed from the gastrointestinal tract.[21] Tranylcypromine has a peak concentration of 25 μg per ml 2.5 hours after a 20-mg dose,[22] with a serum half-life of 3 hours.[23] After inactivation by acetylation, metabolites are excreted by the kidneys. MAO inhibitors may have an enhanced effect in patients who are slow acetylators[24] and should be used cautiously in individuals at risk by either family history or ethnic background.

CLINICAL PRESENTATION OF MAOI OVERDOSE

Acute overdose with MAO inhibitors produces a clinical state resembling that of catecholamine storm, with hyperexcitability, agitation, psychosis, convulsions, hyperpyrexia, cardiac dysrhythmias, hypertension, and dilated pupils. Hypotension, when it occurs, is a poor prognostic sign.

Case Example. An example of a MAO inhibitor overdose is a 32 year old woman who ingested 30 15-mg tablets (7.5 mg/kg) of

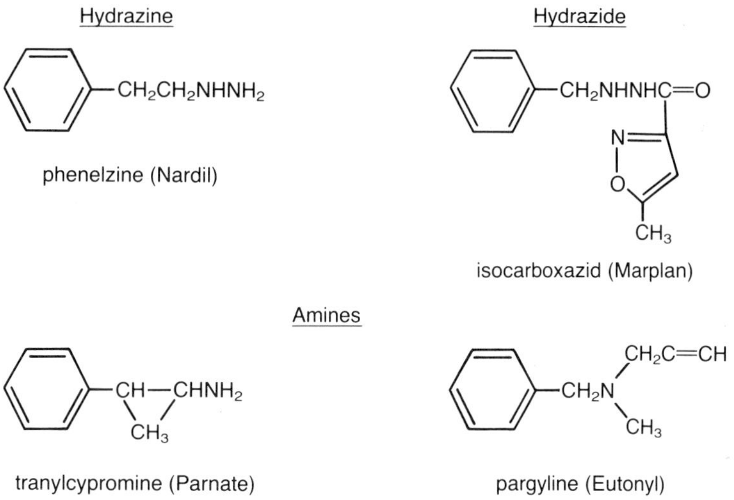

Hydrazine

phenelzine (Nardil) — $CH_2CH_2NHNH_2$

Hydrazide

isocarboxazid (Marplan) — $CH_2NHNHC{=}O$

Amines

tranylcypromine (Parnate)

pargyline (Eutonyl)

Figure 44–4. Classes of monoamine oxidase inhibitors.

phenelzine (Nardil) after her husband confronted her with his desire for a divorce. The patient came to the Emergency Department 6 hours after ingestion, repentant and complaining of an occipital headache. The initial vital signs were blood pressure, 140 over 80 mm Hg; pulse, 102 beats per minute; respirations, 22 per minute; and temperature, 38° C. Gastric lavage revealed only a small amount of pill fragments, and 6 liters of normal saline were used until the return was clear. A 50-gram slurry of charcoal with sorbitol was instilled in the nasogastric tube. The initial physical examination was unremarkable. Admitting laboratory tests, including a CBC, SMA-18, ETOH level, and urinalysis, were all normal. A head CT scan, electrocardiogram, and chest radiograph were also normal. The patient was admitted to the ICU for observation and monitoring.

Eight hours after admission the patient became combative and diaphoretic and required physical restraints. Diazepam (60 mg total) was not effective in sedating the patient, and she was orally intubated after induction with sodium pentothal and vecuronium. Foley catheter drainage contained dark urine positive for myoglobin. The creatine phosphokinase was 42,868 IU/liter. The patient was hydrated with 2 liters of normal saline and 1 ampule of sodium bicarbonate added to each liter. Four hours later a core temperature of 41.4° C was recorded, and she was treated with ice packs and a cooling blanket, which lowered her temperature to 38.5° C. Over the ensuing 6 hours she progressively developed a nodal bradycardia, refractory to atropine, and external pacing, hypotension, metabolic acidosis, oliguria, disseminated intravascular coagulation (DIC), and terminal ventricular fibrillation. The patient died 26 hours after ingestion.

The signs and symptoms of MAO inhibitor overdose are commonly delayed for up to 24 hours.[25–30] After this period of delay, symptoms of neuromuscular excitation and sympathetic hyperactivity occur[25–28, 30–42] (Table 44–5). Later on, signs of CNS and cardiovascular collapse become evident, along with

Table 44–5. CLINICAL SIGNS AND SYMPTOMS OF MONOAMINE INHIBITOR OVERDOSE

MILD		
headache	agitation	mydriasis
nausea	muscle tremors	nystagmus
palpitations	hyperreflexia	flushing
weakness		
MODERATE		
confusion	combativeness	hallucinations
sinus tachycardia	hypertension	tachypnea
atrial flutter	opisthotonos	trismus
muscle rigidity	diaphoresis	vomiting
myoclonus	diarrhea	fever
SEVERE		
bradycardia	hypotension	pulmonary edema
heart block	cardiac arrest	seizures
coma	cerebral edema	hyperthermia
hemolysis	rhabdomyolysis	renal failure
metabolic acidosis	hypoventilation	hypoxemia

various secondary complications, such as DIC, hemolysis, rhabdomyolysis, renal failure, and cardiac arrest.

Both therapy and overdose with MAO inhibitors result in increased levels of dopamine, norepinephrine, and serotonin in the brain. Phenelzine and tranylcypromine are also capable of promoting release of norepinephrine from sympathetic nerve endings.[43] This release of norepinephrine from the presynaptic vesicles may explain the cardiovascular collapse seen late in MAO inhibitor poisoning, since decreased norepinephrine would be available.[28, 44] This same biphasic response is seen with the use of bretylium; an exaggerated biphasic blood pressure response has been similarly reported in a case of bretylium overdose.[45]

Serum levels of MAO inhibitors do not correlate with the degree of observed toxicity.[28] Assays for MAO enzyme activity level are helpful in theory but are difficult to do and are not readily available.[46] Diagnostic confirmation of MAO overdose through detection of increased levels of MAO substrates in blood and urine provides only indirect evidence of MAO inhibitor overdose[35] and may be a relatively nonspecific finding.[47] Currently available drug screens do not detect for the presence of MAO inhibitors, so diagnosis and management must be based on history and clinical presentation.

Adverse Drug Interactions

MAO inhibitor's enzyme inhibition results in increased peripheral stores of norepinephrine. Any of the indirect-acting sympathomimetic drugs can lead to a hypertensive crisis by stimulating release of these stores or, because MAO is inhibited in the liver, the effects of ingested sympathomimetics are not attenuated, leading to an adverse pressor response[48–50] (Table 44–6).

Milder reactions can occur with use of the direct-acting sympathomimetics (epinephrine and norepinephrine), since their breakdown depends on catechol-*O*-methyltransferase (COMT) and not MAO. Still, they should be used only when necessary and with close blood pressure monitoring.[50]

MAO inhibitors also decrease the metabolism of many sedative-hypnotics, chloral hydrate, and barbiturates, thus increasing the risk of respiratory depression.

Antihypertensive agents such as reserpine,

Table 44–6. DRUG RESTRICTION LIST FOR PATIENTS ON MONOAMINE OXIDASE INHIBITORS

ABSOLUTELY CONTRAINDICATED	AVOID
Ephedrine*	Other narcotics
Phenylephrine*	Dextromethorphan*
Phenylpropanolamine*	Reserpine
Metaraminol	Guanethidine
Amphetamines	Beta blockers
Cocaine	Atropine
Meperidine	Thiazide diuretics
L-Dopa	Direct sympathomimetics

*Commonly found in over-the-counter cold remedies.

guanethidine, methyldopa, and the beta-blockers should be avoided for patients taking MAO inhibitors because hypertension may develop, either by peripheral norepinephrine release or unopposed alpha-adrenergic activity.

The use of meperidine has been associated with hyperpyrexia, MAO inhibitor potentiation of primary narcotic effects, and hypertension, and this drug should be avoided.[21]

Adverse Food Interactions

Patients prescribed MAO inhibitors must avoid foods containing tyramine.[51] Older MAO inhibitor food prohibition lists were not accurate in their tyramine content but have been updated and are now more practical and realistic.[6, 52, 53] Adverse food interactions may result in only mild symptoms, like weakness and headache, or can lead to life-threatening hypertensive crisis, intracranial bleeding, and death. Any foods high in tyramine (more than 10 mg), as well as those listed in Table 44–7, are potentially injurious to patients on MAOIs and must be avoided.

Chronic MAOI Side Effects

The chronic use of MAOIs may lead to orthostatic hypotension, weight gain, edema, sexual dysfunction, sedation, excitation, dry mouth, blurred vision, constipation, and (rarely) hepatotoxicity.[6]

Treatment of MAOI Overdose or Toxicity

Patients experiencing MAO inhibitor overdose should be closely monitored for at least 24 hours.[25–27] Ingestion of any amount may be significant, and as little as 2 to 3 mg per

Table 44–7. FOOD RESTRICTION LIST FOR PATIENTS ON MAO INHIBITORS

Unsafe
Any food with a high tyramine content (> 10 mg)
High-protein food that has undergone aging, fermentation, pickling, smoking, or bacterial contamination
Aged cheese
Decayed or spoiled food
Red wine
Fermented products
Pods of broad beans
Fava beans
Safe when fresh and used in moderation
Sour cream
Yogurt
Meat extracts
Chopped liver
Dry sausage
Other alcoholic beverages
Safe when fresh
Cottage cheese
Cream cheese
Processed cheese

kg should be considered potentially life-threatening.[28]

Treatment of MAO inhibitor overdose or toxic reaction is based on the presenting signs and symptoms. Initial attention should focus on establishing and maintaining an adequate airway and ventilations. An intravenous access line should be established and the patient placed on a cardiac monitor. Vital signs should be carefully monitored.

Cardiovascular Complications

Hypertension. Mild-to-moderate hypertension has been successfully treated with sublingual nifedepine.[54] Severe hypertension may be managed with intravenous phentolamine[7, 28] or nitroprusside.[55] Both these agents are relatively short acting and can be used to titrate the blood pressure. Beta-blockers have been used successfully to treat hypertension associated with excessive cardiac stimulation in a case of tranylcypromine toxicity,[56] but because of the possibility of unopposed alpha-adrenergic stimulation, beta-blockers should be used with caution.[57]

Hypotension. Hypotension should be treated initially with a trial of volume expansion. If this is unsuccessful, a direct-acting alpha-adrenergic agent like norepinephrine is recommended,[8] but it must be used cautiously since an enhanced response might occur.[48, 58] Although antishock trousers have been suggested in this setting,[28] their efficacy has yet to be determined. In refractory cases, central hemodynamic monitoring is useful in guiding therapeutic interventions.[41]

Cardiac Dysrhythmias. Dysrhythmias in an MAO overdose are frequently seen in association with other cardiovascular abnormalities[28] and may be difficult to treat.

Supraventricular dysrhythmias, unless hemodynamically significant, can be managed conservatively with careful observation. When intervention is necessary, beta-block-

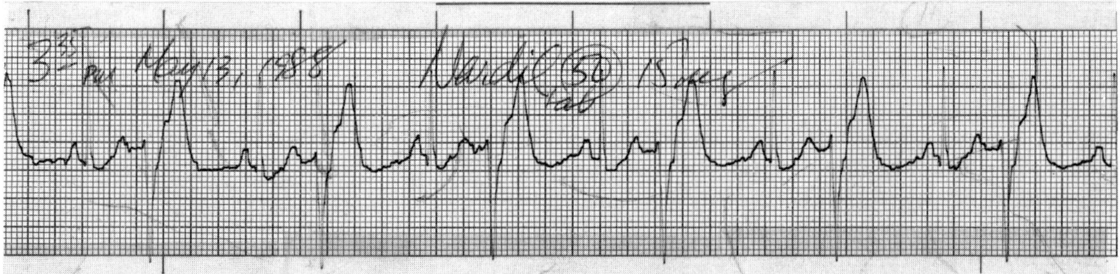

Figure 44–5. The patient is a 26 year old woman who took 50 15-mg tablets of Nardil and went for a walk following a dispute with her husband. She was brought to the emergency department 2 hours later, where she was noted to be in a hyperexcitable state, to have a flushed face and body, and to be hypertensive, with a blood pressure of 180/120. Gastric lavage revealed considerable orange material, and lavage was performed until the return was clear, followed by administration of activated charcoal and sorbitol.

The patient developed a run of ventricular bigeminy (see rhythm strip), which spontaneously subsided in the emergency department. The patient then became hypotensive, with a blood pressure of 80/46 and a pulse of 56. She was treated with intravenous fluids and admitted to the intensive care unit. Arterial blood gas studies on admission showed a PO_2 of 170 (on 2 liters of oxygen per minute), a PCO_2 of 41, and a pH of 7.34.

The patient's hypotension was managed conservatively with fluid resuscitation, and within 12 hours of admission her blood pressure was 90/60 and pulse, 84. Arterial blood gases and all laboratory parameters remained normal throughout her hospital stay. As her physical condition gradually improved over the next 24 hours, she became increasingly despondent. She was transferred to a psychiatric unit 72 hours following admission. (Courtesy of Beaufort Memorial Hospital, Beaufort, South Carolina.)

ers may be effective[56] but should be used cautiously to avoid unopposed alpha-adrenergic stimulation.[57] Calcium channel blockers also may be effective but must be avoided in the presence of hypotension.[28] Digoxin toxicity is enhanced by MAO inhibitors, but it may be utilized with careful monitoring.[59]

Ventricular dysrhythmias should be managed, if clinically indicated, with lidocaine, procainamide, or phenytoin.[28] If they prove refractory, the use of a beta-blocker may be considered. Bretylium is believed to be contraindicated because of its pharmacologic similarity to MAO inhibitors.[45, 60]

Figure 44–5 presents a case report.

Hyperthermia

Hyperthermia should be managed early and aggressively with acetaminophen and, if necessary, external cooling.[28] If the patient's temperature exceeds 40°C, ice baths and paralysis with pancuronium should be considered.

Intravenous dantrolene has been used successfully in a phenelzine overdose–induced hyperthermia.[61] Bromocriptine has been used in cases of malignant hyperthermia and may be of value in MAO inhibitor overdose as well.[62]

CNS Excitation

Agitation may be controlled with intravenous diazepam or amobarbital.[28] Phenothiazines have been reported to cause severe adverse reactions and death in the setting of MAO inhibitor overdose.[63] Narcotics can have an enhanced effect owing to MAO inhibitor suppression of microsomal enzymes.[64] Both should be avoided. Meperidine[65–67] and dextromethorphan[68] have been reported to precipitate paradoxic CNS excitation when administered with MAO inhibitors.

Enhanced Elimination

Acid diuresis has been shown to enhance elimination of MAO inhibitors; however, urinary recovery was only 8 per cent.[69] It is doubtful that this is of any clinical benefit and is not recommended. Further, if rhabdomyolysis is present, acid diuresis may enhance renal precipitation of myoglobin and contribute to renal failure.[70]

Currently, few data support the efficacy of either peritoneal or hemodialysis in the management of MAO inhibitor overdose,[28] although anecdotal reports claiming benefit have been published.[37, 71]

References

1. Zeller EA, Bardsky J: In vivo inhibition of liver and brain monoamine oxidase by 1-isonicotinyl-2-isopropyl-hydrazine. Proc Soc Exp Biol (NY) *81*:459, 1952.
2. Loomer HP, Saunders JC, Kline NS: A clinical and pharmacodynamic evaluation of iproniazid as a psychic energizer. Am Psychiatr Assoc Psychiatr Res Reports *8*:129, 1957.
3. Jarrott B, Vajda FJE: The current status of monoamine oxidase and its inhibitors. Med J Aust *146*:634, 1987.
4. Cole JO: Therapeutic efficacy of antidepressant drugs. JAMA *190*:448, 1964.
5. Medical Research Council: Clinical trial of the treatment of depressive illness. Br Med J *1*:881, 1965.
6. Lippmann S: Monoamine oxidase inhibitors. Am Fam Physician *34*:113, 1986.
7. Tollefson GD: Monoamine oxidase inhibitors: A review. J Clin Psychiatr *8*:280, 1983.
8. Guzzardi L: Monoamine overdose inhibitors. *In* Haddad LM, Winchester JF (eds): Clinical Management of Poisoning and Drug Overdose. Philadelphia, WB Saunders, 1983, p 496.
9. Goldberg LI: Monoamine overdose inhibitors. Adverse reactions and possible mechanisms. JAMA *190*:456, 1964.
10. Ciocatto E, Fagiano G, Boro GL: Clinical features and treatment of overdosage of monoamine oxidase inhibitors and their interaction with other psychotropic drugs. Resuscitation *1*:69, 1972.
11. White K, Pistole T, Boyd JL: Combined monoamine oxidase inhibitor–tricyclic antidepressant treatment: A pilot study. Am J Psychiatr *137*:1422, 1980.
12. Youdim MB: Monoamine oxidase: Its inhibition. Mod Prob Pharmacopsychother *10*:65, 1975.
13. Koplin J, Azelrod J: The role of MAO inhibitors in biogenic amine metabolism. Ann NY Acad Sci *107*:848, 1963.
14. Cawthorn RM, Pinter JE, Haeltime FP, et al: Differences in the structure of A and B forms of human monoamine oxidase. J Neurochem *37*:363, 1981.
15. Liebowitz MR, Quitkin FM, Stewart JW, et al: Antidepressant specificity in atypical depression. Arch Gen Psychiatr *45*:129, 1988.
16. Johnson WC: A neglected modality in psychiatric treatment—the monoamine oxidase inhibitors. Dis Nerv Syst *36*:521, 1975.
17. Shielaih DV, Ballanger J, Jacobsen G: Treatment of endogenous anxiety with phobic, hysterical and hypochondriacal symptoms. Arch Gen Psychiatr *37*:51, 1980.
18. Lipman S, Baldwin M, Manshadi M: Combined trimipramine/phenelzine treatment of depression: Case report. J Clin Psychiatr *43*:430, 1982.
19. Fein S, Paz V, Rao N, et al: The combination of lithium carbonate and an MAOI in refractory depression. Am J Psychiatr *145*:245, 1988.
20. AMA Drug Evaluations. 5th ed. Chicago, American Medical Association, 1983, pp 253, 264, 704.

21. Gilman AG, Goodman LS, Rall TW, et al (eds): Goodman and Gilman's The Pharmacologic Basis of Therapeutics. 7th ed. New York, Macmillan, 1985, pp 423, 443.
22. Lang A, Geissler HE, Mutschler E: Fluorimetrische Bestimmung von tranylcypromin in plasma als 1-Dimethylamino-naphthalin-5-sulfonsäure-Derivat durch direkte quantitative Dünnschichtchromatographie (Eng abs). Arzneimittelforschung *28*:575, 1978.
23. Youdim MBH, Aronson JK, Blau K, et al: Tranylcypromine (Parnate) overdose: Measurement of tranylcypromine concentrations and MAO inhibitory activity and identification of amphetamines in plasma. Psychol Med *9*:377, 1979.
24. Marshall EF, Mountjoy CQ, Campbell IC, et al: The influence of acetylator phenotype on the outcome of treatment with phenelzine, in a clinical trial. Br J Clin Pharmacol *6*:247, 1978.
25. Mawdsley JA: "Parstelin;" A case of fatal overdose. Med J Aust *2*:292, 1968.
26. Mattell G, Thorstrand C: A case of fatal nialamide poisoning. Acta Med Scand *181*:79, 1967.
27. Reid DD, Kerr WC: Phenelzine poisoning responding to phenothiazine. Med J Aust *2*:1214, 1969.
28. Linden CM, Rumack BM, Strehike C, Prairie G: Monoamine oxidase inhibitor overdose. Ann Emerg Med *13*:1137, 1984.
29. Davis JM, Barlett MD, Termini BA: Overdosage of psychotropic drugs: A review. Dis Nerv Syst *29*:246, 1968.
30. Meredith TJ, Vale JA: Poisoning due to psychotropic agents. Adverse Drug React Acute Poisoning Rev *4*:83, 1985.
31. Mackell MA, Case ME, Poklis A: Fatal intoxication due to tranylcypromine. Med Sci Law *128*:354, 1979.
32. Sandler SA: Iproniazid used in attempted suicide. Dis Nerv Syst *20*:79, 1959.
33. Solberg CO: Phenelzine intoxication. JAMA *572*:102, 1961.
34. Bacon GA: Successful suicide with tranylcypromine sulfate. Am J Psychiatr *119*:585, 1962.
35. Baldridge ET, Miller LV, Haverback BJ, et al: Amine metabolism after an overdose of a monoamine oxidase inhibitor. N Engl J Med *267*:421, 1962.
36. Platts MM, Usher A, Stentiford NH: Phenelzine and trifluoperazine poisoning. Lancet *2*:738, 1965.
37. Matter BJ, Donate PE, Brill ML, et al: Tranylcypromine sulfate poisoning. Successful treatment by hemodialysis. Arch Intern Med *116*:18–20, 1965.
38. Marra JP, Minter DL, Hobbins TE: Suicide by the ingestion of tranylcypromine. JAMA *192*:1004, 1965.
39. Lipkin D, Kuslmick T: Pargyline hydrochloride poisoning in a child. JAMA *201*:135, 1967.
40. Robertson JC: Recovery after massive MAOI overdose complicated by malignant hyperpyrexia, treated with chlorpromazine. Postgrad Med J *48*:64, 1972.
41. Breheny FX, Dobb GJ, Clarke GM: Phenelzine poisoning. Anaesthesia *41*:53, 1986.
42. Crome P: Antidepressant overdosage. Drugs *23*:431, 1982.
43. Lee WC, Shin YH, Shideman RD: Cardiac activities of several monoamine oxidase inhibitors. J Pharmacol Exp Ther *133*:180–185, 1961.
44. Goldberg ND, Shideman FE: Species differences in the cardiac effects of a monoamine oxidase inhibitor. J Pharmacol Exp Ther *136*:142, 1963.
45. Bodnar T, Nowak R, Tomlanovich MC: Massive intravenous bolus of bretylium tosylate. Ann Emerg Med *9*:630, 1980.
46. Levine RJ, Sjoerdsma A: Estimation of monoamine oxidase activity in man: Techniques and applications. Ann NY Acad Sci *107*:966, 1963.
47. Von Euler US, Helliver S: Excretion of noradrenaline and adrenaline in muscular work. Acta Physiol Scand *26*:183, 1952.
48. Boakes AJ, Laurence DR, Teoh PC, Barar FS, Benedikter LT, Prichard BN: Interactions between sympathomimetic amines and antidepressant agents in man. Br Med J *1*:311, 1973.
49. Stockley IH: Monoamine oxidase inhibitors. Part I: Interactions with sympathomimetic amines. Pharm J *6*:590, 1973.
50. Zisook S: A clinical overview of monoamine oxidase inhibitors. Psychosomatics *26*:240, 1985.
51. Folks DG: Monoamine oxidase inhibitors: Reappraisal of dietary consideration. J Clin Psychopharmacol *3*:249, 1983.
52. Lippmann SB: Practical MAOI food and drug avoidances (letter). Psychosomatics *28*:591, 1987.
53. Jenike MA: The use of monoamine oxidase inhibitors in the treatment of elderly, depressed patients. J Am Geriatr Soc *32*:571, 1984.
54. Clary C, Schweizer E: Treatment of MAOI hypertensive crisis with sublingual nifedepine. J Clin Psychiatr *48*:249, 1987.
55. Brown TCK, Cass NM: Beware—the use of MAO inhibitors is increasing again. Anaesth Intensive Care *7*:65, 1979.
56. Shepard JT, Whiting B: Beta-adrenergic blockade in the treatment of MAOI self poisoning. Lancet *2*:1021, 1974.
57. Frieden J: Propranolol as an antiarrhythmic agent. Am Heart J *74*:283, 1967.
58. Cuthbert MF, Vere DW: Potentiation of the cardiovascular effects of some catecholamines by a MAOI. Br J Pharmacol *43*:471, 1971.
59. Bohruian JS, Thompson EB: Cardiovascular effects of digoxin-phenelzine interactions in rabbits. J Pharm Sci *62*:1876, 1973.
60. Gessa GL, Cuenca E, Costa E: On the mechanism of hypotensive effects of MAO inhibitors. Ann NY Acad Sci *107*:935, 1963.
61. Kaplan RF, Feinglass NG, Webster W, et al: Phenelzine overdose treatment with dantrolene sodium. JAMA *255*:642, 1986.
62. Mueller PS, Vester JW, Fermaglich J: Neuroleptic malignant syndrome: Successful treatment with bromocryptine. JAMA *249*:386, 1983.
63. Robertson JC: Recovery after massive MAOI overdose complicated by malignant hyperpyrexia treated with chlorpromazine. Postgrad Med J *48*:64, 1972.
64. Stack CG, Rogers P, Linter SPK: Monoamine oxidase inhibitors and anaesthesia. Br J Anaesth *60*:222, 1988.
65. Mitchell RS: Fatal toxic encephalitis occurring during iproniazid therapy in pulmonary tuberculosis. Ann Intern Med *42*:417, 1955.
66. Palmer M: Potentiation of pethidine. Br Med J *2*:944, 1960.
67. Shee JC: Dangerous potentiation of pethidine by iproniazid and its treatment. Br Med J *2*:507, 1960.
68. Rivers N, Horner B: Possible lethal reaction between Nardil and dextromethorphan. Can Med J 103, 1970.

69. Turner P, Young JM, Paterson J: Influence of urinary pH on the excretion of tranylcypromine sulphate. Nature *215*:881, 1967.
70. Eneas JF, Schonfield PY, Humphreys MH: The effect of mannitol–sodium bicarbonate infusion on the clinical course of myoglobinuria. Arch Intern Med *139*:801, 1979.
71. Versaci AA, Nakamoto S, Kolff WJ: Phenelzine intoxication. Report of a case treated by hemodialysis. Ohio State Med J *60*:770, 1964.

CHAPTER 45
BENZODIAZEPINES

James R. Roberts, M.D.
John A. Tafuri, M.D.

The first commercially marketed benzodiazepine was accidentally synthesized in 1955 by Roche Laboratories in Nutley, New Jersey, but the scope of its pharmacologic properties and its clinical applications were not appreciated until 1957.[1] That drug, chlordiazepoxide (Librium), was noted to possess clinically effective sedative, hypnotic, and anticonvulsant properties. When it became available in 1960 it ushered in an era of widespread benzodiazepine use that persists today. Diazepam, perhaps the best known and most commercially successful of all the benzodiazepines, was synthesized in 1959 and marketed as Valium in 1963. Since that time, over 3000 benzodiazepines have been developed,[2] over 120 have been tested for biologic activity, and 28 are currently in clinical use throughout the world.[3, 4] Thirteen benzodiazepines are approved for use in the United States (Table 45–1). Benzodiazepines have varying sedative, hypnotic, amnestic, anxiolytic, anticonvulsant, and muscle relaxant properties. Alprazolam, a newer benzodiazepine, may also have significant antidepressant activity. Individual drugs are FDA approved and marketed for specific indications on the basis of these characteristics, although current evidence indicates that all benzodiazepines are effective for the treatment of anxiety and insomnia.[5]

Since their introduction, the benzodiazepines have enjoyed a meteoric rise in popularity and have largely replaced other sedative-hypnotics. Their extraordinary acceptance in clinical medicine has been based on their safety, efficacy, minimal side effects, low addiction potential, and the medical and public demand for sedative and anxiolytic agents.[6] It has been estimated that 500 million people worldwide have taken benzodiazepines during the last 25 years.[7, 8] The prevalence of benzodiazepine use in the United States in 1979 and 1981 was estimated to be 11 and 13 per cent, respectively. However, long-term use (greater than 1 year) occurs in only 1 to 2 per cent of adults in the general population.[9–19]

Worldwide sales of benzodiazepines exceed 1 billion dollars per year.[20] Annual prescriptions for benzodiazepines in the United States peaked in 1972 at 77 million, but use has subsequently declined by almost one third, largely because of widespread negative publicity and concern over their potential misuse, abuse, and long-term side effects.[1] Despite these concerns, benzodiazepines remain extremely popular, accounting for 5 of the 50 most frequently prescribed drugs in the United States in 1987. Xanax (alprazolam) is currently the most widely used benzodiazepine and is the fourth most prescribed drug in the United States. Halcion (triazolam), Valium (diazepam), and Ativan (lorazepam) are also frequently prescribed, ranking 18th, 19th, and 34th, respectively[21] (Fig. 45–1).

Because of their widespread availability, benzodiazepines are also among the most frequently misused drugs. Many investigators, however, emphasize that dependence and abuse by the general population are largely overstated by the media and are minor compared with alcohol, cocaine, or opiate

Table 45–1. BENZODIAZEPINES AVAILABLE IN THE UNITED STATES

GENERIC NAME	TRADE NAME	YEAR OF INTRODUCTION	RECOMMENDED ADULT DOSE*	AVAILABLE DOSAGE FORMS	FDA-APPROVED INDICATIONS	RATE OF ORAL ABSORPTION
alprazolam	Xanax	1981	Oral: 0.75–4 mg/day divided TID	0.25, 0.5, 1 mg tablets	Anxiety Anxious depression	intermediate
chlordiazepoxide	Librium	1960	Oral: 15–100 mg/day divided TID to QID	5, 10, 25 mg tablets or capsules	Alcohol withdrawal Anxiety Pre-op sedation	intermediate
clonazepam	Klonopin	1974	Oral: 7.5–20 mg/day divided TID	0.5, 1, 2 mg tablets	Seizure disorder	intermediate
clorazepate	Tranxene	1972	Oral: 7.5–60 mg/day divided q D to QID	2.75, 7.5, 15 mg capsules	Anxiety Alcohol withdrawal	rapid
diazepam	Valium	1963	Oral: 6–40 mg/day divided q D to QID IV: 0.1 mg/kg/dose	2, 5, 10 mg tablets	Anxiety/insomnia Alcohol withdrawal Muscle spasm/ seizures Pre-op sedation	rapid
flurazepam	Dalmane	1970	Oral: 15–30 mg/day q HS	15, 30 mg capsules	Insomnia	rapid
halazepam	Paxipam	1981	Oral: 80–160 mg/day divided TID to QID	20, 40 mg capsules	Anxiety	intermediate to slow
lorazepam	Ativan	1977	Oral: 1–10 mg/day divided BID to TID IM: 0.05 mg/kg IV: 0.05 mg/kg	0.5, 1, 2 mg tablets	Anxiety/insomnia Anxious depression Pre-op sedation	intermediate
midazolam	Versed	1986	Oral: not available IM: 0.07–0.08 mg/kg IV: Begin 1–2.5 mg, titrate to effect		Pre-op sedation Anesthesia induction Conscious sedation	rapid†
oxazepam	Serax	1963	Oral: 30–120 mg/day divided TID to QID	10, 15, 30 mg capsules 15 mg tablets	Anxiety Alcohol withdrawal Anxious depression	slow
prazepam	Centrax	1977	Oral: 20–60 mg/day divided BID	5, 10 mg capsules 10 mg tablets	Anxiety	ultraslow
temazepam	Restoril	1981	Oral: 15–30 mg q HS	15, 30 mg capsules	Insomnia	slow
triazolam	Halcion	1983	Oral: 0.125–0.5 mg q HS	0.125, 0.25, 0.5 mg capsules	Insomnia	intermediate

*Maximum dose not established.
†Oral form of midazolam is not yet commercially available.

abuse. It has been estimated that 40 to 50 per cent of drug abusers also use benzodiazepines. As a class, benzodiazepines are not powerful euphoriants and are therefore not frequently abused primarily. Secondary drug abuse is common, however, usually in the form of self-medication to decrease the adverse side effects of stimulants or hallucinogens, to ameliorate the unpleasant symptoms of withdrawal from more highly addictive substances, or to substitute for the drug of primary dependence when it is not available.

Diazepam is the fourth most common drug involved in drug-related visits to the emergency department, mainly as a consequence of intentional overdose.[22] Since the selection of a drug for overdose is highly influenced by its availability,[23–25] it is not surprising that benzodiazepines are commonly taken in overdose.[24, 26] Data from the National Data Collection System of the American Association of Poison Control Centers System showed that benzodiazepines had the highest number of toxic exposures in patients over 17 years of age, both as a single agent and in combination with other drugs and alcohol.[27] In contrast to the sedative-hypnotic drugs they replaced, benzodiazepines are less addictive, possess less potential for abuse, and are remarkably safe.

STRUCTURE

The benzodiazepines are organic bases (Figs. 45–1 and 45–2). All benzodiazepines share a structure composed of a six-membered benzene ring which is attached to a

alprazolam (Xanax)

triazolam (Halcion)

diazepam (Valium)

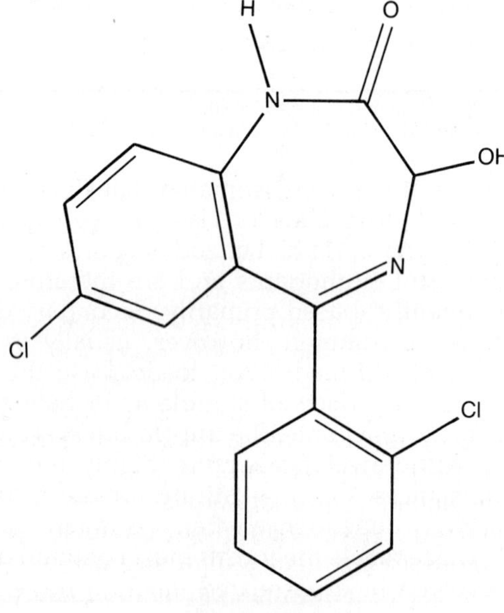

lorazepam (Ativan)

Figure 45–1. The four most prescribed benzodiazepines in the United States.

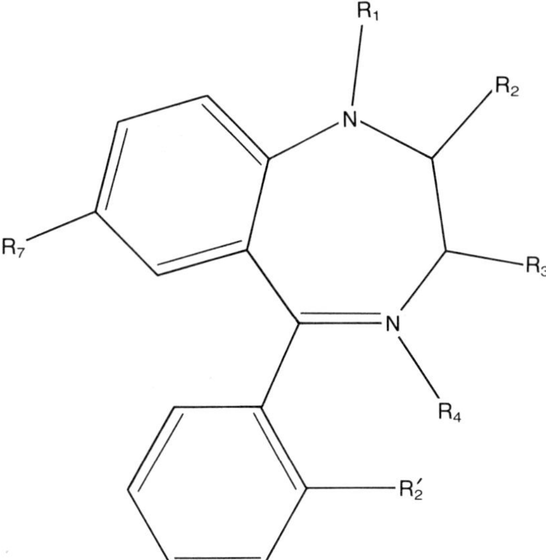

Figure 45–2. The general chemical structure of benzodiazepines.

seven-membered diazepine ring with a benzene ring substituted at the number five position. Specific benzodiazepines are formed by varying the substitutions at the R_1, R_2, R_3, R_4, R_7, and R_2' positions. Despite the myriad benzodiazepine compounds available, all derivatives can be expected to have similar qualitative pharmacologic and clinical effects when adjusted for differences in potency.[28, 29] However, various compounds have significant differences in onset and duration of action and metabolism, which theoretically makes them more suitable for certain indications.

PHARMACOKINETICS

Absorption

Although some benzodiazepines form water-soluble salts at acidic pH, at physiologic pH all are moderately to highly lipid-soluble molecules that are rapidly and completely absorbed from the proximal small bowel[4, 28] (Table 45–2). Significant differences in lipid solubility affect the rate of gastrointestinal absorption and subsequent distribution. Highly lipophilic benzodiazepines (diazepam, flurazepam, midazolam) are rapidly absorbed, and less lipophilic compounds (oxazepam, temazepam) are more slowly absorbed.[2, 30, 31]

The parent forms of two benzodiazepines, clorazepate and prazepam, do not reach the circulation of the system in clinically significant amounts. The active metabolite is formed in the gastrointestinal tract or liver prior to systemic absorption and appears in the serum as desmethyldiazepam.[28, 31] Desmethyldiazepam is rapidly formed from clorazepate after acid hydrolysis within the stomach and is slowly formed from prazepam after first-pass metabolism in the liver.[3, 4, 6, 30, 32]

The rate of oral absorption may be influenced by several factors other than lipid solubility. Absorption is enhanced by taking the drugs on an empty stomach or by the coingestion of alcohol[3, 33, 34] and is slowed by the coadministration of food[35, 36] or aluminum- or magnesium hydroxide–containing antacids.[37, 38] Absorption also may be altered by manipulating the pharmaceutical preparation, such as slow-release diazepam (Valium CR).[39]

Benzodiazepine absorption from intramuscular (IM) injection is variable. Lorazepam and midazolam are the only benzodiazepines adequately absorbed following intramuscular administration.[40, 41] Chlordiazepoxide absorption is particularly slow and erratic, and

Table 45–2. ABSORPTION RATES OF ORALLY ADMINISTERED BENZODIAZEPINES

	TIME OF PEAK PLASMA CONCENTRATION
Rapid	less than 1.2 hours
desmethyldiazepam [from clorazepate (Tranxene)]	
diazepam (Valium)	
flurazepam (Dalmane)	
midazolam* (Versed)	
Intermediate	1.2 to 2.0 hours
alprazolam (Xanax)	
chlordiazepoxide (Librium)	
clonazepam (Klonopin)	
halazepam (Paxipam)	
lorazepam (Ativan)	
triazolam (Halcion)	
Slow	2.0 to 3.0 hours
oxazepam (Serax)	
temazepam (Restoril)	
Ultraslow	greater than 3.0 hours
desmethyldiazepam [from prazepam (Centrax)]	
diazepam CR (slow release)	

*Oral form of midazolam not yet commercially available.

plasma concentration may not peak for 6 to 12 hours.[40, 42] Diazepam is inconsistently absorbed after intramuscular administration.[6, 43, 44] Serum levels of both chlordiazepoxide and diazepam are more rapidly achieved by the oral route than by intramuscular administration.[45]

Following absorption, benzodiazepines are more than 70 per cent protein bound, but the degree of protein binding varies significantly. Protein binding is greatest with diazepam (99 per cent) and least with alprazolam (70 per cent). Only unbound drug is available to cross the blood-brain barrier and interact at CNS receptors. Drug concentrations in the CSF are generally 2 to 4 per cent of plasma levels, or roughly parallel to the concentration of free drug in the plasma. Increased protein binding decreases the concentration of free drug in equilibrium with sites of action and elimination, causing a decrease in intensity of effects and slowing the drug's rate of elimination. Hypoalbuminemia increases the concentration of active drug and may increase clinical effects. There is little or no glomerular filtration of protein-bound benzodiazepines.[6, 45]

Distribution

Following gastrointestinal absorption or intravenous administration, benzodiazepines are rapidly distributed to highly perfused organs, particularly the central nervous system. All benzodiazepines are widely distributed, and tissue concentrations within the brain, liver, and spleen typically exceed that of the serum. The volume of distribution of various benzodiazepines ranges from 0.3 to 5.5 liters per kg. Benzodiazepines are lipophilic and quickly penetrate the blood-brain barrier via passive diffusion to reach their sites of action within the CNS. Since the penetration into the CNS is rapid, the onset of clinical effects is limited more by the rate of systemic absorption of individual compounds rather than by their rate of distribution.

Pharmacologically, the serum and CNS are termed the "central compartment" of drug distribution.[30] Following initial distribution within this compartment, benzodiazepines are slowly *redistributed* to more poorly perfused sites (such as adipose tissue and muscle), collectively termed the "peripheral compartment." Highly lipid-soluble benzodiazepines will undergo more rapid and extensive redistribution.[3, 30]

Duration of Action

Benzodiazepine activity is terminated by at least three mechanisms. Two of these are pharmacokinetic and the third involves a functional change of the benzodiazepine receptor. The rate of *redistribution* of drug from the central compartment (CNS) to the peripheral compartment is the most important determinant of duration of clinical effect.[30] The second mechanism responsible for the duration of action is hepatic *metabolism* and renal *excretion*. The third mechanism is *acute tolerance* or *acute adaptation*, terms used to describe the clinical observation that benzodiazepine receptors appear to become less sensitive to drug effects with continued exposure.

Redistribution

It may seem paradoxic that a drug's measured plasma half-life does not predict its duration of action, but such is the case with benzodiazepines. The duration of action of benzodiazepines is a function of the CNS elimination half-life. The most lipophilic benzodiazepines have the shortest duration of action in the CNS because they are rapidly and extensively redistributed. They have the longest calculated plasma half-lives following redistribution because they remain in clinically inactive peripheral storage compartments (fat, muscle) for prolonged periods of time. Drugs that are less lipophilic have shorter plasma half-lives yet a longer duration of action, because redistribution from the CNS to the peripheral compartment is more limited and occurs more slowly.[46, 47] The rapid egress of highly lipid-soluble benzodiazepines from the central compartment to the peripheral compartment results in a duration of action of less than their respective plasma half-lives might suggest. This is illustrated by comparing the clinical anticonvulsant activity of lorazepam and diazepam. Lorazepam (half-life: 10 to 20 hours), a drug of relatively low lipophilicity, has more prolonged antiseizure activity than the highly lipophilic diazepam (half life: 20 to 70 hours). The benzodiazepine midazolam is extremely lipophilic and also rapidly biotransformed by the liver. It has an extremely short duration of action because both redistribution and

Table 45–3. CLASSIFICATION OF BENZODIAZEPINES ACCORDING TO PLASMA HALF-LIFE

Short	
flurazepam (Dalmane)	1 to 4 hours
midazolam (Versed)	2 to 5 hours
triazolam (Halcion)	2 to 6 hours
Intermediate	
alprazolam (Xanax)	6 to 20 hours
chlordiazepoxide (Librium)	5 to 20 hours
halazepam (Paxipam)	10 to 20 hours
lorazepam (Ativan)	10 to 20 hours
oxazepam (Serax)	5 to 15 hours
temazepam (Restoril)	5 to 20 hours
Long	
clonazepam (Klonopin)	20 to 30 hours
diazepam (Valium)	20 to 70 hours
Very Long	
clorazepate† (Tranxene)	30 to 200 hours
desalkylflurazepam*	45 to 300 hours
desmethyldiazepam*	30 to 200 hours
prazepam† (Centrax)	30 to 200 hours

*Active metabolite of primary benzodiazepine compounds.

†Prodrug or drug precursor which does not reach the system circulation in clinically significant amounts. Compounds are metabolized in GI tract or liver prior to systemic absorption and appear in the serum as desmethyldiazepam.

metabolism contribute significantly to the termination of clinical effects and plasma clearance[3, 4, 28, 31, 48] (Table 45–3).

Metabolism

Hepatic biotransformation via oxidation or conjugation accounts for virtually all benzodiazepine metabolism and clearance in humans[28] (Fig. 45–3). Hepatic metabolism can be divided into two phases: *Phase I metabolism* consists of oxidative pathways, either aliphatic hydroxylation by the cytochrome P-450 enzyme system or *N*-dealkylation. Phase I biotransformation produces pharmacologically active metabolites or intermediates. *Phase II metabolism* consists of hepatic conjugation of hydroxyl and amino groups to form inactive glucuronides, sulfates, and acetylated compounds that are rapidly excreted in the urine. Hepatic metabolism differs among benzodiazepines, and compounds may undergo both Phase I and Phase II metabolism (diazepam, chlordiazepoxide, flurazepam, halazepam, clorazepate, prazepam, triazolam, alprazolam, midazolam, and clonazepam) or only Phase II metabolism (lorazepam, oxazepam, and temazepam).[7]

Phase I oxidation is termed a "susceptible pathway" since the rate of activity may be altered by several factors. Phase I metabolism is inhibited or decreased by increasing age, pre-existing liver disease (including cirrhosis or hepatitis), or the coadministration of estrogens, isoniazid, disulfiram, phenytoin, alcohol, or cimetidine.[3, 49–56] Phase I metabolism is stimulated or induced by cigarette smoking[57] or by the chronic administration of substances that induce the cytochrome P-450 system, such as phenobarbital and alcohol. Benzodiazepines are very weak inducers of hepatic microsomal[61] systems and do not significantly alter their own metabolism.

Phase II conjugation is considered a "nonsusceptible pathway" since those factors that alter benzodiazepine oxidation usually have little or no effect on conjugation.[28, 52, 58–61] Agents undergoing Phase II metabolism may be preferred in patients with liver impairment, in the elderly, or in the presence of drugs that affect Phase I hepatic metabolism.[51, 62] Since the therapeutic indices of all benzodiazepines are very large, it is unclear whether the effects of higher blood concentrations resulting from decreased metabolism are clinically significant.[41]

Several benzodiazepines are biotransformed to active metabolites that contribute to their pharmacologic activity. In some cases the metabolites possess half-lives that far exceed those of the parent compound. In such instances, persistent clinical effects are more likely a consequence of the metabolic products than of the parent compound itself. Flurazepam has a plasma metabolic half-life of 1 to 4 hours, but its pharmacologically active metabolite, desalkylflurazepam, has a serum half-life of 45 to 300 hours. The primary metabolite of diazepam, desmethyldiazepam, is also pharmacologically active, and its half-life exceeds that of diazepam. Theoretically, benzodiazepines with long elimination half-lives or active metabolites may accumulate in the body with repeated dosing, resulting in excess sedation or significant performance-impairing effects. However, significant adaptation or tolerance usually offsets the effect of increasing serum level, and cumulative toxicity is uncommon.

Tolerance

Tolerance develops rapidly to the sedative but not the anxiolytic effects of benzodiazepines.[63] Tolerance to the anticonvulsant and muscle relaxation properties of benzodiazepines has not been extensively studied. It is

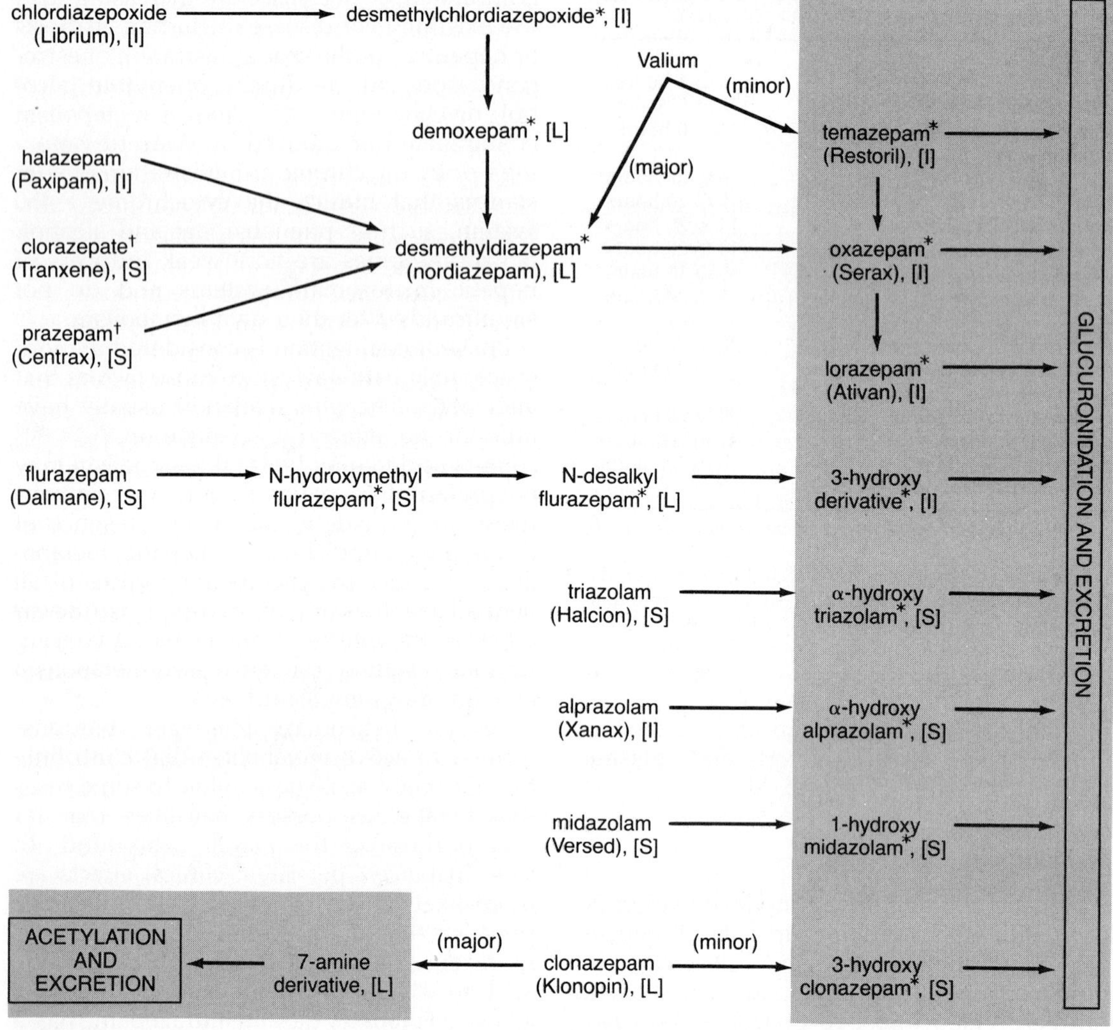

Figure 45–3. Major metabolic pathways of benzodiazepines approved for use in the United States. [S] = conversion half-life of less than 6 hours; [I] = conversion half-life of 6 to 20 hours; [L] = conversion half-life of greater than 20 hours. * = active metabolite. † = prodrug or drug precursor, which does not reach the systemic circulation in clinically significant amounts. Shaded areas denote processes that proceed via Phase II metabolism.

speculated that tolerance is a result of a biologic adaptation of the benzodiazepine receptor complex to constant concentrations of drug. Thus, even if the benzodiazepine concentration within the CNS is constant, the sedative effects are decreased with time. Some patients can tolerate the equivalent of 400 to 500 mg of diazepam per day yet still be awake and functional. Other factors that may influence tolerance include the "drug experience" or "drug sophistication" phenomenon that occurs in patients familiar with pharmacologic actions of the medication. It appears that the tolerance phenomenon occurs with all benzodiazepines.[28, 64, 65]

MECHANISM OF ACTION

Benzodiazepines appear to produce their sedative, hypnotic, anxiolytic, and anticonvulsant actions by binding to specific pharmacologic receptors in the central nervous system (Fig. 45–4). These high-affinity binding sites are stereospecific for all benzodiazepines and do not bind narcotics, barbiturates, or other sedative hypnotics.[66, 67] Benzodiazepine receptors are most concentrated in the cerebral cortex but are also found in the cerebellum, amygdala, hippocampus, hypothalamus, and spinal cord. Receptors have also been identified outside the CNS, although peripheral receptors do not appear to have significant physiologic effects. The molecular receptor for the benzodiazepine molecule is a glycoprotein located on the lipid membranes of both neural and glial cells. It is speculated that there are at least two classes of benzodiazepine receptor believed to mediate different specific effects.[6, 66, 68–72] Type I receptors predominate in the cerebellar cortex, and both type I and type II receptors are found in the cerebral cortex and hippocampus. Type I receptors are postulated to mediate anxiolytic effects, and type II receptors mediate the sedative and other actions of benzodiazepines. No endogenous ligand or neurotransmitter for these receptors has been identified. Benzodiazepine receptors are not influenced by norepinephrine, acetylcholine, dopamine, histamine, or serotonin.[4, 72–79]

DRUG INTERACTION

As a group, the benzodiazepines have little or no propensity to significantly augment or inhibit the activity of most other drugs. This lack of interaction is one reason why benzodiazepines have all but replaced barbiturates as the standard sedative-hypnotics.[80] Probably the most significant drug interaction occurs in the presence of alcohol or other CNS depressants and accounts for the ability of benzodiazepines to enhance the sedation produced by these substances.

The specific mechanism of benzodiazepine interaction with ethanol is complex and not completely understood. The combination is generally believed to produce additive effects rather than actual potentiation as defined in the true pharmacologic sense. The CNS effects are extremely variable and have not been quantified, but the ability of benzodiazepines to enhance the detrimental effects of ethanol on psychomotor skills (e.g., automobile driving) is well documented. Alcohol-induced liver injury tends to decrease the metabolism of benzodiazepines, but the clinical effect depends on the specific benzodiazepine and is difficult to predict. For example, in alcoholics, the elimination half-life of chlordiazepoxide is longer and the clearance slower, but clearance of the major active metabolite, desmethyldiazepoxide, is increased.

A number of other drugs have been reported to have a possible interaction with various benzodiazepines, but many of these interactions are poorly studied and remain theoretical, unconfirmed, or without clinical significance.

BENZODIAZEPINES IN ELDERLY PATIENTS

Benzodiazepines may produce paradoxic excitation in elderly patients, but there are also clinically relevant age-related differences in sedative effects, particularly during the early stages of therapy. No specific information is available that documents an increased sensitivity of benzodiazepine receptors in the brain, but elderly people may lack the phenomenon of acute tolerance. There is clearly an increased sensitivity to benzodiazepine-induced CNS depression that rises steadily with age.

Some of the differences in clinical response have been attributed to the changes in benzodiazepine pharmacokinetics noted with aging. Aging is associated with an increased volume of distribution, an increased plasma half-life, and a decreased hepatic clearance of some benzodiazepines, particularly diazepam and chlordiazepoxide. Pharmacokinetics appear unaltered with drugs exclusively cleared by Phase II metabolism. Increased sensitivity is, however, not strictly related to changes in serum levels, and current knowledge does not explain many of the age-related differences.

If excess sedation, confusion, agitation or other signs of cognitive impairment develop in an elderly patient taking benzodiazepines, it is prudent to immediately discontinue the drug pending further clinical investigation. Larson recently reported that benzodiazepines, particularly the long-acting ones such as diazepam, were the most common drugs associated with cognitive impairment in elderly people, often producing confusion, forgetfulness, slowing of the thought processes, and loss of the ability to care for oneself.[81] This occurred even if the drugs had been well tolerated for years. Benzodiazepines may also cause increased morbidity in patients with dementia from other causes, such as Alzheimer's disease. Often the benzodiazepine effect is overlooked by family and physicians and wrongly attributed to senility or a worsening of the underlying process.

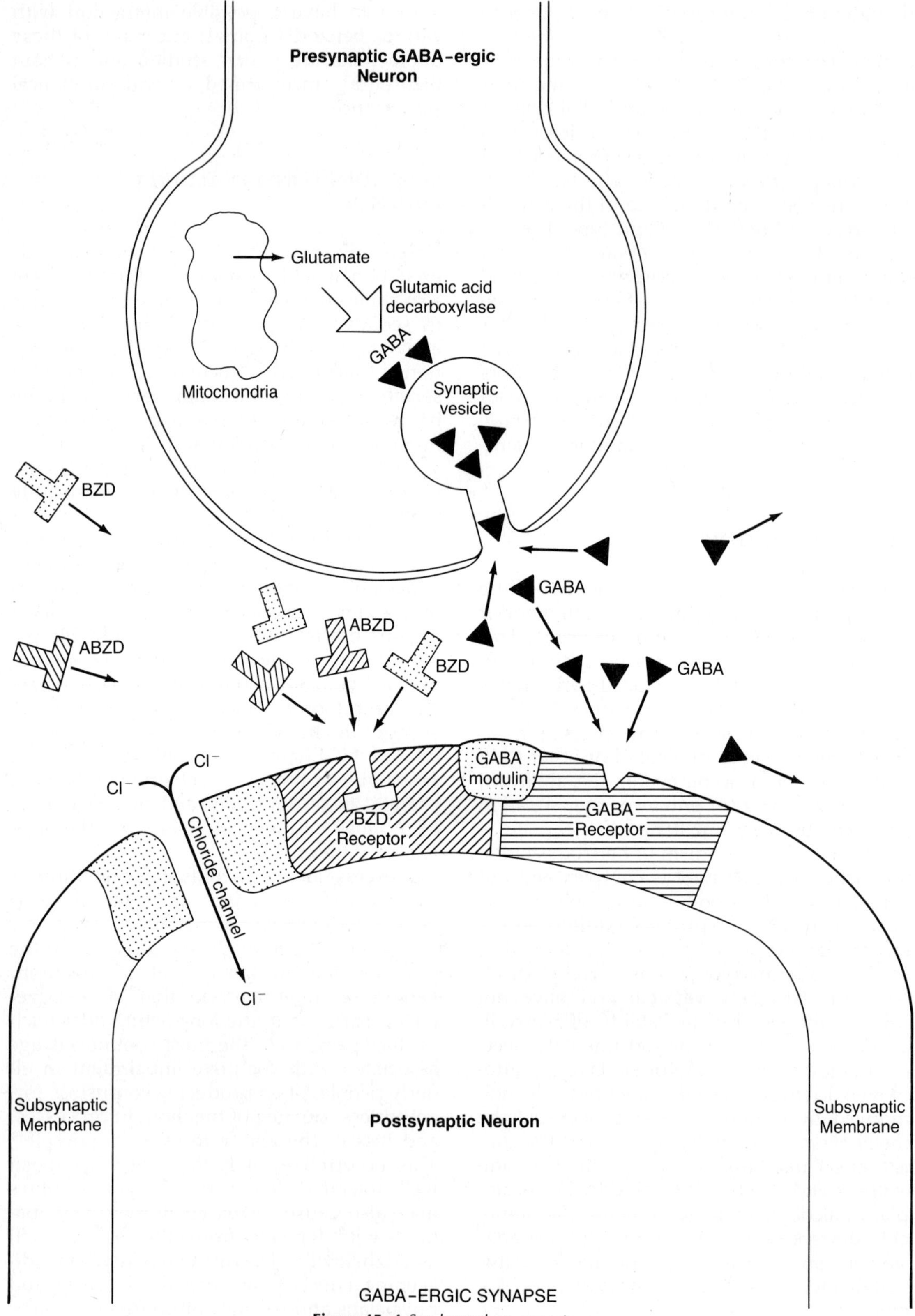

Figure 45–4 *See legend on opposite page*

TOXICITY OF BENZODIAZEPINES

Clinical Toxicity and Untoward Reactions

Therapeutic doses of benzodiazepines cause varying degrees of sedation, drowsiness, lightheadedness, lethargy, and lassitude in virtually all patients, especially when therapy is initiated.[82–84] Dysarthria, ataxia, motor incoordination, impairment of cognition, and amnesia may also be noted. Uncommonly, fatigue, headache, blurred vision, vertigo, nausea and vomiting, diarrhea, arthralgias, chest pain, and incontinence may occur.[3] The frequency and severity of side effects appear to increase with age.[46, 85]

Benzodiazepines may rarely cause aberrant or paradoxic effects. These reactions occur most frequently in patients with overt or latent psychoses and organic brain syndrome, and in elderly patients.[11, 86, 87] The anxiolytic benzodiazepines have been noted to unmask bizarre, uninhibited behavior in some patients, as well as hostility, rage, paranoia, and depression. Triazolam frequently has been noted to produce psychosis,[88] delirium,[89] coma,[90] and complete, transient global amnesia[91–95] when taken in normal oral doses or in minimal overdose. The stronger doses of this drug have recently been taken off the market in Europe.[5] Flurazepam has been associated with nightmares, euphoria, hallucinations, and restlessness.[3, 96] Paradoxic effects are most common in the first one to two weeks of therapy and usually subside spontaneously or with a decreased dose.[7]

Although benzodiazepines exert their therapeutic action within the central nervous system, there is no direct toxicity to the brain. If administered in sufficiently large amounts, benzodiazepines may depress the respiratory and cardiovascular systems indirectly through CNS depression. However, when given alone, benzodiazepines are relatively benign; even if the overdose is sufficient to produce deep coma, only minimal degrees of cardiovascular and respiratory depression occur.[3, 97–100] Other side effects, such as coronary vasodilation[101] and neuromuscular blockade can occur after the intake of extremely large doses[3] but rarely become clinically significant. Hematologic, renal, and hepatic toxicity, as well as acute rhabdomyolysis,[102] anaphylaxis,[3] dermatitis,[7] and acute respiratory distress syndrome,[103, 104] have been noted, but such adverse reactions are unusual and actually may be related to factors other than benzodiazepine overdose.

Uncommon side effects noted to occur after the *intravenous* administration of benzodiazepines include respiratory arrest, cardiac arrest, hypotension, and phlebitis at the site of injection. There is enormous variation in patients' response to intravenous diazepam.[105] Cardiorespiratory toxicity is probably secondary to the rapid administration of too large a dose for a particular individual. Life-threatening adverse reactions occur with a frequency of 1.7 per cent with intravenous diazepam and may be related in part to the use of propylene glycol as a parenteral vehicle in the formulation.[106] The intravenous use of midazolam, a benzodiazepine four to five

---

Figure 45–4. Benzodiazepine receptors and the GABAergic synapse. CNS neurotransmission occurs via a complex circuitry consisting of multiple connections, pathways, feedback mechanisms, and inhibitory/disinhibitory neurons, all under the control of neurotransmitters and neuroinhibitors. The body's most important *neuroinhibitor*, gamma-aminobutyric acid (GABA), is synthesized in nerve endings of presynaptic GABAergic neurons from glutamate, under the influence of the enzyme glutamic acid decarboxylase. GABA is stored in synaptic vesicles located in presynaptic nerve endings and is released into the synapse to function as a neuroinhibitor. GABA activity is terminated by diffusion out of the synapse or reuptake into presynaptic nerve endings.

Specific GABA receptors have been identified on the subsynaptic membrane of postsynaptic neurons. GABA receptors are adjacent to and coupled with chloride ion channels in such a way that activation of GABA receptor "opens" the associated channel, increasing chloride ion flux. The end result is hyperpolarization of the cell membrane, and decreased neuronal excitability.[28, 68, 78, 79] The activity of GABA or its functional relationship to GABA receptors may be related to GABA modulin, an endogenous peptide located in synaptic membranes.

Benzodiazepine receptors are located spatially adjacent to both GABA receptors and chloride ion channels. Benzodiazepines do not directly activate GABA receptors. Activation of the benzodiazepine receptors somehow facilitates or increases GABAergic activity, presumably by increasing chloride ion (and possibly also sodium and potassium) conduction via the GABA-dependent ion channels.[1, 69, 73–77] Benzodiazepine *antagonists* competitively block specific benzodiazepine receptor sites and either block the benzodiazepine binding or displace already bound drug, thereby offsetting any benzodiazepine-mediated GABAergic transmission. (GABA = gamma-aminobutyric acid; BZD = benzodiazepine; ABZD = benzodiazepine antagonist.)

times more potent than diazepam, has been associated with respiratory depression and fatal cardiorespiratory arrest when used for conscious sedation. Patients at particular risk for severe adverse reactions include elderly people, those patients with severe pulmonary or cardiac disease, and patients who have received other cardiorespiratory depressant medications.[6]

Toxicity in Overdose

One of the most remarkable properties of benzodiazepines is their relative safety following overdose. In contrast to the sedative-hypnotic drugs of the past, such as barbiturates, chloral hydrate, meprobamate, glutethimide, and ethchlorvynol, benzodiazepines have a high therapeutic index. Deaths attributable to benzodiazepines taken alone are extremely rare.[1, 23, 26, 33, 49, 82, 86, 96, 99, 107–110] Deaths, when they do occur, are almost always due to benzodiazepines taken in combination with other drugs. When the popularity and widespread use and misuse of benzodiazepines are considered, the paucity of documented fatalities secondary to benzodiazepines alone is a remarkable tribute to their safety.

Central nervous system depression is common in benzodiazepine overdose. Patients will usually become acutely drowsy, stuporous, and ataxic or may present in low-grade coma without focal neurologic abnormalities. The patient can generally be aroused from this state with verbal or painful stimulation. Profound coma, significant hypotension, respiratory depression, or hypothermia is extremely uncommon in oral overdose unless other drugs have also been ingested.[26, 33, 41, 110–112] For example, of the 38 patients with pure benzodiazepine overdose reported by Jatlow, 16 were awake and none were more symptomatic than grade 0 coma (asleep but arousable).[110] No patient required hospitalization despite blood levels considered to be in the toxic range (1 to 9 μg/ml).[57] Although there have been reported cases of prolonged deep coma,[113, 114] prolonged cyclic coma,[115] and benzodiazepine overdose presenting with focal neurologic signs,[116] such clinical scenarios are unusual. Most overdosed patients will become easily arousable or awaken within 12 to 36 hours, secondary to drug redistribution and the development of acute tolerance.[50] The duration of coma in elderly patients may be prolonged.[41, 112] Beyond their transient CNS depression and possible complications secondary to prolonged coma, pulmonary aspiration, or other indirect effects, benzodiazepines are not known to cause any specific injury or long-term toxicity to organ systems.[112, 117]

Although the recovery to consciousness is relatively rapid following benzodiazepine overdose, it is typical for the overdosed patient to be dizzy, depressed, and apathetic for an extended period. Clinically, the patient is noted to have CNS depression with hypotonia, motor retardation, slowed voluntary movements, and decreased reaction times.[112]

Numerous clinical studies testify to the safety of benzodiazepine overdose. In a study by Finkle and associates of 1239 cases of diazepam-associated deaths, only 2 (0.2 per cent) were possibly attributed to diazepam alone.[33] The investigators concluded that the toxicity of diazepam was low and its role in fatal overdoses was minimal. A study conducted by Busto and colleagues evaluated 1071 patients with drug overdose who presented to emergency departments in Toronto.[23] They noted that the effects of benzodiazepine overdose were usually mild, requiring only supportive therapy. The patients were rarely unconscious on presentation and were only infrequently admitted to the hospital. Greenblatt and associates studied 773 admissions for drug overdose to Massachusetts General Hospital in which 99 involved benzodiazepines, either alone or in combination with other agents.[26] Of the 12 admissions that were due to benzodiazepines alone, only one patient reached stage III coma (minimal response to painful stimuli), and one patient suffered significant cardiac or respiratory depression. In a study of 93 cases of diazepam overdose, Jatlow and associates found that patients required only supportive therapy, and no patient who ingested benzodiazepines alone required hospital admission. Numerous other case reports also attest to benzodiazepines' minimal toxicity, even in massive overdose.[28, 50, 118–120]

Analysis of recent national data also supports the safety of benzodiazepines in overdose. In the 4 years during which the National Data Collection System of the American Association of Poison Control Centers has been in operation, 2,980,643 poison exposure cases have been associated with 1122 fatalities. Of these, in only 66 were benzodiazepines involved, and in only 5 were they alone implicated. These five cases, and two fatalities reported recently,[121] all involved the newer, short-acting benzodiazepines (triazolam, alprazolam, temazepam). It is possible that these compounds may have greater potential for toxicity than the older benzodiazepines.[27, 121–125]

Coingestions

The toxicity of benzodiazepines may be significantly enhanced when they are taken in combination with other agents.[108] The study of Greenblatt and associates demonstrated that the coingestion of benzodiazepines with any other drug, including ethanol, analgesics, other sedative-hypnotics, tricyclic antidepressants, phenothiazines, or barbiturates, substantially increased the potential for serious toxicity.[26] The combination of benzodiazepines and barbiturates was noted to be particularly dangerous, with 50 per cent of patients studied requiring mechanical ventilation. Ethanol, identified as a coingestant in 38 per cent of benzodiazepine overdoses in one study,[33] enhances CNS toxicity of these agents directly because of its depressant characteristics and by increasing benzodiazepine absorption and decreasing phase I metabolism.[96, 126] Case reports, clinical studies, and subject reviews have suggested that synergistic toxicity exists between benzodiazepines and tricyclic antidepressants,[127–129] cimetidine,[130] phenothiazines,[128, 131] narcotics,[33, 128, 131] antihistamines,[131] barbiturates,[128] and alcohol.[33, 126, 128, 132]

LABORATORY TESTING AND ANALYSIS

Plasma concentrations of benzodiazepines have been shown to correlate very poorly with the severity of toxic effects, the degree of central nervous system depression, or final outcome. Quantitative plasma measurements are not available in most hospitals, and they provide no significant therapeutic direction to the treating physician.[6, 7, 23, 45, 50, 110, 119, 132, 133] A lethal dose has not been established for any benzodiazepine.

Blood concentrations and clinical effects of diazepam have been studied in some detail. Daily 10-mg doses of diazepam usually produce serum levels of less than 1 μg per ml. Chronic daily doses of 150 to 200 mg per day will produce levels of 5 to 6 μg per ml. Therapeutic levels range between 0.5 and 2 μg per ml but vary widely. When measured for academic or forensic purposes, diazepam levels commonly reach 2 to 5 μg per ml in overdose cases but may reach 10 to 15 μg per ml. Diazepam levels of 5 to 20 μg per ml are generally regarded as toxic, but many patients with serum concentrations in this range manifest only minimal clinical effects. No reliable or interpretable data exist regarding therapeutic or toxic levels for most newer benzodiazepines.

Quantitative measurement of serum benzodiazepine levels (parent compound and metabolite) may be useful to differentiate acute from chronic ingestions or may be of value in medicolegal or forensic situations. For example, diazepam's principal metabolite, desmethyldiazepam, has a half-life that exceeds that of diazepam. In acute ingestion, the level of diazepam should exceed that of desmethyldiazepam; with chronic ingestion, concentrations of desmethyldiazepam should exceed that of diazepam. Although some research toxicology laboratories have the capability to measure these levels, its application is not useful in the management of acute overdose.

The use of *qualitative* urine screening to ascertain the presence or absence of parent benzodiazepines or their metabolites may provide rapid, useful information in the evaluation of patients with an unknown cause of CNS depression. Although thin layer chromatography is used most frequently for general toxicology screening,[134] its ability to detect benzodiazepines or their metabolites in urine is poor. Most laboratories perform initial screens for benzodiazepines with diagnostic immunoassay tests that identify the presence of benzodiazepines or benzodiazepine metabolites in the urine. When a positive result is obtained with a screening immunoassay study, the laboratories should perform confirmatory tests with gas or high-pressure liquid chromatography, or mass spectrometry.

A variety of immunoassay tests are available and are standardized against the detection of a particular single benzodiazepine compound (usually oxazepam). Other structurally similar benzodiazepines are subsequently detected through immunologic cross-reactivity with the compound that is used as a standard in the screening test. The sensitivities for detection of an individual benzodiazepine may differ significantly. For example, the EMIT screen is known to cross-react with chlordiazepoxide, clonazepam, demoxepam, desalkylfurazepam, desmethyldiazepam, flurazepam, lorazepam, oxazepam, prazepam, and temazepam.[135] However, this assay has not been demonstrated to detect consistently several of these compounds unless they are found in extremely high concentrations. Triazolobenzodiazepine derivatives, such as alprazolam or triazolam,[136, 137] may be particularly difficult to detect in small (but clinically significant) ingestions because they possess poor immunologic cross-reactivity with oxazepam since they are administered and excreted in very small quantities. The radioimmunoassay (RIA) screening test Abuscreen will identify alprazolam, chlordiazepoxide, demoxepam, clorazepate, diazepam, temazepam, desmethdiazepam, desalkylflurazepam, halazepam, lorazepam, midazolam, and prazepam but will not detect clonazepam or flurazepam.[138] The latest commercially available immunoassay, based on the technique of fluorescence polarization (Abbott Diagnostics, Chicago) offers detection capabilities similar to that of radioimmunoassay with somewhat improved detection of the triazolobenzodiazepines. It is important to recognize that the laboratory detection of benzodiazepines depends upon the particular toxicologic screen used and the amount and type of benzodiazepine ingested. Some commonly used screens may indicate negative results in spite of a clinically significant benzodiazepine ingestion.

TERATOGENICITY AND BREAST EXCRETION

Benzodiazepines readily cross the placenta[139] and may accumulate in the fetus, with levels that exceed the maternal serum concentration. Several animal studies have suggested that occasional congenital malformations may occur and the incidence of fetal loss may increase when benzodiazepines are used during pregnancy. A possible association between the development of fetal oral clefts in humans and diazepam use in the first trimester of pregnancy had been suggested by several studies in the early 1970s,[140, 141] but a larger, well-controlled study performed in 1983 failed to support this association.[142]

High doses of benzodiazepines taken immediately prior to or during labor may produce the characteristics of floppy baby syndrome in newborn infants, including lethargy, poor feeding, hypothermia, hypotonia, apnea, and low Apgar scores. The occurrence of floppy baby syndrome is associated with the persistence of long-acting benzodiazepine metabolites in the serum of the neonate.[3, 143–145] The incidence appears to be decreased when benzodiazepines that are metabolized by only Phase II metabolism (lorazepam, oxazepam, and temazepam) are administered.[7, 30, 146]

Benzodiazepines and their metabolites are excreted in breast milk in clinically significant amounts[147] and may sedate the nursing neonate. This can result in poor feeding, lethargy, and failure to thrive. Since the metabolic capability of the neonate is immature,[148] the benzodiazepines metabolized by Phase I pathways may persist for extended periods of time. Breast feeding should be avoided if benzodiazepines are to be administered to lactating women.

DEPENDENCE AND THE WITHDRAWAL SYNDROME

Physiologic addiction, characterized by somatic withdrawal symptoms after cessation of the therapy, occurs with benzodiazepines.[19, 149–153] Clinically, the benzodiazepine withdrawal syndrome is similar to barbiturate or alcohol withdrawal; however, benzodiazepine withdrawal occurs less frequently and is usually less severe. Withdrawal is more likely to occur if (1) the duration of therapy is greater than 4 months, (2) high doses have been taken, (3) the drug is abruptly discontinued, and (4) a short-acting drug is used.[150] The exact mechanism of dependency is unknown.

"High-dose" and "low-dose" benzodiazepine dependency states with their subsequent withdrawal syndromes have been identified. High-dose dependency is similar to that classically seen with barbiturate and other sedative-hypnotics and can occur within one month if two to four times the maximum daily recommended dose is administered. The intensity of withdrawal is dose and time related and tends to be severe yet short lived.

Low-dose dependency can occur after therapeutic doses are given for prolonged periods. Withdrawal symptoms are less severe but may last for weeks. However, the validity of the low-dose withdrawal syndrome is somewhat controversial since many individuals take benzodiazepines chronically for years without any sign of overt withdrawal when the drug is abruptly discontinued. Some experts believe that the incidence and severity of benzodiazepine withdrawal has been overestimated. Rickels estimates the incidence to be as low as 1 to 3 per cent following long-acting benzodiazepine use for up to 1 year and 5 to 10 per cent following termination of short, rapidly acting drugs that have been administered for up to 1 year.[154] However, withdrawal symptoms may rarely occur following treatment regimens as short as 4 to 6 weeks[153, 155] and between 15 and 45 per cent of long-term benzodiazepine users may experience some withdrawal symptoms.[3, 156, 157]

The onset and severity of symptoms will vary with the type of benzodiazepine involved. Typically, withdrawal symptoms from long-acting benzodiazepines such as diazepam will be evident between 3 and 7 days after termination of therapy. Symptoms may persist for up to several months.[151, 158] Complete elimination of benzodiazepine is not required to produce overt withdrawal, and symptoms may occur following a rapid reduction in dosage. It is speculated that the serum or tissue levels in people taking benzodiazepines with long half-lives or long-acting metabolites decrease more slowly, thereby minimizing the severity of withdrawal symptoms. With chronic use of short-acting benzodiazepines, withdrawal symptoms can occur less than 24 hours following termination of therapy, and the symptoms are usually more severe than those associated with withdrawal from benzodiazepines with longer half-lives.[6, 150, 152, 159–162] Alprazolam may cause a particularly difficult withdrawal syndrome.[5]

Symptoms of Withdrawal

Since most patients undergoing long-term benzodiazepine therapy have underlying psychiatric disturbances, it may be difficult to distinguish withdrawal symptoms from an exacerbation or reappearance of the underlying psychiatric illness. Unsuspected concurrent withdrawal from alcohol or other sedative-hypnotics may exacerbate the symptoms of benzodiazepine withdrawal. Typically, benzodiazepine withdrawal includes increased anxiety and apprehension, agitation, insomnia, tremors, nightmares, photophobia, headache, myalgias, and a heightened sensorium (hyperacusis). More severe and less common symptoms include nausea and vomiting, diaphoresis, hyperpyrexia, palpitations, vertigo, and psychosis.[151, 163, 164] Seizures rarely have been reported and may occur up to 2 weeks following cessation of therapy.[165] One death secondary to benzodiazepine withdrawal has been documented.[166]

Treatment of Withdrawal

The treatment of withdrawal includes the administration of long-acting benzodiazepines or occasionally barbiturates, followed by a gradual tapering of dosage, preferably over a period of at least 4 weeks.[152, 155] A gradual reduction in dosage is recommended whenever benzodiazepines are electively discontinued in patients who have had long-term therapy. Most clinicians prefer to discontinue the short-acting benzodiazepines and replace them with equivalent doses of diazepam. Withdrawal may then be prevented or minimized by decreasing the daily dose by an equivalent of 0.5 to 2.5 mg of diazepam or a maximum of one quarter of the daily dose every 1 to 2 weeks. However, individual sensitivity is quite varied, and it is best to titrate the dose and rate of reduction to the patient's symptoms. Clonidine,[167, 168] propranolol,[169, 170] and tricyclic antidepressants[158] also have been used successfully as adjunctive therapy to decrease some of the somatic symptoms of benzodiazepine withdrawal. Withdrawal usually can be accomplished on an outpatient basis in the compliant and motivated patient.

Fetal Dependency

Women who take benzodiazepines during pregnancy may cause intrauterine benzodiazepine dependency in the fetus and benzodiazepine withdrawal in the neonate. The syndrome resembles neonatal narcotic withdrawal; symptoms include hypertonicity, irritability, tremors, hyperreflexia, tachypnea, and weight loss. Although these infants may feed vigorously, they frequently vomit.[171] Symptoms usually begin 2 to 6 days after delivery but may be delayed up to 10 days because of decreased benzodiazepine clearance in the neonate. The withdrawal syndrome in neonates is usually treated with phenobarbital.

DIAGNOSIS OF BENZODIAZEPINE OVERDOSE

The patient with a pure benzodiazepine overdose will display mild-to-moderate sedation, often with dysarthria and ataxia, without serious neurologic, cardiovascular, or respiratory impairment. The diagnosis is usually made entirely by history or laboratory results since there are no diagnostic clinical features or specific toxidromes. Clinical clues that suggest an alternative diagnosis or a concomitant ingestion include deep coma, hyperreflexia or clonus, cardiovascular instability, and respiratory depression requiring assisted ventilation. Associated trauma, underlying medical disorders, or the concomitant ingestion of other drugs may make the clinical diagnosis of benzodiazepine overdose quite difficult. In obtaining the history or analyzing any toxicologic laboratory data, particular attention should be paid to the possible ingestion of any compounds that may potentiate the toxicity of benzodiazepines. It is emphasized that significant ingestions of the newer benzodiazepines may escape the detection of an unsophisticated toxicology laboratory.

TREATMENT

Current therapy for benzodiazepine overdose is conservative and supportive. The coingestion of other toxic substances, concurrent trauma, or other underlying medical conditions may alter significantly the diagnostic and therapeutic approach. One should always be cognizant of conditions that may mimic a benzodiazepine ingestion, such as head trauma, ethanol intoxication, hypoglycemia, carbon monoxide poisoning, or cardiovascular attack (CVA).

Gastric emptying by either ipecac or gastric lavage may be undertaken, with standard precautions based on the patient's level of consciousness and adequacy of airway protection. Gastric emptying should be followed by oral activated charcoal and a cathartic. In pure benzodiazepine overdose, gastric emptying has not been demonstrated to decrease mortality and is not routinely required. Minimally symptomatic patients or those with ingestions more than 2 hours prior to evaluation can safely be observed and closely monitored without gastric emptying, although activated charcoal should be routinely administered. Very few patients with a pure benzodiazepine overdose will require treatment beyond activated charcoal and observation. Patients without complications who are able to ambulate without ataxia after treatment and 4 to 6 hours of observation can be discharged after appropriate psychiatric consultation. In instances of respiratory depression or cardiovascular compromise, airway protection and mechanical ventilation should be instituted. Circulatory support should consist of the administration of intravenous crystalloid fluids and, rarely, vasopressors.

There are no practical ways to enhance benzodiazepine elimination significantly. Forced diuresis is of no proven value. Hemoperfusion, hemodialysis, and peritoneal dialysis are relatively ineffective in removing clinically significant amounts of benzodiazepines from the serum because of extensive protein binding.[41, 112] More importantly, under normal circumstances the potential toxicity of benzodiazepine overdose is not sufficient to warrant the use of such aggressive intervention.

Several currently available drugs have been noted to reverse some of the effects of benzodiazepines in overdose. Doxapram appeared to reverse diazepam sedative effects in one report[172] but may be associated with potentially serious side effects. Naloxone has been reported anecdotally to partially reverse the respiratory depressant and sedative effects of benzodiazepine overdose,[90, 173, 174] although a controlled study has failed to demonstrate any significant benefit.[175] Although the mode of action is unclear, physostigmine occasionally has been noted to reverse the central nervous system and respiratory depression induced by benzodiazepines.[176–179] Because of the potential for cholinergic toxicity from physostigmine, its routine use in an uncomplicated benzodiazepine overdose is seldom warranted.

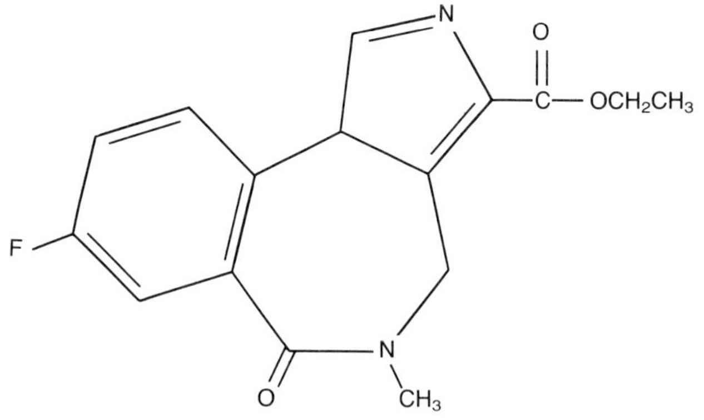

Figure 45–5. The chemical structure of flumazenil (Ro 15–1788), a specific benzodiazepine antagonist.

Benzodiazepine Antagonists

Imidazobenzodiazepine derivatives recently have been developed. They competitively and reversibly bind CNS benzodiazepine receptors while possessing no significant benzodiazepine agonist activity.[180, 181] The most promising of these investigational antagonists, flumazenil (Ro 15–1788, Fig. 45–5), is undergoing a multicenter clinical trial in the United States for treatment of overdose patients. This agent is currently available in Europe under the trade name Anexate. In studies performed to date, flumazenil has been noted to reverse rapidly and completely the sedative, anxiolytic, anticonvulsant, amnestic, ataxic, anesthetic, and muscle relaxant effects of benzodiazepines in animals and humans.[181, 183] It also has been shown to restore an EEG to the baseline waking state in patients who have previously been administered benzodiazepines,[184] and it has been demonstrated to be an effective antidote in cases of benzodiazepine overdose.[185, 186] In studies of coma secondary to benzodiazepines,[180, 187, 188] patients respond dramatically in 1 to 5 minutes after the administration of flumazenil. The duration of the antagonist effects is short lived due to a half-life of approximately 1 hour. Repeated doses may be required to maintain the desired clinical effects.

The most common side effects of flumazenil administered to normal volunteers are dizziness, facial erythema, anxiety, and headache. Symptoms are mild and disappear within several minutes. Flumazenil has been noted to precipitate convulsions in epileptic patients taking benzodiazepines for seizure control and in patients with the coingestion of drugs that lower the seizure threshold (e.g., tricyclic antidepressants). Seizures may be controlled by the readministration of benzodiazepines or barbiturates. As with naloxone use for opiate intoxication, flumazenil has the potential to precipitate withdrawal symptoms in benzodiazepine-dependent individuals.[189] In animal studies, the severity of withdrawal depends on the specific benzodiazepine used, the dose and duration of treatment, and the dose of flumazenil administered.[190] Although withdrawal symptoms are usually more severe with flumazenil than when benzodiazepines are simply discontinued, they rarely become clinically serious.[189, 191]

Although the potential toxicity of benzodiazepines is relatively low, and aggressive therapy for pure overdose is rarely required, flumazenil offers several important potential uses in clinical medicine. Since it reverses only benzodiazepine-induced CNS depression, it is diagnostic as well as therapeutic. The antagonist can confirm a suspected diagnosis of benzodiazepine overdose or exclude benzodiazepine intoxication as a cause of CNS depression in an undiagnosed patient.[181, 185, 192] In coma secondary to multiple drug overdose, removing the benzodiazepine component may avoid the need for intubation and mechanical ventilation.[183, 193, 194] Flumazenil may be useful postoperatively to reverse the effects of preoperative sedation,[195] or to reverse an inadvertent overdose when benzodiazepines are used for conscious sedation in outpatients.[192] The current status of flumazenil for the routine treatment of polydrug or benzodiazepine overdose in the emergency department is uncertain but should be clarified in the near future.

References

1. Greenblatt DJ, Shader RI: Drug therapy. Benzodiazepines. N Engl J Med *291*:1011–1015, 1974.

2. Sternbach LH: Benzodiazepines: Today and Tomorrow. Lancaster, MTP Press, 1980.
3. Harvey SC: Hypnotics and sedatives. *In* Gilman AG, Goodman LS, Rall TW, et al: The Pharmacological Basis of Therapeutics. 7th ed. New York, Macmillan, 1985.
4. Smith DE, Wesson DR: The Benzodiazepines: Current Standards for Medical Practice. Lancaster, MTP Press, 1985.
5. Choice of benzodiazepines. Med Lett *30*(760):26–28, 1988.
6. Sellers EM: Anxiolytics, hypnotics, and sedatives. *In* Kalant H, Roschlau WHE, Sellers EM (eds): Principles of Medical Pharmacology. New York, Oxford University Press, 1985.
7. Lader M: Clinical pharmacology of benzodiazepines. Annu Rev Med *38*:19–28, 1987.
8. Lewis D: The physician's contribution to the drug abuse scene. Tufts Med Alumni Bull *30*:36, 1971.
9. Balter MB, Manheimer DI, Mellinger GD, et al: A cross-national comparison of anti-anxiety/sedative drug use. Curr Med Res Opinion *8*:5–20, 1984.
10. Mellinger GD, Balter MB: Prevalence and pattern of use of psychotherapeutic drugs: Results from a 1979 national survey of American adults. *In* Tognini G, Bellantriono C, Lader M (eds): Proceedings of the International Seminar of Epidemiological Impact of Psychotropic Drugs. New York, Elsevier, 1981.
11. Laux G, Puryear D: Benzodiazepine—misuse, abuse and dependency. Am Fam Physician *30*:139–147, 1984.
12. Balter MD, Levine J, Manheimer DI: Cross-national study of the extent of anti-anxiety–sedative drug use. N Engl J Med *290*:769–774, 1974.
13. Fox R: Abuse of benzodiazepines (letter). Lancet 2:681–682, 1978.
14. Lader M: Benzodiazepines—the opium of the masses? Neuroscience *3*:159–165, 1978.
15. Skegg DC, Doll R, Perry J: Use of medicines in general practice. Br Med J *1*:1561–1563, 1977.
16. Woody GE, O'Brien C, Greenstein R: Misuse and abuse of diazepam: An increasingly common medical problem. Int J Addiction *10*:843–848, 1975.
17. Morgan K, Gilleard C, Reive A: Hypnotic usage in residential homes of the elderly: A prevalence and longitudinal analysis. Age Aging *11*:229–234, 1982.
18. Mellinger GD, Balter MB, Uhlenhuth EH: Prevalence and correlates of the long-term regular use of anxiolytics. JAMA *251*:375–379, 1984.
19. Marks J: The benzodiazepines—use and abuse. Arzneimittelforsch *30*:898–901, 1980.
20. Lader MH, Higgitt AC: Management of benzodiazepine dependence—update 1986. Br J Addiction *81*:7–10, 1986.
21. Simonsen LLP: The top 200 drugs of 1987. Pharmacy Times *54*(3):38–46, 1988.
22. Macdonald DI: Cocaine heads ED drug visits. JAMA *258*:2029, 1987.
23. Busto U, Kaplan HL, Sellers EM: Benzodiazepine-associated emergencies in Toronto. Am J Psychiatr *137*:224–227, 1980.
24. Kessel N: Self-poisoning. Br Med J *2*:1336–1340, 1965.
25. Oliver RG, Hetzel BS: Rise and fall of suicide rates in Australia: Relation to sedative availability. Med J Aust 2:919–923, 1972.
26. Greenblatt DJ, Allen MD, Noel BJ, et al: Acute overdosage with benzodiazepine derivatives. Clin Pharmacol Ther *21*:497–514, 1977.
27. Litovitz TL, Normann SA, Veltri JC: Annual report (1985) of the American association of poison control centers national data collection system. Am J Emerg Med *4*:427–458, 1986.
28. Greenblatt DJ, Shader RI, Abernethy DR: Current status of benzodiazepines: Part I. N Engl J Med *309*:354–358, 1983.
29. Greenblatt DJ, Divoll M, Abernethy DR, et al: Benzodiazepine hypnotics: Kinetic and therapeutic options. Sleep *5*:S18–S27, 1982.
30. Van Rooyen JM, Offermeier J: Pharmacokinetics of the benzodiazepines. S Afr Med J *69*:S14–S22, 1985.
31. Greenblatt DJ, Shader RI, Divoll M, et al: Benzodiazepines: A summary of pharmacokinetic properties. Br J Clin Pharmacol *11*:11S–16S, 1981.
32. Kaplan SA, Jack ML: Metabolism of the benzodiazepines: Pharmacokinetic and pharmacodynamic considerations. *In* Costa E: The Benzodiazepines: From Molecular Biology to Clinical Practice. New York, Raven Press, 1983.
33. Finkle BS, McCloskey KL, Goodman LS: Diazepam and drug-associated deaths: A survey in the United States and Canada. JAMA *242*:429–434, 1979.
34. Hayes SL, Pablo G, Radomski T, et al: Ethanol and oral diazepam absorption. N Engl J Med *296*:186–189, 1977.
35. Greenblatt DJ, Allen MD, MacLaughlin DS, et al: Diazepam absorption: Effect of antacids and food. Clin Pharmacol Ther *24*:600–609, 1978.
36. Divoll M, Greenblatt DJ, Ciraulo DA, et al: Clobazam kinetics: Intra-subject variability and effect of food on absorption. J Clin Pharmacol *22*:69–73, 1982.
37. Greenblatt DJ, Shader RI, Harmatz JS, et al: Influence of magnesium and aluminum hydroxide mixture on chlordiazepoxide absorption. Clin Pharmacol Ther *19*:234–239, 1976.
38. Shader RI, Georgotas A, Greenblatt DJ, et al: Impaired absorption of desmethyldiazepam from clorazepate by magnesium aluminum hydroxide. Clin Pharmacol Ther *24*:308–315, 1978.
39. Gustafson JH, Weissman L, Weinfeld RE, et al: Clinical bioavailability evaluation of a controlled release formulation of diazepam. J Pharmacokin Biopharmaceut *9*:679–691, 1981.
40. Greenblatt DJ, Shader RI, Frankle K, et al: Pharmacokinetics and bioavailability of intravenous, intramuscular, and oral lorazepam in humans. J Pharm Sci *68*:57–63, 1979.
41. Greenblatt DJ, Divoll M, Harmatz JS: Pharmacokinetic comparison of sublingual lorazepam with intravenous, intramuscular and oral lorazepam. J Pharm Sci *71*:248–252, 1982.
42. Greenblatt DJ, Shader RJ, Koch-Weser J, et al: Slow absorption of intramuscular chlordiazepoxide. N Engl J Med *291*:1116–1118, 1974.
43. Kortilla K, Linnoila M: Absorption and sedative effects of diazepam after oral administration and intramuscular administration into the vastus lateralis muscle and the deltoid muscle. Br J Anaesth *47*:857–862, 1975.
44. Greenblatt DJ, Koch-Weser J: Intramuscular injection of drugs. N Engl J Med *295*:542–546, 1976.
45. Norman TR, Graham BD: Plasma concentrations of benzodiazepines—a review of clinical findings and implications. Prog Neuro-Psychopharmacol Biol Psychiat *8*:115–126, 1984.
46. Swift CG, Stevenson IH: Benzodiazepines in the elderly. *In* Costa E: The Benzodiazepines: From

Molecular Biology to Clinical Practice. New York, Raven Press, 1983.
47. Klotz U, Avant GR, Hoyumpa A, et al: The effect of age and liver disease on the disposition and elimination of diazepam in adult man. J Clin Invest *55*:347–359, 1975.
48. George KA, Dundee JW: Relative amnesic action of diazepam, flunitrazepam and lorazepam in man. Br J Clin Pharmacol *4*:45–50, 1977.
49. Shader RI, Ciraulo DA, Greenblatt DJ: Drug interactions involving psychotropic drugs. Psychosomatics *19*:671–681, 1978.
50. Robins AH: The other side of the benzodiazepines. S Afr Cont Med Educ *2*:43–48, 1984.
51. Ruffalo RL, Thompson RF, Segal J: Diazepam-cimetidine drug interaction: A clinically significant effect. South Med J *74*:1075–1078, 1981.
52. Dobb GJ, Ukich A, Ilett KF: Does cimetidine inhibit the clearance of temazepam after an overdose? [letter] Med J Aust *145*:58–59, 1986.
53. Greenblatt DJ, Abernethy DR, Morse DS, et al: Clinical importance of the interaction of diazepam and cimetidine. N Engl J Med *310*:1639–1642, 1984.
54. Klotz U, Reiman I: Influence of cimetidine on the pharmacokinetics of desmethyldiazepam and oxazepam. Eur J Clin Pharmacol *34*:227–230, 1983.
55. Somogi A, Gugler R: Drug interactions with cimetidine. Clin Pharmacokinet *7*:23–41, 1982.
56. Abernethy DR, Greenblatt DJ, Divoll M, et al: Interaction of cimetidine with the triazolobenzodiazepines alprazolam and triazolam. Psychopharmacology *80*:275–278, 1983.
57. Boston Collaborative Drug Surveillance Program, 1973: Clinical depression of the central nervous system due to diazepam and chlordiazepoxide in relation to cigarette smoking and age. N Engl J Med *288*:277–280, 1973.
58. Greenblatt DJ, Abernethy DR, Divoll M, et al: Noninteraction of temazepam and cimetidine. J Pharm Sci *73*:399–401, 1983.
59. Patwardhan RV, Yarborough GW, Desmond PV, et al: Cimetidine impairs the glucuronidation of lorazepam and oxazepam. Gastroenterology *79*:912–916, 1980.
60. Greenblatt DJ: Clinical pharmacokinetics of oxazepam and lorazepam. Clin Pharmacokinet *6*:89–105, 1981.
61. Greenblatt DJ, Sellers EM, Shader RI: Drug disposition in old age. N Engl J Med *306*:1081–1088, 1982.
62. Schentag JJ, Cerra FB, Calleri G, et al: Pharmacokinetic and clinical studies in patients with cimetidine associated mental confusion. Lancet *1*:177–181, 1979.
63. Rickels K: Benzodiazepines: Use, overuse, and abuse. Br Med J *11*:71S–83S, 1981.
64. Greenblatt DJ, Woo E, Allen DM, et al: Rapid recovery from massive diazepam overdose. JAMA *240*:1872–1874, 1978.
65. Braestrup C, Nielsen M: Anxiety. Lancet *2*:1030–1034, 1982.
66. Mohler H, Okada T: Demonstration of benzodiazepine receptors in the central nervous system. Science *198*:849–851, 1977.
67. Squires RF, Braestrup C: Benzodiazepine receptors in rat brain. Nature *266*:732–734, 1977.
68. Eadie MJ: Currently available benzodiazepines. Med J Aust *141*:827–831, 1984.
69. Braestrup C, Nielsen M: Benzodiazepine receptors. Arzneimittelforschung *30*:852–857, 1980.
70. Skolnick P, Paul SM: Benzodiazepine receptors in the central nervous system. Int Rev Neurobiol *23*:103–140, 1982.
71. Pieri L: Neuropharmacology of benzodiazepines. *In* Tiengo M, Cousins MJ (eds): Pharmacological Basis of Anesthesiology, Clinical Pharmacology of New Analgesics and Anesthetics. New York, Raven Press, 1983.
72. Klepner CA, Lippa AS, Denson DI, et al: Resolution of two biochemically and pharmacologically distinct benzodiazepine receptors. Pharmacol Biochem Behav *11*:457–462, 1979.
73. Costa E, Guidotti A, Mao CC: Evidence for involvement of GABA in the action of benzodiazepines: Studies on rat cerebellum. *In* Costa E, Greengard P (eds): Mechanism of Action of Benzodiazepines. New York, Raven Press, 1975.
74. Polc P, Haefely W: Effects of two benzodiazepines, phenobarbitone, and ooclofen on synaptic transmission in the cat cuneate nucleus. Naunyn Schmiedebergs Arch Pharmacol *294*:121–131, 1976.
75. Sepinwall J, Cook L: Mechanism of action of the benzodiazepines: Behavioral aspect. Fed Proc *39*:3024–3031, 1979.
76. Toffano G, Leon A, Massotti M, et al: GABA modulin, a regulatory protein for GABA receptors. *In* Pepeu G, Kuhar MJ, Enna SJ (eds): Receptors for Neurotransmitters and Peptide Hormones. New York, Raven Press, 1980.
77. Haefely W, Kulcsar A, Mohler H, et al: Possible involvement of GABA in the central actions of benzodiazepines. *In* Costa E, Greengard P (eds): Mechanism of Action of Benzodiazepines. New York, Raven Press, 1975.
78. Stahmer SD: Pharmacodynamics of benzodiazepines. S Afr Med J *69*:S14–S20, 1985.
79. Paul S, Marangos PJ, Skolnick P: The benzodiazepine-GABA-chloride ionphore receptor complex: Common site of minor tranquilizer action. Biol Psychiatr *16*:213–229, 1981.
80. Breckenridge A: Interactions of benzodiazepines with other substances. *In* Costa, E: The Benzodiazepines: From Molecular Biology to Clinical Practice. New York, Raven Press, 1983.
81. Larson EB, Kukill WA, Buchner D, et al: Adverse drug reactions associated with global cognitive impairment in elderly persons. Ann Intern Med *107*:169–173, 1987.
82. Greenblatt DJ, Shader RI: Benzodiazepines in Clinical Practice. New York, Raven Press, 1974.
83. Rickels K: Use of anti-anxiety agents in anxious outpatients. Psychopharmacology *58*:1–17, 1978.
84. Hollister LE: Valium: A discussion of current issues. Psychosomatics *18*:1–15.
85. Meyer BR: Benzodiazepines in the elderly. Med Clin North Am *66*:1017–1035, 1982.
86. Palmer GC: Use, overuse, misuse and abuse of benzodiazepines. Ala J Med Sci *15*:383–392, 1978.
87. Hollister LE: Benzodiazepines—an overview. Br J Clin Pharmacol *11*:117S–119S, 1981.
88. Einarson TR, Yoder ES: Triazolam psychosis—a syndrome? Drug Intell Clin Pharmacol *16*:330, 1982.
89. Trappler B, Bezeredi T: Triazolam intoxication (letter). Can Med Assoc J *126*:893–894, 1982.
90. Olson KR, Yin K, Osterloh J: Coma caused by trivial triazolam overdose. Am J Emerg Med 3:210–211, 1985.
91. Morris HH, Estes ML: Traveler's amnesia: Transient global amnesia secondary to triazolam. JAMA *258*:945–946, 1987.

92. Ewing JA: Traveler's amnesia (letter). JAMA *259*:350, 1988.
93. Elliot WJ: Traveler's amnesia (letter). JAMA *259*:350–351, 1988.
94. DiMaio L: Traveler's amnesia (letter). JAMA *259*:351, 1988.
95. Radack HB: Traveler's amnesia (letter). JAMA *259*:351, 1988.
96. Greenblatt DJ, Shader RI, Abernethy DR: Current status of benzodiazepines. N Engl J Med *309*:410–416, 1983.
97. Rao S, Sherbaniuk RW, Prasad K, et al: Cardiopulmonary effects of diazepam. Clin Pharmacol Ther *14*:182–189, 1973.
98. Hollister LE: Clinical Pharmacology of Psychotherapeutic Drugs. New York, Churchill Livingstone, 1978.
99. Greenblatt DJ, Shader RI, Koch-Weser J: Flurazepam hydrochloride. Clin Pharmacol Ther *17*:1, 1975.
100. Benowitz NI, Rosenburg J, Becker CE: Cardiopulmonary catastrophes in drug overdosed patients. Med Clin North Am *63*:267, 1979.
101. Ikram H, Rubin AP, Jewkes RF: Effect of diazepam on myocardial blood flow of patients with and without coronary artery disease. Br Heart J *35*:626–630, 1973.
102. Caruana RJ, Dilworth LR, Williford PM: Acute rhabdomyolysis associated with an overdose of lorazepam, perphenazine and amitriptyline. NC Med J *44*:18–19, 1983.
103. Stringer MD: Adult respiratory distress syndrome associated with flurazepam overdose (letter). J R Soc Med *78*:74–75, 1985.
104. Richman S, Harris RD: Acute pulmonary edema associated with librium use. Radiology *103*:57–58, 1972.
105. Reidenberg MM, Levy M, Warner H, et al: Relationship between diazepam dose, plasma level, age, and central nervous system depression. Clin Pharmacol Ther *23*:371–374, 1978.
106. Greenblatt DJ, Koch-Weser J: Adverse reactions to intravenous diazepam: A report from the Boston Collaborative Drug Surveillance Program. Am J Med Sci *266*:261–266, 1973.
107. Katz RL: Sedatives and tranquilizers. N Engl J Med *286*:757–760, 1972.
108. Benzodiazepine overdosage. Med Lett *18*:60, 1976.
109. Bank RL: Overdose of benzodiazepines (letter). JAMA *247*:304, 1982.
110. Jatlow P, Dobular K, Bailey D: Serum diazepam concentrations in overdose: Their significance. Am J Clin Pathol *72*:571–579, 1979.
111. Strong JM: Changing trends in drug overdose over a six year period. Milit Med *148*:17–20, 1984.
112. Prescott LF: Safety of benzodiazepines. *In* Costa E: The Benzodiazepines: From Molecular Biology to Clinical Practice. New York, Raven Press, 1983.
113. Ruff RL, Kutt H, Hafler D: Prolonged benzodiazepine coma. NY State Med J *81*:776–777, 1981.
114. Zileli MS, Teletar F, Deniz S, et al: Oxazepam intoxication simulating non-keto-acidotic diabetic coma (letter). JAMA *215*:1986, 1971.
115. Welch TR, Rumack BH, Hammond K: Clonazepam overdose resulting in cyclic coma. Clin Toxicol *10*:433–436, 1977.
116. Deleu D, Keyser J: Flunitrazepam intoxication simulating a structural brainstem lesion. J Neurol Neurosurg Psychiatry *50*:236–237, 1987.
117. Goldfrank LR, Bresnity EA: Sedative-hypnotics (the deep sleep). *In* Goldfrank LR (ed): Toxicologic Emergencies. East Norwalk, CT, Appleton-Century-Crofts, 1982.
118. Solomon K: Safety of oxazepam. NY State J Med *78*:91–92, 1978.
119. Allen-Divoll M, Greenblatt DJ, Lacasse Y: Pharmacokinetic study of lorazepam overdosage. Am J Psychiatr *137*:1414–1415, 1980.
120. McCormick SR, Nielsen J, Jatlow PI: Alprazolam overdose: Clinical findings and serum concentrations in two cases. J Clin Psychiatr *46*:247–248, 1985.
121. Martin CD, Chan SC: Distribution of temazepam in body fluids and tissues in lethal overdose. J Anal Toxicol *10*:77–78, 1986.
122. Litovitz T: Fatal benzodiazepine toxicity (letter). Am J Emerg Med *5*:472–473, 1987.
123. Litovitz TL, Veltri JC: Annual report (1983) of the American association of poison control centers national data collection system. Am J Emerg Med *2*:420–443, 1983.
124. Veltri JC, Litovitz TL: Annual report (1984) of the American association of poison control centers national data collection system. Am J Emerg Med *3*:423–450, 1984.
125. Litovitz TL, Martin TG, Schmitz BF: Annual report (1986) of the American association of poison control centers national data collection system. Am J Emerg Med *5*:405–445, 1987.
126. Sellers EM, Busto U: Benzodiazepines and ethanol: Assessment of the effects and consequences of psychotropic drug interactions. J Clin Pharmacol *22*:249–262, 1982.
127. Goethe JW, Edelman SL: Chlordiazepoxide toxicity in limbitrol overdose. Am J Psychiatr *142*:774, 1985.
128. Forrest ARW, Marsh I, Bradshaw C, et al: Fatal temazepam overdoses (letter). Lancet *2*:226, 1986.
129. King LA: Synergistic effect of benzodiazepines in fatal amitriptyline poisonings (letter). Lancet *2*:982–983, 1982.
130. Hiss J, Hepler BR, Falkowski AJ, et al: Fatal bradycardia after intentional overdose of cimetidine and diazepam. Lancet *2*:982, 1982.
131. Lader M, Pettursson H: Rational use of anxiolytic/sedative drugs. Drugs *25*:514–528, 1983.
132. Bailey DN: Blood concentrations and clinical findings following overdose of chlordiazepoxide alone and chlordiazepoxide plus ethanol. Clin Toxicol *22*:433–446, 1984.
133. Divoll M, Greenblatt DJ, Lacasse Y, et al: Benzodiazepine overdosage: Plasma concentration and clinical outcome. Psychopharmacology *73*:381–383, 1981.
134. Kellermann AL, Fihn SD, LoGerto JP, et al: Impact of drug screening in suspected overdose. Ann Emerg Med *16*:1206–1216, 1987.
135. Package insert, EMIT · Urine Immunoassay. Sylva Company, Palo Alto, CA, August 1985.
136. Weddington WW, Carney AC: Alprazolam abuse during methadone maintenance therapy (letter). JAMA *257*:3363, 1987.
137. Fraser AD: Urinary screening for alprazolam, triazolam and their metabolites with the EMIT(R) d.a.u.(TM) benzodiazepine metabolite assay. J Anal Toxicol *11*:263–266, 1987.
138. Package insert, Abuscreen—Radioimmunoassay for benzodiazepines. Roche Diagnostic Systems, Nutley, NJ, July 1987.

139. Kanto J, Erkkola R, Sellman R: Accumulation of diazepam and *N*-desmethyldiazepam in the fetal blood during labor. Am Clin Res *5*:375–379, 1973.
140. Saxen I: Associations between oral clefts and drugs taken during pregnancy. Int J Epidemiol *4*:37, 1975.
141. Safra MJ, Oakley GP: Valium: An oral cleft teratogen. Cleft Palate J *13*:198, 1976.
142. Rosenberg L, Mitchell AA, Parsels JL, et al: Lack of relation of oral clefts to diazepam use during pregnancy. N Engl J Med *309*:1281, 1983.
143. Cree JE: Diazepam in labour: Its metabolism and effect on the clinical condition and thermogenesis of the newborn. Br Med J *4*:251, 1973.
144. Spreight ANP: Floppy-infant syndrome and maternal diazepam and/or nitrazepam. Lancet 2:878, 1977.
145. Whitelaw AGL, Cummings AJ, McFadyen IR: Effect of maternal lorazepam on the neonate. Br Med J *282*:1106–1108, 1981.
146. Drury KAD: Floppy-infant syndrome: Is oxazepam the answer? Lancet *2*:1126, 1977.
147. Cole AP, Hailey DM: Diazepam and active metabolites in breast milk and their transfer to the neonate. Arch Dis Child *50*:741–742, 1975.
148. Kaplan SA: Pharmacokinetics of the benzodiazepines. *In* Priest RG, Vianna Filho U, Amrein R, Skreta M (eds): Benzodiazepines Today and Tomorrow. Lancaster, MTP Press, 1980.
149. Ashton H: Benzodiazepine withdrawal: An unfinished story. Br Med J *288*:1135–1140, 1984.
150. Owen RT, Tyler P: Benzodiazepine dependence: A review of the evidence. Drugs *25*:385–398, 1983.
151. Petursson H, Lader MH: Withdrawal from long-term benzodiazepine treatment. Br Med J *283*:643–645, 1981.
152. Busto U, Sellers EM, Naranjo CA: Withdrawal reaction after long-term therapeutic use of benzodiazepines. N Engl J Med *315*:854–859, 1986.
153. Power KG, Jeffom DWA, Simpson RJ, et al: Controlled study of withdrawal symptoms and rebound anxiety after six week course of diazepam for generalised anxiety. Br Med J *290*:1246–1248, 1985.
154. Rickels K: Benzodiazepines in the treatment of anxiety: The North American experience. *In* Costa E: The Benzodiazepines: From Molecular Biology to Clinical Practice. New York, Raven Press, 1983.
155. Murphy SM, Owen RT, Tyrer PJ: Withdrawal symptoms after six weeks' treatment with diazepam. Lancet 2:1389, 1984.
156. Tyrer P, Owen R, Dawling S: Gradual withdrawal of diazepam after long-term therapy. Lancet *1*:1402–1406, 1983.
157. Hallstrom C, Lader M: The incidence of benzodiazepine dependence in long-term users. J Psychiat Treat Eval *4*:293–296, 1982.
158. Higgitt AC, Lader MH, Fonagy P: Clinical management of benzodiazepine dependence. Br Med J *291*:688–690, 1985.
159. Tien AY, Gujavarty KS: Seizure following withdrawal from triazolam (letter). Am J Psychiatr *142*:1516–1517, 1985.
160. Jerkovich GS, Preskorn SH: Failure of buspirone to protect against lorazepam withdrawal symptoms (letter). JAMA *258*:204–205, 1987.
161. Noyes R, Clancy J, Coryell WH, et al: A withdrawal syndrome after abrupt discontinuation of alprazolam. Am J Psychiatr *142*:114–116, 1985.
162. Tyrer PJ: Benzodiazepines on trial. Br Med J *288*:1101–1102, 1984.
163. Drury WM: Benzodiazepines—a challenge to rational prescribing. J R Coll Gen Pract *35*:86–88, 1985.
164. Lader M, Petursson H: Long-term effects of benzodiazepines. Neuropharmacology *22*:527–533, 1983.
165. Breier A, Charney DS, Nelson JC: Seizures induced by abrupt discontinuation of alprazolam. Am J Psychiatr *141*:1606–1607, 1984.
166. Relkin R: Death following withdrawal of diazepam. NY State J Med *66*:1770–1772, 1966.
167. Vinogradov S, Reiss AL, Csernansky JG: Clonidine therapy in withdrawal from high dose alprazolam treatment (letter). Am J Psychiatr *143*:1188, 1986.
168. Keshavan MS, Crammer JL: Clonidine in benzodiazepine withdrawal. Lancet *1*:1325–1326, 1985.
169. Tyrer P, Rutherford D, Juggett A: Benzodiazepine withdrawal symptoms and propranolol. Lancet *1*:520–522, 1981.
170. Gauche WG: Propranolol for the treatment of diazepam withdrawal symptoms (letter). S Afr Med J *66*:870, 1984.
171. Smith DE, Wesson DR: Benzodiazepine dependency syndromes. *In* Smith DE, Wesson DR: The Benzodiazepines: Current Standards for Medical Practice. Lancaster, MTP Press, 1985.
172. Allen CJ, Gough KR: The effect of doxapram on heavy sedation produced by intravenous diazepam in a patient with tetanus. Br Med J *286*:1181–1182, 1983.
173. Bell EF: The use of naloxone in the treatment of diazepam poisoning. J Pediatr *87*:803–804, 1975.
174. Jordan C, Lehaue JR, Jones JG: Respiratory depression following diazepam: Reversal with high dose naloxone. Anesthesiology *53*:293–298, 1980.
175. Forster AF, Morel DM, Bachmann M, et al: Respiratory depressant effects of different doses of midazolam and lack of reversal with naloxone—a double-blind randomized study. Anesth Analg *62*:920–924, 1983.
176. Avant GR, Speeg KV, et al: Physostigmine reversal of diazepam-induced hypnosis: A study in human volunteers. Ann Intern Med *91*:53–55, 1979.
177. Nagy J, Decsi L: Physostigmine, a highly potent antidote for acute experimental diazepam intoxication. Neuropharmacology *17*:469–475, 1978.
178. Brashares ZA, Conley WR: Physostigmine in drug overdose. Ann Emerg Med *4*:46–48, 1975.
179. DiLiberti L, O'Brien ML, Turner T: The use of physostigmine as an antidote in accidental diazepam intoxication. J Pediatr *86*:106–107, 1975.
180. Scollo-Lavizzari G: First clinical investigation of the benzodiazepine antagonist Ro 15–1788 in comatose patients. Eur Neurol *22*:7–11, 1983.
181. McGonigal P, Schofield CN: Antagonists to the benzodiazepines. Br Dental J *157*:392–393, 1984.
182. Darragh A, Lambe R, Kenny M, et al: Ro 15–1788 antagonises the central effects of diazepam in man without altering diazepam bioavailability. Br J Clin Pharmacol *14*:677–682, 1982.
183. Darragh A, Lambe R, Scully M, et al: Investigation in man of the efficacy of a benzodiazepine antagonist, Ro 15–1788. Lancet *2*:8–10, 1981.
184. Laurian S, Gailard M, Le PK, et al: Effects of a benzodiazepine antagonist on the diazepam-induced electrical brain activity modifications. Neuropsychobiology *11*:55–58, 1984.
185. Hofer P, Scollo-Lavizzari G: Benzodiazepine antagonist Ro 15–1788 in self-poisoning: Diagnostic and

therapeutic use. Arch Intern Med *145*:663–664, 1985.
186. Lheureux P, Askenasi R: Benzodiazepine antagonist Ro 15–1788 in self-poisoning (letter). Arch Intern Med *146*:1241, 1986.
187. Geller E, Niv D, Silbiger A, et al: Ro 15–1788, a benzodiazepine antagonist, in the treatment of 34 intoxicated patients (abs). Anesthesiology *63*:A157, 1985.
188. Geller E, Niv D, Rudick V, et al: The use of Ro 15–1788, a benzodiazepine antagonist, in the diagnosis and treatment of benzodiazepine overdose (abs). Anesthesiology *61S*:A135, 1984.
189. Cumin R, Bonetti EP, Scherschlicht R, et al: Use of the specific benzodiazepine antagonist, Ro 15–1788, in studies of physiological dependence on benzodiazepines. Experientia *38*:833–834, 1982.
190. Intravenous flumazenil (Ro 15–1788): Investigational drug brochure. Hoffmann-La Roche, Nutley NJ, March 1987.
191. Lukes SE, Griffiths RR: Precipitated withdrawal by a benzodiazepine receptor antagonist (Ro 15–1788) after 7 days of diazepam. Science *217*:1161–1163, 1982.
192. Amrein R, Leishman B, Bentzinger C, et al: Flumazenil in benzodiazepine antagonism: Actions and clinical use in intoxications and anaesthesiology. Med Toxicol *2*:411–429, 1987.
193. Ashton CH: Benzodiazepine overdose: Are specific antagonists useful? Br Med J *290*:805–806, 1985.
194. Mendelson WB, Cain M, Cook JM, et al: A benzodiazepine receptor antagonist decreases sleep and reverses the hypnotic actions of flurazepam. Science *219*:414–416, 1983.
195. Martinez-Aguirre E, Navarro T: Ro 15–1788, a highly specific benzodiazepine antagonist: Preliminary clinical experience. *In* Boulton TB (ed): Sixth European Congress of Anaesthesiology Abstracts. London, Academic Press, 1982.

CHAPTER 46

ANTIHISTAMINES AND OTHER SEDATIVES

Günter Seyffart, M.D.

A. Antihistamines

The histamine-blocking activity of various drugs, the so-called "antihistamines," was detected around 1940. Earlier some of these drugs were employed frequently for relief of "common cold"–like symptoms. Their effect in this kind of usage was and still is variable, and the effective mechanism is unknown.[1] Antihistamines are found in various classes of drugs, but not all drugs of a class possess histamine-antagonizing properties. Additionally, many of the antihistamines have other pharmacologic properties that are largely independent of antihistamine activity. Finally, none of the antihistamines block all the many effects of histamine.

Terminology

By occupying receptor sites in effector cells to the exclusion of histamine, antihistamines diminish or abolish the main physiologic actions of histamine but do not prevent the production and the existence of histamine. Two sets of receptors are considered to mediate the effects of histamine-terminal H_1 and H_2 receptors. In general, antihistamines are divided into two groups, H_1-receptor antagonists and H_2-receptor antagonists. H_1-antagonists include various drugs in the ethanolamine, ethylenediamine, alkylamine, piperazine, phenothiazine, and piperidine classes; the pyrrolidine clemastine and a few others belong to other classes (Table 46–1). H_2-antagonists include burimamide, cimetidine, metiamide, ranitidine, and famotidine.

The pharmacologic properties, as well as the adverse effects and major toxic manifestations of the antihistamines, are discussed here to enable understanding and treatment of toxic symptoms.

Table 46–1. ANTIHISTAMINES (TYPE H_1-RECEPTOR ANTAGONISTS) USED WORLDWIDE

ETHANOLAMINES	**PHENOTHIAZINES**
bromodiphenhydramine	alimemazine
carbinoxamine, racemic	chlorpromazine
carbinoxamine, D-form	dimethothiazine
dimenhydrinate	isothipendyl
diphenhydramine	mequitazine
doxylamine	methdilazine
phenyltoloxamine	oxomemazine
ETHYLENEDIAMINES	oxypendyl
antazoline	promethazine
chlorothen	pyrathiazine
chlorpyramine	trimeprazine
clemizole	**PIPERIDINES**
mepyramine	astemizole
methapyrilene	bamipine
pyrilamine	cyproheptadine
thenyldiamine	diphenylpyraline
thonzylamine	piprinhydrate
tripelennamine	pizotifen
ALKYLAMINES	terfenadine
brompheniramine, racemic	thenalidine
brompheniramine, D-form	**PYROLIDINE**
chlorpheniramine, racemic	clemastine
chlorpheniramine, D-form	**MISCELLANEOUS**
dimethindene	azatidine
pheniramine	benztropine
pyrrobutamine	chlortropbenzyl
triprolidine	histapyrrodine
PIPERAZINES (CYCLINES)	mebhydrolin
buclizine	meclastine
chlorcyclizine	medrylamine (topical)
cinnarizine	phenindamine
cyclizine	tolpropamine (topical)
hydroxyzine	trimethobenzamide
meclizine	tritoqualine
oxatomide	

Pharmacologic and Toxicologic Properties of H_1-Antagonists

Immediate hypersensitivity reactions to allergens, such as (foreign) proteins and chemical substances, are predominantly the result of histamine release, causing hay fever, allergic asthma, urticaria, contact dermatitis, and other allergic or anaphylactic conditions. By administering antihistamines, some phenomena, including edema formation and itching, are fairly well controlled. For example, antihistamines inhibit histamine-induced capillary permeability and formation of edema and wheals. However, topical as well as enteral and parenteral administration of antihistamines occasionally may cause allergic reactions, such as skin sensitization with eczematous eruptions and blood disorders, including agranulocytosis, hemolytic anemia, and thrombocytopenia.

One of the most important properties of the H_1-antagonists, besides prevention of allergic reactions, is their influence on the central nervous system. The drugs produce depression and stimulation, but the mechanisms by which various antihistamines accomplish these effects is largely unknown. Moreover, the action on the central nervous system varies with different antihistamines and may reflect antagonism of endogenous histamine released by central histaminergic neurons.

The most common effect is central nervous system depression. This is common to all antihistamines in therapeutic dose or overdosage, and ranges from sedation, varying from slight drowsiness to deep sleep and coma, to inability to concentrate, lassitude, dizziness, and ataxia. These manifestations are more prominent with various ethanolamines and phenothiazines and are less pronounced with alkylamines and piperazines (Table 46–1). Hypotension and muscle weakness may be due to central nervous depression but may also be influenced by inhibition of contraction of the smooth muscles (discussed later).

Stimulation of the central nervous system (CNS) is occasionally encountered in patients after administration of conventional doses of antihistamines. Manifestations are restlessness, nervousness, insomnia, tachycardia, muscle itching, and tremors.[2] CNS stimulation after ingestion of large doses or after overdose, common to all H_1-antagonists, may be exhibited by excitement, hallucinations, toxic psychosis, delirium, tremors, and convulsions. Convulsions often occur after a very short latent period and may be followed by postictal depression, terminating in respiratory failure or cardiovascular shock.

H_1-antagonists inhibit most smooth muscle responses to histamine, mainly the contraction of smooth muscle, including constriction of respiratory smooth muscle, vasoconstriction of the vascular tree, and, to a certain degree, the more important vasodilator effect. These actions cause muscle weakness, heaviness, difficulty in micturition, and predominantly systemic blood pressure variation in the form of hypotension.[3]

Some H_1-antagonists in therapeutic doses or overdose are involved in the dysfunction of the gastrointestinal tract. Common side effects include loss of appetite, nausea, epigastric distress and pain, constipation, and diarrhea, but no vomiting.

By antagonizing the effect of histamine on nerve endings, some antihistamines have local anesthetic properties. H_1-antagonists variably suppress histamine-evoked salivary, lacrimal, and other secretions. They also have atropine-like properties that reduce the secretion of cholinergically innervated glands. Both effects may result in dryness of the mouth and the respiratory tree, fixed pupils, flushed face, and fever.

H_1-antagonists also act by suppressing the vestibular end-organ receptors through inhibiting activation of the central cholinergic pathways and through suppressing vestibular pathways. Because of these actions, they are used in the treatment of motion sickness, vertigo, and vomiting. H_1-antagonists also exhibit adrenaline-enhancing, adrenaline-antagonizing, and/or serotonin-antagonizing effects.

Absorption, Fate, and Excretion

H_1-antagonists are administered topically, orally, and by deep intramuscular or slow intravenous injection. Given orally, these antihistamines in general are readily absorbed from the gastrointestinal tract, converted in the liver to more or less active or, finally, inactive metabolites, and excreted mainly in the urine, predominantly as metabolites. Little of the drug is found in feces. The duration of action varies but is in the range of 4 to 6 hours for most of the agents.

Acute Poisoning

H_1-antihistamines are rarely ingested in overdosage for suicide purposes, probably because of their low toxicity.[4] However, antihistamines with pronounced central nervous system depression effects are often sold as sedatives, unfortunately, alone or combined with sedatives sui generis or even combined with antitussives (diphenhydramine, methapyrilene). Accordingly, physicians treating patients intoxicated with sedatives often have to deal not only with those but also with antihistamines and anticholinergics. This calls for close attention and experience. Because antihistamines often are used uncritically and are available in large amounts and not well protected in households, accidental intoxications in children are common. For small children, one or two tablets may be dangerous; fatalities have been observed after ingestion of two to five tablets.[4]

In children, symptoms of central nervous *stimulation* are prominent. Excitement is often the first evidence of poisoning, followed by hallucinations, tremors, anxiety, insomnia, toxic psychosis, and convulsions. Convulsions indicate a poor prognosis, because the convulsant dose lies near the lethal one. Careful but aggressive treatment measures, therefore, are indicated. In adults, symptoms of central nervous *depression* are prominent, and convulsions are the exception. However, initial sedation is often followed by central nervous hyperexcitability. In contrast, respiratory depression may follow convulsions.

Minor toxic symptoms and adverse reactions after chronic use or abuse have been discussed under pharmacologic and toxicologic properties (see foregoing).

In summary, symptoms of severe intoxication with antihistamines, which call for immediate and different treatments, are

1. Central nervous depression (dominant in adults)
2. Central nervous hyperexcitability (dominant in children)
3. Dangerous hyperpyrexia (dominant in children)
4. Gastrointestinal disturbances
5. In the terminal phase, severe central nervous depression with death from respiratory arrest and/or cardiovascular shock.

Treatment

Because of the relatively low toxicity of most antihistamines, mild and moderate poisonings, in general, do not need intensive treatment but need careful clinical management. Most symptoms, if any, disappear within a few hours, because antihistamines are rapidly converted to less active or inactive metabolites. This may not be the case, however, in elderly patients and those with hepatic and renal disease. Severe poisonings in adults and all intoxications in children call for immediate and different therapy.

In all cases, immediate gastric lavage should be initiated, followed by instillation of activated charcoal to avoid further absorption. Induced vomiting should not be attempted, since most antihistamines have antiemetic properties, and emesis is severely repressed.

Forced diuresis is of little value since antihistamines are rapidly metabolized, and only small amounts of unchanged drug are recovered in the urine.

The patient should be placed in a quiet, dark room if excited and stimulated. In a state of central nervous stimulation, central nervous depressants (short-acting barbiturates and diazepam) should be used with caution to avoid hastening or deepening postconvulsive respiratory depression. Analeptics are inadvisable in the early phases because of the danger of precipitating convulsions.

In respiratory depression or failure, central nervous or respiratory stimulants that may cause convulsions should be avoided. In respiratory failure, especially in the postconvulsive state, artificial respiration and oxygen are required.

Blood pressure should be maintained but not by administration of epinephrine (adrenaline), since it may paradoxically enhance any hypotensive effect. Levarterenol, dopamine, or phenylephrine may be used. If signs of cerebral edema are present as evidence of high cerebrospinal fluid pressure, measures to decompress the brain may be worthwhile.

In hyperthermia, cold water packs or other measures should be considered, including cooling of the central compartment through peritoneal dialysis. Probably salicylates should be avoided here. Extracorporeal detoxification methods may be used if severe intoxications cannot be controlled over a longer period. Exchange transfusions have been used with varying effects[5, 6] and may not be practical in the short term. Peritoneal dialysis is not effective (low clearance). Hemodialysis has been used in diphenhydramine intoxications, but the drug could not be detected in the dialysate.[7] Hemodialysis probably has little effect because most antihistamines have high plasma protein-binding and a relatively large volume of distribution. In vitro experiments have shown that hemoperfusion through activated charcoal or resins allows complete elimination of antihistamines; however, the efficacy of in vivo hemoperfusion is limited by the relatively high volume of distribution. Hemodialysis also may be useful and necessary in case of antihistamine rhabdomyolysis and subsequent acute renal failure.[8] The use of an antidote, physostigmine, has been reported, but its value has not been established, and it is not a true antidote.

In no instance does histamine have any place in the treatment of antihistamine poisonings.

Pharmacologic and Toxicologic Properties of H_2-Antagonists

In 1972, a new and chemically distinct class of drugs was described, which selectively blocked the stimulant effect of histamine on gastric acid secretion.[9, 10] Because these agents suppressed histamine activities that were refractory to the older antihistamines, the existence of a second population of histamine receptors, H_2-receptors, was established, and a new major class of antihistamines arose.[11] These antihistamines are reversible, competitive antagonists of the action on H_2-receptors, but are virtually without any effect on H_1-receptors. Even though H_2-receptors are widely distributed throughout the body, H_2-antagonists interfere remarkably little with physiologic functions other than gastric acid secretion, which led to the hypothesis that extragastric H_2-receptors are of minor physiologic importance.

H_2-receptor antagonists inhibit gastric acid secretion elicited by histamine or other H_2-agonists, as well as gastric secretion elicited by muscarine agonists or gastrin. They have become an important group of drugs in modern medicine for the effective and safe treatment of gastrointestinal diseases such as gastric and duodenal ulcers, Zollinger-Ellison syndrome, reflux esophagitis, stress ulcer, upper gastrointestinal bleeding, and others. To date, the main H_2-antagonists are cimetidine and ranitidine. Data from these two drugs only are examined here.

The list of adverse reactions that have been reported is long. However, in comparison and in contrast to the H_1-antagonists, it is evident that the incidence of adverse reactions is low and that reactions encountered are generally minor. This is partly due to the relative absence of physiologically important H_2-receptors in organs other than the stomach, but also partly due to poor penetration of such drugs across the normal blood-brain barrier. Moreover, some side effects are directly attributable to specific H_2-receptors, since some side effects of cimetidine have not been observed with ranitidine. Some of the adverse and toxic effects of cimetidine and ranitidine can be explained and understood from their pharmacology, as has been demonstrated for those of the H_1-antagonists. Side effects of both agents that are hard to explain are headache, dizziness, malaise, myalgia, nausea, vomiting, diarrhea, and constipation.

Cimetidine decreases libido and causes impotence, since the drug is bound to androgen receptors and contributes to sexual dysfunction and to gynecomastia. Ranitidine, in contrast, lacks antiandrogenic activity and, when it is substituted for cimetidine, gynecomastia and sexual dysfunction may disappear.[12]

Cimetidine binds to cytochrome P-450 and thus diminishes the activity of the hepatic microsomal mixed-function oxidase. Because of this action, other drugs may accumulate owing to inhibition of their metabolism when given concurrently. This is important for warfarin, phenytoin, theophylline, phenobarbital, diazepam and other benzodiazepines, propranolol, and imipramine.[13] Ranitidine, in contrast, seems not to interfere with liver function; therefore, significant drug interactions are unknown.

Cimetidine can cause various central nervous system disorders, especially in elderly patients and those with hepatic and renal disease.[14] As mentioned, these symptoms are not fully understood but may be enhanced by diminished metabolism and renal clearance of the drug (accumulation). The effects include somnolence, lethargy, restlessness, confusion, disorientation, agitation, hallucinations, and seizures. Such reactions are less common or prominent with ranitidine, possibly because this drug has much less ability to pass the blood-brain barrier. Cimetidine administration is rarely associated with hematologic disturbances and hepatic and renal toxicity. Slightly elevated serum creatinine levels may reflect competition between cimetidine and creatinine for renal excretion. However, severe renal damage has been reported anecdotally.[15] Whether or not cimetidine is nephrotoxic is still unclear and controversial. In several other observations with large overdoses of cimetidine, no renal disturbances have been reported.[15] Rapid intravenous injections of both cimetidine and ranitidine occasionally may produce profound bradycardia and cardiotoxic effects.

Absorption, Fate, and Excretion

Given orally, cimetidine and ranitidine are almost completely absorbed. Because of first-pass metabolism in the liver, the bioavailability is 50 to 60 per cent. Both drugs are little bound to plasma proteins (10 to 20 per cent). The duration of action of cimetidine is a few hours; that of ranitidine is 8 to 12 hours. Both drugs are mainly excreted in urine—cimetidine up to 90 per cent within 24 hours (50 to 75 per cent unchanged) and ranitidine up to 60 per cent within 24 hours (about 40 per cent unchanged). The apparent volume of distribution is quite large, in the range of 1.5 liters per kg of body weight, demonstrating that nearly all drug exists outside the intravascular space.

Acute Poisoning and Treatment

Suicide attempts, serious intoxications, and fatalities have not been reported with cimetidine and ranitidine. Available data regarding overdosage are limited.[15] Ingestion of 12 grams of cimetidine daily for 5 days produced no toxic signs, and after single doses of 12 to 20 grams, mild-to-moderate toxic manifestations have been observed.[15] As mentioned, symptoms of acute intoxication with both cimetidine and ranitidine are bradycardia and tachycardia; central nervous system disturbances, including confusion, delirium, drowsiness, slurred speech, flushing, and sweating; dermatologic lesions; endocrine abnormalities; gastrointestinal disorders; and liver dysfunction.

Treatment of overdose is symptomatic. Emesis should be induced, followed by gastric lavage and then activated charcoal. Insignificant transient liver enzyme elevation may occur which does not require discontinuation of the drug. Hypersensitivity reactions leading to severe liver dysfunction require immediate withdrawal of the drug. Impaired renal function following cimetidine may disappear on its discontinuation, but the condition also may require transient dialysis therapy. In ranitidine overdosage, impaired renal function has not been reported. Hemodialysis clearance has been determined for both drugs, ranging from 20 to 85 ml per min (removal in the range of 15 per cent of a dose during one treatment); removal through peritoneal dialysis is negligible (less than 2 per cent of a dose during one treatment);[16–19] but removal through hemoperfusion seems to be significant.[18] These measures are of doubtful value since the drugs possess large volumes of distribution. Moreover, both drugs are converted to less active or inactive metabolites, which are not worthwhile to remove.

In principle, antihistamine overdose does not persist for a long time. Toxic symptoms normally decline within a few hours or a day without residual disorders. Secondary complications, such as pneumonitis, toxic hepatitis, rhabdomyolysis and acute renal failure, are extremely rare and observed in late poisoning or inadequate treatment.

References

1. West S, Brandon B, Stolley P, Rumrill R: A review of antihistamines and the common cold. Pediatrics *56*:100, 1975.
2. Hestand HE, Teske DW: Diphenhydramine hydrochloride intoxication. J Pediatr *90*:1017, 1977.
3. Simpson FO: Combination antihypertensive therapy. Cardiovasc Clin *2*:38, 1970.
4. Würmli K: Vergiftungen mit Antihistaminica. Pharm Acta Helv *48*:200, 1973.
5. Diekmann L, Hosemann R, Dibbern HW: Pheniramin (Avil)-Intoxication bei einem Kleinkind. Arch Toxicol *29*:317, 1972.
6. Huxtable RF, Landwirth J: Diphenhydramine poisoning treated by exchange transfusions. Am J Dis Child *106*:496, 1963.
7. Caridis DT, McAndrew GM, Matheson NA: Haemodialysis in poisoning with methaqualone and diphenhydramine. Lancet *1*:51, 1967.
8. Koppel C, Ibe C, Tenczer J: Clinical symptomatology of diphenhydramine overdose: An evaluation of 136 cases in 1982 to 1985. Clin Toxicol *25*:53, 1987.
9. Black JW, Duncan WAM, Durant CJ, Ganellin CR, Parsons EM: Definition and antagonism of histamine H_2-receptors. Nature *236*:385, 1972.
10. Zeldis JB, Friedman LS, Isselbacher AJ: Ranitidine: A new H_2-receptor antagonist. N Engl J Med *309*:1368, 1983.
11. Ganellin CR, Parsons ME (eds): Pharmacology of Histamine Receptors. Bristol, England, Wright/PSG, 1982.
12. Jansen RT, Collen MJ, Pandol SJ, Allende HD, Raufman JP, Bissonette BM, Duncan WC, Durgan PL, Gillin JC, Gardner JD: Cimetidine-induced impotence and breast changes in patients with gastric hypersecretory states. N Engl J Med *308*:883, 1983.
13. Sedman AJ: Cimetidine—drug interactions. Am J Med *76*:109, 1984.
14. McMillan MA, Ambis D, Siegel JH: Cimetidine and mental confusion. N Engl J Med *298*:284, 1978.
15. Sawyer D, Conner CS, Scalley R: Cimetidine: Adverse reactions and acute toxicity. Am J Hosp Pharm *38*:188, 1981.
16. Garg DC, Baltodano N, Perez GO, Oster JR, Jallad NS, Weidler DJ: Pharmacokinetics of ranitidine after intravenous administration in hemodialysis patients. Pharmacology *31*:189, 1985.
17. McGonigle RJS, Williams LC, Amphlett GE, England RJ, Parsons V: The pharmacokinetics of ranitidine in renal disease. *In* Misiewicz G, Wormsley K (eds): The Clinical Use of Ranitidine. Oxford, Medicine Publ Foundation, Series 5. 1982, p 41.
18. Pizella KM, Moore MC, Schultz RW, Walshe J, Schentag JJ: Removal of cimetidine by peritoneal dialysis, hemodialysis, and charcoal hemoperfusion. Ther Drug Monitor *2*:273, 1980.
19. Sica DA, Comstock T, Harford A, Eshelman F: Ranitidine pharmacokinetics in continuous ambulatory peritoneal dialysis. Eur J Clin Pharmacol *32*:587, 1987.

B. Ethchlorvynol

Ethchlorvynol (β-chlorovinyl ethyl ethynyl carbinol, 1-chloro-3-ethylpent-1-4-yn-3-ol) is a chlorinated acetylenic carbinol that was introduced in 1955 under the trade name of Placidyl.[1] In some respects it may be considered to be a condensation product of chloral hydrate, and clinically it is a useful sedative-hypnotic agent that also possesses anticonvulsant and muscle relaxant properties. With a rapid onset and a short duration of action, it has competed with barbituric acid derivatives as a sleep-inducing agent. It does not induce microsomal liver enzymes, and impaired liver function does not influence its metabolism. The physiologic and biochemical mechanisms responsible for its effects have not yet been elicited.

Pharmacology and Pharmacokinetics

Despite several investigations,[2–12] the characteristics and biochemical pathways of ethchlorvynol elimination have not yet been fully defined. Ethchlorvynol (C_7H_9ClO, molecular weight = 144.6 daltons) ingested in a therapeutic dose is rapidly and completely absorbed from the gastrointestinal tract. Its activity becomes manifest within 15 to 30 minutes, and maximal blood concentrations are attained within 60 to 90 minutes, when absorption ceases. In therapeutic doses, little or none can be detected in blood 3 to 6 hours after ingestion. Ethchlorvynol is rapidly and completely distributed to body tissues, particularly to adipose tissues where it is stored for a prolonged time.[7, 8]

Because of its fat solubility, it concentrates in the brain at higher levels than in serum,[10, 13] although cerebrospinal fluid concentrations are found to be only 50 per cent of that of the serum.[2, 10, 14]

Ethchlorvynol exhibits biphasic pharmacokinetics; after an initial high serum concentration following absorption, ethchlorvynol disappears rapidly from blood, to be followed by an increase in blood level at around 7 to 14 hours. The observed serum elimination half-time after therapeutic doses is 10 to 25 hours,[4] and after overdosage varies from 21 to 105 hours.[4, 11] Ingestion of greater than 15 gm has been associated with 102 to 288 hours of duration of coma.[11] In view of its high affinity to lipid-containing tissues, there is some evidence that the rate of elimination is dose dependent.

After therapeutic doses, the duration of action is 4 to 6 hours and the blood:plasma ratio varies between 0.9[38] and 2.[15] Metabolism in liver originally was assumed to be negligible,[9] but this has been somewhat disproved since it was later found that ethchlorvynol is readily metabolized in liver.[3, 4, 8] Although metabolites have not yet been identified, it would appear that glucuronide conjugation occurs as well as hydroxylation with reduction of unsaturated bonds in the chemical structure. Little unchanged drug is excreted, and approximately 90 per cent of the drug will undergo biotransformation, probably in the liver, since ethchlorvynol is concentrated in bile to three times as much as in serum.[6]

Plasma protein binding in man is not fully known, but has been demonstrated in dogs.[16] Excretion of unchanged ethchlorvynol is accomplished first through the kidneys, second through the feces, and possibly also through the lungs, since ethchlorvynol is volatile and a peculiar odor of the breath is noticed in patients with ethchlorvynol intoxication. It has not been proven whether ethchlorvynol or one of its metabolites is responsible for the odor. The effectiveness of renal excretion is doubted by some investigators since there are variable reports in the literature.[4, 12, 13, 17] A value of 10 per cent of an ingested dose excreted in the urine within 24 hours has been reported,[12, 18] whereas Schultz and associates have reported 27 per cent of an ingested dose being excreted within 3 days in the urine.[10] Cummings and associates found that only 0.025 per cent of an ingested dose was excreted in the unchanged form or as glucuronide in the urine.[4] In addition, renal ethchlorvynol clearances have been found to vary widely in different studies. Renal ethchlorvynol excretion varies from 1.9 ml/min (1.0 to 4.0 ml/min) with urine volumes greater than 500 ml/hr,[13] and other values such as 6.4 ml/min,[18] 8.5 ml/min,[9] and 23 ml/min[11] have been reported. The different values reported for renal ethchlorvynol clearance probably reflect several factors: different analytic techniques were used to determine ethchlorvynol;[2, 4, 12, 19] the writers do not report whether forced diuresis or spontaneous renal excretion was occurring;[10, 18] and the highest value for renal clearance of 23 ml/min was in a patient with a urine volume of 500 ml/hr.[20] In addition, it is not clear whether renal clearance depends upon high blood levels.

Action and Use

Ethchlorvynol is a central nervous system depressant, similar in action to the barbiturates. Although the drug is said to produce less initial excitement than do the barbiturates, clinical confirmation is required. The electroencephalogram (EEG) pattern following ethchlorvynol resembles that seen after barbiturates. In two patients who were given ethchlorvynol for 2 weeks, there was decreased sleep latency and wake time, and rapid eye movement sleep. Decreased stage 4 sleep and increased stage 2 sleep with an increase in total sleep time also occurred.[21] On withdrawal of ethchlorvynol, there was a return of normal sleep latency, rapid eye movement wake time, and time spent in stage 2 sleep, but not in rapid eye movement sleep or in stage 4 sleep.

Ethchlorvynol usually takes effect within 15 to 30 minutes after ingestion, and its hypnotic action lasts for about 5 hours. It is used for the treatment of simple insomnia in patients without pain, and, if ingested along with ethanol, an exaggerated hypnotic effect can be seen. The usual hypnotic dose is 500 mg (range: 250 mg to 1 gm), and, as a sedative, the usual dose is 100 to 250 mg two or three times daily. A dose of 770 mg is approximately equivalent to 100 mg of secobarbital.[4] The transient dizziness and the ataxia occasionally observed with ethchlorvynol may be reduced by concomitant ingestion with milk, which slows its absorption and partitions ethchlorvynol in fat. Ethchlorvynol can be administered without reduction of dose to patients with impaired liver function and chronic renal disease; however, its continued use in patients with impaired renal function may necessitate a reduction in dosage since it accumulates in plasma to cause prolonged drowsiness,[5] although serum ethchlorvynol concentrations are altered by hemodialysis. Ethchlorvynol is contraindicated in patients with porphyria and has been reported to decrease the effects of coumarin and other anticoagulants.

Overdosage

A variable clinical response to ethchlorvynol in overdosage has been observed. The lethal dose and lethal serum levels have not been adequately determined. After ingestion of 50 gm and following early gastric lavage, a patient survived; others with ingestions of 25 gm, 30 gm, and 45 gm also survived.[11] Coma lasting 6 days was observed in a patient who ingested 25 gm,[2] and one patient survived after a 14-hr hemodialysis that removed 14 gm of ethchlorvynol after ingestion of 100 to 125 gm.[22] Fatalities have been reported after an ingestion of 10 gm (156 mg/kg),[19] 27 gm, and 49.5 gm.[11] Known lethal serum levels have been reported at 13.0 mg/dl, 14.0 mg/dl, and 14.8 mg/dl,[19] which are approximately ten times the concentrations reached after therapeutic doses of 1 gm. It must be pointed out that patients have survived following serum levels of 13.5 mg/dl, 16.6 mg/dl, and 21.6 mg/dl.[11] *Prolonged coma is the hallmark of Placidyl overdose.*

Addiction and withdrawal symptoms have been seen with ethchlorvynol. Prolonged use of ethchlorvynol leads to dependence of the barbiturate-alcohol type, and abusers may ingest up to 4 gm daily. They usually show only mild signs of intoxication, and chronic abuse gives rise to drug tolerance. Withdrawal of ethchlorvynol in chronic abusers produces convulsions, hypertonicity, hyperreflexia, and a syndrome resembling delirium tremens and also suggestive of a schizophrenic reaction. In elderly patients, such symptoms can be especially severe. Toxic effects of ethchlorvynol include an unpleasant aftertaste, dizziness, and gastric discomfort with nausea and vomiting. In addition, reductions of blood pressure may be observed. Skin rashes, blurred vision, facial numbness, drowsiness, fatigue, headache, mental confusion, ataxia, grand mal seizures, and peripheral neuropathy have been observed.

Severe acute intoxication is characterized principally by deep coma (with up to 288 hours having been reported), severe respiratory depression, hypotension, bradycardia, hypothermia, and pulmonary edema.[23] In 13 of 19 intoxicated patients, coma lasted an average of 102 hours,[11] which is considerably longer than the average of 40 hours with barbiturate intoxication,[14] and 48 hours with glutethimide intoxication.[20] A patient was described with anuria and renal failure,[17] who on autopsy had a 40 per cent higher ethchlorvynol concentration in renal tissues than in other body tissues.[19] Despite this case report, there is still no good evidence that ethchlorvynol is nephrotoxic. A preliminary report on the effects of gestational exposure to ethchlorvynol is available,[24] and another group has reported that cutaneous bullous eruptions have occurred with ethchlorvynol.[25]

Ethchlorvynol activity may be enhanced by alcohol or barbiturates. In alcoholics, a dose of 0.5 to 1.0 gm is sufficient to cause blood pressure reduction and coma for many hours.[26] The suggestion has been made that alcoholics are particularly sensitive to intoxication, even with therapeutic doses, on the basis that the drug is concentrated three times more in liver (bile) than in serum.[6]

Treatment of Ethchlorvynol Intoxication

Gastric lavage is the first line of treatment and is particularly useful shortly after ingestion of ethchlorvynol. It also may be of value some time later, since it has been demonstrated that substantial amounts of ethchlorvynol have been removed by lavage as late as 5 hours after ingestion.

General management is similar to that for barbiturate intoxication, with attention being paid to monitoring respiration, pulse rate, and blood pressure. It must be stressed that barbiturates should be avoided and that hypotension requiring pressor and intravenous fluid therapy may appear.

Forced diuresis has been used in the past for ethchlorvynol intoxication,[10, 11] but, as noted, unchanged ethchlorvynol is excreted in the urine in very small quantities and accordingly will not respond to either forced diuresis or alkalinization. For these reasons, forced diuresis is not recommended.

In severely intoxicated patients, ethchlorvynol can be actively removed using extracorporeal detoxification procedures.

Hemodialysis has been used in the past with variable clinical results.[6, 11, 13, 16, 18, 22, 27–29] Ethchlorvynol is relatively well dialyzable, despite early reports that showed hemodialytic removal of ethchlorvynol was negligible,[6] probably due to minimal plasma levels at the time of determination. Several investigators have demonstrated substantial reductions in plasma ethchlorvynol levels using hemodialysis; the plasma level fell from 21.6 mg/dl to 9.05 mg/dl after a 10-hr hemodialysis with removal of 5.5 gm of an ingested 15- to 25-gm dose[18] and removal of 2.45 gm of an ingested 11 gm during a 14-hr hemodialysis.[13] In some reports, however, the investigators have commented that the coma has been prolonged despite dialytic removal of substantial amounts of drug, with coma lasting 52 to 288 hrs.[11, 13, 22] In other reports, the serum half-life of ethchlorvynol was reduced from 70 hours to an average of 22 hours (range: 10 to 54 hours), with dialysance values for ethchlorvynol averaging 50 ml/min (range: 40 to 80 ml/min). As for other lipophilic substances such as camphor and glutethimide, *lipid hemodialysis* has been employed for ethchlorvynol detoxification. Despite effective removal of drug, the clinical picture did not, however, improve.[16, 30] Lipid hemodialysis in modern times has been superseded by hemoperfusion.

The effect of hemodialysis on duration of coma in ethchlorvynol intoxication appears to be minimal. However, in most severe and potentially fatal intoxications treated with hemodialysis, only one patient has succumbed.[11]

Peritoneal dialysis has also been used for the treatment of ethchlorvynol intoxication but appears to be of low efficiency, with dialysance values of around 20 ml/min.[10–12, 31, 32]

For severely intoxicated patients, *sorbent hemoperfusion* for drug removal appears to be superior to all other techniques. *Charcoal hemoperfusion* has been used with some success, with ethchlorvynol clearances of 110 to 170 ml/min being reported and up to 30 per cent of an ingested dose being removed.[29, 33–37] Clinical response has been excellent, and patients, even in stage 4 coma, have awakened after hemoperfusion.[29, 34, 35] *Resin hemoperfusion* appears to give the most favorable results. Amberlite XAD-4, an uncharged exchange resin, has been used with some success in severe ethchlorvynol poisoning.[1, 33, 36, 38–42] Approximately 100 per cent of ethchlorvynol in plasma is removed on passage through the resin cartridge, with reported clearances of 184 ml/min at blood flow rates of 200 ml/min being reported.[1, 38] It also has been demonstrated that ethchlorvynol is removed not only from plasma but also from red blood cells, often at a rate faster than the liver can detoxify ethchlorvynol. It must be pointed out that release of ethchlorvynol from tissues and rebound in plasma levels have been demonstrated and contribute to the duration of coma. Since the pharmacokinetic handling of ethchlorvynol exhibits a biphasic pattern, the quantities of ethchlorvynol removed during hemoperfusion decrease because of less availability of drug in plasma and complications of prolonged coma that still occur.[1, 33, 38] Rebound of plasma ethchlorvynol levels occurs 4 to 8 hours following cessation of hemoperfusion, and it has been suggested that prolonged or repeated hemoperfusion (every 6 to 12 hours) should be employed. Indications for hemoperfusion or hemodialysis in severe ethchlorvynol intoxication are

(1) ingestion of a potentially fatal dose (greater than 10 gm);

(2) ingestion of greater than 100 mg/kg/body weight;

(3) serum levels greater than 10 mg/dl in the first 12 hours, or greater than 7 mg/dl at a later time; and

(4) prolonged coma with life-threatening complications despite intensive supportive therapy.

References

1. Lynn RI, Honig CL, Jatlow PI, Kliger AS: Resin hemoperfusion for treatment of ethchlorvynol overdose. Ann Intern Med *91*:549, 1979.
2. Andryanskas S, Matusiak W, Broich JR, et al: Ethchlorvynol in toxicologic analysis. Int Microfilm J Legal Med *2*:154, 1967.
3. Carr DJ, Crampton RF: Ethchlorvynol (correspondence). Br Med J *1*:262, 1963.
4. Cummings LM, Martin YC, Scherfling EE: Serum and urine levels of ethchlorvynol in man. J Pharm Sci *60*:261, 1971.
5. Dawborn JK, Turner A, Pattison G: Ethchlorvynol

as a sedative in patients with renal failure. Med J Aust *2*:702, 1972.
6. Maher JF, Schreiner GE: Editorial review: The clinical dialysis of poisons. Trans Am Soc Artif Intern Organs *9*:385, 1963.
7. Maynert EW: Sedatives and hypnotics. *In* DiPalma JV (ed): Drill's Pharmacology in Medicine. New York, McGraw-Hill, 1971, p 250.
8. American Medical Association: New and Nonofficial Drugs 1963. Philadelphia, J. B. Lippincott, 1963.
9. P'An SY, Kodet MJ, Gardocki JF, McLamore WM, Bavley A: Pharmacologic studies on the hypnotic and anticonvulsant actions of ethyl-beta-chlorovinyl ethynyl carbinol. J Pharmacol Exp Ther *114*:326, 1955.
10. Schultz JC, Crowder DG, Medart WS: Excretion studies in ethchlorvynol (Placidyl) intoxication. Arch Intern Med *117*:409, 1966.
11. Teehan BP, Maher JF, Carey JJH, Flynn PD, Schreiner GE: Acute ethchlorvynol (Placidyl®) intoxication. Ann Intern Med *72*:875, 1970.
12. Wallace JE, Wilson WJ, Dahl EV: A rapid and specific method for determining ethchlorvynol. J Forensic Sci *9*:342, 1964.
13. Westervelt FB: Ethchlorvynol (Placidyl®) intoxication: Experience with five patients, including treatment with hemodialysis. Ann Intern Med *64*:1229, 1966.
14. Setter JG, Maher JF, Schreiner GE: Barbiturate intoxication. Evaluation of therapy including dialysis in a large series selectively referred because of severity. Arch Intern Med *117*:224, 1966.
15. Hedley-Whyte J, Laasberg LH: Ethchlorvynol poisoning: Gas-liquid chromatography in management. Anesthesiology *30*:107, 1969.
16. Welch LT, Bower JD, Ott CE, Hume AS: Oil dialysis for ethchlorvynol intoxication. Clin Pharmacol Ther *13*:745, 1972.
17. Harenko A: One special trait of acute ethchlorvynol poisoning. Acta Neurol Scand *43* (Suppl 31):141, 1967.
18. Ogilvie RI, Douglas DE, Lochead JR, Moscovich MD, Kaye M: Ethchlorvynol (Placidyl) intoxication and its treatment by hemodialysis. Can Med Assoc J *95*:954, 1966.
19. Algeri EJ, Katsas GG, Luongo MA: Determination of ethchlorvynol in biologic mediums, and report of two fatal cases. Am J Clin Pathol *38*:125, 1962.
20. Maher JF, Schreiner GE, Westervelt FB: Acute glutethimide intoxication. I. Clinical experience (twenty-two patients) compared to acute barbiturate intoxication (sixty-three patients). Am J Med *33*:70, 1962.
21. Kripke DF, Lavie P, Hernandez J: Polygraphic evaluation of ethchlorvynol (14 days). Psychopharmacology *56*:221, 1978.
22. Klock JC: Ethchlorvynol poisoning (letter). Ann Intern Med *81*:131, 1974.
23. Glauser FL, Smith WR, Caldwell A: Ethchlorvynol (Placidyl®)-induced pulmonary edema. Ann Intern Med *84*:46, 1976.
24. Peters MA, Hudson PM: Preliminary report on the effects of totigestational exposure to ethchlorvynol. Environ Health Perspect *21*:85, 1977.
25. Brodin MB, Redmond WJ: Bullous eruption due to ethchlorvynol. J Cutan Pathol *7*:326, 1980.
26. Kuenssberg EV: Side effects of ethchlorvynol. Br Med J *2*:1610, 1962.
27. Bower JD, Hume AS: Use of artificial kidney in cases of poisoning. J Miss State Med Assoc *11*:639, 1970.
28. Gibson PF, Wright N: Ethchlorvynol in biological fluids: Specificity of assay methods. J Pharm Sci *61*:169, 1972.
29. Widdop B, Medd RK, Braithwaite RA, Rees AJ, Goulding R: Experimental drug intoxication. Treatment with charcoal haemoperfusion. Arch Toxikol *34*:27, 1975.
30. Hume A, Welch L, Bower J: Lipid dialysis in ethchlorvynol intoxication. Clin Res *18*:62, 1970.
31. Barry KG, Schwarz FD: Peritoneal dialysis. Current status and future applications. Pediatr Clin North Am *11*:593, 1964.
32. Hyde AG, Lawrence AG, Moles JB: Ethchlorvynol intoxication; successful treatment by exchange transfusion and peritoneal dialysis. Clin Pediatr *7*:739, 1968.
33. Dua SJ, Nagrawala J, Thompson R: Letter to the editor. Ann Intern Med *92*:436, 1980.
34. Ehlers S, Stern E, Zaske D, Kjellstrand C: Extracorporeal treatment of ethchlorvynol intoxication. Abstr Eur Dialysis Transpl Assoc *16*:41, 1979.
35. Gelfand MC, Winchester JF, Knepshield JH, Hanson KM, Cohan SL, Strauch BS, Geoly KL, Kennedy AC, Schreiner GE: Treatment of drug overdosage with charcoal hemoperfusion. Trans Am Soc Artif Intern Organs *23*:599, 1977.
36. Koffler A, Bernstein M, LaSette A, Massry S: Fixed-bed charcoal hemoperfusion. Treatment of drug overdose. Arch Intern Med *138*:1691, 1978.
37. Kolthammer J: The in vitro adsorption of drugs from horse serum onto carbon coated with an acrylic hydrogel. J Pharm Pharmacol *27*:801, 1975.
38. Benowitz N, Abolin C, Tozer T, Rosenberg J, Rogers W, Pond S, Schoenfeld P, Humphreys M: Resin hemoperfusion in ethchlorvynol overdose. Clin Pharmacol Ther *27*:236, 1980.
39. Kliger AS: Letter to the editor. Ann Intern Med *92*:436, 1980.
40. Rosenbaum JL, Winsten S, Kramer MS, Moros J, Raja R: Resin hemoperfusion in the treatment of drug intoxication. Trans Am Soc Artif Intern Organs *16*:134, 1970.
41. Rosenbaum JL, Kramer MS, Raja R, Boreyko C: Resin hemoperfusion: A new treatment for acute drug intoxication. N Engl J Med *284*:874, 1971.
42. Zmuda MJ: Resin hemoperfusion in dogs intoxicated with ethchlorvynol (Placidyl®). Kidney Int *17*:303, 1980.

C. Meprobamate and Carisoprodol

This section discusses poisoning with meprobamate and its related compound carisoprodol.

MEPROBAMATE (Miltown, Equanil, Milpath, Equagesic, Pathibamate)

Meprobamate (2-methyl-2n-propyl-propane-1,3-diol-dicarbamate) is a nonbarbiturate tranquilizer used in many psychiatric conditions requiring control of anxiety states. It was developed in 1946, being synthesized originally for possible use as a muscle relaxant, and it was subsequently found to be an important anticonvulsant and to exhibit a marked taming effect when administered to monkeys. The observed behavior in these animals suggests that they lost fear, hostility, and aggressiveness, without markedly impairing their appetite or interest in their surroundings.

Meprobamate was widely acclaimed on its introduction as a tranquilizer into clinical practice around 1954. Its popularity led to its use in a multitude of psychopathologic states, both alone and in combination with many other types of drugs, particularly along with drugs used in chronic and debilitating diseases. Meprobamate's wide availability on prescription to depressed and mentally disturbed patients invited its frequent use as an instrument of accidental poisoning or, more commonly, in attempted suicide. Shortly after its introduction, reports of self-poisoning with fatalities after ingestion of massive doses began to appear in the clinical literature.[1–5]

Pharmacology and Pharmacokinetics

Meprobamate ($C_9H_{18}N_2O_4$, with a molecular weight of 218.3 daltons) is rapidly absorbed from the gastrointestinal tract, with the highest blood concentrations occurring at 1 to 2 hours after ingestion. Meprobamate is eliminated from blood at the rate of 8.5 per cent/hr and, therefore, after therapeutic doses, more than 10 hours is required for blood concentrations to reach a very low level. It is widely distributed in body tissues. The elimination half-life of meprobamate is 8 to 12 hours,[6, 7] and plasma protein binding is approximately 15 per cent;[8] excretion is mainly renal (90 per cent), with less than 10 per cent appearing in the feces. Thirty minutes after ingestion, meprobamate is readily detectable in the urine. Urinary excretion in 24 hours consists of 10 to 11 per cent of unchanged meprobamate, with the rest appearing as glucuronide, a hydrolyzed metabolite, and oxidized derivatives.[8–11] Renal meprobamate clearance is 4 to 28 ml/min.[12]

Pharmacologic Actions and Use

Meprobamate was the first modern (safe and rapidly acting) tranquilizer—an innovative drug that is active centrally but lacks prominent effects on the autonomic nervous system such as those seen after other tranquilizers like reserpine and chlorpromazine. Meprobamate exerts a selective action on the thalamus and also appears to inhibit multineuronal spinal reflexes. It is mildly tranquilizing and has some anticonvulsant and muscle relaxant properties. For this reason it is used in the treatment of anxiety and tension, in which its activity appears to be less effective than that of the benzodiazepines. It is used also in petit mal epilepsy.

Standard doses of meprobamate consist of 0.6 to 1.2 gm daily, in divided doses for outpatient management, or up to 3 gm daily for inpatients under hospital observation. Since renal excretion of meprobamate is fairly substantial, dosage intervals should be increased from 6 hours in patients with normal renal function to 9 to 12 hours in those with renal failure. Similarly, the dosage should be adjusted in patients receiving hemodialysis or peritoneal dialysis to maintain a therapeutic blood concentration.

Contraindications

Because of some degree of drug interaction, an increased effect may be seen with ethanol, sedatives, analgesics, and psycho-

$$H_2N-\overset{O}{\overset{\|}{C}}-OCH_2-\underset{CH_3}{\underset{|}{\overset{C_3H_7}{\overset{|}{C}}}}-CH_2O-\overset{O}{\overset{\|}{C}}-NH_2$$

MEPROBAMATE

tropic drugs. An increased effect also may be seen in myasthenia gravis, ataxia, or acute intermittent porphyria. Meprobamate per se may induce convulsions in patients with a history of epilepsy.

Overdose

Meprobamate intoxication exhibits a variable but probably dose-related duration of coma. For instance, coma with intoxications of 36 to 38 gm is reversed after 18 hours;[13] with 38.4 gm, coma reversal occurred after 44 hours.[14] Intoxication with 14 to 16 gm of meprobamate was associated with coma reversal beginning after 24 hours with forced diuresis, while with 10 to 12 gm, coma reversal began after 10 hours with forced diuresis.[15] Poisoning with 8.4 gm of meprobamate was associated with coma reversal beginning after only 4 hours with forced diuresis.[15] Ehlers reported his experience with 363 patients with pure meprobamate intoxication in which 78 patients were in various stages of coma; coma duration ranged between 1 and 73 hours.[16]

Profound meprobamate intoxication correlates with plasma levels of 20 mg/dl or greater. Most patients enter coma with plasma levels of meprobamate above 10 mg/dl, whereas wakefulness occurs at levels below 5 mg/dl. For comparison, it is worthwhile bearing in mind that therapeutic blood levels are around 1 mg/dl.

The quantity of meprobamate needed to constitute a lethal dose is unknown, but a survey of the literature shows the following: Ehlers reported four deaths in patients who had ingested more than 40 gm of meprobamate, the causes of death being irreversible shock and pulmonary edema.[16] Powell and associates reported on 11 intoxications without fatal outcome, with ingested doses between 10 and 40 gm; however, 2 further cases were fatal from 12 gm (240 mg/kg) and 20 gm (350 mg/kg) and the patients being found dead at home.[4] Schou reported a death after the ingestion of 12 gm of meprobamate, with the death probably being due to overzealous therapy with fluid overload after fluid administration to treat hypotension.[17] Several investigators have observed that fatal intoxication is more common in patients with mixed drug intoxications, and that the death rate in pure meprobamate intoxication is fairly low, even with severe overdosage.[12, 18]

Addiction and Drug Withdrawal

Of all the nonbarbiturate tranquilizers, meprobamate is the most likely to produce euphoria even with therapeutic doses. A daily intake of 1.2 gm or more often may lead to physical dependence. In chronic abuse, symptoms of withdrawal occur 12 to 48 hours following cessation of meprobamate. Avoidance of this syndrome occurs with a gradual dose reduction over a period of 10 days. The syndrome of withdrawal manifests itself in anxiety, restlessness, confusion, and convulsions—all of which should suggest physical dependence caused by heavy drug consumption over a long period of time.

Toxicology

Drowsiness is the most frequent side effect of meprobamate. Other effects include stupor, nausea, vomiting, diarrhea, paresthesia, weakness, and respiratory depression. More central effects are headaches, excitement, ataxia, and disturbance of vision. Acute intoxication produces coma, convulsions, respiratory arrest, and hemodynamic disturbances (hypotensive shock)—the latter being through toxic effects on the myocardium. Arrhythmias, tachycardia, bradycardia, and reduced venous return through general venous dilatation may be observed.[19] The profound and persistent hypotension in human beings after large doses of meprobamate (10 to 40 gm) has been emphasized as an unexpected hazard by several investigators.[2, 5, 14, 15, 20–24] Such hypotension seems to be caused by the direct action of meprobamate on the vasomotor center.[15] In contrast to acute barbiturate intoxication, the fall in blood pressure can appear unexpectedly in mildly comatose patients.

Meprobamate also may be associated with excessive oronasal secretion or relaxation of the pharyngeal wall or both, which may present problems in terms of airway obstruction. Meprobamate does not seem to be nephrotoxic; however, sensitivity reactions even at low doses of the drug have been reported and include stomatitis, proctitis, pronounced anaphylactic reaction, fatal allergic shock, and fatal aplastic anemia—all of which should be considered adverse drug reactions.[25–31]

Treatment of Meprobamate Poisoning

Depending on the severity of the intoxication and the clinical condition of the patient, the physician should select one of the treatment modalities discussed next.

Gastric Lavage. Since meprobamate is rapidly absorbed from the gastrointestinal tract, gastric lavage (and induced vomiting in a conscious patient) may be of value only if carried out shortly after ingestion. However, note that the assumption may not be true that rapid absorption of meprobamate from the gastrointestinal tract occurs when gastric emptying is complete (within 4 hours after ingestion). Jenis and associates reported that a patient with a massive overdose had a favorable response to fluid therapy with return of complete consciousness, to be followed by sudden death; autopsy revealed that the stomach contained 25 gm of meprobamate in a conglomerate mass.[32] Schwartz encountered a similar patient, who ingested 36 gm of meprobamate but remained unconscious despite therapy, even with hemodialysis. Gastroscopy showed a large, gelatinous mass within the stomach, which did not appear to decrease in size on gastroscopy following hemodialysis. Gastrotomy performed 40 hours after admission revealed a tarry mass, which was removed from the stomach. It weighed 140 gm. Eight hours after removal and continued hemodialysis, the patient began to respond.[33]

The reason for development of such masses in the stomach after the ingestion of large amounts of meprobamate is not known. However, such observations are common in carbromal and bromisoval poisoning (see Chapter 46F). In addition, improvement in circulatory function by fluid administration may facilitate further absorption of meprobamate in lethal quantities.

In summary, with large ingested doses of meprobamate, gastric lavage should be continued for some hours. Additionally, gastroscopy is probably indicated and, if the suspected mass is observed, this should be broken through the endoscope and extracted or removed by gastrotomy. Using this method, Hoy and associates observed fragments of meprobamate pills in the gastric aspirate, but on gastroscopy there was no further drug-containing mass.[34] Figure 46–1 demonstrates an approach to removing masses of ingested drugs through the gastroscope and gastric lavage tube.

Management of Hypotension. The importance of frequent measurements of vital signs in meprobamate intoxication cannot be overemphasized. Hypotension may appear rapidly and become persistent unless expansion of blood volume is achieved. However, in view of the pathogenesis of hypotension in meprobamate poisoning, fluid overload should be avoided. Deaths from pulmonary edema have been reported, and administration of pressor agents to support arterial blood pressure may prove more effective than volume replacement. If there is any degree of respiratory embarrassment, then respiratory assistance may be required. The use of *caffeine, sodium benzoate,* and other analeptic drugs has been popular in the past for treatment of severe respiratory depression. In modern clinical toxicology, such measures are not encouraged, but the experimental evaluation of the use of doxapram hydrochloride (Dopram) is under way.

Barbiturates should be avoided or used sparingly for the treatment of epileptiform convulsions, because the combination of barbiturates and meprobamate may lead to intense central nervous system depression. Convulsions after symptomatic recovery usually indicate a withdrawal reaction, and in this case barbiturates are both useful and, in general, safe.

Dialysis. There is no known antidote for meprobamate. In serious intoxication, measures for drug removal in addition to those just outlined have been suggested. Forced diuresis may be of some value when maximal excretion of meprobamate—of about 20 to 30 per cent of the glomerular filtration rate—can be achieved. However, in the presence of hypotensive shock, forced diuresis may not be associated with prompt excretion of meprobamate. It is re-emphasized that pulmonary edema must be avoided.

Peritoneal dialysis,[4, 12, 35–40] giving a dialysance of 2.5 to 11 ml/min,[12, 37, 38] is accordingly equal to or less effective than forced diuresis and for this reason is probably only of value if other methods of drug removal are not available. Maddock and Bloomer calculated that, in a 70-kg man poisoned with 10 gm of meprobamate, with a serum level of 20 mg/dl 3 hours after ingestion, one could eliminate 300 mg/hr using forced diuresis, with 60 per cent of meprobamate being reabsorbed. With peritoneal dialysis, the rate would be 130 mg/hr, using dialysate exchanges every 60 min. With hemodialysis, 1200 mg/hr of meprobamate could be removed.[8]

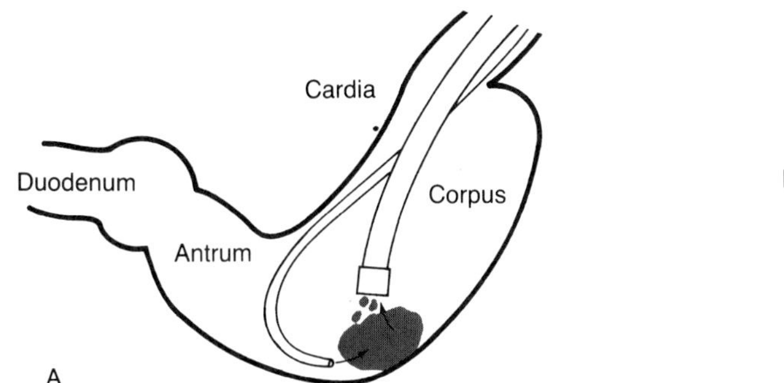

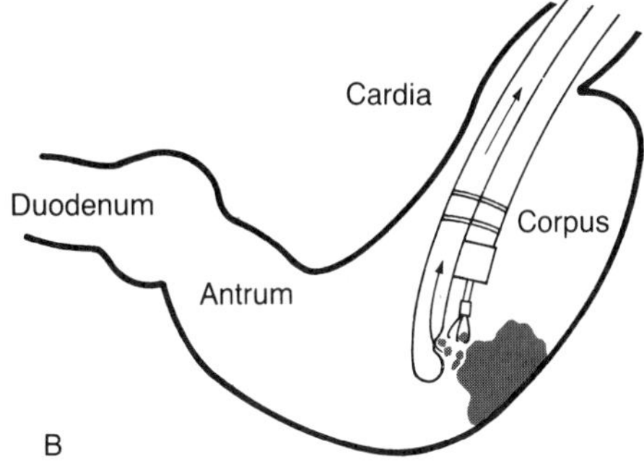

Figure 46–1. Drug conglomerate removal from the stomach by endoscopic gastric lavage. *A*, Removal of conglomerate with gastric tube and suction through the endoscope. *B*, Destroying the conglomerate with the endoscope and removal of fragments with the gastric tube.

Hemodialysis is effective in meprobamate poisoning.[8, 38, 41–45] Meprobamate is well dialyzable (it is only 15 per cent protein bound) with an approximate meprobamate dialysance or clearance of up to 100 ml/min. However, very few data are available about in vivo hemodialysis. In one patient, hemodialysis was performed for 24.5 hours after ingestion of 60 gm of meprobamate; the serum meprobamate fell from 23.6 mg/dl to 15.2 mg/dl, with a total of 5.7 gm being recovered in the dialysate. Dialysance was about 20 ml/min, since a dialyzer (Kiil) of low efficiency was used. Meprobamate dialysance using low efficiency dialyzers is equivalent to renal clearance; these results have been confirmed by Maher and associates[44] and Powell and associates.[4] With the technical advances in hemodialysis since 1960, increased elimination of meprobamate has been reported. Hagstam and colleagues[43] demonstrated reduction in serum meprobamate from 17 mg/dl to 10 mg/dl (41 per cent), while Maddock and Bloomer,[8] in a patient with a serum level greater than 20 mg/dl, observed a meprobamate removal of up to 1200 mg/hr, with meprobamate dialysance values of 100 ml/min.

Simon and Krumlovsky have suggested that hemodialysis is indicated since sometimes a dramatic and unpredictable onset of severe meprobamate intoxication occurs.[46] In the less severe cases, forced diuresis alone should be used.

If the condition of the patient deteriorates despite assisted respiration, forced diuresis, and pressor agents, then hemodialysis should be instituted. Remember that hemodialysis may be possible only if blood pressure allows the performance of hemodialysis, and the patient may require pressor agents to sustain such a blood pressure. In addition, hemodialysis should be considered if the patient has ingested more than 30 to 40 gm of meprobamate.

Hemoperfusion. Recently hemoperfusion has been used in the treatment of meprobamate poisoning and offers some advantages over hemodialysis.

Activated Charcoal Hemoperfusion. In vitro, adsorption of meprobamate to activated charcoal approximating 100 per cent can be demonstrated.[47] Similarly, with horse serum containing meprobamate, it has been found in vitro that both uncoated charcoal and biocompatible acrylic hydrogel-coated carbon adsorb considerable quantities of meprobamate; after 30 minutes, 30 per cent of the initial meprobamate dose remained in the serum, while after 1 hour, 9 per cent remained. After 3 hours, none remained.[48]

In subsequent animal experiments, Widdop and associates observed a plasma meprobamate clearance of 180 ml/min using acrylic hydrogel–coated hemoperfusion.[49] After 3 hours of hemoperfusion, the plasma level had fallen from 27.8 mg/dl to 10.4 mg/dl (a 62 per cent drop), with an estimated 2.7 gm (13 per cent) of the 20-gm ingested dose being eliminated by hemoperfusion.[49] Barbour and associates demonstrated in a patient with severe meprobamate intoxication, who was treated with uncoated charcoal hemoperfusion 14 hours after hospital admission, a dramatic response to hemoperfusion; the patient had areflexia and fixed pupils but spontaneously began to move and had spontaneous respirations 1 hour and 40 minutes after hemoperfusion began, and he subsequently survived.[50] With only a few publications on the use of activated charcoal hemoperfusion, the results appear to be substantially better than those obtained with hemodialysis.[11, 41, 50]

Resin Hemoperfusion. Hemoperfusion through neutral (unchanged) exchange resins is another effective and alternative method for meprobamate removal. Hoy and associates used resin hemoperfusion in one patient with severe meprobamate intoxication who had ingested 300 gm of meprobamate in addition to other drugs.[34] Although the patient had respiratory arrest and a systolic blood pressure of 50 mm Hg, hemoperfusion was employed and blood pressure rose within 20 minutes. The patient awoke and breathed spontaneously 1.5 hours after resin hemoperfusion was initiated. Plasma meprobamate extraction by the resin (Amberlite XAD-4) was 100 per cent during the first two hemoperfusions and was never lower than an 82 per cent extraction during the second procedure. Resin hemoperfusion may be the most efficient method available for removing meprobamate; however, it must be pointed out that this method is reported in only one publication. No clinical results are available for the use of *plasmapheresis* in meprobamate intoxication.

CARISOPRODOL
(Soma, Reia)

Carisoprodol (*N*-isopropyl-2-methyl-2-propyl-1,3-propanediol dicarbamate, $C_{12}H_{24}N_2O_4$, molecular weight = 260.3 daltons) is an *N-isopropylmeprobamate*. It is used mainly as a muscle relaxant to relieve pain, stiffness, and spasm associated with muscle joint disorders and additionally has minor tranquilizing properties.

In the dog, carisoprodol is excreted in the urine as hydroxycarisoprodol; small quantities of hydroxymeprobamate and meprobamate are also present, while traces of unchanged carisoprodol are also excreted in the urine. After intravenous injection, the major circulating compound in the plasma is the unchanged drug, although hydroxycarisoprodol, hydroxymeprobamate, and meprobamate are also present.[51]

```
              C3H7
              |
        H3C—C—CH2—O—CO—NH—C3H7
              |
              CH2—O—CO—NH2
```

CARISOPRODOL

The therapeutic dose is up to 1.4 gm daily and the intraperitoneal LD_{50} in mice is 790 ± 75 mg/kg. Unlike meprobamate, carisoprodol has only minor anticonvulsant activity, and side effects in clinical trials are drowsiness, dizziness, and occasional nausea. Toxic effects and treatment are similar to those of meprobamate.

References

1. Allen MD, Greenblatt DJ, Noel BJ: Meprobamate overdose: A continuing problem. Clin Toxicol *11*:501, 1977.
2. Blumenberg AG, Rosett GHL, Dobrow A: Severe hypotensive reactions following meprobamate overdosage. Ann Intern Med *51*:607, 1959.
3. Kamin J, Shaskan DA: Death due to massive overdose of meprobamate. Am J Psychiat *115*:1123, 1959.
4. Powell LW, Mann GT, Kaye S: Acute meprobamate poisoning. N Engl J Med *259*:716, 1958.
5. Shane AM, Hirsch S: Three cases of meprobamate poisoning. Can Med Assoc J *74*:908, 1956.
6. Bennet WM, Singer J, Coggins C: Guide to drug usage in adult patients with impaired renal function. JAMA *223*:991, 1973.
7. Hollister LE, Levy G: Kinetics of meprobamate elimination in humans. Chematherapie (Basel) *9*:2, 1964.
8. Maddock RK, Bloomer HA: Meprobamate overdosage. Evaluation of its severity and methods of treatment. JAMA *201*:99, 1967.
9. Berger FM: The pharmacological properties of 2-methyl-1,3-propanediol dicarbamate (Miltown), a new interneuronal blocking agent. J Pharmacol Exp Ther *112*:413, 1954.
10. Berger FM: Side-effects of meprobamate. Br Med J *3*:936, 1963.
11. Tremoliere F, Vachon F, Amoudry C, Bourdon R, Givert C: Intérêt de l'epuration par hémo-perfusion sur colonne de charbon active lors d'une intoxication massive par le méprobamate. Nouv Presse Méd *6*:3225, 1977.
12. Gaultier M, Fournier E, Bismuth C, Rapin J, Frejaville JP, Gluckman JC: Les intoxications aigues par le méprobamate. A propos des 141 cas. Soc Méd Hôp Paris *119*:675, 1968.
13. Hiestand EC: Attempted suicide with meprobamate: Presentation of a case. Ohio State Med J *52*:1306, 1956.
14. Woodward MG: Attempted suicide with meprobamate. Northwest Med *56*:321, 1957.
15. Ferguson MJ, Germanos S, Grace WJ: Meprobamate overdosage. Arch Intern Med *106*:237, 1960.
16. Ehlers H: Poisoning with psychopharmaca and barbiturate-free hypnotics. Dan Med Bull *10*:117, 1963.
17. Schou J: Psychosedative drugs, ataractics: With special references to the use and misuse of meprobamate (Equanil, Miltown, Restenil). Ugeskr Laeg *121*:649, 1959.
18. Goulon M: Akute Vergiftungen durch Tranquilizer. Münch Med Wschr *114*:573, 1972.

19. Longchal J, Tenaillon A, Trunet P, Labrousse J, Lissac J: Intoxication par le méprobamate avec incompétence myocardique. Traitement par le dobutamine. Nouv Presse Méd *7*:1408, 1978.
20. Algeri EJ, Katsas GG, Luongo MA: Determination of ethchlorvynol in biologic mediums, and report of two fatal cases. Am J Clin Pathol *38*:125, 1962.
21. Belaval GS, Widen AI: Meprobamate toxicity. US Armed Forces Med J *9*:1691, 1958.
22. Briggs GW: Meprobamate toxicity. Med Bull US Army Europe *16*:137, 1959.
23. Deisher JB: Ingestion of 12 grams of meprobamate with recovery. Northwest Med *55*:1083, 1956.
24. Scott PA, Grimshaw L, Molony JMP: Hypotensive episodes following treatment with meprobamate. Lancet *2*:1158, 1956.
25. Adlin EV, Sher PB, Berk NG: Fatal reaction following the ingestion of meprobamate. Arch Intern Med *102*:484, 1958.
26. Brachfeld J, Bell E: Stomatitis and proctitis as manifestations of meprobamate idiosyncrasy. JAMA *169*:1321, 1959.
27. Carmel WJ, Dannenberg T: Nonthrombocytopenic purpura due to Miltown (2-methyl-2n-propyl-1,3-propanediol dicarbamate). N Engl J Med *255*:255, 1956.
28. Charkes ND: Meprobamate idiosyncrasy: Report of a case and review of the literature. Arch Intern Med *102*:584, 1958.
29. Corley BL, Brundage F: Reaction following ingestion of 400 mg. of meprobamate. Calif Med *86*:183, 1957.
30. Meyer LM, Heeve WL, Bertscher RW: Aplastic anemia after meprobamate (2 methyl-2n-propyl-1,3-propanediol dicarbamate) therapy. N Engl J Med *256*:1232, 1957.
31. Nevins DM: Anaphylactoid reaction following administration of one meprobamate tablet. Ann Intern Med *53*:192, 1960.
32. Jenis EH, Payne RJ, Goldbaum LR: Acute meprobamate poisoning: A fatal case following a lucid interval. JAMA *207*:361, 1969.
33. Schwartz HS: Acute meprobamate poisoning with gastrotomy and removal of a drug-containing mass. N Engl J Med *295*:1177, 1976.
34. Hoy WE, Rivero A, Marin MG, Rieders F: Resin hemoperfusion for treatment of a massive meprobamate overdose. Ann Intern Med *93*:455, 1980.
35. Anderson WE: Peritoneal dialysis in private practice. Curr Ther Res *8*:598, 1966.
36. Castell DO, Sode J: Meprobamate intoxication treated with peritoneal dialysis. Illinois Med J *131*:298, 1967.
37. Dyment PC, Curtis DD, Gourrich GE: Meprobamate poisoning treated by peritoneal dialysis. J Pediatr *67*:124, 1965.
38. Graae J, Ladefoged J: Svaer meprobamatforgiftung behandelt med haemo-og peritonealdialyse. Nord Med *81*:601, 1969.
39. Hardy W, Ten Pas A, Nixon RK: Meprobamate intoxication treated by peritoneal dialysis: Report of a case. Henry Ford Hosp Med Bull *11*:347, 1963.
40. Mouton DE, Cohen RJ: Meprobamate poisoning, successful treatment with peritoneal dialysis. Am J Med Sci *253*:706, 1967.
41. Daumal M, Dunaud JL, Halgain JP, Nadin T: Intoxication massive au méprobamate traitée par hémodialyse à l'aide d'une membrane à haute perméabilité. Nouv Presse Méd *8*:43, 1979.
42. Decker WJ, Combs HF, Freuting JJ, Baney RJ: Dialysis of drugs against activated charcoal. Toxicol Appl Pharmacol *18*:573, 1971.
43. Hagstam K-E, Lindholm T: Treatment of exogenous poisoning with special regard to the need for artificial kidney in severe complicated cases. Acta Med Scand *175*:507, 1964.
44. Maher JF, Schreiner GE: Editorial review. The clinical dialysis of poisons. Trans Am Soc Artif Intern Organs *9*:385, 1963.
45. Pogglitsch H, Zeichen R: Über die Anwendung der extrakorporalen Hämodialyse bei akuten Schlafmittelvergiftungen. Wien Med Wschr *115*:308, 1965.
46. Simon NM, Krumlovsky FA: The role of dialysis in the treatment of poisoning. Am Soc Pharm Exp Ther *5*:1, 1971.
47. Armstrong C, Edwards KDG: Multifactorial design for testing oral ion exchange resins, charcoal, and other factors in the treatment of aspirin poisoning in the rat. Efficacy of cholestyramine. Med J Aust *2*:301, 1967.
48. Kolthammer JC: The in vitro adsorption of drugs from horse serum onto carbon coated with an acrylic hydrogel. J Pharm Pharmacol *27*:801, 1975.
49. Widdop B, Medd RK, Rees AJ, Braithwaite RA: Treatment of drug intoxication in dogs by haemodialysis and haemoperfusion. Trans Eur Soc Artif Organs *1*:72, 1974.
50. Barbour BH, Koffler A, Hill J: Fixed-bed charcoal hemoperfusion as a treatment of drug overdose. Abstract No. 878. Sixth International Congress on Nephrology, Firenze, 1975.
51. Douglas JF, Ludwig BJ, Schlosser A: The metabolic fate of carisoprodol in the dog. J Pharmacol Exp Ther *138*:21, 1962.

D. Chloral Hydrate

Three chloral derivatives are in clinical use. They are *chloral hydrate* (Noctec), *chloral betaine*, and *triclofos sodium* (Triclos). (The latter is no longer commercially available.) The pharmacology and uses of all three chloral derivatives are essentially the same, since they are all converted in vivo to the same active intermediate. The discussion of chloral hydrate, which is preferred clinically, applies equally well to the other compounds.

Chloral hydrate (2,2,2-trichlorethane-1,1-diol) is one of five sedative-hypnotic drugs which were used before 1900. The others are *paraldehyde*, *bromide*, *urethane*, and *sulfonal*. Barbiturates were introduced in 1903. A synonym for chloral hydrate is *trichloroacetalde-*

hyde, while chloral betaine is a chemical complex of chloral and betaine, and triclofos sodium is the monosodium salt of trichloroethanol phosphate ester. Trichloroethanol, the metabolite of chloral hydrate, is itself an excellent hypnotic agent but is not often used as such due to its physical and irritant properties. Street names for chloral hydrate principally reflect its mixture with alcohol, which enhances its action, so we have such well-known terms as "knock-out drops" and "Mickey Finn."

Pharmacology and Pharmacokinetics

Chloral hydrate ($C_2H_3Cl_3O_2$, molecular weight = 165.4 daltons) is rapidly absorbed from the gastrointestinal tract and exerts its action within 30 minutes. It is widely distributed throughout the body and is quickly and almost completely metabolized within the liver and other tissues such as kidney and red blood cells. Chloral hydrate possesses a half-life of only a few minutes, and significant blood levels have not been demonstrated after its oral administration.

Chloral hydrate is converted by hepatic alcohol dehydrogenase to trichloroethanol, which in turn is conjugated to form the inactive glucuronide (urochloralic acid).[1] A small but variable amount of chloral hydrate and a larger fraction of trichloroethanol are also oxidized to *trichloroacetic acid,* mainly in the smooth endoplasmic reticulum of the liver and kidney—an action that rapidly takes place since trichloroacetic acid appears in the plasma shortly following absorption. Trichloroacetic acid is considered to be an inactive compound, and its half-life is more than 30 hours. Chloral hydrate and trichloroethanol are highly lipid soluble and permeate plasma membranes to enter cells throughout the body. Chloral hydrate has been detected in cerebrospinal fluid, milk, and fetal blood, and it may be found in unchanged form in the liver, stomach contents, and upper gastrointestinal tract shortly after drug overdose death.

```
   Cl  OH
   |   |
Cl—C—CH—OH
   |
   Cl
```

CHLORAL HYDRATE

Chloral hydrate possesses a half-life of only a few minutes, whereas trichloroethanol has a half life of 4 to 14 hours;[2–4] the central nervous system concentration of these two active agents correlates with hypnotic response in mice.[5] Chloral hydrate is a potent hypnotic agent with a short duration of action that is limited by its rapid reduction to trichloroethanol, which in turn is responsible for the continuous hypnotic action of the drug.[6]

Since chloral hydrate is undetectable in plasma, determination of plasma trichloroethanol concentrations can be useful in estimating the quantity of drug ingested and the severity of overdose. In vitro, using human plasma, plasma protein binding for trichloroethanol is 35 to 41 per cent, while trichloroacetic acid is 71 to 88 per cent protein bound.[5] The distribution of trichloroethanol between red blood cells and plasma, after a therapeutic dose, is approximately equal (that is, the red blood cell to plasma ratio is 1).

Chloral hydrate is excreted in the urine as free trichloroethanol, trichloroethyl glucuronide (urochloralic acid), and trichloroacetic acid. The principal urinary metabolite is trichloroacetic acid, which is excreted relatively slowly over 24 to 48 hours. Sixteen to 35 per cent of the loading dose is recovered in 24 hours as trichloroacetic acid and its glucuronide, while 5 per cent of the dose is found in the form of free trichloroethanol. A small proportion of urochloralic acid is excreted in the bile.

Concomitant ingestion of ethanol leads to a marked alteration in chloral hydrate metabolism, since ethanol itself accelerates reduction of chloral hydrate to trichloroethanol. After concomitant ingestion of ethanol and chloral hydrate, serum trichloroethanol concentrations peak at an earlier and higher level and remain elevated for considerably longer than does a therapeutic dose taken alone. This means that there is an increased action of the drug, and, consequently, its toxicity is also increased. Chloral hydrate appears to have both inhibitory and enhancing actions on metabolism of some drugs. It may either potentiate or decrease the activity of oral anticoagulants like coumarin.[6–7] While hypothrombinemia has been observed, the clinical significance of interaction between chloral hydrate and coumarin is still in dispute. Chloral hydrate is reported not to induce microsomal enzymes, but it does appear to accelerate the biotransformation of amitriptyline.

Action and Use

Chloral hydrate is a central nervous system depressant; its main activity is in the cerebral hemispheres. It produces drowsiness and sedation promptly, to be followed by a quite sound sleep within 1 hour. At therapeutic doses, blood pressure and respiration are only slightly depressed, while reflexes are not greatly impaired. In contrast to other sedatives, "hangover" and depressant after effects are only rarely encountered. Chloral hydrate is a local irritant to the skin and mucous membranes, a feature that explains its gastrointestinal side effects. It is a safe nocturnal sedative for most patients, and in adults the usual dose is 500 mg to 1 gm. For sedation, a dosage of 250 mg three times daily, not exceeding 2 gm, is usually sufficient. For children, the usual hypnotic dosage is 50 mg/kg of body weight. For sedation in children, half the hypnotic dose should be used, and daily dosage should not exceed 1 gm. Chloral hydrate is available as tablets for oral administration or as suppositories for rectal administration.

Chloral hydrate should not be given to patients with known chloral hydrate sensitivity, and caution must be taken in patients with severe heart disease as well as severe renal or hepatic impairment. As mentioned, possible interaction between oral anticoagulants and ethanol exists.

Addiction and Withdrawal Symptoms

Prolonged and habitual use of chloral hydrate may result in tolerance, physical dependence, and addiction. Drug addiction often results in the taking of enormous doses of the drug, and renal damage has been demonstrated in dependent persons. Chloral hydrate addiction is similar to ethanol addiction, and sudden withdrawal can result in delirium and seizures with a high death rate when unrecognized and untreated.

Overdosage

Doses greater than 2 gm produce toxic symptoms. The reported lethal dose is 5 to 10 gm, but this varies greatly. Fatalities have been reported following ingestion of 1.25 gm and 3 gm, while recovery has been reported after an ingestion of 36 gm.[8] The oral LD_{50} dose in rats is 200 to 500 mg/kg. The known human lethal serum levels are 5 to 10 mg/dl.

The toxicity of chloral hydrate varies markedly in its manifestations, as has been reported from several centers. Basically, in overdose the drug exerts its toxic action in three main ways: as a central nervous system depressant; as a skin and mucous membrane–corrosive agent; and through its toxic action on some organs.[8–20]

Central nervous system manifestations of acute poisoning by chloral hydrate principally consist of deep stupor and coma occurring within 30 minutes of ingestion. Death may occur in a few hours or more promptly from sudden cardiovascular collapse. In addition to the deep narcosis, respiration may be slow and shallow, and the body temperature may be reduced to subnormal levels. Additionally, hypotension and mottling of the skin with cyanosis may be observed. Initially the pupils may be contracted, but later they may be dilated—a manifestation similar to that of deep barbiturate narcosis.

The corrosive action of chloral hydrate may be exhibited by gastritis with nausea and vomiting, especially after ingestion on an empty stomach. During the recovery period from overdosage, severe hemorrhagic gastritis, gastric necrosis, enteritis, and esophagitis with strictures may be observed.[11, 20] Allergic skin reactions may be observed occasionally, occurring from several hours to 10 days after an overdose.

Hepatic damage with jaundice and renal damage with albuminuria may be demonstrated. Parenchymal organ damage is similar to that observed in chloroform poisoning, but it is uncertain whether the toxicity is due to a corrosive or a direct toxic effect of the agent. Prolonged nephrotoxicity with chloral hydrate seems unlikely.

Direct cardiac toxicity of chloral hydrate has been discussed since cardiac complications commonly occur following overdoses of chloral hydrate. A variety of ventricular and atrial arrhythmias have been reported, commonly occurring in patients with preexisting heart disease.[10–12, 15, 16]

Treatment of Chloral Hydrate Poisoning

Treatment of chloral hydrate–intoxicated patients is essentially similar to that of other narcotic agents—for example, phenobarbital.

Gastric lavage may be of value only if carried out shortly after chloral hydrate ingestion, because of its rapid absorption from the gastrointestinal tract. Induction of vomiting in a conscious patient also may be attempted. Activated charcoal ingestion also may prevent drug absorption. It has been suggested that gastric and esophageal irritation should be treated prophylactically with oral demulcent agents.

General treatment consists of standard management for respiratory and blood pressure control. Fluid balance and intravenous glucose to prevent hypoglycemia from liver damage and appropriate rewarming should form the basis of standard therapy. Treatment of arrhythmias, including cardioversion when appropriate, should be provided when indicated.

Active drug removal techniques in serious cases can form an additional measure to those outlined above. Since there is no known antidote to chloral hydrate, several techniques have been suggested. Forced diuresis may be of limited value. Peritoneal dialysis has not yet proved to be a useful technique.

Hemodialysis appears to be of some importance in the effective treatment of chloral hydrate overdosage.[8, 13, 14, 19] Dialysance of trichloroethanol ranges from 120 to 160 ml/min, and its half-life has been reduced to approximately 4 to 6 hours.[14, 19] In one patient, after an ingestion of approximately 38 gm of chloral hydrate, 5.8 gm of trichloroethanol was removed by hemodialysis, and the patient survived.[8] While these interesting and beneficial clinical results have been observed, the clinical response is not explicable when one considers the pharmacokinetic handling of chloral hydrate. Trichloroethanol is equally distributed between the red blood cells and plasma, and its dialysance is therefore limited. In addition, trichloroethanol may be protein bound up to 40 per cent, and this also limits its dialytic removal.

Hemoperfusion using sorbent materials also has been successful in chloral hydrate intoxication. Activated *charcoal hemoperfusion*[21] and *resin hemoperfusion*[22] using uncharged resins have been used with some success both in animals and in human beings. In animal experiments, Widdop and associates demonstrated a trichloroethanol clearance of 93 to 108 ml/min.[21] In a patient with repeated cardiac arrest from chloral hydrate poisoning, Heath and colleagues demonstrated a dramatic improvement with resin hemoperfusion, with recovery of the patient and extubation within 50 minutes of beginning hemoperfusion.[22] If available, hemoperfusion appears to be superior to hemodialysis and should be used if a severely intoxicated patient is encountered.

References

1. Marshall EL Jr, Owens AH Jr: Absorption, excretion, and metabolic fate of chloral hydrate and trichloroethanol. Bull Johns Hopkins Hosp *95*:1, 1954.
2. Berry DJ: Determination of trichloroethanol at therapeutic and overdose levels in blood and urine by electron capture gas chromatography. J Chromatogr *107*:107, 1975.
3. Sellers EM, Lang M, Koch-Weser J, Leblanc E, Kalant H: Interaction of chloral hydrate and ethanol in man. I. Metabolism. Clin Pharmacol Ther *13*:37, 1972.
4. Sellers EM, Lang ML, Cooper SD, Koch-Weber J: Chloral hydrate and trichlofos metabolism. Clin Pharmacol Ther *14*:147, 1973.
5. Mackay FJ, Cooper JR: A study of the hypnotic activity of chloral hydrate. J Pharmacol Exp Ther *135*:27, 1962.
6. Breimer DD: Clinical pharmacokinetics of hypnotics. Clin Pharmacokin *2*:93, 1977.
7. Udall JA: Clinical implications of warfarin interactions with five sedatives. Am J Cardiol *35*:67, 1975.
8. Stalker NE, Gambertoglio JG, Fukumitsu CJ, Naughton JL, Benet L: Acute massive chloral hydrate intoxication treated with hemodialysis: A clinical pharmacokinetic analysis. J Clin Pharmacol *18*:136, 1978.
9. Bonnichsen R, Maehly AC: Poisoning by volatile compounds. II. Chlorinated aliphatic hydrocarbons. J Forensic Sci *11*:414, 1966.
10. DiGiovanni AJ: Reversal of chloral hydrate–associated cardiac arrhythmia by a beta-adrenergic blocking agent. Anesthesiology *31*:93, 1969.
11. Gleich GJ, Mongan ES, Vaules DW: Esophageal stricture following chloral hydrate poisoning. JAMA *201*:266, 1967.
12. Lansky LL: An unusual case of childhood chloral hydrate poisoning. Am J Dis Child *127*:275, 1974.
13. Locket S: Haemodialysis in the treatment of acute poisoning. Proc Roy Soc Med *63*:427, 1970.
14. Loeser WD, Fisher CJ, Boulis G: Forty-three dialyses in a community hospital. JAMA *192*:809, 1965.
15. Muller SA, Fisch C: Cardiac arrhythmia due to use of chloral hydrate. J Indiana Med Assoc *49*:38, 1956.

16. Nordenberg A, Delisle G, Izukawa T: Cardiac arrhythmia in a child due to chloral hydrate ingestion. Pediatrics *47*:134, 1971.
17. Shapiro S, Slone D, Lewis GP, Jick H: Clinical effects of hypnotics. II. An epidemiologic study. JAMA *206*:2016, 1969.
18. Silverman HJ: The adverse effects of commonly used systemic drugs on the human eye. II. Am J Optom *49*:335, 1972.
19. Vaziri ND, Kumar KP, Mirahmadi K, Rosen SM: Hemodialysis in treatment of acute chloral hydrate poisoning. South Med J *70*:377, 1977.
20. Vellar IDA, Richardson JP, Doyle JC, Keating M: Gastric necrosis: A rare complication of chloral hydrate intoxication. Br J Surg *59*:317, 1972.
21. Widdop B, Medd RK, Braithwaite RA, Rees AJ, Goulding R: Experimental drug intoxication. Treatment with charcoal haemoperfusion. Arch Toxicol *34*:27, 1975.
22. Heath A, Delin K, Eden E, Martensson E, Selander D, Wickstrom J, Ahlmen J: Hemoperfusion with Amberlite resin in the treatment of self-poisoning. Acta Med Scand *207*:455, 1980.

E. Glutethimide

Glutethimide (3-ethyl-3-phenyl-2,6-piperidinedione) was introduced as a sedative-hypnotic drug in 1954, being an outgrowth of the development of sedative-hypnotic drugs of the *piperidinedione* and *glutaric acid* groups. The clinically useful piperidinedione derivatives are *methyprylon, pyrithyldione,* and glutethimide (α-phenyl-α-ethyl-glutarimide). Although structurally related to *thalidomide* and *phenobarbital*, glutethimide has metabolic and dispositional pathways quite different from both those drugs.

Developed as a nonbarbiturate sedative-hypnotic with very few side effects, with little or no respiratory depression and a low abuse potential,[1–3] the drug rapidly gained popularity. By 1956, glutethimide was the sixth most frequently prescribed sedative.[4]

Despite its theoretically low toxicity, first reports on acute intoxications indicated that glutethimide could be abused and, moreover, was toxic to humans at comparable doses that were considerably lower than those previously determined from animal experiments.[5–7] By the mid 1960s, it was clear that glutethimide would not replace the barbiturates as an all-purpose sedative-hypnotic drug. It still appears to be prescribed commonly enough to be the cause of severe comas. Mortality from glutethimide ingestion is consistently greater than that for other drugs in the sedative-hypnotic-tranquilizer group. In some of the studies, a larger percentage of patients with glutethimide overdose resulting in stage 4 coma died when compared with similar presentations from overdose of other agents.

Several investigators have reported a variable clinical picture following glutethimide intoxication. In addition, the treatment of glutethimide intoxication may be difficult, as pointed out by Smith in 1969: "Glutethimide intoxication is one of the most difficult drug intoxications to manage . . ."[8] and Knepshield and associates in 1973: "The management of glutethimide poisoning continues to be a vexing problem."[9]

Furthermore, the metabolism of glutethimide in human beings only recently has been fully elucidated. Recently, new metabolites have been described, which are pharmacologically active and which contribute to the poisoning.[10]

Despite some questionable properties, an intravenous preparation of glutethimide became available for trial in 1959 for use as an anesthetic agent;[11] however, its use seems to have been abandoned as a result of central nervous system side effects.

In Europe, glutethimide is not a common agent in self poisoning, whereas in the United States it is still fairly common. The drug is well known under the trade name Doriden.

Pharmacology and Pharmacokinetics

Glutethimide ($C_{13}H_{15}NO_2$, molecular weight = 217.3 daltons) is highly soluble in oil, alcohol, and chloroform, but poorly soluble in water. After oral ingestion it is very slowly and irregularly absorbed from the gastrointestinal tract because of its poor water solubility. Absorption can be significantly enhanced by ingestion of alcohol.[12–14] After ingestion of a therapeutic dose (500 mg), peak plasma levels of glutethimide are reached in 1 to 6 hours.

Once absorbed, glutethimide quickly becomes concentrated in organs containing fat such as brain and adipose tissues, with a volume of distribution larger than that of whole body water. The drug recirculates from fat stores and is carried to the liver where it undergoes biotransformation, somewhat reminiscent of redistribution of ultra-short-acting barbiturates like thiopental.

The biotransformation that takes place in the liver has not yet been fully elucidated, despite a large number of research reports.[1, 15–25] Glutethimide has an asymmetric carbon atom and gives two optical isomers, both of which are metabolized in a different fashion. The D-isomer is hydrolyzed at the glutarimide ring, loses water, and breaks down into α-phenyl-α-ethyl glutaconimide, which is excreted in the urine as a nonconjugated metabolite in approximately 2 per cent of the administered dose. A major portion of the hydrolyzed D-isomer is combined with glucuronic acid and is excreted in the urine in approximately 45 per cent of the administered dose. The L-isomer is hydrolyzed with release of acetaldehyde from α-phenyl glutarimide. This metabolite is isolated in the urine in approximately 4 per cent of the administered dose. The remaining major portion is also combined with glucuronic acid and is excreted in the urine in approximately 45 per cent of the administered dose. Both glucuronides are water soluble but not fat soluble and no longer possess sedative activity. The glucuronides are excreted by the kidney, but about 70 per cent enters the enterohepatic circulation and will then be reabsorbed from the gastrointestinal tract before final excretion by the kidneys. Approximately 30 per cent of glucuronides are excreted directly into the urine.

Alpha-ethyl glutaconimide from the D-isomer is active in animals but does not appear to contribute to the sedative effect of therapeutic doses in human beings, although it appears to be a less active component of glutethimide in severe intoxication. Alpha-phenyl glutarimide possesses no sedative properties.

Approximately 14 usual and unusual metabolites have been identified, either in urine or synthesized in the laboratory.[10, 19] Two metabolites are known to accumulate in plasma and urine of intoxicated patients: 4-hydroxy-2-ethyl-2-phenyl-glutarimide (4-HG) and alpha-phenyl-gamma-butyrolactone.[16, 17, 19, 26] These compounds are not usually associated with the normal metabolic metabolites of glutethimide, but 4-HG has been found to possess twice the pharmacologic activity of the parent drug in mice. In a case report of a patient who had been in coma for 48 hours after glutethimide overdose, it was observed that while serum levels of glutethimide fell, the patient remained in coma long after known subtoxic levels were present. The degree of coma, however, correlated better with levels of 4-HG, and clinical recovery more closely approximated the time course of reduction of 4-HG concentrations in plasma.[27] Thus, a contributory effect of 4-HG either alone or synergistically with the parent compound in prolonging coma must be considered. Alpha-phenyl-gamma-butyrolactone is a nonpolar and highly lipid-soluble compound that appears to cross the blood-brain barrier, is eliminated from body tissues very slowly, and contributes to the half-life activity of the parent compound. Moderate levels of this metabolite have been found to cause significant respiratory problems in animals. In addition, enterohepatic circulation of metabolites and the unpredictable release of glutethimide from lipid stores probably contributes to the fluctuating clinical course often seen in severely intoxicated patients.

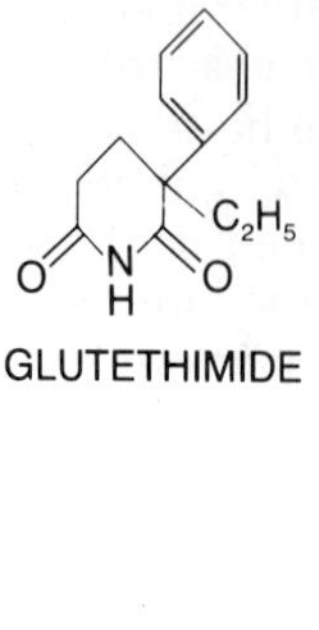

C_2H_5 O N H O

GLUTETHIMIDE

While plasma levels of glutethimide may fall, increasing levels of active metabolites that are capable of entering the central nervous system may add their effects; from a clinical standpoint, a patient who is apparently recovering, is responsive, and has spontaneous respirations may suddenly become apneic and lapse again into coma. Other explanations for "rebound" have been postulated;[28] one mechanism is that recovery of depression from gastrointestinal motility promotes further drug absorption; however, transport of drugs across the intestine proceeds even when gut tissue is denervated or excised and makes this postulate less tenable.

The two active metabolites are always in equilibrium with glutethimide in the fat stores,[21] while enterohepatic circulation and systemic recirculation for these two metabolites exist as just noted.

The total quantity of unchanged glutethimide excreted in the urine is somewhat controversial, since values from 0 to 2 per cent have been detected within 24 hours, and renal glutethimide clearances vary from 0.5 to 1.0 ml/min.[29] Using radiolabeled glutethimide, it has been shown that approximately 1 to 2 per cent of radioactivity is excreted in the stool and probably consists of glutethimide and metabolites.[30]

The spontaneous decline of glutethimide blood levels follows a biphasic curve, with an initial rapid phase and a later slow phase. During the initial rapid phase, a mean serum half-life of 3.8 hr is obtained,[29, 31] the drug being mainly distributed in the (lipid) tissue compartment. The decline in drug concentration during the second, slower phase gives a mean serum half-life of 11.6 hr—this being brought about by loss of drug from tissue compartments and blood (or central compartment) through metabolism and excretion.[29, 31]

However, in a series of patients with glutethimide overdose, mean serum half-life has been found to be prolonged to around 40.1 hr.[32] The definition of biologic half-life for glutethimide is somewhat difficult because of the rapidly appearing inactive metabolites (glucuronides). The half-life of the inactivated dose (effective biologic half-life) and the time when half of the dose is excreted (maximal biologic half-life) are different; the effective biologic half-life is approximately 10 hr, and the maximal biologic half-life is approximately 16 hr.

Glutethimide crosses the placenta and produces similar maternal and fetal plasma concentrations.[29, 33] Glutethimide is 50 per cent plasma protein bound,[34, 35] and the drug also stimulates hepatic microsomal enzyme induction.

Actions and Use

Glutethimide has depressant activity on the central and autonomic nervous systems and has a hypnotic action similar to that of phenobarbital but without analgesic, antitussive, or anticonvulsant actions. It is similar to barbiturates in its effect on the electroencephalogram and in its suppression of rapid eye movement sleep.

The drug exhibits pronounced anticholinergic activity, seen most prominently in the eye, but also manifested by inhibition of salivary secretion and intestinal motility.

As a hypnotic it has a medium duration of action and can be compared with the intermediate-acting barbiturates. Sleep is induced in about 20 minutes and lasts for up to 6 hours. It is used for the treatment of insomnia, but it is not effective in the presence of pain or psychiatric disturbance. The usual dose is 250 to 500 mg at bedtime, and it may be used as a daytime sedative in doses of up to 250 mg, two or three times daily.

In renal failure, glutethimide should be administered in usual doses in patients with mild to moderate renal failure, but it should not be given to patients with severe renal failure without reduction in dosage, since a short hemodialysis or peritoneal dialysis does not significantly alter serum glutethimide concentrations.

Glutethimide is contraindicated in patients with known hypersensitivity to the drug and should not be administered with alcohol since its effect is enhanced by alcohol. It is also suggested that it should not be administered to patients with porphyria.

Dependence and Withdrawal Symptoms

When glutethimide was introduced, it was believed that it did not cause dependence; however, a number of later reports pointed out chronic abuse and both physical and psychologic dependence.[43–52] The abstinence syndrome resulting from glutethimide withdrawal includes tremulousness, nausea, tachycardia, fever, tonic muscle contractions, and generalized convulsions. Similar symptoms occasionally occur even without abstinence in patients who have been taking regular but moderate doses (0.5 to 3 gm daily) and are also seen in patients recovering from acute intoxication without previous history of drug abuse. In the latter, tonic muscle spasms and infrequently generalized convulsions are seen. Catatonia and dyskinesias may be observed from a combination of glutethimide and antihistamine in drug abusers who abstain. Newborn infants of glutethimide-dependent mothers also may exhibit withdrawal symptoms. In the presence of dependence on glutethimide, dosage should be gradually reduced to avoid the symptoms associated with the abstinence syndrome. Because of the effects of glutethimide on hepatic microsomal enzymes, chronic use may produce osteomalacia.

Overdose

Symptoms of intoxication may appear after ingestion of 3 gm or greater of glutethimide. The lethal dose and lethal serum levels are not precisely known, but in general 10 gm of glutethimide are known to be potentially lethal; however, one patient survived after ingesting 45 gm[36] while another died with 7.75 gm.[37] Of 22 patients with doses between 3 and 30 gm, 4 patients died (having ingested 10 gm, 12 gm, 15 gm, and 20 gm, respectively) with the respective causes of death being irreversible shock, pneumonia, respiratory arrest, and cardiac arrest.[40] A computed lethal dose gives an LD_{50} in mice of approximately 40 gm in humans,[38, 39] and, according to Maher and associates,[40] 10 gm will be lethal in 45 per cent of patients and 12 gm lethal in 70 per cent of patients. A seriously toxic (potentially lethal) serum level of glutethimide is 3 mg/dl or greater,[40] and reported fatal serum levels of glutethimide range between 2 and 88 mg/dl.

There is, however, some controversy in relation to prediction of outcome since Chazan and Cohen reported 17 patients with mild intoxication whose plasma levels averaged 3.6 mg/dl (range, 0.9 to 6.4 mg/dl) and 5 patients with symptoms of mild intoxication and average serum levels of 3.6 mg/dl (range, 2.4 to 4.8 mg/dl), while another 12 patients with severe intoxication had an average serum level of 6.0 mg/dl (range, 2.7 to 111.0 mg/dl). Additionally, Wright and Roscoe reported 31 patients with glutethimide intoxication, 11 of whom had taken more than 12 gm.[42] All patients were treated with intensive supportive therapy without the use of dialysis, and only one patient died, of respiratory arrest and pulmonary and cerebral edema; serum glutethimide was 2.9 mg/dl.[42]

An understanding of the pharmacology and pharmacokinetics of glutethimide partially explains its variability of action in severe intoxication; however, it is re-emphasized that serum levels do not necessarily predict death. Ambre and associates gave a possible explanation for the extremely prolonged coma and the intensely toxic effects of glutethimide with small ingestions or with low serum levels. They showed in 1972[16] that the metabolite 4-HG accumulated in the plasma of intoxicated patients, that it was twice as pharmacologically active as the parent drug[17] on the central nervous system, and that in a patient with severe glutethimide intoxication (after 12 gm) peak 4-HG levels were reached after 24 hours while the half-life of serum glutethimide was 10 hours.[26] The highest concentrations of 4-HG correlated with the most severe symptoms (apnea) of intoxication.

Clinical Features

Glutethimide produces the most variable clinical picture following drug intoxication.

The toxic effects of therapeutic doses include nausea, excitement, hangover, blurred vision, and occasional skin rashes. Acute hypersensitivity reactions are manifested in blood dyscrasias and exfoliative dermatitis (a rare phenomenon). Toxic psychoses, convulsions, cerebellar ataxia, and peripheral neuropathy have all been induced by the prolonged use of glutethimide.

Overdosage with glutethimide produces symptoms similar to those of barbiturate overdosage but with the added problem of fluctuations in the depth of coma. The main complication in acute and severe glutethimide intoxication is *profound and prolonged coma,* which has been stressed in many reports.[5, 27, 33, 40, 53–61] Profound coma may be accompanied by the occasional appearance of lateralized or focal neurologic deficits, accompanied by cyclic variations in these signs. Sudden apnea (often seen during gastric lavage) and convulsions may occur with signs of raised intracranial pressure. Severe hypotension, leading to shock and hypothermia, may occur as well as persistent acidosis, areflexia, pulmonary edema, and cardiac arrest. The anticholinergic action of glutethimide may be manifested by dilated pupils with light reactivity or fixed dilated pupils (unilateral or bilateral)[40, 62] and urinary retention. Persistent hyperthermia, often after a phase of hypothermia and lasting for many hours after the patient regains consciousness, has been observed.[55, 60, 63] It is uncertain whether this is due to an anticholinergic effect or occurs as a toxic fever.

Several investigators have reported that patients requiring endotracheal intubation or tracheostomy have had thick, tenacious bronchial secretions that require constant suctioning, despite the strong anticholinergic activity of glutethimide, which has contributed to death in several patients.[53]

It cannot be overemphasized that complications may appear unexpectedly, with apnea occurring in the face of apparent recovery of the central nervous system.

Maher correlated the elimination half-life with the serum levels of glutethimide and suggested that coma would be unduly prolonged at high serum levels.[32] One explanation for this was that at high serum levels, metabolism of glutethimide may be delayed by rate-limited enzymatic degradation. Maher also suggested that serum half-life was longer in the intoxicated and hypotensive patient compared with the normotensive one. An explanation for this in some instances was that impaired perfusion of tissues, particularly liver, could account for prolonged elevation of serum levels. On the other hand, others have reported little apparent correlation between blood levels of the drug and clinical conditions, but this may be due in part to variable tolerance in individuals because of differences in metabolic degradation with use or abuse of glutethimide.[41, 48] Other investigators have compared serum and cerebrospinal fluid concentrations of glutethimide in order to explain the relationship between them and the unique, fluctuating clinical course observed in comatose patients.[4, 64] Despite cerebrospinal fluid levels not exceeding 0.8 mg/dl, there was considerable variation in blood levels and observed neurologic status.[64] The investigators concluded that the best estimate of the duration of coma was the maximal glutethimide concentration found upon admission to the hospital. There seems to be a definite relationship between the rate of decreasing serum glutethimide with maximum concentrations obtained in the serum; however, this does not explain the contribution of metabolites to the clinical course.

Other less severe but still toxic symptoms of glutethimide overdose include emesis, occasional muscle spasms, twitching, neuropathy,[65] methemoglobinemia,[54] and skin lesions resembling burns.[42, 66–68] Nephrotoxicity and hepatotoxicity are not likely problems.

Treatment of Glutethimide Overdose

Glutethimide intoxication falls into three main categories: mild, moderate, and severe, which are treated accordingly. Mild intoxications can be treated symptomatically in most patients; however, moderate intoxications that may exhibit hypotension along with deep coma require attention to fluid balance and the use of vasopressors to maintain adequate blood pressure. Gastric lavage should be employed, and adequate respiratory exchange must be maintained. As in any prolonged coma, urine output should be monitored and maintained, not for elimination of drug but to monitor the possibility of fluid overload that might contribute to pulmonary or cerebral edema.

Severe intoxication with glutethimide, alone or in combination with other agents (alcohol or barbiturates and so on) is generally characterized by profound, prolonged coma, which requires intensive supportive measures with or without the addition of extracorporeal detoxification techniques. The steps to be outlined, in general, are used for most types of drug-induced coma, but several factors unique to glutethimide and some of the controversies that exist in the treatment of the overdose will be discussed. The first step, however, is directed toward intensive supportive therapy and anticipation of the most common complications.

In patients with severe respiratory depression, a cuffed endotracheal tube should be placed and mechanical ventilation with humidified room air or enriched with oxygen should be available. The patient should be placed in an intensive care setting, and meticulous and constant endotracheal toilet is strongly recommended. Analeptic drugs, although popular in the past for glutethimide poisoning, have no place in modern toxicology for treating respiratory depression. It should be remembered that complications of these agents include seizures, cardiac arrhythmias, hyperpyrexia, and hypoxic brain injury.[69]

Circulatory status should be evaluated as expeditiously as possible. While blood is being drawn for toxicologic study, an intravenous infusion of normal saline solution should be started. If there are signs of hypotension, fluid administration should be continued cautiously since glutethimide is believed to be a vasomotor depressant causing relative hypovolemia secondary to peripheral vasodilatation, as seen with the barbiturates. Pulmonary edema has complicated fluid administration in a significant number of patients whose central venous and arterial blood pressures remained low.[69] Attempts to correct hypotension with *norepinephrine* or *metaraminol* in the past have been successful. Modern vasopressor agents also are likely to be successful in this setting (for example, dopamine and dobutamine).

If there is evidence of raised intracranial pressure or cerebral edema, mannitol infusions might be helpful; however, the use of mannitol is controversial since it has the propensity for producing pulmonary edema. The recording of arterial pH, Po_2, Pco_2, blood pressure, and urine volume should be performed on an hourly basis and appropriate corrections made. Electrocardiographic monitoring is also helpful.

If supportive care is likely to be maintained, prolonged artificial respiration may be accompanied by pneumonia, which contributes to the fatal outcome. Some investigators recommend early administration of prophylactic antibiotics in this case. Similarly, since urinary bladder atony caused by the anticholinergic effect of glutethimide might occur, some suggest that a urinary catheter be placed. However, both these measures are individual choices.

While supportive care alone has been associated with a very low incidence of morbidity and mortality, complications increase in proportion to the duration of coma. For this reason, in very severe intoxication attempts to reduce the duration of coma should be instituted, but only when the patient is stable and receiving adequate respiratory, cardiac, and circulatory support and all fluid and electrolyte imbalances have been corrected.

Active Drug Removal. *Alkaline gastric lavage* has been recommended for glutethimide since it possesses a high pK_a of 9.0, and in the ionized form its passage across the gastrointestinal wall will be impaired. The water solubility of glutethimide is potentiated in alkaline solution, and its strong anticholinergic effect increases its residence time within the lumen of the gastrointestinal tract.[70] A nasogastric tube should be placed for gastric lavage, and the presence of a cuffed endotracheal tube to protect the trachea and lungs is also recommended especially in the unresponsive, comatose patient.[14] Gastric and duodenal aspirates should be sent for toxicologic identification and quantification. As stated, caution is advised since many patients have experienced sudden apnea during the manipulations that gastric lavage entails. Lavage with castor oil (a mixture of 1:1 castor oil and water) may be more effective than previously appreciated.[71–73] Because of its poor water solubility and high lipid solubility, undissolved glutethimide may be taken up preferentially by the lipid perfusate and be more readily removed. In contrast to the barbiturates, the absorption of which is usually rapid (gastric aspiration and lavage are probably ineffective 3 to 4 hours after ingestion), lavage is certainly worth one or two attempts in glutethimide overdose, even if ingestion is presumed to have been earlier than 4 hours previously. Other investigators also have recommended castor oil catharsis, which theoretically will propel the dissolved drug more rapidly through the gastrointestinal tract, thereby diminishing its time for absorption. This has not met with wide acceptance in practice.[71]

Activated charcoal has been used to prevent gastrointestinal absorption of glutethimide,[74] and 1 gram of activated charcoal is capable of adsorbing 50 to 60 mg of glutethimide.[75] Therefore, administration of large amounts of charcoal in an aqueous slurry through the nasogastric tube may be effective even if performed within several hours after ingestion. The enterohepatic circulation of at least some of the metabolites also may be interrupted by activated charcoal. However, the known enterohepatic circulation of glutethimide and the higher mortality in patients with absent bowel sounds have stimulated biliary and intestinal drainage attempts in severely poisoned patients. Gallbladder drainage was attempted in one patient and then interrupted because minimal quantities of unmetabolized glutethimide were found in the bile.[31] It is not yet clearly known whether active components besides the inactive glucuronides are excreted in the enterohepatic circulation, which renders biliary drainage techniques unjustified at present.

Forced diuresis is of little help in removing significant quantities of unchanged glutethimide since renal clearance (0.5 to 1.0 ml/min) is limited. Approximately 0.002 mg/min of unchanged glutethimide is excreted after a therapeutic dose, which results in 8.25 mg (1.6 per cent of the initial dose) being excreted in 24-hr urine.[29] Similarly, alkalinization of the urine is contraindicated since glutethimide is a base. Furthermore, animal experiments showed only minimal excretion of glutethimide after alkalinization of the urine.[78] As mentioned, fluid balance must be adequately controlled and overhydration should be avoided since pulmonary and cerebral edema may complicate glutethimide intoxication.

Hemodialysis. The proportion of glutethimide that is not protein bound is removable from the blood by hemodialysis,[40] and, while it is likely that the active metabolites 4-HG and others also will be eliminated, this has not yet been proved. Many investigators have reported on the success of hemodialysis in severe glutethimide intoxication,[3, 13, 14, 29, 35, 36, 38, 40, 58, 59, 72, 76, 79–104] although this has been a hotly debated issue.[8] One study reported removal of 1.2 gm, and reduction of blood levels from 4.2 to 0.35 mg/dl within 8 hours of hemodialysis[80] and another reported removal of 1.4 gm.[38] Dramatic reduction of blood levels has been achieved by other investigators, with the removal of glutethimide varying from 30 to 155 mg/hr and dialysance varying from 29 to 109 ml/min.[38, 76, 80, 83] Hemodialysis is reportedly 30 to 200 times more effective than endogenous renal elimination.[13, 38, 40, 76] Maher showed that hemodialysis reduced the half-life from 40.1 hours to 14.6 hours;[32] a reduction in mortality rates in a series of severe glutethimide-poisoned patients has been reported to be reduced from 50 to 18 per cent with hemodialysis.[40, 77] Early dialysis appears to be of great importance, because distribution of glutethimide into fat and the enterohepatic circulation may require extended dialysis of 10 to 15 hours.

Many workers have reported that clinical response to hemodialysis for glutethimide poisoning is less dramatic than that seen in barbiturate overdose. Chazan and Cohen reported that hemodialysis in glutethimide poisoning was not more efficacious than conservative management.[41] In a controlled retrospective study of 37 patients, 22 had severe symptoms of intoxication. Of these 22, 17 patients with approximately equal degrees of intoxication were divided into two groups: 5 were hemodialyzed and 12 were conservatively managed. There was no difference in duration of coma (41 hours in the hemodialysis group, 36 hours in the group without hemodialysis) nor in the number of complications such as pneumonia, respiratory depression, and death rate.

In a further study, Chazan and Garella reported a series of 70 patients, 13 of whom had severe intoxication; only one death occurred in the whole group who were not subjected to hemodialysis.[106] Similarly, Wright and Roscoe, in a study of conservative management of 31 severely intoxicated patients, reported only one death (3 per cent) and concluded that hemodialysis was not essential in the management of patients severely poisoned with glutethimide.[42] Chazan and Garella reported that the cerebrospinal fluid concentrations of glutethimide correlated in a linear fashion with blood glutethimide values (being approximately 60 per cent of blood values).[106] However, no relationship was apparent between the duration of coma and glutethimide levels on admission or on subsequent changes in blood levels. Nevertheless, patients in coma on admission sustained considerable morbidity, including hypotension in 42 per cent, respiratory failure in 32 per cent, and pneumonia in 35 per cent.

The lack of correlation between blood glutethimide levels and the degree of coma reported by these investigators can be explained on the basis of several facts. First, the contribution of metabolites to the clinical picture in patients was unknown, and no comment was made on the chronicity of previous glutethimide ingestions, both of which factors might considerably influence the response to glutethimide ingestion. Second, other factors, such as age and pre-existing disease of liver or heart, as well as habituation to glutethimide, also can influence drug response. Third, early hemodialysis would remove that portion of glutethimide not sequestered in adipose tissue and the central nervous system.

Jorgenson and Jensen in Denmark demonstrated that the incidence of pulmonary complications increased with the duration of coma, and that most deaths occurring after more than 36 hours of coma were due to pneumonia consequent on atelectasis.[57] In addition, mortality was higher in elderly patients, which was thought to be caused by the increased incidence of pre-existing heart disease in this group, with hypotension being a major risk factor. In a review of approximately 600 patients with acute drug overdosage, it was found that 59 per cent of fatal cases died not from the toxic substance itself, but from the pulmonary complications.[56]

Lipid Hemodialysis. Since glutethimide is lipophilic, it was suggested that oil mixed with dialysate would increase the elimination of glutethimide into the emulsion.[84, 90, 94, 102, 105] Soybean oil, peanut oil, olive oil, and cottonseed oil have been used to give an emulsion of around 15 per cent. In vitro and in animals it has been shown that lipid hemodialysis achieves a dialysance 3.43 times higher than with aqueous hemodialysis,[101] an effect thought to occur by partitioning of lipid-soluble drugs within the oil. Using peritoneal dialysis containing oil emulsions, investigators have found a five-fold higher dialysance than with aqueous peritoneal dialysate, and it is postulated that peritoneal transfer of glutethimide from fat tissue occurs. It must be pointed out, however, that the use of lipid peritoneal dialysate is not without danger.

Clinical evaluation of lipid hemodialysis has revealed that little advantage can be obtained over aqueous hemodialysis. Leitzell and associates demonstrated in vivo a 42.5 ml/min dialysance with lipid dialysate and a 43.7 ml/min dialysance with aqueous dialysate.[94] Similar results were obtained by Mann and colleagues.[105] An in depth discussion of the value of lipid hemodialysis is out of the scope of this text, since the advent of hemoperfusion overcomes any discussion of dialysis and also is applicable in patients who otherwise would not be considered for hemodialysis (those with severe hypotension).

Peritoneal dialysis also has been used in the treatment of glutethimide intoxication[36, 80, 84, 93, 96–98, 107–111] and has been generally shown to be inferior to other methods of drug removal. With peritoneal dialysis, elimination of glutethimide is approximately 10 to 14 mg/hr.[80, 111]

Hemoperfusion

Charcoal Hemoperfusion. Glutethimide is well adsorbed by activated charcoal up to 100 per cent.[112, 113] Many investigators have shown that glutethimide is well removed from blood by hemoperfusion through activated charcoal, with clearances of glutethimide ranging from 70 to 200 ml/min with this method.[114–125] In addition, serum levels of glutethimide are lowered more rapidly and more significantly than with hemodialysis. De Myttenaere and associates, in animal experiments, demonstrated that with severe glutethimide intoxication (3 to 8 gm of glutethimide ingested) a survival rate of 80 per cent, compared with 0 per cent in a control group, was achieved with hemoperfusion.[116] With fixed-bed uncoated charcoal columns (which contained a small quantity, 95 gm, of activated charcoal), clinical results were inferior to those results quoted above.[117, 119]

Resin Hemoperfusion. Hemoperfusion through neutral (uncharged) exchange resins such as *Amberlite XAD-4* has been used in severe acute glutethimide intoxication.[100, 126–128] The resins have a high adsorptive capacity for lipid-soluble substances, and glutethimide clearances with such columns approximate blood flow through the devices (that is, glutethimide clearance of 300 ml/min at a blood flow of 300 ml/min). Rosenbaum and colleagues described a severely poisoned patient who had ingested 75 gm of glutethimide and who received hemoperfusion on three occasions using Amberlite XAD-4 resin.[128] Treatment on three consecutive days for 9 hours, 10 hours, and 8 hours, respectively, removed a total of 30 gm of glutethimide and produced glutethimide clearance values ranging from 225 to 293 ml/min at a blood flow of 300 ml/min. In the first resin hemoperfusion cartridge, 13.4 gm of glutethimide was eluted, despite a modest decrease in blood glutethimide from 11.0 to 9.5 mg/dl in 9 hours. This demonstrates that tissue removal of glutethimide had occurred, and this patient has the highest known ingested dose from which recovery was obtained.

Both resin and charcoal hemoperfusion provide the highest rates of glutethimide removal from blood, and, in general, clinical results are better than with other detoxification methods. However, hemoperfusion does not guarantee a positive outcome in severe glutethimide intoxication, because of the special human characteristics of drug behavior. Several workers have pointed out that repeated hemoperfusion is required for severe glutethimide intoxication because of rebound of drug levels following hemoperfusion with relapse into coma.[118, 128, 129] Therefore, caution should be exercised in the management of severely poisoned patients, and the following are guidelines in arriving at a decision to use hemoperfusion:

(1) Intoxication with an ingested dose greater than 10 gm or a serum level greater than 3 mg/dl.

Table 46–2. EFFICACY OF DETOXIFICATION METHODS FOR THE REMOVAL OF GLUTETHIMIDE

Renal clearance	0.5–1.0 ml/min (with forced diuresis)
Peritoneal dialysis	Approximately 10 ml/min
Hemodialysis	29–109 ml/min
Activated charcoal hemoperfusion	70–200 ml/min
Resin hemoperfusion	300 ml/min

(2) Prolonged deep coma (stage 3–4 coma, according to Reed and associates[130]) and hypotension resistant to standard therapy.

(3) Progressive deterioration despite intensive supportive management.

(4) A flat line on the EEG.[92, 131]

Table 46–2 summarizes the effectiveness of several detoxification methods in glutethimide poisoning.

References

1. Brobeil A, Härter O, Herrmann E: Klinische Vergleichsuntersuchungen mit Schlafmittein. Dtsch Med Wschr *80*:1654, 1955.
2. Gross F, Tripod J, Meier R: Zur pharmakologischen Charakterisierung des Schlafmittels Doriden. Schweiz Med Wschr *85*:305, 1955.
3. Locket S: Haemodialysis in the treatment of acute poisoning. Proc Roy Soc Med *63*:427, 1970.
4. Gosselin RA: National Prescription Audit (October, 1955). Boston, RA Gosselin, 1955.
5. Eidelman JR: Doriden intoxication. Missouri Med *53*:194, 1956.
6. Ibe K, Neuhaus G, Remmer H: Die akute Doriden-Vergiftung. Internist *2*:247, 1961.
7. McBay AM, Katsas GG: Glutethimide poisoning: A report of four fatal cases. N Engl J Med *257*:97, 1957.
8. Smith EC: Management of drug intoxications: The role of dialysis. Chicago Med School *28*:44, 1969.
9. Knepshield JH, Schreiner GE, Lowenthal DT, Gelfand MC: Dialysis of poisons and drugs—annual review. Trans Am Soc Artif Intern Organs *19*:590, 1973.
10. Andresen BD, Davis FT, Long MD: Identification and synthesis of a methylated catechol metabolite of glutethimide isolated from biological fluids of overdose victims. J Pharm Sci *68*:283, 1979.
11. Stephen CR: Glutethimide (Doriden) as an anesthetic agent. Anesthesiology *20*:137, 1959.
12. Kanter DM: The acute toxicity of Doriden overdosage. Connecticut Med J *21*:314, 1957.
13. Kier LC, Whitehead RW, White WC: Blood and urine levels in glutethimide (Doriden) intoxication. JAMA *166*:1861, 1958.
14. Schreiner GE, Berman LB, Kovach R, Bloomer HA: Acute glutethimide (Doriden) poisoning. The use of bemegride (Megimide) and hemodialysis. Arch Intern Med *101*:899, 1958.
15. Aboul-Enein HY, Schauberger CW, Hansen AR, Fischer LJ: Synthesis of an active hydroxylated glutethimide metabolite and some related analogs with sedative-hypnotic and anticonvulsant properties. J Med Chem *18*:736, 1975.
16. Ambre JJ, Fischer LJ: Glutethimide intoxication: Plasma levels of glutethimide and a metabolite in humans, dogs and rats. Res Commun Chem Pathol Pharmacol *4*:307, 1972.
17. Ambre JJ, Fischer LJ: Identification and activity of the hydroxy metabolite that accumulates in the plasma of humans intoxicated with glutethimide. Drug Metab Dispos *2*:151, 1974.
18. Andresen BD, Templeton JL, Hammer RH, Panzik HL: Synthesis and characterization of a catechol metabolite of glutethimide (Doriden) in human urine. Res Commun Chem Pathol Pharmacol *14*:259, 1976.
19. Andresen BD, Davis FT, Templeton JL, Panzik HL, Hammer RH: Toxicity of alpha-phenyl-gamma-butyrolactone, a metabolite of glutethimide in human urine. Chem Pathol Pharmacol *18*:439, 1977.
20. Bernhard K, Just M, Vuilleumier JP, Brubacher G: Über das Verhalten von α-Phenyl-α-äthyl-glutarimid im Tierkörper. I. Aktivitäts-Verteilung und -Ausscheidung nach Gaben ^{14}C-signierter Verbindungen an Ratten. Helv Chim Acta *39*(Fasc. II):596, 1956.
21. Keberle H, Hoffmann K, Bernhard K: The metabolism of glutethimide (Doriden). Experientia *18*:105, 1962.
22. Keberle J, Hoffmann K: Über den biologischen Abbau von Glutarsäureamiden. Experientia *12*:21, 1956.
23. Remmer H, Neuhaus G, Ibe K: Die Eliminationsgeschwindigkeit von Glutethimid (Doriden) beim Menschen. Naunyn-Schmiedeberg's Arch Exp Pathol Pharmakol *242*:90, 1961.
24. Sheppard H, D'Asaro B, Plummer AJ: The detection of glutethimide (Doriden) and a metabolite in dog urine. J Am Pharm Assoc *45*:681, 1956.
25. Stillwell WG: Metabolism of glutethimide in the human. Res Comm Chem Pathol Pharmacol *12*:25, 1975.
26. Hansen AR, Kennedy KA, Ambre JJ, Fischer LJ: Glutethimide poisoning. A metabolite contributes to morbidity and mortality. N Engl J Med *292*:250, 1975.
27. Orfanakis MG, Galloway WB: Glutethimide poisoning. Rocky Mt Med J *74*:34, 1977.
28. Decker WJ, Thompson HL, Arneson LA: Glutethimide rebound. Lancet *2*:778, 1970.
29. Curry SH, Riddall D, Gordon JS, Simpson P, Binns TB, Rondel RK, McMartin C: Disposition of glutethimide in man. Clin Pharmacol Ther *12*:849, 1971.
30. Butikofer E, Cottier P, Imhof P, Keberle H, Riess W, Schmid K: Die Eliminationsgeschwindigkeit von Glutethimid (Doriden) und die Natur der Ausscheidungsprodukte beim Menschen. Naunyn-Schmiedeberg's Arch Exp Pathol Pharmakol *244*:97, 1962.
31. Charytan C: The enterohepatic circulation in glutethimide intoxication. Clin Pharmacol Ther *11*:816, 1971.
32. Maher JF: Determinants of serum half-life to glutethimide in intoxicated patients. J Pharmacol Exp Ther *174*:450, 1970.
33. Bello GV, Moshirpur J, Sklar GS: Coma caused by drug abuse in pregnancy. Mount Sinai J Med *48*:66, 1981.
34. Decker WJ, Combs HF, Freuting JJ, Baney RF: Dialysis of drugs against activated charcoal. Toxicol Appl Pharmacol *18*:573, 1971.
35. Maher JF, Schreiner GE: Acute glutethimide poisoning. II. The use of hemodialysis. Trans Am Soc Artif Intern Organs *7*:1000, 1961.
36. Phillips WC, Bortin MN: Massive glutethimide (Doriden) intoxication: Successful treatment with dialysis. Wisconsin Med J *64*:440, 1965.
37. Medical Division, Research Department: Acute overdosage of Doriden; Personal communication. CIBA Pharmaceutical Company, Summit, NJ, 1967.
38. Chandler BF, Meroney WH, Czarnecki SW, Her-

man RH, Cheitlin MD, Goldbaum LR, Herndon EG: Artificial hemodialysis in management of glutethimide intoxication. JAMA *170*:914, 1959.
39. Doyle JE: Extracorporeal hemodialysis therapy. *In* Doyle JE (ed): Blood Chemistry Disorders. Springfield IL, Charles C Thomas, 1962.
40. Maher JF, Schreiner GE, Westervelt FB: Acute glutethimide intoxication. I. Clinical experience (twenty-two patients) compared to acute barbiturate intoxication (sixty-three patients). Am J Med *33*:70, 1962.
41. Chazan JA, Cohen JJ: Clinical spectrum of glutethimide intoxication (hemodialysis re-evaluated). JAMA *208*:837, 1969.
42. Wright N, Roscoe P: Acute glutethimide poisoning, conservative management of 31 patients. JAMA *214*:1704, 1970.
43. Bartholomew AA: Intoxication and habituation to glutethimide ("Doriden"). Med J Aust *2*:51, 1961.
44. Battegay R: Sucht nach Abusus von Doriden. Schweiz Rundschau Med *46*:991, 1957.
45. Busch W, Engelmeier M-P: Doriden-Rausch. Nervenarzt *30*:516, 1958.
46. Cohen H: Primary glutethimide addiction. New York J Med *60*:280, 1960.
47. Greve W, Schönberg F: Sucht und Entziehungserscheinungen bei barbiturat-freien Schlafmitteln. Dtsch Med Wschr *86*:1606, 1961.
48. Johnson FA, van Buren HC: Abstinence syndrome following glutethimide intoxication. JAMA *180*:1024, 1962.
49. Lloyd EA, Clark LD: Convulsions and delirium incident to glutethimide withdrawal. A case report. Dis Nerv System *20*:524, 1959.
50. Luby ED, Domino EF: Additional evidence of the addiction liability of glutethimide in man. JAMA *181*:46, 1963.
51. Sadwin A, Glen RS: Addiction to glutethimide (Doriden). Am J Psychiat *115*:469, 1958.
52. Zivin I, Shalowitz M: Acute toxic reaction to prolonged glutethimide administration. N Engl J Med *266*:496, 1962.
53. Arieff AJ, Friedmann EA: Coma following nonnarcotic drug overdose: Management of 208 adult patients. Am J Med Sci *266*:405, 1973.
54. Filippini L: Methämoglobinämie bei Doriden-Intoxikation. Schweiz Med Wschr *95*:1618, 1965.
55. Gerster P, Scholer H, Züger M: Klinische Beobachtungen bei einer akuten Vergiftung mit α-Phenyl-α-äthylglutarimid (Doriden). Schweiz Med Wschr *95*:991, 1955.
56. Ibe K: Lung complications secondary to acute poisoning. Br Med J *3*:532, 1969.
57. Jorgenson EQ, Jensen VB: Acute glutethimide poisoning. Dan Med Bull *22*:263, 1975.
58. Nakamoto S, Kolff WJ: The artificial kidney for acute glutethimide (Doriden) and barbiturate poisoning. Cleveland Clinic Q *27*:58, 1960.
59. Smith BE, Pino DM: Glutethimide (Doriden) therapy and overdosage. A review with report of a case. US Armed Forces Med J *11*:161, 1960.
60. Thiebaut F, Mengus M, Finker L, Dorey R: Un cas de coma par ingestion de glutéthimide. Rev Neurol *100*:786, 1959.
61. Winters WA, Grace WJ: Prolonged coma caused by glutethimide. Clin Pharmacol Ther *2*:40, 1961.
62. Brown DG, Hammill JF: Glutethimide poisoning: Unilateral pupillary abnormalities. N Engl J Med *284*:806, 1971.
63. Blakey HH, Barringer T, Billig O: Acute Doriden intoxication. South Med J *49*:172, 1956.
64. Gold M, Tassoni E, Etzi M: Comparison of glutethimide concentration in the serum and CSF of humans in drug overdose. Clin Chem *19*:1158, 1973.
65. Nover R: Persistent neuropathy following chronic use of glutethimide. Clin Pharmacol Ther *8*:283, 1967.
66. Leavell UW, Loyer JR, Taylor RJ: Dermographism and erythematous lines in glutethimide overdosage. Arch Dermatol *106*:724, 1972.
67. Parrish JA, Arndt KA: Skin lesions in barbiturate poisoning. N Engl J Med *283*:764, 1970.
68. Sørensen BF: Skin symptoms in acute narcotic intoxication. Dan Med Bull *10*:130, 1963.
69. Lang PG, Talman WT, Hunt WB: Drug overdosage due to glutethimide. South Med J *65*:413, 1972.
70. Kamisaka Y, Griffiths DW, Leduc L, Lipsky M, Martin H, Thayer WR: Inhibition of glutethimide absorption. Arch Toxikol *28*:12, 1971.
71. Baron JM, Tritch DL: Castor oil catharsis in acute glutethimide intoxication. JAMA *211*:1021, 1970.
72. Ben-Asher MD: Glutethimide (Doriden) poisoning (Controversies in treatment). Arizona Med *28*:28, 1971.
73. Mann JB: Sedative overdose. Audio Digest (Intern Med) *16*:19, 1969.
74. Corby DG, Fiser RH, Decker WJ: Re-evaluation of the use of activated charcoal in the treatment of acute poisoning. Pediatr Clin North Am *17*:545, 1970.
75. Shubin H, Weil MH: The mechanism of shock following suicidal doses of barbiturates, narcotics and tranquilizer drugs, with observations on the effects of treatment. Am J Med *38*:853, 1965.
76. Caplan HL: Recovery in severe glutethimide poisoning. Postgrad Med J *43*:611, 1967.
77. Hickman B, Caridis DT: Hemodialysis in glutethimide poisoning. Br Med J *3*:532, 1969.
78. Boerner D, Jovanovic UJ, Henschler D: Influence on cerebral function of alkalinization as observed during treatment of hypnotic poisoning by forced diuresis. Z Ges Exp Med *152*:223, 1970.
79. Colombi A, Riess W, Thölen H: Behandlung der akuten Glutethimidintoxication (Doriden) mittels Hämodialyse. Helv Med Acta *35*:145, 1970.
80. De Myttenaere M, Schoenfeld L, Maher JF: Treatment of glutethimide poisoning. A comparison of forced diuresis and dialysis. JAMA *203*:865, 1968.
81. Dittrich P v: Die Behandlung der akuten Vergiftung mit Glutethimid (Doriden) durch extrakorporale Hämodialyse. Dtsch Med Wschr *87*:357, 1962.
82. Dutz H, Eckardt D, Lachhein L, et al: Therapie akuter exogener Vergiftungen mit Hilfe von Hämo- und Peritonealdialyse und Ergebnisse dieser Behandlung in der DDR von 1959–1968. Dtsch Gesundh *25*:1437, 1970.
83. Esmond WC, Strauch M: Successful treatment of severe glutethimide (Doriden) poisoning with an optimized artificial kidney (dialung). Invest Urol *3*:512, 1966.
84. Fletcher G, Coplon NS: In vitro comparison of aqueous and lipid dialysate in hemodialysis of glutethimide, secobarbital and phenobarbital (abstr). Proceedings, Fourth Annual Meeting, American Society of Nephrology, 1970, p 25.
85. Grumer HA, Stannus DG, Stoddard GR: The feasibility of a hemodialysis unit in a community hospital. South Med J *59*:769, 1966.

86. Hoeltzenbein J, Kemper F, Opitz K, Wolf G: Kausale Therapie bei schwerer Glutethimid-Vergiftung durch extrakorporale Hämodialyse. Med Klin *56*:1584, 1961.
87. Ibe K, Bennold I, Burmeister H, Kessel M: Die extrakorporale Hämodialyse bei schweren Schlafmittelvergiftung. Berlin Med *16*:350, 1965.
88. Irvine RDH, Montgomerie JZ, Spence M: Assisted respiration, noradrenaline infusion and the artificial kidney for glutethimide (Doriden) poisoning. Med J Aust *2*:277, 1963.
89. Kallen RJ, Zaltzmann S, Coe F, Metcoff J: Hemodialysis in children: Technique, kinetic aspects related to varying body size, and application to salicylate intoxication, acute renal failure and some other disorders. Medicine *45*:1, 1966.
90. King LH, Decherd JF, Newton JL, Shires DL, Bradley KP: A clinically efficient and economical lipid dialyzer. (Use in treatment of glutethimide intoxication. JAMA *211*:652, 1970.
91. Klinkmann H, Hübel A, Röhring A, Schwartz F, Tredt HJ, Precht K: Hämodialyse bei schweren Intoxikationen (Teil I). Dtsch Ges-Wesen *19*:60, 1964.
92. Kubicki ST, Bennold I, Kessel M: Elektroencephalographische Untersuchungen während extrakorporaler Dialyse bei akuten Schlafmittelintoxikationen. Verh Dtsch Ges Inn Med *72*:620, 1966.
93. Kurtz GG, Michael UF, Morosi HJ, Vaamonde CA: Hemodialysis during pregnancy. Arch Intern Med *118*:30, 1966.
94. Leitzell BJ, Barton LJ, Wilcox HG, Bloomer HA: Comparison of lipid and aqueous dialysis for removing glutethimide from plasma. Clin Res *19*:152, 1971.
95. Lubash GD, Ferrari MJ, Scherr L, Rubin AL: Sedative overdosage and the role of hemodialysis. Arch Intern Med *110*:884, 1962.
96. McDonald DF, Greene WM, Kretchmar L, O'Brien G: Experiences in acute glutethimide (Doriden) intoxication. Superiority of extracorporeal dialysis over peritoneal dialysis. Invest Urol *1*:127, 1963.
97. Özdemir AJ, Tannenberg AM: Peritoneal and hemodialysis for acute glutethimide overdosage. NY State J Med *72*:2076, 1972.
98. Penn AS, Rowland LP, Fraser DW: Drugs, coma, and myoglobinuria. Arch Neurol *26*:336, 1972.
99. Renner E: Die Hämodialyse bei exogenen Vergiftungen und Stoffwechselkrankheiten. Internist *6*:196, 1965.
100. Rosenbaum JL, Winsten S, Kramer MS, Moros J, Raja R: Resin hemoperfusion in the treatment of drug intoxication. Trans Am Soc Artif Intern Organs *16*:134, 1970.
101. Shinaberger JH, Shear L, Clayton LE, Barry KG, Knowlton M, Goldbaum LR: Dialysis for intoxication with lipid-soluble drugs, enhancement of glutethimide extraction with lipid dialysate. Trans Am Soc Artif Intern Organs *11*:173, 1965.
102. Shinaberger JH, Shear L, Clayton LE, Barry KG, Knowlton M, Goldbaum L: Intraperitoneal lipid: Enhancement of glutethimide extraction during peritoneal dialysis. Clin Res *13*:54, 1965.
103. Sonda LP: Treatment of Doriden intoxication by hemodialysis. J Michigan Med Soc *61*:960, 1962.
104. Traeger J, Fries D, Bolot J-F, Pozet N, Laurent G: Le traitement de certaines intoxications aigues par l'epuration extrarénale. Bull Lég Toxic Méd *7*:353, 1964.
105. Mann JB, Ginn HE, Matter BJ, Shinaberger JH: Clinical experience with lipid dialysate. Clin Res *16*:63, 1968.
106. Chazan JA, Garella S: Glutethimide intoxication (A prospective study of 70 patients treated conservatively without hemodialysis). Arch Intern Med *128*:215, 1971.
107. Anderson WE: Peritoneal dialysis in private practice. Curr Ther Res *8*:598, 1966.
108. Barbour BH: Peritoneal dialysis in the management of dialysable poisoning. Clin Res *8*:114, 1960.
109. Ellis KG, Lea RG, Drysdale RD: Peritoneal dialysis. Can Med Assoc J *88*:928, 1963.
110. Flanigan WJ, Henderson LW, Merrill JP: The clinical application and technique of peritoneal dialysis. GP *28*:98, 1963.
111. Frey WG: Acute glutethimide poisoning managed by peritoneal dialysis. J Maine Med Assoc *59*:3, 1968.
112. Armstrong C, Edwards KDG: Multifactorial design for testing oral ion exchange resins, charcoal and other factors in the treatment of aspirin poisoning in the rat. Efficacy of cholestyramine. Med J Aust *3*:301, 1967.
113. Fiser RH, Maetz HM, Treuting JJ, Decker WJ: Activated charcoal in barbiturate and glutethimide poisoning in the dog. J Pediatr *78*:1045, 1971.
114. Barbour BH, Koffler A, Hill J: Fixed-bed charcoal hemoperfusion as a treatment of drug overdose (Abstr 878). Sixth International Congress on Nephrology, Firenze, 1975.
115. Chang TMS, Coffey JF, Lister C, Taroy E, Stark A: Methaqualone, methyprylon, and glutethimide clearance by the ACAC microcapsule artificial kidney: In vitro and in patients with acute intoxication. Trans Am Soc Artif Intern Organs *19*:87, 1973.
116. De Myttenaere MH, Maher JF, Schreiner GE: Hemoperfusion through a charcoal column for glutethimide poisoning. Trans Am Soc Artif Intern Organs *13*:190, 1967.
117. de Torrente A, Rumack BH, Blair DT, Anderson FJ: Fixed-bed uncoated charcoal hemoperfusion in the treatment of intoxications: Animal and patient studies. Nephron *24*:71, 1979.
118. Gelfand MC, Winchester JF, Knepshield JH, Hanson KM, Cohan SL, Strauch BS, Geoly KL, Kennedy AC, Schreiner GE: Treatment of drug overdosage with charcoal hemoperfusion. Trans Am Soc Artif Intern Organs *23*:599, 1977.
119. Koffler A, Bernstein M, LaSette A, Massry SG: Fixed-bed charcoal hemoperfusion; Treatment of drug overdose. Arch Intern Med *138*:1691, 1978.
120. Kolthammer JC: The in vitro adsorption of drugs from horse serum onto carbon coated with an acrylic hydrogel. J Pharm Pharmacol *27*:801, 1975.
121. Vale JA, Rees AJ, Widdop B, Goulding R: Use of charcoal haemoperfusion in the management of severely poisoned patients. Br Med J *1*:5, 1975.
122. Vale JA, Crome P, Meredith T, Goulding R: Charcoal haemoperfusion for hypnotic drug overdose (abstr). Artificial Organs *3*(A):50, 1979.
123. Volans GN, Vale JA, Crome P, Widdop B, Goulding R: The role of charcoal haemoperfusion in the management of acute poisoning by drugs. *In* Kenedi RM, Courtney JM, Gaylor JDS, Gilchrist T (eds): Artificial Organs. London, Macmillan, 1977, p 178.
124. Widdop B, Medd RK, Braithwaite RA, Rees AJ, Goulding R: Experimental drug intoxication. Treat-

ment with charcoal haemoperfusion. Arch Toxikol *34*:27, 1975.
125. Widdop B, Medd RK, Rees AJ, Braithwaite RA: Treatment of drug intoxication in dogs by haemodialysis and haemoperfusion. Trans Eur Soc Artif Organs *1*:72, 1974.
126. Medd RK, Widdop B, Braithwaite RA, Rees AJ, Goulding R: Comparison of haemoperfusion and haemodialysis in the therapy of barbiturate intoxication in dogs. Arch Toxikol *31*:163, 1973.
127. Rosenbaum JL, Kramer MS, Raja R, Boreyko C: Resin hemoperfusion: A new treatment for acute drug intoxication. N Engl J Med *284*:874, 1971.
128. Rosenbaum JL, Kramer MS, Raja R: Resin hemoperfusion for acute drug intoxication. Arch Intern Med *136*:263, 1976.
129. Winchester JF, Gelfand MC, Knepshield JH, Schreiner GE: Dialysis and hemoperfusion of poisons and drugs—update. Trans Am Soc Artif Intern Organs *23*:762, 1977.
130. Reed C, Driggs MF, Foote CC: Acute barbiturate intoxication: A study of 300 cases based on a physiologic system of classification of the severity of the intoxication. Ann Intern Med *37*:290, 1952.
131. Stölzer R: Veränderungen des Hirnstrombildes unter extrakorporaler Dialyse. Inaugural Dissertation, Freie Universität Berlin, 1963.

F. Ethinamate and Other Sedatives

Sedative-hypnotic drugs are used to produce drowsiness and promote sleep. Three major groups of substances are used for this indication: the barbiturates, the benzodiazepines, and a multiplicity of drugs assembled here called the nonbarbiturate sedative-hypnotic drugs and tranquilizers. This section deals with several drugs of the latter group: *ethinamate, methyprylon, methapyrilene, carbromal and bromisoval, the bromocarbamides,* and *diethylpentenamide*. Several other minor substances and miscellaneous agents, like *orphenadrine*, also are discussed. Other nonbarbiturate hypnotics such as methaqualone are treated separately.

ETHINAMATE

Ethinamate (1-ethinyl-cyclohexyl-carbamate) is a mild sedative-hypnotic drug used mainly as a hypnotic in simple insomnia.

Pharmacology and Pharmacokinetics

Ethinamate (Valmid) ($C_9H_{13}NO_2$, molecular weight = 167.2 daltons) is rapidly absorbed from the gastrointestinal tract and is in part metabolized by the liver.[1] The major of three metabolites is *hydroxyethinamate* (yielded by hydroxylation of the cyclohexyl ring), and it is yet unclear whether this metabolite has any pharmacologic effect. Hydroxyethinamate is combined with glucuronide to form approximately equal quantities with free hydroxyethinamate. Maximum blood concentrations are reached within 60 minutes after ingestion, and the biologic half-life is reported as 135 minutes.[2] From the absorbed ethinamate, 10 per cent is metabolized to CO_2 while the rest is excreted by the kidney, mainly as hydroxyethinamate glucuronides (89 per cent), and metabolites (9 per cent); only 2 per cent of free ethinamate is excreted in the urine.[3]

Actions and Use

Ethinamate is a mild sedative-hypnotic drug. Its onset is rapid, and its duration of action is short. Sleep is induced within 20 minutes, and the effect of the drug lasts for 3 to 5 hours. Any effect on rapid eye movement sleep is unknown. Since it is mild in action, its activity is less than that of barbiturates for severe insomnia. It is usually prescribed in a dose of 0.5 to 1 gm; for comparison, 500 mg of ethinamate has less activity than 100 mg of *secobarbital*. Ethinamate is contraindicated in patients with known hypersensitivity to this drug.

Intoxication

Overdoses with a few grams cause central nervous system depression with impairment of respiratory function. If ethinamate is ingested concurrently with alcohol or other central nervous system depressants, the potential hazards of both these agents are increased. The minimum lethal dose is unknown, but fatalities have occurred with ingestion of 15 and 60 gm;[3, 4] however, there

HC≡C—(cyclohexyl)—O—CO—NH_2

ETHINAMATE

have been recoveries with ingestions of 20 gm, 28 gm, and 40 gm.[3–5]

Addiction and withdrawal symptoms have occurred after chronic exposure to ethinamate. Chronic use of larger than recommended doses leads to drug dependence,[6, 7] and withdrawal of ethinamate after chronic abuse has been followed by agitation, syncopal episodes, tremulousness, and hyperactive reflexes, in addition to other CNS manifestations such as convulsions, hallucinations, delusions, and disorientation.[8]

The major toxic effect of ethinamate is the production of deep coma with depression of the respiratory system. Nausea and excitement have occasionally been noted in less severe intoxications. Fever, skin rashes, and rarely thrombocytopenic purpura as well as hypersensitivity reactions have been reported. Ethinamate does not appear to be nephrotoxic.

Treatment. Guidelines for treatment of ethinamate intoxication are the same as those for phenobarbital. Forced diuresis has been suggested for management of ethinamate intoxication; however, the amount of unchanged drug excreted in urine is rather small. Ethinamate and its metabolites are well dialyzable, and hemodialysis has been used in the past.[3, 9] A patient was dialyzed 40 hours following ingestion of 15 gm of ethinamate; after 12 hours of hemodialysis, 805 mg of ethinamate and 430 mg of hydroxyethinamate were detected in dialysate.[3] Since dialysis was instituted 40 hours after ingestion of the drug and may account for only 1.23 gm of the total ethinamate in dialysate, it is likely that earlier treatment would have been associated with a more favorable outcome since this patient died as a result of pulmonary edema. Other extracorporeal drug removal treatments have not yet been reported.

METHYPRYLON

Methyprylon (3,3-diethyl-5-methyl-2,4-piperidinedione) was developed in 1954 and introduced in 1955 as a sedative-hypnotic agent. Methyprylon (Noludar) is one of two major compounds derived from *hydropyridine* and *piperidine* in the search for an alternative to barbiturates. The other major compound is *pyrithyldione* (Persedon).

Between 1955 and 1965, a number of reports of intoxication with this drug were published.[10–14] Despite its use since 1955, the clinical manifestations of intoxication and its pharmacokinetics are not well understood. After ingestion of this drug alone, it appears that death is uncommon, since there is only one case report in the literature.[14]

Pharmacology and Pharmacokinetics

Methyprylon ($C_{10}H_{17}NO_2$, = 183.25 daltons) is partially soluble in water (7 per cent) but is freely soluble in organic solvents such as alcohol.

Gastrointestinal absorption is rapid, with the highest blood concentration being achieved 1 to 2 hours following ingestion. Biologic half-life is not well defined, but varies between 4 and 16 hours, although a longer action has been observed in severely poisoned patients. While the metabolic degradation of methyprylon is known, it is not certain in which organ this takes place. Methyprylon is dehydrogenated to 5-methyl-pyrithyldione (metabolite I), then partially oxidized to hydroxy derivatives (metabolite II), and finally oxidized to 5-carboxy-pyrithyldione (metabolite III). The hydroxy derivatives are bound approximately 38 per cent to human plasma proteins.

Other less important metabolites may arise, but the metabolites are partly conjugated to glucuronide, with approximately 97 per cent of the parent drug being metabolized. Intact methyprylon (3 per cent) and its metabolites (60 per cent) are recovered in the urine, while approximately 20 per cent is found in the feces, demonstrating that enterohepatic circulation of the drug occurs.

The varying half-life of methyprylon can be explained in two ways. In normal dosage, intact methyprylon appears rapidly in the urine; however, the duration of action and the activity of the metabolites are not clearly known. Second, metabolic degradation to dehydrogenated metabolites takes some time, and in patients with methyprylon overdose the plasma half-life of the drug is known

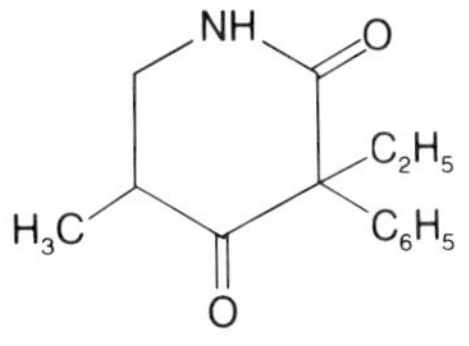

NH, O, C_2H_5, H_3C, C_6H_5, O

METHYPRYLON

to be long, sometimes days. Methyprylon does not accumulate selectively in organ systems.

Actions and Use

Methyprylon is a central nervous system depressant similar to *chloral hydrate* and *secobarbital*, but with less tendency to depress respiration.[15–17] It is used as a sedative-hypnotic agent to induce sleep within 45 minutes and to provide sleep for 5 to 8 hours. It is, therefore, used for the treatment of mild and moderate insomnia, but it has also been used for daytime sedation in anxiety states. In adults the daily intake is 200 to 300 mg, which should not exceed 400 mg since greater amounts do not significantly increase the hypnotic activity. In children the effective dosage varies greatly, but treatment may be initiated with 50 mg and increased up to 200 mg.

Methyprylon is contraindicated in patients with known hypersensitivity to the drug. Caution should be exercised in the use of this drug in the presence of severe hepatic or renal insufficiency, although accumulation is not well recognized. Alcohol potentiates the effect of methyprylon.

Since methyprylon stimulates hepatic microsomal enzymes as well as δ-ALA synthetase, it should be avoided in patients with intermittent porphyria.

Intoxication

The lethal dose of methyprylon is still unknown. Reports of fatalities are rare in the literature.[14, 18–21] However, a lethal outcome has been reported after the ingestion of 6 gm (with coma lasting 120 hrs), with severe hypotension and respiratory failure.[14] On the other hand, patients have survived after ingestion of 9 gm, and one patient survived after the ingestion of 27 gm followed by gastric lavage.[18] The LD_{50} in mice is 900 mg/kg of body weight.[15, 16]

Toxic effects are observed after ingestion of upward of 800 mg. With ingestion of 3 gm of methyprylon, mild and moderate symptoms of intoxication are seen, while with ingestion of 6 gm intoxication is usually severe. At plasma levels of around 3 mg/dl, patients have subsequently wakened, while with levels of methyprylon above 6 mg/dl, respiratory arrest has been observed.[21]

Physical and psychologic dependence on methyprylon has been reported infrequently. However, prolonged use may lead to dependence of the barbiturate-alcohol type,[22] and withdrawal resembles the withdrawal of barbiturates and should be treated in a similar manner. Methyprylon withdrawal symptoms, such as confusion, restlessness, excitement, sweating, and polyuria, have been reported.[23] In addition, generalized convulsions, auditory and visual hallucinations, and psychotic behavior have been observed. For this reason, methyprylon should be cautiously administered to addiction-prone individuals or known drug abusers.

Methyprylon intoxication varies widely in its toxic manifestations. The commonly observed clinical signs are somnolence, confusion, coma, constricted pupils, respiratory depression, and hypotension. In addition, shock and pulmonary edema, increased deep tendon reflexes, and pyrexia all have been observed. In mild intoxication, "hangover," nausea, vomiting, epigastric distress, diarrhea, esophagitis, headache, and rashes have been observed.

Although hepatotoxicity has never been described in detail, jaundice and mild abnormalities in liver function tests have been seen. Hematologic indices are usually normal after overdose or after prolonged intake, although there have been a few isolated reports of neutropenia and thrombocytopenia, and their relationship to methyprylon remains undetermined. While electrocardiographic abnormalities have been reported,[19] they seem to have arisen from hypoxemic myocardial damage, as is observed in barbiturate intoxication. During the recovery phase, abdominal cramps have been reported.

Treatment. General principles of management as for barbiturate poisoning also should be employed in acute methyprylon intoxication. General management consisting of monitoring of respiration, pulse, and blood pressure should be instituted, as well as general supportive measures. Intravenous fluids and proper airway management form the mainstay of therapy. Hypotension, if present, should be treated properly with pressor agents. Analeptic agents have no place in the management of methyprylon overdosage because of their hazardous effects. In the recovery phase of methyprylon overdosage, excitement and convulsions have been observed, and in this setting antiepileptic drugs should be used, but with great caution. Steroids have been used in animals but there is no evidence for their successful human use.[20]

Gastric lavage should be employed for drug removal, with precautions taken to prevent aspiration of gastric contents into the trachea.

Several active drug removal methods have been employed for methyprylon intoxication. Forced diuresis is known not to be very effective,[24, 25] since in one patient, after the ingestion of 22 gm,[24] only 600 mg of methyprylon and its metabolites were collected in a 24-hr urine after forced diuresis.

Hemodialysis also has been employed in the treatment of methyprylon ingestion.[21, 24, 26–28] Methyprylon as intact drug is well dialyzable, and, despite the high plasma protein binding of metabolite II, good results have been obtained with hemodialysis. Dialysance values of 42 ml/min in vitro[28] and 20 to 80 ml/min in vivo have been reported.[21, 24] Hemodialysis has been shown to decrease blood levels from 20.9 mg/dl to 3.0 mg/dl, after 8.5 hours of hemodialysis,[24] or from 4.0 to 0.4 mg/dl after 9 hours of hemodialysis.[29] Elimination with hemodialysis is approximately 500 mg/hr.

Mandelbaum and Simon successfully treated a 57 year old woman after ingestion of 22.5 gm of methyprylon.[24] Through gastric lavage, 4.3 gm (20 per cent of the initial dose) was obtained; with an 8-hr hemodialysis, 3.6 gm (20 per cent of the remaining dose) was obtained; and in a 24-hr forced diuresis urine collection, only 600 mg (5 per cent of the remaining dose) was obtained. General indications for hemodialysis in methyprylon intoxication are ingestion of massive doses or protracted poor clinical state, dramatic deterioration of clinical status despite supportive management, and finally, a flat line on the electroencephalogram with prolonged coma.[12, 29]

It is uncertain whether coma is shortened by hemodialysis, and in some situations hemodialysis may be contraindicated (with severe hypotension).

Peritoneal dialysis also has been utilized in methyprylon poisoning,[10, 27] and a dialysance value of 15 to 20 ml/min has been reported.[10] It appears that peritoneal dialysis is less effective than other active drug removal techniques.

Activated charcoal hemoperfusion also has been used in the treatment of severe methyprylon intoxication. In two procedures, each lasting 2 hours, Chang and associates achieved a good clinical result with activated charcoal hemoperfusion. Clearance values of methyprylon approached 230 ml/min, with reduction of serum methyprylon from 18 mg/dl to 6 mg/dl.[30] Koffler and associates also have obtained good clinical results with the use of uncoated activated charcoal hemoperfusion.[11] Resin hemoperfusion has not yet been reported for the clinical treatment of methyprylon intoxication.

CARBROMAL AND BROMISOVAL

Carbromal (2-ethyl-2-bromo-butyryl-urea) is a mild nonbarbiturate sedative-hypnotic drug that has been available since 1910.[39–43] It was introduced under the trade name Adalin and since then has been widely used in many countries, particularly in Europe, whereas in the United States, as Carbrital, its use has been minimal. Carbromal is a brominated monoureide and has been known under the names of *bromadal, bromodiethylacetурea,* and *uradal.* In central Europe, carbromal was a nonprescription drug until 1978, when it became recognized that it accounted for 30 per cent of all drug intoxications with sedative-hypnotic agents and resulted in a large number of suicidal deaths. The drug then came under prescription.

Bromisoval (N-[2-bromo-3-methylbutyryl]-urea) is also a brominated monoureide with sedative-hypnotic properties, which was introduced in 1905. It has been available in many countries, but not the United States, although it was not as important or as widely used as carbromal. It is known under the trade name *Bromural* and also has the following synonyms: *bromisovalerylurea, bromylum,* and *bromvaletone.*

Pharmacology and Pharmacokinetics

Carbromal ($C_7H_{13}BrN_2O_2$, molecular weight = 237.1 daltons) and *bromisoval* ($C_6H_{11}Br N_2O_2$, molecular weight = 233.1 daltons) exist only in tablet form. After dissolution in the stomach, rapid absorption occurs, possibly facilitated by bromide ions, since debrominization by intestinal bacteria does not occur. Especially in overdosage, carbromal has dangerous properties in the stomach. Tablets

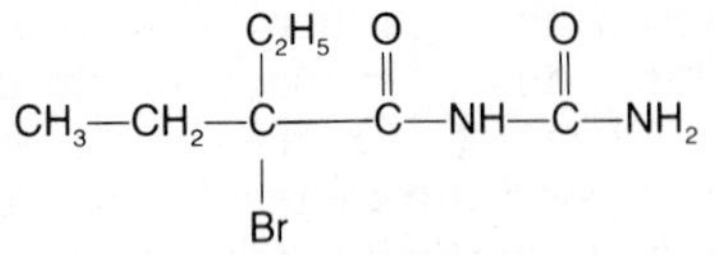

$$CH_3-CH_2-C(C_2H_5)(Br)-C(=O)-NH-C(=O)-NH_2$$

CARBROMAL

often coalesce to form a mass of drug material that prolongs the release of carbromal and prolongs the total absorption, often to several days. This renders therapy ineffective and necessitates the removal of the drug mass, either using gastrotomy or endoscopic removal. (See Chapter 1.) Metabolism of carbromal has been only partially explained,[44–47] despite the fact that in some of the first publications on carbromal clues to its metabolic degradation were given.[40, 42] Metabolism takes place mainly in the liver with the formation of eight carbromal metabolites, of which three are of major importance: bromoethylbutyramide, ethylbutyrylurea, and inorganic bromide. Unchanged carbromal and bromoethylbutyramide are the principal central nervous system depressants whereas ethylbutyrylurea is less important. While the role of inorganic bromide is still controversial, it is unknown whether inorganic bromide influences the narcotic action of the parent substance or acts only on peripheral nerves. Bromisoval biotransformation also occurs in the liver with formation of six metabolites, some of which do not contain bromide.[48]

Most carbromal and bromisoval metabolites are debrominated,[48] with debromination occurring most likely through addition of sulfhydryl-containing substances. It is presumed that bromide cleavage does not occur directly but only after conjugation with cystine.[49]

It is not certain what quantity of bromide is cleaved from the carrier substance,[49–51] but over a 2-week period, after intoxication, a considerable quantity of bromide ions is retained in the body. The clinical picture of chronic bromism differs considerably from acute bromocarbamide intoxication as seen with carbromal and bromisoval; it is probable that in acute bromoureide intoxication the amount of bromide in the drug is not very important and the sedative effect of the substance is not related to bromide effects, although it might be assumed that the bromide atoms influence the distribution behavior of the parent drug. Metabolically split bromide ions are distributed throughout the whole body, and, because of their large ion radius, they displace a portion of intracellular chloride.

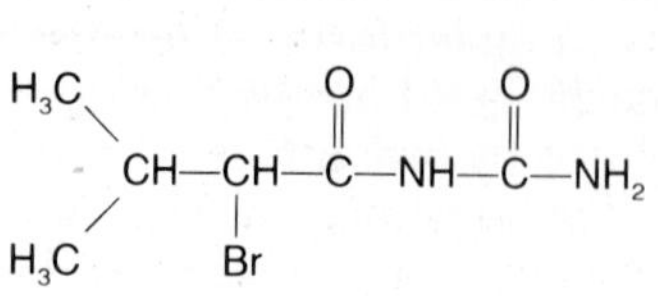

$$(H_3C)_2CH-CH(Br)-C(=O)-NH-C(=O)-NH_2$$

BROMISOVAL

A proportion of carbromal and bromisoval is excreted in an enterohepatic circulation and undergoes continuous reabsorption since only a little is found in the stool.[52] Both monoureides and the metabolites are well distributed to lipid-containing tissues such as brain and spinal cord. The drugs and the metabolites are poorly soluble in water and acid solutions but are highly soluble in alkaline solutions. Only small amounts of the unchanged carbromal and bromisoval are excreted in the urine, whereas the metabolites are predominantly excreted by the kidneys.[53–55]

Actions and Use

Carbromal and bromisoval are central nervous system depressants. Their action begins 30 to 60 minutes after ingestion, and the duration of activity is 6 to 12 hours, a duration comparable to that of phenobarbital. Therapeutic doses are 0.6 to 1.3 gm for carbromal and 0.3 to 0.9 gm for bromisoval.

Intoxication

With carbromal, toxic effects are seen with doses ranging from 3 to 5 gm. In human beings, the lethal dose lies between 10 and 30 gm,[56–62] mainly upward of 20 gm.[59, 61, 63] As for all hypnotic drugs, the absorbed amount is more important than the ingested dose. Mallach and Wirth, in an autopsy study, calculated from tissue concentrations that the lethal quantity absorbed lay between 1.3 and 7.7 gm.[64] After a 20-gm carbromal intoxication in one patient, at autopsy 12-gm masses of tablets, in caked form, were found in the gastrointestinal tract.

Hypothermia and concomitant ingestion of alcohol (which may increase the solubility of carbromal) are also important factors associated with fatalities. Recent experience with modern detoxification methods shows that the quantity of bromocarbamides ingested is less important than the time interval before initiation of therapy.

Prolonged use of carbromal leads to a dependence of the barbiturate-alcohol type.

It cannot be overstressed that the symptomatology in carbromal and bromisoval intoxication is in some respects different from intoxication with other sedative-hypnotic drugs. A particular difference is that even in the fully conscious state the patient may not be out of danger, since sudden cardiac arrest or respiratory failure may ensue. In addition, organ injury different or unknown from that with other substances is known to occur.

In severe intoxication, central nervous system manifestations range from drowsiness to coma. The electroencephalogram shows intermittent flat lines, "burst-suppression," or a completely flat line.[60, 62, 65, 66] Deep tendon reflexes may be normal, can be hyperactive, or can be suppressed. In the respiratory system, a major toxic feature of the poisoning is the development of "shock lung," possibly due to direct toxic action of the substance itself upon lung tissue or to toxic interstitial edema or microthrombosis caused by disseminated intravascular coagulation;[55, 59, 67–72] all these features may result in respiratory insufficiency or respiratory arrest.

Tachycardia is a common feature, in contrast to the bradycardia often observed with barbiturates. Other cardiac abnormalities include toxic cardiac disturbances, myocardial infarction, as well as decreased myocardial contractility (negative inotropic effect), arrhythmias, and increased vascular permeability.[45, 73]

Disseminated intravascular coagulation is fairly common,[74] as is toxic liver injury from hepatocellular necrosis.[74, 75] Renal failure, pancreatitis, transitory hyperglycemia, reduction of immune globulins,[76] ocular disturbances,[77] and nonthrombocytopenic purpura,[78, 79] possibly due to liver injury, have all been reported.

Systemic hypotension may be observed commonly following the development of other toxic symptoms. In almost 90 per cent of patients, hypothermia is seen, and this is often resistant to therapy. Gastric atony and intestinal slowing often prolong the absorption of carbromal or bromisoval.

Fatalities occur with the same frequency after cardiovascular collapse, pulmonary insufficiency, acute renal failure, or hypothermia resistant to the treatment.

Discussion of the toxicology of inorganic bromide is contained in Chapter 61. Briefly, the toxic activity of inorganic bromide is additive to the toxic activity of either carbromal or bromisoval and makes the clinical picture more complex and more confusing.

Treatment. The greatest danger from brominated monoureide intoxication is the development of complications in the late stage of poisoning. It follows, therefore, that early institution of the therapy is of major importance. Some investigators recommend the early administration of heparin (500 to 1000 units/hr) to prevent the effects of disseminated intravascular coagulation. In severely intoxicated patients, early endotracheal intubation and prophylactic artificial respiration utilizing PEEP should be introduced to prevent the development of "shock lung." In addition, prophylactic antibiotics may be in order since pneumonia is a regular feature of poisoning with these agents. The administration of digitalis glycosides may mitigate the negative inotropic effect of carbromal and its metabolites and also of bromisoval.

In view of the dangers of brominated monoureide intoxication, some attempt must be made to remove the drug from the body. *Gastric lavage* is the principal method for such removal. Despite the fact that carbromal and bromisoval in therapeutic doses are rapidly absorbed from the gastrointestinal tract, it is known that, in overdosage, the velocity of absorption is decreased due to both toxic gastrointestinal atony and formation of coalescent tablet masses.[63, 80–82] Carbromal and bromisoval tablets are formulated with a starchlike vehicle that under certain circumstances in acid gastric juice forms an almost insoluble tablet mass. Such a mass in the stomach leads to continuous drug absorption and consequent intoxication. Since both compounds contain inorganic bromide, the tablets are radiopaque; therefore, in patients in whom the suspicion of bromocarbamide ingestion is high, abdominal x-ray studies should be performed. If a plain film of the abdomen shows individual tablets, a prolonged gastric lavage (using 50 to 80 liters of lavage fluid) is recommended, with kneading of the abdomen during efflux of the lavage fluid. With larger drug concretions or masses, it is recommended that the drug masses be removed by endoscopic gastric lavage.[80, 81] This method requires a lot of time

(4 to 8 hours) but in most cases is effective for removing drug concretions. In rare cases, after ingestion of large quantities, the carbromal mass may reach the size of a tennis ball, or even larger; in this case gastrotomy or duodenotomy should be undertaken after a trial period of endoscopic lavage.[68, 80] It is felt that the risk of prolonged drug release from the toxic mass within the stomach is higher than the risk of gastrotomy.

Activated charcoal should be administered after gastric lavage is clear, since activated charcoal strongly absorbs the bromocarbamide left in the intestine. Catharsis may not be as useful as in other drug intoxications, since bromocarbamide produces gastrointestinal atony.

Forced diuresis with alkalinization of the urine has been another method used for removing drug from the body; however, the renal clearance of bromocarbamide and the metabolites is around 6 to 12 ml/min at a urine flow of 500 to 1000 ml/hr.[59, 83] Forced diuresis, therefore, has met with little clinical success.

Extracorporeal detoxification techniques also have been employed in the management of bromoureide intoxication. Hemodialysis has been successfully employed in the management of patients severely intoxicated with carbromal[47, 51, 59, 62, 68–70, 75, 84–89] and also in patients with severe bromisoval intoxication.[58, 75, 88, 90–92] Dialysance values of 85 to 100 ml/min have been reported,[93] and elimination of these bromoureides may reach 1 gm/hr.[59, 93] Hemodialysis is approximately seven times more effective than forced diuresis for drug removal. Grabensee and associates treated a severely intoxicated patient who had ingested 58 gm of carbromal; 2.2 gm of carbromal were eliminated with a 13-hour forced diuresis, and 13 gm were eliminated with two hemodialyses totaling 14 hours.[59]

Peritoneal dialysis also has been used in the treatment of bromoureide intoxication, but it is comparable to forced diuresis and therefore should be used only under certain circumstances.[59, 60]

Sorbent hemoperfusion also has been used successfully in the treatment of severe bromocarbamide ingestion. The bromocarbamide is well adsorbed onto activated charcoal,[94] although bromide itself is not adsorbed.[83, 95] Activated charcoal hemoperfusion has been shown to be an effective method for removing carbromal,[82, 85–87, 96, 97] bromisoval, and bromoethylbutyramide. Carbromal clearances achieved with activated charcoal hemoperfusion range from 110 ml/min to 150 ml/min, while bromoethylbutyramide clearance is about 130 ml/min; all these clearances are superior to those achieved with hemodialysis. Resin hemoperfusion, using the neutral resins Amberlite XAD-2 and XAD-4 also have been used in bromoureide poisoning.[44, 86] Carbromal clearances range from 160 to 250 ml/min, while bromoethylbutyramide clearances are approximately 170 ml/min. In contrast to activated charcoal, it is possible that organic bromide compounds are also adsorbed to the resin. The indications for hemoperfusion or hemodialysis are: (1) ingestion of a potentially lethal dose (greater than 20 gm); (2) deterioration in clinical status despite intensive supportive management;[101] (3) highly abnormal electroencephalogram;[60, 62, 66] (4) impairment of normal drug excretory mechanisms; and (5) the presence of drug concretion in the stomach with the potential for relapse into coma.

In summary, the effectiveness of the various detoxification methods—resin hemoperfusion, charcoal hemoperfusion, hemodialysis, peritoneal dialysis, and forced diuresis—is in the order of the following ratio: 20:13:10:1:1. Such techniques should be employed perhaps more aggressively in bromocarbamide intoxication since the possible complications develop more commonly from poisoning with these agents than with other drugs.

HYDROXYZINE (Atarax, Cartrax, Marax, Sedaril, Vistaril)

Hydroxyzine (piperazine) ($C_{21}H_{27}ClN_2O_2$, molecular weight = 374.9 daltons) is a tranquilizer closely related to the antihistamine *chlorcyclizine*. In recommended doses (25 mg), few side effects have been observed. The daily intake is normally up to 400 mg.

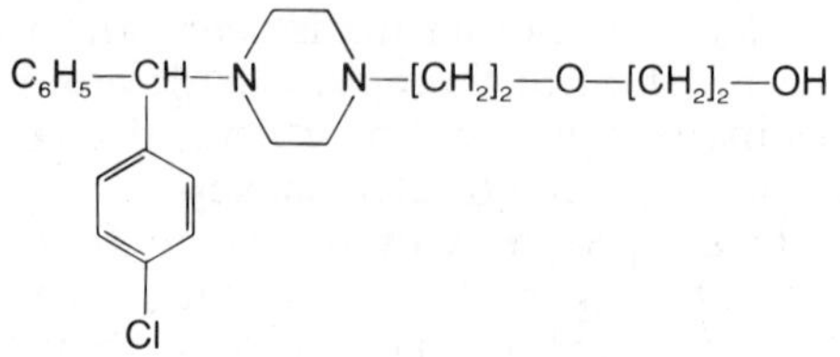

C_6H_5—CH—N(piperazine)N—$[CH_2]_2$—O—$[CH_2]_2$—OH (with 4-Cl-phenyl on CH)

HYDROXYZINE

Overdosage with 1 to 2 gm in adults has led to drowsiness and coma but with rapid recovery and without recognized sequelae. The oral LD_{50} in mice is 515 mg/kg and the estimated human lethal dose is between 25 and 250 mg/kg of body weight.

ORPHENADRINE (Myophen, Norflex, Norgesic, Norgesic Forte)

Orphenadrine (*N,N*-dimethyl-2-[α-o-tolylbenzoloxy]-ethylamine) is a drug that possesses weak anticholinergic and antihistaminic activity. It is claimed to have antispasmodic activity and produces slight euphoria. Its common preparations are as the citrate and as the hydrochloride. The use of orphenadrine in many countries is increasing, along with the increasing use of neuroleptic agents for psychotic and neurotic conditions. Although it was regarded as a "safe" drug, acute intoxication with orphenadrine has become commoner, and deaths have been reported.

Pharmacology and Pharmacokinetics

Orphenadrine ($C_{18}H_{23}NO$, molecular weight = 269.1 daltons; as hydrochloride, $C_{18}H_{23}NO$ HCl, molecular weight = 305.8 daltons; and as citrate, $C_{18}H_{23}NO$ $C_6H_8O_7$, molecular weight = 461.5 daltons) is readily and quickly absorbed from the gastrointestinal tract, with about 50 per cent of the drug being absorbed in 30 minutes and rapidly distributed to the tissues. Most of orphenadrine is metabolized, and eight metabolites are known. Within 3 days, 60 per cent of orphenadrine is excreted in the urine as metabolites, while approximately 8 per cent is excreted as unchanged drug.[99, 100]

Orphenadrine acts centrally (at the brain stem) and has been demonstrated in animals selectively to block facilitatory functions of the reticular activating system. It does not reduce myoneural block, nor does it affect crossed extensor reflexes. Through its anticholinergic, antihistaminic, and antispasmodic effects it reduces muscular rigidity. Though it has little effect on tremor, it reduces excessive salivation and perspiration. In daily doses of 200 to 400 mg, it is used to treat both the arteriosclerotic, idiopathic, and postencephalitic forms of paralysis agitans (Parkinson's disease). The drug is usually used in conjunction with other drugs.

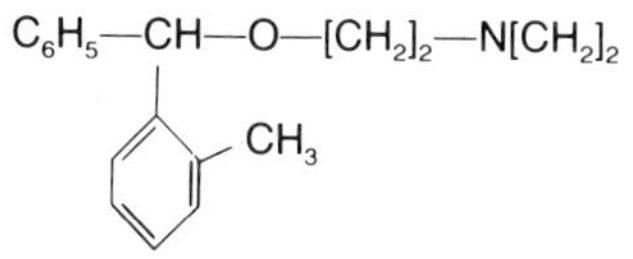
C6H5—CH—O—[CH2]2—N[CH2]2
CH3

ORPHENADRINE

Contraindications

In view of its mild anticholinergic action, orphenadrine should not be used in patients with glaucoma, pyloric and duodenal obstruction, achalasia, prostatic hypertrophy, or obstruction of the bladder neck. It is also contraindicated in patients with myasthenia gravis. In patients concomitantly receiving *propoxyphene*, mental confusion, anxiety, and tremor have been reported, and the combination of orphenadrine and propoxyphene is best avoided. Some preparations contain *orphenadrine, aspirin, phenacetin*, and *caffeine*; these combinations should be avoided in patients with sensitivity to these substances.

Intoxication

A number of papers have reported on acute intoxication with orphenadrine, including several deaths.[101–117] In mice, the LD_{50} is 25 to 200 mg/kg of body weight, while in adult humans, the LD_{50} of orphenadrine is thought to be around 2 to 3 gm,[115] or at plasma levels of 0.4 to 0.8 mg/dl. Death usually occurs 3 to 5 hours after the ingestion of a lethal dose. A dose of 1 gm is felt to induce toxicity and a plasma concentration of 0.2 mg/dl has been reported to be toxic;[117] however, a patient ingesting 100 mg/kg has survived.[116]

Toxic symptoms appear rapidly (2 to 4 hours after ingestion). The major toxic effects are in the central nervous system, cardiovascular system, and parenchymatous organs. Central nervous system symptoms and signs are spasticity, seizures, coma with or without hypoventilation, and shock. Additionally, epileptiform seizures, mydriasis, tremor, and nystagmus have been observed.

Cardiac toxicity is manifested by disturbances in cardiac rhythm and conduction,[102, 109–111, 114, 115] supraventricular tachycardia with a high rate, nonspecific changes in repolarization, and induction of high systemic blood pressure. The etiology of these disturbances is controversial; some think them due to changes in autonomic nervous system activity, while direct cardiotoxicity of orphenadrine has also been discussed.

Hepatic injury is known to occur, with hepatotoxicity being manifested in rises in serum transaminases, reduction of fibrinogen, and prolongation of prothrombin time.[104, 105, 109, 112] Histologically, centrilobular fatty degeneration and necrosis are observed. There are no known renal toxic effects.

Treatment. Treatment is similar to that of *atropine* poisoning. Gastric lavage should be employed but will be of benefit only shortly after ingestion because of the drug's rapid absorption—50 per cent of the therapeutic dose will be absorbed within 30 minutes. General treatment must be commenced as soon as possible. If respiratory insufficiency is present, assisted or controlled respiration should be instituted. Convulsions should be managed symptomatically with *diazepam*; in this context, slow-acting barbiturates are not recommended because of their effects on circulatory and respiratory function. Antiarrhythmic agents may be required for the management of supraventricular tachycardia. If there is evidence of hepatotoxicity, some investigators recommend steroids and standard management for potential liver failure.

Some have recommended forced diuresis; however, little evidence supports the use of forced diuresis in orphenadrine poisoning, since renal excretion of a therapeutic dose may take almost 3 days. Additionally, the pK_a for orphenadrine is 9.8, the drug is a base, and forced acid diuresis is appropriate. However, no clinical data are available on its efficacy. Since its molecular weight is low, orphenadrine removal by hemodialysis has been attempted. A 7-hr hemodialysis in a child who had ingested 3 gm demonstrated no clinical improvement, and no orphenadrine could be detected in the dialysate despite a high plasma level.[116] This may reflect the rapid distribution of drug to tissues within a short time after drug ingestion.

References

1. Langecker H, Schümann HJ, Junkmann K: Chemische und pharmakologische Eigenschaften des Aethinylcyclohexylcarbaminsaüreesters. Arch Exp Pathol Pharmakol *219*:130, 1953.
2. Clifford JM, Cookson JH, Wickham PE: Adsorption and clearance of secobarbital, heptabarbital, methaqualone, and ethinamate. Clin Pharmacol Ther *16*:376, 1974.
3. Davis RP, Blythe WB, Newton M, Welt LG: The treatment of intoxication with ethynyl carbamate (Valmid®) by extracorporeal hemodialysis: A case report. Yale J Biol Med *32*:192, 1959.
4. Kölwel E, Schrag G: Das klinische Bild der Valamidvergiftung. Münch Med Wschr *97*:1486, 1955.
5. Current concepts in therapy. Sedative hypnotic drugs. V. The nonbarbiturates. N Engl J Med *256*:314, 1957.
6. Greve W, Schönberg F: Sucht und Entziehungserscheinungen bei barbituratfreien Schlafmitteln. Dtsch Med Wschr *86*:1606, 1961.
7. Ellinwood CH, Ewing JA, Hoaken PCS: Habituation to ethinamate. N Engl J Med *266*:185, 1962.
8. Essig CF: Newer sedative drugs that can cause states of intoxication and dependence of barbiturate type. JAMA *196*:714, 1966.
9. Langecker H, Neuhaus G, Ibe K, Kessel M: Ein Suizid-Versuch mit Valamin mit einem Beitrag zur Elimination und Therapie. Arch Toxikol *19*:293, 1962.
10. Knepshield JY, Schreiner GE, Lowenthal DT, Gelfand MC: Dialysis of poisons and drugs—annual review. Trans Am Soc Artif Intern Organs *19*:590, 1973.
11. Koffler A, Bernstein M, La Sette A, Massry S: Fixed-bed charcoal hemoperfusion. Treatment of drug overdose. Arch Intern Med *138*:1691, 1978.
12. Kubicki ST, Bennhold I, Kessel M: Elektroencephalographische Untersuchungen während extrakorporaler Dialyse bei akuten Schlafmittelintoxikationen. Verh Dtsch Ges Inn Med *72*:620, 1966.
13. Pribilla O: Studien zur Toxikologie der Schlafmittel aus der Tetrahydropyridin- und Piperidin-Reihe. Arch Toxikol *18*:1, 1959.
14. Reidt WN: Fatal poisoning with methyprylon (Noludar), a non-barbiturate sedative. N Engl J Med *255*:231, 1956.
15. Loughlin EH, Mullin WGJ, Schwimmer J, Schwimmer M: Clinical studies on toxicity and on hypnotic and sedative effects of Ro 1-6463, Noludar. Int Rec Med *168*:52, 1955.
16. Pellmont B, Studer A, Jürgens R: Noludar, ein neues Schlafmittel der Piperidin-reihe. Schweiz Med Wschr *85*:350, 1955.
17. Schallek W, Kuehn A, Seppelin DK: Central depressant effect of methyprylon. J Pharmacol Exp Ther *118*:139, 1956.
18. Bernstein N, Strauss HK: Attempted suicide with methyprylon. JAMA *194*:1139, 1965.
19. Pellegrino ED, Henderson RR: Clinical toxicity of methyprylon (Noludar): Case report and review of 23 cases. J Med Soc New Jersey *54*:515, 1957.
20. Selye H: Protection against methyprylon overdosage by catatonic steroids. Can Anaesth Soc J *17*:107, 1970.
21. Xanthaky YG, Freireich AW, Matusiak W, Lukash L: Hemodialysis in methyprylon poisoning. JAMA *198*:1212, 1966.
22. Berger H: Addiction to methyprylon. Report of case of a 24-year-old nurse with possible synergism with phenothiazine. JAMA *177*:13, 1961.
23. Essig CF: Nonnarcotic addiction. Newer sedative drugs that can cause states of intoxication and dependence of barbiturate type. JAMA *196*:714, 1966.

24. Mandelbaum JM, Simon NM: Severe methyprylon intoxication treated by hemodialysis. JAMA *216*:139, 1971.
25. Simon NM, Krumlovsky FA: The role of dialysis in the treatment of poisoning. Am Soc Pharm Exp Ther *5*:1, 1971.
26. El-Badry A, Hassaballa A, El Ayadi A: Treatment of a nonbarbiturate hypnotic poisoning—methyprylon—by extra-corporeal haemodialysis (a description of a case). J Egypt Med Assoc *48*:605, 1965.
27. Maher JF, Schreiner GE: The dialysis of poisons and drugs. Trans Am Soc Artif Intern Organs *13*:369, 1967.
28. Yudis M, Swartz C, Onesti G, Ramirez O, Snyder D, Brest A: Hemodialysis for methyprylon (Noludar poisoning). Ann Intern Med *68*:1301, 1964.
29. Stölzer R: Veränderungen des Hirnstrombildes unter extrakorporaler Dialyse. Inaugural Dissertation, Freie Universität Berlin, 1963.
30. Chang TMS, Coffey JF, Lister C, Taroy E, Stark A: Methaqualone, methyprylon, and glutethimide clearance by the ACAC microcapsule artificial kidney: In vitro and in patients with acute intoxication. Trans Am Soc Artif Intern Organs *19*:87, 1973.
31. Basalt RC, Wright JA, Cravey RH: Therapeutic and toxic concentrations of more than 100 toxicologically significant drugs in blood plasma, or serum: A tabulation. Clin Chem *21*:44, 1975.
32. Epstein E: Allergy to dermatologic agents. JAMA *198*:517, 1966.
33. Fatteh A, Dudley JB: Letter to the editor. JAMA *219*:756, 1972.
34. O'Dea AE, Liss M: Suicidal poisoning by methapyrilene hydrochloride with documentation by paper chromatography. N Engl J Med *249*:566, 1953.
35. Rives HF, Ward BB, Hicks ML: Fatal reaction to methapyrilene (thenylene). JAMA *140*:1022, 1949.
36. Ulman KC, Groh RH: Identification and treatment of acute psychotic states secondary to the usage of over-the-counter sleeping preparations. Am J Psychiat *128*:1244, 1972.
37. Allin TG, Pogge RC: The use of azacyclonol and pipradrol in general practice. Intern Record Med Gen Pract Clin *169*:222, 1956.
38. Brown BB, Braun DL, Feldman RG: The pharmacologic activity of alpha-(4-piperidyl)-benzhydrol hydrochloride (azacyclonol hydrochloride): An ataractive agent. J Pharmacol Exp Ther *118*:153, 1956.
39. Hoppe J, Seegers K: Das Verhalten des Adalins im menschlichen Körper. Ther Gegenwart 456, 1911.
40. Impens E: Über die physiologische Wirkung eines bromhaltigen Hypnotikums, das Adalin. Med Klin *6*:1861, 1910.
41. Kwan J: Vergleichende Studien über hypnotische Wirkung und intravitale Zersetzung von Adalin, Bromural und Neuronal. Arch Intern Pharmacodyn *22*:331, 1912.
42. Schaefer P: Über Klinische Erfahrungen mit einem neuen Schlafmittel, dem Adalin. Münch Med Wschr *57*:2695, 1910.
43. Takeda S: Untersuchungen über das Bromural in Bezug auf seine Verteilung und Zersetzung im tierischen Organismus. Arch Intern Pharmacodyn *21*:203, 1911.
44. Butler TC: The metabolic fate of carbromal (2-bromo-2-ethyl-buturyl-urea). J Pharmacol Exp Ther *143*:23, 1964.
45. Vohland HW, Hadisoemarto S, Wanke B: Zur Toxikologie von Carbromal. I. Erfassung von Carbromal und wirksamen Metaboliten bei Ratte und Mensch. Arch Toxicol *36*:31, 1976.
46. Vohland HW, Hadisoemarto S, Wanke B: Zur Toxikologie von Carbromal. II. Pharmakokinetik von Carbromal und einigen wirksamen Metaboliten in der Ratte. Arch Toxicol *37*:275, 1977.
47. Vohland HW, Schirop Th, Barckow D, Kreutz G, Streichert B: Zur Toxikologie von Carbromal. III. Beteiligung wirksamen Metaboliten an der akuten Carbromalvergiftung des Menschen. Arch Toxicol *40*:211, 1978.
48. Rackwitz R, Lani K, Kiefhaber P, Halbritter R, Jahrmärker H: Röntgennachweis und Entfernung von Tablettenkonglomeraten bei Intoxikation mit bromhaltigen Hypnotika. Dtsch Med Wschr *102*:1181, 1977.
49. Alha AR: Debromination compounds of bromisoval and carbromal in poisoning. Ann Med Exp Fenn *41*:95, 1963.
50. Goodman LS, Gilman A, Goodman A: The Pharmacological Basis of Therapeutics. New York, Macmillan, 1980.
51. Gruska H, Beyer KH, Grosse G, Wolbergs E: Toxikologie einer mit extrakorporaler Hämodialyse behandelten Carbromalvergiftung mit letalem Ausgang. Arch Toxikol *28*:149, 1971.
52. Grosse-Brockhoff F: Pathologische Physiologie. 2nd ed. Berlin, Springer, 1969.
53. Deisel K: Untersuchungen zur Frage der Ausscheidung von Bromdiäthyl-acetylcarbamid im Harn. Inaugural Dissertation, Universität Erlangen, 1955.
54. Hauck G: Nachweis und Bestimmung von bromhaltigen Medikamenten in Blut, Urin, und Geweben. Arch Toxikol *23*:273, 1968.
55. Kisser W: Über den Nachweis und die quantitative Bestimmung bromierter Harnstoffderivate in der Toxikologie. Arch Toxikol *22*:404, 1967.
56. Benka A: Zwei Fälle von Vergiftung mit Monoureiden. Wien Klin Wschr *80*:715, 1968.
57. Degkwitz R: Leitfaden der Psychopharmakologie. Stuttgart, Wiss Verlagssgesellschaft, 1967.
58. Gibitz H-I, Homma H: Über einen Fall von tödlicher Bromuralvergiftung. Arch Toxikol *17*:295, 1959.
59. Grabensee B, Hofmann K, Jax W, Königshausen T, Schnurr E, Schröder E: Klinik und Therapie der Brom-carbamid-Vergiftung. Dtsch Med Wschr *97*:1911, 1972.
60. Gruska H, Becker V, Beyer K-H, Hüsten J, Kubicki ST, Weiss D: Klinik, Toxikologie und Therapie einer schweren Carbromalvergiftung mit letalem Ausgang. Arch Toxikol *26*:149, 1970.
61. Klimanek G: Vergiftungen durch Adalin und ihre Beziehungen zur gerichts-ärztlichen Praxis. Inaugural Dissertation, Universität Breslau, 1926.
62. von Baeyer H, Kunst H, Freiberg J, Grosser KD, Sieberth HG: Hämodialyse bei Schlafmittelvergiftungen. Dtsch Med Wschr *99*:189, 1974.
63. Steger F: Diagnostische Probleme um ein altbekanntes Schlafmittel: akute Carbromalvergiftung. Fortschr Med *83*:969, 1965.
64. Mallach JH, Wirth E: Über tödliche Vergiftungen mit Carbromal und Bromisoval. Med Welt *24*:212, 1973.
65. Königshausen T, Grabensee B: Das EEG als Routineuntersuchung im Verlaufe schwerer Schlafmittelvergiftungen. Akt Probl Intensivmed *2*(Suppl):220, 1976.

66. Kubicki ST, Bennhold I, Kessel M: Elektroencephalographische Untersuchungen während extrakorporaler Dialyse bei akuten Schlafmittelintoxikationen. Verh Dtsch Ges Inn Med *72*:620, 1966.
67. Barchow D, Schirop T, Zimmermann D, Loddenkemper R, Ohlmeier H, Korsukewitz J: Möglichkeiten zur Beeinflussung pulmonaler Komplikationen bei schweren Schlafmittelvergiftungen. Akt Probl Intensivmed 2(Suppl):204, 1976.
68. Blank HJ, Brinkmann OH, Berndt V: Differential therapie der Bromcarbamid-Vergiftungen. Münch. Med Wschr *120*:693, 1978.
69. Grabensee B, Hofmann K, Herms W, Schröder E, Goeckenjan G, Jax T, Königshausen T: Dialysebehandlung bei schweren Carbromalvergiftungen. Intensivmedizin *9*:344, 1972.
70. Grosse G, Hofer W, Gruska H, Beyer K-H, Kubicki ST, Schirop TH: Zur Klinik der schweren Carbromal-Intoxikation. Klin Wschr *52*:39, 1974.
71. Hoefer WG, Grosse G, Schirop TH, Gahl F, Fehr V: Klinisch-pathologische Aspekte der Carbromal-Intoxikation. *In* Tombergs HP: Poison Control/Engiftungsprobleme. Darmstadt, Steinkopf, 1974, p 88.
72. Mittermayer C, Hagdorn M, Böttcher D, Vogel W, Neuhof H, Mittermayer U: Bromcarbamidvergiftung, ein Modell der Schocklunge. Klin Wschr *50*:467, 1972.
73. van Essen EJ, Csanky-Treels IC, de Krom MC, Tjoeng MM: An acute bromisoval intoxication. Arch Toxicol *44*:299, 1980.
74. Königshausen TH, Förster H, Trobisch H, Borchard F, Grabensee B, Hausamen T-U: Toxisches Leberzerfallskoma mit Verbrauchskoagulopathie nach Carbromalintoxikation. Med Welt *21*(NF):330, 1976.
75. Mittermayer CH, Böttcher D: Lebercoma bei Bromcarbamidvergiftung. Med Welt *28*:1871, 1977.
76. Füsgen I: Eiweissveränderungen bei Bromcarbamidvergiftungen. Diagnostik *10*:721, 1977.
77. Berndt K, Piper HF: Augenveränderungen durch Intoxikation mit bromcarbamidhaltigen Schlafmitteln. Klin Monatsbl Augenheilkd *174*:123, 1979.
78. Feuerman EJ, Brodsky F: Nonthrombocytopenic purpura induced by carbromal. Cutis *23*:486, 1979.
79. van Ketel WG: Purpura door gebruik van carbromal. Ned T Geneesk *111*:252, 1967.
80. Feustel P, Kschowak U, Püschel K: Gastrotomie bei Bromcarbamidvergiftungen—eine zusätzliche Detoxikationsmassnahme. Med Welt *31*:1675, 1980.
81. Rauws AG: The comparison of bromisoval and carbromal in the rat. J Pharm Pharmacol *21*:287, 1969.
82. Voigtmann R, von Bayer H, Sieberth H-G: Hämoperfusion über Aktivkohle—eine wesentliche therapeutische Bereicherung bei schweren Intoxikationen. Med Welt *27*:752, 1976.
83. Wronski R, Butte W, Vollnberg W: In vivo und in vitro Untersuchungen zur Bromureid-Entgiftung durch forcierte Diurese. Hämodialyse und Hämoperfusion. A. Klinischer Teil. Intensivmedizin, *13*(Suppl):62, 1976.
84. Braun L, Backmann L: Indikationen zur Anwendung der extrakorporalen Hämodialyse der sogenannten künstlichen Niere. Landarzt *39*:1373, 1963.
85. Butte W, Vollnbeerg W, Wronski R: In vivo und in vitro Untersuchungen zur Bromureid-Entgiftung durch forcierte Diurese, Hämodialyse und Hämoperfusion. B. Experimenteller Teil. Intensivmedizin *13*(Suppl):63, 1976.
86. Castro LA, Fernandez JC, Müller-Jensen J, Samtleben W: Efficiency of different detoxification methods in removal of carbromal. Symposium on Hemoperfusion, Dialysate, and Diafiltrate Purification. Tutzing (GFR), Sept, 1978.
87. Graben N, Klöppel H-A: Metabolismus von Carbromal unter der Entgiftung mittels kombinierter Hämoperfusion und Hämodialyse. Med Klin *74*:229, 1979.
88. Ibe K, Bennhold I, Burmeister H, Kessel M: Die extrakorporale Hämodialyse bei schweren Schlafmittelvergiftungen. Berlin Med *16*:350, 1965.
89. Merrill JP, Weller JM: Treatment of bromism with the artificial kidney. Ann Intern Med *37*:186, 1952.
90. Edwards KDG, Whyte HM: Therapeutic uses of an artificial kidney. Med J Aust *1*:417, 1959.
91. Klinkmann H, Hübel A, Röhring A, Schwanz F, Tredt HJ, Precht K: Hämodialyse bei schweren Intoxikationen (Teil I). Dtsch Ges-Wesen *19*:60, 1964.
92. Schindera F, Gädecke R, Ross C, Höhmann H, Pohl KD, Sauer M, Bischoff W: Klinik und Therapie einer erfolgreich behandelten schweren Bromisovalerinyl-carbamid-, Methaqualon-, und Meprobamatvergiftung bei einem 12 Jahre alten Kind. Arch Toxikol *30*:95, 1973.
93. Grabensee B, Hofmann K, Jax W, Königshausen T, Schnurr E, Schröder E: Behandlungsmöglichkeiten bei Bromcarbamidintoxikationen. Med Welt *24*:693, 1973.
94. Armstrong C, Edwards KDG: Multifactorial design for testing oral ion exchange resins, charcoal and other factors in the treatment of aspirin poisoning in the rat. Efficacy of cholestyramine. Med J Aust *2*:301, 1967.
95. Lesch P, Blume U, Barthels M, Okonek S, Schmidt FW, Scheibe G, Sussmann P: Hämoperfusion durch verkapselte Aktivkohle zur Therapie exogener und endogener Intoxikationen. Klin Wschr *54*:509, 1976.
96. Grabensee B, Königshausen TH, Schnurr E: Behandlung schwerer Schlafmittelvergiftungen durch extrakorporale Hämoperfusion. Dtsch Med Wschr *101*:158, 1976.
97. Keusch-Beck M, Keusch G, Bammatter F, Schiffl H, Baumann PC, Binswanger U: Hämoperfusion mit Aktivkohle zur Behandlung von Intoxikationen. Schweiz Med Wschr *110*:1566, 1980.
98. Leber HW, Geissler RH, Faber M, Post D: Experimentelle Untersuchungen zur Frage der Effektivität von Dialyse und Hämoperfusion bei Bromcarbamidintoxikationen. Klin Wschr *54*:517, 1976.
99. Ellison T, Snyder A, Bolger J, Okun R: Metabolism of orphenadrine citrate in man. J Pharmacol Exp Ther *176*:284, 1971.
100. Hespe W, de Roos AM, Nauta WT: Investigation into the metabolic fate of orphenadrine hydrochloride after oral administration to male rats. Arch Intern Pharmacodyn *159*:180, 1965.
101. Editorial. Br Med J *3*:410, 1966.
102. Bijlsma UG, Harms AF, Funke ABH, et al: Pharmacology of beta-dimethylaminoethyl-2 methylbenzhydrylether hydrochloride (BS 5930). Arch Intern Pharmacodyn *106*:332, 1956.
103. Blomquist M, Bonnichsen R, Schubert B: Lethal orphenadrine intoxications: A report of five cases. Z Rechtsmed *68*:111, 1971.
104. Bosche J, Mallach HJ: Über anatomische und chemisch-toxikologische Befunde bei einer tödlichen Vergiftung durch Orphenadrin. Arch Toxicol *25*:76, 1969.

105. Bozza-Marrubine ML, Frigerio A, Ghezzi R: Two cases of severe orphenadrine poisoning with atypical features. Acta Pharmacol Toxicol *41*:137, 1977.
106. Buckle RM, Guillebaud J: Hypoglycaemic coma occurring during treatment with chlorpromazine and orphenadrine. Br Med J *4*:599, 1967.
107. Curry AA: Twenty-one uncommon cases of poisoning. Br Med J *1*:687, 1962.
108. Deceuninck F, Silberman RM, Veltman JGL: Een patiente met een psychose na intoxicatie met orfenadrine (Disipal). Ned T Geneesk *117*:25, 1973.
109. De Mercurio D, Chiarotti M, Giusti GV: Lethal orphenadrine intoxication: Report of a case. Z Rechtsmed *82*:349, 1979.
110. Heinonen J, Heikkila J, Mattila MJ, Takki S: Orphenadrine poisoning; A case report supplemented with animal experiments. Arch Toxicol *23*:264, 1968.
111. Malizia E, Sarcinelli L, Pascarella M, Ambrosini M, Smeriglio M, Russo A: Cardiotoxicity from orphenadrine intoxications in humans. Arch Toxicol (Suppl 4):425, 1980.
112. Monti GB, Cirulli A, Andreucci G, Malizia E: Su un caso di intossicazione grave da Orfenadrina e Reserpina. Riv Tossicol Sper Clin *1*:47, 1978.
113. Im Obersteg I, Im Baumler J: Über Suizide mit Psychopharmaka. Münch Med Wschr *106*:969, 1964.
114. Reboa E, Galetti A, Tarateta A, Soliani M: L'intossicazione acuta de orfenadrina nell'infanzia. Minerva Pediatr *30*:167, 1978.
115. Sangster B, van Heijst ANP, Zimmermann ANE: Vergiftiging door orfenadrine (Disipal). Ned T Geneesk *122*:988, 1978.
116. Stoddart JC, Parkin JM, Wynne NA: Orphenadrine poisoning; A case report. Br J Anaesth *40*:789, 1968.
117. Winek CL: Injury by chemical agents. *In* Tedeschi CG, Eckert WG, Tedeschi LG (eds): Forensic Medicine. Philadelphia, WB Saunders, 1977, p 1568.
118. Feuss CD, Gragg L: Quiactin: an adjunct in the treatment of chronic psychoses. Dis Nerv System *18*:29, 1957.
119. Warren MR, Thompson CR, Werner HW: Pharmacological studies on the hypnotic 2-ethyl-3-propyl-glycidamide. J Pharmacol Exp Ther *96*:209, 1949.

CHAPTER 47
ANTICHOLINERGICS

Mark Kirk, M.D.
Ken Kulig, M.D.
Barry H. Rumack, M.D.

The clinical syndrome of anticholinergic poisoning is one of the commonest and most easily recognized. A vast array of medications with significant anticholinergic properties exists. Many over-the-counter (OTC) cough and cold preparations as well as several classes of prescription medications have anticholinergic properties. A large number of common plants and mushrooms, some of which are deliberately ingested for their mind-altering effects, contain anticholinergic alkaloids. Early recognition of the toxic anticholinergic syndrome and prompt treatment based primarily on supportive care should bring a satisfactory conclusion, with a low incidence of morbidity.

PHARMACOLOGY

Acetylcholine is a neurohumoral transmitter found in a variety of neuroeffector junctions and synaptic sites. It is a neurotransmitter in the cerebral cortex and lower centers, such as the reticular activating system, in the postganglionic parasympathetic nervous system (muscarinic sites), and in the skeletal muscle motor end-plate and autonomic ganglia (nicotinic sites). The neurotransmitter is inactivated when metabolized at the synaptic cleft by the enzyme acetylcholinesterase.[1]

Anticholinergic drugs block the action of acetylcholine by competitive inhibition of the neurotransmitter for its receptor sites. In most cases of anticholinergic poisoning, the postganglionic cholinergic nerves are primarily affected, resulting in classic peripheral anticholinergic findings. This has been described as the parasympatholytic or muscarinic blocking effect.

Nicotinic and muscarinic receptors have been isolated in the central nervous system.

The central anticholinergic syndrome refers to an acute psychosis or delirium resulting from inhibition of central cholinergic transmission,[2–4] frequently accompanied by signs of peripheral muscarinic blockade. The autonomic ganglia are affected to a much smaller degree, and the nicotinic receptors at the motor end-plates are unaffected by drugs that block muscarinic sites.[1]

Agents That May Produce the Anticholinergic Syndrome

Both pharmaceutical agents and plants may cause significant anticholinergic toxicity. The most common classes of drugs with anticholinergic properties, along with representative examples, are listed in Table 47–1. For many of these medications—for example, the gastrointestinal antispasmodics or the local mydriatics—the anticholinergic properties are considered the desired therapeutic responses to the drug. Hence, many of the primary pharmacologic effects are not considered "toxic."

On the other hand, the desired therapeutic effects of many other medications—for example, the antipsychotics and the antiparkinsonism drugs—are less clearly related to peripheral anticholinergic symptoms. Thus mydriasis, constipation, tachycardia, and dry mouth are frequently considered manifestations of "toxicity." In addition to the anticholinergic toxicity exhibited by the cyclic antidepressants and antipsychotics in an overdose, these medications exhibit toxicity by additional pharmacologic actions. This makes the clinical presentation and management of the patient much more complicated. The more serious manifestations of an overdose may not be related to the anticholinergic effects. This should be kept in mind when considering treatment options.

Also of note is the possible synergism between medications with anticholinergic properties. Combined use of anticholinergic drugs results in an exponential summation of anticholinergic effects.[2, 19, 20] For example, antiparkinsonism medications, when given in combination with phenothiazines to prevent the occurrence of undesirable extrapyramidal reactions, greatly increase the incidence of toxic confusional states.[21] Small changes in the dose of either drug may precipitate the central anticholinergic syndrome in a previously unaffected individual.[22]

Table 47–1. CLASSES AND EXAMPLES OF PHARMACEUTICALS WITH ANTICHOLINERGIC PROPERTIES

ANTIHISTAMINES
chlorpheniramine (Chlor-trimeton)
cyclizine (Marezine)
dimenhydrinate (Dramamine)
diphenhydramine (Benadryl, Caladryl lotion)
ANTIPARKINSONISM MEDICATION
benztropine mesylate (Cogentin)
biperiden (Akineton)
trihexyphenidyl (Artane)
ANTIPSYCHOTICS
chlorpromazine (Thorazine)
chlorprothixene (Taractan)
haloperidol (Haldol)
prochlorperazine (Compazine)
thiothixene (Navane)
thioridazine (Mellaril)
trifluoperazine (Stelazine)
BELLADONNA ALKALOIDS AND RELATED SYNTHETIC COMPOUNDS
atropine sulfate
glycopyrrolate (Robinul)
scopolamine (including transdermal patches)
GASTROINTESTINAL AND GENITOURINARY ANTISPASMODICS
clidinium bromide (Librax)
dicyclomine (Bentyl)
hyoscyamine (Cystospaz)
hyoscyamine hydrobromide (Pyridium plus)
hyoscyamine sulfate (Donnatal)
L-hyoscyamine (Levsin)
propantheline bromide (Pro-Banthine)
LOCAL MYDRIATICS
cyclopentolate (Cyclogyl)
homatropine hydrobromide
tropicamide (Mydriacyl)
OTC ANALGESICS
cinnamedrine HCl (Midol)
OTC COLD REMEDIES
OTC SLEEP AIDS
diphenhydramine (Sominex)
doxylamine (Unisom)
CYCLIC ANTIDEPRESSANTS
amitriptyline (Elavil)
amoxapine (Ascendin)
desipramine (Norpramine)
doxepin (Sinequan)
imipramine (Tofranil)
nortriptyline (Pamelor)
protriptyline (Vivactil)
SKELETAL MUSCLE RELAXANTS
cyclobenzaprine (Flexeril)
orphenadrine (Norflex)

An unusual form of toxicity involves the use of transdermal scopolamine patches. Accidental instillation of the drug into the eye has occurred following manipulation of the patch. This has resulted in a unilateral fixed dilated pupil or bilateral fixed dilated pupils without focal neurologic changes.[23–25] Several cases of the central anticholinergic syndrome have been reported in adults and children utilizing the patches for treatment of motion sickness.[17, 26, 27] An additional method of systemic anticholinergic toxicity involves the absorption of ophthalmologic agents or nasal decongestants through the conjunctiva, nasal mucosa, or gastrointestinal tract.[5]

Scopolamine eye drops allegedly have been used to deliberately disorient subsequent victims of theft. Victims have been found naked, disoriented, hallucinating, and amnestic to the events prior to hospitalization. Scopolamine was believed to have been placed in a beverage ingested by the victim.[10] Many toxicologic laboratories do not routinely screen for scopolamine, therefore these patients had negative toxicologic screens.[10]

Both anticholinergic pharmaceuticals and plants may be abused. Intentional ingestion may produce euphoria and hallucinogenic effects. It has been proposed that a physiologic dependency and the development of withdrawal symptoms exist when the agent is withheld.[4] Among the most frequently reported anticholinergic drugs abused are the antiparkinsonism agents.[28] Drug seekers may feign extrapyramidal symptoms in order to receive additional anticholinergic agents.[4, 29–33]

A great many types of plants contain alkaloids that cause anticholinergic symptoms in humans (Table 47–2). Most of these are found in the family Solanaceae, which includes the genera *Atropa, Datura, Hyoscyamus, Lycium,* and *Solanum*. The principal alkaloids found in these plants include solanine, atropine (a racemic mixture of D- and L-hyoscyamine, of which only the levorotatory isomer is pharmacologically active), and scopolamine (L-hyoscine). The alkaloid content of each species and each plant varies greatly and depends on such parameters as the time of year, the available moisture, and the temperature. For this reason it is very difficult to determine predicted toxicity in relation to the amount and the origin of the plant material. Recreational abusers of anticholinergic mushrooms and *Datura stramonium* (jimson weed), for example, are unable to titrate the dose of ingested substance because of this tremendous biologic variability and therefore are prone to severe anticholinergic poisoning.

Table 47–2. EXAMPLES OF PLANTS CONTAINING ANTICHOLINERGIC ALKALOIDS[34–40]

Amanita muscaria (fly agaric)
Amanita pantherina (panther mushroom)
Atropa belladonna (deadly nightshade)
Cestrum nocturnum (night-blooming jessamine)
Datura sawolens (angle's trumpet)
Datura stramonium (jimson weed)
Hyoscyamus niger (black henbane)
Lantana camara (wild sage)
Lycium halimifolium (matrimony vine)
Myristica fragrans (nutmeg)
Physalis heterophylla (ground cherry)
Solanum carolinensis (wild tomato)
Solanum dulcamara (bittersweet)
Solanum nigrum (black nightshade)
Solanum pseudocapsicum (Jerusalem cherry)
Solanum tuberosum (potato)

Table 47–3. PERIPHERAL SYMPTOMS/SIGNS OF ANTICHOLINERGIC TOXICITY (MUSCARINIC BLOCKADE)

Tachycardia
Dry, flushed skin
Dry mucous membranes
Dilated pupils (variable)
Hyperpyrexia
Urinary retention
Decreased bowel sounds
Hypertension
Hypotension (may be late finding)

Symptoms/Signs of Anticholinergic Toxicity

The most commonly seen effects of anticholinergic poisoning can be conveniently divided into peripheral (Table 47–3) and central toxicity (Table 47–4).

The peripheral manifestations are the result of a receptor blockade of the postganglionic cholinergic nerves.[1] As a result, there is inhibition of secretions from the salivary glands, bronchioles, and sweat glands. Vasodilation occurs in peripheral blood vessels, especially those of the face. These changes produce dry mucous membranes and dry,

Table 47–4. CENTRAL ANTICHOLINERGIC SYNDROME

Confusion
Disorientation
Loss of short-term memory
Ataxia
Incoordination
Psychomotor agitation
Picking or grasping movements
Extrapyramidal reactions
Visual/auditory hallucinations
Frank psychosis
Coma
Seizures
Respiratory failure
Cardiovascular collapse

hot flushed skin. Elevated body temperature is related to the inability to sweat. Alteration of temperature regulation in the CNS probably also plays a role.[1] Blocking the response of the pupillary sphincter muscles and ciliary muscles of the lens results in markedly dilated pupils and inability to accommodate.[1] In a mixed ingestion, the pupillary findings may be variable and confuse the clinical picture. The vagal effects of the heart are blocked, producing a sinus tachycardia that is frequently but not always seen as one of the earliest and most reliable signs of muscarine blockade.[41] Arrhythmias other than sinus tachycardia are infrequently seen in patients poisoned by anticholinergic agents.[16] Parasympathetic control of the urinary bladder and the gastrointestinal tract is inhibited, causing urinary retention and hypoactive or absent bowel sounds. This altered peristalsis may result in prolonged symptoms secondary to reduced drug absorption.

Anticholinergic delirium, or the central anticholinergic syndrome, is commonly seen but frequently misdiagnosed because the physician may not look for the associated peripheral signs. The presentation is characteristically that of an acutely developing organic brain syndrome with disorientation, agitation, impairment of short-term memory, nonsensical or incoherent speech, meaningless motor activity such as repetitive picking at bed clothes or grabbing at nonexistent objects, and hallucinations.[2, 17, 19, 20, 42] The hallucinations are frequently visual, although tactile and auditory hallucinations occur.[43]

In overdose, both central and peripheral anticholinergic signs are commonly present. However, on occasion the central anticholinergic syndrome may be seen without peripheral signs being evident.[13, 38, 44, 45] This seems more likely to occur in the elderly and those with underlying organic brain syndrome.[20] The syndrome has been seen even when therapeutic doses of anticholinergic drugs have been administered to these risk groups.[13, 20] In several instances, other diagnoses were initially obtained, including dementia[44] and psychotic depression in elderly patients.[13] In a child, varicella encephalitis was considered prior to the diagnosis of central anticholinergic syndrome.[9, 19]

Because of the extreme degree of disorientation, a history of ingestion is frequently impossible to obtain. For this reason a thorough physical examination for common peripheral anticholinergic findings is of vital importance. All medications available to the patient should be inspected, if possible, and any history obtainable from friends or relatives concerning drug abuse or abuse of hallucinogenic plants (particularly jimson weed and mushrooms) may be of value. A history of recent travel and the use of scopolamine patches should be sought. The diagnosis of acute poisoning in the acutely psychotic patient can only be made if it is thought of, and the presence of classic peripheral anticholinergic findings is frequently the key.

As with many other ingestions, the toxicology screen has limited value. Agents producing anticholinergic toxicity may not be part of a routine screen, resulting in a significantly toxic patient and a negative toxicologic screen.[10] Quantitative levels of many anticholinergic agents are usually unobtainable and do not correlate well with symptoms. It takes time to obtain results from a toxicologic screen, therefore the tests are useful for confirmation of the presence of a drug and not as a tool for determining treatment. Treatment should be based on information obtained from the clinical evaluation.

Treatment

The majority of patients poisoned by anticholinergic agents will be adequately treated with supportive care.

Because of inhibitory effects of the anticholinergics on gastrointestinal motility, gastric emptying procedures theoretically may be effective even when patients present many hours after an ingestion. Charcoal is effective for preventing further drug absorption for many of these drugs. Because of the inhibition of gastrointestinal motility, continued and delayed drug absorption may occur. Multiple doses of activated charcoal may play a key role in preventing continued absorption. However, the development of an ileus may limit the use of multiple doses of activated charcoal.

The major controversy surrounding the treatment of the anticholinergic syndrome concerns the use of physostigmine. Physostigmine is a naturally occurring alkaloid obtained from the West African vine *Physostigma venenosum*.[1] It is a reversible cholinesterase inhibitor. After a single dose of physostigmine, the action of acetylcholine is potentiated at the postganglionic parasympathetic and the central cholinergic neuroreceptors, reversing in part the action of anticholinergic agents. Physostigmine crosses the blood-brain barrier and is capable of reversing coma, delirium, seizures, and the extrapyramidal signs of the central anticholinergic syndrome.[2, 6, 8, 11, 16, 40, 46–48] Peripherally, physostigmine may reverse the tachycardia, mydriasis, ileus, and urinary retention seen secondary to muscarine blockade.[16, 35]

One must be cautious, however, about the indiscriminate use of physostigmine,[49, 50] which may precipitate seizures, cholinergic crisis, or bradyarrhythmias and asystole. In one series of 26 patients receiving intravenous physostigmine, 3 (12 per cent) suffered seizures thought to be secondary to this medication (although 17 had ingested a tricyclic antidepressant), and one had bradycardia.[50]

A series of 41 patients taking intentional overdoses of maprotiline showed that 6 of 7 patients treated with physostigmine developed seizures.[51] The investigators concluded that the use of physostigmine should be abandoned in overdosages of maprotiline and other cyclic antidepressants. In a similar series, 2 of 21 patients receiving physostigmine had seizures after administration, and 2 developed cholinergic symptoms (hypersalivation in one patient, bradycardia and hypotension in the other). The investigator concluded that because patients with anticholinergic symptoms usually do well with supportive therapy alone, physostigmine has "little part to play in routine management."[52] Another case report describes a patient poisoned by *Datura stramonium* (jimson weed), who developed atrial fibrillation and a short run of ventricular tachycardia 45 minutes after administration of physostigmine.[39] Similar case reports in two patients ingesting tricyclic antidepressants suggest that physostigmine was responsible for the ultimate development of asystole in two complicated resuscitative efforts.[53] This conclusion has been challenged, however.[54] In an additional case report, an 85 year old man developed ventricular ectopy 30 minutes after receiving 1 mg of physostigmine.[55]

Although the use of physostigmine has been proposed in the treatment of cyclic antidepressant poisoning,[8, 50, 56] there may be dangers associated with its use. In addition to anticholinergic effects on the myocardium, the cyclic antidepressants prolong AV conduction, have a strong myocardial depressant action, and prevent the re-uptake of norepinephrine.[8, 57] These additional effects are thought to contribute to the severe cardiovascular compromise often seen with an overdose of these drugs. The anticholinergic effects of cyclic antidepressants are unlikely to produce cardiovascular compromise in and of themselves. Therefore treatment with physostigmine would be of limited value in cyclic antidepressant toxicity, and evidence exists that it may worsen toxicity.[51, 53, 58, 59] The potential risks associated with physostigmine are greater than the benefits gained from its use in cyclic antidepressant toxicity.[50]

Therefore, there is little question that physostigmine can be dangerous if given inappropriately (that is, in the absence of severe anticholinergic findings) or too quickly.[16] The relative contraindications to the use of physostigmine include asthma, gangrene, cardiovascular disease,[61] and mechanical obstruction of the gastrointestinal or urogenital tract.[1, 16] It has been suggested that atropine be available and given in one half the dose of physostigmine should cholinergic toxicity develop.[16, 62]

The use of glycopyrrolate, a pure peripheral anticholinergic agent, has been proposed as an alternative treatment to the cholinergic toxicity of physostigmine.[3]

The suggested doses of physostigmine are

- For children: A range of 0.02 to 0.06 mg/kg as a therapeutic dose;[62, 63]
- For adults: 1 to 2 mg slowly IV; may be repeated every 10 minutes until cessation of the life-threatening condition. The maximum dose should not exceed 4 mg in a half hour.

The indications for the use of physostigmine in cases of anticholinergic poisoning should be restricted to

- Pronounced hallucinations and agitation in which patients may be dangerous to themselves or others;
- Supraventricular arrhythmias clearly resulting in hemodynamic instability when other attempts to control heart rate (i.e., beta-blockers) have failed or are felt to be too risky in a particular patient;
- Intractable seizures.

Whenever physostigmine is used it should

(1) be given very slowly (over 5 minutes) intravenously; (2) not be given merely to "wake the patient up"; (3) be used only in a setting where advanced life support is available; (4) be used only when definite severe anticholinergic findings are present; and (5) always be preceded and followed by good supportive care.

SUMMARY

Anticholinergic poisoning is common and should be included in the differential diagnosis of any patient with an altered mental status. Evaluation of the vital signs and finding physical signs associated with the anticholinergic syndrome are often the clues to the diagnosis. The majority of patients with anticholinergic poisoning will have a good outcome with simple observation and meticulous attention to supportive care. It is important to emphasize that physostigmine must be used cautiously. Treatment with physostigmine should be limited to severe cases.

References

1. Gilman AG, Goodman LS, Rall TW, et al: The Pharmacological Basis of Therapeutics. 7th ed. New York, Macmillan, 1985.
2. Hall RC, Fox J, Stickney SK, Gardner ER, Perl M: Anticholinergic delirium: Etiology, presentation, diagnosis and management. J Psychedel Drugs *10*:237–241, 1978.
3. Granacher RB, Baldessarini RJ: Physostigmine: Its use in anticholinergic syndrome with antidepressant and antiparkinson drugs. Arch Gen Psychiat *32*:375, 1975.
4. Dilsaver SC: Antimuscarinic agents as substances of abuse: A review. J Clin Psychopharmacol *8*:14–22, 1988.
5. Adler AG, McElwain GE, Merli GJ, Martin JH: Systemic effects of eye drops. Arch Intern Med *142*:2293–2294, 1982.
6. Bergman KR, Pearson C, Waltz GW, et al: Atropine-induced psychosis. An unusual complication of therapy with inhaled atropine sulfate. Chest *78*:891, 1980.
7. Bernstein S, Leff R: Toxic psychosis from sleeping medicine containing scopolamine. N Engl J Med *277*:638, 1967.
8. Callaham M: Tricyclic antidepressant overdose. J Am Coll Emerg Phys *8*:413–425, 1979.
9. Filloux F: Toxic encephalopathy caused by topically applied diphenhydramine. J Pediatr *108*:1018–1020, 1986.
10. Goldfrank L, Flomenbaum N, Lewin N, Weisman R, Howland M, Kaul B: Anticholinergic poisoning. J Toxicol Clin Toxicol *19*:17–25, 1982.
11. Granacher RP, Baldessarini RJ, Messner E: Physostigmine treatment of delirium induced by anticholinergics. Am Fam Phys *13*:99, 1976.
12. Hooper RG, Conner CS, Rumack BH: Acute poisoning from over-the-counter sleep preparations. J Am Coll Emerg Phys *8*:98, 1979.
13. Johnson AL, Hollister LE, Berger PA: The anticholinergic intoxication syndrome: Diagnosis and treatment. J Clin Psychiatry *42*:313–316, 1981.
14. Lumpkin J, Watanabe AS, Rumack BH, Peterson RG: Phenothiazine-induced ventricular tachycardia following acute overdose. J Am Coll Emerg Phys *8*:476, 1979.
15. Manoguerra AS, Ruiz E: Physostigmine treatment of anticholinergic poisoning. J Am Coll Emerg Phys *5*:125, 1976.
16. Rumack BH: Anticholinergic poisoning: Treatment with physostigmine. Pediatrics *52*:449–451, 1973.
17. Wilkinson JA: Side effects of transdermal scopolamine. J Emerg Med *5*:389–392, 1987.
18. Woodward GA, Baldassano RN: Topical diphenhydramine toxicity in a five year old with varicella. Pediatr Emerg Care *4*:18–20, 1988.
19. Hall RC, Feinsilver DL, Holt RE: Anticholinergic psychosis: Differential diagnosis and management. Psychosomatics *22*:581–587, 1981.
20. Hvizdos AJ, Bennett JA, Wells BG, Rappaport KB, Mendel SA: Anticholinergic psychosis in a patient receiving usual doses of haloperidol, desipramine, and benztropine. Clin Pharm *2*:174–178, 1983.
21. Cole J: Atropine-like delirium and anticholinergic substances. Am J Psychiatry *128*:898, 1972.
22. Forrester PA: An anticholinergic effect of general anesthetics on cerebrocortical neurons. Br J Pharmacol *55*:275, 1975.
23. Price BH: Anisocoria from scopolamine patches. JAMA *253*:1561, 1985.
24. Patterson JH, Ivest J, Greganti MA: Transient bilateral pupillary dilation from scopolamine discs. Drug Intell Clin Pharm *20*:986–987, 1986.
25. McCrary JA, Webb NR: Anisocoria from scopolamine patches. JAMA *248*:353–354, 1982.
26. Klein BL, Ashenburg CA, Reed MD: Pediatr Emerg Care *1*:208, 1985.
27. Sennhauser J: Toxic psychosis from transdermal scopolamine in a child. Lancet *2*:1033, 1986.
28. Smith JM: Abuse of the antiparkinson drugs: A review of the literature. J Clin Psychiatry *41*:351–354, 1980.
29. MacVicar R: Abuse of antiparkinsonian drugs by psychiatric patients. Am J Psychiatry *134*:809–811, 1977.
30. Craig DH, Rosen P: Abuse of antiparkinsonian drugs. Ann Emerg Med *10*:98–100, 1981.
31. Kaminer Y, Munitz H, Wijsenbeek H: Trihexyphenidyl (Artane) abuse: Euphoriant and anxiolytic. Br J Psychiatry *140*:473–474, 1982.
32. Pullen GP, Best NR, Maquire J: Anticholinergic drug abuse: A common problem. Br Med J *289*:612–613, 1984.
33. Crawshaw JA, Mullen PE: A study of benzhexol abuse. Br J Psychiatry *145*:300–303, 1984.
34. Faquet RA, Rowland KF: "Spice cabinet" intoxication. Am J Psychiatry *135*:860, 1978.
35. Goldfrank L, Melinek M: Locoweed and other anticholinergics. Hosp Phys *8*:18, 1979.
36. Gowdy JM: Stramonium intoxication. Review of symptomatology in 112 cases. JAMA *221*:585, 1972.
37. Hall RC, Popkin MK, McHenry LE: Angel trumpet

psychosis: A central nervous system anticholinergic syndrome. Am J Psychiatry *134*:312, 1977.
38. Klein-Schwartz W, Oderda GM: Jimson weed intoxication in adolescents and young adults. Am J Dis Child *138*:737–739, 1984.
39. Levy R: Arrhythmias following physostigmine administration in jimson weed poisoning. J Am Coll Emerg Phys *6*:107, 1977.
40. Mikolich RJ, Paulson GW, Cross CJ: Acute anticholinergic syndrome due to jimson seed ingestion. Ann Intern Med *83*:321, 1975.
41. Greenblatt DJ, Shader RI: Anticholinergics. N Engl J Med *288*:1215, 1973.
42. Pall H, Czech K, Kotzaurek R, et al: Experiences with physostigmine salicylate in tricyclic antidepressant poisoning. Acta Pharmacol Toxicol *41*:171, 1977.
43. Perry PJ, Wilding DC, Juhul RP: Anticholinergic psychosis. Am J Hosp Pharm *35*:725–727, 1978.
44. Moreau A, Jones BD, Banno V: Chronic central anticholinergic toxicity in manic depressive illness mimicking dementia. Can J Psychiatry *31*:339–340, 1986.
45. Richmond M, Seger D: Central anticholinergic syndrome in a child: A case report. J Emerg Med *3*:453–456, 1985.
46. Burks JS, Walker JE, Rumack BH, Oh JE: Tricyclic antidepressant poisoning. Reversal of coma, choreoathetosis, and myoclonus by physostigmine. JAMA *230*:1405, 1974.
47. Duvoisin RC, Katz R: Reversal of central anticholinergic syndrome in man by physostigmine. JAMA *206*:1963, 1968.
48. Nattel S, Bayne L, Ruedy J: Physostigmine in coma due to drug overdose. Clin Pharmacol Ther *25*:96, 1979.
49. Mofenson HC, Greensher J: Physostigmine as an antidote: Use with caution. Pediatrics *87*:1011, 1978.
50. Walker WE, Levy RC, Henenson IB: Physostigmine—its use and abuse. J Am Coll Emerg Phys *5*:335, 1976.
51. Knudsen K, Heath A: Effects of self poisoning with maprotiline. Br Med J *288*:601–603, 1984.
52. Newton RW: Physostigmine salicylate in the treatment of cyclic antidepressant overdosage. JAMA *231*:941, 1975.
53. Pentel P, Peterson CD: Asystole complicating physostigmine treatment of tricyclic antidepressant overdose. Ann Emerg Med *9*:588, 1980.
54. Kulig K, Rumack BH: Physostigmine and asystole. Ann Emerg Med *10*:228, 1981.
55. Dysken MW, Janowsky DS: Dose-related physostigmine-induced ventricular arrhythmia: Case report. J Clin Psychiatry *46*:446–447, 1985.
56. Munoz RA, Kuplic JB: Large overdoses of tricyclic antidepressants treated with physostigmine salicylate. Psychosomatics *16*:77–78, 1975.
57. Sullivan JB, Rumack BH, Peterson RG: Management of tricyclic antidepressant toxicity. Top Emerg Med *1*:67, 1979.
58. Vance MA, Ross SM, Millington WR, Blumberg JB: Potentiation of tricyclic antidepressant toxicity by physostigmine in mice. Clin Toxicol *11*:413–421, 1977.
59. Wiezorek WD, Kastner I: Effects of physostigmine on acute toxicity of tricyclic antidepressants and benzodiazepines in mice and rats. Arch Toxicol *5*(suppl):133–135, 1982.
60. Pentel PR, Benowitz NL: Tricyclic antidepressant poisoning: Management of arrhythmias. Med Toxicol *1*:101–121, 1986.
61. Nilsson E, Meretoja OA, Neuvonen P: Hemodynamic responses to physostigmine in patients with a drug overdose. Anesth Analg *62*:885–888, 1983.
62. Daunderer M: Physostigmine salicylate as an antidote. Int J Clin Pharmacol *18*:523–535, 1980.
63. Lagerfelt J: Atropine poisoning in early infancy due to Eumydrin drops. Br Med J *285*:300, 1982.

CHAPTER 48
CAFFEINE AND NICOTINE

Kenneth V. Iserson, M.D., MBA, FACEP

Caffeine and nicotine are two of the most widely used drugs in the United States today. Caffeine is perhaps the most prevalent psychotropic drug in the United States and Canada. Approximately 20 per cent to 30 per cent of people surveyed who use caffeine state they use more than 500 to 600 mg (5 to 10 cups of coffee) daily. And, although only 56 per cent of Americans 10 years or older drink coffee (down from 77 per cent in 1957), it is still estimated that over 1 billion kilograms of coffee are consumed in the United States annually.[1, 2]

The history of caffeine use generally parallels that of coffee use, which appears to have developed in Arabia. After early, unsuccessful attempts to suppress its use, coffee quickly spread to Ethiopia, Turkey, the Near

East, and North Africa. Finally, it reached Europe and from there spread to North and South America. Other sources of caffeine arose somewhat simultaneously. These included tea in China, the kola nut in West Africa, the cocoa bean in Mexico, and the ilex plant (maté) in Brazil. During the Civil War, cassina, also known as the Christmas berry tree, yaupon, or the North American tea plant, was very popular as a coffee substitute in the Confederacy during the blockade.[3]

The history of nicotine use in modern times parallels that of the use of tobacco. The earlier history of tobacco is generally obscure. Cigarettes, the most common form of tobacco used in the United States, have shown a progressive decrease in use. In 1976, 37 per cent of American adults smoked cigarettes, whereas in 1985 only 30 per cent smoked.

Coincident with Americans' increasing concern over the health risks of cigarettes, the nicotine content per cigarette has declined in the United States from an average of 2.3 mg per cigarette in 1950 to an average of 1.3 mg per cigarette in 1980.[4]

CAFFEINE

Sources

Caffeine is found in many different preparations, including beverages such as coffee, tea, and cola drinks; prescription medications such as Cafergot and Darvon compound; over-the-counter (OTC) analgesics, many cold preparations, and OTC stimulants. Caffeine also enters the diet, although in a relatively insignificant amount, in other foods, such as coffee-flavored ice creams, chocolate bars, and foods with chocolate flavoring. Caffeine also can be secreted in breast milk. One medical indication for caffeine has been neonatal apnea; in this situation, caffeine is being replaced with theophylline and theobromine compounds.

The amount of caffeine in each dietary or drug source can vary considerably (Table 48–1). Although instant coffee has been reported to contain between 60 and 99 mg of caffeine per cup, brewed coffee has been reported to contain between 85 and 139 mg per cup. Tea is reported to have between 30 and 75 mg per cup, and cola drinks between 40 and 60 mg per glass. In prescription medications such as Cafergot, caffeine ranges up to 100 mg per tablet.

Chocolate contains both caffeine and the caffeine-like agent theobromine. One average-sized 1.55-oz milk chocolate bar contains about 10 mg of caffeine and 70 mg of theobromine.[5] Theobromine has many of the same physiologic effects as caffeine. Ingestion of excess chocolate has been reported to produce headaches and trigger migraines.

In OTC stimulant preparations, 100 mg of caffeine per tablet is in the low range; these preparations often contain up to 200 mg per tablet. Although the "look-alike" drugs—those designed to resemble prescription amphetamines and containing combinations of caffeine, phenylpropanolamine, and/or ephedrine—were banned by the FDA in 1983, they are still available illicitly and are still causing deaths.[6]

The estimated average daily intake of caffeine for American adults is approximately 211 mg. This approximates two cups of regular coffee per day.[1, 7, 8]

Pharmacology and Pharmacologic Use of Caffeine

Caffeine is an alkaloid structurally identified as 1,3,7-trimethylxanthine. It is a naturally occurring xanthine derivative that can be found in tea leaves, kola nuts, cocoa beans, and coffee beans. A white, odorless crystalline powder, it was first extracted from plants in 1820 by Friedlieb Runge.

Caffeine is quickly absorbed from the oral, rectal, and subcutaneous routes, all of which test almost equally toxic in cats, rats, and dogs. It is rapidly metabolized and excreted in the urine in almost equal parts as 1-methyluric acid and 1-methylxanthine. About 10 per cent of the caffeine is excreted unchanged. The half-life of caffeine is about 3.5 hours. In patients who have overdosed, elimination appears to be nonlinear.[9] The half-life in an overdosed adult patient can be as long as 9 hours.[10] The half-life of caffeine is reduced by smoking and prolonged by pregnancy.[11, 12]

Caffeine appears to stimulate the synthesis and release of catecholamines, especially norepinephrine. A mild decrease in glucose tolerance following caffeine ingestion may be due to the catecholamine and subsequent cyclic adenosine monophosphate increase.

Table 48–1. APPROXIMATE AMOUNTS OF CAFFEINE PER COMPOUND

SOURCES	AMOUNT (*mg*)	DOSE
Beverages		
Brewed coffee	85–139	Cup
Instant coffee	60–99	Cup
Decaffeinated coffee	1–4	Cup
Tea	30–75	Cup
Cola drinks	40–60	Glass
Cocoa	6–60	Cup
Prescription medications		
Cafergot	100	Tab
Darvon compound	32	Tab
Fiorinal	40	Tab
Tri-Aqua	92	Tab
OTC analgesics		
Anacin, aspirin compound, Bromo-Seltzer, Cope, Empirin compound, Midol, Vanquish	32	Tab
Excedrin	65	Tab
OTC cold preparations	15–65	Tab
OTC stimulants	100–200	Tab

(Adapted from Syed IB: The effects of caffeine. J Am Pharm Assoc *16*:568, 1976; and Wells SJ: Caffeine: Implications of recent research for clinical practice. Am J Orthopsychiatr *54*:375–389, 1984.)

Caffeine also induces hepatic drug-metabolizing enzymes. The significance of this action in humans is not known at this time.

In neonates, it is known that the pharmacokinetics of caffeine differs markedly from that in normal adults. Until an infant is 5 to 6 months of age, caffeine has a markedly lengthened half-life. In the child under 3 weeks of age, the half-life is approximately 100 hours, which is almost 30 times that of the adult. At 1 to 2.5 months of age, half-life is reported to be approximately 20 hours, whereas at 3 to 4.5 months it is approximately 15 hours. This is certainly a contributing factor to some of the reported cases of caffeine toxicity in neonates.[13–15]

Whether tolerance to the stimulant effects of caffeine occurs is questionable. Alcohol and caffeine reportedly have no interaction.

Normal Uses/Biologic Effects

Caffeine is used in beverages; prescription medications, including those used for migraine headaches and analgesic relief; OTC analgesics and cold preparations; and OTC stimulants. It is also used widely as a respiratory stimulant in the treatment of idiopathic apnea in the premature neonate.

Caffeine has wide-ranging physiologic effects (Table 48–2). It is distributed throughout all organ systems in proportion to body water. Passing the blood-brain barrier as well as the placental barrier readily, caffeine is known to stimulate the medullary, respiratory, vasomotor, and vagal centers. At high doses, caffeine stimulates the spinal cord. Whether regular consumption of caffeine diminishes its stimulant effects is a significant question.

Caffeine stimulates the parietal cells, resulting in increased gastric secretion. However, the "heartburn" associated with coffee intake is thought to be due to gastrointestinal reflux in persons with a diminished lower esophageal sphincter pressure. Although a link has been suggested through the years, there is no good evidence associating caffeine or coffee with any form of cancer.[16–18] There appears to be an increased risk for late spontaneous abortions in women who consume more than 151 mg of caffeine daily in all forms.[19]

Of the xanthines, caffeine is the least effective in terms of cardiac stimulation, coronary artery dilation, diuresis, and smooth muscle relaxation. However, one study suggests that

Table 48–2. PHYSIOLOGIC EFFECTS OF CAFFEINE

Cardiac muscle stimulant
Central nervous system stimulant
Diuretic
Plasma free fatty acid and glucose elevation
Smooth muscle relaxant
Stimulant of gastric acid secretion

caffeine may have a ventricular dysrhythmogenic effect.[20] Skeletal muscles, however, are stimulated more by caffeine than by the other xanthines.

Chronic Toxicity

As noted, patients with caffeine-induced psychosis, whether it be delirium, manic depression, schizophrenia, or merely an anxiety syndrome, in most cases will be hard to differentiate from patients who have the other organic or nonorganic psychoses. The differential diagnosis also is important in hyperkinetic children who have been exposed to caffeine.

A common presentation in office practice or ambulatory hospital patients is the complaint of an "irregular heartbeat and nervousness." An electrocardiogram usually documents frequent premature ventricular contractions. Cessation of caffeine intake "cures" the patient.

Caffeine toxicity can be both acute or, more commonly, chronic or can be evidenced in a withdrawal state. Despite caffeine's wide use, few deaths have been reported in the literature (Table 48–3). This may be due to both the emetic effect of caffeine and general ignorance among lay people concerning the lethal effect of caffeine.

Although no fatalities have been reported from coffee drinking, some of the first reports of toxicity from caffeine were reported by Curschmann in 1873,[21] Fort in 1883,[22] and Lewin in 1897.[23] Some reports dealt with ingestions of a high-strength, coffee-like preparation of coffee beans containing up to 5 gm of caffeine. The acute oral lethal dose of caffeine in the adult is considered to be greater than 10 gm, or more than 1750 mg per kg. The toxic dose is considerably lower in children. Toxic symptoms can be produced in the adult with 1 gm or more of oral caffeine.

The spectrum of clinical toxicity of caffeine poisoning is rather wide. Many of the symptoms are based on the stimulatory effect on the central nervous and circulatory systems. Initial effects may include insomnia, dyspnea, and excitement progressing to a mild delirium. There may be alternating states of consciousness and muscle twitching. Subsequent symptoms may include diuresis; arrhythmias, including tachycardias and extrasystoles; palpitations; and photophobia. Severe pulmonary edema is common. The terminal event, which in some cases has been the initial presentation, is normally seizures. Hyperglycemia, hypokalemia, and ketonuria also have been reported.

Children show differing symptoms by age. Neonates appear to show hyperirritability,

Table 48–3. DATA FROM KNOWN CAFFEINE FATALITIES

AGE	(REFERENCE)	SEX	ESTIMATED DOSE (*gm*)	ROUTE OF ADMINISTRATION	BLOOD LEVEL (*mg/dl*)	CONCURRENT DRUGS
15 mo	77	M	18.0	PO	104.0	
5 yr	78	F	3.0	PO	15.85	
Teenager	79	M		PO	1.1	(at 20 hr)
19 yr	80	F	18.0	PO	18.1	
19 yr	81	F		PO	13.0	Ephedrine
20 yr	82	F		PO	18.2	Ethanol; phenobarbital; phenylpropanolamine; ephedrine
21 yr	83	F		PO	24.0	Ethanol
21 yr	81	M		PO	34.4	Ephedrine
21 yr	81	M		PO	14.7	Ephedrine
21 yr	81	F		PO	25.1	Ethanol
23 yr	84	F		PO	18.9	Ethanol; ephedrine
23 yr	81	M		PO	18.4	Ethanol; benzodiazepine
27 yr	85	F	6.5–12.0	PO		Ethanol
34 yr	86	F		PO	10.6	Phenobarbital
35 yr	87	F	3.2	IV		
42 yr	88	F		PO	11.4	
44 yr	82	F		PO	26.4	Ethanol; ephedrine
45 yr	89	F	50.0	PO	7.9	
47 yr	90	F	19.0	PO		
61 yr	91	M	18.0	PO		

opisthotonos, muscular hypertonicity alternating with hypotonicity, upward ocular deviation, rigidity, and purposeless lip movements. Older children show alternating levels of consciousness with intermittent agitation, muscle fasciculations, hypertension, tachycardia, hyperirritability with tonic posturing, hyperglycemia with ketonuria, and emesis or hematemesis. In children, it appears that the most significant initial finding is the hyperirritability. Complete recovery after acute toxicity, at least in the adult, has occurred within 6 hours.[24, 25]

Subacute or chronic toxicity has been reported in a number of cases. One cola drinker became "eccentric and stubborn, and at times exhilarated and depressed and would show lapses of memory and deportment with indifference to the usual conventionalities and proprieties."[26] One cola-induced psychosis has been reported.[27] Twenty cases of "syndrome of coffee" have been described, with symptoms including tinnitus, nausea, projectile vomiting, arrhythmia, and inability to walk.[28] Cases of caffeine-induced manic depression and coffee-induced exacerbation of schizophrenic processes also have been observed.[28, 29] Caffeine can exacerbate anxiety or trigger panic attacks in some agoraphobics.[30] Caffeine-induced psychoses have ranged from increased agitation and insomnia to frank psychosis. The psychoses have appeared to relate to previous underlying psychiatric disease. This has been shown in some cases to be improved, and antipsychotic or antidepressant agents have been shown to be more effective when caffeine intake is reduced or discontinued.[31] In acute states, discontinuance of caffeine relieved the psychiatric symptoms.

An association of caffeine with an increase in anxiety and depressive symptoms also has been reported. These appeared to respond well simply to elimination of caffeine.

The most chronic type of caffeine toxicity is the drug-dependent state associated with subsequent caffeine withdrawal headaches, increased sleepiness, and decreased alertness.[32] The exact mechanism of this headache type is not clear. Caffeine also has been reported as possibly arrhythmogenic in a small portion of the population. However, its relationship to coronary artery disease is still unclear.

Acute Toxicity

Acute toxicity is initially manifested by abdominal cramps, nausea, diarrhea, and vomiting. This will often cause the elimination of part of the ingested substance. In severe cases, arrhythmias are frequently seen.

The cause of death in acute toxicity is not clear. However, it is known that a number of deaths have occurred after seizures. Normal antiseizure medications should be used to control seizures if they occur. Some cases of significant pulmonary edema also have been noted. Whether this was an initial causative factor of death or occurred subsequent to arrhythmias is unknown.

Laboratory findings include hyperglycemia, glycosuria, ketonuria, hypokalemia, and leukocytosis. Analysis of caffeine levels is usually performed by either gas-liquid chromatography or high-pressure liquid chromatography. Some reports have indicated that analysis by the latter method is preferable because the lower quantities that would be sought in human toxicity are better measured by high-pressure liquid chromatography.[33] However, unless the method is modified to separate out the levels of the various metabolites, a falsely elevated theophylline level (one metabolite) can result.[9]

Management of Caffeine Overdose

In most adult and pediatric cases of acute caffeine toxicity in which the patient survived, only symptomatic and supportive therapy was used. It appears that if advanced life support techniques are needed in resuscitation, the prognosis is extremely grave. However, if only seizure control is needed, diazepam (Valium) and phenobarbital appear to work well. Beta-blockers may be useful for managing tachyarrhythmias but may unmask alpha-mediated hypertension. Removal of any caffeine still in the gastrointestinal tract is beneficial, as is the administration of activated charcoal and a cathartic.[34] In one severe case, resin hemoperfusion was effective.[35] Exchange transfusions eliminated the CNS symptoms and markedly lowered the serum caffeine level in a premature infant who had a severe iatrogenic overdose.[15]

NICOTINE

Sources

Nicotine is now most commonly used in the form of tobacco, as an animal tranquilizer, and in insecticides. Its use in insecticides has greatly diminished in the past several decades. Lobeline, an alkaloid similar to nicotine, is found in antismoking tablets and lozenges. This alkaloid has similar physiologic actions to nicotine but is less potent.

Common blends of tobacco vary in their nicotine content. The average cigarette contains 15 to 25 mg of nicotine. However, the smoke contains less than 3 mg per cigarette; the smoke of most nonfiltered brands contains 1.2 to 2.4 mg, and filtered brands contain between 0.2 and 1.0 mg. Up to 90 per cent of the nicotine in "mainstream smoke" will be absorbed by the smoker.

Other related alkaloids are found in cigarette smoke. However, the most potent and most prevalent is nicotine. It appears to be responsible for virtually all the pharmacologic effects of cigarettes.[36, 37]

The nicotine in cigar smoke appears to be absorbed more readily through oral mucosa because of the increased pH of the smoke. The total nicotine absorbed, however, appears to be considerably less than for cigarettes.[38, 39] The amount of nicotine absorbed from the new smoke-free cigarettes is about one-eighth that of regular cigarettes. Most nicotine is absorbed through the oral mucosa.[40]

Chemistry, Pharmacology, and Pharmacologic Uses of Nicotine

Nicotine is an alkaloid obtained from the dry leaves and stems of the *Nicotiana* species. These include *N. tabacum* (cultivated tobacco), *N. attenuata* (wild tobacco), *N. glauca* (tree tobacco), and *N. trigonophylla* (desert tobacco). Lobeline, the chief constituent of Indian tobacco, is obtained from the leaves and tops of *Lobelia inflata*.[41]

Nicotine is 1-methyl-2-(3-pyridyl) pyrolidine. It is a colorless, strongly alkaline, volatile liquid and is responsible for the brown color and the classic odor of tobacco. Nicotine is water soluble and is readily absorbed through the oral mucosa, from the GI tract and respiratory system, and through the intact skin. It is 80 to 90 per cent detoxified in the body—mainly in the liver but also in the kidneys and lungs. The major metabolic product of nicotine is cotinine. Lesser amounts of nitrosamines, which have been implicated as carcinogens, are produced during the tobacco-aging process.[42] These metabolites, as well as the nonmetabolized nicotine, are excreted in the urine. Elimination is complete in about 16 hours. An acid urine increases urinary excretion approximately fourfold. Nicotine is also excreted in the milk of lactating women.[39, 43]

Sex-dependent differences in the metabolism of nicotine in nonsmokers as well as changes in the metabolism of smokers have been found. This may be a basis of tolerance to nicotine.[6]

Considerable evidence that nicotine is a highly addictive substance exists. Nicotine withdrawal symptoms can be prolonged and highly debilitating.[44]

Normal Uses of Nicotine

Nicotine is used in tobacco in multiple ways. It is commonly used to smoke, as snuff, and to chew. However, nicotine has also been used in tobacco form as enemas and poultices.

Nicotine is no longer used as a constituent of commercial agricultural insecticides. Now less than 1 per cent of current home garden insecticides are nicotine-based, and these are usually found in powder form. Black Leaf-40 (Black Leaf Products Company, Elgin, IL) is the most common nicotine-containing insecticide in use.

More recently, nicotine sulfate has been used as a dog control agent. It contains approximately 285 mg of nicotine per ml; nicotine sulfate is also used in animal-tranquilizing darts, at a strength of 240 mg of nicotine per ml.[45, 46]

Adverse Effects of Cigarette Smoking

There are many adverse health effects from cigarette smoking. Some of these may be caused by the nicotine content. However, others may be due to the multiple effects from the hundreds of components of cigarette smoke. Nicotine itself stimulates antidiuretic hormone secretion in the posterior pituitary; this action may enhance fluid retention and antagonize diuretic medications. Other elements in the cigarette smoke stimulate microsomal liver enzymes and can increase the dosage requirements of many medications.

Cigarette smoking appears to increase the risk of developing tardive dyskinesia in patients who receive chronic neuroleptics. This increased risk cannot be completely explained by the increased dosages often required for patients who take neuroleptics.[47] Cigarette smoking has also been shown to increase both the time to healing and the recurrence of duodenal ulcers.[48]

Overall, cigarette smoking has been identified as the chief avoidable cause of death in the United States. It is estimated that in 1984 alone, there were 315,120 deaths in the United States attributable to smoking. This number totaled nearly 1 million years of potential life lost, even though it did not include the 100,570 deaths due to cigarette-initiated fires.[49]

Specific diseases for which cigarette smoking is a significant factor in mortality include cancer of the trachea, lung, bronchus, pharynx, larynx, esophagus, lip, oral cavity, bladder, cervix,[49] and pancreas.[17, 18] Cigarette smoking also contributes significantly to deaths from cardiac arrest, aortic aneurysms, chronic bronchitis, emphysema, and chronic airways obstruction.[49]

Toxic States

Nicotine is one of the most lethal poisons known. However, despite its common use, there is a very low incidence of reported toxicity. The incidence was much higher in the 1920s and 1930s when nicotine insecticides were more commonly used. This low incidence of reported poisonings may be due to the strong emetic effect of nicotine as well as the slow absorption rate when oral nicotine (chewing tobacco) is ingested.[50–52]

At present, virtually all acute toxicity from nicotine is being reported from the ingestion of cigarettes. In the United States, more than 90 per cent of toxic exposures from cigarettes are reported in children under 5 years of age. A recent report from Germany states that most of that country's nicotine poisoning cases are in the 7 month to 2 year old age range. In Nigeria, a herbal drug containing nicotine used to treat acute seizures has been shown to increase morbidity and mortality in the pediatric age group.[53, 54]

More than 95 per cent of reported cigarette toxicity is either "asymptomatic" (70 per cent) or "mild" (25 per cent).[55] Most of the recently reported serious toxic states from nicotine have been experienced by animal handlers who have been accidentally exposed to animal control agents.[45, 46] However, there have been suicide attempts with nicotine.[56] No nicotine-related deaths have been reported in recent years.

The constellation of symptoms in nicotine poisoning can be quite varied. In oral ingestion, there is often a burning sensation in the mouth and throat, followed by increased and sometimes profuse salivation, nausea, vomiting, abdominal pain, and sometimes diarrhea. These symptoms can also appear but are less prominent when exposure is by means other than oral ingestion. Other cholinergic signs such as profuse diaphoresis, miosis, and transient cardiac standstill or paroxysmal atrial fibrillation may occur. Headache, dizziness, auditory and visual disturbances, confusion, weakness, and incoordination also have been reported.[57, 58]

Excitement of the CNS is often evidenced by tremors and eventually tonic-clonic convulsions. A later stage develops accompanied by mydriasis, hypotension, and coma. If death occurs, it is usually due to respiratory arrest and will normally occur in less than 1 hour. Often, less than 5 minutes elapses from the time of ingestion to respiratory arrest. It has been hypothesized that, in lower doses, respiratory paralysis is a peripheral effect and in higher doses, it is a central effect.[34, 45, 51, 59–61]

Although a "lethal" dose of nicotine in humans is estimated to be between 30 and 60 mg (0.5 to 1.0 mg/kg), survival following ingestions of 2 gm and 4 gm has been reported.[62] On the other hand, toxic effects have occurred with doses as small as 2 mg.[63]

Acute use of nicotine gum may cause alterations in the oral mucosae such as sore mouth and blistering, hiccups, and various disturbances of the gastrointestinal system.[64] Hiccups, nausea, and flatulence are due to rapid gum chewing and swallowing of nicotine. Chronic ingestion of nicotine gum is often associated with atrial fibrillation. This often occurs with higher than normal doses or more rapid chewing than is recommended.[65, 66] Chronic nicotinism, including tolerance and psychiatric symptoms, can occasionally be seen in bulimics and schizophrenics.[67, 68]

A milder form of nicotine toxicity is the so-called green-tobacco sickness, a condition that occurs in young, nonsmoking tobacco workers who handle uncured tobacco when it is wet. Symptoms are subjectively described as being like those of seasickness.[69, 70] Wearing gloves while harvesting tobacco seems to reduce the prevalence of this syndrome.[71] A mild, reversible neuromuscular syndrome has also been reported with standard recreational use of both smoking and chewing tobacco.[72]

Postmortem examinations of patients who have succumbed often have revealed congestion and hyperemia of the brain, meninges, and many visceral organs. In some cases, hemorrhages have been described in the gastrointestinal tract and lungs.[57, 58]

Clinical Recognition of Toxicity/Differential Diagnosis

Patients presenting with nicotine poisoning may have a variety of symptom complexes. They may be having violent emesis, be actively seizing, or be in respiratory arrest. The history, if it can be obtained, may make the diagnosis. However, treatment will be successful if oriented toward the symptom complex. Strong cholinergic physical findings will be present and may be a major guide to treatment.

Nicotine levels can be routinely identified by urine chromatographic toxicology screens. Also, blood level determinations for nicotine are available in some centers. It has been reported that in smokers, nicotine blood levels are usually less than 0.03 mg per dl. In cases of fatality, 1 mg per dl or more of nicotine has been found.

A method reported to be accurate for determining nicotine levels in plasma is the rapid gas-liquid chromatographic method of Feyerabend and coworkers;[73] however, apparently a naturally occurring substance similar to nicotine interferes with exact determination.[73]

Management of Toxicity

Initial treatment of a patient who has ingested a nicotine substance will depend on the stage of toxicity at examination. If a relatively minor ingestion has occurred without emesis (rare), emesis should be induced. Charcoal definitely should be administered following emesis because this agent is very effective in treating nicotine poisoning. If gastric lavage is to be carried out, a 1:5000 solution of potassium permanganate should be used. Water also could be used for lavage. If respiratory arrest has ensued, artificial ventilation should be continued until spontaneous ventilation resumes. Seizures can be controlled with diazepam or barbiturates or both. Early cholinergic symptoms like excess salivation and diarrhea can be reversed with the judicious use of atropine.

The excretion of nicotine and its metabolites can be increased by acidifying the urine.

Patients who live 4 hours after ingestion usually will survive, although a few deaths have occurred as late as 2 days after ingestion. In both experimental and reported cases, respiratory support for patients who are not in cardiac arrest when they are first seen is successful in saving most victims of nicotine poisoning.

Because significant poisonings have occurred through skin exposure, it is important to remove all the chemical from contact with the skin and flush the skin thoroughly.[13, 74, 75]

Even in mild cases of nicotine poisoning, late symptoms such as ileus and urinary retention may need to be treated with appropriate drainage and supportive therapy. Green-tobacco sickness usually responds to antihistamines/antiemetics and time.

References

1. Greden JF, Fontaine P, Lubetsky M, Chamberlin K: Anxiety and depression associated with caffeinism among psychiatric in-patients. Am J Psychiatr *135*:963, 1978.
2. International Coffee Organization: United States of America: Coffee Drinking Study—Winter 1982. London, International Coffee Organization, 1982.
3. Graham DM: Caffeine–Its identity, dietary sources, intake and biological effects. Nutr Rev *36*:97, 1978.
4. The health consequences of smoking—The changing cigarette. MMWR *30*:48, 1981.
5. Spiller GA (ed): The Methylxanthine Beverages and Foods: Chemistry, Consumption, and Health Effects, New York, Alan R. Liss, 1984, p 171.
6. Beckett AH, Gorrod JW, Genner P: The effect of smoking on nicotine metabolism in vivo in man. J Pharm Pharmacol *23*:62S, 1971.

7. Gilbert RM: Caffeine consumption. Prog Clin Biol Res *158*:185–213, 1984.
8. Syed IB: The effects of caffeine. J Am Pharm Assoc *16*:568, 1976.
9. Fligner CL, Opheim KE, Ainardi V: Caffeine and its metabolites in caffeine overdose cause falsely elevated serum theophylline measurements. Vet Hum Toxicol *26*(suppl 2):11–28, 1984.
10. Shaul PW, Farrell MK, Maloney MJ: Caffeine toxicity as a cause of acute psychosis in anorexia nervosa. J Pediatr *105*:493–495, 1984.
11. Parsons WD, Neims A: Effect of smoking on caffeine clearance. Clin Pharmacol Ther *24*:40–45, 1978.
12. Parsons WD, Pelletier JG, Neims AH: Caffeine elimination in pregnancy. Clin Res *24*:625, 1976.
13. Kulkarmi PB, Dorand RP: Caffeine toxicity in a neonate. Pediatrics *64*:254, 1979.
14. Warszawski D, Gorodischer R, Kaplanski J: Comparative toxicity, caffeine and aminophylline in young and adult rats. Biol Neonate *34*:68, 1978.
15. Perrin C, Debruyne D, Lacotte J, Laloum D, Bonte J-B, Moulin M: Treatment of caffeine intoxication by exchange transfusion in a newborn. Acta Paediatr Scand *76*:679–681, 1987.
16. Pozniak PC: The carcinogenicity of caffeine and coffee: A review. J Am Diet Assoc *85*:1127–1133, 1985.
17. Norell SE, Ahlbom A, Erwald R, Jacobson G, Lindberg-Navier I, Olin R, Tornberg B, Wiechel K-L: Diet and pancreatic cancer: A case-control study. Am J Epidemiol *124*:894–902, 1986.
18. Gorham ED, Garland CF, Garland FC, Beneson AS, Cottrell L: Coffee and pancreatic cancer in a rural California county. West J Med *148*:48–53, 1988.
19. Srisuphan W, Bracken MB: Caffeine consumption during pregnancy and association with late spontaneous abortion. Am J Obstet Gynecol *154*:14–20, 1986.
20. Sutherland DJ, McPherson DD, Renton DW, Spencer CA, Montague TJ: The effect of caffeine on cardiac rate, rhythm, and ventricular repolarization. Chest *87*:319–324, 1985.
21. Curschmann H: Ein Fall von Kaffee-intoxication. Deutsche Klin *11*:377, 1873.
22. Fort JA: Des effects physiologiques du cafe; d'apres des experiences faites sur l'auteur. Bull Gen Therap Paris 1883, p 550.
23. Lewin L: Coffea arabica L. In Lehrbuch der Toxikologie. Berlin, Urban and Schwarzenberg, 1897, p 311.
24. Banner W, Czajka P: Acute caffeine overdose in the neonate. Am J Dis Child *134*:495, 1980.
25. Mace J: Toxicity of caffeine. J Pediatr *92*:354, 1978.
26. Orendorff O: Letter to the editor. JAMA *62*:1828, 1920.
27. Shen WW, D'Souza TC: Cola-induced psychotic organic brain syndrome. Rocky Mountain Med J *76*:312–313, 1979.
28. McManamy MC, Schube PG: Caffeine intoxication. Report of a case the symptoms of which amounted to a psychosis. N Engl J Med *215*:616, 1936.
29. Mikkelsen EJ: Caffeine and schizophrenia. J Clin Psychiatr *39*:732, 1978.
30. Breier A, Charney DS, Heninger GR: Agoraphobia with panic attacks. Arch Gen Psychiatr *43*:1029–1036, 1986.
31. Neil JF, Himmelhoch JM, Mallinger AG, Mallinger J, Hanin I: Caffeinism complicating hypersomnic depressive episodes. Compr Psychiatr *19*:377, 1978.
32. Griffiths RR, Bigelow GE, Liebson IA: Human coffee drinking: Reinforcing and physical dependence producing effects of caffeine. J Pharmacol Exp Ther *239*:416–425, 1986.
33. Bonati M, Castelli D, Latini R, Garattini S: Comparison of gas-liquid chromatography with nitrogen-phosphorus selective detection in high performance liquid chromatography methods for caffeine determination in plasma and tissues. J Chromatogr *164*:109, 1979.
34. Pentel P: Toxicity of over-the-counter stimulants. JAMA *252*:1898–1903, 1984.
35. Zimmerman PM, Pulliam J, Schwengels J, MacDonald SE: Caffeine intoxication: A near fatality. Ann Emerg Med *14*:1227–1229, 1985.
36. Armitage AK, Dollery CT, George CF, et al: Absorption and metabolism of nicotine from cigarettes. Br Med J *4*:313, 1975.
37. Clark MSG, Rand MJ, Vanov S: Comparison of pharmacological activity of nicotine and related alkaloids occurring in cigarette smoke. Arch Int Pharmacodyn Ther *156*:363, 1965.
38. Armitage AK, Turner DM: Absorption of nicotine in cigarette and cigar smoke through the oral mucosa. Nature *226*:1231, 1970.
39. Gosselin RE, et al: Nicotine. In Gosselin RE, et al (eds): Clinical Toxicology of Commercial Products. Baltimore, Williams & Wilkins, 1976, p 246.
40. Russell MAH, Jarvis MJ, Sutherland G, Feyerabend C: Nicotine replacement in smoking cessation. JAMA *257*:3262–3265, 1987.
41. Lampe KF: Systemic plant poisoning in children. South Pediatr *54*:347, 1974.
42. Hoffmann D, Lavoie EJ, Hecht SS: Nicotine: A precursor for carcinogens. Cancer Lett *26*:67–75, 1985.
43. Benowitz NL: Clinical pharmacology of nicotine. Annu Rev Med *37*:21–32, 1986.
44. Brecher EM: Nicotine as an addicting drug. In Brecher EM (ed): Licit and Illicit Drugs; The Consumers Union Report on Narcotics, Stimulants, Depressants, Inhalants, Hallucinogens and Alcohol. Boston, Little, Brown, 1972.
45. Brady ME, Ritschel WA, Saelinger DA, et al: Animal model and pharmacokinetic interpretation of nicotine poisoning in man. Int J Clin Pharmacol Biopharm *17*:12, 1979.
46. Haigh JC, Haigh JM: Immobilizing drug emergencies in humans. Vet Hum Toxicol 22:1–5, 1980.
47. Ramzy Y, Samarthji L, Korpassy A, Ally J: Nicotine exposure and tardive dyskinesia. Biol Psychiatr *22*:67–72, 1987.
48. Bretzke VG: Einflus des Nikotins auf das Ulcus duodeni. Z Gesamte Inn Med *42*:82–84, 1987.
49. CDC: Smoking-attributable mortality and years of potential life lost—United States, 1984. MMWR *36*:693–697, 1987.
50. Lockhard LP: Nicotine poisonings. Br Med J *1*:246, 1933.
51. McNally WD: A report of five cases of poisoning by nicotine. J Lab Clin Med *8*:83, 1922.
52. McNally WD: A report of seven cases of nicotine poisoning. J Lab Clin Med *8*:83–85, 1922.
53. Oyebola DDO, Elegbe RA: Cow's urine poisoning in Nigeria. Trop Geogr Med *27*:194, 1975.
54. Wagner IU: Nikotinvergiftung im Kindesalter. Paediatr Paedol *14*:191, 1979.
55. National Poison Center Network: Computer System for Documenting Data on Poison Exposures. Pittsburgh, December, 1980.

56. Saxena K, Scheman A: Suicide plan by nicotine poisoning: A review of nicotine toxicity. Vet Hum Toxicol *27*:495–497, 1985.
57. von Ahn B: Paroxysmal auricular fibrillation in acute nicotine poisoning. Cardiologia *21*:765, 1952.
58. von Ahn B: A further case of paroxysmal auricular fibrillation in acute nicotine poisoning. Acta Med Scand *145*:28, 1953.
59. Feurt SD, Jenkind JH, Hayes FA, Crockford HA: Pharmacology and toxicology of nicotine with special reference to species variation. Science *127*:1054, 1958.
60. Garcia-Estrada H, Fischman CM: An unusual case of nicotine poisoning. Clin Toxicol *10*:391, 1977.
61. Gold H, Brown F: A contribution to the pharmacology of nicotine. J Pharmacol Exp Ther *54*:463, 1935.
62. Franke FE, Thomas JE: The treatment of acute nicotine poisoning. JAMA *106*:507, 1936.
63. Mensch AR, Holden M: Nicotine overdose after a single piece of nicotine gum. Chest *86*:801, 1984.
64. Tonnesen P, Fryd V, Hansen M, Helsted J, Gunnersen AB, Forchammer H, Stockner M: Effect of nicotine chewing gum in combination with group counseling on the cessation of smoking. N Engl J Med *318*:15–18, 1988.
65. Rigotti NA, Eagle KA: Atrial fibrillation while chewing nicotine gum. JAMA *255*:1018, 1986.
66. Stewart PM, Catterall JR: Chronic nicotine ingestion and atrial fibrillation. Br Heart J *54*:222–223, 1985.
67. Neil JF, Horn TL, Himmelhoch JM: Psychotic pica nicotinism and complicated myocardial infarction. Dis Nerv Syst *38*:724–726, 1977.
68. Short DD, Blinder BB: Nicotine used as emetic by a patient with bulimia. Am J Psychiatr *142*:272, 1985.
69. Gehlbach, SH, Williams WA, Perry LD, et al: Nicotine absorption by workers harvesting green tobacco. Lancet *1*:478, 1975.
70. Kingsbury JM: Poisonous Plants of the United States and Canada. Englewood Cliffs, NJ, Prentice-Hall, 1964, p 284.
71. Ghosh SK, Gokani VN, Parikh JR, Doctor PB, Kashyap SK, Chatterjee BB: Protection against "green symptoms" from tobacco in Indian harvesters: A preliminary intervention study. Arch Environ Health *42*:121–124, 1987.
72. Patten BM: Neuromuscular disease due to tobacco use. Texas Med *80*:47–51, 1984.
73. Feyerabend C, Levitt T, Russell MAH: A rapid gas-liquid chromatographic estimation of nicotine in biological fluids. J Pharm Pharmacol *27*:434, 1975.
74. Faulker JM: Nicotine poisoning by absorption through the skin. JAMA *100*:1664, 1933.
75. Wilson GJB: Nicotine poisoning by absorption through the skin. Br Med J *2*:601, 1930.
76. Wells SJ: Caffeine: Implications of recent research for clinical practice. Am J Orthopsychiatr *54*:375–389, 1984.
77. Farago A: Fatal accidental caffeine poisoning of a child. Bull Int Assoc Forensic Toxicol *5*:2, 1968.
78. DiMaio VJM, Garriott JC: Lethal caffeine poisoning in a child. Forensic Sci *3*:275, 1947.
79. Mack RB: A tasteless proposal. NC Med J *48*:368–370, 1987.
80. McGee MB: Caffeine poisoning in a 19 year old female. J Forensic Sci *25*:29, 1980.
81. Garriott JC, Simmons LM, Poklis A, Mackell MA: Five cases of fatal overdose from caffeine-containing "look-alike" drugs. J Anal Toxicol *9*:141–143, 1985.
82. Hanzlick R, Gowitt GT, Wall W: Deaths due to caffeine in "look-alike drugs." J Anal Toxicol *10*:126, 1986.
83. Winek CL, Wahba W, Williams K, Blenko J, Janssen J: Caffeine fatality: A case report. Forensic Sci Int *29*:207–211, 1985.
84. Rejent T, Michalek R, Krajewski M: Caffeine fatality with coincident ephedrine. Bull Int Assoc Forensic Toxicol *16*:18–19, 1981.
85. Alstott RL, Miller AJ, Forney RB: Report of a human fatality due to caffeine. J Forensic Sci *18*:135, 1973.
86. Turner JE, Cravey RH: A fatal ingestion of caffeine. Clin Toxicol *10*:341, 1977.
87. Jokela S, Vartiainen A: Caffeine poisoning. Acta Pharmacol (Kbh) *15*:331, 1959.
88. Bryant J: Suicide by ingestion of caffeine. Arch Pathol Lab Med *105*:685–686, 1981.
89. Grusz-Hardy E: Lethal caffeine poisoning. Bull Int Assoc Forensic Toxicol *10*:6, 1973.
90. Khodesevick AP: Fatal caffeine poisoning (case from practice). Farmakol Toksikol *19*:62, 1956.
91. Borkowski T: Lethal caffeine poisoning. Bull Int Assoc Forensic Toxicol *8*:13, 1972.

CHAPTER 49
PHENYTOIN AND OTHER ANTICONVULSANTS

Donna Seger, M.D.

PHENYTOIN

Phenytoin is used for the acute and chronic management of all seizure disorders except absence seizures.[1, 2] Nine million annual prescriptions for children and adults rank phenytoin as the most frequently prescribed anticonvulsant drug. Additionally, phenytoin is used to treat cardiac arrhythmias secondary to digitalis intoxication,[3] tricyclic antidepressant overdose with prolonged QRS,[4] trigeminal neuralgias, and certain behavioral disorders.[5]

In 1908, Blitz synthesized phenytoin, but its anticonvulsant activity was not discovered until 1938 when Merritt and Putnam examined the structural relatives of phenobarbital. They discovered phenytoin—a drug that suppressed electroshock-induced convulsions but did not sedate laboratory animals.[2]

The mechanism of phenytoin's anticonvulsant activity is not entirely elucidated. Phenytoin limits the development of maximal seizure activity and decreases the spread of the seizure process from its active focus. It decreases the abnormally increased neuronal membrane excitability[2] but does not affect normal neuronal membrane excitability.[6] It does not increase the seizure threshold for convulsant drugs. One proposed mechanism of phenytoin's anticonvulsant activity is folate depletion. Folic acids and their derivatives appear to have convulsant properties. Phenytoin decreases cerebrospinal fluid (CSF) and red blood cell (RBC) folate levels.[7]

Noted for its antiarrhythmic efficacy in patients with digoxin toxicity, phenytoin's electrophysiologic effects are similar to those of lidocaine. Like lidocaine, phenytoin has little effect on the electrocardiogram. Phenytoin also reverses the sinoatrial block and decreases the efferent impulses in sympathetic cardiac nerves caused by digoxin toxicity. Phenytoin is effective in the treatment of the following digoxin-induced arrhythmias: ventricular arrhythmia, paroxysmal atrial tachycardia, atrial fibrillation, and supraventricular arrhythmia. The drug is ineffective in the treatment of arrhythmias caused by ischemic heart disease.[3]

Toxicity can be caused by acute ingestion, chronic therapeutic ingestion, or IV administration of phenytoin. Understanding the unique pharmacokinetics of phenytoin is prerequisite to the comprehension of phenytoin toxicity.

Pharmacokinetics

Phenytoin is a weak acid with a pKa of 8.3. Following ingestion, the solid dosage form dissolves and the salt precipitates in the acidic medium of the stomach. The size of the acid precipitate determines the rate and extent of gastrointestinal (GI) absorption.[8] Absorption of oral phenytoin is slow, variable, and occasionally incomplete. Peak serum levels do not occur for 3 to 12 hours after ingestion.[2, 8, 9]

Phenytoin is 90 per cent bound to plasma protein, primarily albumin. It has a large volume of distribution, 0.6 to 0.7 L/kg. The degree of protein binding, and therefore the concentration of free drug, varies from person to person. Once absorbed, phenytoin is largely un-ionized[5] and highly lipid soluble. It freely diffuses into all tissues, including those of the central nervous system (CNS). Phenytoin is firmly tissue bound.[9]

Ninety-five per cent of the drug is metabolized by the hepatic microsomal enzyme system. The major metabolite, a parahydroxyphenyl derivative, is inactive. There is marked genetic variability in the rate of phenytoin metabolism.[2, 5] Generally, children rapidly metabolize the drug and therefore have a shorter drug half-life than adults.[6, 8] The metabolites are conjugated with glucuronide and excreted in the bile and, subsequently, the urine.[10] Renal excretion is minor, as only 5 per cent of the drug is excreted unchanged in the urine.[2, 9]

In the adult, the mean half-life of phenytoin is 22 hours. Half-life is extremely variable and ranges from 4 hours to many days. Half-life variation may be caused by hepatic dysfunction, enzyme self-induction, or genetic factors affecting substrate saturation.[7] However, as the serum level of phenytoin approaches toxic value, half-life increases markedly. Increased half-life is caused by phenytoin elimination switching from first order kinetics to zero order kinetics.

Phenytoin has a unique pharmacokinetic pattern. At therapeutic serum levels, phenytoin elimination follows first order (exponential) kinetics. The *rate* at which the drug is eliminated increases as the concentration of the drug increases. There is a predictable, linear relationship between the daily dose and the steady state (dynamic equilibrium). Half-life and time to reach steady state remain constant.[2, 5, 8]

In the upper therapeutic and toxic ranges, phenytoin elimination changes from first order to zero order kinetics. Now, the rate of phenytoin metabolism and the rate of phenytoin excretion remain constant even as the concentration of the drug increases. As phenytoin accumulates, serum phenytoin levels and half-life increase with disproportionate rapidity. The shift to zero order kinetics may be a consequence of saturation of the hydroxylation reaction or inhibition of the reaction by its metabolites. Zero order kinetics occurs when the rate of the hydroxylation reaction reaches maximum velocity.[2, 5, 6, 9]

When the phenytoin serum level is in the therapeutic range, the expected time to reach steady state is approximately 5 days (four to five half-lives). But when phenytoin elimination shifts from first order to zero order kinetics, the time to reach steady state increases. Therefore, a small increase in dose may result in toxic serum phenytoin levels 2 to 3 weeks after the initial dose increase. Phenytoin toxicity may not be recognized owing to the time lag between increased dose and appearance of clinical signs and symptoms of toxicity. Once phenytoin administration is discontinued, toxic phenytoin serum levels will decrease slowly as elimination follows zero order kinetics. As the serum level approaches the therapeutic range, serum levels decrease more rapidly because elimination follows first order kinetics.[2, 5, 6]

Pharmacokinetic Implications: Loading and Route of Administration

Phenytoin may be administered by oral, intravenous, or intraosseous routes. Intramuscular administration is not recommended owing to slow and erratic absorption caused by crystallization at the injection site.[2, 7, 9, 11]

If phenytoin administration is initiated with standard oral maintenance doses of 300 to 400 mg/day, therapeutic concentrations will be reached in 3 to 4 days.[12, 13] Steady state will be attained in 7 to 10 days.[14] Oral "loading" (dose administered to rapidly attain steady state) is not acceptable in many situations owing to the time delay until seizure control is attained. Oral loading may be indicated in patients in whom immediate activity of the drug is not deemed necessary. A single dose of 15 to 18 mg/kg will result in therapeutic serum levels 8 to 30 hours after oral administration.[6, 13, 15] Three to four divided doses over a 12-hour period may increase absorption and decrease the GI side effects of a single large oral dose.[6, 13] Most patients will achieve steady state by 96 hours.[14]

Rapid attainment of therapeutic serum phenytoin levels is required in patients with status epilepticus, acute repetitive seizures, tricyclic antidepressant overdose with prolonged QRS complex, and arrhythmias caused by digitalis toxicity. An IV loading dose of phenytoin is the only method of administration that will rapidly produce therapeutic steady state. If the pretreatment serum level of phenytoin is zero, an intravenous loading dose of 15 to 18 mg/kg will produce serum concentrations within the therapeutic range lasting 18 to 24 hours in most adult patients.[16–18] The loading dose for children is 1.5 mg/kg every 30 minutes to a maximum dose of 6 mg/kg.[7] Each 100 mg of IV phenytoin will increase serum concentration 1.3 μg/ml if the serum level is known.[19] Anticonvulsant activity occurs 3 to 5 minutes after IV infusion. Distribution to the brain is so rapid that plasma and CSF concentrations are equal 10 minutes after initiation of an IV loading dose.[20] Solution and administration rate are discussed in the section on IV phenytoin.

There is a report of intraosseous administration in a child in whom emergency vascular access failed.[21] Absorption from bone was rapid. Pharmacodynamic effects of intraosseous administration may approximate those of intravenous administration.[21] Further investigation is necessary.

Preparations and Dosage

Phenytoin sodium (diphenylhydantoin sodium: Dilantin) is available in 30- and 100-mg capsules. Fifty-mg tablets are also available for oral suspensions. A sterile solution of 50 mg/ml with a special solvent is available for IV administration.[2]

The maintenance oral dose for adults is 3 to 5 mg/kg/day; 4 to 7 mg/kg/day in divided doses is recommended for children. Long half-life and slow absorption indicate that a single daily oral dose is appropriate. But variable product bioavailability (absorption and half-life) may cause fluctuations in plasma phenytoin levels.[2,7,9] Tablets are better absorbed than capsules.[22] Gastric intolerance may also dictate the need for divided doses. Therefore, the Food and Drug Administration (FDA) recommends a single daily oral dose only for Dilantin Kapseals. Dosage increments may be made at 1-week intervals when dosage is less than 300 mg/day. Increments should not occur more frequently than every 2 weeks when dosage exceeds 300 mg/day. Phenytoin serum levels must be monitored.[2]

Drug Interactions

Drugs such as isoniazid (INH), disulfiram,[16] and dicumarol inhibit phenytoin metabolism, causing serum phenytoin levels to increase; toxicity may occur.[6] Toxic phenytoin levels have also been reported after administration of co-trimoxazole,[24] diazepam,[25] sulfonamides,[2] chloramphenicol,[2,6] phenothiazines,[7] chlorpromazine, chlordiazepoxide, estrogens, and trimethadone.[6] Occasionally, increased phenytoin levels have occurred after administration of sulfisoxazole, phenylbutazone, salicylates, and valproate.[2]

Phenobarbital, carbamazepine, diazepam, ethanol, folic acid, antacid, and calcium may cause a decrease in serum phenytoin level. These drugs decrease absorption, increase biotransformation through enzyme induction, or increase excretion. The result is a decrease in phenytoin serum half-life. Phenobarbital and ethanol may increase or decrease the serum phenytoin level.[6]

Many patients with seizure disorders have coexisting psychiatric problems, specifically schizophrenia or depression. Administration of antidepressants causes a decrease in the seizure threshold. Therefore, dosages of antiepileptic medication are increased to maintain seizure control. Serum phenytoin levels need to be closely monitored in these patients.[26]

Side Effects of Chronic Phenytoin (Dilantin) Therapy

Nonfatal side effects occur in up to 45 per cent of patients who require maintenance phenytoin therapy.[27] Serum phenytoin levels frequently do not correlate with side effects. However, levels of less than 15 μg/ml are rarely associated with side effects.[28] Gingival hyperplasia occurs in 20 per cent of patients on chronic Dilantin therapy. Gingival hyperplasia can be minimized by good oral hygiene. Withdrawal of the drug is not necessary.[2] Children may develop a mild transient maculopapular rash within 2 weeks of phenytoin administration. These children may have a higher serum level than children who do not develop a rash. When the drug is discontinued, the exanthem remains for 3 to 5 days and does not reappear when the drug is reinstituted.[28] Phenytoin may inhibit thyroid function or unmask occult hypothyroidism. Decreased thyroid function inhibits hepatic metabolism of phenytoin. Consequently, serum phenytoin levels increase.[29] Hirsutism may occur in young females but can be improved by dosage adjustment. Other reported side effects include hypertrichosis, carbohydrate intolerance, folic acid deficiency, benign intracranial hypertension,[30] peripheral neuropathy,[2,6] osteomalacia, and increased alkaline phosphatase due to altered metabolism of vitamin D.[2] Although mild hypocalcemia has been reported to occur in patients on chronic therapy, recent reports indicate that the incidence is probably very small. Isolated reports of metabolic abnormalities [e.g., antidiuretic hormone (ADH) inhibition and secondary hypernatremia] are rare.[31] Metabolic abnormalities rarely occur in patients on chronic phenytoin therapy.[32]

Many manifestations are reversible with cessation of the drug. Phenytoin induces liver enzyme synthesis, which increases serum liver function tests (LFTs). LFTs should be monitored. Increased LFTs do not require discontinuation of the drug.[2, 6]

Two to three weeks after initiation of therapy, phenytoin may induce a hypersensitivity angiitis manifested by fever, rash, lymphadenopathy, and eosinophilia.[33, 34] Less common features include renal failure, granulocytopenia, myositis, CSF pleocytosis, encephalopathy, and acute pulmonary disease.[34, 35] The association of hepatitis with the hypersensitivity reaction has been designated phenytoin syndrome. Fatal hepatic necrosis may be a consequence of continued phenytoin administration.[33, 36] Fatal hepatic necrosis may occur more frequently than reported because phenytoin therapy has not been commonly associated with hepatic necrosis.

Phenytoin should be withdrawn if manifestations of a hypersensitivity angiitis occur.[33, 35] Prognosis depends on the severity of the syndrome and the time from onset of syndrome to discontinuance of the drug. Reinstitution of the drug may cause more severe sequelae. Owing to structural similarities to phenytoin, phenobarbital should not be initiated as an alternative anticonvulsant. Valproic acid and carbamazepine are better alternatives.[33, 36]

Hepatotoxicity has also been reported when Dilantin and valproate were simultaneously administered. Signs of Dilantin toxicity heralded the onset of liver damage. Either valproate or Dilantin may cause hepatotoxicity. As a result of the liver damage, metabolism of Dilantin may decrease and result in Dilantin toxicity.[37]

The use of Dilantin during pregnancy is associated with fetal malformations, most frequently cleft lip and palate. Since uncontrolled seizures are also associated with malformations, the use of Dilantin is not contraindicated during pregnancy. During the last trimester, decreased absorption may cause a decrease in serum levels. Dilantin levels should be monitored throughout pregnancy.[6]

Interpretation of Phenytoin Serum Levels

Control of seizures and alleviation of cardiac arrhythmias occur when serum levels are between 10 and 20 μg/ml.[9] Toxic effects may develop when serum levels are greater than 20 μg/ml. Serum levels may not accurately predict clinical effectiveness or toxicity, as they measure both protein bound and unbound ("free") drug. Clinical effects are determined by unbound drug, as only unbound drug can cross the cell membrane to reach sites of action and biotransformation.[2, 7, 20]

Free phenytoin may be increased by drugs that displace phenytoin from serum proteins. Free phenytoin is also increased by disorders that decrease albumin (e.g., hepatic dysfunction, cirrhosis, chronic renal failure, and uremia). In these conditions, free phenytoin may be increased by 50 per cent, even when the serum level is "therapeutic."[2, 7, 20]

Efficacy and toxicity correlate with free serum phenytoin levels.[9] Toxic effects occur when free phenytoin levels are greater than 5 μg/ml, however, serum levels of unbound phenytoin are not readily available. Current methods that separate bound and unbound drug are costly, time consuming, and irreproducible.[2]

Current assay methods include spectrophotometry, colorimetry, gas-layered chromatography (GLC), high pressure liquid chromatography (HPLC), radioimmunologic assay (RIA), and enzyme-mediated immunoassay (EMIT). GLC is the most common procedure used for routine monitoring.[8, 9] An assay error of ± 20 per cent must be assumed. A measured value of 20 μg/ml should be considered to be 16 to 24 μg/ml.[9]

Phenytoin Toxicity and Phenytoin Serum Level

Dosage, route of administration, and duration of exposure determine the toxic effects of phenytoin.[2] Acute or chronic ingestion or IV administration of phenytoin may cause clinical signs of toxicity. Hepatic dysfunction, a genetic defect in phenytoin metabolism, inhibition of metabolism by concurrently ingested drugs, or other drug interactions may also precipitate phenytoin toxicity.[20]

Phenytoin concentrations are higher in neural tissue than in serum. Owing to the firm tissue binding of phenytoin, serum levels may not accurately reflect the level of CNS bound drug causing neurologic symptoms. Consequently, neurologic symptoms do not correlate well with serum level.[9]

Varying CNS phenytoin concentrations explain the progression of symptoms that usually occurs during phenytoin intoxication. The cerebellum and brain stem have higher phenytoin levels than the cerebral cortex. Therefore, cerebellar signs of nystagmus and ataxia usually precede the cortical signs of drowsiness, delirium, and stupor.[8]

Fifteen per cent of patients with serum phenytoin levels of 20 to 30 μg/ml will have symptoms. Eighty per cent of patients with serum levels of 30 to 60 μg/ml will also be symptomatic.[8] When serum levels approach 20 μg/ml, nystagmus may occur on lateral gaze. As levels increase, spontaneous, horizontal nystagmus may occur.[38] As serum levels approach 30 μg/ml, vertical nystagmus, ataxia, slurred speech, and drowsiness may occur. Initial ataxia may progress to a lurching gait and subsequent inability to walk or stand. As serum levels reach 40 μg/ml, mentation is affected, more frequently in elderly patients than in younger patients.[8] An etiologic factor may be increased free phenytoin secondary to decreased plasma protein binding in the elderly. Confusion, disorientation, lethargy,[2] hyperactivity, or manic behavior may occur as serum levels increase. Coma and respiratory depression are unusual,[38] but both have been reported.[39] At levels greater than 50 μg/ml, paradoxic seizures may occur.[7, 12]

Nystagmus is not consistently the initial sign of phenytoin toxicity. Nystagmus may not be present at high serum phenytoin levels.[27] Even if nystagmus is not present, phenytoin toxicity should be considered in patients with unusual involuntary muscle movements, mental status changes, and ataxia. Asterixis,[40] dystonic reactions,[41] and symptoms of parkinsonism have been reported as a result of phenytoin intoxication. These symptoms resolve with the resolution of phenytoin toxicity.[42]

Ataxia, nystagmus, drowsiness, and behavior disturbances are the most frequent presenting symptoms of phenytoin toxicity in children. Increased or decreased deep tendon reflexes, slurred speech, diplopia, headache, dizziness, and blurred vision have also been reported.[43] Poor school performance and ataxia without nystagmus may be the initial signs of phenytoin toxicity.[44]

Acute Ingestion

Since seizure control often requires ingestion of multiple anticonvulsant drugs, drug interactions frequently complicate acute phenytoin ingestion.[8] Symptoms occur 1 to 2 hours after phenytoin ingestion. Toxic manifestations are usually relatively brief, but manifestations may be present for 4 to 5 days. The duration of toxic effects does not appear to be dose related.[45, 46] Prolonged toxicity and protracted low plasma levels[45] may occur as a result of prolonged phenytoin absorption. The prolonged absorption may be due to limited phenytoin solubility and decreased intestinal motility.[47] The dissolution rate decreases as the ingested dose of phenytoin increases in the GI tract. Dissolution and absorption may occur throughout the GI tract for up to 60 hours.[48] Peak serum levels have occurred as late as 4 days after ingestion.[47]

Typical clinical features of a patient who has acutely overdosed on phenytoin consist of the triad of nystagmus, ataxia, and drowsiness. The most frequent symptoms of acute phenytoin toxicity are manifestations of cerebellar dysfunction.[38] Acute ingestions have not caused irreversible cerebellar symptoms or findings compatible with Purkinje cell degeneration or atrophy.[8]

Clinical signs and symptoms of phenytoin toxicity have been discussed in the previous section. However, owing to protein binding variations, age, drug interactions, and many other variables, serum levels following an acute overdose may not correlate well with symptoms. A patient may be alert with a serum phenytoin level of 80 μg/ml or comatose and apneic with a level of 65 μg/ml.[13] Symptoms that have been reported as a result of an acute Dilantin overdose include dilated pupils, urinary incontinence, hyperglycemia secondary to inhibition of insulin release,[16, 49] hyperkinesia, asterixis, and transient hemiparesis.[8] Coma, seizures, and apnea[45] have occurred following an acute ingestion.[8]

Treatment of Acute Dilantin Toxicity

Phenytoin intoxications are rarely fatal even when large amounts of phenytoin (100 to 160 mg/kg) are ingested. The initial treatment of an acute overdose includes minimizing absorption from the GI tract. This includes the usual modalities of gastric emptying and administration of charcoal and cathartics. Gastric dialysis (repeated administration of charcoal) may be especially important owing to prolonged absorption.[7, 8]

Once GI absorption has been minimized,

treatment is primarily supportive. Oxygenation and fluid requirements should be monitored. Serum electrolytes and successive phenytoin levels should be obtained.[8] Appreciation of phenytoin kinetics is mandatory for interpretation of results. Metabolic abnormalities or sympathetic response (increased glucose, white cell count, and heart rate and decreased potassium) rarely occur as a result of phenytoin toxicity.[41]

Forced diuresis or modification of urine pH is of no benefit. Hemodialysis, charcoal hemoperfusion, exchange transfusion, and peritoneal dialysis are ineffective owing to phenytoin's protein binding.[8, 39, 50, 51] Plasmapheresis by centrifugation has yielded discouraging results. Plasmapheresis using a hollow-fiber plasmaseparator may warrant further investigation.[39] However, potential complications of plasmapheresis must be carefully considered if it is to be used for an intoxication that rarely causes death.[50]

Chronic Intoxication

As in acute ingestion, toxic effects of chronic phenytoin ingestion are primarily serum level–related cerebellar vestibular symptoms. However, the classic signs (nystagmus, ataxia, and drowsiness) are not always present. Signs and symptoms of coexisting disease or the onset of phenytoin toxicity with previously tolerated doses increases diagnostic confusion.[52] Not surprisingly, the elusive diagnosis of phenytoin toxicity during chronic phenytoin therapy may be delayed.

When classic signs are not present, particularly in young children, other manifestations of toxicity assume importance. CNS effects, behavioral changes, increased frequency of seizures, and GI effects may be the heralding signs of chronic phenytoin toxicity.[2] Hypotonia, pupillary dilatation, incontinence, increased CSF protein, progressive mental and/or neurologic impairment, behavior disorders, psychosis, transient hemiparesis, peripheral neuropathy, and seizures have been reported as the first signs of phenytoin intoxication.[52] Extrapyramidal signs such as dystonic posturing, tremor, tongue protrusion, lip smacking, head nodding, fish mouthing, and facial grimaces may occur in both children and adults. Such presentations may be mistaken for a phenothiazine reaction.[8]

Movement disorders occur most frequently as a result of chronic therapy, although they have been reported after a single large phenytoin ingestion. Phenytoin is postulated to precipitate movement disorders in patients with pre-existing structural or organic disease. The most commonly described movement disorder is choreoathetosis, but orofacial or orobuccal dyskinesias, bradykinesia, tremor, and dystonia have also been described. The disorder is usually mild, self-limited, and associated with levels greater than 20 μg/ml. Decreasing the dose so the serum level falls into therapeutic range usually eliminates the disorder. Discontinuation of the drug may be required in some patients.[1]

During chronic phenytoin intoxication, cerebellar signs (ataxia, nystagmus) occur much more frequently than basal ganglia signs (movement disorders). Studies using cats with chronic phenytoin intoxication have revealed that the cerebellar phenytoin concentration is higher than the basal ganglia concentration. Because phenytoin is usually discontinued when cerebellar signs occur, the basal ganglia seldom attain the high phenytoin levels necessary to produce movement disorders. Serum levels associated with movement disorders are usually much higher than those associated with nystagmus and ataxia,[20] confirming this gradation in levels.[27]

The extent to which Dilantin can produce chronic cerebellar abnormalities is controversial.[53, 54] Animals with chronic phenytoin intoxication demonstrate lesions in the cerebellum, especially the Purkinje cells.[8] Seizures also cause cerebellar degeneration and atrophy. Degeneration caused by phenytoin is difficult to differentiate from that caused by seizures.[8] Computerized axial tomography (CT) has documented cerebellar atrophy and loss of cerebellar tissue following Dilantin therapy.[53, 55] Yet patients with Dilantin-induced cerebellar symptoms demonstrate almost complete symptomatic recovery. The cerebellum functionally compensates for cell loss induced by acute or chronic Dilantin intoxication. The etiology of compensatory changes is yet to be elucidated.[53]

An exact correlation between serum phenytoin levels and symptoms caused by chronic phenytoin toxicity does not exist.

Treatment is supportive. The drug should be withdrawn and serum levels monitored.[38] Phenytoin should be reinstituted when serum levels have reached the therapeutic range.[7]

Intravenous Phenytoin

Owing to phenytoin's lack of solubility and stability in unbuffered aqueous solutions,[3, 4] the FDA recommends IV phenytoin administration only by manual IV push at a rate less than 50 mg/min.[4, 18] This method has many disadvantages. Most hospitals require physicians to administer IV phenytoin over 20 to 30 minutes.[25] Pain at the infusion site is caused by the high concentration of the alcohol-propylene glycol diluent. Additionally, cardiorespiratory depression has been associated with this mode of injection and appears to be related to the variable drug delivery rate.[4, 18] If a stable solution can be administered by controlled infusion, a constant rate of drug delivery may alleviate potential side effects.[4, 56]

Many investigators have attempted to discover the pH and volume of an IV preparation that would maintain phenytoin in solution and reduce the variability of phenytoin delivery. Phenytoin is dissolved in a solvent that contains 40 per cent propylene glycol, 10 per cent alcohol, and 50 per cent water. The solution is adjusted with sodium hydroxide to a pH of 12 to maintain phenytoin solubility. If the pH is less than 11.7, phenytoin sodium becomes phenytoin acid, hydrolyzes, and precipitates.[2]

Solvent pH affects the solution pH.[2, 7] The pH of 5 per cent dextrose in water (D_5W) is 9.44 to 10.15. When D_5W is used as the diluent, the relatively low solution pH causes phenytoin degradation and crystallization. Similar problems occur when lactated Ringer's (LR) solution is used as a diluent. The pH of normal saline (NS) is 9.81 to 10.81, which makes it the diluent of choice with regard to pH.[2, 7, 56]

Propylene glycol solubilizes phenytoin. The resultant solution must contain enough propylene glycol to maintain phenytoin solubility.[2, 3, 25, 46, 56] Therefore, a small solution volume is optimal to maintain propylene glycol concentration as well as appropriate pH. But the resultant phenytoin concentration must also be part of the volume consideration, as administration of high phenytoin concentrations is associated with increased incidence of cardiovascular (CV) complications.[14, 57]

Based on solubility, crystallization, pH, and constant delivered concentration, experimental evidence reveals that 100 mg of phenytoin sodium can be added to 15 to 25 ml of NS for IV administration.[2–4, 25, 46, 56] Crystallization will occur at approximately 1 hour even with this concentration, but the degree of crystallization is not harmful. The solution should be made immediately prior to use and infused within 1 hour.[17, 58] Research has not revealed an appreciable difference in delivered phenytoin concentrations when using filtered versus nonfiltered solutions.[2, 56]

Owing to reports of apnea, cardiac arrhythmias, and cardiac arrest occurring during IV phenytoin administration,[59–64] animal studies were performed. They revealed that propylene glycol caused hypotension, bradycardia, and apnea. Large doses of propylene glycol injected rapidly caused sinoatrial node depression, asystole, and QRS and T wave amplification. Interestingly, deleterious effects were partially prevented by the addition of phenytoin.[10]

Animal studies further revealed that large doses of IV phenytoin could cause PR prolongation, atrioventricular nodal block, bradycardia, peripheral vasodilatation, and cardiac arrest. Myocardial performance was impaired in direct proportion to the total phenytoin dose and rate of administration. The two most clinically relevant CV effects appear to be impairment of myocardial contractility and peripheral vasodilatation.[58]

Fatalities attributed to IV phenytoin have been reported in elderly patients with preexisting heart disease during the treatment of cardiac arrhythmias.[17, 19, 57–64] These patients may be at high risk for cardiotoxicity during the IV administration of phenytoin.[17, 58] However, conclusions regarding the safety of IV administration should not be made based on this high-risk group. IV phenytoin has been reported to cause hypotension and bradycardia in young people when administered at generally accepted rates (35 to 40 mg/min).[65] But the factors associated with CV complications include administration of high concentrations at rates greater than 40 mg/min.[1] Therefore, IV administration of high phenytoin concentration may be potentially dangerous. Recent clinical studies have demonstrated the solution and rate of administration by which diphenylhydantoin can be safely administered intravenously.

Clinical studies have demonstrated that 500 mg of phenytoin diluted in 50 to 75 ml of NS can be safely administered intravenously at a rate of 20 to 40 mg/min.[4] IV piggyback delivery should be monitored by a constant infusion pump.[16, 57] Use of a 0.22-μm inline filter will prevent the possibility of microcrystal formation.[2, 56] Patients should be placed on a cardiac monitor[57] and frequent vital signs recorded. If the patient is 70 years or older or if any side effects occur, the rate should be decreased to 20 mg/min. Patients with the following signs and symptoms should not receive phenytoin: marked bradycardia, second or third degree atrioventricular conduction block, active severe arteriosclerotic heart disease, hypotension, alcohol withdrawal seizures without underlying seizure disorder or repetitive seizures, and seizures due to electrolyte abnormalities or hypoglycemia.[4]

CNS depression is a prominent side effect when treating cardiac arrhythmias. If CNS depression or any sign of toxicity occurs, phenytoin administration should be discontinued. Increasing the dose will have no further effect on the arrhythmia.[3]

Ataxia, confusion, and dizziness have also occurred during IV phenytoin administration. These symptoms are not caused by high drug concentration or rapid rate of administration but usually occur in patients receiving large total doses (greater than 1 gm).[2, 57]

A less serious side effect of IV administration is burning and aching in the arm at or near the IV site. These symptoms may be due to the highly alkaline oily solvent in which phenytoin is dissolved. If the rate is slowed or the concentration decreased, the sensation resolves.[57] A recent report revealed a local reaction to IV phenytoin occurring approximately 2 hours after infusion. A bluish discoloration of tissue distal to the IV site occurred, but there was no evidence of infiltration. Six hours after the infusion, erythema and edema occurred and spread circumferentially and proximal to the elbow. Bullae and vesicles appeared 10 hours after the infusion. Complete resolution occurred in 3 weeks.[66, 67] Phenytoin solution is alkaline (pH 10 to 12.3); when an alkaline solution is infused into a small vein with comparatively low blood volume, the buffer capacity of the blood may be exceeded. The alkalinity may be responsible for the local reaction.[68]

Conclusion

Supportive therapy is the treatment for either an acute overdose of phenytoin or chronic phenytoin toxicity. Toxicity due to IV phenytoin is related to phenytoin concentration and rate of delivery. Research has shown that phenytoin can be safely administered intravenously.

VALPROATE

Valproic acid (VA) was first prescribed for the treatment of absence seizures in 1978.[69] Subsequently, VA has been administered alone and in combination with other anticonvulsants to control myoclonic and tonic clonic seizures; VA does not control partial seizures.[70] Originally, VA administration was considered to be innocuous,[10] but a number of toxic effects have been reported. Currently, the American Academy of Pediatrics' Committee on Drugs does not recommend VA as the initial antiepileptic drug.[71]

Mechanism of Action

As is the case with most antiepileptic drugs, VA's mechanism of action is unknown. The popular gamma-aminobutyric acid (GABA) hypothesis proposes that VA increases total brain and cerebellar synaptosomal GABA concentrations.[10, 72, 73] GABA is a neurotransmitter that inhibits synaptic action and would therefore inhibit propagation of epileptogenic foci. Other possible actions include decreased brain aspartate, production of fatty acids, and hyperpolarization of neurons by increased potassium conductance.[73] When VA is discontinued following chronic administration, the anticonvulsant effect continues after plasma drug levels are no longer measurable. Long-lived active metabolites or adaptive changes in neuronal function may be important facets of VA's action.[70]

Preparations and Dosage

VA (Depakene) is available in 250-mg capsules and as a syrup containing 250 mg/5 ml of sodium valproate. Usual daily doses are 1000 to 3000 mg in adults and 15 to 60 mg/kg in children.[70, 73] Depakote contains equal proportions of VA and sodium valproate.[70]

Pharmacokinetics

VA is rapidly and completely absorbed after oral administration. Peak serum concentrations occur 1 to 4 hours after ingestion of capsules and 15 minutes to 2 hours after ingestion of syrup.[73] Food and enteric coating of the tablet delay peak serum concentration.[70, 72, 73] The drug is 90 per cent bound to plasma proteins and has a small volume of distribution (0.13 to 0.23 L/kg).[10, 70, 74] Although VA is metabolized via several metabolic pathways, anticonvulsant activity of the metabolites is negligible. Steady state concentrations are reached after 1 to 4 days of oral administration.[73] Serum half-life is 15 hours, but half-life is decreased in patients ingesting multiple antiepileptic drugs.[70] Less than 3 per cent of the drug is excreted unchanged in the urine and feces.[10, 70]

Serum Concentration and Laboratory Analysis

Correlation between serum concentration and either seizure control or toxicity is poor.[70] Therapeutic serum concentrations of VA are between 50 and 100 μg/ml. Children may have a lower therapeutic range than adults; childhood seizures may be controlled with less than therapeutic serum levels. Because cognitive function is impaired at higher doses, the lowest dose possible should be used. Once a response occurs, there is no therapeutic gain with higher serum levels. Adverse side effects increase at concentrations greater than 120 μg/ml.[75]

The EMIT assay will yield higher values of serum VA than will the GLC assay. Serum levels must be monitored by the same analytic method. Free VA concentration is not more useful than total VA concentration in determining seizure control.[73]

VA is eliminated partly as ketone bodies and may cause a false-positive test for ketones in the urine. VA may also decrease serum values for total thyroxine and thyronine.[73]

Drug Interactions

VA interacts with numerous drugs, including all the major antiepileptic drugs.[74] Carbamazepine, phenobarbital, phenytoin, or any combination of these drugs lowers the serum VA level. These antiepileptic drugs induce hepatic microsomal enzymes and thereby increase VA clearance.[76] VA half-life is correspondingly decreased, and therapeutic VA levels may not occur.[72, 74]

VA decreases the metabolism of phenobarbital and may increase serum phenobarbital concentrations by 40 per cent.[10, 70, 74] VA does not cause hepatic microsomal enzyme induction.[72]

Because VA can either decrease or increase serum phenytoin levels, serum phenytoin concentrations should be closely monitored.[70, 73, 74]

Adverse Side Effects

Fifteen per cent of patients with therapeutic concentrations of VA will have GI disturbances, which include anorexia, nausea, vomiting, diarrhea, and abdominal pain.[69, 70, 73] Enteric coated tablets decrease the incidence of GI disturbances.[75] Depakote has the lowest incidence of GI side effects.[70] CNS side effects of sedation, ataxia, and tremor may be mitigated by decreasing the dosage.[69, 70, 73] VA-induced pancreatitis may occur weeks to years after initiation of VA therapy and should be considered in patients who develop vomiting and abdominal pain. Transient asymptomatic hyperamylasemia may also occur.[71] Less frequent side effects include aggressive behavior, alopecia, asterixis, confusion, dementia, dizziness, hallucination, headache, hyperactivity, irritability, myoclonic jerks, paresthesias, seizure exacerbation, sleep disorder, speech impairment, stupor, and tremor.[77] Major hematologic side effects include inhibition of platelet aggregation, decreased fibrinogen, neutropenia, thrombocytopenia, prolonged partial thromboplastin time, and prolonged prothrombin time (PT).[69, 73] Bruises, hematomas, and epistaxis may occur secondary to decreased platelet count or abnormal clotting function.[73, 75] Chronic ingestion of VA induces diurnal arterial hyperammonemia in 50 per cent of patients.[78] Hyperammonemia is not related to liver disease,[65] as it occurs in patients with either normal or abnormal LFTs.[79] Hyperammonemia occurs most frequently in patients ingesting multiple anticonvulsants and appears to be related to eating. The clinical relevance of the hyperammonemia is not understood.[78, 79]

Although most patients with hyperammonemia are asymptomatic, an increase in serum ammonia may cause the abrupt onset of somnolence, lethargy, and coma. Concurrent serum VA levels may be therapeutic, subtherapeutic, or toxic.[79] Severe hyperammonemia can be precipitated in children with congenital disorders of the urea cycle.[80–82]

Soon after the initiation of VA, liver enzymes increase in 30 to 66 per cent of patients with therapeutic VA serum levels.[70] Serum bilirubin is the only LFT that increases as VA levels increase.[78] Increased LFTs seem to occur in patients receiving a large mg/kg dose.[81, 82] Dose reduction or discontinuation of the drug results in normalization of the LFTs.[72]

The most serious adverse effect of VA administration is hepatotoxicity with fulminant hepatic failure.[81, 82] Fatal hepatic failure has occurred in children and adolescents during their first 6 months of treatment.[72, 83] There was no dose dependency. Seventy per cent of the cases occurred in children younger than 10 years of age. Eighty-five per cent of the patients were on multiple anticonvulsant drugs.[70, 72, 81, 82, 84] Most children had pre-existing medical problems in addition to epilepsy.[84] Two-thirds had prodromal symptoms of anorexia, vomiting, seizures, decreased level of consciousness, and ataxia.[81, 82] One-third of the patients developed symptoms of liver damage with fever, jaundice, ascites, edema, and bruising. Reye's-like syndrome was reported in a few patients.[10, 79] Terminal hepatic coma developed in all the patients.[81, 82] Lack of clinical signs of hypersensitivity (fever, rash, eosinophilia) indicates that hepatic failure may be an idiosyncratic reaction in children who have a metabolic aberration or other predisposition.[72, 84–86] Pathologically, the majority of the cases revealed microvascular steatosis without evidence of inflammation or hypersensitivity.[10, 70, 72, 84] Originally thought to be a rare occurrence, the incidence may be severely underestimated.[83]

Children in their first 6 months of VA therapy who present with unexplained symptoms of lethargy, vomiting, or general deterioration or any signs of liver damage should be assessed for hepatotoxicity. The drug should be discontinued. Routine monitoring of LFTs cannot predict those patients who will develop life-threatening hepatotoxicity.[81, 82]

Overdose and Toxicity

During chronic VA therapy, lethargy, confusion, and disorientation may indicate a VA serum concentration greater than 100 mg/ml.[69] The same symptom complex may occur after a single large ingestion with normal serum VA concentrations.[69, 87] The toxicity of acute VA ingestion is low,[10, 72, 88] although fatalities have occurred following VA ingestion.[12] Decreased level of consciousness, coma, respiratory depression, and hypertonia have been reported after poisoning.[75, 87, 88] Although LFTs may increase slightly, acute VA ingestion has not been associated with hepatotoxicity.[10, 88, 89]

Standard treatment and supportive care are indicated for a toxic ingestion. GI decontamination by emesis or lavage followed by charcoal and cathartic administration is recommended.[10, 90] Narcan has been reported to reverse VA-induced coma and should be administered if CNS depression is present.[91] If serum levels increase for 3 days following an ingestion, absorption may be prolonged or VA may be reaching saturable kinetics. Repeated administration of charcoal and cathartic may be indicated.[69] The literature contains few reports of extracorporeal detoxification, and its usefulness is probably limited.[87, 92]

Prenatal Exposure

Major and minor malformations are two to three times more frequent in children of epileptic women than in those of nonepileptic women. Exposure to VA during the first trimester increases the risk of fetal neural tube defects.[72, 94, 95] Studies indicate that infants born to women on VA have low Apgars. Free VA increases in the third trimester, and neonatal distress may be secondary to the increase in free VA. Prenatal counseling and amniocentesis are advised.[72, 86, 95]

SUCCINIMIDES

The succinimide anticonvulsants include phensuximide (Milontin), ethosuximide (Zarontin), and methsuximide (Celontin). Most frequently prescribed, ethosuximide is the prototype of the succinimides.[10, 62]

Ethosuximide is well absorbed and reaches a peak level 1 to 4 hours after oral administration. Protein binding is negligible. Although metabolism results in many major metabolites, 25 per cent of the drug is excreted unchanged in the urine. Rate of metabolism and half-life vary with the age of the patient. The average half-life is 30 hours in children and 50 hours in adults.[62, 96]

Dose-related toxic effects include nausea, vomiting, lethargy, anorexia, fatigue, dizziness, and headache. These effects may respond to reduced dosage.[62] Skin rash, blood dyscrasias, allergic reactions, and systemic lupus erythematosus are not dose related.[62, 96, 97]

Treatment for acute intoxication is primarily supportive. Metabolites may play a role in causing prolonged coma.[98] Charcoal clearance of the desmethyl metabolite suggests that repeated charcoal administration and/or charcoal hemoperfusion may be indicated.[99]

OXAZOLIDINEDIONES

Trimethadione (Tridione) was the anticonvulsant drug of choice in the late 1940s. It was replaced by the succinimides in the 1950s. The oxazolidinediones (trimethadione, paramethadione, and dimethadione) are now of limited usefulness.[100]

Trimethadione is rapidly absorbed from the GI tract. Peak plasma concentrations occur in 1/2 to 2 hours after ingestion. It is not significantly bound to plasma proteins. Metabolism is via the hepatic microsomal enzyme system. The active metabolite, dimethadione, is excreted unchanged in the urine and has a half-life of 6 to 13 days. Metabolite accumulates and produces the anticonvulsant effect.[101]

The most frequent side effects are sedation and hemeralopia (blurring of vision in bright light). Other reported side effects include metabolic acidosis, dermatologic reactions, blood dyscrasias, hepatitis, nephrosis, pancytopenia, aplastic anemia, lupus erythematosus, and myasthenic syndrome. Fatalities have been reported.[100, 101]

Treatment for intoxication is supportive. There are no data on the effectiveness of repeated charcoal administration, dialysis, or hemoperfusion.

CARBAMAZEPINE

In 1960, carbamazepine (CBMZ) was first introduced into the United States for pain control of trigeminal neuralgia.[102] In 1974, CBMZ was approved for use as an antiepileptic agent and is now used in the treatment of all epilepsies except absence seizures. CBMZ is also used for the treatment of manic depressive patients in whom lithium is not effective.[103] CBMZ has been considered in the treatment of neurogenic diabetes insipidus, alcohol withdrawal, glossopharyngeal neuralgia, and lightning tabetic pain.[104]

Mechanism of Action

The mechanism of action of CBMZ is unknown. Theories include decreased conduction of sodium ions across nerve cell membrane, which reduces cAMP and elevates levels of brain serotonin; decreased turnover of GABA;[105] increased rate of firing of adrenergic neurons in the locus cereleus; and/or action as a partial agonist at adenosine receptors.[104]

Preparations and Dosage

CBMZ (Tegretol) is available as 100- and 200-mg tablets for oral administration. There are no commercially available suspensions in the United States. There are no available formulations for IV or intramuscular injection.[104, 105]

Pharmacokinetics

CBMZ is an iminostilbene derivative that is chemically related to imipramine, a tricyclic antidepressant (TCA) drug.[2] Although structurally related to TCA, CBMZ shares few of its pharmacologic properties.[106]

CBMZ is absorbed slowly and erratically

after oral administration. Peak serum levels occur 4 to 8 hours after ingestion but may be delayed 24 hours. The drug is 75 per cent bound to plasma protein. Its volume of distribution is 0.79 to 1.40 L/kg. CBMZ is hepatically metabolized to the epoxide, which is as active as the parent compound. Because CBMZ induces drug-metabolizing enzymes, the half-life of the drug after a single dose (18 to 54 hours) is much longer than the half-life of the drug with chronic therapy (10 to 20 hours). CBMZ follows first order elimination kinetics.[107] The epoxide is metabolized to inactive compounds, which are excreted in the urine. Only 3 per cent of the parent compound is excreted unchanged in the urine.[104]

Serum Concentration

There is no simple relationship between the dose of CBMZ and the plasma drug concentration.[104] Children eliminate CBMZ faster than adults and thus require comparatively higher doses.[108] Therapeutic serum concentrations are 4 to 12 μg/ml. If dose-related side effects do not occur, the upper therapeutic range may be exceeded when necessary for seizure control. Some individuals tolerate CBMZ levels of 16 μg/ml without side effects.[105] CNS side effects frequently occur at concentrations greater than 9 μg/ml. A single early morning sample, collected after an overnight fast, gives an accurate estimate of trough levels.[108]

Drug Interactions

Phenobarbital and phenytoin increase the metabolism of CBMZ, causing a reduction of CBMZ half-life to approximately 10 hours.[104] Phenytoin predictably decreases the mean plasma CBMZ level 0.9 μg/ml for each 2 mg/kg of phenytoin ingested daily.[109]

The effects of CBMZ on phenytoin, phenobarbital, and primidone are variable. Anticonvulsant serum levels may increase, decrease, or stay the same after CBMZ is administered. Concomitant VA and CBMZ therapy will probably result in decreased VA levels, whereas CBMZ levels will increase, decrease, or stay the same. Anticonvulsant serum levels should be monitored.[109]

Erythromycin and CBMZ are both metabolized by hepatic microsomal enzymes. Erythromycin competitively inhibits CBMZ metabolism and decreases the clearance of CBMZ. Therefore, CBMZ levels may rise. These two drugs are frequently prescribed independently by the pediatrician and neurologist. CBMZ toxicity should be considered when the two drugs are simultaneously administered.[110]

CBMZ interacts with many drugs. Propoxyphene inhibits CBMZ metabolism, which increases CBMZ levels. Increased risk of neurotoxicity occurs when lithium and CBMZ are administered simultaneously. CBMZ stimulates warfarin metabolism and may result in a decreasing PT. PT should be monitored in all patients receiving CBMZ and warfarin concurrently. Cimetidine administration may increase CBMZ levels, which may subsequently return to preadministration serum levels with continued cimetidine therapy.[109]

Adverse Side Effects

Early concern of fatal hematologic toxicity dampened enthusiasm for the use of CBMZ. This concern for hematologic toxicity was unfounded; CBMZ is a safe and well-tolerated anticonvulsant medication.[105] Rarely, CBMZ may cause aplastic anemia. The prevalence of aplastic anemia is 1 in 50,000 patients who are treated with CBMZ.[104, 105] Less than 25 cases have been reported, but fatalities occurred in 50 per cent. The majority of patients were taking multiple drugs. A mild transient leukopenia may occur in 10 per cent of patients during their first month of treatment, but spontaneous resolution usually occurs despite continued administration of the drug. Persistent leukopenia resolves after discontinuation of the drug. Recommendations for hematologic monitoring are varied and range from weekly laboratory monitoring to monitoring every 3 months.[105]

Mild elevation of LFTs unassociated with clinical signs may occur with CBMZ administration. Discontinuation of the drug is not indicated. Fatal hepatic toxicity has occurred but is very rare. LFTs should be checked periodically in patients taking CBMZ.[111, 112]

Cardiac conduction disturbances may rarely occur in elderly patients.[113–116] A defective conduction system may be a prerequisite for the development of conduction abnormalities. Conduction disturbances may occur shortly after initiation of CBMZ therapy or after long-term therapy. Conduction disturbances are not dose related.[117]

Anorexia, weight loss, and diarrhea are transient GI disturbances that may appear after a dosage increase. Tolerance to these transient side effects usually occurs.[105]

CBMZ may rarely cause the inappropriate secretion of antidiuretic hormone (SIADH). The mechanism of this action is unknown. Transient unrecognized water intoxication has been theorized to occur on initiation of CBMZ therapy. It may be responsible for some early common side effects such as dizziness, headache, mental confusion, and GI upset. Serum electrolytes (specifically serum sodium) should be checked when patients complain of these symptoms.[105, 109, 118]

Hypersensitivity reactions (skin rashes, agranulocytosis, fever, and abnormal LFTs) occur in about 5 per cent of patients. Rarely, CBMZ induces skin reactions, which include a number of rashes, lupus erythematosus, exfoliative dermatitis, Stevens-Johnson syndrome, and cutaneous vasculitis.[119, 120]

In the first few weeks of treatment, neurologic side effects are common. Diplopia is the most common single neurologic side effect. Other neurologic side effects include drowsiness, ataxia, slurred speech, headache, tremor, asterixis, and dystonic reactions. These side effects usually abate over time.[105]

Adverse side effects occur in up to 25 per cent of patients receiving CBMZ. Compared with other anticonvulsants, CBMZ has the advantage of relative freedom from cosmetic, behavioral, and cognitive side effects. CBMZ is a safe and well-tolerated medication.[105, 121]

Overdose

Ingestion of a large amount of CBMZ produces an unpredictable clinical course. Seizures; slurred speech; myoclonus; coma; respiratory depression; apnea; abnormal deep tendon reflexes; nystagmus; ataxia; encephalopathy; hypertension or hypotension; prolonged PR, QRS, and QT intervals; dystonia; and ballistic and athetoid posturing have been reported. A waxing and waning sensorium, seemingly corresponding to plasma CBMZ levels, may occur for days following CBMZ overdose. Cyclic CNS depression and a protracted clinical course should be expected.[106, 107, 122]

The cyclic clinical course is explained by the anticholinergic properties and low water solubility of CBMZ. Decreased GI motility and low water solubility cause prolonged and delayed absorption.[107, 122, 123] Peak levels may not occur for 72 hours after ingestion.[106, 107, 124] Delayed peak levels are not caused by metabolic changes, as the enzymes responsible for oxidative metabolism are not saturable and serum CBMZ half-life after an overdose is not prolonged beyond the therapeutic half-life.[107] Neither the peak serum CBMZ level nor any serum level drawn during the clinical course can be used as a prognostic indicator. The seriousness of toxicity is determined by clinical status, not serum CBMZ level.[103]

Although CBMZ has a similar structure to TCA drugs, the degree to which the clinical course of CBMZ overdose resembles that of TCA overdose is uncertain.[102] As in TCA overdose, prolonged PR, QRS, and QT intervals have been reported in CBMZ overdose.[107] (For a discussion of treatment of CBMZ-induced cardiac arrhythmias see Chapter 34.) There are no reports on the effect of bicarbonate administration to patients with CBMZ-induced cardiac arrhythmias.

Owing to structural similarities between TCA and CBMZ, physostigmine has been administered to patients with CBMZ toxicity. However, dystonic reactions are the only toxic effect that has responded. Cardiac arrhythmias and decreased sensorium are not affected by administration of physostigmine. Dystonias are not life-threatening and will spontaneously resolve. Since physostigmine may cause cholinergic crisis, its use is not indicated.[102, 125]

Delayed, prolonged absorption and reports of gastric concentrations of pills dictate the need for gastric emptying.[106, 107, 122] Once gastric emptying has occurred, administration of multiple doses of activated charcoal will decrease the half-life and increase elimination of CBMZ.[102, 122, 124, 126] Although data are limited, charcoal hemoperfusion may also decrease the half-life of both CBMZ and the epoxide.[123, 124, 127–129] There are no data comparing the efficacy of charcoal hemoperfusion with the administration of multiple doses of activated charcoal. However, a worsening of clinical condition in a patient treated with multiple doses of activated charcoal may be an indication for charcoal hemoperfusion.[124, 127, 129] Owing to the high protein binding, hemodialysis and peritoneal dialysis are ineffective.[124] Since only 2 per cent of CBMZ and 1 per cent of the epoxide metabolite are excreted in the urine, forced diuresis is of no benefit.[124]

Although there are few reports of CBMZ intoxications, serious toxicity is possible. Supportive care is the mainstay of therapy for seriously poisoned patients. Intensive care unit monitoring is indicated until the patient has remained clinically stable for 24 hours.

References

PHENYTOIN

1. Howrie D, Cumrine P: Phenytoin-induced movement disorder associated with intravenous administration for status epilepticus. Clin Pediatr *24*:467–469, 1985.
2. Rall T, Schlerfer L: Drugs effective in the therapy of the epilepsies. *In* Gilman A, Goodman L, Rall T, Murad F (eds): Goodman and Gilman's Pharmacologic Basis of Therapeutics. New York, Macmillan, 1985, pp 450–454.
3. Bigger J, Hoffman B: Antiarrhythmic drugs. *In* Gilman A, Goodman L, Rall T, Murad F (eds): Goodman and Gilman's Pharmacologic Basis of Therapeutics. New York, Macmillan, 1985, pp 450–454.
4. Carducci B, Hedges J, Beal J, Levy R, Martin M: Emergency phenytoin loading by constant intravenous infusion. Ann Emerg Med *13*:1027–1031, 1984.
5. Woo E, Greenblatt J: Choosing the right phenytoin dosage. Drug Ther *7*:131–139, 1977.
6. Penry J, Newmark M: The use of antiepileptic drugs. Ann Intern Med *90*:207–218, 1979.
7. Goldfrank L, Bresnitz E: Phenytoin. *In* Goldfrank L, Flomenbaum N, Lewin N, Weisman R, Howland MA, Kulberg A (eds): Goldfrank's Toxicologic Emergencies. Norwalk, Appleton-Century-Crofts, 1986, pp 326–335.
8. Burckart G, Ternullo S: Management of anticonvulsant overdoses. Clin Toxicol Consult *2*:88–99, 1980.
9. Tozer T, Winter M: Phenytoin. *In* Evans W, Schentag J, Jusko W (eds): Applied Pharmacokinetics. Spokane, Applied Therapeutics, 1980, pp 275–314.
10. Louis S, Kult H, McDowell F: The cardiocirculatory changes caused by intravenous Dilantin and its solvent. Am Heart J *74*:523–529, 1968.
11. Cloyd J, Gummit R, McLain W: Status epilepticus—the role of intravenous phenytoin. JAMA *244*(13):1479–1481, 1980.
12. Salem R, Wilder B, Yost R, Doering P, Lee C: Rapid infusion of phenytoin sodium loading doses. Am J Hosp Pharmacol *38*:354–357, 1981.
13. Record K, Rapp R, Young B, Kostenbauder H: Oral phenytoin loading in adults: Rapid achievement of therapeutic plasma levels. Ann Neurol *5*:268–270, 1979.
14. Wilder B, Serrano E, Ramsay R: Plasma DPH levels after loading and maintenance doses. Clin Pharmacol Ther *14*:797–801, 1973.
15. Osborn H, Zisfein J, Sparano R: Single-dose oral phenytoin loading. Ann Emerg Med *15*:407–412, 1987.
16. Holcomb R, Lynn R, Harvey B, Sweetman B: Intoxication with Dilantin. J Pediatr *4*:627–632, 1972.
17. Cranford R, Leppik I, Patrick B, et al: Intravenous phenytoin: Clinical and pharmacokinetic aspects. Neurology *28*:874–880, 1978.
18. Cloyd J, Bosch D, Sawchuk R: Concentration time profile of phenytoin after admixture with small volumes of intravenous fluids. Am J Hosp Pharmacol *35*:45–48, 1978.
19. Goldschlager A, Karliner J: Ventricular standstill after intravenous diphenylhydantoin. Am Heart J 1967;*74*:410–412, 1967.
20. Brown C, Kaminsky M, Feroli E, Gurley H: Delerium with phenytoin and disulfiram administration. Ann Emerg Med *12*(5):310–313, 1983.
21. Walsh-Kelly C, Berens R, Glaeser P, Losek J: Intraosseous infusion of phenytoin. Am J Emerg Med *4*:523–524, 1986.
22. Kirshner H: Phenytoin toxicity when tablets substituted for capsules. N Engl J Med *303*:1106, 1983.
23. Sachlter G: Dilantin for IV use (letter). Drug Intell Clin Pharm *7*:418–419, 1973.
24. Gillman M, Sandyk R: Phenytoin toxicity and cotrimoxazole. Ann Intern Med *102*:559, 1985.
25. Rogers H, Haslam R, Longstreth J, Lietman P: Phenytoin intoxication during concurrent diazepam therapy. J Neurol Neurosurg Psychiatry *40*:890–895, 1977.
26. Dorn J: A case of phenytoin toxicity possibly precipitated by trazadone. J Clin Psychiatry 2:89–90, 1986.
27. Kooker J, Sumi S: Movement disorder as a manifestation of diphenylhydantoin intoxication. Neurology *24*:68–71, 1974.
28. Wilson J, Hojer B, Tomson G, et al: High incidence of a concentration-dependent skin reaction in children treated with phenytoin. Br Med J *1*:1583–1586, 1978.
29. Kushner M, Weinstein R, Landau B: Hypothyroidism and phenytoin intoxication. Ann Intern Med *102*:341–342, 1985.
30. Kalanie H, Niakan E, Harati Y, Rolak L: Phenytoin induced benign intracranial hypertension. Neurology *36*:443, 1986.
31. Luscher T, Siengenltraler-Zuber G: Severe hypernatremic coma due to DPH intoxication. Clin Nephrol *20*:268–269, 1983.
32. Wagner K, Leikin J: Metabolic effects of phenytoin toxicity. Ann Emerg Med *15*:509–510, 1986.
33. Flowers F, Araujo O, Hanm K: Phenytoin hypersensitivity syndrome. J Emerg Med *5*:103–108, 1987.
34. Engel J, Mellue V, Goodman D: Phenytoin hyper-

sensitivity. A case of severe acute rhabdomyolysis. Am J Med *81*:928–930, 1986.
35. Michael J, Rudin M: Acute pulmonary disease caused by phenytoin. Ann Intern Med *95*:452–454, 1981.
36. Aaron J, Bank S, Ackert G: Diphenylhydantoin-induced hepatotoxicity. Am J Gastroenterol *80*:200–202, 1985.
37. Palm R, Selsith C, Alvan G: Phenytoin intoxication as the first symptom of fatal liver damage induced by sodium valproate. Br J Clin Pharmacol *17*:597–598, 1984.
38. Mack R: Medical exorcism—acute Dilantin intoxication. North Carolina Med J *45*:99–100, 1984.
39. Larsen L, Sterett J, Whitehead B, Marcus S: Adjunctive therapy of phenytoin overdose—a case report using plasmapheresis. Clin Toxicol *24*:37–49, 1986.
40. Murphy M, Goldstein M: Diphenylhydantoin-induced asterixis. JAMA *229*:538–540, 1974.
41. Choonara I, Rosenbloom L: Focal dystonic reaction to phenytoin. Dev Med Child Neurol *26*:677–680, 1984.
42. Goni M, Jumeniz M, Feijoo M: Parkinsonism induced by phenytoin. Clin Neuropharmacol *8*:383–384, 1985.
43. Hughes F, Simon J: Introgenic diphenylhydantoin (Dilantin) intoxication. Texas Med *71*:49–52, 1975.
44. Zinsmeister S, Marks R: Acute athetosis as a result of phenytoin toxicity in a child. Am J Dis Child *130*:75–76, 1976.
45. Wilson J, Huff G, Kilroy A: Prolonged toxicity following acute phenytoin overdose in a child. J Pediatr *95*:135–138, 1979.
46. Gill M, Kern J, Kaneko J, et al: Phenytoin overdose kinetics. Western J Med *128*:246–248, 1978.
47. Chaikin P, Adir J, Crouthamel W: Unusual absorption profile of phenytoin in a massive overdose case. Clin Res *27*:541, 1979.
48. Jung D, Powell R, Walson P, Perrier D: Effect of dose on phenytoin absorption. Clin Pharmacol Ther *28*:479–485, 1985.
49. Banner W, Johnson D, Walson P, Jung D: Effects of single large doses of phenytoin on glucose homeostasis—a preliminary report. J Clin Pharmacol *22*:79–81, 1982.
50. Czajka P, Anderson W, Christoph R, Banner W: A pharmacokinetic evaluation of peritoneal dialysis for phenytoin intoxication. J Clin Pharmacol *20*:565–569, 1980.
51. Lindahl S, Westerling D: Detoxification with peritoneal dialysis and blood exchange after diphenylhydantoin intoxication. Acta Paediatr Scand *71*:665–666, 1982.
52. Logan W, Freeman J: Pseudodegenerative disease due to diphenylhydantoin intoxication. Arch Neurol *21*:631–639, 1969.
53. Lindvall O, Nilsson B: Cerebellar atrophy following phenytoin intoxication. Ann Neurol *16*:258–260, 1984.
54. Baier W, Beck U, Hirsch W: CT findings following diphenylhydantoin intoxication. Pediatr Radiol *15*:220–221, 1985.
55. McLain L, Martin T, Allen J: Cerebellar degeneration due to chronic phenytoin therapy. Ann Neurol *7*:18–23, 1980.
56. Bridges S, Ebersole J: Incidence of seizures with phenytoin toxicity. Neurology *35*:1167–1168, 1985.
57. Earnest M, Marx J, Drury L: Complications of intravenous phenytoin for acute treatment of seizures. JAMA *249*:6, 1983.
58. Voigt G: Death following intravenous Dilantin. Johns Hopkins Med J *128*:153–157, 1968.
59. Russel M, Bousvaros G: Fatal results from diphenylhydantoin administered intravenously. JAMA *206*:2118–2119, 1968.
60. Unger A, Sklaroff H: Fatalities following intravenous use of sodium diphenylhydantoin for cardiac arrhythmias. JAMA *200*:335–336, 1967.
61. Zoneraich S, Zoneraich O, Siegel J: Sudden death following intravenous sodium diphenylhydantoin. Am Heart J *92*:375–377, 1976.
62. Goldschlager A, Karliner J: Ventricular standstill after intravenous diphenylhydantoin. Am Heart J *74*:410–412, 1967.
63. Gellerman G, Martinez C: Fatal ventricular fibrillation following intravenous sodium diphenylhydantoin therapy. JAMA *200*:337–338, 1967.
64. Voigt G: Death following intravenous sodium diphenylhydantoin. Johns Hopkins Med J *123*:153–157, 1968.
65. Barron S: Cardiac arrhythmias after small IV dose of phenytoin. N Engl J Med *295*:678, 1976.
66. Kilarski D, Buchanan C, Behren L: Soft tissue damage associated with intravenous phenytoin. N Engl J Med *311*:1186–1187, 1984.
67. Reeme P, Day D: Phenytoin injection precautions. Clin Pharmacol *4*:618–620, 1985.
68. Paul W: Phenytoin injection precautions. Clin Pharmacol *5*:370–371, 1986.

VALPROIC ACID

69. Wason S, Savitt D: Acute valproic acid toxicity at therapeutic concentrations. Clin Pediatr *24*:466–467, 1985.
70. Rail T, Schlerfer L: Drugs effective in the therapy of the epilepsies. *In* Gilman A, Goodman L, Rall T, Murad F (eds): Goodman and Gilman's Pharmacologic Basis of Therapeutics. New York, Macmillan, 1985, pp 461–463.
71. Isom J: On the toxicity of valproic acid. Am J Dis Child *138*:901–903, 1984.
72. Gram L, Bentsen K: Valproate: An updated review. Acta Neurol Scand *72*:129–139, 1985.
73. Koch-Weser J: Valproic acid. N Engl J Med *302*:661–666, 1980.
74. Levy R, Koch K: Drug interactions with valproic acid. Drugs *24*:543–556, 1982.
75. Schmidt D: Adverse effects of valproate. Epilepsia *25* (Suppl 1):544–549, 1984.
76. May T, Rambeck B: Serum concentrations of valproic acid: Influence of dose and co-medication. Ther Drug Monitor *7*:387–390, 1985.
77. Zaret B, Cohen R: Reversible valproic acid induced dementia: A case report. Epilepsia *27*:234–240, 1986.
78. Ralnaike R, Schapel G, Purdie G, Rischbieth R, Hoffman S: Hyperammonaemia and hepatotoxicity during chronic valproate therapy: Enhancement by combination with other antiepileptic drugs. Br J Clin Pharmacol *22*:100–103, 1986.
79. Gaskins J, Holt R, Postelnick M: Non dosage-dependent valproic acid-induced hyperammonemia and coma. Clin Pharmacol *3*:313–316, 1984.
80. Zaccara G, Campostrini R, Paganini M, et al: Acute changes of blood ammonia may predict short-term

adverse effects of valproic acid. Neurology *34*:1519–1521, 1984.
81. Powell-Jackson P, Tredger T, Williams R: Hepatotoxicity to sodium valproate: A review. Gut *25*:673–681, 1984.
82. Farrell K, Abbott F, Orr J, Applegarth D, Jan J, Wong P: Free and total serum valproate concentrations: Their relationship to seizure control, liver enzymes, and plasma ammonia in children. Can J Neurol Sci *13*:252–255, 1986.
83. Scheffner D: Fatal liver failure in children on valproate. Lancet 2:511, 1986.
84. Green S: Sodium valproate and routine liver function tests. Arch Dis Child *59*:813–814, 1984.
85. Schnabel R, Rambeck B, Janssen F: Fatal intoxication with sodium valproate. Lancet *1*:221–222, 1985.
86. Jeavens P: Non-dose related side effects of valproate. Epilepsia *25* (Suppl 1):S50–55, 1984.
87. Pedersen B, Jensen P: Electroencephalographic alterations during intoxication with sodium valproate: A case report. Epilepsia *25*:121–124, 1984.
88. Karlsen R, Kett K, Henriksin O: Intoxication with sodium valproate. Acta Med Scand *213*:405–406, 1983.
89. Karlsen R, Kett K, Henriksen O: Intoxication with sodium valproate. Acta Med Scand *213*:405–406, 1983.
90. Eeg-Olafsson O, Lindskog U: Acute intoxication with valproate. Lancet *1*:1306, 1982.
91. Steiman G, Woerpel R, Sherard E: Treatment of accidental sodium valproate overdose with an opiate antagonist. Ann Neurol *6*:224, 1979.
92. Mortensen P, Hansen H, Pedersen B, et al: Acute valproate intoxication: Biochemical investigations and hemodialysis treatment. Int J Clin Pharm Therapy Toxicol *21*:64–68, 1983.
93. Merwe A, Albrecht C, Brink M, Coetzee A: Sodium valproate poisoning. S Afr Med J *67*:735–736, 1985.
94. Lindhout D, Schmidt D: In vitro exposure to valproate and neural tube defects. Lancet *1*:1392–1393, 1986.
95. Jager-Roman E, Diechl A, Jakob S, et al: Fetal growth, major malformations, and minor anomalies in infants born to woman receiving valproic acid. J Pediatr *108*:997–1004, 1986.

SUCCINIMIDES

96. Rail T, Schlerfer L: Drugs effective in the therapy of the epilepsies. *In* Gilman A, Goodman L, Rall T, Murad F (eds): Goodman and Gilman's Pharmacologic Basis of Therapeutics. New York, Macmillan, 1985, pp 459–461.
97. Wallace S: Use of ethosuximide and valproate in the treatment of epilepsy. Neurol Clin *4*:601–606, 1986.
98. Karch S: Methsuximide overdose. JAMA *223*:1463–1465, 1973.
99. Baehler R, Work J, Smith W, Dominic J: Charcoal hemoperfusion in the therapy for methsuximide and phenytoin overdose. Arch Intern Med *140*:1466–1468, 1980.

OXAZOLIDINEDIONE

100. Porter R, Pitlick W: Antiepileptic drugs. *In* Katzung B (ed): Basic and Clinical Pharmacology. Los Angeles, Appleton and Lange, 1987, pp 262–278.
101. Rail T, Schlerfer L: Drugs effective in the therapy of the epilepsies. *In* Gilman A, Goodman L, Rall T, Murad F (eds): Goodman and Gilman's Pharmacologic Basis of Therapeutics. New York, Macmillan, 1985, pp 463–464.

CARBAMAZEPINE

102. O'Neal W, Whitten K, Baumann R, et al: Lack of serious toxicity following carbamazepine overdosage. Clin Pharmacol *3*:545–547, 1984.
103. Berrettini W: Erythromycin-induced carbamazepine toxicity. J Clin Psychiatry *47*:147, 1986.
104. Rall T, Schleifer L: Drugs effective in the therapy of the epilepsies. *In* Gilman A, Goodman L, Rall T, Murad F (eds): Goodman and Gilman's Pharmacologic Basis of Therapeutics. New York, Macmillan, 1985, pp 457–459.
105. Clancy R: New anticonvulsants in pediatrics. Carbamazepine and valproate. Curr Probl Pediatr 139–209, 1987.
106. Rockoff S, Baselt R: Severe carbamazepine poisoning. Clin Toxicol *18*:935–939, 1981.
107. Sullivan J, Rumack B, Peterson R: Acute carbamazepine toxicity resulting from overdose. Neurology *31*:621–624, 1981.
108. Pena M, Lope E: Can a single measurement of CBMZ suffice for therapeutic monitoring? Clin Chem *6*:812–813, 1987.
109. Baciewicz A: Carbamazepine drug interactions. Ther Drug Monitor *8*:305–317, 1986.
110. Woody R, Kearns G, Bolyard K: Carbamazepine intoxication following the use of erythromycin in children. Pediatr Inf Dis *6*:578–579, 1987.
111. Galeone D, Lamontanara G, Torelli D: Acute hepatitis in a patient heated with carbamazepine. J Neurol *232*:301–303, 1985.
112. Zucker P, Dawm F, Cohen M: Fatal carbamazepine hepatitis J Pediatr *91*:667–668, 1977.
113. Steiner C, Wit A, Weiss M, Damato A: The antiarrhythmic actions of carbamazepine. J Pharmacol Exp Ther *173*:323–335, 1970.
114. Beermann B, Edhag O: Depressive effects of carbamazepine or idioventricular rhythm in man. Br Med J *2*:171–172, 1978.
115. Durelli L, Mutani R, Sechi P, et al: Cardiac side effects of phenytoin and carbamazepine. Arch Neurol *42*:1067–1068, 1985.
116. Herzberg L: Carbamazepine and bradycardia. Lancet *1*:1097–1098, 1978.
117. Heweston K, Ritch A, Watson R: Sick sinus syndrome aggravated by carbamazepine therapy for epilepsy. Postgrad Med J *62*:497–498, 1986.
118. Ashton M, Ball S, Thomas T, Lee M: Water intoxication associated with carbamazepine treatment. Br Med J *1*:1134–1135, 1977.
119. Harat N, Shalit M: Carbamazepine induced vasculitis. J Neurol Neurosurg Psychiatry *50*:1241–1243, 1987.
120. Alballa S, Fritzler M, Davis P: A case of drug induced lupus due to carbamazepine. J Rheumatol *14*:599–600, 1987.
121. Silverstein F, Parrish M, Johnston M: Adverse behavioral reactions in children treated with CBMZ. J Pediatr *5*:785–787, 1982.
122. May D: Acute CBMZ intoxication. South Med J *77*:24–27, 1984.
123. Vree T, Janssen T, Hekster Y, et al: Clinical pharmacokinetics of CBMZ and its epoxy and hydroxy metabolites in humans after an overdose. Ther Drug Monitor *8*:297–304, 1986.

124. Groot G, Van Heijst A, Maes R: Charcoal hemoperfusion in the treatment of two cases of acute CBMZ poisoning. Clin Toxicol *4*:349–362, 1984.
125. Lehrman S, Bauman M: CBMZ overdose. Am J Dis Child *135*:768–769, 1981.
126. Neuvonen P, Olkkola K: Oral activated charcoal in the treatment of intoxications. Med Toxicol *3*:33–58, 1988.
127. Gary N, Byra W, Eisinger R: Carbamazepine poisoning: Treatment by hemoperfusion. Nephron *27*:202–203, 1981.
128. Nilsson C, Sterner G, Idvall J: Charcoal hemoperfusion for treatment of serious carbamazepine poisoning. Acta Med Scand *216*:137–140, 1984.
129. Chan K, Aguanno J, Jansen R, Dietzler D: Charcoal hemoperfusion for treatment of carbamazepine poisoning. Clin Chem *27*:1300–1302, 1981.

SECTION C

Analgesics

CHAPTER 50

ACETAMINOPHEN

Barry H. Rumack, M.D.
W. Lynn Augenstein, M.D.

MECHANISMS OF ACETAMINOPHEN TOXICITY

Acetaminophen is metabolized primarily by sulfation and glucuronidation of the para-hydroxyl group.[1–3] Neither unchanged acetaminophen nor its glucuronide and sulfate conjugates are toxic. Thus acetaminophen is a remarkably safe drug when used at usual therapeutic doses. Acetaminophen use has markedly increased in the United States; some over-the-counter products that contain acetaminophen are Tylenol, Tempra, Anacin-3, Datril, and Panadol.

A small fraction of an administered dose of acetaminophen is converted to a reactive metabolite by the cytochrome P-450–dependent, mixed-function oxidase enzymes present in hepatic cells.[3–6] After normal doses of acetaminophen, the small amount of reactive metabolite produced is detoxified by preferential conjugation with cellular glutathione and excreted in the urine as cysteine and mercapturic acid metabolites (Fig. 50–1).[2, 3]

In the overdosed patient, the amount of reactive metabolite formed through the cytochrome P-450 pathway is increased because of the greater total amounts of drug presented to the liver. When the increase is large enough to deplete glutathione by 70 per cent or more, the reactive metabolite can no longer be adequately detoxified by that pathway, and covalent binding of excess metabolites to cellular protein macromolecules occurs.[3, 6–10] The covalently bound reactive metabolite arylates the cellular nucleophiles and produces hepatocellular necrosis.[2–4, 6, 11, 12]

Experimental evidence has shown that pretreatment of human subjects with inducers of cytochrome P-450 enzymes, such as phenobarbital,[12] increases the formation of the toxic acetaminophen metabolite. A retrospective study of patients with acetaminophen toxicity suggested that hepatic injury also may be enhanced by previous consumption of barbiturates and large amounts of ethanol.[13] Prospective studies in both animals[13a] and humans[13b] have shown, however, that ethanol taken simultaneously with an acetaminophen overdose is hepatoprotective. Diphenhydramine is also a probable inducer of the enzyme systems.[14]

It has also been suggested that poor nutrition leading to reduced glutathione stores may enhance acetaminophen toxicity, since rats fed a protein-deficient diet were found to be more sensitive to high doses of the drug.[15] Alternatively, it has been postulated that malnutrition may have a net protective effect by producing a decrease in P-450 enzyme activity and thus a reduction in the

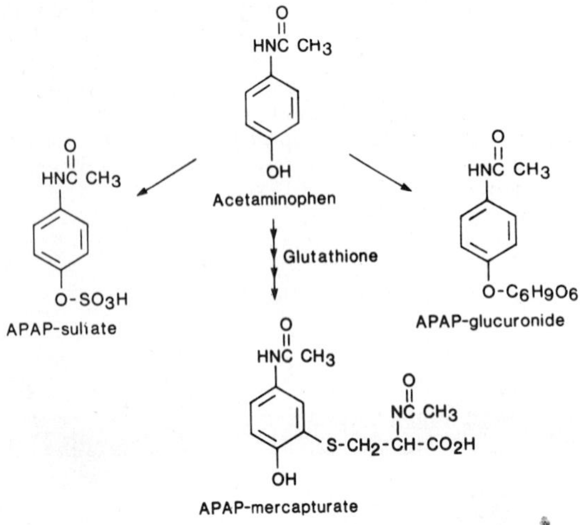

Figure 50–1. Metabolic pathways for acetaminophen. Minor metabolites formed by P-450 mixed-function oxidase (middle) pathway are believed to cause hepatotoxicity.

conversion of acetaminophen to its reactive metabolite.[16]

EVOLUTION OF TREATMENT STRATEGY

The first case of liver damage associated with acetaminophen was reported in the United Kingdom by Davidson in 1966.[17] This was followed by several additional reports describing small numbers of cases over the next 4 years.[18–20] Beginning in 1970, a number of papers reporting on larger patient series appeared in the British literature, including those of Proudfoot and Wright (37 patients),[21] Clark and associates (60 patients),[22] James and associates (54 patients),[23] and Crome and associates (31 patients).[24] Most of the acetaminophen poisonings documented were the result of suicide attempts. In following up 107 patients hospitalized for acetaminophen overdose, Gazzard and colleagues found evidence of deliberate ingestion with suicidal intent in all cases.[25]

Until 1975, there was only one published case of acetaminophen hepatotoxicity due to overdose in the United States.[26] However, in that year it was suggested that this situation was largely a result of failure to accurately diagnose these ingestions.[14] Although the number of reported cases of acetaminophen overdosage rose considerably thereafter in the United States, the mortality rate has been remarkably low. The significant advances achieved in the management of acetaminophen overdose are clearly important factors in this favorable morbidity and mortality picture.

Initially, acetaminophen toxicity was treated primarily with supportive measures, but, as the overdose experience increased, additional management techniques were attempted. Forced diuresis,[19] hemodialysis,[27] and charcoal column hemoperfusion[28] were tried, but none was shown to provide a substantial benefit.[14, 29] The use of antihistamines and corticosteroids was advocated,[19] but animal experiments later suggested that hydrocortisone has no hepatoprotective effects, and antihistamines may even enhance acetaminophen toxicity.[30] Penicillamine also was of questionable efficacy and possibly contributed to nephrotoxicity,[31] and dimercaprol (BAL) was of no value.[32]

Following publication of the important mechanistic findings of Mitchell and colleagues,[5] nucleophilic sulfhydryl compounds, including cysteamine[29, 31] and L-methionine,[31, 33] were administered with encouraging results. These experiments led to trials with N-acetylcysteine, which had the additional benefit of broad availability as a commercial product.

N-ACETYLCYSTEINE

N-Acetylcysteine (NAC) is the *N*-acetyl derivative of the naturally occurring amino acid L-cysteine. NAC constitutes the central portion of the glutathione molecule, and it is known to have chelating,[34] nucleophilic,[35] and weak anti-inflammatory[36] properties. This agent has been marketed in the United States and abroad as a mucolytic, principally for the treatment of respiratory disorders. NAC also has been utilized in the treatment of intestinal impactions[37] and cystinuria[38] and as a chelating agent in the management of toxic gold accumulation in patients with rheumatoid arthritis receiving chrysotherapy.[34] In animals, NAC is reported to be an effective antidote for cyclophosphamide,[39, 40] isophosphamide,[41] and acetaldehyde poisonings[42] and, in conjunction with pyridoxine, an antagonist to the hepatotoxic effects of carbon tetrachloride.[43]

The antidotal mechanism of NAC in acetaminophen overdosage is not completely understood. NAC is metabolized to cysteine, a glutathione precursor.[44] Therefore, one possible mechanism is the maintenance of protective levels of glutathione, which can detoxify the reactive acetaminophen metabolite by conjugation. In mice overdosed with acetaminophen, cysteine has been shown to replenish hepatic glutathione.[45] A direct antidotal effect is also possible, since in vitro experiments have shown that NAC and cysteine, as well as glutathione, will form conjugates with the reactive acetaminophen metabolite.[46]

Other factors may be influential as well. The treatment of acetaminophen-overdosed mice with NAC produces increased survival even when covalent binding of the toxic metabolite to hepatic macromolecules is not prevented.[47, 48] This finding suggests that sulfhydryl compounds such as NAC may act in part by stabilizing cell constituents against the deleterious effects of covalent binding[49, 50] and is consistent with the clinical observation that NAC affords some degree of hepatoprotection even on relatively late administration. In addition, recent findings of Galinsky and Levy suggest that NAC may enhance the metabolic conversion of acetaminophen to its sulfate conjugate, thereby reducing the formation of other metabolites, including the toxic agent.[51]

Because NAC is a broadly available sulfhydryl-containing compound, an effort to determine its efficacy in the treatment of acetaminophen overdosage was undertaken. Piperno and colleagues conducted a series of experiments with NAC in acetaminophen-overdosed CF-1 mice.[52–55] In this animal model, acetaminophen overdosage generally results in debilitation within 1 hour and death within 24 hours. Early oral single-dose NAC treatment (1 hour after overdosage) conferred dramatic hepatoprotection. A dose response profile was obtained for single oral NAC doses between 100 and 1200 mg/kg, with 100 per cent survival documented at the highest dose tested.

Mortality in acetaminophen-overdosed mice was examined following multiple-dose as well as single-dose NAC administration. This study showed that the cumulative mortality incidence was 77.5 per cent for overdosed mice treated with placebo, 27.5 per cent for the group treated with a single dose of NAC, and 12.5 per cent for the group receiving a multiple-dose NAC regimen. When deaths were categorized as "early" (less than 10 hours after overdosage) or "late" (more than 10 hours after overdosage), the NAC multiple-dose regimen was found to be statistically superior ($p < 0.05$) to the single-dose treatment in the prevention of late deaths.

In other oral administration studies in mice, NAC was compared with reference compounds that have been used in acetaminophen overdosage. NAC was more effective than cysteamine regardless of the time interval between overdosage and antidote administration. In contrast to NAC, cysteamine afforded no protection after late administration. The positive effect of NAC on survival of late-treated mice was quite apparent, although hepatoprotection was not confirmed by transaminase levels.

Like NAC, methionine was found to be an effective antidote; however, survival rates were lower with methionine. Also, methionine exhibited a bell-shaped dose-response curve that differed markedly from the linear pattern observed with NAC.

THE NAC MULTICENTER STUDY (ROCKY MOUNTAIN POISON AND DRUG CENTER)

Protocol

To assure the accumulation of a significant number of cases within a reasonable period of time, the NAC Multicenter Study was designed as a national program. Since current literature suggests that supportive treatment alone is not sufficient to minimize acetaminophen toxicity in high-risk patients, the inclusion of an untreated control group in this study was considered ethically unjustifiable.[56] Furthermore, because other possible antidotes, such as cysteamine and L-methionine, were not readily available throughout the United States, the use of a reference drug was not feasible. The study, therefore, was conducted as an open trial.

The existence of the NAC study was made known to emergency departments, poison centers, and hospitals throughout the United States, thus providing the entry of patients from any geographic area. Telephone supervision of physicians reporting cases was accomplished by the investigators and a staff of specially trained nurses. Data on each patient studied were obtained by telephone, confirmed by review copies of hospital records, and entered on case report forms under the investigators' supervision.

The study protocol required that patients be over 12 years of age, with a history of known or suspected acute ingestion of 7.5 gm or more of acetaminophen. Only those patients who could be given their initial dose of NAC within 24 hours following the overdose ingestion were entered.

Supportive Measures

Appropriate emergency and general supportive measures were instituted for each patient. When overdosage of more than one agent was known or suspected, treatment of the most immediately life-threatening component was undertaken first. For acetaminophen overdosage, gastric aspiration and lavage were implemented. If the use of activated charcoal or a cathartic such as sodium sulfate was required because of mixed poisoning, the stomach was lavaged with water or saline prior to NAC administration. This procedure was necessary to prevent adsorption of the NAC by the other agents.

Other supportive measures included maintenance of fluid and electrolyte balance, administration of plasma or clotting factor concentrate if the prothrombin time ratio became abnormal, and administration of IV glucose solution if hypoglycemia developed. Antihistamines, CNS depressants, forced IV fluids, diuretics, and drugs having hepatotoxic potential were avoided.

NAC Administration

NAC was prepared from commercially available, 30-ml vials of 20 per cent acetylcysteine (Mucomyst). One part of the commercial Mucomyst solution was diluted with three parts of cola-type or other soda, grapefruit juice, or plain tap water to provide a 5 per cent NAC solution for administration.

The NAC solution was given orally in a loading dose of 140 mg/kg, followed by a maintenance dose of 70 mg/kg every 4 hours thereafter, over a period of 72 hours (total of 17 maintenance doses). If a patient vomited within 1 hour following a loading or maintenance dose, the dose was repeated. If plasma acetaminophen levels showed a patient to be below the study nomogram (Fig. 50–2), NAC was discontinued. NAC therapy was also terminated if evidence of hepatic encephalopathy appeared, although there is no evidence to suggest that continued administration of NAC in this circumstance would be harmful.

Laboratory Measurements

Immediately following institution or during the course of required supportive measures, blood was drawn for assay of the plasma acetaminophen level. Three additional samples were drawn at 4-hour intervals and three more at 8-hour intervals, for a total of seven additional specimens. All samples were frozen and sent to a single laboratory (University of Colorado Health Sciences Center) for analysis of acetaminophen levels. Initial blood levels were occasionally done at the local hospital, but all eight blood levels reported were done in our laboratory.

In addition, a complete battery of liver and kidney function tests was performed three times on the first day of treatment, twice daily through the fifth day, then once daily until discharge. Other tests, including serum electrolyte and other hematology determinations, urinalysis, and electrocardiogram (ECG), were done at least once daily throughout the period of hospitalization.

Statistical Methods

Objectives

The three basic objectives of the collection of data pertaining to the efficacy of NAC were (1) to demonstrate any reduction in mortality resulting from NAC treatment; (2) to determine whether laboratory measurements show less liver damage or liver function among NAC-treated patients than would be expected if no specific antidote had been given; and (3) to assess the effect of the time interval between overdose and initiation of NAC treatment on laboratory test results and clinical outcome.

Patient Categorization

For purposes of statistical analysis, the study population was partitioned into a num-

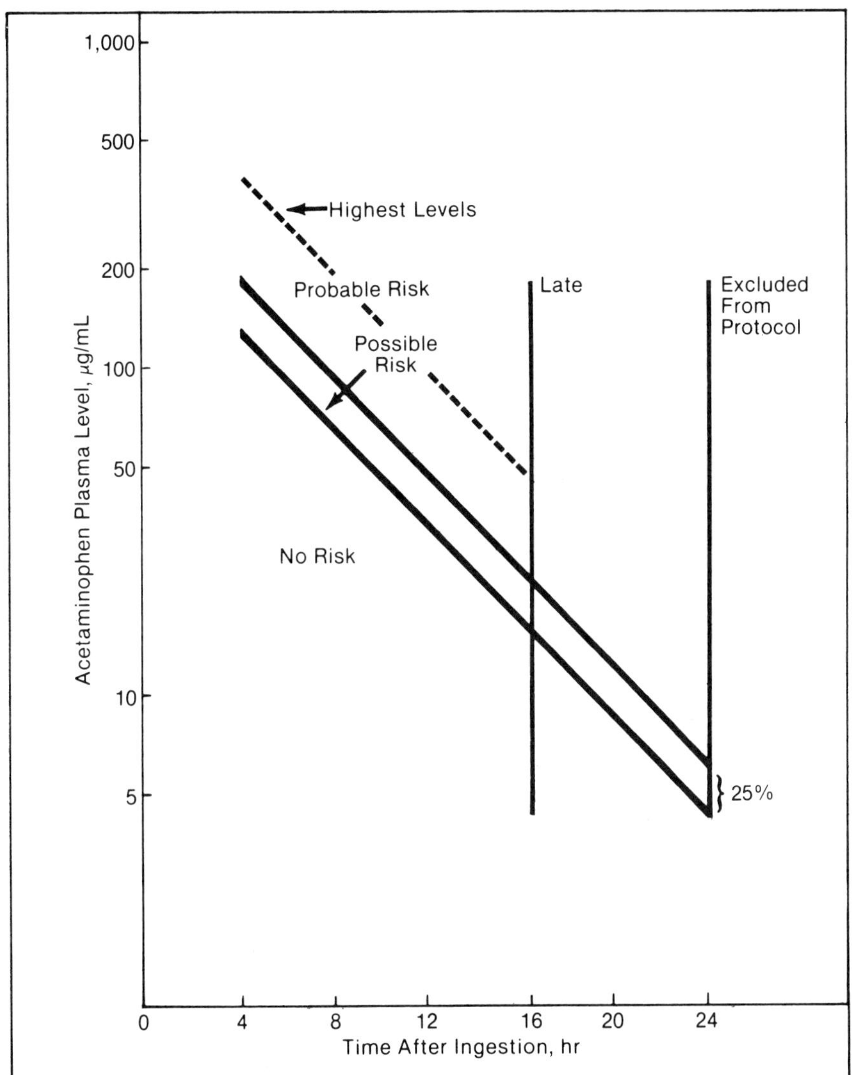

Figure 50–2. Study design nomogram. Possible risk is 25 per cent below nomogram for multiclinic open-study. (From Rumack BH, Peterson RG, Koch GG, Amara IA: Acetaminophen overdose: 662 cases with evaluation of oral acetylcysteine treatment. Arch Intern Med *141*:380, 1981. © 1981, American Medical Association.)

ber of subgroups based on plasma acetaminophen level, time delay from ingestion to treatment, protocol exclusion factors, and number of NAC doses administered. An *exclusion* category was also constructed for NAC-treated patients who lacked usable serum acetaminophen assays or who otherwise did not meet critical protocol criteria.

The basic risk category assignment was determined on the basis of serum acetaminophen levels (Table 50–1). The study design nomogram (see Fig. 50–2) was used as a tool to determine risk. This nomogram contained a safety zone 25 per cent under the originally published nomogram (Fig. 50–3).

The following additional study population partitioning measures were taken prior to data analysis:

1. The *probable risk* group in the NAC-treated population was separated into two segments: those patients who received 16 or more doses of NAC, and those who received fewer than 16 NAC doses. This division was accomplished to allow separate statistical analyses for those high-risk patients who received a full course of NAC therapy and those who did not.
2. The *probable risk with 16 or more doses of NAC* groups in both the U.S. NAC-treated population and the Prescott historical control group were further subdivided into those patients with a predicted 12-hour postingestion serum acetaminophen level of 100 μg/ml or more and those with a predicted level of less than 100 μg/ml. This was done to provide subgroups for statistical evaluation that were less heterogeneous with respect to this important variable.

Table 50–1. RISK CATEGORY ASSIGNMENT BASED ON SERUM ACETAMINOPHEN LEVELS

RISK ASSIGNMENT	PREDICTED SERUM ACETAMINOPHEN LEVEL		
	4-hr	*OR 8-hr*	*OR 12-hr*
Slight Risk	≤120 μg/ml	≤60 μg/ml	≤30 μg/ml
Possible Risk	>120 μg/ml and <200 μg/ml	>60 μg/ml and <100 μg/ml	>30 μg/ml and <50 μg/ml
Probable Risk	≥200 μg/ml	≥100 μg/ml	≥50 μg/ml

(From Rumack BH, Peterson RG, Koch GG, Amara IA: Acetaminophen overdose: 662 cases with evaluation of oral acetylcysteine treatment. Arch Intern Med *141*:380, 1981. © 1981, American Medical Association.)

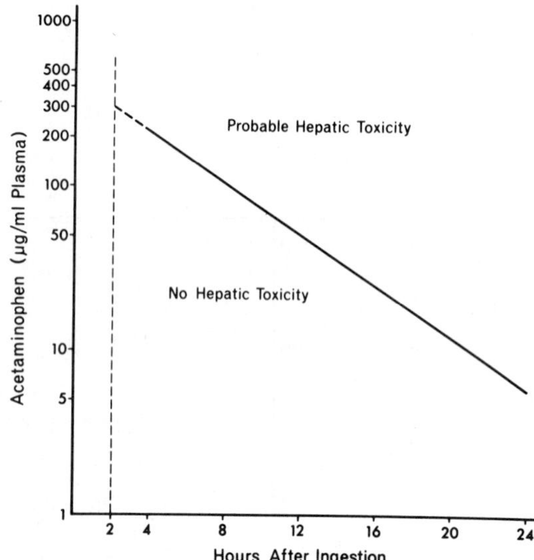

Figure 50–3. The original nomogram. (From Rumack BH, Matthew H: Acetaminophen poisoning and toxicity. Pediatrics *55*:871, 1975.)

3. The *slight risk* group in the NAC-treated population was further subdivided into those patients who received six or more doses of NAC and those who were administered fewer than six NAC doses. It was considered that the *slight risk with six or more doses of NAC* group would yield the most valuable data regarding the safety of NAC for this indication.

Efficacy Evaluation

The peak values of serum glutamic oxaloacetic transaminase (SGOT), serum glutamic pyruvic transaminase (SGPT), serum bilirubin, and prothrombin time were considered to be the most appropriate summary indicators of liver damage or liver function. To deal with the variation in the normal range of transaminase values among the large number of individual laboratories conducting these tests, SGOT and SGPT ratios were calculated by dividing the maximum value recorded for each patient by the upper limit of the normal range for the laboratory performing the test. For all patients in the historical control group and all patients for whom normal ranges were not recorded, the upper limits of normal were considered to be 40 units for SGOT and 35 units for SGPT.

The statistical significance of the relationships between various possible patient risk factors and laboratory measures of hepatotoxicity was evaluated in terms of chi-square statistics, calculated for pertinent sets of two-way contingency tables. Possible risk factors considered were (1) demographic characteristics (age, sex, weight), (2) alleged ingestion dose of acetaminophen, (3) mixed ingestion, (4) alcohol or drug usage history and history of liver disease or other significant disease, (5) emergency treatment measures (forced emesis, lavage, catharsis, activated charcoal, other), (6) number of doses of NAC retained, (7) change in NAC administration schedule, and (8) time delay to first medical encounter, first serum acetaminophen level assay, and first dose of NAC.

Laboratory measures of hepatotoxicity included transaminase, bilirubin, and prothrombin time ratios. Relationships between the possible risk factors and the laboratory measures of hepatotoxicity were then analyzed for the various risk category populations that were previously partitioned.

Safety Evaluation

Assessments of the safety of NAC for the indication under investigation were of three main types: adverse experiences manifested as symptoms and signs, laboratory abnormalities, and electrocardiographic changes.

Acetaminophen in overdose quantities acts as an antidiuretic,[57] and NAC has the potential for producing gastrointestinal disturbances at high oral dosages.[58] It was therefore considered that if NAC caused or aggravated nausea or diarrhea to a significant degree, the possibility of fluid and electrolyte imbalances could be increased. Conversely, it was considered that NAC could reduce the occurrence or severity of these adverse effects by preventing liver damage or protecting liver function.

Specific safety measures included documentation of all adverse experiences observed among patients receiving one or more doses of NAC. The case report provided for entry of information regarding the severity and chronicity of each adverse experience, the action taken and result of the action, and the treating physician's opinion of the relationship of the adverse experience to NAC therapy. Treating physicians were specifically questioned concerning symptoms related to hepatic encephalopathy. All adverse experiences were coded and transformed to summary indexes for statistical purposes.

Clinical laboratory measures in addition to liver function tests were to be obtained at least once daily during each patient's hospitalization. The test battery included blood glucose, serum creatinine, blood urea nitrogen (BUN), serum electrolytes, and complete blood count (CBC) with platelet estimate. Statistical treatment of these results was similar to that utilized for the liver function tests described earlier in the section on Efficacy Evaluation.

The protocol also specified that an ECG be taken daily during the first 5 days of each patient's hospitalization, with a follow-up ECG on the 14th day postingestion. This procedure was commonly modified by the treating physicians. An effort was made to obtain as many tracings as possible, and those received were read by a consulting cardiologist. For statistical analysis, results were coded as "normal," "abnormal-trivial," or "abnormal-nontrivial." In addition, the relationship of ECG abnormalities, serum potassium level, and diarrhea or vomiting was examined when sufficient data were available.

PHARMACOKINETICS

Acetaminophen is a weak acid with a pK_a of 9.5 due to its aromatic hydroxyl group. Absorption is rapid and usually complete by 1 hour in therapeutic dosages, with slightly faster absorption of liquid preparations. In the overdose state, absorption, unless retarded by agents that reduce gastric emptying, is complete by 4 hours, which is when the nomogram begins. Plotting plasma data before this is of no value. Absorption can be retarded by administration of propantheline and accelerated by metoclopramide.[59]

Urinary recovery of acetaminophen and its metabolites is shown in Table 50–2. Additionally, the work of Miller and associates has shown a switch in predominance of sulfate to glucuronide occurring between the ages of 9 and 12.[60] The change in metabolite predominance is consistent with the change from the childhood to the adult pattern of acetaminophen toxicity.[61] Half-life data have been used in the past to describe the toxicity of acetaminophen. It was considered that a

Table 50–2. URINARY RECOVERY OF TRITIATED ACETAMINOPHEN

	% RECOVERED RADIOACTIVITY
Tritiated acetaminophen (unchanged)	2.1
Sulfate conjugate	52.1
Glucuronide conjugate	42.0
Mercapturic acid conjugate	3.8

(From Mitchell JR, Thorgeirsson SS, Potter WZ, et al: Acetaminophen-induced hepatic injury: Protective role of glutathione in man and rationale for therapy. Clin Pharmacol Ther *16*:676, 1974.)

half-life of more than 4 hours was potentially hepatotoxic. Since these half-lives really reflect the inactive sulfate and glucuronide metabolite and not the relatively small amount made of the toxic metabolite, half-life has been abandoned as a predictor of outcome.

Acetaminophen has noncomplex, noncumulative log linear kinetics of the first-order type. This is in contrast to salicylates, which have cumulative kinetics of the zero-order type and exceed metabolic capacity, becoming dependent on urine flow and pH for elimination.

Protein binding of acetaminophen is about 10 per cent and its volume of distribution (VD) slightly higher than that of body water. The VD is generally accepted as 1 L/kg. Although acetaminophen is a metabolite of phenacetin, it does not have the capacity to go backward through this chain (Fig. 50–4). Consequently, neither the renal papillary necrosis nor the methemoglobinemia seen with phenacetin toxicity is seen in humans with acetaminophen toxicity.[62]

Chronic toxicity from accumulation of acetaminophen in the body in a manner similar to that seen with salicylate does not occur. Chronic excessive use of acetaminophen (greater than 4 gm/day), by reducing glutathione stores, eventually may lead to transient hepatotoxicity. Since glutathione turnover is continuous, it is likely that a dose much higher than the recommended therapeutic limit would have to be consumed on a continuous basis before hepatotoxicity could develop.

With these factors in mind, the therapy of acetaminophen overdose has been based upon the use of *N*-acetylcysteine rather than on any attempts at removal by extracorporeal or diuretic means.

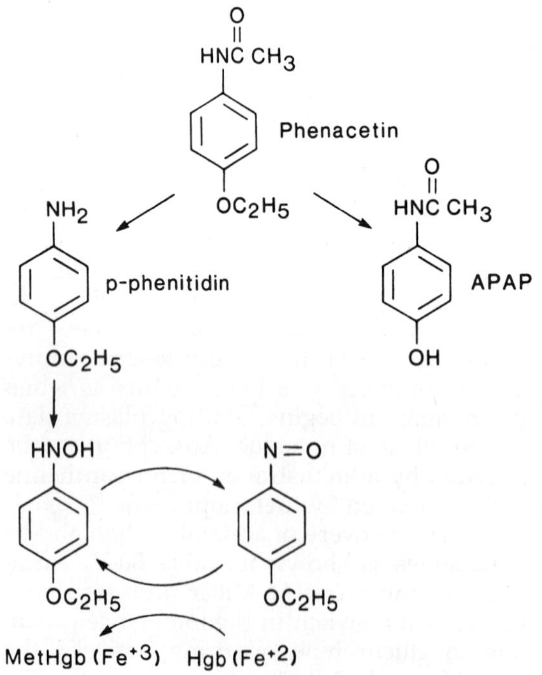

Figure 50–4. Metabolic pathways from phenacetin to acetaminophen and to *p*-phenitidin. Further metabolism from *p*-phenitidin results in products causing methemoglobin. (From Peterson RG, Rumack BH: Pharmacokinetics of acetaminophen: Absorption, distribution, metabolism, excretion. Pediatrics 62:877, 1978. © American Academy of Pediatrics 1978.)

ETHANOL AND ACETAMINOPHEN

Although it had been assumed that the consumption of ethanol, especially on a chronic basis, would produce a situation predisposing to increased risk for acetaminophen hepatotoxicity in overdose, this has been shown not to be true (Table 50–3).[13a, 13b]

PEDIATRIC ACETAMINOPHEN OVERDOSE

(Tables 50–4, 50–5, and 50–6)

The child under age 9 years has a different picture following an acetaminophen overdose from that seen in the adult. Children with very high levels of acetaminophen, well into the toxic range, and who even have been treated late with NAC still show remarkably minor rises in serum hepatic enzymes.[56]

Although it is known that the preponderance of metabolite changes from sulfate to

Table 50–3. ALCOHOL AND ACETAMINOPHEN*

TOXIC BLOOD LEVEL	HISTORY OF CHRONIC ALCOHOL USE	HISTORY OF ACUTE ALCOHOL INGESTION	ELEVATION OF SGOT OR SGPT RATIO†	MAXIMUM SERUM BILIRUBIN RATIO >3.0	MAXIMUM PROTHROMBIN RATIO 2.0
No (332)	No (303)	No (243)	5/229	2/232	0/213
		Yes (60)	5/282 (1.7%)	3/282 (1%)	0/262 (0%)
			0/53	1/50	0/49
	Yes (29)	No (5)	0/5	0/5	0/5
		Yes (24)	0.29 (0%)	1/28 (3.5%)	0/26 (0%)
			0/24	1/23	0/21
Yes (123)	No (112)	No (91)	26/91	7/91	4/89
		Yes (21)	28/112 (25%)	7/112 (6.3%)	4/109 (3.6%)
			2/21	0/21	0/20
	Yes (11)	No (5)	2/5	2/5	2/5
		Yes (6)	3/11 (27%)	3/11 (27%)	2/11 (18%)
			1/6	1/6	0/6

*History of acute or chronic alcohol use or lack of use could be ascertained only in 455 of the 662 patients. No history was obtainable in the remaining patients.

†Number of patients with SGOT or SGPT ratio in toxic range/total number of patients in group having the laboratory test performed.

(From Rumack GH, Peterson RG, Koch GG, Amara IA: Acetaminophen overdose: 662 cases with evaluation of oral acetylcysteine treatment. Arch Intern Med *141*:380, 1981. © 1981, American Medical Association.)

Table 50–4. CHILDHOOD ACETAMINOPHEN TOXICITY (AGE < 6 YEARS)

AGE/SEX	DOSE *(gm)*	DOSE *(mg/kg)**	LEVEL†	SGOT LEVEL *(IU/L)*	PT *(% C)*‡	BILIRUBIN LEVEL (mg/dl)	THERAPY§	COMMENTS
13 mo/M	13	1530	Severe toxicity	244	110	0.28	Acetylcysteine	Plus narcotic; 16.5 hr to acetylcysteine
21 mo/M	3.2	250	Toxic	37	110	0.6	Acetylcysteine	10 hr to acetylcysteine
23 mo/M	4	294	Toxic	39	110	0.8	Acetylcysteine	15.5 hr to acetylcysteine
4 yr/M	11 to 26	700 to 1600	Severe toxicity	138	140	1.3	Acetylcysteine	Plus narcotic and antihistamines; 15 hr to acetylcysteine
6 yr/M	6.5	283	Toxic	198	130	0.6	Acetylcysteine	Plus narcotic, diazepam, and phenobarbital; 20 hr to acetylcysteine

*Dose ingested (by history) as a function of body weight.

†Severe toxic reaction is severely toxic range on nomogram.

‡Prothrombin time (PT) as percentage of a control (C) value.

§Oral acetylcysteine, as described by Rumack and Peterson.[13b]

(From Peterson RG, Rumack BH: Age as a variable in acetaminophen overdose. Arch Intern Med *141*:390, 1981. © 1981, American Medical Association.)

Table 50–5. CHILDHOOD ACETAMINOPHEN TOXICITY (AGE 7 TO 12 YEARS)

AGE/SEX	DOSE (gm)	DOSE *(mg/kg)**	LEVEL	SGOT LEVEL *(IU/L)*	PT *(% C)*†	BILIRUBIN LEVEL *(mg/dl)*	THERAPY‡	COMMENTS
10/M	13	650	Toxic	1660	120	2.5	Acetylcysteine	20 hr to acetylcysteine
11/F	15	341	Toxic	48	N	0.7	Acetylcysteine	11 hr to acetylcysteine
11/M	16	378	Toxic	43	N	1.8	Acetylcysteine	12 hr to acetylcysteine
12/F	11	282	Toxic	196	N	0.7	Acetylcysteine	19 hr to acetylcysteine

*Dose ingested (by history) as a function of body weight.
†Prothrombin time (PT) as percentage of a control (C) value. Normal value is N.
‡Oral acetylcysteine as described by Rumack and Peterson.[13a]
(From Peterson RG, Rumack BH: Age as a variable in acetaminophen overdose. Arch Intern Med *141*:390, 1981. ©1981, American Medical Association.)

glucuronide at about age 9 to 12 years, the relationship of this to hepatotoxicity is unclear. Phenytoin, another drug metabolized by the P-450 system, has a much shorter half-life in the child than in the adult. Isoniazid reactions do not occur with as much frequency in children as in adults, and it has been suggested that perhaps a more efficient glutathione system removes the isoniazid metabolite in a fashion similar to that of acetaminophen.

Therapeutic doses of acetaminophen in children at a rate of 10 mg/kg every 4 hours rarely produce levels considered therapeutic in adults (10 to 20 μg/ml). Children develop levels of 7 or more μg/ml and have a therapeutic response at this lower level.[58]

Emesis is another factor in pediatric cases of acetaminophen overdose. Children tend to vomit spontaneously quite early in the course of an ingestion, thereby leading to reduced absorption and a decreased risk for hepatotoxicity. In fact, even children who demonstrate toxic acetaminophen levels are much less likely than their adult counterparts to develop hepatotoxicity. When directly compared, adults had an incidence of hepatotoxicity more than five times greater than that of children less than 12 years old.[63]

CLINICAL COURSE OF ACETAMINOPHEN OVERDOSE

The therapeutic dose of acetaminophen is 10 to 20 mg/kg every 4 hours. *Toxicity is likely to occur after a minimum acute ingestion of 140 mg/kg or 10 gm in a 70-kg adult*. The toxic dose may vary as a function of individual variation in glutathione levels. The course of acetamin-

Table 50–6. CHILDHOOD ACETAMINOPHEN INGESTIONS (AGE < 6 YEARS)

AGE/SEX	DOSE *(gm)*	DOSE *(mg/kg)**	PLASMA LEVEL† *μg/ml (Time, hr, determination was made)*	SGOT LEVEL *(IU/L)*	PT *(% C)*‡	BILIRUBIN LEVEL *(mg/dl)*	THERAPY§	COMMENTS
12 mo/M	36	2571	0 (7)	—	—	—	Acetylcysteine	Vomited at 2 hr
19 mo/M	14	1400	0 (7)	—	—	—	None	Vomited at 30 min; clinically normal
2.0 yr/M	36	2571	0 (7)	45	N	1.3	Acetylcysteine	Vomited at 45 min
2.0 yr/F	11	1000	NT	—	—	—	Acetylcysteine	No problems
2.5 yr/F	14	1200	1 (4)	—	—	—	Acetylcysteine	Vomited at 60 min
2.5 yr/M	10	800	0 (4)	14	—	—	Acetylcysteine	Vomited at 15 min
3.0 yr/M	7	469	0 (4)	31	—	0.3	Acetylcysteine	Vomited at 60 min
3.0 yr/M	4	294	NT	82	N	0.3	Acetylcysteine	Vomited at 2 hr

*Dose ingested (by history) as a function of body weight.
†Nontoxic on nomogram is NT.
‡Prothrombin time (PT) as percentage of a control (C) value. Normal value is N.
§Oral acetylcysteine as defined by Rumack and Peterson.[13]
(From Peterson RG, Rumack BH: Age as a variable in acetaminophen overdose. Arch Intern Med *141*:390, 1981. ©1981, American Medical Association.)

ophen poisoning is divided into four clinical stages:

Stage 1: 12 to 24 hours postingestion—nausea, vomiting, diaphoresis, anorexia
Stage 2: 24 to 48 hours—clinically improved; SGOT, SGPT, bilirubin, and prothrombin levels begin to rise
Stage 3: 72 to 96 hours—peak hepatotoxicity, SGOT of 20,000 not unusual
Stage 4: 7 to 8 days—recovery

Patients who are treated late or who are untreated and eventually die maintain high levels of enzymes beyond 72 to 96 hours.

Treatment

Oral NAC is clearly the agent of choice. Although IV NAC has been used, it is only permissible in the United States under the Investigational New Drug regulations; in fact, when given intravenously it has caused anaphylaxis.[64] Clinical trials using IV NAC to treat acetaminophen overdose in the United States are currently being done. Preliminary evidence shows that a 48-hour treatment protocol using IV NAC may be more effective and is at least as effective as the 72-hour oral treatment protocol in preventing hepatotoxicity, with minimal side effects.[65] In addition patients taking oral NAC often vomit the medication, which is not a problem when the drug is given intravenously. Until IV NAC is approved for general usage, oral NAC will continue to be the treatment of choice.

The first use of NAC in a human with proven blood levels of acetaminophen was reported in May, 1977.[66] Since that time over 11,000 cases have been treated under protocol in the United States. Mortality has been rare, with 27 deaths directly due to acetaminophen.[67] Of these 27 patients, all adults, 17 either received no NAC treatment or the first NAC dose was later than 24 hours after admission. Of the remaining ten fatalities, eight received NAC at 16 to 24 hours after ingestion. Two patients who received NAC treatment at less than 16 hours after ingestion died. One of these did not receive full supportive care because of end stage lung disease. The other patient's initial SGOT was 4000 IU/L, making the time of ingestion suspect. Thus death is exceedingly rare in acetaminophen overdose, especially if NAC therapy is begun prior to 16 hours after ingestion. Table 50–7 presents a detailed review of 662 patients in the NAC open study.

It has been shown clearly that treatment with NAC should be initiated within the first 16 hours post ingestion.[13b, 68] Since in many cases the patient will not be totally accurate about the time of ingestion, it is acceptable to treat patients any time during the first 24 hours post ingestion. It is most effective the earlier it is begun. In fact, a recent study shows that delays in treatment up to 8 hours after ingestion do not adversely affect outcome. However, NAC efficiency does decrease progressively from 8 to 16 hours after ingestion.[68] Furthermore, even patients with extremely high acetaminophen levels do as well as patients with lower levels when NAC therapy is begun within 8 hours of ingestion.[69] If NAC therapy is delayed beyond 8 hours, however, higher acetaminophen levels were associated with a higher incidence of liver toxicity.[69] Oral NAC does not produce any adverse reactions and, consequently, even when given late in the course does not aggravate encephalopathy, as does cysteamine or methionine.

The following treatment protocol has become the standard approach to acetaminophen overdose:

1. Treat any other coingestants (sedatives and so on) with the standard approach, i.e., lavage, charcoal, and so on. Even if the ingestion is purely acetaminophen, administration of activated charcoal is appropriate to prevent a subsequent toxic plasma acetaminophen level.
2. Draw blood for an acetaminophen level determination 4 hours post ingestion. If the laboratory can process it rapidly, wait for results and plot blood level versus time on the nomogram (see Fig. 50–2) to determine whether treatment is necessary. If a blood level test cannot be performed in a timely manner, then treatment should be instituted and terminated if the blood level is below the nomogram line. Only the *initial* blood level is used. *A 4-hour acetaminophen blood level of 150 μg/ml or greater is an indication to begin treatment with NAC.* Subsequent blood levels that may fall below the line are not an indication to terminate treatment. If the initial acetamin-

Table 50–7. ORAL ACETYLCYSTEINE MULTICLINIC OPEN STUDY: SUMMARY OF 662 PATIENTS

TREATMENT GROUP*	NO. OF PATIENTS	NO. OF DEATHS	PATIENTS WITH TOXIC REACTIONS (%)†	MEAN MAXIMUM SGOT LEVEL (IU/L)	MEDIAN MAXIMUM SGOT LEVEL (IU/L)
I. Probable risk and late probable risk					
A. <10 hr to acetylcysteine therapy	57	0	7	229	43
B. 10–16 hr to acetylcysteine therapy	52		29	1557	168
C. 16–24 hr to acetylcysteine therapy	39	0	62	2695	1915
D. >24 hr to acetylcysteine therapy or no therapy	7	0	43	1869	270
II. Possible risk‡	76	1§	5	390	32
III. No risk‡	297	0	0.4	47	26
IV. Unknown risk‡	111	1‖	18	1313	36
V. Aged <13 yr‡	23	0	6	199	82
Total	662	2	—	—	—

*Probable- and late-probable-risk patients all had plasma acetaminophen levels above the nomogram line in Figure 50–2, with "late" designating those with the initial assay after 16 hours. These patients have been further partitioned according to the time they received the loading dose of acetylcysteine (with group ID including some patients with no therapy). For statistical purposes, the no-risk patients were those with plasma acetaminophen levels below the line from 150 μg/ml at 4 hours to 37.5 μg/ml at 12 hours; the possible-risk patients were those with available plasma acetaminophen levels who were neither probable risk nor no-risk; the unknown-risk patients were those without sufficient plasma acetaminophen level information to assess their risk status; and patients younger than 13 years were a group outside the investigation protocol.

†Toxicity equals SGOT ratio greater than 25.

‡Some of these patients did not receive any acetylcysteine.

§This patient died of respiratory problems associated with the propoxyphene in the combination ingested and is also an alleged homicide.

‖This patient died after initially seen in hepatic failure 72 hours after ingestion. No acetylcysteine was given.

(From Rumack BH, Peterson RG, Koch GG, Amara IA: Acetaminophen overdose: 662 cases with evaluation of oral acetylcysteine treatment. Arch Intern Med *141*:380, 1981. © 1981, American Medical Association.)

ophen level is an 8-hour level, then a level of 75 μg/ml or greater is an indication to start treatment. Likewise, an initial acetaminophen level at 12 hours of 37.5 μg/ml is an indication to begin treatment with NAC.

3. If charcoal was previously given, then lavage the stomach to clear it *before* administering the first NAC dose. Various in vitro and in vivo studies have shown that NAC is adsorbed to charcoal to some degree.[70–74] However, there is no known correlation between serum NAC levels and NAC efficacy in acetaminophen overdose. Therefore, it is probably not necessary to increase the dose of NAC if charcoal has been given. If multiple-dose charcoal is used because of a coingestant, then NAC and charcoal should be alternated, with at least a 2-hour interval between the two. Again, the charcoal should be lavaged from the stomach prior to each NAC dose.
4. NAC should be prepared as a 5 per cent solution in water, grapefruit juice, or a cola beverage. It will taste and smell terrible. If the patient vomits within 1 hour after administration, then the dose should be repeated. If emesis becomes a constant problem, a weighted tube, such as a Cantor or Miller-Abbott tube, should be passed and the drug instilled directly into the duodenum.
5. The initial dose of NAC is 140 mg/kg, and each subsequent dose is 70 mg/kg. Patients should be treated for 17 doses beyond the loading dose at 4-hour intervals.
6. SGOT, SGPT, bilirubin, and prothrombin time determinations should be followed on a daily basis.

Figure 50–5 shows the natural course of acetaminophen hepatotoxicity (solid line) and the modified course when treated with NAC. No sequelae occur after recovery, which is usually complete by day 8.

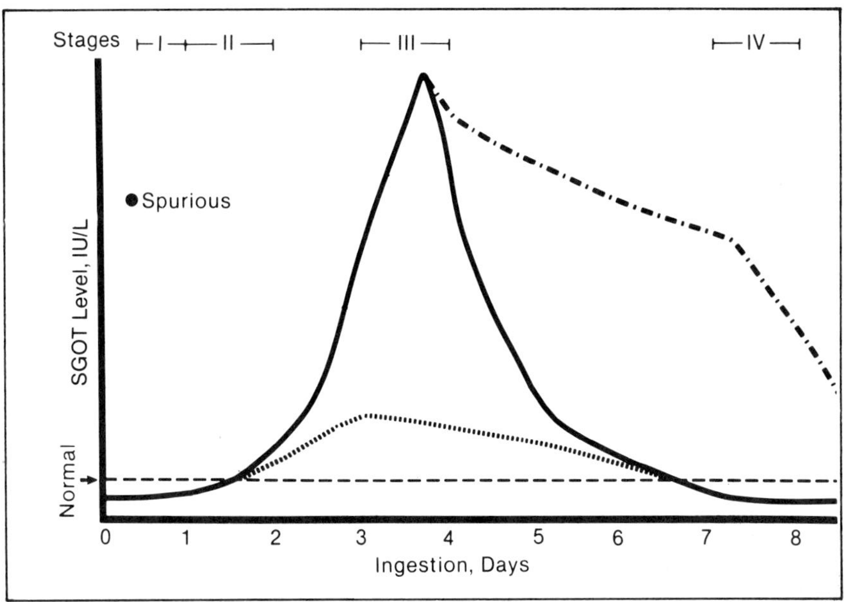

Figure 50–5. Treatment of acetaminophen hepatotoxicity. Dotted line represents the courses of those who received acetylcysteine; solid line, natural courses; and dotted and dashed line, severe courses. (From Rumack BH, Peterson RG, Koch GG, Amara IA: Acetaminophen overdose: 662 cases with evaluation of oral acetylcysteine treatment. Arch Intern Med *141*:380, 1981. © 1981, American Medical Association.)

ACETAMINOPHEN OVERDOSE DURING PREGNANCY

Both the mother and fetus are at risk for hepatotoxicity from acetaminophen overdose during pregnancy.[75] Hepatic necrosis and elevated acetaminophen levels have been reported in stillborn infants whose mothers took acute overdoses of acetaminophen.[76–78] A review of 59 women with acetaminophen overdose during pregnancy showed no malformations attributable to NAC therapy during pregnancy.[78] The authors conclude that pregnant women with acetaminophen overdose be treated with NAC according to the same guidelines as nonpregnant patients. Furthermore, delivery of the fetus should not be induced, as it is easier to treat the fetus with NAC in utero than after birth.

RENAL FAILURE AND ACUTE ACETAMINOPHEN OVERDOSE

Renal dysfunction and acute renal failure have been reported in association with acute overdose of acetaminophen. Renal failure in association with acute acetaminophen overdose has been reported in the following four settings:

1. Severe hepatic failure with encephalopathy or death.[17, 19, 79–82]
2. Hepatic toxicity present but not severe (SGOT or SGPT greater than 1000 IU/L).[19, 21, 26, 79, 82–87]
3. Mild hepatic toxicity (SGOT or SGPT elevated but less than 1000 IU/L).[85, 88]
4. No hepatic toxicity (normal SGOT, SGPT).[86]

Transient renal failure is often present in patients with severe hepatic necrosis from causes other than acetaminophen toxicity, such as viral hepatitis.[82, 89] However, there are many case reports and series of patients, as cited previously, in which patients developed acute renal failure after acetaminophen overdose in the absence of fulminant hepatic failure. In fact, some patients had only mild elevations, or even no elevation, of hepatic enzymes and still developed renal failure that was apparently related to their overdose.

Further evidence of a direct toxic effect of acetaminophen on the kidney comes from animal data.[90, 91] The damage appears to occur by a mechanism in the kidney that is similar to that in the liver. A toxic intermediate formed in situ in the kidney from a cytochrome P-450 pathway is covalently bound to renal macromolecules, causing necrosis of renal cells. This occurs only after depletion of renal glutathione stores and can be prevented in animals by administering a glutathione precursor such as cysteine. Thus NAC probably affords protection against renal damage as well as hepatic damage when given early after an overdose of acetaminophen.

The renal dysfunction is usually secondary to acute tubular necrosis. The renal findings in patients usually occur later than the hepatic dysfunction, with BUN and creatinine levels beginning to elevate at 3 to 4 days after the overdose and peaking at 5 to 10 days. This may be accompanied by decreased urine output. The renal problems may be heralded by proteinuria and hematuria occurring 2 to 4 days after the overdose. Survivors usually recover normal renal function by 2 to 3 weeks after ingestion, although some patients have required temporary hemodialysis or peritoneal dialysis.

The incidence of renal failure in patients with acetaminophen overdose is not known. One series reported renal failure in 1 per cent of all cases of acetaminophen overdose.[85] In patients who develop fulminant hepatic failure from acetaminophen overdose, the incidence of renal failure has been reported as high as 53 per cent.[82] The same study found a 5 per cent incidence of renal failure in acetaminophen overdose patients who did not develop fulminant hepatic failure.

UNUSUAL COMPLICATIONS OF ACETAMINOPHEN OVERDOSE

Occasional reports of myocardial abnormalities associated with acute acetaminophen overdose have appeared. These reports have described various electrocardiographic abnormalities, cardiac arrhythmias, myocardiopathy, and myocardial necrosis.[19, 92–97] It is not clear from these few case reports whether there is a direct toxic effect of acetaminophen on the heart in certain susceptible individuals or whether the cardiac abnormalities are secondary to severe hepatic damage and multisystem failure.

There are also rare reports of pancreatitis,[98–100] metabolic acidosis,[101, 102] and nonhepatic coma[102] associated with acute overdose of acetaminophen.

References

1. Brodie BB, Axelrod I: The estimates of acetanilide and its metabolic products, aniline, *N*-acetyl-*p*-aminophenol and *p*-aminophenol (free and total conjugated) in biological fluids and tissues. J Pharmacol Exp Ther *94*:22, 1948.
2. Mitchell JR, Thorgiersson SS, Potter WZ, et al: Acetaminophen-induced hepatic injury: Protective role of glutathione in man and rationale for therapy. Clin Pharmacol Ther *16*:676, 1974.
3. Jollow DJ, Thorgiersson SS, Potter WZ, et al: Acetaminophen-induced hepatic necrosis. VI. Metabolic disposition of toxic and nontoxic doses of acetaminophen. Pharmacology *12*:251, 1974.
4. Potter WZ, Davis DC, Mitchell JR, et al: Acetaminophen-induced hepatic necrosis. III. Cytochrome P-450–mediated covalent binding in vitro. J Pharmacol Exp Ther *187*:203, 1973.
5. Mitchell JR, Jollow DJ, Potter WZ, et al: Acetaminophen-induced hepatic necrosis. I. Role of drug metabolism. J Pharmacol Exp Ther *187*:185, 1973.
6. Mitchell JR, Jollow DJ, Potter WZ, et al: Acetaminophen-induced hepatic necrosis. IV. Protective role of glutathione. J Pharmacol Exp Ther *187*:211, 1973.
7. Jollow DJ, Mitchell JR, Potter WZ, et al: Acetaminophen-induced hepatic necrosis. II. Role of covalent binding in vitro. J Pharmacol Exp Ther *187*:195, 1973.
8. Davis M, Labadarios D, Williams RS: Metabolism of paracetamol after therapeutic and hepatotoxic doses in man. J Int Med Res *4*(Suppl 4):40, 1976.
9. Davis M, Harrison NG, Ideo G, et al: Paracetamol metabolism in the rat: Relationship to covalent binding and hepatic damage. Xenobiotica *6*:249, 1976.
10. Williams R, Davis M: Clinical and experimental aspects of paracetamol hepatotoxicity. Acta Pharmacol Toxicol *41*(Suppl 2):282, 1977.
11. Potter WZ, Thorgiersson SS, Jollow DJ, et al: Acetaminophen-induced hepatic necrosis. V. Correlation of hepatic necrosis, covalent binding, and glutathione depletion in hamsters. Pharmacology *12*:129, 1974.
12. Mitchell JR, Nelson SD, Thorgiersson SS, et al: Metabolic inactivation: Biochemical basis for many drug-induced liver injuries. *In* Popper H, Schaffner F (eds): Progress in Liver Diseases. New York, Grune & Stratton, 1976, p 259.
13. Wright N, Prescott LF: Potentiation by previous drug therapy of hepatotoxicity following paracetamol overdosage. Scot Med J *18*:56, 1973.

13a. Sato C, Lieber CS: Prevention of acetaminophen-induced hepatotoxicity by ethanol in the rat. Pharmacologist *22*:227, 1980.

13b. Rumack BH, Peterson RG, Koch GG, Amara IA: Acetaminophen overdose: 662 cases with evaluation of oral acetylcysteine treatment. Arch Intern Med *141*:380, 1981.

14. Rumack BH, Matthew H: Acetaminophen poisoning and toxicity. Pediatrics *55*:871, 1975.
15. McLean AEM: Nutrition and the intracellular site of toxic injury. World Rev Nutr Diet *29*:124, 1978.
16. Newman TJ, Bargman GJ: Acetaminophen hepatotoxicity and malnutrition. Am J Gastroenterol *72*:647, 1979.
17. Davidson DGD: Acute liver necrosis following overdose of paracetamol. Br Med J *2*:497, 1966.

18. Thompson JS, Prescott LF: Liver damage and impaired glucose tolerance after paracetamol overdosage. Br Med J *2*:506, 1966.
19. Mclean D, Peters TJ, Brown RAG, et al: Treatment of acute paracetamol poisoning. Lancet 2:849, 1968.
20. Rose PG: Paracetamol overdosage and liver damage. Br Med J *1*:381, 1969.
21. Proudfoot AT, Wright N: Acute paracetamol poisoning. Br Med J *3*:557, 1970.
22. Clark R, Borirakchanyavat V, Davidson AR, et al: Hepatic damage and death from overdose of paracetamol. Lancet *1*:66, 1973.
23. James O, Roberts SH, Douglas AP, et al: Liver damage after paracetamol overdose: Comparison of liver function tests, fasting serum bile acids, and liver histology. Lancet *2*:579, 1975.
24. Crome P, Dobst RCOG, Volans GN, et al: The use of methionine for acute paracetamol poisoning. J Int Med Res *4*(Suppl 4):105, 1976.
25. Gazzard BG, Davis M, Spooner JB, et al: Why paracetamol? J Int Med Res *4*(Suppl 4):25, 1976.
26. Boyer TD, Ruoff SL: Acetaminophen-induced hepatic necrosis and renal failure. JAMA *218*:440, 1971.
27. Farid NR, Glynn JP, Kerr DNS: Hemodialysis in paracetamol self-poisoning. Lancet *2*:396, 1972.
28. Gazzard BG, Wilson RA, Weston MJ, et al: Charcoal haemoperfusion for paracetamol overdose. Br J Clin Pharmacol *1*:271, 1974.
29. Prescott LF, Swainson CP, Forrest ARW, et al: Successful treatment of severe paracetamol overdosage with cysteamine. Lancet *1*:588, 1974.
30. Nimmo J, Dixon MF, Prescott LF: Effects of mepyramine, promethazine, and hydrocortisone on paracetamol-induce hepatic necrosis in the rat. Clin Toxicol *6*:75, 1973.
31. Prescott LF, Sutherland GR, Park J, et al: Cysteamine, methionine, and penicillamine in the treatment of paracetamol poisoning. Lancet *2*:109, 1976.
32. Prescott LF, Wright N: BAL in paracetamol poisoning. Lancet *2*:833, 1974.
33. Crome P, Volans GR, Vale JA, et al: Oral methionine in the treatment of severe paracetamol (acetaminophen) overdose. Lancet *2*:829, 1976.
34. Lorber A, Baumgartner WA, Bovy RA, et al: Clinical application for heavy metal complexing potential for *N*-acetylcysteine. J Clin Pharmacol *13*:332, 1973.
35. Chasseaud LF: Reaction with electrophiles after enzyme-catalysed deacetylation of *N*-acetylcysteine. Biochem Pharmacol *23*:1133, 1974.
36. Bailey KR, Sheffner AL: The reduction of experimentally induced inflammation by sulfhydryl compounds. Biochem Pharmacol *16*:1175, 1967.
37. Meeker IA, Kincannon WN: Acetylcysteine used to liquefy inspissated meconium causing intestinal obstruction in the newborn. Surgery *56*:419, 1974.
38. Mulvaney WP, Quiltes T, Montera A: Experience with acetylcysteine in cystinuric patients. J Urol *14*:107, 1975.
39. Botta JA, Nelson LW, Weikel JH: Acetylcysteine in the prevention of cyclophosphamide-induced cystitis in rats. J Natl Cancer Inst *51*:1051, 1973.
40. Levy L, Harris R: Effect of N-acetylcysteine on some aspects of cyclophosophamide-induced toxicity and immunosuppression. Biochem Pharmacol *26*:1015, 1977.
41. Kline I, Gang M, Woodman RJ, et al: Protection with *N*-acetylcysteine against isophosphamide toxicity and enhancement of therapeutic effect in early murine L1210 leukemia. Cancer Chemother Rep *57*:299, 1973.
42. Sprince H, Parker CM, Smith GC, et al: Protective action of ascorbic acid and sulfur compounds against acetaldehyde toxicity: Implications in alcoholism and smoking. Agents Actions *5*:164, 1975.
43. Republicatique Francaise Patent No. 7.688M (Institut National de la Propriete Industrielle). Issued to Societe D'Etudes et de Recherches Pharmaceutiques (E.R.P.H.A.R.), February 16, 1970.
44. Boyland E, Chasseaud LF: Enzyme-catalyzed conjugations of glutathione with unsaturated compounds. Biochem J *104*:95, 1967.
45. Strubelt O, Siegers A, Schutt A: The curative effects of cysteamine, cysteine and dithiocarb in experimental paracetamol poisoning. Arch Toxicol *33*:55, 1974.
46. Rollins DE, Buckpitt AR: Liver cytosol-catalyzed conjugation of reduced glutathione with a reactive metabolite of acetaminophen. Toxicol Appl Pharmacol *47*:331, 1979.
47. Gerber JG, MacDonald JS, Harbison RI, et al: Effect of *N*-acetylcysteine on hepatic covalent binding of paracetamol (acetaminophen). Lancet *1*:657, 1977.
48. Smith RB, Piperno E: Covalent binding and tissue distribution of ^{14}C-acetaminophen in overdosed mice: Effects of *N*-acetylcysteine treatment. Toxicol Appl Pharmacol *47*:A103, 1979.
49. Williams R, Davis M: Clinical and experimental aspects of paracetamol hepatotoxicity. Acta Pharmacol Toxicol *41*(Suppl 2):282, 1977.
50. Labadarios D, Davis M, Portmann B, et al: Paracetamol-induced hepatic necrosis in the mouse—relationship between covalent bindings, hepatic glutathione depletion and the protective effect of L-mercaptopropionylglycine. Biochem Pharmacol *26*:31, 1977.
51. Galinsky RE, Levy G: Effect of *N*-acetylcysteine on the pharmacokinetics of acetaminophen in rats. Life Sci *25*:693, 1979.
52. Piperno E, Berssenbruegge DA: Reversal of experimental paracetamol toxicosis with *N*-acetylcysteine. Lancet *2*:738, 1976.
53. Piperno E, Mosher AH, Berssenbruegge DA, et al: Pathophysiology of acetaminophen overdosage toxicity: Implications for management. Pediatrics *62*:880, 1978.
54. Piperno E, Winkler JD, Berssenbruegge DA: Antidotal profile of *N*-acetylcysteine in the acetaminophen-overdosed mouse. Clin Toxicol *12*:616, 1978.
55. Piperno E, Berssenbruegge DA: Toxicological Research Report No. 495 (761012). Fort Washington, Pa, McNeil Laboratories, 1976.
56. Koch-Weser J: Drug therapy: Acetaminophen. N Engl J Med *295*:1297, 1976.
57. Msynowitz ML, Forsham PH: The antidiuretic action of acetaminophen. Am J Sci *252*:429, 1966.
58. Data on file. Chronic Human Toxicity Study of Orally Administered Acetylcysteine, 1970. Evansville, Ind, Mead-Johnson Research Center, 1970.
59. Nimmo J, Heading RC, Tothill P, et al: Pharmacological modification of gastric emptying: Effects of propantheline and metoclopramide on paracetamol absorption. Br Med J *1*:587, 1973.
60. Miller RP, Roberts RJ, Fischer LJ: Kinetics of acetaminophen elimination in newborns, children, and adults. Clin Pharmacol Ther *19*:284, 1976.
61. Peterson RG, Rumack BH: Age as a variable in

acetaminophen overdose. Arch Intern Med *141*:390, 1981.

62. Peterson RG, Rumack BH: Pharmacokinetics of acetaminophen: absorption, distribution, metabolism, excretion. Pediatrics *62*:877, 1978.
63. Rumack BH: Acetaminophen overdose in young children. AJDC *138*:428–433, 1984.
64. Walton NG, Mann TAN, Shaw KM: Anaphylactoid reaction to N-acetylcysteine. Lancet *2*:1298, 1979.
65. Bronstein AC, Linden CH, Hall AH, Kulig KW, Rumack BH: Intravenous N-acetylcysteine for acute acetaminophen poisoning (abst). Vet Hum Toxicol *28*:316, 1985.
66. Peterson RG, Rumack BH: Treatment of acute acetaminophen poisoning with N-acetylcysteine. JAMA *237*:2406, 1977.
67. Smilkstein MJ, Kulig KW, Rumack BH: Acetaminophen overdose: Incidence of death in 11195 cases (abs). Vet Hum Toxicol *29*:471, 1987.
68. Smilkstein MJ, Knapp GL, Kulig KW, Rumack BH: Acetaminophen overdose: How critical is the delay to *N*-acetylcysteine? (abs). Vet Hum Toxicol *29*:486, 1987.
69. Smilkstein MJ, Knapp GL, Kulig KW, Rumack BH: Acetaminophen overdose: Do levels predict outcome? (abs). Vet Hum Toxicol *29*:469, 1987.
70. Klein-Schwartz W, Oderda GM: Adsorption of oral antidotes for acetaminophen poisoning (methionine and *n*-acetylcysteine) by activated charcoal. Clin Toxicol *18*:283–290, 1981.
71. Rybolt TR, Burrell DE, Shults JM, Kelley AK: In vitro coadsorption of acetaminophen and *N*-acetylcysteine onto activated carbon powder. J Pharm Sci *75*:904–906, 1986.
72. North DS, Peterson RG, Krenzelok EP: Effect of activated charcoal administration on acetylcysteine serum levels in humans. Am J Hosp Pharm *38*:1022–1024, 1981.
73. Renzi FP, Donovan JW, Martin TG, Morgan L, Harrison EF: Concomitant use of activated charcoal and *n*-acetylcysteine. Ann Emerg Med *14*:568–572, 1985.
74. Ekins BR, Ford DC, Thompson MIB, Bridges RR, Rollins DE, Jenkins RD: The effect of activated charcoal on *n*-acetylcysteine adsorption in normal subjects. Am J Emerg Med *5*:483–487, 1987.
75. Rollins DE, Vonbarber C, Glaumann H, Moldens P, Rane A: Acetaminophen: potentially toxic metabolite formed by human fetal and adult liver microsomes and isolated fetal liver cells. Science *205*:1414–1416, 1979.
76. Haibach H, Akhten JE, Muscato MS, Cary PL, Hoffman MF: Acetaminophen overdose with fetal demise. Am J Clin Pathol *82*:240–242, 1984.
77. Roberts I, Robinson MJ, Mughal MZ, Ratcliffe JG, Prescott LF: Paracetamol metabolites in the neonate following maternal overdose. Br J Clin Pharmol *18*:201–206, 1984.
78. Bronstein AC, Rumack BH: Acute acetaminophen overdose during pregnancy: A review of fifty-nine cases (abs). Vet Hum Toxicol *26*:44, 1984.
79. Prescott LF, Roscoe P, Wright N, Brown SS: Plasma paracetamol half-life and hepatic necrosis in patients with paracetamol overdose. Lancet *1*:519–522, 1971.
80. Dixon MF: Paracetamol hepatotoxicity. Lancet *1*:35, 1976.
81. McJunkin B, Barwick KW, Little WC, Winfield JB: Fatal massive hepatic nerosis following acetaminophen overdose. JAMA *236*:1874–1875, 1976.
82. Wilkinson SP, Moodie H, Arroyo VA, Williams R: Frequency of renal impairment in paracetamol overdose compared with other causes of acute liver damage. J Clin Pathol *30*:141–143, 1977.
83. Jeffrey WH, Lafferrty WE: Acute renal failure after acetaminophen overdose: Report of two cases. Am J Hosp Pharm *38*:1355–1358, 1981.
84. Curry RW, Robinson JD, Sughrue MJ: Acute renal failure after acetaminophen ingestion. JAMA *247*:1012–1014, 1982.
85. Cobden I, Record CO, Ward MK, Kerr DNS: Paracetamol-induced acute renal failure in the absence of fulminant liver damage. Br Med J *284*:21–22, 1982.
86. Prescott LF, Proudfoot AT, Cregeen RJ: Paracetamol induced acute renal failure in the absence of fulminant liver damage. Br Med J *284*:421–422, 1982.
87. Dabbaugh S, Chesney RW: Acute renal failure related to acetaminophen (paracetamol) overdose without fulminant hepatic disease. Int J Pediatr Nephrol *6*:221–224, 1985.
88. Pillans P, Hall C: Paracetamol-induced acute renal failure in the absence of severe liver damage. S Afr Med J *67*:791–792, 1985.
89. Wilkinson SP, Blendis LM, Williams R: Frequency and type of renal and electrolyte disorders in fulminant hepatic failure. Br Med J *1*:186–189, 1974.
90. Mitchell JR, McMurtry RJ, Statham CN, Nelson SD: Molecular basis for several drug-induced nephropathies. Am J Med *62*:518–526, 1977.
91. McMurtry RJ, Snodgrass WR, Mitchell JR: Renal necrosis, glutathione depletion, and covalent bindings after acetaminophen. Toxicol Appl Pharmacol *46*:87–100, 1978.
92. Pimstone BL, Uys CJ: Liver necrosis and myocardiopathy following paracetamol overdosage. S Afr Med J *42*:259–262, 1968.
93. Sanerkin NG: Acute myocardial necrosis in paracetamol poisoning. Br Med J *3*:478, 1971.
94. Will EJ, Tomkins AM: Acute myocardial necrosis in paracetamol poisoning. Br Med J *4*:430–431, 1971.
95. Weston MJ, Williams R: Paracetamol and the heart. Lancet *1*:536, 1976.
96. Weston MJ, Talbot IC, Howorth PJN, Mant AK, Capildeo R, Williams R: Frequency of arrhythmias and other cardiac abnormalities in fulminant hepatic failure. Br Heart J *38*:1179–1188, 1976.
97. Benson RE, Boleyn T: Paracetamol overdose: Plan of management. Anaesth Intens Care *4*:334–339, 1974.
98. Gilmore IT, Tourvas E: Paracetamol-induced acute pancreatitis. Br Med J *1*:753–754, 1977.
99. Coward RA: Paracetamol-induced acute pancreatitis. Br Med J *1*:1086, 1977.
100. Caldarola V, Hassett JM, Hall AH, Bronstein AB, Kulig KW, Rumack BH: Hemorrhagic pancreatitis associated with acetaminophen overdose. Am J Gastroenterol *81*:579–582, 1986.
101. Zabrodski RM, Schnurr LP: Anion gap acidosis with hypoglycemia in acetaminophen toxicity. Ann Emerg Med *13*:956–959, 1984.
102. Flanagan RJ, Mant TGK: Coma and metabolic acidosis early in severe acute paracetamol poisoning. Human Toxicol *5*:179–182, 1986.

CHAPTER 51
SALICYLATES AND SALICYLAMIDE

A. T. Proudfoot, B.Sc., FRCPE

Salicylic acid was first isolated from willow bark (*Salix alba*) in 1838, but it was not until 1899 that aspirin (acetylsalicylic acid) was introduced into clinical practice. Aspirin and some chemically related compounds—known as salicylates—have since been prescribed widely by the medical profession and purchased over the counter by the public. Few if any drugs or groups of drugs in the history of therapeutics can rival the scale on which they were consumed until the last few years. Inevitably, acute and chronic poisoning have been important consequences of their extensive use and availability.

THE SALICYLATES

Only a few salicylates are in common use. They are acetylsalicylic acid (aspirin), sodium salicylate, and salicylic acid itself. Methyl salicylate (oil of wintergreen) was formerly very popular but is now rarely encountered. Until recently, there were numerous different aspirin-containing products available in many countries, but two factors have greatly reduced their use. The first is the longstanding concern over their adverse effects, particularly on the gastrointestinal tract in adults, and the second is anxiety over a causal relationship between therapeutic doses of aspirin and Reye's syndrome in children. Indeed, the latter has led to consideration of prohibiting the use of aspirin in that age group. Restriction of the therapeutic indications for salicylates will inevitably reduce their availability and, consequently, the prevalence of acute poisoning with them.

Aspirin is frequently formulated with other drugs such as codeine, caffeine, and acetaminophen (paracetamol) in a variety of proprietary preparations; significant opioid toxicity may rarely be a feature of overdosage with codeine and salicylate combinations.[1]

More recently, benorylate, a conjugate of aspirin and acetaminophen, and diflunisal, a derivative of salicylic acid, have been marketed. The former is hydrolyzed to its parent drugs after absorption, but serious poisoning with it is very uncommon. Similarly, information on acute overdosage with diflunisal in humans is limited.

Salicylates are also contained in a variety of preparations for topical application and can lead to poisoning through percutaneous or transmucosal absorption. Salicylic acid ointment, usually in concentrations of up to 5 per cent, is still commonly used as a keratolytic agent for removing the scales of psoriasis. Salicylates are also contained in some teething gels and corn solvents.

CLASSIFICATION OF SALICYLATE POISONING

Classification of salicylate poisoning is usually straightforward in the majority of cases, but occasionally the nomenclature and overlap between some classes create confusion. Five types can be recognized.

Congenital

Salicylates readily cross the placenta from mother to child, and maternal overdosage, depending on the stage of pregnancy at which it occurs, may lead to intrauterine death of the fetus[2] or, rarely, to the child being born with salicylate poisoning. Only sporadic cases have been reported, including one of hyperventilation and vomiting in a 20-hour-old baby whose mother had ingested 15 to 18 gm of aspirin 27 hours before giving birth. The mother's blood salicylate concentration 20 hours before delivery was 38 mg/dl, whereas the admission serum level in the infant was 35 mg/dl.[3]

Therapeutic Overdosage

Therapeutic overdosage is usually the result of well-intentioned but misguided overtreatment of febrile illnesses in childhood. The kinetics of salicylate elimination in young children are such that the metabolic pathways are soon saturated by repeated excessive doses, causing plasma salicylate concentrations to increase to toxic levels.[4–6] Moreover, the hyperpyrexia and hyperventilation that sometimes complicate the resulting intoxication may be interpreted as indicating the need for further treatment. Less commonly, salicylate abuse or chronic therapeutic overdosage leads to intoxication in adults.[7–10]

Frequent applications of teething gels[11] or the extensive application of ointments containing salicylic acid also can lead to poisoning, even in adults.[12]

Accidental Poisoning

Accidental ingestion of excessive quantities of salicylates was formerly one of the most common types of poisoning in childhood and was probably the single most frequent cause of salicylate intoxication. It usually occurred between the ages of 1 and 4 years, the period at which children gain independent mobility and explore their environments, using their mouths as well as their fingers and eyes, and may have been facilitated by the attractive color and flavor of some pediatric aspirin preparations.[13] However, the pediatric situation has changed considerably in recent years. The introduction of effective safety packaging has reduced the prevalence of accidental overdosage (see hereafter), and this is likely to be accelerated by the withdrawal of pediatric aspirin products because of their possible etiologic role in Reye's syndrome.

Nonaccidental Poisoning

Although therapeutic poisoning is "nonaccidental," this term is now seemingly reserved for the type of poisoning in which a parent deliberately and covertly administers a drug to a child to induce illness.[14] Salicylates have been used for this purpose. It is a form of child abuse and is complex in etiology. Frequently the objective is to inflict suffering on the spouse or to bring the parents together through mutual concern for the ill child. The real incidence of nonaccidental poisoning is unknown.

Self-Poisoning

Deliberate ingestion of massive amounts of salicylate is common. Its peak incidence is in individuals between the ages of 15 and 35 years, but it is also common in older age groups and rarely may be encountered in those 8 to 10 years of age. Self-poisoning is usually an impulsive act that occurs against a background of adverse interpersonal, social, and economic factors and is often precipitated by a disagreement with a key person in the victim's life; depression is present in a significant percentage of such patients.

EPIDEMIOLOGY

For many years salicylates have been among the most important drugs ingested in overdosage, and a recent report from Maryland indicates that in 1980 aspirin and aspirin substitutes still comprised the single most important group of drugs involving children under the age of 5 years and teenagers.[15] Aspirin, alone or in combination with other drugs, was involved in 22,067 of 1,368,748 poison exposures reported to the American Association of Poison Control Centers National Data Collection System in 1988.[16] However, the incidence of poisoning with salicylates appears to be decreasing. Comparison of the 1968 and 1977 reports of the National Clearinghouse for Poison Control Centers shows that the proportion of poisonings contributed by salicylates to all poisonous ingestions in those below the age of 5 years fell from 21.7 to 3.4 per cent. Similarly, the percentage of all drug overdoses with salicylates in older age groups decreased from 14 to 4.6 per cent. Other reports indicate the declining popularity of salicylates for self-poisoning in Australia[17] and Britain.[18]

Deaths from salicylate overdosage still occur.[19, 20] Thirty-four of the aspirin ingestions reported to the Poison Control Centers National Data Collection System in 1988 were fatal.[16] In the United States, however, the number of salicylate deaths in children under the age of 5 years fell from 140 in 1962 to 12 in 1980.[21] This improvement has in part been attributed to the introduction of child-resistant containers.[22] The number of accidental childhood deaths from salicylate poisoning in Britain has also fallen, but this antedated the introduction of safety packaging in that country.[23]

SALICYLATE PHARMACOKINETICS AFTER OVERDOSAGE

The pharmacokinetic characteristics of salicylates taken in overdosage have important implications for the genesis and treatment of poisoning.

Absorption

Salicylates are rapidly and completely absorbed from the jejunum and small bowel when administered in aqueous solutions. However, ingestion of excessive doses does not always occur in the fasting state, so absorption and the attainment of peak plasma salicylate concentrations may be delayed by the presence of food in the stomach and prolonged gastric emptying. It has also been suggested that salicylates cause pyloric spasm, thus delaying gastric emptying and absorption, but variability in the rates of disintegration and dissolution of different formulations is probably more important. About 10 per cent of adults who ingest overdoses show a rise in plasma salicylate concentrations after gastric lavage, almost certainly due to the flushing of salicylate from the stomach into the small bowel, thus facilitating absorption.

When enteric-coated aspirin formulations are taken, the onset of toxic features and the attainment of peak plasma concentrations may be delayed for 12 or more hours.[24]

Salicylates are rapidly hydrolyzed during absorption through the intestinal mucosa and first-pass hepatic metabolism. Acetylsalicylic acid can only be detected in the plasma for a few hours after an overdose, whereas plasma concentrations of salicylic acid, the principal product of hydrolysis, decline slowly with a half-life on the order of 20 to 30 hours.

Protein Binding

Salicylates are extensively bound to two receptor sites on plasma albumin, one of which has a high affinity and is saturated at low plasma salicylate concentrations, whereas the other has a less marked affinity and only contributes significantly as plasma concentrations increase. It has been calculated that a total concentration of about 800 mg/L is required before free and bound salicylate concentrations would be equal.[25] However, the extent of protein binding is variable even between individuals with comparable plasma albumin concentrations. In one girl, free salicylate decreased from 60 to 17 per cent as total plasma concentrations fell from 925 to 83 mg/L.[26]

Volume of Distribution

The volume of distribution of salicylate is reported to be about 10 L after therapeutic doses[27, 28] but may increase with increasing plasma concentrations.[28]

Metabolism and Excretion

Therapeutic doses of salicylic acid are mainly eliminated by conjugation with glycine and glucuronic acid to form salicyluric acid and salicylphenolic and acyl glucuronides, respectively. A small proportion is also hydroxylated to gentisic acid. However, overdose patients with plasma salicylate concentrations in the range of 250 to 699 mg/L have been found to eliminate a significantly smaller proportion of their salicylate load as salicyluric acid than volunteers taking therapeutic doses.[29] This has been attributed to saturation of the metabolic pathway, but recent evidence from acutely poisoned adults suggests that glycine depletion may be the explanation.[30] Whatever the truth, repeated administration of salicylate, particularly in children, may lead to accumulation and intoxication within a few days.

Renal excretion is the most important mechanism for salicylate elimination as plasma concentrations rise.

Kinetics in Children

Neonates absorb salicylate as rapidly as any other age group but metabolize it more slowly than young teenagers because of comparatively immature hepatic function. Renal excretion is also slower, and neonates therefore attain higher plasma concentrations. Reduced plasma albumin concentrations in this age group may increase the volume of distribution, particularly as plasma concentrations increase.[31]

Kinetics in the Elderly

Absorption of therapeutic doses of salicylate is not impaired in the elderly, but the elimination half-life and volume of distribution may be significantly increased. These observations may be explained by impaired hepatic and renal function despite the normal results of conventional laboratory function tests.[32]

CLINICAL FEATURES

Salicylism

The pharmacologic actions of salicylates are almost entirely the result of inhibition of the cyclo-oxygenase enzyme of the prostaglandin synthetase complex. Acute salicylate poisoning causes a wide variety of features, but tinnitus, some degree of deafness, profuse sweating, and flushing, with warm extremities and bounding pulses, are almost invariably present. There is usually obvious hyperventilation, with both the rate and depth of respiration being increased. Nausea and vomiting may result from direct gastrointestinal irritation.

The mechanisms whereby these features are produced are incompletely understood and occasionally controversial. Electrocochleographic recordings in two overdose patients showed an elevation of hearing threshold (most marked in the 30- to 60-db range), which was completely and rapidly reversible.[33] Uncoupling of oxidative phosphorylation has traditionally been held to account for the increases in heat production, basal metabolic rate, oxygen consumption, and carbon dioxide output, with the resulting increased cardiac output and hyperpyrexia. Some animal studies have suggested that the hyperventilation of salicylism is probably also secondary to increased body metabolism rather than to inhibition of prostaglandin synthetase, whereas others indicate that it is due to a mechanism other than the ability to inhibit oxidative phosphorylation. Studies of plasma concentrations of Krebs cycle organic acids in poisoned humans (see hereafter) have also cast doubt on the role of uncoupling of oxidative phosphorylation.

Acid-Base Disturbances

Characteristic Changes

Acid-base disturbances in salicylate poisoning are common and complex. Hyperventilation leads to respiratory alkalosis, whereas uncoupling of oxidative phosphorylation and interference with glycolysis are thought to be reponsible for some degree of metabolic acidosis. Both cause a reduction in plasma bicarbonate concentrations, and the latter cannot be interpreted as indicating only one of them. Some degree of respiratory alkalosis and metabolic acidosis is present in virtually every moderate or severe poisoning and alters arterial hydrogen ion concentration (pH) in opposing directions. The age of the patient seems to be the most important factor in determining which predominates. In children under the age of 4 years the metabolic component is usually the more important, and these patients almost invariably have acidemia.[34] In contrast, the respiratory component tends to dominate the acid-base change in older children and most adults, who, as a result, usually have either normal or reduced arterial hydrogen ion concentrations.[35] Occasionally, adults have been observed to have a dominant metabolic acidosis. The arterial hydrogen ion concentration resulting from these complex changes is undoubtedly more important in determining the severity of poisoning and outcome than the nature of the acid-base disturbance per se.[20]

Evolution of the Acid-Base Disturbance

It is commonly held that in human salicylate poisoning a dominant metabolic acidosis follows an initial respiratory alkalosis. However, the evidence for this sequence of events is less than satisfactory, and as long ago as 1959 Winters and colleagues commented that in children this sequence did not always occur and that the phase of alkalosis may be very brief.[34] They found acidemia in all of their patients who had intoxication of longer than 24 hours duration but were unable to say that the two observations were causally related since nearly all these children developed intoxication in the course of treatment of an underlying illness. Similarly, it has been shown that adults may develop severe and fatal acidemia within as little as 3 or 4 hours of massive aspirin overdosage.

Causes of Acidemia

The reasons for the development of acidemia are far from clear. Salicylates are weak acids, but, with the concentrations commonly encountered in acute poisoning and extensive protein binding, it is unlikely that this contributes significantly. Increased urinary excretion of keto acids and Krebs cycle organic acids in poisoned children was reported many years ago[36] but has not been confirmed, and plasma concentrations of these acids have not been measured often enough to warrant firm conclusions about their importance. Bartels and Lund-Jacobsen found that although increased blood lactate and ketone body concentrations were demonstrated in 15 out of 45 adults with acute intoxication (serum salicylate concentrations 207 to 815 mg/L, mean 470 mg/L), it was considered that their quantitative importance in respect to the acid-base changes was modest.[37] Moreover, they also concluded that the hyperlactatemia was more probably due to inhibition of liver lactate elimination than to overproduction secondary to hyperventilation or uncoupling of oxidative phosphorylation.

Both salicylate in the cerebrospinal fluid and acidemia are powerful stimuli to respiration, and the latter facilitates the former.[38] The combination of the two might therefore be expected to cause greater hyperventilation than is seen in patients with normal or low arterial hydrogen ion concentration. Chapman and Proudfoot, however, found that the mean $PaCO_2$ was higher in fatal cases (most of whom were acidemic) than in the survivors (most of whom had normal or low arterial hydrogen ion concentrations), and although the difference was not statistically significant they considered that failure to hyperventilate commensurate with the magnitude of the stimuli may be a factor in the development of acidemia.[20] In most of their cases relative hypoventilation could not be ascribed to concomitant ingestion of central nervous system (CNS) depressant drugs. This contrasts with the findings off Gabow and associates[35] of a lower incidence of alkalosis and a higher incidence of respiratory acidosis in salicylate-poisoned patients who had also ingested CNS depressant drugs.

Differential Diagnosis of a High Anion Gap Acidosis

Salicylate poisoning may be the final diagnostic consideration in the lengthy investigation of a complex acidosis in patients who do not give a history of aspirin ingestion. Salicylates produce a high "anion gap" acidosis, which also occurs with poisons such as ethylene glycol, methanol, and paraldehyde. In addition, a high anion gap is also observed in diabetic ketoacidosis, lactic acidosis (which may occur in iron, ethanol, isoniazid, or phenformin overdosage), starvation, alcoholic ketoacidosis, nonketotic hyperosmolar coma, and acute and chronic renal failure. (See Chapter 7 for a fuller discussion of anion gap acidosis.)

Central Nervous System Features

CNS toxicity is an important indicator of severe salicylate poisoning. Serious depression of consciousness is rare, and patients are more often agitated, restless, and uncommunicative before coma supervenes. These features are most commonly encountered in children under the age of 5 years in whom acidemia is the usual acid-base disturbance.[34, 39] Adults seldom show CNS toxicity, but when they do it is again usually associated with acidemia.[20, 35] Animal studies have provided a rational basis for the CNS toxicity of salicylates in the presence of acidemia by showing that the latter facilitates the shift of salicylates from the extracellular fluid into cells, particularly the brain.[38] This, in turn, is due to the pH-dependent ionization of salicylates, which are un-ionized to a greater extent when blood pH falls. They are then more lipid soluble and able to cross cell membranes. Studies in children have confirmed that the more severe the acidemia, the more salicylate is present in the cerebrospinal fluid. However, altered consciousness in salicylate poisoning has not always occurred in patients who have been acidemic. Some have been alkalemic, but in many of these cases plasma salicylate concentrations have been very high, and it seems possible that this alone may allow sufficient salicylate to enter the brain.

The concomitant ingestion of CNS depressant drugs reduces the respiratory stimulant effect of salicylates and encourages the development of acidemia and neurologic features.[35] It has been known for many years that CNS depressants increase the mortality from salicylates in animals.

Convulsions may occur in severe salicylate poisoning but are uncommon. Animal studies suggest that they may be the result of hyperventilation or reduced brain glucose concentrations, both of which may occur in the absence of hypoglycemia. Cerebral edema also has been reported on rare occasions.

Fluid Retention and Pulmonary Edema

Vomiting, sweating, and hyperventilation, perhaps accentuated by coexistent hyperpyrexia, produce some degree of dehydration in salicylate poisoning and could conceivably account for the common observation that urinary output lags behind the rate of fluid administration when attempts are made to force a diuresis. However, fluid retention and oliguria despite apparently adequate hydration have been reported in two children and were thought to be the result of inappropriate secretion of antidiuretic hormone, although other mechanisms were not excluded.[40] Moreover, hypoxia and hypocapnia can be present with or without clinical or radiologic signs of pulmonary edema before any attempt is made to force a diuresis.

The mechanism of fluid retention is of considerable importance, since attempts to force a diuresis may lead to pulmonary edema. The finding of normal pulmonary capillary wedge pressures in most cases suggests that the pulmonary edema is noncardiac in origin and not the result of fluid overload. This view is supported by observations from two other sources. First, studies in sheep showed that salicylates increased the rate of pulmonary lymph flow and lymph protein clearance, indicating increased lung vascular permeability, perhaps as the result of impaired platelet function, a direct toxic effect on capillary epithelium, or inhibition of prostaglandin synthesis.[41] Second, measurement of the protein content of plasma, pulmonary edema fluid, and urine in two poisoned adults also supports the concept of increased vascular permeability and confirms that pulmonary edema is noncardiac despite administration of intravenous fluids.[42]

Radiologic studies in salicylate intoxication indicate that pulmonary edema occurs in about 35 per cent of patients over the age of 30 years and that cigarette smoking, chronic ingestion of the drug, metabolic acidosis, and the presence of neurologic features on admission are major risk factors.[43] However, there is controversy over how frequently pulmonary edema complicates salicylate intoxication in children. In the study by Walters and colleagues,[43] none of the 55 patients under the age of 16 years developed pulmonary edema, but in that by Fisher and coworkers, 2 out of 20 children of similar age developed the complication.[44] A high anion gap acidosis was again noted to be a predisposing factor.

Rarely, oliguria may be due to acute tubular necrosis and not dehydration. Urinalysis may not be helpful in the diagnosis since hyaline casts and excessive tubular cells may be observed in the urine of nonoliguric patients who have been poisoned with salicylate.

Purpura

Some patients, particularly young women, develop petechial hemorrhages during the course of acute salicylate poisoning. They are most commonly seen on the eyelids and may spread to the rest of the face and neck but not to the trunk or limbs. There may be associated subconjunctival hemorrhages. The purpura is probably due to a combination of increased capillary permeability, decreased platelet stickiness, and a marked rise in venous pressure during retching or struggling in the course of gastric emptying. The patient and her relatives can be reassured that the unsightly rash is of no serious significance and that the lesions will disappear within a few days. Investigation is clearly unnecessary.

Hyperpyrexia

Hyperpyrexia is said to be a common complication of salicylate intoxication in children. It could be the result of metabolic stimulation due to uncoupling of oxidative phosphorylation but may more simply reflect the illness for which the salicylate was prescribed in the first place. Hyperpyrexia is a very uncommon complication of salicylate poisoning in adults but a serious prognostic sign.[20] The possibility that it is due to other drugs taken concomitantly, particularly monoamine oxidase inhibitors, must also be considered.

Plasma Electrolyte Changes

Robin and colleagues reported six patients aged between 5 and 52 years who presented with neuromuscular abnormalities, electrocardiographic changes, and hypokalemia as features of severe salicylate poisoning.[45] In most cases hypokalemia was present within a few hours of ingestion of the drug. Every patient was alkalemic owing to a predominant respiratory alkalosis, and it was postulated that the hypokalemia resulted from a subsequent shift of potassium into cells and excessive loss in urine. Severe hypokalemia may also complicate the treatment of salicylate poisoning by forced alkaline diuresis but is readily corrected by the administration of adequate potassium supplements.[46] Similarly, hypocalcemia complicates attempts at alkalinization.[47] Transient hypercalcemia, possibly due to the calcium carbonate content of the tablets, has been reported after overdosage with soluble aspirin.[48]

Hypoprothrombinemia and Gastrointestinal Hemorrhage

Despite the importance attributed to therapeutic doses of salicylates as an etiologic factor in upper alimentary hemorrhage, severe bleeding from the stomach or duodenum is a rare complication of acute massive overdosage. Chronic administration of large doses of salicylates undoubtedly inhibits the synthesis of factors II, V, VII, and X, but clinically significant hypoprothrombinemia (as assessed by prolongation of the prothrombin time) in acute poisoning is most uncommon. Therapeutic administration of vitamin K should rarely be necessary.

Gastric Perforation

Gastric perforation has been reported after acute salicylate overdosage[49] but is exceedingly rare. More surprisingly, it has also been reported after overdosage with enteric-coated aspirin preparations,[50] one of the major objectives of which is to minimize gastric irritation. Such formulations are designed to disintegrate in an alkaline rather than an acid medium.

Poisoning Complicating Gastric Outlet Obstruction

Several reports indicate that enteric-coated aspirin tablets may be retained in the stomach for long periods in the presence of pyloric stenosis. Salicylate poisoning may or may not complicate gastric retention of such tablets, which can often be seen as filling defects on barium meal examination.[51]

DIAGNOSIS

Clinical

In the majority of cases it is not difficult to make a diagnosis of acute salicylate poisoning. Many children poisoning themselves accidentally will be found ingesting the tablets. Adults seldom lose consciousness with salicylates alone and are usually so miserable with salicylism that they are only too ready to admit to what they have taken. On other occasions, however, diagnosis may be much more difficult, particularly when CNS depressant drugs have been ingested simultaneously or with therapeutic or nonaccidental poisoning in childhood. In such circumstances hyperventilation, diaphoresis, and the associated acid-base abnormalities are the most important diagnostic clues. Anderson and colleagues made a detailed study of adults in whom the diagnosis of salicylate intoxication was delayed from 6 to 72 hours after admission to hospital.[52] In these patients poisoning was usually therapeutic rather than due to acute massive overdosage, and the patients tended to be older, with a high incidence of chronic medical conditions that often were the reason for taking the salicylates. Many had altered consciousness, which prevented disclosure of salicylate ingestion; this, together with features such as convulsions and hallucinations, led to many being subjected to detailed neurologic investigations before the diagnosis of salicylate poisoning was established. Delayed diagnosis was associated with a high morbidity and a mortality of about 25 per cent. In retrospect, it was apparent that the common clinical and laboratory features of poisoning had not always been appreciated. It is not uncommon to refer a patient for psychiatric evaluation only to discover that in fact he or she has salicylate intoxication.[10]

Plasma Salicylate Concentrations

Once the possibility of salicylate intoxication is considered, it is easily confirmed by measurement of the plasma salicylate concentration. Several analytical techniques are available,[53] but most hospital laboratories use a simple colorimetric method that estimates total plasma salicylate concentrations. The disadvantages of using a nonspecific method that also measures the very low concentrations of metabolites are more than counterbalanced by the ease and speed with which it can be carried out and by the fact that there is no simple assay that will measure unbound salicylic acid, the most important component. Acetylsalicylic acid and salicylic acid and its metabolites can be readily measured by high-performance liquid chromatography. Indiscriminately requested drug screens yield a low proportion of salicylate intoxications.[54]

A plasma salicylate level greater than 30 mg/dl or 30 mg per cent (or 300 mg/L) is usually associated with clinical toxicity.

ASSESSMENT OF THE SEVERITY OF POISONING

The severity of salicylate poisoning clearly dictates the urgency and invasiveness of therapeutic intervention but cannot be assessed from only one type of observation. The patient's clinical state is by far the most important single factor but in the majority is unlikely to show features other than those commonly referred to as salicylism. In these situations, assessment of severity is based on the plasma salicylate concentration interpreted in the context of the patient's clinical state and, particularly, the knowledge of the arterial hydrogen ion concentration.

As noted previously, CNS features are the most important indicators of severe salicylate intoxication, but they are rarely encountered in older children and adults. Unfortunately, plasma salicylate concentrations correlate poorly with features of acute toxicity, although clinically serious poisoning and most deaths occur in patients with the highest plasma concentrations.[20] Patients with normal hearing usually experience tinnitus with concentrations greater than 30 mg/dl, and few are likely to complain of tinnitus below 20 mg/dl, whereas those with pre-existing hearing loss may fail to notice tinnitus despite plasma salicylate concentrations well in excess of the accepted therapeutic range. Nor is the acid-base disturbance or degree of hyperventilation (as assessed by arterial carbon dioxide tension) related to salicylate concentrations. This is hardly surprising, since toxicity is presumably related to the concentration of free drug, which, in turn, depends on a number of factors including the total plasma concentration and a variable degree of protein binding. The concentration of free salicylate is likely to comprise less than half the total plasma concentration in most cases of acute intoxication. Done attempted to circumvent these difficulties by relating the severity of poisoning to a theoretic plasma salicylate concentration at the moment of ingestion, calculated by extrapolation backward from the plasma half-life determined 6 or more hours after the single dose taken.[55] Measurements made before 6 hours were considered misleading since the drug may still be being absorbed. The Done nomogram has enjoyed wide popularity among pediatricians but perhaps has not been as widely adopted for the assessment of adult poisoning.

The concentration of salicylate in cerebrospinal fluid reflects the concentration of unbound drug in plasma; studies in children and animals have shown that the severity of intoxication is closely related to cerebrospinal fluid salicylate concentrations. These, in turn, were related to the total plasma concentration and the arterial hydrogen ion concentration. Although the latter does not influence protein binding of salicylates, high hydrogen ion concentrations reduce ionization and thereby facilitate the shift of salicylate into cells.

In practice, however, it is unthinkable that measurement of cerebrospinal fluid salicylate concentrations should ever be allowed to assist the management of acute salicylate poisoning.

TREATMENT

As with any form of poisoning, treatment of acute salicylate poisoning is directed toward preventing further absorption of the drug, enhancing its elimination, and reducing its toxicity.

Preventing Further Absorption

If intoxication has developed as a result of percutaneous absorption, it is clearly imperative to clean the skin thoroughly and withhold further applications of salicylic acid ointment.

Gastric Emptying

When a large overdose of salicylates has been ingested, consideration should be given to emptying the stomach. The time interval between ingestion and admission that allows recovery of a toxicologically significant amount of drug is a matter of considerable uncertainty. Some investigators have suggested that salicylates in overdosage inhibit gastric emptying and that gastric aspiration and lavage are useful up to 12 hours after ingestion. However, the evidence for this is limited, and it seems more appropriate to advise gastric emptying up to 8 hours after ingestion. An obvious exception to this recommendation is the gastric retention of enteric-coated formulations, for which lavage is probably indicated up to 12 hours postingestion.

Administration of syrup of ipecacuanha (ipecac) is the method of choice for gastric emptying in conscious children. In adults, the choice lies between emesis and gastric aspiration and lavage and is made according to the doctor's personal experience and belief in the relative efficacy of the two techniques. If lavage is chosen, it is essential to use a large-diameter tube and to aspirate as much of the gastric contents as possible at the outset, since the introduction of water into the stomach may wash salicylate through the pylorus into the small bowel, leading to rapid absorption. Lavage should be carried out using as much tepid water (in aliquots of 300 to 400 ml) as is necessary to produce a clear gastric effluent. The efficiency of the procedure may be increased by gentle massage over the left hypochondrium during lavage. The addition of alkali to the lavage fluid may facilitate dissolution of retained enteric-coated tablets but may also accelerate gastric emptying and absorption of any form of salicylate.

Activated Charcoal

Activated charcoal is indicated in the management of salicylate poisoning to reduce salicylate absorption. It is most effective if given immediately after ingestion and declines rapidly in value as the time from ingestion increases. There is probably little effect after about 2 hours. Unfortunately, most adults who take overdoses of salicylates are seen too late for activated charcoal to be of any value, and its major role is in the management of accidental poisoning in childhood. Nevertheless, plasma salicylate concentrations continue to increase in some patients despite gastric aspiration and lavage, and it is possible that activated charcoal left in the stomach after lavage might reduce subsequent absorption. Coadministration of cathartics does not affect the absorptive capacity of charcoal for salicylate.[56]

Indications for Enhancing Elimination

Measures to enhance elimination are clearly justified in very severely poisoned patients with acidemia, impaired consciousness, pulmonary or cerebral edema, and cardiac or renal failure. They also should be used when plasma salicylate concentrations are high (greater than 100 mg/dl [100 mg per cent]). Whereas a relatively small proportion of patients falls into these categories, very large numbers may be unwell with protracted symptoms of salicylism although not at risk of dying. It is generally recommended that plasma salicylate concentrations exceeding 50 mg/dl in adults and 35 mg/dl in children are indications for enhancing elimination, the lower value for children being a reflection of their tendency to acidemia and, therefore, CNS toxicity. However, although plasma drug concentrations provide a working guideline for management, they are hardly sacrosanct. It is more important to consider the severity of symptoms and biochemical abnormalities in each individual and to judge whether they could be ameliorated more rapidly by attempting to increase the rate of elimination of salicylate.

Techniques for Increasing Elimination

Several techniques have been used to enhance the elimination of salicylate from the body. They include forced alkaline diuresis, administration of alkali alone, exchange transfusion, peritoneal dialysis, hemodialysis, charcoal hemoperfusion, and, most recently, administration of repeated doses of oral activated charcoal.

Forced Alkaline Diuresis

The rationale for forced alkaline diuresis to enhance salicylate elimination is simple. As discussed earlier, the metabolic pathways for salicylates are saturated with therapeutic doses, and renal excretion becomes increasingly important as plasma salicylate concentrations reach toxic levels. Even then, only the relatively small percentage of plasma salicylate that is unbound is available to be filtered by the glomeruli, and this amount cannot be altered. However, renal tubular reabsorption of filtered salicylate can be reduced, and urinary excretion consequently increased, by two maneuvers. First, since salicylates are weak acids, alkalinization of the urine keeps them in an ionized, nonreabsorbable state. Second, a brisk diuresis increases the rate of flow down the nephron and reduces the urine:tubular cell gradient for reabsorption. Forced alkaline diuresis has the obvious advantages of not requiring special equipment or particular expertise. There is no doubt that it shortens the plasma half-life of salicylate, and it is not surprising that it has been widely adopted as the treatment of choice for salicylate poisoning. However, it must be appreciated that forced alkaline diuresis is a metabolically invasive procedure and its progress must be carefully monitored, both clinically and biochemically.

Although the objectives of forced alkaline diuresis are simple in theory, they are more difficult to achieve in practice. As mentioned, most patients with salicylate intoxication of several hours duration are dehydrated, and, despite the administration of large volumes of intravenous fluid, the onset of diuresis may be delayed by 2 or more hours, causing concern about circulatory overload. The urine pH in patients poisoned with salicylates is usually in the range of 5.5 to 6.5, and it may be difficult to make it alkaline. Preoccupation with attaining an alkaline urine may lead to the administration of excessive sodium bicarbonate and produce potentially dangerous alkalemia. Despite these drawbacks, forced alkaline diuresis is, and is likely to remain, the treatment of choice for enhancement of salicylate excretion.

To a large extent, the amount of fluid and alkali to be given to achieve forced alkaline diuresis is a matter of choice for the individual physician. Diuresis can be induced by the intravenous administration of isotonic dextrose and saline alone but the onset may be delayed; administration of a loop diuretic such as furosemide may be helpful if there is concern about fluid retention and pulmonary edema. Fortunately, salicylate poisoning occurs predominantly in children and young adults, who are well able to cope with the considerable fluid load this treatment imposes. Patients often incur a positive fluid balance of 2 to 4 liters before the onset of diuresis, but this seldom gives rise to problems. However, the rate of fluid administration may have to be reduced in elderly patients or those with cardiac or renal disease. Pulmonary edema may complicate the use of forced diuresis in acidemic adults, and in such cases the acid-base abnormality must be corrected before attempting to induce a diuresis.

The method of alkalinizing the urine is no longer a source of controversy; intravenous sodium bicarbonate is the method of choice. Acetazolamide, a carbonic anhydrase inhibitor, effectively alkalinizes the urine but may exacerbate metabolic acidosis and should not be used.

Alkali Administration Alone

The plasma salicylate half-life can also be satisfactorily reduced by alkalinization without forcing a diuresis and avoiding the risks of fluid overload.[57] Although to date this approach has been studied only in mild and moderate intoxication, there is no reason to doubt that it would be effective, particularly if used in conjunction with repeated administration of oral activated charcoal. It may be the treatment of choice in older patients with pre-existing diseases that might compromise their ability to handle the fluid load of conventional forced diuresis. Further assessment is required, but the approach merits consideration.

Repeated-Dose Oral Activated Charcoal

The realization that repeated doses of oral activated charcoal can considerably enhance the elimination of drugs that have already been absorbed is one of the most exciting therapeutic advances in clinical toxicology in recent years. Repeated oral charcoal can reduce the plasma half-life of salicylates more effectively than conventional forced alkaline diuresis in mild to moderately poisoned patients[58, 59] and should be offered to any patient with salicylate intoxication.

Exchange Transfusion and Peritoneal Dialysis

These techniques are relatively inefficient and have been superseded by forced alkaline diuresis and hemodialysis. Despite this, peritoneal dialysis has a role in the management of severely poisoned patients who are geographically remote from hemodialysis centers.

Hemodialysis

Hemodialysis is a very efficient method of eliminating salicylate from the circulation, but its use should be reserved for severely poisoned patients and those who are at particular risk of pulmonary edema if attempts are made to induce a diuresis. It is probably the treatment of choice when plasma salicylate concentrations are very high (greater than 100 mg/dl [1000 mg/L]) or when the patient is acidemic and unresponsive to bicarbonate therapy with features of CNS toxicity. Not only does it remove salicylate rapidly but it also permits control of electrolyte and fluid balance[60] should signs of circulatory overload develop.

Charcoal Hemoperfusion

Hemoperfusion has been used relatively infrequently for the treatment of salicylate poisoning, but the evidence indicates that it is as effective as hemodialysis in removing salicylates. However, although it is now generally accepted that charcoal hemoperfusion is technically simpler than hemodialysis, it clearly does not allow adequate control of fluid or electrolyte balance unless a conventional dialyzer is used in series with the column. Hemodialysis is therefore preferred.

Other Measures

Vitamin K (intravenously) rarely may be necessary for the correction of hypoprothrombinemia. The patient with severe salicylate poisoning who has CNS toxicity and high plasma concentrations presents a formidable clinical problem. The critical nature of the condition is usually all too obvious, and cardiac arrest may occur without warning or be precipitated by convulsions or preceded by dysrhythmias. Therefore, considerable urgency exists in initiating treatment aimed at correction of the metabolic abnormalities and eliminating salicylate from the circulation.

References

1. Leslie PJ, Dyson EH, Proudfoot AT: Opiate toxicity after self poisoning with aspirin and codeine. Br Med J *292*:96, 1986.
2. Rejent TA, Baik S: Fatal in utero salicylism. J Forens Sci *30*:942, 1985.
3. Earle R: Congenital salicylate intoxication—report of a case. N Engl J Med *265*:1003, 1961.
4. Allen MD, Greenblatt DJ: Accidental salicylate poisoning. Pediatrician *6*:244, 1977.
5. Mitchell I: "Therapeutic" salicylate poisoning in children. Br Med J *1*:1081, 1979.
6. Fiscina S: Death associated with aspirin overdose. Milit Med *151*:499, 1986.
7. Vivian AS, Goldberg IB: Recognizing chronic salicylate intoxication in the elderly. Geriatrics *37*:91, 1982.
8. Schwartz JE: Chronic aspirin intoxication. Ariz Med *41*:799, 1984.
9. Skiendzielewski JJ, Parrish G, Harrington TM: Mental confusion in an elderly, chronically ill patient. Ann Emerg Med *15*:571, 1986.
10. Steele TE, Morton WA: Salicylate-induced delirium. Psychosomatics *27*:455, 1986.
11. Paynter AS, Alexander FW: Salicylate intoxication caused by teething ointment. Lancet *2*:1132, 1979.
12. Davies MG, Briffa DV, Greaves MW: Systemic toxicity from topically applied salicylic acid. Br Med J *1*:661, 1979.
13. Howrie DL, Moriarty R, Breit R: Candy flavoring as a source of salicylate poisoning. Pediatrics *75*:869, 1985.
14. Pickering D: Salicylate poisoning as a manifestation of the battered child syndrome. Am J Dis Child *130*:675, 1976.
15. Trinkoff AM, Baker SP: Poisoning hospitalizations and deaths from solids and liquids among children and teenagers. Am J Public Health *76*:657, 1986.
16. Litovitz TL, Schmitz BF, Holm KC: 1988 Annual Report of the American Association of Poison Control Centers National Data Collection System. Am J Emerg Med *7*:495, 1989.
17. Hardwicke C, Holt L, James R, Smith AJ: Trends in self-poisoning with drugs in Newcastle, New South Wales, 1980–1982. Med J Aust *144*:453, 1986.

18. Proudfoot AT: Clinical toxicology, past, present and future. Hum Toxicol *7*:481, 1988.
19. McGuigan MA: A two-year review of salicylate deaths in Ontario. Arch Intern Med *147*:510, 1987.
20. Chapman BC, Proudfoot AT: Adult salicylate poisoning: deaths and outcome in patients with high plasma salicylate concentrations. (In press.)
21. Brancato DJ, Nelson RC: FDA poison control notes. Vet Hum Toxicol *26*:273, 1984.
22. Clarke A, Walton WW: Effect of safety packaging on aspirin ingestion by children. Pediatrics *63*:687, 1979.
23. Fraser NC: Accidental poisoning deaths in British children, 1958–77. Br Med J *280*:1595, 1980.
24. Wortzman DJ, Grunfeld A: Delayed absorption following enteric-coated aspirin overdose. Ann Emerg Med *16*:434, 1987.
25. Wosilait WD: Theoretical analysis of the binding of salicylate by human serum albumin: the relationship between free and bound drug and therapeutic levels. Eur J Clin Pharmacol *9*:285, 1976.
26. Alván G, Bergman U, Gustafsson LL: High unbound fraction of salicylate in plasma during intoxication. Br J Clin Pharmacol *11*:625, 1981.
27. Needs CJ, Brooks PM: Clinical pharmacokinetics of the salicylates. Clin Pharmacokinet *10*:164, 1985.
28. Rubin GM, Tozer TN, Øie S: Concentration-dependence of salicylate distribution. J Pharm Pharmacol *35*:115, 1983.
29. Notarianni LJ, Ogunbona FA, Oldham HG, Patel DK, Bennett PN, Humphries SJ: Glycine conjugation of salicylic acid after aspirin overdose. Br J Clin Pharmacol *15*:587P, 1983.
30. Bennett PN, Notarianni LJ, Patel DK, Ho SG: Evidence for glycine depletion after aspirin overdose. Br J Clin Pharmacol *16*:219P, 1983.
31. Buchanec J, Galanda V, Višňovský P, Haláková E: Effect of age on pharmacokinetics of salicylate. J Pediatr *99*:833, 1981.
32. Cuny G, Royer RJ, Mur JM, Serot JM, Faure G, Netter P, Maillard A, Penin F: Pharmacokinetics of salicylates in elderly. Gerontology *25*:49, 1979.
33. Ramsden RT, Latif A, O'Malley S: Electrocochleographic changes in acute salicylate overdosage. J Laryngol Otol *99*:1269, 1985.
34. Winters RW, White JS, Hughes MC, Ordway NC: Disturbances of acid-base equilibrium in salicylate intoxication. Pediatrics *23*:260, 1959.
35. Gabow PA, Anderson RJ, Potts DE, Schrier RW: Acid-base disturbances in the salicylate-intoxicated adult. Arch Intern Med *138*:1481, 1978.
36. Schwartz R, Landy G: Organic acid excretion in salicylate intoxication. J Pediatr *66*:658, 1965.
37. Bartels PD, Lund-Jacobsen H: Blood lactate and ketone body concentrations in salicylate intoxication. Hum Toxicol *5*:363, 1986.
38. Hill JB: Salicylate intoxication. N Engl J Med *288*:1110, 1973.
39. Gaudreault P, Temple AR, Lovejoy FH: The relative severity of acute versus chronic salicylate poisoning in children: a clinical comparison. Pediatrics *70*:566, 1982.
40. Temple AR, George DJ, Done AK, Thompson JA: Salicylate poisoning complicated by fluid retention. Clin Toxicol *9*:61, 1976.
41. Bowers RE, Brigham KL, Owen PJ: Salicylate pulmonary edema: The mechanism in sheep and review of the clinical literature. Am Rev Resp Dis *115*:261, 1977.
42. Hormaechea E, Carlson RW, Rogrove H, Uphold J, Henning RJ, Weil MH: Hypovolemia, pulmonary edema and protein changes in severe salicylate poisoning. Am J Med *66*:1046, 1979.
43. Walters JS, Woodring JH, Stelling CB, Rosenbaum HD: Salicylate-induced pulmonary edema. Radiology *146*:289, 1983.
44. Fisher CJ, Albertson TE, Foulke GE: Salicylate-induced pulmonary edema. Clinical characteristics in children. Am J Emerg Med *3*:33, 1985.
45. Robin ED, Davis RP, Rees SB: Salicylate intoxication with special reference to the development of hypokalemia. Am J Med *26*:869, 1959.
46. Lawson AAH, Proudfoot AT, Brown SS, Macdonald RH, Fraser AG, Cameron JC, Matthew H: Forced diuresis in the treatment of acute salicylate poisoning in adults. Q J Med *38*:31, 1969.
47. Fox GN: Hypocalcemia complicating bicarbonate therapy for salicylate poisoning. West J Med *141*:108, 1984.
48. Reid IR: Transient hypercalcemia following overdoses of soluble aspirin tablets. Aust NZ J Med *15*:364, 1985.
49. Robins JB, Turnbull JA, Robertson C: Gastric perforation after acute aspirin overdose. Hum Toxicol *4*:527, 1985.
50. Farrand RJ, Green JH, Haworth C: Enteric-coated aspirin overdose and gastric perforation. Br Med J *4*:85, 1975.
51. Kwong TC, Laczin J, Baum J: Self-poisoning with enteric coated aspirin. Am J Clin Pathol *80*:888, 1983.
52. Anderson RJ, Potts DE, Gabow PA, Rumack BH: Unrecognized adult salicylate intoxication. Arch Intern Med *85*:745, 1976.
53. Kwong TC: Salicylate measurement: clinical usefulness and methodology. CRC Crit Rev Clin Lab Sci *25*:137, 1987.
54. Krenzelok EP, Guharoy SL, Johnson DR: Toxicology screening in the emergency department: Ethanol, barbiturates and salicylates. Am J Emerg Med *2*:331, 1984.
55. Done AK: Aspirin overdosage: Incidence, diagnosis and management. Pediatrics *62* (Part 2 Suppl):890, 1978.
56. Czajka PA, Konrad JD: Saline cathartics and the adsorptive capacity of activated charcoal for aspirin. Ann Emerg Med *15*:548, 1986.
57. Prescott LF, Balali-Mood M, Critchley JAJH, Johnstone AF, Proudfoot AT: Diuresis or urinary alkalinisation for salicylate poisoning? Br Med J *285*:1383, 1982.
58. Hillman RJ, Prescott LF: Treatment of salicylate poisoning with repeated oral charcoal. Br Med J *291*:1472, 1985.
59. Mofenson HC, Caraccio TR, Greensher J, D'Agostino R, Rossi A: Gastrointestinal dialysis with activated charcoal and cathartic in the treatment of adolescent intoxications. Clin Pediatr *24*:678, 1985.
60. Jacobsen D, Wiik-Larsen E, Bredesen JE: Haemodialysis or haemoperfusion in severe salicylate poisoning? Hum Toxicol *7*:161, 1988.

CHAPTER 52

NONSTEROIDAL ANTI-INFLAMMATORY DRUGS AND COLCHICINE

Robert P. Kimberly, M.D.

General Properties

Nonsteroidal Anti-Inflammatory Drugs

Nonsteroidal anti-inflammatory drugs (NSAIDs) inhibit prostaglandin synthesis and possess both analgesic and antipyretic properties. They are usually rapidly absorbed after oral administration, although food may retard absorption in some instances. Little drug may remain for recovery from gastric contents within 1 to 2 hours after ingestion. Renal excretion is usually the dominant route of elimination, although several agents have a substantial enterohepatic circulation with fecal excretion. NSAIDs are potent inhibitors of prostaglandin synthesis, which may result in marked side effects. However, the available experience with acute overdosage suggests that NSAIDs possess a reasonable margin of safety.

NSAIDs fall into several subgroups based on chemical structure (Table 52–1).

Arylalkanoic acid derivatives [ibuprofen (Motrin), naproxen (Naprosyn), fenoprofen (Nalfon), flurbiprofen (Ansaid), ketoprofen (Orudis), suprofen (Suprol)] are rapidly absorbed and usually well tolerated. Ibuprofen shows the least protein binding. In animal studies, both naproxen and fenoprofen are associated with nephritis after chronic high-dose administration. Naproxen has a significantly longer half-life than the other compounds (Table 52–2). Both naproxen and its more rapidly absorbed sodium salt (Anaprox) circulate in the blood as the naproxen anion.

Carbo- and heterocyclic acetic acid derivatives and similar compounds [diclofenac (Voltaren), indomethacin (Indocin), sulindac (Clinoril), and tolmetin sodium (Tolectin)] may be clinically effective when response to drugs of another subgroup has been suboptimal. Indomethacin, an indole acetic acid, may have prominent gastrointestinal (GI) tract and central nervous system (CNS) side effects. Nausea, abdominal pain, both occult and frank GI bleeding, and peptic ulceration may occur with all NSAIDs. Indomethacin may cause headache and aggravate psychiatric disturbances, producing mental confusion, depression, and psychotic episodes. Since the drug has been associated with corneal deposits during prolonged therapy, attention to visual signs and symptoms has been recommended during therapy with all NSAIDs. Tolmetin, a pyrrole derivative, does not seem to be associated with the psychiatric effects seen with indomethacin. Sulindac, an indene acetic acid derivative, requires hepatic conversion of the parent compound to the active sulfide metabolite. This metabolite has a comparatively long half-life, similar to that of naproxen but much shorter than that of either phenylbutazone (Azolid, Butazolidin) or oxyphenbutazone (Oxalid, Tandearil). Sulindac and indomethacin have a substantial enterohepatic circulation.

The derivatives of *anthranilic acid,* the amine analogue of salicylic acid, include meclofenamate sodium (Meclomen) and mefenamic acid (Ponstel). They have a propensity to cause diarrhea, which may be bloody and severe. Autoimmune hemolytic anemia has been associated with prolonged use of mefenamic acid. Anthranilic acid derivatives may potentiate the effects of coumarin-type anticoagulants. The use of mefenamic acid, released in the United States as an analgesic, has been restricted because of toxicity. Meclofenamate sodium appears to have greater anti-inflammatory potential.

Pyrazolone derivatives [phenylbutazone (Azolid, Butazolidin), oxyphenbutazone (Oxalid, Tandearil); also aminopyrine, antipyrine] are poorly tolerated by some patients and have toxic effects that have included agranulocytosis, thrombocytopenia, aplastic

Table 52–1. NONSTEROIDAL ANTI-INFLAMMATORY DRUGS

CHEMICAL CLASS	COMPOUND	TRADE NAME
I. Carboxylic Acids		
Arylalkanoic acid derivatives	fenoprofen calcium	Nalfon
	flurbiprofen	Ansaid
	ibuprofen	Motrin, Rufen, Advil, Medipren, Nuprin
	ketoprofen	Orudis
	naproxen	Naprosyn, Anaprox
	suprofen	Suprol
Carbo- and heterocyclic acetic acid derivatives	diclofenac	Voltaren
	indomethacin	Indocin
	sulindac	Clinoril
	tolmetin sodium	Tolectin
Anthranilic acid derivatives	meclofenamate sodium	Meclomen
	mefenamic acid	Ponstel
II. Enolic Acids		
Pyrazolone derivatives	phenylbutazone	Azolid, Butazolidin
	oxyphenbutazone	Oxalid, Tandearil
	sulfinpyrazone*	Anturane
Oxicam derivatives	piroxicam	Feldene

*Primarily a uricosuric and platelet-active agent.

anemia, and death. Reported instances of renal failure with phenylbutazone have been due to renal papillary necrosis, precipitation of uric acid stones with tubular or ureteral obstruction, and idiosyncratic reactions after both short- and long-term drug administration. The toxic effects of these drugs are more pronounced in elderly patients. Sulfinpyrazone (Anturane), a chemically related compound used as a uricosuric agent in gout and as a platelet-active compound, does not possess significant anti-inflammatory activity. It is rarely associated with the adverse effects observed with other pyrazolone congeners.

Members of the *oxicam family* [piroxicam (Feldene)] are enolic, not carboxylic, acids but share the property of prostaglandin synthesis inhibition with other NSAIDs. Piroxicam has a mean half-life of approximately 50 hours, with a wide range of at least 30 to 86 hours. Peak drug plasma concentrations occur 3 to 5 hours after drug administration. Steady state blood levels on a once daily dosage schedule are reached in 1 to 2 weeks.

Table 52–2. DRUG EXCRETION

DRUG	MEAN HALF-LIFE (hr)	MAJOR EXCRETORY ROUTE	SERUM PROTEIN BINDING (%)
diclofenac	2	65% renal, 35% fecal	99*
fenoprofen	3	90% renal	99
flurbiprofen	3–4		99
ibuprofen	2	45–79% renal	99
indomethacin	4.5	60% renal, 33% fecal	99
ketoprofen	3	60% renal	99
meclofenamate	3.3	66% renal, 33% fecal	High
naproxen	13	95% renal	99
oxyphenbutazone	70–80	61% renal, 27% fecal	High
phenylbutazone	72–84	61% renal, 27% fecal	98
piroxicam	50	66% renal, 33% fecal	High
sulindac (sulfide metabolite)	7.8 (16.4)	50% renal, 25% fecal	High
suprofen	3	90% renal	99
tolmetin	1	100% renal	High
colchicine	(0.5%)†	30% renal, 70% renal	Moderate

*Drugs with a high degree of protein binding are not available for efficient removal by dialysis or hemoperfusion.

†Although the plasma half-life is short, the intracellular half-life is considerably longer owing to strong intracellular binding.

As with many other NSAIDs, GI symptoms are the most prominent side effects and may include GI bleeding and peptic ulceration.

Colchicine

Colchicine is unlike other NSAIDs in that its anti-inflammatory effectiveness is manifest primarily in acute attacks of pseudogout and gouty arthritis. Colchicine, a phenanthrene derivative, is the active alkaloidal principle derived from various species of the plant *Colchicum* (e.g., *Colchicum autumnale*, or the meadow saffron). Like the NSAIDs, the drug is rapidly and almost completely absorbed after oral administration. Colchicine is actively taken up intracellularly; the drug half-life is considerably longer within the cell than in the plasma.

The mechanisms of at least some of colchicine's actions are related to the formation of a reversible covalent complex between colchicine and a subunit protein of intracellular microtubules. All actions, however, may not be related to interaction with microtubules. Colchicine does not appear to inhibit prostaglandin synthesis. Colchicine's role in the management of familial Mediterranean fever and Behçet's syndrome may not depend upon an "anti-inflammatory" capacity. Colchicine is neither antipyretic nor analgesic; however, it is an antimitotic agent that can interfere with cell division.

CLINICAL FINDINGS

General Side Effects

These can be considered in two categories: drug-drug interactions (Table 52–3) and direct side effects (Table 52–4).

NSAIDs[1, 2]

Potentiation of protein-bound drugs, including coumarin-type oral anticoagulants, phenytoin, sulfonamides, and oral antidiabetic drugs (sulfonylureas, and acetohexamide for phenylbutazone) constitutes the drug interaction of greatest significance. NSAIDs also affect coagulation by altering platelet function, measured as bleeding time and/or platelet aggregation. Therefore, use of these drugs with warfarin should be approached with caution.

NSAIDs can cause fluid retention with oliguria and an increase in blood pressure. The response to furosemide and propranolol, medications that might be used in the management of these clinical signs, is often blunted, and dosage should be altered ac-

Table 52–3. SIGNIFICANT DRUG INTERACTIONS

INTERACTION	POTENTIAL		
	High	*Uncertain*	*Low*
1. Displacement/potentiation of protein-bound drugs, e.g.: warfarin* phenytoin sulfonamides sulfonylureas	meclofenamate phenylbutazone oxyphenbutazone	fenoprofen flurbiprofen naproxen piroxicam sulindac suprofen	indomethacin ibuprofen ketoprofen tolmetin
2. Hepatic microsomal enzyme induction	phenylbutazone oxyphenbutazone		
3. Altered renal tubular secretion of drugs, e.g.: probenecid	indomethacin naproxen ketoprofen		sulindac
4. Altered diuretic and antihypertensive effects of: furosemide propranolol captopril	indomethacin phenylbutazone		All NSAIDs have a modest potential
5. Increased lithium levels	ibuprofen indomethacin		

*NSAIDs also may affect coagulation by altering platelet function.

Table 52–4. PRINCIPAL ADVERSE REACTIONS WITH THERAPEUTIC DOSES

NSAID	COLCHICINE
Group Reactions	
GI intolerance, including peptic ulcer	GI intolerance, including bloody diarrhea and reversible malabsorption syndrome
Hepatic dysfunction	Myoneuropathy (vascular damage with shock)*
Fluid retention	
Altered platelet function	(Bone marrow suppression)
Tinnitus/decreased auditory acuity	
(Oliguria/anuria)	
(Renal papillary necrosis/ nephritis)	(Disseminated intravascular coagulation)
Idiosyncratic Reactions	
Agranulocytosis (aminopyrine, phenylbutazone)	
Exfoliative dermatitis (phenylbutazone)	
Aseptic meningitis in systemic lupus (ibuprofen, sulindac, tolmetin)	
Allergic interstitial nephritis (fenoprofen and others)	
Hypersensitivity hepatitis (sulindac)	

*Adverse reactions in parentheses are rare and probably occur only in a specifically susceptible host.

cordingly. The antihypertensive response to captopril, but not to enalapril or lisinopril, may also be blunted by NSAIDs.[3] Probenecid, and perhaps penicillin, can decrease tubular secretion of indomethacin, naproxen, ketoprofen, and, to a lesser extent, sulindac, leading to a longer elimination half-life. The active sulfide metabolite of sulindac is not affected. Similarly, lithium levels may be increased by concomitant administration of indomethacin and should, therefore, be carefully monitored.

Some drug side effects are characteristic of all NSAIDs. GI irritation with dyspepsia, increased occult GI blood loss, GI bleeding, and possible peptic ulceration occur with all NSAIDs, although with lesser frequency with some of the newer agents. Administration with nonabsorbable antacids and food often will alleviate symptoms. Hepatic dysfunction with elevated transaminases and modest elevations of alkaline phosphatase can occur. Although the mechanism is unknown for the majority of cases, a hypersensitivity reaction has been suggested for several instances of hepatic dysfunction seen with phenylbutazone and sulindac. Phenylbutazone and other pyrazolones have been associated with hepatic failure.

All NSAIDs may cause fluid retention with decreased urine flow and elevation of blood pressure. Indomethacin and phenylbutazone appear more potent in this regard. Concomitant elevation of serum creatinine and blood urea nitrogen also may occur, although patients with renal insufficiency or stimulation of the renin-angiotensin system (sodium depletion, congestive heart failure, cirrhosis with ascites) are more likely to show a large change in renal function. Several cases of reversible renal failure requiring dialysis have been reported with therapeutic doses of these agents. Hyperkalemia with hyporeninemia and hypoaldosteronism may occur with or without changes in creatinine or blood urea nitrogen (BUN). Although it may be of large magnitude, the elevation of serum potassium is usually small and may be overlooked.

Renal parenchymal effects may include renal papillary necrosis, chronic interstitial nephritis, and allergic interstitial nephritis. Although animal studies suggest that the first two manifestations are dose dependent, allergic interstitial nephritis may occur with dosages in accepted therapeutic ranges. It is probable that susceptibility to any of these effects varies with the individual patient. Although parenchymal damage is more common, phenylbutazone may also precipitate uric acid stones because of its uricosuric properties; evaluation of acute renal dysfunction induced by phenylbutazone should consider ureteral blockage. All NSAIDs may cause tinnitus and decreased auditory acuity. These effects are reversible and not of major concern in the management of drug overdose.

Idiosyncratic reactions to nonsteroidal anti-inflammatory drugs are numerous. Despite the relatively brief clinical experience with the newer agents, aseptic meningitis in systemic lupus erythematosus (ibuprofen, tolmetin, sulindac), allergic interstitial nephritis (fenoprofen), and hypersensitivity hepatitis (sulindac) have been described. Phenylbutazone is associated with a range of severe idiosyncratic reactions, including agranulocytosis and aplastic anemia, exfoliative dermatitis, and hepatic necrosis.

Colchicine

Colchicine affects cell populations with rapid turnover and, therefore, frequently affects the GI tract, especially if taken orally.

Anorexia, nausea, vomiting, abdominal pain, and diarrhea may occur with doses within the therapeutic range. Diarrhea may be severe and, at times, bloody. Uncommon side effects include alopecia involving the scalp and axillary and pubic hair areas, liver dysfunction, mental depression, and myopathy. Hematopoietic dysfunction [bone marrow failure, disseminated intravascular coagulation (DIC)] tends to be dose related. Side effects due to colchicine are more likely to occur in the presence of hepatic and renal dysfunction and in elderly patients. With overdosage, generalized vascular damage with hypotension and shock may occur.

Acute Poisoning[4–6]

Acute poisoning with NSAIDs other than the pyrazolones generally does not result in significant morbidity and mortality. Serious toxicity, including a few deaths, however, has been reported.[4–20] The increased availability of ibuprofen preparations as over-the-counter analgesics may influence this clinical spectrum with regard to ibuprofen overdose since the risk of serious toxicity is dose related.[20] Currently available information indicates that mefenamic acid overdosage appears to be associated with a higher incidence of neuromuscular irritability and convulsions than are other NSAIDs.[21–26] Members of the pyrazolone group (phenylbutazone, oxyphenbutazone) are associated with a significantly greater degree of toxicity with concomitant fatalities.[27–32]

Acute poisoning with NSAIDs presents with few specific clinical findings (Table 52–5). GI symptoms may include nausea, vomiting, indigestion, dyspepsia, and epigastric pain. Patients may report decreased auditory acuity and tinnitus. Confusion, disorientation, dizziness, drowsiness, and even stupor progressing to coma may occur. Blurred vision, diplopia, and seizures have been described. Physical findings can include altered body temperature with either hyper- or hypothermia, abnormal respiration ranging from hyperventilation to profound respiratory depression, changes in cardiovascular status usually with sinus tachycardia and hypotension, renal dysfunction with oliguria or anuria, and abnormal neurologic and neu-

Table 52–5. MANIFESTATIONS OF NSAID OVERDOSE

ORGAN SYSTEM	MANIFESTATION	MANAGEMENT
Gastrointestinal	Anorexia, nausea, vomiting	
	Abdominal pain	Nonabsorbable antacids
	Gastric mucosal irritation	H2-receptor antagonists
Hepatobiliary	Hepatic dysfunction, hyperamylasemia	
Respiratory	Hyperventilation	
	Respiratory depression	Mechanical ventilation
Cardiovascular	Sinus tachycardia	
	Hypotension	Fluids
	Cardiovascular collapse*	Pressors, hemodynamic monitoring
	Cardiac arrest	
Renal	Hematuria, proteinuria	
	Acute renal failure	Dialysis
Hematologic	Hypoprothrombinemia, granulocytosis,† leukopenia, thrombocytopenia*	Vitamin K
Metabolic	Hyper- and hypothermia	
	Electrolyte abnormalities	Replacement
Neuromuscular	Confusion, disorientation, drowsiness, headache, tinnitus, dizziness, blurred vision, nystagmus, diplopia, ataxia, hypertonia, hyper-reflexia, muscle twitching, convulsions‡	Anticonvulsants (e.g., diazepam)
	Coma	

*Cardiovascular collapse and cytopenias are described primarily in association with pyrazolones (phyenylbutazone, oxyphenylbutazone).

†Granulocytosis is reported with sulindac; leukocytosis is occasionally reported with pyrazolones.

‡Convulsions have been reported with many NSAIDs but appear to be much more frequent with mefenamic acid ingestion.

romuscular activity with ataxia, nystagmus, muscular irritability, and seizure activity. Later findings can include clinical evidence of bleeding due to hypoprothrombinemia and thrombocytopenia.

Acute poisoning with colchicine is potentially life-threatening, with death occurring in a large percentage of cases reported in the literature.[33–50] Although this risk may be overstated because of a strong reporting bias, the potential seriousness of colchicine overdose cannot be overemphasized. Correlation of outcome with total ingested dose is imperfect, since death has been reported with doses as small as 7 to 8 mg.[34, 35, 49, 51] The risk of serious complications with colchicine overdose is magnified in the elderly and in the presence of renal or hepatic dysfunction. Very large doses of colchicine (greater than 0.8 mg/kg) are associated with a high probability of death.[34, 35, 49]

Acute poisoning with colchicine most commonly presents with GI symptoms (nausea, vomiting, abdominal pain, and diarrhea) and a peripheral leukocytosis that includes early myeloid forms (Table 52–6). Hemorrhagic gastroenteritis may lead to profuse and bloody diarrhea. Hypotension with hypovolemia and profound muscle weakness may also occur in the early stages of colchicine poisoning.

Within 24 to 72 hours after significant colchicine ingestion, evidence of multiorgan dysfunction may become evident.[49] Diffuse interstitial edema of pulmonary parenchyma with normal or elevated pulmonary capillary wedge pressures may accompany increasing hypoxemia and respiratory distress.[42, 52] Myocardial depression accompanied by shock may evolve to frank cardiovascular collapse. Arrhythmias and cardiac arrest may occur precipitously. Muscle necrosis may lead to both clinically significant weakness and myoglobinuria. Neurologic abnormalities may range from confusion to seizures, papilledema, or coma. An ascending paralysis of the CNS may also occur. Potential metabolic abnormalities include hyponatremia, hypo-

Table 52–6. MANIFESTATIONS OF COLCHICINE OVERDOSE

ORGAN SYSTEM	MANIFESTATION	MANAGEMENT
Early Clinical Phase (within 24 hours of ingestion)		
Gastrointestinal	Anorexia, nausea, vomiting	
	Abdominal pain, cramping	
	Diarrhea	Fluid replacement
Cardiovascular	Hypovolemia	Fluid replacement
	Hypotension	Hemodynamic monitoring
Hematologic	Leukocytosis	
Phase of Multiorgan Dysfunction (24–72 hours after ingestion)		
Gastrointestinal	Bloody diarrhea, ileus	
Respiratory	Hypoxemia, respiratory depression, pulmonary edema (cardiogenic or noncardiogenic)	
	Adult respiratory distress syndrome	Mechanical ventilation
Cardiovascular	Shock, cardiovascular collapse	Fluids, pressors
	Ventricular depression	Hemodynamic monitoring
	Cardiac arrest	
Renal	Hematuria, proteinuria	
	Oliguric renal failure	Dialysis
Hematologic	Marrow suppression with pancytopenia	Appropriate transfusions
	Disseminated intravascular coagulation, hypoprothrombinemia	Plasma, vitamin K
Metabolic	Metabolic acidosis	
	Hyponatremia, hypocalcemia, hypokalemia, hypophosphatemia	Appropriate replacement
Neuromuscular	Lethargy, confusion, stupor, coma	
	Papilledema, seizures, muscle weakness, rhabdomyolysis	Anticonvulsants
Late Clinical Phase (> 7 days after ingestion)		
Hematologic	Rebound leukocytosis	
Integumentary	Alopecia	

kalemia, hypocalcemia,[40] and metabolic acidosis. Oliguric renal failure, at times with hematuria and proteinuria, may result from several factors including hypotension and myoglobinuria. Hematologic complications may include DIC, granulocytopenia, and thrombocytopenia.[44, 53]

Chronic Toxicity

Late sequelae of an acute overdosage of NSAIDs have not been identified. Two major concerns regarding the adverse effects of prolonged administration are peptic ulceration and chronic nephritis. Both ulceration and renal damage may result from acute poisoning; there is no evidence that prolonged use in the recommended dose range will lead to renal parenchymal damage. Although some effects of NSAIDs depend on the total daily dose, evidence for cumulative dose toxicity in a clinical setting is available only for corneal deposits and retinal disturbances reported with prolonged indomethacin therapy.

Chronic colchicine administration has been associated with bone marrow depression, thrombocytopenia, aplastic anemia, peripheral neuritis, myopathy,[54–57] and depilation.

Laboratory Findings

Although no laboratory findings are diagnostic of the etiologic agent in either acute or chronic poisoning with NSAIDs or colchicine, they are of great importance in assessing clinical status. With NSAIDs, serum creatinine and BUN may be elevated. Hyperkalemia may be present as a result of either relative renal insufficiency or hyporeninemic hypoaldosteronism; hypokalemia has also been described. Electrolytes may show decreased total CO_2, reflecting a metabolic acidosis; arterial blood gases may reveal respiratory acidosis when respiratory depression is present. Urinalysis may show hematuria, pyuria, proteinuria, or casts. Tolmetin sodium may cause a false-positive test for urine protein when the sulfosalicylic acid method is used.

Liver enzymes [serum glutamic oxaloacetic transaminase (SGOT), serum glutamic pyruvic transaminase (SGPT), lactic dehydrogenase (LDH), alkaline phosphatase] may be elevated. Hematologic evaluation may reveal either a dyscrasia (low white blood cell count, platelet count, or red cell count) or elevated white blood cells with eosinophilia associated with some idiosyncratic reactions. Hypoprothrombinemia may be reflected in a prolonged prothrombin time. Methemoglobinemia may occur with antipyrine poisoning but less so than with phenacetin.

Laboratory findings with colchicine include hyponatremia, hypokalemia, and hypocalcemia.[40] Metabolic acidosis with an increased anion gap may reflect shock with lactic acidosis or acute renal dysfunction. Both serum creatinine and BUN may be elevated. Oliguric renal failure, hematuria, myoglobinuria, and proteinuria may accompany renal dysfunction. After a leukocytosis characterized by early myeloid forms and manifested usually within hours of the ingestion, lymphopenia, granulocytopenia, and thrombocytopenia of severe magnitude may ensue.[53] Varying degrees of DIC with decreased fibrinogen and platelets, elevated fibrin split products, prolonged prothrombin time, and schistocytes on the peripheral smear may develop with colchicine poisoning.

TREATMENT

Acute Poisoning (see Tables 52–4 through 52–6)

NSAIDs

The approach to acute poisoning with NSAIDs is the same as that for all compounds.[4–6] The stomach contents are emptied by emesis in the conscious patient or by lavage in the semiconscious patient provided the airway is protected. Since most NSAIDs achieve peak plasma levels within 2 to 3 hours (naproxen, piroxicam, and sulindac up to 4 hours), effective gastric emptying must be achieved within several hours of ingestion. Activated charcoal may be administered to decrease absorption.

Further therapy is supportive and directed toward specific clinical signs and symptoms. Respiratory depression, although rare, may require respiratory support; renal shutdown may require either peritoneal dialysis or hemodialysis. GI irritation may respond symptomatically to oral nonabsorbable antacids, such as magnesium aluminum hydroxide; seizures can be managed with diazepam or barbiturates.

Since arylalkanoic acid, anthranilic acid, and indole, pyrrole, and indene acetic acid derivatives are acidic, they have the theoretical potential for increased urinary excretion with alkalinization and diuresis. Oxicams are also acidic by virtue of the enolic 4-hydroxy substituent. Studies in rats have demonstrated increased urinary tolmetin excretion with alkalinization, but human data are not available. All NSAIDs are protein bound (see Table 52–2) and are not accessible for effective removal by dialysis or hemoperfusion.

Colchicine

Colchicine is rapidly absorbed, but gastric emptying and lavage to remove any residual colchicine from the GI tract are important. Activated charcoal instilled into the gut may bind any remaining colchicine and reduce its absorption.[58] Since colchicine is bound intracellularly, hemodialysis and hemoperfusion play no role in removing colchicine from the blood and reducing drug levels.[59]

Attentive supportive management is essential with colchicine overdose.[49] Respiratory compromise (cardiogenic or noncardiogenic pulmonary edema, central respiratory depression) may require intubation and mechanical ventilation to maintain proper oxygenation. Renal failure may require dialysis, whereas careful attention to electrolytes, calcium, and phosphorus is necessary to guide appropriate replacement. Severe marrow depression may necessitate antibiotic coverage for fever in the face of granulocytopenia, platelet transfusions for clinically significant bleeding, and fresh frozen plasma for management of DIC.

Shock is usually a significant factor in severe colchicine overdose and often the cause of death. The clinical picture of shock is complicated, since some patients may have an increased cardiac index whereas others may have a decreased cardiac index.[52] The mechanisms contributing to shock may include hypovolemia, bacterial sepsis resulting from the loss of GI mucosal integrity, and a direct myocardial depressant action of colchicine. Direct hemodynamic monitoring is critical since the contributions of hypovolemia and ventricular dysfunction to the net circulatory status will vary from patient to patient. Fluid replacement and the use of pressors are guided by clinical status and hemodynamic monitoring.

Chronic Poisoning

Cumulative poisoning, such as that seen with heavy metals, does not appear to occur with NSAIDs. Chronic usage may make certain adverse effects, such as peptic ulceration, more likely. It is not clear that renal papillary necrosis or interstitial nephritis occurs as a result of cumulative-dose exposure in humans as opposed to a result of either an acute large-dose exposure or an idiosyncratic reaction. Renal parenchymal lesions have been demonstrated in animal toxicity studies as a result of cumulative high-dose administration.

Colchicine, in chronic high dosage, may lead to blood dyscrasias, peripheral neuritis, myopathy, and depilation. Since colchicine may induce reversible malabsorption of vitamin B_{12}, prolonged usage may lead to relative deficiency.

CAUTIONS AND PREVENTIONS

The potential for cross-reactivity to induce the syndrome of asthma, rhinitis, and urticaria exists among all NSAIDs. As mentioned, NSAIDs may cause GI bleeding, which may be severe and without premonitory symptoms, exacerbate hypertension, and induce cardiac decompensation by fluid retention in the setting of pre-existent compromised function. Renal function should be checked periodically.

The pyrazolone derivatives phenylbutazone and oxyphenbutazone should be used sparingly, especially in the elderly, and for limited periods of time. Frequent hematologic evaluation should be performed, but, since toxicity may occur suddenly, such monitoring does not completely ensure against blood dyscrasias or other idiosyncratic reactions.

Colchicine should be used with caution in patients with renal, hepatic, GI, or cardiac disease. Dosage should be decreased if loss of appetite, nausea, vomiting, diarrhea, or weakness occurs.

As with all potent medications, the optimal use of NSAIDs and colchicine requires careful monitoring. Supplies dispensed should not exceed those necessary to maintain the patient between periods of reasonable follow-up evaluations. All medications should be kept out of the reach of children.

References

1. Clive DM, Stoff JS: Renal syndromes associated with nonsteroidal anti-inflammatory drugs. N Engl J Med *310*:563, 1984.
2. Simon LS, Mills JA: Nonsteroidal anti-inflammatory drugs. N Engl J Med *302*:1179, 1237, 1980.
3. Zusman RM: Effects of converting-enzyme inhibitors on the renin-angiotensin-aldosterone, bradykinin, and arachidonic acid-prostaglandin systems: correlation of chemical structure and biologic activity. Am J Kidney Dis *10* (Suppl 1):13, 1987.
4. Court H, Volans GN: Poisoning after overdose with nonsteroidal anti-inflammatory drugs. Adv Drug React Acute Poisoning Rev *3*:1, 1984.
5. Prescott LF: Clinical features of management and analgesic poisoning. Hum Toxicol *3*:75S, 1984.
6. Vale JA, Meredith TJ: Acute poisoning due to nonsteroidal anti-inflammatory drugs. Clinical features and management. Med Toxicol *1*:12, 1986.
7. Appleby DH: Fenoprofen (Nalfon) overdose. Drug Intell Clin Pharm *15*:129, 1981.
8. Barry WS, Meinzinger MM, Howse CR: Ibuprofen overdose and exposure in utero: results from a postmarketing voluntary reporting system. Am J Med Symposium July 13:35, 1984.
9. Brogden RN, Heel RC, Speight TM, Avery GS: Piroxicam. A reappraisal of its pharmacology and therapeutic efficacy. Drugs *28*:292, 1984.
10. Court H, Streete P, Volans GN: Acute poisoning with ibuprofen. Hum Toxicol *2*:381, 1983.
11. Fredell EW, Strand LJ: Naproxen overdose. JAMA *238*:938, 1977.
12. Freestone S, Critchley JAJH: Self-poisoning with sutoprofen. Br Med J *289*:470, 1984.
13. Gross GE: Granulocytosis and sulindac overdose. Ann Intern Med *96*:793, 1982.
14. Hunt DP, Leigh RJ: Overdose with ibuprofen causing unconsciousness and hypotension. Br Med J *281*:1458, 1980.
15. Lo GCC, Chan JYW: Piroxicam poisoning. Br Med J *2*:798, 1983.
16. MacDougall LG, Taylor-Smith A, Rothberg AD, Thomson PD: Piroxicam poisoning in a two-year-old child. S Afr Med J *66*:31, 1984.
17. Mosvold J, Mellem H, Stave R, Osnes M, Laufen H: Overdosage of piroxicam. Acta Med Scand *216*:335, 1984.
18. Runkel R, Chaplin MD, Sevelius Ortega E, Segre E: Pharmacokinetics of naproxen overdoses. Clin Pharmacol Ther *20*:269, 1976.
19. Waugh PK, Keatinge DW: Hypoprothrombinaemia in naproxen overdosage. Drug Intell Clin Pharm *17*:549, 1983.
20. Hall AH, Smolinske SC, Conrad FL, Wruk KM, Kulig KW, Dwelle TL, Rumack BH: Ibuprofen overdose: 126 cases. Ann Emerg Med *15*:1308, 1986.
21. Balali-Mood M, Critchley JAJH, Proudfoot AT, Prescott LF: Mefenamic acid overdosage. Lancet *1*:1354, 1981.
22. Gossinger H, Hruby K, Haubenstock A, Jung M, Zwerina N: Coma in mefenamic acid poisoning. Lancet *2*:384, 1982.
23. Kingswell RS: Mefenamic acid overdose. Lancet *2*:307, 1981.
24. Robson RH, Balali-Mood M, Critchley JAJH, Proudfoot AT, Prescott LF: Mefenamic acid poisoning and epilepsy. Br Med J *2*:1438, 1979.
25. Shipton EA, Muller FO: Severe mefenamic acid poisoning: A case report. S Afr Med J *67*:823, 1985.
26. Young RJ: Mefenamic acid poisoning and epilepsy. Br Med J *2*:672, 1979.
27. Berlinger WG, Spector R, Flanigan MJ, Johnson GF, Groh MR: Hemoperfusion for phenylbutazone poisoning. Ann Intern Med *96*:334, 1982.
28. Bury RW, Mashford ML, Glaun BP, Saaroni G: Acute phenylbutazone poisoning in a child. Med J Aust *1*:478, 1983.
29. Inman WHW: Study of fatal bone marrow depression with special reference to phenylbutazone and oxyphenbutazone. Br Med J *1*:1500, 1977.
30. Okonek A: Intoxication with pyrazolones. Br J Clin Pharmacol *10*:385S, 1980.
31. Prescott LF, Critchley JAJH, Balali-Mood M: Phenylbutazone overdosage: Abnormal metabolism associated with hepatic and renal damage. Br Med J *281*:1106, 1980.
32. Strong JE, Wilson J, Douglas JF, Coppel DL: Phenylbutazone self-poisoning treated by charcoal haemoperfusion. Anaesthesia *34*:1038, 1979.
33. Allender WJ: Colchicine poisoning as a mode of suicide. J Foren Sci *27*:944, 1982.
34. Baum J, Meyerowitz S: Colchicine: Its use as a suicidal drug by females. J Rheumatol *7*:124, 1980.
35. Bismuth C, Baud F, Dally S: Standardized prognosis evaluation in acute toxicology: Its benefit in colchicine, paraquat and digitalis poisonings. J Toxicol Clin Exp (France) *6*:33, 1986.
36. Caplan YH, Orloff KG, Thompson BC: A fatal overdose with colchicine. J Anal Toxicol *4*:153, 1980.
37. Dobbs AJ, Lawrence PJ, Biggs JC: Colchicine overdose. Med J Aust *2*:91, 1978.
38. Dominguez de Villota E, Galdos P, Mosquera JM, Tomas MI: Colchicine overdose: An unusual origin of multi-organ failure. Crit Care Med *7*:278, 1979.
39. Ellwood MG, Robb GH: Self-poisoning with colchicine. Postgrad Med J *47*:129, 1971.
40. Frayha RA, Tabbara Z, Berbir N: Acute colchicine poisoning presenting as symptomatic hypocalcemia. Br J Rheumatol *23*:292, 1984.
41. Heaney D, Derghazarian CB, Pineo GF, Ali MAM: Massive colchicine overdose: A report on the toxicity. Am J Med Sci *271*:233, 1976.
42. Hill RN, Spragg RG, Weldel MK, Moser KM: Adult respiratory distress syndrome associated with colchicine intoxication. Ann Intern Med *83*:523, 1975.
43. Hobson CH, Rankin AP: Fatal colchicine overdose. Anaesth Intensive Care *14*:453, 1986.
44. Liu YK, Hymowitz R, Carroll MG: Marrow aplasia induced by colchicine: a case report. Arthritis Rheum *21*:731, 1978.
45. Murray SS, Kramlinger KG, McMichan JC, Mohr DN: Acute toxicity after excessive ingestion of colchicine. Mayo Clin Proc *58*:528, 1983.
46. Naidus RM, Rodvien R, Mielke CH, Jr: Colchicine toxicity: A multisystem disease. Arch Intern Med *137*:394, 1977.
47. Stahl N, Weinberger A, Benjamin D, Pinkhas J: Fatal colchicine poisoning in a boy with familial Mediterranean fever. Am J Med Sci *278*:77, 1979.
48. Stanley MW, Taurog JD, Snover DC: Fatal colchicine toxicity. Clin Exp Rheumatol *2*:167, 1984.
49. Stapczynski JS, Rothstein RJ, Gaye WA, Neimann JT: Colchicine overdose: Report of two cases and review of the literature. Ann Emerg Med *10*:364, 1981.
50. Stemmermann GN, Hayashi T: Colchicine intoxica-

tion: A re-appraisal of its pathology based on a study of three fatal cases. Hum Pathol 2:321, 1971.

51. Jarvie D, Park J, Stewart MJ: Estimation of colchicine in a poisoned patient by using high performance liquid chromatography. Clin Toxicol *14*:375, 1979.
52. Sauder P, Kopferschmitt J, Jaeger A, Mantz JM: Haemodynamic studies in eight cases of acute colchicine poisoning. Hum Toxicol 2:169, 1983.
53. Powell HC, Wolf PL: Neutrophilic leukocyte inclusions in colchicine intoxication. Arch Pathol Lab Med *100*:136, 1976.
54. Editorial: Colchicine myoneuropathy. Lancet 2:668, 1987.
55. Krontos HA: Myopathy associated with chronic colchicine toxicity. N Engl J Med *266*:38, 1962.
56. Kuncl RW, Duncan G, Watson D, Alderson K, Rogawski MA, Peper M: Colchicine myopathy and neuropathy. N Engl J Med *316*:1562, 1987.
57. Riggs JE, Schochet SS, Gutman L, Crosby TW, DiBartolomeo AG: Chronic human colchicine neuropathy and myopathy. Arch Neurol *43*:521, 1986.
58. Neuvonen PJ: Clinical pharmacokinetics of oral activated charcoal in acute intoxications. Clin Pharmacokinet *7*:465, 1982.
59. Bismuth C, Fournier PE, Galliot M: Biological evaluation of hemoperfusion in acute poisoning. Clin Toxicol *18*:1213, 1981.

SECTION D

Antimicrobial/ Anticancer Agents

CHAPTER 53

ANTIMICROBIAL AGENTS AND ANTHELMINTHICS

A. Antimicrobial Agents

Johanna Goldfarb, M.D.
Jeffrey L. Blumer, Ph.D., M.D.

Antimicrobial agents are substances that suppress the growth of microorganisms (Table 53–1). Many are produced by bacteria, fungi, or actinomycetes and are called antibiotics. Recently, a number of agents have been synthesized or designed, and these synthetic antimicrobials have greatly broadened the spectrum of drugs available to treat infectious diseases.

An ideal antimicrobial agent would affect only the pathogen or pathogens for which it was prescribed and not the host at all; however, no such agent exists. All have some effect on the host. We will discuss the untoward effects of antimicrobial agents prescribed to treat infecting pathogens. These adverse effects in the host are incidental and often completely unrelated to the chemotherapeutic effect. Thus, in selecting an antimicrobial agent, the efficacy and potential toxicities must be considered within the context of the severity of the infection and the availability, safety, and efficacy of alternative agents.

In general, the side effects of antimicrobials are reversible when the drug is discontinued. Many of these effects are mild, and even those that occur frequently are usually well

Table 53–1. ANTIMICROBIAL AGENTS

Penicillins
amoxicillin
ampicillin
bacampicillin
benzathine penicillin
cyclacillin
hetacillin
penicillin G, crystalline and oral
procaine penicillin

β-Lactamase Inhibitors
clavulanic acid: Augmentin (ampicillin/clavulanic acid)
sulbactam: Unasyn (ampicillin/sulbactam)

Antipseudomonal Penicillins
azlocillin
carbenicillin
mezlocillin
piperacillin
ticarcillin
timentin (ticarcillin/clavulanic acid)

Antistaphylococcal Penicillins
cloxacillin
dicloxacillin
flucloxacillin
methicillin
nafcillin
oxacillin

Cephalosporins
First Generation
cefadroxil
cefazolin
cephalothin
cephapirin
cephradine

Second Generation
cefaclor
cefamandole
cefoxitin
cefuroxime
cefonicid
cefotetan

Third Generation
cefixime
cefoperazone
cefotaxime
cefpiramide
ceftazadime
ceftriaxone
ceftizoxime
moxalactam

Other β-Lactams
aztreonam
imipenem/cilastatin

Aminoglycosides
amikacin
gentamicin
kanamycin
neomycin
netilmicin
streptomycin
tobramycin

Tetracyclines
chlortetracycline
demeclocycline
methacycline
minocycline
oxytetracycline
tetracycline

Macrolides
clindamycin
erythromycin base
erythromycin estolate
erythromycin ethyl succinate
erythromycin gluceptate
erythromycin lactobionate
erythromycin stearate
lincomycin

Glycopeptides
vancomycin
teicoplanin

Miscellaneous
chloramphenicol
metronidazole
trimethoprim-sulfamethoxazole
trimethoprim

Sulfonamides
Fansidar (sulfadoxine/pyrimethamine)
sulfacytine
sulfadiazine
sulfadoxine
sulfamethizole
sulfamethoxazole
sulfasalazine
sulfisoxazole
triple sulfa (sulfadiazine/sulfamerazine/sulfamethazine)

Urinary Tract Agents
methenamine mandelate
nitrofurantoin

Quinolones
cinoxacin
ciprofloxacin
nalidixic acid
norfloxacin
oxolinic acid

Antimycobacterial Agents
ansamycin
capreomycin
clofazimine
ethambutol
ethionamide
isoniazid (INH)
para-amino salicylic acid
pyrazinamide
rifampin
streptomycin
viomycin

Antiparasitic Agents
dapsone
furazolidine

Antifungal Agents
amphotericin B
flucytosine
griseofulvin
ketoconazole
miconazole
nystatin

Antiviral Agents
acyclovir
amantadine
azidothymidine (AZT)
dihydroxy-propoxymethylguanine (DHPG)
ribavirin
vidarabine

tolerated through the short course of therapy needed to treat most infections. It may not be necessary to change therapy when these side effects occur. Minor toxicity, however, may become more significant during a longer course of therapy.

Some antimicrobials have potentially permanent or life-threatening side effects. These should be used only when clearly indicated for a severe or potentially severe infection, and they should be used in a manner least likely to predispose the patient to the particular toxicity. When other equally efficacious agents are available, it may be preferable to employ the safer alternative.

Underlying disease states may affect the incidence and severity of antimicrobial side effects. Thus, an understanding of drug clearance and metabolism is crucial to judging the safety of a particular agent in a patient with liver or renal functional impairment. A reversible toxic effect may become irreversible in the presence of a renal or hepatic disease that delays or inhibits drug clearance. Moreover, adverse effects readily handled by the normal host may prove disastrous to the critically ill patient.

Antimicrobial pharmacology and toxicology is a rapidly changing field in which an understanding of drug biodisposition, along with mechanisms of potential toxicity, have increasingly helped guide clinical decisions about antimicrobial therapy. The ability to monitor serum concentrations of some agents with narrow therapeutic indices has greatly enhanced their safe use in individual patients.

Knowledge of each drug's potential side effects is essential to safely monitor therapy. Since most side effects are reversible when identified quickly, it is important to monitor patients prospectively for signs of toxicity. Therapy often can be modified or discontinued, avoiding serious outcomes. Drugs with not easily reversible side effects may need extremely close monitoring, including laboratory evaluation of target organ function, to avoid missing the earliest evidence of a developing toxicity.

This section is organized by organ system and addresses mechanisms of individual drug side effects in the context of clinical situations.

Table 53–2. ANTIMICROBIALS ASSOCIATED FREQUENTLY WITH PHLEBITIS

amphotericin B
cephalosporins
clindamycin
erythromycin
penicillins: nafcillin*
trimethoprim-sulfamethoxazole
tetracyclines
vancomycin
vidarabine

*Nafcillin has been implicated significantly more frequently than other penicillins.

DRUG ADMINISTRATION

Parenteral administration is necessary for antimicrobial agents, which are either not well absorbed from the gastrointestinal tract or liable to breakdown by gastric acid. In general, parenteral administration results in higher serum concentrations than does oral or intramuscular therapy. In the severely ill or vomiting patient, parenteral therapy may be necessary to ensure attainment of adequate serum concentrations, even with drugs that normally are well absorbed orally. An intrathecal or intraventricular route may be chosen to treat a central nervous system infection caused by an organism that requires drugs that would not attain adequate cerebrospinal fluid concentrations another way. Each of these routes of administration has attendant adverse events. The safety and risk of toxicity associated with the route of administration of a drug often will influence the selection of one antimicrobial over another.

Parenteral Therapy

Drugs given parenterally frequently cause local irritation. Phlebitis occurs consistently with the intravenous administration of vancomycin, erythromycin, and amphotericin B. These are among the most sclerosing antimicrobial agents available, and intramuscular administration of these drugs is not safe. Cephalosporins vary in the frequency of their local toxicity, but phlebitis has been reported with virtually all these agents. Because of their longer elimination half-lives, the third generation cephalosporins can be given less frequently, resulting in a lower incidence of phlebitis (Table 53–2).

Intramuscular Injection

Although the cephalosporins and penicillins may be administered by intramuscular injection, this route is painful and can result in sterile abscesses, especially with repeated injections. Pentamadine also is frequently associated with abscesses. Intramuscular injection of penicillin, including procaine and benzathine penicillin, is always associated with pain at the injection site that may last for several days. Although this local pain is a universal side effect, it is not associated with long-term sequelae (except perhaps the emotional fear of injections).

Rarely, very serious complications may result from intramuscular penicillin therapy. These include the inadvertent injection of the drug into a nerve or artery. Injection into the sciatic nerve with subsequent nerve damage and retarded limb growth was seen more frequently when penicillin was regularly administered into the buttock of young children. Avoiding this site and using the thigh for intramuscular injections in young children can eliminate this complication. Accidental injection of an intramuscular dose of penicillin into an artery is still a risk and is associated with ischemia and potential loss of the limb.[1] This complication is more often seen with the use of depot forms of penicillin administered via a Tubex delivery system. To avoid this complication, one must always test the site of injection by withdrawing on the syringe and never injecting if there is blood return. In general, intramuscular injections are painful and probably best avoided whenever possible. If it is necessary to employ this route of administration, pretreatment of the skin surface with a topical local anesthetic or use of an anesthetic diluent may ameliorate some of the discomfort.

The "red-man (neck) syndrome" is associated with the rapid intravenous administration of vancomycin.[2] The patient is noted to be flushed, with reddening of the face and neck. There may be pruritus or tingling of the face and neck, accompanied by a rapid fall in blood pressure; the resultant shock can be fatal. Vancomycin doses should be infused over 45 to 60 minutes, and patients receiving vancomycin should be monitored closely during drug administration. If the syndrome occurs, the infusion should be stopped immediately and the blood pressure supported with fluids and pressors if necessary. A rapid improvement in the blood pressure is usual once the infusion is stopped. This reaction may be due to histamine release, as it can be blocked in an animal model with antihistamines.[3] In adults given 1000 mg of vancomycin over 1 hour, there was an infusion rate–dependent increase in plasma histamine concentration, with a correlation between histamine release and reaction severity.[4] The reaction has been frequently associated with the perioperative period.[16] It is not an allergic reaction nor a contraindication to further doses and does not require desensitization. A similar syndrome has been described with high dose rifampin.[5] The acute fall in blood pressure that can occur with a too rapid intravenous infusion of pentamadine may have a similar etiology and can likewise be avoided by slow administration.

Intrathecal and Intraventricular Administration

The intrathecal route of drug administration, once standard therapy for gram-negative meningitis, has become less popular and is now less frequently indicated. Many of the newer cephalosporins readily penetrate into the cerbrospinal fluid and are increasingly part of the standard therapy for meningitis caused by sensitive gram-negative enteric bacteria. In contrast, the treatment of cerebrospinal fluid shunt infections may still require intraventricular therapy. Organisms resistant to the penicillins and cephalosporins, such as the methicillin-resistant staphylococci, are sometimes not eradicated easily with intravenous therapy alone. The aminoglycosides are used frequently in this setting. Although the intrathecal administration of these agents is most often well tolerated, it is occasionally associated with signs of local inflammation. This is manifested by cerebrospinal fluid pleocytosis with pronounced eosinophila. More serious inflammation may present as a radiculitis associated with intralumbar administration.[6] Although there is far less experience with it, vancomycin can also be given by the intrathecal route. Vancomycin appears to be less well tolerated than the aminoglycosides. The penicillins and cephalosporins are not usually indicated for intrathecal therapy, as adequate doses almost always can be obtained by intravenous administration. Intrathecal administration of the penicillins has been associated with seizures, arachnoiditis, and severe and fatal encephalopathy.[7]

Oral Therapy

Lack of compliance with oral therapy is often considered a disadvantage to its use. Many outpatient studies have documented poor compliance with oral protocols and suggest that parenteral therapy may at times be more effective. The palatability of an antimicrobial preparation and its gastrointestinal side effects do affect compliance and are a factor in selecting therapy.

NEUROTOXICITY OF ANTIBIOTICS

Nervous system toxicity may be divided into central and peripheral effects. Central nervous system side effects include nonspecific complaints such as sleepiness, headache, and behavioral abnormalities. Specific central nervous system effects, such as seizures, and optic toxicity and ototoxicity also occur. Peripheral effects include peripheral neuropathy and neuromuscular effects.

Central Nervous System Effects

The penicillins and cephalosporins are generally very safe, with few serious side effects. However, seizures, myoclonus, and problems with mentation and level of consciousness have been reported, particularly with penicillins.[8] Most often this toxicity is seen in the setting of renal failure, which may allow drug accumulation. The precise mechanism responsible for these neurologic side effects is unclear, but it is known that direct application of penicillin to the brain is associated with seizures. In contrast, neurotoxicity related to the cephalosporins is much less common. It occurs almost exclusively in the setting of renal failure and very high serum concentrations.

Unusual and bizarre behavioral and neurologic reactions that pass quickly have been reported after intramuscular injection of procaine penicillin. Reactions include a fear of imminent death, dizziness, auditory and visual disturbances, violent behavior, and generalized seizures. Rapid release of procaine appears to be responsible for these immediate and transient side effects.[9]

Seizures also may occur with the administration of a number of different agents. They are seen with isoniazid when it is taken in very high doses and are noted regularly with the therapeutic administration of cycloserine and piperazine (which should be avoided in patients with seizure disorders).[10] Seizures have occurred during very-high-dose therapy with metronidazole.[11] The pathogenesis of the seizures associated with these drugs is uncertain. Coadministration of pyridoxine with high doses of isoniazid prevents seizures and attenuates the fall in GABA levels thought to predispose to these events.[12] Large doses of pyridoxine have been used successfully to stop seizures in human overdoses of isoniazid.[13]

Cinchonism, a spectrum of symptoms including tinnitus, blurred vision, nausea, headache, and a loss of hearing acuity, occurs with the high doses of quinine used to treat acute malaria. Permanent damage to vision, balance, and hearing may occur.[14]

Generalized central nervous system toxicity manifested as an encephalopathy is reported occasionally with cycloserine, ethionamide, metronidazole, and isoniazid.[10, 11] Dizziness and sleepiness as well as visual disturbances are rare side effects of rifampin therapy.[15]

Rarely, metronidazole administration is associated with cerebellar dysfunction and ataxia. Ethionamide occasionally may cause psychiatric disturbances, which are alleviated by pyridoxine and nicotinamide. Memory loss and psychosis can occur with isoniazid.[10] Acyclovir is associated with lethargy, obtundation, tremor, confusion, hallucinations, and coma in rare patients.[16] Among the other antiviral agents, amantadine has been found to cause nervousness, lightheadedness, and insomnia,[17] whereas adenine arabinoside has been associated with hallucinations, psychosis, ataxia, tremor, and dizziness at high doses.[18]

Pseudotumor Cerebri. Benign intracranial hypertension, or pseudotumor cerebri, is a clinical diagnosis of unknown etiology. The diagnosis requires the presence of increased intracranial pressure in the absence of a structural etiology. The ventricles may be seen to be decreased in size with computed tomography, but no lesions explain the increased pressure. An association of this poorly understood syndrome with tetracycline has been made in both adults and children. The occurrence of a bulging fontanel temporally related to tetracycline therapy in infants was reported in the 1960s when this drug was still used in young children.[19] These clinical case reports lack sophisticated evaluation (structural confirmation) but are convincing, as there was rapid improvement when the drug was discontinued. No mechanism has been proposed for this association with the tetracyclines, nor is there a known etiology for pseudotumor associated with other drugs or with infections.

Peripheral Neurotoxicites

Neuromuscular Blockade. Neuromuscular blockade is a rare but potentially life-threatening toxicity as it can affect the muscles of respiration. The aminoglycosides are the agents most frequently associated with this side effect.[20] In the presence of very high concentrations of aminoglycoside at the neuromuscular junction, there is interference with neuromuscular transmission, resulting in the potential for paralysis and respiratory arrest. Excessive serum concentrations can occur during rapid intravenous administration. This side effect also has been described after instillation of an aminoglycoside in high concentration directly into the pleural or peritoneal spaces.

The mechanism of the paralysis may involve both an inhibition of the presynaptic release of acetylcholine and a blunting of the response of the postsynaptic receptor sites to acetylcholine.[21] The aminoglycosides inhibit the uptake of calcium into the presynaptic region of the axon and prevent the release of acetylcholine. Local application of calcium reverses the effect in in vitro models, and calcium can be administered clinically to treat this side effect when it occurs.[21]

Curare and curare-like drugs, such as succinylcholine and magnesium, all enhance the neuromuscular blocking activity of the aminoglycosides and should be used with care in the patient receiving an aminoglycoside.[22] Babies with infantile botulism, neonates with hypermagnesemia, and patients with myasthenia gravis also are at increased risk for respiratory compromise and may have a clinically significant increase in weakness when placed on aminoglycosides.[22–24]

Muscle Stimulation. In high dose, quinine can cause significant uterine muscle contraction.[25] The association of quinine with abortion has caused many to avoid using this drug in pregnancy. However, in areas of the world where chloroquine-resistant malaria is common, quinine is the mainstay of effective therapy. In this setting, quinine has been given by slow infusion successfully during pregnancy.[26] A loading dose of 20 mg/kg over 4 hours was used, followed by 10 mg/kg every 4 hours infused over 4 hours. A 7-day course was completed orally as tolerated.

Neuropathy. A peripheral neuropathy has been described with the long-term use of nitrofurantoin, tetracycline, chloramphenicol, metronidazole, ethambutol, cycloserine, ethionamide, and isoniazid.[10, 27, 28] Isoniazid-associated neuropathy occurs especially with the high doses that may be used early in the course of therapy for tuberculosis. This toxicity is less frequent when conventional doses are prescribed but still occurs in about 1 per cent of recipients at standard doses (3 to 5 mg/kg/day). Alcoholic patients, malnourished individuals, and those who are slow acetylators appear to be at special risk. Numbness and tingling occur in the legs, at times with paresthesias in the hands and fingers. Weakness and ataxia may occur at rest, while myalgias may increase with activity. If the precipitating drug is not promptly stopped, residual effects may continue for months. Pyridoxine replacement (100 mg/day) is effective in treating isoniazid-associated neuropathy and should be prescribed prophylactically for those patients at risk.[10]

The Eye. The retrobulbar neuritis associated with ethambutol is of considerable clinical significance, occurring in about 1 per cent of patients on a regime of 25 mg/kg daily for 60 days, followed by a maintenance dose of 15 mg/kg per day.[29] If the drug is not discontinued promptly, this toxicity may become irreversible and cause blindness. High doses of ethambutol (50 mg/kg/day) are associated with blindness and should be avoided.

The most common presentation is loss of central vision and color discrimination. Funduscopic examination will be normal. Color perception should be evaluated every 4 to 6 weeks in patients receiving ethambutol in order to identify early manifestations. Children who cannot cooperate with eye testing and who cannot communicate early signs of visual difficulties are best treated with alternative drugs whenever possible.

Ocular toxicities also occur with chloroquine.[10] These may be temporary, such as reversible blurring of vision, but severe damage leading to blindness can occur with large doses. Chloroquine binds to melanin and can localize in the melanin of the eye.[30] The patients may present with ring lesions, which consist of hyperpigmentation of the macula with surrounding alternating rings of hyperpigmentation and depigmentation.

Optic neuritis has been described with prolonged courses of chloramphenicol. This side effect is usually reversible when the drug is discontinued.[31] Since chloramphenicol is now rarely used for long-term therapy, this is a very rare occurrence.

Ototoxicity. Ototoxicity is an important side effect of clinical concern with the aminoglycosides and vancomycin. It has been less frequently reported with erythromycin and with doses of chloroquine usually reserved for diseases other than malaria.[32]

About 2 per cent of patients treated with aminoglycosides experience changes in vestibular or auditory function.[33] Auditory toxicity is the major toxicity associated with neomycin, kanamycin, and amikacin, whereas vestibular side effects are greater with streptomycin and gentamicin. Toxicities with tobramycin are split equally. Although netilmicin may have less auditory toxicity than tobramycin, it is very difficult to show significant clinical differences in the occurrence of this side effect among the aminoglycosides gentamicin, tobramycin, or amikacin[33] (Table 53–3). (Spectinomycin is an aminocyclotol antibiotic and is not associated with oto- or nephrotoxicity).

Table 53–3. QUALITATIVE ASSESSMENT OF RELATIVE VESTIBULAR AND AUDITORY TOXICITY IN HUMANS AND LABORATORY ANIMALS FOR VARIOUS AMINOGLYCOSIDES*

ANTIBIOTIC	RELATIVE TOXICITY†	
	Vestibular	*Auditory*
streptomycin	+ + +	+
gentamicin	+ +	+
tobramycin	+	+
amikacin	+	+ + +
kanamycin	+	+ + +
dihydrostreptomycin	+	+ +
neomycin	+	+ + + +

*Values for tobramycin, amikacin, and gentamicin are our added estimates.

†+ + + + equals a maximum effect.

(Adapted from Hawkins JE Jr: Antibiotics and the inner ear. Trans Am Acad Ophthalmol Otolaryngol *63*:206–218, 1959, by Bendush CL: Ototoxicity: Clinical considerations and comparative information. *In* Whelton A, Neu HC (eds): The Aminoglycosides. New York, Marcel Dekker, 1982, p 467.)

The mechanism for both auditory and vestibular toxicity appears to involve direct drug damage to the hair cells. Clinically, detection of the earliest damage from the aminoglycosides requires screening for high-frequency losses. If therapy is continued, there is further destruction of hair cells, and deafness occurs as speech frequency perception is lost. Toxicity may be cumulative with repeated courses of aminoglycosides.[76]

Vestibular dysfunction, like the damage to the auditory apparatus, appears to be caused by damage to and scarring of the hair cells of the vestibular apparatus and the semicircular canals.[34] Clinically, vestibular side effects present as nystagmus and ataxia.

Risk factors for ototoxicity include the duration of aminoglycoside therapy, bacteremia, fever, liver disease, and hypovolemia.[35] Another independent risk factor appears to be the concurrent use of ethacrynic acid.[36]

The importance of these effects in children is less clear, as most studies are of adult populations. Notable is the lack of significant toxicity in children with cystic fibrosis who are frequently treated with repeated courses of aminoglycosides.

Tinnitus and a feeling of fullness in the ears may herald aminoglycoside-related hearing loss, but often there is no clear warning. Vestibular toxicity may begin with nausea, vomiting, vertigo, dizziness, and unsteady gait.

Prevention of aminoglycoside-associated ototoxicity, like prevention of nephrotoxicity, involves limiting use of these drugs as much as possible, measuring serum aminoglycoside concentrations, monitoring for auditory and vestibular function in all patients in whom this is possible, avoiding the concomitant use of other ototoxic drugs, maintaining hydration and urinary output, monitoring renal function, and adjusting aminoglycoside doses as necessary.

Although ototoxicity may occur with vancomycin therapy, this association has been questioned as a true entity.[3] Vancomycin does not appear to be ototoxic in various animal models.[37] Case reports suggest that ototoxicity occurs only in the presence of very high serum concentrations or in the presence of other ototoxic drugs such as the aminoglycosides. It appears prudent to follow serum concentrations and to appropriately modify doses of vancomycin in patients with renal failure who may develop very high levels if doses are not carefully adjusted.

In contrast to the ototoxicity of aminoglycosides, the sudden bilateral loss of hearing that has been reported with erythromycin therapy is quite unusual.[38] Prompt return of hearing occurred in reported cases when the drug was discontinued. Risk factors for this effect appear to be age and dose. It has occurred most frequently after intravenous or peritoneal doses. Pre-existing renal or liver disease also seemed to be predisposing factors in the younger patients with this toxicity. This side effect usually occurs early in the course of drug therapy. It may not occur, or is exceedingly rare, in childhood.

PULMONARY TOXICITIES

Pulmonary toxicity is unusual with antimicrobial therapy. Primary lung fibrosis is perhaps the most dramatic lung effect and is strongly associated with nitrofurantoin. A direct toxic effect of the drug is postulated.[39] Prominent lung involvement also occurs as part of an immunologic response to some antimicrobial agents.

Acute drug-associated pneumonitis often begins with the sudden onset of fever, chills, cough, dyspnea, chest pain, and, very rarely, cyanosis.[40] Infiltrates on chest radiograph and a peripheral eosinophilia may be present. Permanent damage and fibrosis occur if therapy is continued. An increased incidence of asthma may be a sign in patients with a history of asthma. Although the symptoms reverse quickly when the drug is stopped, severe cases have been treated with corticosteroid therapy.[41]

The pulmonary toxicity associated with nitrofurantoin therapy occurs commonly as part of a presumed hypersensitivity reaction. The toxicity occurs more quickly on re-exposure to the drug and may be accompanied by a rash, both of which suggest an immunologic mechanism.[42] Subacute and chronic forms exist, with the latter occurring only with very prolonged therapy.[43] At times presentation may be severe and acute and may be difficult to separate from an anaphylactic reaction. Similar toxic pulmonary reactions have been described with the tetracyclines and minocycline.[44, 45]

The acute adult respiratory distress syndrome (ARDS) has been described in association with amphotericin B infusion in the immunocompromised patient who is also receiving white blood cell infusions.[46] This association is not universally accepted, as most of the reported patients had complicating factors that might have contributed to the development of ARDS.[47]

The use of ribavirin for inhalation must be monitored closely as lethal malfunctions of the mechanical ventilator can occur if the drug is allowed to precipitate on ventilator tubing.[48] It is possible to arrange an aerosol in a circuit that avoids this possible complication of therapy.

CARDIAC TOXICITIES

The Gray Baby Syndrome

A possible association of chloramphenicol with cardiac effects was made early in the clinical experience with the drug.[49, 50] The occurrence of the gray baby syndrome, a frequently fatal form of cardiovascular collapse, was first described and associated with chloramphenicol therapy in neonates in 1959 by Sutherland. Confirmed by others, it appeared to be reversible if the drug was discontinued and the child given support.[51] Epidemiologic evidence suggested the association of high-dose chloramphenicol therapy with a sudden rise in the infant mortality rate that occurred with the advent of routine therapy with chloramphenicol.[52, 53]

Older children and adults are also at risk for this toxicity, which appears in relation to elevated serum concentrations of the drug (greater than 20 μg/ml).[54] The apparently increased susceptibility of the newborn infant to this severe side effect may be related to their decreased ability to clear the drug. Neonates vary in their ability to metabolize chloramphenicol, making individual dosing necessary. With the development of safer and more efficacious antimicrobials for neonatal infections, chloramphenicol should no longer be used routinely in the neonate.

The rapid onset of the syndrome suggests a direct toxic effect of the drug on the heart. In a newborn pig model, isolated perfused hearts exposed to chloramphenicol showed reversible reductions in cardiac output at concentrations of 25 μg/ml or more.[55] This correlates with the marked myocardial dysfunction described clinically in children with the gray syndrome.[56] A study of isolated heart mitochondria suggests that impaired mitochondrial respiration and abnormal oxidation of fatty acids and carbohydrates occur in the presence of high chloramphenicol concentrations and correlate in the animal model with cardiac dysfunction.

Other antimicrobials with direct effects on the heart include quinidine, emetine, and clindamycin. Emetine is associated with electrocardiographic changes, hypotension, tachycardia, and precordial pain, which may occur during or shortly after treatment with therapeutic doses of the drug. Emetine appears to have a negative inotropic effect, and may, like quinidine, affect the rate of phase 0 depolarization of the cardiac action potential.[57]

GASTROINTESTINAL TOXICITIES

Gastrointestinal side effects related to antimicrobial therapy include local effects of drugs on the gastrointestinal mucosa and the antimicrobial effects on the bacterial flora in the intestine. Nausea and vomiting, the most frequent gastrointestinal side effects associated with antimicrobial agents, are often related to the direct effect of drugs on the gastric mucosa but may be due to central nervous system effects as well.

Antimicrobial therapy is most frequently associated with gastrointestinal upset when drugs are administered orally. Nausea, vomiting and/or diarrhea occur with many antimicrobial agents (see Table 53–4). Some oral agents cause pain by a direct effect on the gastric mucosa. The incidence of gastrointestinal side effects can be as high as 45 per cent with erythromycin ethylsuccinate. The estolate in another study had only a 5 per cent rate of these symptoms, but clearly gastrointestinal upset is common with the erythromycins and appears to be a direct effect.[58] The tetracyclines are also regularly associated with stomach pain. Both tetracycline and doxycycline have been associated with esophageal ulceration presenting as retrosternal pain, apparently due to a direct effect of drug on the mucosa.[59] Gastritis and actual ulceration have also been described with clindamycin.[60] These compounds need to be taken with water and should not be taken at bedtime.

Diarrhea may be related to malabsorption of an oral agent or to changes in microbial flora caused by the spectrum of activity of the antimicrobial agent. Broad-spectrum tetracyclines frequently cause diarrhea. This side effect is less often experienced with doxycyline, which is said to be related to its better absorption.[61] Similarly, amoxicillin, which is better absorbed than ampicillin, also causes less diarrhea. Diarrhea appears to be a direct effect of drugs such as ampicillin, tetracycline, chloramphenicol, penicillin, lincomycin, and clindamycin; it occurs in a significant percentage of patients. Usually this is tolerated during the relatively brief course of an antimicrobial treatment. Sometimes, however, a nonspecific mild diarrhea may become severe enough to interfere with absorption of the antimicrobial agent and to cause significant morbidity (Table 53–4).

Antimicrobial-associated diarrhea accompanied by blood and mucus in the stools may indicate mucosal involvement. Therapy needs to be re-evaluated and, if possible, changed. The resulting dehydration occasionally may necessitate intravenous rehydration. Often, however, discontinuation of the drug is all that is necessary.

The gastrointestinal complication of most concern is the development of pseudomembranous enterocolitis. Although this may begin without prior gastrointestinal complaints, diarrhea in a patient on antimicrobial therapy must be followed closely. The acute development of fever and pain in a patient with copious diarrhea and bloody or mucous stools strongly suggests this diagnosis.[64] Pseudomembranous enterocolitis is diagnosed when proctoscopic examination discloses pseudomembranes (small, yellow-white plaques) along the colonic mucosa. Lesions may become confluent, but no true ulcerations are present. Overlying mucus often covers an erythematous and slightly friable colonic mucosa. Pseudomembranes consist of epithelial cell debris, fibrin, and polymorphonuclear leukocytes. "Thumbprinting" on a plain abdominal radiograph or on a barium enema should suggest the possibility of this diagnosis.

Various causes have been proposed, and multiple host factors appear to be important. However, much data suggest that an alteration in bowel flora induced by the offending antimicrobial may allow the emergence of resistant organisms such as *Clostridium difficile*. Such organisms can produce cytotoxic

Table 53–4. GASTROINTESTINAL SIDE EFFECTS OF ANTIMICROBIAL THERAPY

DRUG	DIARRHEA	NAUSEA/ VOMITING	EPIGASTRIC, ABDOMINAL PAIN	STOMATITIS, GLOSSITIS
acyclovir	—	+	+	—
amantadine	—	+		
amphotericin B	+	+	+	
ampicillin/clavulinic acid	+ +	+	+	—
cephalosporins	+			+
chloramphenicol	+		+	+
clavulanic acid	+ +	+	+	+
clofazamine		+	+	
dapsone	+			
emetine	+	+ +	—	—
erythromycin	+ −	+ +	+ +	
ethionamide		+		
flucytosine	+			
fusidic acid		+	+	
ketoconazole	+ +	+ +	+ +	—
mendelamine	+			
metronidazole	+	+	+	+
minocycline	+	+ +	+ +	
nalidixic acid	+	+ +	+	
niridazole	+ +	+ +	+ +	
nitrofurantoin	+	+ +	+	
nystatin	+			
para-aminosalicyclic acid		+		
penicillins	+		+	+
ampicillin	+ +	+	+	+
amoxicillin	+ +	+	+	+
pentamadine		+		
piperazine	+	+	+	
praziquantel		+	+	
pyrimethamine		+	+	
quinine	+	+	+	
spiramycin	+	+	—	—
suramin		+		
tetracycline	+ +	+ +	+	+
thiabendazole	+ +	+ +	+ +	
Alcohol Intolerance (Disulfiram-Like Reactions)*				
cefamandole				
cefoperazone				
metronidazole				
moxalactam				
Pancreatitis				
pentamadine				
sulfonamides				
tetracyclines				

*Adapted from Neu HC: The new beta-lactamase-stable cephalosporins. Ann Intern Med *97*:408–419, 1982, and Eneanya DI, Bianchine JR, Duran DO, Andresen BD: The actions and metabolic fate of disulfiram. Ann Rev Pharmacol Toxicol *21*:575–596, 1981.

substances that affect mucosal function and integrity. Overgrowth of staphylococci may be seen in the stool in some cases, and a toxin has been isolated from the staphylococci that is capable of causing tissue destruction and cell damage.[65] The role of the staphylococci in causing pseudomembranous enterocolitis is debated, but most cases appear to be associated with *C. difficile.* A heat-labile toxin can be isolated from patients with antimicrobial-associated pseudomembranous colitis.[66] Colonic damage and death occur in a hamster model when the animals are exposed to this toxin.[67] The toxic effects of the toxin can be neutralized by antiserum that includes specific *C. difficile* antiserum.[64] A toxin with similar characteristics has been isolated from cultures of strains of *C. difficile* obtained from patients with colitis.[68]

Although pseudomembranous colitis is most often associated with oral therapy, parenteral exposure also may be a predisposing factor. Most cases occur during a course of antimicrobial therapy, often a week or two after therapy begins. However, cases have occurred up to 4 weeks after discontination of an antimicrobial agent. Once the disease is diagnosed, the offending drug should be discontinued immediately.

The course of the disease after stopping the drug may last days to weeks and requires careful monitoring of the patient's fluid and electrolyte status. In severe cases, and when broad-spectrum antimicrobial therapy continues to be required, consideration should be given to treatment with oral vancomycin.[69]

A definitive diagnosis requires proctoscopy. This procedure probably is indicated in all patients with severe inflammatory diarrhea (fecal leukocytes) that has not responded to discontinuation of antimicrobials or in the patient in whom other diagnostic possibilities exist that would alter the choice of therapy. Pseudomembranous enterocolitis is potentially lethal, due to fluid and electrolyte abnormalities, and is related to secondary sepsis.

Although clindamycin is the drug most commonly associated with pseudomembranous colitis, almost every antimicrobial, even metronidazole, has been shown to have a connection. Clindamycin has been associated with rates as high as 46 per cent and as low as 0.1 per cent of courses of therapy.[70, 71] This association may reflect the characteristics of the patients likely to be treated with clindamycin in addition to any property of the drug. In an epidemiologic study from Sweden, about half the cases of pseudomembranous colitis were associated with penicillins, about one third with cephalosporins, and about 14 per cent with lincosamides (mostly clindamycin), reflecting the more frequent use of the penicillins and cephalosporins.[72] The clustering of cases in some studies has suggested possible nosocomial transmission of *C. difficile*.[73]

Liver

Antibiotic-associated hepatic reactions are manifested mainly as hepatocellular toxicity or cholestasis and less frequently a mixed pathologic and clinical picture.

Hepatocellular Toxicities. Reversible, nonspecific liver enzyme elevations occur in from 1 to 4 per cent of patients treated with the various penicillins, notably with the ureidepenicillins, carbenicillin, ticarcillin, and oxacillin, as well as with the new beta-lactams imipenem and aztreonam. Nonspecific mild elevations may also occur with many antimicrobials (Table 53–5).

Whereas 15 per cent of isoniazid-treated patients will have transient minor elevations in liver enzymes (two times upper limit of normal), a much smaller group will have serious, potentially fatal hepatic reactions.[74] This toxicity is correlated with age: it rarely occurs in patients under 20 years, occurs in 0.3 per cent of those 20 to 34 years, in 1.2 per cent of those 35 to 49 years old, and in 2.3 per cent of those over 50 years.[75] Alcoholic patients with liver damage are especially prone, and the drug must be used with care in anyone with pre-existing liver disease.[76]

Patients should be warned to report symptoms including anorexia, malaise, fatigue, and jaundice. Such symptoms should be evaluated promptly with liver function tests. This complication rarely occurs until 1 to 2 months after the initiation of therapy. The drug should be stopped immediately in any patient with liver enzyme elevations above five times normal. Two of nineteen patients with isoniazid-induced hepatitis died in a series of 2321 recipients of the drug.[77]

Isoniazid-related hepatitis is believed to be caused by a drug metabolite, hydrazine.[74] Rapid acetylators may be at an increased risk for this toxicity because of an increase in free hydrazine seen in these individuals. The role of added toxicity when rifampin is used with isoniazid remains unresolved but may be significant in patients with pre-existing liver disease.[75] Toxic hepatitis also occurs with para-aminosalicylic acid (PAS),[78] and isonia-

Table 53–5. DROGS ASSOCIATED WITH LIVER DYSFUNCTION

PRIMARILY CHOLESTATIC
erythromycin
nalidixic acid
nitrofurantoin
sulfamethoxazole
PRIMARILY HEPATOCELLULAR
amphotericin B (?)
griseofulvin
isoniazid
nitrofurantoin
pyrazinamide
quinidine
rifampin
sulfonamides

zid toxicity may be increased in the presence of this drug.

Nonspecific reversible elevations in SGOT occur in 5 per cent of patients receiving ethionamide.[79] Pyrazinamide is associated with liver toxicity that is potentially fatal. This complication is less frequent with the lower doses currently used,[80] but as with the other metabolically cleared antituberculous drugs, liver function should be monitored closely and the drug stopped if hepatitis occurs. Pre-existing liver disease also increases risks of hepatitis with pyrazinamide.

Tetracycline has been associated with acute fatty necrosis of the liver.[81] This complication is very rare but is frequently fatal when it occurs. It is most often seen with high doses given parenterally. Pregnant women may be at increased risk, but since tetracycline is best avoided during pregnancy and alternative therapy is almost always available, this should now rarely be a concern.[82] Flucytosine hepatitis occurs, frequently with a rash, and requires stopping the drug.[83]

Ketoconazole is associated with liver function abnormalities in 2 to 5 per cent of recipients. About 1 in 15,000 patients have a symptomatic and serious hepatitis that begins at least a week or 10 days into treatment. Liver biopsy shows hepatocellular or cholestatic damage and at times a mixture of both. After stopping the drug, recovery is usually complete.[84]

Cholestatic Liver Disease. Liver toxicity from erythromycin originally was believed to occur exclusively with the estolate; however, it is now clear that it can occur with the other formulations of erythromycin as well. This side effect is rare, occurring in less than 1 per cent of adults and in an even smaller percentage of children treated with erythromycin.[85] Pregnant women may be at increased risk.[86]

The mechanism of the cholestatic hepatitis appears to be a hypersensitivity reaction. The syndrome usually occurs after 2 to 3 weeks of therapy in patients who are exposed to the drug for the first time, but it occurs after only 1 to 2 days in patients who are reexposed after a recent course of erythromycin therapy. Nausea and epigastric pain occur first and may be severe enough to suggest acute gallbladder pain. Fever, transaminasemia, and a picture of cholestatic jaundice follow. Eosinophilia and leukocytosis may be present also, and liver biopsy usually demonstrates cholestasis with periportal infiltration.[87]

The occurrence of liver toxicity is an absolute indication to stop the drug and is a contraindication to further exposure to the erythromycins. Recovery is prompt and usually complete when the drug is discontinued.

Cholestatic jaundice also has been reported in association with nitrofurantoin therapy.[88] The mechanisms are unclear. The role of the patient's acetylator phenotype has not been confirmed.

Pancreatitis

Pancreatitis has been associated with tetracycline,[89] pentamidine,[90] and trimethoprim-sulfamethoxazole[91] (see Table 53–4).

RENAL TOXICITY

Renal function and nephrotoxic potential are important considerations when choosing antimicrobials. Most antimicrobials are eliminated from the body by the kidney. When renal disease is present, dosage adjustment may be required, especially for those antimicrobial agents with a narrow therapeutic index. In addition, certain antimicrobial side effects may be exacerbated in the patient with renal functional impairment.

The kidneys regulate extracellular fluid volume, osmolality, pH, and the electrolyte content of the blood. Receiving roughly 25 per cent of the cardiac output each minute, the kidneys eliminate antimicrobials by glomerular filtration and by tubular secretion. Glomerular filtration produces an ultrafiltrate of plasma. Small-molecular-weight drugs, such as the aminoglycosides and vancomycin, are filtered freely. The glomerular ultrafiltrate is protein free, and thus protein-bound drugs are retained. Bound drug remains in the vascular space to be cleared later by the tubules or at other body sites.

Antimicrobials excreted unchanged in the urine, such as vancomycin and the aminoglycosides, require dosage adjustments in renal disease to avoid drug accumulation. Penicillins, which are cleared by both filtration and secretion, also accumulate in renal failure if dosages are not adjusted. The acylureidopenicillins are about 60 to 75 per cent excreted by tubular secretion.[92] This secretory mechanism is saturable, and at higher concentrations nonrenal elimination pathways may become important in their clearance. Thus, the half-lives of these drugs are dose dependent. Dose-dependent kinetics is also characteristic of the other antipseudomonal penicillins, azlocillin and piperacillin.[93, 94] In contrast, nafcillin, unlike the other penicillins, is cleared by the liver. It, therefore, requires no dosage adjustment in renal failure.

The older cephalosporins are almost all cleared by the kidney. The third-generation cephalosporins, except for cefoperazone and ceftriaxone, which show significant hepatic elimination, are mainly cleared by glomerular filtration. Like the penicillins, these antimicrobials will accumulate in renal failure unless doses are decreased. The lack of toxicity associated with the cephalosporins, even at high serum concentrations, makes these drugs especially attractive in patients with renal failure.

The nephrotoxic effects of antimicrobials are most often related to their direct cytotoxic effects on the epithelial cells of the proximal and distal tubules. Glomerular lesions are much less frequent but do occur either associated with immune complex deposition in the glomeruli or as part of a vasculitis, such as may occur with serum sickness.[95] Finally, crystalluria, due to drug precipitation in tubular urine, may also occur and cause renal damage.[96]

Nephrotoxicity is often defined clinically in terms of abnormal laboratory parameters. However, significant renal toxicity, especially due to tubular damage, may go undetected until glomular filtration is affected. Creatinine clearance measurements are a good reflection of glomerular filtration but may be difficult to obtain. Serum creatinine levels, therefore, are often used as a crude measure of renal function. Creatinine levels may remain normal until the glomerular filtration rate has fallen by 30 to 50 per cent.

Tubular Toxins

Aminoglycosides

Nephrotoxicity, as demonstrated by a significant rise in serum creatinine concentration, occurs in from 5 to 20 per cent of adult patients finishing a therapeutic course of an aminoglycoside.[97–98] Estimates of the risk of nephrotoxicity vary considerably. Differences in the reported incidence among these studies are due to such factors as the variability in the doses used, the vigor of the drug monitoring, and the ages of the patients studied. All aminoglycosides have some potential for nephrotoxicity, even with careful therapeutic drug monitoring.[99]

The aminoglycosides are normally cleared unchanged by glomerular filtration, and protein binding of these agents is insignificant. The serum half-life of these drugs depends on both renal clearance and tissue concentrations (accumulated dose). A single large overdose, therefore, is unlikely to cause severe damage in the presence of normal renal function, whereas chronic moderate overdosage continued over time likely will be associated with significant toxicity. The relative risk for nephrotoxicity among the aminoglycosides appears to be related to the number of ionizable amino groups on the specific agents. Neomycin, for example, invariably causes nephrotoxicity whereas toxicity with streptomycin is rare. Neomycin nephrotoxicity is so substantial and frequent that this drug is now limited to use in topical and oral therapies. Even so, oral therapy must be monitored closely as absorption does occur and may cause significant toxicity in the patient with pre-existing renal disease. The incidences of nephrotoxicity with gentamicin, tobramycin, netilmicin, and amikacin—the aminoglycosides most often used in clinical practice—lie between those of neomycin and streptomycin. Studies comparing these drugs for their relative safety are difficult to interpret as variables are difficult to match. A clearly significant difference in clinical nephrotoxicity among these agents is hard to demonstrate.

Possible predisposing factors for toxicity with all the aminoglycosides include the presence of prior renal disease, elevated trough concentrations of the aminoglycoside, decreased creatinine clearance, long duration of therapy, volume depletion, the presence of liver failure, and congestive heart failure.[100] Renal disease may be a significant risk factor in part because of difficulties with drug dosing in these patients. Elevated serum concentrations may not be good predictors of impending toxicity as often these are evidence of the presence of existing renal functional impairment. Monitoring serum concentrations is helpful, however, in limiting permanent nephrotoxicity and in guiding dosing, especially in patients with renal disease.

Methods of predicting which patients will have significant nephrotoxicity have been sought (Fig. 53–1).[101] The presence of renal cell enzymes in the urine has been found to reflect renal cell damage and death. These enzymes are specific to their particular cell site. Alanine aminopeptidase, for example, is a brush border enzyme that rises early but nonspecifically in patients with renal toxicity from the aminoglycosides.[102] These tests, however, have not been clinically useful in predicting or controlling aminoglycoside toxicity.[103]

The excretion of β_2-microglobulin, a protein catabolized by the proximal tubule cells, is a sensitive and specific sign of proximal tubule dysfunction. Levels rise in most patients on aminoglycosides, but elevations are

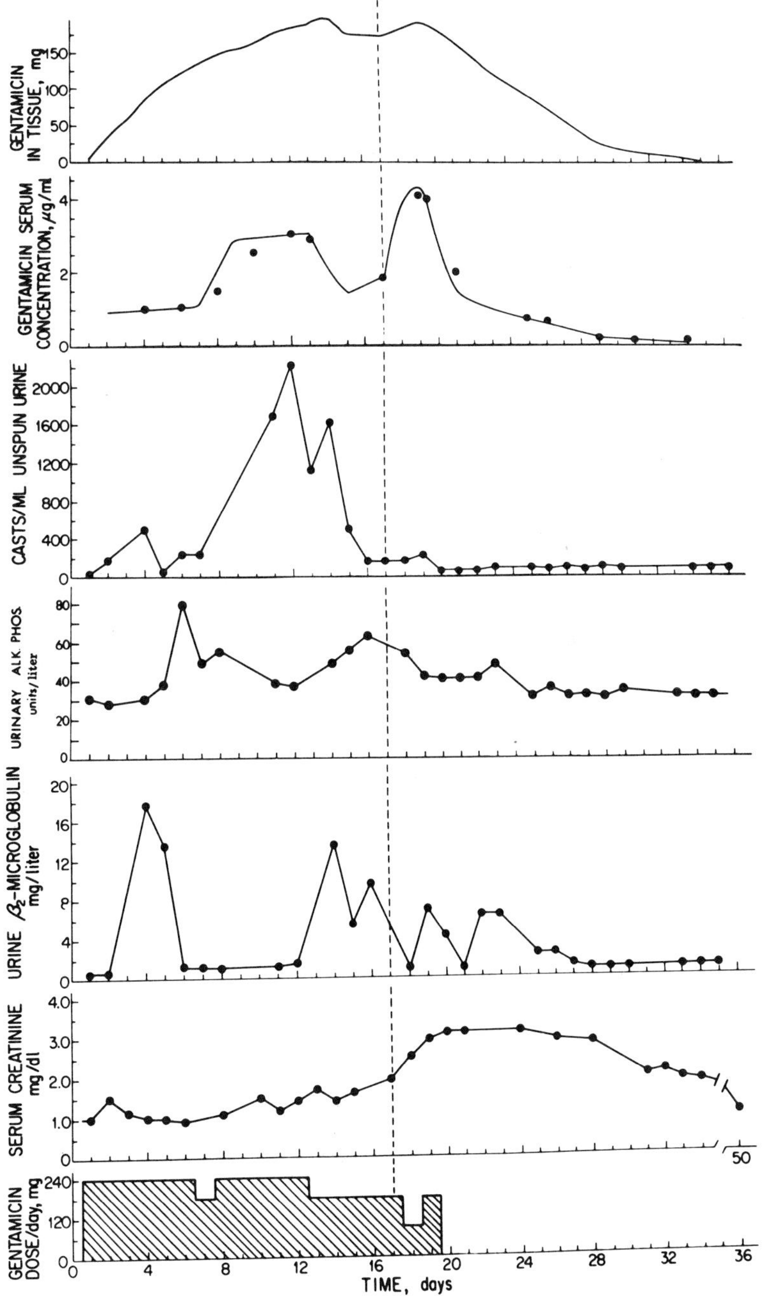

Figure 53–1. Dosing, serum creatinine, urinary β_2-microglobulin, urinary alkaline phosphatase, urinary cast excretion, serum trough concentrations measured (●) versus predicted (—), and predicted tissue accumulation plotted versus time for a typical nephrotoxic patient. The dashed vertical line marks the day of first significant serum creatinine rise as a reference point. The order of elevation of these indices was tissue accumulation, β_2-microglobulin. (From Schentag JJ: Aminoglycoside pharmacokinetics as a guide to therapy and toxicity. *In* Whelton A, Neu HC (eds): The Aminoglycosides. New York, Marcel Dekker, 1982, pp 143–167.)

much higher in patients who are nephrotoxic than in those who are not.[101] Beta$_2$-microglobulin excretion has been used experimentally as an indicator of tubule damage but has not been useful in clinical situations.

Perhaps the only clinically useful method of detecting early aminoglycoside nephrotoxicity is to follow serial urinalyses. Granular casts in the urine reflect cellular debris from tubular damage. An increasing number of casts in concentrated acidic urine specimens appear to be an early sign of tubular damage, preceding the rise in serum creatinine by 2 to 9 days.[104] Following serial first-voided urine specimens for casts appears to be an important method of detecting impending, more serious nephrotoxicity.[101]

Clinical findings of aminoglycoside toxicity include loss of urinary concentrating ability, a tubular function. Nonoliguric renal failure is seen frequently with aminoglycoside toxicity and may also correspond to the tubular damage. The origin of the reduced glomerular filtration rate that occurs late in the course of nephrotoxicity is unclear and difficult to relate to the tubular cell damage alone. Tubular obstruction with cellular debris may be, in part, the cause of the falling glomerular filtration rate and acute renal failure seen in severe aminoglycoside nephrotoxicity.[105]

In animal studies, salt depletion, prerenal azotemia, and acidosis each increase the risk of nephrotoxicity by aminoglycoside antibiotics. A human correlate is the reported enhancement of aminoglycoside nephrotoxicity by loop diuretics. This is thought to result from depletion of vascular volume and subsequent decreased renal perfusion.

Aminoglycoside doses should be calculated on the basis of renal function. Ongoing renal damage, such as may occur in a critically ill patient or from aminoglycoside toxicity itself, sometimes makes it necessary to reconsider aminoglycoside dosing on a daily basis. The first dose of an aminoglycoside should be a full dose, to ensure attainment of therapeutic concentrations. Dosage reduction in renal failure may be achieved by either extending the dosing interval, which maintains peak concentrations, or lowering each dose at the normal dosing interval. Patients on aminoglycosides must have peak and trough concentrations determined, and these should be followed closely during periods of changing renal function.

Rising trough concentrations suggest drug accumulation and sometimes herald the onset of nephrotoxicity. Serum creatinine and blood urea nitrogen (BUN) levels should also be followed. A rise in the creatinine level generally indicates that significant tubular damage has occurred and that there is a need to decrease the dose and or to lengthen the dosing interval. This should be done immediately, even prior to obtaining drug levels.

Toxicity usually occurs after the first week of therapy. The creatinine and BUN levels may continue to rise even after the drug is stopped; ongoing damage may in part reflect release of drug from tissue stores.[101, 106] The aminoglycosides cause nephrotoxicity in all patients given excessive doses. Nephrotoxicity, however, is also seen in individuals dosed appropriately and monitored with therapeutic levels of drug. Unusually high tissue accumulation appears to be the responsible factor in these patients.[101] Although renal function usually returns to normal or close to normal levels, this may take several weeks. At times, permanent renal damage remains and baseline creatinine levels may remain elevated, especially in the patient with underlying renal disease. Healing appears to involve regeneration of tubules.[107]

Amphotericin B and clindamycin may increase the risk of aminoglycoside toxicity when given concurrently.[108, 109] It is unclear whether concomitant use of an aminoglycoside with vancomycin increases the toxicity of the aminoglycoside,[2] but careful monitoring of both drugs is appropriate in the patient who is on dual therapy. A synergistic toxicity between the aminoglycosides and the cephalosporins is suggested by several studies[110] but has not been substantiated in others.[111] Animal models do not support an additive toxicity and in fact show a protective effect, probably due to decreased aminoglycoside uptake by the tubular cells in the presence of a cephalosporin.[112]

Nephrotoxicity has been studied in the newborn puppy as a model for the neonate. In the neonatal mammal, the renal cortex is incomplete and continues to develop after birth. Glomerular filtration is correspondingly reduced in the neonate, and renal clearance of most antimicrobials is also reduced. Aminoglycoside toxicity appears to affect areas of the inner cortex of the newborn animal and to move outward in the experimental model. The maturing cortex may allow regeneration in the developing kidney of the neonate.[113]

Cephalosporins

Cephaloridine, a first-generation cephalosporin, is now rarely used because of its renal toxicity.[114] Cephalothin is the only other cephalosporin reported to cause tubular failure, and this is very rare compared with the incidence associated with cephaloridine. Cephaloridine is an organic anion and is taken up by the proximal tubular cells, where it appears to accumulate. The active transport of this drug into the proximal tubular cells is blocked competitively by other organic anions such as probenecid, suggesting that the drug is actively transported into renal tubular cells by the organic anion secretory carrier of the tubule.

As a class, the cephalosporins, other than cephaloridine, are rarely nephrotoxic and are well tolerated in very ill patients, including patients with renal failure. Although a decrease in dose is appropriate in renal failure, the margin of safety with these drugs is very great, and even very high serum concentrations are well tolerated without toxicity. This is a major advantage of this class of drugs and makes them very useful in the patient with renal disease.

Tetracycline

In the past, out-of-date tetracycline was noted to cause renal toxicity. Proximal tubule damage and a Fanconi syndrome occurred in patients who took such preparations.[115] This effect appears to be due to citric acid degradation of the tetracycline to anhydro-4-epitetracycline. Citric acid is no longer used to stabilize the drug, to avoid this problem.[116]

Distinct from this effect is an "antianabolic effect," which is a defect in amino acid utilization,[117] as well as a direct nephrotoxic effect of high-dose tetracycline. Nephrotoxicity is especially likely to occur in the presence of prior renal disease.[118] Animal studies suggest that disruption of organelles in renal tubular cells precedes the development of acute renal failure in dogs treated with high doses of tetracycyline.[119]

Doxycycline is eliminated by the liver and can be used more safely in patients with renal failure who require tetracycline therapy, avoiding the potential side effects of the other tetracyclines in patients with renal disease.[120]

Amphotericin B

Amphotericin B is extremely nephrotoxic, causing some detectable renal impairment in about 80 per cent of treated adults.[121] The glomerular filtration rate (GFR) may initially fall up to 40 per cent and usually remains depressed throughout therapy. Mild renal tubular acidosis, hypokalemia, and hypomagnesemia are very common. Recovery occurs in the months after cessation of therapy, but levels of the GFR 50 per cent below normal may persist for prolonged periods after a course of amphotericin B.[122]

Amphotericin is rapidly bound to cell membranes after infusion, especially those with a high cholesterol:phospholipid ratio. The binding of the drug to cell membranes results in increased ion permeability and a decrease in electrical resistance across the membrane.[123] This is lytic for kidney lysosomes at acid pH.[124] Necrosis of tubular epithelial cells with calcium deposits is seen on renal biopsy of patients with amphotericin B nephrotoxicity.

In animal studies, an additional effect has been observed. There is an immediate fall in inulin clearance and urine output during the acute infusion of amphotericin B. This is consistent with renal vasoconstriction, which occurs during the infusion.[125] This causes decreased renal blood flow and may cause tubular damage, further potentiated by the membrane effects of the drug.

Free water clearance and diluting ability are normal during amphotericin B therapy, but reabsorption of water and maximal urine osmolality are decreased. Significant amounts of potassium are lost in the urine, and large quantities of potassium often are required to maintain serum levels within the normal range.

Patients receiving amphotericin B must be monitored closely, with frequent checks of the hematocrit, serum potassium, blood urea nitrogen, and creatinine levels; and urinalysis. Hypokalemia occurs in about one fourth of patients and may be severe and life threatening. Sometimes very large amounts of potassium supplementation are required to maintain normal serum values and to keep up with urinary losses. The total body clearance of amphotericin B is poorly understood, but renal clearance does not appear to be important in drug elimination.[126] Thus, there is no rationale for altering amphotericin B dosing in the face of renal functional impairment caused by the drug, but other renally cleared drugs will be affected and doses should be modified.

Glomerulonephritis

Glomerulonephritis caused by drug allergy is usually seen as part of a serum sickness. Deposition of antigen-antibody complexes occurs nonspecifically along the glomeruli. The nephrotic syndrome has occurred with drug allergy but is rarely associated with antimicrobials, except for penicillin. More commonly, the adverse immunologic response to the antimicrobial agents is an interstitial nephritis.[127]

Interstitial Nephritis

Immune interstitial nephritis can occur with penicillin G, the sulfonamides, ampicillin, methicillin, and rifampin, and less frequently with carbenicillin, cephalexin, cephalothin, trimethoprim/sulfamethoxazole, erythromycin, nafcillin, oxicillin, and trimethoprim.[128] Rash, fever, arthralgias, and eosinophilia frequently accompany the hematuria and proteinuria. Eventually azotemia and oliguria occur. Eosinophils are usually present in the urine.[129]

Methicillin is the penicillin most frequently associated with this reversible complication occurring in up to 10 per cent of patients.[130] The prompt recurrence of nephritis in patients re-exposed to a drug previously associated with nephritis supports an immunologic hypothesis. Renal biopsy in affected patients shows interstitial edema with leukocytes, predominately lymphocytes, plasma cells, and monocytes, although eosinophils and polymorphonuclear cells may also be present. The finding of linear deposits of IgG along the basement membranes of renal tubules in affected patients is reported by some but not all researchers.

The interstitial nephritis associated with rifampin toxicity may be accompanied by acute cortical necrosis. Deposits of immunoglobulins around and in the tubule in rifampin nephritis again suggest an immunologic mechanism for this potentially permanent toxicity.[131]

Patients receiving antimicrobial agents associated with interstitial nephritis must be followed prospectively for signs of toxicity. Urinalyses to check for hematuria should be obtained at least weekly during long courses of therapy. Signs of eosinophilia should be sought if erythrocytes appear. The drug should be discontinued immediately once nephritis occurs. Most often there will be quick reversal and no permanent damage.

Crystalluria

Sulfonamides

Sulfonamides are metabolized primarily in the liver, but each specific sulfonamide and its liver metabolites are eliminated by the kidneys, by differing routes. Glomerular filtration with tubular reabsorption occur with sulfamethoxazole, whereas sulfathiazole is excreted by tubular secretion. The acetylated metabolites of the sulfonamides are excreted primarily by tubular secretion.[132]

Crystalluria occurs when sulfonamides precipitate out of solution in the kidney; this may result in significant renal damage. Triple-sulfas (combinations of different sulfonamides) were developed to reduce this complication, by allowing high total doses of sulfonamide to be administered while keeping the solubility of each drug below the range of precipitation expected in the urine. Crystalluria is less common now with the newer sulfonamides which are more soluble; it is estimated to occur in 0.2 to 0.3 per cent of patients.[132] It is still recommended that patients treated with the sulfonamides be advised to maintain large fluid intakes to ensure solubility of the drugs. Abnormal renal function makes sulfonamides less safe to use as this complication is more likely to occur.

A reversible crystalline nephropathy has been associated with acyclovir in about 5 per cent of treated patients. This appears to be from crystal formation, which can be avoided by avoiding dehydration and by slow infusion rates and dosage reduction in the face of renal functional impairment. This effect is reversible when the drug is discontinued.[133]

The quinolone antibiotic norfloxacin has

been associated with crystalluria, but this has not been associated with significant human renal impairment as yet.[134] Maintaining adequate hydration may be important when administering these agents.

Urate Clearance

Urate clearance is decreased in the presence of certain antimicrobials.[135] This predisposes patients with gout to exacerbations. Drugs with this side effect include pyrazinamide and ethambutol.[136]

Vancomycin

Early formulations of vancomycin appeared highly nephrotoxic. This now appears to have been related to impurities in these early preparations.[2, 3] With improved purification of vancomycin, the apparent nephrotoxic effects have all but disappeared. In several series, renal abnormalities were rare, unless vancomycin was administered concomitantly with an aminoglycoside. Vancomycin is normally cleared unchanged by glomerular filtration. In the setting of aminoglycoside nephrotoxicity, vancomycin levels will rise rapidly unless the dose is reduced and/or the dosing interval lengthened. In the presence of renal failure, the serum half-life of vancomycin is greatly extended, and the dosing interval may be increased up to 7 days. Vancomycin is not cleared by peritoneal dialysis or hemodialysis.[137] Renal toxicity may occur at very high drug concentrations but appears to reverse quickly when doses are adjusted, even with continuation of the drug. Vancomycin serum concentrations and renal function (creatinine and BUN) should be followed in patients receiving the drug.

ENDOCRINE TOXICITY

Endocrine effects of the antimicrobials are unusual but do occur. Gynecomastia had been noted as a side effect in a significant per cent of male patients treated with ketoconazole.[138] A blunted cortisol response to adrenocorticotropin in human volunteers also has been noted.[139] The clinical significance of this is unclear, but a case report suggests that adrenal insufficiency can occur with very-high-dose ketoconazole therapy.[140]

Rifampin is associated with the enhanced metabolism of many drugs and has been associated with the decreased efficacy of oral contraceptives.[141] Hyperglycemia, possibly due to increased gastrointestinal glucose absorption, also has been described with rifampin therapy.[142] A transient decrease in sperm counts is reported with high-dose nitrofurantoin therapy in about one third of patients.[143] Another rare endocrine effect is the decrease in diabetic control reported with ethionamide.[10]

CUTANEOUS REACTIONS[144]

Nonspecific skin reactions during a course of antimicrobial therapy occur occasionally and must be differentiated from true allergic reactions to specific agents. Ampicillin, for example, is associated with a nonspecific, apparently nonallergic, maculopapular rash. Almost all patients treated with the drug during an Epstein-Barr virus infection will develop this rash.[145] Other similar viral exanthems also may occur during or after antimicrobial therapy and are not an indication of drug allergy. These rashes, like the ampicillin rash with Epstein-Barr infection, do not require changing therapy.

Urticarial rashes are of special concern. When these occur with the first dose of a drug, an IgE-mediated allergic response possibly associated with anaphylaxis is suggested. The presence of urticaria, or a history of urticaria soon after a dose of an antimicrobial, should warn the clinician that the drug, as well as other drugs of the same class, may be contraindicated. Desensitization prior to any further doses is indicated if the drug is absolutely essential (Table 53–6). This topic is further discussed in the section on Immunotoxicity later in this chapter.

Rashes occurring in the first hours after a dose are late allergic reactions resulting from IgM antibody. Therapy can be continued, and at times the rash may disappear, possibly as a result of blocking IgG antibody. However, the clinician must be aware that the rash may progress in some patients, with development of an exfoliative dermatitis or Stevens-Johnson syndrome, which is a definite indication to stop therapy.

Table 53–6. ADVERSE CUTANEOUS REACTIONS TO ANTIMICROBIALS

	MORBILLIFORM	MACULAR	URTICARIA	PURPURA/ VESICLES	STEVENS-JOHNSON EXFOLIATION	SEROSITIS	ANGIOEDEMA/ ANAPHYLAXIS
amphotericin B	+						+
cephalosporins	+	+	+		+		+
chloramphenicol		+		+			
clindamycin	+	+			+		
erythromycin	+	+					
ethambutol	+	+			+		+
ethionamide	+	+		purpura		+	
INH	+	+	+	purpura			
nalidixic acid	+	+	+				
penicillins	+	+	+		+		+
rifampin	+	+					
spectinomycin			+				
sulfones					+		
sulfonamides	+	+	+	purpura	+		
tetracyclines	+		+		+	+	+
TMP/SMX	++	++	++		+	+	+
vancomycin	+						+

Sun-Related Toxicities (Photosensitivity)

Phototoxicity is an epidermal response of sun-exposed skin in the presence of the sensitizing drug. It is a "sunburn" and may be followed by secondary pigmentation. The photosensitizing drug absorbs photons and provokes an electron excitation leading to the appearance of free radicals or peroxides and heat, which cause cell damage.[144] In photoallergic reactions, light transforms the sensitizing drug into a reactive hapten that can combine with skin proteins to form a new antigen. Skin lesions occur on re-exposure to the drug and to sunlight.[144]

HEMATOLOGIC TOXICITY

Antimicrobial agents frequently affect the hematopoietic system. These effects may be due to direct effects on stem cells in the bone marrow or on the formed cells in the blood stream. Thus, suppression of each of the three cell lines can occur independently or in combination (Table 53–7). Most often suppression is reversible when the offending drug is discontinued. However, some drugs are associated with irreversible toxicity, such as the aplastic anemia associated with chloramphenicol. Thus, it is important to be aware of the potential for myelotoxicity when using antibiotics and to conduct surveillance for these side effects. Those agents associated with irreversible toxicity are best reserved for the treatment of severe infections and should be used only when alternative therapy is not as effective or is not available.

Effects on the Erythrocyte

Anemia. Anemia may occur by suppression of bone marrow production (aplasia) or by peripheral destruction (hemolysis). Initially, a falling hemoglobin level can be investigated with a reticulocyte count and a review of the peripheral blood smear. Anemia from bone marrow suppression will show a falling reticulocyte count and a normal smear. A hemolytic anemia will show an abnormal smear with evidence of hemolysis, such as erythrocyte fragments (burr cells, spherocytes, schistocytes) and an elevated reticulocyte count. Significant hemolysis is also associated with elevation in direct bilirubin levels and a fall in the serum haptoglobin to zero.

Table 53–7. HEMATOLOGIC TOXICITY

Effects on the erythrocyte (RBC)
Peripheral destruction—hemolysis due to immune mechanisms and to RBC abnormalities
Marrow suppression
Effects on the leukocytes
Antibody-mediated peripheral destruction
Marrow suppression
Effects on the platelets
Peripheral destruction
Marrow suppression
Platelet dysfunction
Aplastic anemia

Bone marrow aspiration is usually not required to differentiate between these processes. In rare cases which are unclear, or where other diagnostic possibilities exist, bone marrow aspiration may be performed to define the process and rule out other serious diagnoses. In aplasia, bone marrow elements are suppressed and decreased in number, whereas in hemolysis there is often hyperplasia of the marrow elements as the marrow attempts to compensate for peripheral losses.

Hemolytic anemia is probably most frequently associated with the penicillins and the cephalosporins but also occurs occasionally with the sulfonamides, rifampin, tetracycline, isoniazid, and nitrofurantoin.[127] A Coombs-positive reaction with or without hemolysis occurs with the penicillins.[146] Specific IgG antibodies that react with penicillin–red blood cell complexes can be identified. This occurs in less than 1 per cent of patients treated with penicillins. Coombs antibody is present in from 5 to 25 per cent of patients treated with a cephalosporin, with rates depending on the particular compound studied. These antibodies are caused by binding of the cephalosporin with the red blood cell as well as by nonselective adsorption of plasma proteins such as immunoglobulins, complement, albumin, and fibrinogen to the red cell membrane.[147] Hemolysis rarely occurs despite the frequency with which these antibodies are expressed (Table 53–8).

Patients with glucose-6-phosphate dehydrogenase deficiency (G6PD), are at risk for hemolysis when exposed to certain antimicrobials, including the sulfonamides, primaquine, nitrofurantoin, furazolidine, and nalidixic acid.[148] Dapsone-associated hemolysis occurs in the normal host at levels above 100 mg per day and at 50 mg per day if G6PD deficiency is present.[149] Sulfonamides should be avoided in patients with hemoglobin Zurich and H, who also may hemolyze when exposed to these drugs.[150]

Table 53–8. DRUGS ASSOCIATED WITH HEMOLYTIC ANEMIA

cephalosporins
isoniazid
penicillins
quinine
quinidine
rifampin
sulfonamides
tetracyclines

Severe hemolysis, as may occur in the patient with a hemolytic anemia, may present clinically with nausea, fever, and jaundice.

Methemoglobinemia is also common with dapsone and occurs with primaquine in patients with congenital deficiency of NADH methemoglobin reductase.[151]

Anemia Secondary to Bone Marrow Suppression. Suppression of erythropoiesis frequently occurs during chronic illnesses but may be additionally affected by some antimicrobials. Amphotericin B therapy is usually associated with a fall in hemoglobin. The anemia is normochromic and normocytic and appears to be caused by marrow suppression.[152] Hemoglobin values should be followed closely as transfusion occasionally may be required.

The antiviral agent azidothymidine (AZT) is the first that has been useful in the treatment of human immunodeficiency viral (HIV or AIDS) infection and disease. AZT frequently will cause a fall in hemoglobin, which may require a decrease in drug dosage or transfusions to treat the resulting anemia or both.[153] Associated illnesses may contribute to the etiology, and evaluation of anemia in a patient with HIV infection should include a search for other infectious causes before ascribing it to drug therapy alone.

Agranulocytosis

Drug-related immunologic destruction of granulocytes usually develops after the second week of therapy but may be delayed and occur weeks or months into a course of therapy. It is characterized by a sudden fall in the peripheral neutrophil count; fever may be present. Absolute neutropenia can be severe and may place the patient at increased risk of infection. Neutrophil counts of less than 1000 per mm^3 should be taken very seriously, and the offending drug should be discontinued immediately. Fevers in patients with drug-induced neutropenia should be evaluated fully and treated rapidly and broadly.

Drug-induced neutropenia may be due to antibodies to the neutrophil. In this context, the fall in the neutrophil count may occur within minutes on repeat exposure to an offending drug. This observation is consistent with peripheral destruction of mature cells.

The neutropenia seen with prolonged high-dose therapy with penicillins and cephalosporins is of uncertain etiology, but it may not have an immunologic basis as rechallenge is not associated with an accelerated recurrence of the neutropenia and the neutrophil count may fall more slowly.[154] In at least a subset of these cases, however, rash and drug-dependent leukoagglutinins have been described, and an immune mechanism may be responsible.[155]

Direct bone marrow toxicity appears to be responsible for the gradual falls in neutrophil count associated with sulfonamides, flucytosine, chloramphenicol, trimethoprim/sulfamethoxazole, and nitrofurantoin. Flucytosine-caused bone marrow suppression affects platelets as well as neutrophils at high serum concentrations. This occurs most often in the setting of renal failure, in which amphotericin B therapy may be responsible for the fall in creatinine clearance. Neutropenia is a very frequent side effect of AZT; 24 per cent of the treated patients have granulocyte counts below 1000 cells/mm^3 by the twelfth week.[153] These effects are usually reversible, with normal counts occurring within 2 weeks of stopping the offending drug.

Gancyclovir [dihydroxy-propoxymethyl guanine (DHPG)], a congener of acyclovir, has been used experimentally to treat or at least to suppress cytomegaloviral infections in the immunocompromised host with some limited success. However, this antiviral agent also has major bone marrow suppressive effects. Neutropenia and leukopenia occur in up to 50 per cent of treated patients.[156]

Thrombocytopenia

Reversible drug-related thrombocytopenia, like neutropenia, is usually immunologic in origin.[127] Platelet antibody activity can be demonstrated in vitro using serum from affected individuals to catalyze lysis or agglutination of platelets. Re-exposure to an offending drug causes an immediate fall in platelet count, suggesting peripheral destruction of the mature cells in the vascular space. Antibodies can be demonstrated in cases associated with quinine and quinidine, with a megakaryocytic bone marrow and peripheral thrombocytopenia.[157] Thrombocytopenia occurs also with the sulfonamides, trimethoprim/sulfamethoxazole, and nitrofurantoin.

Intermittent administration of high-dose rifampin has been associated with a clinically significant thrombocytopenia and a hemolytic anemia. This appears to be due to rifampin-dependent antibodies. Other manifestations may include systemic signs such as hypotension, shortness of breath, and renal failure. A second course of rifampin in a patient who tolerated the primary exposure should be monitored carefully, as hypersensitivity reactions may occur.[158]

An antibody-induced immune thrombocytopenia has been described with the penicillins and cephalosporins. These are reversed quickly when the particular drug is discontinued. Trimethoprim/sulfamethoxazole (TMP/SMX) and isoniazid are each associated with a reversible bone marrow suppression.

Coagulation Defects

Platelet Dysfunction. Platelet dysfunction has been described with penicillins and is concentration related.[159] The penicillins, especially carbenicillin and ticarcillin, bind to adenosine diphosphate receptor sites on the platelet and can interfere with platelet aggregation. This effect is reversible, unlike the effect of aspirin on platelets. With very-high-dose therapy, significant bleeding may occur.[160]

Clotting Abnormalities. A bleeding diathesis has been described with moxalactam, cefamandole, and cefoperazone.[161] Moxalactam (but not cefamandole or cefoperazone), like the penicillins, can inhibit ADP-dependent platelet aggregation. The prolongation of the prothrombin time associated with the three cephalosporins is thought by some to be due to a drug-induced hypoprothrombinemia. Hypoprothrombinemia may occur secondary to the inhibition of the microsomal vitamin K-dependent carboxylase activity by the tetrazole side chain. This prevents activation of prothrombin.[162] Cefamandole, moxalactam, and cefaperazone all have a 1-methyl-5-thiotetrazole group at the 3 position of the thiazolidine ring (Fig. 53–2).

Bleeding during therapy with these drugs is unusual and may not occur in children. In adults, the presence of malnutrition and other causes of platelet dysfunction, such as aspirin, heparin, oral anticoagulants, renal

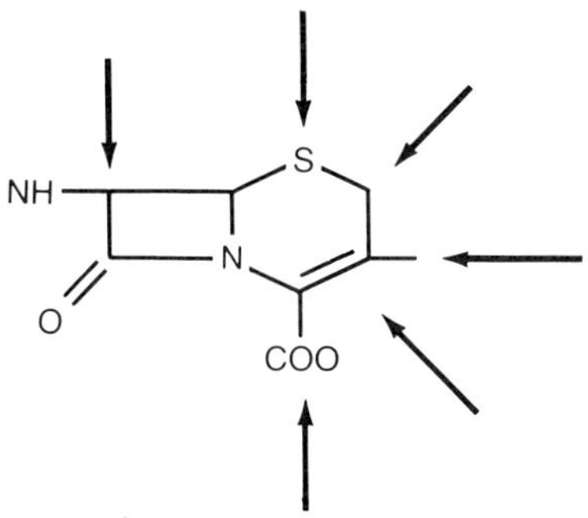

Basic chemical structure of cephalosporin molecules. Potential points of chemical modification of the cephalosporin nucleus are noted by arrows

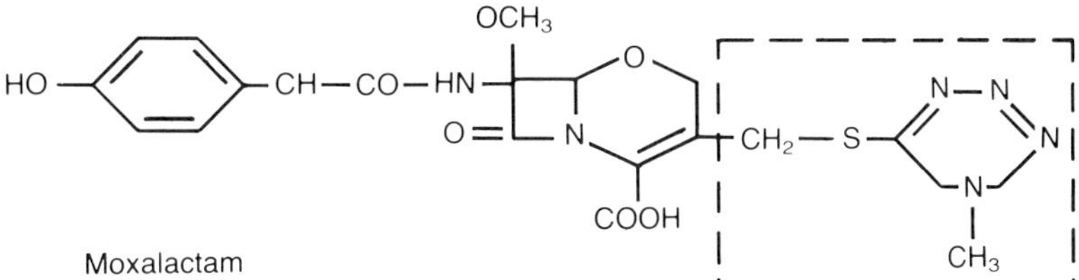

Moxalactam

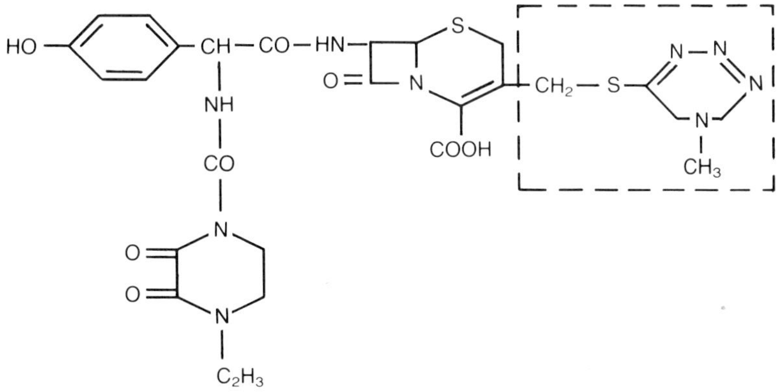

Cefoperazone

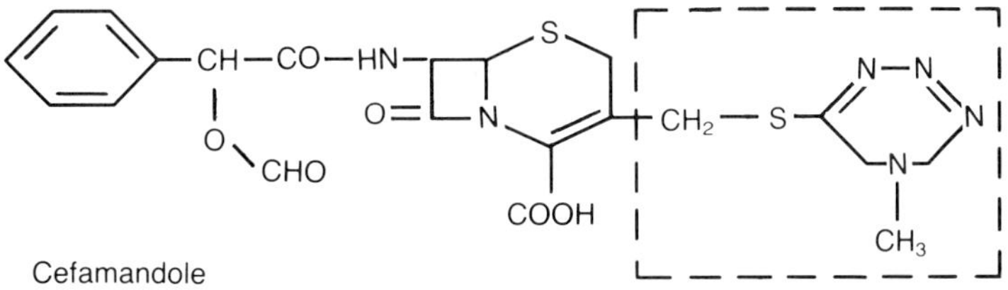

Cefamandole

Figure 53–2. Cephalosporin nucleus. Arrows depict sites for chemical modification leading to alterations in pharmacokinetics and pharmacodynamics. The thiomethyltetrazole ring, which appears in the box on structures of moxalactam, cefoperazone and cefamandole, has been implicated as a cause of the hypoprothrombinemia occasionally seen with these drugs.

failure, and sepsis, increases the risk of this side effect.[163] Vitamin K should be given weekly as prophylaxis to patients requiring therapy with one of these cephalosporins, especially those considered at special risk. Bleeding time and prothrombin time should be monitored. Moxalactam therapy warrants special monitoring and dosage adjustment according to renal function to avoid the platelet dysfunction associated with high-dose therapy.

Aplastic Anemia

The most serious hematologic toxicity associated with antimicrobial therapy is aplastic anemia. This usually permanent and irreversible complication most often is fatal. The drug most frequently associated with aplastic anemia is chloramphenicol, but the sulfonamides also have been implicated.

The mechanism of chloramphenicol-induced aplastic anemia has been most intensively studied. Chloramphenicol causes a nondose-related, idiosyncratic, and usually latent aplastic anemia, often presenting weeks to months after exposure to the drug. Fortunately, this is a rare complication, occurring in perhaps 1 in 40,000 patients exposed to the drug.[164] The occurrence in twins, as well as an apparent predisposition to this side effect in family members of victims, suggests a genetic predisposition.[165] There is no way at present to screen for or diagnose the likelihood of this complication prior to its occurrence.

The presumed mechanism of this side effect is the production of the nitroso- derivative of chloramphenicol by susceptible individuals.[166] Nitrosochloramphenicol can be synthesized by mammalian cells as demonstrated in vitro.[167] In vitro, nitrosochloramphenicol is very toxic to human myeloid precursor cells.[168] Exposure of stem cells in vitro causes irreversible inhibition of DNA synthesis and cell death. No such effect is seen with exposure to chloramphenicol.

A controversy about the relative risks of developing aplastic anemia after oral versus intravenous chloramphenicol remains unsettled. At first, all cases of aplastic anemia were described after at least some oral exposure to the drug, and almost no cases were related to the intravenous drug alone. With time, however, a case has been reported following intravenous therapy[169] and even after exposure to eye drops.[170] However, the possibility that exposure to the gastrointestinal tract may somehow predispose to the permanent drug toxicity remains unresolved.

High serum concentrations (>25 μg/ml) of chloramphenicol are associated with a reversible bone marrow suppression expressed as a reticulocytopenia, anemia, leukopenia, thrombocytopenia, or any combination of these abnormalities. Patients with bone marrow suppression from chloramphenicol have ultrastructural abnormalities of stem cell mitochondria, visible by elecron microscopy, which reverse when the drug is discontinued.[171] Increases in stainable marrow iron are seen in patients that correlate with the rise in free serum erythrocyte protoporphyrin. Toxicity appears to be due to damage to the mitochondrial membrane.

The reversible myelotoxicity of chloramphenicol both in vitro and in vivo is also seen with the chloramphenicol analogue thiamphenicol. This analogue cannot be metabolized into a nitroso- compound because it lacks an NO_2 group.[172] As might be expected by the mechanisms discussed for chloramphenicol toxicity, thiamphenicol can and does cause the reversible marrow suppression seen with chloramphenicol but is not associated with aplastic anemia despite its extensive use in Europe and Japan.[173]

Patients on high doses of chloramphenicol should be monitored closely for bone marrow effects, and the drug should be stopped or the dose reduced if toxicity occurs. Serum concentrations should be followed in patients requiring prolonged courses of therapy and in any patient with liver disease in whom serum concentrations may be difficult to predict.

IMMUNOTOXICITY

Immunologic reactions to antibiotics cause symptoms that can affect every organ system in the body (Table 53–9). Thus, important contraindications to therapy with an individual agent must include a history of a hypersensitivity reaction to that agent or other agents in that class. The mechanisms of these diverse reactions include all aspects of the immune system (Table 53–10).

It has been estimated that up to 10 per cent of patients treated with a penicillin will experience a hypersensitivity reaction to the

Table 53–9. IMMUNOTOXIC REACTIONS

Systemic
Anaphylactic shock
Serum sickness/vasculitis
Fever, eosinophilia
Hematologic
Hemolytic anemia
Agranulocytosis
Thrombocytopenia
Hepatic
Hepatitis
Renal
Interstitial nephritis
Respiratory
Asthma
Eosinophilic pneumonia
Autoimmune Reactions
SLE syndrome
Skin
Maculopapular/maculovesicular rash
Contact dermatitis
Fixed drug eruptions
Erythema multiforme
Stevens-Johnson syndrome
Phototoxicity/photoallergy

drug. This figure may be up to 40 per cent in those who have a prior history of an adverse reaction to penicillin.[174] These reactions may vary from a minor rash to fatal anaphylaxis. In one series, 0.04 to 0.2 per cent of all acute allergic reactions to penicillin were severe, and 0.001 per cent of these had a fatal outcome.[175]

The penicillins and their metabolites are potent immunogens because of their ability to combine with proteins and act as haptens for acute antibody-mediated reactions. The most frequent (about 95 per cent) or "major" determinant of penicillin allergy is the penicilloyl determinant produced by opening the β-lactam ring of the penicillin. This allows

Table 53–10. MECHANISMS OF DRUG-INDUCED IMMUNOTOXICITY

Antibody-Mediated Reactions
Anaphylaxis (immediate penicillin reactions)
Cell-Mediated Reactions
Contact dermatitis
Cytotoxic
Activation of complement by specific antibodies that react with target cell surface antigen (Coombs + hemolytic anemia)
Immune Complex Reaction
Serum sickness (example, Cefaclor)

linkage of the penicillin to protein at the amide group. "Minor" determinants (less frequent) are the other metabolites formed, including native penicillin and penicilloic acids. These metabolites may be formed in vivo or in vitro when reconstituted penicillins in solution break down (Fig. 53–3).

These determinants act as haptens: substances that react with specific antibody. Hapten-protein conjugates are very immunogenic. Most anaphylactic penicillin reactions are due to IgE that is specific to the minor determinants.[174] The IgE antibody is present on most cells, and basophils and the antigen-antibody reaction trigger mediator release.

Anaphylaxis

Anaphylaxis presents clinically as the acute onset of peripheral vascular collapse and shock. This may begin minutes after contact with the precipitating allergen. It is the most feared and serious of the allergic reactions and carries with it a significant risk of death. Skin and mucosal lesions, including urticaria and angioedema, may immediately precede the onset of anaphylaxis. Nausea, vomiting, diarrhea, and bronchospasm may occur as part of the acute reaction to the drug. These end-organ responses are initiated by the release of histamine, serotonin, bradykinin and other vasoactive substances released by the basophils and mast cells (Fig. 53–4).

Penicillins, cephalosporins, and sulfonamides are the antimicrobials most often associated with anaphylactic reactions. A history of prior exposure and prior allergic reactions, especially to those that are more frequently associated with anaphylactic reactions, should be sought before administering any antimicrobial therapy. The history of an urticarial rash within minutes up to 1 hour after exposure to a drug is suggestive of an IgE-mediated reaction. It should raise concern for the possibility that a severe reaction, including anaphylaxis, might occur with subsequent exposures to the offending drug and other drugs of the same class. A history of anaphylaxis or exfoliative dermatitis should preclude rechallenge with the same or related drugs (Table 53–11).

Not every rechallenge in patients with a history of drug allergy will result in an allergic response.[176] However, it is impossible to predict who may safely be retreated and

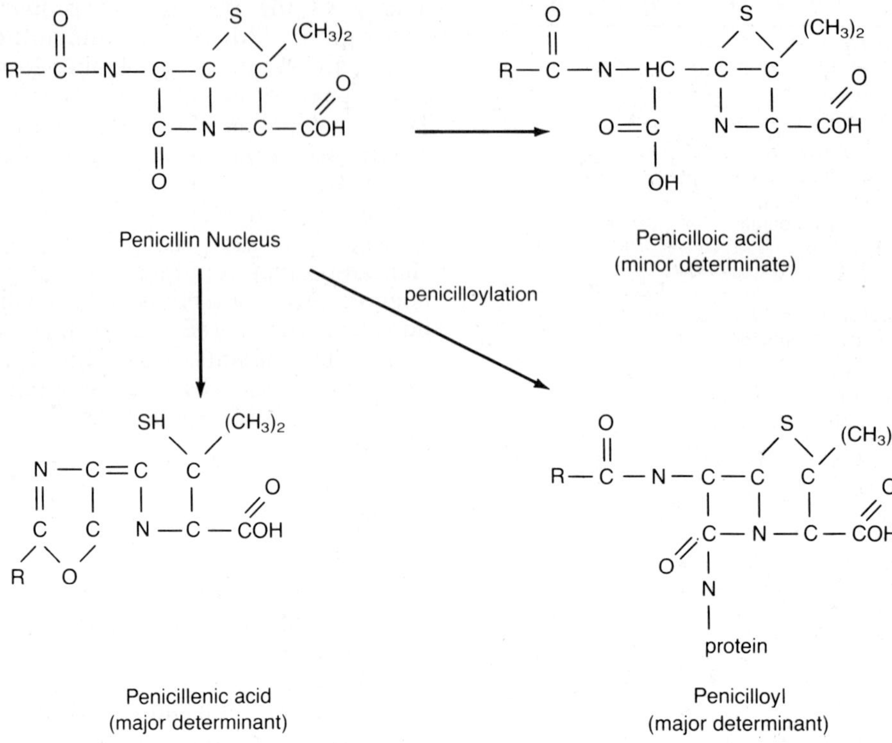

Figure 53–3. Antigenic determinants implicated in hypersensitivity reactions to penicillin.

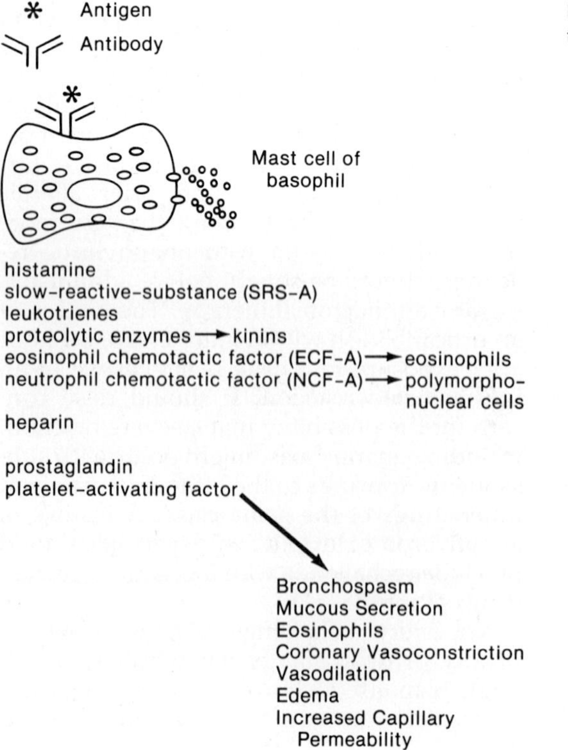

Figure 53–4. Pathophysiology of an anaphylactic reaction to a drug.

Table 53–11. DRUGS ASSOCIATED WITH ANAPHYLACTIC REACTIONS

aminoglycosides
amphotericin B
cephalosporins
clindamycin
ethambutol
lincomycin
penicillins
sulfonamides
tetracyclines
vancomycin

who is still at great risk for life-threatening sequelae. If the drug is absolutely indicated and an effective alternative agent is not available, then desensitization should be undertaken. Most experience with desensitization techniques has been with penicillin. Skin testing before initiating therapy may help indicate the likelihood of a persisting allergy. A commercial skin test called PrePen is available for penicillin but it must be combined with a test for the minor penicillin determinants because these may also mediate anaphylaxis. Even with a negative response to these skin tests, desensitization may be the safest way to administer penicillin or a related drug in a patient with a clear history of acute penicillin allergy. Once desensitization is completed, the therapeutic doses must be given without interruption. If the drug is stopped, desensitization must be repeated prior to using the drug again, as blocking antibodies may fade and anaphylaxis may be possible again (Table 53–12).

Cross-reactivity between the cephalosporins and the penicillins occurs and may reflect the structural similarities (β-lactam ring) of these classes of drugs. Up to 20 per cent, but probably closer to 5 to 10 per cent, of patients who are allergic to penicillin will be allergic to the cephalosporins. A patient with a history of a severe reaction to a penicillin, such as anaphylaxis or exfoliative dermatitis, probably should not be treated with a cephalosporin. When this class of drugs is absolutely necessary, desensitization probably should be performed. Cross-reactivity between penicillin and the newer cephalosporins occurs, and these must be used with care in patients with a history of penicillin allergy. Aztreonam, a monobactam, appears to have little cross-reactivity with the penicillins and cephalosporins and has been used in allergic patients.[177]

Serum Sickness

Serum sickness is a rare complication of antimicrobial therapy, caused by a delayed hypersensitivity reaction. It usually begins approximately 7 to 10 days after the initiation of therapy. It may occur after the drug has already been stopped. The rash associated with serum sickness may include urticaria and angioneurotic edema. Palpable skin lesions consistent with a vasculitis are often present and are very suggestive of the diagnosis. This IgG-mediated toxicity also may cause gastrointestinal signs, pericarditis, myocarditis, polyneuritis, and, rarely, myelitis. The skin lesions of serum sickness most often begin after the first week of therapy but may occur even later, up to 3 weeks after first exposure to the allergen. Fever is common, and red blood cell casts in the urine confirm the presence of a vasculitis. The offending drug should be stopped and avoided in the future. The penicillins, the sulfonamides, and especially the cephalosporin cefaclor[178] are most frequently associated with serum sickness (Table 53–13).

Table 53–12. PENICILLIN DESENSITIZATION

The patient must be admitted to a critical care site. A secure intravenous line is started. In the presence of professionals trained and prepared to treat acute anaphylaxis, desensitization can be started by either of the following protocols:

A. Cutaneous[193]
   1. 5 units of crystalline penicillin is injected intracutaneously into the lower forearm
   2. At 60–90 minute intervals: 10, 100, 1000 units are given intracutaneously.
   3. This is followed by 10,000 units and then 50,000 units subcutaneously.
   4. Begin intravenous penicillin at the same dose and continue increasing doses until the therapeutic dose is reached or:

B. Oral[176]
   1. 100 units of penicillin V elixir is given PO.
   2. Double each oral dose and give a dose every 15 min until about 1,300,000 units are given.
   3. Begin intravenous penicillin.

Note:
1. No prior therapy with hydrocortisone or diphenhydramine.
2. Mild cutaneous reactions are allowed to resolve spontaneously or may be treated with diphenhydramine, 25 mg IV.
3. Life-threatening reactions should be managed appropriately.

Table 53–13. ANTIBIOTICS ASSOCIATED WITH SERUM SICKNESS

aminoglycosides
cephalosporins—cefaclor
griseofulvin
isoniazid
lincomycin
nitrofurantoin (?)
p-aminosalicylic acid
penicillins
sulfonamides
tetracyclines (?)

Allergic Vasculitis
ethionamide
isoniazid
penicillins
quinidine
sulfonamides
tetracyclines

Cutaneous Reactions

Cutaneous reactions can occur with most antimicrobial agents and are perhaps the most common adverse reaction. Most are mild and self-limited and, as described earlier, are frequently not an indication to stop therapy. Reactions that do suggest a drug reaction begin within 1 or 2 weeks of beginning the drug. These cutaneous reactions are symmetric and frequently pruritic. Morbilliform and erythematous macules are most usual. A hypersensitivity reaction has been suggested because of the presence of IgM immunocomplexes in the skin.[179] These rashes disappear quickly when the inciting drug is discontinued. Therapy can be continued through these late-onset allergic rashes, but the patient must be followed closely. Progression of the rash and the development of systemic signs suggest the need to stop the antimicrobial agent.

Certain rashes clearly indicate the need to stop drug therapy and are described here.

Erythema multiforme may begin as a rash of nonspecific macules or papules. These develop into "target" or "iris" lesions that are diagnostic of erythema multiforme. These lesions may be accompanied by vesicles and coalescence of the macules into plaques or other confluent lesions, often with urticaria. Lesions appear in crops and persist for as long as 1 to 3 weeks. Recovery is usually complete and uneventful once the lesions begin to heal.[180] In more severe cases, however, systemic signs are prominent and there are accompanying mucosal lesions. Painful mucosal ulcers occur in the mouth, eyes, vagina, and anus. Skin lesions may coalesce into generalized erythema and vesicles, which may be hemorrhagic. Desquamation of the epidermal layer can follow. The patients appear toxic and are critically ill as fluid loss, dehydration, and sepsis are not infrequent; they are life-threatening complications. This severe form of erythema multiforme is called the Stevens-Johnson syndrome. Stevens-Johnson syndrome occurs so frequently with the antimalarial drug Fansidar (sulfadoxine/pyrimethamine) that therapy with this drug is recommended only for the treatment of malaria and no longer for chronic prophylaxis, even in areas with endemic chloroquine-resistant disease. Streptomycin and quinine also may cause this reaction infrequently.

Trimethoprim/sulfamethoxazole is associated with a very high frequency of neutropenia, thrombocytopenia, severe skin rash, and Stevens-Johnson syndrome in patients with acquired immunodeficiency syndrome (AIDS). This severely limits the usefulness of this drug for these patients.[181]

Obviously, the appearance of erythema multiforme or the Stevens-Johnson syndrome in a patient taking an agent associated with these reactions is an indication to stop the drug immediately and to avoid it in the future.

These syndromes occur in association with certain infections, such as herpes simplex. The mechanism is unknown, but a hypersensitivity or immune complex reaction has been suggested, as the reaction occurs 7 to 14 days after exposure to a precipitating drug.

Erythema nodosum, distinguished by the presence of painful subcutaneous nodules predominately over the lower legs, has a prolonged course and is associated with systemic signs. An Arthus or mixed form of allergic reaction is suggested. Sulfonamides, especially trimethoprim-sulfamethoxazole, and penicillins are associated with erythema nodusum reactions, as well as various viral and bacterial infections.

Other Immunologic Effects

Many studies have examined the effects of the antimicrobial agents on immunologic function.[182] The data available involve in vitro or animal studies, which may not pertain to the situation in the human host. Rifampin, tetracycline, and chloramphenicol have been shown to have depressive effects in various in vitro immunologic tests. No evidence suggests any clinical significance of these findings.

Chloroquine is effective as an anti-inflammatory agent in certain connective tissue disorders, suggesting an immunomodulatory activity. In vitro chloroquine inhibits some monocyte and lymphocyte functions and responses, including the generation of immunoglobulin-secreting cells.[183] The clinical relevance of these in vitro observations is suggested by the observation that Peace Corps volunteers taking chloroquine prophylaxis developed lower antibody titers to human diploid cell rabies vaccine than a control group not on prophylaxis.[184]

MISCELLANEOUS REACTIONS

Dental and Skeletal

Irreversible dental discoloration and enamel dysplasia have occurred after intrauterine or early childhood exposure to tetracyclines.[185] This appears to be dose related and due to deposition of the tetracyclines in calcifying areas of bone and teeth. Discoloration usually occurs with prolonged or repeated exposure but may occur even after a single course of therapy. Doxycycline and oxytetracycline may cause less discoloration and should be used preferentially when absolutely needed in the child under 7 years of age who requires a tetracycline for treatment.

Joints

In immature animals the quinolone antibiotics are associated with an arthropathy. Because of concern for this side effect in humans, these drugs are not recommended for use in childhood.[186]

Drug Fever

Drug fever is a common sign of drug allergy. It may occur alone or in combination with other signs of allergy, such as rash. Fever may precede the development of other more serious signs of drug allergy, such as serum sickness. The penicillins and cephalosporins lead the list of antimicrobial agents associated with drug fever. The mechanism

Table 53–14. DRUGS FREQUENTLY IMPLICATED IN DRUG FEVER

cephalosporins
chloramphenicol
dapsone
erythromycin
isoniazid
nitrofurantoin
penicillins
pyrazinamide
quinidine
quinine
streptomycin
sulfonamides
tetracycline

of drug fever is uncertain. Fever may be produced through the formation of antigen-antibody complexes; alternatively, other antibody-mediated mechanisms may be responsible.[187] A cell-mediated hypersensitivity reaction has also been suggested. Drug fevers are usually sustained, occur at least daily, and often are unassociated with any other complaints (Table 53–14).

The fever and chills associated with amphotericin B infusions occur only during drug infusion and therefore are different from the usual drug fever. Fever and chills may be due to a direct toxic effect of the drug, possibly mediated through prostaglandin E_2 synthesis.[188] Based on this hypothesis, a double-blind placebo/controlled study of ibuprofen (a single dose of 10 mg/kg) given 30 minutes before the start of amphotericin B infusion decreased chills from 87 per cent to 48 per cent.

The Jarisch-Herxheimer reaction consists of fever, chills, flushing, and at times hypotension; it occurs in association with the onset of antibacterial treatment. It was first described with penicillin treatment of syphilis. A similar reaction also has been described with treatment of acute Lyme disease.[189] The cause is believed to be the release of endotoxins from rapidly dying bacteria.[190]

Mononucleosis-like syndromes with fever, lymphadenopathy, and generalized fatigue occur with dapsone and rifampin and may be immunologic in origin (Table 53–15).[191]

Electrolyte Abnormalities Associated with Antimicrobials

Electrolyte abnormalities may occur with antimicrobials that contain large salt loads.

Table 53–15. DRUGS ASSOCIATED WITH AUTOIMMUNE OR SLE-LIKE REACTIONS*

Autoimmune Reaction
isoniazid†

SLE-Like Reaction
griseofulvin
quinidine
para-aminosalicylic acid
penicillin
streptomycin
sulfonamides
tetracycline

*Arthritis, fever, skin rash, lymphadenopathy, serositis, anti-DNA antibody.
†Anti-DNA antibodies without other signs.

The penicillins may cause sodium overload with subsequent fluid retention. This may be very significant clinically, especially in the patient with underlying cardiac disease. Carbenicillin, for example, contains 4.7 mEq of sodium per gram of drug. When the dosage is 20 to 30 gm per day, this drug may make a significant contribution to sodium metabolism. This may be sufficient reason to use one of the more expensive but lower salt-containing ureidepenicillins (Table 53–16).

Another side effect resulting from the electrolyte content of the penicillin salt is the rapid rise in serum potassium that may occur with a large intravenous bolus of the potassium salt of crystalline penicillin. Cardiac arrest has been precipitated by the rapid infusion of very large doses of aqueous penicillin potassium. In renal failure, the use of potassium penicillin is usually best avoided; even slow infusions here may result in rises of serum potassium to toxic levels. Using the sodium salt avoids this potentially severe side effect.

Table 53–16. SODIUM CONTENT OF THE PARENTERAL PENICILLINS

	mEq/gm	MAXIMUM DOSE	TOTAL Na mEq/Day
ampicillin	3	12	36
azlocillin	2.17	24	52
carbenicillin	4.7–5	40	188–200
methicillin	3	12	36
mezlocillin	1.85	24	44.4
oxacillin	2.8	12	34
piperacillin	1.85	24	44.4
nafcillin	2.9	12	35

(From Drug Facts and Comparisons. Philadelphia, JB Lippincott, 1986.)

Hypokalemia may occur during penicillin therapy owing to competition of the penicillin at the distal renal tubule and excessive potassium excretion.[192]

References

1. Stroller KP, Losey R: Inadvertent intra-arterial injection of penicillin: An unseen danger. Pediatrics *75*:785–786, 1985.
2. Farber BF, Moellering RC: Retrospective study of the toxicity of preparations of vancomycin from 1974–1981. Antimicrob Agents Chemother *23*:138–141, 1983.
3. Cooper GL, Given DB: Vancomycin: A Comprehensive Review of 30 Years of Clinical Experience. New York, John Wiley, 1986, pp 1–84.
4. Polk RE, Healy KP, Schwartz LB, Rock DT, Garson ML, Roller K: Vancomycin and the red-man syndrome: Pharmacodynamics of histamine release. J Infect Dis *157*:502–507, 1988.
5. Bolan G, Laurie RE, Broome CV: Red man syndrome: Inadvertent administration of an excessive dose of rifampin to children in a day care center. Pediatrics *77*:633–635, 1986.
6. Kaiser AB, McGee ZA: Aminoglycoside therapy of Gram-negative bacillary meningitis. N Engl J Med *293*:1215–1220, 1975.
7. Mandel GL, Sande MA: Penicillins and cephalosporins. *In* Gilman AG, Goodman LS, Rall TW, Murad F (eds): The Pharmacological Basis of Therapeutics. 7th ed. New York, Macmillan, 1985, pp 1115–1149.
8. Oldstone MBA, Nelson E: Central nervous system manifestations of penicillin toxicity in man. Neurology *16*:693–700, 1966.
9. Green RL, Lewis JE, Kraus J, Frederickson EL: Elevated plasma procaine concentrations after administration of procaine penicillin G. N Engl J Med *291*:223–226, 1974.
10. Pratt WB: Chemotherapy of tuberculosis. *In* The Chemotherapy of Infection. New York, Oxford University Press, 1977, pp 231–262.
11. Frytak S, Moertel CG, Childs DS, Albers JW: Neurologic toxicity associated with high dose metronidazole therapy. Ann Intern Med *88*:361–362, 1978.
12. Wood JD, Peesker SJ: The effect on GABA metabolism in brain of isonicotinic acid hydrazide and pyridoxine as a function of time after administration. J Neurochem *19*:1527–1537, 1972.
13. Katz GA, Jobin GC: Large doses of pyridoxine in the treatment of massive ingestion of isoniazid. Am Rev Resp Dis *101*:991–992, 1970.
14. Pratt WB: The chemotherapy of malaria. *In* The Chemotherapy of Infection. New York, Oxford University Press, 1977, pp 307–345.
15. Band JD, Fraser DW: Adverse effects of two rifampicin dosage regimens for the prevention of meningococcal infection. Lancet *1*:101–102, 1984.
16. Kenney RE, Kirk LE, Bridgen D: Acyclovir tolerance in humans. Am J Med *73S*:176–181, 1982.
17. Hayden FG, Gwaltney JM, Van de Castle RL, Adams KF, Giordani B: Comparative toxicity of amantadine hydrochloride and rimantadine hydrochloride in healthy adults. Antimicrob Agents Chemother *19*:226–233, 1981.

18. Lauter CB, Bailey EJ, Lerner AM: Microbiologic assays and neurological toxicity during use of adenine arabinoside in humans. J Infect Dis *134:*75–79, 1976.
19. Fields JP: Bulging fontanel: A complication of tetracycline therapy in infants. J Pediatr *58:*74–76, 1961.
20. Pittinger C, Adamson R: Antibiotic blockade of neuromuscular function. Annu Rev Pharmacol *12:*169–184, 1972.
21. Wright JM, Collier B: The effects of neomycin upon transmitter release and action. J Pharmacol Exp Ther *200:*576–587, 1977.
22. L'Hommedieu CS, Huber PA, Rasch DK: Potentiation of magnesium-induced neuromuscular weakness by gentamicin. Crit Care Med *11:*55–56, 1983.
23. L'Hommedieu CS, Stough R, Brown L, Kettrick R, Polin R: Potentiation of neuromuscular weakness in infant botulism by aminoglycosides. J Pediatr *95:*1065–1070, 1979.
24. Hokkanen E: The aggravating effect of some antibiotics on the neuromuscular blockade in myasthenia gravis. Acta Neurol Scand *40:*346–352, 1964.
25. Stirling H, Hodge CH: Quinine as an adjuvant to surgical induction of labour. J Obstet Gynecol *68:*939–943, 1961.
26. Phillips RE, Looareesuwan S, White NJ, Silamut K, Kietinun C, Warrell DA: Quinine pharmacokinetics and toxicity in pregnant and lactating women with *Falciparum* malaria. Br J Clin Pharmacol *21:*677–683, 1986.
27. Holmberg L, Boman G, Bottiger LE, Eriksson B, Spross R, Wessling A: Adverse reactions to nitrofurantoin. Am J Med *69:*733–738, 1980.
28. Sinclair D, Phillips C: Transient myopathy apparently due to tetracycline. N Engl J Med *307:*821–822, 1983.
29. Leibold JE: The ocular toxicity of ethambutol and its relation to dose. Ann NY Acad Sci *135:*904–909, 1966.
30. Bernstein H, Zvaifler N, Rubin M, Mansour AM: The ocular deposition of chloroquine. Invest Ophthalmol *2:*384–392, 1963.
31. Joy RJT, Scaletter LR, Sodee DLB: Optic and peripheral neuritis: Probable effect of prolonged chloramphenicol therapy. JAMA *173:*1731–1734, 1960.
32. Toone EC, Hayden GD, Ellman HM: Ototoxicity of chloroquine. Arthritis Rheum *8:*475–476, 1965.
33. Bendush CL: Ototoxicity: Clinical considerations and comparative information. *In* Whelton A, Neu HC (eds): The Aminoglycosides. New York, Marcel Dekker, 1982, pp 453–486.
34. Koeda T, Umemura K, Yokota M: Toxicology and pharmacology of aminoglycoside antibiotics. *In* Umezawa H, Hooper IR: Aminoglycoside Antibiotics. New York, Springer-Verlag 1982, pp 293–356.
35. Moore RD, Smith CR, Lietman PS: Risk factors for the development of auditory toxicity in patients receiving aminoglycosides. J Infect Dis *149:*23–30, 1984.
36. Mathog RH, Klein WJ: Ototoxicity of ethacrynic acid and aminoglycoside antibiotics in uremia. N Engl J Med *280:*1223–1224, 1969.
37. Wold JS, Turnsipseed SA: Toxicology of vancomycin in laboratory animals. Rev Infect Dis *3* suppl:S224–229, 1981.
38. Haydon RC, Thelin JW, Davis WE: Erythromycin ototoxicity: Analysis and conclusions based on 22 case reports. Otolaryngol Head Surg *92:*678–84, 1984.
39. Spielberg SP, Gordon GB: Nitrofurantoin cytotoxicity. J Clin Invest *67:*37–41, 1981.
40. Dawson RB: Pulmonary reactions to nitrofurantoin. N Engl J Med *274:*522, 1966.
41. Murray MJ, Kronenberg R: Pulmonary reactions simulating cardiac pulmonary edema caused by nitrofurantoin. N Engl J Med *273:*1185–1187, 1965.
42. Pearsall HR, Ewalt J, Tsoi MS, Sumida S, Backus D, Winterbauer RH, Weber DR, Jones H: Nitrofurantoin lung sensitivity: Report of a case with prolonged nitrofurantoin lymphocyte sensitivity and interaction of nitrofurantoin stimulated lymphocytes with alveolar cells. J Lab Clin Med *83:*728–737, 1974.
43. Resenow EC, DeRemee RA, Dines DE: Chronic nitrofurantoin pulmonary reactions. Report of five cases. N Engl J Med *279:*1258–1262, 1968.
44. Ho D, Tashkin DP, Bein ME, Sharma O: Pulmonary infiltrates with eosinophilia associated with tetracycline. Chest *76:*33–36, 1979.
45. Allen J: Minocycline. Ann Intern Med *85:*482–487, 1976.
46. Wright DG, Robichaud KJ, Pizzo PA, Deisseroth AB: Lethal pulmonary reactions associated with the combined use of amphotericin B and leukocyte transfusions. N Engl J Med *304:*1185–1189, 1981.
47. Forman SJ, Robinson J, Wolf JS, Spruce WE, Blume KG: Pulmonary reactions associated with amphotericin B and leukocyte transfusions. N Engl J Med *305:*584–585, 1981.
48. Demers RR, Parker J, Frankel LR, Smith DW: Administration of ribaviron to neonatal and pediatric patients during mechanical ventilators. Resp Care *31:*1188–1195, 1986.
49. Patel JC, Banker PE, Modi CJ: Chloramphenicol in typhoid fever: Preliminary report of clinical trials in six cases. Br Med J *2:*908–909, 1949.
50. Chatterjee PK, Roy BB: Vasomotor collapse after chloramphenicol. Br Med J *2:*1334, 1950.
51. Sutherland JM: Fatal cardiovascular collapse of infants receiving large amounts of chloramphenicol. Am J Dis Child *97:*761–767, 1959.
52. Buetow KC: An epidemiological approach to the problem of rising neonatal mortality in Baltimore. Am J Public Health *51:*217–227, 1961.
53. Lischner H, Seligman SJ, Krammer A, Parmalee AH: An outbreak of neonatal deaths among term infants associated with administration of chloramphenicol. J Pediatr *59:*21–34, 1961.
54. Thompson WL, Anderson SE, Lipsky JJ, Lietman PS: Overdoses of chloramphenicol. JAMA *234:*149–150, 1975.
55. Werner JC, Whitman V, Schuler LG, Fripp RR, et al: Acute myocardial effects of chloramphenicol in newborn pigs: A possible insight into the gray baby syndrome. J Infect Dis *152:*344–350, 1985.
56. Fripp RR, Carter MC, Werner JC, Schuler HG, et al: Cardiac function and acute chloramphenciol toxicity. J Pediatr *103:*487–490, 1983.
57. Yang WCT, Dubick M: Mechanism of emetine cardiotoxicity. Pharmacol Ther *10:*15–26, 1980.
58. Ginsburg CM, McCracken GH, Crow SD: Erythromycin therapy for Group A streptococcal pharyngitis: Results of a study of estolate and ethylsuccinate formulations. Am J Dis Child *138:*536–539, 1984.
59. Stillman AE, Martin RJ: Tetracycline-induced

esophageal ulcerations. Arch Dermatol *115:*1005, 1979.
60. Sutton DR, Gosnold JK: Oesophageal ulceration due to clindamycin. Br Med J *1:*1598, 1977.
61. Hinton NA: The effect of oral tetracycline HCl and doxycycline on the intestinal flora. Curr Ther Res *12:*341–352, 1970.
62. Neu HC: The new beta-lactamase-stable cephalosporins. Ann Intern Med *97:*408–419, 1982.
63. Eneanya DI, Bianchine JR, Duran DO, Andresen BD: The actions and metabolic fate of disulfiram. Annu Rev Pharmacol Toxicol *21:*575–596, 1981.
64. Bartlett JG, Chang TW, Gurwith M, Gorback SL, Onderdonk AB: Antibiotic-associated pseudomembranous colitis due to toxin-producing clostridia. N Engl J Med *298:*531–534, 1978.
65. Dearing WH, Baggenstoss AH, Weed LA: Studies on the relationship of *Staphylococcus aureus* to pseudomembranous enteritis and to postantibiotic enteritis. Gastroenterology *38:*441, 1960.
66. Larson HE, Parry JV, Price AB, Davies DR, Dolby J, Tyrrell DAJ: Undescribed toxin in pseudomembranous colitis. Br Med J *1:*1246–1248, 1977.
67. Bartlett JG, Chang TW, Taylor N, Onderdonk AB: Colitis induced by *Clostridium difficile.* Rev Infect Dis *1:*370, 1979.
68. George RH, Symonds JM, Dimock F, et al: Identification of *Clostridium difficile* as a cause of pseudomembranous colitis. Br Med J *1:*695, 1978.
69. Neu HC, Prince A, Neu CO, Garvey GJ: Incidence of diarrhea and colitis associated with clindamycin therapy. J Infect Dis *135:*S120–135, 1977.
70. Keighley MRB, Burdon DW, Arabi Y, et al: Randomized controlled trial of vancomycin for pseudomembranous colitis and postoperative diarrhoea. Br Med J *2:*1667–1673, 1978.
71. Colitis associated with clindamycin. Med Lett *16:*73–74, 1974.
72. Aronsson B, Mollby R, Nord CE: Antimicrobial agents and *Clostridium difficile* in acute enteric disease. Epidemiologic data from Sweden, 1980–1982. J Infect Dis *151:*476–481, 1985.
73. Kabins SA, Spira TJ: Outbreak of clindamycin-associated colitis. Ann Intern Med *83:*830–831, 1975.
74. Mitchell JR, Zimmerman HJ, Ishak KG, Thorgeirsson UP, Timbrell JA, Snodgrass WR, Nelson SD: Isoniazid liver injury: Clinical spectrum of pathology and probable pathogenesis. Ann Intern Med *84:*181–192, 1976.
75. Public Health Service, US Department of Health, Education, and Welfare: Isoniazid-associated hepatatis; Summary of the report of the Tuberculosis Advisory Committee and special consultants to the Director, Centers for Disease Control. MMWR *23:*97–98, 1974.
76. Gronhagen-Riska C, Hellstrom PE, Froseth B: Predisposing factors in hepatitis induced by INH-rifampin treatment of tuberculosis. Am Rev Resp Dis *118:*461–466, 1978.
77. Kopanoff DE, Snider DE, Caras GJ: Isoniazid-related hepatitis. A US Public Health Service Cooperative Surveillance Study. Am Rev Resp Dis *117:*991–1001, 1978.
78. Simpson DG, Walker JH: Hypersensitivity to para-aminosalicylic acid. Am J Med *29:*297–306, 1960.
79. Simon E, Verus E, Banki G: Changes in SGOT activity during treatment with ethionamide. Scand J Resp Dis *50:*314–322, 1969.
80. Girling DJ: The hepatic toxicity of antituberculous regimens containing isoniazid, rifampicin and perazinamide. Tubercle *59:*13–32, 1978.
81. Schultz JC, Adamson JS, Workman WW, Norman TD: Fatal liver disease after intravenous administration of tetracycline in high doses. N Engl J Med *269:*999–1004, 1963.
82. Whalley PJ, Adams RH, Combes B: Tetracycline toxicity in pregnancy: Liver and pancreatic dysfunction. JAMA *189:*357–362, 1964.
83. Cohen J: Antifungal chemotherapy. Lancet *2:*532–536, 1982.
84. Janssen PAJ, Symoens JE: Hepatic reactions during ketoconazole treatment. Am J Med *74:*80–85, 1983.
85. Ginsburg CM: A prospective study on the incidence of liver function abnormalities in children receiving erythromycin estolate, erythromycin ethylsuccinate or pencillin V for treatment of pneumonia. J Pediatr Infect Dis *5:*151–154, 1986.
86. McCormack WM, George H, Donner A, Kodgis LF, Alpert S, Lowe EW, Kass EH: Hepatotoxicity of erythromycin estolate during pregnancy. Antimicrob Agents Chemother *12:*630–635, 1977.
87. Sande MA, Mandel GL: Antimicrobial agents: Tetracyclines, chloramphenicol, erythromycin and miscellaneous antibacterial agents. *In* Gilman AG, Goodman LS, Rall TW, Murad F (eds): The Pharmacological Basis of Therapeutics. 7th ed. New York, Macmillan, 1985, pp 1170–1198.
88. Bhagwat AG, Warren RE: Hepatic reaction to nitrofurantoin. Lancet *2:*1369, 1969.
89. Elmore MF, Rogge JD: Tetracycline-induced pancreatitis. Gastroenterology *81:*1134–1136, 1981.
90. Webster LT: Drugs used in the chemotherapy of protozoan infections. *In* Gilman AG, Goodman LS, Rall TW, Murad F (eds): The Pharmacological Basis of Therapeutics. 7th ed. New York, Macmillan, 1985, pp 1058–1065.
91. Brockner J, Boisen E: Fatal multisystem toxicity after co-trimoxazole. Lancet *1:*831, 1978.
92. Meyers BR, Hirschman SZ, Strougo L, Srulevitch E: Comparative study of piperacillin, ticarcillin and carbenicillin pharmacokinetics. Antimicrob Agents Chemother *17:*608–611, 1980.
93. Leroy A, Humbert G, Godin M, Fillastre JP: Pharmacokinetics of azlocillin in subjects with normal and impaired renal function. Antimicrob Agents Chemother *17:*344–349, 1980.
94. Thompson MIB, Russo ME, Matsen JM, Atkin-Thor E: Piperacillin pharmacokinetics in subjects with chronic renal failure. Antimicrob Agents Chemother *19:*450–453, 1981.
95. Appel GB, Neu HC: Nephrotoxicity of antimicrobial agents. N Engl J Med *296:*663–670, 1977.
96. Lehr D: Clinical toxicity of sulfonamides. Ann NY Acad Sci *69:*417–447, 1957.
97. Smith CR, Lietman PS: Comparative clinical trials of aminoglycosides. *In* Whelton A, Neu HC (eds): The Aminoglycosides: Microbiology, Clinical Use, and Toxicology. New York, Marcel Dekker, 1982, pp 497–511.
98. Bennett WM: Aminoglycoside nephrotoxicity. Nephron *35:*73–77, 1983.
99. Matzke GR, Lucarotti RL, Shapiro HS: Controlled comparison of gentamicin and tobramycin nephrotoxicy. Am J Nephrol *3:*11–17, 1983.
100. Moench TR, Smith CR: Risk factors for nephrotoxicity. *In* Whelton A, Neu LHC (eds): The Aminoglycosides: Microbiology, Clinical Use, and Toxi-

cology. New York, Marcel Dekker, 1982, pp 401–417.
101. Schentag JJ: Aminoglycoside pharmacokinetics as a guide to therapy and toxicity. *In* Whelton A, Neu HC (eds): The Aminoglycosides: Microbiology, Clinical Use, and Toxicology. New York, Marcel Dekker, 1982, pp 143–167.
102. Mondorf AW: Urinary enzymatic markers of renal damage. *In* Whelton A, Neu HC (eds): The Aminoglycosides: Microbiology, Clinical Use, and Toxicology. New York, Marcel Dekker, 1982, pp 283–301.
103. Reed MD, Vermeulen MW, Stern RC, Cheng PW, Powell SH, Boat TF: Are measurements of urine enzymes useful during aminoglycoside therapy? Pediatr Res *15:*1234–1239, 1981.
104. Schentage JJ, Gengo FM, Plaut ME, Danner D, Mangione A, Jusko WJ: Urinary casts as an indicator of renal tubular damage in patients receiving aminoglycosides. Antimicrob Agents Chemother *16:*468–474, 1979.
105. Neugarten J, Aynedjian HS, Bank N: Role of tubular obstruction in acute renal failure, due to gentamicin. Kidney Int *24:*330–335, 1983.
106. Bertino JS, Kliegman RM, Myers CM, Blumer JB: Alterations in gentamicin pharmacokinetics during neonatal exchange transfusion. Dev Pharmacol Ther *4:*205–215, 1982.
107. Elliott WC, Bennett WM: Acquired gentamicin insensitivity. Rate of functional recovery with continued drug administration. Clin Res *29:*461A, 1981.
108. Churchill DN, Seely J: Nephrotoxicity associated with combined gentamicin-amphotericin therapy. Nephron *19:*176–181, 1977.
109. Butkus DB, deTorrente A, Terman DS: Renal failure following gentamicin and combination with clindamycin. Nephron *17:*307–313, 1976.
110. Wade JC, Smith CR, Petty BG, Lipsky JJ, Conrad G, Ellner J, Leitman PS: Cephalothin plus an aminoglycoside is more nephrotoxic than methicillin plus an aminoglycoside. Lancet *2:*604–606, 1978.
111. Fanning WL, Gump D, Jick H: Gentamicin, and cephalothin-associated rises in blood urea nitrogen. Antimicrob Agents Chemother *10:*80–82, 1976.
112. Dellinger P, Murphy T, Pinn V, Barza M, Weinstein L: Protective effect of cephalothin against gentamicin-induced nephrotoxicity in rats. Antimicrob Agents Chemother *9:*172–178, 1976.
113. Cowan RH, Jukkola F, Arant BS: Pathophysiologic evidence of gentamicin nephrotoxicity in neonatal puppies. Pediatr Res *14:*204–211, 1980.
114. Barza M: The nephrotoxicity of cephalosporins: An overview. J Infect Dis *137:*S60–73, 1978.
115. Fulop M, Drapkin A: Potassium depletion syndrome secondary to nephropathy apparently caused by "outdated tetracycline." N Engl J Med *272:*986–989, 1965.
116. Benitz KF, Diermeier HF: Renal toxicity of tetracycline degradation products. Proc Soc Exp Biol Med *115:*930–935, 1964.
117. Shils ME: Renal disease and the metabolic effects of tetracycline. Ann Intern Med *58:*389–408, 1963.
118. Kuzucu EY: Methoxyflurane, tetracycline and renal failure. JAMA *211:*1162–1164, 1970.
119. Clausen G, Nagy Z, Szalay L, Aukland K: Mechanisms in acute oliguric renal failure induced by tetracycline infusion. Scand J Clin Lab *35:*625–633, 1975.
120. Whelton A: Tetracyclines in renal insufficiency: Resolution of a therapeutic dilemma. Ann NY Acad Med *54:*223–236, 1978.
121. Butler WT, Bennett JE, Alling DW, Wertlake PT, Utz JP, Hill GJ: Nephrotoxicity of amphotericin B: Early and late effects in 81 patients. Ann Intern Med *61:*175–187, 1964.
122. Medoff G, Kobayashi GS: Strategies in the treatment of systemic fungal infections. N Engl J Med *302:*145–155, 1980.
123. Andreoli TE: On the anatomy of amphotericin B–cholesterol pores in lipid bilayer membranes. Kidney Int *4:*337–345, 1973.
124. Weissmann G, Pras M, Hirschhorn R: A common mechanism for the fungicidal and nephrotoxic effects of amphotericin B. J Clin Invest *45:*1084, 1966.
125. Bathena DB, Bullock WE, Nuttall CE, Luke RG: The effect of amphotericin B therapy on the intrarenal vasculature and renal tubules in man. Clin Nephrol *9:*103–107, 1978.
126. Maddux MS, Barriere SL: A review of complications of amphotericin B therapy: Recommendations for prevention and management. Drug Intell Clin Pharm *14:*177–181, 1980.
127. de Weck AL: Immunopathological mechanisms and clinical aspects of allergic reactions to drugs. *In* de Weck AL, Bundgaard J (eds): Allergic Reactions to Drugs. New York, Springer-Verlag, 1983, pp 73–133.
128. Linton AL, Clark WF, Driedger AA, Turnbull DI, Lindsay RM: Acute interstitial nephritis due to drugs. Ann Intern Med *93:*735–741, 1980.
129. Nolan CR III, Anger MS, Keheller SP: Eosinophiluria: A new method of detection and definition of the clinical spectrum. N Engl J Med *315:*1516–1519, 1986.
130. Ditlove J, Weidmann P, Bernstein M, Massry SG: Methicillin nephritis. Medicine *56:*483–491, 1977.
131. Poole G, Stradling P, Worlledge S: Potentially serious side effects of high dose twice-weekly rifampicin. Br Med J *3:*343–346, 1971.
132. Mandell GL, Sande MA: Antimicrobial agents: Sulfonamides, trimethoprim-sulfamethoxazole and agents for urinary tract infections. *In* Gilman AG, Goodman LS, Rall TW, Murad F (eds): The Pharmacological Basis of Therapeutics. 7th ed. New York, Macmillan 1985, pp 1095–1114.
133. Balfour HH, Bean B, Laskin OL, et al: Acyclovir halts progression of herpes zoster in immunocompromised patients. N Engl J Med *308:*1448–1453, 1983.
134. Swanson BN, Boppana VK, Vlasses PH, Rotmensch HH, Ferguson BK: Norfloxacin disposition after sequentially increasing doses. Antimicrob Agents Chemother *23:*284–288, 1983.
135. Khanna BK: Acute gouty arthritis following ethambutol therapy. Br J Dis Chest *74:*409–414, 1980.
136. Jenner PJ, Ellard GA, Allan WGL, Singh D, Girling DJ, Nunn AJ: Serum uric acid concentrations and arthralgia among patients treated with pyrazinamide-containing regimens in Hong Kong and Singapore. Tubercle *62:*175–179, 1981.
137. Magera BE, Arroyo JC, Rosansky SJ, Postic B: Vancomycin pharmacokinetics in patients with peritonitis on peritoneal dialysis. Antimicrob Agents Chemother *23:*710–714, 1983.
138. Restrepo A, Stevens DS, Utz JP (eds): First international symposium on ketoconazole. Rev Infect Dis *2:*519–562, 1980.
139. Pont A, Williams PL, Williams DS, Loose E, Feld-

man RE, Reitz C, Bochra C, Stevens DA: Ketoconazole inhibits adrenal steroid synthesis. Ann Intern Med *97:*370–372, 1982.
140. Tuchker WS, Snell BB, Island DP, Gregg CR: Reversible adrenal insufficiency induced by ketoconazole. Arch Intern Med *253:*2413–2414, 1985.
141. Orme MLE: The clinical pharmacology of oral contraceptive steroids. Br J Clin Pharmacol *14:*31–42, 1982.
142. Takasu N, Yamada T, Miura H, Sakamoto S, Korenaga M, Nakajima K, Kanayama M: Rifampicin-induced early phase hyperglycemia in humans. Am Rev Resp Dis *125:*23–27, 1982.
143. Nelson WO, Bungle RG: The effect of therapeutic dosages of nitrofurantoin upon spermatogenesis in man. J Urol *77:*275–281, 1957.
144. Schulz KH: Cutaneous manifestations of drug allergy. *In* de Weck AL, Bundgaard H (eds): Allergic Reactions to Drugs. New York, Springer-Verlag, 1983, pp 135–162.
145. Bierman CW, Pierson WE, Zeitz SJ, Hoffman LS, VanArsdel PP: Reactions associated with ampicillin therapy. JAMA *220:*1098–1100, 1972.
146. Kerr RO, Cardamone J, Dalmasso AP, Kaplan ME: Two mechanisms of erythrocyte destruction in penicillin-induced hemolytic anemia. N Engl J Med *287:*1322–1325, 1972.
147. Parry MF: Toxic and adverse reactions encountered with new beta-lactam antibiotics. Bull NY Acad Med *60:*358–368, 1984.
148. Beutler E: Hemolytic anemia in disorders of red cell metabolism *In* Disorders of Red Cell Metabolism. New York, Plenum Publishers, 1978.
149. DeGowin RL: A review of the therapeutic and hemolytic effects of dapsone. Arch Intern Med *120:*242–248, 1967.
150. Weinstein L, Dalton AC: Host determinants of response to antimicrobial agents. N Engl J Med *279:*467–473, 1968.
151. Cohen RJ, Sachs JR, Wicker DJ, Conrad ME: Methemoglobinemia provoked by malaria chemoprophylaxis in Vietnam. N Engl J Med *279:*1127–1131, 1968.
152. McGregor RR, Bennett JE, Ersley AJ: Erythropoietin concentrations in amphotericin B-induced anemia. Antimicrob Agents Chemother *14:*270–273, 1978.
153. Richman DD, Fischl MA, Grieco MH, et al: The toxicity of AZT in the treatment of patients with AIDS and AIDS-related complex. N Engl J Med *317:*192–196, 1987.
154. Homayouni H, Gross PA, Setia U, et al: Leukopenia due to penicillin and cephalosporin homologues. Arch Intern Med *139:*827–828, 1979.
155. Rouveix B, Lassoued K, Vittecoq D, Regnier B: Neutropenia due to beta-lactamine antibodies. Br Med J *287:*1832–1834, 1983.
156. Laskin OL, Cederberg DM, Mills J, Eron LJ, Mildvan D, Spector SA: Gancyclovir for the treatment and suppression of serious infections caused by cytomegalovirus. Am J Med *83:*201–207, 1987.
157. Libman LG, Goldsmith KLG: Quinidine-induced thrombocytopenia. Proc R Soc Med *65:*590, 1972.
158. Grosset J, Leventis S: Adverse effects of rifampin. Rev Infect Dis *5S:*440–446, 1983.
159. Hochman R, Clark J, Rolla A, et al: Bleeding in patients with infections. Are antibiotics helping or hurting? Arch Intern Med *142:*1440–1442, 1982.
160. Brown CH, Natelson EA, Bradshaw W, Williams TW, Alfrey CP: The hemostatic defect produced by carbenicillin. N Engl J Med *291:*265–270, 1974.
161. Weitekamp MR, Aber RC: Prolonged bleeding times and bleeding diathesis associated with moxalactam administration. JAMA *249:*69–71, 1983.
162. Kerremans AL, Lipsky JJ, Van Loon J, Gallego MO, Weinshilboum RM: Cephalosporin-induced hypoprothrombinemia: Possible role for thiol methylation of 1-methyltetrazole-5-thiol and 2-methyl-1,3,4-thiadiazole-5-thiol. J Pharmacol Exp Ther *235:*382–388, 1985.
163. Panwalker AP, Rosenfield J: Hemorrhage, diarrhea, and superinfection associated with the use of moxalactam. J Infect Dis *147:*171–172, 1983.
164. Yunis AA: Chloramphenicol-induced bone marrow suppression. Sem Hematol *10:*225–234, 1973.
165. Dameshek W: Chloramphenicol aplastic anemia in identical twins—a clue to pathogenesis. N Engl J Med *281:*42–43, 1969.
166. Yunis AA, Miller AM, Salem Z, Arimura GK: Chloramphenicol toxicity: Pathogenetic mechanisms and role of the *p*-NO_2 in aplastic anemia. Clin Toxicol *17:*359–373, 1980.
167. Fonts JR, Brodie BB: The enzymic reduction of chloramphenicol, *p*-nitrobenzoic acid and other aromatic nitro compounds in mammals. J Pharmacol Exp Ther *119:*197, 1957.
168. Murray KT, Downey KM, Yunis AA: Degradation of isolated deoxyribonucleic acid mediated by nitroso-chloramphenicol. Biochem Pharmacol *31:* 2291–2296, 1982.
169. Alavi JB: Aplastic anemia associated with intravenous chloramphenicol. Am J Hematol *15:*375–379, 1983.
170. Fraunfelder FT, Bagby GC, Kelly DJ: Fatal aplastic anemia following topical administration of ophthalmic chloramphenicol. Am J Ophthalmol *93:*356–360, 1982.
171. Yunis AA, Smith US, Restrepo A: Reversible bone marrow suppression from chloramphenicol. Arch Intern Med *126:*272–275, 1970.
172. Yunis AA: Chloramphenicol toxicity and the role of the *p*-NO_2 in aplastic anemia. *In* Najean Y, Tognoni G, Yunid A (eds): Safety Problems Related to Chloramphenicol and Thiamphenicol therapy. New York, Raven Press, 1981, pp 17–29.
173. Tomoeda M, Yamamoto K: The hematologic adverse reaction experience with thiamphenicol in Japan. *In* Najean Y, Tognoni G, Yunid A (eds): Safety Problems Related to Chloramphenicol and Thiamphenicol. New York, Raven Press, 1981.
174. Levine BB: Immunologic mechanisms of penicillin allergy. N Engl J Med *275:*1115–1125, 1966.
175. Idsoe O, Guthe T, Willcox RR, DeWeck AL: Nature and extent of penicillin side reactions with particular reference to fatalities from anaphylactic shock. Bull WHO *38:*159, 1968.
176. Green GR, Peter GA, Geraci JE: Treatment of bacterial endocarditis in patients with penicillin hypersensitivity. Ann Intern Med *67:*235–249, 1967.
177. Adkinson NF Jr, Saxon A, Spence MR, Swabb EA: Cross-allergenicity and immunogenicity of aztreonam. Rev Infect Dis *7:*S613–S621, 1985.
178. Levine LR: Quantitative comparison of adverse reactions to cefachlor vs. amoxicillin in a surveillance study. Pediatr Infect Dis *4:*358–361, 1985.
179. Cream JJ, Turk JL: A review of the evidence for immune complex deposition as a cause of skin disease in man. Clin Allergy *1:*235–247, 1971.

180. St Clair K, Duvic M: Erythema multiforme. Intern Med *8*:113–125, 1987.
181. Gordin F, Simon GL, Wofey CB, et al: Adverse reactions to trimethoprim-sulfamethoxazole in patients with the acquired immunodeficiency syndrome. Ann Intern Med *100*:495–499, 1984.
182. Descotes J: Immunotoxicology of drugs and chemicals. New York, Elsevier Science Publishers, 1986.
183. Salmeron G, Lipsky PE: Immunosuppressive potential of antimalarials. Am J Med *74*:19–24, July 18, 1983 Suppl.
184. Pappaioanou M, Fishbein DB, Dreesen EW, et al: Antibody response to preexposure human diploid-cell rabies vaccine given concurrently with chloroquine. N Engl J Med *314*:280–284, 1986.
185. Grossman ER, Walcheck LA, Freedman H: Tetracyclines and permanent teeth. The relation between dose and tooth color. Pediatrics *17*:567–570, 1971.
186. Christ W, Lehnert T, Ulbrich B: Specific toxicologic aspects of the quinolones. Rev Infect Dis *10S*:141–146, 1988.
187. Cluff LE, Johnson JE: Drug fever. Prog Allergy *8*:149, 1964.
188. Gigliotti F, Shenep JL, Lott L, Thornton D: Induction of prostaglandin synthesis as the mechanism responsible for the chills and fever produced by infusing amphotericin B. J Infect Dis *156*:784–789, 1987.
189. Steere AC, Hutchinson GJ, Rahn DW, Sigal LH, Craft JE, DeSanna ET, Malawista SE: Treatment of early manifestations of Lyme Disease. Ann Intern Med *99*:22–26, 1983.
190. Gelfand JA, Elin RJ, Berry FW, Frank MM: Endotoxemia associated with the Jarisch-Herxheimer reaction. N Engl J Med *295*:211–213, 1976.
191. Leiker DL: The mononuclear syndrome in leprosy patients treated with sulfones. Int J Leprosy *24*:402–405, 1956.
192. Tattersal MHN, Battersby G, Spiers ASD: Antibiotics and hypokalemia. Lancet *1*:630–631, 1972.
193. Parker CW: Drug allergy. N Engl J Med *292*:511, 732, 957, 1975.

B. Anthelminthics

Shawn Gazaleh, M.D., FACEP
Terry Branson, M.D., FACEP

Helminthiasis is a most common disease worldwide. Billions of people are affected by it. Although many of the parasites are more or less unique to certain global areas, our shrinking world and rising immigration have insured them a place in the medical vocabulary of physicians worldwide. Other helminthic diseases are cosmopolitan, and their recognition and treatment are a part of any general medical practice.

However, we will not discuss the recognition and treatment of helminthic disease but instead the adverse effects of anthelminthics (or "antihelminthics"). Reports of actual poisoning by such drugs are few, but their adverse effects are protean and may be mistaken for the disease itself. In many cases, the adverse effects are temporary and require only "tincture of time." In other cases, the adverse effects may be cumulative and indeed fatal if not promptly recognized.

Two drugs in this group, diethylcarbamazine, and ivermectin, are sometimes accidentally ingested as they are found in the home as dog heartworm medicine. Treatment of overdose is primarily symptomatic and supportive.

Diethylcarbamazine

(Banocide, Hetrazan, Caricide, Carbilazine)

Diethylcarbamazine (1-diethylcarbamyl-4-methylpiperazine) is the drug of choice for the treatment of filariasis, including that caused by *Wuchereria bancrofti*, *W. malayi*, and *Loa loa*. It also may kill the adult filarial worm. It is found in the home as medicine for dog heartworm (*Dirofilaria immitis*).

It is effective against the microfilaria of *Onchocerca volvulus;* however, it has little action against the adult *O. volvulus*.

Diethylcarbamazine is highly soluble in water. It is readily absorbed from the gastrointestinal tract. It also has been used as a lotion for treatment of onchocerciasis.

Toxicity and Side Effects. The toxicity of diethylcarbamazine is very low. No deaths have been attributed to it.[1]

Untoward reactions believed to result directly from the drug include anorexia, nausea, vomiting, headache, weakness, and arthralgias.

In patients with onchocerciasis, a violent reaction may occur 16 hours after initiation of treatment, characterized by severe pruritus, tenderness and enlargement of lymph nodes, swelling and edema of skin, fever, headache, tachycardia, and occasionally a fine papular rash. These symptoms usually persist for a few days and then subside. After that, large doses can be tolerated without further reaction.

Encephalitis occurring during infection with *Loa loa* may be aggravated by treatment with diethylcarbamazine. A combination with steroids or the use of steroids initially may be preferable.

Changes in visual function and in the posterior segment of the eye may occur during treatment of onchocerciasis with diethylcarbamazine. Transient pigment lesions, optic disc leakage, and visual loss have occurred during therapy.[2] Transient proteinuria has been observed in some patients, the mechanism for which is uncertain. The possibility that circulating immune complexes are involved is being investigated.[3, 4]

Treatment. Treatment is symptomatic. Antihistamines are generally of no value. Betamethasone has been recommended for severe reactions that may occur during the treatment of onchocerciasis.

Ivermectin

(Ivomec, Eqvalan)

Ivermectin is a member of the family of compounds known generically as avermectins. They are macrocyclic lactones obtained from the fermentation broth of *Streptomyces avermetalis.* Given orally or parenterally, they are active against a broad range of nematode and arthropod parasites of domestic animals, as well as *Onchocerca volvulus,* causing human onchocerciasis (river blindness).[5, 6] Ivermectin is now used to treat dog heartworm and is found in the home.

Ivermectin appears to paralyze the parasite by potentiating the release and binding of gamma-aminobutyric acid (GABA) in certain nerve synapses and thereby blocking GABA-mediated postsynaptic transmission of nerve impulses.[7–10]

Toxicity and Side Effects. Adverse reactions to ivermectin are rare. They include pruritus, arthralgia, and dizziness.

Treatment. Symptomatic and supportive.

Antimony Compounds

Antimonial compounds are no longer recommended for the treatment of helminthiasis. They have been replaced with newer, less toxic agents.

Trivalent antimonial compounds exert their anthelminthic effect via inhibition of phosphofructokinase.[11] Phosphofructokinase is an enzyme that catalyzes the rate-limiting step in glycolysis. Antimony compounds are administered parenterally only because they irritate the gastrointestinal tract. The trivalent compound leaves the plasma rapidly but remains in circulation as a result of binding by the erythrocytes. Consequently, renal excretion is slow, and the compound tends to accumulate. It may be detected in the urine for several weeks to months after therapy.

Several antimonial compounds are useful against schistosomiasis. Antimony potassium tartrate is the drug of choice against *Schistosoma japonicum.* Antimony sodium dimercaptosuccinate is a drug of choice against *S. haematobium* and *S. japonicum.* Stibophen is a useful alternative to niridazole or antimony sodium dimercaptosuccinate in the treatment of *S. mansoni.*[12] The dosage and schedule for treatment, as well as the duration of therapy, vary according to the disease and which compound is being used.

Toxicity and Side Effects. The use of trivalent antimonial compounds is contraindicated in hepatic disease unless such disease is a result of schistosomiasis. Electrocardiographic changes may occur but usually are not clinically relevant. However, when bradycardia occurs, the drug may need to be discontinued. Other observed adverse effects include pneumonia—especially after the use of tartrates, severe coughing, arthralgias, arthritis and myalgias, headaches, fainting, dyspnea, apnea, abdominal pain, vascular collapse, facial edema, and skin rashes. Hepatic function may be depressed, and the possible, although rare, complication of hepatitis will contraindicate further use of the compound. Anaphylactoid reaction may occur during the treatment.

Particular side effects associated more specifically with certain antimonial compounds are shown in Table 53–17. Pentavalent antimonial compounds are used to treat protozoal infections. Their side effects are similar to those of trivalent antimonials, but they are

Table 53–17. ADVERSE EFFECTS OF ANTIMONY COMPOUNDS

Dimercapto-succinate	Fever, fatigue, rashes, vomiting. Contraindicated in the presence of bacterial infection or infection of herpes simplex or zoster
Stibophen	Hemolytic anemia, thrombocytopenia, vomiting, albuminuria. Discontinue drug if any of these or complicating febrile infection occur
Tartrates—especially potassium tartrates	Phlebitis, cough, vomiting. Maybe fatal reactions from too rapid injection

less toxic and and are cleared much more rapidly via the kidneys.

Treatment. Treatment is symptomatic and consists of discontinuing the trivalent or pentavalent antimonial if the reaction is severe. Supportive care may be required.

Bephenium Hydroxynaphthoate

Bephenium hydroxynaphthoate is a quaternary ammonium compound introduced by Coop and associates for the treatment of hookworm infections.[13]

Goodwin and colleagues in 1958 showed that it compared favorably in effectiveness with tetrachloroethylene, had no toxic side effects, and was also effective against roundworm.[14]

It is minimally absorbed from the gastrointestinal tract.

The dosage for adults is 5 gm twice daily for 1 day for *Ancylostoma duodenale* and for 3 days for *Necator americanus.*

Toxicity and Side Effects. Bephenium hydroxynaphthoate has no serious side effects. It has a bitter taste and may cause nausea and vomiting.

Treatment. Symptomatic and supportive. In severe cases, the drug should be withdrawn.

Bithionol

Bithionol (2,2′-thio,bis[4,6-dichlorophenol]) is the treatment of choice for human fascioliasis. The usual dose is 30 to 50 mg per kg of body weight per day for 10 to 15 days. A single dose of 45 gm for an adult and half that for children was successful in one outbreak.[15]

For the treatment of paragonimiasis, it is given orally in a dose of 30 mg per kg of body weight on alternate days for 20 days.[16]

Toxicity and Side Effects. Skin reactions and gastrointestinal irritation are rarely severe enough to interrupt treatment.

Treatment. Symptomatic and supportive.

Flubendazole

Flubendazole (methyl [5-*p*-fluorobenzoyl]-2-benzimidazole carbamate) is a member of the benzimidazole family and is a parafluoro analogue of mebendazole. It is a relatively new anthelminthic produced by Janssen Pharmaceuticals, Belgium. A recent study of its efficacy and side effects pointed toward its usefulness in the treatment of hookworm, *Trichuris trichiura* (whipworm), and *Ascaris lumbricoides* (roundworm).

Toxicity and Side Effects. Side effects are vague and include nausea, abdominal pain, abdominal rumbling, the passage of soft stools and diarrhea, dyspepsia, mild fatigue, and breathlessness.[17]

Unlike mebendazole, flubendazole has not been shown to be teratogenic in animals.

Treatment. Symptomatic and supportive. In severe cases, the drug should be withdrawn.

Hycanthone

(Etronol)

Hycanthone (1-[[2-(diethylamino)ethyl]-amino]-4-(hydroxmethyl)-9H-thioxanthen-9-one) is a metabolite of lucanthone.[18] It is effective against *Schistoma haematobium* and *S. mansoni.* The mechanism of action is unknown.

Enteric hycanthone tablets are well absorbed from the gastrointestinal tract; however, a single intramuscular injection of 200 mg may suffice for the entire treatment.

The drug is not marketed in the United States.

Toxicity and Side Effects. Untoward reactions to hycanthone are very frequent but self-limiting. They include gastrointestinal disturbances with nausea, vomiting, abdominal pain, generalized weakness, dizziness, headache, and myalgias.

A very serious but infrequent adverse effect is hepatic necrosis.

Hycanthone exhibits mutagenic,[19] carcinogenic,[20] and teratogenic effects in animals.[21] The importance of these effects in the treatment of human schistosomiasis is not clear.

Its use should be avoided in pregnant women and for at least 1 month after a woman has given birth.

It should not be administered to children, young adults, or patients with liver damage.

Treatment. Treatment is symptomatic. The use of concomitant drugs that may affect the liver should be avoided.

Levamisole or Tetramisole

(Anthelvet, Ripercol, Ketrax)

Levamisole and tetramisole are racemics. Levamisole, the L-isomer, is more nematocidal and is available separately as Ketrax. The action of levamisol is due to ganglionic stimulation, which produces a rapid and reversible muscular paralysis in the helminth. At higher concentrations, it also inhibits the fumarate reductase enzyme system of the helminth, and some of its nematocidal activity may be due to this. The drug is rapidly absorbed and extensively metabolized.[22]

Levamisole is effective against various nematodes, but it is useful most specifically in the treatment of ascariasis. (Mebendazole and pyrantel pamoate, however, are the drugs of choice against this parasite.)[12]

Treatment for ascariasis requires only a single dose of 120 to 150 mg. There are few adverse effects, and the cure rate is high when this regimen is followed.

Toxicity and Side Effects. Levamisole has also been shown to be an immunostimulant, and many of its adverse effects have been exposed during its experimental use in regard to rheumatoid arthritis, other collagen vascular diseases, and malignancies. A study of patients with Sjögren's syndrome who were treated with levamisole was abandoned because of the side effects attributed to this drug, which included confusion, insomnia, weakness, pruritus, rash, headache, muscular pain, and increase in articular pain and swelling.[23] Levamisole also has been shown to produce agranulocytosis when used over a prolonged period and at high dosage.[24]

Treatment. Symptomatic and supportive. The drug should be withdrawn.

Mebendazole

(Vermox)

Mebendazole (methyl *N*-[5(6)-benzoyl-2-benzimidazol-yl] carbamate) is a member of the benzimidazole family and is the parent compound of flubendazole. It selectively and irreversibly blocks the glucose uptake by nematodes and cestodes. However, it does not affect blood glucose levels in treated patients.[25]

Mebendazole is a drug of choice against *Enterobius vermicularis* (pinworm), *Necator americanus* and *Ancylostoma duodenale* (North American and European hookworm), *Trichuris trichiura* (whipworm), and *Ascaris lumbricoides* (roundworm).[12] For trichuriasis, ascariasis, and hookworm infection, the dosage is 100 mg twice daily for 3 days. For enterobiasis, one 100-mg tablet is sufficient.[25]

Mebendazole is also quite effective against certain nematodes (e.g., *Capillaria phillippinensis*) and may be a useful adjunct to surgery in the management of hydatid disease.[26]

Toxicity and Side Effects. Mebendazole is poorly absorbed from the gastrointestinal tract,[27] and, when compared with the other anthelminthics, it is well tolerated. On occasion, it may cause diarrhea and abdominal pain.[25] Pyrexia may be observed when mebendazole is used in the treatment of hydatid disease, but this likely represents tissue necrosis in the cyst rather than a toxic effect of the drug.[28] Mebendazole is teratogenic and embryotoxic in animals; therefore, its use is contraindicated during pregnancy.[12] Its use is not recommended in children under 2 years of age because of limited experience with the age group.

Treatment. Symptomatic.

Metrifonate

(Bilarcil)

Metrifonate (0,0-dimethyl-Cl-hydroxy-2,2,2-trichloroethyl phosphonate) is an organophosphorus compound that was introduced in 1951 as an insecticide[29] and in 1960 as a drug for the treatment of schistosomiasis.[30]

Metrifonate, also called trichlorfon, is an inhibitor of plasma cholinesterase activity. Erythrocyte acetylcholinesterase is inhibited to a lesser degree.

The drug is very effective in the treatment of *Schistosoma haematobium* infections.

The dosage is 5 to 15 mg per kg given orally three times at intervals of 2 weeks.

Toxicity and Side Effects. Toxic doses of metrifonate produce symptoms that are typical of cholinergic drugs.

Several cases of suicide attempts with metrifonate were reported from the Soviet Union, Poland, Rumania, and Japan. Polyneuropathy was seen in approximately 24 per cent of the patients.[31, 32]

Treatment. Treatment is symptomatic. Atropine has been used in severe cases.

Niclosamide

(Yomesan)

Niclosamide (N-2[2′-chlorosalicylamide]) is considered the most effective agent for the treatment of cestodes. It is not absorbed from the gastrointestinal tract and is excreted in the feces.[33]

Toxicity and Side Effects. Niclosamide is well tolerated by patients, with almost no side effects. An occasional patient may have gastrointestinal symptoms. It has no toxic effect on the bone marrow or on hepatic or renal function.[34]

Treatment. Symptomatic.

Niridazole

(Ambilhar)

Niridazole, 1-(5-nitro-2-thiazol-yl)-2-imidazolidinone, is used in the treatment of schistosomiasis. It has also been used in the treatment of amebiasis.

Niridazole also has been shown to be a potent long-acting suppressant of cellular hypersensitity[35] and possibly is carcinogenic.[36]

The drug is absorbed from the gastrointestinal tract. It is excreted in the urine and feces. Its presence confers a dark color in the urine.

Toxicity and Side Effects. Niridazole may cause slight electrocardiographic and electroencephalographic changes, vomiting, abdominal pain, dizziness, agitation, hallucinations, seizures, headache, insomnia, and rash.

Less frequently, it may cause psychosis and hemolytic anemia in glucose-6-phosphate dehydrogenase-deficient individuals.[37]

Niridazole should not be used in patients with seizure disorders or liver disease.

Treatment. Symptomatic and supportive.

Oxamniquine

(Vansil, Mansil)

Oxamniquine is an antischistosomal drug mainly effective against *S. mansoni.*[38] It is readily absorbed after oral administration. Most of an administered dosage is excreted in the urine. A very small portion is excreted unchanged. It may give the urine a dark orange or reddish color on the second day of treatment; a metabolite of the drug is suspected of being responsible for this.

The dosage of oxamniquine depends upon the geographic location and strain of *S. mansoni.* It varies from 12 mg per kg given as a single dose to 60 mg per kg given over 3 days.

Toxicity and Side Effects. Oxamniquine is well tolerated by the oral route. Side effects include dizziness, headache, vague abdominal pain, nausea, and vomiting.

Liver function studies may show mild elevation of the transaminase levels in older patients, but such elevations are transient.

Fever has been reported. Its cause is uncertain.[39] It could be related to higher dosages of oxamniquine.[40]

Treatment. Symptomatic.

Piperazine

(Antepar, Vermizine)

Piperazine is effective against *Enterobius (oxyuris) vermicularis* and *Ascaris lumbricoides.* It is readily absorbed from the gastrointestinal tract and excreted essentially unchanged in the urine within 24 hours.

Piperazine, administered orally, causes flaccid paralysis of the helminth and, as a result, expulsion of the worm from the intestine.

In ascariasis, the usual dosage is 75 mg per kg, with a maximum of 3.5 gm as a single daily dose for 2 consecutive days.

In oxyuriasis, the usual daily dosage is

65 mg per kg, with a maximum of 2.5 gm given for 7 days.

Toxicity and Side Effects. Adverse reactions to piperazine are rare. They include nausea, vomiting, abdominal pain, diarrhea, rash, fever, weakness, seizures, electroencephalographic abnormalities, visual disturbances, and cerebellar ataxia (wobble worm).[41]

The drug is contraindicated in patients with hepatic or renal dysfunction and in those with seizure disorders. Its safety in pregnancy has not been established.

Treatment. Discontinue medication. Administer antihistamines. Treat the patient symptomatically.

Poquil

Poquil is a cyanine dye known as 6-dimethylamino-2[2-(2,5-dimethyl]-1-phenyl-3-pyrryl) vinyl[-1-methyl]-1-unolinium chloride dihydrate. In a dose of 1.5 mg per kg per 24 hr for 8 days, it has been shown to be effective in the treatment of oxyuriasis.[42]

Toxicity and Side Effects. Poquil is well tolerated. It leaves a slightly bitter aftertaste. Occasionally, it may cause nausea and vomiting. It does not appear to be hepatotoxic or nephrotoxic.

Treatment. Symptomatic and supportive. In severe cases, the drug should be withdrawn.

Praziquantel

(Droncit)

Praziquantel is a compound effective against cestodes and schistosomes.[43–45] It is readily absorbed from the gastrointestinal tract.

The drug and its metabolites are excreted by the kidneys. It is administered in a single oral dose of 25 mg per kg.

Toxicity and Side Effects. No untoward effects from proziquantel have thus far been reported.

Pyrantel Pamoate

(Combantrin, Antiminth)

Pyrantel pamoate is effective in the treatment of enterobiasis, *Ascaris lumbricoides,* and *Necator americanus.* It acts as a depolarizing neuromuscular blocking agent, which results in spastic neuromuscular paralysis in the parasite and thus expulsion from the host's intestine.[46]

The drug is poorly absorbed from the gastrointestinal tract. More than 40 per cent is excreted in the feces. Small amounts of the drug and its metabolites are detected in the urine.

Pyrantel pamoate is administered in a dosage of 11 mg per kg.

Toxicity and Side Effects. Pyrantel pamoate is generally well tolerated. The most frequent side effects are nausea, vomiting, abdominal pain, headache, dizziness, insomnia, drowsiness, tenesmus, fever, nasal congestion, and rash.

Transient elevation of SGOT has been seen, and the drug should be used with caution in patients with liver disease. It should not be used in pregnant women and in children less than 1 year old.

Treatment. Symptomatic and supportive.

Pyrvinium Pamoate

(Povan, Vanquin)

Pyrvinium pamoate is effective in the treatment of oxyuriasis and strongyloidiasis.

It is minimally absorbed from the gastrointestinal tract and will color the stool red.

Toxicity and Side Effects. Untoward side effects are minimal. Occasionally, a patient may complain of nausea, vomiting, and abdominal pain. It rarely may cause a photosensitivity skin reaction.

Treatment. Symptomatic and supportive.

Thiabendazole

(Mintezol)

Thiabendazole (2-[4-thiazolyl]-H-benzimidazole), like mebendazole and flubendazole, is a member of the benzimidazole group of compounds. It mechanism of action is unknown, but its anthelminthic activity may derive from its inhibition of the helminth-specific enzyme fumarate reductase system. Thiabendazole is rapidly absorbed and is metabolized by the liver. Most of it is excreted within the first 24 hours by the kidneys.

Thiabendazole is a drug of choice against cutaneous larva migrans (creeping eruption), visceral larva migrans, *Strongyloides stercoralis,* and *Trichostrongylus* species.[12] It is also effective against *Necator americanus* (hookworm) and has been used in conjunction with corticosteroids and other anti-inflammatory agents against *Trichinella spiralis.* However, examinations of deltoid biopsy specimens from patients treated with thiabendazole for trichinosis have revealed motile larvae, casting some doubt upon its usefulness in this disease.[12]

Recent research suggests that topical thiabendazole may be efficacious in the treatment of cutaneous larva migrans.[47]

Toxicity and Side Effects. Adverse reactions to thiabendazole therapy are numerous and may limit the usefulness of this drug. Loss of appetite and nausea often may occur. Other adverse effects include dizziness, headache, drowsiness, weakness, tinnitus, blurred vision, diarrhea, epigastric discomfort, and pruritus. Hypotension, bradycardia, crystalluria, and malodorous urine also have been noted, as well as self-limited leukopenia. SGOT elevation, jaundice, elevated blood glucose, and cholestasis also have been observed. Nephrotoxicity is possible.[48]

A recent report linked theophylline toxicity with thiabendazole and suggested that thiabendazole may somehow inhibit hepatic metabolism of theophylline.[49] Hypersensitivity reactions associated with thiabendazole therapy occur frequently and include fever, chills, skin rashes, angioedema, erythema multiforme, Stevens-Johnson syndrome, and anaphylaxis.

Treatment. Most of the adverse effects of thiabendazole are transient and should require only symptomatic management. In regard to its metabolism by the liver and the occasional rise of the SGOT seen during its use, one should avoid this drug in persons with liver disease. It also seems reasonable to monitor the levels of concomitant drugs that are metabolized by the liver when thiabendazole is in use. The safety of thiabendazole has not been established in pregnancy or during lactation. Also, since this medication may cause drowsiness, patients should be warned against driving, operating machinery, and so forth, while under treatment.

References

1. Hawkings F: Diethylcarbamazine and new compounds for the treatment of filariasis. Adv Pharmacol *16:*129, 1979.
2. Bird AC, Hadi EL Sheikh, Anderson J, Fuglsang H: Changes in visual function and in the posterior segment of the eye during the treatment of onchocerciasis with diethylcarbamazine citrate. Br J Ophthalmol *64:*191, 1980.
3. Ngu JL, Mate A: Proteinuria associated with diethylcarbamazine. Lancet *1:*710, 1980.
4. Greene BM, Taylor HR, Humphrey RL: Proteinuria associated with diethylcarbamazine treatment of onchocerciasis. Lancet *1:*254, 1980.
5. Aziz MA, Diallo S, Diop IM, Lariviere M, Porta M: Efficacy and tolerance of ivermectin in human onchocerciasis. Lancet *2:*171, 1982.
6. Awadzi K, Dadzie KY, Shulz-Key H, Haddock DRW, Gilles HM: The chemotherapy of onchocerciasis X. An assessment of four single-dose treatment regimes of MK-933 (ivermectin) in human onchocerciasis. Ann Trop Med Parasitol 79-1:63, 1985.
7. Wang CC, Pong SS: Actions of avermectin B_{1a} on GABA nerves. Prog Clin Biol Res *97:*373, 1982.
8. Campbell WC, Fisher MH, Stapley EO, et al: Ivermectin, a new potent antiparasitic agent. Science *221:*823, 1983.
9. Campbell WC: An introduction to the avermectins. NZ Vet J *29:*174, 1981.
10. Pong SS, Wang CC, Fritz LC: Studies on the mechanism of action of avermectin $B_{1a:}$ Stimulation of release of gamma-aminobutyric acid from brain synaptosomes. J Neurochem *34:*351, 1980.
11. Katz M: Anthelmintics. Drugs *13:*124, 1977.
12. Drugs for Parasitic Infections. Med Lett *20:*17, 1978.
13. Coop FC, Standen OD, Scarnell J, Rawes DA, Burrows RB: A new series of anthelmintics. Nature (Lond) *181:*183, 1958.
14. Goodwin LG, Hayewarden LG, Standen OD: Clinical trials with bephenium hydroxynaphthoate against hookworm in Ceylon. Br Med J *2:*1572, 1958.
15. Hardman EW, Jones RLH, David HA: Fascioliasis; A large breakout. Br Med J *2:*502, 1971.
16. Yokogawa M, Okwa T, Tsuji M, Iwaski M, Shigeyasu M: Chemotherapy of paragonimiasis with bithionol. The follow-up studies for one year after treatment with bithionol. Jap J Parasitol *11:*103, 1962.
17. Bunnag D, Haunasuta T, Jarupakorn U, Chindanond D, Desakorn V: Clinical trial of flubendazole on hookworm, *Trichuris trichiura* and *Ascaris lumbricoides* infections. Southeast Asian J Trop Med Public Heatlh *2:*363, 1980.
18. Rosi D, Peruzotti G, Dennis EW, Bebberian D, Freeze H, Archer S: A new active metabolite of "Miracil D." Nature (Lond) *208:*1005, 1965.
19. Batzinger RP, Buedine E: Mutagenic activity in vitro and in vivo of five antischistosomal compounds. J Pharmacol Exp Ther *200:*1, 1977.
20. Vulay O, Urman H, Kashirath P, Clayson D, Shubik P: Carcinogenic potential of hycanthone in mice and hamsters? Int J Cancer *23:*97, 1979.
21. Moore JA: Teratogenicity of hycanthone in mice. Nature (Lond) *239:*107, 1972.

22. Adams JG: Pharmacokinetics of levamisole. J Rheumatol *137*(Suppl 4):142, 1978.
23. Tangsrud SE, Golf S: Sjögren's syndrome: A contraindication to levamisole treatment? Br Med J *2*:1386, 1977.
24. Thompson KS, Herbrick JM, Klassen LW, Severson CD, Overlin LV, Blaschke JW, Silverman MA, Vogel CL: Studies on levamisole-induced agranulocytosis. Blood *56*:388, 1980.
25. Keystone JS, Murdoch JK: Mebendazole: Diagnosis and treatment, drugs five years later. Ann Intern Med *91*:582, 1979.
26. Bekhti A, Schaaps J-P, Capron M, Dessaint J-P, Santoro F, Capron A: Treatment of hepatic hydatid disease with mebendazole: Preliminary results in four cases. Br Med J *2*:1047, 1977.
27. Brugmans JP, Thienport DC, Wingaarden I, Vanparijs OF, Schremans VL, Lauvers HL: Mebendazole in enterobiasis; Radiochemical and pilot clinical study in 1278 subjects. JAMA *217*:313, 1971.
28. Beach RC, Clayden GS, Ekyn SJ: Complications of mebendazole treatment for hydatid disease. Br Med J *2*:1111, 1979.
29. Lorenz W, Henglein A, Schrader G: The new insecticide 0,0-dimethyl-2,2,2,trichloro-1-hydroxy ethyl phosphate. J Am Chem Soc *77*:2254, 1955.
30. Lebrun A, Cerf J: Note preliminair sur la toxicité (Dipterex). Bull WHO *22*:579, 1960.
31. Lobzin VS, Tsimovol PE: Neurological disorders in chlorophos poisoning. Zh Nevropat Psikhiat *69*:679, 1967.
32. Akimov GA, Buchko VM, Kremleva RV: Neurological disorders in chlorophos poisoning. Klin Med (Mosk) *5*:65, 1975.
33. Keeling JED: The chemotherapy of cestode infections. Adv Chemother *3*:109, 1968.
34. Abdallah A, Saif M: The efficacy of N-2'-chloro-4'-nitrophenyl-5-chlorosalicylamide in the treatment of taeniasis. J Egypt Med Assoc *44*:379, 1961.
35. Mahmoud AA, Mandel MA, Warren KW, Webster LT: Niridazole, a potential long-acting suppressant of cellular hypersensitivity. J Immunol *114*:279, 1975.
36. Bulay O, Patil K, Wilson R, Shubik P: Kidney tumors induced in rats by the antischistosomal drug niridazole. Cancer Res *39*:4996, 1979.
37. Doyen A, Lèonard J, Mbendi S, Sonnet J: Influence des doses therapeutiques du CIBA 32644-Ba sur l'hematopoiése des patients atteints de bilharziose et d'amibiase. Acta Trop (Basel) *24*:59, 1967.
38. daSilva LC, Sette H Jr, Obamone DAF, Saozalequezar A, Pumskas JA, Raia S: Further clinical trials with oxamniquine (UK4271), a new anti-schistosomal agent. Rev Inst Med Trop Sao Paulo *17*:307, 1975.
39. Higashi GI, Farid Z: Oxamniquine fever—drug induced or immune complex reaction? Br Med J *2*:830, 1979.
40. Jordon P: Oxamniquine and fever. Br Med J *2*:1366, 1979.
41. Parsons AC: Piperazine neurotoxicity: "Worm wobble." Br Med J *4*:792, 1971.
42. Roger A: Preliminary report on a new antioxyuritic, poquil. Can Med Assoc J *74*:297, 1956.
43. Thomas H, Andrews P: Praziquantel—A new cestodicide. Pesticide Sci *8*:556, 1977.
44. Katz N, Rocha RS, Chaves A: Preliminary trials with praziquantel in human infections due to *Schistosoma mansoni*. Bull WHO *57*:781, 1971.
45. McMahon JE, Kolstrup N: Praziquantel—A new schistosomicide against *Schistosoma haematobium*. Br Med J *2*:1396, 1979.
46. Greenwood R: Drug evaluation data. Pyrantel pamoate. Drug Intel Clin Pharmacol *6*:226, 1972.
47. Davis CM, Asrael RM: Treatment of creeping eruption with topical thiabendazole. Arch Dermatol *97*:325, 1968.
48. Clark RG, Lewis KHC: Death in sheep after overdose with thiabendazole. NZ Vet J *25*:187, 1977.
49. Sugar AM, Kearns PJ, Haulk AA, Rushing JL: Possible thiabendazole-induced theophylline toxicity. Am Rev Resp Dis *122*:501, 1980.

CHAPTER 54
ISONIAZID

Michael W. Shannon, M.D., M.P.H.
Frederick H. Lovejoy, Jr., M.D.

Isoniazid (INH) was introduced in 1952 and remains the most common antibiotic used in the treatment of tuberculosis.[1] Recently, because of an increase in the incidence of tuberculosis, INH has become more widely prescribed.[2–4] With this expanded use has come a greater frequency of INH poisoning.[3] Fortunately, a greater understanding of the biochemical mechanisms underlying its effects has led to the development of effective strategies for the treatment of INH intoxication.[1–3]

PHARMACOLOGY

Isoniazid, which contains a pyridine nucleus, is structurally related to the nutrients nicotinic acid (niacin, vitamin B_3), nicotinamide adenine dinucleotide (NAD), and pyridoxine (vitamin B_6) (Fig. 54–1). Its complete name, isonicotinic acid hydrazide, identifies INH as a congener of nicotinic acid.[1] Isoniazid has a primary pKa of 1.9.[5]

Isoniazid is rapidly absorbed from the gastrointestinal tract (primarily the small intestine), with peak serum concentrations achieved within 1 to 2 hours.[5] Absorption is delayed by the concomitant administration of antacids.[1] Once absorbed, INH is distributed throughout body water, having an apparent volume of distribution of 0.6 L/kg.[5] INH has negligible binding to plasma proteins.[5]

The primary metabolic pathway for INH is acetylation by the enzyme *N*-acetyltransferase. This enzyme is located in the liver and intestinal mucosa. Acetyltransferase has been identified as a polymorphic enzyme whose pharmacokinetic activity follows Michaelis-Menten (saturable) kinetics. Additionally, the activity of this enzyme is under the control of genetic (autosomal dominant) inheritance.[5] Phenotypically, slow and fast acetylators have been described. The slow acetylation enzyme is found in 50 to 60 per cent of American whites and blacks. Acetylator activity is responsible for a number of the pharmacokinetic differences observed in slow versus fast acetylators: (1) slow acetylators have a smaller first-pass effect than fast acetylators, (2) average serum INH concentrations are 30 to 50 per cent lower in fast versus slow acetylators, and (3) fast acetylators metabolize INH five to six times faster than slow acetylators. The elimination half-life of INH in fast acetylators is approximately 70 minutes compared with a mean of 3 hours in slow acetylators. The major metabolic products of INH metabolism are acetylisoniazid, isonicotinic acid, and hydrazine.[1, 5, 6]

Isoniazid and its (inactive) metabolites are excreted in the urine, with 75 to 95 per cent of a single dose being eliminated within 24 hours. Twenty-seven per cent of INH is excreted unchanged in slow acetylators in contrast to 11 per cent in fast acetylators.[5] The clearance of INH averages 46 ml/min.[5]

Isoniazid has a significant effect on several biochemical pathways (Table 54–1).

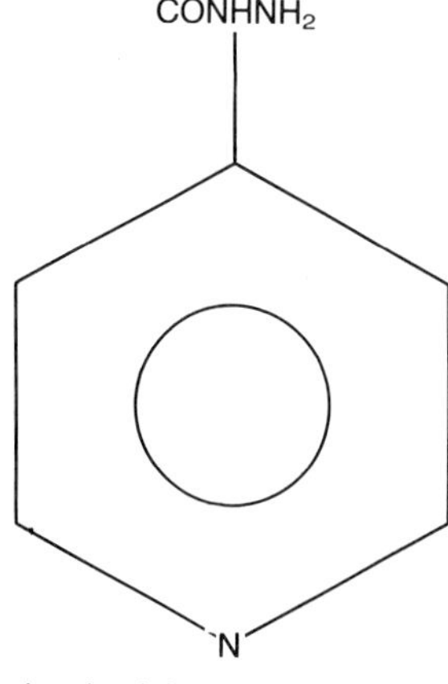

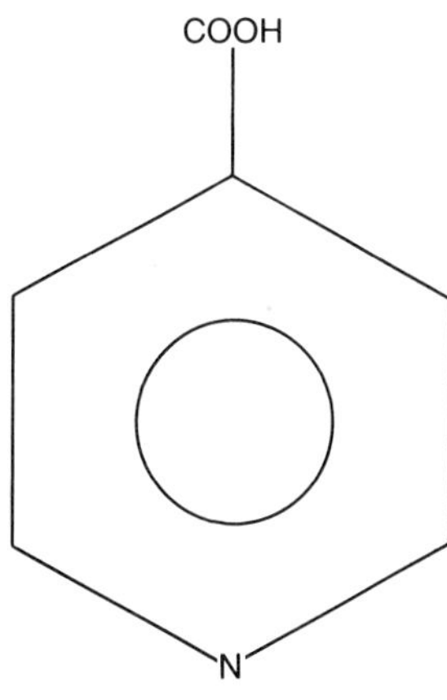

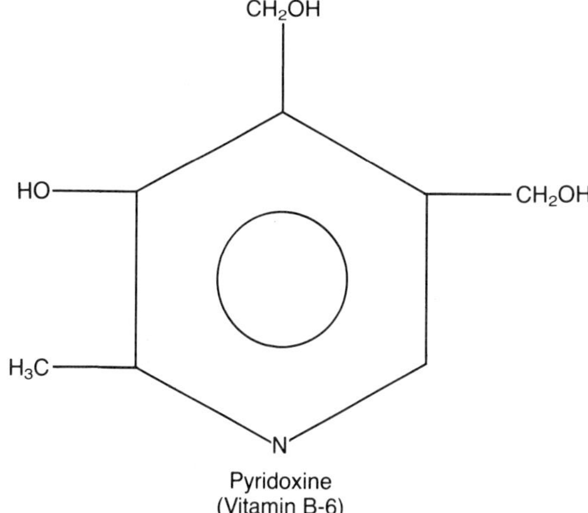

Figure 54–1. Structural relationships of isoniazid.

Table 54–1. METABOLIC ACTIONS OF ISONIAZID

BIOCHEMICAL EFFECT	CLINICAL EFFECT	REF
Inhibition of enzymes:		
P-450	↓ Metabolism of other drugs	8
Monoamine oxidase	Mood elevation	2
	↑ Sensitivity to tyramine	8
Glutamate decarboxylase	↓ GABA levels	9, 11, 18
GABA aminotransferase	↑ GABA levels	10
Apotryptophanase	Neuritis	2
Histaminase	↑ Sensitivity to scombroid spp.	8
Pyridoxine phosphokinase	↓ Conversion of pyridoxine to pyridoxal phosphate	9, 13
Transaminases	↓ Catecholamine synthesis	13
Decarboxylases		
Binds pyridoxal phosphate	↓ Pyridoxine activity	13
Replaces nicotinic acid, producing inactive NAD	Impaired glucose and fatty acid oxidation, metabolic acidosis	13–15, 18

Isoniazid is an inhibitor of several cytochrome P-450–mediated functions, particularly demethylation, oxidation, and hydroxylation.[7] INH also affects the enzymes involved in the metabolism of the central nervous system (CNS) neurotransmitter gamma-aminobutyric acid (GABA). GABA is the primary neurotransmitter at the motor inhibitory neurons of the CNS. GABA levels are regulated by two enzymes, glutamic acid decarboxylase (GAD) and GABA aminotransferase. GAD catalyzes the synthesis of GABA, whereas GABA aminotransferase promotes GABA breakdown. INH is an inhibitor of both enzymes but has a greater inhibitory effect on GAD, leading to reduced GABA levels.[8, 9] Reduction in GABA has been directly associated with the development of seizures.[10] Monomethylhydrazine, a constituent of mushrooms from the Gyromitra species, has a similar pharmacologic action.

Isoniazid's effect on pyridoxine metabolism is *pivotal* in the drug's toxicity. Pyridoxine activity is markedly reduced by INH, ultimately leading to clinical pyridoxine depletion. At least two mechanisms are responsible for this loss of pyridoxine activity: (1) INH inhibition of the enzyme pyridoxine phosphokinase, which converts pyridoxine to its active form, pyridoxal phosphate,[8, 11, 12] and (2) INH binding to pyridoxal phosphate, forming an inactive hydrazone complex that is excreted in the urine.[5, 12] Daily urinary excretion of pyridoxine is doubled with INH doses of 3 to 5 mg/kg and is quadrupled with INH doses of 20 mg/kg.[5] The consequences of pyridoxine depletion include impaired activity of pyridoxine-dependent transaminases and decarboxylases (including GAD). Inhibition of these enzymes also leads to a decrease in catecholamine synthesis.

Because of INH's structural similarity to nicotinic acid, it may replace nicotinic acid in the synthesis of NAD, forming an inactive compound.[5, 12–15]

Isoniazid readily crosses the placenta and enters breast milk. No teratogenic or mutagenic effects have been identified with INH use during pregnancy.[5]

CLINICAL TOXICOLOGY

Chronic Intoxication

Because of its biochemical effects, INH is associated with a myriad of adverse reactions when taken in therapeutic doses. The overall incidence of adverse drug reactions with INH is 5.4 per cent.[1] The most common of these are rash, fever, and abnormal liver function with the appearance of jaundice. INH-induced hepatotoxicity occurs in as many as 10 to 22 per cent of patients and is age dependent, appearing more often in older patients.[1, 5, 16–18] INH hepatotoxicity may result from the generation of hepatotoxic hydrazines.[1, 18] Less commonly, autoimmune phenomena occur, associated with the appearance of antinuclear antibodies. Autoimmune manifestations may include hemolytic anemia, thrombocytopenia or agranulocytosis, arthritis, vasculitis, and polyserositis.[5]

Peripheral or optic neuritis may also occur with INH use. Optic neuritis generally appears as decreased visual acuity (often unilateral).[1, 2] Symptoms of peripheral neuritis include paresthesias in a stocking-glove distribution, which may progress proximally.[2] Although primarily a sensory neuritis, myalgias, weakness, and ataxia may occur.[2] Neuritis is usually reversible and may be due to INH inhibition of the neuronal enzyme apotryptophanase.[2] The coadministration of pyridoxine with INH prevents the occurrence of neuritis.

Isoniazid may precipitate seizures in those with seizure disorder. In patients without a seizure history, an INH dose of 14 mg/kg is associated with a 1 to 3 per cent incidence of seizures.[1, 2] INH doses of 35 to 40 mg/kg uniformly produce seizures.

Significant drug interactions exist with INH.[2, 7] An effect on the anticonvulsant phenytoin has been well described; altered mental status (occasionally coma) has occurred in patients who were simultaneously prescribed INH and phenytoin, associated with the development of toxic serum phenytoin concentrations. Phenytoin toxicity has a frequency of up to 27 per cent and results from INH inhibition of cytochrome P-450 hydroxylases.[1, 7, 16] This decrease in phenytoin clearance tends to occur in the second week of combined treatment.[16] Other drugs whose elimination is reduced by concomitant administration of INH are carbamazepine, anticoagulants and rifampin.[7]

Isoniazid use also may have a significant effect on diet. Inhibition of the enzyme monoamine oxidase has been associated with an increased sensitivity to tyramine-containing foods; flushing, palpitations, and hypertension have been reported after such an ingestion. An inhibitory effect on the enzyme histaminase has led to adverse reactions after the ingestion of fish from the scombroid species.[2, 7]

Acute Intoxication

The acute ingestion of more than 1.5 gm of INH leads to minor toxicity, whereas ingestion of more than 6 to 10 gm is usually fatal without aggressive treatment.[2] *Severe INH toxicity correlates with serum INH concentrations of greater than 30 mcg/ml.*

Clinical manifestations of INH intoxication may appear as soon as 30 minutes after an ingestion.[2, 19, 20] Early signs and symptoms include nausea, vomiting, slurred speech, dizziness, mydriasis, and tachycardia. Subsequently, a cascade of biochemical events soon leads to the striking clinical features that characterize INH intoxication, namely, *recurrent seizures, severe metabolic acidosis, and coma* (Fig. 54–2).

Seizures after INH overdose are episodic and tend to occur at regular intervals; either hyper- or areflexia precedes their onset.[2] Improvement in consciousness may occur between seizures.[13] Once they begin, seizures are difficult to control despite the use of anticonvulsants.

Severe metabolic acidosis is another prominent feature of INH overdose. Although pH ranges of 6.8 to 7.3 are common, surviving victims may present with a systemic pH as low as 6.49.[19] The etiology of metabolic acidosis appears to be an increase in the generation of lactic acid as a result of the muscular activity of recurrent seizures. Experimental data have demonstrated that paralyzed animals with INH overdose do not develop severe metabolic acidosis.[11] However, other theories of metabolic acidosis have been proposed including (1) the generation of acidic INH metabolites, (2) an increase in ketoacids due to enhanced fatty acid oxidation, and (3) the formation of inactive NAD, leading to impairment of both glucose and fatty acid metabolism. The last-named theory has led to the suggestion that nicotinic acid be administered in INH overdose.[5, 12–15, 20]

Coma may be protracted after INH overdose (lasting more than 24 hours) and may continue after seizures have abated and metabolic acidosis has been corrected. This profound CNS depression has been attributed to CNS catecholamine depletion.[19]

Other clinical effects of acute INH intoxication are severe hypotension, hyperglycemia, acetonuria, abnormal liver function tests, and renal failure.[2, 13, 19] INH-induced renal failure is often exacerbated by the myoglobinuria, which develops from seizure-induced rhabdomyolysis.[15]

DIAGNOSIS

In the absence of history, INH overdose may be suspected in patients who present with the characteristic symptoms complex, particularly those in whom a high incidence of tuberculosis has been reported (e.g.,

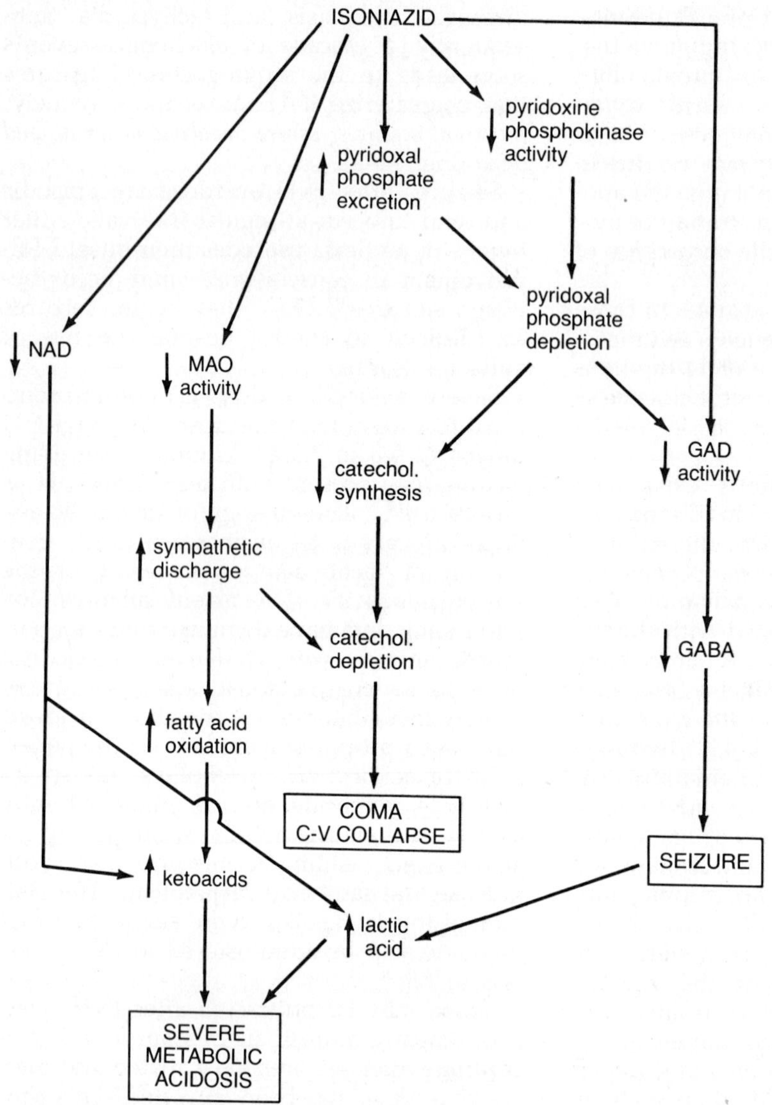

Figure 54–2. Proposed mechanisms of isoniazid toxicity.

Southwestern native Americans, recently immigrated Indochinese, those with AIDS).[2–4] The differential diagnosis of severe metabolic acidosis includes diabetic ketoacidosis and the ingestion of methanol, ethylene glycol, iron, ibuprofen, or salicylates. Of these, only INH overdose has recurrent seizures as its hallmark.

The toxic screen generally does not detect the presence of INH, although serum INH concentrations may be measured if intoxication is suspected. Other important laboratory tests are an arterial blood gas, electrocardiogram, electrolytes, liver function tests, creatine phosphokinase, and urinalysis.

MANAGEMENT (Table 54–2)

The initial management of INH intoxication requires stabilization of vital signs with provision of a patent airway and oxygen,

Table 54–2. SUMMARY OF TREATMENT STRATEGIES FOR ISONIAZID OVERDOSE

Supportive Care
- Ventilatory support
- Intravenous access
- Fluids and vasopressors

Gastrointestinal Decontamination
- Gastric lavage
- Activated charcoal
- Cathartic (osmotic or saline)

Pharmacologic Treatment
- Sodium bicarbonate to correct metabolic acidosis
- Benzodiazepines (diazepam or lorazepam)
- Pyridoxine: gram for gram per dose ingested, 5 gm if INH dose unknown; may be repeated if necessary
- Furosemide

Enhanced Elimination
- Forced diuresis
- ? Repetitive activated charcoal
- Hemodialysis

administration of sodium bicarbonate, and cardiovascular support with intravenous fluids and vasopressors.

If emergency department arrival is within 4 hours of ingestion, gastrointestinal decontamination with gastric lavage followed by the administration of activated charcoal with a cathartic is indicated. Ipecac-induced emesis is relatively contraindicated owing to the potentially rapid onset of seizures. Delayed absorption of INH after an overdose has not been observed, suggesting that late gastrointestinal decontamination may be ineffective. Interestingly, however, INH has a small volume of distribution and low protein binding, pharmacokinetic features which are found in drugs (e.g., aspirin, phenobarbital, theophylline) whose elimination is enhanced by multiple-dose activated charcoal.[21] Although speculation at this point, perhaps multiple-dose activated charcoal may be found effective for INH intoxication as well.

Intravenous pyridoxine has been shown to be highly effective for INH intoxication and should be administered to all symptomatic patients.[22] The milligram dose of pyridoxine should *equal* the ingested dose of INH. Pyridoxine (given as pyridoxine hydrochloride) has been shown to terminate seizures, correct metabolic acidosis, and abbreviate the duration of coma.[2, 23] The efficacy of pyridoxine is directly correlated with the administered dose; in one study, recurrent seizures occurred in 60 per cent of patients who received no pyridoxine, 47 per cent of those who received 10 per cent of the ideal pyridoxine dose, and 0 per cent of those who received a full dose of pyridoxine.[23] When the quantity of ingested INH is unknown, a pyridoxine dose of 5 gm is given. Repeated doses of pyridoxine may be required based on the resolution of signs and symptoms. Large doses of pyridoxine (up to 5 gm/kg) are tolerated without adverse effect.[3] Of note, pyridoxine is commonly dispensed in vials of 1 gm. A significant INH overdose may be sufficient to deplete the local supply of pyridoxine. Contingency plans should be created for access to pyridoxine in the event of multiple INH exposures within a brief period.

Conventional anticonvulsants remain important in the early treatment of seizures.[24] The benzodiazepines (e.g., intravenous diazepam) are agents of choice because they have a synergistic effect with pyridoxine as well as inherent GABA agonist activity.[2, 23–26] The prophylactic administration of benzodiazepines has no proven efficacy. Several authors have recommended against the use of phenytoin because of an apparent lack of efficacy and the potential for phenytoin intoxication.[2, 13] However, impaired phenytoin metabolism has only been documented after its use in chronic INH ingestion, not acute intoxication. Phenytoin may be an acceptable anticonvulsant, although its efficacy remains in question.[25] Phenobarbital, like the benzodiazepines, is a potent GABA agonist that may be effective in the treatment of seizures. However, phenobarbital may worsen CNS depression, especially if administered after a benzodiazepine.

Forced diuresis with furosemide or mannitol enhances the elimination of INH.[2, 14] Similarly, hemodialysis and peritoneal dialysis are effective in the treatment of INH intoxication. Seventy-five per cent of an INH dose may be removed within 5 hours by hemodialysis with clearance rates as high as 120 ml/min.[5] Hemodialysis should be reserved for patients who develop INH-induced renal failure.

References

1. Mandell GL, Sande MA: Isoniazid. *In* Gilman AG, Goodman LS, et al (eds): The Pharmacological Basis of Therpeutics. 7th ed. New York, Macmillan Publishing, 1985, pp 1199–1202.
2. Holdiness MR: Neurological manifestations and tox-

icities of the antituberculosis drugs—a review. Med Toxicol 2:33–51, 1987.
3. Blanchard PD, Yao JDC, McAlpine DE, et al: Isoniazid overdose in the Cambodian population of Olmstead County, Minnesota. JAMA *256*:3131–3133, 1986.
4. Anon: Tuberculosis and acquired immunodeficiency syndrome (AIDS)—New York City. MMWR *36*:785–794, 1987.
5. Weber WW, Hein DW: Clinical pharmacokinetics of isoniazid. Clin Pharmacol *4*:401, 1979.
6. Boxenbaum HC, Riegelman S: Pharmacokinetics of isoniazid and some metabolites in man. J Pharmacokinet Biopharm *287*:325, 1976.
7. Baciewicz AW, Self TH: Isoniazid interactions. South Med J *78*:714–718, 1985.
8. Holtz P, Parm D: Pharmacological aspects of Vitamin B-6. Pharm Rev *16*:113–178, 1964.
9. Wood JD, Paesker SJ: The effect on GABA metabolism in brain of isonicotinic acid hydrazide and pyridoxine as a function of time after administration. J Neurochem *19*:1527–1537, 1972.
10. Wood JD, Peesker SJ: A correlation between changes in GABA metabolism and isonicotinic acid hydrazide induced seizures. Brain Res *45*:489–498, 1972.
11. Chin L, Sievers ML, Herrier HE, et al: Convulsions as the etiology of lactic acidosis in acute isoniazid toxicity in dogs. Toxicol Appl Pharmacol *49*:377–384, 1979.
12. Mailler J, Robinson A, Percy AKL: Acute isoniazid poisoning in childhood. Am J Dis Child *134*:290–292, 1980.
13. Orlowski JP, Paganini EP, Pippenger CE: Treatment of a potentially lethal dose isoniazid ingestion. Ann Emerg Med *17*:73–76, 1988.
14. Pahl MV, Vaziri ND, Ness R, et al: Association of beta-hydroxybutyric acidosis with isoniazid intoxication. Clin Toxicol *22*:167–176, 1984.
15. DiAugustine RP: Formation in vitro and in vivo of the isonicotinic acid hydrazide analogue of nicotinamide adenine dinucleotide by lung nicotinamide adenine dinucleotide glycohydralase. Mol Pharmacol *12*:291–298, 1976.
16. Miller RR, Porter J, Greenblatt DJ: Clinical importance of the interaction of phenytoin and isoniazid. Chest *75*:356–358, 1979.
17. Byrd RB, Hom BR, Solomon DA, et al: Toxic effects of isoniazid in tuberculosis chemoprophylaxis. JAMA *241*:1239–1241, 1979.
18. Mitchell JR, Zimmerman HJ, Ishak KG, et al: Isoniazid liver injury: Clinical spectrum, pathology and probable pathogenesis. Ann Intern Med *84*:181–192, 1976.
19. Hankins DG, Saxena K, Faville RJ, et al: Profound acidosis caused by isoniazid ingestion. Am J Emerg Med *5*:165–166, 1987.
20. Terman DS, Teitelbaum DT: Isoniazid self-poisoning. Neurology *20*:299–304, 1970.
21. Levy G: Gastrointestinal clearance of drugs with activated charcoal. N Engl J Med *307*:676–678, 1982.
22. Sievers ML, Herrier RN: Treatment of acute isoniazid toxicity. Am J Hosp Pharmacol *32*:202–206, 1975.
23. Wason S, Lacouture PG, Lovejoy FH: Single high-dose pyridoxine treatment for isoniazid overdose. JAMA *246*:1102–1104, 1981.
24. Boehnert MT, Lewander WJ, Gaudreault P, et al: Advances in clinical toxicology. Pediatr Clin North Am *32*:193–211, 1985.
25. Chin L, Sievers ML, Herrier RN, et al: Potentiation of pyridoxine by depressants and anticonvulsants in the treatment of acute isoniazid intoxication in dogs. Toxicol Appl Pharmacol *58*:504–509, 1981.
26. Chin L, Sievers ML, Laird HE, et al: Evaluation of diazepam and pyridoxine as antidotes to isoniazid intoxication in rats and dogs. Toxicol Appl Pharmacol *45*:713–722, 1978.

CHAPTER 55
CHEMOTHERAPEUTIC AGENTS

Edith P. Mitchell, M.D.
Philip S. Schein, M.D.

Antineoplastic agents are distinguished by a low therapeutic index, reflecting their relative inability to discriminate effectively between normal and target tissues. As a generalization, they function preferentially against rapidly proliferating tissues, such as those of the bone marrow and gastrointestinal tract. Acutely, overdosage with most of the agents may cause leukopenia, granulocytopenia, thrombocytopenia, and hypoplasia of all elements of bone marrow. With repeated insult, the bone marrow eventually may develop a chronic hypoplastic state associated with a low-grade pancytopenia. This form of drug effect is readily measured during treatment with simple clinical and laboratory techniques, thus allowing for dose reduction, or cessation of therapy, before toxicity becomes severe.

The acute consequences and management of these complications are of special concern, since none of the agents are easily removed, once introduced into the body. Antidotes are not available, except in the case of methotrexate. The long-term consequences of antineoplastic treatment are now increasingly appreciated, particularly cumulative organ toxicity of insidious onset manifested clinically after the damage has become severe and irreversible.[1] These considerations have arisen in part because of the widespread use of this class of drugs, both for the treatment of cancer and as immunosuppressive and anti-inflammatory agents for non-neoplastic conditions.[2–5] As a result of recent advances in cancer chemotherapy, patients with specific forms of cancer have now benefited from intensive cytotoxic drug treatment to the extent that an approximately normal projected life expectancy has been achieved. An increasing number of patients who have undergone "curative" surgical treatment of cancer receive cytotoxic drugs as adjuvant therapy. In addition, many patients receive chemotherapy prior to surgical resection of tumor, or in combination with other therapy. As a result of widespread use of such antineoplastic and immunosuppressive drugs, an increasingly large population of patients is at risk of direct or indirect acute and long-term complications.

Although intentional overdoses of chemotherapeutic agents are rarely reported, inadvertent errors in dosage or administration have occurred. Attempts to increase excretion of the drugs, for the most part, have been unsuccessful except in the case of methotrexate, which is primarily eliminated by renal excretion. Increasing the excretion of other drugs is inhibited by a short half-life, as with nitrogen mustard; binding to albumin or other serum proteins; binding to tissues; active transport into cells; and high lipid solubility. These factors also account for the poor removal of the agents by dialysis or hemoperfusion techniques.[6] Thus the mainstay of management of either intentional or inadvertent overdoses is supportive care.

Management of the Patient with Methotrexate Overdose. Methotrexate toxicity is a common problem. Since its management is not only critical but also serves as a model for other anticancer drug toxicity, this will be discussed in detail. Methotrexate (MTX) is the only chemotherapeutic agent for which therapy significantly alters drug concentration or elimination; however, these measures require early diagnosis and rapid medical intervention for maximum benefit to prevent stomatitis, esophagitis, and oral ulceration. Furthermore, MTX is excreted primarily by the kidneys and in high doses may induce renal failure by its precipitation in renal tubules and collecting ducts.[7, 8] Immediate hydration with saline and sodium bicarbonate is necessary, to establish urinary flow in excess of 250 ml per hr, at a pH of 7 or above, for enhancement of MTX excretion.[9] Citrovorum rescue (Leucovorin, 15 to 100 mg per m^2) should be administered intravenously or orally and repeated every 6 hours for eight doses. For greatest effectiveness, this should be given within 42 hours of methotrexate administration. If possible, methotrexate plasma levels should be measured at 24 and 48 hours after the methotrexate dose. If the level exceeds 2.0×10^{-5} M at 24 hours or 9×10^{-7} M at 48 hours, then citrovorum factor should be continued an additional 48 hours or until the plasma measurement is below the critical level.[10]

Other investigational rescue methods that are not presently in general clinical use include administration of thymidine, which increases intracellular pools of thymidine triphosphate, carboxypeptidase G_1,[5] an enzyme that hydrolyzes and inactivates methotrexate.[11] Hemodialysis and hemoperfusion, although not particularly effective,[6] may be attempted in the presence of excessive methotrexate concentrations, especially if renal function is poor or deteriorates subsequent to methotrexate.[12, 13] Ventriculolumbar perfusion was reported beneficial in a patient following an inadvertent intrathecal dosage of 624 mg.[14]

Significant refinements in the use of antibiotics and blood products should lessen the infectious and bleeding complications.

GENERAL ANTICANCER DRUG TOXICITY AND ITS MANAGEMENT

An analysis of chronic toxicity is made complex by several factors. In many cases in which a drug-specific effect has become recognized, there are few estimates of the frequency of the toxic effect, or quantitative assessment of its severity, in relation to dose and duration of treatment. In addition, the drugs in question are largely employed in diseases that are in themselves systemic in nature and can produce specific organ complications that may be misinterpreted as drug-induced. It is also recognized that some of the observed late effects of treatment may not have resulted from a direct action of the drug on the specific tissue but could have arisen from the accompanying immunosuppression and enhanced predisposition toward specific pathogens, including, perhaps, carcinogenic change.

Pharmacology

The effective clinical use of cancer chemotherapeutic agents and the management of the unique problems consequent to their use require a general understanding of their pharmacology and the factors that alter absorption, transport, distribution, metabolism, and excretion. It is well recognized that these agents have a narrow therapeutic index and that in clinical practice toxicity is the rule rather than the exception. The result is adverse reactions in many organs, with the more rapidly dividing cell systems, in general, being more vulnerable.

Table 55–1 presents the basic pharmacology of the commonly used cancer chemotherapeutic agents, and Table 55–2 gives the more important toxic effects of the major anticancer drugs.

Gastrointestinal Toxicity

Chemotherapeutic drugs often profoundly affect the gastrointestinal tract, which may contribute significantly to the cachexia and malnutrition of the host. The rapid proliferation of the cell population in the crypt epithelium makes the gastrointestinal tract extremely vulnerable to direct toxicity from chemotherapeutic agents. In addition, other indirect effects, such as anorexia, nausea, vomiting, and diarrhea, are extremely common.

Nausea and Vomiting

Chemotherapy-induced nausea and vomiting are mediated by the vomiting center in the medullary reticular formation.[15, 16] The vomiting center lies close structurally to the chemoreceptor trigger zone (CTZ) in the area postrema of the fourth ventricle. Emesis results when the vomiting center is stimulated from the CTZ or afferent fibers located in the cerebral cortex, gastrointestinal tract (particularly the duodenum), heart, and vestibular apparatus.[17] Vomiting induced by various chemicals, drugs, and toxic substances, including apomorphine, cytotoxic agents, and radiation, is mediated through the CTZ.[15, 18, 19] The mechanisms by which compounds interact with the CTZ or how afferent vagal impulses are initiated are not known.[20]

Nausea and vomiting are the most common early manifestations of toxicity from antineoplastic therapy and may result in dehydration, electrolyte imbalance, weakness, and weight loss, depending on the severity and duration. There is great variability in the emetogenic properties of anticancer drugs, although specific agents such as cisplatin, imidazole carboxamide, DTIC, nitrogen mustard, and streptozocin produce vomiting in virtually all patients to whom they are administered.

Management of nausea and vomiting associated with chemotherapy requires judicious use of various classes of antiemetics by the most effective and convenient route. Compounds that exert an effect on the CTZ, such as the phenothiazines, have shown the greatest potential and are the most commonly used antiemetics. Corticosteroids and benzodiazepines are increasingly used. Antihistamines, which may be beneficial in motion sickness, have shown limited effectiveness in emesis associated with cancer chemotherapy,[21, 22] but may potentiate effectiveness or decrease toxicity when used in combination with other drugs.[23, 24] Table 55–3 lists commonly used antiemetics and recommended doses.

The psychologic effect of treatment, however, is emphasized by studies that have shown that placebo treatment may be effective. In a controlled double-blind study, Moertel and associates compared the effectiveness of several antiemetic drugs with placebo in patients receiving intravenous 5-fluorouracil.[25] The phenothiazine derivatives thiopropazate (Dartal), 10 mg, and prochlorperazine (Compazine), 5 mg, given orally three times daily, demonstrated superior antiemetic effect over placebo. Trimethobenza-

Table 55–1. PHARMACOLOGY OF CANCER CHEMOTHERAPEUTIC AGENTS

	Metabolism and Excretion	*Mechanism of Action*
ANTIMETABOLITES		
cytosine arabinoside	Deaminated to the corresponding uridine arabinoside in the liver and excreted in the urine. Some deamination occurs in the kidney	Competitive inhibitor of DNA polymerase
hydroxyurea	Urinary excretion	Inhibition of ribonucleotide reductase
5-fluorouracil	Detoxified by liver	Inhibits thymidylate synthetase
methotrexate	90% excreted in urine as intact compound	Inhibits dihydrofolate reductase
6-mercaptopurine excreted in urine; methylation of sulfur group	Converted to 6-thiouric acid in liver by xanthine oxidase—this enzyme is inhibited by allopurinol	Inhibits conversion of phosphoribosylpyrophosphate to the amine
6-thioguanine		
ANTIBIOTICS		
actinomycin D	Biliary	Intercalates DNA and inhibits RNA polymerases
doxorubicin and daunorubicin	Metabolized by soluble hepatic enzymes and excreted in bile	Intercalates DNA and inhibits RNA polymerases
bleomycin	Degraded by aminopeptidase and excreted in urine	Reacts with DNA, causing release of free bases
ALKYLATING AGENTS		
nitrogen mustard	Immediately reactive; rapidly decomposed	All introduce alkyl groups into DNA, RNA, and protein and cause cross-linking of DNA molecule
cyclophosphamide	Must be activated by liver microsomal oxidase system; metabolites excreted in urine	
phenylalanine mustard		
chlorambucil	Generally slow acting	
thiotepa	Formation of ethylenimonium ion is initial reaction	
busulfan	Slow urinary excretion	
chloroethyl nitrosoureas (BSNU), CCNU, MeCCNU, chlorozotocin	Highly lipid-soluble except chlorozotocin; metabolized by microsomal enzymes and excreted in the urine	
DTIC (dacarbazine)	Activated by liver microsomal system; 50% excreted unchanged by the kidney	
cis-dichlorodiamine II (cisplatin)	Rapidly bound to plasma proteins; primarily excreted by the kidney	

mide (Tigan) showed only slight advantage over placebo. In further investigations,[26] these researchers reported superior therapeutic effectiveness of thiethylperazine (Torecan), 10 mg, and thiopropazate (Dartal), 10 mg, over placebo. Chlorprothixene (Taractan) showed significant antiemetic activity but clinically intolerable sedative effects. Metoclopramide, which increases lower esophageal sphincter pressure and enhances gastric emptying, showed no therapeutic advantage. The investigators concluded that thiopropazate (Dartal), prochlorperazine (Compazine), and thiethylperazine (Torecan) are effective antiemetics when administered orally in standard doses. These agents, however, are associated with extrapyramidal and sedative effects that do not correlate with their antiemetic activity. Other agents with demonstrated efficacy in treating the nausea and vomiting associated with cancer chemotherapy include corticosteroids[27] and lorazepam,[28] droperidol,[29] haloperidol,[30] scopolamine,[31] metoclopramide,[47] and delta-tetrahydrocannabinol (THC).[32]

In 1975, Sallan and coworkers pursued reports from patients who described *decreased* nausea and vomiting from cancer chemo-

Table 55–2. MAJOR TOXICITIES OF CHEMOTHERAPEUTIC AGENTS

Generic Name	*Brand Name*	*Usual Single Dosage and Administration*	*Major Toxicity*
ALKYLATING AGENTS			
cyclophosphamide	Cytoxan	600–1500 mg/m² IV; 50–400 mg/m²/day PO	Moderate nausea, vomiting, and bone marrow suppression with higher doses. Occasional hemorrhagic cystitis
mechlorethamine	Mustargen	8–16 mg/m² IV	Severe nausea and vomiting, moderate bone marrow suppression; is a severe vesicant
melphalan (phenylalanine mustard, L-FAM)	Alkeran	2–10 mg/day PO	Bone marrow suppression
busulfan	Myleran	2–6 mg/day PO	Prolonged bone marrow suppression, may last weeks to months
chlorambucil	Leukeran	6–12 mg/day PO	Moderate bone marrow suppression
triethylenethiophosphamide	Thiotepa	0.2–1.0 mg/kg IV	Moderate bone marrow suppression
carmustine (BCNU)	BiCNU	100–130 mg/m² PO	Moderate nausea and vomiting; delayed myelosuppression
lomustine (CCNU)	CeeNu	100–200 mg/m² PO	Moderate nausea and vomiting; delayed myelosuppression
semustine (MeCCNU)		120–150 mg/m² PO	Moderate nausea and vomiting; delayed myelosuppression
dimethyl triazeno imidazole carboxamide (DTIC, dacarbazine)	Dacarbazine	2–10 mg/kg IV	Severe nausea and vomiting
streptozocin		1–2 gm IV	Severe nausea and vomiting; renal tubular dysfunction
VINCA ALKALOIDS			
vincristine	Oncovin	0.015–0.05 mg/kg IV	Alopecia, peripheral neuritis, paralytic ileus, constipation; is a severe vesicant
vinblastine	Velban	0.1–0.2 mg/kg	Same as vincristine. Bone marrow depression; a vesicant
EPIPODOPHYLLOTOXINS			
etoposide (VP-16)	Ve Pesid	100–200 mg/m² IV	Myelosuppression, alopecia, peripheral neuropathy
teniposide (VM-26)			Myelosuppression, alopecia, peripheral neuropathies
ANTIMETABOLITES			
methotrexate (amethopterin, MTX)	Methotrexate	2–5 mg/day PO 25–50 mg IV (conventional) 200 mg–10 gm IV (high dose)	Mucositis, myelosuppression. Renal failure, nausea, and vomiting with high dosage
5-fluorouracil (5-FU)	Fluorouracil	300–750 mg/m² IV	Mucositis, which may have a high mortality if bloody diarrhea occurs; myelosuppression
cytarabine (cytosine arabinoside, Ara-C)	Cytosar	1–3 mg/kg/day IV	Myelosuppression, moderate nausea and vomiting
6-mercaptopurine (6-MP)	Purinethol	100 mg/m²/day PO	Myelosuppression, hepatitis
6-thioguanine	Thioguanine	70–80 mg/kg/day	Myelosuppression
ANTIBIOTICS			
bleomycin	Blenoxane	10 mg/m² IV or SQ	Moderate nausea and vomiting, fever, chills, mucositis with ulcerations, pulmonary fibrosis
dactinomycin, actinomycin D (Act D)	Cosmegan	0.01–0.04 mg/kg IV	Mucositis with ulcerations, myelosuppression, moderate nausea and vomiting, alopecia
daunorubicin, doxorubicin	Adriamycin	30–45 mg/m² IV 60 mg/m² IV	Moderate nausea and vomiting, mucositis, alopecia, and myelosuppression. Cardiac toxicity with cumulative doses above 500 mg/m²; is a severe vesicant

Table 55–2. MAJOR TOXICITIES OF CHEMOTHERAPEUTIC AGENTS *Continued*

Generic Name	*Brand Name*	*Usual Single Dosage and Administration*	*Major Toxicity*
ANTIBIOTICS *(Continued)*			
mithramycin	Mithracin	25–50 μg/kg IV	Moderate nausea and vomiting, hypocalcemia, coagulation abnormalities, myelosuppression
mitomycin-C	Mutamycin	0.02–0.06 mg/kg IV	Mild nausea and vomiting, prolonged myelosuppression, TTP-like syndrome
MISCELLANEOUS			
cisplatin	Platinol	1–3 mg/kg IV	Severe nausea and vomiting, renal failure deafness
hydroxyurea	Hydrea	20–40 mg/kg PO	Myelosuppression
diethylstilbestrol (DES)		1–15 mg/day PO	Fluid retention, uterine bleeding, feminization in males, increase in serum calcium
fluoxymesterone	Halotestin	10–20 mg/day PO	Masculinization in females. Fluid retention
tamoxifen	Novaldex	10–30 mg/day	Increase in serum calcium
mitotane (op'DDD)	Nutitabe	1–10 gm/day	Diarrhea, tremors, mild nausea and vomiting
procarbazine	Matulane	50–300 mg/day	Myelosuppression, CNS depression, alcohol withdrawal syndrome
allopurinol	Zyloprim	100–300 mg/day	Skin rash, mild nausea and vomiting

therapy while being "high" after smoking marijuana. Subsequently this group reported the effectiveness of delta-9-tetrahydrocannabinol (THC), the major ingredient in marijuana, in relieving chemotherapy-associated nausea and vomiting.[32] Orally administered THC (15 or 20 mg) demonstrated superior activity compared with placebo. Complete or partial alleviation of symptoms was noted in 14 of 20 patients treated with THC, but in none of 22 treated with placebo. Chang and colleagues reported less nausea and vomiting in osteogenic sarcoma patients treated with high-dose methotrexate given with THC (10 mg PO q 3 h) compared with placebo.[33] Antiemetic activity correlated with increasing THC plasma concentrations. Plasma concentrations of 5.0, 5.0 to 10.0, and 10.0 ng/ml were associated with incidences of nausea, vomiting, or both of 44, 21, and 6 per cent respectively. The incidence of nausea and vomiting after the use of placebo cigarettes was 96 per cent, and the incidence of these symptoms was 83, 38, and 0 per cent, which corresponded to plasma concentrations of 5.0, 5.0 to 10.0, and 10.0 ng/ml respectively when marijuana cigarettes were used. Other patients receiving cyclophosphamide and doxorubicin, however, did not respond well to THC.

Lucas and Laszlo reported on the effectiveness of THC for patients with nausea and vomiting refractory to standard antiemetics.[34] Of 53 patients treated at doses of 5 to 10 mg per m^2 every 4 to 6 hours, 19 per cent reported complete alleviation of nausea and vomiting, 53 per cent reported a 50 per cent reduction of symptoms, and 28 per cent experienced no relief. Patients receiving chemotherapy with cisplatin did not respond well in general. A synthetic cannabinoid, nabilone, given orally also demonstrated antiemetic effectiveness superior to prochlorperazine in patients receiving cancer chemotherapy.[35]

We have conducted a randomized study comparing THC with prochlorperazine (Compazine) in patients refractory to standard antiemetic therapy.[36] Twenty-three of 36 (64 per cent) patients reported THC superior to prochlorperazine, and nine (25 per cent) experienced complete relief of symptoms with THC.

Side effects of THC, which included dizziness, somnolence, euphoria, and paranoid ideation, were acceptable to the patients in most studies. However, Frytak and associates reported that THC was no more effective than prochlorperazine and found that it had a greater incidence of unpleasant side effects.[37] This latter group was older than in former trials, and it is now accepted that the

Table 55–3. ANTIEMETICS

	Trade Name	*Common Dosage and Administration*
PHENOTHIAZINES		
chlorpromazine	Thorazine	10–20 mg PO q 4–6 hr 25–50 mg IM q 3–4 hr 50–100 mg by suppository q 6–8 hr
prochlorperazine	Compazine	5–10 mg PO q 4–6 hr 5–10 mg IM q 3–4 hr 25 mg by suppository q 4 hr
thiethylperazine	Torecan	10 mg PO q 4–6 hr 10 mg IM q 3–4 hr 10 mg by suppository q 4 hr
BUTYROPHENONES		
droperidol	Inaptine	2.5–10 mg IM q 4–6 hr 1.0–2.5 mg IV q 1 hr
haloperidol	Haldol	1.0–2.0 mg PO q 4–6 hr
CANNABINOIDS		
tetrahydro-cannabinol		5–15 mg/m² PO q 4 hr
nabilone		2 mg PO q 6–12 hr
CORTICOSTEROIDS		
dexamethasone	Decadron	4–20 mg IV q 6–8 hr 10–40 mg PO q 4–6 hr
methyl-prednisolone	Medrol	125–250 mg IV q 6 hr
ANTIHISTAMINES		
trimethobenzamide	Tigan	100 mg PO q 4–6 hr 100 mg IM q 4–6 hr
dephenhydramine	Benadryl	50 mg IV q 4–6 hr
SUBSTITUTED BENZAMIDES		
metoclopramide	Reglan	1–3 mg/kg IV
BENZODIAZEPINES		
diazepam	Valium	5 mg PO q 4–6 hr 2–5 mg IV q 4–6 hr
lorazepam	Ativan	1–4 mg IV q 6–8 hr 2–4 mg PO q 4–6 hr

Dosages may need adjusting depending on individual side effects and severity of symptoms.

elderly are at greater risk for adverse reactions.

The mechanisms for the antiemetic effect of THC are unknown.[38] It is clear that THC can be used effectively as an antiemetic in patients who experience nausea and vomiting from cancer chemotherapy.[39–41] Because of problems with the bioavailability of orally administered tablets, dosages and routes of administration deserve further study.

High-dose intravenous metoclopramide is an effective agent in controlling nausea and vomiting associated with chemotherapy.[42–44] In a randomized double-blind trial of patients treated with cisplatin, Gralla and colleagues reported that metoclopramide was superior to placebo and to prochlorperazine in reducing the frequency, volume, severity, and duration of nausea and vomiting.[44] Results are even better with the combination of metoclopramide, dexamethasone, and lorazepam.[45–48]

Mucositis

Gastrointestinal toxicity occurring as stomatitis, glossitis, esophagitis, and oral ulceration may severely decrease dietary intake. This form of toxicity is most commonly caused by methotrexate, methylglyoxal-bisguanylhydrazone, 5-FU, the antibiotic antitumor agents, and the vinca alkaloids. Single doses of methotrexate, 30 mg per m², rarely produce mucositis,[49] whereas larger doses, or repeated smaller doses, may produce moderate-to-severe symptoms. Mucositis caused by 5-FU may be associated with bloody diarrhea and a high mortality.[50]

The toxicity of methotrexate to the gastrointestinal epithelium and other normal tissue depends on the duration of exposure to cytotoxic concentrations of the drug rather than to peak levels achieved.[10] The plasma concentration and time thresholds for gastrointestinal epithelium are approximately 2×10^{-8} M and 42 hours, respectively.[10, 51–53] Disappearance of methotrexate from plasma following an intravenous injection is triphasic.[51, 54] Studies have shown that the terminal half-life, which begins 6 to 24 hours following high-dose therapy, is a major contributor to gastrointestinal and bone marrow toxicity.[10, 54, 55]

Toxicity to the gastrointestinal tract can be diminished if citrovorum factor rescue is given within 42 hours of administration of methotrexate.[56] Monitoring of methotrexate plasma concentrations may help identify those patients at risk for increased toxicity. Continuation of citrovorum rescue factor at standard doses, 6 to 12 mg per m² every 3 to 6 hours for those patients with prolonged time thresholds, and augmentation of the dose to match the elevated plasma level of methotrexate, may be necessary.[57–59] Intrathecal injection of methotrexate[60] and distribution of this drug into third-space compartments, such as ascitic fluid and pleural effusions, result in prolonged plasma levels because of slow drug removal from these reservoirs.[61]

Mucositis may preclude adequate oral nutrition. Treatment is usually conservative and symptomatic, including warm saline mouth rinses, topical corticosteroids, topical anesthetics such as viscous xylocaine prior to fluid and food ingestion, and nystatin if moniliasis is evident. Fluid intake with a straw and intravenous nutritional support may be indicated.

Diarrhea and Constipation

Autonomic nerve dysfunction manifested as colicky abdominal pain, constipation, and adynamic ileus is frequently associated with vincristine treatment.[62, 63] The elderly are particularly predisposed to these toxicities. Symptoms occur within 3 days of administration of the drug and may be unaccompanied by other evidence of peripheral nerve dysfunction. Holland and coworkers reported the presence of constipation in one third of patients treated with vincristine, with greater frequency, severity, and earlier onset in the group receiving the highest doses (range, 12.5 to 75 μg/kg).[64] If treated conservatively, this condition usually resolves over a 2-week period.

Profuse diarrhea may complicate treatment with 5-FU[65] and methyl-GAG.[66]

Gastrointestinal Bleeding

Gastrointestinal bleeding, unless resulting from severe thrombocytopenia, is rarely a complication of chemotherapy. Hemorrhagic gastritis may be caused by exogenous irritants, such as corticosteroids; however, bleeding usually ends concomitantly with discontinuation of the steroid.[65]

Hepatic Toxicity

Liver damage is most frequently associated with the use of methotrexate and 6-mercaptopurine and may be seen with methyl-GAG.[66] In addition, azathioprine, an immunosuppressive agent widely used in maintenance of transplant allografts, is metabolized in vivo to 6-MP,[67] and its hepatic toxicity is similar to that of 6-MP.

Methotrexate. Hepatic toxicity resulting from methotrexate was initially appreciated in patients being treated for acute lymphocytic leukemia and psoriasis. One of the earliest reports described extensive hepatic fibrosis in five patients who had each received several hundred milligrams of amethopterin (methotrexate) for leukemia therapy over periods of 6 to 14 months.[68] The introduction of antifolates and steroids in the period 1948 to 1951 and the additional use of antipurines in 1952 to 1957 brought about a marked increase in the incidence of hepatic fibrosis found at autopsy in leukemic children treated with these agents. It was concluded that risk factors in the pathogenesis of hepatic fibrosis included both drug therapy and the duration of survival. Those children with hepatic fibrosis lived, on the average, twice as long as those with no fibrosis.

Hersh and colleagues carried out a prospective study of 22 patients who received methotrexate for leukemia and other disorders.[69] Abnormalities of serum enzymes SGOT, SGPT, and LDH and prolongation of bromsulphthalein retention were particularly associated with intensive methotrexate treatment and less so with an intermittent drug schedule. Furthermore, abnormalities occurring during intermittent therapy tended to be reversible with discontinuation of the drug. Histologic abnormalities included portal inflammation and fatty changes. It also has been observed that methotrexate can exacerbate pre-existing cirrhotic liver damage, with potential hepatic coma.[70]

Following the initial use of methotrexate for psoriasis and with the use of the drug for its long-term management, reports of liver damage began to appear.[71–73] The primary association of cirrhosis and fibrosis was with prolonged small-dosage schedules, such as 2.5 mg per day for 2 to 5 days with a corresponding rest period. There was significantly less cirrhosis in those treated with intermittent large dosages, such as 10 to 25 mg every 1 to 4 weeks, even though the total monthly dose schedule was higher. In addition, the speed of onset of liver damage appeared to be dose-dependent.[71]

These findings have been confirmed and reported in an international cooperative study, consisting of 550 patients with severe psoriasis who underwent percutaneous liver biopsy while being treated with methotrexate.[74] The dosage schedule was important.

Daily oral methotrexate was associated with significantly greater nuclear variability, necrosis, and fibrosis compared with more intermittent schedules, even at an equivalent total cumulative dose. However, the total cumulative dose was also important, and increasing the drug dose is correlated with significant worsening of the biopsy findings. In addition to schedule and total dose of drug, alcohol ingestion significantly was associated with periportal inflammation, fibrosis, and cirrhosis. Age, sex, and severity of psoriasis did not correlate with abnormal histologic changes.

Methotrexate at present is used in high dosage (100 to 400 mg/kg) followed by citrovorum factor rescue in certain chemotherapeutic applications.[75] Liver damage may result from use of the drug in this manner, but, to date, this subject has not been systematically studied and conclusions remain unclear. The duration of infusion may be an important variable, with less toxicity seen for a 6-hour infusion than for a 24-hour infusion. The effect of citrovorum factor rescue upon long-term liver damage is not clear.

Although liver function tests may be abnormal during a course of methotrexate, there may not be a direct relationship between these abnormalities and the production of fibrosis. Furthermore, the incidence of false-negatives makes routine liver function tests rather insensitive indicators of slowly progressive disease.[69, 75, 76] When chronic therapy is used, the schedule should be intermittent and alcohol intake minimized. It is pertinent to follow serum enzyme levels as indicators of hepatic disease, but percutaneous liver biopsy is the only reliable means for accurately assessing severity of hepatotoxicity.

The clinical characteristics of 6-mercaptopurine and azathioprine hepatotoxicity differ from those seen with methotrexate; onset is more rapid, usually occurring 1 to 2 months after treatment. However, a range of 1 week to 2 or more years of treatment has been reported.[77–81] Liver damage is manifested by elevated serum transaminase levels, at times also with elevations in alkaline phosphatase and bilirubin. In many cases, these abnormalities resolve upon cessation of therapy but may reappear after rechallenge with the drug.[78] The histologic picture is that of hepatocellular necrosis and intrahepatic cholestasis and may resemble that of chlorpromazine damage.[79] Severe hepatic decompensation may occur with the use of 6-MP in the presence of pre-existing liver disease,[79] under which circumstances it should be used cautiously, if at all.

The incidence of liver damage secondary to 6-MP is not known, but there have been estimates that 10 to 40 per cent of patients treated for acute leukemia with 6-MP may raise difficult questions as to its etiology, which may be resolved only by empiric adjustments of drug dosage. In patients in whom azathioprine is used to control chronic active hepatitis, the complication rate is low, but toxicity may go undetected because it closely resembles the natural course of the disease.

Mithramycin. Among all the chemotherapy drugs currently available, much higher elevations of LDH, SGOT, and SGPT are seen with mithramycin. Approximately 50 per cent of patients receiving 25 to 50 μg per kg per day for 5 days will show changes within 1 to 4 days.[82] Microscopically, hepatic necrosis is visualized, with fatty changes and vacuolization. In addition, synthesis of albumin and clotting factors II, V, VII, and X is depressed. Thus a coagulopathy with transient prolongation of prothrombin time is fairly common. Significant drug-induced thrombocytopenia also may occur, resulting in a severe bleeding diathesis. Abnormalities usually occur within 24 hours following drug administration, peak in 2 to 3 days, and return to baseline levels in 4 to 21 days. Both the hepatotoxicity and the coagulopathy may be reduced by decreasing the dose of drug or by using an alternate-day treatment regimen.[83, 84]

Other Agents. Acute hepatoxicity from chemotherapeutic agents, as evidenced by mild transient elevations in enzymes, may be seen with cytosine arabinoside,[85] DTIC,[86] the nitrosoureas,[87] streptozocin,[88] and L-asparaginase,[89] amsacrine,[90–92] and busulfan.[93] In cases of pre-existing hepatic disease, enhanced toxicity may be observed in drugs that are metabolized in the liver or primarily excreted into the bile. These include doxorubicin,[94] daunorubicin,[95] vincristine,[96, 97] vinblastine,[97] etoposide,[98] and procarbazine.[99]

Pulmonary Toxicity

Busulfan. Several cases of diffuse pulmonary disease associated with busulfan treatment have been reported, so that the syndrome of "busulfan lung" has been recognized as a distinct clinical entity.[100–103]

Clinically, an insidious onset of cough, dyspnea, and low-grade fever occurs. These symptoms may appear 8 months to 10 years after initiation of therapy, with an average of 4 years. Chest roentgenograms show diffuse interstitial and intra-alveolar infiltrates. Pulmonary function studies reveal diminished diffusing capacity, as well as the changes of restrictive lung disease. The differential diagnosis of this clinical presentation requires that the syndrome be distinguished from opportunistic infections or leukemic infiltration of the lungs. Appropriate sputum cultures, viral serology/cytology determinations, and biopsy are necessary to demonstrate the characteristic pathologic features of the syndrome and to exclude a potential infection.

Microscopically, atypical alveolar and bronchiolar cells with large hyperchromatic nuclei are seen. Occasionally, these dysplastic cells in sputum are identified, by cytologic examination, as being malignant.[101] Of special interest in this regard are two case reports.[104, 105] They describe patients with chronic granulocytic leukemia, treated with long-term busulfan, who developed diffuse interstitial pulmonary fibrosis, atypical alveolar cell hyperplasia, and bronchiolar cell carcinoma.

The histologic findings associated with busulfan are similar to those seen with pulmonary irradiation, except for the absence of vascular-proliferative changes. Both conditions give rise to atypical alveolar lining cells and pulmonary fibrosis. The radiomimetic property of the alkylating agent may be responsible for damaging the alveolar lining cells and capillary endothelium. An increase in capillary permeability results in the development of interstitial and intra-alveolar fibrinous edema and hyaline membranes; the end result is progressive fibrosis.[106] The injury to the endothelium appears to result in proliferation and dysplasia of the large, type II granular pneumocyte, as documented by electron microscopy.[107]

Clinically, the course of busulfan lung is characterized by progressive deterioration in pulmonary function, with evidence of arterial hypoxemia, decreased vital capacity, carbon monoxide diffusing capacity, and total lung capacity. Forced expiratory volume in 1 second (FEV_1) frequently remains normal. The abnormalities of pulmonary function progress in spite of withdrawal of busulfan and administration of corticosteroids. In the majority of cases the patients have died within 6 months of the establishment of the diagnosis.[105]

Cyclophosphamide. The pulmonary abnormalities associated with busulfan may not be unique to this compound, but potentially are common to the alkylating agents as a group. In a discussion of drug-induced pulmonary disease, Rosenow comments on a cyclophosphamide-induced pulmonary syndrome characterized by bronchioloalveolar lining hyperplasia similar to that produced by busulfan.[105] Case reports have documented cyclophosphamide-associated pulmonary toxicity in a patient treated with high doses (40 mg/kg IV) and in a patient treated with prolonged low doses (50 to 150 mg/day PO for 27 months).[108, 109] Although cyclophosphamide pulmonary toxicity is unusual in human beings, it is still important for the physician to be aware of the potential toxicity of this very commonly used antineoplastic agent.

Bleomycin. Pulmonary toxicity is characteristically the most serious side effect of bleomycin. The onset, which may be delayed for more than 1 month after withdrawal of the drug, frequently is insidious and characterized by nonproductive cough, dyspnea, and tachypnea. Fine inspiratory rales in both lungs may be an early finding.[110] Blood gases show arterial hypoxemia, and pulmonary function studies show a decreased diffusion capacity and restrictive pulmonary disease. Roentgenography shows a pattern of diffuse interstitial disease with patchy basilar infiltrates, whereas pleural effusion and mediastinal or hilar adenopathy are unusual. Lung biopsy specimens show a variety of findings, including atypical alveolar cells, fibrinous exudate, and hyaline membranes during the acute stages. These changes may progress to diffuse interstitial and intra-alveolar fibrosis, similar to the pattern observed with busulfan.

Clinical toxicity is difficult to characterize in its earliest stages because of the insensitivity of prevailing diagnostic tests. Furthermore, changes in pulmonary function are nonspecific and, as a result, are of little assistance in predicting or detecting the onset of pulmonary toxicity, or in distinguishing it from either opportunistic infections or progression of disease.[111]

The incidence of clinical toxicity is estimated to be 5 to 10 per cent in patients receiving a total dose of less than 450 mg.[112] When a total dose of 550 mg is exceeded, current data indicate that fatal bleomycin pulmonary toxicity will occur in 10 per cent of patients. We have reported a 30 per cent incidence of bleomycin pulmonary toxicity in 13 patients with lymphoma treated with a combination of five drugs (cyclophosphamide, Adriamycin, vincristine, prednisone, and bleomycin-BACOP), who received a relatively low dose of bleomycin, 15 mg per m^2 (two patients).[113] The clinical syndrome of toxicity was manifested by fever, dyspnea, hypoxia, decreased diffusing capacity, and increased interstitial markings on chest films. Pulmonary fibrosis was proved at autopsy in one patient receiving 165 mg per m^2 and by open lung biopsy in one patient receiving 45 mg per m^2, total doses. Two patients with bleomycin toxicity developed diffusely positive pulmonary toxicity by gallium scans at the time of pulmonary symptoms. Peptide analyses of the bleomycin used as a single agent and in BACOP demonstrated no significant difference in peptide composition.

Because of the pulmonary toxicity seen in the first 13 patients treated with BACOP, the regimen was changed and bleomycin reduced to 5 mg per m^2 twice a month. Subsequent patients have been treated with this modified BACOP without signs or symptoms of pulmonary toxicity. It is indeed possible that bleomycin pulmonary toxicity may be enhanced when this agent is used in combination with other drugs, particularly alkylating agents and cisplatin. Concomitant treatment with prednisone does not prevent this complication.

In patients older than 70 years, who appear to be at increased risk for bleomycin pulmonary toxicity, there is no correlation between this complication and route of administration, nor with the type of tumor undergoing treatment.[112] Although a systematic study has not been conducted, it is the clinical impression of several investigators that bleomycin, like other specific antibiotic antitumor agents, has the capacity to enhance or exacerbate prior irradiation damage in previously irradiated sites.[112, 114–117] Since bleomycin is eliminated primarily by the kidney, enhanced toxicity is observed in renal failure.[118] Additionally, a synergistic effect is seen between previous bleomycin administration and high-dose oxygen therapy.[119] Therefore, high concentrations of oxygen should be avoided during anesthesia subsequent to bleomycin. The treatment of bleomycin toxicity includes withdrawal of the drug and the administration of corticosteroids; the efficacy of the latter has not been adequately documented.[111, 112]

Methotrexate. Several cases of diffuse pulmonary disease have been reported in association with intermittent therapy with methotrexate.[120–123]

Clinically, there is an abrupt onset of fever, a nonproductive cough, dyspnea, and hypoxemia. The chest roentgenogram shows patchy intra-alveolar and interstitial infiltrates; hilar and mediastinal adenopathy has also been observed.[121] Peripheral eosinophilia has been a feature in some patients not receiving corticosteroids.[120, 122] In childhood leukemia, this syndrome invariably appears when the patient is in remission and receiving maintenance therapy with intermittent methotrexate.[120, 123] In this setting it is frequently misinterpreted as leukemic infiltration of the lung or an opportunistic pulmonary infection. The disorder usually occurs 2 weeks to 3 months after initiation of therapy and does not appear to be related to total cumulative dose.

The histologic examination of the lung shows diffuse interstitial lymphocytic infiltrates, eosinophils, giant cells, and noncaseating granulomas, which serve to distinguish this form of toxicity from busulfan and bleomycin pulmonary toxicity.[122, 123] Because of the peripheral eosinophilia, the process has been considered to represent an allergic granulomatous pneumonitis. This process is usually reversible with the use of corticosteroids and withdrawal of methotrexate.

Other chemotherapy drugs associated with pulmonary toxicity include mitomycin C,[124, 125] BCNU and other nitrosoureas,[126–130] cyclophosphamide,[131] chlorambucil,[132] melphalan,[133] azathioprine,[134] Ara-C,[135] and procarbazine.[136] No specific therapy exists for the pulmonary disease. Response to corticosteroids is variable; however, progressive respiratory insufficiency usually occurs.

Cardiac Toxicity

Aside from myelosuppression, the principal drug effect limiting treatment with daunomycin and doxorubicin is cardiac toxicity. Isolated transient electrocardiographic changes without other evidence of cardiac abnormalities have been observed in 11 per cent of patients receiving Adriamycin.[137, 138] These have been nonspecific and include sinus tachycardia, ST-segment depression, T wave flattening, and occasional premature ventricular beats. These abnormalities appear not to be related to the total dose of the drug administered and can occur during or after intravenous administration. Upon withdrawal of the drug, the electrocardiogram usually returns to the pretreatment pattern. This is an acute reversible form of cardiac toxicity and has not been associated with any long-term sequelae.

A cumulative dose-dependent, drug-induced cardiomyopathy resulting in congestive heart failure is a second dose-related form of cardiac toxicity, characterized by the onset of the classic symptoms and signs of biventricular failure. The electrocardiogram shows a generalized diminution of QRS (ventricular complex) voltage, and cardiac function tests show findings typical of decreased myocardial contractility.[137, 139, 140] In one study, congestive heart failure occurred only once in the 366 patients who received less than 500 mg per m^2 of body surface area of Adriamycin.[137] However, when this total dose was exceeded, 10 to 33 patients (30 per cent) developed cardiac failure. A similar dose relation has been reported for children receiving daunomycin in the treatment of acute lymphocytic leukemia.[141] The onset of congestive failure may occur within 2 weeks after therapy has been discontinued but is commonly delayed 1 to 6 months following completion of treatment.[137, 141] When congestive failure develops, it is sometimes irreversible but often responds to standard treatment with digitalis and diuretics. Early recognition and treatment have improved morbidity and mortality. Prior mediastinal (cardiac) radiation, and possibly concomitant treatment with cyclophosphamide, can potentiate the cardiotoxic properties of Adriamycin.

Histologic and ultrastructural studies of the hearts of patients who had received large doses have shown foci of damaged and degenerating muscle cells, mitochondrial swelling and inclusion bodies, and alterations of nuclear chromatin.[140] Lethal cardiac toxicity can be avoided in the majority of patients by limiting the total dose to less than 500 mg per m^2 of body surface area. Using the ratio of pre-ejection period to left ventricular ejection time as an index of toxicity, Rinehart and associates found eight of nine patients who received between 310 and 540 mg per m^2 of body surface area of Adriamycin to have a decrease in left ventricular function.[140]

Adriamycin and daunomycin are important antitumor agents; however, their dose-related cardiac toxicity limits their usefulness in maintaining remissions of patients who respond to these agents. At present, it is recommended that a total dose of 500 mg per m^2 of body surface not be exceeded, in order to prevent serious or lethal cardiac toxicity. When there has been prior mediastinal or direct cardiac irradiation, the total dose should not exceed 400 mg per m^2.[142]

The schedule of Adriamycin administration may influence the incidence of cardiomyopathy. A reduced weekly dose or a continuous intravenous infusion may decrease the incidence of drug-associated changes demonstrated by cardiac biopsy. The risk of development of cardiomyopathy is enhanced in patients with advanced stages, pre-existing hypertension, previous or concurrent radiotherapy to the heart, and concurrent cyclophosphamide administration.[143–145]

Whereas systolic time intervals,[146, 147] the QRS-Korotkoff interval,[148] electrocardiography,[149] echocardiography,[150] and percutaneous endomyocardial biopsy[151–153] are among the diagnostic tests useful in predicting Adriamycin-induced cardiomyopathy, radionuclide cineangiography is clinically the most useful. Pathologically, there is dilatation with degeneration of myofibrils, and myocyte vacuolization, and mitochondrial and nuclear degeneration can be demonstrated.[153, 154] Aggressive treatment with inotropic drugs, diuretics, digitalis, bed rest, and salt restriction is indicated, since the cardiac dysfunction is frequently refractory to medical management.[146]

Other chemotherapeutic agents with cardiotoxicity include cyclophosphamide,[155] 5-FU,[156, 157] cisplatin,[158] mitoxantrone,[267] amsacrine,[268] vinca alkaloids,[269] and high-dose interleukin therapy.[270]

Neurotoxicity

Neurotoxicity is most frequently associated with the vinca alkaloids,[159–161] procarbazine,

L-asparaginase, and intrathecal administration of methotrexate.[159] In addition, 5-FU, cisplatin, and the nitrosoureas may result in adverse effects on the nervous system, but with a much reduced frequency.[159]

Vincristine. The earliest and most consistent clinical findings of vincristine neurotoxicity are the diffuse loss of cutaneous sensation of the toes and fingertips and loss of the Achilles tendon reflex without demonstrable abnormalities of tests of discrimination, position, or vibratory sense.[161] Depression of other deep tendon reflexes, progressing to complete areflexia, may occur. Maximal depression of reflexes usually occurs 17 days following administration, with return toward normal after 1 to 3 months. Cranial nerve neuropathies may also occur.

Profound motor weakness is one of the most serious manifestations of vincristine neurotoxicity. Objective clinical findings characteristically reveal impairment of the extensors of the fingers, toes, and wrists.[160, 161] Foot or wrist drop and a broad-based gait occur, which may be severe but are in some cases completely reversible over several months. Cranial nerve dysfunction may result in ptosis, optic atrophy, and facial palsies. The earliest manifestation of autonomic nervous system disorder is usually abdominal colic and constipation, which may be accentuated in the elderly. Other neurologic abnormalities associated with vincristine administration include rare instances of seizures and, more frequently, myalgias of the jaw or throat. Inadvertent intrathecal injection of vincristine results in rapid neurologic deterioration with peripheral neuropathies, cranial nerve palsies, paralytic ileus, bladder atony, hypertension or hypotension, seizures, and inappropriate ADH secretion, progressing to death.[160, 161]

All these manifestations of vincristine neurotoxicity are usually more profound in the elderly and are dose related, being more severe with doses in excess of 1.5 mg per m^2.

Methotrexate. Intrathecal administration of methotrexate may be accompanied by symptoms of meningeal irritation, transient or permanent paraparesis, and encephalopathy.[162] Sterile arachnoiditis with stiff neck, headache, vomiting, and cerebrospinal fluid (CSF) pleocytosis has been reported in 10 to 40 per cent of patients.[162, 163] The symptoms usually begin 2 to 4 hours after the dose of intrathecal methotrexate and last 12 to 72 hours.[159, 162, 163] Meningoencephalopathy can develop several months following therapy and may occur during high-dose intravenous therapy. Cerebral atrophy is evident in approximately 50 per cent of patients given intrathecal methotrexate and cranial irradiation.[164]

L-Asparaginase. Cerebral dysfunction manifested as lethargy, somnolence, confusion, disorientation, hallucinations, and depression commonly occurs subsequent to administration of L-asparaginase. These changes, reported in 30 to 60 per cent of patients,[165] usually resolve following cessation of therapy. In addition to the acute toxicity, a delayed encephalopathy beginning approximately 1 week after therapy and lasting several weeks has been reported.[159, 165]

5-Fluorouracil (5-FU). Reversible cerebellar ataxia has been reported in less than 5 per cent of patients receiving intravenous doses.[166] Clinically, dizziness, gross dysmetria, coarse nystagmus, slurred speech, and truncal ataxia may occur. The syndrome appears unrelated to the sex or age of the patient or the total dose of 5-FU received. The incidence, however, does increase with higher single doses and usually ends 1 to 6 weeks after therapy is discontinued. These symptoms are more frequent with intravenous administration of tegafur (Ftorafur), a furanyl analogue.[159]

Procarbazine. Central nervous system depression, often progressing to profound stupor, is common with oral procarbazine therapy and is accentuated greatly with intravenous therapy.[167] In addition, peripheral neuropathy; enhancement of barbiturates, narcotics, and phenothiazines; and monoamine oxidase inhibition have been observed. Alcohol intolerance similar to that seen with disulfiram (Antabuse) has been reported, and consequently patients should be warned of this complication.[159, 167]

Other Agents. Irreversible ototoxicity may occur with cisplatin. Tinnitus, which occurs early, may be followed by high-frequency hearing loss.[168] Other agents with known neurotoxicity are hexamethylmelamine,[169] BCNU,[170] ara-C,[171] etoposide,[172] dacarbazine,[173] and methyl G.[174]

Cutaneous Reactions

Alopecia. Diffuse thinning of the hair or patchy alopecia may occur with many antineoplastic agents, including oral and intravenous cyclophosphamide.[175] This hair loss is almost never permanent, and partial or even total regrowth frequently occurs despite continued chemotherapy. However, virtually all patients receiving therapeutic doses of Adriamycin, daunomycin, and vincristine experience significant alopecia. With continued therapy, hair growth may resume at a slower rate in some patients, but frequently total alopecia remains until cessation of therapy.

Miscellaneous. Diffuse melanosis of the nailbed or transverse pigmented bands are frequently noted with 5-FU[176] and Adriamycin therapy.[177] Hyperpigmentation that resembles the melanosis of Addison's disease is seen frequently with chronic busulfan therapy.[178] Urticaria, rash, and proctitis may occur with bleomycin therapy,[111, 112] whereas folliculitis is found with actinomycin D.[179]

Extravasation of vesicants like nitrogen mustard,[180] Adriamycin,[177] daunomycin,[181] vincristine,[182] vinblastine,[183] and actinomycin D[184] may result in painfully severe local reactions, with subsequent necrosis, tissue slough, fibrosis, and joint contracture. Should extravasation occur, the infusion should be discontinued immediately and the infusion set removed. Infiltration of the local area with 1 mg of dexamethasone or methylprednisolone, or sodium thiosulfate if nitrogen mustard was extravasated,[180] followed by cold compresses, may provide some therapeutic benefit and symptomatic relief. Surgery may be required to debride devitalized tissue and to provide improved function and cosmesis.[185, 186]

Fever

Hyperpyrexia, frequently severe and associated with shaking chills, occurs in approximately half of patients receiving bleomycin.[111] It usually develops within 12 hours following administration and may persist for up to 48 hours. Antipyretics and antihistamines may provide symptomatic relief. Rare febrile reactions have been reported with DTIC[187] and mithramycin.[82, 188] In addition, fever with chills, dyspnea, hypotension, and cardiovascular collapse may occur with L-asparaginase,[165] a bacterially derived enzyme. Epinephrine given immediately usually causes resolution of the symptoms.

Hypersensitivity

Anaphylactic reactions occur after administration of various chemotherapy agents. Acute reactions are reported more commonly with L-asparaginase,[189] cytarabine,[190] bleomycin,[191] and dacarbazine.[192] Other drugs with less reported frequency are cisplatin,[193] cyclophosphamide,[194] methotrexate,[195] etoposide,[196] and doxorubicin.[197]

Hematologic Complications

Most cancer chemotherapeutic agents cause some degree of bone marrow toxicity. Bleeding caused by thrombocytopenia or infection due to leukopenia should be treated with appropriate platelet transfusions, antibiotics, and granulocyte transfusions when indicated. Bleomycin,[111] streptozocin,[88] and vincristine[64] usually are not associated with bone marrow toxicity except in patients whose marrow is already compromised by prior cytotoxic or radiation therapy.

White blood cell and platelet depression usually begins 4 to 5 days following administration of most chemotherapeutic agents, with the nadir appearing at 10 to 14 days. Recovery as shown by peripheral blood counts is usually rapid and complete by 21 to 28 days. With the chloroethyl nitrosoureas, and mitomycin,[87] myelotoxicity is more profound, with delayed nadirs at 4 to 7 weeks and a much slower recovery. With repeated courses of treatment, there is cumulative toxicity. Recovery from busulfan-induced myelosuppression may require several months after initial severe toxicity.

Infectious complications following chemotherapeutic agents are related to the absolute number of polymorphonuclear leukocytes, with a significant increase in the risk of sepsis with granulocyte counts below 1000 per mm^3. Fever with or without documented bacterial infection may occur. The diagnosis of infection in patients with granulocytopenia may be difficult because the usual signs and symptoms may be absent as a result of lack of an adequate inflammatory response. Despite the negative clinical findings, a careful history should be taken, and a physical examination with close attention to the oropharynx and anorectal area should be done. Chest x-ray films, urinalysis, and cultures of blood, stool, throat, and urine are essential for elucidating the etiology of the fever.[198]

Empiric broad-spectrum antibiotic therapy should be initiated in the febrile and leukopenic patient after appropriate cultures have been obtained.[198, 199] Granulocyte transfusions should be given only to those patients who have proved bacteremia and an inadequate response to antibiotics.[200] Since prolonged antibiotic therapy may predispose to other serious infections, the antibiotics may be discontinued following recovery of granulocytes above 1000 to 2000 per mm^3 if no source of infection is found and the fever is diminished.

Patients with thrombocytopenia following chemotherapy should receive platelet transfusions when platelet counts measure fewer than 20,000 per mm^3. If bleeding is evident, platelet transfusions should be given at a higher platelet count.[201]

Anemia

Moderate anemia and striking changes in red blood cell morphology and peripheral smears are frequent consequences of chemotherapeutic agents.[202] Macrocytosis and megaloblastic changes in the bone marrow occur. If severe anemia occurs, other causes should be excluded.[203, 204] A microangiopathic hemolytic anemia with renal failure has been reported in association with mitomycin C.[205]

Myelodysplastic Syndrome

Pancytopenia associated with a high incidence of cytogenetic abnormalities and other myelodysplastic changes is reported with increasing frequency following chemotherapy treatment.[206–208] The process may evolve into bone marrow failure or overt acute myelogenous leukemia. Both phases are associated with a poor response to therapy and frequent death.[209, 210]

Treatment

Myelosuppression induced by chemotherapy drugs is usually limited and generally reversible. Judicious use of transfusion support, antibiotics, and other supportive care will allow prompt management of problems and reversal of potentially lethal situations.[202]

Fluid and Electrolytes

Hyponatremia associated with the syndrome of inappropriate ADH secretion has been reported with vincristine therapy.[211] The syndrome usually lasts for 1 to 2 weeks following cessation of therapy. Hyperkalemia may follow rapid cell lysis, especially if there is renal compromise. Hypocalcemia may accompany mithramycin therapy.[87]

Urinary Tract Toxicity

A number of drugs used in the treatment of cancer are associated with complications to the kidney and urinary tract. Management may be further complicated by tumor lysis and the concomitant use of other nephrotoxic drugs, such as nonsteroidal anti-inflammatory agents and antibiotics.

Cyclophosphamide. In 1959, Coggins and associates first reported the complication of hemorrhagic cystitis in patients who were treated with cyclophosphamide.[212] This acute cystitis is ordinarily a frequent complication of therapy, particularly in patients who are insufficiently hydrated when receiving large, intermittent intravenous doses. The incidence of cystitis has been reported to range from 4 to 36 per cent in patients treated with cyclophosphamide. Dysuria, frequency, and urgency occur, and evidence of gross or microscopic hematuria and pyuria may be seen on urinalysis. The onset is extremely variable; it may occur early after the first dose,[212, 213] or it may be delayed until several weeks after the drug has been withdrawn.[214] Cystoscopic examination shows a variety of changes, including mucosal hyperemia, telangiectatic blood vessels, focal or diffuse subepithelial bleeding sites, and mucosal ulceration and necrosis.[215–217] Histologic examination of the urinary bladder by biopsy or at autopsy has shown numerous thin-walled vessels with capillary budding; the epithelium is edematous and scattered areas of necrosis may be present. Urinary cytology commonly shows atypical epithelial cells, which may be misinterpreted as evidence of malignancy.[218]

Acute cystitis usually resolves spontaneously with hydration and cessation of chemotherapy, but microscopic hematuria may persist for several months. Infrequently, the bleeding is massive and life-threatening, and in such cases urologic intervention may be required. In reviewing the role of surgical management in patients with hemorrhagic cystitis, Berkson and associates point out that diverting urine from the bladder mucosa may be quite successful in controlling major bladder hemorrhage in patients who do not respond to conservative management.[219] Urinary diversion bypasses the bladder epithelium and prevents further alkylation in patients still receiving the drug. In patients who develop cystitis long after withdrawal of the drug, the continued flow of urine may prevent adequate healing and hemostasis in the damaged bladder epithelium.

Long-term treatment with cyclophosphamide has the potential for causing the development of chronic bladder fibrosis and vesicoureteral reflux.[216, 220, 221] Histologic examination of the bladder shows alterations similar to those seen after radiotherapy: capillary dilatation, edema, inflammatory cells, and proliferating fibroblasts in the adjacent stroma. The telangiectatic vessels are predisposed to bleeding after minimal trauma. In the most systematic study of this problem, urinary bladder fibrosis was found at autopsy in 10 of 40 patients who had received long-term treatment with cyclophosphamide.[221] Patients whose bladders were affected had received the largest total doses—in excess of 6.0 gm per m^2 of body surface area—over the longest period of time. In approximately 50 per cent of cases, the process was entirely asymptomatic.

Patients receiving cyclophosphamide should be instructed to maintain a high urinary output during therapy. In addition, regular examination of the urine should be performed to detect evidence of microscopic hematuria. If cystitis develops, it is recommended that cyclophosphamide therapy be discontinued and an alternative alkylating agent, such as chlorambucil or melphalan, which does not carry the risk of toxicity, be utilized.

An unusual renal toxicity has been described in association with high-dose cyclophosphamide treatment: impaired water excretion has been observed after administration of intravenous doses in excess of 50 mg per kg of body weight per day.[222] This syndrome is characterized by hyponatremia, decreased urine volume, and inappropriately concentrated urine, without associated glomerular or proximal tubular abnormalities. The damage is reversible after cessation of cyclophosphamide. This effect has been attributed to the alkylating metabolites of cyclophosphamide and their direct action on the distal renal tubule.

The clinical usefulness of *cis*-diamminedichloroplatinum is limited by its dose-dependent nephrotoxicity.[223–225] A reduction in renal blood flow and glomerular filtration rate that is usually reversible commonly occurs in patients following a dose exceeding 50 mg per mm^2. More severe abnormalities may be observed with higher doses or prolonged therapy, and multiple courses. The incidence decreases with pre- and postinfusion hydration and concomitant mannitol therapy and/or furosemide. Urinary β-glucuronidase activity may serve as a measure of nephrotoxicity.[223]

Electrolyte abnormalities with increased salt and water excretion, hypomagnesemia, and hypocalcemia may develop acutely and persist long after treatment. Whereas asymptomatic hypomagnesemia is a common finding in patients receiving cisplatin, magnesium wasting may produce symptomatic weakness and tetany. Pathologically, the primary finding is coagulative necrosis of the distal tubular epithelium and collecting ducts. With appropriate hydration, most patients tolerate multiple courses of therapy without clinically significant impairment of renal function.

Nitrosoureas. Renal tubular damage, resulting in a full Fanconi-like syndrome and renal failure, is the major dose-limiting toxic effect of streptozocin.[226] We noted renal abnormalities in 28 per cent of 106 patients treated. Nephrotoxicity was the major contributing factor of death in four of these patients. Hypophosphatemia is usually seen as the earliest abnormality and may appear after only one dose of drug. Acetonuria, aminoaciduria, glycosuria, and hyperchloremia are a part of the syndrome.[227] In addition, evidence for glomerular damage with elevations in BUN and creatinine has been reported.[228] Renal function may return to normal if the drug is stopped early after abnormalities appear; however, irreversible nephrotoxicity will occur with continued treatment.

Although renal toxicity with chlorethyl nitrosoureas is uncommon, an increased incidence is seen in prolonged therapy resulting in high cumulative doses.[229–233] Harmon and associates reported nephrotoxicity in six of

17 patients treated with methyl-CCNU.[229] All patients received total doses greater than 1500 mg per m^2, and none developed renal insufficiency during nitrosourea treatment. During therapy, a progressive decrease in the size of the kidneys was noted, which continued despite cessation of therapy. Irreversible renal failure occurred after completion of the 2-year course of treatment. Pathologically, thickening of glomerular basement membranes and tubular atrophy were observed. In a retrospective review of patients treated with methyl-CCNU, Nichols and Moertel reported nephrotoxicity in 4 of 857 patients.[230] Three of these patients had received a cumulative dose greater than 1700 mg per m^2. Fourteen per cent of the patients whose total cumulative dose was over 1000 mg per m^2 had evidence of renal impairment. Schacht and colleagues reported renal dysfunction in six patients treated with BCNU.[233] Total cumulative doses in all were greater than 1500 mg.

The nephrotoxic potential of the nitrosoureas appears to be well established, with the insidious progressive development of renal dysfunction months to years after cessation of chemotherapy. Initially, the urinalysis, serum BUN, and creatine may all be normal, with abnormalities detected only by more sophisticated tests such as the glomerular filtration rate and renal plasma flow. If therapy with chlorethyl nitrosourea is continued for more than 15 months, or if the cumulative dose is greater than 1000 mg per m^2, one should suspect the possibility of nephrotoxicity and discontinue therapy if renal size decreases or if substantial diminution of the glomerular filtration rate occurs.

Methotrexate. When used in small intravenous doses of 40 to 60 mg per m^2, methotrexate has not been associated with appreciable nephrotoxicity. However, there are now extensive trials of high-dose treatment with citrovorum factor rescue. At these larger doses of 100 mg per kg and more, several investigators have reported severe kidney damage, with oliguria, azotemia, and fatal renal failure.[10] This is a particularly ominous situation, since at least 90 per cent of administered methotrexate is normally excreted as intact drug in the urine. Nephrotoxicity is thought to be due to precipitation of drug in the renal tubules. The solubility characteristics of methotrexate may compound the problem, since the drug is ten times less soluble at a pH of 5.5 than at a pH of 7.5.[10, 54] Methotrexate renal toxicity is far more likely to occur in older patients, and Pittman and associates reported greater than 50 per cent increases in serum creatinine in 19 of 33 (60 per cent) adults receiving high-dose methotrexate without an intensive hydration and alkalinization regimen.[234]

Jacobs and colleagues demonstrated that 10 per cent or more of administered high-dose methotrexate is metabolized to 7-hydroxymethotrexate and excreted in the urine as this metabolite; 7-hydroxymethotrexate is three to five times less soluble than the parent compound.[60]

In our experience, high-dose methotrexate therapy can be safely administered under certain scrupulously honored conditions:

1. Patients must be monitored closely before, during, and after methotrexate infusion to ensure adequate hydration, urine output, urine alkalinization, and citrovorum factor rescue. Sodium bicarbonate administration is necessary to ensure a urinary pH of 7.0 or higher.
2. Patients must have normal creatinine clearances before each course of therapy.
3. A urine output of 125 ml per m^2 per hour and a urine pH of 7.5 must be attained before drug administration is begun, and these values must be maintained for a full 24 hours after methotrexate infusion.

These principles are based on the clinical pharmacology of high-dose methotrexate. If followed carefully, they allow one to administer this therapy with minimal nephrotoxicity.

Other Drugs. Other chemotherapy drugs with renal complications include mitomycin,[235] mithramycin,[236] and azacytidine.[237, 238]

Fertility

Testicular Function. Azoospermia has been reported in patients receiving alkylating agents.[239–242] Richter and associates studied the effect of chlorambucil on spermatogenesis in eight patients with malignant lymphomas.[241] They observed dose-dependent oligospermia, which progressed to azoospermia when total doses of 400 mg were exceeded. Recovery from oligospermia occurred in one patient when the drug was withdrawn after this total dose was reached. Similar findings were reported in five patients who recovered spermatogenesis either partially or totally after withdrawal of chlorambucil.[239] Alterations in testicular function in 31 patients who received daily cyclophosphamide for more than 6 months were reported: 18 (60 per cent) had azoospermia.[242] Testicular biopsy specimens showed tubular atrophy with markedly diminished or absent spermatogenesis. The problem is complex because of the potential influence of the specific disease state on testicular function.

Sherins and DeVita analyzed the effect of intensive combination chemotherapy on reproductive function in 16 men with malignant lymphoma.[243] Combination chemotherapy involving mechlorethamine or cyclophosphamide, vincristine, prednisone, and procarbazine had been completed 6 months to 7 years previously; all patients were considered to be in complete remission. All had normal libido and potency. Only four of the men had normal spermatogenesis. The remainder showed partial or complete testicular failure, as evidenced by biopsy-proved spermatogonial arrest associated with elevated levels of follicle-stimulating hormone. Within each treatment group, the men with normal spermatogenesis were those who had been experiencing remission, without chemotherapy, for the longest period of time. One patient observed at regular intervals over a period of 3.5 years experienced a rise in sperm count from almost zero to 15 million per ml and was able to impregnate his wife. These findings, and those reported after chemotherapy with alkylating agents alone, indicate that return of normal spermatogenesis is possible in rare cases, but it may take several years after discontinuation of therapy.[240, 241, 243] In a follow-up study of 26 men with cyclophosphamide-related azoospermia, 12 patients experienced a return of spermatogenesis within 15 to 49 months (median duration, 30 months). There was no significant association of recovery with age, duration of cyclophosphamide therapy, or total dose administered.[244]

It is of interest that the toxic effect of chemotherapy on the testis is specific for the tubular epithelium. The Sertoli and Leydig cells remain histologically and functionally normal, as evidenced by normal levels of testosterone and luteinizing hormone.[245]

Ovarian Function. Alterations in menstrual function have been associated with the administration of cytotoxic agents such as busulfan,[246] chlorambucil,[247] cyclophosphamide,[248] and vinblastine.[249] Uldall and coworkers reported a series of 34 women with glomerulonephritis treated with daily cyclophosphamide for an average of 18 months.[248] Eighteen (53 per cent) of the women developed amenorrhea an average of 17 months from the onset of therapy. Urinary estrogens were low and urinary gonadotropins were elevated, suggesting primary ovarian failure as the cause of the amenorrhea. Only 10 per cent of patients observed for one year after withdrawal of cyclophosphamide experienced a return of menstrual periods. In a similar group of patients, ovarian biopsies were performed on several women with ovarian failure following long-term treatment with cyclophosphamide.[250] Histologic findings included absence of ova with no evidence of follicular maturation. Sobrinho and associates described nine women with Hodgkin's disease who developed oligomenorrhea or amenorrhea shortly after beginning chemotherapy with vinblastine.[249] All nine had findings consistent with primary ovarian failure. It is probable that both total dose and duration of administration are important determinants of the reversibility of this complication.

Fetal Abnormalities

Widespread use of antineoplastic agents has caused increasing concern that these drugs will produce adverse effects on fetal development, especially when administered to pregnant women during the first 4 months of gestation.[251, 252] Since chemotherapeutic agents significantly affect rapidly dividing tissues, the fetus is at significant risk for development of untoward effects. Approximately 13 per cent of over 300 documented pregnancies with a history of exposure to chemotherapy during the first 4 months of gestation now have reported associated malformations.[253] Low birth weight may occur following exposure at any gestational age.[254] However, the accurate number of abnormalities cannot be ascertained because of the number of spontaneous abortions and inaccurate reporting.

Folic Acid Antagonists. The antifolate agents are the chemotherapeutic drugs that have been consistently implicated as fetal toxins in women, to the extent that these agents have been used as abortifacients in some centers. Thiersch reported successful termination of pregnancy in 10 of 12 cases in which aminopterin was used specifically for this purpose.[255] Three of the fetuses in his series had malformations, including cleft palate, hydrocephalus, and meningoencephalocele.

Nicholson reviewed the literature dealing with the effects of cytotoxic agents in pregnancy.[247] Of 52 patients who were reported to have received aminopterin during the first trimester of pregnancy—in most cases as an abortifacient—34 eventually aborted. The state of the fetus was described in 12 cases, and in 10 of these macroscopic malformation was detected, with a predilection for the central nervous system. In three pregnancies during which women had received aminopterin after the first trimester, no fetal abnormalities were detected, although one fetus died from spontaneous abortion at the 26th week. In the latter case, the mother had been receiving concomitant treatment with 6-mercaptopurine and desacetylmethylcolchicine. Five women had received methotrexate after the first trimester; they delivered six normal babies.

6-Mercaptopurine and Azathioprine. Similar fetal abnormalities have been reported with other drugs. Of 20 women who received 6-mercaptopurine during the first trimester of pregnancy, 8 aborted.[256] There were one stillbirth and one abortion in 28 pregnancies treated after the first trimester, and no cases of macroscopic fetal abnormality.

Abortions are reported less frequently with azathioprine, a drug that is commonly used to prevent renal transplant rejection and to treat systemic lupus erythematosus. In 1970, the Human Kidney Transplant Registry had on record 29 women who became pregnant while receiving azathioprine and corticosteroids,[257] and 18 normal children were delivered. Seven women had spontaneous abortions, five of which occurred early in pregnancy. There was no evidence of fetal abnormality. Penn and associates reported eight women with renal homografts who became pregnant ten times, and eight pregnancies were allowed to come to term.[258] One premature infant died from hyaline membrane disease. Of the surviving infants, one had pulmonary valvular stenosis, two had transient adrenocortical insufficiency and lymphopenia, and one had the respiratory distress syndrome.

Alkylating Agents. Aside from isolated case reports, this class of chemotherapeutic compounds does not appear to be a consistent cause of fetal abnormality but does have the potential for terminating early pregnancy. In Nicholson's review of 60 pregnant women who had received alkylating agent chemotherapy—34 during the first trimester—only four cases of fetal malformation were reported.[247]

Other Agents. Fetal abnormalities have occurred after a combination of nitrogen mustard, vincristine, procarbazine, and prednisone was given in the first trimester to treat Hodgkin's disease.[259] We have seen one single exception. The overall problem of drug-induced congenital abnormalities is extremely complex. With the exception of methotrexate, the teratogenic potential of human anticancer immunosuppressive therapy appears lower than one might have predicted from animal studies. Moreover, the overall risk of fetal malformation after cytotoxic therapy during the second and third trimesters does not appear to be greater than normal. Nevertheless, women should be encouraged to take measures to avoid becoming pregnant while receiving chemotherapy. A decision to allow an established pregnancy to continue or to interrupt therapy during the first trimester cannot be made using available criteria; it must obviously take into account the wishes of the patient after she has been fully informed of the possible risks. In addition, the effect of in utero exposure to cytotoxic drugs on subsequent fertility needs clarification, particularly for women, since the formation of ova takes place during fetal development.

Carcinogenesis

Many of the drugs in use, specifically the alkylating agents and procarbazine, are potent mutagens and have carcinogenic potential.[258] Epidemiologists have been watching for the emergence of second cancers in patients receiving chemotherapy, and there are now data to suggest an association.

Acute leukemia has been reported following treatment of multiple myeloma, Hodgkin's disease, lymphoma, CLL, and carcinomas of the breast, colon, and ovary.[260–266] Further studies are needed to understand the relationship between chemotherapeutic agents and the development of second malignancies.

The relatively low incidence may reflect in part the relatively poor survival rate of patients who were treated with chemotherapy in the past; they may not have lived a sufficiently long period of time to express drug-related genetic injury. With the present improvements in survival and the use of these agents in non-neoplastic conditions, this situation may change.

References

1. Schein PS, Winokur SH: Immunosuppressive and cytotoxic chemotherapy: Long-term complications. Ann Intern Med *82*:84, 1975.
2. Hall TC: Use of cancer chemotherapeutic agents in non-neoplastic diseases. Cancer *31*:1256, 1973.
3. Kaplan SR, Calabresi P: Drug therapy: Immunosuppressive agents. N Engl J Med *289*:952, 1973.
4. Skinner MD, Schwartz RS: Immunosuppressive therapy. N Engl J Med *287*:221, 1972.
5. Steinberg AD, Plotz PH, Wolff SM, Wong VG, Augus SG, Decker JL: Cytotoxic drugs in treatment of non-malignant disease. Ann Intern Med *76*:619, 1972.
6. Winchester JF, Rahman A, Tilstone WJ, Bregman H, Mortensen LM, Gelfand MC, Schein PS, Schreiner GE: Will hemoperfusion be useful for cancer chemotherapeutic drug removal? Clin Toxicol *17*:557, 1980.
7. Hande KR, Donehower RC, Chabner BA: Pharmacology and pharmacokinetics of high-dose methotrexate in man. *In* Pinedo HM (ed): Clinical Pharmacology of Antineoplastic Drugs. New York, Elsevier/North Holland, 1978, p 97.
8. Fox RM: Methotrexate nephrotoxicity. Clin Exp Pharmacol Physiol (5)(Suppl):43, 1977.
9. Condit PT, Chanes RE, Joll W: Renal toxicity of methotrexate. Cancer *23*:126, 1969.
10. Bleyer WA: The clinical pharmacology of methotrexate. Cancer *41*:36, 1978.
11. Bertino JR, Condos S, Horvath C, et al: Immobilized carboxypeptidase GI in methotrexate removal. Cancer Res *38*:1936, 1978.
12. Ahmad S, Shen F, Bleyer WA: Methotrexate-induced renal failure and ineffectiveness of peritoneal dialysis. Arch Intern Med *138*:1146, 1978.
13. Hande KR, Balow JE, Drake JC, et al: Methotrexate and hemodialysis. Ann Intern Med *87*:495, 1977.
14. Spiegel RJ, Cooper PR, Blum RH, et al: Treatment of massive intrathecal methotrexate overdose by ventriculolumbar perfusion. N Engl J Med *311*:386, 1984.
15. Borison HL, Wang WC: Physiology and pharmacology of vomiting. Pharmacol Rev *5*:193, 1953.
16. Borison HL: Area postrema: Chemoreceptor trigger zone for vomiting. Is that all? Life Sci *14*:1807, 1974.
17. Scogna D, Smalley R: Chemotherapy-induced nausea and vomiting. Am J Nurs *79*:1562, 1979.
18. Borison HL, Brand ED, Askind RK: Emetic action of nitrogen mustard (mechloroethamine hydrochloride) in dogs and cats. Am J Physiol *192*:410, 1958.
19. Wang SC, Rinz AA, Chinn HI: Mechanism of emesis following irradiation. Am J Physiol *193*:335, 1958.
20. Mitchell EP, Schein PS: Gastrointestinal toxicity of chemotherapeutic agents. Semin Oncol *9*:52–64, 1982.
21. Harris JG: Nausea, vomiting and cancer treatment. Cancer *29*:1941, 1978.
22. Wang SC: Emetic and antiemetic drugs. Physiol. Pharmacol. Vol. II Academic Press, New York, 1965, p. 255.
23. Gay LN, Carliner PE: The prevention and treatment of motion sickness. Bull Johns Hopkins Hosp *84*:470, 1949.
24. Jaju BP, Wang SC: Effects of diphenhydramine and dimenhydrinate on vestibular neuronal activity of cat. A search for the locus of their antimotion sickness action. J Pharmacol Exp Ther *176*:718, 1971.
25. Moertel CG, Reitemeir RJ, Gage RP: A controlled clinical investigation of antiemetic drugs. JAMA *186*:116, 1963.
26. Moertel CG, Reitemeir RJ: Controlled clinical studies of orally administered antiemetic drugs. Gastroenterology *57*:262, 1969.
27. Bruera ED, Roca E, Cedaro L, et al: Improved control of chemotherapy-induced emesis by addition of dexamethasone to metoclopropramide in patients resistant to metoclopropramide. Cancer Treat Rep *67*:381, 1983.
28. Plezia PM, Alberb DS, et al: Immediate termination of intractable vomiting induced by cisplatin combination chemotherapy using intensive five-drug antiemetic regimen. Cancer Treat Rep *68*:1493, 1984.
29. Grossman B, Lessin LS, Cohen P: Droperidol prevents nausea and vomiting from cis-platinum. N Engl J Med *301*:47, 1979.
30. Plotkin DA, Plotkin D, Okien R: Haloperidol in the treatment of nausea and vomiting due to cytotoxic drug administration. Curr Ther Res *15*:599, 1973.
31. Shaw JE, Bayne W, Schmidt LG: Clinical pharmacology of scopolamine. Clin Pharmacol Ther *19*:115, 1976.
32. Sallan S, Zinsberg N, Frei EM: Antiemetic effect of delta-9-tetrahydrocannabinol in patients receiving cancer chemotherapy. N Engl J Med *293*:795, 1975.
33. Chang AE, Shilling DJ, Stillman RC, Goldberg NH, Seipp CA, Barofsky I: Delta-9-tetrahydrocannabinol as an antiemetic in cancer patients receiving high-dose methotrexate. Ann Intern Med *91*:819, 1979.
34. Lucas VS, Laszlo J: Delta-9-tetrahydrocannabinol for refractory vomiting induced by cancer chemotherapy. JAMA *243*:1241, 1980.
35. Herman TS, Einhorn L, Jones SE: Superiority of nabilone over prochlorperazine as an antiemetic in patients receiving chemotherapy. N Engl J Med *300*:1295, 1979.
36. McCabe M, Smith FP, Goldberg D, McDonald J, Wooley PV, Warren R, Brodeur R, Schein PS, Simon RM, Rosenberg SA: Comparative trial of oral delta-9-tetrahydrocannabinol (THC) and prochlorperazine (PCZ) for cancer chemotherapy-related nausea and vomiting. Proc Am Soc Clin Oncol *22*:4161, 1981.
37. Frytak S, Moertel CG, O'Fallon JR: Delta-9-tetra-

hydrocannabinol as an antiemetic for patients receiving chemotherapy. Ann Intern Med *91*:815, 1979.
38. Sallan SE, Cronin CM, Zellen M, et al: Antiemetics in patients receiving chemotherapy for cancer. N Engl J Med *302*:134, 1980.
39. Davis GH, Weatherstone RM, et al: A pilot study of orally administered tetrahydrocannabinol in the management of patients undergoing radiotherapy for carcinoma of the bronchus. Br J Clin Pharmacol *1*:301, 1974.
40. Chang AE, Shiling DJ, Stillman RC, et al: A prospective evaluation of delta-9-tetrahydrocannabinol as an antiemetic in patients receiving Adriamycin and Cytoxan chemotherapy. Cancer *47*:1746, 1981.
41. Dobkins A, Evers W, Israel J: Double-blind study of trimethobenzamide, and a placebo as postanesthetic antiemetics following methoxyflurane anaesthesia. Can Anaesth Soc J *15*:80, 1968.
42. Strum SB, McDermed JE, Opfell RW, et al: Intravenous metoclopramide. An effective antiemetic in cancer chemotherapy. JAMA *247*:2683, 1982.
43. Swann IL, Thompson EN, Zureshi K: Droperidone or metoclopramide in preventing chemotherapeutically induced nausea and vomiting. Br Med J *2*:1188, 1979.
44. Gralla RJ, Itri LM, Pisko SE, et al: Antiemetic efficacy of high-dose metoclopramide randomized trials with placebo and prochlorperazine in patients with chemotherapy-induced nausea and vomiting. N Engl J Med *305*:905, 1981.
45. Drapkin RL, Sokol GH, Paladine WJ, et al: The antiemetic effect and dose response of dexamethasone in patients receiving cisplatinum. Proc Am Soc Clin Oncol *199*:61, 1982.
46. Cassileth PA, Lusk EJ, Torri S, et al: Antiemetic efficacy of dexamethasone therapy in patients receiving cancer chemotherapy. Arch Intern Med *143*:1347, 1983.
47. Kris MG, Gralla RJ, et al: Improved control of cisplatin-induced emesis with high-dose metoclopramide and with combinations of metoclopramide, dexamethasone, and diphenhydramine. Results of consecutive trials in 255 patients. Cancer *55*:527, 1985.
48. Krebs HB, Myers MG, et al: Combination antiemetic therapy in cisplatin-induced nausea and vomiting. Cancer *55*:2645, 1985.
49. Acute Leukemia Group B: Acute lymphocytic leukemia in children. JAMA *207*:923, 1969.
50. Hoston J, Olson KB, Sullivan J, Reilly C, Schneider B, Eastern Cooperation Oncology Group: 5-Fluorouracil in cancer: An improved regimen. Ann Intern Med *73*:897, 1970.
51. Young RC, Chabner BA: An in vivo method for determining differential effects of chemotherapy on target tissues in animals and man: Correction with plasma pharmacokinetics. J Clin Invest *52*:92A, 1973.
52. Chabner BA, Myers CE, Oliverio VT: Clinical pharmacology of anticancer drugs. Semin Oncol *2*:165, 1977.
53. Chabner BA, Young RC: Threshold methotrexate concentration for in vivo inhibition of DNA synthesis in normal and tumorous target tissues. J Clin Invest *52*:1104, 1973.
54. Stoller RG, Jacobs SA, Drake JC, Lutz RS, Chabner BA: Pharmacokinetics of high-dose methotrexate (NSC-740). Cancer Chemother Rep *6*:19, 1975.
55. Huffman DH, Wan SH, Azarnoff DL, Hoogstraten B: Pharmacokinetics of high-dose methotrexate (NSC-740). Clin Pharmacol Ther *14*:572, 1973.
56. Stoller RG, Hane KR, Jacobs SA: Use of plasma pharmacokinetics to predict and prevent methotrexate toxicity. N Engl J Med *297*:630, 1977.
57. Chabner BA, Johns DG, Bertino JR: Enzymatic cleavage of methotrexate provides a method for prevention of drug toxicity. Nature *239*:395, 1972.
58. Isacoff WH, Townsend CM, Eilber FR, Forster T, Morton DL, Block JB: High-dose methotrexate therapy of solid tumors: Observations relating to clinical toxicity. Med Pediatr Oncol *2*:319, 1976.
59. Bleyer WA: Methotrexate: Clinical pharmacology, current status, and therapeutic guidelines. Cancer Treat Rep *4*:87, 1977.
60. Jacobs SA, Bleyer WA, Chabner BA, Johns DG: Altered plasma pharmacokinetics of methotrexate administered intrathecally. Lancet *1*:455, 1975.
61. Wan SH, Huffman DH, Azarnoff DL, Stephens R, Hoogstraten B: Effect of route of administration and effusions on methotrexate pharmacokinetics. Cancer Res *34*:3487, 1974.
62. Weiss H, Walker M, Wiernik P: Neurotoxicity of commonly used antineoplastic agents. N Engl J Med *291*:75, 1974.
63. Rosenthal S, Kaufman S: Vincristine neurotoxicity. Ann Intern Med *80*:733, 1975.
64. Holland JF, Scharlau C, Gailani S, Krant MJ, Olson KB, Horton J, Schnider BJ, Lynch JJ, Owens A, Carbone PP, Colsky J, Grab D, Miller SP, Hall TC: Vincristine treatment of advanced cancer: A cooperative study of 392 cases. Cancer Res *33*:1258, 1973.
65. Sherlock P: Effect of cancer treatment on nutrition and gastrointestinal function (editorial). Clin Bull *9*:136, 1979.
66. Killen J, Mitchell EP, Woolley PV: Phase II studies of methylglyoxal-bis-guanylhydrazone. Cancer *50*:1258, 1982.
67. Elion GB: Biochemistry and pharmacology of purine analogues. Fed Proc *26*:898, 1967.
68. Colsky J, Greenspan EM, Warren TN: Hepatic fibrosis in children with acute leukemia after therapy with folic acid antagonists. Arch Pathol *39*:191, 1955.
69. Hersh EM, Wong VG, Henderson ES, Freirich EJ: Hepatotoxic effects of methotrexate. Cancer *19*:600, 1966.
70. Hansen HH, Selawry OS, Holland JF, McCall OB: The variability of individual tolerance to methotrexate in cancer patients. Br J Cancer *25*:298, 1971.
71. Dahl MGC, Gregory MM, Schever PJ: Methotrexate hepatotoxicity in psoriasis—comparison of different dose regimens. Br Med J *1*:654, 1972.
72. Muller SA, Farrow GM, Martalock DL: Cirrhosis caused by methotrexate in the treatment of psoriasis. Arch Dermatol *100*:523, 1969.
73. Roenigk HH Jr, Bergfield WF, St Jacques R, Owens FJ, Hawk WA: Hepatotoxicity of methotrexate in the treatment of psoriasis. Arch Dermatol *103*:250, 1971.
74. Weinstein G, Roenigk H, Maibach H, Cosmides J, Halprin K, Millard M: Psoriasis-liver-methotrexate interactions. Arch Dermatol *108*:36, 1973.
75. Bertino JR, Leavitt M, McCullough JL, Chabner BA: New approaches to chemotherapy with folate antagonists: Use of leucovorin "rescue" and enzy-

matic folate depletion. Ann NY Acad Sci *186*:486, 1971.
76. Dahl MGC, Gregory MM, Scheur PJ: Liver damage due to methotrexate in patients with psoriasis. Br Med J *1*:625, 1971.
77. Clarke PA, Hsia YE, Huntsman RG: Toxic complications of treatment with 6-mercaptopurine: Two cases with hepatic necrosis and intestinal ulceration. Br Med J *1*:393, 1960.
78. Einhorn M, Davidsohn I: Hepatotoxicity of mercaptopurine. JAMA *188*:802, 1964.
79. Kravitt EL, Stein JH, Kirkendall WM, Clifton JA: Mercaptopurine hepatotoxicity in a patient with chronic active hepatitis. Arch Intern Med *120*:729, 1967.
80. McIlvaine SK, MacCarthy JD: Hepatitis in association with prolonged 6-mercaptopurine therapy. Blood *14*:80, 1979.
81. Zarday J, Veith IJ, Gliedman ML, Soberman R: Irreversible liver damage after azathioprine. JAMA *222*:690, 1972.
82. Kennedy BJ: Metabolic and toxic effects of mithramycin during tumor therapy. Am J Med *49*:494, 1070.
83. Brown JH, Kennedy BJ: Mithramycin in the treatment of disseminated testicular neoplasms. N Engl J Med *272*:111, 1965.
84. Yarbro JW, Kennedy BJ: A comparison of the rate of recovery from inhibition of RNA synthesis in mouse liver and transplantable glioma. Cancer Res *27*:1779, 1967.
85. Bodey GP, Coltman CA, Freireich EJ, Lackland AB, Bonnet JD, Gehan EA, Haut AB, Hewlet JS, McCredit KB, Saiki JH, Wilson HE: Chemotherapy of acute leukemia: Comparison of cytarabine alone and in combination with vincristine, prednisone, and cyclophosphamide. Arch Intern Med *133*:260, 1974.
86. Gottlieb JA, Serpick AA: Clinical evaluation of 5-(3,3,-dimethyl-1-triazone) imidazole-4carboxamide in malignant melanoma and other neoplasms: Comparison of twice-weekly and daily administration schedules. Oncology *25*:225, 1971.
87. Young RC, Walker MD, Canellos GP, Schein PS, Chabner BA: Initial clinical trials with methyl-CCNU 1-(2-chlorethyl) 3-(4-methylcyclohexyl)-1-nitrosourea (MeCCNU). Cancer *31*:1164, 1973.
88. Schein PS, O'Connell MJ, Blom J: Clinical antitumor activity and toxicity of streptozotocin (NSC 85998). Cancer *34*:993, 1974.
89. Haskell CM, Canellos GP, Leventhal BG, Carbone PP, Block JB, Serpick AA, Selawry OS: Therapeutics and toxic effects in patients with neoplastic disease. N Engl J Med *281*:1028, 1969.
90. Arlin ZA, Flomenberg N, Gee TS, et al: Treatment of acute leukemia with 4'-(9-acridinylamino)methanesulfon-m-anisidide (AMSA) in combination with cytosine arabinoside and thioguanine. Cancer Clin Trials *4*:317, 1981.
91. Laurence MJ, Ries CA, Reynolds RD, et al: AMSA—A promising new agent in refractory acute leukemia. Cancer Treat Rep *66*:1475, 1982.
92. Applebaum FR, Shulman HM: Fatal hepatotoxicity associated with AMSA therapy. Cancer Treat Rep *66*:1863, 1982.
93. Amronin GD, Delman RM, Shanbran E: Liver damage after chemotherapy for leukemia and lymphoma. Gastroenterology *42*:401, 1962.
94. Benjamin RS: A practical approach to Adriamycin (NSC 123127) toxicity. Cancer Chemother Rep *6*:191, 1975.
95. Menard DB, Gisselbrecht C, Marty M, et al: Antineoplastic agents and the liver. Gastroenterology *78*:142, 1980.
96. Van den Berg HW, Desai ZR, Wilson R, et al: The pharmacokinetics of vincristine in man. Reduced drug clearance associated with raised serum alkaline phosphatase and dose-limited elimination. Cancer Chemother Pharmacol *8*:215, 1982.
97. Desai ZR, Van den Berg HW, Bridges JM, et al: Can severe vincristine neurotoxicity be prevented? Cancer Chemother Pharmacol *8*:211–214, 1982.
98. Issel BF, Crooker ST: Etoposide (VP-16-216). Cancer Treat Rev *107*:124, 1979.
99. Robert J, Barbier P, Manaster J, et al: Hepatotoxicity of cytostatic drugs evaluated by liver function tests and appearance of jaundice. Digestion *1*:229, 1968.
100. Feingold ML, Kass LG: Effects of long-term administration of busulfan. Arch Intern Med *124*:66, 1969.
101. Kass LG, Melamed MR, Mayer K: The effect of busulfan on human epithelia. Am J Clin Pathol *44*:385, 1965.
102. Leake E, Smith WG, Woodliff HJ: Diffuse interstitial pulmonary fibrosis after busulfan therapy. Lancet *2*:432, 1963.
103. Podall LN, Winbler S: Busulfan lung. Am J Roentgenol *120*:151, 1974.
104. Min K, Gyorkey F: Interstitial fibrosis, atypical epithelial changes and bronchiolar cell carcinoma following busulfan therapy. Cancer *22*:1027, 1968.
105. Rosenow EC III: The spectrum of drug-induced pulmonary disease. Ann Intern Med *77*:977, 1972.
106. Heard BE, Cooke RA: Busulfan lung. Thorax *23*:187, 1968.
107. Littler WA, Kay JM, Hasleton PS: Busulfan lung. Thorax *24*:639, 1969.
108. Robin AE, Haggard ME, Travis LB: Lung changes and chemotherapeutic agents in childhood: Report of a case associated with cyclophosphamide therapy. Am J Dis Child *129*:337, 1970.
109. Topilow AA, Rothenberg SP, Cottrell TS: Interstitial pneumonia after prolonged treatment with cyclophosphamide. Am Rev Resp Dis *108*:114, 1973.
110. DeLena M, Guzzon A, Monfardini S, Bonadonna G: Clinical, radiological, and histopathologic studies on pulmonary toxicity induced by treatment with bleomycin. Cancer Chemother Rep *56*:343, 1972.
111. Yagoda A, Mukhirji B, Young C, Etcubanas E, Lamonte C, Smith JR, Tan CTC, Krakoff IA: Bleomycin, an antitumor antibiotic: Clinical experiment in 274 patients. Ann Intern Med *77*:861, 1972.
112. Blum RH, Carter SK, Agre K: A clinical review of bleomycin—new antineoplastic agent. Cancer *31*:903, 1973.
113. Macdonald JS, Schein PS, Hubbard S, DeVita VT: Severe bleomycin pulmonary toxicity at low total doses in patients treated with combination chemotherapy. Clin Res *23*:341A, 1975.
114. Samules ML, Johnson DE, Holoye PY, et al: Large-dose bleomycin pulmonary toxicity. A possible role of prior radiotherapy. JAMA *235*:1117, 1976.
115. Einhorn LH, Krause M, Hornback N, et al: Enhanced pulmonary toxicity with bleomycin and radiotherapy in oat cell lung. Cancer *37*:2414, 1976.
116. Skarin A, Lokich J, Goodman R, et al: Combined

intensive chemotherapy and radiotherapy in oat cell carcinoma of the lung. Proc Am Soc Clin Oncol *16*:264, 1975.
117. Holman KE, Bleehan NM, Brewin TB: Clinical studies with bleomycin. Br Med J *4*:635, 1972.
118. Krakoff IH, Cortikovic E, Currie V, et al: Clinical, pharmacologic and therapeutic studies of bleomycin given by continuous infusion. Cancer *40*:2027, 1977.
119. Goldiner PL, Carlon GC, Cortikovic E, et al: Factors influencing postoperative morbidity and mortality in patients treated with bleomycin. Br Med J *1*:1664, 1978.
120. Clarysse AM, Cathey WJ, Cartwright GE, Wintrobe MM: Pulmonary disease complicating intermittent therapy with methotrexate. JAMA *209*:1861, 1969.
121. Filip DJ, Logue GL, Harle TS, Farrar WH: Pulmonary and hepatic complications of methotrexate therapy of psoriasis. JAMA *216*:881, 1971.
122. Goldman GC, Moschella SL: Severe pneumonitis occurring during methotrexate therapy. Arch Dermatol *103*:194, 1971.
123. Schwartz JR, Kajani MK: Methotrexate therapy and pulmonary disease. JAMA *210*:1924, 1969.
124. Orwall ES, Kiessling P, Patterson R: Interstitial pneumonia from mitomycin. Ann Intern Med *89*:352, 1978.
125. Buzdar AU, Legha SS, Luna MA, et al: Pulmonary toxicity of mitomycin. Cancer *45*:236, 1980.
126. Holoye PY, Jenkin DE, Brenberg SD: Pulmonary toxicity in long-term administration of BENU. Cancer Treat Rep *60*:1691, 1976.
127. Durant JR, Norgord MJ, Murad TM, et al: Pulmonary toxicity associated with bischloroethyl nitrosourea (BCNU). Ann Intern Med *90*:191, 1979.
128. Weiss RB, Poster DS, Penta JS: The nitrosoureas and pulmonary toxicity. Cancer Treat Rep *8*:111, 1981.
129. Lee W, Moore RP, Wampler GL: Interstitial pulmonary fibrosis as a complication of prolonged methyl-CCNU therapy. Cancer Treat Rep *62*:1355, 1978.
130. Ahlgren JD, Smith FP, Kerwin DM, et al: Pulmonary disease as a complication of chlorozotocin chemotherapy. Cancer Treat Rep *65*:223, 1981.
131. Spector JI, Zimbler H: Cyclophosphamide pneumonitis. N Engl J Med *307*:251, 1982.
132. Cole SR, Myers TJ, Klatsky AU: Pulmonary disease with chlorambucil therapy. Cancer *41*:455, 1978.
133. Goucher G, Rowland V, Hawking J: Melphalan-induced pulmonary interstitial fibrosis. Chest *77*:805, 1980.
134. Weisenburger DD: Interstitial pneumonia associated with azathioprine therapy. Am J Clin Pathol *69*:181, 1978.
135. Haupt HM, Hutchins GM, Moore GW: Ara-C lung: Noncardiogenic pulmonary edema complicating cytosine arabinoside therapy of leukemia. Am J Med *70*:256, 1981.
136. Lokich JJ, Moloney WC: Allergic reaction to procarbazine. Clin Pharmacol Ther *13*:573, 1972.
137. Lefrok EA, Pitha J, Rosenheim S: A clinico-pathologic analysis of Adriamycin cardiotoxicity. Cancer *3*:302, 1973.
138. Molpas J, Scott R: Daunomycin in acute myelocytic leukemia. Lancet *1*:469, 1969.
139. Bonadonna G, Monfardini S: Cardiotoxicity of daunomycin. Lancet *1*:837, 1969.
140. Rinehart J, Lewis R, Bolcerzak SP: Adriamycin cardiotoxicity in man. Ann Intern Med *81*:475, 1974.
141. Halazun JF, Wagner HR, Gaeta JF, Sinks LF: Daunorubicin cardiac toxicity in children with acute lymphocytic leukemia. Cancer *33*:545, 1974.
142. Von Hoff DD, Layard MW, Basa P, et al: Risk factors for doxorubicin-induced congestive heart failure. Ann Intern Med *91*:710, 1979.
143. Minow RA, Benjamin RS, Gottlieb JA: Adriamycin (NSC 123127) cardiomyopathy—an overview with determination of risk factors. Cancer Chemother Rep (Part 3)*6*:195, 1975.
144. Weiss AJ, Metter GE, Fletcher WS, et al: Studies on Adriamycin using a weekly regimen demonstrating its clinical effectiveness and lack of cardiac toxicity. Cancer Treat Rep *60*:813, 1976.
145. Chlebowski R, Pugh R, Paroly W, et al: Adriamycin on a weekly schedule: Clinically effective with low incidence of cardiotoxicity. Clin Res *27*:53A, 1979.
146. Rinehart J, Lewis RP, Balerzak SP: Adriamycin cardiotoxicity in man. Ann Intern Med *81*:475, 1974.
147. Henderson IC, Sloss LJ, Jaffe N, et al: Serial studies of cardiac function in patients receiving Adriamycin. Cancer Treat Rep *62*:923, 1978.
148. Greco FA: Subclinical Adriamycin toxicity. Detection by timing the arterial sounds. Cancer Treat Rep *62*:901, 1978.
149. Jones SE, Evy GA, Grove BM: Electrocardiographic detection of Adriamycin heart disease. Proc Am Soc Clin Oncol *16*:228, 1975.
150. Bloon KR, Bini RM, Williams CM, Sonley MJ, Gribben MR: Echocardiography in Adriamycin toxicity. Cancer *41*:1265, 1978.
151. Singer JW, Narahare KA, Ritchie JL, et al: Time and dose-dependent changes in ejection fraction determined by radionuclide angiography after anthracycline therapy. Cancer Treat Rep *62*:945, 1978.
152. Bristow MR, Mason JW, Billingham ME, Daniels JR: Doxorubicin cardiomyopathy evaluation by phonocardiography, endomyocardial biopsy, and cardiac catheterization. Ann Intern Med *88*:168, 1978.
153. Billingham ME, Mason JW, Bristow MR, et al: Anthracycline cardiomyopathy monitored by morphologic changes. Cancer Treat Rep *62*:865, 1978.
154. Ferrans VJ: Overview of cardiac pathology in relation to anthracycline cardiotoxicity. Cancer Treat Rep *62*:955, 1978.
155. O'Connell TX, Berenbaum MC: Cardiac and pulmonary effects of high-dose cyclophosphamide and isophosphamide. Cancer Res *34*:1568, 1974.
156. Moertel CG, Reitemeir RJ: Experience with 5-fluorouracil in the palliative management of advanced carcinoma of the gastrointestinal tract. Staff Meet Mayo Clin *37*:520–529, 1962.
157. Roth A, Kolaric K, Popovic S: Cardiotoxicity of 5-fluorouracil (NSC 19893). Cancer Chemother Rep *59*:1051, 1975.
158. Wiltshaw E, Carr B: Cis-platinum II diamminedichloride. Recent Results Cancer Res *48*:178, 1974.
159. Weiss H, Walker M, Wiernik P: Neurotoxicity of commonly used antineoplastic agents. N Engl J Med *291*:75, 1974.
160. Rosenthal S, Kaufman S: Vincristine neurotoxicity. Ann Intern Med *80*:733, 1975.
161. Sandler SG, Tobin W, Henderson ES: Vincristine-induced neuropathy: A clinical study of fifty leukemia patients. Neurology *19*:367, 1969.

162. Bleyer WA, Drake JC, Chabner BA: Neurotoxicity and elevated cerebrospinal fluid methotrexate concentration in meningeal leukemia. N Engl J Med *289*:770, 1973.
163. Geiser CF, Bishop Y, Jaffe N, Furman L, Traggis D, Frei E: Adverse effects of intrathecal methotrexate in children with acute leukemia in remission. Blood *45*:189, 1975.
164. Ochs JJ, Burger P, Brecher ML, et al: Computed tomography brain scans in children with acute lymphocytic leukemia receiving methotrexate alone as central nervous system prophylaxis. Cancer *45*:2274, 1980.
165. Haskell CM, Canellos GP, Levanthal BG: L-Asparaginase toxicity. Cancer Res *29*:974, 1969.
166. Moertel CG, Reitemeir RJ, Hahn RG: Fluorinated pyrimidine therapy of advanced gastrointestinal cancer. Gastroenterology *46*:371, 1964.
167. Brunner KW, Young CW: A methyl-hydrazine derivative in Hodgkin's disease and other malignant neoplasms. Ann Intern Med *63*:69, 1965.
168. Higby DJ, Wallace HJ Jr, Holland JF: Diamminedichloroplatinum (NSC-119875): A Phase I study. Cancer Chemother Rep *57*:459, 1973.
169. Johnson BL, Fisher RI, Bender RA, et al: Hexamethylmelamine in alkylating agent–resisting ovarian carcinoma. Carcinoma *42*:2157, 1978.
170. Madajewicz S, West CR, Park HC, et al: Phase II study—intra-arterial BCNU therapy for metastatic brain tumors. Cancer *47*:653, 1981.
171. Russell JA, Powles RL: Neuropathy due to cytosine arabinoside. Br Med J *4*:652, 1974.
172. Falkson G, Van Dyke JJ, Van Eden EB, et al: A clinical trial of the oral form of 4-demethylepipodophyllotoxin-D-ethylidene glucoside (NSC-141540) (VP-16-213). Cancer *35*:114, 1975.
173. Paterson AHG, McPherson TA: A possible neurologic complication of DTIC. Cancer Treat Rep *61*:105, 1977.
174. Killen JY, Mitchell EP, Hoth DF, et al: Phase II studies of methylglyoxal bisguanylhydrazone (NSC 32946) in carcinoma of the colon and lung. Cancer *50*:1258, 1982.
175. Buckner KW, Rudolph RH, Fefer A, Clift RA, Epstein RB, Funk DD, Neiman PE, Slichter SG, Storb R, Thomas ED: High-dose cyclophosphamide therapy for malignant disease: Toxicity, tumor response, and the effects of autologous marrow. Cancer *29*:357, 1972.
176. Kennedy BJ, Theologides A: The role of 5-fluorouracil in malignant disease. Ann Intern Med *55*:719, 1961.
177. Tan C, Etcubanos E, Wollner N, Rosen G, Gilladoga A, Showell J, Murphy ML, Krakoff IH: Adriamycin—an antitumor antibiotic in the treatment of neoplastic diseases. Cancer *32*:9, 1973.
178. Haut A, Abbott WS, Wintrobe MM, Cartwright GE: Busulfan in the treatment of chronic myelocytic leukemia. The effect of long-term intermittent therapy. Blood *17*:1, 1961.
179. Epstein EH Jr, Lutzner MA: Folliculitis induced by actinomycin-D. N Engl J Med *281*:1094, 1069.
180. Wintrobe MM, Huguley CM Jr: Nitrogen-mustard therapy for Hodgkin's disease, lymphosarcoma, the leukemias, and other disorders. Cancer *1*:357, 1948.
181. Holton CP, Vietti TJ, Nora AH, Donaldson MH, Stuckey WJ, Watkins WL, Lane DM: Clinical study of daunomycin and prednisone for induction of remission in children with advanced leukemia. N Engl J Med *208*:171, 1963.
182. Selawry OS, Hananian J: Vincristine treatment of cancer in children. JAMA *183*:741, 1963.
183. Wright TL, Hurley R, Korst DR, Monte RW, John RJ, Will JJ, Louis J: Vinblastine in neoplastic disease. Cancer Res *23*:169, 1963.
184. Frei E III: The clinical use of actinomycin-D. Cancer Chemother Rep *58*:49, 1974.
185. Laughlin RA, Landeen JM, Habal MB: The management of inadvertent subcutaneous Adriamycin infiltration. Am J Surg *137*:408, 1979.
186. Ignoffo RJ, Friedman MA: Therapy of local toxicities caused by extravasation of cancer chemotherapeutic drugs. Cancer Treat Rep *64*:17, 1980.
187. Falkson G, Van der Merwe AM, Falkson HC: Clinical experience with 5-(3,3-bis(2-chlorethyl)-1-triazeno) imidazole-4-carboxamide (NSC 82196) in the treatment of metastatic malignant melanoma. Cancer Chemother Rep *56*:67, 1972.
188. Kennedy BJ: Mithramycin therapy in advanced testicular neoplasms. Cancer *26*:755, 1970.
189. Evans WE, Tsiatis A, Rivera G, et al: Anaphylactoid reactions to *Escherichia coli* and *Erwinia* asparaginase in children with leukemia and lymphoma. Cancer *49*:1378, 1982.
190. Weiss RB, Burno S: Hypersensitivity reactions to cancer chemotherapeutic agents. Ann Intern Med *94*:66, 1981.
191. Dinarello CA, Ward SB, Wolff SM: Pyrogenic properties of bleomycin (NSC-125066). Cancer Chemother Rep *57*:393, 1973.
192. Movsesian MA, Merrill JM: Eosinophilia with DTIC chemotherapy. Ann Intern Med *93*:642, 1980.
193. Gralla RJ, Casper ES, Kelsen DP, et al: Cisplatin and vindesine combination chemotherapy for advanced carcinoma of the lung. A randomized trial investigating two dosage schedules. Ann Intern Med *95*:414, 1981.
194. Lakin JD, Cahill RA: Generalized urticaria to cyclophosphamide: Type I hypersensitivity to an immunosuppressive agent. J Allergy Clin Immunol *58*:160, 1976.
195. Klimo P, Ibrahim E: Anaphylactic reaction to methotrexate in high doses as adjuvant treatment of osteogenic sarcoma. Cancer Treat Rep *65*:725, 1981.
196. O'Dwyer PJ, Weiss RB: Hypersensitivity reactions induced by etoposide. Cancer Treat Rep *68*:959, 1984.
197. Wortman JE, Lucas VS, Schuster E, et al: Sudden death during doxorubicin administration. Cancer *44*:1588, 1979.
198. Schimpff SC: Therapy of infection in patients with granulocytopenia. Med Clin North Am *61*:1101, 1977.
199. Love LS, Schimpff SC, Schiffer CA, Wiernik PH: Improved prognosis in patients with gram-negative bacteremia. Am J Med *68*:643, 1980.
200. Herzig BH, Herzig GP, Bull MI, Graw RC, Ray KK: Granulocytic transfusions; Therapy for gram-negative septicemia. N Engl J Med *296*:701, 1977.
201. Aisner J: Platelet transfusion therapy. Med Clin North Am *61*:1133, 1977.
202. Door RT, Fortz WL: Cancer Chemotherapy Handbook. New York, Elsevier/North Holland, 1980.
203. McGrath BP, Ibels LS, Raik E, et al: Erythroid

toxicity of azathioprine: Macrocytosis and selective marrow hypoplasia. Q J Med *44*:57, 1975.

204. Kennedy BJ: Hydroxyurea therapy in chronic myelogenous leukemia. Cancer *29*:1052, 1972.
205. Gulnti SC, Sordillo P, Kempin S, et al: Microangiopathic hemolytic anemia observed after treatment of epidermoid carcinoma with mitomycin C and 5-fluorouracil. Cancer *45*:2252, 1980.
206. Foucar K, McKenna RW, Bloomfield CD, Bowers TK, Brunning RD: Therapy-related leukemia: A panmyelosis. Cancer *43*:1285, 1979.
207. McKenna RW, Parkin J, Foucar R, Brunning RD: Ultrastructural characteristics of therapy-related acute nonlymphocytic leukemia. Evidence for a panmyelosis. Cancer *48*:725, 1981.
208. Rowley JD, Golomb HM, Vardiman JW: Nonrandom chromosome abnormalities in acute leukemia and dysmyelopoietic syndromes in patients with previously treated malignant disease. Blood *58*:759, 1981.
209. Pedersen-Bjergaard J, Philip P, Pedersen NI, Hon-Jensen K, Svejgaard A, Jensen G, Nissen NI: Acute nonlymphocytic leukemia, preleukemia, and acute myeloproliferative syndrome secondary to treatment of other malignant diseases. II. Bone marrow cytology, cytogenetics, results of HLA-typing, response to antileukemic chemotherapy, and survival in a total series of 55 patients. Cancer *54*:452, 1984.
210. Michels SD, McKenna RW, Arthur DC, Brunning RD: Therapy-related acute myeloid leukemia and myelodysplastic syndrome. A clinical and morphologic study of 65 cases. Blood *65*:1364, 1985.
211. Robertson GL, Bhoopatam N, Zelkoitz LJ: Vincristine neurotoxicity and abnormal secretion of antidiuretic hormone. Arch Intern Med *132*:717, 1973.
212. Coggins PF III, Ravdin RG, Eisman EM: Clinical pharmacology and preliminary evaluation of Cytoxan. Cancer Chemother Rep *3*:9, 1959.
213. Host H, Nissen-Meyer R: A preliminary clinical study of cyclophosphamide. Cancer Chemother Rep *9*:47, 1960.
214. George P: Hemorrhagic cystitis and cyclophosphamide. Lancet *2*:942, 1963.
215. Anderson EF, Cobb OE, Glenn JF: Cyclophosphamide hemorrhagic cystitis. J Urol *97*:857, 1967.
216. Marsh FP, Vince FP, Pollock DJ, Path MC, Blandy JP, Chir M: Cyclophosphamide necrosis of bladder causing calcification contracture and reflux; Treated by colocystoplasty. Br J Urol *43*:324, 1971.
217. Riggenbach R, Barrett O, Shown T: Hemorrhagic cystitis due to cyclophosphamide. South Med J *61*:139, 1968.
218. Wall RL, Clausen KP: Carcinoma of the urinary bladder in patients receiving cyclophosphamide. N Engl J Med *296*:271, 1975.
219. Berkson BM, Lome LG, Shapiro I: Severe cystitis induced by cyclophosphamide. N Engl J Med *293*:271, 1975.
220. Bennett AH: Cyclophosphamide and hemorrhagic cystitis. J Urol *111*:603, 1974.
221. Johnson WW, Meadows DC: Urinary bladder fibrosis and telangiectasia associated with long-term cyclophosphamide therapy. N Engl J Med *284*:290, 1971.
222. De Fronzo RA, Braine H, Colvin OM, Davis PJ: Water intoxication in man after cyclophosphamide therapy. Ann Intern Med *78*:861, 1973.
223. Kuhn JA, Argy WP, Rakowski TA, Moriarity JJ, Schreiner GE, Schein PS: Nephrotoxicity of cis-diamminedichloroplatinum II as measured by urinary glucuronidase. Cancer Treat Rep *64*:1083, 1980.
224. Korvach JS, Moertel CG, Schutt AJ, Reitemeier RG, Hahn RG: Phase II study of cis-diamminedichloroplatinum (NSC 119875) in advanced carcinoma of the large bowel. Cancer Chemother Rep *57*:357, 1973.
225. Talley PN, O'Bryan RM, Gutterman JU, Brownlee KW, McCredie KB: Clinical evaluation of toxic effects of cis-diamminedichloroplatinum II (NSC 119875)—Phase I study. Cancer Chemother Rep *57*:465, 1973.
226. Schein PS, DeLellis RA, Kahn CR, et al: Islet cell tumors: Current concepts and management. Ann Intern Med *79*:239, 1973.
227. Sadoff L: Nephrotoxicity of streptozotocin (NSC-85998). Cancer Chemother Rep *54*:457, 1970.
228. Broder LE, Carter SK: Pancreatic islet cell carcinoma. II. Results of therapy with streptozotocin in 52 patients. Am J Med *79*:108, 1973.
229. Harmon WE, Cohen HS, Schneeberger EE, Grupe WG: Chronic renal failure in children treated with methyl CCNU. N Engl J Med *300*:1200, 1979.
230. Nichols WC, Moertel CG: Nephrotoxicity of methyl CCNU. N Engl J Med *301*:1189, 1979.
231. Silver HKB, Morton DL: CCNU nephrotoxicity following sustained remission in oat cell carcinoma. Cancer Treat Rep *63*:226, 1979.
232. Micetich KC, Jensen AM, Mandard JC, et al: Nephrotoxicity of semustine (methyl-CCNU) in patients with malignant melanoma receiving adjuvant chemotherapy. Am J Med *71*:967–972, 1981.
233. Schacht RG, Feiner HD, Gallo GR, et al: Nephrotoxicity of nitrosoureas. Cancer *48*:1328, 1981.
234. Pittman SW, Parker LM, Tattersall MHN, Jaffe W, Frei E: Clinical trial of high-dose methotrexate (NSC 740) with citrovorum factor (NSC 3590); Toxicologic and therapeutic observations. Cancer Chemother Rep *6*:43, 1975.
235. Kressell BR, Ryan KP, Duong AT, et al: Microangiopathic hemolytic anemia, thrombocytopenia, and renal failure in patients treated for adenocarcinoma. Cancer *48*:1738, 1981.
236. Kennedy BJ: Metabolic and toxic effects of mithramycin during tumor therapy. Am J Med *85*:494, 1970.
237. Von Hoff DD, Slavik M, Muggia FM: 5-Azacytidine. A new anticancer drug with effectiveness in acute myelogenous leukemia. Ann Intern Med *85*:237, 1976.
238. Peterson BA, Collins AJ, Vogelzang NJ, Bloomfield CD: 5-Azacytidine and renal tubular dysfunction. Blood *57*:182, 1981.
239. Cheviakoff S, Calamera JC, Morgenfeld M, Mancini RE: Recovery of spermatogenesis in patients with lymphoma after treatment with chlorambucil. J Reprod Fertil *33*:155, 1973.
240. Zuereshi M, Goldsmith H, Pennington J, Cox PE: Cyclophosphamide therapy and sterility. Lancet *2*:1290, 1972.
241. Richter P, Calamera JC, Morganfeld MC, Kierszenbaum AL, Lavieri JC, Manai RE: Effects of chlorambucil on spermatogenesis in the human with malignant lymphoma. Cancer *25*:1026, 1970.
242. Fairley KF, Barrie TU, Johnson W: Sterility and testicular atrophy related to cyclophosphamide therapy. Lancet *1*:568, 1972.

243. Sherins RJ, DeVita VT Jr: Effect of drug treatment for lymphoma on male reproduction capacity. Studies on men in remission after therapy. Ann Intern Med *79*:216, 1973.
244. Brickanan JD, Fairley KF, Barrie JU: Return of spermatogenesis after stopping cyclophosphamide therapy. Lancet *2*:156, 1975.
245. Van Thiel DH, Sherins RJ, Myers GH Jr, et al: Evidence for a specific seminiferous tubular factor affecting follicle-stimulating hormone secretion in man. J Clin Invest *51*:1009, 1972.
246. Galton DAG, Till M, Wiltshaw E: Busulfan: Summary of clinical results. Ann NY Acad Sci *68*:967, 1958.
247. Nicholson HO: Cytotoxic drugs in pregnancy. J Obstet Gynaecol Br Comm *75*:307, 1968.
248. Uldall PK, Kerr DNS, Tacchi D: Sterility and cyclophosphamide. Lancet *1*:693, 1972.
249. Sobrinho LG, Levine RA, DeConti RC: Amenorrhea in patients with Hodgkin's disease treated with antineoplastic agents. Am J Obstet Gynecol *109*:135, 1971.
250. Warne GL, Fairley KF, Hobbs JB, et al: Cyclophosphamide-induced ovarian failure. N Engl J Med *289*:1159, 1973.
251. Pastore G, Antonelli R, Fine W, et al: Late effects of treatment of cancer in infancy. Med Pediatr Oncol *105*:369, 1982.
252. Holmes GE, Holmes FF: Pregnancy outcome of patients treated for Hodgkin's disease: A controlled study. Cancer *41*:1317, 1978.
253. Schardein JL: Chemically induced birth defects. *In* Cancer Chemotherapeutic Agents. New York, Marcel Dekker, 1985, Chapter 27.
254. Nicholson HO: Cytotoxic drugs in pregnancy. Review of reported cases. J Obstet Gynaecol Br Comm *75*:307, 1968.
255. Thiersch JB: Therapeutic abortions with a folic acid antagonist, 4-amino pteroylglutamic acid, administered by the oral route. Am J Obstet Gynecol *63*:1298, 1952.
256. Skinner MD, Schwartz RS: Immunosuppressive therapy. N Engl J Med *287*:221, 1972.
257. Golby M: Fertility after renal transplantation. Transplantation *10*:201, 1970.
258. Penn I, Makowski E, Droegmueller W, Halgrimson CG, Starzl TE: Parenthood in renal homograft recipients. JAMA *216*:1755, 1971.
259. Garrett MJ: Teratogenic effect of combination chemotherapy. Ann Intern Med *80*:667, 1974.
260. Kapadia SB, Krause JR, Ellis LD, Pan SF, Wald N: Induced acute nonlymphocytic leukemia following long-term chemotherapy. A study of 20 cases. Cancer *45*:1315, 1980.
261. Grunwald HW, Rosner F: Acute myeloid leukemia following treatment of Hodgkin's disease—A review. Cancer *50*:676, 1982.
262. Greene MH, Boice JD, Greer BE, Blessing JA, Dembo AJ: Acute nonlymphocytic leukemia after therapy with alkylating agents for ovarian cancer—A study of five randomized clinical trials. N Engl J Med *307*:1416, 1982.
263. Boice JD, Greene MH, Killen JY, Ellenberg SS, Keehn RJ, McFadden E, Chen TT, Fraumeni JF: Leukemia and preleukemia after adjuvant treatment of gastrointestinal cancer with semustine (methyl-CCNU). N Engl J Med *309*:1079, 1983.
264. Bartolucci AA, Liu C, Durant JR, Gams RA: Acute myelogenous leukemia as a second malignant neoplasm following the successful treatment of advanced Hodgkin's disease. Cancer *52*:2209, 1983.
265. Coltman GA, Dixon DO: Second malignancies complicating Hodgkin's disease: A Southwest Oncology Group 10-year followup. Cancer Treat Rep *66*:1023, 1982.
266. Glicksman AS, Pajak TF, Gottlieb A, Nissen N, Stutzman L, Cooper MR: Second malignant neoplasms in patients successfully treated for Hodgkin's disease: A Cancer and Leukemia Group B study. Cancer Treat Rep *66*:1035, 1982.
267. Shenkenberg TD, Van Hoff DD: Mitoxantrone; A new anticancer drug with significant clinical activity. Ann Intern Med *105*:67–70, 1986.
268. Lindpainter K, Lindpainter LS, Wentworth M: Acute myocardial necrosis after administration of amsacrine. Cancer *57*:1284–1286, 1986.
269. Mandel EM, Lewinski U, Djaldeti M: Vincristine-induced myocardial infarction. Cancer *36*:1979–1982, 1975.
270. Nora R, Abrams J, Silverman HJ: Myocardial infarction in patients receiving high-dose interleukin. Proc Am Soc Clin Oncol *6*:245, 1987.

SECTION E

Heavy Metals and Inorganic Agents

CHAPTER 56

MERCURY

Regine Aronow, M.D.

Mercury is a commonly found substance in the environment.[1] Its greatest industrial use is in chlor-alkali production and in the manufacture of electrical apparatus (such as batteries, switches, and bulbs). It is used as an antifouling agent and as a pigment in some paints, as a slimicide in paper production, as a working fluid in instruments, as a fungicide in agriculture, as a catalyst or building block in the manufacture of some plastics and other chemicals, and in a number of other processes. Mercury is used in medicine as a germicidal and a bactericidal agent and serves as a weight in Miller-Abbott decompression tubes. In dentistry, it is used in the making of amalgam fillings. Discharges from chemical plants, refuse containing any of the above-described products, the burning of fossil fuels, and the natural release from geologic formations, as well as during the mining and the extraction of ores, all contribute to the diffusion of mercury into the environment.[2] The more common sources of occupational exposure to mercury are listed in Table 56–1.

Little known is the fact that mercury is used as a bactericidal and fungicidal agent in some paints, especially to maintain the shelf life of latex paints and coatings; this is not *required to be stated on the label.*[2a]

Over the last 60 years, the outstanding number of cases of mercury poisoning described in the literature has been in the form of acrodynia (pink disease) from exposure to mercurous chloride (calomel) teething preparations or diaper powders, acute poisoning from the intentional or accidental ingestion of organic mercury salts, inhalation exposure from heating various mercury compounds, the release of the vapor from elemental mercury and from various alkyl mercury compounds in industrial and agricultural settings, or ingestion of organic mercury in food such as in Japan and Canada from contaminated fish, in Iraq, Pakistan, Ghana, and Guatemala from mercury fungicide-treated grain being made into flour for bread, in New Mexico from pigs fed mercury fungicide-treated grain,[3] and the use of alkyl mercurials as a commercial germicidal diaper rinse in Argentina.[65]

Mercury poisoning presents in many diverse ways, depending on the type (oral, inhalation, dermal, ingestion, aspiration), duration (acute, chronic), and intensity (cumulative) of the exposure, and the chemical (elemental, inorganic, or specific organic) form of the mercury.[4] Additionally, animal and environmental evidence indicates that the elemental form can be converted within biologic systems to an inorganic salt, some organic forms to inorganic forms, and possibly under certain conditions inorganic forms to organic forms.[5] This may account for mixed symptomatology occurring in some patients. A high index of suspicion on the part of the physician and a detailed history of exposure may be almost as important as laboratory indices to establish the diagnosis. Microenvironmental acute exposures to mercury vapor have been shown not to correlate with standard measuring techniques.[66] This concept has not yet been reported in application to chronic exposures.

Mercury is generally classified as occurring in an inorganic form (elemental mercury,

Table 56–1. COMMON OPERATIONS IN WHICH EXPOSURE TO MERCURY MAY OCCUR

ORGANIC MERCURY	INORGANIC MERCURY	
During mining, extraction, and processing of mercury ore During manufacture of fungicides and slimicides During treatment and utilization of seeds and bulbs During use as a wood, timber, and paper preservative and slimicide During use in laboratories (histology, pathology) During use in medicine	During use as a liquid cathode in electrolytic production of chlorine and caustic soda from brine During manufacture of inorganic and organic compounds for use as pesticides, antiseptics, germicides, and skin preparations. Also miscellaneous applications as chemical intermediator, preservatives, and pigments During preparation of amalgams in dentistry, chemistry processing, molding operations, and jewelry making During manufacture of mildew-proof paints and marine antifouling agents During manufacture of organic mercurials; batteries, lamps (fluorescent and mercury ore), power tubes, tungsten-molybdenum wire and rods During manufacture of inorganic salts for use as catalysts in production of urethanes, vinyl chloride monomers, anthraquinone derivatives, and other miscellaneous chemicals	During use as a chemical intermediate and in the manufacture of felt; as a flotation agent in manufacture of bowling balls; or as a laboratory reagent During use or manufacture of instruments (thermometers, barometers, manometers) with mercury as a working fluid During manufacture of explosives and fireworks During use as a conductor during construction and maintenance of military and nuclear power systems, in mercury-stem boilers, and in air rectifiers During use and manufacture of compounds for pulp and paper industry as controls for biologic growths During roasting and smelting operations and extraction of silver and gold During mining and subsequent refining of ore containing cinnabar

Adapted from OSHA documents.

mercurous and mercuric salts) or in an organic form (alkyls and aryls). Elemental mercury can volatilize slowly at room temperature and rapidly with heat.[5] Inhalation of mercury vapor is very hazardous and almost 100 per cent is absorbed, with an average of 75 per cent retained.[6] Ingestion of elemental mercury, such as from a broken thermometer bulb, is relatively harmless unless there is an inordinate delay in passage through the gastrointestinal tract. It can be converted to mercuric oxide within the body.[5] When injected intravenously or distributed from subcutaneous deposits or lacerations, conversion to the mercuric form may gradually take place from the embolization (visible on x-ray films), resulting in mercurialism as well as abscess formation and ischemia.[7] The significance of the release of mercury from dental amalgam is still being evaluated.[67]

The mercurous salts are less toxic than the mercuric salts. Both can be corrosive to the eyes, skin, and mucous membranes.[5] Approximately 15 per cent of a given dose of inorganic salts may be absorbed from the gastrointestinal tract.[1] Accidental ingestion of disk batteries containing mercury salts has rarely resulted in corrosion of the mucosa and/or mercury poisoning.[68]

Inorganic mercury can cross the placental barrier.[8] Exposure of children of thermometer plant workers to elemental mercury also has been reported.[10]

The organic forms of mercury involve mostly short-chain alkyls, such as a methyl mercury, which has metabolically stable bonds and causes unique symptomatology, and the phenyl aryls, which rapidly are converted to inorganic compounds in the body.[5] Methyl mercury appears to be completely absorbed from the gastrointestinal tract, and phenyl mercury 80 to 100 per cent absorbed.[1]

Methyl mercury crosses the placental barrier and concentrates in the fetus, as evidenced by fetal blood levels higher than the mother's and also concentrates in breast milk at levels lower than in the mother's blood.[8–12]

Pathophysiology

The definition of the mechanisms by which various mercurials exert their toxic effects in the body is still under study. Generally, mercurials are attracted to sulfhydryl radicals in the body and are bound to proteins, onto membranes, and into enzymes, altering their normal functioning.[5] Short-chain alkyl mercurials, especially methyl mercury, penetrate the red blood cell membrane and bind to hemoglobin.[13] Elemental mercury and methyl mercury readily cross the blood-brain barrier and are distributed in the central nervous system.[14] Mercury becomes sequestered in lysosomal dense bodies of neurons;[69] the ultimate significance of this is yet to be defined.

Inorganic mercury accumulates primarily in the kidneys and in the liver, spleen, bone marrow, red blood cells, intestine, skin, and respiratory mucosa. It is excreted mostly through the kidneys (glomerular filtration and tubular secretion) and, to a lesser degree, the gastrointestinal tract. Following vapor inhalation, about 7 per cent is expelled through respiration.[15] In human beings, the half-life of elemental mercury is about 58 days, and of inorganic mercury about 40 days.[16]

Methyl mercury accumulates in the central nervous system and the liver. It undergoes metabolism (acetylation or conjugation) in the liver and is excreted through the bile and reabsorbed from the gastrointestinal tract. About 1 per cent of the body burden is excreted per day through the feces and to a limited degree through the urine. Its half-life in human beings has been calculated to be from 52 to 70 days.[13, 16, 17]

Laboratory Assessment

The use of the laboratory to establish blood and urine mercury levels and to monitor the effectiveness and duration of therapy can be very helpful in some kinds of mercury poisoning. Many factors, however, have to be considered.

There are no firmly established diagnostic levels. Population surveys of adults have revealed that 90 per cent had blood levels below 2 to 4 μg/dl and urine levels below 10 to 20 μg/L.[16, 19, 20] There is marked variation between investigators as to what constitute diagnostic levels. Mercury levels above 4 μg/dl in blood and 20 μg/L in urine probably should be considered abnormal (much lower levels would be expected in infants and young children). Blood levels are not always reliable indicators of excessive mercury exposure as the mercury may distribute in the body within a few days and in chronic exposure take several weeks to arrive at a steady state level.[1, 2, 4] Symptoms usually are not evident with urine mercury levels under 300 μg/L and generally do not correlate well with the level.[21] A chelation challenge with BAL or penicillamine may bring about a significant increase that may aid in establishing the diagnosis and decision about specific treatment.

There is no way, however, to measure the amount of mercury in the brain.

Methyl mercury is excreted primarily through the feces and to a lesser degree through the urine, so urine levels may be in the normal range. Blood levels remain in the same range for all mercurials but the ratios of red blood cell to plasma concentrations vary, most significantly in methyl mercury exposure, with the red blood cell to plasma ratio being about 10:1.[13, 18]

Heavy metal-free glassware must be used for both blood and urine collections. Mercury is volatile and easily lost. It diffuses through plastic materials, adsorbs on surfaces, and absorbs into plastics, silicone, and rubber. Also, bacterial activity can break down the mercurial present with loss of mercury vapor. If specific organic mercurials are to be identified, an entirely different methodology will be needed, which is not universally available. It is important to check with the laboratory before obtaining the samples so proper collection, storage, transport, and handling occurs,[22] and how proficient the laboratory or its referral agency is at mercury determinations.

Mercury is excreted in sweat and in salivary (parotid gland) secretions. Concentration in sweat is reportedly higher than in urine, and parotid fluid concentration is about two fifths of that in blood.[23]

Hair analyses for mercury under well-controlled conditions may reflect the total exposure to methyl mercury but not from mercury vapor exposrure, since hair is very porous and can absorb mercury from the atmosphere. Hair concentrations of 400 to 500 μg/gm or more may be associated with symptoms of neurotoxicity.[24]

Clinical Effects

The clinical effects most commonly associated with the different kinds of mercury exposure are described next.

Mercury Vapor

Acute Exposure. Within a few hours from the beginning of exposure, the patient may develop cough, dyspnea, a tight feeling in the chest, chills, fever, weakness, salivation, nausea, vomiting, diarrhea, and a metallic taste in the mouth. This may subside completely or progress to an interstitial pneumonitis with patchy bilateral infiltrates and areas of emphysema and atelectasis seen on chest radiograph, a necrotizing bronchiolitis, and pulmonary edema.[25–30] (Infants and young children seem particularly susceptible to such exposures, often with associated pneumothorax and death resulting after a few days of apparent improvement.)[31–33] While most cases recover, interstitial fibrosis of the lungs has resulted and some psychoneurologic symptoms associated with chronic mercury poisoning have been reported.[26, 34]

Chronic Exposure. Mercury is cumulative and may take weeks, months, or years to produce a recognizable clinical picture. In industry, the allowable threshold limit value (TLV) for an 8-hour working day is only 0.05 mg/m^3. Repeated short exposures to levels of 100 mg/m^3 over time will result in symptoms. Since elemental mercury vapor passes easily into the blood and crosses the blood-brain barrier into the brain where it is slowly converted to mercuric oxide and stored, psychologic and neurologic symptoms are prominent. Tremors (static or intentional), erethism (anxiety, emotional instability, irritability, depression, forgetfulness, insomnia, regressive behavior), excessive salivation, gingivostomatitis, nausea, vomiting, diarrhea, discoloration of lens capsules, constriction of visual fields, fatigue, muscular weakness, anorexia, anosmia, headache, vertigo, peripheral neuritis, proteinuria, polyuria, anuria, chronic pneumonitis with low grade fever, and dermatitis may occur.[26, 27, 35] Percutaneous absorption of mercury vapor also occurs.[70]

Inorganic Mercury Salts

Acute Exposure. The lethal dose of mercuric chloride for an adult is between 1 and 4 grams, with as little as half a gram causing fatality. Following ingestion, within a few minutes the corrosive qualities of the salt may produce severe nausea, vomiting, hematemesis, tenesmus, abdominal pain, a metallic taste in the mouth, bloody diarrhea, colitis, and necrosis of the intestinal mucosa. Dehydration and cardiovascular collapse may ensue. There are red blood cells, casts, and protein in the urine; oliguria and uremia develop; and then shutdown from acute tubular necrosis may occur as the mercury is being excreted through glomerular filtration and tubular secretion. This may progress very rapidly.[37–39]

Chronic Exposure. Similar to symptoms of chronic mercury vapor exposure, tremors, erethism, ataxia, slurring of speech, gingivostomatitis, excessive salivation, loosening of teeth, anxiety, insomnia, and mental deterioration may be seen.[37, 38] Intrauterine exposure to inorganic mercury may result in tremors and involuntary movements in the infant.[36] Mercury intoxication from chronic exposure to elemental mercury simulating amyotrophic lateral sclerosis (ALS) has recently been described.[40] Cases simulating mucocutaneous lymph node syndrome have also been described.[71] Some patients with Kawasaki disease have been found to have elevated urine mercury levels without explanation.[72] The significance of this relationship has not been pursued.

Following the use for many years of mercurous chloride as a laxative, colitis, chronic renal failure, and dementia have been reported.[39] Children exposed to mercurous chloride in teething lotions and diaper powders developed acrodynia. This also has been described following the use of mercuric chloride as a diaper rinse,[39] from the heating of paint containing a mercurial fungicide,[44] and from mercury exposure from broken fluorescent light bulbs.[43] The symptom complex of acrodynia (pink disease) includes redness of the palms and soles, edema of the hands and feet, skin rashes, diaphoresis, tachycardia, hypertension, photophobia, irritability, anorexia, insomnia, poor muscle tone—especially of the pectoral and pelvic girdles—and constipation or diarrhea.

The chronic use of ointments containing mercurials has caused the nephrotic syndrome[45] and renal tubular acidosis.[46]

Organic Mercury Salts

The Alkyls. Symptoms from methyl mercury exposure may occur weeks to months later and are primarily neurologic, with ataxia, constricted visual fields (tunnel vision), scotomata, paresthesias, neurasthenia, loss of libido, teratospermia, hearing loss, arthralgia, memory loss, depression, mental deterioration, emotional instability, incoordination, involuntary movements including static tremor, chorea, athetosis and myoclonus, paralysis, and coma.[20, 47, 48] Some patients have died.

Ethyl mercury may produce gastrointestinal symptoms and renal damage in addition to the central nervous symptoms described for methyl mercury.[20]

The alkyl mercury halides are irritating to the eyes, mucous membranes, and skin and may cause dermatitis and burns.[49]

Intrauterine exposure to methyl mercury has resulted in impairment of motor and mental development of various degrees, with cerebral palsy, deafness, blindness, microcephaly, fretfulness, irritability, and excessive crying described.[9–12]

The Aryls. Phenyl mercury produces the symptoms of inorganic mercury exposure.

A much smaller dose is required to cause poisoning through ingestion, as phenyl mercury is absorbed at least four times more effectively from the gastrointestinal tract than are the inorganic salts.[1]

Chronic exposure to the vapors of a mercurial fungicide in paint[44] and to repeated injections of gamma globulin containing sodium ethylmercurithiosalicylate (merthiolate, thimerosal) as a bacteriostatic agent[50] has been associated with acrodynia. Elevated urine mercury levels have been found in asymptomatic individuals whose home interiors were painted with latex paint containing phenylmercuric acetate (used to maintain shelf life).[73] A cluster of patients with neuromyasthenia in an industrial setting appeared to be related to the use of paints containing an organomercurial fungicide.[74]

Exposure to organomercurials may cause a sensitizing dermatitis.

Treatment

In all cases of mercury poisoning, there must be cessation of further exposure, maintenance of respiration and circulation by appropriate supportive care, and (except in short-chain alkyl mercury exposure) a chelating agent administered immediately to increase excretion and relieve target organs of any mercury burden.[51–54]

In acute mercury vapor exposure, pulmonary toxicity should be anticipated and serial blood gases and chest radiographs monitored. Oxygen and even positive end-expiratory pressure (PEEP) may be needed. The use of prophylactic antibiotics, bronchodilators, and steroids should be considered. Chelation therapy with BAL, 4 mg/kg/dose given deep intramuscularly, should be given immediately and then every 4 hours for several days.[26–30, 35] Decisions on tapering the dose or ending administration will depend on blood and 24-hour urine mercury levels. Since there is no recognized need for mercury in the body, as much should be removed as possible.

Chronic mercury vapor exposure may respond slowly to chelation. BAL (dimercaprol) has dithiol groups that compete with binding sites in the body for mercury. It increases mercury excretion through the bile into the feces as much as through the kidneys into the urine.[26, 27, 35] Side effects of BAL are nausea, vomiting, headache, tachycardia, fever, conjunctivitis, blepharospasm, and lacrimation.

After an initial course of BAL, the oral chelating agent, penicillamine may be used.[55] One hundred mg/kg/24 hr (up to 1 gram) in four divided doses may be given on an empty stomach, for 7 to 10 days. If treatment is to continue longer, the dose should be reduced to 35 mg/kg/24 hr (up to 1 gram). Toxic effects include fever, rash, leukopenia, eosinophilia, and thrombocytopenia. Animal experiments and limited clinical experience indicate that the chemical *N*-acetyl-D,L-penicillamine (NAP) (Aldrich Chemical Company, Milwaukee, WI) is a more specific chelating agent for mercury.[39, 41, 56–58] The dose regimen and side effects are the same as those of penicillamine. (For infants and children, these agents may be put in an ounce of fruit juice or put on Karo syrup at the time of administration.) Based on experience with chronic occupational vapor exposure, some investigators recommend heat or sauna treatment to increase mercury excretion through sweating, but no comparative studies with chelation therapy are available.[59]

In acute ingestions of inorganic salts, decontamination of the gastrointestinal tract to prevent further absorption and corrosion should be accomplished as rapidly as possible. The patient's condition dictates whether syrup of ipecac or lavage should be used to empty the stomach. A protein solution to bind the mercury, such as egg whites, or 5 per cent salt-poor albumin or 5 per cent sodium formaldehyde sulfoxylate to reduce mercuric ion to the less soluble mercurous ion may be used as lavage fluid. This should be followed by a saline cathartic (unless diarrhea has already ensued) and 20 to 50 grams of activated charcoal. Start BAL administration, 4 mg/kg/dose intramuscularly immediately and then give it every 4 hours for 7 to 10 days.

Monitor electrolytes, fluid balance, and renal function carefully. Obtain blood and urine mercury levels, collecting all urine in appropriate containers in timed aliquots. When potentially toxic doses have been taken, peritoneal dialysis (with 5 per cent salt-poor albumin added) or hemodialysis established early in the course concurrent with BAL administration may remove 10 to 15 per cent of the ingested mercury and, even more importantly, relieve the kidneys and treat any uremia caused by the reversible kidney damage. It has been the practice to wait until the almost inevitable (since the kidney is the primary site of deposition) anuria occurs to start dialysis. Limited experience suggests an advantage of instituting dialysis within the first 24 hours before maximal renal mercury concentrations can occur on the second day. This also may assist in controlling fluid and electrolyte imbalance as circulatory collapse accentuates the toxic tubular lesions. Dialysis may have to be continued over several days.[39, 51–54] If blood and urine mercury levels are still elevated following the course of BAL and return of renal function, a course of the oral chelating agent *N*-acetyl-D,L-penicillamine or, if this is not available, penicillamine, 35 to 100 mg/kg/24 hr (not to exceed 1 gram/24 hours) divided into four doses a day, may be given on an empty stomach.[60] Urine mercury levels should be monitored to determine when to stop chelation.

Therapy for short-chain alkyl organic mercury compounds from acute or chronic exposure has been less than dramatically effective. *N*-Acetyl-D,L-penicillamine decreased brain and blood mercury levels, and increased urinary and fecal excretion, with a marked decrease in the half-life of methyl mercury.[61] Human experience with *N*-acetyl-D,L-penicillamine has shown reduced blood levels and increased urinary excretion with only limited clinical improvement in those severely poisoned. Those patients with mild or moderate poisoning improved but so did some not given the treatment.[47]

Another approach has been to administer orally a polythiol nonabsorbable resin (8 gm/day) to trap the mercury secreted in the bile, thus interfering with reabsorption and increasing fecal excretion. Blood mercury levels decreased.[37]

Limited experience with a regional hemodialyzer system utilizing L-cysteine as a chelating agent removed considerable mercury in two patients,[62] and exchange transfusion in three children removed a small amount of their total body burden of mercury with some clinical improvement.[63]

The earlier in the course of poisoning any of these treatment modalities can be instituted, the more chance they have of being effective. The prognosis following severe neurologic involvement is generally poor. Even so, increased excretion and a decrease of blood levels and half-life should be attempted. Other treatment is symptomatic.

In acute or chronic poisoning from long-chain alkyl or aryl mercurials, therapy should be approached the same as for inorganic mercury except *N*-acetyl-D,L-penicillamine (or if not available, penicillamine) as an oral chelator appears to be more effective than BAL. The prognosis is better than in short-chain alkyl poisoning.[1, 4, 5]

Acrodynia usually responds to oral chelation therapy with *N*-acetyl-D,L-penicillamine.[39, 44] Several weeks of treatment may be needed. Blood and urine mercury levels should be monitored to determine when to stop chelation therapy. As the body burden of mercury declines, symptoms resolve.[39, 44] Infection and electrolyte imbalance (sodium loss) may require specific treatment.

Successful treatment of two patients with inorganic mercury poisoning with the investigational drug 2,3-dimercaptopropane-1-sulfonate has recently been reported.[64]

DMSA, 2-3-dimercaptosuccinic acid (available as an orphan drug through Johnson and Johnson), has been used successfully as an oral chelating agent in a limited number of patients with mercury poisoning;[75] it has been shown in animals to decrease tissue levels and enhance excretion of both inorganic and organic mercurials.[76]

References

1. Chisolm JJ: Poisoning from heavy metals (mercury, lead and cadmium). Pediatr Ann *9*:458, 1980.
2. Levin M, Jacobs J, Polos PG: Acute mercury poisoning and mercurial pneumonitis from gold ore purification. Chest *94*:554, 1988.

2a. Federal Register: Vol 41, Number 76. April 19, 1976, pp 16497–16516.

3. Zepp EA, Thomas JA, Knotts GR: The toxic effects of mercury. Clin Pediatr *13*:783, 1974.
4. McIntyre AR: The toxicities of mercury and its compounds. J Clin Pharmacol *11*:397, 1971.
5. Petering HG, Tepper LB: Pharmacology and toxicology of heavy metals: Mercury, Pharmacol Ther *1*:131, 1976.
6. Cherian MG, Hursh JB, Clarkson TW, Allen J: Radioactive mercury distribution in biological fluids and excretion in human subjects after inhalation of mercury vapor. Arch Environ Health *33*:109, 1978.
7. Murray KM, Hedgepeth JC: Intravenous self-administration of elemental mercury: Efficacy of dimercaprol therapy. Drug Intell Clin Pharm *22*:972, 1988.
8. Suzuki T, Matsumoto N, Miyama T, Katsunuma H: Placental transfer of mercuric chloride, phenyl mercury acetate and methylmercury acetate in mice. Ind Health *5*:149, 1967.
9. March DO, Myers GJ, Clarkson TW, Amin-Zaki L, Tikriti S: Fetal methyl mercury poisoning: New data on clinical and toxicological aspects. Trans Am Neurol Assoc *102*:69, 1977.
10. Hudson PJ, Vogt RL, Brondum J, Witherell L, Myers G, Paschal DC: Elemental mercury exposure among children of thermometer plant workers. Pediatrics *79*:935, 1987.
11. Amin-Zaki L, Elhassani S, Majeed MA, Clarkson TW, Doherty RA, Greenwood MR: Intra-uterine methylmercury poisoning in Iraq. Pediatrics *54*:587, 1974.
12. Pierce PE, Thompson JF, Likosky WH, Nickey LN, Barthel WF, Hinman AR: Alkyl mercury poisoning in humans. JAMA *220*:1439, 1972.
13. Kershaw TG, Dhahir PH: The relationship between blood levels and dose of methylmercury in man. Arch Environ Health *35*:28, 1980.
14. Rabenstein DL: The chemistry of methylmercury toxicology. J Chem Ed *55*:292, 1978.
15. Hursh JB, Magos L: Clearance of mercury (Hg-197, Hg 203) vapor inhaled by human subjects. Arch Environ Health *31*:302, 1976.
16. Magos L: Mercury, an environmental and dietary hazard. J Hum Nutr *32*:179, 1978.
17. Al-Shahristani H, Shihab KM: Variation of biological half-life of methylmercury in man. Arch Environ Health *28*:342, 1974.
18. Berlin M, Taylor A, Marks V: Dose-dependence of methylmercury metabolism. Arch Environ Health *30*:307, 1975.
19. Jacobs MB, Ladd AC, Goldwater LJ: Absorption and excretion of mercury in man. Arch Environ Health *9*:454, 1964.
20. Dales LG: The neurotoxicity of alkyl mercury compounds. Am J Med *53*:219, 1972.
21. Taylor A, Marks V: Diagnostic value of urine mercury measurements. Ann Clin Biochem *14*:297, 1977.
22. Clarkson TW, Greenwood MR: Mercury, biological specimen collections. The Use of Biological Specimens for the Assessment of Humans to Exposures of Environmental Pollutants. Martinus Nijhoff, The Hague, 1979, p 109.
23. Joselow MM, Hallee TJ: Absorption and excretion of mercury in man. Salivary excretion of mercury and its relationship to blood and urine mercury. Arch Environ Health *17*:35, 1968.
24. Giovanoli-Jakubczak T, Berg GG: Measurement of mercury in human hair. Arch Environ Health *28*:139, 1974.
25. Jaffe KM, Shurtleff DB, Robertson WO: Survival after acute mercury vapor poisoning. Am J Dis Child *137*:749, 1983.
26. Hallee TJ: Diffuse lung disease caused by inhalation of mercury vapor. Am Rev Resp Dis *99*:430, 1969.
27. Vroom FQ, Greer M: Mercury vapor intoxication. Brain *95*:305, 1972.
28. Natelson EA, Matthes FT, Kirschner R, Yow MD, Brennan JC: Acute mercury vapor poisoning in the home. Chest *59*:677, 1971.
29. Burke WJ, Quagliana JM: Acute inhalation mercury intoxication. J Occup Med *5*:157, 1963.
30. Jung RC, Aaronson J: Death following inhalation of mercury vapor at home. West J Med *132*:539, 1980.
31. Matthes FT, McFarland RB, Reigel H: Acute poisoning associated with inhalation of mercury vapor. Pediatrics *22*:675, 1958.
32. Campbell JS: Acute mercurial poisoning by inhalation of metallic vapour in an infant. Can Med Assoc J *58*:72, 1948.
33. Moutinho ME, Koos BJ, Longo LD: Acute mercury vapor poisoning. Am J Dis Child *135*:42, 1981.
34. McFarland RB, Reigel H: Chronic mercury poisoning from a single brief exposure. J Occup Med *20*:332, 1978.
35. Sunderman FW: Clinical response to therapeutic agents in poisoning from mercury vapor. Ann Clin Lab Sci *8*:259, 1978.
36. Koos BJ, Longo LD: Mercury toxicity in the pregnant woman, fetus and newborn infant. Am J Obstet Gynecol *126*:390, 1976.
37. Winek CL, Fochtman FW, Bricker JD, Wecht CH: Fatal mercuric chloride ingestion. Clin Toxicol *18*:261, 1981.
38. Kahn A, Denis R, Blum D: Accidental ingestion of mercuric sulphate in a 4-year-old child. Clin Pediatr *16*:956, 1977.
39. Aronow R, Fleischmann LE: Mercury poisoning in children. Clin Pediatr *15*:936, 1976.
40. Adams CR, Ziegler DK, Lin JT: Mercury intoxication simulating amyotrophic lateral sclerosis. JAMA *250*:642, 1983.
41. Kark RAP, Poskanzer DC, Bullock JD, Boylen G: Mercury poisoning and its treatment with *N*-acetyl-D,L-pencillamine. N Engl J Med *285*:10, 1971.
42. Wands JR, Weiss SW, Yardley JH, Maddrey WC: Chronic inorganic mercury poisoning due to laxative abuse. Am J Med *57*:92, 1974.
43. Tunnessen WW, McMahon KJ, Baser M: Acrodynia: Exposure to mercury from fluorescent light bulbs. Pediatrics *79*:786, 1987.
44. Hirschman SZ, Feingold M, Boylen G: Mercury in house paint as a cause of acrodynia. N Engl J Med *269*:889, 1963.
45. Barr RD, Smith H, Cameron HM: Tissue mercury levels in the mercury-induced nephrotic syndrome. Am J Clin Pathol *59*:515, 1973.
46. Husband P, McKellar WJD: Infantile renal tubular acidosis due to mercury poisoning. Arch Dis Child *45*:264, 1970.

47. Bakir F, Rustam H, Tikriti S, al-Damluji SF, al-Shahristani H: Clinical and epidemiological aspects of methyl-mercury poisoning. Postgrad Med J *56*:1, 1980.
48. Snyder RD: The involuntary movements of chronic mercury poisoning. Arch Neurol *26*:379, 1972.
49. Fisher AA: Contact Dermatitis. 2nd ed. Lea & Febiger, Philadelphia, 1973, p 109.
50. Matheson DS, Clarkson TW, Gelfand EW: Mercury toxicity (acrodynia) induced by long-term injection of gammaglobulin. J Pediatr *97*:153, 1980.
51. Batson R, Peterson JC: Acute mercury poisoning; Treatment with BAL and in anuric states with continuous peritoneal lavage. Ann Intern Med *29*:278, 1948.
52. Maher J, Schreiner GE: The dialysis of mercury and mercury-BAL complex. Clin Res *7*:298, 1959.
53. Sanchez-Sicilia L, Seto DS, Nakamoto S, Kolff WJ: Acute mercurial intoxication treated by hemodialysis. Ann Intern Med *59*:692, 1963.
54. Lowenthal DT, Chardo F, Reidenberg MM: Removal of mercury by peritoneal dialysis. Arch Intern Med *134*:139, 1974.
55. Aposhian HV: Penicillamine and its analogues: Metabolic properties and oral activities against the lethal effects of mercuric chloride, in Metal Binding in Medicine. J. B. Lippincott, Philadelphia, 1960.
56. Aposhian HV, Aposhian MM: *N*-acetyl-D,L-penicillamine; A new oral protective agent against the lethal effects of mercuric chloride. J Pharmacol Exp Ther *126*:131, 1959.
57. Smith ADM, Miller JW: Treatment of inorganic mercury poisoning with *N*-acetyl-D,L-penicillamine. Lancet *1*:640, 1961.
58. Markowitz L, Schaumberg HH: Successful treatment of inorganic mercury neurotoxicity with *N*-acetyl penicillamine despite an adverse reaction. Neurology *30*:1000, 1980.
59. Wheater RH: Evaluation of mercury vapor exposure hazards. Questions and Answers. JAMA *243*:165, 1980.
60. Swaiman KF, Flayler DG: Mercury poisoning with central and peripheral nervous system involvement treated with penicillamine. Pediatrics *48*:639, 1971.
61. Aaseth J: Mobilization of methylmercury in vivo and in vitro using *N*-acetyl-D,L-penicillamine and other complexing agents. Acta Pharmacol Toxicol *39*:289, 1976.
62. Kostyniak PJ, Clarkson TW, Cestero RV, Freeman RB, Abbasi AH: An extracorporeal complexing hemodialysis system for the treatment of methylmercury poisoning. 1. In vitro studies of the effects of four complexing agents on the distribution and dialyzability of methylmercury in human blood. J Pharm Exp Ther *192*:260, 1975.
63. Elhassani SB, Amin-Zaki L, Majeed MA, Clarkson TW, Doherty RA, Greenwood MR, Kilpper RW: Exchange transfusion treatment of methylmercury-poisoned children. J Environ Sci Health *C13*:63, 1978.
64. Campbell JR, Clarkson TW, Omar MD: Therapeutic use of 2,3-dimercaptopropane-1-sulfonate in two cases of inorganic mercury poisoning. JAMA *256*:3127, 1986.
65. Gotelli CA, Astolfi E, Cox C, Cernichiari E, Clarkson TW: Early biochemical effects of an organomercury fungicide in infants: "Dose makes the poison." Science *227*:638, 1985.
66. Stofford W, Bundy SD, Goldwater LJ, Bittikofer JA: Microenvironmental exposure to mercury vapor. Am Ind Hyg Assoc J *39*:378, 1978.
67. Eley BM, Cox SW: Mercury poisoning from dental amalgam—an evaluation of the evidence. J Dent *16*:90, 1988.
68. Mant TGK, Lewis JL, Mattoo TK, Rigden SPA, Volans GN, House IM, Wakefield AJ, Cole QRS: Mercury poisoning after disc-battery ingestion. Hum Toxicol *6*:179, 1987.
69. Cavanagh DB: Long persistence of mercury in the brain (editorial). Br J Indust Med *45*:649, 1985.
70. Hursh JB, Clarkson TW, Miles EF, Goldsmith LA: Percutaneous absorption of mercury vapor by man. Arch Environ Health *44*:120, 1989.
71. Adler R, Boxstein D, Schaff P, Kelly D: Metallic mercury vapor poisoning simulating mucocutaneous lymph node syndrome. J Pediatr *101*:967, 1982.
72. Orlowski JP, Mercer RD: Urine mercury levels in Kawasaki disease. Pediatrics *66*:633, 1980.
73. Aronow R: Communication at Centers for Disease Control meeting, Atlanta, December 20, 1989.
74. Miller G, Chamberlain R, McCormack WM: An outbreak of neuromyasthenia in a Kentucky factory—the possible role of a brief exposure to organic mercury. Am J Epidemiol *86*:756, 1967.
75. Fournier L, Thomas G, Garnier R, Buisine A, Houze P, Pradier F, Dally S: 2,3-Dimercaptosuccinic acid treatment of heavy metal poisoning in humans. Med Toxicol *3*:499, 1988.
76. Aposhian HV: DMSA and DMPS: Water-soluble antidotes for heavy metal poisoning. Annu Rev Pharmacol Toxicol *23*:193, 1983.

CHAPTER 57
IRON

Teddi F. Eisen, M.D.
Peter G. Lacouture, Ph.D
Frederick H. Lovejoy, Jr., M.D.

Iron ingestions are common, with 17,350 cases reported in 1986.[1] Roughly 95 per cent of these exposures occurred in children and were accidental. Iron is a common toxic ingestion because (1) most preparations are available over the counter and thus are accessible in large quantities; (2) they are often brightly colored and sugar coated, making them attractive to curious children; (3) they are not considered harmful by many parents; and (4) iron compounds are often used during and after pregnancy and are therefore common in families with young children.

Iron salts are ubiquitous compounds, occurring in hematinics, multivitamins, prenatal vitamins, and some oral contraceptives. Most of these preparations contain one of three ferrous salts: fumarate, gluconate, or sulfate.

PHARMACOLOGY

Iron is widely distributed in tissue. The total body burden is normally 4 to 5 gm. Serum iron reflects the amount of iron bound to transferrin. Normal concentrations are 50 to 150 μg per dl. Iron in the blood is bound by a specific iron-binding B-globulin called transferrin. Serum transferrin concentrations range from 300 to 400 μg per dl. The total iron binding capacity (TIBC) indicates the available binding potential of transferrin for iron. It is normally one-third saturated. Ferritin is the chief iron-storage protein in the body. Serum concentrations reflect reticuloendothelial storage of iron and range from 90 to 110 μg per dl in adults and are generally 30 μg per dl in children.

Iron is absorbed into the mucosal cells of the duodenum and jejunum in the ferrous form, where it is oxidized to its ferric state and complexed to ferritin. Iron in the ferric state is then released from ferritin into the plasma, where it is rapidly bound to transferrin. This transferrin-iron complex attaches to the reticuloendothelial cells in the bone marrow and transfers the ferric molecule necessary for erythropoiesis. Any additional iron is stored in the liver or spleen as ferritin or hemosiderin. When the TIBC is exceeded, a small amount of iron attaches to albumin, and the remainder circulates in its free form. Iron has been shown to cross the placenta and accumulate in the fetus. A distinctive feature of iron metabolism is the absence of a specific mechanism for excretion. Natural elimination is limited to 1 to 2 mg per day and occurs by menstrual blood loss and desquamation of gastrointestinal mucosa. In the overdose state, iron accumulates in target organs because its excretion cannot exceed 2 mg/day.

PATHOPHYSIOLOGY

Iron toxicity occurs most commonly by the oral route. However, absorption has occurred through aspiration and burned skin.[2]

Iron poisoning occurs when serum iron concentrations exceed the TIBC, resulting in free circulating iron. This causes (1) massive postarteriolar dilatation, thought to be due to a direct effect of ferritin release (a potent vasodepressant) and serotonin/histamine release, with subsequent venous pooling and increased total peripheral resistance; (2) increased capillary permeability due to direct iron effect, with attendant plasma loss and decreased blood volume; (3) acidosis due to the release of hydrogen ions associated with both the oxidation of ferrous iron to the ferric state and the subsequent hydration of the ferric ion; and (4) mitochondrial poisoning, particularly of the hepatocytes, once transferrin has become saturated. This may result from the known action of iron as a potent catalyst of lipid peroxidation, altering mitochondrial membrane permeability and steric configuration, leading to mitochondrial dysfunction.[3] Alternatively, it may be due to the ability of iron to act as an electron sink, shunting electrons away from the electron transport system.[3]

Acute iron overload exerts its primary pathologic effects on the gastrointestinal tract, liver, and cardiovascular system.

The Gastrointestinal Tract

Iron has a direct corrosive action on the gut mucosa, causing early as well as late pathologic findings. Hemorrhagic necrosis of the proximal gastrointestinal tract is a common finding at autopsy. Two types of lesions are readily identified: corrosive mucosal lesions of the stomach and proximal small bowel (which occur early), and segmental infarction of the distal small bowel (which occurs later). Histologic examination of these areas shows mucosal necrosis and intraluminal hemorrhage. Mucosa, submucosa, basement membrane (veins, capillaries, and lymphatics), cytoplasm, and nuclear tissue show heavy iron staining.[4] Pyloric stenosis and intestinal obstruction are rare late complications.

The Liver

Changes in the liver have ranged from no change to cloudy swelling, hemorrhagic periportal necrosis, and fatty degeneration with Kupffer or parenchymal cell deposition of iron.[5] Peripheral (periportal) portions of the liver are affected to a greater extent than the central hepatic cells, probably because of their proximity to the portal vein. On a subcellular basis, severe mitochondrial injury in liver cells and histochemical alterations in a number of oxidative enzymes of the Krebs cycle have been demonstrated.[6] Liver damage may lead to hepatic failure with hypoglycemia and hypoprothrombinemia. Coagulopathy may result because free iron inhibits the thrombin-induced conversion of fibrinogen to fibrin.[7]

The Cardiovascular System

The myocardium shows evidence of fatty degeneration in iron poisoning. Iron acts on the vascular system, causing massive postarteriolar dilatation and increased capillary permeability leading to venous pooling, decreased blood volume, and reduced cardiac output. Ultimately, hypotension, tissue hypoperfusion, and metabolic acidosis result.

Secondary Systemic Pathophysiologic Effects

Metabolic acidosis can result from the release of hydrogen ion with the oxidation of ferrous iron to its ferric state and its subsequent hydration to ferric hydroxide, interference with oxidative enzymes, and the accumulation of lactic acid from anaerobic metabolism.

Additional, less consistent secondary systemic effects involve the central nervous system, kidneys, lungs, and pancreas. Cerebral hypoperfusion results in shock. Hemorrhage in the lungs and kidneys, along with focal pulmonary atelectasis and fatty degeneration of the renal tubules, may occur.[8] Degenerative changes may occur in the pancreas, resulting in elevation of serum amylase levels. Even though the gastrointestinal mucosa, liver, and spleen demonstrate positive staining for iron, the heart, brain, lungs, and kidneys are often negative. This suggests that many changes in these organs may be secondary to other events such as severe hypotension, acidosis, or coagulopathies.

CLINICAL PRESENTATION

The clinical presentation of the acutely poisoned patient can be divided into four stages.

During the *first phase*, up to 6 hours post ingestion, gastrointestinal symptoms initially predominate. Vomiting and diarrhea, often bloody, occur owing to the local corrosive effects of iron on the stomach and small bowel. *Vomiting* has the most sensitive as well as the highest negative predictive value with serious iron ingestion.[9] There may be associated nausea and abdominal pain. In severe cases, the various hemodynamic alterations previously described lead to severe hypotension and compensatory tachycardia, with diminished tissue perfusion and metabolic acidosis. Effects such as depressed sensorium, ranging from lethargy to coma, and hypotonia may develop. Other serious manifestations during the first phase include fever and leukocytosis reflecting mucosal damage, hyperglycemia secondary to hepatic or pancreatic changes, and dyspnea caused by pulmonary alveolar exudation.[10] Patients with mild or moderate iron poisoning generally experience only gastrointestinal symptoms with eventual recovery and do not progress beyond this phase.

During the *second phase*, 6 to 24 hours post ingestion, the patient with a serious iron ingestion shows apparent clinical stabilization, presumably as free circulating iron is taken up by the reticuloendothelial system. This remission is transient, and progression to severe complications may ensue.

Only a small number of patients proceed to the *third phase*, 12 to 24 hours post ingestion. During this phase there is recurrence of the gastrointestinal symptoms, profound shock, metabolic acidosis, seizures, severe lethargy and coma, hepatic necrosis with jaundice, hypoglycemia and coagulation defects, oliguria or frank renal failure due to shock, and pulmonary edema and hemorrhage. Serum iron concentrations may be normal during this phase. Fever may be a manifestation of septicemia due to *Yersinia enterocolitica*, resulting from a combination of gut mucosal damage and bacterial growth stimulated by iron.[11]

The *fourth phase* occurs late, 2 to 6 weeks post ingestion. There may be gastric obstruction and pyloric stenosis. Although cirrhosis of the liver is more common in chronic iron overload, postnecrotic changes after acute exposure are more commonly seen as fine diffuse fibrotic changes with fatty degeneration.

EVALUATION

Assessment of the severity of poisoning is important in determining appropriate management. This is based on a variety of factors, including an estimation of the ingested dose, the patient's clinical status, the physical examination, laboratory parameters, and abdominal radiographs.

History

An estimation of the ingested dose of elemental iron is useful in determining who is at significant risk for serious intoxication. Iron poisoning is determined based on the amount of *elemental* iron ingested: the amount of the iron salt (in mg) is multiplied by the percentage of elemental iron in each tablet (Table 57–1). Doses less than 20 mg per kg are considered to be nontoxic. The toxic dose of iron is greater than 30 to 60 mg per kg. The usual estimated lethal dose is 200 to 250 mg per kg. However, these measurements are often difficult to obtain and therefore unreliable.

Clinical Status

Another index of severity is the patient's clinical status. Most patients are asymptomatic or exhibit symptoms of mild gastrointestinal irritation, including nausea, vomiting, and abdominal colic. Hematemesis or bloody stools may occur with more severe ingestions. Patients with spontaneous vomiting and diarrhea within 6 hours of ingestion are more likely to have a serum iron concentration greater than 300 mcg/dl. Anyone remaining asymptomatic for 6 hours post ingestion would not be expected to develop toxicity and may be sent home with instructions to return if symptoms develop.[9]

Physical Examination

In severe iron ingestions, the physical examination may reveal unstable vital signs, with shock and coma. However, most patients have an unremarkable physical examination except for possible abdominal tenderness.

Laboratory Parameters

Peak serum iron concentrations occur at 2 to 4 hours post ingestion and should be drawn during this time to best estimate the risk of toxicity. Serum iron concentrations obtained more than 6 hours after ingestion may underestimate toxicity, since iron is rapidly cleared from the blood into the tissues. A serum iron concentration exceeding the TIBC, indicating free circulating iron, is another useful index of potential toxicity. Generally, a peak serum iron concentration below 300 μg per dl is nontoxic. Concentrations between 300 and 500 μg per dl indicate mild poisoning, concentrations between 500 and

Table 57–1. PRODUCTS CONTAINING IRON

	MANUFACTURER	IRON COMPLEX	TOTAL ELEMENTAL IRON PER DOSAGE UNIT
Chocks Bugs Bunny Plus Iron	Miles Laboratories, Inc.	Fumarate	18 mg
Chocks Plus Iron	"	"	18 mg
Feminins Tablets	Mead Johnson Nutritional Division	"	18 mg
Femiron with Vitamins	J. B. Williams	"	20 mg
Feosol Elixir	Menley & James (formerly SKF)	Sulfate	44 mg/5 ml
Feosol Plus Capsules	"	Sulfate (desiccated)	65 mg
Feosol Spansule Capsules	"	"	50 mg
Feosol Tablets	"	"	65 mg
Fergon Capsules	Breon Laboratories Inc.	Gluconate	50 mg
Fergon Elixir 6%	"	"	35 mg/5 ml
Fergon Tablets	"	"	36 mg
Fer-In-Sol Capsules	Mead Johnson Nutritional Division	Sulfate	60 mg
Fer-In-Sol Drops	"	"	15 mg/0.6 ml
Fer-In-Sol Syrup	"	"	18 mg/5 ml
Filibon Capsules	Lederle Laboratories	Fumarate	30 mg
Filibon OT Tablets	"	"	30 mg
Flintstones Plus Iron Multivitamin	Miles Laboratories, Inc.	"	18 mg
Geriplex Kapseals	Parke-Davis	Sulfate	6 mg
Geriplex FS Liquid	"	Ammonium citrate	15 mg/30 ml
Geritonic Liquid	Geriatric Pharm. Corp.	"	35 mg/5 ml
Gevrabon Liquid	Lederle Laboratories	Gluconate	20 mg/30 ml
Golden Bounty Multivitamin	E. R. Squibb & Sons	Fumarate	18 mg
Iberet Filmtab	Abbott Laboratories	Sulfate	105 mg
Iberet-Liquid	"	"	26 mg/5 ml
Iberol Filmtab	"	"	105 mg
Monster Vitamins with Iron	Bristol Myers	Fumarate	12 mg
Myadec Capsules/Tablets	Parke-Davis	"	20 mg
Natabec Kapseals	"	Sulfate	30 mg
Natalins Rx Tablets	Mead Johnson Pharmaceutical Division	Fumarate	60 mg
Natalins Tablets	"	"	45 mg
One-A-Day Vitamins Plus Iron	Miles Laboratories, Inc.	"	18 mg
One-A-Day Vitamins Plus Minerals	"	"	18 mg
Pals Plus Iron Chewable	Bristol-Myers	"	12 mg
Poly-Vi-Flor Tablets with Iron	Mead Johnson Nutritional Division	"	12 mg
Poly-Vi-Flor Drops with Iron	"	Sulfate	10 mg/ml
Poly-Vi-Sol Tablets with Iron	"	Fumarate	12 mg
Poly-Vi-Sol Drops with Iron	"	Sulfate	10 mg/ml
Spiderman Vitamins with Iron	Hudson	not specified	18 mg
Stuart Formula (tablets)	Stuart Pharmaceuticals	Fumarate	18 mg
Stuart Formula (liquid)	"	"	5 mg/5 ml
Stuart Hematinic Tablets	"	"	22 mg
Stuart Hematinic Liquid	"	"	22 mg/5 ml
Stuartinic Tablets	"	"	100 mg
Stuart Prenatal Tablets	"	"	60 mg
Theragran-M Tablets	E. R. Squibb & Sons	Carbonate	12 mg
Tri-Vi-Sol Drops with Iron	Mead Johnson Nutritional Division	Sulfate	10 mg/ml
Unicap M Plus Iron	The Upjohn Company	"	10 mg
Unicap Plus Iron	"	"	18 mg

(Adapted from Krenzelok EP, Hoff JV: Accidental childhood iron poisoning: A problem of marketing and labeling. Pediatrics 63:591, 1979.)

1000 μg per dl indicate moderate poisoning, and concentrations over 1000 μg per dl indicate severe intoxication.

Other laboratory parameters useful in predicting a serum iron concentration above 300 μg per dl, when a concentration is not immediately available, are a leukocytosis over 15,000 per mm^3 and a blood glucose greater than 150 mg per dl.[9] If below the stated levels, these measures are not predictive of toxicity. Blood should also be obtained for routine electrolytes, arterial blood gas, hemoglobin, hematocrit, complete blood count, coagulation studies, serum hepatic transaminases, renal function tests, and cross match and blood type. Stool and gastric contents should be tested for blood.

Radiographs

Radiographs of the abdomen have proved useful in the presence of ingested iron, if obtained within 2 hours of ingestion, and may document the success or failure of gastrointestinal evacuation techniques.[12] Serial radiographs may be necessary to identify persistent bezoars. Negative radiographs, however, do not exclude iron ingestion. Radiopacity depends upon the time since ingestion, the content of elemental iron, and the type of formulation. For example, chewable vitamins with iron are not likely to be visualized.

Abdominal films are also useful in predicting the severity of iron ingestion. One retrospective study revealed that 60 per cent of patients with a positive radiograph also had a serum iron concentration above 300 μg per dl.[9]

MANAGEMENT

Gastrointestinal Decontamination

Removal of iron from the stomach is best accomplished with syrup of ipecac if the patient is alert or gastric lavage using the largest tube possible if the patient is obtunded or lacks a gag reflex. There exists considerable controversy as to the optimal lavage solution. Lavage with 1 to 1.5 per cent bicarbonate solution has been advocated. However, the use of large volumes of sodium bicarbonate in the lavage fluid may theoretically lead to hypernatremia. Lavage with normal saline is generally sufficient. However, since bicarbonate promotes the formation of insoluble ferrous carbonate salt, which is less irritating than iron, it seems reasonable that a small amount (100 ml) of 1 per cent sodium bicarbonate may be instilled into the stomach either *before* or *after* lavage without substantial risk.

The use of Fleet's or other phosphate-containing preparations has been previously recommended, but reports of life-threatening hyperphosphatemia, hypocalcemia, and hypernatremia have argued against their use.[13,14] Also, these solutions appear less efficacious in vitro than bicarbonate preparations in complexing free iron.[15] Thus, phosphate-containing solutions are not recommended.

The use of deferoxamine, a chelator of iron, in the lavage solution is also controversial because its efficacy has not been established and it is unclear whether the absorbed iron-deferoxamine complex (ferrioxamine) is toxic.

Although activated charcoal does not bind iron alone, it does absorb ferrioxamine with an affinity similar to that for salicylates.[16] Thus, administration of activated charcoal and oral deferoxamine may prove effective in eliminating iron from the gastrointestinal tract pending further investigation.

Some have advocated the use of whole bowel irrigation with polyethylene glycol electrolyte lavage solution.[17,18] This solution is considered optimal because it results in negligible gastrointestinal fluid and electrolyte fluxes. Its use may be considered if a slow-release iron preparation has been ingested or an abdominal radiograph after gastric decontamination reveals the persistence of tablets in the stomach or proximal small bowel.[19]

Iron tablets may form concretions in the stomach and duodenum, leading to continued iron release and adherence of the mass to the gut mucosa resulting in severe hemorrhagic infarction, with subsequent perforation, peritonitis, and death.[20–22] Survivors may develop scarring leading to pyloric stenosis and small bowel obstruction.[23] Gastrotomy, for removal of bezoars from the gastrointestinal tract, has been reported to reduce the toxic effects of iron ingestion and prevent perforation.[24–26] Such extreme measures are indicated if conventional methods of decontamination are ineffective in removing the bezoar, if a large number of opacities are identified in a single location on abdominal radiograph without progression through the gastrointestinal tract, or if evidence of a perforated viscus is present.

Supportive Care

The first and most important aspect of supportive care is to ensure a patent airway and adequate ventilation. Reliable venous access should also be established. Since an early manifestation of iron poisoning is gastrointestinal hemorrhage, the patient should be observed for signs of blood loss, and vital signs should be carefully monitored for evidence of hypovolemia. Fluid volume loss should be treated aggressively with normal saline. Administration of blood products may be necessary in cases of life-threatening hemorrhage. Monitoring of urine output, central venous pressure, and heart rate should guide fluid therapy. Although large fluid volumes may be necessary in severe iron overdoses during the first 24 hours, fluid balance should be carefully monitored to avoid pulmonary edema. Metabolic acidosis should be monitored by serial arterial blood gas determinations and treated with intravenous sodium bicarbonate. Hypoglycemia, if present, should be managed with intravenous glucose. Recurrent or prolonged seizures can be suppressed with intravenous diazepam.

Chelation

In patients requiring chelation therapy, deferoxamine, a chelator produced by the bacteria *Streptomyces pilosus*, should be utilized.[27] Deferoxamine is a specific chelator that binds free serum iron in the ferric state. Iron of ferritin and hemosiderin from hepatic and splenic stores and transferrin-bound iron is minimally affected, and iron of cytochromes and hemoglobin is unaffected.[27] A dose of 100 mg of deferoxamine will bind approximately 9 mg of elemental iron.[28]

Deferoxamine is believed to work by binding free circulating iron in the plasma. Some hypothesize that it enters cells, exerting a protective effect at the mitochondrial and intracellular levels, perhaps by binding iron in the cytoplasm so that it does not interfere with mitochondrial enzyme systems and mitochondrial membranes.[3]

Deferoxamine is poorly absorbed from intact gut mucosa.[29, 30] It has a volume of distribution of about 60 per cent of body weight and a plasma half-life in humans of 10 to 30 minutes[31] and is rapidly metabolized to inactive products by plasma and other tissues.[3, 32] Ferrioxamine, however, has a smaller volume of distribution of about 20 per cent and remains in the extracellular space.[33] It is water soluble and rapidly excreted unchanged in the urine. Therapy with deferoxamine is based on the severity of symptoms and serum iron concentrations. Peak serum iron concentrations below 300 μg per dl are not likely to produce significant symptoms, so the value of deferoxamine in these cases is minimal.

However, if the serum iron concentration is greater than the TIBC, a deferoxamine challenge test may be warranted. This involves the intramuscular administration of 40 to 50 mg per kg, up to 1 gm, of deferoxamine. The occurrence of a characteristic "vin rose" urine indicates the presence of unbound circulating iron and the need for continued chelation. Clear guidelines do not exist for asymptomatic patients whose iron concentrations are 300 to 500 μg per dl. Any symptomatic patient with an iron concentration in this range should be given deferoxamine. All patients with a peak serum iron concentration above 500 μg per dl should receive deferoxamine. Any significantly symptomatic patient (hypotension, altered mental status, or bleeding) should be treated with deferoxamine without waiting for an iron concentration. Deferoxamine may be given by the intramuscular route in patients showing no signs of hypotension. The dose is 50 to 100 mg per kg up to 2 gm every 4 to 8 hours to a maximum of 6 gm per 24 hr.[34] While the minimal effective dose of deferoxamine has not yet been established, doses up to 37.1 gm over 52 hours have been tolerated in an adult without adverse effects.[35] Intravenous deferoxamine is preferred if the patient is hypotensive. The recommended maximum infusion rate is that which the patient can tolerate without hypotension. Poor perfusion of skeletal muscle during shock may result in potentially less effective muscle absorption.

Therapy with deferoxamine should be continued until the vin rose coloring of the urine clears. Some authors recommend continuing treatment for 24 hours after the urine color returns to normal.[3] Alternatively, therapy may be continued until the serum iron level falls below the TIBC. Ferrioxamine, however, interferes with the colorimetric assay of iron but not with atomic absorption spectrophotometry.[36]

The most common adverse reactions to deferoxamine include gastrointestinal distress and hypotension, both of which usually respond to slowing of the infusion. Fluids and, less frequently, vasopressors may be necessary to maintain blood pressure. Rashes[37] and anaphylaxis[34] have been occasionally reported. Rapid desensitization protocols have been developed for sensitive patients with serious iron intoxication.[38]

Deferoxamine has been administered to pregnant women without adverse effect to the fetus.[39, 40] Conversely, death due to iron poisoning occurred in a pregnant woman after deferoxamine therapy was withheld for fear of producing fetal damage.[41]

Elimination Enhancement

Hemodialysis is not effective in removing free iron. Ferrioxamine, however, is somewhat dialyzable, with up to 2.2 per cent of iron excreted in 5 hours.[42] Renal shutdown is an indication for hemodialysis, since ferrioxamine is eliminated primarily by the kidneys.

Exchange transfusion has been demonstrated to increase the rate of iron removal as much as 30-fold compared with deferoxamine therapy alone.[43] This approach, which removes free and bound iron, may be useful in severe iron intoxications when conservative measures have failed.

Charcoal hemoperfusion would appear to be of little value, given the poor affinity of charcoal for iron. Nevertheless, since charcoal binds ferrioxamine, this method offers a possible therapeutic modality.[16]

DISPOSITION

Criteria for admission include (1) any patient requiring chelation; (2) any patient with a positive deferoxamine challenge test; and (3) any patient who develops symptoms within 6 hours of iron ingestion.

Most patients will survive iron ingestions without significant sequelae. Outcome is closely correlated with the early onset of shock and coma. Untreated patients who develop shock and coma have a mortality rate close to 100 per cent; with general supportive care it drops to 50 per cent, and with chelation therapy it approaches 10 per cent. Those who never manifest shock or coma have a mortality rate of essentially 0 per cent. Overall, the prognosis is excellent for survivors of acute iron ingestion.

References

1. Litovitz TL, Martin TG, Schmitz B: 1986 Annual Report of the American Association of Poison Control Centers National Data Collection System. Am J Emerg Med *5*:405–445, 1987.
2. Doolin EJ, Drueck C: Fatal iron intoxication in an adult. J Trauma *20*:518–522, 1980.
3. Robotham JL, Leitman PS: Acute iron poisoning—a review. Am J Dis Child *134*:875–879, 1980.
4. Reissmann KR, Coleman TJ: Acute intestinal iron intoxication. II. Metabolic, respiratory, and circulatory effects of absorbed iron salts. Blood *10*:46–51, 1955.
5. Witzelben CL, Chaffey NJ: Acute ferrous sulfate poisoning. A histochemical study of its effect on the liver. Arch Pathol *82*:454–460, 1966.
6. Luongo MA, Bjornson SS: The liver in ferrous sulphate poisoning: a report of three fatal cases in children and an experimental study. N Engl J Med *25*:995–999, 1954.
7. Rosenmund A, Haeberli A, Struab PW: Blood coagulation and acute iron toxicity. J Lab Clin Med *103*:524–533, 1984.
8. Smith RP, Jones CW, Cochran WE: Ferrous sulfate toxicity. N Engl J Med *243*:641, 1950.
9. Lacouture PG, Wason S, Temple AR, et al: Emergency assessment of severity in iron overdose by clinical and laboratory methods. J Pediatr *99*:89–91, 1981.
10. Brown RJK, Gray JD: The mechanism of acute ferrous sulphate poisoning. Can Med Assoc J *73*:192–197, 1955.
11. Melby K, Slordahl S, Gutteberg TJ, Nordbo SA: Septicaemia due to *Yersinia enterocolitica* after oral overdoses of iron. Br Med J *285*:467–468, 1982.
12. Hosking CS: Radiology in the management of acute iron poisoning. Med J Aust *1*:576–579, 1969.
13. Geffner ME, Opas LM: Phosphate poisoning complicating treatment for iron ingestion. Am J Dis Child *134*:509–510, 1980.
14. Bachrach L, Correa A, Levin R, Grossman M: Iron poisoning: Complications of hypertonic phosphate lavage therapy. J Pediatr *94*:147–149, 1979.
15. Czajka PA, Konrad JD, Duffy JP: Iron poisoning: An in vitro comparison of bicarbonate and phosphate lavage solutions. J Pediatr *98*:491–494, 1981.
16. Yonker J, Banner W, Picchionie A: Absorption characteristics of iron and deferoxamine onto charcoal (abstract). Vet Hum Toxicol *22*:361, 1980.
17. Bock GW: Whole blood irrigation for iron overdose (letter). Ann Emerg Med *16*:137, 1987.
18. Tenenbein M: Whole blood irrigation in iron poisoning. J Pediatr *111*:142–145, 1987.

19. Proudfoot AT, Simpson D, Dyson EH: Management of acute iron poisoning. Med Toxicol *1*:83–100, 1986.
20. Gezernik W, Schaman A, Chappell JS: Corrosive gastritis as a result of ferrous sulphate ingestion. S Afr Med J *57*:151–154, 1980.
21. Knott LH, Miller RC: Acute iron intoxication with intestinal infarction. J Pediatr Surg *13*:720–721, 1978.
22. Ross FGM: Pyloric stenosis and fibrous structure of the stomach due to ferrous sulphate poisoning. Br Med J *2*:1200–1202, 1953.
23. Henretig FM, Karl SR, Weintraub WH: Severe iron poisoning treated with enteral and parenteral deferoxamine. Ann Emerg Med *12*:306–309, 1983.
24. Landsman I, Bricker TJ, Reid BS, Bloss RS: Emergency gastrotomy. Treatment of choice for iron bezoar. J Pediatr Surg *22*:184–185, 1987.
25. Foxford R, Goldfrank L: Gastrotomy—a surgical approach to iron overdose. Ann Emerg Med *14*:1223–1226, 1985.
26. Peterson CD, Fifield GC: Emergency gastrotomy for acute iron poisoning. Ann Emerg Med *9*:262–264, 1980.
27. Moeschlin S, Schnider U: Treatment of primary and secondary haemochromatosis and acute iron poisoning with a new potent iron-eliminating agent (desferoxamine-B). N Engl J Med *269*:57–61, 1963.
28. McEnery JT, Greengard J: Treatment of acute iron ingestion with deferoxamine in 20 children. J Pediatr *68*:773–779, 1966.
29. Lovejoy FH: Chelation therapy in iron poisoning. J Clin Toxicol *19*:871–874, 1982–1983.
30. Leikin S, Vossough P, Mochir-Fatemi F: Chelation therapy in acute iron poisoning. J Pediatr *71*:425–430, 1967.
31. Propper R, Nathan D: Clinical removal of iron. Ann Rev Med *33*:509–519, 1982.
32. Keberle H: The biochemistry of desferrioxamine and its relation to iron metabolism. Ann NY Acad Sci *119*:758–768, 1964.
33. Peters G, Keberle H, Schmid K, Brunner H: Distribution and renal excretion of desferrioxamine and ferrioxamine in the dog and in the rat. Biochem Pharmacol *15*:93–109, 1966.
34. Westlin WF: Desferrioxamine as a chelating agent. Clin Toxicol *4*:597–602, 1971.
35. Peck MG, Rogers JF, Rivenbark JF: Use of high doses of desferoxamine (Desferal) in an adult with acute iron overdosage. J Toxicol *19*:865–869, 1982.
36. Heffer RE, Rodgerson DO: The effect of deferoxamine on the determination of serum iron and iron-binding capacity. J Pediatr *68*:804–806, 1966.
37. Westlin WF: Desferrioxamine in the treatment of acute iron poisoning: Clinical experience with 172 children. Clin Pediatr *5*:531–535, 1966.
38. Miller KB, Rosenwasser LJ, Bessett JM, et al: Rapid desensitization for deferoxamine anaphylactic reaction. Lancet *1*:1059, 1981.
39. Blanc P, Hryhorczuk D, Danel I: Deferoxamine treatment of acute iron intoxication in pregnancy. Obstet Gynaecol *64*:125–145, 1984.
40. Rayburn WF, Donn SM, Wulf ME: Iron overdose during pregnancy: Successful therapy with deferoxamine. Am J Obstet Gynecol *147*:717–718, 1983.
41. Strom RL, Schiller P, Seeds AE, Bensel RT: Fatal iron poisoning in a pregnant female. Minn Med *59*:483–489, 1976.
42. Whitten CF, Chen Y, Gibson G: Studies in acute iron poisoning: II. Further observations on desferrioxamine in the treatment of acute experimental iron poisoning. Pediatrics *38*:102–110, 1966.
43. Movassaghi N, Puruggnan GG, Leiken S: Comparison of exchange transfusion and deferoxamine in the treatment of acute iron poisoning. J Pediatr *75*:604–608, 1969.

CHAPTER 58
LEAD

Lorne K. Garrettson, M.D.

In this chapter, lead poisoning is divided into three categories: (1) inorganic lead poisoning with acute symptoms; (2) inorganic lead poisoning without symptoms, occurring during childhood; and (3) organic lead poisoning. This classification comes primarily from consideration of symptoms, diagnostic procedures, and steps taken in the identification of patients at risk. Specific therapeutic agents are similar in all three groups of patients.

Pathophysiology

Lead's effects on cells are thought to be due to its ability to combine with sulfhydryl groups on proteins. Yet the anatomic alterations of lead poisoning are more limited than would be expected from such a general mode of toxicity. The primary organs of attack are the brain and peripheral nervous system, bone marrow, kidney, and liver. Lead effects on the bone marrow have been well characterized.[1] Several enzymes in the heme synthetic pathway are partially inhibited. The result is anemia. Assay of the substrates of these enzymes has been used in diagnosis, and the result of the inhibition of the last enzyme in the heme synthetic pathway is important in screening of children. Lead also inhibits pyrimidine 5′-nucleotidase, which is active in the breakdown of ribonucleic acid (RNA).[2] Blockade of this enzyme leads to clumping of ribosomal RNA, which is seen as stippling. Lead blocks the production of 1,25-dihydroxyvitamin D.[3]

Lead's effect on the brain has been reviewed.[4] An arterial lesion was observed. Schwann cells and neurons may be affected. The mechanism of the learning disability seen in school children who had asymptomatic lead absorption in the preschool years is also unresolved. Renal tubular function is altered so that aminoaciduria, glycosuria, and proteinuria are seen.

Pharmacokinetics

The absorption of lead from the gut has been reviewed.[5] The mechanisms and rates of lead absorption are poorly characterized. In the adult, 10 per cent of an administered dose is absorbed. In the child, it is estimated that up to 50 per cent of ingested lead may be absorbed. Calcium and zinc appear to block absorption and iron to enhance it, yet the clinical relevance of these observations is unclear. Some salts of lead, including some oxides (red lead), the naphthenate, and acetate, are rapidly and more completely absorbed and may lead to rapid, acute disease. Metallic lead embedded in tissue is generally poorly absorbed. However, lead near joints, where it is in contact with the relatively acid synovial fluid, may lead to systemic lead toxicity.[6]

Data on the accumulation and elimination of lead in subjects administered lead have been simulated by a multiple compartment, first-order model, which predicts a half-life of 2 months following cessation of administration and a terminal half-life of over 30 years.[7] When exposure was stopped for operatives in a lead industry, the decline of blood lead after therapy with edetic acid (EDTA) had a median half-life of 619 days for those with normal renal function and 1907 days (range, 1658 to 7185) for those with impaired function.[8] In workers removed from the workplace for elevated lead levels, 50 per cent achieved levels of less than 40 μg per dl in 180 days and 75 per cent in 460 days.[9]

The importance of the large burden of lead in the deep bony compartments is still unsettled. Chelating agents clearly have access to part of the lead in bone and hasten its removal. Chelation can reduce blood lead in the face of large bone burdens. Whether the deep bone lead is physiologically inert because the rate of unstimulated movement from bone to blood is so slow is still in question. Heavily leaded persons with wasting disease may be at unusual risk.

Sources of Lead

Common sources of large amounts of lead include paint, putty, and some folk remedies. Industrial fallout can poison workers, workers' children through contaminated work clothing, and others by the contamination of dirt and air. Lower amounts are found in water drawn from systems with lead pipe or lead-soldered joints, air, and lead leached from improperly glazed pots. Ingested lead sinkers and retained bullets may produce toxic levels of lead. The ingestion of whiskey cooled in leaded condensers, such as old car radiators, can lead to toxicity. Indoor firing ranges have been a source of lead poisoning.

Industrial sources of lead include lead smelters, battery reclamation processes, radiator repair activities, and lead paint on ships and bridges when underlying metal is cut with an acetylene torch.

Environmental Considerations

Except in suicidal lead administration, an environmental source is always involved. Referral to a health department, an occupational hygienist, or the Occupational Safety and Health Administration or its state counterpart is an essential part of the medical management of all lead-poisoned patients.

INORGANIC LEAD POISONING WITH ACUTE SYMPTOMS

The majority of lead poisoning occurs from the absorption of inorganic lead and requires an extended absorptive period to achieve levels sufficient to cause symptoms. Symptoms may arise acutely, but the poisoning is, in fact, chronic. Suicidal administration of soluble lead salts produces an acute syndrome.[10]

Clinical Presentation

Symptoms of lead poisoning, at all ages, are not specific.[11] Clusters of symptoms are suggestive. In the toddler, anorexia is the earliest symptom, which may not be recognized until the appetite improves following chelation therapy. Other prodromal signs include occasional vomiting, irritability, and refusal to play. More serious signs include persistent vomiting, stupor, peripheral nerve weakness, convulsions, and coma.

In the preschool-aged child, adolescent, and adult, colicky or constant abdominal pain, nausea and vomiting, anorexia, a metallic taste, constipation, limb and joint pain, irritability, fatigue, and insomnia are all early symptoms. Hypertension may be present. Anemia and convulsions can occur with prolonged and high exposure. Peripheral neuropathy, with wrist drop as the classic sign, may occur. In the adult, nerve conduction velocity may be a useful laboratory test if blood tests are to be delayed.

Patients who have ingested or injected soluble lead salts will show an acute onset of symptoms. The sensorium may be depressed within hours. In addition to the symptoms seen with more slowly absorbed lead poisoning, hemolysis and hepatic injury may occur. Specific therapy is the same, but supportive care includes blood transfusion when required.

Laboratory Findings

In suspected lead poisoning with acute symptoms, the diagnosis must be confirmed with haste. The blood lead level (BLL) must be used for confirmation that lead is the cause of symptoms. Whether performed by flame ionization spectroscopy or anodic stripping voltametry, the BLL, when performed by an experienced laboratory, is accurate, reproducible, and reasonably precise (± 5 μg/dl). The turn-around time for a single assay, when performed routinely, is 5 to 10 minutes.

The erythrocyte protoporphyrin (EP, also called ZnPP or FEP) level is found in all cases except the acute administration of soluble salts. It is supportive but does not make the diagnosis. The primary use of the EP level has been the screening of children at risk. It is inexpensive and rapid. The EP level is measured directly in whole blood without sample preparation, and the turn-around time is 1 or 2 minutes.

Significant delays in obtaining these assays may occur because laboratories performing the tests are in central state locations; assays may not be available in even the largest hospital centers. Physicians confronted with symptomatic patients require prompt answers and, perhaps, special arrangements for specimen transportation and telephoned reports.

If the blood lead and EP levels are not available for rapid confirmation of the diagnosis of lead poisoning, nonspecific laboratory tests must be used. Examination of the blood smear for stippling can be done rapidly and is positive in most cases. The bone marrow has a larger percentage of stippled cells and should be examined when the peripheral smear leaves the examiner in doubt. Stippling suggests, but does not confirm, lead poisoning.

Assays of coproporphyrin, δ-aminolevulinic acid, and δ-aminolevulinic acid dehydrase in the red cell have been used as confirmatory tests. When available, they are useful. These tests are all more costly than the EP test and are being replaced by it.

X-ray films of long bones in the preschool-aged child may show densities at the ends of long bones or ribs.[12] Such lines support a diagnosis of chronic lead absorption and usually indicate the need for chelation. Lead lines do not show up readily in older children and adults.

X-ray examination of the abdomen may show radiopaque material, an indication for catharsis. If the patient is acutely ill, chelation therapy may begin before catharsis has been accomplished.

Treatment[13]

If the patient is convulsing, administer diazepam, 0.1 mg/kg IV, to a maximum dose of 10 mg. To maintain seizure control, phenytoin and/or phenobarbital may be indicated.

After the acute phase is past, begin chronic anticonvulsant medication with either phenobarbital or phenytoin and continue for at least 1 year.

If the patient is in coma or convulsing, increased intracranial pressure can be assumed. Neurosurgical support is recommended. Care in a nursing unit that can monitor intracranial pressure is advised. Mannitol, steroids, and hypothermia may be employed.

Establish urine flow with normal saline. This is essential as chelated lead is cleared in the urine. After urine flow is established, restrict fluids to basal maintenance plus losses, as cerebral edema is always a concern.

In all symptomatic patients or patients with BLLs above 70 gm/dl, chelation therapy should include both dimercaprol (BAL) and calcium disodium edetate (calcium disodium versenate, EDTA). On the first day of EDTA therapy, more lead may be mobilized from bone than is excreted, and a worsening of symptoms may occur. BAL is a small molecule that can cross into cells and protect against these increases of central compartment lead, which cause this worsening. Also, combined therapy causes a greater total excretion of lead. BAL is given intramuscularly every 4 hours in a dose of 4 mg/kg to children and 2.5 mg/kg to adults.

The preferred route of administration of EDTA is intravenous, but it may be given intramuscularly in the child. The dose is 50 mg/kg/day in two divided doses in the nonconvulsing child and 1 to 2 gm/day in the adult. As the compound is painful on injection, the volume to be injected into muscle is mixed with 0.5 ml of 1 per cent procaine. Multiple sites may be used, and these should be recorded so rotation of sites can be planned. If the patient is convulsing or in coma, the dose is increased to 75 mg/kg/day in the child and 3 to 4 gm/day in the adult. After a delay of 2 days following the completion of the first 5-day course, a second course can be given. A third course should be delayed, if clinical circumstances permit, for 5 to 7 days following the second course of therapy.

Side effects of EDTA, given for 5 days at a dose of 50 mg/kg, are uncommon. Acute renal shutdown can occur. Resolution is usual in 1 to 5 days. BAL may cause local pain, paresthesia, lacrimation, salivation, vomiting, and neutropenia. Antihistamines may relieve some of the side effects of BAL. The patient should be monitored for the moderate hypertensive effect that is common following BAL injection; treatment is rarely indicated.

Symptomatic operatives and those with lead levels above 60 μg/dl must be removed from the workplace until levels fall below 40 μg/dl.

LEAD POISONING WITHOUT SYMPTOMS IN THE DEVELOPMENTAL YEARS

Clinical Presentation

Asymptomatic children with elevated lead levels may require chelation therapy to protect them from developmental deficits. Screening programs to detect such children are required.[14] Physicians seeing children for acute medical care can obtain the necessary laboratory screening values if suspicion is high and environmental and behavioral information suggests that the patient is at risk. Categories of children at risk who should be tested by EP, with a confirmatory blood lead assay if the EP is elevated, are listed in Table 58–1. Testing of children with pica is important. Anemia in children may be due, in part, to the block of heme synthesis by lead. Pica is more frequent in iron-deficient children, so they are at greater risk of undue lead exposure. All children of lead operatives need to be screened periodically, as they are at increased risk of exposure.

The developmental syndrome, involving cognitive and behavioral delays, becomes recognizable several years after the exposure to lead.[15] Children show a three- to ten-point drop in I.Q. In the subsets of the tests for intellectual functions, auditory and visual associative difficulties have been most frequently identified. Behavior changes include distractibility, impulsiveness, and hyperki-

Table 58–1. CHILDHOOD POPULATIONS TO TEST FOR UNDUE LEAD ABSORPTION

All children
During the second year of life
With a lead-poisoned sibling
With pica
With anemia
With hyperkinetic behavior
With neurologic disease, including seizures
Living in houses built before 1950
Whose parents work in a lead industry

netic behavior. Teachers' ratings of these behaviors in children have shown a remarkably close correlation with tooth lead, which serves as an indicator of past exposure. Although these symptoms are not life-threatening, the impact on the social and intellectual development of children is pervasive.

Laboratory Findings

Screening is best done by obtaining both blood lead and EP levels. If only one is to be obtained, the EP level is the more important test. The EP level is elevated in all chronic lead ingestions in which the lead has reached significant levels, it is not subject to contamination during collection of the specimen, and it also detects iron deficiency, which is important in itself and in the treatment of lead poisoning. Thus, an elevated EP level requires further testing to determine cause in all instances.

BLLs to be used in determining therapy requirements must be drawn from a venipuncture. Specimens obtained from a finger prick are easily contaminated.

Treatment and the Need to Treat[16]
(Table 58–2)

Patients whose BLLs are above 70 gm/dl should be admitted and chelated with both EDTA (50 mg/kg/day) and BAL. Patients whose BLL is 55 to 69 gm/dl should be admitted and chelated with EDTA alone.

With a BLL of 55 gm/dl or less, other tests should be used to determine the need for chelation therapy. X-ray of the long bones and an EDTA provocative test will assist in this decision.

The EDTA provocative (or 8-hour mobilization) test for patients in the potentially high-risk category does not require hospitalization. A child is brought to the office or clinic in the early morning. EDTA is given in a single dose of 50 mg/kg (maximum dose, 1000 mg) in multiple sites, with 0.5 ml of 1 per cent procaine. Urine flow is maintained by an augmented oral fluid intake. Urine is collected for 8 hours in a plastic container. If the ratio of lead excreted (in μg) divided by the dose of EDTA (in mg) is greater than 0.7, the child is admitted to the hospital and treated. When the ratio is between 0.6 and 0.7 and the child is less than 3 years of age, the child is treated for 3 days. Ratios not meeting these criteria indicate the need to remove the sources of lead and monitor BLL monthly. We treat all children in this BLL category who have lead lines in their bones. If long bones are radiologically positive, lead ingestion has occurred over an extended period and chelation is indicated for this patient at moderate risk.

After hospitalization and when the patient

Table 58–2. DRUGS USED IN THE TREATMENT OF LEAD-POISONED PATIENTS

	GENERIC/OTHER NAMES	DOSE	ADMINISTRATION	(A) ADVERSE REACTIONS (C) CONTRAINDICATIONS
EDTA	Calcium disodium edetate, calcium disodium versenate	50 mg/kg/24 hr (child) 75 mg/kg/24 hr (child severe) Maximum 1 gm/24 hr (mobilization test) 2–4 gm/24 hr (adult)	IM or IV, q 6–12 h	(A) Use for more than 5 days may lead to loss of other ions and cardiac arrhythmias (C) The sodium salt must never be used, as hypocalcemia rapidly ensues
BAL	Dimercaprol, British antilewisite	4 mg/kg/dose	IM q 4 h	(A) Allergic reactions may be treated with antihistamines
Penicillamine	Cuprimine	20 mg/kg/24 hr	PO, bid or tid	(A) Allergic rashes, eosinophilia, neutropenia, aplastic anemia, nephropathy, hepatitis
Iron	Ferrous sulfate	5 mg/kg/24 hr (as elemental iron)	PO	(A) Gastric irritation (C) Should not be given at the same time of day with penicillamine; must not be given during BAL therapy

is in a lead-free environment, the use of penicillamine may be considered. Patients who present with lead levels between 40 and 55 μg per dl may also be treated with penicillamine. The dose is 20 mg/kg/day given in divided doses on an empty stomach. Food and milk must be withheld for a short period after administration. Therapy may continue until the child has normal BLLs or side effects occur.

The side effects of penicillamine can usefully be divided into three categories: (1) allergic/pseudoallergic, (2) chelation, and (3) antimetabolic. The pseudoallergic response to penicillamine is a rash indistinguishable from an ampicillin rash. It is a fine, light-pink morbilliform rash that appears on the third or fourth day of therapy, disappears with cessation of therapy, and will not recur with reinstitution of therapy. It will fade even if therapy continues. Ampicillin causes a similar rash.

True allergic responses are common. The drop in platelet count, frequent in the first week of therapy, may be allergic. Eosinophilia counts usually do not exceed 1000 cells/mm^3, although values as high as 5000 have been seen. Neither transient thrombocytopenia nor eosinophilia is an indication to discontinue therapy—both will abate. Allergic skin reactions characteristically associated with IgG and IgE occur. Toxic erythema and erythema multiforme may occur and are indications to discontinue penicillamine and test for cross reactivity before further administration of penicillin or ampicillin.

The common chelation side effect is limited to the loss of taste, or hypogeusia, attributed to a depletion of zinc. Taste may return without cessation of therapy or specific replacement. Hypocalcemia has been reported only after prolonged use in the treatment of Wilson's disease.

The antimetabolite action of penicillamine is the most dangerous side effect. Most common is the production of neutropenia. We discontinue therapy whenever neutrophils drop below 1500/mm^3. Following this precaution, neutrophils of most patients will be normal within 1 week, and we have not seen a case in which abnormally low values were present for more than 4 to 6 weeks. If therapy continues, aplastic anemia has been reported. Caution demands that a white blood cell count and differential determination be performed weekly for 1 month, biweekly for the next month, then monthly for the duration of therapy.

Other side effects of penicillamine include proteinuria, which is evidence of a glomerular toxicity. This is uncommon in children. Serious nephropathy and acute hepatitis have been reported.

All patients should be referred to a public health agency for inspection of the home and other environs to determine the source of the lead.

Biweekly and then monthly or bimonthly blood specimens for lead analysis must be obtained on all patients who have been hospitalized. Patients who have not been treated should be followed with BLL assay monthly.

When the EP level is elevated but the BLL is normal, iron deficiency should be presumed. The population of children who have lead poisoning frequently have iron deficiency. Treatment with iron should be instituted. In the presence of elevated lead, a ferritin assay or the transferrin saturation should be used to determine the need for iron therapy. Iron, in a dose of 5 to 6 mg/kg/day, is given in divided doses for 90 days.

ORGANIC LEAD POISONING

Organic lead poisoning is essentially limited to exposure to tetraethyl lead (TEL). Two circumstances lead to most exposures. Workers cleaning tanks used for leaded gasoline storage have been overcome. The repeated inhalation of leaded gasoline as a drug of abuse has led to intoxication.[17] The manufacturing of TEL has declined markedly recently, but the process has had a good safety record in recent years, and few poisonings are expected in operatives. Dermal absorption occurs, and poisoning from this route is possible. TEL itself is not the primary toxin but is converted to triethyl lead and inorganic lead, which accounts for the disease.

Clinical Presentation

Symptoms occur after approximately 1 week of heavy exposure. Central nervous system symptoms predominate. Insomnia, nausea, vomiting, irritability, restlessness, and anxiety have been reported. During this stage, bradycardia, hypotension, and brisk reflexes may be observed. With continued exposure, tremor, weakness, confusion, chorea, mania, convulsions, and ataxia may ensue. Muscle, hepatic, and renal damage as identified by elevated serum creatinine phosphokinase (CPK), lactic dehydrogenase (LDH), and serum glutamic oxaloacetic transaminase (SGOT) levels and by protein in the urine has been reported in severe cases.

Laboratory values differ from those seen with inorganic lead toxicity. Anemia is uncommon. Specific substrates in the heme synthetic pathway, such as EP, are not always elevated. Blood lead is elevated as is urinary excretion of lead, although this may be less than expected for the degree of clinical illness.

Treatment

Treatment is symptomatic in the acute phase. Chelation has been used to lower the inorganic lead produced in the body. There is no antidote for triethyl lead intoxication.

References

1. Piomelli S, Seaman C, Zullow D, Curran A, Davidow B: Threshold for lead damage to heme synthesis in urban children. Proc Natl Acad Sci *79*:3335, 1982.
2. Cook LR, Angle CR, Stohs SJ: Erythrocyte arginase, pyrimidine 5′-nucleotidase (P5N), and deoxypyrimidine 5′-nucleotidase (dP5N) as indices of lead exposure. Br J Ind Med *43*:387, 1986.
3. Rosen JF, Chesney RW, Hamstra A, DeLuca HF, Mahaffey KR: Reduction in 1,25 dihydroxyvitamin D in children with increased lead absorption. N Engl J Med *302*:1128, 1980.
4. Hirano A, Iwata M: Neuropathology of lead intoxication. *In* Vinken PJ, Bruyn GW (eds): Handbook of Clinical Neurology. Vol 36. New York, North-Holland Publishing Company, 1979, Chap 2.
5. Moore MR: Diet and lead toxicity. Proc Nutr Soc *38*:243, 1979.
6. Switz DM, Elmorshidy ME, Deyerle WM: Bullets, joints, and lead intoxication. Arch Intern Med *136*:935, 1976.
7. Marcus AH: Multicompartment kinetic models for lead. Linear kinetics and variable absorption in humans without excessive lead exposure. Environ Res *85*:459, 1985.
8. Hryhorczuk DO, Rabinowitz MB, Hessl SM, et al: Elimination kinetics of blood lead in workers with chronic lead intoxication. Am J Ind Med *8*:33, 1985.
9. O'Flahery EJ: The rate of decline of blood lead in lead industry workers during medical removal. The effect of job tenure. Fund Appl Toxicol *6*:372, 1986.
10. Sixel-Dietrick F, Doss M, Pfeil C-H, Solcher H: Acute lead intoxication due to intravenous injection. Hum Toxicol *4*:301, 1985.
11. Graef JW: Clinical aspects of lead poisoning. *In* Vinken PJ, Bruyn GW (eds): Handbook of Clinical Neurology. Vol 36. Amsterdam, North-Holland Publishing Company, 1979, p 1.
12. Blickman JG, Wilkinson RH, Graef JW: The radiologic "lead band" revisited. AJR *146*:245, 1986.
13. Chisolm JJ: Treatment of lead poisoning. Mod Treat *8*(3):593, 1971.
14. Preventing Lead Poisoning in Young Children. A statement by the Centers for Disease Control, USDHHS, PHS, Center for Environmental Health, Chronic Disease Division, Atlanta, GA 30333, January 1985.
15. Needleman AL, Gunnoe C, Leviton A, et al: Deficits in psychological and classroom performance of children with elevated dentine lead levels. N Engl J Med *300*:689, 1979.
16. Piomelli S, Rosen JF, Chisolm JJ, et al: Management of childhood lead poisoning. J Pediatr *105*:523, 1984.
17. Edminster SC, Bayer MJ: Recreational gasoline sniffing: Acute gasoline intoxication and latent organolead poisoning. Case reports and literature review. J Emerg Med *3*:365, 1985.

CHAPTER 59
ARSENIC AND OTHER HEAVY METALS

Alan H. Hall, M.D.
William O. Robertson, M.D.

Arsenic

Consider arsenic as a prototype for this group of toxic agents. Its history predates the time of Christ. Because arsenic is nearly tasteless and resembles sugar, its popularity as a political poison for homicidal use during the Middle Ages was renowned. By the middle 1800s, it gained favor as an ingredient of paints and wallpapers in the form of "Paris green." Subsequently, it became extensively employed as a pesticide, being largely replaced by modern halogenated hydrocarbons and anticholinesterases only in the mid 20th century. Arsenic-containing rodenticides and ant poisons, however, are still responsible for a large number of exposures and poisonings yearly, with the majority being accidental and occurring in young children. Suicidal and homicidal arsenic poisonings also continue to be frequently reported.[1–3] Even intravenous injection of arsenic in suicide attempts has been noted.[4] Although medicinal uses have virtually disappeared, arsenic continues to be widely employed within industry, agriculture, and the ceramic trades.

As with other metals, arsenic exists in multiple forms. In contrast to lead, iron, and mercury, a "metallic" form of arsenic is not known to exist; instead, arsenic is found in two main valence states. The pentavalent form (able to form five bonds with other atoms) once enjoyed popularity as a trypanocidal and spirocheticidal agent; this practice has been abandoned because of its visual side effects. Pentavalent arsenic has been shown to be converted to trivalent arsenic by cell cultures in vitro and in experimental animals,[5, 6] and some or all of its in vivo toxicity may be due to this conversion. The trivalent form (able to form three bonds with other atoms) is considered more toxic, even though current concepts consider both forms to be similarly active at the cellular level. Nonetheless, in experimental animals fed equal amounts of arsenic, one group receiving sodium arsenate (pentavalent) and the other sodium arsenite (trivalent), the latter group uniformly was more severely afflicted. The mechanisms of arsenic toxicity are thought to be inhibition of sulfhydryl group–containing cellular enzymes and replacement of phosphate atoms in "high energy" compounds, so-called arsenolysis.[7] Inorganic arsenic compounds are considered to be more toxic than organic arsenicals. The range of toxicity in humans may vary widely for different arsenic compounds. Toxic doses have been estimated at between 1 mg and 10 gm. An arsenic trioxide dose of 9 to 14 mg caused characteristic poisoning in a child,[8] and ingestion of as much as 2150 mg of arsenic oxide has been survived with aggressive treatment.[1] From 1 to 4 mg/kg has been estimated to be a potentially fatal human dose.

ACUTE EXPOSURE

In humans, acute ingestions of either form characteristically make an impact on the gastrointestinal tract. Although "noncorrosive" (in contrast to mercury), such ingestion leads to oral irritation and a sensation of burning in the mouth and thorax, followed by the development of nausea, vomiting, and significant diarrhea. Hemorrhagic gastroenteritis may occur in serious cases. Arsenic causes dilation of blood vessels and damages the vascular lining tissue, resulting in fluid leakage into the interstitial space ("third spacing"), which can lead to intravascular volume depletion and severe shock if adequate fluid replacement is not rapidly accomplished.

A garlic-like odor may be noted on the breath. Seizures have occurred in some cases.[9] Muscular twitches and spasms may ensue. Hepatic involvement later becomes evident, with multiple abnormalities in the liver profile. This is followed by kidney involvement and subsequent renal failure. Delirium, coma, and death may occur. Peripheral neuropathy and bone marrow depression with anemia may be late sequelae of acute arsenic poisoning. Cardiac irregularities can include a variety of electrocardiogram (ECG) abnormalities and arrhythmias (see Chapter 5). Visual disturbances including "dimness" of vision, photophobia, and conjunctivitis have been described in some cases.[4, 9]

Inorganic arsenic crosses the placental barrier, and neonatal death has been reported following acute maternal arsenic intoxication.[10] Arsenic is a teratogen in experimental animals.[11, 12]

Most acute arsenic poisonings are seen following exposure by the oral route. However, serious acute arsenic poisoning with peripheral neuropathy has been noted on rare occasions following inhalation and dermal exposure.[13]

CHRONIC EXPOSURE

Symptomatic systemic poisoning is seldom seen in industrial settings, despite wide arsenic use.[14] Attempted homicides and deliberate long-term self-poisoning for the purpose of malingering have resulted in chronic toxicity.[3] Chronic exposure causes a metallic taste in the mouth; gastrointestinal disturbances; multiple skin afflictions, especially hyperkeratosis of the palms of the hands; anemia, with occasional basophilic stippling; and peripheral neuropathy. Mee's lines (transverse white striae of the fingernails) may be seen with chronic arsenic exposure. Anemia is frequently associated with chronic arsenic intoxication, and aplastic anemia with subsequent fatal myelogenous leukemia has been reported.[15]

About 7 per cent of patients with cutaneous cancers have been exposed to arsenic.[16] Arsenical keratosis and carcinoma tend to localize in areas of chronic irritation. Carcinomas of the mucous membranes, including tracheal and bronchogenic carcinomas, have been associated with chronic occupational arsenic exposure.[7, 16] Hepatic hemangiosarcomas have been noted in vineyard workers chronically exposed to arsenic.[17]

CLINICAL MANAGEMENT OF ACUTE ARSENIC POISONING

The initial step in management is a suspicion of the possibility of arsenic poisoning. This may be a feat in itself: the exposure may not be known to the patient, as in cases of attempted homicide. Patients who present with gastrointestinal, neurologic, and subsequent renal involvement and have a history of possible exposure should have a determination of urinary arsenic. If no etiology for such a clinical picture can be ascertained, an arsenic level may uncover an unsuspected diagnosis. Similarly, the symptoms of chronic exposure are also mimicked by other toxic agents; here, too, when such symptoms are combined with a known or suspected exposure, urinary arsenic determination is warranted.

Measurement by a reliable, experienced laboratory is absolutely essential. Laboratories are much more often requested to screen for heavy metals in asymptomatic, occupationally exposed workers. It is frequently necessary for the physician to communicate directly with the laboratory technician to establish that a rapid turnaround time is needed in cases of symptomatic arsenic exposure. The normal blood arsenic value is less than 7 mcg/dl.[18] Blood arsenic levels have been shown to be less useful than timed urinary arsenic excretions for following the course of acute poisoning.[1] In fatal cases, postmortem blood arsenic levels have been between 10 and 48 times greater than the upper limit of normal.[18] Falsely elevated values may be reported not uncommonly by inexperienced laboratories.

Urine arsenic levels may be measured as "spot" (i.e., concentration in a single voided urine specimen, reported in mcg/L) or in a timed urine collection (i.e., concentration in all pooled urine collected for a 12- to 24-hour period, reported in mcg/12 or 24 hours). Timed collections are usually felt to be more accurate, as they average out variations in urine concentration and volume. Normal urinary arsenic levels may vary but are seldom greater than 50 to 100 mcg/L and only rarely greater than 200 mcg/L, unless an unusual arsenic exposure has occurred.[18] Excretion of more than 50 to 100 mcg of arsenic/24 hr may be considered abnormal.[9] An exception may sometimes be noted shortly after ingestion of large quantities of shellfish, especially lobster, which can contain high concentrations of organically bound arsenic. Urinary arsenic levels as high as 1500 to 1700 mcg/L may be transiently observed after a large shellfish meal.[18]

In questionable cases without acute, life-threatening symptomatology, the diagnosis may be confirmed by a chelation challenge test. A baseline 24-hour urine arsenic excretion is measured. Then chelation therapy is administered for 24 hours while a second 24-hour arsenic excretion is collected. A substantial increase in urinary arsenic excretion during chelation confirms the diagnosis, indicates the presence of an elevated total body burden of "mobilizable" arsenic, and suggests that a course of chelation therapy may be of value.

Under no circumstances should any credence be paid to hair analysis of an individual patient, unless perhaps it is conducted as part of an epidemiologic investigation of a group of patients. Such results ought to be applied only to the group. Pubic hair is less likely to be contaminated with environmental arsenic and may be the preferable sample. If hair analysis has prompted concerns and reasoning fails to persuade the patient differently, obviously little alternative exists other than to attempt to confirm or refute the existence of increased arsenic excretion by measurement of urinary arsenic levels.

SPECIFIC MANAGEMENT

Once a diagnosis of arsenic poisoning is firmly established or considered most likely, treatment is initiated by two avenues: (1) supportive measures, and (2) specific measures. Although perhaps self-evident, elimination of further exposure to the arsenic is critical.

Supportive Measures

Traditional supportive measures are employed; evacuation of stomach contents via emesis or lavage ought to be considered if the ingestion has been relatively recent. Activated charcoal is considered beneficial. The use of cathartics, particularly in the face of gastrointestinal symptoms, is of dubious value at best. In contrast, careful assessment of the intravascular volume and administration of appropriate replacement fluids and electrolytes are mandatory and may be lifesaving in severe cases. Should any bleeding occur, blood replacement ought to be considered. Otherwise, it has no place in therapy. Of course, in acute arsine poisoning, exchange transfusion is of primary importance to overcome the hemolytic response. Baseline complete blood count, urinalysis, and liver and renal function tests should be obtained and followed periodically in cases of significant poisoning. Vital signs and ECG should be closely monitored.

Although most authorities recommend beginning chelation therapy as soon as possible, there is no good evidence that this will modify the initial course of the poisoning where shock due to intravascular volume losses is the major cause of death. Early chelation therapy may prevent late development of peripheral neuropathy in some, but not all, patients. For chronic poisoning or when late sequelae follow acute exposure, additional symptomatic therapy will be warranted. Particularly for patients with neurologic symptoms, physical and occupational therapy are used to assure optimum recovery.

Chelation Therapy

Specific therapy currently centers on the use of "chelators," relatively simple organic compounds with remarkable selective affinities for arsenic (or other metals). Resultant bonding eliminates arsenic from the active metabolic pool. The metal-chelator complex, being water soluble, can be excreted in the urine or removed by hemodialysis. Injectable British antilewisite [dimercaprol (BAL)] has been the initial arsenic chelating agent of choice for many years. More recently, *D*-penicillamine, a chelator for oral administration, has been reported to also be efficacious in arsenic poisoning,[9] although some animal studies have questioned its efficacy.[19]

Acute Poisoning

At present, recommended therapy for significant *acute* arsenic poisoning is as follows:

1. Administration of BAL in its oil vehicle intramuscularly (3 to 5 mg/kg initially as a single dose), followed by 3 to 5 mg/kg/dose every 6 to 12 hours for a 24-hour period and thereafter every 12 to 24 hours for 5 to 10 days. Naturally, the course of BAL therapy can be shortened if laboratory determinations refute or

modify the initial diagnosis. Some experts advise substituting oral *D*-penicillamine, 100 mg/kg/24 hr to a maximum of 1 to 2 gm daily divided into four oral doses and administered for 5 to 10 days *after* the initial 12 to 48 hours of intramuscular BAL therapy.

BAL therapy causes such side effects as hypertension, tachycardia, fever, burning or painful sensations, and gastrointestinal upsets. The intramuscular injections are quite painful, a moderately severe dysphoric reaction often occurs, and the medication has a most unpleasant sulfur-like "rotten eggs" odor.

Common side effects of *D*-penicillamine are gastrointestinal upsets (nausea, vomiting, diarrhea) and skin rashes. More serious adverse effects noted during prolonged administration for other indications such as rheumatoid arthritis are not usually seen during metal chelation. *D*-penicillamine should not be administered to penicillin-allergic patients, as cross-sensitivity may occur. The only available preparation is for oral administration, and it cannot be used when patients are vomiting.

2. If renal failure should ensue (regardless of cause), hemodialysis is able to remove both free and chelated arsenic.[20] The contribution of hemodialysis to arsenic clearance is presently unclear, however, and the amount removed may be small compared with both ingested dose and total body burden.[2] As chelated arsenic is relatively inactive, the criterion for hemodialysis should be renal failure per se as a first order of priority.

Chronic Poisoning

For *chronic* poisoning, unless symptoms are particularly explosive, most authorities favor initial and subsequent use of *D*-penicillamine for 5 to 10 days in the doses described previously, followed by a period of 2 to 7 days of no chelation therapy (during which time residual tissue arsenic appears to become "mobilized" and susceptible to further removal). After this delay, a second course of oral *D*-penicillamine is initiated. Chelation therapy may be repeated several times in a similar fashion if urinary arsenic elimination increases accordingly when each course is initiated. Monitoring of timed urinary arsenic excretions during the initial chelation, between courses, and on resumption of chelation therapy can provide valuable information about therapeutic efficacy. When resumption of chelation no longer provokes an increase in arsenic excretion, it is likely that maximum therapeutic benefit has been achieved and chelation therapy can be terminated.

Some clinicians begin therapy with *both* BAL and *D*-penicillamine in cases of particularly severe arsenic poisoning, continuing with oral *D*-penicillamine alone after several days. For emphasis, in all instances, removing the patient from further arsenic exposure may be the most significant intervention undertaken; it cannot be ignored.

N-acetylcysteine (NAC, Mucomyst) has been utilized as an arsenic chelating agent in experimental animals with conflicting results.[21, 22] NAC cannot be recommended for use in human arsenic poisoning at this time.

Dimercaptosuccinic acid (DMSA), a water-soluble chelating agent for oral administration, has been used in Europe (and in the United States on an investigational basis) to treat both acute and chronic arsenic poisoning with good results.[23, 24] Although DMSA therapy must currently be considered experimental, it has been effective in some cases in which BAL or *D*-penicillamine was not efficacious.

To summarize: when arsenic poisoning is a possibility, seek to confirm the diagnosis, initiate supportive measures (especially adequate fluid and electrolyte replacement) as well as chelation therapy, begin hemodialysis if renal failure occurs, and preclude the patient from any further arsenic exposure. In many instances, local public health officials as well as industry physicians can prove particularly helpful. If the source has been occupational, ensuring that the employer and appropriate local, state, or federal authorities are notified may prevent further exposure of both the index patient and coworkers.

ARSINE

When metals containing arsenic are exposed to acids, arsine (AsH_3), a gaseous form of arsenic (arsenous hydride), is formed. A considerable number of arsine poisonings have occurred from metal refining, but other industrial processes such as galvanizing, lead plating, and soldering have also been implicated. Arsine gas is also heavily utilized in the production of microelectronic components.

Arsine poisoning causes a rapid and severe Coombs'-negative hemolytic anemia, a unique and characteristic clinical syndrome. Hematuria and mild hemolysis occur only rarely in arsenic poisoning.[9, 25] Arsine exposure results in a variable onset of symptoms, initially abdominal pain, nausea, and vomiting. Excretion of dark red urine frequently develops 4 to 6 hours after exposure, followed in 24 to 48 hours by jaundice. *The triad of abdominal pain, hematuria, and jaundice is characteristic of arsine poisoning, with subsequent development of acute renal failure secondary to kidney damage from red blood cell breakdown products.* Pulmonary edema may occasionally occur. ECG abnormalities have been noted, and delayed neurologic sequelae such as polyneuropathy and psycho-organic syndromes have been described.

The treatments of choice for acute arsine poisoning are exchange transfusion and hemodialysis in the event of renal failure. The place of chelation therapy in arsine poisoning is uncertain. Increased urinary arsenic excretion may be produced by administration of chelating agents, but BAL does not protect against the development of hemolysis, even if administered soon after exposure.[26] If chelation therapy is considered, the dosing regimens described previously may be utilized.

Other Heavy Metals

Virtually all such heavy metal exposures are a result of industrial exposures. A few heavy metals, such as thallium and antimony, had been used as pesticides in the past, but this use has been virtually abandoned. Today several metals are purposefully used in medications, among them gold, aluminum, potassium, zinc, copper, and selenium; others appear inadvertently, e.g., nickel[27] and aluminum,[28–30] during renal dialysis.

Fortunately, many reach the patient's gastrointestinal tract in a relatively nonabsorbable form—few, if any, consequences will ensue. In contrast, if the metal is highly ionizable ($CuSO_4$), the typical corrosive gastrointestinal symptoms will follow; subsequent absorption is evidenced by hepatic, renal, or other system impairment.

A number of metals can be volatilized; inhalation will produce the syndrome of "metal fume fever." Metal fume fever is an acute illness that occurs upon inhalation of certain fumes from metals, primarily zinc, copper, magnesium, cadmium, nickel, aluminum, manganese, beryllium, silver, and vanadium.[31] It is an occupational hazard to workers in foundries, marinas, and shipyards. Metal fume fever is characterized by abrupt onset of fever, shaking chills, excessive salivation, headache, cough, and respiratory distress. In the absence of pulmonary involvement, the disease is usually self-limited and subsides spontaneously within 24 to 48 hours. Treatment is supportive.

In those patients with pulmonary involvement, acute chemical pneumonitis may be severe and sometimes fatal, especially with acute exposure to beryllium, cadmium, and nickel.[31, 32] Acute pulmonary edema can develop rapidly. Intravenous steroids, particularly with cadmium exposure, are recommended to reduce the amount of respiratory tract injury.[32] Aminophylline to treat bronchospasm may be indicated. Critically ill patients may require management as outlined in Chapter 10.

In coping with heavy metal poisonings, several caveats are to be kept in mind:

1. Although most such problems are the result of chronic industrial exposures, single acute exposures can and do occur—and may be either accidental or purposeful in origin.
2. Reliable laboratory confirmation of toxicity is critical—from the patient's perspective as well as from the vantage point of society, other exposed persons, liability issues, and so on. Unfortunately, such confirmation often appears long after the treatment has been completed and signs and symptoms have cleared. Technologic equipment advances, plus the emergence of reliable toxicology laboratories, are rapidly overcoming this delay.
3. As a generalization, hair analysis is totally valueless—although many patients and some health professionals accept these determinations with a religious fervor. Blood

levels, too, particularly for recent acute exposures, may prove deceiving; initial peaks may be missed and subsequent tissue bonding can cause serum levels to plummet. By and large, quantitative urinary levels are preferred when absorption has been an issue.

4. Treatment is primarily supportive and always includes elimination of further exposures.

Arising as they do on relatively rare occasions, poisonings or exposures to these substances warrant a quick search for any possible recent advances in the field. Contact your local or regional Poison Center or local or state toxicologist or seek out the assistance of your regional medical library to update your information base accordingly.

A review of the common heavy metals that produce human toxicity follows.

ALUMINUM

Aluminum has a major use as a building material when light weight and corrosion resistance are important. Aluminum hydroxide gel has long been employed as a gastric antacid and is known to cause constipation. Recent concerns have stemmed from its detection in infant formulas,[33] particularly soy-based preparations; significant concentrations of aluminum occur during the household preparation of the formula from utensils and so on. To date, no specific consequences have been attributed to the "contamination." Aluminum cookware is not known to cause human toxic effects.

The association between aluminum and dialysis encephalopathy has been well documented.[28–30] A recent review by Hughes[34] provides clear evidence, however, that such encephalopathic changes are separate and distinct from those seen in Alzheimer's disease, virtually eliminating any consideration of aluminum as etiologic for the latter condition. A comprehensive review of the topic by Monteagudo and colleagues[35] has just appeared.

Inhalation of bauxite (aluminum ore) may result in weakness, fatigue, and respiratory distress; fibrosis, emphysema, and spontaneous pneumothorax are known complications.[36]

Treatment involves the use of deferoxamine mesylate to mobilize aluminum from bone to serum, with subsequent removal from serum by hemofiltration or hemodialysis.[36a]

ANTIMONY

Antimony was once used medically as an emetic, but this use has been abandoned because of toxicity. Tartar emetic (antimony potassium tartrate), a trivalent antimony compound, was also used as an insecticide.[37] Antimony has several industrial uses, as in the production of storage batteries. It is highly toxic, and symptoms resemble those of arsenic poisoning.[37] Cardiac arrhythmias may be a more prominent feature of antimony than of arsenic poisoning. Treatment is similar to that of arsenic poisoning; chelation therapy with BAL[37, 38] may be effective when treating poisoning with the trivalent forms of the metal.

BERYLLIUM

Beryllium is a light metal used in the manufacture of light-weight alloys and nuclear reactors as well as ceramics.[36] Beryllium is a well-known cause of pulmonary disease; chronic berylliosis is a chronic granulomatous lung disease that may be indistinguishable from sarcoidosis and miliary tuberculosis. Its prime use in the manufacture of fluorescent light bulbs has been abandoned, but chronic effects are still emerging. Skin lesions, usually dermatitis, ulceration, and granulomas, are generally the most common signs of the industrial disease. Hypercalcemia may be induced. Acute chemical pneumonitis may occur from beryllium, and treatment is supportive; steroid therapy may be useful.[38]

CADMIUM

Over the past decade, cadmium has received considerable attention in the medical literature as a cause of human toxicity. This is partly attributed to the purported association of essential hypertension with low-level, long-term exposure to cadmium.[39, 40] Acute ingestion of cadmium can cause severe gastroenteritis. Inhalation of cadmium can cause severe and sometimes fatal pulmonary edema.[32, 41, 42] Prolonged inhalation of cadmium oxide can result in pulmonary dysfunction and emphysema. Prolonged industrial exposure can produce renal dysfunction characterized by tubular proteinuria, glycosuria, and aminoaciduria.[39] A syndrome known as *itai-itai* ("ouch-ouch" disease) was described in Japan, resulting from cadmium contamination of rice; it is characterized by severe bone pain and osteomalacia, occurring especially in parous women with calcium and vitamin D deficiency.[36–39]

Finally, the death rate in cadmium workers has been found to be higher than expected. Workers exposed to cadmium oxide may have an increased incidence of prostatic cancer.[39]

Acute poisoning from cadmium usually results from the inhalation of cadmium dust and fumes, generally cadmium oxide. It is characterized by a metallic taste in the mouth, cough, dyspnea, substernal and pleuritic chest pain, fever, and, in severe cases, fulminant pulmonary edema. Treatment involves removing the patient from the source, supportive therapy for pulmonary edema, and chelation therapy with calcium disodium edetate.[32, 42] Calcium disodium edetate for acute cadmium poisoning may also produce nephrotoxicity.[42a] BAL is contraindicated in cadmium poisoning; although it increases renal excretion of cadmium, it has been found to increase nephrotoxicity.[32, 36–38, 42] Steroid therapy may be indicated in the management of acute cadmium pneumonitis.[32, 42]

CHROMIUM

The major use of chromium is in chromium plating, as in the automobile industry. Chromium is now considered an essential trace metal and is required, for example, for the maintenance of normal glucose tolerance.[43] Chromium deficiency can result in impaired glucose tolerance particularly in malnourished children.[43]

Acute chromium poisoning from chromium trioxide or chromate salts, if ingested, is characterized by fulminant gastroenteritis, thrombocytopenia, shock, and toxic nephritis. Treatment of acute toxicity involves gastric lavage, alkaline diuresis, chelation therapy with calcium disodium edetate or BAL, hemodialysis in the event of renal failure, and supportive therapy.[37, 38]

Chromium trioxide causes local burns, which may be treated with calcium disodium edetate ointment. Chronic industrial exposure via dust or fumes can cause ulceration, subsequent perforation of the nasal septum, and hepatitis with or without jaundice.[36] The incidence of respiratory tract cancer in chromium workers is 15 to 20 times greater than in the general population.[36]

COBALT

Cobalt is an essential trace metal incorporated in vitamin B_{12}, which is essential in the prevention of pernicious anemia. Cobalt and its salts are useful in paint dryers, as catalysts, and in permanent magnets.

During the 1960s, cobalt was added to some beers as a foam restorative and stabilizer, which resulted in epidemic cardiomyopathy among heavy beer drinkers in Canada, the United States, and Belgium.[37] Chronic administration of cobalt salts has resulted in goiter and reduced thyroid activity. Acute poisoning is rare, but gastrointestinal, respiratory, and nephrotoxic effects have been observed; supportive therapy and chelation therapy with BAL may be warranted.[37]

COPPER

Copper is a trace metal in humans and is essential to several human enzymes, such as cytochrome C oxidase. Human copper deficiency, usually associated with an inherited abnormality in its carrier protein as opposed to a dietary problem, results in anemia, and infants may suffer the fatal Menkes' kinky hair syndrome, which is a progressive infantile brain disease transmitted by x-linked recessive inheritance.[44–46]

Wilson's disease is an autosomal recessive disorder that results from abnormal deposition of excessive copper, primarily in the liver, brain, and kidneys, ending in chronic active hepatitis; renal tubular abnormalities with proteinuria, aminoaciduria, and glycosuria; and neurologic abnormalities.[46] Copper deposition at the periphery of the cornea results in the rusty-brown Kayser-Fleischer ring, which is pathognomonic for Wilson's disease and occurs in all untreated patients with neurologic manifestations; it may occur in asymptomatic patients as well.[46]

Copper sulfate was once used as an emetic in the management of drug poisoning but has been replaced because of its marked toxicity.[47]

Acute copper sulfate poisoning is common in India, and copper is commonly employed as a suicidal poison among the people of India.[48] Copper sulfate causes a metallic taste in the mouth, epigastric pain, vomiting, and, in severe cases, diarrhea, shock, jaundice, and hepatic and renal failure. Treatment is supportive and symptomatic; chelation therapy with BAL may be indicated,[48] as well as dialysis in the event of renal failure.[49]

Penicillamine is presently the treatment of choice for Wilson's disease and also has a role in the management of acute copper poisoning.[46]

GOLD

The therapeutic use of gold in the management of selected patients with rheumatoid arthritis has made gold one of the more common causes of heavy metal toxicity. Gold is available to rheumatologists and physicians who manage rheumatoid arthritis as gold sodium thiomalate, in a solution for intramuscular injection (myochrysine). The therapeutic use of gold must be carefully monitored, as it is quite toxic. Allergic reactions, dermatitis, gastrointestinal symptoms, the nephrotic syndrome, nephritis, peripheral neuritis, hepatitis, and hematologic abnormalities are all possible adverse reactions.

Treatment of gold toxicity includes discontinuation of therapy, chelation therapy with BAL, administration of steroids, and supportive therapy.[37]

MAGNESIUM

Magnesium is one of the most important of the trace elements and is the second most abundant intracellular metallic element. Magnesium is essential to numerous human enzyme systems, including the synthesis of adenosine triphosphate (ATP). Discussions of magnesium metabolism and states of magnesium deficiency and excess are numerous and are found elsewhere.[50–52]

With respect to poisoning, magnesium oxide inhalation is one of the more common causes of metal fume fever. Of note are several recent well-documented reports[53, 54] of hypermagnesemia, plus associated symptoms, developing following "excessive" administration of $MgSO_4$ by those who advocate cathartic management of acute ingestions. Apparently, abnormal hosts—anorectics, the very aged, and so on—are particularly susceptible.

MANGANESE

Manganese is an essential trace metal in humans and is important to certain enzyme systems; the enzyme adenyl cyclase is involved in the formation of cyclic adenosine monophosphate (AMP).[44, 55, 56]

Acute toxic inhalation of manganese is known to produce the syndrome of metal fume fever. Chronic manganese poisoning is found chiefly among miners, in whom inhalation of dust gives rise primarily to psychiatric and neurologic disturbances.[57] The psychiatric disturbance is usually self-limited and is believed by some to resemble schizophrenia.[57] The neurologic illness resembles the clinical picture of parkinsonism. It is interesting that the neurologic picture has responded to therapy by levodopa and other antiparkinsonian drugs.[58]

NICKEL

Nickel causes little human toxicity other than dermatitis, but nickel carbonyl is extremely toxic. Nickel carbonyl is a colorless liquid formed when nickel combines with carbon monoxide.[38] Acute inhalation of nickel carbonyl causes severe pulmonary edema, which is often delayed in onset, and liver necrosis. Therapy is supportive; chelation therapy with BAL and perhaps sodium diethyldithiocarbamate trihydrate (dithiocarb) may be effective.[38] Inhalation poisoning with nickel carbonyl is highly fatal.[32] Chronic excess industrial exposure to nickel carbonyl is associated with an increased incidence of nasal and lung carcinoma.[36, 38]

SELENIUM

Selenium has been found to be an essential trace element in humans and warm-blooded animals. Selenium is an active catalyst in peroxide metabolism and is essential to glutathione peroxidase; it is an essential constituent of Factor 3.[59] Selenium deficiency has been reported to be associated with congestive cardiomyopathy.[60] Selenium is used medically in the treatment of dandruff.

Acute selenium poisoning produces primarily central nervous system effects, including convulsions. As sodium selenate, selenium is highly toxic; it bonds sulfhydryl enzymes and produces a clinical syndrome similar to that of arsenic.[37] Treatment is supportive; the use of BAL may be contraindicated.[37]

SILVER

Silver has many uses in jewelry, coins, silverware, and electrical wiring.[36] In years gone by, silver found its way into many nostrums; injectable forms were often associated with argyria. Today medical uses for silver are primarily in the form of silver nitrate, which is used as prophylaxis for ophthalmia neonatorum; silver nitrate sticks are used as a cauterizing agent in the treatment of nose bleeds. Acute ingestion of silver nitrate causes severe gastrointestinal symptoms, as it is highly caustic; management resembles that for caustic ingestion.[37] The topical use of silver nitrate in the management of burns has produced methemoglobinemia.[37] Silver may be a cause of metal fume fever. Chronic exposure to silver causes argyria or silver-blue discoloration of the skin; this is primarily of cosmetic concern.[36, 37] Treatment of silver toxicity is primarily supportive; chelation therapy with BAL has been ineffective in curing argyria and is not indicated.[36–38]

THALLIUM

Thallium is an extremely toxic metal and at one time was widely used as an insecticide/rodenticide and depilatory agent. In 1965, it was removed from the market because of the high incidence of poisoning and death.[38] Thallium is still used in industry in the manufacture of optical lens and in scintillation counters.[36]

Ingestion of thallium salts results in a severe hemorrhagic gastroenteritis followed by delirium, coma, convulsions, hepatic and renal failure, bone marrow depression, and often death. In those patients who survive the initial insult, alopecia develops, which is considered pathognomonic for thallium poisoning.[38] Permanent neurologic damage and mental retardation were observed in a high percentage of patients who survived.[38]

Treatment involves the use of Prussian blue (potassium ferric ferrocyanide) and hemodialysis.[61] Prussian blue binds thallium and prevents its absorption from the gastrointestinal tract. Soluble ferric ferrocyanide, 125 mg/kg twice a day with 50 ml of 15 per cent mannitol, is given by duodenal tube; therapy should be continued until urinary excretion of the thallium is 0.5 mg/day or less.[38] Prussian blue is presently approved only for use in Europe.

Long-term hemodialysis is the only other treatment modality that may be of benefit and should be employed in significant cases.[61]

TIN

Because tin is relatively safe, it is the element of choice for containers of canned foods. Although tin is safe, organic tin compounds such as triethyl tin are considerably more toxic; as a contaminant of an oral medication used for skin disorders, triethyl tin was responsible for an epidemic of poisoning in France in which more than 100 victims died.[37] Chronic exposure to triethyl tin causes cerebral edema and results in headache, vomiting, psychic disturbances, and convulsions.[37] Treatment is supportive.

TITANIUM

Titanium is relatively inert. Titanium tetrachloride is one of the few compounds that reacts violently with water to liberate heat and produce hydrochloric acid.[37] The tendency in most hazardous chemical spills is to wash off the liquid or powder with water. In the case of titanium tetrachloride (which is a liquid), as with certain forms of phosphorus, this would prove disastrous. Dry wiping of the chemical is indicated. Titanium tetrachloride fumes can cause chemical pneumonitis, and titanium tetrachloride liquid can lead to blindness if splashed in the eye.[37] Treatment of all injuries is supportive and symptomatic.

VANADIUM

Vanadium is now considered a trace metal essential to human life. Vanadium is an important ubiquitous metal that has multiple uses in industry.[36] Inhalation of vanadium dust among industrial workers is a common cause of metal fume fever. Gastrointestinal disturbance, renal dysfunction, and psychiatric disturbances may occur. Chronic overexposure to vanadium can cause a greenish-black discoloration of the tongue, which is considered characteristic.[37] Therapy of acute poisoning is supportive; chelation therapy with calcium disodium edetate is considered effective.[37, 38]

ZINC

Zinc is an important trace metal that is essential to human existence.[44] More than 70 human enzyme systems depend on zinc for their function, and they span a broad range of biologic activities, including RNA and DNA synthesis and other biochemical and morphologic events of the cell cycle.[62] Zinc is essential to human growth.[63]

Zinc has many uses in manufacturing processes, paints, and enamels and is a wood preservative. Zinc phosphide is presently a popular rodenticide. Zinc oxide is formed during the melting or heating of metallic zinc in the presence of air and is the classic cause of metal fume fever.[31, 32, 36–38, 44, 64] Therapy is supportive.

Acute zinc toxicity causing death has been reported following the accidental infusion of 7.4 gm of zinc sulfate from a parenteral hyperalimentation solution in a patient being treated for enterocutaneous fistula.[65]

Ingestion of elemental zinc has been shown to cause lethargy.[66] Ingested liquid zinc chloride solutions are quite caustic and produce erosive pharyngitis and esophagitis with nausea, vomiting, and abdominal pain as well as hypocalcemia.[67] Chelation therapy with either edetic acid (EDTA) or BAL has been shown to be effective and may be indicated.

Zinc can cause corneal abrasions on eye contact. Irrigation and ophthalmology consultation are indicated.

References

1. Fesmire FM, Schauben JL, Roberge RJ: Survival following massive arsenic ingestion. Am J Emerg Med *6*:602, 1988.
2. Levin-Scherz JK, Patrick JD, Weber FH, Garabedian C: Acute arsenic ingestion. Ann Emerg Med *16*:702, 1987.
3. Hutton JT, Christians BL, Dippel RL: Arsenic poisoning. N Engl J Med *307*:1080, 1982.
4. DiNapoli J, Hall AH, Drake R, Rumack BH: Cyanide and arsenic poisoning by intravenous injection. Am J Emerg Med *18*:308, 1989.
5. Bertolero F, Pozzi G, Sabbioni E, Saffiotti U: Cellular uptake and metabolic reduction of pentavalent to trivalent arsenic as determinants of cytotoxicity and morphological transformation. Carcinogenesis *8*:803, 1987.
6. Tsukamoto H, Parker HR, Peoples SA: Metabolism and renal handling of sodium arsenate in dogs. Am J Vet Res *44*:2331, 1983.
7. Schoolmeester WL, White DR: Arsenic poisoning. South Med J *73*:198, 1980.
8. Watson WA, Veltri JC, Metcalf TJ: Acute arsenic exposure treated with oral D-penicillamine. Vet Hum Toxicol *23*:164, 1981.
9. Peterson RG, Rumack BH: D-penicillamine therapy of acute arsenic poisoning. J Pediatr *91*:661, 1977.
10. Lugo G, Cassady G, Palmisano P: Acute maternal arsenic intoxication with neonatal death. Am J Dis Child *117*:328, 1969.
11. Ferm VH, Saxon A, Smith BM: The teratogenic profile of sodium arsenate in the golden hamster. Arch Environ Health *22*:557, 1971.
12. Morrissey RE, Mottet NK: Arsenic-induced exencephaly in the mouse and associated lesions occurring during neurulation. Teratology *28*:399, 1983.
13. Hessl SM, Berman E: Severe peripheral neuropathy after exposure to monosodium methyl arsenate. J Toxicol Clin Toxicol *19*:281, 1982.
14. ACGIH: Documentation of the Threshold Limit Values and Biological Exposure Indices. 5th ed. Cincinnati, OH, American Conference of Governmental Industrial Hygienists, 1986.
15. Kjeldsberg CR, Ward HP: Leukemia in arsenic poisoning. Ann Intern Med *77*:935, 1972.
16. Rees I, Adelman M, Pratilas V: Chronic arsenic poisoning. Anesthesiology *51*:84, 1979.
17. Popper H, Thomas LB, Telles NC, Falk H: Development of hepatic angiosarcoma in man induced by vinylchloride, thorotrast, or arsenic. Am J Pathol *92*:349, 1978.
18. Baselt RC: Arsenic. *In* Disposition of Toxic Drugs and Chemicals in Man. 2nd ed. Davis, CA, Biomedical Publications, 1982.
19. Kreppel H, Reichl FX, Forth W, Fichtl B: Lack of effectiveness of D-penicillamine in experimental arsenic poisoning. Vet Hum Toxicol *31*:1, 1989.
20. Winchester JF, Gelfand MC, Knepshield JH, Schreiner GE: Dialysis and hemoperfusion of poisons and drugs—Update. Trans Am Soc Artif Intern Organs *23*:762, 1977.
21. Shum S, Skarbovig J, Habersang R: Acute lethal arsenite poisoning in mice: Effect of treatment with N-acetylcysteine, D-penicillamine and dimercaprol in survival time. Vet Hum Toxicol *23*(Suppl):39, 1981.
22. Riggs BS, Kulig K, Knapp G, Rumack BH: Arsenic poisoning: Comparison of IV NAC vs IM BAL vs PO D-penicillamine (abs). Vet Hum Toxicol *30*:359, 1988.
23. Kosnett MJ, Becker CE: Dimercaptosuccinic acid as a treatment for arsenic poisoning (abs). Vet Hum Toxicol *29*:462, 1987.
24. Kosnett MJ, Becker CE: Dimercaptosuccinic acid:

Utility in acute and chronic arsenic poisoning (abs). Vet Hum Toxicol *30*:369, 1988.
25. Kersjes MP, Maurer JR, Trestrail JH, McCoy DJ: An analysis of arsenic exposures referred to the Blodgett Regional Poison Center. Vet Hum Toxicol *29*:75, 1987.
26. Fowler BA, Weissberg JF: Arsine poisoning. N Engl J Med *291*:1171, 1974.
27. Webster JD, Parker TF, Alfrey AC, Smythe WR, Kubo H, Neal G, Hull AR: Acute nickel intoxication by dialysis. Ann Intern Med *92*:631, 1980.
28. Alfrey AC, LeGendre GR, Kaehny WD: The dialysis encephalopathy syndrome: Possible aluminum intoxication. N Engl J Med *294*:184, 1976.
29. Poisson M, Marshaly R, Lebkiri B: Dialysis encephalopathy: Recovery after interruption of aluminum intake. Br Med J *2*:1610, 1978.
30. Arieff AI, Cooper JD, Armstrong D, Lazarowitz VC: Dementia, renal failure, and brain aluminum. Ann Intern Med *90*:741, 1979.
31. Dula DJ: Metal fume fever. J Am Coll Emerg Phys *7*:448, 1978.
32. Braunwald E, Isselbacher KJ, Petersdorf RG, Wilson JD, Martin JB, Fauci AS: Harrison's Principles of Internal Medicine. 11th ed. New York, McGraw-Hill, 1987.
33. Fisher CE, Knowles ME, Massey RC, McWeeny DT: Levels of aluminum in infant formulae. Lancet *1*:1024, 1989.
34. Hughes JT: Aluminum encephalopathy and Alzheimer's disease (letter). Lancet *1*:490, 1989.
35. Monteagudo FSE, Cassidy MJD, Folb PI: Recent developments in aluminum toxicology. Med Toxicol *4*:1, 1989.
36. Goyer RA: Toxic effects of metals. *In* Klaassen CD, Amdur MO, Doull CD (eds): Casarett and Doull's Toxicology: Basic Science of Poisons. 3rd ed. New York, Macmillan, 1986.
36a. Wills MR, Savory J: Aluminum poisoning: Dialysis and encephalopathy, osteomalacia, and anemia. Lancet *2*:29–33, 1983.
37. Gosselin RE, Smith RP, Hodge HC: Clinical Toxicology of Commercial Products. 5th ed. Baltimore, Williams & Wilkins, 1984.
38. Arena JM, Drew RH: Poisoning. Toxicology, Symptoms, Treatment. 5th ed. Springfield, IL, Charles C Thomas, 1986.
39. Perry HM, Thind GS, Perry EF: Biology of cadmium. Med Clin North Am *60*:759, 1976.
40. Carruthers M, Smith B: Evidence of cadmium toxicity in a population living in a zinc-mining area. Lancet *1*:845, 1979.
41. Baker EL, Peterson WA, Holtz JL, Coleman C, Landrigan PJ: Subacute cadmium intoxication in jewelry workers: An evaluation of diagnostic procedures. Arch Environ Health *173*, May/June, 1979.
42. Toxicological profile for cadmium. Prepared by Life Systems Inc. for Agency of Toxic Substances Disease Registry, March, 1989.
42a. Klaassen CD, Waalkes MP, Catilena LR: Alteration of tissue deposition of cadmium by chelating agents. Environ Health Perspect *54*:233–242, 1984.
43. Mertz W: Chromium and its relation to carbohydrate metabolism. Med Clin North Am *60*:739, 1976.
44. Burch RE, Sullivan JF: Diagnosis of zinc, copper and manganese abnormalities in man. Med Clin North Am *60*:655, 1976.
45. O'Dell B: Biochemistry of copper. Med Clin North Am *60*:687, 1976.
46. Scheinberg IH: Effects of heredity and environment on copper metabolism. Med Clin North Am *60*:705, 1976.
47. Stein RS, Jenkins D, Korns ME: Death after use of cupric sulfate as emetic. JAMA *235*:801, 1976.
48. Chuttani JK, Gupta PS, Gulati S, Gupta DN: Acute copper sulfate poisoning. Am J Med *39*:849, 1965.
49. Cole DEC, Lirenman DS: Role of albumin-enriched peritoneal dialysate in acute copper poisoning. J Pediatr *92*:955, 1978.
50. Wacker WEC, Parisi AF: Magnesium metabolism. N Engl J Med *278*:658, 1968.
51. Wacker WEC, Parisi AF: Magnesium metabolism—concluded. N Engl J Med *278*:772, 1968.
52. Geiderman JM, Goodman SL, Cohen DB: Magnesium—the forgotten electrolyte. J Am Coll Emerg Phys *8*:204, 1979.
53. Garrelts JC, Watson WA, Holloway KD, Sweet DE: Mg toxicity secondary to catharsis during management of theophylline poisoning. Am J Emerg Med *7*:34, 1989.
54. Gren J, Woolf A: Hypermagnesemia associated with catharsis in a salicylate-intoxicated patient with anorexia nervosa. *In* Braunwald E (ed): Harrison's Textbook of Internal Medicine. 11th ed. New York, McGraw-Hill, 1987.
55. Utter MF: Biochemistry of manganese. Med Clin North Am *60*:713, 1976.
56. Cotzias GC, Miller ST, Papavasiliou PS, Tang LC: Interactions between manganese and brain dopamine. Med Clin North Am *60*:729, 1976.
57. Cook DG, Fahn S, Brait KA: Chronic manganese intoxication. Arch Neurol *30*:59, 1974.
58. Mena I, Court J, Fuenzalida S, Papavasiliou PS, Cotzias GC: Modification of chronic manganese poisoning. N Engl J Med *282*:5, 1970.
59. Schwarz K: Essentiality and metabolic functions of selenium. Med Clin North Am *60*:745, 1976.
60. Johnson RA, Baker SS, Fallon JT, Maynard EP, Ruskin JN, Wen Z, Ge K, Cohen HJ: An Occidental case of cardiomyopathy and selenium deficiency. N Engl J Med *304*:1210, 1981.
61. Pedersen RS, Olesen AS, Freund LG, Solgaard P, Larsen E: Thallium intoxication treated with long-term hemodialysis, forced diuresis and Prussian blue. Acta Med Scand *204*:429, 1978.
62. Riordan JF: Biochemistry of zinc. Med Clin North Am *60*:661, 1976.
63. Gordon EF, Gordon RC, Passal DB: Zinc metabolism. J Pediatr *99*:341, 1981.
64. Burch RE, Sullivan JF: Clinical and nutritional aspects of zinc deficiency and excess. Med Clin North Am *60*:675, 1976.
65. Brocks A, Reid H, Glazer G: Acute intravenous zinc poisoning. Br Med J *1*:1390, 1977.
66. Murphy JV: Intoxication following ingestion of elemental zinc. JAMA *212*:2119, 1970.
67. Chobanian SJ: Accidental ingestion of liquid zinc chloride. Ann Emerg Med *10*:91, 1981.

CHAPTER 60
SODIUM AND SODIUM CHLORIDE

Howard Mofenson, M.D.
Thomas Caraccio, Pharm.D.

Sodium chloride (NaCl) is ubiquitous in nature and essential to all life. It is the basic milieu of mammals. Sodium chloride occurs as colorless cubic crystals or as white crystalline powder. Salt intoxication and death have occurred when it is used as an emetic.[1–3] Other causes of salt poisoning are the ingestion or aspiration of sea water,[4] incorrectly prepared electrolyte solutions or infant milk formulas,[5–9] excess dark Karo syrup[10] or improper dilution of broth,[11] baking soda used as home remedies,[12, 13] saline nose drops causing nasal obstruction,[14] hypertonic saline used to empty the uterus,[15, 16] saline enemas, especially in Hirschsprung's disease,[17] and intentional poisoning in child abuse.[18, 19] The Chinese used saturated salt solution for suicide and the "Chinese restaurant syndrome" has been blamed on the high content of sodium in Chinese food. In 1988, the American Association of Poison Control Centers National Database reported 1331 toxic exposures (0.1 per cent) to sodium chloride.[20]

Physiology and Kinetics

The atomic weight of Na is 23 and that of Cl is 35.5. Since sodium is monovalent, 1 mEq of sodium equals 1 mmol. One gram of salt equals 17.2 mEq or mmol. Sodium maintains osmotic stability and is responsible for greater than 90 per cent of the osmolality of extracellular fluid.[21] In association with chloride and bicarbonate, it regulates acid-base equilibrium. Sodium functions as a preservative of normal irritability of muscles, which is essential for the generation of the action potential in excitable tissues and regulates the permeability of cells. In the United States, adults consume 5 to 15 grams of salt daily. The sodium intake of children is less; the sodium needed for growth is 0.5 mEq/kg from birth to 3 months of age, which decreases to 0.1 mEq/kg at 6 months.[22] The average content of sodium in human milk is 7 mEq/L and that in cow milk is 21 mEq/L. The maximum tolerated sodium intake is 250 mEq/M^2/24 hr.[23]

Absorption. Sodium is rapidly absorbed throughout the gastrointestinal tract—maximally from the jejunum and ileum by way of the sodium-potassium–activated ATPase system, which is augmented by aldosterone and desoxycorticosterone acetate. It is also absorbed by rectal enema, and absorbed subcutaneously by clysis.

Distribution. Sodium, the major cation of extracellular fluid, is present in concentrations of 135 to 145 mEq/L. It accounts for only 10 mEq/L of intracellular fluid. The volume of distribution is 0.64 L/kg.

Excretion. Sodium excretion occurs in the urine, sweat, and feces. The kidney is the principal organ for regulation of sodium output. The kidney filters sodium at the glomerulus, but 60 to 70 per cent is reabsorbed in the proximal tubules, along with bicarbonate and water. Another 25 to 30 per cent is reabsorbed in the loop of Henle, along with chloride and more water. In the distal tubules, aldosterone modulates the reabsorption of sodium and, indirectly, chloride. The renal threshold for sodium is 110 to 130 mEq/L. Less than 1 per cent of the filtered sodium is excreted in the urine.

Chloride, the other component of salt, is also essential for water balance, acid-base balance, and serum osmolality. It plays a role in the chloride shift and in excretion as hydrochloric acid. Abnormalities in sodium metabolism are accompanied by abnormalities in chloride metabolism.

TOXICITY

Hypernatremia exists when the proportion of sodium to water exceeds normal or when the water loss is greater than the sodium loss, as in profuse sweating; prolonged hyperpnea; severe vomiting or diarrhea; polyuria; diabetes insipidus, either primary (decreased antidiuretic hormone) or nephrogenic (decreased tubular sensitivity to ADH); osmotic diuresis; and high salt intake without corresponding intake of water. Elderly pa-

Table 60–1. CLINICAL DISORDERS OF SODIUM METABOLISM CAUSING HYPERNATREMIA

CLINICAL DISORDER	MECHANISM
Cushing's disease	Hyperactivity of adrenal cortex and salt retention
High environmental temperature	Excess loss of hypertonic sweat
Diarrhea	Loss of sodium and excess water
Salt poisoning	Excess intake without water
Postobstructive diuresis	Excess renal water loss
Nephrogenic diabetes insipidus	Excess water loss
Diabetes insipidus	Excess water loss
Hypercalcemic nephropathy	Excess water loss
Sickle cell nephropathy	Excess water loss
Aldosteronism	Hypersecretion of aldosterone

(Modified from Chan JC: Fluid and electrolyte and acid-base disorders in children. Curr Prob Pediatr II (10):6, 1981.)

tients with an altered thirst mechanism may develop hypernatremia. Cushing's disease, excess aldosteronism, or excess production of other mineralocorticoids is a rare cause of hypernatremia (Table 60–1).

Salt poisoning increases both the plasma sodium concentration, the total body sodium, and the extracellular fluid volume, whereas the hypernatremia from other causes, such as dehydration, increases the plasma sodium but decreases the body sodium and the extracellular fluid volume.

Acute poisoning has been reported from the use of salt in the following situations:

As simple salt eating—Easy accessibility of salt to children has resulted in ingestions of significant magnitude.

As acute poisoning from salt used as an emetic—Advice to physicians and parents in the past often recommended the use of salt solutions as an emetic. This practice has been condemned because of the number of deaths resulting from hypernatremia. Salt is a dangerous emetic, with only one quarter the emetic effect of syrup of ipecac.[1–3]

Seawater—Ingesting or aspirating seawater, which contains 350 to 400 mg/dl or 152 to 173 mEq or mmol per liter of sodium may produce hypernatremia. The Dead Sea contains 387 mg/dl (168 mEq/L or mmol/L) and the Great Salt Lake in Utah, 882 mg/dl (383.4 mEq/L or mmol/L) of sodium.[4]

As errors in formulating infant diets—Infant formula preparation with salt mistakenly substituted for carbohydrate has resulted in individual and mass accidental poisonings.[5–9] Excessive Karo syrup (35 mEq/L of sodium) has produced hypernatremia.[10] One of the first reported instances of mass salt poisoning occurred in Binghamton, New York, in March, 1962. The case fatality rate was 6 of 14 exposed infants.[5]

As a homemade salt solution—Giving poorly absorbed sugars or solutions containing more than 40 mEq/L of sodium chloride may lead to an increase in stool volume and a lower concentration of sodium in the stool in proportion to water.[7, 8] The treatment of diarrhea with bouillon prepared by dissolution of cubes or powder in water can cause significant hypernatremia if there is inadequate dilution.[11] Errors in the treatment of diarrhea with home-prepared solutions have resulted in tragic cases of hypernatremia. Verbal instructions were frequently misunderstood or forgotten by anxious parents. Carefully written instructions and commercially prepared solutions are necessary to prevent this pitfall. A subtle salt intoxication can result in ill infants from continuous use of skim milk, which has considerable natural sodium and chloride.

Misuse of baking soda for the treatment of "gas" in infants has produced metabolic alkalosis and hypernatremia.[12, 13]

Saline solution nose drops in infants—Homemade saline nose drops are commonly recommended to loosen up nasal secretions in infants and children. Improper preparation has resulted when mothers misunderstood or received inadequate instructions. Even the persistent use of saline is irritating and interferes with cilia action. Hypertonic nasal salt solutions can result in irritated nasal mucosa, edema, inflammation, complete nasal obstruction, and respiratory distress in infants and small children.[14]

As an injectable—Overzealous intravenous use of saline or hypertonic solutions and intra-amniotic injections to induce abortions or empty the uterus (in the case of removal of hydatidiform mole) can result in symptomatic hypernatremia and permanent damage to the nervous system.[15, 16]

As an enema solution—Salt poisoning has occurred from the use of salt in enemas to treat high fevers, chronic constipation, and Hirschsprung's disease.[17]

As a form of child abuse—Cases of acute hypernatremia have been reported from administration of excess salt and the combination of excess salt and water deprivation as a means of child abuse.[18, 19]

CLINICAL PRESENTATION

The clinical presentation in infants can be quite deceptive. Irritability, lethargy, and/or tachypnea may be the only finding(s), especially in infants.

The patient may have gastrointestinal symptoms and complain of abdominal cramps. Thirst, irritability, weakness, headache, and altered mental status may be present. Coma or convulsions, when present, are a grave sign. Pulmonary edema, especially with marked fluid overload, may be the presenting picture. Hypertension and tachycardia may be evident. Shock indicates severe fluid loss. Salt poisoning may cause acute renal tubular necrosis.[24–27]

A sodium concentration of greater than 150 mEq/L indicates hypernatremia. Although altered mental status and convulsions are occasionally seen with serum sodiums of 150 to 160 mEq/L, they are more common in the 160 to 185 mEq/L range. Death usually occurs at serum sodium values of greater than 185 mEq/L, especially when untreated.

The toxic oral dose of salt is 0.5 to 1.0 gm/kg. The estimated fatal amount is about 1 to 3 gm/kg. For each additional 140 mEq of sodium in the body, 1 liter of water is retained.

The patient who has ingested enough salt to elevate the serum sodium more than 10 mEq/liter in a child or 15 mEq/liter in an adult should have gastrointestinal decontamination and medical evaluation.

To calculate the approximate increase in serum sodium in mEq/liter:

1. One teasponful of salt is approximately 5000 mg or 86 mEq.

2. $$\frac{\text{Amount ingested in mg}}{\text{molecular weight of NaCl (58 Daltons)}} = \text{mEq NaCl}$$

3. $$\frac{\text{mEq NaCl}}{\text{body weight} \times \text{Vd (0.64 kg)}} = \text{Serum increase Na in mEq/liter}$$

MANAGEMENT

The management of the hypernatremic patient should be directed toward *slow* correction of the fluid deficit, the elevated serum sodium, and the elevated serum osmolality.

If the patient presents in shock, a fluid bolus of intravenous normal saline, 10 to 20 ml/kg is indicated.[22] It is important to keep in mind that normal saline has 154 mEq/L of sodium and 154 mEq/L of chloride, and this may well be relatively hypotonic compared with the patient's serum sodium. An alternative to normal saline is Ringer's lactate solution (130 mEq/L of sodium, 109 mEq/L of chloride, and 28 mEq/L of lactate). Intravenous normal saline is probably indicated as well in the face of dehydration.

Slow correction of the serum sodium over 24 to 72 hours is essential, as too rapid administration of water leads to intracellular uptake and resultant cerebral edema, with its attendant complications. Pulmonary edema also may occur. Osmotic diuresis with mannitol may be indicated with cerebral edema, and digitalization and diuresis with furosemide may be appropriate for cardiac failure.

A general rule of thumb is to lower the serum sodium 10 mEq/L/day.

Once shock and dehydration are corrected with intravenous normal saline, as evidenced by improvement in vital signs and adequate urine flow, then hydration can proceed with 0.20 per cent saline intravenous solution. If acidosis is present, sodium bicarbonate also may need to be added to the intravenous solution. Since these patients may be hyperglycemic and hypocalcemic, monitoring serum calcium and glucose is important. Calcium replacement also may be necessary.

Serum sodium, calcium, osmolality, electrolytes, BUN, and glucose; arterial blood gases; and urine flow will need monitoring frequently throughout hospitalization, as well as other parameters, especially in the event of complications. Neurosurgical consultation to monitor the intracranial pressure may be appropriate in the event of seizures secondary to cerebral edema. Serum sodium should be determined every 4 to 6 hours initially until the patient becomes stabilized. Potassium replacement with potassium phosphate is indicated once urine flow is established.

With acute salt ingestion, gastric decontamination with ipecac or gastric lavage is indicated. Activated charcoal does not adsorb sodium effectively. A cathartic is probably not advisable, since it may promote increased fluid loss and exacerbate the serum hypernatremia.

Seizures should be controlled with diazepam or phenobarbital. Patients with a serum sodium level greater than 200 mEq/L or patients who are moribund in spite of conservative therapy should be considered for hemodialysis, and nephrology consultation is indicated. Supportive care with critical care monitoring in an intensive care unit is indicated for all critically ill patients.

References

1. DeGenaro F, Nyhan WL: Salt—a dangerous antidote. J Pediatr *78*:1048–1049, 1971.
2. Barer J, Hill LL, Hill RM, et al: Fatal poisoning from salt used as an emetic. Am J Dis Child *125*:889, 1973.
3. Roberts CJ, Noakes MJ: Fatal outcome from administration of a salt emetic. Postgrad Med *50*:513–515, 1974.
4. Porath A, Mosseri M, Harman I, et al: Dead sea water poisoning. Ann Emerg Med *18*:187–191, 1989.
5. Finberg L, Kiley J, Luttrell CN: Mass accidental poisoning in infancy. JAMA *184*:187, 1963.
6. Rostad R, Blystad W, Knuturd O: Sodium chloride intoxication in newborn infants. Clin Pediatr *3*:1, 1964.
7. Hansted C: Alimentary salt poisoning. Arch Pediatr *77*:457, 1960.
8. Calvin ME, Knepper R, Robertson WO: Hazards to health: Salt poisoning. N Engl J Med *270*:625–626, 1964.
9. Saunders N, Balfe JW, Laski B: Severe salt poisoning in an infant. J Pediatr *88*:268, 1976.
10. Hopp R, Woodruff C: Sodium overload from Karo syrup. J Pediatr *93*:883, 1978.
11. Nomura FM Jr. Broth edema in infants. N Engl J Med *274*:1077, 1966.
12. Fuchs S, Listernick R: Hypernatremia and metabolic alkalosis as a consequence of the therapeutic misuse of baking soda. Pediatr Emerg Care *3*:242–243, 1987.
13. Puczynski MS, Cunningham DG, Mortimer JC: Sodium intoxication caused by the use of baking soda as a home remedy. Can Med Assoc J *128*:821–822, 1983.
14. Utin LS, Bartlett GL Jr: Iatrogenic acute nasal obstruction in an obligate nasal breather. JAMA *243*:1657, 1980.
15. Frost AC: Death following intrauterine injection of hypertonic saline solution with hydatidiform mole. Am J Obstet Gynecol *101*:342, 1968.
16. Cameron JM, Dayan AD: Association of damage with therapeutic abortion induced by amniotic fluid replacement: Report of 2 cases. Br Med J *1*:1010–1013, 1966.
17. Moseley PK, Segar WE: Fluid and electrolyte disturbances as a complication of enemas in Hirshsprung's disease. Am J Dis Child *115*:714, 1968.
18. Pickel S, Anderson C, Holliday MA, et al: Thirsting and hypernatremic dehydration—A form of child abuse. Pediatrics *45*:54–59, 1970.
19. Rodgers D, Tripp D, Bentouim A, et al: Non-accidental poisoning: An extended syndrome of child abuse. Br Med J *1*:793, 1976.
20. Litovitz TL, Schmitz BF, Holm KC: 1988 Annual report of the American Association of Poison Control Centers Data Collection System. Am J Emerg Med *7*:495–545, 1989.
21. Williams K, Lovejoy FH Jr: Sodium chloride. Clin Toxicol Rev *6*(10), 1984.
22. Chameides L (ed): Textbook of Pediatric Advanced Life Support (PALS). Dallas, American Heart Association, 1988.
23. Bennett DR: Daily dose of sodium bicarbonate. JAMA *239*:2385, 1978.
24. Finberg L, Rush BF Jr, Chueng CS: Renal excretion of sodium in hypernatremia. Am J Dis Child *107*:483, 1964.
25. Simpson FO: Sodium intake, body sodium, and sodium excretion. Lancet *1*:25–28, 1988.
26. Feig PU: Hypernatremia and hypertonic syndromes. Med Clin North Am *65*:271, 1981.
27. Elton NW, Elton WJ, Nazareno JP: Pathology of acute salt poisoning in infants. Am J Pathol *39*:252, 1963.
28. Habbick BF, Hill A, Tchang SPK: Computerized tomography in an infant with salt poisoning: Relationship of hypodense areas in the basal ganglia to serum sodium concentration. Pediatrics *74*:1123–1125, 1984.
29. Finberg L: Hypernatremia (hypertonic) dehydration in infants. N Engl J Med *289*:196, 1973.

CHAPTER 61
BROMIDES AND BROMATES

Lydia Baltarowich, M.D.
Regine Aronow, M.D.

BROMIDES

Bromide (Br) is ubiquitous in nature and is found in all biologic materials. Human exposure to bromide occurs through dietary intake, industrial-occupational exposures, and pharmaceutical use. Medicinal bromide-containing compounds can be subdivided into inorganic bromide salts (NaBr, KBr, NH_4 Br, and $CaBr_2$) and organic bromides that release bromide ion during their metabolism. Since the mid 1800s, bromides have been used as sedative-hypnotics and anticonvulsants.[1-3] They were readily prescribed by physicians and widely distributed in pharmacies as over-the-counter sleep and "nerve" remedies. Their chronic use frequently resulted in neuropsychiatric symptoms that produced some of the more colorful case reports in toxicology. The most popular and often misused remedies were Bromo-Seltzer and Miles Nervine; both are still marketed but since 1975 no longer contain bromide.[2, 4] Old products, however, may be stocked in a home or pharmacy.

At present, bromide intoxication from medicinal use is rare. Current formulations containing bromide are largely confined to antihistamine preparations such as brompheniramine and dextromethorphan, both of which are contained in a variety of cough and cold products;[5-7] triple bromides used occasionally as anticonvulsants; and potassium bromide solution as contrast media for retrograde pyelography.[8] The 1988 nonprescription *Physicians' Desk Reference* no longer lists any "sleep aids" containing bromide salts.[7] As of February 1989, nonprescription "sleep aids" containing KBr, NaBr, and scopolamine hydrobromide "have to be reformulated."[9]

The organic bromides carbromal and bromisoval, known as bromureides, have been easily available abroad as over-the-counter sedative-hypnotics and thus are responsible for a large number of suicide intoxications in Europe. Several carbromal preparations, such as Obral and Carbrital, contain barbiturates. Their prolonged abuse can result in bromism, but acute intoxication results from the central nervous system (CNS) depressant effects of the barbiturate and the carbromal itself.[1, 2, 10, 11] Paxarel (acetylcarbromal) is currently marketed in the US.[12] Chronic bromisoval use may result in cerebellar atrophy and a severe cerebellar syndrome.[13]

The popular anesthetic halothane is an organic bromide that releases bromide ion. Studies have shown that peak plasma bromide concentrations occur within 2 to 3 days after anesthesia, are dose dependent, and can remain elevated for 9 to 22 days. This may contribute in some degree to postanesthetic sedation and appears to be unrelated to hepatotoxicity.[2, 14]

Bromocriptine and pancuronium bromide in therapeutic doses liberate bromide in clinically insignificant amounts.[1]

Industrial uses of bromide are extensive, particularly in agriculture and photography. Photographic chemicals, such as activators and developers, contain sodium, potassium, and ammonium salts.[3, 15] Methyl bromide is an organic bromide used as a fumigant in agriculture. Although it releases bromide ion, the primary toxic agent is probably methyl bromide itself and involves enzyme inactivation by combining with sulfhydryl groups in molecules. Methyl bromide fumigation leaves bromide residues in foodstuffs, such as vegetables and fruit, thus increasing our dietary bromide intake.[1-3] Ethylene dibromide has also been used as a fumigant, but contact with it today is usually as a lead-scavenger in gasoline. It has been shown to be mutagenic, carcinogenic, and teratogenic.[1, 3]

Pharmacology

Bromide salts are rapidly and completely absorbed in the gastrointestinal tract and, like chloride, are distributed primarily in extracellular water. Their oral bioavailability is 96 per cent, peak blood levels occur within

2 hours, and their volume of distribution is 0.35 to 0.48 L/kg, which is slightly greater than that of chloride. In body tissues, the main physiologic action of bromide is displacement of chloride. A 40 to 50 per cent replacement of chloride by bromide is considered fatal. The bromide:chloride ratio in body tissues varies. The major intracellular pool of bromide are erythrocytes. The RBC:serum bromide ratio is greater than the equivalent chloride ratio. On the other hand, chloride is more readily transported into cerebrospinal fluid (CSF) than bromide, and therefore the CSF:serum ratio for chloride is greater than that for bromide.[1, 3, 16] Bromide crosses the placenta and easily accumulates in fetal tissue. It is also secreted in breast milk. Although minimal amounts of bromide are excreted in sweat, tears, and feces, primary excretion is by kidney tubular filtration and reabsorption. Renal bromide clearance is 26 ml/kg/day. Renal excretion of bromide is slow, resulting in a half-life of 12 days following oral administration. The kidney differentiates between chloride and bromide, preferentially reabsorbing bromide and excreting chloride to maintain a halide ion equilibrium. Thus, with prolonged use, significant accumulation of bromide ion results in loss of chloride ion. The bromide half-life is significantly affected by chloride intake. When dietary chloride is high, bromide excretion increases. Salt-restricted states prolong the half-life. Pharmacologically, bromide may produce its CNS depressant effect by disturbing the active and passive transport of chloride across neuron cell membranes.[1, 3, 16]

Laboratory Findings

Although total body chloride is decreased with chronic bromide intake, measured serum chloride levels may be reported as elevated. The range for normal serum chloride is 98 to 106 mEq/L. An indirect indicator of bromism is an elevated serum chloride level, since all laboratory methods for chloride determination show positive interference from other halides. The most commonly used methods to quantify chloride are potentiometric (Kodak-Ektachem) and colorimetric [Dupont ACA (automatic clinical analyzer)]. These show the greatest positive interference by bromide. The coulometric procedure (Beckman ASTRA) is the reference method for chloride quantitation and is therefore least influenced by other halides. It is not possible to estimate bromide levels by the degree of chloride elevation.[17–19]

Since measurement of serum chloride is necessary to calculate the anion gap, pseudohyperchloremia results in a low anion gap calculation (less than 10 mEq/L). Other causes of low anion gap hyperchloremic states include hypoalbuminemia and the presence of unmeasured nonsodium cations such as calcium, magnesium, multiple myeloma cationic proteins, and lithium. In summary, the presence of hyperchloremia and a low anion gap supports the diagnosis of bromism.

Serum bromide levels can be measured by a gold chloride colorimetric procedure with a detectability limit of 50 mg/L as well as gas chromatography. Normal bromide levels in adults are about 3 to 4 mg/L (3 to 4 mcg/ml) and come primarily from bromide residues in fumigated foodstuffs.[2] Although serum bromide levels do not consistently correlate with the severity of intoxication, there are generally accepted ranges of toxicity. Levels less than 50 mg/dl (500 mg/L) are considered therapeutic. Levels greater than 100 mg/dl (1000 mg/L) may produce toxic symptoms, and serious toxicity usually occurs when levels exceed 200 mg/dl. A level of 300 mg/dl may be lethal. The significance of bromide levels must be correlated with the clinical status of the patient. Elderly and debilitated patients, especially those on salt-restricted diets, with chronic heart failure or hypertension and chronic renal failure, manifest toxicity at much lower levels. A dosage of 3 to 5 mg/day is considered therapeutic in adults.[1–5, 15]

Clinical Toxicity

Gastrointestinal irritation with nausea and vomiting limits absorption of large bromide doses; therefore, acute overdose is seldom seen unless it is superimposed on chronic abuse. Bromide intoxication nearly always takes the form of chronic intoxication known as bromism, which is characterized by neuropsychiatric, dermatologic, and gastrointestinal symptoms.[1, 13] Some of the more striking and clinically challenging cases of bromism have presented as abnormal behavior. An organic brain syndrome or "dementia" is frequent, but a spectrum of manifestations can occur, such as agitation, delirium, auditory and visual hallucinations, depression, schizophrenic and manic-depressive psychoses, and even hallucinosis with clear consciousness.[20–24] At one time, it was not uncommon for patients with bromism to be misdiagnosed and placed in psychiatric facilities. In two series of patients reviewed from a psychiatric hospital, 10 to 20 per cent had detectable bromide levels and 2 to 10 per cent had clinical bromism.[15, 25, 26] Bromism may also be superimposed on psychiatric illness, anxiety-prone personalities, dementia, and other drug abuse.[27]

Objective neurologic findings include slurred speech, tremor, ataxia, and generalized incoordination, much as in alcohol intoxication. With continued exposure, CNS depression and encephalopathy may progress to coma.[1, 3, 20]

Resolution of CNS symptoms is slow and usually lags behind decreasing bromide levels. A transient amnesia may follow recovery.[15] Bromism should be part of the differential diagnosis in patients presenting with altered mental status, along with structural causes and infectious, toxic-metabolic, and psychiatric etiologies.

Mydriasis is the most frequent objective ocular finding in bromide intoxication. Subjectively, patients complain of color disturbances, blurring of vision, apparent movement of objects, micropsia (rarely macropsia), and visual hallucinations.[24, 28] Ocular bobbing that resolved was described in a patient with bromide encephalopathy.[29]

Bromoderma is the primary dermatologic manifestation of systemic bromism and occurs in 25 to 30 per cent of patients.[5, 15] The severity of bromoderma and the level of serum bromide do not correlate. The most common lesion is an acneiform eruption on the face and upper trunk. In addition, erythema nodosum–like lesions on the lower extremities, pemphigus-like vesicles containing bromide, erythema multiforme, pyoderma gangrenosum, and nonspecific morbilliform dermatitis have also been described. Bromoderma tuberosum is a tumor-like lesion.[30, 31] The bromide content of affected skin is increased.[5]

Neonatal bromism is described in several cases of in utero exposure from maternal bromide abuse and one occupational exposure to bromide-containing photographic chemicals. Consistent features are CNS depression and hypotonia, with a weak suck and cry, which slowly resolve as bromide levels decrease. Two siblings with significant growth retardation were born to a mother who abused Bromo-Seltzer throughout the pregnancies, and dysmorphic features were present in the child whose mother worked in a photography lab. Definitive teratogenicity of bromide has not been proved.[32–35]

Although most other sedative-hypnotics produce dependency and a withdrawal syndrome, withdrawal delirium from bromide is described only rarely. It seems to begin soon after therapy for bromide intoxication is initiated.[1, 20]

Bromism distinguishes itself with CNS symptoms, usually insidious in onset and suggestive of an organic brain syndrome or dementia, skin lesions, and an elevated serum chloride level producing a normal or low anion gap. In this setting bromide levels should be obtained and an intense historical reassessment begun regarding the patient's medications, including over-the-counter remedies often considered unimportant, such as old "nerve tonics" and sleep aids. Only a high index of suspicion will lead to a correct diagnosis.

Assessment and Management

Patients who are comatose or have unstable vital signs should receive general supportive treatment. Blood should be sent for glucose, electrolytes, blood urea nitrogen (BUN), creatinine, complete blood count (CBC), arterial blood gases (ABG), and an alcohol level. Blood and urine toxicologic screen, urinalysis (UA), urinary chorionic gonadotropins (UCG), electrocardiogram (EKG), and chest x-ray are also indicated. As with other overdoses, the physician must search for associated pathology such as head trauma, vascular or infectious CNS pathology, and the possibility of multiple drug ingestions. A computed axial tomography (CAT) scan of the head and/or a lumbar puncture may be necessary.

In acute bromide intoxication, ipecac-induced emesis, or gastric lavage in the comatose or seizing patient, is indicated. In chronic bromism, gastrointestinal decontamination is necessary only in unstable patients in whom an acute ingestion of bromide and a mixed intoxication are superimposed. Charcoal does not effectively bind cations and anions, i.e., bromide, and therefore should be given only in a mixed ingestion or when organic bromides are involved. Cathartics may be given.[4, 15]

Stopping bromide intake and accelerating excretion are key in the treatment of bromism. Therapy is based on the chloride-bromide relationship in body fluids and the preferential renal excretion of bromide when chloride loading occurs. Chronic poisoning in cooperative adult patients can be treated with oral sodium chloride: 2 to 3 gm, 3 to 4 times/day, supplemented with 4 to 10 L fluid/day to maintain a urine output of 3 to 6 ml/kg/hr. Ammonium chloride can be used when a sodium load is undesirable. Symptoms usually improve within 1 to 4 weeks, when bromide levels fall to less than 100 mg/dl.[4, 5, 15]

More severely intoxicated and uncooperative patients are treated with IV 0.9 per cent saline or D5 1/2 normal saline (NS) in conjunction with a diuretic, usually furosemide (1 mg/kg), or a total dose of 40 mg, to maintain a urine flow rate of 3 to 6 ml/kg/hr. Fluid, electrolyte, and acid-base status must be carefully monitored during therapy. Therapy ends with an improvement of symptoms and a serum bromide concentration of less than 50 to 100 mg/dl.[4, 5]

The serum half-life of bromide in relation to various treatment modalities has been compared. Sodium chloride loading reduced the normal bromide half-life from 12 days to 2 to 3 days. Furosemide and lactated Ringer's solution decreased it to 1 day (26 hr). Hemodialysis results in a half-life of 2 hours, which is comparable to that produced by ethacrynic acid plus mannitol. Because chloride loading and diuretics effectively accelerate bromide excretion, more aggressive treatment such as hemodialysis is only rarely necessary. Therefore, hemodialysis should be reserved for situations in which chloride loading is impossible, such as chronic heart failure and renal failure, or in very severe poisoning that does not respond to therapy.[25, 30, 36]

BROMATES

Bromates ($KBrO_3$, $NaBrO_3$) are distinct from bromides and have no medicinal use. They are used solely in industry as a flour bleach and as "neutralizers" in cold wave hair permanent kits, which can contain either 2 per cent potassium bromate or 10 per cent sodium bromate.[37, 38] In the US in the late 1940s and early 1950s, these were widely available in home permanent wave kits, resulting in ten reported cases of accidental bromate poisonings, primarily in children under the age of 4. After manufacturers began substituting less toxic neutralizers, case reports decreased; only one case was reported in 1975. In the 1980s, case reports of bromate poisoning have again appeared.[37, 39–41] Six cases of childhood exposure are reported from ingestion of "professional-use-only" products sold to the public but not regulated by packaging and labeling standards.[37, 39, 40] The largest series of adult bromate poisoning is found in the Japanese literature, where in the 1960s and 1970s suicide attempts by hairdressers ingesting bromate neutralizers accounted for 20 case reports.[38]

Pharmacology/Kinetics

Potassium bromate is a colorless, odorless, tasteless compound that is absorbed unchanged in the gastrointestinal tract, is very stable in plasma, and is excreted essentially unchanged in urine. A very slow reduction of bromate to bromide may occur, which can minimally elevate bromide levels.[40, 41]

Based on cases in the literature, seriously toxic to lethal doses of $KBrO_3$ are estimated at 240 to 500 mg/kg. $KBrO_3$ is more toxic than $NaBrO_3$. For a 5- to 10-kg child this would be 2 to 4 oz of a 2 per cent $KBrO_3$ solution (1500 to 3000 mg). In a 70-kg adult, this is equivalent to 16 to 35 gm bromate.[37, 38]

Bromate blood levels are not available. Although the detection of bromide or its levels does not correlate with the severity of bromate intoxication, in young children bromide levels may be a clue that actual ingestion of bromate took place. Additionally, serial bromide levels may be indicative of bromate to bromide conversion during thiosulfate therapy.[41] Adults, however, may have a blood bromide level above the estimated normal of 3 to 4 mg/L without ingesting a bromate.[2, 37, 39, 40]

Clinical Toxicity

Bromates can produce serious toxicity and even death. Symptoms usually begin within

2 hours of ingestion, with gastrointestinal manifestations of nausea/vomiting, diarrhea, and abdominal pain, all of which are thought to be caused by the caustic hydrobromic acid produced when bromate reacts with gastric juice. Although anemia and hemolysis are described, it is not clear whether these are a direct bromate effect or related to renal failure. A prominent feature in chlorate poisoning, methemoglobinemia, has not been detected in humans with bromate poisoning.[37, 39] Hypotension has been variably reported.

CNS depression can occur, and generalized seizures have been described in a few pediatric cases with significant renal failure and uremia.[37–39] The nephrotoxicity of bromates accounts for their major morbidity and mortality. Acute renal failure usually occurs 1 to 3 days after ingestion, presenting as oliguria or anuria. It has been documented in 12 of 17 pediatric cases and 20 of 22 adult cases. One child and nine adults died from complications of renal failure.[37, 38] In the majority of pediatric patients, acute renal failure resolved within 3 to 9 days.[40] However, recovery of renal failure was not complete in many adults, and some went on to chronic renal failure.[37, 42] Pathologic findings in the kidney consist of acute tubular necrosis with glomerular sparing.[37]

Bromate ototoxicity results in permanent sensorineural hearing loss with intact vestibular function. Deafness appears to be documented best in the adult series from Japan;[38] 17 of 20 adults developed deafness between 4 and 16 hours post ingestion. Only two pediatric cases were reported. In children, deafness may have been clinically overlooked owing to the presence of life-threatening acute renal failure, or it may have gone unnoticed in the infant group. The exact mechanism of ototoxicity has not been established. Of interest is that several other substances can produce nephrotoxicity and ototoxicity: aminoglycoside antibiotics, ethacrynic acid, and furosemide.[37, 38, 40]

Management

General principles of assessment and management in unstable poisoned patients apply to bromate intoxication.[43] Physicians must not overlook the possible presence of other substances and associated hypoglycemia. The patient's fluid, acid-base, and electrolyte status, particularly potassium elevations secondary to renal failure, are critical in these cases. If present, acute renal failure should be appropriately treated with fluids and a trial of diuretics.

To prevent bromate absorption and hydrobromic acid production, gastric lavage with 2 per cent $NaHCO_3$ is immediately recommended instead of ipecac-induced vomiting, which may mask the onset of gastrointestinal symptoms. Although bromate adsorption by activated charcoal has not been documented, when multiple or unknown substances are suspected it should be given.[4, 37]

Administration of intravenous sodium thiosulfate promotes reduction of bromate to the less toxic bromide. Although its clinical efficacy has not been fully determined, its most important role may be its early administration to prevent serious renal injury if significant ingestion has occurred. Either 10 to 50 ml of a 10 per cent solution or 100 to 500 ml of a 1 per cent solution (1.5 to 3 ml/kg), given as an IV drip over 30 to 60 minutes at a maximum rate of 3 ml/min, is recommended.[37, 39]

Prophylactic dialysis to eliminate bromate and prevent nephrotoxicity and ototoxicity has not been sufficiently researched. Theoretically, hemodialysis or peritoneal dialysis may be considered in a severe intoxication if it can be performed within several hours of ingestion.[39, 41] If pretreated with sodium thiosulfate, its effectiveness may be gauged by serum bromide and dialysate bromide recovery.[41] Hemodialysis may be necessary to treat renal failure that does not begin to resolve within 2 to 3 days or for complications such as intractable hyperkalemia, acidosis, or fluid overload.

References

1. Van Leewen FXR, Sangster B: The toxicology of bromide ion. Crit Rev Toxicol *18*:189–213, 1987.
2. Baselt RC (ed): Disposition of Toxic Drugs and Chemicals in Man. 2nd ed. Davis, CA, Biomedical Publications, 1982.
3. Seiler MG, Sigel M (eds): Handbook on Toxicity of Inorganic Compounds. New York, Marcel Dekker, 1988, pp 143–154.
4. Rumack BH (ed): Poisindex Information System. Denver, Micromedex, Inc. (ed expires 5/31/89).
5. Ellenhorn MJ, Barceloux DG (eds): Medical Toxicology: Diagnosis and Treatment of Human Poisoning. New York, Elsevier, 1988, p 503.

6. Physicians' Desk Reference. 43rd ed. Oradell, NJ, Medical Economics Co., Inc., 1989.
7. Physicians' Desk Reference for Non-Prescription Drugs. 9th ed. Oradell, NJ, Medical Economics Co., Inc., 1989.
8. Joyce DA, Matz LR, Saker BM: Renal failure and upper urinary tract obstruction after retrograde pyelography with potassium bromide solution. Hum Toxicol *4*:481–490, 1985.
9. Night Time Sleep Aid Drug Products for OTC Human Use. Federal Register, Department of Health and Human Services FDA 21 CFR Part 338. February 14, 1989.
10. Butte W, Meyer GJ, Volluberg W: Detoxication methods for bromureide poisoning. Arch Toxicol *41*:61–67, 1978.
11. Maes V, Huyghens L, Dekeyser J, Sevens C: Acute and chronic intoxication with carbromal preparations. Clin Toxicol *23*:341–346, 1985.
12. Oral hypnotic drugs. Med Lett *31*:24, 1989.
13. Van Balkom AJLM, Van de Wetering BJM, Tavy DLJ, Hekster REM, Van Wderkom TCAM: Cerebellar atrophy due to chronic bromisovalum abuse demonstrated by computed tomography. J Neurol Neurosurg Psychiatr *48*:342–347, 1985.
14. Tinker JH, Gandolfi AJ, Van Dyke RA: Elevation of plasma bromide levels in patients following halothane anesthesia. Anesthesiology *44*:194–196, 1976.
15. Shannon M: Bromides. Clin Toxicol Rev 8, 1986.
16. Vaiseman N, Koren G, Pencharz P: Pharmacokinetics of oral and intravenous bromide in normal volunteers. Clin Toxicol *24*:403–413, 1986.
17. Henry JB (ed): Todd, Sanford, Davidson: Clinical Diagnosis and Management by Laboratory Methods. 17th ed. Philadelphia, WB Saunders, 1984, p 127.
18. Elin RJ: Bromide interferes with determination of chloride by each of four methods. Clin Chem *27*:778–779, 1981.
19. Komaiko W, Hussain S, Brecher M, Bissell M: Positive interference with EKTACHEM chloride and carbon dioxide methods by bromide-containing drugs. Clin Chem *34*:429–430, 1988.
20. Carney MWP: Five cases of bromism. Lancet *2*:523–524, 1971.
21. Dominquez RA: Bromide intoxication: A persistent problem. J Ky Med Assoc *76*(9):438–440, 1978.
22. Sayed AJ: Mania and bromism: A case report and a look to the future. Am J Psychiatr *133*:228–229, 1976.
23. Battin DG, Varkey TA: Neuropsychiatric manifestations of bromide ingestion. Postgrad Med J *58*:523–524, 1982.
24. Levin M: Eye disturbances in bromide intoxication. Am J Ophthalmol *50*:478–483, 1960.
25. Adamson JS, Flanigan WJ, Ackermann GL: Treatment of bromide intoxication with ethacrynic acid and mannitol diuresis. Ann Intern Med *65*:749–752, 1966.
26. Hanes FM, Yates A: An analysis of four hundred instances of chronic bromide intoxication. Southern Med J *31*:667–670, 1938.
27. McDanal CE, Owens D, Bolman W: Bromide abuse: A continuing problem. Am J Psychiatr *131*:913–915, 1974.
28. Grant WM (ed): Toxicology of the Eye. 3rd ed. Springfield, Charles C Thomas, 1986, p 156.
29. Paty DW, Sherr H: Ocular bobbing in bromism. Neurology *22*:526–527, 1972.
30. Millins JL, Rogers RS: Furosemide as an adjunct in the therapy of bromism and bromoderma. Dermatologica *156*:111–119, 1978.
31. Baer RI, Harris H: Types of cutaneous reactions to drugs. JAMA *202*:710–713 (150–153), 1967.
32. Mangurten HH, Ban R: Neonatal hypotonia secondary to transplacental bromism. J Pediatr *85*:426–428, 1974.
33. Finken R, Robertson W: Transplacental bromism. Am J Dis Child *106*:Z224–226, 1963.
34. Mangurten HH, Kaye CI: Neonatal bromism secondary to maternal exposure in a photographic laboratory. J Pediatr *100*:596–598, 1982.
35. Opitz JM, Grosse FR, Haneberg B: Congenital effects of bromism. Lancet *1*:91–92, 1972.
36. Wieth JO, Funder J: Treatment of bromide poisoning: Comparison of forced halogen turnover and hemodialysis. Lancet *2*:327–329, 1963.
37. Lue JN, Johnson CE, Edwards DL: Bromate poisoning from ingestion of professional hair-care neutralizer. Clin Pharmacol *7*:66–70, 1988.
38. Matsumoto I, Morizono T, Paparella MM: Hearing loss following potassium bromate: Two case reports. Otolaryngol Head Neck Surg *88*:625–629, 1980.
39. Warshaw BL, Carter MC, Hymes LC, Brunner BS, Rauber AP: Bromate poisoning from hair permanent preparations. Pediatrics *76*:975–978, 1985.
40. Gradus D, Rhoads M, Bergstrom LB, Jordan SC: Acute bromate poisoning associated with renal failure and deafness presenting as hemolytic uremic syndrome. Am J Nephrol *4*:188–191, 1984.
41. Lichtenberg R, Zeller WP, Gatson R, Hurley RM: Bromate poisoning. J Pediatr *114*:891–894, 1989.
42. Kuwahara T, Ikehara Y, Kanatsu K, Doi T, Nagai H, Nakayashiki H, Tamura T, Kawai C: 2 cases of potassium bromate poisoning requiring long-term hemodialysis therapy for irreversible tubular damage. Nephron *37*:278–280, 1984.
43. Gosselin RE, Smith RP, Hodge HC (eds): Clinical Toxicology of Commercial Products. 5th ed. Baltimore, Williams & Wilkins, 1984, p III74–77.

CHAPTER 62
IODINE

Daniel Carl Postellon, M.D.
Regine Aronow, M.D.

Discovered by Courtois in 1812, iodine was originally prepared from the ashes of kelp and other seaweeds. At the present time, the major sources of iodines in the United States are natural and oil field brines, from which they are separated by ion exchange chromatography.[1] Iodine is the heaviest of the halogens of industrial interest. Iodine is used in the manufacture of organic chemicals, especially pharmaceuticals such as x-ray contrast media, antiseptics, germicides, medicinal soaps, dyes, and inks and catalysts and chemicals for photography, process engraving, and lithography.[2]

Iodine is an essential element in nutrition, being required by the thyroid gland for the production of thyroxine. The daily requirement of iodine is 5 μg/100 kcal, or about 150 μg/day in adults, of which the thyroid gland takes up about 70 μg. Iodine is rapidly converted to iodide and is stored in the thyroid gland as thyroglobulin. Iodine is converted to thyroxine by, first, conversion from iodide to iodine, formation of monoiodotyrosine and diiodotyrosine, and then coupling to form thyroxine or tetraiodothyronine.

Iodine is a strong oxidizing agent and may react with a variety of reagents used to monitor health status. Both povidone-iodine and tincture of iodine have been shown to cause a false-positive test for blood using orthotolidine (Hematest) or guaiac reagents.[3] The use of povidone-iodine or tincture of iodine as a skin disinfectant prior to obtaining a capillary blood sample for glucose monitoring can give a false elevation of blood glucose by some strip methods.[4] These interactions may cause difficulties in managing patients being treated for iodine poisoning.

IODINE

Solid iodine, sheets, or granules, such as may be encountered in an industrial setting, sublime readily at ordinary temperatures to form a violet-colored vapor. Iodine vapors are intensely irritating to the eyes, mucous membranes, and skin. In the United States, the maximum allowable concentration in the workplace is 0.1 ppm (1 mg/m^3). However, at that concentration (meant to prevent systemic effects from iodine exposure), some people may experience eye irritation. Higher concentrations may lead to excessive tearing, tightness in the chest, sore throat, headaches, irritation of the respiratory tract, and pulmonary edema similar to that seen with chlorine gas exposure.[5]

For commercial uses, bulk iodine is transported in 45- to 90-kg drums. Iodine is available as a pharmacologic agent in aqueous and alcoholic solutions (Table 62–1). (Iodophors, organically bound iodine compounds, and iodides will be discussed later.)

Symptoms from acute or chronic exposure to iodine may occur through inhalation, dermal or ocular contact, or ingestion. Iodine vapor may cause brown staining of the corneal epithelium and subsequent spontaneous loss of this layer of cells, with complete spontaneous healing.[6] A 7 per cent solution of iodine is corrosive to the eye and the skin. Owing to its strong oxidizing action, iodine acts directly as an acid corrosive, precipitating cell proteins. Lesser concentrations have been popular as skin disinfectants and have occasionally been reported to cause hypersensitivity reactions. Although the stronger solutions of iodine are less available than previously, old solutions of lesser percentages may concentrate through evaporation.

Ingestions, either accidental or suicidal, may potentially cause severe corrosion of the gastrointestinal tract and possible delayed strictures of the esophagus or stomach. Any food present may convert the iodine to the less toxic iodide and form a blue-black complex often seen as blue emesis, the pathognomonic sign of iodine ingestion. The reported lethal range in adults is a few tenths of a gram to more than 20 gm.[5] The probable mean lethal dose is about 2 to 4 gm of free iodine or 1 to 2 oz of strong tincture.

Table 62–1. IODINE CONTENT OF COMMERCIAL PRODUCTS

PRODUCT	% IODINE	% Na IODIDE	% K IODIDE	SOLUTE
Tincture of iodine, USP	2	2.4		47% ETOH
Strong iodine tincture, USP	7		5	83% ETOH
Strong iodine solution (Lugol's solution or compound iodine solution)	5		10	Water
Iodine topical solution, USP	2	2.4		Water
SSKI Tabs			130 mg/tab	
SSKI Solution			1 gm/ml (100 mg/0.1 ml)	

Note: ETOH = ethyl alcohol.

Management

Patients exposed to large amounts of iodine solutions, or to smaller amounts of solid iodine, may present in shock due to corrosive poisoning. Such patients may require intensive support, including establishment of an artificial airway, assisted ventilation, and vigorous fluid resuscitation. Caustic injury to the oropharynx and esophagus requires endoscopic evaluation. Ingestion involving smaller amounts of iodine is treated by converting the iodine to noncorrosive iodides or other iodine complexes. Immediate treatment with a 1 to 5 per cent solution of starch or flour in water or, if not available, milk, can reduce corrosive injury through the formation of starch-iodine complexes.[1] Sodium thiosulfate, 100 ml of a 1 per cent solution taken orally, can reduce iodine to iodide in animal and in vitro studies. The optimum dose is not established.[5] Ipecac-induced emesis or gastric lavage is contraindicated if possibly caustic injury to the esophagus has occurred. If starch was given prior to emesis or lavage, the emesis or gastric aspirate will be blue or blue-black, confirming the presence of iodine in the stomach.

IODOPHORS

Iodophors are compounds of iodine linked to surfactants that act as carriers or solubilizing agents for iodine. The most widely used iodophor is a complex of povidone (polyvinyl pyrrolidone) and 1 per cent iodine (Betadine), although other iodophors are available. Iodophors liberate small quantities of free iodine in solution and have a substantial antiseptic effect. Nevertheless, bacterial contamination with *Pseudomonas* is known to occur.[8] The direct irritation to skin or mucous membranes is less than that of available iodine solutions and tinctures. Caustic injury from ingestion of iodophors is unlikely, and such ingestions are of low toxicity.

Iodophors do contain substantial quantities of iodine, which may be absorbed across skin or mucous membranes. This is particularly a hazard where the integrity of the skin is compromised and may lead to systemic toxicity. One hundred–fold elevations of serum inorganic iodine levels can be seen in patients with burns[9, 10] or decubitus ulcers[7] treated with topical povidone-iodine, leading to metabolic acidosis. As iodine is excreted readily in the urine, the risk of toxicity may be greater in patients with pre-existing renal failure. Acidosis may occur in such patients by the following reaction:

$$6\,NaHCO_3 + 3I_2 \rightarrow NaIO_3 + 5NaI + 6CO_2 + 3H_2O$$

The apparent high serum chloride concentration with a negative anion gap, which is often seen in such patients, may be a laboratory artifact. Technicon STAT/ION Auto Analyzers[11] and other chloride-selective electrodes may give falsely elevated chloride readings, even in the presence of minimally elevated iodide levels.[12] It is not clear if iodine, by itself, can cause renal failure in humans.[7] Although it is reassuring to know that iodide can be readily removed by dialysis,[13] this is rarely necessary, except in anuric patients. Vaginal douching with povidone-iodine leads to absorption of significant quantities of iodine across the vaginal mucosa, with increases in serum total iodine levels.[14, 15] In Safran and Braverman's study,[14] changes in thyroid hormone levels were subtle, and overt hypothyroidism did not occur.

Infants may be more susceptible to the effects of elevated iodine levels. Vaginal disinfection with 1 and 2 per cent povidone-iodine solutions prior to delivery was associated with transient hypothyroidism [elevation of thyroid-stimulating hormone (TSH)] in newborn infants.[16] Iodine is concentrated in breast milk,[17] and elevated serum iodine levels were found in a breast-fed infant whose mother used a povidone-iodine vaginal gel.[18] Neonates absorb iodine readily from topical povidone-iodine, and total plasma iodine levels may remain elevated for 3 days after a single application.[19] Goiter and hypothyroidism can occur in neonates with prolonged or intensive exposure to iodine or povidone-iodine.[20–22] Such infants usually have normal T4 (levothyroxine) levels and elevated TSH levels. Thyroid function returns to normal after povidone-iodine is discontinued. Even transient hypothyroidism can complicate the care of a sick neonate, and such infants may be falsely diagnosed as having permanent congenital hypothyroidism by neonatal screening programs.

In summary, iodophors are generally safe when used as antiseptics and are less irritating than solutions of iodine or iodides. In certain situations, significant amounts of iodine may be absorbed from iodophors, leading to acidosis or hypothyroidism. In patients with normal renal function, treatment consists of removing exposure to the iodophor.

IODIDES

Acute ingestions of iodide salts are generally considered benign and do not require treatment. Treatment of iodine ingestion involves converting the iodine to the much less toxic iodides. Iodine deficiency, causing goiter and endemic cretinism, is still a major world health problem, affecting more than 400 million people in Asia alone.[23] Although iodine deficiency is no longer a public health problem in the United States, there is a reverse concern that iodine intakes are excessive.[24] Milk and dairy products are the major sources of iodine in the American diet, probably owing to the use of iodophors as bactericidal agents in the dairy industry.[25, 26] Besides the generally recognized sources such as seafood and iodized salt, iodinated compounds are used in baked goods,[27] algin-based food thickeners, and erythrosine (FD & C Red No. 3), a red food coloring.[1, 24] Excessive intake of iodine can be a cause of hypo- or hyperthyroidism.[28] Japanese populations, by consumption of edible seaweeds,[29] have reached iodine intakes of 200 mg/day, with resulting goiter and hypothyroidism. Iodide-induced thyrotoxicosis has been extensively reviewed by Fradkin and Wolff.[30] Iodide-induced thyroid disease usually requires the presence of underlying chronic iodine deficiency or pre-existing thyroid disease. Besides dietary intake, such patients often have additional exposure to iodine-containing medication, including amiodarone, benziodarone, diiodohydroxyquin, iodinated glycerol, topical antiseptics, and radiocontrast agents.[28] Hypothyroidism is easily treated by replacement therapy with *L*-thyroxine. Iodide-induced thyrotoxicosis is difficult to treat but may respond to a short course of thiouracils.[28] When iodine is added to a population's diet as a prophylaxis against iodine-deficiency goiters, there is usually an increase in the incidence of thyrotoxicosis, particularly in individuals over 40 years of age.[26, 31]

A number of unusual conditions have been described as allergic reactions to iodides or iodinated medication. These include iododerma, a protean group of skin lesions that includes urticarial lesions, acneiform papules and pustules, vesicles, bullae, vegetating lesions, nodules, and tumors.[32] Chronic exposure to potassium iodide has been described as a cause of fever.[33] A hypersensitivity mechanism has been postulated in which activated iodine combines with a protein to produce an immunogenic molecule. Such allergic reactions to iodides usually respond to discontinuation of the offending compound. They may reappear years later in response to any major source of iodide exposure, including radiocontrast materials.

SUMMARY

Iodine and solutions of iodine may act as corrosive poisons.[34] Fatalities have been described.[34] Ingestions of iodine may be treated by complexing the iodine with a starch solution or converting the iodine to iodides with thiosulfate. Iodides and other iodinated compounds are much less toxic and may be tolerated in large doses. In susceptible individuals, they can cause hypothyroidism, thyrotoxicosis, goiter, and hypersensitivity reactions.

References

1. Bulman RA: Iodine. *In* Seiler HG, Sigel H (eds): Handbook on Toxicity of Inorganic Compounds. New York, Marcel Dekker, 1988, p 327.

2. Gosselin RE, Smith RP, Hodge HC: Clinical Toxicology of Commercial Products. Vol III, 5th ed. Baltimore, Williams & Wilkins, 1984, pp 213–214.
3. Hait WN, Snepar R, Rothmen C: False-positive Hematest due to povidone-iodine. N Engl J Med *297*:1350–1351, 1977.
4. Feingold KR, Sater B, Engle B: Iodine-induced artifacts in home blood glucose measurements. Diabetes Care *6*:317–318, 1983.
5. Rumack BH: Iodine. *In* Rumack BH (ed): Poisindex Information System. Denver, CO, Micromedex, Inc, 1989.
6. Grant WM: Toxicology of the Eye. 3rd ed. Springfield, IL, Charles C Thomas, 1986, pp 519–520.
7. DelaCruz F, Harper Brown D, Leikin JB, Franklin CH, Hryhorczuk DO: Iodine absorption after topical administration. West J Med *146*:43–45, 1987.
8. Siegel JD, Duer PN, Haley CE, Thomassen KA, Perrotta DM: Contaminated povidone-iodine solution—Texas. MMWR *38*:133–134, 1989.
9. Alexander NM, Nishimoto M: Protein-linked iodotyrosines in serum after topical application of povidone-iodine (Betadine). J Clin Endocrinol Metab *53*:105–108, 1981.
10. Lavelle KJ, Doedens DJ, Kleit SA, Forney RB: Iodine absorption in burn patients treated topically with povidone-iodine. Clin Pharmacol Ther *17*:355–362, 1975.
11. Fischman RA, Fairclough GF, Cheigh JS: Iodide and negative anion gap. N Engl J Med *298*:1035–1036, 1978.
12. Baker C, Bermes EW, Brooks M: The response of chloride-selective electrodes to iodide. Clin Chem *23*:1126, 1977.
13. Blum M, Spinowitz B, Gombos EA: Dialysance of iodide. N Engl J Med *299*:154, 1978.
14. Safran M, Braverman LE: Effect of chronic douching with polyvinyl pyrrolidone—iodine absorption and thyroid function. Obstet Gynecol *60*:35–40, 1982.
15. Vorherr H, Vorherr UF, Mehta P, Ulrich JA, Messer RH: Vaginal absorption of povidone-iodine. JAMA *23*:2628–2629, 1980.
16. L'Allemand D, Gruters A, Heidemann P, Schurnbrand P: Iodine-induced alterations of thyroid function in newborn infants after prenatal and perinatal exposure to povidone iodine. J Pediatr *102*:935–938, 1983.
17. Gushurst CA, Mueller JA, Green JA, Sedor F: Breast milk iodide: Reassessment in the 1980s. Pediatrics *73*:354–357, 1984.
18. Postellon DC, Aronow R: Iodine in mother's milk. JAMA *247*:463, 1982.
19. Pyati SP, Ramamurthy RS, Krauss MT, Pildes RS: Absorption of iodine in the neonate following topical use of povidone-iodine. J Pediatr *91*(5):825–828, 1977.
20. Chabrolle JP, Rossier A: Goiter and hypothyroidism in the newborn after cutaneous absorption of iodine. Arch Dis Child *53*:495–498, 1978.
21. Jackson HJ, Sutherland RM: Effect of povidone-iodine on neonatal thyroid function. Lancet *2*:992, 1981.
22. Lyen KR, Finegold D, Orsini R, Herd JE, Parks JS: Transient thyroid suppression associated with topically applied povidone-iodine. Am J Dis Child *136*:369–370, 1982.
23. Hetzel BS: Iodine deficiency disorders (IDD) and their eradication. Lancet *2*:1126–1129, 1983.
24. Taylor F: Iodine going from hypo to hyper. FDA Consumer April 1981, pp 15–18.
25. Wheeler SM, Fleet GH, Ashley RJ: The contamination of milk with iodine from iodophors used in milking machine sanitation. J Sci Food Agric *33*:987–995, 1982.
26. Stewart JC, Vidor GI: Thyrotoxicosis induced by iodine contamination of food—a common unrecognized condition? Br Med J *1*:372–375, 1976.
27. London WT, Vought RL, Brown FA: Brief recording: Bread a dietary source of large quantities of iodine. N Engl J Med *273*:381, 1965.
28. Braverman LE: Iodine-induced thyroid disease. *In* Ingbar SH, Braverman LE (eds): Werner's The Thyroid, A Fundamental and Clinical Text. 5th ed. Philadelphia, JB Lippincott, 1986, p 738.
29. Suzuki H, Higuchi T, Sawa K: Endemic coast goiter in Hokkaido Japan. Acta Endocrinol (Kobh) *50*:161–176, 1965.
30. Fradkin JE, Wolff J: Iodide-induced thyrotoxicosis. Medicine *62*:1–20, 1983.
31. Barker DJP: Rise and fall of Western diseases. Nature *338*:371–372, 1989.
32. Bishop ME, Garcia RL: Iododerma from wound irrigation with povidone-iodine. JAMA *240*:249–250, 1978.
33. Kurtz SC, Aber RC: Potassium iodide as a cause of prolonged fever. Arch Intern Med *142*:1543–1544, 1982.
34. Clark MN: A fatal case of iodine poisoning. Clin Toxicol *18*(7):807–811, 1981.

CHAPTER 63
FLUORINE AND FLUORIDE

Howard C. Mofenson, M.D.
Thomas R. Caraccio, Pharm.D.

Fluorine is of general interest because of its toxic properties and the effect of its compound, fluoride, on dental enamel and bone. Fluoride is well established in the prophylaxis of dental caries and is under investigation for treatment of osteoporosis. Fluorine is widely distributed in nature and gains access to plants from the soil as well as from atmospheric sources. The sources of atmospheric fluorine include the burning of soft coal and the manufacture of materials such as superphosphate, aluminum, steel, lead, copper, and nickel.[1] Fluorine is used in organic synthesis. Hydrogen fluoride (hydrofluoric acid—see next chapter) is used in the petroleum industry and in etching glass. Cryolite (sodium aluminum fluoride) is used in aluminum reduction and many other processes.

Poisoning from both organic and inorganic fluorine was recognized as a clinical entity in the early part of this century. Over 112 fatal cases were reported in 1935, most occurring from suicide attempts with rodenticides or when sodium fluoride was mistaken for sugar, salt, or baking soda.[2] Such errors have occasionally led to massive poisonings, the largest of which was in 1943 when 163 inmates of a state prison were poisoned, resulting in 47 fatalities.[3] Today, children are the usual victims of fluoride exposures. In 1988, the American Association of Poison Control Centers reported that 92.5 per cent of 6127 fluoride exposures occurred in children less than 6 years of age.[4] A cause of this prevalence in pediatrics has been attributed to fluoride's attractive dosage forms, which are available in many flavors, and the dispensing of them in nonchild-resistant containers. Pediatric exposures, however, rarely result in intoxications or fatalities.

This chapter reviews the many sources, pharmacology, toxicology, and management of fluoride poisoning.

Sources

The insoluble inorganic forms used in industry, such as cryolite and fluorespatite (found in bone meal), are poorly absorbed and nontoxic when ingested. Fluorides are used as an anticariogenic agent in humans in areas of low fluoride in the water supply. Fluoride is combined in vitamin formulations that are prescribed for children. The soluble organic forms, such as stannous fluoride, sodium fluoride, and insecticides, are toxic by all routes.[5, 6]

Fluorine ion content (the toxic component) is determined by the molecular weight of fluorine (18.99) divided by the molecular weight of the compound. Table 63–1 shows the amount of fluorine ion in various sources.

Toxicity

Chronic endemic fluoride toxicity, usually expressed as mottled teeth, was discovered in 1931. The therapeutic dose of sodium fluoride in caries prevention is 0.25 to 0.5 mg a day, which gives a serum blood concentration of 0.4 to 2.0 μg/ml. See Table 63–2.

Guidelines for the average fluoride intake in water is 0.05 to 0.07 mg/kg/24 hours. Some patients get gastrointestinal upset at 6 mg/kg of sodium fluoride, but under 16 mg/kg, fluoride appears to be relatively safe. Potentially lethal amounts are greater than 30 mg/kg of elemental fluorine. The safe and adequate dietary intake varies with age; 0.1 to 0.5 mg in infants and 1.5 to 4.0 mg in adults. The average-sized 2 year old can safely ingest 60 mg of sodium fluoride, or 120 fluoride tablets of 0.5 mg each. Toxicity is associated with a serum fluoride concentration of greater than 2 μg/ml. The maximum amount of sodium fluoride in a tube of toothpaste should be less than 260 mg. The maximum amount of elemental fluorine to be prescribed is 120 mg, or 240 mg of sodium fluoride. If ingested by a small child, this amount would not produce acute toxicity. The threshold limit volumes for fluorine derivatives are given in Table 63–3.

Mechanism of Toxicity

Fluoride is a protoplasmic poison that binds with calcium, inhibits enzyme systems,

Table 63–1. AMOUNT OF FLUORINE IN VARIOUS SOURCES

SOURCE	TYPE OF FLUORIDE	ELEMENTAL FLUORIDE
Water	elemental	1 mg/L (1 ppm)
Rinses (0.005%)	sodium fluoride	9.1 mg/mL
Toothpaste	stannous fluoride	260 mg/tube maximum
Tablet	stannous fluoride	0.25 to 4.0 mg/tablet
Vitamin drops	sodium fluoride	0.25 to 1.0 mg/mL
Vitamin tablet	sodium fluoride	0.5 mg/tablet
Roach powder (30–90%)	sodium fluoride	300–900 mg/gram

1 mg elemental fluoride = 2.2 mg sodium fluoride
= 4.0 mg stannous fluoride
= 7.6 mg monophosphate fluoride

1 gram sodium fluoride = 452 mg elemental fluoride ion

1 gram stannous fluoride = 242 mg elemental fluoride ion

1 gram monophosphate fluoride = 130 mg elemental fluoride ion

and activates glycolytic and proteolytic mechanisms. There are four major pathophysiologic methods through which ingestion of fluoride compounds may cause acute intoxication.[9, 10] (1) Sodium fluoride reacts with gastric hydrochloric acid to form hydrofluoric acid (HF) ($NaF + HCl \rightarrow NaCl + HF$), which has a direct corrosive effect on the gastric mucosa, especially when gastric acidity is high. (2) The fluoride ion chelates calcium and lowers serum ionized calcium concentration. Paresthesias, tetany, convulsions, and cardiac dysrhythmias may occur. (3) Fluoride interferes with many enzymes, particularly the cholinesterases, and enzymes in which magnesium and manganese are present. (4) Fluoride impairs the formation of collagen tissue and also has a direct action on muscle and nerve tissue, which has been reported to cause many neurologic disturbances.[10]

Kinetics

The ingested fluoride is readily absorbed from the gastrointestinal tract. It is also absorbed by inhalation. Calcium and magnesium salts, antacids, and dairy products interfere with the absorption of ingested fluoride. The peak plasma concentration occurs in 30 to 60 minutes. Approximately 75 per cent of fluoride is immobilized in bone and teeth in children, and 50 per cent in adults. The plasma contains 70 per cent of the whole blood fluoride. Removal of the body burden may take up to 8 years. The serum half-life is 2 to 9 hours. Elimination is renal. Fluoride is a weak acid with a pKa of 3.3. Ninety per cent of fluoride is reabsorbed at a urine pH of 5.0. At a urine pH of 7, only 27 per cent is reabsorbed.

Table 63–2. SUPPLEMENTAL FLUORIDE DOSAGE SCHEDULE VERSUS THE FLUORIDE CONCENTRATION OF DRINKING WATER

PROPHYLAXIS AGE	FLUORIDE IN WATER SUPPLY *(mg/F/day)*		
(Years)	*(<0.3)*	*(0.3 to 0.7)*	*(>0.7 ppm)*
0–2	0.25	none	none
2–3	0.50	0.25	none
3–16	1.00	0.50	none

(Modified from Forbes CB, Woodruff CA [eds]: Handbook of Nutrition. Elk Grove Village, IL, American Academy of Pediatrics, 1985, p 171.)

Table 63–3. EXPOSURE LIMITS FOR FLUORINE AND DERIVATIVES

FLUORINE DERIVATIVE	LIMIT (PPM)
Fluorine	1
Hydrogen fluoride	3
Fluoride salts	2.5 mg/m^3
Boron trifluoride	1
Bromine pentafluoride	0.1
Carbonyl fluoride	2
Chlorine trifluoride	0.1
Nitrogen trifluoride	10
Oxygen difluoride	0.05
Perchloryl fluoride	5
Selenium hexafluoride	0.05
Sulfur hexafluoride	1000
Sulfur pentafluoride	0.025
Sulfur tetrafluoride	0.1
Sulfuryl fluoride	5
Tellurium hexafluoride	0.02

Manifestations

(1) *Low-overdose ingestion* produces local gastrointestinal upset, salivation and a metallic taste that may last 48 hours.[5, 6]

(2) *High-overdose ingestion,* in addition to causing more severe local manifestations, may produce systemic symptoms of convulsions, coma, dysrhythmias, hypotension without compensatory tachycardia, acidosis, paresthesias, and coagulation disturbances. Hypocalcemia can develop very rapidly. Coagulopathies can develop as result of hypocalcemia. Hyperkalemia may be present.[5, 6]

(3) *Chronic fluoride ingestion* of 1 ppm of fluoride in drinking water can cause mottling of the teeth. Exposure to 1.7 ppm will produce mottling in 30 to 50 per cent of patients. Chronic poisoning may cause osteosclerosis, calcification of ligaments and tendons, bony exostoses, and renal calculi.[10]

(4) *Inhalation of fluoride* can produce both acute and chronic toxicity. Acute severe inhalations can lead to respiratory distress, headache, nausea, polyuria, and polydipsia.[1]

Chronic low-grade inhalation, such as has been reported in aluminum workers, can produce fluorosis.[1, 5] Fluorosis is characterized by weakness, marked increase in bone density, and calcification of the soft tissues.

Laboratory Tests and Monitoring Parameters

The normal concentration of plasma fluoride ranges from 10 to 370 ng/ml: 450 ng/ml in erythrocytes and 0.2 to 1.9 mg/L in urine. The concentrations depend on fluorine in water supply.[11, 12]

In *acute* poisonings, blood levels for fluoride are useful only within the first hour after ingestion because of their rapid absorption. Urine levels may be more useful but should be obtained within the first hour after exposure. Urine levels in some cases may remain elevated for days, especially in overfluorinated dialysis patients. Levels of fluoride over 5 mg/L in urine indicate possible chronic toxicity.[11]

For chronic exposures, radiographs of the long bones may show evidence of fluorohydroxyapatite disposition. Radiologic evidence of aortic calcium deposits also has been reported. Fluoride concentrations in bone ash from bone biopsies are useful confirmatory findings of chronic exposure.[11]

In general, all patients with fluoride intoxication should undergo monitoring of the calcium level and electrolytes, especially potassium, and have an electrocardiogram.

Management

(1) In any severely compromised patient, the maintenance of vital functions should be of first consideration. Stabilizing the patient may necessitate securing an artificial airway, assisted ventilation, cardiac massage, and re-establishing vascular volume and tissue perfusion. Specific treatment for fluoride poisoning should be directed toward reducing the corrosive action of hydrogen fluoride on the gastrointestinal mucosa, preventing fluoride absorption, counteracting hypocalcemia and hyperkalemia, and managing cardiac or metabolic abnormalities. These managements will be described later.

(2) Gastrointestinal decontamination is best accomplished with gastric lavage. AVOID emesis since fluoride can form corrosive hydrogen fluoride in the stomach. Lime water (calcium chloride, 10 per cent, 5 ml in 1 liter of saline) has been recommended to bind fluoride. Activated charcoal or a cathartic may be effective, but there are no data about their effectiveness.

(3) If a patient has a history of ingesting *caries-preventive* fluoride in amounts less than 3 mg/kg of *elemental* fluoride, milk

and observation at home are advised. If symptoms develop, refer the patient for medical evaluation. If over 5 mg/kg is ingested, administer milk and refer the patient for medical evaluation.

(4) In fluoride insecticide or rodenticide exposure, administer milk and refer the patient for medical evaluation. Gastric lavage with 0.15 per cent calcium hydroxide, 5 ml in 1 liter of water or aluminum hydroxide gel (Maalox) is recommended.

(5) Monitor calcium and potassium. If a significant amount was ingested (over 30 mg/kg), administer calcium gluconate, 10 ml of 10 per cent intravenously in adults or 0.2 to 0.3 ml/kg of 10 per cent intravenously in children, with electrocardiographic and blood pressure monitoring, even if no hypocalcemia appears. If hypocalcemic tetany develops, follow the initial calcium with infusion at the rate of 15 gm/m^2/24 hours in adults or 500 mg/kg/24 hours in children. The need for treatment of hyperkalemia is urgent if the serum potassium level is greater than 7 mEq/liter or if the electrocardiogram shows changes of hyperkalemia. Therapeutic modalities directed at net removal of potassium from the body should be initiated at the same time as the acute short-term measures *a* through *c* listed next:

   (a) Calcium gluconate dose: see number 5 for hypocalcemia.
   (b) Sodium bicarbonate (generally 1 to 2 mEq/kg of intravenous sodium bicarbonate with the usual precautions[12] and frequent monitoring of arterial blood gases and potassium levels are indicated).
   (c) Dextrose/insulin for adult: 5 to 10 per cent glucose with 0.2 U/kg of insulin for each 200 to 400 mg/kg of glucose administered; child: 0.5 to 1 gm/kg of dextrose IV (insulin is not required).
   (d) Sodium polystyrene sulfonate (SPS) (Kay-Exelate). SPS acts too slowly to be of immediate value but it may be administered to further reduce the body burden of potassium. The oral adult dose of SPS is 15 to 30 grams, mixed in 50 to 100 ml of 20 per cent sorbitol, every 4–6 hours if potassium is elevated; in children, 1 gram of SPS/kg/dose every 6 hours. The rectal enemas of SPS are less effective than the oral route but can be utilized if the oral route is not tolerated or an ileus is present. The rectal SPS may be repeated every 2 to 6 hours if potassium is still elevated and the enema has been evacuated.
   (e) Hemodialysis is reserved for severe cases of hyperkalemia in which more conservative measures have failed or are inappropriate.

(6) Treat acidosis with IV sodium bicarbonate, 1 to 3 mEq/kg as needed, to keep the blood pH at 7.5. Repeated monitoring of arterial blood gases is appropriate; the usual precautions for use of sodium bicarbonate have already been outlined (see Chapter 7). It is also beneficial to alkalinize the urine to a pH of 7 with sodium bicarbonate. Diuresis is effective and can be accomplished by administering large amounts of IV fluids at a rate to keep the urine flow at 3 to 6 ml/kg/hour.

(7) Hemodialysis should be reserved for situations in which there is renal compromise or severe hyperkalemia, as described previously.

(8) Cardiac monitoring and management of dysrhythmias with lidocaine and other antiarrhythmics or temporary pacing are important in intoxications by fluoride.

Summary

Fluorine is used in both organic and inorganic forms. Inorganic forms, used primarily in industry, are nontoxic when ingested, though toxic when inhaled. Organic forms include stannous fluoride and sodium fluoride. These are used in mouthwashes, water fluoridation, or insecticides and may cause toxicity.

Fluoride is a protoplasmic poison that binds with calcium, inhibits enzyme systems, and activates glycolic and proteolytic mechanisms. Management consists of symptomatic and supportive care, plus the administration of calcium and the treatment of hyperkalemia. Hemodialysis may be useful in severe cases. Prognosis is largely dictated by the clinical course over the first several hours. Survival beyond 4 hours is generally associated with a favorable outcome.

Most exposures reported today involve children under 6 years of age who ingest fluoride in vitamin preparations used for prophylaxis against dental caries. These rarely result in intoxication or fatalities.

References

1. Haynes AC, Murad F: Agents affecting calcification: Calcium, parathyroid hormone, calcitonin, vitamin D and other compounds. *In* Gilman AG, Goodman LS, Rall TW (eds): The Pharmacological Basis of Therapeutics. 7th ed. New York, Macmillan, 1985, pp 1538–1545.
2. Yolken R, Konecny P, McCarthy P: Acute fluoride poisoning. Pediatrics *58*:90–93, 1976.
3. Lidbeck WL, Hill TB, Beeman JA: Acute sodium fluoride poisoning. JAMA *14*:862, 1943.
4. Shannon M: Fluoride. Clin Toxicol Rev *8*(2):91, 1985.
5. Mack RB: Fluoride ingestion—cavity emptor. Contemp Pediatr *5*:115–124, 1988.
6. Heifetz SB, Horowitz HS: Amounts of fluoride in self-administered dental products. Pediatrics *77*:876, 1986.
7. Fluorine, hydrogen fluoride, and derivatives. *In* Dreisbach RH (ed): Handbook of Poisoning: Prevention, Diagnosis and Treatment. Los Altos, CA, Lange Medical Publications, 1983, pp 236–239.
8. Baltazar RF, Mower MM, Reider R, et al: Acute fluoride poisoning leading to fatal hyperkalemia. Chest *78*:660, 1980.
9. Cummings CC, McIvor ME: Fluoride-induced hyperkalemia: The role of Ca(+2)-dependent K(+) channels. Am J Emerg Med *6*:1–3, 1988.
10. Fluoride intoxication in a dialysis unit—Maryland. MMWR *29*:134–136, 1980.
11. Hodge HC, Smith FA: Occupational fluoride exposure. J Occupat Med *19*:12–39, 1977.
12. Chameides L (ed): Pediatric Advanced Life Support. Dallas, American Heart Association, 1988.

CHAPTER 64
HYDROFLUORIC ACID

Michael McGuigan, M.D.

Hydrofluoric acid (HF or fluohydric acid), a solution of hydrogen fluoride gas in water, is a nearly colorless, fuming liquid. Because hydrofluoric acid attacks glass or stoneware by dissolving the silica, it is usually stored in plastic containers. The available commercial forms of hydrofluoric acid are listed in Table 64–1.

PATHOPHYSIOLOGY

HF vapor or liquid produces tissue dehydration and necrosis similarly to other mineral acids. In contrast, however, HF is able to penetrate deeply into tissues. Additionally, at the cell membrane, free fluoride ions bind calcium, increase potassium permeability, and alter membrane electrical potential, resulting in spontaneous depolarization of nervous tissue.[1] Severe HF poisoning may result in systemic fluoride poisoning.

HF toxicity occurs after ingestion, inhalation, or ocular or dermal contact. *Ingestion* of HF produces pain and corrosion of the oral mucous membranes, esophagus, and stomach. Fatalities have occurred.[2]

Inhalation of the fumes of concentrated (60 to 100 per cent) HF solution results in oropharyngeal irritation, coughing, and retrosternal burning. More severe exposures may produce laryngeal edema, bronchospasm, and pulmonary edema. Evidence of respira-

Table 64–1. AVAILABLE FORMS OF HYDROFLUORIC ACID

SOURCE	CONCENTRATION (%)
Industrial	
Allied Chemical	
Anhydrous	100
Aqueous	70
Electronic/reagent grades	5–52
Dow Corning	100
Fisher Scientific	52
	49
Stauffer	
Anhydrous	100
Aqueous	70
Household	
Wisk Products	8

tory tract injury may be delayed as long as 24 hours.[3] Pulmonary aspiration of HF liquid may produce severe, rapidly progressive hemorrhagic pulmonary edema.

Ocular exposure to HF produces irritation of the conjunctiva and eyelids. Exposure to highly concentrated fumes or liquid forms of HF may result in opacification of the cornea with subsequent perforation. Corneal abnormalities may develop over several days.[4]

Dermal contact is the most frequently reported route of HF toxicity. The rapidity with which initial symptoms of pain and burning begin is influenced by the concentration of the HF. Solutions of less than 20 per cent HF can produce pain and erythema up to 24 hours after exposure; 20 to 50 per cent HF produces pain and erythema within 8 hours of exposure; solutions of more than 50 per cent HF produce immediate burning, erythema, and vesicle formation.

The clinical course of HF skin burns is characterized by a variable delay in the amount of local pain, erythema, and edema.[5] With time the severity of the pain increases and the involved skin appears pale and blanched. Severe burns develop vesicles (which may be hemorrhagic) or bullae. The final stages are tissue necrosis, skin sloughing, and scar formation. Involvement of the nails or nail beds may lead to permanent disfigurement.[6] Rarely, HF will penetrate to the bone and cause local demineralization. The involvement of a large surface area may result in acute systemic fluoride poisoning.[7–10]

TREATMENT

Ingestion. Patients who ingest HF should receive milk or water to remove residual acid from the esophagus. Milk is preferable because the calcium will inactivate the fluoride ion. Further evaluation and treatment are similar to those for the management of other caustic acid ingestions.

Inhalation. Asymptomatic patients with a history of exposure to HF fumes should be observed carefully for 24 hours. Symptomatic patients should receive humidified oxygen. Upper airway irritation and bronchial spasm should be treated symptomatically. Pulmonary edema will respond to positive pressure ventilation.

Ocular. Eye contact should be treated with immediate water irrigation. Because of the potential for perforation, ophthalmology consultation is advised.

Dermal (Fig. 64–1). Therapy for skin burns has included topical therapy, intradermal infiltrations, and intra-arterial infusions. Many topical therapies have been proposed.[11] A rational approach to the first aid therapy of HF skin burns is to flush the contaminated area with cool running water to dilute and

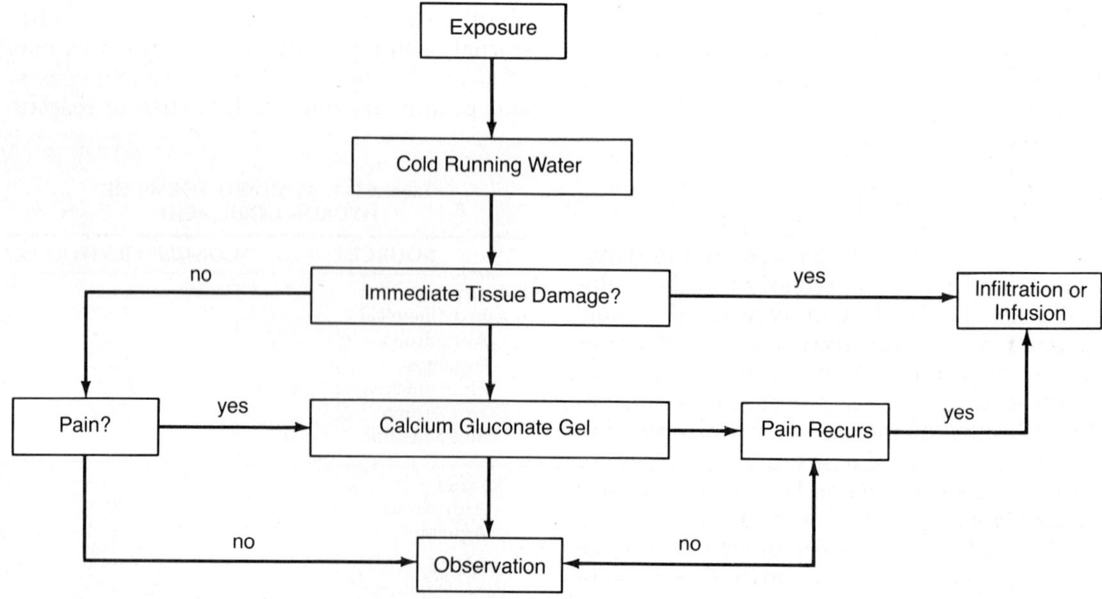

Figure 64–1. Management algorithm for skin burns with hydrofluoric acid.

remove residual acid from the skin. Subsequent application of gels or aqueous solutions of calcium salts will result in the formation of insoluble fluoride complex.[12] The topical use of ice, corticosteroids, sodium bicarbonate, or quaternary ammonium salts (benzalkonium, benzethonium) appears to be ineffective in reducing morbidity.

Because all topical therapies have limited tissue penetration, the successful treatment of dermal contact with HF that has penetrated the skin requires either intradermal infiltration with calcium gluconate or intra-arterial infusions of calcium gluconate or chloride.

Intradermal infiltration with calcium gluconate is indicated when HF produces immediate tissue damage or when symptoms do not respond to or recur following topical therapy.[3, 11]

The infiltration technique utilizes a 30-gauge needle to inject 0.5 ml of 10 per cent calcium gluconate into each square centimeter of painful dermis and subcutaneous tissue. Doses can be repeated as needed to avoid pain. There are some disadvantages to local calcium gluconate infiltration. Multiple injections cause pain and tissue trauma. The injection of large volumes of fluid may result in compromised tissue perfusion. The gluconate salt may contain insufficient quantities of calcium to neutralize large amounts of fluoride (0.5 ml of 10 per cent calcium gluconate has only enough calcium to neutralize 0.025 ml of 20 per cent HF[11]). Finally, to treat subungual burns successfully, it is necessary to remove the nail.

The intra-arterial infusion of calcium salts (gluconate or chloride) is effective for treating HF skin burns.[13–15] Intra-arterial infusion fluid consists of 10 ml of 10 to 20 per cent calcium gluconate mixed in 40 ml of saline or 5 per cent dextrose in water.[13–15] The volume is infused using a pump apparatus through an arterial catheter over 4 hours. The infusion may be repeated if pain returns within 4 hours after the calcium infusion has been stopped.

Important advantages of infusion over infiltration are the ability to deliver more calcium to the burn site and the theoretically better calcium distribution to tissues. In addition, arterial infusion avoids the repeated painful injections required for infiltrate therapy. Disadvantages to intra-arterial infusions include the risks associated with an invasive vascular procedure, local arterial spasm, and long duration of in-hospital therapy (up to 24 hours). Theoretically, intra-arterial calcium is irritating to vascular endothelium.

The management of HF skin burns can be summarized as follows: immediately following exposure, the site should be flushed for 15 minutes with cool running water. The site should then be inspected for tissue damage. If tissue damage is evident, the patient should receive calcium gluconate, either by infiltration or infusion. If there is no obvious tissue damage, further therapy depends on the presence or absence of pain. If there is no pain, no therapy is needed. If pain develops, a calcium gluconate gel should be applied. If pain does not recur, no further therapy is indicated. If pain recurs, infiltration or infusion is indicated.

References

1. Klauder JV, Skelanski L, Gabriel K: Industrial uses of compounds of fluorine and oxalic acid. Arch Indust Health *12*:412–419, 1955.
2. Manoguerra AS, Neuman TS: Fatal poisoning from acute hydrofluoric acid ingestion. Am J Emerg Med *4*:362–363, 1986.
3. Tintinalli JE: Hydrofluoric acid burns. J Am Coll Emerg Phys *7*:24–26, 1978.
4. Hatai JK, Weber JN, Doizaki K: Hydrofluoric acid burns of the eye: report of possible delayed toxicity. J Toxicol Cut Ocular Toxicol *5*:179–184, 1986.
5. Shewmake SW, Anderson BG: Hydrofluoric acid burns. A report of a case and review of the literature. Arch Dermatol *115*:593–596, 1979.
6. Dibbell DG, Iverson RE, Jones W, et al: Hydrofluoric acid burns of the hand. J Bone Joint Surg *52*:931–936, 1970.
7. Mayer TG, Gross PL: Fatal systemic fluoride due to hydrofluoric acid burns. Ann Emerg Med *14*:149–153, 1985.
8. Mullett T, Zoeller T, Bingham N, et al: Fatal hydrofluoric acid cutaneous exposure with refractory ventricular fibrillation. JBCR *8*:216–219, 1987.
9. Tepperman PB: Fatality due to acute systemic fluoride poisoning following a hydrofluoric acid skin burn. J Occup Med *22*:691–692, 1980.
10. McIvor ME, Cummings CE, Mower ME, et al: Sudden cardiac death from acute fluoride intoxication: The role of potassium. Ann Emerg Med *16*:777–781, 1987.
11. Carney SA, Hall M, Lawrence JC, et al: Rationale of the treatment of hydrofluoric acid burns. Br J Indust Med *31*:317–321, 1974.
12. Bracken WM, Cuppage F, McLaury RL, et al: Comparative effectiveness of topical treatment for hydrofluoric acid burns. J Occup Med *27*:733–739, 1985.
13. Velvart J: Arterial perfusion for hydrofluoric acid burns. Hum Toxicol 2:233–238, 1983.
14. Pegg SP, Siu S, Gillett G: Intra-arterial infusion in the treatment of hydrofluoric acid burns. Burns *11*:440–443, 1985.
15. Vance MV, Curry SC, Kunkel DB, et al: Digital hydrofluoric acid burns: treatment with intra-arterial calcium infusion. Ann Emerg Med *15*:890–896, 1986.

CHAPTER 65
ALKALI INJURY

A. Alkali Injury and Esophageal Burns

Kathryn D. Anderson, M.D.

Even the most conscientious parent is no match for the enterprising toddler who wishes to get at the content of cupboards, whether they are locked, theoretically above reach, or even when materials are discarded in the garbage can. Free enterprise has dictated that there is a plethora of caustic alkalies available to the American consumer (Table 65–1).

Materials to unplug drains, clean ovens, and generally sanitize the home are freely available in an astonishing variety on supermarket shelves. Children are subjected, therefore, to burns of the skin, eyes, and esophagus when they come in contact with or ingest chemicals such as sodium or potassium hydroxide in solid or liquid form. Esophageal burn results in an injury that may lead to repeated hospitalizations, multiple surgical procedures, and, possibly, eventual loss of the esophagus. Long-term outcome depends on sound therapy and appropriate management decisions.

The consequences of caustic injection are related to the form of the material. The solid crystalline products commonly cause burns confined to the oropharynx, since crystals adhere to the oral mucosa and the extreme pain may prevent the toddler from continuing the ingestion of caustic material.[1–3] Liquid caustic products, such as lye or sodium carbonate, for instance, washing soda, are easily swallowed by the small child who gulps liquids without tasting. Esophageal burns are more likely to follow ingestion of caustic liquids and may occur in the absence of mouth or pharyngeal burns. Although Clinitest tablets are solid, a significant burn of the esophagus can occur following their ingestion.[4] Hearing aid batteries contain 7 per cent potassium hydroxide and can leak alkali, producing a burn if lodged in the esophagus. Bisphenol A is contained in the resin portion of epoxy glue and is also caustic. Most of the other household products, such as ammoniacal cleaning liquids and bleaches, produce superficial burns with no long-term consequences.

Esophageal burn is the result of direct contact of the substance with the esophagus.

Table 65–1. COMMON HOUSEHOLD CAUSTICS

	MANUFACTURER	CAUSTIC	PERCENTAGE (%)	pH	USE
Red Devil drain opener	Pennwalt	sodium hydroxide (lye)	96–100	14	Unplugs drains, cuts grease
Red Devil lye Lewis lye	Rasco	sodium hydroxide	96–100	14	Unplugs drains, cuts grease
Crystalline Dran-O	Drackett	sodium hydroxide	57	14	Unplugs drains, cuts grease
Liquid Dran-O	Drackett	sodium hydroxide	1.8–10	14	Pours through standing water
Liquid Plumr	Clorox	sodium hydroxide	3–5	14	For toilet use, cannot cut grease
Electrasol dishwasher detergent	Economics Lab	sodium carbonate sodium silicate sodium tripolyphosphate	100 (total)	10.5	Dishwasher detergent
Clinitest reagent tablets	Ames	sodium hydroxide	54	14	Test for urine sugar
Easy-off oven cleaner	Boyle-Midway	sodium hydroxide	1.8–10	14	Oven cleaner
Ammonia	Parsons	ammonium hydroxide	3.6	12	Cleaning agents

(Updated and adapted from Haddad LM: Caustic alkalis. *In* Tintinalli JE (ed): A Study Guide in Emergency Medicine. Dallas, American College of Emergency Physicians, 1980.)

Alkalis combine with proteins and fats, resulting in liquefaction necrosis of the esophageal wall. In addition, these materials are intensely hygroscopic and rapidly absorb the water available to them in the tissues, producing adherence to the esophageal wall. Classification of injury is based on the depth of the burn. Burns are classified as first degree when they involve only the mucosa, second degree when they are transmural, and third degree when the necrosis extends into the periesophageal tissue in the mediastinum or pleural or peritoneal cavity.[3] If only a small amount of material is ingested with a first degree burn, mucosal healing occurs with minimal scarring. More severe forms of burn produce strictures in the esophagus.

Transmural injury to the esophagus can heal but will result in stricture more often than not. Stricture at the site of the burn can be documented within days of ingestion but may be noted weeks, months, or even years later.[5, 6] Sites of stricture are anatomically narrow areas of the esophagus, namely the cricopharyngeal muscle, aortic arch, carina, and diaphragmatic hiatus. There are frequently two or more areas of stricture. A second consequence of stricture is the increased risk of development of carcinoma in the damaged esophagus.[7]

EMERGENCY DEPARTMENT EVALUATION

History

A history of ingestion is difficult to elicit, since the child is rarely observed swallowing the caustic substance. The parent will most often bring the child to the emergency department because he or she is crying, is in pain, may be drooling, has developed swelling of the lips with blister formation on the mucous membrane, and refuses to drink. The parent should be questioned closely about caustics available both inside and outside the home. The emergency department physician should be familiar with the forms of caustics and their trade names, since the parent may not be aware that common household goods contain strong alkalis. The presence of a diabetic family member or babysitter should also be ascertained.

Aspiration of alkali in children is infrequent but can result in laryngeal or epiglottic edema. This will give rise to hoarseness, stridor, or severe respiratory distress. It is difficult to elicit a history of chest pain or abdominal pain in the toddler, but if these are present, perforation of the esophagus must be carefully sought. Subcutaneous emphysema is usually a late phenomenon and is rarely seen in the emergency department. Damage to the stomach in the child is rare, since the child will usually stop swallowing the noxious material once it begins to burn. Adults or teens who attempt suicide, however, may continue their ingestion, and they are extremely vulnerable to gastric perforation.

Physical Examination

Swelling of the lips, drooling, and white plaque formation on the mucous membranes are readily observed in the young child. The rest of the skin should be carefully examined, especially the eyes. Young children who are in distress will often rub their eyes, and if they have had their hands in the caustic material may transfer it to the conjunctiva. Observation of the child's cry, careful auscultation of the chest, and examination of the abdomen are also extremely important. One should also listen for any extraneous sounds during inspiration or expiration that might suggest involvement of the respiratory tract.

Laboratory Work-Up

Complete blood counts and electrolytes are drawn for routine baseline values. Since the caustic alkali is usually neutralized by the acid in the stomach, it is not readily absorbed, and metabolic disturbance is not common. After initiation of treatment, a chest radiograph is appropriate, followed by soft tissue neck films if respiratory symptoms exist. If perforation is suspected, it is appropriate to obtain an early contrast study of the esophagus to observe for any leak. Metrizamide is water soluble, nontoxic, and now readily available for this purpose.

EMERGENCY MANAGEMENT

Administration of antidote for alkali ingestion after the child arrives in the emergency department is probably inadvisable. Since the burn is immediate, by the time the child reaches the emergency department it is too late for the antidote to be effective.[5, 8] And since the child will probably require general anesthesia for evaluation of the esophagus, it is better to have the stomach as empty as possible. If the parent calls the emergency department prior to arriving and immediately after ingestion, he or she can be advised to give the child *MILK*, although it is extremely doubtful if the child will swallow anything because of the intense pain. *Emetics and gastric lavage are contraindicated.*

Rapid evaluation of the airway immediately after the child enters the emergency department is paramount. If there is any respiratory difficulty, arterial blood gases should be drawn and the need for endotracheal intubation determined.

Any caustic material on the skin should be washed off using water or normal saline. Washing should continue for at least 15 minutes. Alkali will give a somewhat silky feel to the skin, which should be irrigated until this feeling disappears. An intravenous infusion of 5 per cent dextrose with lactated Ringer's or 1/4 normal saline is started in the emergency department and can be run at maintenance values, as there is no necessity for overhydration of the patient. Temperature is carefully checked for baseline and repeated every 15 minutes. Antibiotics are administered immediately. A broad-spectrum antibiotic such as a second generation cephalosporin or a combination of ampicillin and gentamicin may be given. The administration of steroids is controversial.[9] A prospective study performed in my institution over the past 17 years has shown no statistical difference in the development of stricture in those patients who were treated with steroids and antibiotics versus those treated with antibiotics alone.

Appropriate radiographs are then obtained and the patient admitted to the hospital.

HOSPITAL MANAGEMENT

The establishment of the diagnosis is the most important aspect of the early care of the child who has ingested caustic alkali. Because of the possibility of esophageal injury in the absence of mouth or pharyngeal burns, all patients should undergo esophagoscopy. It is important that the child be completely still during this procedure; therefore, I recommend general anesthesia and esophagoscopy in the operating room. The risk of perforation of the esophagus is extremely high in inexperienced hands, and the child who is thrashing about is at tremendous risk of compounding the esophageal injury. Rigid or flexible endoscopy is performed at the discretion of the surgeon. The high risk of perforation requires that the examination be confined to the upper esophagus and extend only to and not beyond the first site of burn.[3, 6] The appearance of a damaged esophagus will vary from scattered white plaques adherent to the mucosa (type 1), to reddened, friable tissue, not circumferential (type 2), to the extreme of friable tissue with circumferential plaques and partial occlusion of the lumen (type 3).[10] Some physicians are proponents of delayed esophagoscopy 24 to 48 hours following admission and believe that immediate esophagoscopy may miss visualization of the burn. We have not missed any significant burns by esophagoscoping within 12 hours of ingestion, and, by adhering to the rule that the entire esophagus is left alone once a burn is seen, there have been no instances of perforation in our institution. It is especially important if steroids are to be used that the diagnosis be established early, rather than giving the child steroids if no burn is present. Children ingesting mild alkalis such as ammonia or bleaches do not require esophagoscopy, since the burns produce only mucosal damage and heal without scarring. Electric dishwasher detergents, particularly the new liquid automatic dishwashing detergents (LADDs), are potentially caustic. Esophagoscopy is, therefore, indicated in children who have ingested these products.

Barium swallow is also performed routinely within several days after ingestion following the diagnosis by endoscopy. This study serves as a baseline and gives information about the extent and severity of the injury.[10] Radiologic features of a severe burn (Fig. 65–1) include (1) blurred esophageal margins, suggesting mucosal ulceration, (2) collection of contrast material in plaques, suggesting necrosis, and (3) motility disturbance. Strictures can later be identified by barium swallow and the length documented at that time. For evaluation of the length of the stricture, a technique that we have found

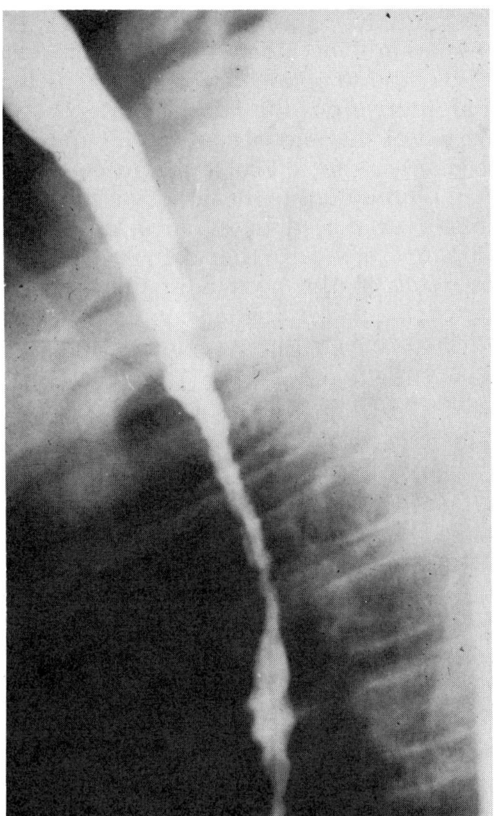

Figure 65–1. Severe stricture requiring esophageal substitution.

useful[11] involves filling a Penrose drain with barium, passing it either via nasogastric tube or a string through the esophagus with the child under general anesthesia (such as at the time of dilatation), and obtaining an x-ray.

The patient is treated with broad-spectrum antibiotics for 3 weeks. These are administered intravenously prior to esophagoscopy and continued parenterally until the child is able to swallow. After this time, antibiotics are given orally. If steroids are used, prednisolone (2 mg/kg/day) is administered intravenously and continued as oral prednisone in an appropriate dosage following resumption of oral intake. The steroid is tapered over a 3-week period and discontinued concomitantly with the antibiotics.

On rare occasions, for example, after ingestion of industrial-strength lye, the esophagus is so badly damaged that stricture is inevitable. In these instances, retrograde dilatation is safest. During the initial esophagoscopy, therefore, a length of string is attached to a urethral filiform and follower and gently passed through the esophagus into the stomach. A gastrostomy is performed, and the string is retrieved and drawn out through the gastrostomy stoma in the abdominal wall. The proximal end of the string is transferred to the nostril and the ends tied together.

After the child demonstrates the ability to swallow saliva, fluids are begun by mouth, avoiding acid liquids such as cola, fruit juice, or carbonated beverages. The child progresses to a regular diet as tolerated. Foods with sharp edges, such as pretzels, potato chips, and French fries, are avoided. The child with a severely burned esophagus and inability to swallow requires gastrostomy feedings.

The child who is able to resume oral feedings and in whom a baseline barium swallow shows prompt passage of contrast into the stomach has sustained a mild injury. With reliable parents, the child does not need to be hospitalized through the entire 3 weeks of antibiotic and steroid therapy. Esophagoscopy and barium swallow are performed 3 weeks after ingestion if a type 2 or 3 burn was present. If no stricture is documented, the patient is followed clinically, and barium swallow is performed as needed at 1, 2, and 6 months post ingestion. Rarely are esophagoscopy and dilatation needed in mild cases. If there are only a few plaques of type 1 burn initially, the patient is followed clinically.

If a stricture is observed after 3 weeks, dilatation is performed. Graduated sizes of tapered, mercury bougies are introduced through the stricture up to the point at which the stricture "grabs" the dilator. No attempt is made to force larger dilators through the stricture, as this maneuver cracks the fibrous tissue and results in a tighter stricture. Following each dilatation, the dilator is wiped with gauze. Dilatation is discontinued if any blood appears. If a dilatation cannot be safely performed from above, a string is passed and gastrostomy performed. If the string is already in place, the stricture is dilated by drawing graduated dilators through the esophagus in a retrograde fashion. Dilatation is usually performed over a 6-month period and continued until it is no longer necessary or until lack of progress dictates that the esophagus be abandoned. The frequency of dilatation is determined by the child's ability to eat a normal diet. This may be required as often as every 10 to 14 days. As progress is made with dilating the stricture, the interval between dilatations is increased.

Long-term follow-up is necessary even in relatively mild strictures. Following growth spurts, such as that seen with the onset of puberty, a stricture may again become manifest and require gentle dilatation.

ESOPHAGEAL REPLACEMENT

Indications for esophageal replacement are (1) patient's inability to swallow saliva with persistent aspiration, spitting, or drooling; (2) persistent stricture after sequential dilatation (see Fig. 65–1); (3) frequency of dilatation requiring indefinite hospitalization; and (4) perforation of the stricture during dilatation resulting in a large, irreparable tear.

Esophageal replacement is to be avoided if at all possible, since no substitute is ever as satisfactory as the native esophagus. However, once the decision is made that this will be necessary, a cervical esophagostomy and gastrostomy are performed. Since scarring in the cervical esophagus may continue for 6 months or more following ingestion, esophageal replacement is deferred for at least this time to avoid stricture formation at the cervical anastomosis. The entire esophagus is resected to avoid the risk of carcinoma.

Choice of Esophageal Substitute

The colon is the most common esophageal substitute,[12, 13] although I prefer a reverse gastric tube.[14–16] If colon is used, the esophageal substitute may be chosen from the right or left colon. In some institutions, the jejunum is the organ of choice,[17] and most recently microvascular surgery has permitted free replacement of the portion of the strictured esophagus by transposing a segment of jejunum.[18] The techniques for replacement of the esophagus with the left colon and the reverse gastric tube are briefly described.

Left Colon

A barium enema is performed to rule out colon anomalies that would preclude its use. After standard bowel preparation and preoperative administration of parenteral antibiotics, the entire colon is exposed and its blood supply inspected. The midcolic artery is temporarily occluded to ensure that collateral blood flow is adequate through the marginal artery from the left colic artery. After division of the midcolic artery, an appropriate length of the left colon is transected. The colon is brought into the neck by a substernal tunnel[12] or placed in a retrohilar position through a standard thoracotomy incision.[13] The route to the neck is at the surgeon's discretion. A cervical anastomosis is performed between the esophageal stoma and the upper end of the colon. The distal end of the transverse colon is sutured to the stomach in a dependent position. Colon continuity is re-established by an end-to-end anastomosis.

Gastric Tube

I prefer the gastric tube for several reasons. There is never a problem with vascularity since the stomach has better submucosal collateral vessels than does the colon. The transposed gastric tube will retain its inherent mucous barrier and is therefore less vulnerable to ulceration from gastric acid. The precise length of gastric tube to reach the cervical esophagus can be measured as the tube is formed.

The vascular pedicle for the reversed gastric tube is based on the left gastroepiploic artery, and the right gastroepiploic artery is divided proximal to the pylorus. A flap of greater curvature of the stomach is separated by staples, and the staple lines in both tube and stomach are reinforced with serosal sutures (Figs. 65–2 and 65–3). The gastric tube, like the colon, can be placed behind either the sternum or the lung or in the esophageal bed following blunt transmediastinal removal of the diseased esophagus.[19] Cervical anastomosis is as described for the colon.

Postoperatively, antibiotics are continued for 72 hours, and gastrostomy feedings are resumed when peristalsis returns. After 10 days, the integrity of the transposed colon or gastric tube is demonstrated by barium swallow, and the child is allowed to begin oral feedings.

Complications are encountered with both techniques. Salivary fistulas at the cervical anastomosis are usually minor, and most heal spontaneously. Scarring may produce anastomotic strictures that may require dilatation and, occasionally, surgical revision.

Reflux of acid into the esophageal conduit may produce ulceration with anemia, especially if stasis prevents prompt drainage.[20, 21] Reflux esophagitis is usually more of a problem in the transposed colon since the gastric tube is protected by its own mucous barrier. Massive bleeding has been reported in the transposed colon.[22] The most catastrophic complications are ischemia and loss of colon conduit from damage to the vascular pedicle. These are not reported with the gastric tube, which retains its excellent blood supply in its transposed position.

Long-term follow-up supports both methods of esophageal substitution as satisfactory for growth and development. The children can be expected to lead essentially normal lives following esophageal replacement.

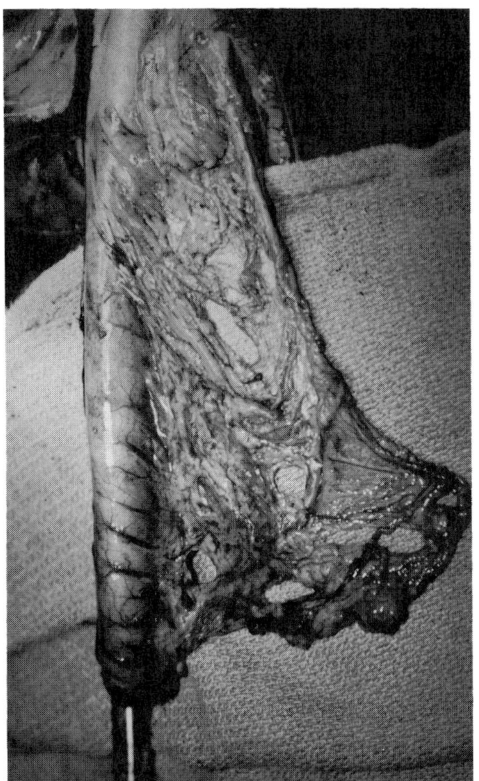

Figure 65–3. Completed gastric tube.

COMMENTS

National attention was drawn to the danger of lye ingestion by Leape and coworkers.[1] Subsequent legislation required safety caps on containers of lye of more than 2 per cent concentration. This has resulted in a marked decrease in the incidence of accidental ingestions in the home. Legislation, however, cannot prevent carelessness in the home itself; the practice of leaving toxic products exposed in uncapped containers, such as drinking cups or cola bottles (obviously attractive to toddlers), is quite common. At present, physician education of parents remains the best defense against the devastating effects of caustic products on the esophagus. My advice to parents is that if they must have these caustic products in the home, they should use them once, rinse the container with plenty of water, and discard the container immediately.

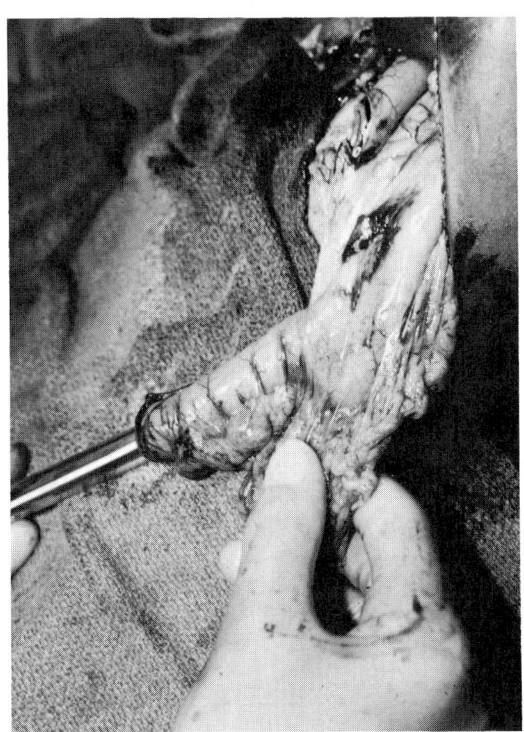

Figure 65–2. Separation of flap of greater curvature of stomach, based on left gastroepiploic artery.

References

1. Leape LL, Ashcraft KW, Scarpellie DG, Holder TH: Hazard to health: Liquid lye. N Engl J Med *284*:578, 1971.
2. Ashcraft KW, Padula RT: The effects of dilute corrosives on the esophagus. Pediatrics *53*:226, 1974.
3. Cardona JD, Daly JF: Current management of corrosive esophagitis. Ann Otol *80*:521, 1971.

4. Burrington JD: Clinitest burns of the esophagus. Ann Thorac Surg *20*:400, 1975.
5. Krey H: Treatment of corrosive lesions in the esophagus. Acta Otolaryngol (Stockh) (Suppl) *102*:1, 1952.
6. Kirsh MM, Ritter F: Caustic ingestion and subsequent damage to the oropharyngeal and digestive passages. Ann Thorac Surg *21*:74, 1976.
7. Appelqvist P, Salmo M: Lye corrosion carcinoma of the esophagus. Cancer *45*:2655, 1980.
8. Leape LL: New liquid lye drain cleaners. Clin Toxicol *7*:109, 1974.
9. Campbell AS, Barnett HF, Ranson JM, Williams GD: Treatment of corrosive burns of the esophagus. Arch Surg *112*:495, 1977.
10. Martel W: Radiologic features of esophagogastritis secondary to extremely caustic agents. Radiology *103*:31, 1973.
11. Tunell WP, Rosser S, Anderson KD: Esophagram with a barium filled Penrose drain. J Pediatr Surg *6*:667, 1971.
12. Gross RE, Firestone FN: Colonic reconstruction of the esophagus in infants and children. Surgery *61*:955, 1967.
13. German JC, Waterston DJ: Colonic interposition for replacement of the esophagus in children. J Pediatr Surg *11*:227, 1976.
14. Ein SH, Shandling B, Simpson JS, Stephens CA: A further look at the gastric tube as an esophageal replacement in infants and children. J Pediatr Surg *8*:859, 1973.
15. Anderson KD, Randolph JG: The gastric tube for esophageal replacement in children. J Thorac Cardiovasc Surg *66*:333, 1973.
16. Anderson KD: *In* Welch KJ, Randolph JG, Ravitch MM, O'Neill JA, Rowe MI (eds): Replacement of the Esophagus in Pediatric Surgery. Chicago, Year Book Medical Publishers, 1986, pp 704–707.
17. Ring WS, Varco RL, L'Heureux PR: Esophageal replacement with jejunum in children: An 18 to 33 year follow-up. J Thorac Cardiovasc Surg *83*:918, 1982.
18. McCaffrey TV, Fisher J: Repair of traumatic cervical esophageal stenosis using microvascular full jejunum transfer. Ann Otorhinolaryngol *93*:512, 1984.
19. Rodgers BM, Ryckman FC, Talbert JL: Blunt transmediastinal total esophagectomy with simultaneous substernal colon interposition for esophageal strictures in children. J Pediatr Surg *16*:189, 1981.
20. Malcolm JA: Occurrence of peptic ulcer in colon used for esophageal replacement. J Thorac Cardiovasc Surg *55*:763, 1968.
21. Anderson KD, Randolph JG, Lilly JR: Peptic ulcer in children with gastric tube interposition. J Pediatr Surg *10*:701, 1975.
22. Stanley-Brown EG: Massive hemorrhage after colon interposition: Early and late. J Pediatr Surg *9*:235, 1974.

B. The Miniature Battery Hazard

Toby Litovitz, M.D.

DEFINITION OF THE PROBLEM: DEMOGRAPHICS

More than 2500 disc battery ingestions are estimated to occur annually in the United States, based on extrapolations from the 1276 reports to the American Association of Poison Control Centers National Data Collection System in 1987.[1] The vast majority of exposure cases reported to date involve button cell ingestions, with their attendant favorable prognosis in the absence of esophageal lodgement. Infrequent cases of battery placement in the nose or ear also occur and are nearly always followed by a severe outcome, especially where lodgement persists owing to delayed diagnosis.

Analysis of a series of 125 button cell ingestion cases demonstrates that adults comprise only 8.1 per cent of cases. The ingestion scenario in these adults frequently involves mistaking the battery for a tablet of medication; very occasionally a suicidal motivation is implicated. Children under 6 years of age account for 71.2 per cent of battery ingestion cases, 6 to 12 years olds for 16.2 per cent, and 13 to 17 year olds for 4.5 per cent.[2] In adolescents and older children, button cell ingestions often follow use of the cells in play, such as tossing the battery in the air and catching it with the mouth. In the younger child, concomitant hearing impairment is a recurrent problem, with ingestion of batteries removed from the child's own hearing aids.

MECHANISM OF BATTERY-INDUCED TISSUE INJURY

The multifactorial mechanism of button battery–induced injury includes the following:

1. Electrolyte (potassium or sodium hydroxide, concentration up to 45 per cent) leakage from the cell, especially at the site of

the battery seal. Corrosive dissolution of the crimp region surrounding the button cell seal increases the risk of leakage.

2. An external current generated between cathode and anode across the battery crimp area can pass through tissue, causing hydrolysis of tissue fluids and local hydroxide generation. Bathing a button cell in an electrolyte-rich fluid, such as occurs when ear drops are placed in the ear with a battery lodged in it, increases the external current and subsequent hydroxide formation.
3. Pressure necrosis of an impacted battery on adjacent tissue may occur, as with ingested pennies. This is assumed to be the least important contributing mechanism.

Both the external electrical current mechanism and the leakage theory have a final common denominator of alkaline-type injury to the tissue. Leakage of the strongly alkaline electrolyte and subsequent chemical burns to surrounding tissue were long accepted as the major mechanisms. Recently, however, the external current generated between cathode and anode across the battery crimp area has been implicated as an alternate, and possibly primary, cause of injury.

The role of heavy metal leakage from button cells in subsequent injury has proved insignificant. Despite the tens of thousands of button cell ingestions that have occurred over the years, symptomatic cases of heavy metal poisoning following battery ingestion have not been reported. The medical literature cites two asymptomatic cases of modestly elevated mercury levels following battery ingestion when button cell disassembly occurred in the gastrointestinal tract.[3, 4] The theoretical mercury hazard is minimized by the reduction of toxic mercuric oxide released from a split button cell to nearly nontoxic elemental mercury in the presence of gastric acid and iron dissolved from the corroding steel battery can. In addition, battery discharge causes mercuric oxide reduction to elemental mercury. Thus, spent batteries contain mercury predominantly in the less toxic elemental form.

CLINICAL PRESENTATION AND PROGNOSTIC FACTORS

Battery lodgement, be it in the esophagus or nasal or aural cavities, is the sole consistent predictor of a severe clinical outcome. Esophageal lodgement generally follows ingestions of larger cells (20 mm or more in diameter), although many of these will pass to the stomach without consequence. Occasionally esophageal lodgement is reported following the ingestion of batteries with diameters as small as 15 mm in very young children (under 1 year of age) owing to their expectedly smaller esophageal diameter. Severe injuries, ranging from esophageal burns occurring only 4 to 6 hours after ingestion to permanent esophageal injury requiring surgical intervention or recurrent dilatation, may occur. Two pediatric fatalities following battery lodgement in the esophagus have been reported following 24-hour to 4-day delays in diagnosis.[5, 6]

In contrast, the vast majority of button battery ingestions are associated with a benign clinical outcome and involve the more common 7- to 12-mm cells. These ingested button cells pass to the stomach rapidly and traverse the entire gastrointestinal tract without complications. Nonetheless, all patients who ingest batteries must be evaluated by a physician immediately to allow radiographic location of the cell and exclusion of an esophageal position. Symptoms associated with esophageal lodgement may include vomiting, fever, dysphagia, odynophagia, and tachypnea. Prompt removal of batteries in the esophagus is essential to prevent severe consequences, including tracheoesophageal fistula, tension pneumo- or hemothorax, perforation through the aortic arch or its branches, and massive exsanguination and cardiac arrest. Second degree esophageal burns have followed battery lodgement in the esophagus for as little as 4 hours. Esophageal rupture has occurred after battery lodgement for only 6 hours.

Batteries placed in the ear or nose and not promptly removed routinely damage surrounding tissue. Observed injuries include tympanic membrane perforation or destruction, necrosis of the dermis of the external ear canal, destruction of the ossicles, hearing impairment, nasal septal perforation, nasal turbinate destruction, and atrophic rhinitis.[7, 8] When batteries are lodged in the nares, the patient often presents with unilateral nasal discharge or pain. Batteries in the ear are likely to be discovered when otic discharge or pain is experienced. Both of these clinical presentations warrant a thorough examination to exclude a foreign body, although sinusitis, mastoiditis, acute perforation of the tympanic membrane in otitis media, and external otitis may have similar clinical findings.

PATIENT EVALUATION, MANAGEMENT, AND DISPOSITION

When button cell ingestion is suspected, a chest x-ray must be obtained urgently (even in the asymptomatic patient) to exclude an esophageal battery position. When a foreign body in the ear or nose is suspected based on history, pain, or discharge, complete visualization of the implicated cavity is essential.

Batteries lodged in the esophagus must be removed expeditiously by endoscopy. Alternate removal techniques, such as attaching a magnet to the end of a nasogastric tube or passing a balloon-tipped catheter beyond the battery, then inflating the balloon and retracting the catheter, have been proposed. Neither of these blind techniques are recommended. Direct esophageal visualization allows a determination of the degree of injury, clearly influencing subsequent management. In addition, direct visualization may prevent esophageal perforation following blind esophageal intubation.

If on initial evaluation the battery is found beyond the esophagus and the patient is asymptomatic, hospitalization is unnecessary. Instead, follow-up at home with resumption of a regular diet and normal activity is advised to promote gastrointestinal transit. Each stool is checked by the patient or parent for the battery to document passage and the patient or parent advised to report any symptoms. Most batteries (85.4 per cent) pass within 72 hours, although passage has been documented to require as long as 73 days. Often, an x-ray obtained 1 week following ingestion indicates that passage occurred unnoticed. In uncomplicated cases, more frequent x-rays are not recommended. In the absence of significant symptoms, batteries that appear "hung up" in the bowel do not require removal despite their persistence in a single location. These batteries nearly always pass (eventually) without complications. The single exception is the infrequent ingestion of a relatively large battery (usually greater than 20 mm) in a small child. These cells are likely to lodge in the esophagus but may pass to the stomach without problem, then fail to negotiate the pylorus. In these unusual cases, should passage from the stomach fail to occur following a trial of metoclopramide, endoscopic removal is advised. Cimetidine has also been advocated in patients with prolonged gastric retention of the battery, as corrosion occurs more slowly in an alkaline medium. In routine cases, cathartics, cimetidine, and metoclopramide are withheld, as no significant therapeutic effect has been demonstrated in the dog model.[8] The single most common error in the treatment of button battery ingestion cases is excessively aggressive therapeutic intervention. Surgical or endoscopic battery retrieval in asymptomatic patients when the battery has passed beyond the esophagus is rarely appropriate.

Batteries lodged in nasal or aural cavities also mandate urgent retrieval. Prior to battery removal, nasal and otic drops must be avoided to slow corrosion.[9] Removal may require patient sedation and direct visualization through an operating microscope. A magnetized instrument may prove a real asset during this process. Alternately, a 1-mm 90° pick can be positioned beyond a button cell in the ear canal, rotated, then retracted.

Battery imprint codes allow identification of the electrochemical system (mercuric oxide, silver oxide, lithium, manganese dioxide) and battery size. Following ingestion, the imprint code may be obtained from an identical replacement cell or the product instructions. Interpretation of the imprint code and assistance with patient management can be obtained from the National Button Battery Ingestion Hotline (202-625-3333).

References

1. Litovitz TL, Schmitz BF, Matyunas N, Martin TG: 1987 Annual Report of the American Association of Poison Control Centers National Data Collection System. Am J Emerg Med *6*:479, 1988.
2. Litovitz TL: Battery ingestions: Product accessibility and clinical course. Pediatrics *75*:469–476, 1985.
3. Kulig K, Rumack CM, Rumack BH, et al: Disk battery ingestion: Elevated urine mercury levels and enema removal of battery fragments. JAMA *249*:2502–2504, 1983.
4. Mofenson HC, Greensher J, Caraccio T, et al: Ingestion of small flat disc batteries. Ann Emerg Med *12*:88–90, 1983.
5. Blatnik BS, Toohill RJ, Lehman RH: Fatal complications from an alkaline battery foreign body in the esophagus. Ann Otol *86*:611–615, 1977.
6. Shabino CL, Feinberg AN: Esophageal perforation

secondary to alkaline battery ingestion. J Am Coll Emerg Phys *8*:360–362, 1979.
7. Kavanagh KT, Litovitz T: Miniature battery foreign bodies in auditory and nasal cavities. JAMA *255*:1470–1472, 1986.
8. Skinner DW, Chui P: The hazards of "button-sized" batteries as foreign bodies in the nose and ear. J Laryngol Otol *100*:1315–1318, 1986.
9. Litovitz T, Butterfield AB, Holloway RR, et al: Button battery ingestion: Assessment of therapeutic modalities and battery discharge state. J Pediatr *105*:868–873, 1984.

CHAPTER 66
ACIDS AND ANTACIDS

James F. Winchester, M.D.

ACID INGESTION

The principal acids to be discussed in this chapter are listed in Table 66–1. Most mineral acids are corrosive in nature and are found in many homes in the form of automobile battery acid (28 per cent sulfuric acid); toilet bowl cleaners (sodium bisulfate—which on hydration forms sulfuric acid, hydrochloric acid, or isocyanic acid) and other cleaning agents containing hydrochloric or phosphoric or oxalic acids; soldering fluxes [often compounds of zinc chloride and hydrochloric acid or ammonium chloride and hydrochloric acid (sal ammoniac)]; and antirust compounds, hydrochloric or oxalic acids.[1] Many of these acids are found in industry but also may be used in certain hobbies (aqua regia, a combination of hydrochloric and nitric acid that will dissolve precious metals such as gold and silver). Organic acids are usually low molecular weight compounds and present hazards similar to those of the corrosive mineral acids. These are also listed in Table 66–1.

Many other acidic substances exist either in the form of free halogens, such as iodine or bromine; bleach products (sodium hypochlorite), which may release chlorine gas in the stomach; and other substances, such as boric acid, carbolic acid (phenol), hydrocyanic acid (cyanide), hydrofluoric acid, oxalic acid, and salicylate. For discussion of these latter compounds, see the appropriate sections of this book.

Table 66–1. ACIDS

CORROSIVE (INORGANIC)	ORGANIC
Hydrochloric acid	Formic acid
Sulfuric acid	Acetic acid
Nitric acid	Lactic acid
Phosphoric acid	Trichloroacetic acid
Hydrofluoric acid	

Ingestion of many other substances is associated with systemic acidosis (see Chapter 7). Important substances that produce systemic acidosis are shown in Table 66–2, and these will not be discussed further.

Toxicology

Most of the toxicity from acids is in the form of corrosive burns to the skin after accidents in the home, school, college, or industrial plant. These are rarely reported, except in the case of particularly severe burns and when there are particular treatment recommendations.[2] Most acid poisoning results from inhalation of acid fumes, from fuming acid vapors (for example, hydrochloric acid, sulfur dioxide, chlorine, and so on), or from the ingestion of strong acids. After respiratory exposure, chemical pneumonitis supervenes, and this may also be seen after tracheal aspiration of ingested acids.[1] Chemical pneumonitis resulting from inhalation of fuming acid vapors is managed along the lines of nitrogen oxide poisoning, which is discussed in Chapter 87.

Ingestion of acid solutions differs from that of alkali solutions. The majority of chemical

Table 66–2. SUBSTANCES PRODUCING SYSTEMIC ACIDOSIS

METABOLIC ACIDOSIS	LACTIC ACIDOSIS
salicylate	salicylate
ammonium chloride	nalidixic acid
arginine/lysine	biguanides
ethylene glycol	tetracycline (in conjunction with biguanides)
ethanol	drug-associated coma (e.g., heroin)
methanol	goat milk acidosis
acetazolamide	D-lactic acidosis
ketogenic diet	formaldehyde
nitroprusside resistance	isoniazid
percutaneous salicylic acid	iron intoxication
Vacor	carbon monoxide
vasopressors	ethanol
glue sniffing	
insulin	
toluene	
amiloride	
lithium	
salbutamol-induced diabetic ketoacidosis	
ascorbic acid	
tienilic acid	
ketamine	
fructose	
hydrogen sulfide/sulfur	
formaldehyde	

burns after ingestion are caused by alkalis and only rarely by acid. At the time of writing, less than 100 cases of acid ingestion had been reported,[3, 4] in contrast to many reports of alkali ingestion. Putting aside the numeric differences between acid and alkali ingestion, there are several important differences between the effects of acids and alkalis on the gastrointestinal tract. Strong acids produce immediate pain in the buccal cavity after ingestion and, probably because of this, are less often swallowed than are the corrosive alkalis. Alkalis tend to have their primary effect on the esophagus, with gastric involvement in only 20 per cent of the reports, by producing a rapidly penetrating liquefactive necrosis, unless the compound is sufficiently neutralized or diluted.[5, 6] Strong acids may be less often swallowed, but, when they are, they produce less local injury in the esophagus. Their major effects are in the stomach, where they produce a coagulative necrosis.[4, 7–9] Esophageal involvement after acute acid ingestion is estimated at around 6 to 20 per cent,[10] but it is perhaps more common than initially thought if careful radiologic examination is made.[11] Esophageal perforation from acid ingestion has not been reported in any patient, and most esophageal injuries respond well to conservative measures, in contrast to alkali ingestion. When associated with gastric injuries, the esophageal injuries are generally severe.[3, 6, 11]

The extent of damage is related most importantly to the molar concentration of the acids and to the duration of superficial contact with the epithelial surface. It has been stated that sulfuric acid is more hazardous than the other mineral acids,[12] but on balance it appears that they all produce lesions of similar severity, in relation to the molar (M) concentration of the acid. The lethal dose of acids is approximately 30 ml when taken as sulfuric acid 95 per cent (18 M), nitric acid 69 per cent (15 M), and hydrochloric acid 36 per cent (12 M).[13] On the other hand, less than 5 ml of mineral acid has produced a fatality,[14] and in animal experiments intralaryngeal instillation of 2 to 3 ml/kg of 0.1 normal hydrochloric acid in dogs produced death as a result of pulmonary consolidation.[15] Low molecular weight acids like acetic acid are also strong irritants, although they are probably less corrosive than mineral acids. Of several reported cases of acetic acid, trichloroacetic acid, and lactic acid poisoning, all caused esophageal strictures and gastric lesions similar to those produced by the mineral acids.[1] Their management is similar to that of the mineral acids.

Pathophysiology of Acid Ingestion

Although the acids are probably less often swallowed than are corrosive alkalis, this may not be the case in certain strong-willed, distraught, retarded, or inebriated individuals. The acids exert only a superficial effect on the esophageal squamous epithelium as they pass rapidly down the esophagus, but acids in the stomach follow a well-defined pattern of being transported along the major rugal folds (magenstrasse)[7] in the lesser curvature of the stomach to produce a rapid coagulative necrosis. The acids are then pooled by spasm of the pylorus and antrum of the stomach at the site where the acid produces the greatest damage.[9] Diffuse acid damage also may be seen after ingestion on a full stomach. Pyloric stenosis is the most frequent characteristic complication of acid ingestion in patients who survive this acute episode, manifesting itself usually after several weeks but sometimes after several years, with an incidence approaching 80 per cent.

Occasionally, small bowel lesions, due to passage of unneutralized acid through the pylorus, and gastric perforation may be observed. Late complications less commonly seen are antral stenosis, hourglass deformity of the stomach, corrosive-induced obstruction, achlorhydria, and several other less well-defined abnormalities.[1, 15]

Manifestations of Acid Intoxication

The major causes of death in acid ingestion, which appears to have a more fulminating course than that of alkali ingestion, are circulatory shock, asphyxia due to glottic or laryngeal edema, perforation of the stomach or esophagus, intercurrent infections, or, later, the results of stricture formation or bowel resection.

The principal early manifestations are pain in the buccal, pharyngeal, and esophageal areas, associated with dysphagia. The necrotic areas are gray in color but rapidly change to black, except in the case of nitric acid, in which the color is yellow. Nausea and vomiting, along with epigastric pain, with or without hematemesis, may occur. One of the features is an intense thirst, which may be the result of circulatory collapse with its usual manifestations of clammy skin, weak and rapid pulse, shallow respirations, scanty urine, and so on. Uncorrected, this may lead to renal failure and ischemic lesions in the liver and the heart. Glottic edema will be manifested by upper respiratory stridor and should be anticipated in any patient reporting with acid ingestion. Ulceration of necrotic tissues may lead to perforation and to its associated complications, such as peritonitis.

Late complications of acid poisoning may produce esophageal, gastric, and pyloric strictures and stenosis, and these may require surgical repair. Permanent scarring also may appear in any tissue subject to acid corrosive burns, such as cornea, skin, and mouth. Gastric carcinoma may also be a delayed complication of acid ingestion.[16] Hydrochloric acid infusions or ingestion of the noncorrosive ammonium chloride can produce systemic acidosis. Laboratory manifestations are infrequent, but leukocytosis is commonly observed, and, if renal involvement from circulatory collapse occurs, then there will be evidence of acute renal failure. Phosphoric acid ingestion has produced hyperphosphatemia, hypocalcemia, and metabolic acidosis, with mild local caustic activity.[17] Disseminated intravascular coagulation has been observed in one patient after ingestion of glacial acetic acid.[18]

Treatment

As with alkali ingestion, treatment is controversial.[4] Topical acid burns should be immediately irrigated with copious amounts of water. In the case of hydrofluoric acid burns, however, the fluoride ion immobilizes calcium at the cell membrane and increases the permeability to potassium, leading to spontaneous depolarization of nervous tissue and the production of pain. In this case, iced magnesium sulfate applied topically, if the concentration of hydrofluoric acid is greater than 20 per cent, should be a temporizing measure and later should be followed by subcutaneous injection of 10 per cent calcium gluconate in a volume of 0.5 ml/cm^2. Also, with hydrofluoric acid burns from greater than a 20 per cent concentrate, one should anticipate pulmonary edema.[2] Acid burns should be followed by surgical debridement and standard management.

The treatment of acid ingestion remains controversial in that many investigators have used or recommended neutralizing agents, such as the standard antacids of magnesium oxide, Milk of Magnesia, calcium hydroxide, and aluminum hydroxide gel.[4] Although all agree that it is better to avoid antacids that will release carbon dioxide after acid contact, thereby reducing the possibility of gastric distention and rupture, there is no uniform or standardized method for treatment of this very serious condition, as Penner has pointed out.[4] Dilution is desirable, but many have outlined, and Penner has highlighted, that dilution of strong acids with water produces considerable heat, with the possibility that the exothermic reaction will compound the chemical injury of the stomach and other gastrointestinal areas. Emesis is understandably contraindicated, as is the administration of soap,[19, 20] which in most instances results only in emesis rather than the desired neutralization.

While many of the treatment regimens remain unsubstantiated, many lean to conservative measures.[21] The following recommendations can be made until more evidence is available:[4] (1) Nasogastric intubation with suction of gastric contents should be instituted as rapidly as possible after the diagnosis of acid ingestion is made. It appears from the literature that concerns expressed about perforation of the stomach with nasogastric and orogastric intubation have not been substantiated. If ingestion is recent, some studies show that contact damage may occur up to 90 minutes after ingestion. Gastric suction should prevent additional contact necrosis, as well as providing gastric decompression. The nasogastric tube should be of adequate caliber, and repositioning of the nasogastric tube under fluoroscopy may be required in order to remove all the acid ingested. (2) After the acid is extracted, large-volume cold water lavage or cold milk lavage should be followed by antacid lavage (aluminum hydroxide). Recent evidence on the neutralizability of acids with antacids shows that antacids like aluminum hydroxide and aluminum phosphate may require considerable volumes to achieve maximal acid-neutralizing capacity.[22] (3) Appropriate management of respiration and shock should be provided as required. (4) Theoretically, it appears that the risks of laparotomy with gastric resection with or without small bowel resection may not be greater than the risks of perforation of a viscus from acid ingestion, but emergency laparotomy probably should be performed only in selected cases, although some have advocated gastric resection early after ingestion.[23] (5) No evidence supports the use of prophylactic antibiotics or steroids to prevent esophageal or gastric fibrosis.

Since 1960, 25 cases of acid ingestion have been reported, in whom there was a 28 per cent mortality rate, a 16 per cent esophageal stricture rate, and a 60 per cent rate of pyloric stenosis. There was also a 32 per cent emergency laparotomy rate for peritonitis after perforation of a viscus.[4] Systemic fluoride toxicity with a fatal outcome has been reported after a hydrofluoric acid burn to the skin.[24]

ANTACID INGESTION

Probably much more common than acid ingestion is the ingestion of excessive quantities of antacids that usually do not give rise to clinical problems, except in such syndromes as the milk-alkali syndrome in patients with peptic ulcer disease and prolonged exposure to antacids.

The antacids range from the simple alkalis, such as sodium bicarbonate, to the more complex inorganic hydroxides of magnesium, aluminum, phosphate, and calcium. The antacids carry varying capacities for neutralizing the major test substrate hydrochloric acid and, as such, vary in their capacity to induce a metabolic alkalosis. Sodium bicarbonate is most commonly associated with a metabolic alkalosis by neutralizing hydrochloric acid in the stomach.

In a single patient with end-stage renal disease, requiring dialysis, ingestion of aluminum hydroxide, magnesium hydroxide, neutral phosphate, and sodium polystyrene sulfonate resin (a non-absorbable antacid) produced a profound metabolic alkalosis, with seizures.[25] The investigators suggest that to avoid such a situation the resin not be ingested together with the other antacids.

The constituents of the antacid itself may give rise to clinical syndromes: renal stones (magnesium-ammonium-phosphate) with acute renal failure,[26] or pure silicon bladder stones,[27] after long-term ingestion of magnesium trisilicate antacids.

Certain preparations may contain substances that give rise to unexpected intoxications: bromide intoxication from bromide-containing antacids,[28] and methemoglobinemia from an antacid-containing subnitrate.[29]

Occasionally, deficiency (other than calcium) states may result from ingestion of antacids, as has been reported for copper (which was adsorbed onto a mixture of antacids and also rendered insoluble for absorption by the high gastric pH).[30]

Excessive antacid ingestion rarely gives rise to clinical problems, but the common manifestations are listed in Table 66–3. In a study by Peterson and associates, the stool frequency was highest in the large-dose antacid group (66 per cent) in patients undergoing high-dose antacid therapy for peptic ulcer disease.[31]

The management of antacid overdose, for the most part, consists of withdrawing the

Table 66–3. COMMON SYMPTOMS OF EXCESSIVE ANTACID INGESTION

Metabolic alkalosis
Diarrhea (magnesium salts)
Constipation (aluminum salts)
Hypercalcemia (calcium carbonate)
Hypophosphatemia (aluminum hydroxide)

antacid, then either allowing the metabolic alkalosis to recover spontaneously or, if severe, instituting appropriate therapy with either hydrochloric acid intravenously or, in less severe cases, ammonium chloride by mouth. Only in the most severe cases is it necessary to resort to hemodialysis for correction of the alkalosis. For further management of alkalosis, see Chapter 7.

References

1. Gosselin RE, Smith RP, Hodge HC (eds): Acids. *In* Clinical Toxicology of Commercial Products. 5th ed. Baltimore, Williams & Wilkins, 1984, p III-8.
2. Tintinalli JE: Hydrofluoric acid burns. J Am Coll Emerg Phys *7*:24, 1978.
3. Hawkins DB, Demeter MJ, Barnett TE: Caustic ingestion—controversies in management—review of 214 cases. Laryngoscope *90*:98, 1980.
4. Penner GE: Acid ingestion: Toxicology and treatment. Ann Emerg Med *9*:374, 1980.
5. Ritter RN, Newman MH, Newman DE: Clinical and experimental study of corrosive burns of the stomach. Ann Otol Rhinol Laryngol *77*:830, 1968.
6. Ashcraft KW, Padula RT: The effect of dilute corrosives on the stomach. Pediatrics *53*:226, 1974.
7. Waldeyer W: Die Magenstrasse. Sitzungsber Preuss Akad Wissensch Ges *29*:595, 1908.
8. Testa GF: Contribito radiologio o sperimentale allo studio della lesiont esofage e gastrich nelle caustticazioni da alcali. Radiol Med (Torino) *25*:25, 1938.
9. Chong GC, Beahrs OH, Payne WS: Management of corrosive gastritis due to ingested acid. Mayo Clin Proc *49*:861, 1974.
10. Boikan WS, Singer HA: Gastric sequelae of corrosive poisoning. Arch Intern Med *46*:342, 1930.
11. Muhletaler CA, Gerlock AJ, Soto LD, Halter SA: Acid corrosive esophagitis—radiographic findings. Am J Roentgenol Radiother Nucl Med *134*:1137, 1980.
12. Gray HK, Holmes CL: Pyloric stenosis caused by ingestion of corrosive substances: Report of a case. Surg Clin North Am *28*:1041, 1948.
13. Polson CJ, Tattersall RN: Clinical Toxicology. Philadelphia, JB Lippincott, 1959.
14. Gonzales TA, Vance M, Helpern M, Umberger CJ: Legal Medicine: Pathology and Toxicology. 2nd ed. New York, Appleton-Century-Crofts, 1954.
15. Greenfield LJ, Singleton RF, McCaffree DR, Coalson JJ: Pulmonary effects of experimental graded aspiration of hydrochloric acid. Ann Surg *170*:74, 1969.
16. O'Donnell CH, Abbott WE, Hirshfeld JW: Surgical treatment of corrosive gastritis. Am J Surg *78*:251, 1949.
17. Caravati EM: Metabolic abnormalities associated with phosphoric acid ingestion. Ann Emerg Med *16*:904, 1987.
18. Greif F, Kaplan O: Acid ingestion: Another cause of disseminated intravascular coagulopathy. Crit Care Med *14*:990, 1986.
19. Rumack BH: Soap solution contraindicated in acid ingestion (letter). J Am Coll Emerg Phys *8*:124, 1979.
20. Siotis LJ, Peterson CD, Kreuzelok EP: Acid ingestion neutralizing agents (letter). J Am Coll Emerg Phys *8*:124, 1979.
21. Di Costanzo J, Nouclerc M, Jouglard J, Escoffier JM, Cano N, Martin J, Gauthier A: New therapeutic approach to corrosive burns of the upper gastrointestinal tract. Gut *21*:370, 1980.
22. Martin WJ, Lloyd CW: Antacids (letter). Ann Intern Med *95*:118, 1981.
23. Scher LA, Maull KI: Emergency management and sequelae of acid ingestion. J Am Coll Emerg Phys *7*:206, 1978.
24. Tepperman PB: Fatality due to systemic fluoride poisoning following a hydrofluoric skin burn. J Occup Med *20*:691, 1980.
25. Madias NE, Levey AS: Metabolic alkalosis due to absorption of "nonabsorbable" antacids. Am J Med *74*:155, 1983.
26. Millette CH, Snodgrass GL: Acute renal failure associated with chronic antacid ingestion. Am J Hosp Pharm *38*:1352, 1981.
27. Anon: Silicon overdosage in man. Nutr Rev *40*:208, 1982.
28. Deleu D, De Keyser J, Ebinger G: Bromide intoxication due to chronic intake of a bromide-containing antacid. Acta Gastroenterol Belg *48*:509, 1985.
29. Jacobsen JB, Huttel MS: Methemoglobinemia after excessive intake of subnitrate-containing antacid. Ugeskr Laeger *144*:2349, 1982.
30. van Kalmthout PM, Engels LG, Bakker HA, Burghouts JT: Severe copper deficiency due to excessive use of an antacid combined with pyloric stenosis. Dig Dis Sci *27*:859, 1982.
31. Peterson WL, Sturdevant RAL, Franke HD: Healing of duodenal ulcer with an antacid regimen. N Engl J Med *297*:341, 1977.

CHAPTER 67
BLEACH, SOAPS, AND DETERGENTS

Anthony R. Temple, M.D.

BACKGROUND AND EPIDEMIOLOGY

Until about 1950, cleaning products for home laundry, household maintenance, and personal hygiene were usually some form of soap. However, soap has the disadvantage of combining with the minerals in hard water to form an insoluble precipitate or "soap curd," which clings to whatever surface it contacts—skin, bathtub, clothes, dishes, and so on. To achieve a product that cleans like soap but does not form troublesome precipitates, most products now use synthetic detergents.[1]

Although the term soap is loosely applied to a variety of cleaning materials, a true soap is specifically a salt of a fatty acid, usually made by the reaction of alkali with natural fats and oils or with the fatty acids obtained from animal or vegetable sources. Soap, then, is one type of surface active agent, or surfactant.

Strictly speaking, a "detergent" is any cleansing agent. In common usage, however, the phrase "synthetic detergent" and its abbreviation "detergent" have come to mean the household cleaning products that are based on nonsoap surfactants, primarily used for laundering and dishwashing. Other household cleaning products include disinfectant cleaners, bleaches, drain cleaners, oven cleaners, ammonia, and toilet bowl cleaners.

The safety of soaps, detergents, and household cleaning products is of considerable concern to toxicologists and others. From a poison control/toxicologic perspective, these agents receive attention because they are frequently involved in human exposures, they are high-use consumer products, and they are in the home in areas accessible to children. In addition, animal studies and clinical experience have shown certain products within this broad category to be irritating to human tissues.

Statistics from the American Association of Poison Control Centers (AAPCC) indicate that annually about 6 per cent of reported accidental ingestion cases involve "soaps, detergents, cleaners," 2 to 3 per cent "household bleaches," and 1 to 2 per cent "corrosive acids and alkalis" (ammonia, drain cleaners, and so on). In 60 to 70 per cent of the reports of accidental exposures involving cleaning products, children less than 5 years old are the victims. Only 48 per cent of the AAPCC victims involving poisoning by soaps, detergents, and cleaners are reported to become symptomatic, and less than 1 per cent have major symptoms. With household bleaches, 59 per cent of the reported victims are symptomatic, and less than 1 per cent have major symptoms.[2] In a survey reviewing the epidemiologic characteristics of household cleaning product exposures reported to the Utah regional poison control center, 92.5 per cent involved children aged 5 years or younger, 2.7 per cent involved children aged 6 to 17, and 4.8 per cent involved adults (aged 18 years and above); 53.6 per cent of the victims were male and 46.4 per cent, female. The majority of the cases (95.3 per cent) occurred inside the home, principally in the kitchen and bathroom, whereas 3.3 per cent occurred outdoors, 0.4 per cent in the workplace, and 1.0 per cent in various other locations.[3]

One particularly interesting finding from the Utah study was *the high frequency of exposures that occurred while the product was in use*—72.1 per cent versus only 23.8 per cent of products that were in storage. In 2.6 per cent of the cases, the product had been discarded. *Only 54 per cent of the exposures involved a product in its original container; of the remainder, in over half the contents were diluted or dissolved.* It was common for children to swallow a product their parents had just placed on the sink or washbasin while using it or for children to get into products after they had been placed in the dispensing cup of the dishwasher or other appliance.[3]

TOXICOLOGY OF INDIVIDUAL PRODUCT CATEGORIES

Product Composition

Household detergents are mixtures of organic and inorganic ingredients. Composition varies within as well as between product types.[1] The principal organic ingredient is a surfactant, a substance that lowers the surface tension of water to enable it to "wet" surfaces more effectively, remove dirt, disperse soil, and emulsify oil or grease. Surfactants are chemically classified as anionic, cationic, nonionic, and amphoteric. The electrical charge of the chemical moiety determines the ionic classification of a given surfactant. Amphoteric surfactants contain both anionic and cationic moieties. Nonionic surfactants have no positive or negative moieties, and the molecule is electrically neutral. Household detergents generally contain anionic or nonionic surfactants or mixtures of these types. Cationic and amphoteric surfactants are used in consumer products, but to a lesser extent.

Table 67–1 lists examples of each class of surfactant. Table 67–2 lists examples of common household cleaning products and their active chemical ingredient(s).

The *anionic surfactants* most widely used in detergents are straight-chain alkylbenzene sulfonates, also referred to as linear alkylate sulfonates (LAS), and alcohol ether sulfates, also referred to as alcohol ethoxy sulfates or sulfated alcohol ethoxylates. Commonly used *nonionic surfactants* are alcohol ethoxylates, also referred to as ethyoxylated alcohols or alkoxylated alcohols. Nonionic surfactants are found in heavy-duty laundry liquids and nonphosphate granular products. *Cationic surfactants* include quaternary ammonium compounds, such as benzalkonium chloride, benzethonium chloride, and cetylpyridinium chloride and substituted alkyl quaternary compounds. They are frequently used as disinfectants and are found in fabric softeners.

Most detergents also contain *"builders,"* usually inorganic salts, which inactivate calcium and other minerals that interfere with detergency and which also are used to maintain the proper pH of the washing solution. Phosphates, carbonates, silicates, and aluminosilicates are commonly used as builders. Phosphates have been the principal builders used, but phosphate use in detergents has been curtailed since it was suggested that limiting phosphate entry into drainage water—from detergents, along with phosphorus from fertilizer, human and animal wastes, vegetation, and other sources—might help reduce eutrophication in lakes. As a result, low and nonphosphate granular laundry detergents have been developed that contain higher levels of surfactants and carbonates, silicates, aluminosilicates, or sulfates to offset the reduction in phosphate content. Detergent formulations also may contain various other functional ingredients at low levels, such as soil-redeposition inhibitors, fluorescent whitening agents, fabric softeners, suds-controlling agents, enzymes, bleaches, perfumes, and colorants.

Household bleaches contain varying concentrations of sodium peroxide, sodium perborate, or sodium hypochlorite. The most commonly used household bleaches contain approximately 3 to 6 per cent solutions of sodium hypochlorite in water. Granular bleaches may have higher concentrations. Commercial bleaches contain peroxides or perborates. As with bleaches, most *household ammonias* contain weak solutions of ammonia. Industrial ammonias may be much more concentrated.

Table 67–1. COMMONLY AVAILABLE CHEMICALS USED IN HOUSEHOLD CLEANING PRODUCTS

Synthetic Detergents
- Anionic
  - alkyl sodium sulfates
  - alkyl sodium sulfonates
  - dioctyl sodium sulfosuccinate
  - linear alkyl benzene sulfonate (sodium)
  - sodium lauryl sulfate
  - tetrapropylene benzene sulfonate (sodium)
- Nonionic
  - alkyl ethoxylate
  - alkyl phenoxy polyethoxy ethanols
  - polyethylene glycol stearate
- Cationic
  - alkyl dimethyl 3,4-dichlorobenzene ammonium chloride
  - benzalkonium chloride
  - benzethonium chloride
  - cetylpyridinium chloride
- Amphoteric

Builders
- sodium carbonate
- sodium metasilicate
- sodium sulfate
- sodium tripolyphosphate

Bleaches
- sodium hypochlorite
- sodium perborate
- sodium percarbonate

Ammonia
- anhydrous ammonia

(Courtesy of the Soap and Detergent Association, New York, NY.)

Table 67–2. SELECTED HOUSEHOLD CLEANING PRODUCTS

BRAND NAME	CHEMICALS	TYPE
Ajax Cleanser	sodium alkyl benzene sulfonate	Anionic detergent
ALL Condensed Phosphate Laundry Detergent	nonionic detergent, sodium polyphosphate, sodium sulfate	Nonionic detergent
Big Wally Foam Cleaner	ammonia, ethyl alcohol	Ammonia
Bold Granular Laundry Detergent	sodium alkyl benzene sulfonate, sodium tripolyphosphate, sodium sulfate	Anionic detergent
Calgonite Electric Dishwasher Detergent	complex sodium phosphates, chlorinated trisodium phosphate, sodium silicate	Strong irritant; potentially caustic
Cascade Electric Dishwasher Detergent	chlorinated trisodium phosphate, sodium silicate	Strong irritant; potentially caustic
Cheer Granular Laundry Detergent	sodium alkyl benzene sulfonate	Anionic detergent
Clorox	sodium hypochlorite	Bleach
Comet Cleanser with Chlorinol	dodecyl benzene sulfonate, sodium hypochlorite	Anionic detergent; bleach
Dash Laundry Detergent	sodium alkyl benzene sulfonate, sodium alkyl ethoxylate sulfate	Anionic/nonionic detergent
Downy Fabric Softener	alkyl dimethyl ammonium chloride	Cationic detergent
Dran-O Drain Cleaner	sodium hydroxide	Caustic
Dynamo Laundry Detergent	sodium alkyl benzene sulfonate	Anionic detergent
Easy-Off Oven Cleaner	sodium hydroxide	Caustic
Electrasol Electric Dishwasher Detergent	sodium carbonate, sodium silicate sodium tripolyphosphate	Strong irritant; potentially caustic
ERA Laundry Detergent	sodium alkyl ethoxylate sulfate	Nonionic detergent
Fab Granular Laundry Detergent	sodium alkyl benzene sulfonate	Anionic detergent
Future Acrylic Floor Finish	acrylic polymers	Nontoxic floor wax
Gain Enzyme Laundry Detergent	sodium alkyl ethoxylate sulfate, sodium sulfate, sodium tripolyphosphate	Nonionic detergent
Glass Plus	isopropyl alcohol, glycol ether	Isopropyl alcohol
Glory Concentrated Rug Shampoo	sodium lauryl sulfate	Anionic detergent
Ivory Snow, Liquid	ammonium alkyl ethoxylate sulfate	Nonionic detergent
Joy Dish Detergent	sodium alkyl ethoxylate sulfate	Nonionic detergent
Lysol Toilet Bowl Cleaner	hydrochloric acid	Acid
Mr. Clean Liquid Household Cleaner	sodium alkyl ethoxylate sulfate	Nonionic detergent
Mr. Muscle Oven Cleaner	sodium hydroxide	Caustic
Mop & Glo Wax	acrylic copolymer, alkyl phenyl ethoxylate	Nonionic detergent, floor wax
Oxydol	sodium alkyl benzene sulfonate, sodium perborate	Anionic detergent
Palmolive Crystal Clear*	sodium tripolyphosphate, sodium carbonate, sodium sulfate	Strong irritant, potentially caustic
Pine Sol Disinfectant	pine oil, isopropyl alcohol	Hydrocarbon
Purex Fabric Softener	quaternary ammonium compounds	Cationic detergent
Red Devil Lye Drain Cleaner	sodium hydroxide	Caustic
Sani-Flush Toilet Bowl Cleaner	sodium bisulfate	Acid
Spic & Span Household Cleaner	sodium sesquicarbonate	Strong irritant; potentially caustic
Sta-Puf Fabric Softener	quaternary ammonium compounds	Cationic detergent
Sunlight*	sodium carbonate, sodium polyphosphates, sodium sulfate, sodium silicate	Strong irritant, potentially caustic
Tide Laundry Detergent	sodium alkyl benzene sulfonate	Anionic detergent
Top Job	tetrapotassium pyrophosphate sodium carbonate	Strong irritant; potentially caustic
Vanish Toilet Bowl Cleaner	sodium acid sulfate	Acid
Windex Window Cleaner	isopropyl alcohol	Isopropyl alcohol
Wisk Nonphosphate Laundry Detergent	anionic detergent	Anionic detergent
Woolite Rug Cleaner	sodium lauryl sulfate	Anionic detergent

*LADD (liquid automatic dishwashing detergent).

Product Toxicology

Because cleaning agents present in the home are generally mixtures of ingredients, the biologic effects of formulated cleaning agents are not always predictable from the chemical and physical properties of the individual ingredients.[4] Fortunately, the acute systemic oral toxicity of most ingredients and the cleaning products themselves is not high. However, the topical effects may range from mild irritation to corrosive-like effects. Irritation or burns of the mucosa of the oral cavity, esophagus, and stomach may result from accidental ingestion of some household cleaning products. The mucous membranes of the eye also are susceptible to injury by cleaning products. Most household soaps and detergents do not cause substantial harm and are not similar to lye or other corrosive substances.[1, 4] However, they are irritants and will cause erythema, superficial erosion, and resultant inflammation if left in contact with mucosal surfaces for an extended period of time.[5] Long-term sequelae are a function of the extent and depth of damage, which in most cases is not severe, with damaged mucosal tissue regenerating and normal function being restored within a few days. On the other hand, it is important to note that selected laundry products, automatic dishwasher detergents, household cleaners for walls and hard surfaces, and some specialty products (for example, drain cleaners and oven cleaners) are sufficiently strong to injure the oral, esophageal, and gastric mucosa. As a rule, these products can be identified by their pH (very alkaline) or warnings on the label. Cleaning products that have been shown to cause substantial injury to mucous membranes following toxicology testing are required to carry appropriate warning labels and may require child-resistant packaging.[1]

Many of the products containing noncorrosive substances also induce vomiting. It is interesting to note that the emetic effects of some of these substances are similar to those of syrup of ipecac and are reasonably prompt in action. It would be unusual if appreciable quantities of most common soaps and detergents were accidentally ingested without induction of vomiting. As a result, one should be aware that spontaneous vomiting may occur.

In the Utah study, the medical outcome of the cases indicated a low percentage of exposures in which symptoms occurred and only a few patients who needed medical care other than a call to the poison center.[3] The types of symptoms reported all were related to the irritant effects of the products on the gastrointestinal system. The most common symptom was nausea or vomiting or both, followed by diarrhea, mucosal (oral) irritation, and only occasional abdominal pain. There was no vomiting of blood, passing of blood in bowel movements, pain or difficulty with swallowing, or indication of esophageal injury.

Soaps. The toxicity of soaps is generally quite low. Exposure to soaps, as to other mild irritants, may produce cutaneous, ocular, oral, or gastrointestinal irritation without erosion. Ingestion of large amounts of soap may induce emesis or produce mild diarrhea.

Surfactants. Surfactants are generally of low toxicity, except those formulations characterized by a relatively high degree of alkalinity. Anionic or nonionic surfactants when used alone have low toxicity, causing local irritation to skin, eye, or oral or gastrointestinal mucosa. Ingestions may result in emesis or mild diarrhea. Cationic detergents are more toxic than anionic or nonionic detergents. Concentrated solutions have caustic qualities, whereas more dilute solutions have marked irritant effects. In addition to these local or topical effects, systemic absorption may produce more generalized toxic symptoms, especially central nervous system symptoms, including restlessness, confusion, convulsions, respiratory paralysis, muscle weakness, and cyanosis.

Bleaches. Household bleaches are mild to moderate irritants and are generally not associated with any degree of tissue destruction. They result in skin or eye irritation, mild oral or esophageal burns, or gastrointestinal irritation. They may produce emesis in higher concentrations. In one study of 393 patients, no esophageal strictures or perforations developed after the ingestion of chlorine bleach.[6] Similar results were found in another study of 129 cases.[7] It is our experience that burns and scarring do not occur with household hypochlorite bleaches.[3] Other bleaches contain sodium peroxide or sodium perborate. Sodium peroxide has low toxicity. It decomposes in the gastrointestinal tract, releasing oxygen, and may cause gastritis. Sodium perborate decomposes to peroxide and borate. This type is more alkaline and irritating and may have the toxic systemic effects of boric acid. Solid-form bleaches have potentially greater toxicity because they are concentrated.

Ammonia Compounds. Weak ammonia solutions are mild irritants, whereas very concentrated solutions may be caustic. Ingestion of household ammonia produces erythema and superficial erosion, with attendant symptoms. Its vapors are irritating to the eyes, respiratory tract, and mucous membranes. The inhaled fumes from more concentrated ammonia may produce marked irritation of the eyes, with profuse tearing, and irritation of the upper respiratory tract. Severe inhalation may produce a feeling of tightness on the chest and delayed-onset pulmonary edema or persistent cough or both for several days. Industrial-strength ammonia in very high concentrations behaves as a caustic.

Builders. The addition of builders to a detergent plays a significant role in the product's actual toxicity. The phosphates add somewhat to the general irritant and emetic quality of the detergent. However, the use of silicates and carbonates, as in "low-phosphate" detergents, or certain phosphates, such as trisodium phosphate, may raise the alkalinity of the product and significantly increase its irritant quality.[8, 9] Highly alkaline detergent products may produce severe ocular irritation, oral burns, esophageal burns, and bloody gastritis.

Electric dishwashing detergents typically have a much higher alkalinity because of the addition of alkaline builders, such as sodium carbonate, sodium silicates, and sodium tripolyphosphates. Electric dishwashing detergents are sold in granular form (Electrasol, Cascade) and liquid form (Sunlight, Palmolive Crystal Clear). The pH of the new liquid automatic dishwashing detergents (LADDs)[10] ranges from 11.8 to 12.7. Concern has been expressed that dishwashing detergents may have toxic effects similar to those of caustics, especially the liquid form. A recent study[10] indicates that ocular exposure to LADDs is associated with a high incidence of toxicity, and these patients require emergency department evaluation and treatment of these exposures.

Caustics. Strong alkalis and acids cause tissue destruction. Acids produce a coagulation necrosis that tends to cause a superficial type of damage, rather than a deep, penetrating type of burn. Alkalis tend to cause a deep and penetrating necrosis, which often results in severe effects such as esophageal perforation. These deeper burns are associated with more severe scarring and stricture formation. Some household cleaning products may contain alkalis or acids but generally in concentrations too small to produce causticity.

Mixing Chemicals. As a note of interest, mixing hypochlorites with other household cleaning agents can result in the release of gases that are irritating to the pulmonary tract and may result in pulmonary edema if the exposure is severe enough. Hypochlorite mixed with strong acids releases *chlorine* gas. Hypochlorite mixed with ammonia releases *chloramine* gas.

MANAGEMENT OF EXPOSURES

In all cases of *ingestions* involving soaps, detergents, or household cleaning agents, immediate dilution with water or milk should be instituted. When irritation is prominent or anticipated, demulcents may be used. Emesis rarely need be induced. Since delayed spontaneous emesis may occur, the person who has ingested a cleaning product should be kept in an upright or prone position and observed for at least 2 hours. For products that are highly alkaline, all mucosal surfaces should be examined. Esophagoscopy is not indicated unless the product is indeed caustic. Discomfort should be treated with mild analgesics. If diarrhea or excessive vomiting occurs, symptomatic treatment and measures to maintain fluid and electrolyte balance should be instituted. Figure 67–1 summarizes a basic approach to the emergency management of household cleaning product ingestions.

In all cases of *eye contact,* irrigation should be initiated immediately, and the eye should be gently flushed with water until the material is completely removed. This may be accomplished best by holding the head back and gently pouring copious amounts of slightly cool to lukewarm water from a container into the eye. The eye should be rinsed continuously for 15 to 30 minutes, especially if the package label indicates that the product is injurious or corrosive to eyes. For any product identified as corrosive to the eye, an ophthalmologist should be consulted as soon as possible for a thorough eye examination.

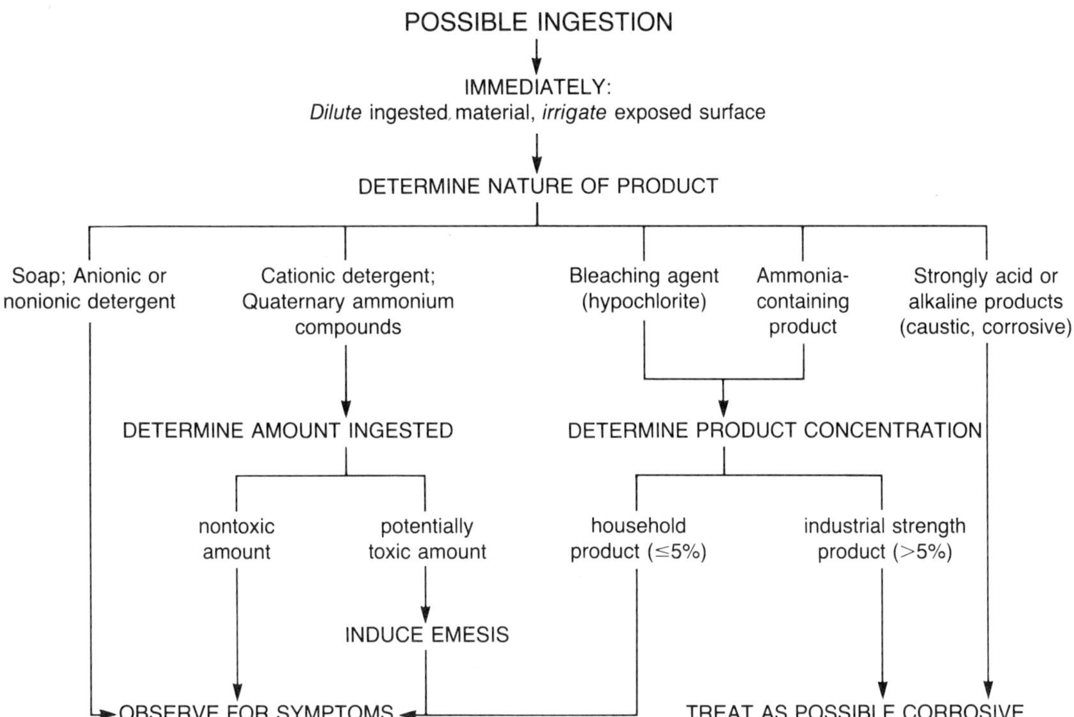

Figure 67–1. Emergency management outline for household cleaning product ingestion. (From Temple AR, Lovejoy FH Jr: Household Cleaning Products and Their Accidental Ingestion. SDA Scientific and Technical Report No. 5R. Soap and Detergent Association, New York, 1980. Reproduced with permission.)

For *skin contact,* simple rinsing with water should be used to prevent extended contact. Obviously, limiting contact is not generally a problem.

For *inhalation* of fumes, removal from contaminated air is the essential first aid measure. Observation for acute and latent pulmonary manifestations should be made in all symptomatic cases or cases of clearly severe exposures.

For products characterized by caustic qualities, additional measures appropriate to caustic management (see Chap. 65) should be undertaken.

References

1. Temple AR, Lovejoy FH Jr: Household cleaning products and their accidental ingestion. SDA Scientific and Technical Report No. 5R. Soap and Detergent Association, New York, 1980.
2. Litovitz TL, Schmitz BF, Holm KC: 1988 Annual Report of the American Association of Poison Control Centers National Data Collection System. Am J Emerg Med *7*:495, 1989.
3. Temple AR, Veltri JC: Outcome of accidental ingestions of soaps, detergents, and related household products. Vet Hum Toxicol *21*:9, 1979.
4. Seabaugh VM, Bayard SP, et al: Detergent toxicity survey. Am J Public Health *67*:367, 1977.
5. Berenson MM, Temple AR: Detergent toxicity: Effects on esophageal and gastric mucosa. Clin Toxicol *8*:399, 1975.
6. Landau GD, Saunders WH: Effect of chlorine bleach on the esophagus. Arch Otolaryngol *80*:174, 1964.
7. Pike DG, et al: Re-evaluation of the dangers of Clorox ingestion. J Pediatr *63*:303, 1963.
8. Scharpf LG, Hill ID, Kelly RE: Relative eye-injury potential of heavy-duty phosphate and non-phosphate laundry detergents. Food Cosmet Toxicol *10*:829, 1972.
9. Lee JF, Simonowitz D, Block GE: Corrosive injury of the stomach and esophagus by non-phosphate detergents. Am J Surg *123*:6529, 1972.
10. Krenzelok EP: Liquid automatic dishwashing detergents: A profile of toxicity. Ann Emerg Med *18*:60, 1989.

Pesticides

CHAPTER 68
ORGANOPHOSPHATES AND OTHER INSECTICIDES

Lester M. Haddad, M.D., FACEP

THE ORGANOPHOSPHATE INSECTICIDES

The organophosphate insecticides are the insecticide group of choice in the agricultural world and are the most common cause of poisoning among the pesticides. The Environmental Protection Agency[1] (EPA) has reported that over 80 per cent of all hospitalizations from pesticide poisoning were due to the organophosphate group; primarily involved were farmers, skilled and unskilled laborers, and children. The 1987 Annual Report of the American Association of Poison Control Centers (AAPCC) National Data Collection System listed 9032 exposures to organophosphate insecticides resulting in 2646 patients managed at a health care facility and 3 deaths.[2] The highest incidence of poisoning from these agents in the United States occurs in California and in states in the farm belt and the South.

The organophosphates have achieved great popularity because of their effectiveness as insecticides and their lack of persistence in the environment. Because of their unstable chemical structure, they disintegrate into harmless radicals within days after application. Thus, they do not persist in body tissues or the environment, as do chlorophenothane (DDT) and the organochlorines, and subsequently have replaced DDT as the insecticide group of choice.[3]

As a group, the organophosphate insecticides are highly toxic chemicals rapidly absorbed by all routes—respiratory, gastrointestinal, ocular, and dermal. In spite of extensive regulation, careful labeling, and educational efforts, the public persists in being unaware that minute quantities of any chemical can be harmful or even fatal and that a chemical can penetrate intact skin without producing sensation. Herein lies the danger of these highly toxic compounds. To give this concept clinical relevance, I am reminded of a 4-year-old farm boy who died after his foot and lower leg plunged through the top of a rusty tin containing Disyston when he was climbing in the barn. He played for about an hour, then went inside after he began vomiting. His mother changed his clothes and washed his leg but his condition worsened. In spite of hospitalization, he ultimately succumbed.

Individual organophosphates exhibit wide ranges of difference in their ability to penetrate skin, their oral absorption, and their toxicity. Tetraethylpyrophosphate (TEPP) was the first organophosphate; synthesized in 1854, it came into use in Germany during World War II as an agricultural substitute for nicotine and for possible use as a nerve gas in chemical warfare. Since TEPP is water soluble and directly acting, its absorption and onset of action are the most rapid by either the oral or dermal route; it is also the most highly toxic of the organophosphate insecticides.

Parathion [0,0 diethyl 0-(paranitrophenol phosphorothioate)], an organic derivative of phosphoric acid, was recognized shortly after World War II as the most effective of the 50 or more organophosphates for insecticidal use. Since parathion must first be converted to paraoxon by substitution of an oxygen for a sulfur to be physiologically active, symptoms from parathion intoxication are often delayed from 6 to 24 hours. Of the organophosphate group, parathion is the most common cause of human poisoning and fatality.[1, 2, 4]

The highly toxic group of organophosphates is used primarily for agricultural purposes. An intermediate group exists, used primarily as an insecticide for animals. At the lower end of the spectrum are agents used for golf courses and for the house and garden, such as malathion. Malathion is poorly absorbed through skin, its oral toxicity is low, and it can be metabolized.[5] Table 68–1 lists some representative organophosphate compounds and their usages.

Pathophysiology

The organophosphate insecticides produce a specific biochemical lesion, that of acetylcholinesterase inhibition, thus producing a striking physiologic picture in human poisoning.

Acetylcholine is the most important chemical transmitter at synaptic junctions; acetylcholinesterase breaks down acetylcholine by hydrolysis into its two primary fragments, acetic acid and choline, both of which are essentially inert.

The two principal human cholinesterases are acetylcholinesterase and pseudocholinesterase. Acetylcholinesterase (true cholinesterase) is found primarily in nervous tissue and erythrocytes; pseudocholinesterase is found in the liver and the serum. The organophosphates are powerful inhibitors of the cholinesterases and act by eventual irreversible binding of the active sites of the enzymes with phosphate radicals, forming phosphorylated enzymes.[6]

The toxicologic effects of the organophosphates are almost entirely due to the inhibition of acetylcholinesterase in the nervous system, resulting in accumulation of acetylcholine at synapses and myoneural junctions. Thus, organophosphate poisoning is more accurately assessed in the laboratory by measurement of the red cell (true) cholines-

Table 68–1. ORGANOPHOSPHATE INSECTICIDES

COMMON NAME	PRODUCT EXAMPLE	CHEMICAL NAME
AGRICULTURAL INSECTICIDES (high toxicity)		
TEPP	Miller Kilmite 40	Tetraethylpyrophosphate
phorate	Thimet (American Cyanamid)	O,O-diethyl S-(ethylthio)methyl phosphorodithioate
parathion	Niagara Phoskil Dust	O,O-diethyl 0-p-nitrophenyl phosphorothioate
mevinphos	Phosdrin (Shell)	dimethyl-O-(1-methyl-2-carbomethoxyvinyl) phosphate
disulfoton	Disyston	diethyl-S-2-ethyl-2-mercaptoethyl phosphorodithioate
ANIMAL INSECTICIDES (intermediate toxicity)		
coumaphos	Co-Ral Animal Insecticide	diethyl-0 (3-chloro-4-methyl-7-coumarinyl) phosphorothioate
Chlorpyrifos (Dursban)	Rid-A-Bug (Kenco)	0,0-diethyl-0-(3,5,6-trichloro-2-pyridyl) phosphorothioate
trichlorfon	Trichlorfon Pour On (Hess & Clark)	dimethyl trichlorohydroxyethyl phosphonate
ronnel	Korlan Livestock Spray (Dow)	0,0-dimethyl 0-(2,4,5-trichlorophenyl) phosphorothioate
HOUSEHOLD USE OR GOLF COURSE SPRAY (low toxicity)		
diazinon	Security Fire Ant Killer (Woolfolk)	diethyl-0-(2-isopropyl-4-methyl-6-pyrimidyl) phosphorothioate
malathion	Ortho Malathion 50 Insect Spray	dimethyl-S-(1,2-bis-carboethoxy) ethyl phosphorodithioate
vapona (dichlorvos, DDVP)	Shell No-Pest Strip	0,0-dimethyl-0-2,2-dichlorovinyl phosphate
acephate	Chevron Orthene	0,S-dimethylacetylphosphoramidothioate

terase rather than the serum (pseudo-) cholinesterase.

The overabundance of acetylcholine initially excites and then paralyzes transmission in cholinergic synapses, which include (1) the central nervous system, (2) the parasympathetic nerve endings and a few sympathetic nerve endings such as sweat glands (muscarinic effects), and (3) the somatic nerves and the ganglionic synapses of autonomic ganglia (nicotinic effects). The signs and symptoms of organophosphate poisoning are thus expressions of these three effects caused by excess acetylcholine (Table 68–2).

Smith[6] has described the reaction between paraoxon and acetylcholinesterase:

1. The initial attachment occurs by electrostatic attraction.
2. The paranitrophenol, or the "leaving" group, separates from the parent molecule and is metabolized. The diethylphosphate that remains reacts chemically and becomes firmly attached. This "second stage" is still reversible by the specific antidote pralidoxime.
3. After approximately 24 to 48 hours (the "critical interval"), if antidote is not administered, one of the ethyl groups leaves the phosphate moiety, and cholinesterase is irreversibly destroyed. If this 24- to 48-hour critical interval is passed without administration of antidote, enzyme resynthesis must occur to restore acetylcholinesterase; this takes weeks.[6] During this time the patient requires complete pulmonary support until enzyme resynthesis occurs. Recovery has occurred after weeks of such therapy.[6]

Clinical Presentation and Evaluation

Organophosphate poisoning, in our experience, seems to occur in three main circumstances: accidental exposure among adult farm workers; accidental poisoning of children by pesticides present in home or garage or by ingestion of pet flea and tick killers; and suicide attempts, this last-named group accounting for a slightly higher percentage in the United States. These categories parallel those from other reports.[1, 4, 7, 8]

The time interval between exposure and onset of symptoms varies with the chemical, route of entry, and degree of exposure and symptoms almost always occur within 24 hours.[8]

Symptoms (see Table 68–2) initially are usually gastrointestinal and resemble a flu-like syndrome: abdominal pain and vomiting, headache, and dizziness. Diarrhea is not as common.[4, 7] In fact, it is not uncommon for those patients that do not give an adequate history to be misdiagnosed as having acute gastroenteritis and discharged from the emergency department, only to return later in serious condition. In one study, 16 of 20 transfer patients who were toxic from organophosphate insecticides were incorrectly diagnosed as having other conditions.[9] The

Table 68–2. CLINICAL EFFECTS OF ORGANOPHOSPHATE POISONING (ACETYLCHOLINE EXCESS)

ANATOMIC SITE OF ACTION	PHYSIOLOGIC EFFECTS
Muscarinic Effects	
Sweat glands	Sweating
Pupils	Constricted pupils
Lacrimal glands	Lacrimation
Salivary glands	Excessive salivation
Bronchial tree	Wheezing
Gastrointestinal	Cramps, vomiting, diarrhea, tenesmus
Cardiovascular	Bradycardia, fall in blood pressure
Ciliary body	Blurred vision
Bladder	Urinary incontinence
Nicotinic Effects	
Striated muscle	Fasciculations, cramps, weakness, twitching, paralysis, respiratory embarrassment, cyanosis, arrest
Sympathetic ganglia	Tachycardia, elevated blood pressure
Central Nervous System Effects	Anxiety, restlessness, ataxia, convulsions, insomnia, coma, absent reflexes, Cheyne-Stokes respirations, respiratory and circulatory depression

presence of excessive salivation, miosis, lacrimation, and weakness during the initial phase is more indicative of organophosphate poisoning.

The development of coma, pulmonary edema, ataxia, confusion or psychosis, dyspnea or cyanosis, fasciculations, convulsions, pancreatitis, bradycardia or cardiac arrhythmia, and/or weakness or paralysis indicates severe poisoning, and aggressive emergency management must be instituted. Routine exposure to the organophosphate animal insecticides and to those for house and garden may or may not result in critical poisoning.[8]

Pancreatitis is an uncommon but definite presentation of organophosphate insecticide poisoning,[10, 11] with reports of acute pancreatitis with hyperamylasemia and hyperglycemia recently described in the literature. Organophosphates produce an increase in the secretion rate of acinar pancreatic glands because of their cholinergic innervation.[10]

Organophosphate poisoning outside the United States has been associated with Q-T interval prolongation and polymorphous ventricular arrhythmia of the "torsades de pointes" type.[12] This complication may lead to delayed, sudden death after the patient appears to be well on the way to recovery from respiratory and neurologic involvement.[12] Onset of arrhythmia 5 days after exposure has been described.[12]

Clinical evaluation includes a detailed history of occupational background and possible exposure and may be difficult to elucidate.

A history of exposure is most helpful but often not available, as the family may not recognize exposure or the depressed patient may not reveal the agent. On physical examination the presence of diaphoresis; miosis (and occasionally mydriasis); lacrimation; excessive salivation; respiratory distress with wheezes, rhonchi, and rales; bradycardia or irregular heartbeat; disturbances in consciousness or orientation; weakness or paralysis; extensor plantar responses; and muscle fasciculations may be noted.

Emergency Management

A comatose patient who is diaphoretic, has pinpoint pupils and the odor of an insecticide on clothing or breath, and is noted to have muscle fasciculations represents the classic presentation of organophosphate poisoning.[8] Respiratory distress may be present. This patient should be managed as such until proven otherwise; therapy is never to be delayed until return of laboratory values.

Following initial assessment of vital signs and insertion of an intravenous line, appropriate blood studies should be drawn, both to confirm the diagnosis of organophosphate poisoning and to rule out other causes of metabolic coma. The patient should be examined and also evaluated for possible evidence of trauma.

Specific steps in management include the following.

1. Decontamination. If the patient is awake and ambulatory on arrival to the emergency department and has insecticide on the clothes or skin, have him or her shower immediately for 30 minutes, with an attendant near by. If he or she is unable to shower, then this must be performed by nursing staff or personnel. Thoroughly wash skin and hair with soap and water. A second washing of skin with ethyl alcohol is also recommended. Ensure that personnel wear gloves to avoid contamination while cleansing a patient.

For gastric decontamination, use ipecac if the patient is fully alert, even if a petroleum distillate is the carrier. If the patient is unconscious, the patient should be intubated prior to gastric lavage. Both activated charcoal and sodium sulfate or sorbitol as a cathartic are indicated.

2. Airway. Establish an airway if necessary. The classic literature[13–15] constantly suggests the importance of adequate oxygenation and ventilation prior to the use of atropine, as atropine is said to precipitate ventricular fibrillation in a poorly oxygenated patient, especially when the patient clinically exhibits cyanosis.

However, adequate oxygenation is not always possible in these patients, as they are often in respiratory distress on arrival in the emergency department.

3. Respiratory Status. Respiratory distress, in fact, is commonly found in these patients from multiple causes. (a) The organophosphate insecticides cause excessive salivation and bronchial secretions as well as bronchospasm and wheezing. (b) Pulmonary edema is not uncommon in these patients. Organophosphate poisoning should be suspected in any child who presents in pulmonary edema, especially if there is no cardiac history. (c) Chemical pneumonitis may develop from the petroleum distillate carrier, or (d) aspiration pneumonia in comatose patients is a possibility. (e) Muscle paralysis obviously contributes to respiratory embarrassment. And finally, (f) the adult respiratory distress syndrome (ARDS) may develop in critical patients.[8]

Nasotracheal or endotracheal intubation with complete respiratory support may be necessary in these patients, and pulmonary consultation, if available, should be obtained. A chest x-ray and arterial blood gases are essential in early assessment of these patients.

Adequate oxygenation may be difficult prior to initiation of atropine/pralidoxime therapy. In fact, by drying secretions, atropine does much to alleviate the respiratory distress and is often indicated primarily for management of pulmonary symptomatology.[8]

Theophylline is considered contraindicated in the management of organophosphate poisoning.[13–15] The use of central nervous system depressants such as morphine or phenothiazines is obviously not warranted.

4. Cardiac Monitoring. An electrocardiogram and cardiac monitoring are indicated in all significant cases of organophosphate poisoning. In patients who are comatose and/or have pulmonary edema, cardiac monitoring for dysrhythmias such as heart block or "torsades de pointes" ventricular tachycardia is a necessity.[12] "Torsades de pointes" ventricular tachycardia has been reported to date only outside the United States in critical patients who had been comatose or had pulmonary edema;[12] electrical pacing in such cases was successful in management of ventricular tachyarrhythmias.[12] Cardiac monitoring during atropine therapy or dopamine administration for hypotension is indicated.

5. Cholinesterase Level. Cholinesterase levels are helpful in securing a diagnosis of organophosphate poisoning but have no relation to management. Although the red cell cholinesterase level is a more accurate assessment of organophosphate poisoning, most hospital laboratories perform the serum cholinesterase level, which measures pseudocholinesterase found in liver and the serum.

In addition to organophosphate poisoning, the serum cholinesterase may be depressed in parenchymal liver disease, including viral hepatitis, cirrhosis, congestion secondary to congestive heart failure, and metastatic carcinoma.[16] Low values[16] may also be noted in patients with malnutrition, acute infections, anemias, myocardial infarction, and dermatomyositis, particularly in those who exhibit a low serum albumin. A depressed serum cholinesterase may be due to a genetic variant in 3 per cent of patients. The serum cholinesterase level is depressed before red cell cholinesterase and is a sensitive indicator of exposure to organophosphates.[17–20]

Twenty-five per cent or greater depression of the red cell cholinesterase level is a true indicator of poisoning.

Red cell cholinesterase levels may take up to 90 to 120 days to return to normal values, whereas the serum cholinesterase recovers in days to weeks. Other laboratory studies in addition to routine laboratory studies should include a serum amylase and thin-layer or gas chromatography for confirmation.

6. Pralidoxime. Pralidoxime is the treatment of choice for organophosphate poisoning and should be used for nearly all patients with clinically significant organophosphate poisoning, particularly those patients with muscular fasciculations and weakness. Pralidoxime is produced by Ayerst in the United States as 2-PAM Chloride or Protopam, and its administration should be begun as soon as possible upon clinical recognition of poisoning.

Pralidoxime and the other oximes comprise one of the few classes of drugs that correct a biochemical lesion.[20] Other oximes that have the capability of reactivating cholinesterase include obidoxime chloride (pINN) or Toxogonin (common in Europe); pralidoxime iodide (2-PAM iodide); and pralidoxime mesylate (P_2S), the methanesulfonate salt.

Hayes[21] describes three desirable effects of pralidoxime chloride in the management of organophosphate poisoning: (1) the primary effect of cleaving the phosphorylation-acetylcholinesterase bond, thus freeing and reactivating acetylcholinesterase; (2) directly reacting with and detoxifying the organophosphorus molecules; and (3) having an anticholinergic "atropine-like" effect.[21]

Pralidoxime is given intravenously at an initial dose of 1 gm, or 25 to 50 mg/kg to children, usually over a 15- to 30-minute period. The effect is often dramatic, with disappearance of coma (often temporary) and fasciculations and a return of strength and well-being. This dose may be repeated often, generally 1 gm every 6 hours for 48 hours; in fact, up to 500 mg/hr has been given to critical adult patients.[7, 8] To be effective, it should be given during the "48-hour critical interval."

The package insert for Protopam (Ayerst) states that pralidoxime is ineffective or marginally effective against poisoning by ciodrin, dimefox, dimethoate, methyl diazinon, methyl phencapton, phorate, shradan, and wepsyn.

Pralidoxime is of low toxicity. The early use of pralidoxime in my experience obviates the need for high-dose atropine therapy.[8] Pralidoxime was once administered prophylactically to workers exposed to organophosphates.

Pralidoxime reduces the incidence of Wadia's "type II or late-onset paralysis" (onset of paralysis and/or respiratory depression 24 hours after exposure).

Wadia and associates,[22] who first noticed the occurrence of late-onset paralysis in India, where there was a shortage of pralidoxime, suggested that the lack of late-paralysis descriptions in Western literature was due to the ready availability of pralidoxime and other cholinesterase-reactivating oximes in the Western world. Type II paralysis was not noticed once in a study of 198 reported cases in which oxime therapy was routinely used.[23]

7. Atropine. Atropine is the physiologic antidote for organophosphate poisoning. A trial dose of atropine should be instituted on clinical grounds when one suspects organophosphate intoxication.[7, 8] Atropine should be initiated at the same time as pralidoxime therapy. The ability to administer large doses of atropine without observable adverse effect is virtually diagnostic of organophosphate poisoning.[7] Initial doses of atropine should be given with the physician in constant attendance, with cardiac monitoring and frequent assessment of vital signs.

An initial trial dose of atropine, 2 mg IV, should be given to an adult. Repeat 2 mg in 15 minutes if there is no observable adverse effect. Atropine may then be repeated, or increased in increments, at 15- to 60-minute intervals, or as indicated, until the patient demonstrates signs of atropinization.

Up to 5 mg IV of atropine every 15 minutes may be necessary for the critical adult patient with organophosphate poisoning,[7, 8, 17] for example, the patient with disturbances of vital signs: hypothermia, hypotension, or respiratory arrest.

The initial dose of atropine for children is 0.05 mg/kg IV. Maintenance doses for children range from 0.02 to 0.05 mg/kg.

Signs of atropinization include flushing, dry mouth, and dilated pupils. Dilated or uneven pupils are uncommon but have been described with organophosphate poisoning. Initially pinpoint pupils that become dilated with atropine, however, provide a reliable guide for effective atropinization. Although the literature frequently mentions tachycardia as a sign of atropinization, cholinesterase inhibition will cause either bradycardia or tachycardia, depending on whether cholinergic stimulation is muscarinic (bradycardia) or nicotinic (tachycardia) via the sympathetic ganglia. Bradycardia that becomes tachycardia following the use of atropine, however, can be a reliable sign of atropinization.

Atropine should be used for at least 24 hours as a physiologic antidote to competitively block the effect of acetylcholine while the organophosphate is being metabolized.

Atropine should be tapered in those patients who begin to show signs of improvement, usually after 12 to 24 hours. One can taper both the dose and the time interval. Close observation is necessary, as the effects of organophosphate toxicity may rebound. Delayed pulmonary edema and/or cardiac toxicity has been described.[7, 8, 12–15]

Signs of excessive atropinization include fever, delirium, and muscle twitching. It is not uncommon for these to develop as the effect of organophosphate begins to wear off, and they may be the sign for the physician to begin tapering the dose.

Remember, atropine has ***no*** effect on skeletal muscle and autonomic ganglia.[7, 8, 13–15]

Complications

Both hyper- and hypoglycemia have been reported as acute manifestations[7] of organophosphate poisoning and may require management. Pancreatitis is uncommon but may occur.[9] Cardiac arrhythmia as described may develop.[12] Transient liver function and coagulation abnormalities have been reported.[7]

Chronic neurologic sequelae occur from organophosphate poisoning, including subtle cerebral dysfunction and neurophysiologic disturbances.[24, 25] Reports of peripheral neuropathy, Guillain-Barré syndrome,[26] and polyneuropathy[27] have also been described. A specific syndrome following exposure to the organophosphate-related chemical triorthocresyl phosphate has been described, known as ginger-jake paralysis.[28] Chapter 26F on chronic pesticide poisoning further elaborated on the chronic effects of organophosphate poisoning.

Death usually occurs within 48 hours in those untreated patients who develop pulmonary effects and may occur within 10 to 14 days in treated patients.

Occupational Prevention

The organophosphates are so highly toxic that continuous emphasis on their proper usage is essential. Personal hygiene, cleansing of contaminated clothes, and avoidance of skin contact for all handlers of these agents are mandatory. A cholinesterase level in workers prior to exposure is worthwhile as a parameter for future values. Periodic checks are useful to avoid symptomatic poisoning, since depressions of the serum cholinesterase will occur before symptoms appear.

CARBAMATE INSECTICIDES

The carbamates are a group of insecticides derived from carbamic acid. They have a broad spectrum of uses as agricultural and household garden insecticides. Sevin, Baygon, and Lannate are used most commonly. Table 68–3 lists a group of carbamate insecticides in general order of decreasing toxicity. Aldicarb is the most toxic and is considered a systemic insecticide because it is taken up from the soil and incorporated into the plant and fruit.

Table 68–3. CARBAMATE INSECTICIDES

COMMERCIAL NAME	CHEMICAL
Temik	aldicarb
Matacil	aminocarb
Vydate	oxamyl
Isolan	isolan
Furadan	carbofuran
Lannate	methomyl
Zectran	mexacarbate
Mesurol	methiocarb
Dimetilan	dimetilan
Baygon	propoxur
Sevin	carbaryl

(Adapted from Gleason MN, Gosselin RE, Hodge HC, Smith RP: Clinical Toxicology of Commercial Products. 3rd ed. Baltimore, Williams & Wilkins, 1976.)

The carbamate insecticides are ***reversible*** cholinesterase inhibitors. They cause this effect by reversible carbamylation of the enzyme acetylcholinesterase, allowing accumulation of acetylcholine, as with the organophosphate insecticides. The carbamates are absorbed by all routes, including inhalation, ingestion, and dermal absorption.

The 1987 Annual Report of the AAPCC National Data Collection System[2] reported 4458 exposures to carbamate insecticides with 905 patients treated at a health care facility and 0 deaths. They also reported 2478 joint exposures to organophosphate and carbamate insecticides with 0 deaths.

Carbamates Versus Organophosphates

As both the organophosphate and the carbamate insecticides are cholinesterase inhibitors and the organophosphates have been discussed, contrasting the two groups helps in understanding the carbamates.

1. Although the organophosphate insecticides cause irreversible inhibition of the cholinesterase enzymes, the carbamyl-enzyme complex is ***reversible*** and dissociates far more readily than the organophosphate complex. The clinical syndrome is more benign and of much shorter duration with the carbamate insecticides.
2. Unlike the organophosphates, the carbamates poorly penetrate the central nervous system. Thus, the clinical presentation of carbamate poisoning resembles that of organophosphate poisoning with the exception of prominent central nervous system effects, such as convulsions. Convulsions are uncommon with the carbamate insecticides.
3. Serum and red cell cholinesterase values are not reliable in "capturing" the diagnosis of carbamate poisoning, as they are with the organophosphates, for enzyme activity (as mentioned previously) returns to normal within a few hours. A patient may show symptoms in the emergency department 6 hours after exposure, but the cholinesterase levels may have already returned to normal. The rule that one's judgment must prevail in clinical decision-making is especially true with the carbamate insecticides.

Clinical Presentation and Treatment

The clinical picture of carbamate poisoning is one of cholinergic crisis, as just described.

Treatment of symptomatic carbamate insecticide poisoning includes establishment of airway, stabilization of vital signs, removal of the poison by ipecac or gastric lavage with the usual precautions, and removal of contaminated clothes and thorough cleansing of skin. Activated charcoal and cathartic are indicated in the event of ingestion.

Atropine is the drug of choice in the management of carbamate insecticide poisoning. The dosage for adults is 0.4 to 2.0 mg IV, repeated every 15 to 30 minutes until signs of atropinization appear (dry mouth, flushing, and dilated pupils if pupils were originally pinpoint). Unlike with organophosphate poisoning, large doses of atropine are not usually needed, and atropinization may be necessary for only 6 to 12 hours for the majority of patients. The exception is the critical patient. Patients preferably should be well oxygenated with the use of atropine. Children's dosage of atropine is 0.05 mg/kg initially, repeated as necessary at intervals similar to those for adults. The rationale for the use of atropine is the same as that with the organophosphate insecticides.

Observation for serious cases is recommended for at least 24 hours. Milder intoxications do not require such prolonged observation. As with all insecticide poisonings, the patient must be observed with respect to possible toxicity from the carrier, which may be methyl alcohol.

One is advised not to use morphine, reserpine, phenothiazines, or chlordiazepoxide in the face of carbamate poisoning.[30]

In the critical patient with respiratory arrest and pulmonary edema, sophisticated critical care management with pulmonary consultation is necessary. General supportive care is indicated.

Pralidoxime is ***not*** indicated in the patient with pure carbamate insecticide poisoning, as the cholinesterase-carbamate complex is reversible and readily dissociates. The physiologic antidote atropine, which is competitive to acetylcholine at the neuroreceptor end-plate, is all that is indicated until the enzyme acetylcholinesterase is able to dissociate, recover function, and metabolize overabundant acetylcholine.

The major controversy is whether pralidoxime is contraindicated[13] in carbamate poisoning. Early writers reported that pralidoxime reduced the antidotal effect of atropine in the management of carbamate poisoning, especially with carbaryl.[14, 30]

In two clinical situations pralidoxime may be given to a patient with carbamate insecticide poisoning, even though it is not indicated for carbamate intoxication. One is when a patient presents with symptoms typical of cholinesterase inhibition and the insecticide is either unknown or not definitely known. The other is when a patient suffers from concomitant organophosphate and carbamate intoxication.

The first case, the unknown insecticide poisoning, is rather common. In fact, common sense tells us that several instances surely have occurred over the years when patients with carbamate intoxication were administered pralidoxime by well-intentioned physicians who thought they were faced with organophosphate poisoning. Indeed, failure to administer pralidoxime to a critical patient with organophosphate poisoning can only increase the likelihood of fatality.

When a physician is faced with a critically ill patient exhibiting signs and symptoms of cholinesterase inhibition, either from an unknown insecticide or from concomitant organophosphate and carbamate exposure, it is my belief that a trial of pralidoxime is clearly warranted.

Sequelae

A few reports of delayed neurotoxicity from carbamate poisoning are beginning to appear in the literature,[31–33] although recovery is generally complete in the majority of exposures.

ORGANOCHLORINE INSECTICIDES

Once the most important group of insecticides, the organochlorines have been largely banned in the United States. Table 68–4 lists the organochlorine insecticides in decreasing order of toxicity. In general, they are central nervous system stimulants.

DDT, first introduced in 1942, introduced

Table 68–4. ORGANOCHLORINE INSECTICIDES

endrin
aldrin
endosulfan
dieldrin
toxaphene
lindane
benzene hexachloride (BHC)
DDT
heptachlor
kepone
terpene polychlorinates
chlordane
dicofol (kelthane)
chlorobenzilate
mirex
methoxychlor

(Adapted from Morgan, DP: Recognition and Management of Pesticide Poisonings. 3rd ed. Washington DC, Environmental Protection Agency, 1982.)

modern pesticides in the United States.[34] Malaria has been brought under control worldwide primarily as a result of the efficacy of DDT. The other organochlorines also have been most popular. For example, chlordane has been one of the most effective agents for termite and roach control. Mirex has been one of the primary agents used for red ant control.

In 1948 it was discovered that DDT was stored indefinitely in human tissues; however, not until 1970 did studies reveal that DDT is found in virtually everyone in the general population of the United States. It was found further that six organochlorine insecticides are stored in tissues in the general population: DDT, BHC (benzene hexachloride), DDD (dichlorodiphenyldiethane), heptachlor, aldrin, and dieldrin.[34]

The National Cancer Institute has further shown that heptachlor causes malignant tumors in mice and rats.[13] Chlordane is chemically related, and roughly 10 per cent of it is heptachlor. The chronic effects of organochlorine pesticide poisoning are still being assessed.

DDT was banned in 1972 in the United States. Heptachlor, kepone, mirex, endrin, aldrin, dieldrin, BHC, strobane, chlorobenzilate, and chlordane were subsequently banned by the EPA. The use of toxaphene is now severely restricted by the EPA. Methoxychlor, kelthane, and lindane are still available. Since lindane is used widely, it will represent the organochlorines for clinical discussion.

Lindane

Lindane is the gamma isomer of benzene hexachloride. At present it enjoys wide usage as a general garden insecticide for control of black widow spiders, centipedes, and cotton insects; for control of ticks, scabies, and lice; and for powder-post beetles.

Examples of products containing lindane are Kwell, Isotox lindane garden dust or spray (Chevron), Gammex suspension (Jansen-Salsbery), Ortho lindane borer and leaf miner spray (Chevron), Gammasan (Chipman), Farnam screwworm smear bomb (Farnam), and Gamene.[14]

Lindane is available in ointments, shampoos, creams, dusts, and sprays. Its only restriction is use in vaporizers, since fatal vapor exposures in the home have been reported.[13, 14]

Clinical Presentation

A common clinical presentation is seizures in children who have been using lindane for treatment of scabies or lice for prolonged periods of time.

More insidious presentations may occur; the patient may be apprehensive, confused, dizzy, or comatose. He or she may complain of muscle twitching, tremors, or paresthesias. If the compound is ingested, nausea and vomiting are often presenting complaints. As with all the organochlorine insecticides, significant toxicity produces seizures, and status epilepticus may occur. Death is usually by respiratory failure.

Hepatic and renal compromise is very uncommon. Agranulocytosis and fatal aplastic anemia have been reported.[13, 14]

Treatment

Treatment is symptomatic and supportive. Oils should not be used as either cathartics or dermal cleansing agents, as they increase absorption. Gastric lavage and use of activated charcoal and sodium sulfate are indicated for ingestion. If dermal exposure occurred, contaminated clothes should be removed, and the skin should be thoroughly cleansed with soap and water.

Management of seizures in both children and adults is with Valium or phenobarbital. Respiratory depression and even respiratory arrest, especially with concomitant use of

Valium and phenobarbital in children, may occur. These drugs preferably should be used only in critical care areas where emergency endotracheal intubation can be performed.

Both Gleason and colleagues[14] and Morgan[30] recommend that epinephrine not be utilized in patients with organochlorine poisoning, as the organochlorines induce myocardial irritability and ventricular arrhythmias may occur. However, dopamine may be necessary in the event of hypotension unresponsive to fluid administration, and epinephrine may be necessary in the event of cardiopulmonary arrest.

Laboratory values are of no help in the management of lindane or organochlorine poisoning, as lindane is stored in the tissues of the general population and a positive test does not confirm acute poisoning. Blood level determinations by sophisticated techniques are necessary for confirmation of poisoning but are generally not available.

The organochlorines, including lindane, do ***not*** affect the serum or red cell cholinesterase level.

When a patient with a history of insecticide use has seizures, supportive therapy is appropriate whether the cause is organophosphate, organochlorine, carbamate, or other insecticide agent.

In a critically ill patient with unknown insecticide exposure, a trial of atropine and pralidoxime should ***not*** be withheld until the etiologic agent is discovered, for the use of these agents may prove life-saving in organophosphate poisoning. Atropine must be used with caution, as it can cause ventricular irritability, especially when a myocardial irritant such as an organochlorine is present.

There are no reports of dialysis or hemoperfusion being effective with lindane or other organochlorine insecticides.

Hematologic, hepatic (especially with endrin, which is markedly hepatotoxic), and renal studies as well as cardiopulmonary monitoring should be carried out in acute intoxication from lindane or other organochlorines for at least 48 to 72 hours. Long-term hematologic follow-up is necessary for the patient with lindane intoxication.

As the carrier for these agents may be xylene or a petroleum distillate, management also must include observation and treatment for these entities.

The National Pesticide Telecommunications Network at Texas Tech University has a 24-hour telephone (1-800-858-PEST) to provide helpful information in pesticide-related emergencies.

BOTANICAL INSECTICIDES

The botanical pesticides are pyrethrum, rotenone, ryania, and sabadilla. ***Pyrethrum*** is the most widely used household insect spray; examples of products containing pyrethrum[14] follow:

Hot Shot fly and mosquito insect killer (Conwood)
Black Flag house and garden insect killer (Boyle-Midway)
Raid bug killer (Johnson)
Parsons Fly-Di insect spray (Parsons)
Ortho home and garden insect spray (Chevron)

Over 2000 products contain pyrethrum and its related compounds. It is also one of the oldest insecticides.

Pyrethrum is derived from the flowers of the chrysanthemum, ***Chrysanthemum cineriae folium.*** After the flowers are dried and ground to a fine powder, the residue contains about 1 per cent active material.[14] The six active chemicals in pyrethrum are known collectively as the pyrethrins. Synthetic derivatives of the pyrethrins are known as the pyrethroids, such as allethrin.

Most insecticides containing the pyrethrins usually have a synergist, piperonyl butoxide, which increases their ability and effectiveness. The usual carrier is a petroleum distillate.

The toxicity of pyrethrum products is low, and systemic poisoning is rare. The major problem one may encounter is allergy to pyrethrum. About 50 per cent of those patients who are sensitive to ragweed exhibit cross-reactivity to pyrethrum. Anaphylaxis is a possibility, and acute rhinitis, asthma, dermatitis, and hypersensitivity pneumonitis have been reported.[35]

Rotenone is derived from several plants, particularly the derris root of Malaya, the larchocarpus (cube) of Central and South America, and the tephrisia of Africa. It is widely used as an insecticide. It is available in dust and sprays either alone or in combination with other insecticides, such as pyrethrum.

Examples of products containing rotenone[14] are Acme Quality Paints All-Round Bomb (in combination with pyrethrum) and Noxfish (Penick).

One of the major uses of rotenone has been for the treatment of scabies and chiggers. The fresh derris root in Malaya is much more toxic than other sources and has been used for suicide. Rotenone is highly toxic to birds and fish and is often employed as a fish poison.

Rotenone at normal concentrations is relatively nontoxic to humans. It causes prompt emesis upon ingestion and has a very low gastrointestinal absorption. Usual preparations contain 5 per cent rotenone or less. Rotenone also rapidly decomposes on exposure to light and air and is most unstable. No deaths from rotenone in the United States have been reported.

In massive overdose, principal effects include protracted vomiting, respiratory depression, and hypoglycemia and its symptoms.

In symptomatic overdose, treatment is appropriate supportive therapy.

Ryania, from the American Flacourtiaceae family; and *sabadilla*, or cevadilla or caustic barley, from the dried ripe seeds of the Mexican plant *Schoenocaulon officiale*, are no longer marketed.

INSECT REPELLENTS

Insect repellents are intended for human use so are generally nontoxic with routine usage. By skin application or spraying of clothes, they repel mosquitoes, gnats, or other insects from biting or annoying the user. An example is Avon Skin-So-Soft bath oil, a nontoxic oil that is an excellent gnat repellent.

Two insect repellents that may cause clinical poisoning are N, N-diethyltoluamide (DET) and para-dichlorobenzene.

DET is a highly effective insect repellent used commercially (Off! by Johnson) as a spray. Although clinical poisoning from DET is rare, multiple reports of toxicity and death are scattered throughout the medical literature,[36–40] including a recent report[40] of five cases of ingestion of DET resulting in two deaths.

Common symptoms following ingestion[40] include coma, seizures, and hypotension. Other reports indicate agitation, slurred speech, ataxia, staggering gait, and intractable seizure activity[36–38]; anaphylaxis has also been described.[39]

Although poisoning from insect repellents is rare, treatment is symptomatic in such an event. A thorough differential diagnosis for encephalopathy must be considered, since causes of encephalopathy besides insect repellent poisoning are far more common.

First used as a moth repellent and occasionally as an insecticide, para-dichlorobenzene is now most commonly used as a bathroom deodorant in toilet bowls, diaper pails, and occasionally garbage pails. Its use as a moth repellent persists, and it is the least toxic ingredient found in mothballs.

Ingestion of para-dichlorobenzene among children is very common. A typical poison information phone call involves an infant or toddler who reaches into the toilet bowl and eats a piece of the "white deodorant cake." These ingestions are usually innocuous, and usually only observation is necessary.

Para-dichlorobenzene has occasionally proved to be an irritant to the eyes, nose, and throat, and allergic phenomena have been described. Massive ingestions may produce tremors and hepatic or renal injury or both. Treatment is symptomatic and supportive.

References

1. Information Statistics, the Environmental Protection Agency. Washington, DC, EPA, 1980.
2. Litovitz TL, Schmitz BF, Matyunas N, Martin TG: 1987 Annual Report of the American Association of Poison Control Centers National Data Collection System. Am J Emerg Med *6*:479–515, 1988.
3. Milby TH: Prevention and management of organophosphate poisoning. JAMA *216*:2131–2133, 1971.
4. Hirshberg A, Lerman Y: Clinical problems in organophosphate poisoning. Fund Appl Toxicol *4*:S209–S214, 1984.
5. Palmgren MS, Lee TC: Malathion and diazinon levels in grain dust from New Orleans area grain elevators. Am Ind Hyg Assoc J *45*:168, 1984.
6. Smith PW: Bulletin: Medical Problems in Aerial Applications. Washington, DC, Office of Aviation Medicine, Federal Aviation Administration, Department of Transportation, 1977.
7. Namba T, Nolte CT, Jackrel J, Grob D: Poisoning due to organophosphate insecticides. Am J Med *50*:475–490, 1971.
8. Haddad LM: Organophosphate poisoning. *In* Haddad LM, Winchester JF (eds): Clinical Management of Poisoning and Drug Overdose. Philadelphia, WB Saunders, 1983, pp 704–710.

9. Zwiener RJ, Ginsburg CM: Organophosphate and carbamate poisoning in infants and children. Pediatrics *81*:121, 1988.
10. Dressel TD, Goodale RL, Arneson MA, Borner JW: Pancreatitis as a complication of anticholinesterase insecticide intoxication. Ann Surg *189*:199–204, 1979.
11. Moore PG, James OF: Acute pancreatitis induced by acute organophosphate poisoning. Postgrad Med J *57*:660–662, 1981.
12. Ludomirski A, Klein HO, Sarelli P, Becker B, Hoffman S, Taitelman U, Barzilai J, Lang R, David D, DiSegni E, Kaplinsky E: Q-T prolongation and polymorphous ("torsades de pointes") ventricular arrhythmias associated with organophosphorus insecticide poisoning. Am J Cardiol *49*:1654–1658, 1982.
13. Arena JM: Poisoning: Toxicology, Symptoms, Treatment. 2nd ed. Springfield, Charles C Thomas, 1970.
14. Gleason MN, Gosselin RE, Hodge HC, Smith RP: Clinical Toxicology of Commercial Products. 3rd ed. Baltimore, Williams & Wilkins, 1976.
15. Gilman AG, Goodman LS, Gilman A: The Pharmacological Basis of Therapeutics. 7th ed. New York, MacMillan, 1985.
16. Henry JB: Todd-Sanford-Davidsohn: Clinical Diagnosis by Laboratory Methods. 16th ed. Philadelphia, WB Saunders, 1979.
17. Ducatman AM, Moyer TP: Clinical laboratory role in the evaluation of the patient exposed to acetylcholinesterase-inhibiting pesticides. Am Assoc Clin Chem, July, 1982.
18. Areekul S, Srichairat S, Kirdudom P: Serum and red cell cholinesterase activity in people exposed to organophosphate insecticides. Southeast Asian J Trop Med *12*:94, 1981.
19. Warren M, Spencer HC, Churchill FC, Francois VJ, Hippolyte R, Staiger MA: Assessment of exposure to organophosphate insecticides during spraying in Haiti. Bull WHO *63*:353–360, 1985.
20. Coye MJ, Barnett PJ, Midtling JE, Velasco AR, Romero P, Clements CL, Rose TG: Clinical confirmation of organophosphate poisoning by serial cholinesterase analyses. Arch Intern Med *147*:438, 1987.
21. Hayes WJ: Toxicology of Pesticides. Baltimore, Williams & Wilkins, 1975.
22. Wadia RS, Sadagopan C, Amin RB, Sandesai HV: Neurological manifestations of organophosphorus insecticide poisoning. J Neurol Neurosurg Psychiatr *37*:841–847, 1974.
23. Gadoth N, Fisher A: Late onset of neuromuscular block in organophosphorus poisoning. Ann Intern Med *88*:654, 1978.
24. Schuman SH, Whitlock NH, Caldwell ST, Horton PM: Update on hospitalized pesticide poisonings in South Carolina, 1983–1987. J S Carolina Med Assoc, Feb, 1989, pp 62–66.
25. Savage EP, Keefe TJ, Mounce LM, Heaton RK, Lewis JA, Burcar PJ: Chronic neurological sequelae of acute organophosphate pesticide poisoning. Arch Environ Health *43*:38, 1988.
26. Fisher J: Guillain-Barré syndrome following organophosphate poisoning. JAMA *238*:1950, 1977.
27. DeJager A, van Weerden TW, Houthoff HJ, deMonchy J: Polyneuropathy after massive exposure to parathion. Neurology *31*:603–605, 1981.
28. Morgan JP, Penovich P: Jamaica ginger paralysis. Arch Neurol *35*:530, 1978.
29. Morgan JP: Jamaica ginger paralysis. JAMA *248*:1864, 1982.
30. Morgan DP: Recognition and Management of Pesticide Poisonings. 3rd ed. Washington, DC, Environmental Protection Agency, 1982.
31. Garber M: Carbamate poisoning: The "other" insecticide. Pediatrics *79*:734, 1987.
32. Dickoff DJ, Gerber O, Turofsky Z: Delayed neurotoxicity after ingestion of carbamate pesticide. Neurology *37*:1229, 1987.
33. Branch RA, Jacqz E: Is carbaryl as safe as its reputation? Am J Med *80*:659, 1986.
34. Hayes WJ: Pesticides Studied in Man. Baltimore, Williams & Wilkins, 1982.
35. Carlson JE, Villaveces JW: Hypersensitivity pneumonitis due to pyrethrum. JAMA *237*:1718, 1977.
36. Heick HM, Shipman RI, Norman MG: Reye-like syndrome associated with the use of insect repellent. J Pediatr *97*:471, 1980.
37. Zadicoff CM: Toxic encephalopathy associated with the use of insect repellent. J Pediatr *95*:140, 1979.
38. Gryboski J, Weinstein D, Ordway NK: Toxic encephalopathy related to use of an insect repellent. N Engl J Med *264*:289, 1961.
39. Miller JD: Anaphylaxis associated with insect repellent. N Engl J Med *307*:1341, 1982.
40. Tenenbein M: Severe toxic reactions and death following the ingestion of diethyltoluamide-containing insect repellents. JAMA *258*:1509, 1987.

CHAPTER 69
PARAQUAT AND THE BIPYRIDYL HERBICIDES

James F. Winchester, M.D.

PARAQUAT

Paraquat (1,1-dimethyl-4,4′-bipyridylium chloride) is the most important bipyridyl herbicide in the group of three: paraquat, diquat, and morfamquat (Fig. 69–1). Although paraquat is not a new chemical, it remains widely used in agriculture, acting as a nonselective herbicide with somewhat unique properties. It has caused something of an agricultural revolution in many areas of the world in view of the fact that the chemical can be sprayed from ground level or the air; desiccates crops such as cotton, allowing a single harvest rather than multiple harvests; is totally denatured on contact with the earth; and allows farmers to plant their seed directly into the earth or with minimal tilling of the earth.

Paraquat was introduced as a herbicide in 1962. Toward the end of the 1960s it was realized that the drug posed a serious hazard to humans—usually not associated with its proper use but as a result of drinking of the concentrate after it was decanted into unauthorized and unlabeled containers like soda bottles and so on. Although the initial deaths were accidental, in recent years suicidal deaths predominate. In light of the patients' protracted illness from pulmonary fibrosis, ending in death, the medical profession, aware of treatment difficulties, lobbied to bring about legislation in most countries to limit sales and use of the concentrated solution to licensed agricultural workers. To some extent, this reduced the likelihood of accidental exposure but also drew the attention of potential suicide patients toward the compound.

By 1973, 230 deaths were reported in the world literature; to the end of 1971, 60 recoveries had been reported in the world literature. In the United Kingdom, however, between 1963 and 1978 211 patients had died from paraquat ingestion. Most adult cases were due to deliberate self-poisoning rather than to accidental exposure. Review of the world literature in 1977 by Harley and associates disclosed approximately 600 deaths following accidental or intentional ingestion, with 60 per cent of the fatalities attributed to successful suicides.[1]

Paraquat Preparations and Toxic Action

Paraquat is available in the liquid concentrate form, as granules subsequently dissolved in water, or as an aerosol (Table 69–1). The concentrates are available for agricultural use as dichloride or dimethyl salts, both of which are water soluble. Paraquat is a parasubstituted quaternary bipyridyl cation, and concentrations of paraquat salt should be converted to per cent (weight-weight) of paraquat base, in order not to underestimate the amount of paraquat in the concentrate. For example, the 29.1 per cent liquid concentrate contains 239.6 gm/L of paraquat cations, and the 0.44 per cent aerosol solution contains 0.2 per cent of paraquat cation. Paraquat itself is caustic in nature. The concentrate, in some countries but not in the United States, also may contain a detergent (15 per cent of an aliphatic petroleum solvent) that solubilizes wax on plant leaves, allowing paraquat to enter cells and exert its phytotoxicity. In some countries, both the vehicle and paraquat itself may contribute to the toxicity.

Paraquat exerts its herbicidal activity by interfering with intracellular electron transfer systems, inhibiting reduction of NADP to NADPH during photosynthesis,[2] at which time the superoxide (the reactive form of oxygen) radical is formed. This eventually leads to the destruction of lipid cell membranes by polymerization of unsaturated lipid compounds,[3] with peroxide radicals also being formed. Human toxicity is felt to follow a mechanism similar to that in plants, with depletion of the naturally occurring enzyme superoxide dismutase,[4] a compound responsible for the back conversion to oxygen of naturally formed, small quantities of super-

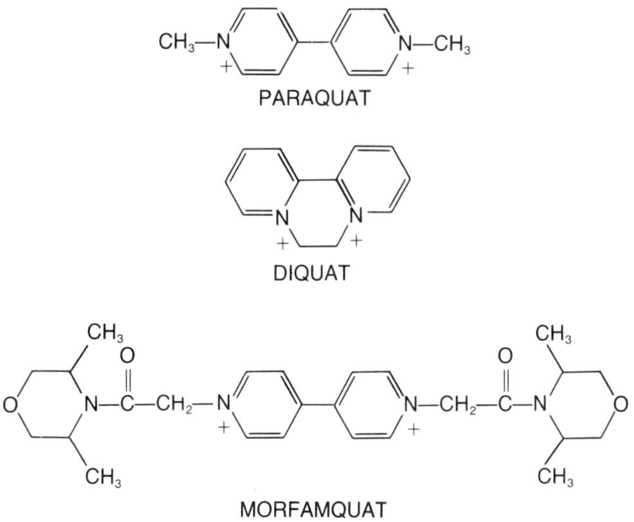

PARAQUAT

DIQUAT

MORFAMQUAT

Figure 69–1. Bipyridyl herbicides.

oxide. In rats, pulmonary prolyl hydroxylase, an enzyme promoting collagen formation, is increased soon after paraquat poisoning.[5] Experiments have shown that an increase in pulmonary prolyl hydroxylase precedes the total increase in collagen formation, which leads to irreversible pulmonary fibrosis.

Oxidative reactions probably account for the toxicity of the bipyridyls, since the major tissue biochemical features are lipid peroxidation[6, 7] and superoxide radical formation.[8–11] These are inextricably linked, but by themselves may not account for all of the toxicity. Vitamin E (alpha-tocopherol), a potent antioxidant, may prevent partially or completely the cytotoxic effects of paraquat in cultured hepatocytes,[12] but in human beings it had no effect on survival from paraquat poisoning. In the latter study, patients with acute lethal toxicity (see later) had no evidence of lipid peroxidation (assessed by serum methyl malondialdehyde determinations), whereas those with subacute toxicity had elevated serum methyl malondialdehyde concentrations compared with controls, which preceded pulmonary fibrosis.[13] Lipid peroxidation may be the consequence of cell damage rather than the cause of it.[14]

Metal ions also may be involved in tissue injury induced by paraquat and its biochemical products. Lipid peroxidation may be enhanced by iron radicals,[15] whereas removal of iron by the chelating agent deferoxamine reduces paraquat toxicity, in bacterial preparations[16] or in normal mice,[15] as well as in vitamin E–deficient rats.[17] The beneficial effect of deferoxamine in preventing paraquat toxicity in rats has not been confirmed

Table 69–1. PARAQUAT PREPARATIONS IN THE UNITED STATES AND THE UNITED KINGDOM

PARAQUAT CONCENTRATION	U.S. TRADE NAME*	U.K. TRADE NAME
20–44% liquid	Paraquat concentrate	Gramoxone
	Gramoxone extra	Gramoxone S
	Gramoxone super	Dextrone X
	Gramoxone paraquat herbicide	
	Surefire (contains diuron)	
	Cyclone	
7–10% liquid	Prelude (contains metalochlor and linuron)	Dexuron (contains diquat)
	Prelude EW (contains metalochlor and linuron)	Gramonol (contains monolinuron)
		Total-Col (contains diuron)
		Cleansweep (contains diquat)
2.5% granules		Weedol (contains 2.5% diquat)
		Pathclear (contains diquat and Simazine)

*Previous compounds in the United States included the concentrates Chevron Industrial Weed and Grass Killer, Ortho-Paraquat-CL, Ortho-Dual-Paraquat, and the 0.44% aerosol Orthospot Weed and Grass Killer.

in one study.[18] On the other hand, addition of selenium to the diet induces some protection against paraquat lethality in chicks, which may be due in part to an increase in Se-dependent glutathione peroxidase.[19] Exogenous glutathione also may protect against injury from paraquat when incubated with type II pneumocytes exposed to paraquat.[20] Dimethylthiourea (another free radical scavenger) given to animals poisoned with paraquat actually increases paraquat toxicity, increases plasma concentrations, decreases whole body clearance, and decreases apparent volume of distribution of paraquat.[21]

Clinical Exposure and Manifestations of Poisoning

Following the first reported death from the concentrated solution, the rate of accidental poisoning rose to give a mortality rate of 33 to 50 per cent. Most early cases were accidental because of the resemblance of paraquat to root beer or a cola drink, especially when decanted into soft drink bottles left unlabeled. The compound also may resemble dark vinegar, and one patient succumbed after sprinkling paraquat on French fried potatoes.

Studies of paraquat sprayers with heavy exposure have revealed that while skin rashes (particularly on scrotal and intergluteal areas, resulting from paraquat trickling down the back from leaking knapsack sprays), cracked nails, and epistaxis occur, systemic reactions are not observed.[22–28] Chest roentgenograms, measures of liver and renal function, and diffusion capacity for carbon monoxide (DL_{CO}) are negative despite the detection of minute quantities of paraquat in the urine.[24] These studies demonstrate that inhalation and dermal absorption of paraquat is poor if paraquat is used in the recommended way, with proper attention being paid to spray equipment and accurate dilution, protective clothing, and protection of pre-existing skin lesions.

There have been several experiments designed to study absorption of paraquat through the skin.[29–33] Early experiments in rabbits, using moderate-to-highly concentrated solutions of paraquat (240 mg cation/kg), demonstrated systemic absorption from occluded dermal sites and fatality from absorption.[29] On the other hand, absorption in mice (from application of 1 mg/kg) is considerably slower than from other pesticides.[30] Of overriding importance, however, is the demonstration in vitro that human skin is much less permeable to paraquat than are the skins of some experimental animals, in factors ranging from 40 times (haired rat) to 1460 times (hairless mouse) greater than human skin, with a human skin permeability constant of 0.73 cm/hr × 10^5.[31] Therefore, it is necessary to examine results of in vivo permeability of skin to paraquat; Wester and associates have demonstrated that only 0.03 μg/cm^2 of a paraquat solution containing 9 μg/cm^2 would be absorbed from intact skin in 24 hours.[32] That this may increase somewhat can be predicted from results of absorption of the closely related chemical diquat; 0.4 per cent of a topical dose is absorbed from an unoccluded site, 1.4 per cent from an occluded site, and 3.8 per cent from an occluded and damaged dermal site.[33] This latter observation is extremely important, for making recommendations to spray workers with pre-existing skin lesions, and for interpreting published cases of poisoning following dermal exposure.

The published cases, in which the skin of patients was felt to be the site of absorption, invariably describe patients with skin ulcers, desquamation, dermal burns, dermatitis, and so on.[34–45] In many cases it is impossible to exclude ingestion fully. One patient who had skin abrasions and frequent exposure to concentrate developed an indolent ulcer and progressive (and fatal) respiratory failure.[42] Another died after a single dermal exposure to paraquat concentrate over a large surface area and pre-existing skin lesions;[43] another (with an indolent skin ulcer) died after repeated exposure to 2.8 per cent paraquat and subsequent development of respiratory failure with pathologic features different from the classic picture after paraquat ingestion.[44] In the latter study, hypertrophic pulmonary artery lesions were seen in the patient; in animal experiments, the same lesions developed in the lungs of rats exposed to dermal contact of 8 mg of paraquat at weekly intervals, up to 9 weeks. Others have mistakenly used paraquat for the treatment of lice or other skin disorders.[35, 36] Putative evidence from these studies suggests that contact exposure to paraquat on the skin might lead to fatal pulmonary disease. Unfortunately, in many of the human fatalities, paraquat identification procedures were not employed in lung (or other) tissues. It must, therefore, be stated that contact exposure (particularly if the skin is not washed immediately after soaking, or if clothing is not changed, or if skin lesions are present) rarely might produce sufficient dermal absorption and subsequent fatal pulmonary lesions. This should prompt identification of paraquat in blood and urine in such exposed patients before instituting therapy. An extensive review of reported cases of purported skin absorption and animal and human experiments supports this view; prolonged exposure to solutions containing more than 5 gm/L concentration might lead to fatal poisoning, and exposure to less concentrated solutions may produce fatalities if there are pre-existing skin lesions.[46] Subcutaneous injection of paraquat has produced a fatality.[47] Corneal exposure to paraquat can result in ulceration and scarring.[48]

Inhalation of spray is unlikely to cause systemic toxicity because of its low vapor pressure and large spray droplets. Moreover, elegant experiments have been conducted using accurate analytic techniques for the detection of significant exposure to paraquat in respirator filter pads and clothing or dermal contamination in field workers spraying paraquat with low-beam spray machines.[22] These studies have suggested that, if paraquat is properly used, the person wearing short-sleeved and open-necked shirts would be exposed to only 0.06 per cent of the acute dermal LD_{50} dose obtained in male white rats.[49] There is some suggestion that the human pulmonary changes could result from ingestion of smaller amounts of paraquat than in the rat; nevertheless, with such low doses, considerable margin for safety exists.

Attention has been directed to possible hazards of inhalation of Mexican paraquat-sprayed marijuana smoke (a program previously supported financially by the United States). In addition, the Drug Enforcement Administration had authorized the spraying of marijuana crops in many states. It appears that significant paraquat inhalation is unlikely, owing first to the low concentration of paraquat used and second to the conversion of paraquat into bipyridines (4,4'-dipyridyl) by smoking marijuana; bipyridines are known pulmonary toxins, but their role in injury associated with paraquat-contaminated marijuana smoking is unknown.[50] The first publication on the risk of paraquat-induced lung damage from smoking contaminated marijuana estimated that the user would have to smoke 5 contaminated marijuana cigarettes (each containing 500 ppm of paraquat) every day for 1 year to lead to lung fibrosis.[51]

Smoking contaminated marijuana with its approximately 60 to 70 per cent conversion of paraquat to bipyridines appears relatively safe, although two studies suggest that there may be a potential for paraquat-induced lung damage. The first was an epidemiologic study that assessed the risk from smoking contaminated marijuana in certain areas of the United States. Paraquat was found on marijuana in concentrations ranging from 3 to 2264 ppm. The assessment was that in states contiguous to Mexico there was a higher chance than in other states of being exposed to more than 500 μg/year of paraquat in inhaled marijuana smoke, and that this constituted a significant risk for pulmonary damage.[52] The assessment of risk was based on the second study, which demonstrated focal lesions of fibrosis (1 mm at the lowest concentration of paraquat used) with direct instillation of as low as 1 pg of paraquat directly into the lung of rabbits.[53] These studies must be interpreted while realizing that no cases of paraquat lung have been encountered in heavy users of contaminated marijuana, nor from inhalation of paraquat vapor. There is still some question of the toxicity of ingested marijuana in cookies or brownies, even though the National Institute for Drug Abuse has suggested that approximately 1 pound of sprayed marijuana, ingested over a short time, would be required to constitute a lethal dose. Paraquat on marijuana is unable to be seen, tasted, smelled, or otherwise detected, except by using very sophisticated gas chromatography or radioimmunoassay. In view of its tastelessness in food, paraquat has been implicated in, or later proved to be responsible for, homicidal deaths in the United Kingdom, the United States, and Japan.

The overriding effect of paraquat is the production of pulmonary toxicity, first because paraquat is concentrated by an energy-dependent process in the lung,[54] and secondly because of the free availability of oxygen to form superoxide radicals in the highest oxygen tensions (alveoli) in the body.

Clinical Features

Acute Toxicity

Local Effects. The major acute local effects result from the caustic properties of paraquat, which produce local ulceration of epithelial surfaces. Blistering of the skin and cracking and even loss of the fingernails have been reported. Corneal ulceration has been reported after the splashing of paraquat concentrate into the eyes.[44] The major local effects, however, are seen in the mouth and esophagus after ingestion of the concentrate. These may include ulcers on the lips (Fig. 69–2) and burning and ulceration of the tongue and pharynx, even to the point of producing a pseudomembrane reminiscent of diphtheria.[55] Esophageal ulceration can proceed to esophageal perforation (Fig. 69–3), with all its attendant problems.[56] All these manifestations will be present within a few minutes to hours of ingestion, but the initial presenting symptoms may be just a burning sensation in the buccal cavity, with ulceration seen within 1 to 2 days.

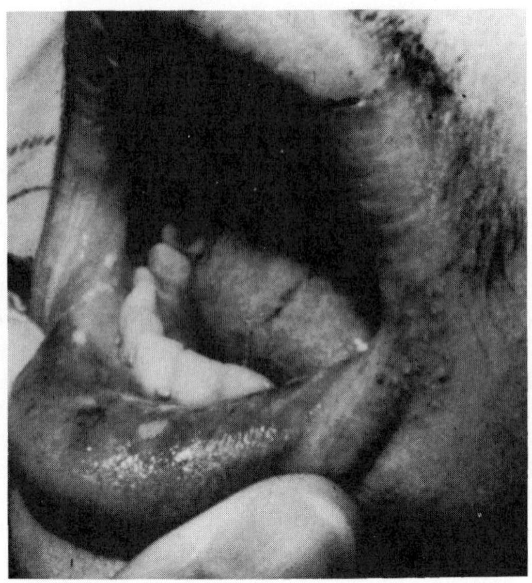

Figure 69–2. Ulceration of buccal mucosa 24 hours after paraquat ingestion.

Systemic Effects. Following massive ingestion (greater than 30 mg/kg or 50 ml of the paraquat concentrate), the patient may have pulmonary edema, cardiac failure, renal failure (which may result within hours of ingestion), hepatic failure, and also convulsions caused by central nervous system involvement. After massive ingestion, death may occur within several hours to a few days as a result of multiple organ failure.

Subacute Toxicity

Ingestion of 4 ml/kg or greater causes the aforementioned symptoms, with development of renal failure within 24 hours of ingestion in those who have consumed significant quantities; although reversible, this

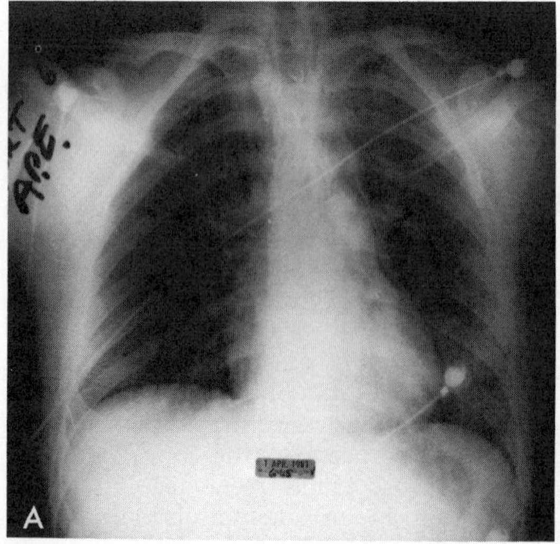

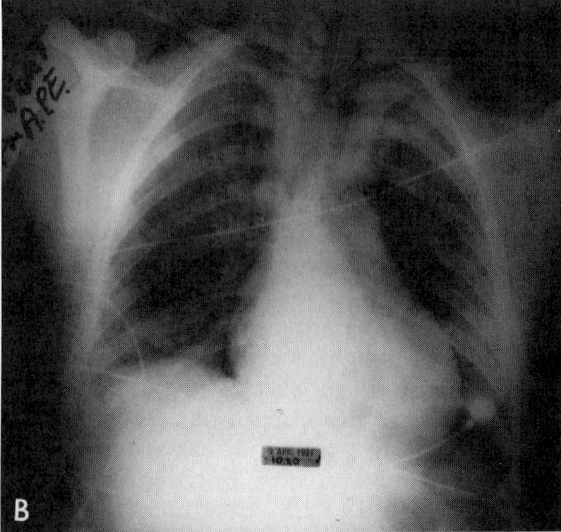

Figure 69–3. Esophageal rupture after fatal paraquat poisoning. Chest radiographs of a man 3 days after ingestion. *A,* Pneumomediastinum (radiolucent shadow, left heart border). *B,* Tracking of air into superior mediastinum 4 hours later.

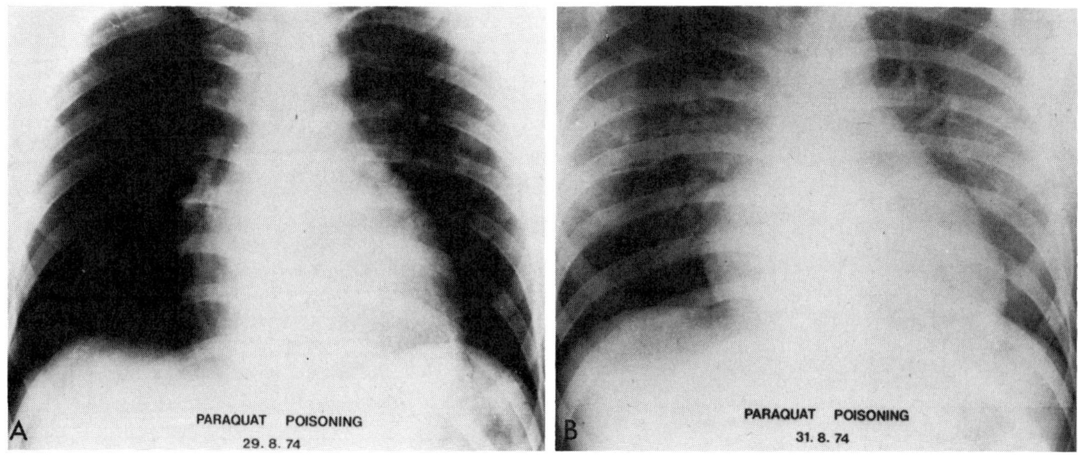

Figure 69–4. Fatal paraquat poisoning. *A*, Radiograph of an 18 year old man 6 hours after paraquat ingestion. *B*, Evidence of pulmonary fibrosis 3 days later.

impairs paraquat excretion and increases the likelihood of death. Renal failure may be manifested by proteinuria and oliguria within 2 to 6 days, with renal tubular functional changes that can produce glycosuria, aminoaciduria, and increased fractional excretion of sodium, urate, and phosphate.[57] Paraquat itself may interfere with the Jaffe reaction for the measurement of creatinine.[58] In sheep, renal tubular secretion of paraquat progressively falls as serum paraquat rises—evidence that paraquat poisons its tubular secretory mechanisms; the glomerular filtration rate, as in humans, is severely impaired.[59] It is imperative that renal function be preserved for as long as possible.

The major effect of paraquat poisoning, however, is pulmonary involvement, which develops initially with pulmonary edema 24 to 48 hours after ingestion to produce the syndrome resembling adult respiratory distress syndrome, and progresses to pulmonary fibrosis over a few days (Fig. 69–4). The respiratory involvement begins with pulmonary hemorrhage and congestion, to be followed by intra-alveolar and obliterative fibrosis, which in most cases is irreversible although there have been isolated reports of full recovery, even with severe pulmonary involvement. Hypoxemia with respiratory distress is the predominant feature, accompanied by severe agitation. Often a metabolic acidosis accompanies the respiratory problem and other manifestations of organ involvement. Myocarditis and epicardial hemorrhage may produce electrocardiographic changes with arrhythmias. Paraquat is one of the few poisons that may produce necrosis of the adrenal glands, and this must be borne in mind if the patient develops hypotension.

The pulmonary changes depend on the quantity of paraquat ingested, which is often 20 ml of concentrate (a mouthful, the volume of which may vary from 4.5 ml in the child,[60] or from 10 ml[61] to 20 ml[60] in the adult), and initially the lesions in the lung may well be reversible. Pulmonary fibrosis develops only in those patients who survive the first few days after ingestion. Although death occurs within 1 to 2 weeks, progressive pulmonary fibrosis and progressive respiratory failure may occur even up to 6 weeks after ingestion of the agent.

Laboratory Abnormalities

Paraquat Estimation. A simple urine test for paraquat, sensitive only to concentrations of 1 μg/ml or above (1 ppm), however, is to add 2 ml of a 1 per cent solution of sodium dithionite in 1 N sodium hydroxide to 10 ml of urine; a blue color indicates the presence of paraquat. Gas chromatography and high-pressure liquid chromatography can detect levels of 0.1 to 0.2 μg/ml with some accuracy.

The introduction of a radioimmunoassay has improved the detectability of paraquat, as well as giving a clearer predictability of survival, since it can detect and measure blood levels well below 0.1 μg/ml.[62] It has been demonstrated that serum levels greater than 0.2 μg/ml at 24 hours and 0.1 μg/ml at 48 hours are usually associated with a fatal outcome[63] (Fig. 69–5*A*), unless the concentrations are kept well below this level with

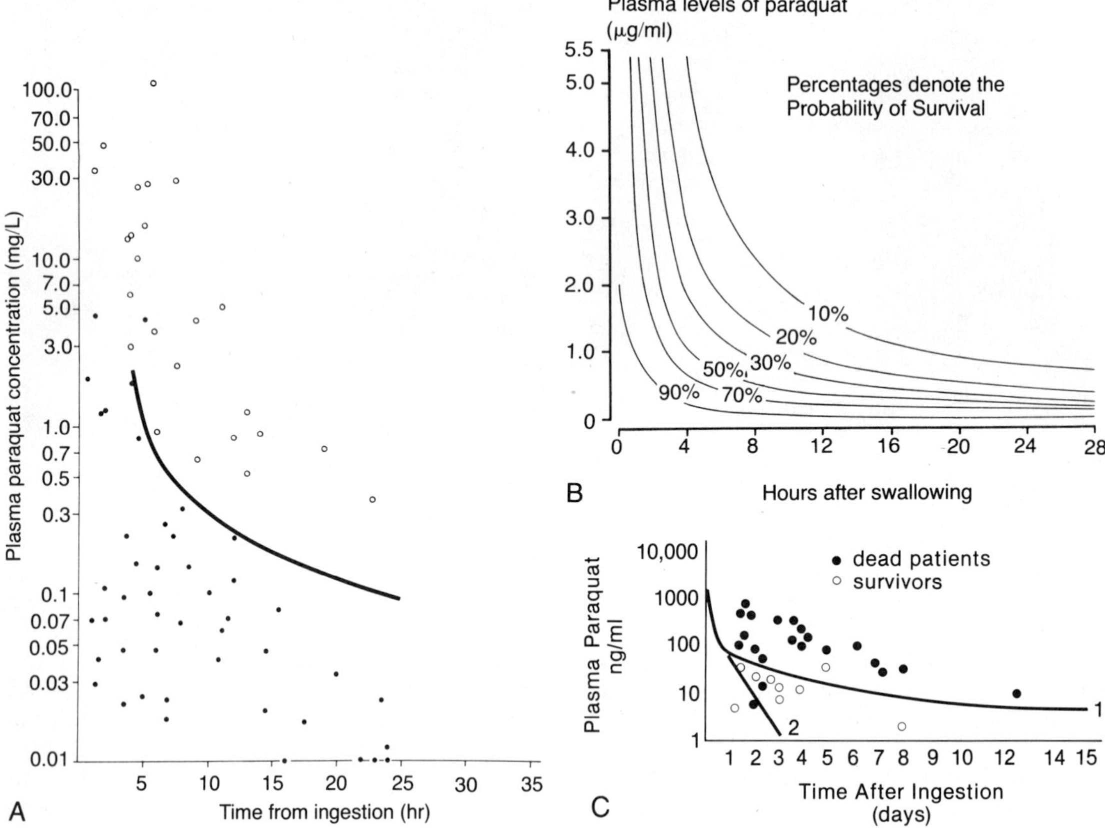

Figure 69–5. Correlation of plasma paraquat concentration and time from ingestion with survival. *A*, Analysis of raw data. *B*, Statistical probability of survival, analyzed from data in *A*. *C*, Probability of survival in late presenters.

(*A* from Proudfoot AT, Stewart MS, Levitt T, Widdop B: Paraquat poisoning: Significance of plasma paraquat concentrations. Lancet 2:330, 1979. *B* from Hart TB, Nevitt A, Whitehead A: A new statistical approach to the prognostic significance of plasma paraquat concentrations. Lancet 2:1222, 1984. *C* from Scherrman JM, Galliot M, Garnier R, Bismuth C: Intoxication aiguë par le paraquat: intérêt prognostique et thérapeutique du dosage sanguin. Toxicol Eur Res 3:141, 1983.)

treatment.[64] A more detailed analysis of blood concentration data has resulted in probability curves for survival related to time after ingestion and blood concentration or paraquat[65] (Fig. 69–5*B*). The predictability of plasma paraquat concentrations on prognosis has been confirmed,[66] extending beyond (Fig. 69–5C) the 35-hour time period of the original analysis (Fig. 69–5*A*).

In addition to detection of paraquat in urine or blood, other organ damage may be manifest, but in general toxicity may be graded by repeated evaluation of pulmonary function. Pulmonary toxicity will be manifested by pulmonary hemorrhage, edema, atelectasis, hyaline membranes, interstitial and alveolar fibrosis, and bronchial epithelial proliferation, as well as pleural effusions. Serial measurements of arterial oxygen tension will indicate a low arterial oxygen tension, as well as an increased alveolar-oxygen tension gradient (A-a/O_2), and these should all be followed in a serial fashion. Additionally, diffusion capacity for carbon monoxide (DL_{CO}), which should also be measured serially, will indicate the severity and progression of the alveolocapillary block that develops when pulmonary fibrosis ensues.[67] A recent study has suggested that the respiratory index (RI = A-aDO_2/PO_2) is a simple method to predict survival; in 51 patients with paraquat poisoning, survivors had an RI consistently less than 1.5, and nonsurvivors had an RI equal to or greater than 1.5 at any time point after ingestion[68] (even in late cases in which graphed plasma paraquat/time of ingestion fell out with the predictive graph).[63] A-aDO_2 is a measure of diffusion capacity for oxygen derived from the expression:

$$A\text{-}aDO_2 = 713 \times FiO_2 - pCO_2 - [FiO_2 + (1 - FiO_2) / R] - pO_2$$

where FiO_2 is inspired oxygen concentration (%), pCO_2 and pO_2 are arterial partial pressures of carbon dioxide and oxygen respectively (mm Hg), and R is the respiratory quotient assumed to be = 0.8.[69]

Treatment

In view of the proposed mechanisms for the production of paraquat toxicity (Fig. 69–6), it is possible at several points to interrupt the pathway for paraquat toxicity, also shown in Figure 69–6. Management is primarily directed at removing paraquat from the gastrointestinal tract,[70] increasing its excretion from blood, and, traditionally, adopting measures aimed at preventing pulmonary damage with anti-inflammatory agents and some newer drugs. Hospitalization is mandatory in all cases suspected (and confirmed by urine or plasma tests) of paraquat poisoning.

Prevention of Absorption from Gastrointestinal Tract

Recommended Treatment. Gastric lavage should be performed, using diatomaceous clays in the lavage solution. The diatomaceous earths are bentonite and Fuller's earth. Lavage must be performed cautiously in view of the ulceration of the pharynx and the esophagus, with rupture possible in the esophagus, and the recovery of paraquat may be small.[71] Bentonite can be poured only in a 6 to 7.5 per cent suspension and should be given if Fuller's earth is not available. On the other hand, Fuller's earth can be administered in a 30 per cent suspension, at which it remains pourable, along with magnesium sulfate, to produce a catharsis. Three hundred grams of Fuller's earth and 50 grams of magnesium sulfate are mixed with 1 liter of sterile water and autoclaved.[72] After lavage using 250 to 500 ml, a dosage of 250 to 500 ml is given every 2 to 4 hours for 2 or 3 days, or until paraquat cannot be detected in any biologic solution. It must be remembered that the omission of magnesium sulfate (or any other cathartic agent) will allow the absorption of water from the suspension and will produce constipation or even intestinal obstruction. If Fuller's earth is not available, activated charcoal may be employed. In fact, it has been shown that activated charcoal adsorbs paraquat as effectively as bentonite or Fuller's earth.[73–75] Recently an ion-exchange resin (Kayexalate or sodium resonium) has been demonstrated to be an effective adsorbent.[76]

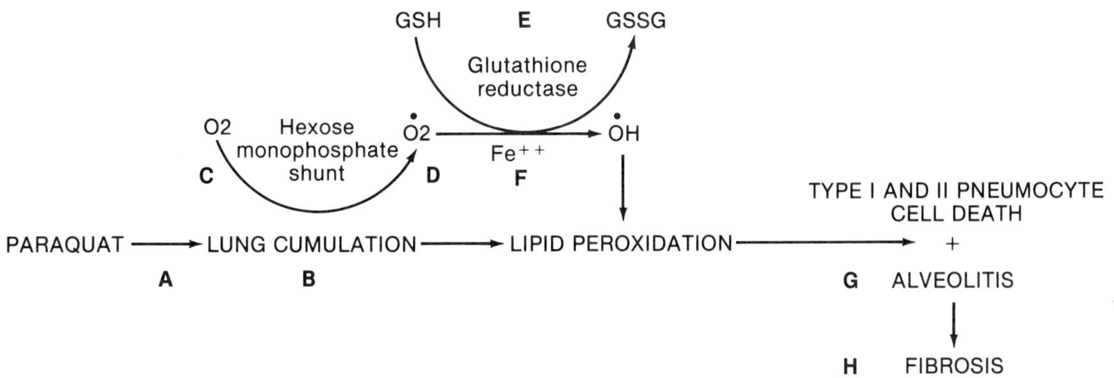

A Fuller's earth, GI decontamination, removal from blood
B Paraquat antibody Fab fragments, D-propranolol
C Low FiO_2, superoxide dismutase
D Free radical scavengers, antioxidants (vitamin E)
E Glutathione
F Deferoxamine
G Cyclophosphamide, prednisone, radiotherapy
H Antifibrotic agents

Figure 69–6. Proposed mechanisms of paraquat toxicity and therapy.

Successes with severe paraquat poisoning have been reported with total gut lavage (irrigation), using a high volume of a specially prepared salt solution through a nasogastric tube with a peristaltic pump for 3 to 4 hours.[77] The solution is that used by gastrointestinal surgeons for preparation of bowel prior to surgery, along the lines suggested by Hewitt and associates: in 1000 ml of distilled water, a warmed solution of sodium chloride, 6.14 gm; KCl, 0.75 gm; and sodium bicarbonate, 2.94 gm. This should be delivered at a rate of 75 ml/min by nasogastric tube and will produce a massive diarrhea. Additionally, it has been suggested that the addition of mannitol to Hewitt's solution will avoid the potential for the absorption of large quantities of fluid with aggravation of pulmonary edema. Okonek and colleagues have shown that this method of treatment will increase the excretion of paraquat to a very significant degree.[63, 77] The technique, however, demands constant supervision and control of electrolyte problems. Moreover, the theoretic risk of paraquat passively accompanying the fluid absorption (0.5 to 1 L) with gut lavage has led some to recommend against gut lavage.[71]

Increasing Excretion from the Blood

Forced diuresis was initially popular in the management of patients with paraquat poisoning. It was felt that this would prevent the renal tubular reabsorption and increase the total renal clearance of paraquat, as well as reduce the concentration of paraquat in the renal tubular lumen. In the rat, paraquat is filtered freely by the rat kidney, and a small, unfiltered component is actively secreted by the tubules.[79] However, at 24 hours after oral doses the clearance of inulin, para-amino hippurate, organic bases, and the bipyridyl itself is reduced. A reduction of para-amino hippurate (PAH) clearance (a marker of renal plasma flow)[80] suggests that bipyridyls may themselves cause profound changes in renal hemodynamics as a result of fluid redistribution from the gastrointestinal tract, and so on.

Therefore, it is unlikely that forced diuresis will increase the elimination of paraquat substantially, since it is not reabsorbed by the tubules. Moreover, the technique is likely to be effective only within the first 24 hours after ingestion, during the period of maximal excretion of urinary paraquat; the onset of renal failure will make this method unlikely to be of any effect. Careful attention must be paid to the maintenance of renal function in the early stages of paraquat poisoning, since ensuing renal failure would allow accumulation of paraquat in other tissues, particularly the lung.

Both peritoneal dialysis and hemodialysis have been suggested as measures for removing paraquat from blood. Peritoneal dialysis seems to be ineffective and is not recommended, since only small amounts of paraquat are removed into the peritoneal dialysate. Hemodialysis or hemoperfusion, on the other hand, has been associated with successful outcomes in paraquat-poisoned patients, usually when the paraquat level or ingested dose has been moderate to low.[64, 77, 81–83] Based on simple measurements of paraquat clearance across extracorporeal devices, it appears that charcoal hemoperfusion is more effective than hemodialysis in removing paraquat, at the same blood levels and blood flow rate through the devices. (For a fuller description of hemoperfusion and hemodialysis, see Chapter 8). Hemodialysis, alone or in combination with hemoperfusion, has been criticized as "ineffective"[84, 85] or a "failure,"[86] whereas continuous arteriovenous hemofiltration, following repeated hemoperfusion, was not associated with a successful clinical outcome although successful in maintaining low plasma paraquat concentrations.[87]

Charcoal hemoperfusion was initially suggested by Maini and Winchester for the treatment of human paraquat poisoning after experiments in dogs had demonstrated that, in comparison with controls, substantial reduction of plasma paraquat levels could be achieved with either charcoal hemoperfusion or Zerolit-221 resin hemoperfusion (an experimental ion-exchange resin).[88] Charcoal hemoperfusion in dogs treated within 12 hours after poisoning with paraquat appeared to reduce the mortality,[89] but its use in severely poisoned humans was not associated with success.[86, 87, 90, 91] However, recent reports of prolonged hemoperfusion or hemodialysis, with almost continuous treatment periods of up to 2 to 3 weeks after an ingestion,[64, 77, 92] have indicated successful clinical outcomes in two patients in whom the plasma paraquat concentration was kept below the "critical borderline" of 0.1 μg/ml,[92] and in others in whom the plasma level indicated a moderate to poor prognosis (Fig. 69–7).[64] Paraquat antibodies immobilized on agarose-polyacrolein spheres enclosed in hemoperfusion devices have been shown experimentally to bind paraquat avidly from animal blood passing through the devices.[93] Plasmapheresis also has been advocated, but further studies are needed before its effectiveness is proved.

Summary Statement. The recommended regimen for increased paraquat excretion from the blood at this point is hemoperfusion or hemodialysis when necessary. In an analysis of 42 patients treated by hemoperfusion or hemodialysis, Hampson and Pond drew attention to the fact that there were no survivors after treatment if the plasma paraquat concentration was greater than 3 mg/L, regardless of time after ingestion.[86] As do others,[14, 94] they suggest that hemoperfusion or hemodialysis is likely to benefit those with a probability of survival of between 20 and 70 per cent (see Fig. 69–5*B*), and within the first 10 to 12 hours after ingestion, since paraquat is rapidly distributed to tissues in the first few hours after ingestion.[95]

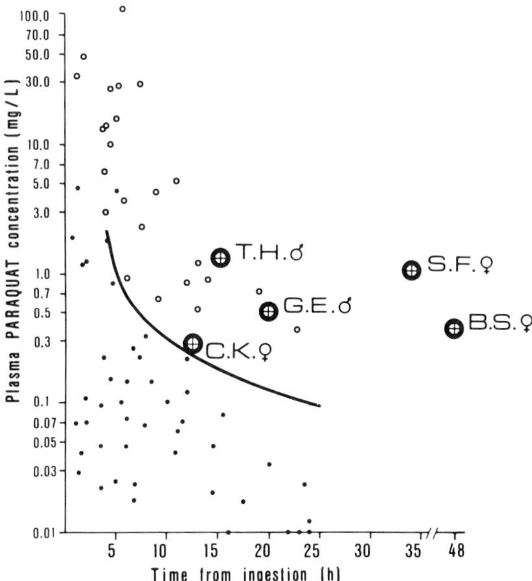

Figure 69–7. Patients (TH, SF, GE, BS, CK) who survived potentially fatal paraquat concentrations after intensive hemoperfusion/hemodialysis. (Reprinted with permission from Okonek S, Weileman LS, Majdanzic J, Setyadharma H, Reinecke HJ, Baldamus C, Lohmann J, Bonzel KE, Thon T: Successful treatment of paraquat poisoning. Activated charcoal per os and continuous "hemoperfusion." J Toxicol Clin Toxicol *19*:807, 1982. Data from Figure 69–5*A* drawn for comparison.)

Prevention of Pulmonary Damage

Paraquat accumulates selectively in lung tissue by an energy-dependent process,[54] and the main efforts of therapeutic intervention have been to prevent this cumulation. The lung changes are similar to the direct toxicity of high alveolar oxygen tension as seen with lung changes in oxygen toxicity. In addition to the measures previously outlined, prevention of superoxide radical formation may be accomplished by employing low-oxygen breathing mixtures with production of therapeutic hypoxemia. It has been shown in animals that paraquat-poisoned rats allowed to breathe normal room air die in a far higher and more significant number than those allowed to breathe low-oxygen mixtures.[96–98] Hyperoxia (100 per cent oxygen) enhances the toxicity of paraquat in rats, compared with those breathing room air.[99] Oxygen administration to patients poisoned with paraquat appears to accelerate the lung changes. Use of low FiO_2 mixtures requires positive end-expiratory pressure and continuous positive pressure breathing, and it is suggested that an inspired oxygen concentration of greater than 21 per cent should be used only when arterial oxygen pressure falls below 40 mm Hg. Although the value of low inspired oxygen has not been established in humans, putative evidence suggests that this should be employed.[100] Other methods of reducing oxygen toxicity, such as cardiopulmonary bypass, also have been proposed,[101] although, again, this method has not been proved.

Immunosuppression

Traditionally, corticosteroids have been used, in addition to these measures, although they have not been proved to be effective. Their role has recently been brought into question. It has been shown, in sheep, that methylprednisolone given before or after paraquat reduces the increase in lymph flow and prostacyclin, but not thromboxane B_2, accumulation in lymph,[102] nor the increase in lung neutrophils induced by the agent alone.[103] Moreover, in rabbits, paraquat pneumonitis was not prevented with prednisone under carefully controlled conditions.[104] Prostanoids are known suppressors of inflammatory reactions, but injections of prostaglandin E_1 have been shown to increase the early respiratory failure–induced mortality.[105]

Other agents, such as azathioprine, beclomethasone, bleomycin, fluorouracil, and fibrinolytic agents (potassium aminobenzoate) have been used without clear-cut benefit being shown.

A great deal of attention has been paid to the use of radiotherapy in the prevention and treatment of paraquat-induced pulmonary fibrosis, following a case report by Webb and associates[106] of successful reversal of pulmonary damage (in a patient who was not improving on cyclophosphamide and methylprednisolone therapy) after radiotherapy. (The patient ingested 3 gm; the plasma paraquat concentration was 80 μg/L at 36 hours.) A further successful outcome was seen in a paraquat-poisoned patient (plasma paraquat concentration of 2.1 mg/L 7.5 hours after ingestion), given an intensive regimen, including hemoperfusion, and 1125 rads to each lung beginning on day 3.[107] More extensive studies of single-dose radiation at different times after paraquat administration in mice have not confirmed that radiotherapy has any benefit on paraquat-induced pulmonary injury.[108] One patient more intoxicated (the patient ingested 10 to 20 gm; the plasma paraquat concentration was 120 μg/L at 36 hours) than the case of Webb and colleagues[106] and five others (four in a follow-up series from Webb's group,[109] with toxic paraquat concentrations, and one in Taiwan,[110] for whom no plasma paraquat data were given) failed to respond to radiation and succumbed.[111] Dextro-propranolol has been used to displace paraquat from lung, in a manner similar to imipramine displacement from isolated perfused rat lungs with chlorpromazine.[112] It has generally been given concomitant with the enzyme superoxide dismutase, and no clear-cut results have been forthcoming. It is possible that dextro-propranolol was infused too late in the course of paraquat poisoning, when lung damage had already occurred; similarly, the same situation exists with the enzyme superoxide dismutase. Superoxide dismutase reverses the formation of superoxide radicals and has been used in several clinical studies with both aerosol and intravenous administration, all without benefit.[57, 113–115]

Cyclophosphamide combined with high dose dexamethasone has been used. Addo and Poon-King reported a 72 per cent survival in 72 patients treated with no increment in oxygen inhalation, forced diuresis, gut decontamination, and dexamethasone and cyclophosphamide intravenously.[116] It was subsequently pointed out that of the 25 patients in whom plasma paraquat concentrations were measured, 18 had high concentrations and 12 died; of the 6 survivors, the chance of survival was 30 per cent,[65] and controlled clinical trials would be necessary to confirm these results.[117, 118]

Lung Transplantation

Lung transplantation in four patients[67, 119–121] has not been entirely successful; when blood levels of paraquat were still high, patients have developed respiratory failure with lung histology consistent with either rejection or paraquat toxicity.[67, 119] Serial lung transplant in one patient resulted in a successful transplant (the first developed paraquat toxicity), but the patient was ventilator dependent due to progressive toxic myopathy (a new feature of paraquat toxicity), and eventually died from bronchopneumonia.[120] The patient reported by Kamholz and associates had a successful transplant but died from complications arising from a ruptured bronchial stump.[121]

Immunotherapy

Monoclonal and polyclonal antibodies to paraquat can be manufactured. Plasma paraquat concentrations rise, in test animals compared with controls, after Fab antibody fragment administration, whether given before,[122] or after[123] paraquat administration. Specific antibodies have been shown to bind paraquat in vitro and to prevent uptake of paraquat into lung slices by pretreatment of the incubation media. However, pretreatment, or treatment after exposure to paraquat, does not influence displacement of paraquat from lung tissue.[124] Moreover, 100-mg monoclonal antibody pretreatment did not prevent mice from paraquat toxicity after an LD_{100} dose 17 hours later, and the investigators predicted that a 100- to 200-gm Fab fragment antibody dose would be required for an adult human, an amount beyond production capabilities.[125] It thus appears that immunotherapy is of limited value in treating paraquat poisoning.

Summary and Conclusions

Ingestion of paraquat concentrate is almost always associated with a fatal outcome, but this should not detract from intensive management of such poisoned patients, since occasional patients, even after massive ingestion with pulmonary involvement, have fully recovered. The mechanisms producing paraquat lung toxicity have been partially elucidated and have given rise to the treatment regimens as outlined in this chapter, with the additional measures required to reduce blood levels below those associated with a fatal outcome. In this regard, intensive, almost continuous hemoperfusion or hemodialysis is recommended, especially within the first few hours after ingestion; additionally, lower inspired oxygen therapy should be employed. The other immunosuppressive and immunotherapy regimens outlined will require further study, until their efficacy is demonstrated.

Because of its dramatic nature, paraquat poisoning often arouses press comment on the availability of the agent. As with many chemicals, however, the overriding public health issue is to insure the proper labeling of containers holding paraquat, not to decant it into soft drink bottles, and to make sure that the compound is not likely to arouse children's interest. Moreover, the unauthorized use of small quantities of concentrate by those who take it home from authorized agricultural depots should be strongly discouraged. Only improper use of the paraquat concentrate results in accidental or suicidal poisoning. Poison information on paraquat can be obtained in the United States from Imperial Chemical Industries (ICI Americas) at 1-800-327-8633, and in the United Kingdom from Imperial Chemical Industries (062-558-2711).

DIQUAT

Diquat (1,1-ethylene-2,2,bipyridylium), closely related to paraquat, exerts the same activity as a herbicide in photosynthesizing plants. The lung is most severely damaged in paraquat toxicity, but there is no histologic evidence of lung damage in animals following diquat administration. Diquat produces more gastrointestinal disturbances, more renal effects, and less pulmonary toxicity than does paraquat. It appears not to accumulate selectively in any organ, except perhaps the kidney, in which event subsequent renal failure is more common. Apparently diquat is reduced by a different electron-transferring agent than paraquat or even morfamquat.[2] Fortunately, diquat is usually ingested in a much lower concentration (see Table 69–1), and it is usually admixed with low concentrations of paraquat. Although it has been stated that lung toxicity with diquat is less than that with paraquat, animal experiments have suggested that in a hyperoxic environment diquat may well be equal to paraquat in its pulmonary toxicity.[99] It has been suggested that diquat as well as paraquat exerts a greater effect on gastrointestinal water content, which can produce hemoconcentration and changes in water distribution so that renal failure ensues.[126] For diquat poisoning, the absence of changes in histology at necropsy in animals may be explained by its greater effect on fluid redistribution.[3] Fluid redistribution, but also cerebral hemorrhage, may be the major determinants of a fatal outcome in diquat poisoning.[127]

Treatment

Treatment is identical to that for paraquat, with removal of diquat from the gastrointestinal tract with adsorbent catharsis or gut lavage or both. Hemoperfusion is more effective than hemodialysis for removal of diquat, but, as renal failure is of prime concern, it may be necessary to employ hemodialysis early in the course of diquat poisoning.

MORFAMQUAT

Morfamquat has found less use than the other two bipyridyls, paraquat and diquat, but can produce mammalian toxicity. Studies by Conning and associates showed that rats fed morfamquat developed renal damage, whereas diquat was the only one of the three bipyridyls that produced bilateral cataracts.[128] No human or animal toxicity has been reported with morfamquat. Its use is limited in the United Kingdom, but the general recommendation can be made that treatment should be along the lines proposed for paraquat poisoning.

References

1. Harley JB, Grinspan S, Root RK: Paraquat suicide in a young woman: Results of therapy directed against the superoxide radical. Yale J Biol Med *50*:481, 1977.

2. Baldwin RC, Past A, MacGregor JT, Hine CH: The rates of radical formation from the dipyridylium herbicides paraquat, diquat and morfamquat in homogenates of rat lung, kidney and liver: An inhibitory effect of carbon monoxide. Toxicol Appl Pharmacol *32*:298, 1975.
3. Burk RF, Lawrence RA, Lane JM: Liver necrosis and lipid peroxidation in the rat as the result of paraquat and diquat administration. J Clin Invest *65*:1024, 1980.
4. Montgomery MR: Paraquat toxicity and pulmonary superoxide dismutase: An enzymic deficiency of lung microsomes. Res Comm Chem Pathol Pharmacol *16*:155, 1977.
5. Hollinger MA, Chvapil M: Effect of paraquat on rat lung prolyl hydroxylase. Res Comm Chem Pathol Pharmacol *16*:159, 1977.
6. Sandy MS, Moldeus P, Ross D, Smith MT: Role of redox cycling and lipid peroxidation in bipyridyl herbicide cytotoxicity. Studies with a compromised isolated hepatocyte model system. Biochem Pharmacol *35*:3095, 1986.
7. Kramer K, Rademaker B, Rozendal WH, Timmerman H, Bast A: Influence of lipid peroxidation on beta-adrenoceptors. FEBS Lett *198*:80, 1986.
8. Fridovich I: Biological effects of the superoxide radical. Arch Biochem Biophys *247*:1, 1986.
9. Krall J, Bagley AC, Mullenbach GT, Hallewell RA, Lynch RE: Superoxide mediates the toxicity of paraquat for cultured mammalian cells. J Biol Chem *263*:1910, 1988.
10. Bagley AC, Krall J, Lynch RA: Superoxide mediates the toxicity of paraquat for Chinese hamster ovary cells. Proc Natl Acad Sci USA *83*:3189, 1986.
11. Ruch RJ, Klaunig JE: Inhibition of mouse hepatocyte intercellular communication by paraquat-generated free oxygen radicals. Toxicol Appl Pharmacol *94*:427, 1988.
12. Watanabe N, Shiki Y, Morisaki N, Saito Y, Yoshida S: Cytotoxic effects of paraquat and inhibition of them by vitamin E. Biochim Biophys Acta *883*:420, 1986.
13. Yasaka T, Okudaira K, Fijito H, Masumoto J, Ohya I, Miyamoto Y: Further studies of lipid peroxidation in human paraquat poisoning. Arch Intern Med *146*:681, 1986.
14. Smith LL: Mechanisms of paraquat toxicity in lung and its relevance to treatment. Hum Toxicol *6*:31, 1987.
15. Ogino T, Awai M: Lipid peroxidation and tissue injury by ferric citrate in paraquat-intoxicated mice. Biochim Biophys Acta *958*:388, 1988.
16. Korbashi P, Kohen R, Katzhendler J, Chevion M: Iron mediates paraquat toxicity in *Escherichia coli*. J Biol Chem *261*:12472, 1986.
17. van Asbeck BS, Hillen FC, Boonen HC, de Jong Y, Dormans JA, van der Wal NA, Marx JJ, Sangster B: Continuous intravenous infusion of deferoxamine reduces mortality by paraquat in vitamin E–deficient rats. Am Rev Respir Dis *139*:769, 1989.
18. Osheroff MR, Schaich MK, Drew RT, Borg DC: Failure of desferrioxamine to modify the toxicity of paraquat in rats. J Free Rad Biol Med *1*:71, 1985.
19. Mercurio SD, Combs GF Jr: Selenium-dependent glutathione peroxidase inhibitors increase toxicity of prooxidant compounds in chicks. J Nutr *116*:1726, 1986.
20. Hagen TM, Brown LA, Jones DP: Protection against paraquat-induced injury by exogenous GSH in pulmonary alveolar type II cells. Biochem Pharmacol *35*:4537, 1986.
21. Fairshter RD, Vaziri ND, Crosby SA, Rosario L, Toohey JA, Ulrich TR: Effect of dimethylthiourea on plasma paraquat concentrations. Toxicology *50*:47, 1988.
22. Staiff DC, Comer SW, Armstrong JR, Wolfe HR: Exposure to the herbicide, paraquat. Bull Environ Contam Toxicol *14*:334, 1975.
23. Howard JK: Paraquat: A review of worker exposure in normal usage. J Soc Occup Med *30*:6, 1980.
24. Swan AAB: Exposure of spray operators to paraquat. Br J Industr Med *26*:322, 1969.
25. Howard JK: A clinical survey of paraquat formulation workers. Br J Industr Med *36*:220, 1979.
26. Chester G, Woollen BH: Studies of the occupational exposure of Malaysian plantation workers to paraquat. Br J Industr Med *38*:23, 1981.
27. Howard JK, Sabapathy NN, Whitehead PA: A study of the health of Malaysian plantation workers with particular reference to paraquat spraymen. Br J Industr Med *38*:110, 1981.
28. Howard JK: The myth of paraquat inhalation as a route for human poisoning. J Toxicol Clin Toxicol *20*:191, 1983.
29. McElligott TF: The dermal toxicity of paraquat: Differences due to techniques of application. Toxicol Appl Pharmacol *21*:361, 1972.
30. Grissom RE Jr, Brownie C, Guthrie FE: Dermal absorption of pesticides in mice. Pesticide Biochem Physiol *24*:119, 1985.
31. Scott RC, Walker M, Dugard PH: A comparison of the in vitro permeability properties of human and some laboratory animal skins. Int J Cosmetic Sci *8*:189, 1986.
32. Wester RC, Maibach HI, Bucks DAW, Aufrere MB: In vivo percutaneous absorption of paraquat from hand, leg, and forearm of humans. J Toxicol Environ Health *14*:759, 1984.
33. Maibach HI, Feldmann R: Systemic absorption of pesticides through the skin of man. Occupational Exposure to Pesticides, report to the Federal Working Group on Pest Management from the task group. 1974, p 120.
34. Fitzgerald GR, Barniville G, Black J, Silke B, Carmody M, O'Dwyer WF: Paraquat poisoning in agricultural workers. Irish Med Assoc J *71*:336, 1978.
35. Ongum VL, Owor R, Tomusanga ET: Paraquat (Gramoxone) used as a pediculocide. *In* Bagshawe AE, Maina G, Magela EN (eds): Use and Abuse of Drugs and Chemicals in Tropical Africa. East African Literature Bureau, 1974, p 229.
36. Binns CW: A deadly cure for lice—a case of paraquat poisoning. Papua New Guinea Med J *19*:105, 1976.
37. Waight JJJ: Fatal percutaneous paraquat poisoning. JAMA *242*:472, 1979.
38. Wohlfahrt D: Fatal paraquat poisonings after skin absorption. Med J Aust *6*:512, 1982.
39. McDonagh BJ, Martin J: Paraquat poisoning in children. Arch Dis Child *45*:425, 1970.
40. Tungsanga K, Israsena S, Chuslip S, Sitprija V: Paraquat poisoning: Evidence of systemic toxicity after dermal exposure. Postgrad Med J *59*:338, 1983.

41. Athanaselis S, Qammaz S, Alevisopoulos G, Koutselinis A: Percutaneous paraquat intoxication. J Toxicol Cut Ocular Toxicol *2*:3, 1983.
42. Jaros F: Acute percutaneous paraquat absorption. Lancet *1*:275, 1978.
43. Newhouse M, McEvoy D, Rosenthal D: Percutaneous paraquat absorption. Arch Dermatol *114*:1516, 1978.
44. Levin PJ, Klaff LJ, Rose AG, Ferguson AD: Pulmonary effects of contact exposure to paraquat: A clinical and experimental study. Thorax *34*:150, 1979.
45. Bismuth C, Garnier R, Dally S, Fournier PE, Scherrman JM: Prognosis and treatment of paraquat poisoning: A review of 28 cases. J Toxicol Clin Toxicol *19*:461, 1982.
46. Smith JG: Paraquat poisoning by skin absorption: A review. Hum Toxicol *7*:15, 1988.
47. Almog C, Tal E: Death from paraquat after subcutaneous injection. Br Med J *3*:721, 1967.
48. Cant JS, Lewis DRH: Ocular damage due to paraquat and diquat. Br Med J *3*:59, 1968.
49. Kimbrough RD, Gaines TB: Toxicity of paraquat to rats and its effect on rat lung. Toxicol Appl Pharmacol *17*:679, 1970.
50. Groce DF, Kimbrough RD: Acute and subacute toxicity in Sherman strain rats exposed to 4,4′- and 2,2′-dipyridyl. J Toxicol Environ Health *10*:363, 1982.
51. Chemistry and toxicology of paraquat-contaminated marijuana. Final report to the National Institutes for Drug Abuse, June 1978.
52. Landrigan PJ, Powell KE, James LM: Paraquat and marijuana: Epidemiologic risk assessment. Am J Public Health *73*:784, 1983.
53. Zavala DC, Rhodes ML: An effect of paraquat on the lungs of rabbits: Its implications for smoking marihuana. Chest *74*:418, 1978.
54. Rose MS, Smith LL, Wyatt I: Evidence for an energy-dependent accumulation of paraquat into rat lung. Nature *252*:315, 1974.
55. Stephens DS, Walker DH, Schaffner W, Kaplowitz LG, Brashear R, Roberts R, Spickard WA: Pseudodiphtheria: Prominent pharyngeal membrane associated with fatal paraquat ingestion. Ann Intern Med *94*:202, 1981.
56. Ackrill P, Hasleton PS, Ralston AJ: Oesophageal perforation due to paraquat. Br Med J *2*:1252, 1978.
57. Vaziri ND, Ness RL, Fairshter RD, Smith WR, Rosen SM: Nephrotoxicity of paraquat in man. Arch Intern Med *139*:172, 1979.
58. Webb DB, Davies CG: Paraquat poisoning and kidney function tests. Lancet *1*:1424, 1981.
59. Webb DB: Nephrotoxicity of paraquat in the sheep and the associated reduction in paraquat secretion. Toxicol Appl Pharmacol *68*:282, 1983.
60. Jones DV, Work CE: Volume of a swallow. Am J Dis Child *102*:427, 1961.
61. Fisher HK, Humphries M, Bails R: Paraquat poisoning: Recovery from renal and pulmonary damage. Ann Intern Med *75*:731, 1971.
62. Levitt T: Determination of paraquat in clinical practice using radioimmunoassay. Proc Anal Div Chem Soc *16*:72, 1979.
63. Proudfoot AT, Stewart MS, Levitt T, Widdop B: Paraquat poisoning: Significance of plasma paraquat concentrations. Lancet *2*:330, 1979.
64. Okonek S, Weileman LS, Majdanzic J, Setyadharma H, Reinecke HJ, Baldamus C, Lohmann J, Bonzel KE, Thon T: Successful treatment of paraquat poisoning. Activated charcoal per os and continuous "hemoperfusion." J Toxicol Clin Toxicol *19*:807, 1982.
65. Hart TB, Nevitt A, Whitehead A: A new statistical approach to the prognostic significance of plasma paraquat concentrations. Lancet *2*:1222, 1984.
66. Schermann JM, Galliott M, Garnier R, Bismuth C: Acute paraquat poisoning: Prognostic significance and therapeutical interest of blood assay. Toxicol Eur Res *3*:141, 1983.
67. Cooke NJ, Flenley DC, Matthew H: Paraquat poisoning: Serial studies of lung function. Q J Med *42*:683, 1973.
68. Suzuki K, Takasu N, Arita S, Maenosono A, Ishimatsu S, Nishima M, Tanaka S, Kohama A: A new method for predicting the outcome and survival period in paraquat poisoning. Hum Toxicol *8*:31, 1989.
69. Goldfarb MS, Ciurej TF, McAslan TC, Sacco WJ, Weinstein MA, Cowley RA: Tracking respiratory therapy in the trauma patient. Am J Surg *129*:255, 1975.
70. Smith LL, Wright A, Wyatt I, Rose MS: Effective treatment for paraquat poisoning in rats and its relevance to treatment of paraquat in man. Br Med J *4*:569, 1974.
71. Meredith TJ, Vale JA: Treatment of paraquat poisoning in man: Methods to prevent absorption. Hum Toxicol *6*:49, 1987.
72. Vale JA, Meredith TJ: Paraquat poisoning. *In* Vale JA, Meredith TJ (eds): Poisoning; Diagnosis and Treatment. London, Update Books, 1981, p 135.
73. Okonek S, Setyadhama H, Burchert A, Krienke EG: Activated charcoal is as effective as Fuller's earth or bentonite in paraquat poisoning. Klin Wschr *60*:207, 1982.
74. Gaudrealt JP, Friedman PA, Lovejoy FH: Efficacy of activated-charcoal and magnesium citrate in the treatment of oral paraquat intoxication. Ann Emerg Med *14*:123, 1985.
75. Gaudrealt JP, Friedman PA, Lovejoy FH: Activated charcoal binding capacity to paraquat in vitro and in vivo. Vet Hum Toxicol *25*:275, 1983.
76. Yamashita M, Naito T, Takagi S: The effectiveness of a cation resin (Kayexalate) as an adsorbent of paraquat; Experimental and clinical studies. Hum Toxicol *6*:89, 1987.
77. Okonek S, Hofmann A, Hennigsen B: Efficacy of gut lavage, haemodialysis in the therapy of paraquat or diquat intoxication. Arch Toxicol *36*:43, 1976.
78. Hewitt J, Reeve J, Rigby J: Whole-gut irrigation in preparation for large bowel surgery. Lancet *2*:337, 1973.
79. Lock EA: The effect of paraquat and diquat on renal function in the rat. Toxicol Appl Pharmacol *48*:327, 1979.
80. DeWardener HE: The Kidney. London, J&A Churchill, 1963.
81. Hendy MS, Williams PS, Ackrill P: Recovery from severe pulmonary damage due to paraquat administered intravenously and orally. Thorax *39*:874, 1984.
82. Hoffman S, Jedeikin R, Korzetzs Z, Shapiro A-L, Kaplan R, Bernheim J: Successful management of severe paraquat poisoning. Chest *84*:107, 1983.

83. Tabei K, Asano Y, Hosoda S: Efficacy of charcoal hemoperfusion in paraquat poisoning. Artif Organs *6*:37, 1982.
84. Mascie-Taylor BH, Thompson J, Davison AM: Haemoperfusion ineffective for paraquat removal in life threatening paraquat poisoning. Lancet *1*:1376, 1983.
85. Van De Vyver FL, Giuliano RA, Paulus J, Verpooten GA, Framke JP, De Zeeuw RA, Van Gaal LF, De Broe ME: Hemoperfusion-hemodialysis ineffective for paraquat removal in life-threatening poisoning? J Toxicol Clin Toxicol *23*:117, 1985.
86. Hampson EC, Pond SM: Failure of haemoperfusion and haemodialysis to prevent death in paraquat poisoning. A retrospective review of 42 patients. Med Toxicol Adverse Drug Exp *3*:64, 1988.
87. Pond SM, Johnston SC, Schoof DD, Hampson EC, Bowles M, Wright DM, Petrie JJ: Repeated hemoperfusion and continuous arteriovenous hemofiltration in a paraquat poisoned patient. J Toxicol Clin Toxicol *25*:305, 1987.
88. Maini R, Winchester JF: Removal of paraquat from blood by haemoperfusion over sorbent materials. Br Med J *3*:281, 1975.
89. Widdop B, Medd RK, Braithwaite RA, Vale JA: Haemoperfusion in the treatment of paraquat poisoning. Proc Eur Soc Artif Organs *2*:244, 1975.
90. Gelfand MC, Winchester JF, Knepshield JH, Hanson KM, Cohan SL, Strauch BS, Geoly KL, Kennedy AC. Schreiner GE: Treatment of severe drug overdosage with charcoal hemoperfusion. Trans Am Soc Artif Intern Organs *23*:599, 1977.
91. Vale JA, Crome P, Volans GN, Widdop B, Goulding R: The treatment of paraquat poisoning using oral sorbents and charcoal haemoperfusion. Acta Pharmacol Toxicol (Suppl II) *41*:109, 1977.
92. Okonek S, Baldamus CA, Hofmann A, Schuster CJ, Bechstein PB, Zoller B: Two survivors of severe paraquat intoxication by "continuous hemoperfusion." Klin Wschr *57*:957, 1979.
93. Azhari R, Margel S, Labes A, Haviv Y: Specific removal of paraquat by hemoperfusion through antiparaquat conjugated agarose-polyacrylein microsphere beads. J Biomed Mater Res *21*:25, 1987.
94. Proudfoot AT, Prescott LF, Jarvie DR: Haemodialysis for paraquat poisoning. Hum Toxicol *6*:69, 1987.
95. Bismuth C, Scherrmann JM, Garnier R, Baud FJ, Pontal PG: Elimination of paraquat. Hum Toxicol *6*:63, 1987.
96. Fisher HK, Clements JA, Wright RR: Enhancement of oxygen toxicity by the herbicide paraquat. Am Rev Respir Dis *107*:246, 1973.
97. Douze JMC, Van Dijk A, Gimbrere JSF, van Heijst ANP, Maes R, Rauws AG: Intensive therapy after paraquat intoxication. Intens Med *11*:241, 1974.
98. Rhodes ML, Zavala DC, Brown D: Hypoxic protection in paraquat poisoning. Lab Invest *5*:496, 1976.
99. Kehrer JP, Haschek WM, Witschi H: The influence of hyperoxia on the acute toxicity of paraquat and diquat. Drug Chem Toxicol *2*:397, 1979.
100. Chollet A, Muszynzky J, Bismuth C, Pham J, El Khouly M, Surugue R: L'hypooxygenation dans l'intoxication par le paraquat a propos de six cas. Toxicol Eur Res *5*:71, 1983.
101. Fisher HK: Two experiments not previously described: (1) non-human, and (2) human based on some previous work. *In* Fletcher K (ed): Clinical Aspects of Paraquat Poisoning. London, Imperial Chemical Industries, 1975, p 74.
102. Kitazawa K, Kobayashi T, Shibamoto T, Hirai K: Effects of methylprednisolone on acute lung paraquat toxicity in sheep. Am Rev Respir Dis *137*:173, 1988.
103. Shibamoto T, Kobayashi T: Acute effect of paraquat on lung fluid balance and prostanoid production in awake sheep. Am Rev Respir Dis *134*:1252, 1986.
104. Seidenfeld JJ: Steroid pretreatment does not prevent paraquat pneumonitis in rabbits. Am J Med Sci *289*:51, 1985.
105. Williams JH Jr, Fairshter RD, Ulich TR, Crosby S, Chen M, Rosario L, Vaziri ND: Adverse effects of (15S)-15-methyl-prostaglandin E_1 in normal and paraquat-exposed rats. Toxicol Appl Pharmacol *92*:330, 1988.
106. Webb DB, Willams MV, Davies BH, James KW: Resolution after radiotherapy of severe pulmonary damage due to paraquat poisoning. Br Med J *288*:1259, 1984.
107. Talbot AR, Barnes MR, Ting RS: Early radiotherapy in treatment of paraquat poisoning. Br J Radiol *61*:405, 1988.
108. Parkins CS, Fowler JF: A cautionary note on the resolution of paraquat lung damage after radiotherapy. Br J Radiol *58*:1137, 1985.
109. Williams MV, Webb DB: Paraquat lung: Is there a role for radiotherapy? Hum Toxicol *6*:7, 1987.
110. Chou MH, Yeh JC, Kuo HT, Chung CH: Low dose radiotherapy of pulmonary complications resulting from paraquat intoxication. J Formosan Med Assoc *86*:452, 1987.
111. Bloodworth LL, Kershaw JB, Stevens PE, Alcock CJ, Rainford DJ: Failure of radiotherapy to reverse progressive pulmonary fibrosis caused by paraquat. Br J Radiol *59*:1037, 1986.
112. Junod AF: Accumulation of ^{14}C-imipramine in isolated perfused rat lungs. J Pharmacol Exp Ther *183*:182, 1972.
113. Connolly ME, Davies DS, Draffan GH, Bennett PN, Dollery CT: Clinical experience with paraquat poisoning. *In* Fletcher K (ed): Clinical Aspects of Paraquat Poisoning. London, Imperial Chemical Industries, 1975, p 1.
114. Fairshter RD, Rosen SM, Smith WR: Paraquat poisoning: New aspects of therapy. Q J Med *45*:551, 1976.
115. Davies DS, Hawksworth GM, Bennett PN: Paraquat poisoning. Proc Eur Soc Toxicol *18*:21, 1977.
116. Addo E, Poon-King T: Leucocyte suppression in treatment of 72 patients with paraquat poisoning. Lancet *1*:1117, 1986.
117. Cyclophosphamide for paraquat poisoning? Lancet *2*:375, 1986.
118. Vale JA, Meredith TJ, Buckley BM: Paraquat poisoning. Lancet *1*:1439, 1986.
119. Matthew H, Logan A, Woodruff MFA, Heard B: Paraquat poisoning—Lung transplantation. Br Med J *3*:759, 1968.
120. Cooper JD, The Toronto Lung Transplant Group: Sequential bilateral lung transplantation for paraquat poisoning—a case report. J Thorac Cardiovasc Surg *89*:734, 1985.
121. Kamholz S, Veith FJ, Mollenkopf F, Montefusco C, Nehlsen-Cannarella S, Kaleya R, Pinsker K, Tellis V, Soberman R, Sablay L, Matas A, Gliedman M, Goldsmith J, Fell S, Brodman R, Merav A, Shander

A, Hollinger I, Nagashima H: Single lung transplant in paraquat intoxication. NY State J Med *84*:82, 1984.
122. Nagao M, Takatori T, Wu B, Terazawa K, Gotouda H, Akabane H: Immunotherapy for the treatment of acute paraquat poisoning. Hum Toxicol *8*:121, 1989.
123. Cadot R, Descotes J, Grenot C, Cuilleron CY, Evreux SC: Increased plasma paraquat levels in intoxicated mice following antiparaquat $F(ab')_2$ treatment. J Immunopharmacol *7*:467, 1985.
124. Wright AF, Green TP, Robson RT, Niewola Z, Wyatt I, Smith LL: Specific polyclonal and monoclonal antibody prevents paraquat accumulation into rat lung slices. Biochem Pharmacol *36*:1325, 1987.
125. Wright AF, Green TP, Daleyyat P, Smith LL: Monoclonal-antibody does not protect mice from paraquat toxicity. Vet Hum Toxicol *29*(suppl 2):102, 1987.
126. Crabtree HC, Lock EA, Rose MS: Effects of diquat on the gastrointestinal tract of rats. Toxicol Appl Pharmacol *41*:585, 1973.
127. Vanholder R, Colardyn F, De Rueck J, Praet M, Lameire N, Ringoir S: Diquat intoxication. Report of two cases and review of the literature. Am J Med *76*:1267, 1981.
128. Conning DM, Fletcher K, Swan AAB: Paraquat and related bipyridyls. Br Med Bull *25*:245, 1969.

CHAPTER 70
CYANIDE

Alan H. Hall, M.D.
Barry H. Rumack, M.D.

Cyanide poisoning may be encountered in a wide variety of settings. Cyanide salts and hydrocyanic acid are used in many common industrial processes such as electroplating, jewelry cleaning, precious metal extraction, laboratory assays, and some photographic processes.[1–5] Cyanide-containing imported metal cleaning solutions have been responsible for poisoning when unintentionally ingested.[6] Hydrogen cyanide gas is a fumigant rodenticide.[5] Criminal tampering by replacement of the ingredients in over-the-counter capsules with cyanide salts has resulted in a number of deaths.[2, 7, 8]

Some victims of closed-space fire smoke inhalation have cyanide toxicity in addition to carbon monoxide poisoning.[9–12] A number of compounds can liberate cyanide on spontaneous or thermal decomposition or by chemical reaction with acids or acid fumes (e.g., cyanogen, cyanogen bromide, cyanogen iodide, cyanogen chloride, calcium cyanide).[1, 2, 5] Some cyanogenic compounds and hydrogen cyanide gas have been considered for military use as chemical warfare agents.[13] At low concentrations, however, the cyanogen halides have primarily lacrimating and pulmonary irritant effects.[5] Other compounds can release cyanide as a byproduct of metabolism or a chemical reaction in the gut, or by bacterial degradation following ingestion (laetrile, amygdalin from plant sources, nitrile compounds such as acetonitrile or propionitrile, aliphatic thiocyanates such as Lethane and Thanate).[2, 5, 14–25]

Acetonitrile (methyl cyanide) is the active chemical in many sculpted nail removers, such as Nailene Glue Remover (84 per cent acetonitrile). Acetonitrile is slowly metabolized to hydrogen cyanide and formic acid and has recently been reported as a cause of pediatric intoxication and death.[20, 20a]

Some pigmented forms of *Pseudomonas aeruginosa* have the capacity to produce cyanide and could conceivably cause intoxication in heavily colonized burn patients.[26] Sodium nitroprusside releases cyanide during its metabolism and can cause elevated blood cyanide levels.[27, 28] Some patients with elevated blood cyanide levels during infusion of nitroprusside have developed clinical manifestations of cyanide poisoning.[28, 29] The frequent lack of correlation between blood cyanide levels and cyanide poisoning symptomatology during nitroprusside administration suggests that the decision to employ antidote therapy must be made more on clinical grounds (presence of metabolic acidosis, signs and symptoms consistent with cyanide poisoning) than on blood cyanide levels alone. Concomitant hydroxocobalamin (low dose, 100 mg) and sodium thiosulfate infusions have been successfully used experimentally to prevent sodium nitroprusside–induced increases in blood cyanide levels.[27, 28]

Compounds such as ferro- or ferricyanide do not commonly release significant amounts of cyanide when ingested and most often cause only gastrointestinal distress.[5] However, ingestion of potassium aurocyanide caused serious poisoning in one reported case.[30] Isocyanate compounds such as methyl isocyanate and toluene diisocyanate do not release cyanide after absorption and are not responsible for cyanide poisonings, being primarily irritant and sensitizing agents.[5]

Chronic exposure to low levels of cyanide has been postulated to cause optic or peripheral ataxic neuropathies in heavy smokers and persons who consume large amounts of cyanogenic foodstuffs (notably cassava).[31–36] The development of these neuropathies seems to require both chronic low-level cyanide exposure and either a deficiency of the endogenous cyanide-detoxifying enzyme rhodanese or protein-calorie malnutrition with a dietary sulfur deficiency.[33, 36] Mild disorders of vitamin B_{12} and folate levels and certain thyroid function abnormalities have been noted in workers with chronic cyanide exposure.[4] Thyroid enlargement and altered I^{131} uptake have also been described in a few workers chronically exposed to cyanide.[5]

Despite the wide use of cyanide and cyanogenic compounds, serious acute cyanide poisoning is rare. Of 2,980,643 cases of human poison exposure reported to the American Association of Poison Control Centers National Data Collection System from 1983 through 1986, only 1142 cases involved cyanide and 8447 involved cyanogenic plants.[37–40] In these patients, only 45 of 9566 survivors developed severe toxicity, and only 23 deaths were recorded.[37–40]

PATHOPHYSIOLOGY

Cyanide poisoning produces histotoxic hypoxia by binding with the ferric ($Fe\ 3+$) iron of mitochondrial cytochrome oxidase, inhibiting this important respiratory enzyme and disrupting the normal functioning of the electron transport chain and the ability of cells to utilize oxygen in oxidative phosphorylation.[41] The result is a shift to anaerobic metabolism, a substantial decrease in adenosine triphosphate (ATP) synthesis, depletion of cellular energy stores, and greatly increased lactic acid production causing an elevated anion gap metabolic acidosis.[1] Numerous iron- or copper-containing enzymes may be inhibited by cyanide, but cytochrome oxidase inhibition is the major intracellular toxic mechanism in cyanide poisoning.[5]

The tissue hypoxia of cyanide poisoning has several etiologies. Those tissues most dependent on oxidative phosphorylation, the heart and brain, are most severely and rapidly affected. Central inhibition of the respiratory centers leads to hypoventilation, producing an additional hypoxic hypoxia. Myocardial depression with decreased cardiac output produces an additional stagnation hypoxia. Cyanide also shifts the oxyhemoglobin dissociation curve to the left,[42] making it more difficult for hemoglobin-bound oxygen to be released to tissues. Some cyanide also binds to the ferrous ($Fe\ 2+$) iron of normal hemoglobin,[43] producing a small amount of cyanhemoglobin, which will not transport oxygen. Until the stage of respiratory depression or arrest the blood is normally oxygenated. However, the tissues are unable to extract and utilize this oxygen, leading to a greater than normal amount on the venous side and an increased central venous O_2 per cent saturation.[44]

Cyanide binding to cytochrome oxidase is a reversible process. The body has a natural defense against cyanide exposure in the form of an endogenous enzyme, namely, rhodanese. This enzyme catalyzes cyanide complexing with sulfur, forming the much less toxic ion thiocyanate (SCN). The body's sulfur pool is small, however, and the availability of sulfur constitutes the rate-limiting factor in natural cyanide detoxification. In the absence of an exogenous source of sulfur, rhodanese activity is too slow to prevent serious toxicity or death in significant cyanide poisoning.

The mechanism by which chronic cyanide exposure might cause neurotoxicity has been poorly understood. Recent studies suggest that increases in intraneuronal calcium levels and lipid peroxidation might be mechanisms by which cyanide can produce nerve injury.[45, 46]

Cyanide Toxicokinetics

The kinetics of cyanide are not well understood. Available data are from either animal experiments or anecdotal human case reports. In dog plasma in vitro, cyanide is approximately 60 per cent protein bound.[47] In vivo, whole blood cyanide levels may be four or more times greater than serum levels owing to the concentration of cyanide in erythrocytes.[48]

The volume of distribution (Vd) of cyanide in dogs is 0.498 L/kg.[49] A similar Vd of 0.41 L/kg was estimated in a single case of human potassium cyanide poisoning treated with sodium nitrite/thiosulfate.[3] In this same case, estimates of other toxicokinetic parameters were as follows: area under the curve (AUC) 48 μg-hr/mL, clearance (Cl) 163 ml/min, and terminal phase elimination half-life (T½) 19 hours.[3] This last-named value is in contrast to half-life values of 20 to 60 minutes often quoted in the literature[5, 9] but consistent with findings in dogs showing only minimal excretion within the first 3 hours after oral administration despite about 95 per cent absorption.[47] In a single patient not treated with specific antidotes, the average urinary cyanide excretion over nearly 40 hours was 0.64 mg/hr following a probable ingestion of between 117 and 511 mg of potassium cyanide.[2]

In this same victim of the 1982 Chicago cyanide-acetaminophen tampering incident (not treated with specific antidotes), the mean whole blood cyanide level 1 hour after ingestion was 8.2 μg/ml. This level rose to a mean of 19.7 μg/ml at 3 hours and 23.4 μg/ml at 9 hours post ingestion. Despite intensive supportive treatment, this patient died about 40 hours after ingestion. In contrast, in a patient who survived an ingestion of 1 gm of potassium cyanide following treatment with sodium nitrite/thiosulfate, the highest whole blood cyanide level was 15.68 μg/ml at 1 3/4 hours after ingestion, falling to 0.82 μg/ml at 5 hours.[3] In another patient who survived cyanide poisoning secondary to dermal and inhalation exposure to propionitrile, treatment with the hydroxocobalamin/sodium thiosulfate antidote kit currently used in France caused a decrease in the whole blood cyanide level from 5.71 μg/ml at 2 hours after exposure to 0.93 μg/ml 30 minutes later.[21] Specific antidote therapy can decrease blood cyanide levels more rapidly than is seen in cases where specific antidotes are not administered.

CLINICAL PRESENTATION

The natural history of severe acute cyanide poisoning is a rapid progression (faster with inhalation than with ingestion) to coma, convulsions, shock, respiratory failure, and death.[1, 41] Patients rendered intensive supportive care only have survived serious poisoning with whole blood cyanide levels as high as 2.3 μg/ml.[41] Patients treated similarly but also administered specific antidotes have survived with whole blood cyanide levels as high as 40 μg/ml.[50] Most patients who recover from acute cyanide poisoning do not have permanent sequelae, although rare cases of parkinsonian-like states or memory deficits and personality changes have been reported.[51–53]

The clinical presentation depends on the route of exposure, the dose, and the elapsed time. Patients with inhalation exposure to high concentrations may experience sudden loss of consciousness after only a few breaths.[5, 54] Patients who ingest potentially fatal amounts may not develop life-threatening symptomatology for up to 1/2 to 1 hour following exposure.[3] Delayed onset of symptoms (1 1/2 to 12 or more hours) may follow exposure to cyanogens such as laetrile, amygdalin, or nitrile compounds.[14, 19, 20]

In patients who do not experience sudden collapse, the initial signs and symptoms can resemble those of anxiety or hyperventilation syndrome.[1] Early signs include those of central nervous system stimulation (giddiness, headache, anxiety), tachycardia, hyperpnea, mild hypertension, and palpitations.

Late signs of poisoning are nausea, vomiting, tachycardia or bradycardia, hypotension, generalized seizures, coma, apnea, dilated pupils (either nonreactive or sluggishly reactive), and a variety of cardiac effects including erratic supraventricular or ventricular arrhythmias, atrioventricular blocks, ischemic electrocardiogram (ECG) changes, and eventual asystole.[1] Noncardiogenic pulmonary edema may occur, even in ingestions.[55] Nearly equally red retinal arteries and veins have been described,[56] although this finding is difficult to appreciate in most patients. The smell of bitter almonds (often described simply as musty) may be appreciated in some cases, but the ability to detect this odor is genetically determined and many people cannot do so.[1] Cyanosis is a late sign, usually only noted at the stage of apnea and circulatory collapse. The absence of cyanosis in spontaneously breathing or artificially ventilated patients having signs compatible with severe hypoxia should suggest the diagnosis.[1]

Although many references state that systemic cyanide poisoning can occur from dermal exposure, it is difficult to find actual reported cases other than those due to serious (20 per cent total body area) burns from molten cyanide salts[57] or total immersion in vats of cyanide solutions (with the potential for ingestion and vapor inhalation as well as dermal exposure).[58, 59] Significant absorption and systemic toxicity can follow direct eye instillation in experimental animals,[60] suggesting that patients with ocular exposure should have copious immediate irrigation with tap water or normal saline and a several-hour period of observation in a controlled setting.

EVALUATION AND TREATMENT

Initial Evaluation

The initial physical examination focuses on the vital signs and the respiratory, cardiovascular, and central nervous systems. Continuous vital sign and ECG monitoring should be done. Whole blood cyanide levels are available but generally take hours to obtain and cannot be used to guide emergent diagnosis or therapy.[1] They can, however, provide documentation of the diagnosis and response to treatment. A rapid automated microdiffusion assay has been developed[61] but is not currently in general use.

Lactic acid levels, serum electrolytes, and arterial blood gases should be monitored as frequently as necessary to guide fluid, electrolyte, sodium bicarbonate, and respiratory therapies. A chest film should be obtained and monitored if pulmonary edema develops.

Screening Laboratory Values

Based on anecdotal case reports and animal experiments, certain screening laboratory values may help suggest the diagnosis when no history is available.[1]

Cyanide produces *lactic acidosis,* which is noted directly on arterial blood gases and is also reflected in an *elevated anion gap* on the serum electrolyte panel [anion gap = Na − (Cl + CO_2); normal < 12 to 16 mEq/L]. If the patient is still breathing or is receiving assisted ventilation, the arterial pO_2 will be relatively normal, resulting in a *normal calculated arterial O_2 per cent saturation* (calculated from a nomogram). Some cyanide, however, binds to normal hemoglobin, producing cyanhemoglobin,[43] which is incapable of carrying oxygen, resulting in a *decreased measured arterial O_2 per cent saturation* (measured directly with a co-oximeter). The difference between the measured and calculated arterial O_2 per cent saturations can be termed the "O_2 per cent saturation gap," and a difference of five percentage points (*not* 5 per cent) may be of significance.

Cyanide inhibits oxygen extraction from the blood at the tissue level. More oxygen than normal is present on the venous side, which may be reflected in an increased (>40 mm Hg) peripheral venous pO_2[14] or a *narrowing* of the difference between the *measured* arterial O_2 per cent saturation and the *measured* central venous or pulmonary artery O_2 per cent saturation.[44] (Normal central venous O_2 per cent saturation is about 70 per cent.) It is presently unclear exactly how these blood gas parameters may be affected by supplemental oxygenation.

Of commonly encountered poisons, only carbon monoxide, hydrogen sulfide, and cyanide are suggested by this constellation of findings. Carbon monoxide and hydrogen sulfide poisoning can frequently be ruled out from the history, and carbon monoxide poisoning can usually be rapidly ruled out with a carboxyhemoglobin level. Patients exposed to hydrogen sulfide may have the odor of sulfur or rotten eggs about the body or clothes or in a freshly drawn tube of blood. Nitrites may also be antidotes for hydrogen sulfide poisoning.[62–66] Sodium thiosulfate is not efficacious in hydrogen sulfide poisoning, but there is no evidence that it will do any harm. Using this screening laboratory scheme may help to raise clinical suspicion to the point where it seems prudent to administer antidotes for suspected cyanide poisoning.[1]

Treatment

Cyanide-exposed patients with only restlessness, anxiety, or hyperventilation do not require antidote therapy.[54, 67] Such patients should be administered supplemental oxygen and carefully monitored. Antidotes should be administered *only* if more serious symptomatology develops.

Rescuers must not enter areas with high cyanide air concentrations without full protective clothing and proper respirators.[68] Mouth-to-mouth breathing should be avoided if at all possible, and care must be taken by rescuers not to inhale the victim's exhaled air. Appropriate prehospital care consists of airway management including endotracheal intubation if required, administration of 100 per cent supplemental oxygen by tight-fitting mask or endotracheal tube, placement of at least one large-bore intravenous line, administration of sodium bicarbonate if shock (with presumed metabolic acidosis) is present, decontamination of exposed skin or eyes, administration of antiarrhythmic or anticonvulsant medications if necessary, and administration of amyl nitrite by inhalation.

Amyl nitrite pearls may be broken in gauze and held close to the nose and mouth of patients who are spontaneously breathing. Alternatively, they may be placed into the lip of the face mask or inside the resuscitation bag in patients with apnea or hypoventilation. Amyl nitrite should be inhaled for 30 sec/min, changing to a fresh pearl every 3 to 4 minutes.

Supportive measures alone may sometimes prove to be satisfactory treatment,[41, 54, 55, 69–72] although patients administered specific antidotes together with supportive therapy have survived with higher whole blood cyanide levels, awakened sooner from coma, and had more rapid correction of acidosis requiring less sodium bicarbonate administration.[2, 3, 14, 16, 50, 73, 74] Standard antiarrhythmic and anticonvulsant therapies are appropriate for cyanide-induced arrhythmias and convulsions. Atropine or vasopressors may be required if symptomatic bradycardia or hypotension is present. Metabolic acidosis should be corrected with sodium bicarbonate.

Although measures to decrease absorption can be valuable, they should not delay required supportive or antidotal treatment. Exposed skin and eyes should be copiously flushed with water or normal saline. Contaminated clothing should be removed and isolated in impervious containers. Inducing emesis is *contraindicated* because of the potential for rapid progression to coma or seizures. Gastric lavage with a large-bore orogastric tube might be beneficial if done soon after an ingestion. Older references suggest using various neutralizing agents in the lavage fluid, but there is no evidence for their efficacy. An in vitro study found that 1 gm of regular activated charcoal bound 35 mg of cyanide,[75] and a rat study using large doses of superactivated charcoal administered shortly after potassium cyanide ingestion produced decreased mortality and morbidity.[76] A single dose of approximately 1 gm/kg body weight of activated charcoal can be instilled after gastric lavage is completed.

Antidotes

Specific therapy is the administration of the antidotes found in the Lilly Cyanide Antidote kit. Amyl nitrite has been discussed previously. Once intravenous access is available, discontinue amyl nitrite inhalation and administer sodium nitrite intravenously. The usual adult dose is 300 mg (one 10-ml ampule of a 3 per cent solution). The pediatric dose for the average child is 0.15 to 0.33 ml/kg. If suspicion or knowledge exists that a child may have significant anemia, the Lilly kit product information should be consulted for modification of the dose based on the known or suspected hemoglobin level.

Sodium nitrite, however, potentially has significant toxicity of its own. It is a potent vasodilator, and overly rapid administration may result in severe hypotension.[50, 77] This can be avoided by initial slow administration either by slow intravenous push over no less than 5 minutes or by dilution of the dose in 50 to 100 ml of normal saline, initially beginning with a slow infusion rate and then increasing to the most rapid rate possible without causing hypotension. Frequent blood pressure monitoring is mandatory during sodium nitrite administration.

Another potentially serious, although rare, adverse effect of sodium nitrite is induction of excessive methemoglobin levels.[17, 50, 67, 77] Induction of some level of methemoglobinemia has long been thought to be the mechanism of action of sodium nitrite, as methemoglobin has a higher affinity for cyanide than cytochrome oxidase. This hypothesis has been recently questioned, and vasodilatation with changes in local capillary blood flow or other mechanisms may play a significant role.[78] Excessive methemoglobin induction occurs most often in patients administered excessive amounts of sodium nitrite, but can sometimes be seen with therapeutic doses.[17, 50, 67, 77] Methemoglobin levels should be monitored, especially when multiple doses of sodium nitrite may be required. Inducing levels greater than 30 to 40 per cent must be avoided in all cases.

Administering enough sodium nitrite to induce a "therapeutic methemoglobin level" of 25 per cent has sometimes been recommended.[9, 79] However, patients have had excellent clinical recovery from acute cyanide poisoning with elevated whole blood cyanide levels even when sodium nitrite–induced methemoglobin levels were as low as 2 per cent.[3] The determination of when "enough" sodium nitrite has been infused is the patient's clinical response. Once satisfactory clinical improvement has occurred, no further sodium nitrite should be administered unless the patient suffers a recurrence of symptomatology.

The administration of sodium nitrite should be immediately followed by intravenous administration of sodium thiosulfate in an adult dose of 12.5 gm (one 50-ml ampule of a 25 per cent solution). The average pediatric dose is 1.65 ml/kg. There have been no reported cases of significant adverse effects from sodium thiosulfate administration in humans despite over 50 years of clinical use.[80] In selected patients with less severe poisoning, sodium thiosulfate alone may be sufficient therapy.[80]

In cases of smoke inhalation with known carbon monoxide and suspected cyanide poisoning, sodium thiosulfate and 100 per cent supplemental oxygen should be administered initially. Sodium nitrite administration should be withheld until the patient is at pressure in a hyperbaric oxygen chamber where dissolved plasma oxygen can adequately compensate for induced methemoglobinemia.[10]

Second doses of sodium nitrite and thiosulfate at one-half the initial amounts may be administered ½ hour after the first doses if there is inadequate clinical response. Administering further "prophylactic" doses to patients who have regained consciousness, spontaneous respirations, and stable vital signs is unnecessary and potentially dangerous. With exposure to certain nitrile compounds, however, continued metabolic release of cyanide may cause a prolonged poisoning requiring multiple doses of antidotes.[20] If producing a satisfactory clinical response, sodium thiosulfate alone could be used in such cases as its inherent toxicity is low.

Alternate antidotes in clinical use in other parts of the world such as hydroxocobalamin, dicobalt-EDTA (Kelocyanor), and 4-dimethylaminophenol (4-DMAP) are not currently available in the United States.[1, 41]

Hyperbaric Oxygen

Supplemental normobaric oxygen is efficacious in treating cyanide-poisoned patients.[59] Hyperbaric oxygen therapy may be even more efficacious in patients not responsive to supportive and antidotal therapy.[81] Reported human experience with this modality is limited, comprising one death and one survival following supportive, antidotal, and hyperbaric oxygen therapies.[73, 81] Animal experiments have both confirmed and refuted the potential greater efficacy of hyperbaric oxygen over 100 per cent normobaric oxygen.[82, 83] Smoke inhalation victims with serious known carbon monoxide poisoning and suspected cyanide toxicity should be treated with hyperbaric oxygen.[10]

Extracorporeal Elimination Techniques

One case of severe acute cyanide poisoning treated with supportive therapy, antidotes, and hemodialysis has been reported.[84] The contribution of the extracorporeal procedure to the clinical outcome is difficult to determine. The cyanide ion is a small charged molecule (molecular weight 26) with a low Vd (0.41 to 0.498 L/kg)[3, 49] and is thus potentially dialyzable, but hemodialysis cannot be considered a standard therapy at this time.

One patient with severe acute cyanide poisoning treated with supportive measures, antidotes, and charcoal hemoperfusion has also been reported.[6] This patient was improving following antidotal and supportive therapy at the time hemoperfusion was begun, and a direct contribution of the procedure to the clinical outcome is questionable. Hemoperfusion would presently seem to have no place in the treatment of acute cyanide poisoning.

Disposition

Asymptomatic patients with apparent minimal exposure should be observed in a controlled setting for at least 4 to 6 hours. If exposure has been to a nitrile compound, the onset of symptoms may be delayed for 12 or more hours,[19, 20] necessitating a longer period of observation and monitoring.

Patients having serious symptomatology (coma, convulsions, shock, metabolic acidosis, arrhythmias, ischemic ECG changes, hypoventilation) and all those administered antidotes should be admitted to an intensive care unit for careful monitoring until all symptomatology has resolved or a minimum of 24 hours. Outpatient follow-up at intervals for a period of weeks to months should be arranged to screen for the development of rare delayed central nervous system effects.[51–53]

References

1. Hall AH, Rumack BH: Clinical toxicology of cyanide. Ann Emerg Med *15*:1067, 1986.
2. Hall AH, Rumack BH, Schaffer MI, Linden CH: Clinical toxicology of cyanide: North American clinical experiences. *In* Ballantyne B, Marrs TC (eds): Clinical and Experimental Toxicology of Cyanides. Bristol, Wright, 1987, p 312.
3. Hall AH, Doutre WH, Ludden T, Kulig KW, Rumack BH: Nitrite/thiosulfate treated acute cyanide poisoning: Estimated kinetics after antidote. Clin Toxicol *25*:121, 1987.
4. Blanc P, Hogan M, Mallin K, Hryhorczuk D, Hessl S, Bernard B: Cyanide intoxication among silver-reclaiming workers. JAMA *253*:367, 1985.
5. Hartung R: Cyanides and nitriles. *In* Clayton GD, Clayton FE (eds): Patty's Industrial Hygiene and Toxicology. Vol 2, Toxicology, 3rd ed. New York, John Wiley and Sons, 1982, p 4845.
6. Krieg A, Saxena K: Cyanide poisoning from metal cleaning solutions. Ann Emerg Med *16*:582, 1987.
7. Wolnik KA, Fricke FL, Bonnin E, Gaston CM, Salzger RD: The Tylenol tampering incident—tracing the source. Anal Chem *56*:466, 1984.
8. Murphy DH: Cyanide-tainted Tylenol: What pharmacists can learn. Am Pharm *NS26*:19, 1986.
9. Jones J, McMullen MJ, Dougherty J: Toxic smoke inhalation: Cyanide poisoning in fire victims. Am J Emerg Med *5*:317, 1987.
10. Hart GB, Strauss MB, Lennon PA, Whitcraft DD: Treatment of smoke inhalation by hyperbaric oxygen. J Emerg Med *3*:211, 1985.
11. Clark CJ, Campbell D, Reid WH: Blood carboxyhemoglobin and cyanide levels in fire survivors. Lancet *1*:1332, 1981.
12. Symington IS, Anderson RA, Thomson I, Oliver JS, Harland WA: Cyanide exposure in fires. Lancet *2*:91, 1978.
13. Barr SJ: Chemical warfare agents. Top Emerg Med *7*:62, 1985.
14. Hall AH, Linden CH, Kulig KW, Rumack BH: Cyanide poisoning from laetrile: Role of nitrite therapy. Pediatrics *78*:269, 1986.
15. Sayre JW, Kaymakcalan S: Cyanide poisoning from apricot seeds among children in central Turkey. N Engl J Med *270*:1113, 1964.
16. Rubino MJ: Cyanide toxicity: Report of a case. Poison Information Bulletin, Connecticut Poison Information Center *3*:1, 1978.
17. Lasch EE, El Shawa R: Multiple cases of cyanide poisoning by apricot kernels in children from Gaza. Pediatrics *68*:5, 1981.
18. Shragg TA, Albertson TE, Fisher CJ: Cyanide poisoning after bitter almond ingestion. West J Med *136*:65, 1983.
19. Amdur ML: Accidental group exposure to acetonitrile: A clinical study. J Occup Med *1*:627, 1959.
20. Caravati EM, Litovitz TL: Pediatric cyanide intoxication and death from an acetonitrile-containing cosmetic. JAMA *260*:3740, 1988.

20a. Kurt TL, Day LC, Reed WG, Gandy W: Cyanide poisoning from sculpted nail remover. Presented at the Annual Meeting of the American Association of Poison Control Centers (AAPCC), Atlanta. Oct. 12–15, 1989.

21. Bismuth C, Baud FJ, Djeghout H, Astier A, Aubriot D: Cyanide poisoning from propionitrile exposure. J Emerg Med *5*:191, 1987.
22. Cameron GR, Doniger CR, Hughes AWM: The toxicity of lauryl thiocyanate and n-butyl-carbitol-thiocyanate (Lethane 384). J Pathol Bacteriol *49*:363, 1939.
23. Coulter E, Creery RDG: "Lethane" poisoning. Report of a fatal case. Br Med J *1*:379, 1953.
24. Guy AG: Aspiration pneumonia due to "Lethane" hair oil. Br Med J *2*:94, 1951.
25. von Oettingen WF, Heuper WC, Deichmann-Gruebler W: The pharmacological action and pathological effects of alkyl rhodanates in relation to their chemical constitution and physical-chemical properties. J Ind Hyg *18*:310, 1936.
26. Contreras AA, Evans BW, Moncrief JA, Lindberg RB, Villarreal Y, Mason AD: Some aspects of cyanide-producing capabilities of *Pseudomonas aeruginosa* strains isolated from infected burn patients. J Trauma *3*:527, 1963.
27. Cottrell JE, Casthely P, Brodie JD, Patel K, Klein A, Turndorf H: Prevention of nitroprusside-induced cyanide toxicity with hydroxocobalamin. N Engl J Med *298*:809, 1978.
28. Schulz V, Gross R, Pasch T, Busse J, Loeschcke G: Cyanide toxicity of sodium nitroprusside in therapeutic use with and without sodium thiosulfate. Klin Wochenschr *60*:1393, 1982.
29. Vesey CJ, Cole PV, Linnell JC, Wilson J: Some metabolic effects of sodium nitroprusside in man. Br Med J *2*:140, 1974.
30. Wright IH, Vesey CJ: Acute poisoning with gold cyanide. Anesthesia *41*:936, 1986.
31. Vincent M, Vincent F, Marka C, Faure J: Cyanide and its relationship to nervous suffering. Physiopathological aspects of intoxication. Clin Toxicol *18*:1519, 1981.
32. Bonnet JL, Yacoub M, Mouillon M: Intret diagnostique et therapeutique du dosage des thiocyanates dans le sang et les urines des malades atteints de

nevrites retrobulbaires toxiques. Bull Mem Soc Franc Ophthalmol *85*:157, 1972.

33. Poole CJM, Kind PRN: Deficiency of thiosulphate sulphurtransferase (rhodanese) in Leber's hereditary optic neuropathy. Br Med J *292*:1229, 1986.
34. Osuntokun BO, Monekessa G, Wilson J: Relationship of a degenerative tropical neuropathy to diet: Report of a field survey. Br Med J *1*:547, 1969.
35. Osuntokun BO, Monekessa G, Wilson J: Plasma amino acids in the Nigerian nutritional ataxic neuropathy. Br Med J *3*:647, 1968.
36. Cliff J, Lundqvist P, Martensson J, Rosling H, Sorbo B: Association of high cyanide and low sulphur intake in cassava-induced spastic paraparesis. Lancet *2*:1211, 1985.
37. Litovitz TL, Martin TG, Schmitz B: 1986 annual report of the American Association of Poison Control Centers National Data Collection System. Am J Emerg Med *5*:405, 1987.
38. Litovitz TL, Normann SA, Veltri JC: 1985 annual report of the American Association of Poison Control Centers National Data Collection System. Am J Emerg Med *4*:427, 1986.
39. Litovitz T, Veltri JC: 1984 annual report of the American Association of Poison Control Centers National Data Collection System. Am J Emerg Med *3*:423, 1985.
40. Veltri JC, Litovitz TL: 1983 annual report of the American Association of Poison Control Centers National Data Collection System. Am J Emerg Med *2*:420, 1984.
41. Vogel SN, Sultan TR, Ten Eyck RP: Cyanide poisoning. Clin Toxicol *18*:367, 1981.
42. Becker CE: The role of cyanide in fires. Vet Hum Toxicol *27*:487, 1985.
43. Yacoub M, Faure J, Morena H, Vincent M, Faure H: L'intoxication cyanhydrique aigue. Donnees actuelles sur le metabolisme du cyanure et le traitement par hydroxocobalamine. J Eur Toxicol *7*:22, 1974.
44. Paulet G: Valeur et mechanisme d'action de l'oxygenotherapie dans le traitement de l'intoxication cyanhydrique. Arch Internat Physiol Biochem *63*:340, 1955.
45. Johnson JD, Meisenheimer TL, Isom GE: Cyanide-induced neurotoxicity: Role of neuronal calcium. Toxicol Appl Pharmacol *84*:464, 1986.
46. Johnson JD, Conroy WG, Burris KD, Isom GE: Peroxidation of brain lipids following cyanide intoxication in mice. Toxicol *46*:21, 1987.
47. Christel D, Eyer P, Hegemann M, Kiese M, Lorcher W, Weger N: Pharmacokinetics of cyanide poisoning in dogs, and the effects of 4-dimethylaminophenol or thiosulfate. Arch Toxicol *38*:177, 1977.
48. Ballantyne B: Artifacts in the definition of toxicity by cyanide and cyanogens. Fundam Appl Toxicol *3*:400, 1983.
49. Sylvester DM, Hayton WL, Morgan RL, Way JL: Effects of thiosulfate on cyanide pharmacokinetics in dogs. Toxicol Appl Pharmacol *69*:265, 1983.
50. Feihl F, Domenighetti G, Perret C: Intoxication massive au cyanure avec evolution favorable. Schweiz Med Wochenschr *112*:1280, 1982.
51. Jouglard J, Nava G, Botta A, Michel-Manuel C, Poyen B, Mattei J-L: A propos d'une intoxication aigue par le cyanure traite par l'hydroxocobalamine. Marseille Medicale *12*:617, 1974.
52. Jouglard J, Fagot G, Deguigne B, Arlaud J-A: L'intoxication cyanhydrique aigue et son traitement d'urgence. Marseille Medicale *9*:571, 1971.
53. Uitti RJ, Rajput AH, Ashenhurst EM, Rozdilsky B: Cyanide-induced parkinsonism: A clinicopathologic report. Neurology *35*:921, 1985.
54. Peden NR, Taha A, McSorley PD, Bryden GT, Murdoch IB, Anderson JM: Industrial exposure to hydrogen cyanide: Implications for treatment. Br Med J *293*:538, 1986.
55. Graham DL, Laman D, Theodore J, Robin ED: Acute cyanide poisoning complicated by lactic acidosis and pulmonary edema. Arch Intern Med *137*:1051, 1977.
56. Buchanan IS, Dhamee MS, Griffiths FED, Yeoman MB: Abnormal fundus appearance in a case of poisoning by a cyanide capsule. Med Sci Law *16*:29, 1976.
57. Bourrelier J, Paulet G: Intoxication cyanhydrique consecutive a des brulures graves par cyanure de sodium fondu. Sur trois cas traites par EDTA cobaltique. Presse Med *22*:1013, 1971.
58. Dodds C, McKnight C: Cyanide toxicity after immersion and the hazards of dicobalt edetate. Br Med J *291*:785, 1985.
59. Bismuth C, Cantineau J-P, Pontal P, Baud F, Garnier R, Poulos L, Bolo A: Priorite de l'oxygenation dans l'intoxication cyanhydrique: A propos de 25 cas. J Toxicol Med *4*:107, 1984.
60. Ballantyne B: Acute systemic toxicity of cyanide by topical application to the eye. J Toxicol Cut Ocular Toxicol *2*:119, 1983.
61. Groff WA, Stemler FW, Kaminskis A, Froehlich HL, Johnson RP: Plasma free cyanide and blood total cyanide: A rapid completely automated microdiffusion assay. J Toxicol Clin Toxicol *23*:133, 1985.
62. Hoidal CR, Hall AH, Robinson MD, Kulig K, Rumack BH: Hydrogen sulfide poisoning from toxic inhalations of roofing asphalt fumes. Ann Emerg Med *15*:826, 1986.
63. Peters JW: Hydrogen sulfide poisoning in a hospital setting. JAMA *246*:1588, 1981.
64. Stine RJ, Slosberg B, Beacham BE: Hydrogen sulfide intoxication: A case report and discussion of treatment. Arch Intern Med *85*:756, 1976.
65. Smith RP, Kruszyna R, Kruszyna H: Management of acute sulfide poisoning: Effects of oxygen, thiosulfate, and nitrite. Arch Environ Health *166*:166, 1976.
66. Scheler W, Kabisch R: Uber die antagonistiche beeinflussung der akuten H2S vergiftung bei der maus durch methamoglobinbildner. Acta Biol Med Ger *11*:194, 1963.
67. Berlin CM: Treatment of cyanide poisoning in children. Pediatrics *46*:793, 1970.
68. Anon: CHRIS Hazardous Chemical Data. Washington, DC, U.S. Department of Transportation, U.S. Coast Guard, 1985.
69. Brivet F, Delfraissy JF, Duche M, Bertrand P, Dormont J: Acute cyanide poisoning: Recovery with non-specific supportive therapy. Intensive Care Med *9*:33, 1983.
70. Ortega JA, Creek JE: Acute cyanide poisoning following administration of laetrile enemas. J Pediatr *93*:1059, 1978.
71. Moertel CG, Ames MM, Kovack JS, Moyer TP, Rubin JR, Tinker JH: A pharmacological and toxicological study of amygdalin. JAMA *245*:591, 1981.
72. Morse DL, Boros L, Findley PA: More on cyanide poisoning from laetrile. N Engl J Med *301*:892, 1979.

73. Litovitz TL, Larkin RF, Myers RAM: Cyanide poisoning treated with hyperbaric oxygen. Am J Emerg Med *1*:94, 1983.
74. Moss M, Khalil N, Gray J: Deliberate self-poisoning with laetrile. Can Med Assoc J *125*:1126, 1981.
75. Andersen AH: Experimental studies on the pharmacology of activated charcoal. I. Adsorption power of charcoal in aqueous solution. Acta Pharmacol *2*:69, 1946.
76. Lambert RJ, Kindler BL, Schaeffer DJ: The efficacy of superactivated charcoal in treating rats exposed to a lethal oral dose of potassium cyanide. Ann Emerg Med *17*:595, 1988.
77. Viana C, Cagnoli H, Cedan J: L'action du nitrite de sodium dans l'intoxication par les cyanures. Compt Rend Soc Biol *115*:1649, 1934.
78. Way JL, Sylvester D, Morgan RL, Isom GE, Burrows GE, Tamulinas CB, Way JL: Recent perspectives on the toxicodynamic basis of cyanide antagonism. Fundam Appl Toxicol *4*:S231, 1984.
79. Birse GS: Cyanide poisoning. J Am Osteopath Assoc *83*:881, 1984.
80. Perrson H, Walter J: Sodium Thiosulfate Monograph: Use in Cyanide Poisoning. Geneva, International Programme on Chemical Safety, 1987.
81. Trapp W: Massive cyanide poisoning with recovery: A Boxing Day story. Can Med Assoc J *102*:517, 1970.
82. Takano T, Miyazaki Y, Nashimoto I, Kobayashi K: Effect of hyperbaric oxygen on cyanide intoxication: In situ changes in intracellular oxidation reduction. Undersea Biomed Res *7*:191, 1980.
83. Way JL, End E, Sheehy MH, De Miranda P, Feitknecht UF, Bachand R, Gibbon SC, Burrows GE: Effects of oxygen on cyanide intoxication. IV. Hyperbaric oxygen. Toxicol Appl Pharmacol *22*:415, 1972.
84. Wesson DE, Foley R, Sabatini S, Wharton J, Kapusnik J, Kurtzman NA: Treatment of acute cyanide intoxication with hemodialysis. Am J Nephrol *5*:121, 1985.

CHAPTER 71
OTHER HERBICIDES AND FUNGICIDES

Betty S. Riggs, M.D., FACEP
Ken Kulig, M.D., FACEP

Although herbicides and fungicides are commonly used chemicals in the United States and abroad, they are uncommonly reported as causes of poisoning. Of 1,166,940 cases reported in the 1987 Annual Report of the American Association of Poison Control Centers, 4167 (0.36 per cent) were due to herbicides and 1325 (0.11 per cent) were due to fungicides. Of these, 201 were due to paraquat or diquat.[1]

A study of admissions to a poison treatment center in Edinburgh from 1981 to 1986 showed that of 9000 admissions, 33 were due to herbicides and only 4 involved fungicides.[2]

CHLOROPHENOXY HERBICIDES
(Fig. 71–1)

Chlorophenoxy herbicides are auxins, or growth regulators, that cause abnormal plant growth and ultimately destroy the plant. They are commonly used for control of broadleaf weeds in cereal crops and pastures.[3]

The clinical presentation in cases of accidental or intentional chlorophenoxy overdose may include irritation of the gastrointestinal tract, muscle twitching, muscle tenderness, myotonia, rhabdomyolysis, metabolic acidosis, fever, tachycardia, hyperventilation, vasodilatation, sweating, coma, convulsions, and abnormal renal and liver function studies.[4]

Chlorophenoxy herbicides can be measured in plasma and urine by radioimmunoassay[5] and gas liquid chromatography.[6] However, the need for treatment is based on findings in the history and physical examination rather than on chlorophenoxy levels. Other laboratory parameters that should be monitored after significant exposures include renal function studies, liver function studies, serum creatine phosphokinase (CPK), complete blood count (CBC), and urinalysis for albumin and myoglobin.

Appropriate decontamination procedures should be performed after exposure to chlorophenoxy compounds. For ingestions, gas-

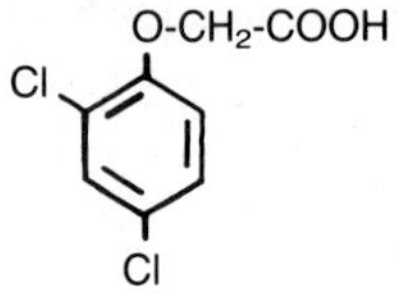

2, 4-D

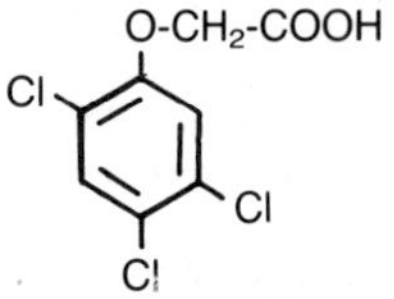

2, 4, 5-T

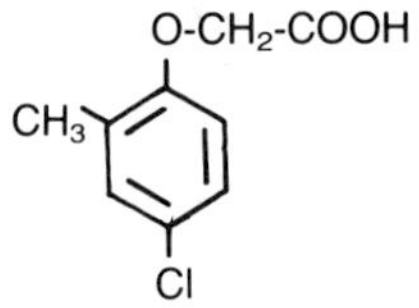

MCPA

Figure 71–1. Chlorophenoxy herbicides.

tric lavage may be performed if done soon after ingestion followed by administration of 30 to 100 gm of activated charcoal in adults (1 gm/kg in children) plus one dose of cathartic.[7] After dermal exposure, the skin should be washed thoroughly with soap and water with attention to decontamination of easily overlooked areas such as the hair, umbilicus, and nails. Contaminated leather articles must be discarded. Aggressive supportive care is equally important and includes correcting respiratory depression, hypotension, arrhythmias, hyperthermia, seizures, and acidosis.

2,4-Dichlorophenoxyacetic Acid (2,4-D)

Studies in human volunteers have demonstrated that 2,4-D is well absorbed from the gastrointestinal tract,[8, 9] but less well absorbed via the dermal route.[10] In a study of six human volunteers who were given a dose of 5 mg/kg orally, 2,4-D was detectable in the plasma in 1 hour and in the urine within 2 hours.[8] The volume of distribution was 10.1 ± 0.3 L/kg, and more than 75 per cent was excreted unchanged in the urine within 96 hours. A second volunteer study using the same oral dose found the average elimination half-life ($T_{1/2}\beta$) to be 11.7 hours.[9] The $T_{1/2}\beta$ in one patient who ingested an overdose of 2,4-D and dicamba was 16.7 hours.[11]

In a patient with disseminated coccidioidomycosis, 2,4-D was given therapeutically in gradually increasing intravenous doses. Although an intravenous dose of 2000 mg (37 mg/kg) produced no side effects, 3600 mg IV (66 mg/kg) resulted in coma, muscle twitching, hyporeflexia, and urinary incontinence. At 24 hours post administration, the patient was awake but complained of profound muscle weakness, which resolved 24 hours later.[12]

Many cases of intentional self-poisoning with 2,4-D have been reported. A 76 year old male who ingested an unknown amount of 2,4-D was found vomiting and combative and was treated with 100 mg of phenobarbital. Twenty hours later he was unarousable and had Cheyne-Stokes respirations, myotonia, and guaiac-positive nasogastric aspirate. The patient died 6 days post ingestion.[13]

In another case of suicidal ingestion of 50 gm of 2,4-D, the patient was comatose, hypotonic, hyporeflexic, and hypotensive 9 hours post ingestion. Treatment included diuresis and supportive care, but the patient died 12 hours post ingestion.[14]

Adverse effects have been reported after exposure to 2,4-D during normal usage. Peripheral neuropathy with painful paresthesias and muscle stiffness has occurred after dermal and inhalational exposure to 2,4-D.[15–17] Iritis that was reversible with treatment was reported in a worker who rubbed his eyes after moving containers of 2,4-D.[18]

Enhanced renal elimination with alkaline diuresis has been reported in a case of 2,4-D and mecoprop ingestion.[19] Renal clearance of 2,4-D increased from 0.14 ml/min at pH 5.1 to 63 ml/min at pH 8.3. Alkaline diuresis can be induced by adding 88 to 132 mEq sodium bicarbonate/L D_5W given at a rate to produce adequate urine output with a pH of 7.5 or more.[7] Furosemide may be required to maintain diuresis. Careful monitoring of fluid and electrolyte balance must be performed to prevent noncardiogenic pulmonary edema.

2,4,5-Trichlorophenoxyacetic Acid (2,4,5-T)

Another selective chlorophenoxy herbicide is 2,4,5-T, which is more effective on woody plant species.[3]

The kinetics of 2,4,5-T have been studied in five human volunteers who ingested a single dose of 5 mg/kg. Good absorption from the gastrointestinal tract was demonstrated, and 88.5 ± 5.1 per cent of the ingested dose was excreted unchanged in the urine within 96 hours.[20] First-order kinetics were described with a Vd of 0.079 L/kg and a $T_{1/2}\beta$ of 23.1 hours.

A 61 year old male who ingested 24 gm of 2,4-D and 7.5 gm of 2,4,5-T in a hydrocarbon solvent was hypertonic, hyperreflexic, hyperthermic, and responsive only to pain by 6 hours post ingestion. By 24 hours post ingestion he was completely unresponsive to pain but normothermic. Although he remained unconscious for 4 days, he recovered by 5 days post ingestion. One month later he had difficulty walking and evidence of a peripheral neuropathy, which resolved 3 months later.[21]

A 48 year old male who drank a mixture of equal parts of 2,4-D; 2,4,5-T butyl ester; and inert ingredients was found drowsy and vomiting. By 3 hours post ingestion he was vomiting, diaphoretic, hypotensive, tachycardic, tachypneic, and responsive only to pain. During 43 hours of hospitalization, the patient developed hyperthermia, oliguria, hemoconcentration, a rising blood urea nitrogen (BUN) level, and shock unresponsive to pressors.[3]

Major uses of 2,4,5-T were banned by the US Environmental Protection Agency in 1979.[22] All remaining uses were subsequently cancelled.[23] 2,3,7,8-Tetrachlorodibenzo-P-dioxin (TCDD) is a byproduct of 2,4,5-T production. Dioxin has been discussed in Chapter 26D.

4-Chloro-2-methylphenoxyacetic Acid (MCPA)

Another chlorophenoxy herbicide, MCPA, is used to control annual and perennial weeds in cereals, grassland, and turf.[3]

Five volunteers given an oral dose of 15 μg/kg body weight of MCPA had a peak plasma concentration of 0.15 μg/ml at 1 hour. During the first 24 hours, 40 per cent of the dose was excreted in urine. Dermal absorption was demonstrated after 1 gm of MCPA emulsion was placed on the skin and washed off after 2 hours. A maximum plasma level of 0.12 μg/ml was reached after 24 hours. Maximal urinary excretion occurred 24 to 48 hours after application, with slow excretion continuing for up to 5 days.[24]

Significant toxicity has been reported after the suicidal ingestion of MCPA. A 61 year old male ingested a weedkiller later identified as MCPA and shortly thereafter developed vomiting, slurred speech, and muscle jerking. By 1.5 hours post ingestion he was unconscious, with copious oral secretions. Physical examination revealed edema of the tongue and fauces, coarse rales at the bases of the lungs, small unreactive pupils, hyporeflexia, generalized fibrillary twitching of the skeletal muscles, and clonic spasms of the limbs. Treatment included intubation, gastric lavage, paraldehyde to control abnormal muscle movements, and pressors for hypotension. The patient remained unconscious for 72 hours but recovered. Laboratory abnormalities included occult fecal blood for 21 days, elevated transaminases, and decreased hemoglobin and platelet counts.[25]

Hypocalcemia complicated the course of one fatal case of ingestion of Herbatox (22.7 per cent MCPA and 9.1 per cent 2,4-D). A 55 year old female became confused and aggressive shortly after ingestion and later became unconscious, hypertonic, areflexic, tachycardic, and hypoxic. Initial treatment included lavage and alkaline diuresis. The hospital course was complicated by hypotension, renal insufficiency, and hypocalcemia requiring calcium infusion. After 15 days, the patient died of multiple organ failure.[26]

MCPA can be detected in blood and tissues. Two fatal cases have been described.[27,28]

2-Methyl,4-chlorophenoxypropionic Acid (MCPP)

MCPP, or mecoprop, has also been involved in cases of human poisoning. Two cases of MCPP ingestion followed a similar clinical course with rapid loss of consciousness, muscle cramps, and hypotension. Laboratory abnormalities included decreased platelets and hemoglobin and elevated CPK and myoglobin. One patient also developed acute renal failure secondary to rhabdomyolysis and required hemodialysis. Both recovered.[29]

UREA-SUBSTITUTED HERBICIDES

These herbicides, which are photosynthesis inhibitors, are used mainly for weed control in noncrop areas.[3] Examples of this class of herbicides include diuron, linuron, monolinuron, and monuron.

Diuron is well absorbed from the gastrointestinal and respiratory systems, but information regarding dermal absorption is lacking.[3] Diuron undergoes hepatic metabolism, and the majority of metabolites are excreted in the urine.[3] Monuron has also been shown to undergo metabolism via the liver microsomes.[30]

Urea-substituted herbicides have low systemic toxicity based on animal feeding studies. Diuron, for example, had a median lethal dose (LD50) of 1017 mg/kg in normal juvenile rats, an LD50 of 437 mg/kg in rats on a low protein diet, and an LD50 of 2390 mg/kg in rats on a high protein diet.[31]

Cases of human ingestion also generally support the idea that these compounds are of low systemic toxicity. A 39 year old female ingested an herbicide containing 56 per cent diuron and 30 per cent amitrole (38 and 20 mg/kg, respectively). The patient showed no clinical evidence of toxicity, but her urine contained metabolites of diuron.[32]

However, in another case significant clinical findings did occur after ingestion of an herbicide containing monolinuron. A 63 year old female drank 1 cup of Gramonol, containing monolinuron 14 per cent and paraquat 10 per cent. Nine hours post ingestion the patient was noted to have a cyanotic appearance. At 43 hours post ingestion she had a 36 per cent methemoglobin level and a 7 per cent sulfhemoglobin level. Hemolysis was also noted. The patient recovered after treatment with 50 mg of methylene blue. The patient's paraquat level was not in the serious risk category, and the patient's methemoglobinemia was attributed to monolinuron, which is metabolized to aniline.[33] Another similar case with methemoglobinemia, hemolysis, and a nontoxic paraquat level following Gramonol ingestion has also been reported.[34]

Plasma levels of these herbicides are not clinically useful. Methemoglobin and sulfhemoglobin levels should be obtained in patients with a history of urea-substituted herbicide ingestions who appear to be cyanotic or who have dyspnea.

Treatment should include decontamination and aggressive supportive care. Additionally, methylene blue, 1 to 2 mg/kg/dose, should be given if significant methemoglobinemia is present. If other evidence of severe toxicity is present, other causes should be sought and appropriate treatment given.[7]

ENDOTHALL

Endothall is an herbicide with significant toxicity. The acute oral LD50 is 51 mg/kg.[4] It is irritating to the eyes, mucous membranes, and skin, and systemic toxicity and death can occur after ingestion.

In one fatal case a 23 year old male ingested 40 ml of Endothall. He vomited spontaneously six times and complained of abdominal pain on arrival in an emergency department 50 minutes post ingestion. The patient was given a charcoal slurry but vomited again. Six hours after presentation he complained of dyspnea and abdominal pain. During the next several hours, the patient developed hematemesis, hypotension, acidosis, anuria, disseminated intravascular coagulation, and cardiovascular collapse. In spite of aggressive supportive care the patient expired 12 hours post ingestion. No toxicology studies were reported to exclude the possibility that other toxins were involved.[35]

Treatment should include appropriate decontamination and aggressive supportive care.

CARBAMATE HERBICIDES AND FUNGICIDES

Carbamate herbicides and fungicides differ from the carbamate insecticides by a substitution on the nitrogen rather than the oxygen moiety (Fig. 71–2). Unlike the carbamate insecticides, these compounds do not produce inhibition of cholinesterase enzymes or a cholinergic syndrome.[3] Toxicity is unusual.

(Mono)thiocarbamates. This group includes cycloate, molinate, pebulate, diallate, and triallate, which are selective herbicides with generally low mammalian toxicity.[3] Molinate, used to control weeds in rice paddies, was implicated in the illness of eight people who were exposed to contaminated well water.[36] After molinate was applied to nearby rice paddies, the well, which was the source of water for four families, developed an odor. Subsequently eight people developed nausea, diarrhea, abdominal pain, fever, weakness, and conjunctivitis, whereas four addi-

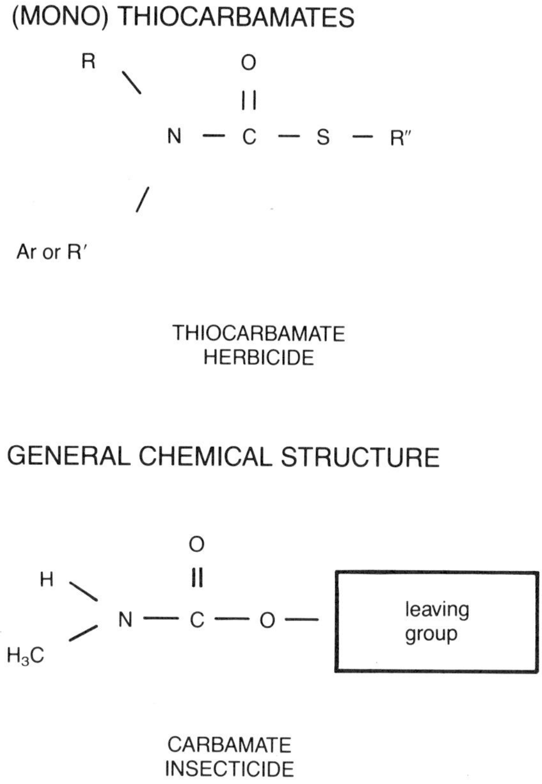

(MONO) THIOCARBAMATES

R \ O || N — C — S — R″ / Ar or R′

THIOCARBAMATE HERBICIDE

GENERAL CHEMICAL STRUCTURE

H \ O || N — C — O — leaving group / H_3C

CARBAMATE INSECTICIDE

Figure 71–2. Structure of carbamate herbicides and cholinesterase-inhibiting carbamate insecticides. (From Morgan DP: Recognition and Management of Pesticide Poisonings. 3rd ed. Washington, DC, US Environmental Protection Agency, 1982.)

tional people developed only abdominal pain. Symptoms resolved when the families stopped using the well water. Analysis of the water 15 days later revealed a molinate concentration of 0.006 ppm.

Bisdithiocarbamates. Thiram belongs to the bisdithiocarbamate class and is used as a fungicide. It is structurally similar to disulfiram, and this compound may produce a disulfiram reaction when ethanol is ingested after a significant exposure to thiram. This reaction is characterized by flushing, sweating, headache, weakness, tachycardia, and hypotension.[37–39] One such case resulted in a fatality 4 days after a 10-hour exposure to thiram.[40] Contact dermatitis with a positive patch test has occurred in a male who bowled on a green treated with thiram[41] and in a male who golfed on a course treated with thiram.[42] Allergic contact dermatitis occurred in four patients treated in the same hemodialysis unit who had positive skin tests to thiram.[43] The source of the thiram was reportedly from rubber parts of the hemodialysis unit that come into contact with the dialysate. There is one reported case of Henoch-Schönlein purpura occurring in a 23 year old male who was exposed to thiram for 1 month while planting seedlings treated with the fungicide. The patient had had nausea and signs of eye, skin, and respiratory tract irritation on the job; however, a causal association between thiram exposure and Henoch-Schönlein purpura was not proven.[44]

Metallobisdithiocarbamates. These comprise a class of carbamate fungicides that includes ziram, nabam, and ferbam.[4] The bisdithiocarbamates are named for the metallic component, e.g., ziram for zinc and ferbam for iron. These compounds are moderately irritating to the skin and respiratory mucous membranes after exposure to sprays or dusts. Nausea, vomiting, and diarrhea may result from ingestion.[4] One case of an ingestion of 500 ml of ziram solution of unknown concentration resulted in a fatality a few hours post ingestion. Autopsy revealed only nonspecific findings such as focal necrosis of the mucosa of the small intestine, congestion of the viscera, acute emphysema, focal atelectasis, and desquamation of alveolar and bronchial epithelia.[45]

Ethylene Bisdithiocarbamate. These fungicides are maneb and zineb. These compounds are irritating to the skin and respiratory tract mucosa.[4] Cases of contact dermatitis have been reported.[3]

A case of acute intoxication with maneb and zineb occurred in a 42 year old man who walked through a field 1 day after it had been sprayed with maneb and zineb.[46] The patient became transiently uncommunicative, nervous, tired, weak, and dizzy. Six days later he again walked through a recently sprayed field and developed headache, nausea, fatigue, weakness, difficulty undressing, unclear speech, decreased level of consciousness, and tonic-clonic seizures. An electroencephalogram (EEG) showed diffuse slowing, and computed tomography (CT) of the brain was normal. The patient was fully recovered 5 days later.

One case of acute renal failure after exposure to maneb has been reported.[47] A 62 year old man with stomach cancer treated for 2 years with fluorouracil (5-FU) applied maneb to his garden on two occasions two days apart using protective clothing. The day following the second application he ate corn from the garden without first washing it and afterward washed his hands with water only. That night he had diarrhea followed by hoarseness and muscle weakness. Five days later he presented with acute renal failure requiring hemodialysis. The patient recovered and later had a normal work-up including intravenous pyelography.

Chronic exposure to maneb purportedly produced a complex of symptoms similar to those of chronic manganese toxicity.[48] After two agricultural workers, a 41 year old woman and a 27 year old man, developed a parkinsonian syndrome following maneb exposure, a formal study of exposed workers was undertaken. Fifty farm workers with more than 6 months' exposure to maneb were compared with 19 rural workers without exposure. The exposed workers displayed a statistically significant increase in headaches, nervousness, memory problems, fatigue, and muscle rigidity with cogwheeling. However, there was no significant difference in manganese levels between the two groups.[48]

HEXACHLOROBENZENE

Hexachlorobenzene, an aromatic hydrocarbon fungicide, has been used since 1945 for seed treatment.[3] Kinetic information in humans is unavailable.

The toxicity of hexachlorobenzene in humans was demonstrated by an outbreak of cutaneous porphyria in Turkey that occurred when seed wheat, which had been treated with a fungicide containing hexachlorobenzene, was used instead for human consumption.[49] From 1955 to 1959 approximately 3000 cases of hexachlorobenzene-induced porphyria occurred in southeastern Turkey.[50] Symptoms included hyperpigmentation, hypertrichosis, weight loss, hepatomegaly, and painless arthritis. The most striking finding was blistering and epidermolysis of exposed parts of the skin. Healing was poor and occurred in winter, leaving pigmented scars and contractures. Relapses occurred in the summer with increased sun exposure.[49] Breast-fed infants of affected mothers were noted to develop "pembe yara," or pink sore, and had a mortality rate of 95 per cent.[50] Treatment of seven patients with 1 to 2 gm of edetic acid (EDTA) daily for up to 1 year resulted in symptomatic improvement. Chelation also resulted in increased excretion of urine uroporphyrins but no change in the excretion of urine coproporphyrins.[50]

Twenty years after hexachlorobenzene exposure, 32 Turkish patients were studied. Clinically, patients were noted to have small stature; hyperpigmentation; hypertrichosis; scars on cheeks, arms, and hands; pinched facies; and arthritis. The most striking finding was that of small hands, with sclerodermoid thickening of the skin, and an abnormal shape secondary to osteoporosis and almost complete atrophy of the terminal phalanges.[51] A hexachlorobenzene level of 0.7 ppm was detected in breast milk from one porphyric patient; none was detected in milk from four controls. Subcutaneous fat from one porphyric patient had a hexachlorobenzene level of 0.21 ppm. Urine and stool uroporphyrin levels were still elevated in 5 of 29 patients in whom levels were obtained.

References

1. Litovitz TL, Schmitz BF, Matyunas N, Martin TG: 1987 Annual Report of the American Association of Poison Control Centers National Data Collection System. Am J Emerg Med *6*:479–515, 1988.
2. Proudfoot AT, Dougall H: Poisoning treatment centre admissions following acute incidents involving pesticides. Hum Toxicol *7*:255–258, 1988.
3. Hayes WJ Jr: Pesticides Studied in Man. Baltimore, Williams & Wilkins, 1982.
4. Morgan DP: Recognition and Management of Pesticide Poisonings. 3rd ed. Washington, DC, US Environmental Protection Agency, 1982.
5. Knopp D, Nuhn P, Dobberkau HJ: Radioimmunoassay for 2,4-dichlorophenoxyacetic acid. Arch Toxicol *58*:27–32, 1985.
6. Rivers JB, Yauger WL, Klemmer HW: Simultaneous gas chromatographic determination of 2,4-D and dicamba in human blood and urine. J Chromatogr *50*:334–337, 1970.
7. Micromedex. Poisindex Information Systems. Denver, Micromedex, 1989.
8. Kohli JD, Khanna RN, Gupta BN, et al: Absorption and excretion of 2,4-dichlorophenoxyacetic acid in man. Xenobiotica *4*:97–100, 1974.
9. Sauerhoff MW, Braun WH, Blau GE, et al: The fate of 2,4-dichlorophenoxyacetic acid (2,4-D) following oral administration to man (abstract). Toxicol Appl Pharmacol *37*:136–137, 1976.
10. Feldmann RJ, Maibach HI: Percutaneous penetration of some pesticides and herbicides in man. Toxicol Appl Pharmacol *28*:126–132, 1974.
11. Young JF, Haley TJ: Pharmacokinetic study of a patient intoxicated with 2,4-dichlorophenoxyacetic acid and 2-methoxy-3,6-dichlorobenzoic acid. Clin Toxicol *11*:489–500, 1977.
12. Seabury JH: Toxicity of 2,4-dichlorophenoxyacetic acid for man and dog. Arch Environ Health *7*:202–209, 1963.

13. Dudley AW Jr, Thapar NT: Fatal human ingestion of 2,4-D, a common herbicide. Arch Pathol *94*:270–275, 1972.
14. deLarrard J, Barbaste M: Fatal suicidal poisoning due to 2,4-D. Arch Mal Prof Med Trav Secur Soc *30*:434, 1969.
15. Berkley MC, Magee KR: Neuropathy following exposure to a dimethylamine salt of 2,4-D. Arch Intern Med *111*:351–352, 1963.
16. Goldstein NP, Jones PH, Brown JR: Peripheral neuropathy after exposure to an ester of dichlorophenoxyacetic acid. JAMA *171*:1306–1309, 1959.
17. Wallis WE, Van Poznak A, Plum F: Generalized muscular stiffness, fasciculations, and myokymia of peripheral nerve origin. Arch Neurol *22*:430–439, 1970.
18. McMillin RB, Samples JR: Iritis after herbicide exposure. Am J Ophthalmol *99*:726–727, 1985.
19. Prescott LF, Park J, Darrien I: Treatment of severe 2,4-D and mecoprop intoxication with alkaline diuresis. Br J Clin Pharmacol *7*:111–116, 1979.
20. Gehring PJ, Kramer CG, Schwetz BA, et al: The fate of 2,4,5-Trichlorophenoxyacetic acid (2,4,5-T) following oral administration to man. Toxicol Appl Pharmacol *26*:352–361, 1973.
21. O'Reilly JF: Prolonged coma and delayed peripheral neuropathy after ingestion of phenoxyacetic weedkillers. Postgrad Med J *60*:76–77, 1984.
22. The Environmental Protection Agency: Rebuttal presumption against registration on 2,4,5-T. Fed Reg *43* (April 21):17116-17157, 1978.
23. Baselt RC: Deposition of Toxic Drugs and Chemicals in Man. 2nd ed. Davis, CA, Biomedical Publications, 1982.
24. Kolmodin-Hedman B, Hoglund S, Swensson A, et al: Studies on phenoxy acid herbicides: II. Oral and dermal uptake and elimination in urine of MCPA in humans. Arch Toxicol *54*:267–273, 1983.
25. Jones DIR, Knight AG, Smith AJ: Attempted suicide with herbicide containing MCPA. Arch Environ Health *14*:363–366, 1967.
26. Kancir CB, Andersen C, Olesen AS: Marked hypocalcemia in a fatal poisoning with chlorinated phenoxy acid derivatives. J Toxicol Clin Toxicol *26*:257–264, 1988.
27. Popham RD, Davies DM: A case of MCPA poisoning. Br Med J *1*:677–678, 1964.
28. Johnson HRM, Koumides O: A further case of MCPA poisoning. Br Med J *2*:629–630, 1965.
29. Meulenbelt J, Zwaveling JH, Van Zoonen P, et al: Acute MCPP intoxication: Report of two cases. Hum Toxicol *7*:289–292, 1988.
30. Ross D, Farmer PB, Gescher A, et al: The formation and metabolism of N-hydroxymethyl compounds-I. The oxidative N-demethylation of N-dimethyl derivatives of arylamines, aryltriazines, arylformamidines and arylureas including the herbicide monuron. Biochem Pharmacol *31*:3621–3627, 1981.
31. Boyd EM, Krupta V: Protein deficiency diet and diuron toxicity. J Agric Food Chem *18*:1104–1107, 1970.
32. Geldmacher-von Mallinckrodt M, Schussler E: Zu stoffwechsel und toxicitaet von 1-(3,4-dichlorophenyl)-3,3-dimethylharnstoff (Diuron) beim menschen. Arch Toxikol *27*:187–192, 1971.
33. Proudfoot AT: Methaemoglobinaemia due to monolinuron—not paraquat. Br Med J *285*:812, 1982.
34. Ng LL, Naik RB, Polak A: Paraquat ingestion with methaemoglobinaemia treated with methylene blue. Br Med J *284*:1445–1446, 1982.
35. Day LC: Delayed death by Endothall, an herbicide (abs). Vet Hum Toxicol *30*:366, 1988.
36. Minakawa O, Ishii S, Konno H: Analytical method of residue of molinate, a herbicide in paddy field, and actions of molinate to living bodies. Jpn J Public Health *25*:645–651, 1978.
37. Barnes BA, Fox LE: Screening some thiuram disulfides and related compounds for acute toxicity and Antabuse-like activity. J Am Pharm Assoc *44*:756–759, 1955.
38. Reinl W: Hypersensitivity to alcohol after exposure to the fungicide tetramethylthiuram disulfide (TMTD). Arch Toxikol *22*:12–15, 1966.
39. Krupa A, Pienkowska H, Tarka Z: Acute poisoning with "thiram." Med Wiejsk *6*:29–31, 1971.
40. Marcinkowski T, Manikowski W: Fatal case of intoxication with "Seed Dressing T." Med Pr *24*:91–95, 1973.
41. Gunther DW: Tetramethylthiuramdisulphide (TMTD) and bowls. Med J Aust *1*:1177, 1970.
42. Shelley WB: Golf-course dermatitis due to thiram fungicide: Cross-hazards of alcohol, disulfiram, and rubber. JAMA *188*:415–417, 1964.
43. Penneys NS, Edwards LS, Katsikas JL: Allergic contact sensitivity to thiuram compounds in a hemodialysis unit. Arch Dermatol *112*:811–813, 1976.
44. Duell PB, Morton WE: Henoch-Schönlein purpura following thiram exposure. Arch Intern Med *147*:778–779, 1987.
45. Buklan AI: Acute poisoning with ziram. Sud Med Ekspert *17*:51, 1974.
46. Israeli R, Sculsky M, Tiberin P: Acute intoxication due to exposure to maneb and zineb: A case with behavioral and central nervous system changes. Scand J Work Environ Health *9*:47–51, 1983.
47. Koizumi A, Shiojima S, Omiya M, et al: Acute renal failure and maneb (manganous ethylenebis [dithiocarbamate]) exposure. JAMA *242*:2583–2585, 1979.
48. Ferraz HB, Bertolucci PHF, Pereira JS, et al: Chronic exposure to the fungicide maneb may produce symptoms and signs of CNS manganese intoxication. Neurology *38*:550–553, 1988.
49. Schmid R: Cutaneous porphyria in Turkey. N Engl J Med *263*:397–398, 1960.
50. Peters HA, Johnson SAM, Cam S, et al: Hexachlorobenzene-induced porphyria: Effect of chelation on the disease, porphyrin and metal metabolism. Am J Med Sci *251*:314–322, 1966.
51. Cripps DJ, Gocmen A, Peters HA: Porphyria turcica: Twenty years after hexachlorobenzene intoxication. Arch Dermatol *116*:46–50, 1980.

CHAPTER 72

PHOSPHORUS, STRYCHNINE, AND OTHER RODENTICIDES

A. Phosphorus

Jay M. Arena, M.D.

Elemental phosphorus exists in two forms: red and yellow. Red phosphorus is nonvolatile, insoluble, and unabsorbable and thus is nontoxic on ingestion. Yellow (or white) phosphorus is extremely toxic and highly volatile, burning on contact with air or water.

No longer used in matches or fireworks, yellow phosphorus is most commonly used in rodenticides, either as powders or pastes. The two most common products are Stearn's Electric Brand Paste (2.5 per cent) and Pearson's Poison Paste (2 per cent). The public uses these pastes on articles such as bread or cheese to attract rats. Unfortunately, children have ingested such articles, often with fatal results. These products also have been used in successful suicide attempts. Even though the percentage of yellow phosphorus contained in these products is low, these products are extremely toxic, and significant ingestions usually have a 50 per cent mortality rate. The lethal dose is considered to be 1 mg/kg, although as little as 3 mg was reported to be fatal to a 2-year-old child.

Symptomatology. Yellow phosphorus is a general protoplasmic poison and produces a characteristic clinical syndrome on ingestion. Initial effects are gastrointestinal, neurologic, and cardiovascular. After a quiescent phase generally described as lasting from 24 to 72 hours, hepatic, renal, hematologic, and metabolic disturbances may ensue. Yellow phosphorus on skin can cause severe second- and third-degree burns, and systemic absorption is possible if the exposure is not treated aggressively.[1]

Symptoms occur rapidly following significant ingestion. Nausea, vomiting, diarrhea, hematemesis, rectal bleeding, and abdominal pain generally occur. Characteristic and diagnostic of phosphorus poisoning is luminescence of the vomitus, flatus, and stool—this is a striking and pathognomonic clinical sign.[2] Also, the patient's breath has a garlic odor. Coma and seizures may be seen early in severe cases. Shock is usually present. Death, when it occurs in the initial phase, is by cardiac arrhythmias, which are generally unresponsive to therapy.[3] Death from cardiac arrest has been observed within 1 hour of ingestion but may occur up to 12 hours post ingestion.

If the patient survives the initial phase, the absorbed phosphorus generally produces effects in from 24 to 72 hours—thus a patient with known symptomatic phosphorus ingestion should be hospitalized for at least 72 hours. Characteristic of the second phase is acute yellow atrophy and hepatic failure, evidenced by hepatomegaly, coma, jaundice with pruritus, hypoglycemia with seizures, and coagulation abnormalities with petechiae and hemorrhage, often gastrointestinal. Renal shutdown and metabolic acidosis also may occur.

Laboratory studies may reveal acidosis; abnormal liver function studies with hyperbilirubinemia, abnormal prothrombin time, and low fibrinogen; hypoglycemia; and elevated blood urea nitrogen (BUN). Urinalysis may reveal casts, hematuria, and albuminuria. Electrocardiograms on patients who survive the initial phase may reveal ST-T changes indicative of myocardial ischemia or infarction.

Chronic phosphorus poisoning in industrial workers is now a rarity; these workers characteristically incurred anemia, cachexia, and necrosis of the mandible ("phossy jaw").

Treatment. Gastric lavage invariably should be done if the patient is seen within the first few hours. Lavage should be performed with potassium permanganate (1:5000 solution) or 2 per cent hydrogen peroxide, as these form harmless oxides of phosphorus, followed by activated charcoal, which should be instilled before the lavage tube is removed. Mineral oil or petrolatum has been given by mouth or nasogastric tube as a solvent to prevent absorption of phosphorus and to hasten elimination; a dose of 200 to 250 ml is given at first and then 1 oz (30 ml) every 3 hours for the first 48 hours. Absorption has been said to be increased by milk, olive oil, and other fats and oils, and these should be avoided. The role of cathartics is not clear.

There is no antidote for phosphorus poisoning. Treatment is symptomatic and supportive. Fresh whole blood; correction of shock, acidosis, and blood loss; cardiac monitoring and management of arrhythmias; and treatment of seizures all may be necessary in the emergency phase. Management of hepatic and renal failure and other complications may be indicated in the secondary phase. Vitamin K is indicated if the blood prothrombin level is low. Vitamin B complex, thiamine, and ascorbic acid are regarded as useful supplements. Cutaneous burns should be washed with copious amounts of water for 15 to 30 minutes or with a 1 per cent solution of cupric sulfate, which forms a coat of black cupric phosphide.

References

1. Rubitsky HJ, Myerson RM: Acute phosphorus poisoning. Arch Intern Med *83*:164, 1949.
2. Simon FA, Pickering LK: Acute yellow phosphorus poisoning—"smoking stool syndrome." JAMA *235*:1343, 1976.
3. Talley RC, Linhart JW, Trevino AJ, et al: Acute elemental phosphorus poisoning in man: Cardiovascular toxicity. Am Heart J *84*:139, 1972.

B. Strychnine

Betty S. Riggs, M.D., FACEP
Ken Kulig, M.D., FACEP

Strychnine, formerly a common component of tonics and aphrodisiacs,[1–3] has few current medical uses. Recently it has been used experimentally in the treatment of selected cases of impotence,[4] nonketotic hyperglycinemia,[5–7] and sleep apnea.[8] However, its efficacy in the treatment of any medical condition remains unproven. Strychnine is used occasionally in veterinary medications, rodenticides, and avicides.

Strychnine poisoning is rare, occurring in only 140 of 1,166,940 cases reported to the American Association of Poison Control Centers in 1987.[9] The majority (87 of 140 cases) resulted from the accidental or intentional ingestion of strychnine-containing rodenticides. An unusual source of poisoning occurs in illicit drug abusers who have mistakenly snorted or injected strychnine as a drug adulterant or a substitute of the purported drug.[10, 11]

Pharmacokinetics. An alkaloid obtained primarily from the seeds of the ***Strychnos nux vomica*** tree, strychnine occurs in the form of odorless, colorless crystals or a white powder with a bitter taste[12] (Fig. 72–1). The estimated potentially lethal dose is difficult to define. As little as 16 mg of strychnine hydrochloride was fatal in a 1 year old infant who also ingested "sublethal" doses of iron and quinine[13]; however, a 13 month old infant survived after ingesting 10 to 20 mg of strychnine hydrochloride.[14] An adult survived after reportedly ingesting 15,000 mg of strychnine sulfate.[15]

After ingestion, strychnine is readily absorbed from the gastrointestinal tract,[1–3] nasal mucosa,[10] and injection sites.[16] It rapidly distributes to tissue, with 50 per cent of an intravenous dose reportedly distributing to tissues within 5 minutes.[17] Only 20 per cent or less is excreted unchanged in the urine.[17,18]

Metabolism of strychnine by the microsomal fraction of liver from various animal species has been demonstrated.[19] More re-

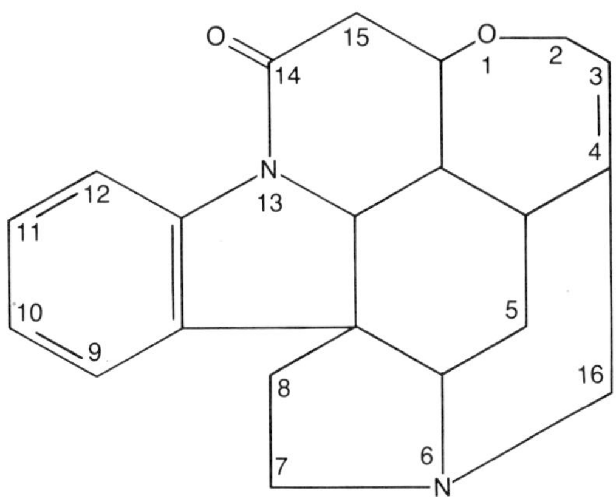

Figure 72–1. Chemical structure of strychnine.

cently, in vitro studies using rat and rabbit livers identified five metabolites, with the major metabolite, strychnine *N*-oxide, accounting for 15 per cent of metabolized strychnine.[20] The major enzyme responsible for metabolism was the cytochrome P-450 mono-oxygenase.

Kinetic studies based on only one case described first-order kinetics with a Kel of 0.07/hr and a half-life of 10 hr.[21]

Mechanism of Toxicity. Glycine, the major postsynaptic inhibitory neurotransmitter in mammalian spinal cord and brain stem, is thought to produce hyperpolarization via an increase in chloride conductance.[22, 23] Strychnine antagonizes this effect of glycine. Specific binding sites for [^{3}H] strychnine have been demonstrated in synaptic membrane preparations from rat brain stem and spinal cord,[24] and these are the pharmacologically active binding sites.[25] Evidence suggests that strychnine and glycine interact at two separate binding sites on the glycine receptor in an allosteric manner; i.e., the binding of one compound at its site lowers the affinity of the glycine receptor for the other compound at its site.[26]

Areas of the central nervous system with the highest density of glycine receptors in rat and human brain have been localized by autoradiography to the gray matter of the spinal cord, with a progressively decreased density of receptors in the more rostral regions of the neuraxis.[27, 28] A correlation between these anatomic findings and the physiologic findings in strychnine poisoning has been postulated (Table 72–1).

Clinical Effects. Within 15 to 20 minutes postexposure, signs and symptoms of strychnine toxicity are usually present[11, 29] (Table 72–2). By antagonizing the inhibitory neurotransmitter glycine, strychnine produces excitation of the central nervous system. Occasionally seizures may be the first manifestation of toxicity,[10] but a prodrome of nervousness, myalgias, and myoclonic jerks is more common.[11]

Strychnine-induced seizures characteristically are tonic and extensor in nature and may be accompanied by opisthotonos.[11, 29, 30] Normally, when an extensor motor neuron is stimulated, collaterals cause excitation of inhibitory interneurons whereby glycine produces hyperpolarization of flexor motor neurons. Thus, flexor muscles are inhibited from contracting simultaneously during contraction of extensor muscles. Strychnine blocks this reciprocal inhibition, allowing a predominance of excitation, which is expressed as convulsions.[23] The pattern of convulsive activity is determined by the strongest muscle acting at each joint, which is typically the extensor. The patient is usually conscious during the seizure, and there is generally no postictal period.[14, 31, 32] Strychnine-associated seizures may be provoked by any sensory stimulus.[11, 29, 30] The experience is usually both terrifying and painful for the patient.

Physical examination may reveal muscle tenderness, myoedema, hypertonicity, hy-

Table 72–1. POSTULATED RELATIONSHIP BETWEEN CLINICAL EFFECTS OF STRYCHNINE AND AREAS WITH STRYCHNINE BINDING SITES

CLINICAL EFFECT	ANATOMIC LOCATION OF STRYCHNINE BINDING SITES
Heightened acuity of perception	
Visual	Retina (inner plexiform layer)
Auditory	Superior olivary nucleus, nuclei of lateral lemniscus
Cutaneous	Dorsal horn of spinal cord, cuneate and gracile nuclei, and analogous portions of trigeminal nuclei
Hyperalgesia and pain associated with seizures	Dorsal horn of spinal cord (especially laminae II and V) and analogous portions of trigeminal nuclei
Hyperreflexia, muscle stiffness or spasm	
Limb and trunk muscles	Dorsal and ventral horns of spinal cord
Masticatory muscles	Sensory and motor portions of trigeminal nuclei
Muscles of facial expression	Sensory portions of trigeminal nuclei and nucleus VII
Increased respiratory rate, bradycardia, and hypertension	Respiratory and cardiovascular centers in medulla and pons
Initiation of seizures by visual and acoustic stimuli	Superior colliculus
Disequilibrium	Vestibular nuclei

(Reprinted with permission from Zarbin MA, Wamsley JK, Kuhnar MJ: Glycine receptor: Light microscopic autoradiographic localization with [^{3}H] strychnine. J Neurosci 1:545, 1981.)

Table 72–2. CLINICAL EFFECTS OF STRYCHNINE

Anxiety	Trismus
Myalgias	Risus sardonicus
Myoclonic jerks	Hyperreflexia
Muscle tenderness	Extensor spasms
Myoedema	Tonic seizures without loss of consciousness
Hypertonicity	Apnea
Hyperesthesia	
Nystagmus	

perreflexia, and clonus.[11, 31] Trismus and risus sardonicus are also frequently observed,[10, 32] whereas bilateral horizontal nystagmus is a rarely reported finding.[32]

Strychnine affects the diaphragm in a manner analogous to its effects on other muscle groups, resulting in respiratory compromise and hypoxia. Thus, death from acute strychnine poisoning is usually the result of respiratory arrest followed by cardiac arrest.[29]

Other clinical sequelae of strychnine toxicity occur as a result of seizure activity. Marked hyperthermia, lactic acidosis, rhabdomyolysis, and myoglobinuria with subsequent acute renal failure have been reported.[11, 29, 30, 33–36]

The differential diagnosis includes other poisonings that may cause myoclonus or seizures, such as overdoses of cyclic antidepressants, theophylline, chlorinated hydrocarbon insecticides, amphetamines, and cocaine among many others. Medical causes of seizures, such as tetanus, idiopathic seizure disorders, drug withdrawal, meningitis, and intracerebral bleeding, should be considered. Strychnine poisoning should be strongly suspected whenever hypertonicity, particularly of extensor muscles, or apparent seizures occur in an awake patient. The diagnosis can be confirmed by detection of strychnine in body fluids.

Laboratory Findings. Strychnine can be detected in blood, urine, and gastric contents as well as tissue samples[37–41] (Table 72–3). Strychnine can be qualitatively detected by thin layer chromatography and quantitated by high-performance liquid chromatography[42] or gas chromatography with a flame ionization detector.[37, 38] Strychnine levels are not useful in determining the need for therapy, which generally must be started before laboratory results return.

Other laboratory data that may be helpful in determining the need for therapy are aimed at diagnosing the sequelae of strychnine poisoning. Arterial blood gases should be obtained to rule out hypoxia and metabolic acidosis. Creatine phosphokinase, myoglobin, and renal function studies should be monitored because of the possibility of rhabdomyolysis, myoglobinuria, and acute renal failure. Other laboratory findings may include abnormal lactate, glucose, and phosphorus levels and white blood cell count.[11, 33]

Treatment. The primary goals of therapy are maintenance of an adequate airway, with assisted ventilation if needed, and control of hypertonicity and seizure activity. Patients should be placed in a quiet, dark room to avoid sensory stimuli.

Neither emesis nor lavage is recommended initially because of the possibility of inducing seizures with resultant aspiration. Activated charcoal, which has been shown to adsorb strychnine very effectively,[43] should be administered as quickly as possible in a dose of 30 to 100 gm in adults or 1 gm/kg in children. If activated charcoal must be given down a nasogastric tube, pretreatment with diazepam is recommended.

Benzodiazepines are the drugs of choice in the treatment of strychnine-induced seizures because they appear to increase inhibitory neurotransmitter effects in the central nervous system.[44] *Benzodiazepines facilitate the inhibitory action of gamma-aminobutyric acid (GABA), producing anticonvulsant and sedative effects.* They also mimic the inhibitory actions of glycine, resulting in anxiolytic and muscle relaxant effects.[44] The potency of benzodiazepines in various pharmacologic and behavioral tests has been shown to correlate with their potency in displacing [^{3}H] strychnine binding.[45]

Table 72–3. STRYCHNINE CONCENTRATIONS IN 12 FATALITIES (mg/L or mg/kg)

	BLOOD	BRAIN	LIVER	KIDNEY	URINE	GASTRIC CONTENTS
Average	26	14	144	54	11	47
(Range)	(0.5–61)	(0.5–26)	(5–257)	(0.07–106)	(1–33)	(7.5–100)

(Reprinted with permission from Baselt RC: Disposition of Toxic Drugs and Chemicals in Man. 2nd ed. Davis, CA, Biomedical Publications, 1982, p 702.)

Diazepam has been used successfully to treat strychnine-induced seizures as well as ameliorate prodromal symptoms.[10, 31, 32, 46] Doses of 5 to 10 mg should be given intravenously initially and repeated as frequently as necessary to control symptoms. A diazepam drip of 5 to 10 mg/hr may be started and the dose increased as necessary. Prior to the availability of benzodiazepines, barbiturates reportedly were used efficaciously.[47] In cases resistant to standard anticonvulsants, intubation and neuromuscular paralysis may be required to prevent hyperthermia, lactic acidosis, and rhabdomyolysis.[21, 33, 48]

Although forced diuresis and peritoneal dialysis have been used in the past to treat strychnine poisoning, data to support the efficacy of these treatment modalities were not presented.[49] In one recent case report, less than 1 per cent of the reportedly ingested dose was recovered in the urine, supporting previous kinetic studies that indicate that the major mechanism of elimination is via hepatic metabolism.[17, 18] Thus, forced diuresis and peritoneal dialysis do not enhance strychnine elimination.

Resolution of severe symptoms generally occurs within 24 hours.[32] Recovery may be complete if seizures are adequately controlled during that period and the patient had not been hypoxemic. However, prolonged muscle hyperexcitability for 72 hours and hypertonicity lasting for 1 week have been reported.[21]

References

1. Hawkins GF: Two cases of strychnine poisoning in children. Br Med J *2*:26, 1962.
2. Haslam MT: Accidental strychnine poisoning. Br Med J *1*:1191, 1965.
3. Muller FO: Availability of medicines containing strychnine (letter). S Afr Med J *51*:652, 1977.
4. Savion M, Segenreich E, Kahan E, et al: Pharmacologic, nonhormonal treatment of impotence: Evaluation of associated factors. Urology *29*:510–512, 1987.
5. Ch'ien LT, Chance P, Arneson D, et al: Glycine encephalopathy. N Engl J Med *298*:687, 1978.
6. Sankaran K, Casey RE, Zaleski WA, et al: Glycine encephalopathy in a neonate: Treatment with intravenous strychnine and sodium benzoate. Clin Pediatr *21*:636–637, 1982.
7. Haan EA, Kirby DM, Tada K, et al: Difficulties in assessing the effect of strychnine on the outcome of nonketotic hyperglycinaemia: Observations on sisters with a mild T-protein defect. Eur J Pediatr *145*:267–270, 1986.
8. Remmers JE, Anch AM, de Groot WJ, et al: Oropharyngeal muscle tone in obstructive sleep apnea before and after strychnine. Sleep *3*:447–453, 1980.
9. Litovitz TL, Schmitz BF, Matyunas N, et al: 1987 Annual Report of the American Association of Poison Control Centers National Data Collection System. Am J Emerg Med *6*:479–515, 1988.
10. O'Callaghan WG, Joyce N, Counihan HE, et al: Unusual strychnine poisoning and its treatment: Report of eight cases. Br Med J *285*:478, 1982.
11. Boyd RE, Brennan PT, Deng JF, et al: Strychnine poisoning: Recovery from profound lactic acidosis, hyperthermia, and rhabdomyolysis. Am J Med *74*:507–512, 1983.
12. Reynolds JEF, Prasad AB (eds): Martindale: The Extra Pharmacopoeia. 28th ed. London, The Pharmaceutical Press, 1982, pp 319–320.
13. Stannard NW: Child death due to Easton's tablets. Practitioner *203*:668–669, 1969.
14. Jackson G, Ng SH, Diggle GE, et al: Strychnine poisoning treated successfully with diazepam. Br Med J *3*:519–520, 1971.
15. Priest RE: Strychnine poisoning successfully treated with sodium amytal. JAMA *110*:1440, 1938.
16. Decker WJ, Baker HE, Tamulinas SH, et al: Two deaths resulting from apparent parenteral injection of strychnine. Vet Hum Toxicol *24*:161–162, 1982.
17. Weiss S, Hatcher RA: Studies on strychnine. J Pharmacol Exp Ther *19*:419–482, 1922.
18. Sgaragli GP, Mannaioni PF: Pharmacokinetic observations on a case of massive strychnine poisoning. Clin Toxicol *6*:533–540, 1973.
19. Adamson RH, Fouts JR: Enzymatic metabolism of strychnine. J Pharmacol Exp Ther *127*:87–91, 1959.
20. Mishima M, Tanimoto Y, Oguri K, et al: Metabolism of strychnine in vitro. Drug Metab Dispos *13*:716–721, 1985.
21. Edmunds M, Sheehan TMT, Van't Hoff W: Strychnine poisoning: Clinical and toxicological observations on a nonfatal case. J Toxicol Clin Toxicol *24*:245–255, 1986.
22. Curtis DR, Hosli L, Johnston GAR, et al: The hyperpolarization of spinal motoneurons by glycine and related amino acids. Exp Brain Res *5*:235–258, 1968.
23. Snyder SH: The glycine synaptic receptor in the mammalian central nervous system. Br J Pharmacol *53*:473–484, 1975.
24. Young AB, Snyder SH: Strychnine binding associated with glycine receptors of the central nervous system. Proc Natl Acad Sci USA *70*:2832–2836, 1973.
25. Mackerer CR, Kochman RL, Shen TF, et al: The binding of strychnine and strychnine analogs to synaptic membranes of rat brainstem and spinal cord. J. Pharmacol Exp Ther *201*:326–331, 1977.
26. Marvizon JCG, Vazquez J, Calvo MG, et al: The glycine receptor: Pharmacological studies and mathematical modeling of the allosteric interaction between the glycine- and strychnine-binding sites. Molecular Pharmacol *30*:590–597, 1986.
27. Zarbin MA, Wamsley JK, Kuhar MJ: Glycine receptor: Light microscopic autoradiographic localization with [^{3}H] strychnine. J Neurosci *1*:532–547, 1981.
28. Probst A, Cortes R, Palacios JM: The distribution of glycine receptors in the human brain: A light microscopic autoradiographic study using [^{3}H] strychnine. Neuroscience *17*:11–35, 1986.
29. Dittrich K, Bayer MJ, Wanke LA: A case of fatal strychnine poisoning. J Emerg Med *1*:327–330, 1984.
30. Lambert JR, Byrick RJ, Hammeke MD: Management of acute strychnine poisoning. Can Med Assoc J *124*:1268–1270, 1981.

31. Maron BJ, Krupp JR, Tune B: Strychnine poisoning successfully treated with diazepam. J Pediatr *78*:697–699, 1971.
32. Blain PG, Nightingale S, Stoddart JC: Strychnine poisoning: Abnormal eye movements. J Toxicol Clin Toxicol *19*:215–217, 1982.
33. Gordon AM, Richards DW: Strychnine intoxication. J Am Coll Emerg Phys *8*:520–522, 1979.
34. Loughhead M, Braithwaite J, Denton M: Life at pH 6.6 (letter). Lancet *2*:952, 1978.
35. Bismuth C, Caramella JP, Rosenberg N: Rhabdomyolyse au cours d'intoxication par la strychnine—A propos de 2 cas. Nouv Presse Med *6*:3549–3550, 1977.
36. Goldstein MR: Recovery from severe metabolic acidosis (letter). JAMA *234*:1119, 1975.
37. Perper JA: Fatal strychnine poisoning—a case report and review of the literature. J Forensic Sci *30*:1248–1255, 1985.
38. Winek CL, Wahba WW, Esposito FM, et al: Fatal strychnine ingestion. J Anal Toxicol *10*:120–121, 1986.
39. Lloyd JTA, Pedley E: Acute strychnine poisoning after a massive dose. Br Med J *2*:429–430, 1953.
40. Cotten MS, Lane DH: Massive strychnine poisoning: A successful treatment. J Miss State Med Assoc *7*:466–468, 1966.
41. Baselt RC: Disposition of Toxic Drugs and Chemicals in Man. 2nd ed. Davis, CA, Biomedical Publications, 1982, pp 701–703.
42. Alliot L, Bryant G, Guth PS: Measurement of strychnine by high-performance liquid chromatography. J Chromatogr *232*:440–442, 1982.
43. Anderson AH: Experimental studies on the pharmacology of activated charcoal: III. Adsorption from gastro-intestinal contents. Acta Pharmacol *4*:275–284, 1948.
44. Richter JJ: Current theories about the mechanism of benzodiazepines and neuroleptic drugs. Anesthesiology *54*:66–72, 1981.
45. Young AB, Zukin SR, Snyder SH: Interaction of benzodiazepines with central nervous glycine receptors: Possible mechanism of action. Proc Natl Acad Sci USA *71*:2246–2250, 1974.
46. Herishanu Y, Landau H: Diazepam in the treatment of strychnine poisoning. Br J Anaesth *44*:747–748, 1972.
47. Kempf GF, McCallum JTC, Zerfas LG: A successful treatment for strychnine poisoning: Report of eleven cases. JAMA *100*:548–551, 1933.
48. Racle JP, Chavagnac B, Brenez M, et al: Intoxication aigue a la strychnine: A propos d'un cas d'evolution favorable sous curarisation et assistance respiratoire. Cah Anesthesiol *35*:413–414, 1987.
49. Teitelbaum DT, Ott JE: Acute strychnine intoxication. Clin Toxicol *3*:267–273, 1970.

C. Other Rodenticides

Brooks C. Metts, Pharm.D.

Rodenticides are used to kill rats, mice, gophers, moles, voles, ground squirrels, and prairie dogs. Populations of these animals are controlled for both economic and health reasons. Rodents damage crops in the field and foods in storage, sometimes host human diseases, bite people, and cause material damage by gnawing.[1, 2]

A wide variety of inorganic and organic compounds have been used as rodenticides (Table 72–4). Early rodenticides were agents derived from plant material, such as strychnine and red squill, or inorganic chemicals, such as arsenic trioxide. Newer agents are primarily synthetic organic compounds. Some rodenticides are nearly as dangerous to man and other animals as they are to rodents. Recently efforts have been made to lessen the danger by restricting the use of some agents and requiring premarketing studies of new agents. Still, there are no rodenticides that cannot cause harm if misused.[1]

Children, suicidal patients, victims of attempted homicide, exterminators, psychiatric or impaired geriatric patients, and those who accidentally ingest rodenticides from containers normally used for edible products may be victims of rodenticide poisoning.[3]

Because there are so many vastly different agents in use as "rat poisons," one must read the entire label of the ingested product to determine the actual chemical exposure. Reading only part of a label can be mislead-

Table 72–4. AGENTS USED AS RODENTICIDES

bromethalin
cholecalciferol
warfarin
second-generation anticoagulants
pyriminil
sodium monofluoroacetate
red squill
strychnine
thallium
arsenic
zinc phosphide
phosphorus
ANTU
norbromide
barium carbonate

ing. For example, one might be told that a patient was exposed to d-Con. There are several products under this name: d-Con Pellets contain warfarin 0.025 per cent, d-Con Mouse Prufe also contains warfarin 0.025 per cent; however, d-Con Mouse Prufe Concentrate contains 0.3 per cent warfarin (12 times the amount found in the others), and d-Con Mouse Prufe II contains the more potent, longer-acting anticoagulant brodifacoum. It is not unusual to see similar names or even the same trade name used for different products. It is often worth the effort to find the container and positively identify the ingredients to know what effects might be expected and how to approach treatment.

Bromethalin

Available Products. Assault, Vengance.

Bromethalin is one of the newest rodenticides. It is available in pellets of 0.01 per cent concentration as a general-use rodenticide. Bromethalin acts as a neurotoxin, its mechanism of action appearing to be the uncoupling of oxidative phosphorylation in the mitochondria of the central nervous system. There is a decrease in the production of adenosine triphosphate (ATP), resulting in fluid accumulation with fluid-filled vacuoles between the myelin sheaths covering the central nerves. Vacuole formation leads to increased cerebrospinal fluid pressure and increased pressure on nerve axons. The result is a decrease in nerve impulse conduction, which can lead to paralysis and death.[4] Bromethalin is a nonselective mammalian poison. All animals, including man, are vulnerable. Its use as a rodenticide is based on the rodent's consumption of larger quantities of food per body weight than larger animals.[5]

To date there have been no toxic human exposures reported. Based on animal studies, signs and symptoms of acute exposure would be expected to include headache, confusion, personality changes, tremors, seizures, coma, and respiratory depression. In animals death occurs within 18 hours following acute exposure.[6] In chronic exposures symptoms might include lethargy and incoordination due to loss of muscle tone, numbness, and confusion.

Purina Assault is available as green pellets in two sizes: 1/8″ mouse size, 45 mg/pellet, 22 pellets/gm, 935 pellets/pack; and 3/16″ rat size, 142 mg/pellet, 7 pellets/gm, 298 pellets/pack. Pellets are packaged in water-proof paper place packs weighing 1.5 oz and 1.5-oz prefilled bait stations.[7]

Treatment for bromethalin poisoning is symptomatic and supportive. One-time exposure to small amounts of bromethalin should not cause serious effects. When exposures exceed 0.1 mg/kg (1 gm of bait/kg), induce vomiting with syrup of ipecac. Follow with administration of activated charcoal. In large exposures, observe for central nervous system (CNS) symptoms: headache, confusion, personality change, tremors, seizures, or coma. Seizures should be treated with diazepam, phenytoin, or phenobarbital. Cerebral edema should be treated with mannitol or dexamethasone. In animal studies, dexamethasone and osmotic agents were effective in treating cerebral edema due to bromethalin ingestion.[8] Toxic effects of bromethalin were completely reversed in animal studies within 3 to 7 days.

Cholecalciferol

Available Products. Rampage, Quintox.

One of the most recently marketed rodenticides, cholecalciferol (vitamin D_3) takes advantage of the fact that rodents are extremely sensitive to small percentage changes in plasma calcium balance. Hypercalcemia produced by cholecalciferol results in calcification of the coronary vessels with subsequent myocardial infarction.[9] Rodenticide baits come in a 0.75 per cent concentration of cholecalciferol as pellets and mouse seed. Pellets come in 30-gm packs and bulk containers. Each pellet contains 0.0577 mg, or 2308 International Units (IU), of vitamin D. There are 13 pellets/gm (30,000 IU).[10]

There is wide individual variation in the amount of cholecalciferol required to produce hypervitaminosis D in humans. Continued ingestion of 50,000 IU or more per day can cause poisoning. Most reported poisonings are a result of chronic excess ingestion of vitamin D.[11] There is no information available on acute exposures. However, owing to the long elimination half-life (> 30 days), a very large single dose might produce chronic effects.

Cholecalciferol toxicity results in hypercalcemia.[11] When plasma calcium rises above 11.5 to 12 mg/dl, symptoms are common. These include confusion, anorexia, headache, fatigue, nausea, vomiting, and diarrhea. Concentrations above 13 mg/dl produce renal insufficiency and calcification of kidneys, skin, vessels, lungs, heart, and stomach. In children, one episode of moderately severe hypercalcemia may interrupt growth completely for at least 6 months or more, with the deficit never being fully corrected.[12]

Several bait pellets or a small amount of the mouse seed should not be toxic, and no treatment is necessary. Larger quantities should be removed from the gastrointestinal tract before absorption occurs. Begin monitoring serum calcium levels 24 hours after ingestion. Levels should be elevated within 24 to 48 hours, at which time hypercalcemia should be treated. Institute a low-calcium diet, and promote forced diuresis to increase elimination of calcium, using furosemide as the preferred diuretic. Oral prednisone, 5 to 15 mg/6 hr, also increases calcium excretion. Calcitonin may also be necessary to reduce serum calcium. Phenobarbital and phenytoin have been used to induce hepatic microsomal enzymes in an infant to hasten vitamin D metabolism.[13] In severe hypercalcemia (> 15 mg/dl) not responding to other measures, mithramycin should be considered.

Warfarin-Type Anticoagulants

Available Products

Hydroxycoumarin (Warfarin, Wincon). Kill-Ko, Rat Busters, Rat Kakes, Rat Doom, Rat Dragon, Rat End, Ratmort, Rat-I-Cide, Rat-Ola, d-Con, Sweeney's Mouse Bait, Mouse-Nots, Mouse Prufe, Rat War, Sla-Rat, Vam-O.

Warfarin + Sulfaquinoxaline. Anchor rat & mouse bait packet, Strike, Sweeney's Ready Mixed, Ratangle II, Rat Bait Meat Bits, Rat-Fix, Rat-O-Cide, Ratorex, Final, Eagle 7.

The introduction of warfarin in the early 1950s revolutionized rodent control. It proved to be an effective rodenticide and was safer than existing agents. Toxicity requires very large single amounts or smaller doses for 4 to 6 days.[14] Some products containing warfarin also add the antibiotic sulfaquinoxaline to reduce vitamin K–producing bacteria in the gut.

Warfarin compounds decrease the activity of the vitamin K–dependent blood clotting factors. When clotting factors are sufficiently reduced, bleeding occurs. Ecchymosis, hematuria, uterine bleeding, melena or hematochezia, epistaxis, hematoma, gingival bleeding, and hematemesis are seen, generally in that order.[15] In adults 5 to 10 mg/day of warfarin produces prothrombin levels about 1.5 to 2.5 times normal. Loading doses of 20 to 60 mg were formerly used, but ingestions exceeding this amount could cause bleeding.

There are no good studies correlating bait formulations and prothrombin activity, although some suggest that warfarin is not completely absorbed in these forms. Four oz (113 gm) of a 0.25 per cent bait would contain 28 mg of warfarin. Even if completely absorbed, this would be unlikely to produce bleeding in an adult with a single acute exposure. Patients on anticoagulants would be at risk with much smaller amounts. Identification of the product is important, since the second-generation anticoagulants are more potent and have longer half-lives.

Mouthful amounts in children present no risk, and treatment is not necessary. Exposure to amounts larger than 0.5 mg/kg and chronic exposures should be evaluated.

Treatment involves the administration of syrup of ipecac to prevent absorption or administration of activated charcoal followed by a cathartic. The prothrombin time (PT) should be checked initially and again in 12 to 24 hours. Patients who are asymptomatic and have normal PTs and no evidence of bleeding may be discharged from the emergency department. They may return as outpatients for follow-up PTs.

When the PT is two or more times normal or there is evidence of bleeding, vitamin K should be given. Vitamin K is rapidly metabolized and has to be given three to five times daily.[16] Blood transfusions may be indicated in the event of major blood loss. Repeated hematocrits and PTs are indicated.

When patients are already on anticoagulants, emesis should be avoided; activated charcoal alone should be given to absorb the toxin. Few deaths have been reported with warfarin compounds, since early treatment can be effective.

Second-Generation Anticoagulants

During the mid to late 1970s a second generation of anticoagulants (Table 72–5) was introduced into the market. These have the same mechanism of action as the warfarin agents. Their main advantages as rodenticides are that they are effective in single or limited feedings (warfarin requires repeated feedings for 4 to 5 days) and are effective against animals who are resistant or more tolerant to older anticoagulants.[17] Although their mechanism of action is the same as that of warfarin, second-generation agents are different in two important ways: they are more potent and have a longer half-life. In dogs the half-life is 120 days.[18] In humans, a single ingestion of 0.12 mg/kg of brodifacoum produces anticoagulation lasting 51 days.[19] Others have reported coagulation defects lasting from 45 days to over 7 months.[18–20]

Unknown quantities and amounts exceeding 0.10 mg/kg should be evacuated from the stomach before they can be absorbed. Ipecac may be given or gastric lavage performed when ipecac is contraindicated, followed by activated charcoal and a cathartic.

Obtain a baseline PT and partial thromboplastin time (PTT), with repeat estimations at 24 and 48 hours and as clinically indicated. If at any point the PT or PTT is increased or there is some risk of bleeding, then vitamin K should be given. In severe ingestions give vitamin K via slow IV infusion. For severe hemorrhaging, whole blood or plasma may be required. Oral vitamin K can be used once the patient is stable. High doses of vitamin K administered for long periods of time with continued monitoring of PT may be indicated.

Table 72–5. SECOND-GENERATION ANTICOAGULANTS

brodifacoum
  Enforcer, Talon, Talon G, Havoc, Ropax, Mouse Prufe II
bromadiolone
  Bromone, Super Caid, Ratimus, Maki, Rat-A-Rest, Just One Bite, Trax-One
chlorophacinone
  Rozol, Caid, Drat
diphacinone
  Diphacin, Ramik, Promar, PCQ, Finis, Thro Pac Pellets, Guardian, Kill-Ko, Formula 163, Rat-Ola, Rodere Paraffinized Rat Bait
diphenacoum
  Ratak
isovaleryl
  Isotrac
Pivalyn
  Purina Rat Kill
Pivalyl
  Black Magic

Pyriminil, PNU

Available Products: Vacor rat bait, DLP 787 tracking powder.

This agent was released in 1975 as a one-feeding (acute) rodenticide. Owing to its severe toxicity, it was withdrawn as a general use pesticide in 1979. Vacor produces destruction of the beta cells of the pancreas, causing diabetes mellitus in survivors. Sensory and motor neuropathies as well as other nervous system dysfunction are seen.[21–23] Death has been reported with a dose of 780 mg, and symptoms have been produced with 390 mg (5.6 mg/kg).[24] The exact mechanism of action of Vacor is unknown, but in animals it seems to act as a niacinamide antagonist.

Recent ingestion should be treated by evacuation of the stomach with ipecac or gastric lavage. Activated charcoal and a cathartic should be administered. Adults should be given 500 mg niacinamide IV (slow push) immediately, followed by 200 to 400 mg every 4 hours for 48 hours, up to a maximum of 3000 mg/day. Children are given one-half the adult dose. When the patient is able to take medication by mouth, the dose of niacinamide is 100 mg orally four times daily for 2 weeks. Blood and urine sugar should be monitored as well as alkaline phosphatase, amylase, lactic dehydrogenase (LDH), serum glutamic oxaloacetic transaminase (SGOT), ketones, electrolytes, and blood urea nitrogen (BUN). Diabetic ketoacidosis should be managed appropriately with insulin as necessary. Diabetes may be brittle and difficult to control and may persist permanently; the patient may become insulin dependent for life.

Sodium Monofluoroacetate

Available Products

Sodium Monofluoroacetate. Sodium Fluoroacetate, Compound 1080, Fratol.

Fluoroacetamide. Compound 1081, Fluorakil, Fussol, Megarox, Yancock.

Sodium fluoroacetate was developed during World War II as an alternative to imported natural rodenticides.[25] This compound is readily absorbed through the gastrointestinal and respiratory tracts, mucous membranes, and broken skin and is highly toxic. In humans, doses of 0.5 to 2 mg/kg should be considered highly dangerous; 5 mg/kg is estimated to be the lethal dose.[26] Sodium fluoroacetate must first be metabolized to fluorocitrate, the active toxin. Some have proposed that toxicity is caused by blockage of the Krebs cycle, thus preventing energy metabolism; however, this mechanism has recently been challenged.[27] Critical effects are produced primarily in the CNS (seizures and respiratory depression) and the heart (tachycardia and ventricular fibrillation).

Fluoroacetamide has essentially the same actions as fluoroacetate but is less toxic.[1] Because it is so highly toxic, the use of sodium monofluoroacetate is restricted to licensed exterminators. Following ingestion, effects are delayed 30 minutes to 2 hours (while metabolism to fluorocitrate occurs). Vomiting is commonly seen. Apprehension, auditory hallucinations, and facial paresthesias often precede convulsions. Cardiac effects often follow and may include ectopic beats, tachycardia, ventricular fibrillation, and cardiac arrest. Diffuse tubular degeneration of the kidneys has been seen in two cases.[1]

Immediately after ingestion the stomach should be emptied, followed by administration of activated charcoal. If it is 30 minutes after exposure or if substantial vomiting has occurred, activated charcoal and cathartic alone should be considered. Continuous cardiac monitoring is indicated. There is no specific therapy for fluoroacetate toxicity. Any symptomatic patient should be admitted to the hospital and provided symptomatic and supportive therapy.

Red Squill

Available Products: Deathdiet, Rat Snax, Rat Squill, Rat Nip, Rat Not, Rodine.

Red squill is a botanic rodenticide derived from the red variety of *Urginea maritima,* or sea onion. Red squill contains two cardiac glycosides, scillaren A and scillaren B.[28] Red squill is very bitter and has a powerful emetic action, hence much of the material may be ejected from the stomach before it is absorbed. The cardiac glycosides produce effects similar to those of digitalis, and treatment is similar to that for digitalis toxicity (see Chapter 90).

Thallium

Available Products: Martin's Rat Stop, Patterson's Mole & Gopher Killer.

Thallium sulfate is a colorless and odorless powder. It was introduced in the US in the 1930s as a rodenticide.[1] Thallium is absorbed rapidly from the gastrointestinal tract. It is also absorbed through the skin and by inhalation. The use of thallium as a pesticide was prohibited in the US in 1965.[30] Fatalities have been seen with adult dosages of 8 mg/kg. The usual lethal dose is 10 to 15 mg/kg.[31] Children under 10 to 12 years of age can tolerate larger amounts.[1]

Ingestion of thallium sulfate often causes nausea, sometimes with occasional vomiting. For the first 3 to 4 days (up to 1 week) following ingestion, the only symptom may be constipation unresponsive to laxatives.[31] Following this latent period patients develop neuropathic pain, starting in the lower extremities. At the same time severe abdominal pain occurs. During the second week tachycardia develops, severe toxic polyneuritis is evident, and hair loss begins.

According to Moeschlin,[31] symptoms essential for diagnosis include dark bands at the hair roots, retrosternal pain, abdominal cramps, constipation, hysteriform behavior, polyneuritis, tachycardia, hair loss, and lunula strips in the nails.

Treatment of thallium poisoning is difficult, and there is no consensus regarding management. Recent reports emanate from Europe, where therapeutic agents used are not available in the US.[32]

Forced potassium diuresis can be used. Potassium chloride has been used to increase the urinary excretion of thallium by competing for reabsorption. It can decrease the half-life from 30 days to 8 to 10 days and has been used with good results.[32–34] Hemoperfusion or hemoperfusion alternating with hemodialysis has been used to increase elimination of thallium.[31, 32, 35]

Prussian blue (Berliner blue) is used in Europe to chelate thallium in the gut and prevent intestinal reabsorption. The drug is not available in the US.

Patients surviving 4 to 5 weeks will probably live, but damage to organ systems may be permanent.

Arsenic

Available Products:

Arsenic Trioxide. S. L. Cowley & Sons Rat and Mouse Poison, Rat Snack.

Sodium Arsenite: Rat Death Liquid.

Arsenious Oxide: Blue Ball Rat Killer.

Although more commonly used as a pesticide or herbicide, arsenic has some limited use as a rodenticide. Arsenites are salts of arsenous acid (from arsenic trioxide). Arsenites are more soluble and more rapidly toxic than other forms of arsenic and thus are used as rodenticides, herbicides, and pesticides.[1] (For effects and treatment of exposure to arsenic see Chapter 59.)

Zinc Phosphide, Aluminum Phosphide, Phosphine Gas

Available Products

Zinc Phosphide: ZP, ZP Tracking powder, ZP AG, Mr. Rat Guard, Gopha Rid, True Grit Tracking Powder, True Grit Gopher Rid, Phosvin, Zinc-Tox.

Aluminum Phosphide: Phostoxin.

Zinc phosphide is a dark gray crystalline powder with an odor similar to that of rotten fish.[1] It is available as powder or pellets and in crimped oat forms. Phosphine gas is formed rapidly in contact with dilute acids or more slowly in contact with water.[36] Aluminum phosphide is used to generate phosphine gas,[37, 38] and virtually all of the effects seen with zinc phosphide[1, 39] can be attributed to phosphine gas. Toxic exposures to phosphine gas by inhalation have also been reported (see Chapter 81).[37] The lethal dose in humans is not known, but patients have died after ingesting as little as 4 to 5 gm and survived following ingestion of 25 to 50 gm zinc phosphide. The threshold limit value for phosphine gas is 0.3 ppm.

Zinc phosphide will cause severe gastrointestinal irritation. Nausea and vomiting can be seen with ingestion of as little as 30 mg and often occur early after toxic exposure. Vomiting can be constant. Other early signs and symptoms include chest tightness, excitement, agitation, thirst, and feeling or being "cold all over." Shock, oliguria, convulsions, and coma have been seen in fatal cases.[36, 37]

Late effects include delayed pulmonary edema, metabolic acidosis, hypocalcemic tetany, circulatory collapse, liver damage, bradycardia and electrocardiogram (ECG) abnormalities, thrombocytopenia, and methemoglobinemia. Pulmonary edema can result in death within a few hours. The majority of deaths occur after approximately 30 hours, probably owing to myocardial damage. Patients who survive 3 days generally recover.

Time is critical following ingestion, since vomiting within the first hour improves the prognosis. If spontaneous vomiting does not occur, vomiting can be induced with syrup of ipecac. Activated charcoal followed by gastric lavage might be considered as an alternative. The use of 1:1000 potassium permanganate as the lavage solution has been suggested. Theoretically this would oxidize the phosphide to phosphate. However, experimental and clinical evidence for benefit cannot be found. It is important to clear zinc phosphide from the entire gastrointestinal tract; therefore, charcoal and a cathartic should be left in the stomach following gastric emptying.

Treatment is symptomatic and supportive. Patients who are symptomatic should be monitored in an intensive care setting for at least 72 hours. The status of pulmonary, cardiac, circulatory, renal, and hepatic systems should be followed closely. No patients have been reported to live if refractory shock had ensued. Those who live for 3 days generally recover.

ANTU (alpha-Naphthyl-Thiourea)

Available Products: Dr. Hess Anturat, Bantu, Rattrach, Kill Kantz, Krysid, Nott's Rat-tu, College brand rodenticide.

ANTU produces pulmonary edema and pulmonary effusion in adult Norway rats. Young Norway rats, roof rats, and most other animals except dogs are resistant.[1] Animal studies suggest that the lethal dose for humans may be about 4 gm/kg. Effects expected include vomiting, dyspnea, cyanosis, and pulmonary rales.

Treatment includes emptying the stomach in large exposures, followed by administration of activated charcoal and a cathartic. Patients should be observed for 72 hours for delayed pulmonary edema. Significant toxicity thereafter is not expected.

Norbromide

Available Products: Shoxin, Raticate.

Norbromide is selectively toxic to Norway rats. Death is caused as a result of intense peripheral vasoconstriction.[40] Other rats, rodents, and animals, including man, are resistant since they do not possess the vascular receptor for this compound. Volunteers given 20 to 300 mg had no symptomatic complaints but at the higher doses demonstrated a slight decrease in temperature and blood pressure. Lowest values were at 1 hour after ingestion, and values returned to normal by 2 hours.[1]

Following large exposures the stomach should be emptied and activated charcoal given. Treatment, if needed, is symptomatic and supportive.

Barium

Available Products: No commercial products in the United States.

Barium carbonate is one of several soluble barium salts, including sulfide, chloride, chlorate, and nitrate. All are toxic. Rodenticides contain 20 to 25 per cent barium carbonate. The lethal dose is estimated to be 2 gm. Acute toxicity may be seen with 200 mg.[1]

Barium apparently produces a depolarizing neuromuscular blockade resulting in weakness of striated, cardiac, and smooth muscle. Symptoms include paresthesias around the mouth that may spread to the hands and feet. Vomiting and diarrhea with colicky abdominal pain may appear 1 to 8 hours after ingestion. Tightness in the throat, dysarthria, headache, muscle twitching, generalized weakness, and paralysis can be seen. Paralysis can range from weakness of one limb to complete paralysis with respiratory failure.[41] Many of the reported cases have resulted from contamination of food. In such cases the rapidity of onset and absence of eye signs can help rule out botulism.[41]

Treatment should start with emptying of the stomach by emesis or lavage unless there has already been substantial vomiting. Sodium sulfate (30 gm in 250 ml of water) should be administered to precipitate the barium by forming insoluble barium sulfate and may be repeated in 1 hour. Fluids and electrolytes should be monitored. Hypokalemia is commonly seen, and plasma potassium should be monitored and hypokalemia corrected.[42, 43] Repeated neurologic assessment is a necessity. Mechanical ventilation may be needed in severe cases and can be life-saving. The prognosis is good if the patient is stabilized and is maintained for 24 hours. Recovery is usually complete.

References

1. Hayes WJ: Pesticides Studied in Man. Baltimore, Williams & Wilkins, 1982.
2. Public Health Study Team: Pest Control and Public Health. Vol V. Washington, DC, National Academy of Sciences, 1976, p 81.
3. Arena JM: Poisoning: Toxicology, Symptoms, Treatment. 4th ed. Springfield, IL, Charles C Thomas, 1979.
4. Dreikorn BA, O'Doherty OP: The discovery of bromethalin, an acute rodenticide with a unique mode of action. ACS Symp Ser *255*:45, 1984.
5. Jackson WB, Spaulding SR, VanLier RBL, Dreicorn BA: Bromethalin—a promising new rodenticide. Proceedings Tenth Vertebrate Pest Conf, University of California, Davis, 1982, p 10.
6. Material Safety Data Sheet: Bromethalin Concentrate 2%. Indianapolis, Elanco Products Co, revised 1987.
7. Technical Bulletin: Assault (Bromethalin). St. Louis, Purina Mills.
8. Cherry JT, Gunnoe MD, VanLier RBL: The metabolism of bromethalin and its effects on oxidative phosphorylation and cerebral fluid pressure. Toxicologist *2*:108, 1982.
9. Product Information: True Grit Rampage Rat and Mouse Bait. Overland Park, KS, Ceva Laboratories, 1986.
10. Product Information: Quintox Rat and Mouse Bait, Quintox Mouse Seed. Rodent Control Product and Label Catalog. Madison, WI, Bell Laboratories, 1985.
11. Paterson CR: Vitamin D poisoning: Survey of causes in 21 patients with hypercalcemia. Lancet *1*:1165, 1980.
12. Haynes RC, Murad F: Agents affecting calcification. *In* Gilman AG, Goodman LS, Rall TW, Murad F (eds): The Pharmacological Basis of Therapeutics. 7th ed. New York, Macmillan, 1985.

13. Lukaszkiewicz J, Proszynska K, Lorenc RS: Hepatic microsomal enzyme induction: Treatment of vitamin D poisoning in a 7-month-old baby. Br Med J *295*:6607, 1987.
14. Holmes RW, Love J: Suicide attempt with warfarin, bishydroxycoumarin-like rodenticide. JAMA *148*:935, 1952.
15. O'Reilly RA: Anticoagulant, antithrombotic and thrombolytic drugs. *In* Gilman AG, Goodman LS, Rall TW, Murad F (eds): The Pharmacological Basis of Therapeutics. 7th ed. New York, Macmillan, 1985.
16. Bjornsson TD, Blaschke TF: Vitamin K1 disposition and therapy of warfarin overdose (letter). Lancet *2*:846, 1978.
17. Kaukeinen D: A review of the secondary poisoning hazard potential to wildlife from the use of anticoagulant rodenticides. Proceedings Tenth Vertebrate Pest Conf, University of California, Davis, 1982, p 123.
18. Lipton RA, Evans MK: Human ingestion of a "superwarfarin" rodenticide resulting in a prolonged anticoagulant effect. JAMA *252*:3004, 1984.
19. Jones EC, Growe GH, Naiman SC: Prolonged anticoagulation in rat poisoning. JAMA *252*:3005, 1984.
20. Barlow AM, Gay AL, Park BK: Difenacoum (Neosorexa) poisoning. Br Med J *265*:541, 1982.
21. Prosser PR, Karam JH: Diabetes mellitus following rodenticide ingestion in man. JAMA *239*:1148, 1978.
22. Pont A, Rubino JM, Bishop D, Peal R: Diabetes mellitus and neuropathy following Vacor ingestion in man. Arch Intern Med *139*:185, 1979.
23. LeWitt PA: The neurotoxicity of the rat poison Vacor. N Engl J Med *302*:73, 1980.
24. LeWitt PA: The rat poison Vacor. N Engl J Med *302*:1147, 1980.
25. Egekeze JO, Oehme FW: Sodium monofluoroacetate (SMFA, compound 1080): A literature review. Vet Hum Toxicol *21*:411, 1979.
26. Proctor NH, Hughes JP: Chemical Hazards of the Workplace. Philadelphia, JB Lippincott, 1978.
27. Kun E: Monofluoroacetic acid (compound 1080), its pharmacology and toxicology. Proceedings Tenth Vertebrate Pest Conf, University of California, Davis, 1982, p 34.
28. Klaassen CD: Nonmetallic environmental toxicants: Air pollutants, solvents and vapors and pesticides. *In* Gilman AG, Goodman LS, Rall TW, Murad F (eds): The Pharmacological Basis of Therapeutics. 7th ed. New York, Macmillan, 1985.
29. Deleted in press.
30. Saddique A, Peterson CD: Thallium poisoning: A review. Vet Hum Toxicol *25*:16, 1983.
31. Moeschlin MD: Thallium poisoning. Clin Toxicol *17*:133, 1980.
32. Nogue S, Mas A, Pares A, Nasal P, Bertran A, Milla J, Carrera M, To J, Pazos MR, Corbella J: Acute thallium poisoning: An evaluation of different forms of treatment. J Toxicol Clin Toxicol *19*:1015, 1982–83.
33. Chamberlain PH, Stavinoha WB, Davis H, Knikwe MD, Panos TC: Thallium poisoning. Pediatrics *22*:1170, 1958.
34. Reed D, Crawley J, Faro SN, Pieper SJ, Kurland LT: Thallotoxicosis. JAMA *183*:516, 1963.
35. DeBaker W, Zachee P, Verpooten GA, Majelyne W, Vanheule A, DeBroe ME: Thallium intoxication treated with combined hemoperfusion-hemodialysis. J Toxicol Clin Toxicol *19*:259, 1982.
36. Stephenson JBP: Zinc phosphide poisoning. Arch Environ Health *15*:83, 1967.
37. Wilson R, Lovejoy FH, Jaeger RJ, Landrigan PL: Acute phosphene poisoning aboard a grain freighter. JAMA *244*:148, 1980.
38. Salmon TP, Bentley WJ: Aluminum phosphide (phostoxin) as a burrow fumigant for ground squirrel control. Proceedings Tenth Vertebrate Pest Conf, University of California, Davis, 1982, p 142.
39. Johnson HD, Voss E: Toxicological studies of zinc phosphide. J Am Public Health Assoc *41*:468, 1952.
40. Morgan DP: Recognition and Management of Pesticide Poisonings. 3rd ed. Washington, DC, EPA, 1982.
41. Lewi Z, Bar-Khayim Y: Food poisoning from barium carbonate. Lancet *2*:342, 1964.
42. Phelan DM, Hagley SR: Is hypokalemia the cause of paralysis in barium poisoning? Br Med J *289*:882, 1984.
43. Bering J: Hypokalemia of barium poisoning (letter). Lancet *1*:110, 1975.

Inhalation Poisoning and Solvents

CHAPTER 73

AIR POLLUTION: AIR QUALITY INDEX AND OZONE

Wayne R. Snodgrass, M.D., Ph.D.

AIR QUALITY INDEX AND OVERVIEW

Air pollution is recognized now to be prevalent throughout the planet Earth. Every one of us with each breath inhales chemicals, some of which are manmade, and some of these at current levels of exposure pose a risk of morbidity and mortality over a period of time. Air pollutants are vast in number and complexity; the best understood and most frequently monitored are sulfur dioxide (SO_2), nitrogen dioxide (NO_2), carbon monoxide (CO), sulfates, particulates (TSP = total suspended particulates), benzopyrene and other polycyclic aromatic hydrocarbons (PAHs), and oxidants such as ozone (O_3), and peroxyacetylnitrate (PAN). Other well-known air pollutants include asbestos, lead, arsenic, cadmium, beryllium, fluoride, mercury, manganese, and plutonium.[1, 2]

National ambient air quality standards (NAAQS) are shown in Table 73–1. The NAAQS levels are maximal or unhealthful levels. Exposure to these levels results in adverse health effects. The 1- to 24-hour averages are not to be exceeded more than once a year. Ambient air levels of this magnitude require a public warning for persons with heart or respiratory disorders to reduce physical activity and outdoor exertion.[3] The NAAQS were determined based on limited data from sea level observations. At high altitudes different standards may be necessary. For example, California uses 6 ppm instead of 9 ppm for the 8-hour standard for carbon monoxide above 1500 meters.[2]

The Pollutant Standards Index (PSI) is an arbitrary scale that rates various levels of individual pollutants to indicate a relative risk for acute exposure. A value of 100 is assigned to the NAAQS level and the PSI ranges from 50 to 500 (Table 73–2).

Susceptibility to the adverse effects of air pollution is greatest among infants, elderly people, individuals with chronic heart and lung diseases, including asthma, and tobacco smokers. Symptoms caused by pollutants may occur at once or may lag behind the peak of exposure by 1 to 2 days. Staying indoors may reduce exposure to certain oxidants, but exposure to NO_2, hydrocarbons, SO_2, CO, and TSPs may or may not be reduced by remaining indoors and depends upon ventilation of the dwelling.[2] Considerable published data document the adverse effects of air pollution.[4–10] In addition to cancer, worsening or outright initiation of chronic obstructive lung disease has been related to air pollutants.[11–13]

Air pollutants occur in the physical forms of gases, liquid droplets, and particulates. The addition of moisture, e.g., in the respiratory tract, tends to enlarge particles. Size determines whether specific components are filtered out in the upper airways (>2.0 microns), are deposited in alveoli (0.05 to 2.0 microns), or are exhaled like a gas (<0.05 micron).[2]

Air pollution is known to alter the rate of hospital admissions. Elevated ozone and aerosol sulfates appeared to cause a 7 per cent or greater increase in respiratory admissions as reported in southern Ontario.[14] Total suspended particulates and sulfur dioxide levels seemed to correlate with emergency department visits in a study done in Ohio.[15]

Table 73–1. NATIONAL AMBIENT AIR QUALITY STANDARDS

POLLUTANT	TIME INTERVAL	CONCENTRATION,* μg/m³	PPM
Carbon monoxide	1 hr	40,000	35
Carbon monoxide	8 hr	10,000	9
Hydrocarbons	3 hr (6–9 AM)	160	0.24
Nitrogen oxide	1 yr†	100	0.05
Ozone	1 hr	160	0.08
Sulfur oxide	24 hr	365	0.14
Sulfur oxide	1 yr	80	0.03
Sulfur oxide	3 hr	1,300	0.05
Particulates	24 hr	260	—
Particulates	1 yr	75	—

*Corrected for standard conditions at sea level and 25° C.

†Short-term standard soon to be adopted. Exposures to concentrations at or below those concentrations are not expected to cause any confirmed adverse health effects in humans, even to those who are highly susceptible.

(From Mitchell RS, Judson FN, Moulding TS, Weiser P, Brock LL, Kelble DL, Pollard J: Health effects of urban pollution. Special consideration of areas at 1500 meters and above. JAMA *242*:1163–1168, 1979.)

Sulfur dioxide (SO_2) and associated particulates in high concentration have been identified clearly as the major pollutants in most severe air pollution disasters.[2] SO_2 results from the burning of coal and oil. It is a severe pulmonary irritant in high concentrations. Sulfate particulates also are quite prevalent in many urban atmospheres; they usually contain ammonium ion as the cation. For inland areas, $(NH_4)_2SO_4$ is the major sulfate form, but in coastal regions, where ammonium is deficient, sulfate ion is bound as NH_4HSO_4. SO_2 is converted to sulfates. There are two types of sulfate particulates: those with a median diameter of 0.2 ± 0.02 μm (micrometers), which are thought to be the result of homogeneous oxidation of SO_2 in air, and those with a median diameter of 0.54 ± 0.07 μm, which are the result of a heterogeneous reaction of SO_2 on particulates.[16]

Air pollution from fossil fuel burning in automobiles, electric power plants, and other industries contributes largely to the predicted *greenhouse effect* warming of the earth. By the year 2025, an average 3°C temperature rise is expected. Oceans will rise from polar ice melting; coastal areas will flood. Prior to the year 1850 the atmospheric carbon dioxide (CO_2) level was 280 ppm or less; this level of CO_2 was not exceeded for many millions of years, as documented by earth core sampling measurements. Between 1950 and 1980, the atmospheric CO_2 in the air we breathe rose from 315 ppm to 340 ppm.[69, 70]

The earth is a closed system. Fossil fuel burning by humans may be short-circuiting the natural carbon cycle on the planet. Approximately 60 per cent of annual CO_2 production remains in the atmosphere, some of which is used in photosynthesis by plants; about 40 per cent of annual CO_2 production eventually equilibrates to the oceans, where some of it becomes calcium carbonate ($CaCO_3$), i.e., rock. Increased dissolved CO_2 may have implications for altering the pH of ocean waters. The lag time for equilibration of these processes may be many years. This would include the lag time for temperature rise due to the high heat capacity of water in the oceans.[17] Infrared-absorbing trace gases, in addition to CO_2, will double the climatic warming resulting from CO_2 alone. One example is nitrous oxide (N_2O), which "leaks" during the process of nitrogen fixation. Intensive agricultural chemical fertilizer use worldwide and other sources now result in a 0.2 to 0.5 per cent (2.8 to 5.6 trillion grams) per year increase in atmospheric nitrous oxide. N_2O via conversion to NO (nitric oxide) reacts with and decreases upper atmospheric ozone, another source of ozone loss.[18] In comparison with fossil fuel and other energy use by humans, solar energy annually reaching land surface areas (1.5×10^{17} kwh) is several thousand times greater.[19]

Indoor air pollution for some chemical exposures poses a greater risk than outdoor air pollution. CO, NO_2, SO_2, tobacco smoke, asbestos, volatile organic compounds, radon, and various allergens, including fungi, are all known indoor air pollutants.[3, 20–24] Sidestream smoke from tobacco smoke contains up to 100 times the mainstream smoke concentrations of some highly toxic compounds, such as carcinogenic nitrosamines, naphthylamine, acrolein, polonium, cadmium, and

Table 73–2. COMPARISON OF POLLUTANT STANDARDS INDEX (PSI) VALUES WITH POLLUTANT CONCENTRATIONS, HEALTH-EFFECT DESCRIPTORS, GENERAL HEALTH EFFECTS, AND CAUTIONARY STATEMENTS

		POLLUTANT LEVELS							
INDEX VALUE	AIR QUALITY INDEX	*TSP* *(24 hr)* $\mu g/M^3$	SO_2 *(24 hr)* $\mu g/M^3$	*CO* *(8 hr)* $\mu g/M^3$	O_3 *(1 hr)* $\mu m/M^3$	NO_2 *(1 hr)* $\mu g/M^3$	HEALTH-EFFECT DESCRIPTOR	GENERAL HEALTH EFFECTS	CAUTIONARY STATEMENTS
500	Significant harm	1000	2620	57.5	1200	3750		Premature death of the ill and the elderly. Healthy people will experience adverse symptoms that affect their normal activity	All persons should remain indoors, keeping windows and doors closed. All persons should minimize physical exertion and avoid traffic
400	Emergency	875	2100	46.0	1000	3000	Hazardous	Premature onset of certain diseases, in addition to significant aggravation of symptoms and decreased exercise tolerance in healthy persons	The elderly and persons with diseases should stay indoors and avoid physical exertion. General population should avoid outdoor activity
300	Warning	625	1600	34.0	800	2260	Very unhealthful	Significant aggravation of symptoms and decreased exercise tolerance in persons with heart or lung disease, with widespread symptoms in the healthy population	The elderly and persons with heart or lung disease should stay indoors and reduce physical activity
200	Alert	375	800	17.0	400	1130	Unhealthful	Mild aggravation of symptoms in susceptible persons, with irritation symptoms in the healthy population	Persons with heart or respiratory ailments should reduce physical exertion and outdoor activity
100	NAAQS*	260	365	10.0	160		Moderate		
50	50% of NAAQS	75	80	5.0	80		Good		

*National Ambient Air Quality Standard.

(Adapted from "Guideline for Public Reporting of Daily Air Quality-Pollutant Standards Index," Environmental Protection Agency. *In* Katz S: On the Air Quality Index. Am Fam Physician, Oct 1978, pp 121–122.)

carbon monoxide.[3] One estimate suggests that FEV_1 lung growth rate in children ages 6 to 10 years is reduced by 0.17 per cent per pack of cigarettes smoked daily by the mother.[3] In an important Centers for Disease Control study, for 28 of 30 cases in which a variety of chemicals were measured, the average indoor concentrations exceeded the outdoor levels.[25] Personal air concentrations (most of the time was spent indoors) exceeded outdoor air concentrations for every chemical, usually by a factor of 2 to 5.[25] For dichlorobenzene (e.g., mothballs) the indoor average air level was 50 $\mu g/m^3$, compared with an average outdoor level of less than 2 $\mu g/m^3$.[25]

Children potentially may be more susceptible to the adverse effects of air pollution than healthy adults. A large number of studies document toxic effects of air pollutants on otherwise healthy children and suggest the need for greater monitoring of this population.[26–47]

Formal attempts at quantifying and predicting risk of toxicity from air pollution, i.e., so-called risk assessment, are being reported in recent years.[48–50] One potential practical outcome of these attempts may be earlier recognition of problems when they occur.

Protective equipment to attempt to treat or decrease the severity of acute exposure to air pollutants is limited usually to face masks, respirators, or self-contained breathing apparatus that may be effective only for dust or particulates or may provide an alternate gaseous atmosphere. Equipment may vary in effectiveness.[51]

OZONE*

A discussion of ozone (O_3) actually involves two subjects: the *depletion* of ozone in the stratosphere (upper atmosphere) of the earth, and the *increase* of ozone in the troposphere (lower atmosphere). Following a brief discussion of the depletion of the "ozone layer," the major focus is on the increase of ozone in the troposphere, as ozone is the most potent ambient respiratory irritant known to occur in ambient air pollution.[52, 53]

Depletion of Ozone in the Stratosphere

The ozone layer is located in the stratosphere, 10 to 30 miles up, and is vital to the well-being of plants and animals. Ozone molecules, consisting of 3 oxygen atoms, absorb most of the ultraviolet radiation of the sun. Increase in ultraviolet radiation has been associated with an increase in skin cancer, cataracts, and possibly immunologic disturbances. Furthermore, research is underway to determine whether an increase in ultraviolet radiation may affect the food chain. There is concern that ultraviolet-B radiation can reach the earth's surface through the ozone "hole," as ultraviolet-B radiation can penetrate several meters below the ocean surface and theoretically damage phytoplankton, which is the beginning of the food chain for all aquatic creatures.[70, 71]

Chlorofluorocarbons (CFCs) have been used as coolants in refrigerators; they are now banned in the United States as propellant gases for spray cans but are standard ingredients in plastic foam materials such as Styrofoam. The release of chlorine molecules on decomposition of the CFC molecule has been associated with destruction of the highly reactive ozone. Not until 1985 was the "hole" in the ozone documented over the Antarctic: it is now known that the Antarctic ozone at certain times has been depleted by as much as 50 per cent. In March, 1988, thinning of the ozone layer over the North Pole was also noted. The half-time for the recovery of the ozone layer is normally 3 to 4 years but it may require 8 to 10 years for reconstitution under abnormal situations.[72]

Nations worldwide are finally cooperating to reduce drastically the worldwide production of CFCs, in order to preserve the protective ozone layer, as evidenced by the Montreal Protocol, signed by 35 countries on September 16, 1987.[70] The Montreal Protocol, while a definite beginning, is hardly sufficient to solve this ominous threat to our human race.

Increase of Ozone in the Troposphere

Ozone (O_3) is a highly reactive chemical species, more chemically reactive than oxygen (O_2) itself. Since it contains two unpaired electrons, it also has free radical potential. In contact with aqueous solutions, including lung and other tissues, ozone can form hydroxyl free radical (OH•), one of the most reactive oxygen chemical species known.[54] Via free radical mechanisms, ozone can cause lipid peroxidation and oxidation of thiols, amines, and proteins—all leading to cell and

*Portions of this section on ozone were excerpted from material originally appearing in reference 70.

tissue toxicity[55] (Fig. 73–1). This oxidant theory of ozone's mechanism of toxicity is supported by animal data documenting the efficacy of selected antioxidant therapy to decrease ozone-induced pneumotoxicity. Dimethylthiourea, a hydrogen peroxide scavenger, protects rats from ozone lung damage.[56]

Controlled human exposure studies and outdoor epidemiologic field health studies have documented impairment of pulmonary function in exercising adults and children exposed to ozone air concentrations of 0.12 ppm or less.[52] The current NAAQS for ozone is 0.12 ppm for a 1-hour period. Thus, adverse human health effects for ozone are known at the level currently designated by the NAAQS. The current OSHA standard TLV (threshold limit value) is 0.10 ppm for 8 hours. Thus, ozone is the only known outdoor air pollutant for which permissible ambient exposures can exceed a workplace exposure limit.[52] In America, the NAAQS is exceeded regularly and frequently in many areas of the country[57] (Fig. 73–2). Violation in any monitored area occurs when, during a 3-year running period, the standard is exceeded for 1 hour in any one of more than 3 days.[58] In California, first, second, and third stage alerts are declared whenever ozone levels reach or exceed 0.20 ppm—1 hour average; 0.35 ppm—1 hour average; and 0.5 ppm—1 hour average, respectively. The TLV guideline represents conditions under which

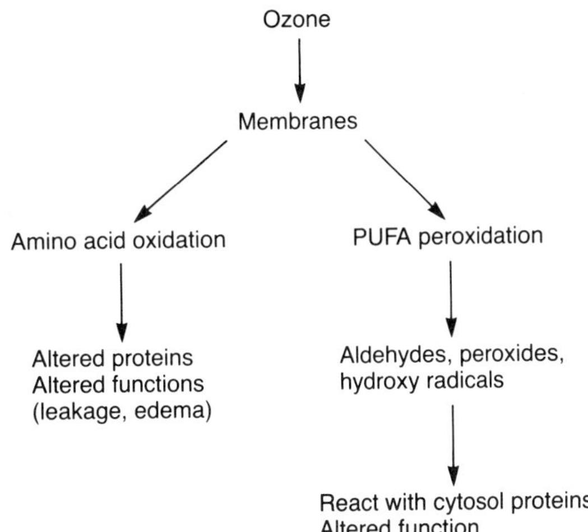

Figure 73–1. Mechanism of cell and tissue toxicity from ozone.

it is believed that nearly all workers may be exposed day after day without adverse effects. The TLV and OSHA limits are not intended to be protective of sensitive subgroups, which is a requirement for an NAAQS.[52]

What are the clinical data that ozone causes harm to humans? Ozone is a principal component in photochemically produced smog, such as that found in the Los Angeles air basin. Studies in the 1960s clearly demonstrated the deleterious effects of smog on Los Angeles residents, especially those individ-

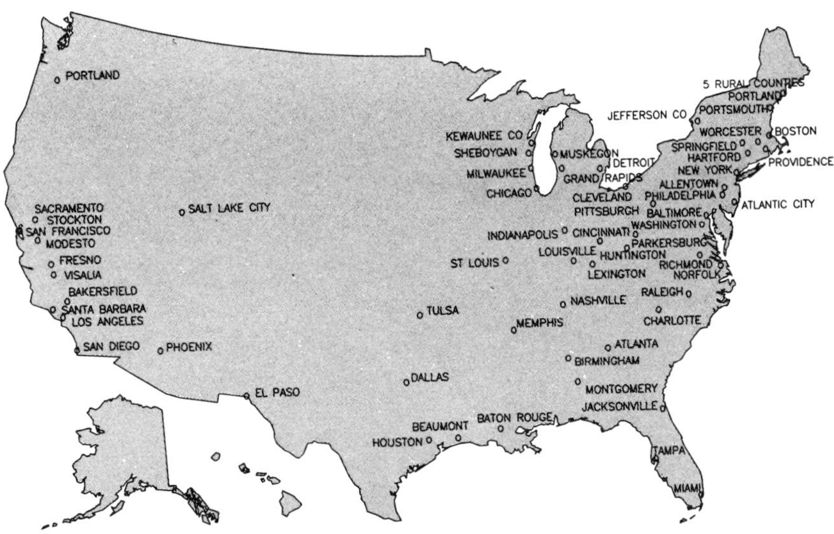

Figure 73–2. Map prepared by the Environmental Protection Agency of areas violating the national ambient air quality standards for ozone.

uals with pre-existing pulmonary disease.[5] More recent clinical work has documented specifically ozone's dose response pulmonary function toxicity. Typical effects of ozone are cough, substernal discomfort, and impaired performance in lung function tests, e.g., decreased forced expiratory volumes and flow rates.

Of more concern are the bronchoconstrictive effects of ozone, which can be seen in some sensitive normal subjects and asthmatic patients after as little as 2 hours of exposure to levels commonly observed on days of poor air quality.[59] In a group of rigorously selected, healthy, young adult nonsmoker men (ages 18 to 33, N = 24) (29 others rejected because of allergies or cold air sensitivity) during exercise at an ozone air level of 0.16 ppm for 2 hours, the FEV_1 decreased from 4114 ml to 4020 ml (2.3 per cent), compared with a baseline increase with time from 4093 ml to 4134 ml (1.0 per cent). A larger (4.3 per cent) decrease occurred in the maximal midexpiratory flow rate.[60] These decrements in lung function in a highly purified atmosphere of an inhalation laboratory occurred at just above the NAAQS level and in a selected group of healthy young nonsmoking subjects. Greater effects would be expected in ambient air containing additional pollutants in a general population, including older individuals and those with pre-existing pulmonary, cardiac, or other physical impairments.

In a different group of healthy young adult nonsmokers studied outdoors, the overall pulmonary effects of ozone (range: 0.021 to 0.124 ppm) were about twice as large as those reported in purified air chamber studies. Furthermore, the magnitude of the decreased lung function was such that a 26 per cent decrease in forced expiratory flow was predicted at an ozone level of 0.12 ppm, the NAAQS.[61]

Children also have been shown to incur pulmonary function impairment with ozone exposure. At 0.12 ppm ozone, an average 17 per cent decrease in peak expiratory flow rate was predicted from lung function data in 91 children.[62] After one outdoor exposure of children to ozone, including a maximal 1-hour exposure of 0.185 ppm, a shift in peak expiratory flow rate persisted approximately 1 week.[63] Persistence of decreased lung function following ozone exposure also has been documented in adults.[64]

One perhaps unique risk for ozone exposure occurs for passengers of commercial airline flights over the northern transatlantic route from February to April during which they may pass through portions of the stratospheric (upper atmosphere) ozone cover. Preliminary data suggest an association between cough and shortness of breath with ozone in individuals with this unique exposure.[65]

Lung cancer related to chronic ozone exposure is suspected, but apparently few published human data directly address this question. In selected strains of laboratory mice, ozone can increase the incidence of lung cancer.[66] This unproved risk for humans clearly deserves more study.

The obvious best treatment for ozone toxicity is prevention, i.e., reduction of environmental tropospheric ozone levels to well below the current NAAQS (it is estimated that the current NAAQS is approximately four times the ozone air level that existed naturally prior to significant manmade pollution). However, in the interim, what can a treating physician recommend to a patient to attempt to decrease ozone exposure? Remaining indoors will reduce ozone exposure. Use of antioxidant compounds may offer some potential treatment in the future. In one group of 14 normal human subjects, partial protection against ozone-induced bronchoconstriction by a combination therapy of vitamin E and vitamin C was reported.[67] Similarly, but working by a different mechanism, indomethacin partially blocked the worsening in FVC and FEV_1 in healthy subjects exposed to ozone.[68]

In summary, because ozone is a pervasive air pollutant, it affects large segments of the population. Short-term pulmonary function abnormalities are associated with ozone exposure above 0.12 ppm for 1 hour (this level is the current NAAQS) or above 0.10 ppm for 8 hours in a single day. In the United States, the urban population potentially exposed to ozone at greater than 0.12 ppm for at least 1 hour a week while participating in moderate exercise is about 13,000,000. For exposure to greater than 0.10 ppm for 1 hour, the number rises to 21,000,000 people.[52] Clearly, ozone is an air pollutant of major concern, and efforts to curtail its tropospheric production deserve adequate resources to attempt to lessen the health hazards of exposure to it.

References

1. Suess MJ, et al: Ambient Air Pollutants from Industrial Sources. New York, Elsevier Science Publishing Company, 1985.
2. Mitchell RS, Judson FN, Moulding TS, et al: Health effects of urban air pollution. Special consideration of areas at 1,500 meters and above. JAMA *242*:1163–1168, 1979.
3. Angle CR: Indoor air pollutants. Adv Pediatr *35*:239–280, 1988.
4. Shumway RH, Azari AS, Pawitan Y: Modeling mortality fluctuations in Los Angeles as functions of pollution and weather effects. Environ Res *45*:224–241, 1988.
5. Brandt JWA, et al: Human respiratory diseases and atmospheric air pollution in Los Angeles, California. Air Water Pollut *8*:259–277, 1964.
6. Brandt JWA: Human cardiovascular diseases and atmospheric air pollution in Los Angeles, California. Air Water Pollut *9*:219–231, 1965.
7. Ozkaynak H, Lippmann M: Associations between 1980 U.S. mortality rates and alternative measures of airborne particle concentration. Risk Anal *7*:449–461, 1987.
8. Finkel J, Duel C: Clinical Implications of Air Pollution Research. Acton, MA, Publishing Sciences Group, 1976, pp 285–303.
9. Stern AC (ed): Fundamentals of Air Pollution. New York, Grune and Stratton, 1977.
10. Magill PL, et al: Air Pollution Handbook. New York, McGraw-Hill, 1956.
11. Stuart BO: Health assessment of environmental pollutants: Proliferative and degenerative diseases. Toxicol Indust Health *4*:461–467, 1988.
12. Hagmar L, Nielsen J, Skerfving S: Clinical features and epidemiology of occupational obstructive respiratory disease caused by small molecular weight organic chemicals. Monogr Allergy *21*:42–48, 1987.
13. Speizer FE: Overview of the risk of respiratory cancer from airborne contaminants. Environ Health Perspect *70*:9–15, 1986.
14. Bates DV, Sizto R: Air pollution and hospital admissions in southern Ontario: The acid summer haze effect. Environ Res *43*:317–331, 1987.
15. Samet JM, Bishop Y, Speizer FE, et al: The relationship between air pollution and emergency room visits in an industrial community. J Air Pollut Control Assoc *31*:236–240, 1981.
16. Gentilizza M, Vadjic V: Size distribution of suspended particulates in different areas and seasons as a function of their sulphate and ammonium content. Sci Total Environ *66*:225–234, 1987.
17. Laurmann JA: Scientific uncertainty and decision making: The case of greenhouse gases and global climate change. Sci Total Environ *55*:177–186, 1986.
18. Banin A: Global budget of N_2O: The role of soils and their change. Sci Total Environ *55*:27–38, 1986.
19. Gerelli E: Entropy and the end of the world. Sci Total Environ *56*:297–300, 1986.
20. Gammage RB, Kaye SV (eds): Indoor Air and Human Health. Chelsea, MI, Lewis Publishers, 1985.
21. Samet JM, Marbury MC, Spengler JD: Health effects and sources of indoor air pollution. Am Rev Respir Dis *137*:221–242, 1988.
22. White LE, Clarkson JR, Chang SN: Health effects from indoor air pollution: Case studies. J Community Health *12*:147–155, 1987.
23. Moschandreas DJ: Indoor air quality controls. Develop Toxicol Environ Sci *15*:201–211, 1987.
24. Kirsch LS: The problem of indoor pollutants. Environment *25*:17–42, 1983.
25. Wallace LA, Pellizzari ED, Hartwell TD, et al: The TEAM (total exposure assessment methodology) study: Personal exposures to toxic substances in air, drinking water, and breath of 400 residents of New Jersey, North Carolina and North Dakota. Environ Res *43*:290–307, 1987.
26. Avol EL, Linn WS, Shamoo DA, et al: Short-term respiratory effects of photochemical oxidant exposure in exercising children. J Air Pollut Control Assoc *37*:158–162, 1987.
27. Charpin D, Kleisbauer JP, Fondarai J, et al: Respiratory symptoms and air pollution changes in children: The Gardanne Coal-Basin Study. Arch Environ Health *43*:22–27, 1988.
28. Goren AI, Hellmann S: Prevalence of respiratory symptoms and diseases in school children living in a polluted and in a low polluted area in Israel. Environ Res *45*:28–37, 1988.
29. Broomhall J, Kovar IZ: Environmental pollutants in breast milk. Rev Environ Health *6*:311–317, 1986.
30. Marty H: The influence of meteorological and air pollution factors on acute diseases of the airways in children as illustrated by the Biel region (Switzerland). Experientia (Suppl) *51*:255–259, 1987.
31. Wedler E, Fegeler U, Moyzes R, Eberhard K: Influences of pollution and weather on obstructive respiratory tract diseases of children in West Berlin. Experientia (Suppl) *51*:25–30, 1987.
32. Weiss B: Environmental contaminants and behavior disorders. Dev Pharmacol Ther *10*:346–353, 1987.
33. Rindel A, Bach E, Breum NO, et al: Correlating health effects with indoor air quality in kindergartens. Int Arch Occup Environ Health *59*:363–373, 1987.
34. Vedal S, Schenker MB, Munoz A, et al: Daily air pollution effects on children's respiratory symptoms and peak expiratory flow. Am J Public Health *77*:694–698, 1987.
35. Arossa W, Spinaci S, Bugiani M, et al: Changes in lung function of children after an air pollution decrease. Arch Environ Health *42*:170–174, 1987.
36. Verplanke AJ, Remijn B, Hoek F, et al: Hydroxyproline excretion in school children and its relationship to measures of indoor air pollution. Int Arch Occup Environ Health *59*:221–231, 1987.
37. Dassen W, Brunekreef B, Hoek G, et al: Decline in children's pulmonary function during an air pollution episode. J Air Pollut Control Assoc *36*:1223–1227, 1986.
38. Schlipköter HW, Rosický B, Dolgner R, Pelech L: Growth and bone maturation in children from two regions of the F.R.G. differing in the degree of air pollution: Results of the 1974 and 1984 surveys. J Hyg Epidemiol Microbiol Immunol *30*:353–358, 1986.
39. Shy CM, Hasselblad V, Burton RM, et al: Air pollution effects on ventilatory function of U.S. schoolchildren: Results of studies in Cincinnati, Chattanooga and New York. Arch Environ Health *27*:124–128, 1973.
40. Chapman RS, et al: Air pollution and childhood ventilatory function: I. Exposure to particulate matter in two southwestern cities, 1971–1972. *In* Finkel J, Duel C (eds): Clinical Implications of Air Pollution Research. Acton, MA, Publishing Sciences Group, 1976, pp 285–303.

41. Collins JJ, Kasap HS, Holland WW: Environmental factors in child mortality in England and Wales. Am J Epidemiol *93*:10–22, 1971.
42. Douglas JWB, Waller RE: Air pollution and respiratory infection in children. Br J Prev Soc Med *20*:1–8, 1966.
43. McMillan RS, Wiseman DH, Hanes B, et al: Effects of oxidant air pollution on peak expiratory flow rates in Los Angeles schoolchildren. Arch Environ Health *18*:941–949, 1969.
44. Lowengart RA, Peters JM, Cicioni C, et al: Childhood leukemia and parents' occupational and home exposures. J Natl Cancer Inst *79*:39–46, 1987.
45. Hager-Malecka B, Lukas A, Szczepanski Z, et al: Granulocyte viability test in children from an environment with heavy metal pollution. Acta Paediatr Hung *27*:227–231, 1986.
46. Paigen B, Goldman LR, Magnant MM, et al: Growth of children living near the hazardous waste site, Love Canal. Hum Biol *59*:489–508, 1987.
47. Sultz HA, Feldman JG, Schlesinger ER, et al: An effect of continued exposure to air pollution on the incidence of chronic childhood allergic disease. Am J Public Health *60*:891–900, 1970.
48. Brown HS, West CR, Bishop DR: Chemical Health Effects Assessment Methodology for airborne contaminants. Risk Anal *7*:389–402, 1987.
49. Somers E: Making decisions from numbers. Reg Toxicol Pharmacol *7*:35–42, 1987.
50. Milvy P: A general guideline for management of risk from carcinogens. Risk Anal *6*:69–79, 1986.
51. Cherrie JW, Howie RM, Robertson A: The performance of nuisance dust respirators against typical industrial aerosols. Ann Occup Hyg *31*:481–491, 1987.
52. Lioy PJ, Dyba RV: Tropospheric ozone: The dynamics of human exposure. Toxicol Indust Health *5*:493–504, 1989.
53. Kinney PL, Ware JH, Spengler JD: A critical evaluation of acute ozone epidemiology results. Arch Environ Health *43*:168–173, 1988.
54. Glaze WH: Reaction products of ozone: A review. Environ Health Perspect *69*:151–157, 1986.
55. Mehlman MA, Borek C: Toxicity and biochemical mechanisms of ozone. Environ Res *42*:36–53, 1987.
56. Warren DL, Hyde DM, Lust JA: Synergistic interaction of ozone and respirable aerosols on rat lungs. IV. Protection by quenchers of reactive oxygen species. Toxicology *53*:113–133, 1988.
57. Marwick C: As nation's long hot summer drags on, so does war against forms of air pollution. JAMA *260*:603–607, 1988.
58. Russell M: Ozone pollution: The hard choices. Science *241*:1275–1276, 1988.
59. Golden JA, Nadel JA, Boushey HA: Bronchial hyperirritability in healthy subjects after exposure to ozone. Am Rev Respir Dis *118*:287–294, 1978.
60. Linn WS, Avol EL, Shamoo DA, et al: A dose-response study of healthy, heavily exercising men exposed to ozone at concentrations near the ambient air quality standard. Toxicol Ind Health *2*:99–112, 1986.
61. Spektor DM, Lippman M, Thurston GD, et al: Effects of ambient ozone on respiratory function in healthy adults exercising outdoors. Am Rev Respir Dis *138*:821–828, 1988.
62. Spektor DM, Lippman M, Lioy PJ, et al: Effects of ambient ozone on respiratory function in active, normal children. Am Rev Respir Dis *137*:313–320, 1988.
63. Lioy PJ, Vollmuth TA, Lippmann M: Persistence of peak flow decrement in children following ozone exposures exceeding the National Ambient Air Quality Standard. J Air Pollut Control Assoc *35*:1068–1071, 1985.
64. Folinsbee LJ, Horvath SM: Persistence of the acute effects of ozone exposure. Aviat Space Environ Med *57*:1136–1143, 1986.
65. Schädeli D, Moser HP, Brubacher G, et al: Effect of inhalation of ozone on healthy people. Int J Vitam Nutr Res *57*:454, 1987.
66. Mustafa MG, Hassett CM, Newell GW, et al: Pulmonary carcinogenic effects of ozone. Ann NY Acad Sci *534*:714–723, 1988.
67. Chatham MD, Eppler JH Jr, Sauder LR, et al: Evaluation of the effects of vitamin C on ozone-induced bronchoconstriction in normal subjects. Ann NY Acad Sci *498*:269–279, 1987.
68. Schelegle ES, Adams WC, Siefkin AD: Indomethacin pretreatment reduces ozone-induced pulmonary function decrements in human subjects. Am Rev Respir Dis *136*:1350–1354, 1987.
69. Brown LR (ed): State of the World, 1989: A Worldwatch Institute Report on Progress Toward a Sustainable Society. New York, WW Norton, 1989.
70. Leaf A: Potential health effects of global climatic and environmental changes. N Engl J Med *321*:1577–1583, 1989.
71. Roberts L: Does the ozone hole threaten Antarctic life? Science *244*:288–289, 1989.
72. National Research Council, Committee on the Atmospheric Effects of Nuclear Explosions. Washington, DC, National Academy Press, 1985.

CHAPTER 74
CARBON MONOXIDE POISONING

Roy A. M. Myers, M.D.

Carbon monoxide poisoning is the leading cause of death from poisoning in the United States, accounting for more than half of the yearly poison deaths.[1,2] Each year, an average of 3800 people die of carbon monoxide poisoning: 1500 by accident and the rest by suicide.[3] It is an extremely difficult diagnosis to make, and the true incidence of the poisoning is unknown. In a retrospective study, Barrett et al.[4] indicated a missed clinical diagnosis in 30 per cent of cases; thus, carbon monoxide poisoning has a major impact on morbidity and mortality, and a greater awareness on the part of the treating physician is essential.

Carbon monoxide is a colorless, odorless, tasteless, and nonirritating gas produced by incomplete combustion of carbon-containing materials. Fires remain the major cause of carbon monoxide deaths and poisoning and present an occupational hazard to firefighters responsible for rescuing victims.[5] Other workers exposed to high carbon monoxide levels include those in the steel industry,[6] miners, auto mechanics, and those involved in warehouse storage and loading facilities where high concentrations of carbon monoxide are produced by the moving equipment, including vehicles with propane engines. The most common sources of carbon monoxide poisoning in the home are fire and malfunctioning heating appliances such as furnaces. Motor vehicles produce carbon monoxide as a result of incomplete combustion. This may affect people either accidentally (by fumes entering the driving cabin through rusted floor boards) or intentionally (by suicide). It is evident that the transportation system so important to commerce, industry, business, and pleasure causes significant exposure to carbon monoxide.

Inadequate ventilation from charcoal, Sterno, wood, and gas fires used for cooking and heating of homes can result in carbon monoxide poisoning.[7] Any form of heating via furnaces can produce carbon monoxide, which through inadequate installation or blockage of vents can accumulate to poisonous levels. The home heating system in Korea, involving the burning of charcoal briquettes, is a major cause of carbon monoxide poisoning. Heat is transmitted through ducts under the floors. Damage to these ducts allows carbon monoxide leakage directly into the sleeping area, with devastating effects. Any form of incompletely burned, carbon-containing material must be ventilated adequately to prevent carbon monoxide poisoning.

Methylene chloride, a hydrocarbon solvent used in household and industrial aerosols and paint strippers, is slowly converted to carbon monoxide in the body. The half-life of carbon monoxide converted in the body is much greater than that of inhaled carbon monoxide.[8] Carbon monoxide is also endogenously produced consequent to the breakdown of hemoglobin and myoglobin, the major heme-containing compounds.

In a structural fire, multiple toxins may be produced by the combustion of building materials, which if inhaled may present a complex clinical picture. The carbon monoxide poisoning may be aggravated by hypoxia as a result of the fire's combustion of oxygen from the environment. Alcohol or drugs may have been ingested prior to a fire, further clouding the picture and making the diagnosis of neurologic impairment and its treatment more complex.

CARBON MONOXIDE KINETICS

Carbon monoxide in inspired air is absorbed rapidly by the lungs and combines with hemoglobin. It has a high affinity for hemoglobin, 230 to 270 times that of oxygen. This affinity is defined by Haldane's first law:

$$M(\mathrm{PCO}/\mathrm{PO_2}) = \mathrm{COHb}/\mathrm{O_2Hb}$$

M is the affinity constant, which is between 230 and 270; PCO and PO_2 are the partial pressures of carbon monoxide and oxygen to which the hemoglobin molecules are exposed; COHb is the concentration of carboxyhemoglobin; and O_2Hb is the oxyhemoglobin concentration. This relationship was first described by Douglas et al.[9] in the early 1900s. They determined that the relative ratio of carboxyhemoglobin to oxyhemoglobin is dependent on the partial pressure of each in the immediate environment.

The workload, a measure of heart rate and ventilation during exercise, reflects the individual's activity. Varying oxygen partial pressures and the length of exposure are intimately related to carboxyhemoglobin uptake. The rate of carbon monoxide uptake is inversely proportional to the partial pressure of oxygen in the environment. To better describe the actual uptake of carbon monoxide, Coburn et al.[10] have developed a mathematical model relating carbon monoxide uptake and metabolism. Nine variables that influence the rate of carboxyhemoglobin reduction are included. In the subject breathing atmospheric air at equilibrium, the carboxyhemoglobin level (over endogenous production) is expressed by the following equation:

$$\%COHb = 0.16 \times CO$$

where the carbon monoxide concentration is expressed in parts per million. A more detailed component of this formula considers the carboxyhemoglobin concentration at a specific time, the background COHb, the rate of endogenous carbon monoxide production, blood volume, arterial oxygen concentration (in mmHg) and oxyhemoglobin concentration (in mmHg), the carbon monoxide/oxygen affinity for hemoglobin, the diffusion rate of carbon monoxide through the lungs in mmHg per minute (per millimeters of mercury), the dry barometric pressure in the lungs, and the ventilation rate. Coburn et al. were able to estimate levels of carboxyhemoglobin for subjects at rest and doing light and heavy work.[10]

Most carbon monoxide uptake variation occurs with ventilation up to a maximum of 20 liters per minute.[11] Above 20 liters per minute, there is actually a 15 per cent reduction from the proportional values. This uptake can vary by up to 25 per cent between individuals, as seen in normal young volunteers. It can also vary under different pathologic conditions, as when a dead space exists where diffusion coefficients are changed. There is up to a three-fold increase in ventilation doing light work compared with a rest period. These variations in uptake are also evident in the elimination rate of carbon monoxide. Inspired concentrations of 0.01 per cent carbon monoxide can result in COHb equilibrium concentrations at 14 per cent. By increasing this concentration to 0.05 per cent, carboxyhemoglobin levels of 44 per cent are noted. If the time of exposure is lengthened to several minutes at 0.1 per cent carbon monoxide, the carboxyhemoglobin level reaches 60 per cent.[7] Carbon monoxide levels of 10 per cent have been recorded in smoke at fire scenes. Firefighters not using face masks and engaged in strenuous activity can have carbon monoxide levels of 75 per cent in less than 1 minute.[12] Cigarette smoking can result in levels of carboxyhemoglobin of up to 10 per cent. Automobile exhaust may contain carbon monoxide levels of up to 9 per cent, and coal gas combustion can produce 10 per cent to 18 per cent carbon monoxide levels.

HYPOXIA

Displacement of oxygen from hemoglobin by carbon monoxide results in hypoxia. Normal hemoglobin carries 20 mL of oxygen per 100 mL of whole blood (20 vol %). For normal cellular function, the delivery of 5 vol % of oxygen is essential: this in reality is the arterial venous oxygen difference (a-vDO_2). Where carbon monoxide binding to hemoglobin has occurred, a relative hypoxemia is produced. To deliver 5 vol % of oxygen at the tissue level, a lower than normal cellular PO_2 is necessary. This is the direct effect on the partial pressure of oxygen as a result of saturation of the hemoglobin molecule with carbon monoxide. The remaining oxygen on the hemoglobin molecule is more tightly bound, producing a leftward shift of the oxyhemoglobin dissociation curve. To release oxygen from the carboxyhemoglobin unit, a lower tissue oxygen level is necessary. Tissue hypoxia is the net result.

Carbon monoxide has an affinity for other iron-containing hemoproteins such as myoglobin, cytochrome oxidase, cytochrome P_{450}, and hydroxyperoxidase, although the major binding is with hemoglobin. Some 15 per cent to 20 per cent of carbon monoxide in extravascular tissue combines with myoglobin and cytochrome.[13–15] Myoglobin is an oxygen reservoir and part of the oxygen transport mechanism. The myoglobin affinity constant for oxygen is 40. When hypoxia exists, oxygen is liberated from the myoglobin.[14] The oxymyoglobin dissociation curve comes into play at a PaO_2 of less than 60 mmHg. Myoglobin also exhibits a leftward shift of the oxygen dissociation curve in the presence of carbon monoxide, as first described by Roughton.[16] Carbon monoxide has a greater affinity for cardiac than skeletal muscle and will shift from the blood into the muscles under hypoxic conditions.[13] Once the tissue oxygen levels are restored to normal, carbon monoxide is liberated from myoglobin and reappears in the blood.

Investigators have demonstrated that increased carboxyhemoglobin levels, found with low levels of carbon monoxide poisoning (such as after smoking or inhalation of heavy atmospheric carbon monoxide), impair exercise performance even in clinically normal subjects.[17–19] Cardiac dysrhythmias may be the cause of death in this situation. Autopsies of 270 cases showed that 45 per cent had acute circulatory failure and myocardial damage when death occurred from carbon monoxide poisoning.[20] Dilatation of the heart, pulmonary edema, and diminished potassium concentrations in the myocardium were evident, as were histologic lesions in the myocardial cells. The cardiac effect of carbon monoxide is further seen in patients with angina, who are particularly sensitive to carbon monoxide and show an earlier onset of angina during physical exertion.[21] A wide range of changes, including conduction defects with dysrhythmias and ventricular fibrillation, low voltages, and depressed ST segments, may be seen.[22] The dysrhythmias and hypotension may further complicate the hypoxic syndrome. Decreased carriage and delivery (transportation and impaired release) result in a deficiency of oxygen in the tissue that is greater than that produced by an equivalent reduction in the ambient PO_2 (altitude increase) or with anemia.[23, 24] The genesis of neurologic injury is a consequence of the anoxia. The precise effects of carbon monoxide poisoning compared with those of severe anoxia are not clearly differentiated.

CELLULAR DYNAMICS

If the carbon monoxide binds directly to the iron-containing hemoproteins, producing cellular anoxia, cells with the highest metabolic rates (in the heart and central nervous system) will be affected primarily in their cellular respiration. Direct competition for oxygen at the receptive site of the cytochrome chain (primarily cytochrome a3 and P_{450}) may induce symptomatology, and this may be of more importance than the absolute carboxyhemoglobin level.[25, 26] The plasma concentration of physically dissolved carbon monoxide is related to the partial pressure of carbon monoxide in blood. It is postulated that the plasma carbon monoxide diffuses to the tissues (namely, the myocardial cells and neurons) and is then responsible for the symptomatology. The COHb level indicates a red cell load. Goldbaum was able to show that the infusion of carboxyhemoglobin-loaded red cells into an animal produced minimal symptomatology.[27] However, with inhalation of carbon monoxide and both red cell and plasma carbon monoxide loading, lethal symptoms of poisoning were evident.[27, 28] At the present stage, we have no means of directly measuring the plasma or cellular loads of carboxymyoglobin. The many discrepancies in the literature between the clinical presentation and the carboxyhemoglobin levels may be a result of this unmeasured tissue concentration of carbon monoxide.

The precise cellular effect of carbon monoxide poisoning remains controversial, with the actual reason for coma states in association with low carboxyhemoglobin levels being the point of dispute. Coburn disputes the involvement of cytochromes, postulating that the coefficient of diffusion of carbon monoxide is so effective that if there is a low red cell level of carbon monoxide, there is then a low tissue and cellular level.[3, 13] Geyer[29] demonstrated that rats with perfluorochemical-type blood substitutes survived indefinitely while breathing carbon monoxide levels of 10 per cent—a level normally rapidly fatal to rats with normal blood constituents. The fluorohydrocarbons transport 7.04 vol % of oxygen in dissolved solution. This enables the tissues to be provided with oxygen for their metabolic needs. Because cytochrome oxidase in myoglobin has an affinity for oxygen nine times greater than that of carbon monoxide and available oxygen in the fluorohydrocarbon solution, there is neither tissue poisoning nor hypoxia, and thus the rats survived.[29]

The importance of the tissue load of carbon monoxide may be indicated indirectly in the work of Cramer, who described a case of fetal death resulting from accidental maternal carbon monoxide poisoning.[30] The mother, with a relatively low level of carboxyhemoglobin (23.7 per cent), presented with minimal symptomatology, but the fetus died in utero. At fetal autopsy, right ventricular blood COHb levels of 25 per cent were noted, whereas the level of carboxyhemoglobin in the spleen and liver was raised to 35.1 per cent. This must represent a tissue deposition of carbon monoxide.

Fetal Toxicity with Maternal Carbon Monoxide Poisoning

Cramer's work[30] has highlighted a problem that is more widespread than anticipated. Fetal COHb levels are usually 10 per cent to 15 per cent higher than maternal levels. This results from simple diffusion[31] or by a carrier-mediated mechanism in the fetal blood and circulation.[31, 32] Placental carbon monoxide diffusion ability increases with gestational age and the weight of the fetus.[33] There is a slow, steady state of diffusion of carbon monoxide through the placenta. At 10 hours of exposure, fetal carboxyhemoglobin level exceeds the maternal level. The longer the mother is exposed to carbon monoxide, the greater will be the fetal carboxyhemoglobin level. Because fetal hemoglobin absorbs oxygen at lower tensions than adult hemoglobin, PaO_2 decreases in fetal blood in proportion to the increasing carboxyhemoglobin concentration. With the normal leftward shift of the oxyhemoglobin dissociation curve in the fetus, there is then a discharge of oxygen in the fetal tissues at lower than normal adult levels. This leftward shift is further exaggerated by carbon monoxide poisoning, which substantially impairs the release of oxygen from the mother to the fetus and from fetal hemoglobin to the fetal tissue. It is thus not uncommon to report the survival of the mother but the death of the fetus[30, 34–36] from carbon monoxide exposure. All reviews indicate a high fetal death rate. When the fetus survived, a variety of psychomotor disturbances existed, including mental retardation, idiocy, and hypotonia of the extremities and neck.

NEUROPATHOLOGIC LESIONS

With the reduction of tissue oxygen supply in carbon monoxide poisoning, cerebral metabolism is adversely affected. Among the postulated mechanisms are arterial hypoxemia,[37] direct cellular action of carbon monoxide,[25, 38, 39] and reduction of cerebral blood flow.[40, 41] The basic cellular mechanism of cerebral damage is unknown. MacMillian noted that cerebral energy homeostasis was maintained until a level of 2 per cent carbon monoxide was reached.[42] At this level, decreases in cerebral adenosine triphosphate and increases in both adenosine diphosphate and adenosine monophosphate were observed. In addition there was an early depletion of tissue citrate and alpha-oxyglutarate. This was a similar pattern to that seen during a state of altered cerebral perfusion such as in cerebral oligemia.[42] There was no basic qualitative nor quantitative difference in the metabolic response of brain tissue to either carbon monoxide–induced changes or those seen with hypoxemia. Carbon monoxide–induced cardiovascular depression and hypotension resulting from its effect on myoglobin and the myocardium may result in reduction of cerebral blood flow, which then becomes the principal factor for cerebral damage.[42] However, the histologic picture in the cerebrum is not completely explained by a hypoxic insult, which generally affects the neocortex, hippocampus, caudate, putamen, and cerebellum. Leukoencephalopathy is an infrequent consequence of cerebral hypoxia. Other systemic factors such as acidosis, hypotension, and loss of cerebral autoregulation may contribute to the cerebral injury induced by carbon monoxide poisoning. The cerebral effects may be manifested by impaired cognitive and psychomotor function (an early sign) or may ultimately lead to coma and death. Patients may recover from this cerebral insult, but recently it has been shown that, without appropriate treatment, relapses or recurrence of neuropsychiatric dysfunction after an apparent complete recovery can occur.[43]

Computed tomography (CT) has been used to further elucidate the degenerative changes in the brain. Patients who had been comatose for at least 6 hours had a CT scan prior to hyperbaric oxygen therapy[44] and a subsequent repeat scan. Two groups of patients could be defined. In the group with no CT abnormalities, normal blood gases, and carboxyhemoglobin in the range of 40 per cent, 9 of 10 patients had good recovery. In the second group, there were reduced tissue densities in the globus pallidus after 2 weeks, which remained at a 3-month follow-up. At a 1-year follow-up, these patients had evidence of marked ventricular dilatation and cortical atrophy. Their outcome was poor, with severe disabilities and a vegetative state. It was postulated that this was a direct effect of carbon monoxide on the brain, producing edema, softening, necrosis, and degenerative demyelination. However, these areas of low density in the globus pallidus are seldom seen in true hypoxic disease. Sawada et al.[44] suggested that carbon monoxide may have special cytotoxicity, and since gray matter has a higher rate of oxygen consumption, it is more susceptible to hypoxia. In carbon monoxide poisoning, however, the white matter is most severely affected. The edema subsequent to carbon monoxide poisoning may be vasogenic in origin, with an increase in the extracellular fluid from increased vascular permeability. Early detection of diffuse brain edema by CT scan may thus be an indicator of a poor prognosis.[45]

Recently the concept of toxic oxygen radicals having a direct effect on nerve tissue has been postulated. Lipid peroxidases inducing peroxidation of polyunsaturated fatty acids in membranes and lipoproteins of nerve tissue may be a consequence of toxic oxygen radicals. These radicals impair the function of the membrane and damage cellular components. The risk of lipid peroxidation in brain tissue is potentially high, because the concentration of polyunsaturated lipids is high, and because there is a relatively low content of catalase and glutathione peroxidase.[46]

CARBON MONOXIDE HALF-LIVES

A range of carbon monoxide half-lives is found in the literature: 3 to 5 hours in air, 30 to 80 minutes in 100 per cent oxygen, and 20 to 30 minutes in hyperbaric oxygen.[7, 47–49] End and Long[19] first showed a dramatic reduction in the half-life under hyperbaric conditions at 3 atmospheres absolute (ATA). They identified a species difference, with dogs eliminating carbon monoxide more rapidly than guinea pigs. Douglas et al.[9] added 5 per cent carbogen with 95 per cent oxygen and increased the rate of clearance of carbon monoxide over that of 100 per cent oxygen alone. Our own work[50] has shown a wide individual variation, as well as a difference in actual groups; at normobaric 100 per cent oxygen, half-life ranged from 31.5 to 149.7 minutes, while at 3 ATA hyperbaric oxygen, ranges from 4.2 to 86.4 minutes were noted. If an individual has a short half-life in one environment, the half-life will be short in another. The most rapid half-life in any of our patients was 4.2 minutes at 3 ATA and 31.5 minutes on surface 100 per cent oxygen. Another patient, however, had a 74.7-minute hyperbaric oxygen half-life, with a 90.8-minute half-life on 100 per cent oxygen at surface. The longest time noted was 86.4 minutes at 3 ATA and 149.7 minutes at surface oxygen. Those patients arriving from fires with short but high concentration exposures of carbon monoxide appeared to have high levels of carbon monoxide, which rapidly declined. In patients exposed for longer intervals at lower levels (as in suicide attempts or warehouse exposures), the initial level of carbon monoxide was lower, but the half-life was longer. The calculation of half-life was based on the formula of $T\frac{1}{2} = 1n\ 2/k$. $T\frac{1}{2}$ represents the half time of kinetic process of carbon monoxide secretion, 1n 2 is the natural logarithm of base 2, and k is the rate constant obtained from plotting the k curve. The fraction of inspired oxygen (FIO_2), minute ventilation, and vital signs of pulse and blood pressure of each patient were monitored, as was the carbon monoxide level taken on a half-hourly basis. This was done during transportation to the hospital, using an estimated FIO_2 of 60 per cent. In the hospital, 100 per cent normobaric oxygen was administered by a tightly fitting aviator-type face mask with a free-flow oxygen demand regulator. A face mask or intubation was used for administering 100 per cent oxygen hyperbaric oxygen conditions at 3 ATA for 46 minutes. Particular attention was given to the inspiratory rate and depth and the heart rate.

CLINICAL PRESENTATION OF CARBON MONOXIDE POISONING

The clinical manifestations of carbon monoxide poisoning vary, depending on factors such as the concentration of carbon monoxide to which the patient is exposed, the duration of the exposure, the depth of breathing, and the heart rate at the time of exposure. In most clinical situations it is not possible to determine the length of time of exposure or the time elapsed from discovery of the patient at the scene to arrival at the hospital. Many hospitals do not have the means to measure carboxyhemoglobin levels from blood samples. In other situations, the physician is unaware that carbon monoxide poisoning is the cause of the symptomatology. In the 1950s, the speed at which the emergency medicine system delivered the patient from the scene of the poisoning to the hospital environment was much slower than in today's emergency transportation systems. Resuscitation methods in earlier days were not like current protocols, in which a highly trained paramedic may give not only oxygen but also drugs and may even intubate a patient for better ventilation. In 1930, Sayers and Davenport[49] indicated minimal symptomatology with concentrations of carboxyhemoglobin at less than 10 per cent. As the concentration of carbon monoxide increased, so did the symptomatology. At levels of 10 per cent to 20 per cent, tightness across the forehead and headache were noted. Between 20 per cent and 30 per cent, a throbbing headache and more severe symptoms became evident. Levels between 30 per cent and 40 per cent were associated with severe headache with generalized weakness, dizziness, dimness of vision, nausea, vomiting, and ultimate collapse. Levels between 40 per cent and 50 per cent resulted in syncope and the additional symptomatology as well as tachycardia and tachypnea. Levels over 50 per cent could lead to coma and intermittent convulsions; above 60 per cent, cardiac and respiratory function was depressed. The characteristic symptoms of various levels could overlap.

Today, a great range of symptoms has been delineated. Patients having low levels of carbon monoxide (under 10 per cent) may present unconscious. Other patients with high levels of carbon monoxide (50 per cent) may have minimal symptomatology: for example, a headache; at the extreme, we have treated patients who had levels of carbon monoxide below 10 per cent but presented in a coma.[51–53] These patients had a history of carbon monoxide exposure and recovered consciousness with hyperbaric oxygen treatments (their level of consciousness was not changed by surface 100 per cent oxygen). The major problem the clinician faces today is distinguishing carboxyhemoglobin from the tissue level of carbon monoxide.

The clinical presentation of carbon monoxide poisoning covers a wide spectrum. Included in the symptoms are headache, nausea, vomiting, lightheadedness, weakness, sleepiness, decreased exercise tolerance, palpitation, visual disturbances, and irritability. Among the acute signs are tachypnea, tachycardia, fever, vomiting, confusion or disorientation, hypotension, arrhythmias, coma, convulsions, and respiratory failure. There may also be retinal hemorrhages, cherry red skin (rarely), pulmonary edema, and rhabdomyolysis.

Chronic or delayed signs and symptoms of carbon monoxide poisoning include personality changes, psychiatric disturbance, apathy, apraxia, aphasia, disorientation, muscular rigidity, gait disturbances, fecal and urinary incontinence, and coma.

The carboxyhemoglobin level is often misleadingly low, particularly if there has been long interval between exposure and the blood test. Another cause of low COHb levels is the administration of oxygen before blood sampling.[54]

Pre-existing Cardiovascular and Respiratory Symptoms in Carbon Monoxide Poisoning

Patients with pre-existing coronary artery disease experience exacerbation of anginal symptoms at low-level (less than 10 per cent) carbon monoxide poisoning.[3, 21, 55] If carboxyhemoglobin rises above 15 per cent, these patients are at increased risk for myocardial infarction,[3] while the ventricular fibrillation threshold can be lowered by carboxyhemoglobin levels as low as 9 per cent.[1] Lowered threshold effects are also observed in intermittent claudication.[56]

Patients with pre-existent chronic obstructive pulmonary disease (COPD) have reduced exercise tolerance with levels of carboxyhemoglobin as low as 9 per cent, which can be reached by a heavy smoker.[57] During a period of high ambient carbon monoxide concentration, COPD patients may present to the emergency department with acute pulmonary decompensation.[58]

Mild to Moderate Carbon Monoxide Intoxication: Symptomatology

Symptoms of mild to moderate carbon monoxide poisoning are often nonspecific and include headaches, dizziness, weakness, nausea, dyspnea, visual disturbance, irritability, and lack of concentration.[59] Physical findings are also nonspecific: tachycardia, tachypnea, mild systolic hypotension, low-grade fever, vomiting, and confusion.[1, 59] Carboxyhemoglobin levels may be in the range of 20 to 30 per cent, and the diagnosis may be missed at this stage. Carbon monoxide intoxication is most commonly misdiagnosed as food poisoning, hysteria, acute delirium tremens, acute ethanol or methanol intoxication, migraine headache, and cerebral vascular disease.[4]

Severe Carbon Monoxide Poisoning: Symptoms and Signs

Carboxyhemoglobin levels in patients with severe carbon monoxide poisoning are usually over 50 per cent.[4] These patients may present with cardiovascular or neurologic complications. Patients without prior coronary heart disease may develop angina or myocardial infarction.[3] Cardiac arrhythmias are the major causes of death from acute carbon monoxide poisoning. In our own experience, patients who die in the admission phase before aggressive treatment can be instituted are those with cardiovascular disturbance and arrhythmias. Premature ventricular contractions are common; idioventricular blocks and atrial fibrillation have also been documented.[1, 3] Patients develop hypotension and syncope following myocardial depression.

Neurologic manifestations are seen at all degrees of carboxyhemoglobin levels. Headache is common, and its intensity varies with the carboxyhemoglobin level.[1] At higher carboxyhemoglobin levels (greater than 50 per cent), patients are more likely to be comatose. In addition to coma, they may also have grand mal seizures. Deep tendon reflexes may be increased, and hyperventilation, generalized muscular rigidity, and agitation may be present.[3] CT scans taken at this time may reveal areas of low density in the globus pallidus. If this is evident in an unconscious patient, the outcome is poor.[44, 60] In these severe cases, other unusual manifestations may also be evident, including dermatologic changes such as cherry red discoloration of the skin[53] or blisters.[61]

Ophthalmologic manifestations include visual field defects, paracentral scotomota, homonymous hemianopia, blindness, papilledema, and retinal hemorrhages.[62, 63] Auditory and vestibular disturbances include damage to the labyrinth, the eighth nerve, or brain stem nuclei. The resultant symptoms and signs are loss of balance, ataxia, nystagmus, hearing loss, and tinnitus.[3]

Pulmonary manifestations include noncardiogenic pulmonary edema, which is often multifactorial in etiology, and congestive cardiac failure. Aspiration may contribute to the pulmonary edema.[3] Renal complications occur with carbon monoxide binding to skeletal muscles, causing rhabdomyolysis and myoglobinuria. Consequently, creatine kinase, lactate dehydrogenase, aspartate, and alanine transferase are elevated 24 to 48 hours after intoxication.[53] Acute tubular necrosis and renal failure occasionally are seen.[3]

Delayed Neuropsychiatric Presentation

The classic history is that the patient loses consciousness and appears to recover with or without treatment (air or surface oxygen), but deteriorates after a lucid interval. The lucid interval could last from 1 to 21 days; the subsequent decline has a fairly rapid onset.[53, 64, 65] The presentation of the delayed syndrome includes aphasia, apraxia, apathy, disorientation, hallucinations, bradykinesia, cogwheel rigidity, gait disturbances, and fecal and urinary incontinence. There may also be evidence of gross neurologic or cognitive defects; personality changes, including impulsiveness, mood changes, violence, and verbal aggressiveness, are evident. The incidence of delayed neuropsychiatric symptomatology following carbon monoxide poisoning ranges from 3 per cent to 40 per cent.[65–67] Because the personality and pathologic changes are often subtle, the true incidence could be much higher.[64] There are no clinical indicators to predict the incidence or occurrence of this syndrome. One of the newer methods of assessing patients for this syndrome, and for neurologic abnormality in general, is the psychometric test.[68–71] If this test is not available, it is essential that patients be followed closely for a minimum of 7 to 10 days after carbon monoxide exposure to determine if any subtle neurologic changes occur.

Carbon Monoxide Poisoning in Children

Symptoms of children exposed to carbon monoxide vary from those of the adult in that earlier gastrointestinal disturbances (nausea, vomiting, and diarrhea) occur. Carboxyhemoglobin levels at presentation are usually lower than in the adult, and the condition is often misdiagnosed.[72] Lethargy and syncope have also been reported as major symptoms in children, and the home is the location of the poisoning in 90 per cent of cases.[73] Because of these differences, the approach to children should be more aggressive than in adults, and they should be treated at lower carbon monoxide levels than in the adult. Treatment is particularly important in the pregnant female exposed to carbon monoxide poisoning.

DIAGNOSTIC TESTS

Because of the wide range of signs and symptoms in carbon monoxide poisoning, it should always be considered as a diagnosis. A range of diagnostic tests are available, the most important of which is determination of the carboxyhemoglobin level. This should be obtained immediately on admission and at timed intervals (every half hour or every 2 hours) to determine the progressive decrement in carbon monoxide levels. Arterial blood gases and lactate acid levels measure the degree of acidosis. Drug screening is essential, particularly if a suicide attempt is suspected or if there has been an associated fire; carelessness resulting from intoxication with ethanol or other drugs is often the cause of the fire. Creatine kinase and lactate dehydrogenase may be elevated, as will serum alanine transferase and aspartate transferase up to 1 to 2 days after severe poisoning. Hyperglycemia has been reported and is considered to be caused by a hormonal "stress" response rather than the poisoning itself.

Electrocardiograms are essential in patients with a history of coronary artery disease or in the presence of arrhythmias or hypotension.[21] Computed cerebral tomography may indicate severe poisoning. Areas of low density may reflect cerebral edema or necrosis.[44] In the late stages of severe poisoning, the CT scan may indicate areas of low density in the white matter and widening of the cerebral sulci as well as atrophy. An electroencephalogram may be helpful in the acute stage, but its wide range of features are nonspecific; these include continuous theta and delta activity, low-voltage activity accompanied by intervals of spiking or silence, and rhythmic bursts of slow waves.

The carbon monoxide neuropsychological screening battery (CONSB), developed at the Maryland Institute for Emergency Medical Services Systems, helps detect subtle cerebral dysfunction and is used as a guideline for determining recovery.[71] It is administered immediately on admission (after appropriate history is obtained and physical examination performed) and then is used in the follow-up period to determine response to treatment and whether the patient has returned to normal. The test can be completed in 20 to 25 minutes and can be administered by an emergency medicine department nurse or hyperbaric medicine nurse while the patient is breathing surface oxygen.

The CONSB is composed of six subtests that help determine a variety of cognitive deficits, including dysgraphia, dysphasia, agnosia, and dyspraxia.[69] The patient's responses are used as criteria for determining the optimal oxygen treatment. Test 1 is used to assess the patient's orientation and to obtain general information about the patient (the patient's name, age, address, the date (month and year), level of education, and location of the hospital). These give the examiner the ability to determine the orientation of the patient.

Test 2, the digit span, measures the patient's attentiveness and short-term memory. A series of digits are recited, and the patient attempts to repeat the series in the exact order. With each set of numbers, an additional digit is added to the series. The highest number of correct digits is the score.

Test 3 is the trails making test (A and B), which detects the temporal/spatial orientation of the patient. Lines must be drawn from consecutive numbers in trails A; in trails B, lines are drawn from numbers to alphabetic characters in a consecutive manner. The time taken to do the test and the number of errors are measured.

Test 4, the digit symbol test, measures visual motor coordination and visual discrimination. Symbols and numerals are displayed, and the patient must complete the appropriate symbol on a chart within a specified amount of time. The number of correct symbols and numerals is measured.

Test 5, the aphasia screening test, measures dysphasia, dyspraxia, and agnosia. The patient is asked to observe, name, and copy a number of figures; do some simple arithmetic; recognize items; and write the answers. In this test, the number of errors is measured.

Test 6, the block design test, measures visual/spatial function. A number of designs are demonstrated in a book, and the patient is asked to build these designs from blocks. The blocks have sides that are either completely red, completely white, or half red and half white. The patient is given a time limit in which to reproduce the design and is scored accordingly.

In our assessment of patients using the CONSB, we have been able to distinguish between patients who are normal and those who have impaired neurologic function. The test is not specific for carbon monoxide and could show abnormal results if the patient is drunk, drugged, or suffering from mental deterioration. The test is used in conjunction with the history and other physical findings to determine whether mental status is appropriate. Following treatment with either normobaric or hyperbaric oxygen, the test is repeated, and improvement in function is assessed. When appropriate treatment has been given, significant improvement is noted. We presently use this test as the end point of our treatment goal and find it to be a more sensitive indicator of neurologic impairment than the general clinical assessment, which is too superficial. Applications of the test are limited; it is not appropriate for unconscious patients, substance abuse patients, or patients with head injury or other forms of cerebral dysfunction. However, it remains our most sensitive test for determining abnormal CNS function following carbon monoxide exposure.

CLINICAL MANAGEMENT OF PATIENTS

At the Scene

At the scene, prehospital care providers retrieve the person from the source of carbon monoxide. After the airway is cleared, a face mask with a reservoir oxygen bag is placed on the patient, and the highest oxygen concentration possible is given. An IV line is established to obtain a blood sample for carboxyhemoglobin and to provide a line for drugs if needed for cardiac arrhythmias. Fundamental care of the acutely traumatized patient is administered in accordance with advanced trauma life support protocols. The standard plastic disposable mask used in the field should be used until arrival at the emergency medicine department, where it should be changed to the aviator-type face mask used for general anesthesia. Standard plastic face masks allow the patient to receive a maximum of 50 per cent to 60 per cent oxygen. The dissociation of carboxyhemoglobin to oxyhemoglobin and carbon dioxide is reduced (normal half-life of 100 per cent oxygen is 80 to 100 minutes). If the patient is comatose or showing evidence of respiratory distress, he or she should be intubated and ventilated by Ambu bag until arrival at a hospital, where the patient is placed on a ventilator.

In the Hospital

In the hospital the patient is treated as having an acute emergency. If the patient is unconscious, the possibility of associated trauma (such as a fall or a subdural hematoma) must be ruled out as the cause of the unconsciousness. For this reason a full neurologic assessment is undertaken. Hypotension and arrhythmias must be treated with lidocaine and dopamine as necessary. A full workup including ECG and cardiology consultation may be necessary to exclude a myocardial infarction as a result of the carbon monoxide insult. If there is concern about raised intracranial pressure, a neurosurgical service assessment is essential. If intracranial pressures are elevated and documented by a Richmond bolt or some other form of intracranial monitoring, the patient should be hyperventilated and treated in an intensive care unit.

The major investigations undertaken on admission include carboxyhemoglobin levels (if available) and toxicology screens. In the critically ill patient, the following blood tests are run: complete blood count, blood urea nitrogen and creatine, creatine phosphokinase (CPK), CPK-MB fraction, lactate dehydrogenase, aspartate, and alanine transferase. The urine is assessed for myoglobin. Arterial blood gases are measured, particularly if smoke inhalation has occurred. There is a weak correlation between pH and percent of carboxyhemoglobin level in the initial arterial blood gases. When tissue hypoxia and acidosis have developed, there is a stronger correlation between high carboxyhemoglobin levels and acidosis. We found that patients presenting with acidosis, alkalosis, or normal blood gases could have equally severe neurologic symptoms at carboxyhemoglobin levels of 1 per cent to 62 per cent.[52] A far more sensitive correlation was found between abnormal psychometric results and carboxyhemoglobin levels than between abnormal psychometric results and blood gases. We do not advocate administration of sodium bicarbonate to patients with acidosis, because we believe that 100% oxygen will allow the acidosis to resolve on its own. Sodium bicarbonate may shift the patient's oxyhemoglobin dissociation curve further to the left.

ECGs and chest x-ray films are obtained on these patients, and the neuropsychologic screening battery is then performed. If the battery is not available, it is essential to perform a detailed mental status assessment of the patient.

It must next be determined whether the patient needs observation in the emergency medicine department or admission to the hospital. The following are appropriate criteria for hospitalizing carbon monoxide victims:

1. Carboxyhemoglobin levels greater than or equal to 25 per cent
2. Ischemic heart disease history and carboxyhemoglobin level greater than 15 per cent
3. Carboxyhemoglobin levels greater than 10 per cent in a pregnant woman
4. Ischemic chest pains and/or ECG evidence of ischemia
5. Metabolic acidosis
6. Abnormal neuropsychological testing
7. History of unconsciousness
8. Patients who remain symptomatic following 4 hours of 100 per cent oxygen treatment
9. Moderately symptomatic conscious patients with clinically suspected CO poisoning (in hospitals without the availability of carboxyhemoglobin level testing)

The majority of patients seen in the emergency department following carbon monoxide poisoning have a mild exposure. If they become asymptomatic after receiving 100 per cent oxygen treatment for 3 to 4 hours, they can be sent home. The guidelines for optimal treatment relate to the initial carboxyhemoglobin level and repeat follow-up levels. It is essential that the carboxyhemoglobin level be below 5 per cent before the patient is sent home. Provided the patient shows no symptoms or neuropsychologic impairment, we advise 1 to 2 days of rest and then return to normal activity. For patients with more severe problems, the follow-up period will be longer and return to work delayed. When patients are discharged home, it is essential that the home and work environment be checked carefully to determine whether the original source of carbon monoxide is still present.

We follow our own patients for 7 to 10 days with follow-up telephone calls and repeat visits as needed. If this is too cumbersome, the patient can be referred back to the primary care physician, who should look for signs of neurologic deterioration, which may indicate recurrent symptomatology. In our experience, patients treated with surface oxygen are likely to develop delayed or recurrent sequelae after apparent resolution. This recurrence may be noted at any time from 1 to 21 days after the original exposure without any new exposure to carbon monoxide.[65]

HYPERBARIC OXYGEN THERAPY

Although there have never been any controlled, double-blind, randomized trials for the use of hyperbaric oxygen in the treatment of carbon monoxide poisoning, there have also never been any controlled, double-blinded, randomized trials comparing the use of oxygen against air in the treatment of this condition. The use of hyperbaric oxygen in the treatment of carbon monoxide poisoning is increasing each year, as evidenced by the statistics in the National Hyperbaric Registry that is kept by the Department of Hyperbaric Medicine at the Maryland Institute for Emergency Medical Services Systems. Over the years, this number has increased dramatically: from 128 patients treated nationwide with hyperbaric oxygen for carbon monoxide poisoning in 1977 to 2166 patients in 1986. The primary rationale for using hyperbaric oxygen is to reduce the half-life of carbon monoxide poisoning and at the same time mobilize carbon monoxide from the tissue as rapidly as possible. The very high plasma-bound level of oxygen caused by hyperbaric pressure results in the availability of oxygen for both neurologic and myocardial tissue and a rapid breakdown of CO.

Few hospitals have hyperbaric facilities; thus, a problem exists in determining who should receive hyperbaric oxygen instead of surface oxygen. Patients who show evidence of severe carbon monoxide poisoning, including cardiac arrhythmias, hypotension, and loss of consciousness, and those who remain unconscious and confused should be transferred for hyperbaric oxygen. The earlier this transfer is effected, the better the outcome.

Goulon et al., reporting from France, described 302 patients with carbon monoxide poisoning treated between 1962 and 1969.[74] Two hundred seventy-three of these cases were considered severe and were treated with hyperbaric oxygen. When hyperbaric oxygen was administered during the first 6 hours, the mortality rate in the severe cases was 13.5 per cent; when treatment was administered after 6 hours, the mortality rate increased to 30.1 per cent. The most common cause of mortality was circulatory failure and pulmonary edema.[74] Because of our successes with late presentations of unconscious patients suspected of having carbon monoxide poisoning, we strongly advocate aggressive hyperbaric treatment in this type of patient.[51] We compared a group of patients who had mild carbon monoxide intoxication (carboxyhemoglobin levels of under 30 per cent and normal or borderline abnormal neuropsychometric test results) with more severely intoxicated patients (carboxyhemoglobin levels greater than 30 per cent and unconsciousness or unable to perform neuropsychologic tests or having grossly abnormal results). The mildly affected patients were treated with surface oxygen for up to 4 hours. The severely affected were treated with hyperbaric oxygen on our standard protocol of 40 minutes on 100 per cent oxygen at 2.8 ATA. Follow-up hyperbaric oxygen was given if the patient had not returned to normal after the original treatment. These follow-up treatments were initially given at 6 hours and then twice daily until normal follow-up psychometric testing was achieved. In this situation, 10 per cent to 12 per cent of the mild cases developed recurrence or delayed neurologic sequelae. None of the patients treated with hyperbaric oxygen had sequelae or delayed symptoms.[65] Over the past 2 years, this incidence has remained constant, with additional cases of subacute recurrent sequelae reported in patients treated with surface oxygen. Similar results have been noted in other reports.[75, 76]

Indications

As we have become more aware of the importance of the neurologic symptomatology in the presentation of carbon monoxide poisoning, we have based our decision making more on the clinical criteria than on the carboxyhemoglobin level.[54] Our indications for hyperbaric oxygen therapy are:

1. All comatose patients
2. Patients with neurologic impairment as evidenced by psychometric testing or by other means
3. Cardiovascular involvement, with ischemic chest pain, ischemic ECG, or cardiac arrhythmias, and a history of carbon monoxide exposure
4. All patients with carboxyhemoglobin levels over 40 per cent
5. Patients who are pregnant and have carboxyhemoglobin levels over 15 per cent
6. Patients with a history of ischemic heart disease and levels of carbon monoxide of 20 per cent and above
7. Patients who have been treated with surface oxygen and develop recurrent symptomatology up to 3 weeks after the original treatment
8. Patients whose symptoms do not resolve after 6 hours of continuous 100 per cent surface oxygen.

Patients with these criteria at a facility that does not have a hyperbaric chamber should be referred if possible to the nearest facility offering hyperbaric oxygen therapy.

The transportation of these patients has been facilitated with the advanced prehospital care available throughout the country. Any advanced cardiac life support system should be able to transport the uncomplicated patient safely when indicated, taking particular care with the securing of an airway if needed and IV line and intravenous infusion to allow administration of medications.

Patients who are critically ill, such as those patients who have sustained cardiac arrest or life-threatening cardiac arrhythmias, have concomitant conditions (such as multiple trauma), or are deemed too unstable for transfer may require in-hospital management and stabilization with 100 per cent oxygen to a carboxyhemoglobin level of 5 per cent or less. Subsequent transfer (if possible) to a hyperbaric chamber may be appropriate. Consultation and coordination with a regional hyperbaric center is helpful.

The decision of whether to treat a patient with 100 per cent oxygen at the local hospital or transfer the patient to a hyperbaric chamber may be quite difficult. Given the variables for each hospital and each community, it may be helpful for each facility and area to establish specific criteria *prior* to the advent of such an emergency.

Complications

The earlier hyperbaric literature indicated concerns about oxygen toxicity, particularly relating to the central nervous and pulmonary systems. These are very uncommon complications within the protocols followed at hyperbaric facilities. In a 6-year period in which 891 patients were treated in 14,966 dives in our multiplace facility, with the patients breathing 100 per cent oxygen by face mask or hood and at various depths ranging from 2 to 6 ATA, we were able to document 137 incidences of acute oxygen toxicity occurring in 90 patients. The frequencies of other complications in this series are listed as follows:

1. Nausea and vomiting, 0.3 per cent
2. Seizures, 0.21 per cent
3. Muscular twitching, 0.13 per cent
4. Anxiety, 0.09 per cent
5. Vertigo, 0.06 per cent
6. Respiratory changes, 0.05 per cent; altered consciousness, 0.05 per cent
7. Sweating, 0.03 per cent; behavior changes, 0.03 per cent
8. Visual changes, 0.02 per cent; auditory changes, 0.02 per cent

Thus the incidence of toxicity is very low. A convulsion is not considered dangerous, because the brain is not anoxic; in fact, the hyperoxia causes the seizure. The seizure is aborted by stopping the 100 per cent oxygen and giving the patient air instead. Another means of reducing the incidence of oxygen seizures is allowing intermittent air breaks during the hyperbaric treatment. A 5-minute air break is given for every 45 minutes of oxygen.

The most common side effect of hyperbaric oxygen is barotrauma, particularly as it relates to the ears and sinuses. Any patient who is unable to clear his/her ears with the routine methods of the Valsalva maneuver, swallowing, or yawning can develop barotrauma with tympanic membrane hemorrhage and possibly rupture. In the unconscious patient, this is prevented by performing bilateral myringotomies. Patients who are intubated and unconscious are unable to clear their ears and are likely to develop barotrauma. Patients suffering from claustrophobia may have problems in the chamber; this can be controlled by drugs and appropriate nursing intervention during the hyperbaric oxygen treatment.

Availability of Facilities

For the past 10 years, we have maintained a registry of the functional hyperbaric facilities throughout the country. The number of hyperbaric facilities has grown from 37 in 1977 to over 220 units in April, 1986. Four states (Montana, Idaho, Wyoming, and Iowa) are without hyperbaric facilities, and the heaviest concentrations of facilities are in California (40), Florida (20), and Texas (18). There are 118 single unit facilities and 85 multiple unit facilities, with 17 facilities being both. Location of hyperbaric facilities can be ascertained by calling the Diver's Alert Network at Duke University (919/684-8111) or the Maryland Institute for Emergency Medical Services Systems (301/328-7814); both resources have information about hyperbaric facilities throughout the continental United States and Canada and operate on a 24-hour basis.

SUMMARY

Carbon monoxide poisoning is far more complex than previously considered. Major deficiencies exist in terms of rediagnosis of the disease and of the measurements used to determine involvement and severity of symptoms. Carboxyhemoglobin concentration is a relatively poor indicator of severity; psychometric testing is more sensitive in assessing poisoning severity. The pathophysiology of the subacute and late and recurrent sequelae of carbon monoxide poisoning is poorly understood, but awareness of such problems is increasing. Psychometric testing for determining severity and as a means of comparing treatment modalities has proved valuable. The need for long-term follow-up is also evident, given that sequelae recur in 10 per cent of patients. Continued coma (a rare entity) treated with hyperbaric oxygen is associated with successful outcomes. Once a basis for assessment of severity has been developed, it will be possible to undertake randomized trials comparing the effects of 100 per cent oxygen with those of hyperbaric oxygen in the treatment of carbon monoxide poisoning. Multicenter trials may more rapidly determine the most effective treatment regimen.

References

1. Dolan MC: Carbon monoxide poisoning. Can Med Assoc J *133:*392, 1985.
2. U.S. Public Health Service: Vital Statistics of the United States. Washington, DC, Government Printing Office, 1976.
3. Mofenson HC, Caraccio TR, Brody GM: Carbon monoxide poisoning. Am J Emerg Med 2:254, 1984.
4. Barret L, Danel V, Faure J: Carbon monoxide poisoning, a diagnosis frequently overlooked. Clin Toxicol *23:*309, 1985.
5. Sammons JH, Coleman RL: Firefighters' occupational exposure to carbon monoxide. J Occup Med *16:*543, 1974.
6. Hovath SM, Dahms TE, O'Hanlon JF: Carbon monoxide and human vigilance. Arch Environ Health *23:*343, 1971.
7. Jackson DL, Menges H: Accidental carbon monoxide poisoning. JAMA *243:*772, 1980.
8. Rioux JP, Myers RAM: Methylene chloride poisoning: A paradigmatic review. J Emerg Med *6:*227–238, 1988.
9. Douglas CG, Haldane JS, Haldane JBS: The laws of combustion of hemoglobin with carbon monoxide and oxygen. J Physiol (Lond) 44:275, 1912.
10. Coburn RF, Forster RE, Kane PB: Consideration of the physiological variables that determine the blood carboxyhemoglobin concentration in man. J Clin Invest *44:*1899, 1965.
11. Forbes WH: Carbon monoxide uptake via the lungs. Ann NY Acad Sci *174:*72, 1970.
12. Stewart RD, Hake CL: Paint-remover hazard. JAMA *235:*398, 1976.
13. Coburn RF: The carbon monoxide body stores. Ann NY Acad Sci *174:*11, 1970.
14. Fabel H: Normal and critical O_2—supply of the heart. *In* Lubbers DW, et al (eds): Oxygen Transport in Blood and Tissues. New York, Grune and Stratton, 1968, p 159.
15. Wittenberg JB: Myoglobin-facilitated oxygen diffusion; Role of myoglobin in oxygen entry into muscle. Physiol Rev *50:*560, 1970.
16. Roughton FJW: Transportation of oxygen and carbon dioxide. *In* Fenn WO, Rahn H (eds): Handbook of Physiology and Respiration, Sec 3, Vol 1. Washington, DC, American Physiology Society, 1964, p 767.
17. Ball EG, Strittmatter CF, Cooper O: The reaction of cytochrome oxidase with carbon monoxide. J Biol Chem *193:*635, 1951.
18. Drinkwater BL, Raven PB, et al: Air pollution, exercise and heart stress. Arch Environ Health *28:*177, 1974.
19. End E, Long CW: Oxygen under pressure in carbon monoxide poisoning. J Ind Hyg *24:*301, 1942.
20. Cosby RS, Bergeron M: Electrocardiographic changes in carbon monoxide poisoning. Am J Cardiol *11:*93, 1963.
21. Aronow WS, Isbell MW: Carbon monoxide effect on exercise-induced angina pectoris. Ann Intern Med *79:*392, 1973.
22. DeBias DA, Banerjee CM, Birkhead NC, et al: Effects of carbon monoxide inhalation on ventricular fibrillation. Arch Environ Health *31:*38, 1976.
23. Forster RE: Reactions of carbon monoxide with heme proteins. Ann NY Acad Sci *174:*10, 1970.
24. Ganong WF: Review of Medical Physiology. Los Altos, CA, Lange Medical Publications, 1965, p 542.
25. Chance B, Erecinska M, Wagner M: Mitochondrial responses to carbon monoxide toxicity. Ann NY Acad Sci *174:*193, 1970.
26. Estabrook RW, Franklin MR, Hildebrandt AG: Factors influencing the inhibitory effect of carbon monoxide on cytochrome P-450-catalyzed mixed function oxidation reactions. Ann NY Acad Sci *174:*218, 1970.
27. Goldbaum LR, Orellano T, Degal E: Mechanism of the toxic action of carbon monoxide. Ann Clin Lab Sci *6:*372, 1976.
28. Goldbaum LR, Ramisez RG, Absalon KB: What is the mechanism of carbon monoxide toxicity? Aviat Space Environ Med *46:*1289, 1975.
29. Geyer RP: Review of perfluorochemical-type blood substitutes. *In* Proceedings of the Tenth International Congress for Nutrition; Symposium on Perfluorochemical Artificial Blood, Kyoto 1975. Igakushobo, Osaka, Japan, 1975, p 3.
30. Cramer CR: Fetal death due to accidental maternal carbon monoxide poisoning. J Toxicol Clin Toxicol *19:*297, 1982.
31. Longo LD: The biological effects of carbon monoxide on the pregnant woman, fetus and newborn infant. Am J Obstet Gynecol *129:*69, 1977.
32. Ginsberg MD, Myers RE: Fetal brain damage following maternal carbon monoxide intoxication; An experimental study. Acta Obstet Gynaecol Scand *53:*309, 1974.
33. Bissonnette JM, Wickham WK, Drummond WH: Placental diffusing capacities at various carbon monoxide tensions. J Clin Invest *59:*1038, 1977.
34. Phillips P: Carbon monoxide poisoning during pregnancy. Br Med J *1:*14, 1924.
35. Muller GL, Graham S: Intrauterine death of the fetus due to accidental carbon monoxide poisoning. N Engl J Med *252:*1075, 1955.
36. Caravati EM, Adams CJ, Joyce SM, Schafer NC: Fetal toxicity associated with maternal carbon monoxide poisoning. Ann Emerg Med *17:*714, 1988.

37. Siesjo BK, Nilsson L: The influence of arterial hypoxemia upon labile phosphates and upon extracellular lactate and pyruvate concentrations in the rat brain. Scand J Clin Lab Invest *27*:83, 1971.
38. Hsu YK, Cheng YL: Cerebral subcortical myelinopathy in carbon monoxide poisoning. Brain *61*:384, 1938.
39. Jakob H: Uber die diffuse hemispharen markerkraukung nach kohlenoxydvergiftung bei fallen nut klinisch intervallarer verlaufsform. 2. Neurol Psychiatr *167*:161, 1939.
40. Eos G, Priestman G: Cerebral vascular changes in carbon monoxide poisoning. J Neuropathol Exp Neurol *1*:158, 1942.
41. Preziosi TJ, Lindenberg R, Levy D, Christenson M: An experimental investigation in animals of the functional and morphologic effects of single and repeated exposures to high and low concentrations of carbon monoxide. Ann NY Acad Sci *174*:369, 1970.
42. MacMillian V: The effects of acute carbon monoxide intoxication on the cerebral energy metabolism of the rat. Can J Pharmacol *53*:354, 1975.
43. Choi IS: Delayed neurological sequelae in carbon monoxide intoxication. Arch Neurol *40*:433–435, 1983.
44. Sawada Y, Ohashi N, Maemura K, et al: Computerized tomography as an indication of long term outcome after acute carbon monoxide poisoning. Lancet *1*:783, 1980.
45. Ikeda T, Kondo T, Mogami H, et al: Computerized tomography in cases of acute carbon monoxide poisoning. Med J Osaka Univ *29*:253, 1978.
46. Mead JF: Free radical mechanism of lipid damage and consequences for cellular membranes. *In* Pryor WA (ed): Free Radicals in Biology. Vol 1. New York, Academic Press, 1976, p 51.
47. Kindwall E: Carbon monoxide poisoning. *In* Davis JC, Hunt TK (eds): Hyperbaric Oxygen Therapy. Bethesda, MD, Undersea Medical Society, 1977, p 177.
48. Peterson JE, Stewart RD: Absorption and elimination of carbon monoxide by inactive young men. Arch Environ Health *21*:165, 1970.
49. Sayers PR, Davenport SJ: Review of carbon monoxide poisoning. Public Health Bulletin 195. Washington, DC, U.S. Government Printing Office, 1930.
50. Myers RAM, Jones DW, Britten JS: Carbon monoxide half life. *In* Proceedings of the VIII International Congress on Hyperbaric Medicine, Long Beach, California, August 20–22, 1984. San Pedro, CA, Best Publishing, 1987, p 263.
51. Myers RAM, Snyder SK, Linberg S, Cowley RA: Value of hyperbaric oxygen in suspected carbon monoxide poisoning. JAMA *246*:2478, 1981.
52. Myers RAM, Britten JS: Do arterial blood gases have value in prognosis and treatment decisions in carbon monoxide poisoning? Crit Care Med (in press).
53. Marzella L, Myers RAM: Carbon monoxide poisoning. Am Fam Physician *34*:186, 1986.
54. Olson KR: Carbon monoxide poisoning; Mechanisms, presentation, and controversies in management. J Emerg Med *1*:233, 1984.
55. Aronow WS, Cassidy J: Effect of carbon monoxide on maximal treadmill exercise; A study in normal persons. Ann Intern Med *83*:496, 1975.
56. Aronow WS, Stemmer EA, Isbell MW: Effect of carbon monoxide exposure on intermittent claudication. Circulation *49*:416, 1974.
57. Caverley PMA, Leggett RJE, Flenley DC: Carbon monoxide and exercise tolerance in chronic bronchitis and emphysema. Br Med J *283*:87S, 1981.
58. Kurt Mogielnicki RP, Chandler JE: Association of the frequency of acute cardiorespiratory complaints with ambient levels of carbon monoxide. Chest *74*:10, 1978.
59. Burney RE, Wu SC, Nemiroff MJ: Mass carbon monoxide poisoning; Clinical effects and results of treatment in 184 victims. Ann Emerg Med *11*:394, 1982.
60. Sawada Y, Sakameto T, Nishide K, et al: Correlation of pathological findings with computed tomographic findings after acute carbon monoxide poisoning. N Engl J Med *308*:1296, 1983.
61. Myers RAM, Snyder SK, Majerus TC: Cutaneous blisters and carbon monoxide poisoning. Ann Emerg Med *14*:603, 1985.
62. Kelley JS, Sophocleus GH: Retinal hemorrhages in subacute carbon monoxide poisoning. JAMA *239*:1515, 1978.
63. Dempsey L, O'Donnell JJ, Hoff JT: Carbon monoxide retinopathy. Am J Ophthalmol *82*:692, 1976.
64. Werner B, Back W, Akerblom H, et al: Two cases of acute carbon monoxide poisoning with delayed neurological sequelae after a "free" interval. Clin Toxicol *23*:249, 1985.
65. Myers RAM, Snyder SK, Emhoff TA: Subacute sequelae of carbon monoxide poisoning. Ann Emerg Med *14*:1163–1167, 1985.
66. Smith JS, Brandon S: Morbidity from acute carbon monoxide poisoning at three-year follow-up. Br Med J *1*:318, 1973.
67. Choi IS: Delayed neurologic sequelae in carbon monoxide intoxication. J Toxicol Clin Toxicol *19*:297, 1982.
68. Myers RAM, Mitchell JT, Cowley RA: Psychometric testing and carbon monoxide poisoning. Disaster Med *1*:279, 1983.
69. Messier LD, Myers RAM: Development of a neuropsychological screening battery for assessment of carbon-monoxide-poisoned patients. Int J Clin Neuropsychol (in press).
70. Myers RAM, Messier LD, Jones DW, Cowley RA: New direction in the research and treatment of carbon monoxide exposure. Am J Emerg Med *2*:226, 1983.
71. Messier LD, Myers RAM: The Carbon Monoxide Screening Battery Manual of Instructions. Baltimore, MD, Maryland Institute for Emergency Medical Services Systems, June 1987.
72. Gemelli F, Cattani R: Carbon monoxide poisoning in childhood. Br Med J *26*:291, 1985.
73. Crocker PJ, Walker JS: Pediatric carbon monoxide poisoning. J Emerg Med *3*:443, 1986.
74. Goulon M, Barois A, Rapin M, et al: Intoxication oxycarbonee et anoxic algue par inhalation de gaz de charbon et d'hydrocarbures; A propos de 302 cas dont 273 traites par oxygene hyperbare a 2 ATA. Ann Med Interne *120*:335, 1969.
75. Norkool DM, Kirkpatrick JN: Treatment of acute carbon monoxide poisoning; A review of 115 cases. Ann Emerg Med *14*:1168, 1985.
76. Ziser V, Shupak A, Halpern P, et al: Delayed hyperbaric oxygen treatment for acute carbon monoxide poisoning. Br Med J *289*:960, 1984.
77. Myers RAM: Hyperbaric medicine U.S.A. 1986. Jap J Hyperbaric Med *22*:1–15, 1987.

CHAPTER 75
GENERAL ANESTHETICS

John Adriani, M.D.*

Anesthetic drugs are central nervous system depressants. By controlling the quantity to which an organism is exposed, it is possible to achieve a reversible depression of the central nervous system (CNS) that is characterized by loss of reflex activity and insensitivity to external stimuli. This state is referred to as *anesthesia* (without feeling). Anesthesia is an adjunct to patient care only and so has therapeutic function. Surgery, as it is now practiced, would hardly be possible without it. Anesthetic agents either act systemically to depress the cortex, subcortical, thalamic, and other nuclei in the brain or locally to block conduction along peripheral nerves when applied directly to their surfaces. Thus, anesthesia is recognized as *general* (systemic) or *local*. Local anesthesia is more precisely referred to as *regional anesthesia*.

To be surgically useful as a sole agent, an anesthetic drug must fulfill two functions: it must abolish reflex responses to painful and other external stimuli so that the patient is immobile, and it must provide muscle relaxation to facilitate performance of the surgical procedure without causing undesirable, serious alterations of other physiologic functions. A third requirement, loss of consciousness for patient comfort, may or may not be desirable. During local anesthesia, anxiolytic or amnesic agents may be administered to provide patient comfort when loss of consciousness is unwanted.[1]

CHARACTERISTICS OF ANESTHETIC AGENTS

General anesthetic agents are either volatile substances that are administered by inhalation or water-soluble nonvolatile drugs that are administered by routes other than inhalation. In most cases the latter are given intravenously; occasionally they are given intramuscularly or rectally. Volatile drugs differ in pharmacologic characteristics from nonvolatile drugs, but each member of both groups, though chemically different, has common characteristics. They are qualitatively similar but quantitatively different. Volatile drugs are "complete" anesthetics (i.e., they establish a blockade along the sensory pathways from the periphery to the thalamus and to the cerebral cortex). Unconsciousness and a decrease in reflex activity result. The number of impulses from the cortex to the periphery is decreased, resulting in a reduction in muscle tone of varying degrees, depending on the potency and quantity of the drug used. Nonvolatile drugs do not effectively block these pathways.[1]

Volatile Anesthetics

Volatile anesthetics are gases or liquids that readily vaporize at room temperature (usually below boiling point, 60°C). With the exception of nitrous oxide, all are organic compounds. Volatile anesthetics are highly lipid soluble and poorly water soluble and do not bind chemically with receptors in the nervous system, as do the nonvolatile CNS depressants. The binding is presumed to be "loose," resulting from attraction of the electrons and protons of the drug with those of the receptors in a process similar to adhesion (Van der Waals' forces). Volatile anesthetics do not bind with plasma proteins and are said to be inert. However, they do undergo varying degrees of biodegradation. The anesthetic effect is caused by the unmetabolized molecules and not by the metabolites. These are exhaled unchanged at the conclusion of anesthesia. The metabolites are nonanesthetic and nonhypnotic.

The useful volatile drugs are aliphatic (straight chain) hydrocarbons, ethers, halogenated hydrocarbons, and halogenated ethers. Halogenation of aliphatic hydrocarbons or ethers with chlorine or bromine increases narcotic potency, decreases volatility, reduces flammability, and decreases stability

*Deceased. This chapter was the last manuscript Dr. Adriani wrote, thus ending a truly lifelong dedication to pharmacology, anesthesiology, and medicine. Dr. John Adriani was nationally recognized as a pioneer in his field, and this chapter is a testimony to his fine work.

in vivo.[2] The older halogenated compounds were chlorinated hydrocarbons; of these, the most extensively used were chloroform, ethyl chloride, and trichloroethylene. Brominated compounds were also used but fell into disuse because they are more toxic than chlorinated hydrocarbons. Halogenated compounds have supplanted the nonhalogenated compounds, because they are more potent and are nonflammable. All halogenated compounds in current use are liquids. Halogenated compounds are, in most cases, more cardiotoxic and hepatotoxic than their unhalogenated counterparts. Toxicity appears to be dose-related.[1–3] Chlorinated ethers were not clinically suitable, because their vapors were pungent and caused lacrimation.

After World War II, a series of brominated and chlorinated hydrocarbons and ethers, the molecular structures of which embody the fluorine atom, made their appearance. Some of these fluorinated compounds, referred to as freons, possess narcotic activity. They were noted to be superior to the nonfluorine-containing halogens. Five of these compounds came into general use; four of them are still used as inhalation anesthetics. The fluorine atom confers stability and increases volatility, but does not enhance narcotic potency.[2] These compounds have less propensity for cardiotoxicity and hepatotoxicity than unfluorinated halogenated compounds. Halogenated hydrocarbons and ethers are less stable in vivo and are metabolized to a greater extent than their nonhalogenated counterparts. Some halogenated hydrocarbons are not compatible with epinephrine, norepinephrine, and other catecholamines; severe cardiac arrhythmias or ventricular fibrillation may occur when they are used concomitantly.[4]

Many gases and volatile liquids possessing CNS depressant activity have been investigated over the years, but only three gases (nitrous oxide, ethylene, and cyclopropane) and a few liquids (among them ethyl ether, vinyl ether, chloroform, ethyl chloride, fluoroxene, trichloroethylene, halothane, methoxyflurane, enflurane, and isoflurane) received acceptance and were used clinically.[1] Because they are flammable, cardiotoxic, or hepatotoxic, all have fallen into disuse, with the exception of nitrous oxide, halothane, enflurane, and isoflurane. Methoxyflurane is still available but is sparingly used.

Nonvolatile Anesthetics

Nonvolatile anesthetics are solids or liquids that do not readily volatilize at room temperature (e.g., alcohol and paraldehyde). Some are water soluble; a few are not. Solvents such as propylene glycol are used to dissolve the nonwater-soluble compounds. They are all lipid soluble in varying degrees, and potency increases as lipid solubility increases. Nonvolatile anesthetics are "incomplete anesthetics" (i.e., they do not effectively block transmission of impulses from the periphery to the thalamus or from the thalamus to the cerebral cortex as do the volatile drugs). Below-therapeutic doses induce a hypnotic state from which a subject may be readily aroused. Larger doses parenterally produce a more profound state of hypnosis accompanied by anterograde amnesia, but not complete abolition of superficial and deep reflex activity. Painful stimuli continue to cause movement. This state of narcosis is commonly referred to as *basal narcosis.* Nonvolatile drugs bind reversibly by ionic bonding or by covalent bonding that resembles ionic bonding, with specific receptors on cells in nervous and other tissues. Generally, pharyngeal and laryngeal reflexes remain active, and pharyngeal and tracheal procedures are not tolerated except when depression of the nervous system is profound.

Unlike the volatile anesthetics, non-volatile anesthetics are nonanalgesic, with the exception of the narcotic analgesics. Few are satisfactory as sole agents for surgical anesthesia unless greater-than-therapeutic doses are used. It is customary to use combinations of nonvolatile and volatile drugs. The nonvolatile drugs provide basal narcosis and render the subject unconscious; the volatile drugs provide analgesia, muscle relaxation, and suppression of reflex activity. One type of drug complements the other.[2] The combination of volatile, nonvolatile, and various adjunctive drugs used to produce general anesthesia is frequently termed *balanced anesthesia.* The term was introduced by Lundy in 1924 when he began to combine thiopental with analgesics. Unfortunately, this term, which has little meaning from a pharmacologic standpoint, has gained widespread usage. The term implies that the objectionable features of each drug in a combination are offset by the others and connotes that multiple drugs are administered with precision, when actually their administration is imprecise and largely a matter of guesswork. The fewer the number of drugs that are administered, the better, because bizarre and not well-understood drug interactions do occur from time to time.

In addition to being incomplete anesthetics, nonvolatile drugs have other disadvantages. They must be metabolized by the liver and other tissues, or, if they are not biodegradable, they must be eliminated unchanged by the kidney into the urine.[1, 5] Once a predetermined dose has been administered, one must rely on the organism's ability to eliminate it, particularly if a dose has been overestimated and respiratory and circulatory depression ensue. Thus, nonvolatile drugs are said to be "noncontrollable"—that is, they cannot be eliminated from the body as can the volatile drugs by "washing" them from the lungs. They accumulate in the tissues, particularly lipid tissues, following continuous infusion or repeated incremental doses, often resulting in a depression of the respiratory and circulatory systems and prolonged somnolence. They bind to plasma proteins, particularly to the albumin fraction. The bound fraction is not bioactive.[1]

The concept that a drug can be "titrated" into the tissues, as is often believed when nonvolatile drugs are infused, is fallacious.[6] Unless a drug exerts its pharmacologic action and is then quickly and completely dissipated and eliminated from the body, it cannot be said that it is "titrated." It and its metabolites accumulate in the various body fluid compartments and produce cumulative effects.[1, 7] In a true titration process one chemical combines irreversibly with another to form an entirely different compound.

TOXICITY OF ANESTHETICS

Anesthetics are protoplasmic poisons possessing three distinctive characteristics: (1) they progressively depress the activity of all types of cells as the intracellular concentration increases; ultimately the cells are totally inactivated and death ensues; (2) they have a special predilection for and selectively depress nerve cells; and (3) the depression is reversible. The cell reverts to its normal state as soon as the drug is eliminated.

In general, the nervous system is depressed from the cortex first, followed by the subcortical areas, midbrain, and the medulla. The spinal cord ordinarily is not significantly depressed. Overdosage of CNS depressants paralyzes the medullary centers. The respiratory center is the most sensitive of these and is affected first. The vasomotor center usually remains active unless overdosage is massive. Volatile drugs can be "washed out" of the lungs with oxygen administered by mechanical ventilation, thereby reducing the blood alveolar concentration, which in turn causes a decrease in blood concentration, which then causes a decrease in brain concentration. Spontaneous respiration returns when the medullary concentration is reduced to the point at which the respiratory center is reactivated.[1, 13] Volatile anesthetics are called "controllable anesthetics," because the alveolar, blood, and tissue concentrations can be varied voluntarily by increasing or decreasing the quantity in the inspired mixture. The blood level correlates well with the brain level.

On the other hand, nonvolatile anesthetics are not controllable. Once administered, a dose is nonretrievable. Medullary paralysis persists, and lung insufflation by some readily available, effective method must be continued until the blood and tissue levels are decreased by biodegradation or renal excretion of the drug or both. The circulatory system may also be depressed in cases of sustained overdosage with nonvolatile drugs. Hypotension usually ensues. The effects on the circulatory system vary with different drugs and are usually dose-related.[1, 2] The plasma level does not necessarily correlate well with the tissue level. Blood levels may be only a fraction of the tissue level.

The medullary paralyzing dose is not necessarily lethal. *A lethal dose exists for each drug, greater than the medullary paralyzing dose, that will cause death even though effective mechanical ventilation is sustained.* The margin between the lethal dose and the medullary paralyzing dose is wide for some drugs and narrow for others. In dogs, the plasma concentration of ethyl ether that depresses the myocardium is several times greater than that which causes respiratory center paralysis. On the other hand, plasma concentrations of chloroform that depress the myocardium are close to those that paralyze the respiratory centers. The levels for human beings are not known. The wider the margin between these two doses, the safer the drug. Overdosage of anesthetics is customarily managed in an operating room setting, usually by experienced anesthesiologists who have the expertise and equipment to manage such emergencies. However, these drugs are also available outside operating room settings. Some volatile drugs, such as ether, chloroform, trichloroethylene, and ethyl chloride, are used as laboratory reagents or as solvents in manufacturing processes. Persons other than surgical patients may be poisoned, and emergency treatment must be rendered by persons other than anesthesiologists, such as emergency physicians or other health professionals. Basic knowledge of the pharmacologic behavior of these drugs is essential for nonanesthesiologists called on to manage such emergencies.

NEUROMUSCULAR BLOCKING AGENTS

Volatile anesthetics, with the exception of nitrous oxide, produce muscle relaxation, but often at undesirable levels. Muscle relaxation with nonvolatile drugs is totally inadequate for abdominal or other types of surgery. To overcome this deficiency and to minimize the doses of both volatile and nonvolatile drugs, neuromuscular blocking agents (e.g., curariform agents and muscle relaxants) are used as adjuncts. These are non-narcotic, nonanalgesic salts of quaternary nitrogenous bases.[1, 7] Because they are used routinely in combination with general anesthetics, neuromuscular blocking agents are discussed in this chapter even though they manifest neither anesthetic nor hypnotic activity.

Neuromuscular blocking agents are highly ionized, hydrophilic (water-soluble), and lipophobic (lipid-insoluble) compounds. They do not readily penetrate blood-brain and placental barriers or other lipid-containing cellular membranes. They bind ionically with receptors on striated muscle. They either compete with the neurotransmitter at the myoneural junction and prevent depolarization of the membrane (thereby inhibiting contraction of skeletal muscle fibers) or they cause sustained depolarization of the membrane (thereby inactivating muscle fibers). The former are referred to as *nondepolarizers* and the latter as *depolarizers*. Depolarizers cause an initial contraction of muscle fibers, followed by relaxation. This stimulation results in undesirable generalized fasciculations, followed by flaccid paralysis. The duration of action of muscle relaxants varies with the chemical nature of the relaxant and the degree and duration of binding at the myoneural junction.

Neuromuscular blocking drugs do not readily penetrate the microsomal reticulum of the liver and are, therefore, not easily metabolized. Unless they undergo biodegradation in plasma they are eliminated unchanged by the kidney into the urine. They do not penetrate the blood-brain barrier and therefore produce no central effects. They do not act on and relax smooth or cardiac muscle. They are administered intravenously in incremental doses to effect the desired degree of relaxation, and they act within several minutes.[4, 5] They are also effective intramuscularly, but the onset of action is slower. Because they are highly ionized and nonlipophilic, they are poorly absorbed from the gastrointestinal tract. They may cause paresis if ingested orally and renal function is impaired; otherwise whatever portion is absorbed is quickly excreted into the urine, unless dosage is massive or they are metabolized in plasma (e.g., succinylcholine and atracurium).

Paresis may be obtained by administering doses that paralyze small but not large fiber in a muscle. Generally, doses that result in total paralysis are used.[1, 7] Intermittent lung inflation, therefore, is required intraoperatively, either by using a ventilator or by compressing the breathing bag of the anesthetic apparatus manually. A nonanesthetized overdosed patient is managed by supplying respiratory support until the blockade is reversed. The sensorium remains clear; the subject is aware of surroundings, perceives painful and other stimuli, and recalls events that transpired. Doses in excess of paralyzing doses do not appear to be organotoxic. The autonomic nervous system continues to function, possibly giving rise to circulatory changes. Occasions have been reported when insufficient dosages of analgesic and hypnotic drugs were administered intraoperatively, and the paralyzed patient recalled experiencing pain, hearing conversations, and being aware of events that transpired in the operating room.[4]

Use of muscle relaxants as adjuncts permits administration of smaller doses of anesthetics and maintenance of anesthesia at lower levels. Fewer side effects, such as arrhythmias and hypotension, occur at lower levels.[5] Volatile anesthetics, particularly the ethers (both halogenated and non-halogenated), the magnesium and lithium ions, and certain antibiotics (particularly the aminoglycosides), augment the action of neuromuscular blocking agents. Decreased doses of relaxant are required when these drugs are used concomitantly.

The paralysis induced by nondepolarizing drugs may be reversed by cholinesterase inhibitors, such as edrophonium (Tensilon), neostigmine (Prostigmin), and pyridostigmine (Regonol, Mestinon). No satisfactory drug is available that reverses depolarizing agents. Tubocurarine (the active alkaloid in curare), pancuronium (Pavulon), vecuronium (Norcuron; a congener of pancuronium with a shorter action), and atracurium (Tracrium) are the most widely used nondepolarizing relaxants in present practice.[5, 7]

The only depolarizing relaxant in use is succinylcholine (Anectine).[1, 7] This is a unique drug in the class of relaxants, because unlike other relaxants, it is an ester of succinic acid and choline, both of which are found in human tissues. It is rapidly hydrolyzed by plasma esterases, particularly pseudocholinesterase, into succinic acid and the nitrogenous base choline. The greater proportion of a single dose is metabolized within 3 to 5 minutes. Because it is rapidly metabolized, it is customarily administered by intravenous drip. Rare patients who have abnormal, slow-acting esterases as a hereditary trait metabolize the drug slowly and develop apnea of many hours duration when given the usual dose. Continuous intermittent pulmonary insufflation with oxygen is required until muscle tone returns. Neostigmine and similar drugs should not be used to attempt to reverse the block, because they actually enhance it. When large doses of succinylcholine are infused over a long period of time, the drug accumulates in the myoneural membrane and alters the membrane so that the drug acts like a nondepolarizer (Phase II block or sensitizing block). Cautious use of neostigmine is permissible under these circumstances. The presence or absence of a blockade may be determined by use of a peripheral nerve stimulator specifically designed for the purpose and used by anesthetists.

SPECIFIC NONVOLATILE AGENTS

Short-Acting Barbiturates

Numerous nonvolatile drugs have been introduced for use as basal narcotics over the past century, but most of them are no longer available because they were unsatisfactory or because they have been supplanted by more efficacious drugs. Chloral hydrate, Hedonal (a carbamate), and paraldehyde were some of the first basal narcotics used. These gave way to the short-acting intravenous barbiturates, such as pentobarbital (Nembutal), secobarbital (Seconal), and amobarbital (Amytal). These were not suitable, because the onset of narcosis was gradual and the degree and duration variable and unpredictable. Incremental doses were necessary to abolish reflex activity. Cumulative effects resulted in prolonged somnolence accompanied by respiratory and circulatory depression. They were, however, widely used and satisfactory in small doses intravenously for sedation during operations performed under local anesthesia and for induction of general anesthesia. Their use virtually ended when they were placed in Schedule II by the Drug Enforcement Agency; they are still available, however.

Ultra-Short-Acting Barbiturates

Ultra-short-acting barbiturates have proved to be far more satisfactory than short-acting barbiturates and are still used today. They are more potent and easily and quickly penetrate the blood-brain barrier. Unconsciousness develops within 1 minute. However, they possess no significant analgesic or anesthetic activity. They must be combined with an analgesic drug to be useful. Hexobarbital (Evipal), an *N*-methyl barbiturate, was among the first of this type to be used (1932). Later it was supplanted by thiopental (Pentothal) and thiosecobarbital (Surital). Both are thiobarbiturates. Later, methohexital (Brevital), an *N*-methyl barbiturate, was introduced. All three are in use today.[5, 7]

Thiopental is the most widely used of the three ultra-short-acting barbiturates. It is more lipophilic than the long- and short-acting barbiturates. A single induction dose of 250 to 300 mg quickly penetrates the blood-brain barrier and induces narcosis within 1 minute or less. As the blood level falls after a single dose, the drug diffuses from the brain back into the plasma. A redistribution occurs, first to the highly perfused tissues, such as the heart, lungs, liver, and kidney, and then to the lesser perfused tissues, such as skeletal muscles. After several hours, most of it equilibrates between the plasma and poorly perfused adipose tissue, from which it is slowly released to be carried to the liver, where it is metabolized. Repeated incremental doses are required to sustain the necessary brain concentration; thus these compounds are seemingly short-acting. If used over a prolonged period, cumulative long-lasting effects occur. The usual 1-gram maximal dose is metabolized in its entirety by the liver at the rate of 10 per cent per hour and requires approximately 24 hours for complete biodegradation. Some renal excretion occurs in cases of overdosage. The intermediate metabolites are also bioactive. Thus the term *short-acting* is, in essence, a misnomer and is misleading.[1, 3] Dose-related respiratory depression occurs after administration of thiopental. The myocardium is depressed, and cardiac output and blood pressure are decreased. Overdosage causes respiratory and circulatory failure. No antagonists are available to reverse barbiturate narcosis.

Narcotic Analgesics

The narcotic analgesics are the only nonvolatile drugs used for anesthesia that manifest analgesic activity in the awake state. Narcotic analgesics are lipophilic basic amines that form salts with acids. They are administered as the nonbioactive salt but are converted to the bioactive base in the body. The bases are poorly ionized and readily penetrate lipid barriers at body pH. They obtund the dull, aching type of pain but are not sufficiently analgesic to abolish sharp pain, such as is experienced during surgical procedures, unless massive doses are administered or they are combined with nitrous oxide or other inhalation agents.[1, 5]

Narcotic analgesics relieve pain by a dual mechanism: (1) they act by elevating the threshold to pain in a manner resembling the non-narcotic analgesics but at different receptor sites and by different mechanisms; and (2) they alter the psychologic response to pain. The pain may still persist, but the patient disregards it or becomes indifferent to it.[1, 8] Thus they are superior to non-narcotic analgesics, because they relieve anxiety. For this reason they are almost routinely used for preanesthetic sedation. Narcotic analgesics have a sedative action that varies in degree among the different chemical types of this class of drug.[1, 5] Narcotic analgesics are sometimes referred to as "strong analgesics," "potent analgesics," "addictive analgesics," and "opioid analgesics." Presently the term *opioid analgesic* is most commonly used to designate these drugs.

Morphine and codeine are alkaloids derived from opium; for this reason they are referred to as opiates.[2] The morphine molecule has been modified by oxidation, esterification, and other chemical reactions to form semi-synthetic opiates, such as heroin, hydromorphone (Dilaudid), hydrocodone (Dicodid), and others. Phenanthrene is the underlying basic structure in the opiate molecule. Analgesic activity in morphine and morphine-like drugs is a result of a specific chemical grouping or side chain consisting of a two-carbon chain with a tertiary amino nitrogen on one end and an electrically positive carbon bearing a benzene ring and a carbon with an oxygen atom on the other end.

This side chain binds to opiate receptors. Numerous narcotics have been synthesized, but few have been found to be serviceable. All fall into one of the chemical groups embodying this chemical side chain. The first group derived from phenanthrene includes levorphanol (Levodromoran), nalbuphine (Nubain), butrophenol (Stadol), and buprenorphine (Buprenex). A second group derived from piperidine includes four drugs widely used pre- and intraoperatively: meperidine (Demerol), alphaprodine (Nisentil), fentanyl (Sublimaze), and two modifications of fentanyl, sufentanyl (Sufenta) and alfentanyl (Alfenta). All four are agonists. A third group derived from a seven-straight-carbon-chain heptane (referred to as the methadone series) includes methadone and propoxyphene (Darvon). These are used only occasionally by anesthesiologists. A fourth group (called the benzmorphan series), derived from a partially ablated phenanthrene nucleus, includes phenazocine (Prinadol) and pentazocine (Talwin). Synthetic narcotics are called opioids because their actions are qualitatively similar to morphine prototypes of analgesics. Most of these have a more rapid onset of action and a shorter duration of action than the opiates, which are longer lasting. Morphine and morphinone are among the long-lasting narcotic analgesics.

Narcotic analgesics undergo biodegradation in the liver. Their action may be prolonged in cases of hepatic insufficiency. Therapeutic doses may lead to overdosage under these circumstances. Unlike most of the nonvolatile CNS depressants, narcotic analgesics have little effect on the myocardium and vascular smooth muscle. Cardiac output, even in the diseased heart, is not significantly decreased. Nitrous oxide, which is used with narcotic analgesics for its additive effects, usually causes a decrease in cardiac output in diseased hearts. Therefore, it is avoided for cardiac surgery. Under these circumstances doses in excess of the therapeutic dose are used. In other words, patients are deliberately overdosed, and vital functions are sustained postoperatively by artificial ventilation and other measures until the drug is metabolized. Under ordinary circumstances, narcotic analgesics are administered in increments together with nitrous oxide or other inhalation anesthetics and a muscle relaxant to obtain satisfactory surgical anesthesia. The intravenous route is employed intraoperatively. Fentanyl and its analogues may cause muscle rigidity that includes the chest wall, causing apnea. This is reversed by naloxone or succinylcholine. Intrathecal and epidural morphine are used for pain control postoperatively. Doses of a fraction of the intramuscular or intravenous dose produce analgesia. Severe respiratory depression reversible by naloxone may occur. In less common usage than the agonists are the mixed agonist-antagonist group of drugs. Psychotomimetic effects sometimes accompany analgesia. Pentazocine (Talwin), nalbuphine (Nubain), butorphenol (Stadol), and buprenorphine (Buprenex) are used less extensively intraoperatively than the agonists. Overdosage with these also causes respiratory depression and failure.

The most prominent, obvious, and serious manifestation of narcotic analgesic overdosage is respiratory depression. This leads to hypoxia, hypercapnia, and respiratory failure, which if not immediately overcome, leads to cardiac arrest. Obstruction of the airway also plays a role because the tongue and muscles supporting it are relaxed. Respiratory depression from the combination of narcotic analgesics with other drugs is one of the most common causes of cardiac arrest in postanesthetic recovery rooms. Patients may "react" after an operation is concluded and appear to be alert while in the operating room but develop respiratory depression that is overlooked after admission to the recovery room. They are apparently alert when first admitted but then become somnolent. This comes about because the mechanical stimulation occurring during operation has ceased. In the absence of tactile, auditory, and other stimuli, the patient reverts to the narcotic state and ceases breathing, becomes obstructed, or both, and asphyxiates if left unattended. Naloxone is used to reverse the action of narcotic analgesics. The patient may become renarcotized unless the dose of naloxone is repeated when successive doses of analgesic have been used. The naloxone concentration at the receptors gradually decreases as a result of uptake and tissue redistribution and elimination. The plasma naloxone level falls, and the subject then becomes renarcotized in the face of a persisting high plasma level of analgesic. The subject may also become renarcotized from enterohepatic redistribution of the analgesic excreted into the bile and from other tissue depots. The plasma level of analgesic rises again after an initial decrease. Proper airway management and continued surveillance and monitoring of patients who have received narcotics is essential to avert a catastrophe that often occurs with amazing suddenness.[5] (See Chapter 38 for further discussion of opiates.)

Psychosedatives

The search for drugs that are superior to those previously described has continued. Numerous non-barbiturate compounds have been introduced, all of which are qualitatively similar to but quantitatively different from the barbiturates. The barbiturates and the drugs that preceded them were nonspecific depressants (i.e., they depressed the cortex and subcortical centers and produced a generalized degree of hypnosis or narcosis).

In recent years, a variety of chemical groups of drugs have been introduced that are specific depressants (i.e., they act on specific nuclei in the subcortex, thalamus, hypothalamus, and limbic system, producing anxiolytic, amnesic, and other psychosedative effects without inducing a hypnotic state when used in therapeutic doses.[8] These are used extensively in the oral dosage form by practitioners in most phases of medicine as anxiolytic and antipsychotic agents (tranquilizers). Overdosage of these agents causes depression of the CNS in the same manner as do the nonselective depressants. Furthermore, they act additively with other CNS depressants and further augment the hypnotic state. A number of psychosedatives are used parenterally for pre-anesthetic medication or for induction of anesthesia and for maintenance intraoperatively. Some have been developed primarily to be used in anesthesiology. When administered in greater than therapeutic doses or with other CNS depressants, as is often the case, respiratory and circulatory failure result. The pharmacologic response of a given dose and the onset of action is more profound and more pronounced when given intravenously than orally. Among the classes of psychosedatives that have been developed and are in current use are benzodiazepines, cyclohexanones, etomidate, phenothiazines, and butyrophenones.

Benzodiazepines

Many benzodiazepines are available. In general most of these are used as anxiolytics by physicians in all phases of medicine. Among the few that are used as adjuncts to anesthesia are diazepam (Valium), flurazepam (Dalmane), lorazepam (Ativan), and midazolam (Versed). Diazepam is combined with a narcotic, usually meperidine, and administered parenterally for minor surgical procedures, sedation during regional block, and for endoscopic and other diagnostic procedures in physicians' offices and areas other than operating rooms. Too often facilities for managing overdosage are lacking in the latter settings. Midazolam, a more recent addition, is more rapid acting and more potent than diazepam. Unless administered slowly in incremental doses, respiratory arrest occurs, particularly when combined with a narcotic analgesic. The amnesic effects are more pronounced than they are with diazepam. Usual doses cause drowsiness and amnesia; larger doses cause a semi-comatose state or coma. Some benzodiazepines have shorter half-lives than others. Diazepam has a half-life of 4 days; lorazepam, less than 24 hours. Midazolam was developed primarily as an adjunct to anesthesia. Flurazepam is orally administered as a hypnotic the night before surgery. The unmetabolized fraction adds to the effects of the anesthetics administered the following day. Elderly and debilitated patients are less tolerant to the benzodiazepines and metabolize them more slowly than youthful healthy subjects; therefore, they require reduced doses. Overdosage causes respiratory depression, coma, and eventually respiratory and circulatory failure.

An antagonist to the benzodiazepines, flumazenil, is presently used clinically in Europe but available only as an investigational drug (RO 15788) in the United States.[9] It acts on receptor sites for benzodiazepines in a manner similar to naloxone (Narcan) at opiate receptors. As is the case with naloxone, the effects of flumazenil may not outlast the effects of the offending drug, and renarcotization occurs if the dose is not repeated. Careful continuous monitoring is, therefore, essential in cases of overdosage.

Cyclohexanones

Two cyclohexanone derivatives have been introduced into anesthesiology: phencyclidine (PCP; better known as "angel dust") and ketamine. The use of phencyclidine in man was abandoned because it manifested too many side effects, particularly psychotomimetic responses. It is available as an anesthetic, for use in veterinary medicine, particularly in primates.

A congener, ketamine (Ketalar), is pharmacologically similar to phencyclidine. When first approved and released, it enjoyed widespread use until its limitations began to be recognized. Subhypnotic doses cause delirium, hallucinations, and sometimes seizures in certain susceptible individuals, particularly the elderly. These same manifestations may occur on emergence as well as on induction. Patients often recall the hallucinatory effects as unpleasant and refuse a repeat administration of the drug at a later date. Hallucinations do not appear to be a problem in children, and for this reason it is used more frequently in children than in adults. Increasing the dose results in an anesthetic state. Some degree of muscle rigidity is present. The patient may vocalize spontaneously during anesthesia. A vertical nystagmus is present, and sometimes the eyes do not close. The pharyngeal and laryngeal reflexes remain active or become hyperactive, thereby increasing the tendency toward laryngospasm. Salivary secretions are increased and may precipitate laryngeal spasm if they come into contact with the hyperactive vocal cords. An anticholinergic drug, either atropine or glycopyrrolate (Robinol), given intravenously decreases secretions. Apnea may develop, but the patient voluntarily breathes when commanded to do so. The anesthetic state obtained with ketamine is sometimes referred to as *disassociation anesthesia*, because the coordination between cerebral centers appears to be disrupted.

The behavior of ketamine in single anesthetic doses is unique and differs from other nonvolatile depressants. However, after repeated doses it causes a hypnotic state similar to other nonvolatile drugs. Combining ketamine with narcotics, barbiturates, and similar-acting drugs causes a more profound respiratory depression than when the drug is used alone. Overdosage results in respiratory and circulatory failure. No antagonist is available to reverse the depression. Delirium and other psychotomimetic effects are treated by administering therapeutic doses of diazepam or one of its congeners or a therapeutic dose of a phenothiazine intravenously.

Etomidate

Etomidate (Amidate) is a non-barbiturate, rapid-acting hypnotic used principally as an induction agent or for very short procedures. Chemically it is the ethyl ester of imidazole carboxylic acid. It manifests no analgesic activity. Induction doses do not appear to cause cardiac depression, but otherwise its effects are similar to thiopental and related ultra-short-acting barbiturates. Onset of action is 1 minute; duration, 3 to 4 minutes. Plasma cortisol levels may be decreased even after single doses. Overdosage is characterized by respiratory depression and failure, which is followed by circulatory failure.[3]

Phenothiazines

The phenothiazines, once popular as adjuncts to anesthesia, have limited use at present. Previously they were combined with narcotics for anesthetic premedication, and prophylactically as antiemetics. They manifest little hypnotic and no analgesic activity. However, when combined with narcotics and hypnotics, they produce a synergistic effect that results in respiratory depression. They may cause a pronounced α-adrenergic blockade. A difficult-to-reverse hypotension is common with combinations of phenothiazines and anesthetics and hypnotics. Alpha-adrenergic stimulants such as ephedrine and phenylephrine are ineffective as a result of the blockade of adrenergic receptors by the phenothiazine. Drugs that act directly on vascular smooth muscle, such as pitressin and angiotensin II (no longer available), are effective but may cause coronary and renal artery constriction. Promethazine (Phenergan) is the most innocuous of the phenothiazines when combined with anesthetics, and is the only one currently used in anesthesia practice. A fixed-ratio combination consisting of equal parts by weight of meperidine and promethazine (Mepergan) is used for preanesthetic sedation and as an adjunct to regional anesthesia. Promethazine has a pronounced hypnotic effect compared to other phenothiazines and a milder adrenergic blocking effect. Overdosage causes respiratory and circulatory depression and hypotension.[7]

Butyrophenones

The butyrophenones are pharmacologically similar to the phenothiazines but are longer lasting. Two are available: haloperidol (Haldol) and droperidol (Inapsine). Of the two, droperidol is used in anesthesia practice with narcotic analgesics, particularly fentanyl. The α-adrenergic blockade is less pronounced than with phenothiazines. The duration of action of droperidol is approximately 8 hours, and it augments the action of narcotics given in incremental doses over this period of time. Overdosage causes marked respiratory depression, followed by respiratory failure accompanied by hypotension.

Neuroleptanalgesia is an old, vague, and ill-defined term used to describe an altered state of consciousness and awareness resulting from use of a combination of the narcotic fentanyl and droperidol. The term was revived to describe the hypnotic state resulting from use of this combination. A fixed-ratio dose combination of droperidol (50 parts) and fentanyl (1 part) was widely promoted under the proprietary name of Innovar.[7, 10] Misconceptions concerning the combination led to its misuse, with disastrous results. The combination was given in increments intraoperatively. As a result overdosage of both ingredients occurred, leading to respiratory and cardiac failure. One single dose of droperidol suffices, and fentanyl is added as needed. It is no better than any other combination of a narcotic and a psychosedative. There is no such pharmacologic entity as "Innovar anesthesia."[7, 10]

Propofol

Propofol is a substituted isopropylphenol that is a new, rapidly acting, intravenous anesthetic. High lipid solubility contributes to a rapid onset of unconsciousness following intravenous administration of 1.5 to 3 mg/kg. Awakening occurs in 4 to 8 minutes, and, in contrast to barbiturates, postoperative sedation is minimal with propofol.

Other than pain on injection and an occasional allergy, complications of propofol use are considered rare, and at the time of this writing, no cases of overdose from propofol have been reported. It must be kept in mind that this is a new agent, and experience with propofol use at this time is minimal.

GENERAL ANESTHETIC EFFECTS OF LOCAL ANESTHETICS

Many clinicians are surprised to learn that local anesthetics are central nervous system depressants capable of producing a state of general anesthesia. However, local anesthetics are not suitable for general anesthesia, because the level is uncontrollable and the anesthetic state is accompanied by severe adverse circulatory effects. The mechanism involved in inducing the CNS depression is entirely different from any of those embodied by inhalational anesthetics, hypnotics, and narcotic analgesics. The concentration of local anesthetic necessary perineurally to effect a block is many times greater than can be tolerated when the drug circulates in the plasma. Unless the drug is confined to and is absorbed slowly from the injection site, an analgetic plasma level is attained, which is in essence an overdose. Overdosage is characterized by convulsions initially, followed by coma, depression of the myocardial tissues, and cardiac arrest. Overdose is avoided by using the least volume of most dilute solution that is effective. Local anesthetics are combined with epinephrine to retard absorption and to prolong the block. Most adverse reactions from local anesthetics are a result of inadvertent intravascular injection, the use of quantities in excess of established limits, or failure to exercise recommended precautions. Local anesthetics are rapidly absorbed from mucous membranes. Plasma levels that simulate those following intravascular injection are quickly attained by application to mucous and serous membranes.

Local anesthetics act by stabilizing membranes of tissues that possess electrophysiologic activity. These membranes are capable of generating electrical impulses that initiate conduction along a nerve or contraction of a muscle fiber. Membranes possessing the attribute of generating electrical potentials do so by allowing the influx and efflux of ions, namely potassium and sodium, through channels contained within them. Sodium ions are present on the exterior of the membrane in a four- or fivefold greater concentration than that of potassium ions present on the interior. The disparity in ionic concentration results in a positive electrical charge on the exterior of the membrane and a negative charge on the interior that generates a potential of approximately 90 mV. Application of a physical, mechanical, or chemical stimulus to the membrane causes the channels to widen so that sodium ions flow inward and potassium ions migrate outward. The potential falls to zero and then becomes positive on the interior and negative on the exterior. This process, called *depolarization,* initiates the electrical impulse that is propagated as an electric current along a nerve or causes a muscle fiber to contract.

Local anesthetics temporarily and reversibly alter the chemical nature of the protein that causes the ionic channels to widen at the time of membrane stimulation. Widening of the channels is inhibited. The ions do not migrate, and depolarization does not take place. No electrical impulse is generated to initiate conduction or contraction.

Organs that contain membranes manifesting physiologic activity that are inactivated by analgetic levels of local anesthetics in plasma are the brain, conducting tissues of the heart, the myocardium itself, and smooth muscle–containing structures, notably the vascular system. Inactivation occurs more or less in the order listed. At first the inhibitory neurons of the cortex are inactivated. The facilitory (excitatory) neurons remain active. Evanescent convulsions occur that are often the first manifestations of local anesthetic overdosage. However, there are prodromal manifestations (such as anxiety, apprehension, metallic taste in the mouth, a feeling of numbness of the face, seeing double, and accentuation of sounds) that are frequently overlooked. The facilitory neurons are inactivated next, and the convulsions subside. The subject becomes comatose, respiration ceases, and the vascular system is depressed. Cardiac output falls as the myocardial tissues become inactivated, the pulse becomes feeble, the blood pressure falls, and ultimately the heart arrests as a result of vasodilatation and decreased cardiac output. Overdosage from local anesthetics can be swiftly fatal. Local anesthetics, with the exception of those used to control arrhythmias in dilute solutions, are unsuitable for use systemically to obtain general anesthesia. Fatalities from overdosage of local anesthetics are by no means rare.

The observation that cocaine caused numbing of the mucous membranes led to its adoption as a local anesthetic, topically in the eye at first, on other mucous membranes later, and finally by perineural injection.[3, 18] Systemic reactions and fatalities occurred frequently. The search for safer drugs began. Hundreds of compounds were synthesized, but few stood the test of time. Most were esters of an organic acid and a tertiary amino alcohol. Finally procaine (Novocaine) emerged as the standard. Later a series of amides were developed that have the same structural configuration responsible for local anesthetic activity as the esters in their molecules. Lidocaine (Xylocaine), the first of these to be used, has supplanted procaine as the standard. The duration of action of both procaine and lidocaine is approximately 1 hour when injected perineurally. However, some operations outlasted the anesthetic time; therefore, longer-lasting drugs were sought. A longer-acting congener of procaine, tetracaine (Pontocaine), emerged and has enjoyed long use for spinal anesthesia. Mepivacaine (Carbocaine), similar chemically and in pharmacologic behavior to lidocaine, is also widely used. Two long-lasting amides, bupivacaine (Marcaine) and editocaine (Duranest), are also available. Their duration of action is more than 3 hours. The entire group of anesthetics named with the suffix *-caine* are qualitatively similar but quantitatively different.

Once a local anesthetic acts systemically and inactivates vital organs, there is little that can be done to reverse the process. Clinicians should maintain the circulation by instituting external cardiac compression so that perfusion is adequate and wait for the drug to leave the tissues. Redistribution of the drug to other tissues occurs, and excretion begins. When the plasma level falls, the drug diffuses, and vital organs resume activity. The patient must also be ventilated artificially during this time. During the convulsive phase, spasm of the jaw muscles occurs, causing the airway to become obstructed. Convulsions are evanescent, but if they persist, they may be counteracted to re-establish the airway by administering diazepam (5–10 mg) or a short-acting barbiturate (secobarbital or pentobarbital, 50–100 mg; or thiopental, if available intravenously, in 50- to 75-mg increments). Hypotension should be overcome with vasopressors. Bradycardia, which often precedes hypotension, is not overcome by atropine, because it is caused by inactivation of myocardial fibers and not by vagal stimulation. Acidosis, which is invariably present, should be corrected with sodium bicarbonate. The longer-lasting local anesthetic drugs are lipophilic and undergo protein binding to a greater degree than the short-acting anesthetics. Elimination from the brain and heart requires a longer period of time than it does with short-acting anesthetics. The heart responds within 10 to 15 minutes when overdosage is caused by a short-acting drug such as lidocaine, but may not respond for 20 to 30 minutes with bupivacaine.

TECHNIQUES OF ADMINISTRATION OF VOLATILE DRUGS

Volatile anesthetics may be administered by inhalation, using one of four techniques: open-drop, insufflation, semiclosed, and closed. The *open-drop technique* is crude and can be used only for highly volatile liquids. It has fallen into disuse and is used only in under-developed areas where anesthesiology has not advanced beyond a primitive state. The liquid, dropped on layers of gauze stretched over a cone-shaped wire screen that fits over the subject's mouth and nose, is volatilized by the inhaled air. The air serves as both a vehicle and a source of oxygen.[1, 5]

In the *insufflation technique,* a stream of an anesthetic mixture, consisting of gases or vapors of volatile drugs mixed with air or oxygen, is insufflated into the oropharynx, nasopharynx, or trachea by means of a catheter or cannula. This technique is seldom used and then only when use of other methods is not feasible.

In the *semiclosed technique,* the subject inhales a mixture of anesthetic gases and vapors mixed with oxygen delivered from flow meters and vaporizers into a 3- to 5-liter rubber reservoir bag connected to a mask. Unidirectional valves placed at the mask–bag junction and at the side or top of the mask assure that exhalations are expelled to the room and that a fresh mixture of constant composition is inhaled from the reservoir with no return of exhaled gases into the reservoir.[1, 2, 5] The semiclosed system is the most widely used system in present practice.[5]

The *closed technique* consists of an airtight system that permits total rebreathing of exhaled gases or vapors. The circle filter apparatus consists of a tight-fitting face mask, a 3- to 5-liter rubber breathing bag, a cannister containing an absorbent (soda lime) for carbon dioxide, and two corrugated tubes with unidirectional valves arranged so that exhaled gases pass from the mask to the cannister and reservoir bag and back to the patient. Oxygen to meet the metabolic requirements of the patient is supplied from cylinders or a central piping system. Flow meters to measure gas flow and vaporizers for volatile liquids are required, as with semiclosed apparatus. Complete enclosure of gases and vapors without escape into the environment can be achieved only by using the closed system. This system is provided with an exhalation valve that can be opened or closed. Opening the valve converts the system from a closed system to a semiclosed.[2]

Interest in the closed system, used extensively several decades ago for flammable anesthetics, is rekindling because of the necessity for reducing contamination of operating room air with traces of anesthetic gases and vapors. There is evidence from data obtained statistically and from animal studies that chronic exposure to traces of inhalational anesthetic drugs may have deleterious effects on exposed hospital personnel. The incidence of abortions and fetal malformations appears to be higher in women who are exposed or whose husbands are exposed than in those who are not.[13, 14] In order to avoid exposure, "scavenging" systems are now required on all anesthetic apparatus, and exhaled and waste gases are aspirated and expelled into the outside atmosphere.[14, 15] The closed system is more difficult to use with halothane and the fluranes, because they are more potent than ether and cyclopropane. Concentrations are difficult to maintain at a safe level within the system.

STAGES OF ANESTHESIA

The progressive depression of the nervous system by volatile anesthetic agents causes a succession of reflex changes that are clinically useful in estimating the drug concentration in the nervous system. The disappearance and appearance of these reflexes, as the inhaled concentration is varied, serve as useful guides for the administration of volatile anesthetics. The manner in which volatile drugs influence these reflex changes differs considerably from that of nonvolatile drugs. The changes caused by volatile drugs are labile and more obvious. Presumably, this is because of the inertness of volatile drugs, since they readily diffuse in and out of cells. Volatile drugs bind to appropriate cell surfaces by electrostatic (adhesive) forces. Intracellular drug levels closely correlate with blood levels. Variations in blood levels are quickly reflected in cellular levels. The blood levels can be varied by varying the alveolar concentration, which, in turn, is varied by varying the inhaled concentration. This is not the case with nonvolatile drugs.[2, 5]

Anesthetic drugs affect all physiologic systems to some degree. However, the changes in the nervous, respiratory, and circulatory systems are the most obvious. Anesthetists monitor these three systems constantly. They are used as sole agents in patients who are breathing spontaneously. The character, rate, and depth of respiration; the pulse and blood pressure; changes in reflex activity; and variations in muscle tone are observed closely.

Four stages of anesthesia can be delineated when administering volatile drugs.[16] One stage gradually merges into the next as the cellular concentrations in the brain increase. No abrupt line of demarcation exists between stages. In Stage I, referred to as the *stage of analgesia,* the patient remains conscious but does not perceive painful stimuli. Reflexes remain active, and subjects attempt to withdraw from noxious stimuli, even though such stimuli are not interpreted as painful. The sensorium remains clear. This stage is of limited usefulness for performing surgery, because the subject moves about and often becomes uncooperative when stimulated painfully. This stage is used by dentists administering nitrous oxide to produce conscious sedation.

In Stage II, called the *stage of delirium,* the cerebral cortex is depressed, and consciousness is lost. Cortical inhibitions are abolished, and control of excitatory centers is lost. Muscular movements become exaggerated. Excitement may occur, and signs of sympathetic stimulation may be present. Salivation and excess mucus secretion may occur. This stage is avoided and should be transcended as quickly as possible. It is exaggerated by fear and apprehension and external stimuli. Fear and apprehension are allayed by prescribing preanesthetic medication consisting of a narcotic, such as morphine, and an anticholinergic drug (atropine) or glycopyrrolate to inhibit secretion of mucus and saliva. All forms of external stimulation—tactile, auditory, or visual—are avoided until Stage III has been attained.[1, 5]

Stage III is the stage of surgical anesthesia. Anesthesia is completely established, and superficial reflexes are abolished. Deep reflexes and those associated with vital functions, particularly those in the medulla, remain active. Voluntary movements are absent. Tapping the eyelid gently no longer evokes the so-called "lid reflex" that causes the subject to wink. The medullary centers remain active. Respiration is automatic and rhythmic and resembles that noted in normal sleep, because the respiratory centers are no longer subject to cortical and subcortical influences. Pulse and blood pressure, which are usually elevated in Stage II, return to preanesthetic levels.

Stage III is broad and divided into substages called planes. The stages are indicated by roman numerals, and planes by arabic numerals. In the first plane, there is little or no loss of muscle tone. Ocular movements continue when the lids are retracted and light enters the pupil. The pupillary size does not change significantly. In plane 2, the smaller muscles throughout the body are relaxed. When plane 3 is attained, intercostal activity is lost, and respiration becomes diaphragmatic in quality. Minute volume exchange and muscle tone are diminished. In plane 4, complete relaxation of the large muscles and loss of reflexes occur. Diaphragmatic activity is diminished, and the pupils are widely dilated.

In Stage IV, the medullary centers are inactive. The respiratory center is completely depressed, and apnea results. Unless respiratory support is promptly instituted, cardiac arrest occurs, and death results from ensuing hypoxia.

The stages of anesthesia apply principally to ether or ether administered with nitrous oxide. They have also been used to follow the depth of cyclopropane and ethylene anesthesia. They are helpful in following levels of anesthesia with halothane but *not* with methoxyflurane, enflurane, and isoflurane. Nonvolatile drugs used in conjunction with volatile anesthetic agents nullify them. These stages cannot be used to follow the levels of narcosis induced by nonvolatile drugs. All anesthetics cause varying degrees of respiratory depression and subsequent hypercapnia, so it is common to assist respiration to avoid hypercapnia. The respiratory pattern, therefore, cannot be used as a guide.[1, 3, 5] Thus, in clinical practice, the stages of anesthesia are primarily of academic interest and are of limited clinical use. They are mentioned here to call attention to the progressive depression caused by volatile agents, the signs and symptoms a patient may present who has been exposed to these agents in cases of poisoning, and the signs that indicate recovery as the agent is eliminated. The volatile liquids are absorbed if ingested orally, and patients present these signs as they become narcotized and recover.

ELECTRICAL ACTIVITY OF THE CEREBRAL CORTEX

Electrical activity of the cerebral cortex is depressed by anesthetic drugs and hypnotics. The reduction in cortical potential is in proportion to the degree of cerebral depression. The variations of potential (voltage) are demonstrable on the electroencephalograph.

During anesthesia, seven typical wave patterns are discernible in the descent from consciousness to overdosage. The pattern is different for each drug. The encephalogram may be used as a guide to determine levels of depression for both volatile and nonvolatile drugs.

There are, however, limitations and pitfalls in the use of the encephalograph for determining levels of anesthesia during surgical operations. Artifacts, technical difficulties, skill in interpretation of the record, and a lag between the times of establishment of the central and circulatory effects of the drug all limit the usefulness of the encephalogram for routine use. It is a useful tool for research purposes and for diagnosis and assessing the prognosis in cases of hypoxic brain damage after anesthetic mishaps and poisoning. In deeply comatose patients, the pattern displayed may simulate that of brain death and lead to an error in diagnosis.[17]

ABSORPTION AND ELIMINATION OF VOLATILE ANESTHETIC AGENTS

The absorption and elimination of volatile anesthetic agents follow the same basic principles and physical laws as do those of inert nonanesthetic gases and vapors like oxygen and nitrogen.[2, 17] Both absorption and elimination are influenced by the following factors:

1. The tension or vapor pressure of the volatile drug in the inspired mixture
2. The tidal exchange
3. The minute volume exchange
4. The functional residual air volume
5. The solubility coefficient (partition of the drug between blood and the alveolar air)
6. The rate of diffusion of the drug molecules through the alveolar membrane
7. The rate of flow of blood through the lungs
8. The rate of flow of blood through the tissues
9. The solubility of partition of the drug between the plasma and tissues.

During induction, a pressure gradient of the gas or vapor is established between the inspired gases and the alveolar gases, between the alveolar gases and the blood, and between the blood and body cells. The drug diffuses inward from the inspired gases, where the concentration is high, to the cells, where it is zero. Obviously, the higher the gas tension in the inspired air, the more rapidly the blood and cells will become saturated. Concentrations greater than the maintenance concentration are used on induction to saturate blood and tissues, particularly in cases of drugs that have a high solubility coefficient. During recovery, the pressure gradient is reversed. The subject inhales room air; the drug moves from the cells, where the gradient is high, to the blood, where it is less, to the alveolar air, where it is still less, and thence to the outside atmosphere, where it is zero.

An adequate tidal exchange is necessary for proper mixing of gases or vapors with functional residual air. The functional residual air volume is an important factor because it represents the total gas volume that comes into contact with the functional alveolar surface and mixes with tidal air. When functional residual air volume and tidal volume approximate each other, abrupt changes may occur in alveolar concentration with each inspiration. A momentary increase or decrease in concentration may be immediately reflected in the blood level, and the level of anesthesia changes. When the functional residual air volume increases and becomes disproportionate to tidal volume, mixing is slowed. Saturation and desaturation of tissues are impaired, and induction and recovery are prolonged. An even level of anesthesia is difficult to achieve during maintenance. An increase in minute volume exchange increases tissue saturation by increasing the total quantity of drug passing into the lungs and blood.[1, 2, 5]

The level of anesthesia depends on the brain drug tension. This, in turn, depends on the alveolar tension. Brain tissue has not only a relatively high lipid content but is also well perfused; therefore, equilibrium between the blood and brain tensions is established before it is in other tissues or organs. Passage of a drug from the blood to the brain is influenced by the cerebral blood flow, the cerebral vascular resistance, and the penetration of the drug through the blood-brain barrier. Once equilibrium is established between the alveolar air and the brain, anesthesia could be maintained at a given level were it not for the uptake of the drug by other nonequilibrated tissues. This necessitates the intermittent addition of drug to the inhaled mixture to replace the portion passing from the arterial blood to various organs, muscles, and adipose and other tissues.[2, 5]

Volatile anesthetics are sufficiently water soluble to readily diffuse through the alveolar membrane and do so in the same manner as do inert nonanesthetic gases such as nitrogen, helium, and oxygen. The drugs cause no physical changes in the membrane; otherwise they would not be suitable for clinical use. Some volatile anesthetics are categorized as being "irritating," the implication being that in some way they injure the alveolar membrane. This is not so. Vapors of some volatile drugs, particularly ethers, stimulate vagal nerve endings in pulmonary tissues and cause varying degrees of exaggerated breathing. Ethyl ether does so more than all other volatile drugs. Also, the mucous glands in the respiratory tract are stimulated, causing excessive salivation and mucous secretion. Both responses are mistakenly interpreted as "irritation."[1, 5]

The process of elimination of volatile anesthetics is the reverse of absorption. The bulk of an unmetabolized portion of an inhalation anesthetic gas or vapor is eliminated through the lungs unchanged. Traces are eliminated into the urine, the intestinal and stomach contents, and saliva and through the skin. Elimination is governed by its solubility in blood, as is the case with absorption. Blood and tissues are more quickly saturated by the less water-soluble gases or vapors than they are by those that are highly soluble. Highly water-soluble drugs are rapidly absorbed by the blood and distributed to highly perfused tissues. As a result, a longer time is required to deliver the number of molecules required to establish anesthesia in the brain, because the drug is being taken up by the other highly perfused watery tissues as well. Induction time is longer than it is with the less water-soluble drugs.

The blood–gas ratio (partition coefficient) is a numeric value that indicates how much of a gas or vapor is taken up by blood and how much remains in the alveolar air when an equilibrium is established between them. Drugs such as nitrous oxide that have relatively small numeric values are rapidly absorbed and eliminated. The blood–gas ratio for nitrous oxide is 0.47; that is, 0.47 part in blood to 1 part in alveolar air at equilibrium. Induction of anesthesia and recovery occur quickly with nitrous oxide. Drugs that have numerically large coefficients, such as ethyl ether 12 (blood, 12 parts; alveolar air, 1 part) or methoxyflurane 13 (blood, 13 parts; alveolar air, 1 part), are characterized by slow induction (15 to 30 minutes) and slow recovery. The longer a drug of this type is administered, the greater will be the uptake (quantity absorbed) by the well-perfused tissues and the longer the period of postoperative somnolence. Induction with halothane, which has a blood–gas coefficient of 2.3, takes longer than induction with nitrous oxide but is far shorter than induction with ether. The blood–gas ratio for a particular drug is not a fixed value applicable to all individuals. It may vary from individual to individual and even in the same individual at different times. Variations are a result of fluctuations in red blood cell mass, body temperature, plasma composition, and other variable factors in a given individual.[1, 2, 6]

Another factor of importance in tissue uptake is lipid solubility. All volatile anesthetics are lipophilic and concentrate in greater quantities in high lipid content cells. Adipose tissue cells contain 90 per cent fat, but they are poorly perfused; therefore, the uptake and release of lipophilic agents from adipose tissues is slow. The oil–water and oil–blood partition coefficients have been used as indices of potency in the past. They are determined by equilibrating a layer of vegetable oil over an equal volume of water or blood containing the drug and determining the partition between the two. The uptake of a drug by the oil will be greater for the more lipophilic drugs. Chloroform has an oil–blood ratio of 100—that is, 100 parts will be found in the layer of oil to every 1 remaining in the blood at equilibrium. Chloroform is classed as being more potent than cyclopropane, which has a ratio of 34.5. The oil–blood ratio is important from the standpoint of uptake of a lipophilic drug by adipose tissues. Methoxyflurane has a partition coefficient of 400. This is greater than that of any other inhalation anesthetic. In view of this, it is not surprising that, after prolonged exposure, a considerable amount is sequestered in lipid tissue, where it remains for days. It is slowly released and metabolized to various fluoride compounds, among which is the fluoride ion. Blood fluoride levels may become elevated to the point that the renal tubules are injured when the fluoride is excreted.[1, 3]

The potency of volatile anesthetic agents

is now assessed by determining the minimum alveolar concentration (MAC) necessary to abolish reflex responses to superficial painful stimuli in 50 per cent of patients tested. MAC values are now listed in the medical literature pertaining to anesthetic drugs. The importance of the MAC has been overemphasized, for the values established are approximate, not fixed. They vary from individual to individual and even in the same individual at different times, since the method of determining reflex activity is imprecise.[18]

PSYCHIC AND PHYSICAL DEPENDENCE

Of all pharmacologic groups of drugs known, the central nervous system stimulants and depressants appear to be the only ones that are abused. Chemical substances, such as commercial solvents and petroleum distillates with similar pharmacologic attributes but which have no therapeutic usefulness, are also subject to abuse by ingestion. The stimulants cause psychic dependence; the depressants cause both psychic and physical dependence.[19, 20] Different drugs or combinations of drugs act in different ways in different individuals. For this reason, some prefer one drug or combination to another. Those who have difficulty in facing reality readily succumb to the habit of taking drugs for nonmedical purposes. The world appears less real under the influence of drugs.[21] At first, psychic dependence develops when depressants are abused; tolerance and physical dependence follow later.[19a] Stimulants, taken in excess, also cause depression. When stimulants are combined with depressants, the two types tend to augment each other, and further depression occurs. Fatalities have been reported from abusing combinations, such as narcotics or alcohol combined with cocaine.

Drugs and chemicals that cause dependence are important from the standpoint of poisoning. Cases of overdosing are common, particularly when nonvolatile drugs are abused.[21] Sniffing of volatile substances by health professionals and ancillary personnel in hospitals and drug and chemical establishments is more common than is believed because health professionals usually have access to these drugs. Inadvertent overdosage with these also has been reported. Nonvolatile depressants almost without exception cause both psychic and physical dependence. Volatile drugs cause psychic dependence, but evidence that they cause tolerance and physical dependence is inconclusive. Dependence on nitrous oxide, ethylene, cyclopropane, ethyl ether, chloroform, trichloroethylene, carbon tetrachloride, halothane, and methoxyflurane has been reported among physicians, nurses, laboratory technicians, and other individuals in hospital and laboratory settings.[22–24]

SPECIFIC AGENTS

Nitrous Oxide

Worldwide, nitrous oxide (N_2O) is used more than any other inhalation anesthetic. Nitrous oxide, the monoxide of nitrogen—once referred to as "laughing gas"—is a nonirritating, sweet-smelling, nonflammable gas of mild narcotic potency. It is dispensed as a liquid under a pressure of 800 or more pounds per square inch in steel cylinders from which it escapes when allowed to volatilize by activating the valve. It maintains its stability at ordinary temperatures under these conditions for years. Its molecule is composed of two nitrogen and one oxygen atoms. Ordinarily, the nitrogen atoms in nitrous oxide undergo no further oxidation. On the other hand, nitrous oxide readily parts with its oxygen atom, thereby acting as an effective oxidizing agent and supporting combustion. Mixtures of flammable volatile anesthetics explode with ease when combined with nitrous oxide, even in the absence of oxygen. It is strongly suspected that this oxidizing capacity may be a factor in alleged adverse reactions associated with chronic exposure to nitrous oxide. Because it is so active chemically, it is highly probable that traces undergo some degree of biodegradation and that metabolites could be involved in adverse reactions.[2, 22]

The oil–water ratio for nitrous oxide is 3.1. This is low compared with 34.5 for cyclopropane, 330 for halothane, and 400 for methoxyflurane. The uptake by adipose tissues is relatively poor, and only insignificant traces circulate in blood after discontinuing inhalation of the gas. Nitrous oxide rarely yields levels of anesthesia below first plane when used as a sole agent. The maximum allowable concentration (MAC) for nitrous oxide is 100, indicating that 100 per cent must be present in the alveoli to attain Stage III. Anesthesia may be obtained, with some suboxygenation, with alveolar concentrations of 85 to 90 per cent (625 to 650 mm Hg). These are not safe concentrations; therefore, the gas is not suitable as a sole agent for surgical anesthesia. Attempts to obtain surgical anesthesia using nitrous oxide without adjunctive drugs often lead to suboxygenation.[5, 6] *Fatalities occurring during its administration are due to asphyxia.* Mixtures containing 20 per cent oxygen must be administered at flow rates equal to minute volume exchange at which the subject breathes, otherwise hypoxia results.

Nitrous oxide has a blood–gas ratio of 0.47. Induction and recovery, therefore, are rapid, requiring approximately 3 minutes. Its effectiveness is enhanced by combining it with other central nervous system depressants such as morphine and other narcotics, with basal narcotics such as thiopental or ketamine, or with halothane, enflurane, or isoflurane. Overdosage does not occur with 20 per cent or more of oxygen in the inhaled mixture at atmospheric pressure, because the number of milligrams per unit volume of blood necessary to paralyze the respiratory center is greater than the amount that actually dissolves in blood at atmospheric pressure.[2, 3]

Nitrous oxide is analgesic when concentrations of 60 per cent or more are inhaled. It is an anxiolytic in concentrations ranging from 25 to 50 per cent (365 to 380 mm Hg); the sensorium remains clear. It is used extensively for this purpose in outpatient surgical and dental procedures. It is administered to dental patients through a nasal inhaler continuously for hours at a time to supplement dental nerve blocks. Dentists refer to its use in this manner as "conscious sedation."[1, 3] Little surgery can be performed effectively with this level of analgesia, because sharp pain is not obtunded.

Nitrous oxide was used at one time as an induction agent for ether. It is used extensively in present anesthesia practice as a carrier gas for the vapors of halothane, methoxyflurane, enflurane, and isoflurane. It is used in obstetrics for analgesia in combination with narcotics and psychosedatives. Semiclosed inhalers must be used to administer the gas in order to eliminate nitrogen from the tissues. Without anoxia, the drug causes little significant disruption of important systemic and vital functions.

Nitrous oxide is 35 times more soluble than nitrogen. The gas diffuses into hollow viscera and potential body spaces containing air (such as the pneumothorax, paranasal sinuses, and pneumoperitoneum) or into the cerebral ventricles following pneumoencephalography, thus increasing already existing pressures in such closed spaces. It should not be used in these situations. When administration is discontinued, the nitrous oxide is released into the alveoli faster than nitrogen dissolves in blood to replace it, diluting the alveolar gases. A reduction in alveolar oxygen tension may result. This state of affairs is referred to as *diffusion anoxia.* It can be avoided by allowing the subject to inhale oxygen instead of air at the conclusion of anesthesia.[1, 3, 5]

Nitrous oxide has several desirable features: it is nonflammable, nonirritating to the respiratory tract, relatively inexpensive, and rapidly absorbed and eliminated. Postanesthetic nausea and emesis are infrequent. Systemic effects are of little significance in nondebilitated subjects. There is no justification for using the drug if anesthesia cannot be obtained without hypoxia. As noted, fatalities caused by nitrous oxide per se result from asphyxia. When administered in nonasphyxial concentrations, there are few contraindications to its use.[1, 5] If ventilation is adequate in areas in which high concentrations may develop or if mixtures are inhaled with sufficient oxygen, there should be no deaths.[22] Impure nitrous oxide may contain traces of nitric and other oxides. These combine with water in the lungs to form nitrous and nitric oxide, which injure the pulmonary epithelium and cause pulmonary edema.

Chronic exposure to nitrous oxide may have adverse effects on rapidly dividing cells, such as those of the bone marrow, germ plasma, and fetal tissues. A transient leukopenia may follow continuous prolonged administration (24 hours or more). Hospital personnel in operating rooms exposed to volatile anesthetics, among them nitrous oxide, are alleged to have a higher proportion of abortions and fetal malformations than nonexposed personnel in similar settings.[14] Suppression of testicular function has been noted in animals.[22] Chronic exposure affects vitamin B_{12} metabolism, resulting in bone marrow and neurologic changes. Neurologic changes in dentists have been reported that are strongly suggestive of combined degeneration of the spinal cord similar to that occurring in pernicious anemia.[22]

Nitrous oxide has the potential for abuse, particularly among hospital personnel. Physical dependency and withdrawal have been demonstrated in mice. Psychic dependency obviously exists in human beings. Deaths have been reported from use for nonmedical purposes or for "entertainment." These have been ascribed to asphyxia from inadequate ventilation of areas in which high concentrations may develop, from inhalation of mixtures with insufficient oxygen, or from suicide. Patients who fail to regain consciousness within several minutes after breathing fresh air after exposure should be suspected of having hypoxic brain damage or having ingested some other central nervous system depressant.

Halothane

Halothane (Fluothane) is a two-carbon halogenated hydrocarbon with three fluorine atoms on one carbon and a bromine, chlorine, and hydrogen atom on the other (F_3C-CBrClH). It is a potent, nonflammable inhalation anesthetic gas resembling chloroform in some respects. At room temperatures, halothane generates a vapor pressure of approximately 240 mm Hg. It has an MAC of 0.77. Concentrations of 0.5 to 2 per cent (7.5 to 15 mm Hg) are generally required for anesthesia.[1, 3] Therefore, it is sufficiently volatile to be used at room temperature. Halothane vapors are nonpungent and easily inhaled. It is poorly analgesic at subanesthetic concentrations[1, 2] and muscle relaxation is not satisfactory if it is not used with a neuromuscular blocking agent as an adjunct. During recovery it is said to manifest *antianalgesia;* that is, exaggerated pain is felt on emergence.[1]

The myocardium is progressively depressed, and as inhaled concentrations are increased, cardiac irritability is enhanced. Spontaneous arrhythmias are common at lower levels of anesthesia.[1, 5] Ventricular tachycardia or fibrillation may result when the drug is used simultaneously with epinephrine and pharmacologically similar catecholamines.[3, 4] Hypotension develops shortly after induction, but usually corrects itself after the incision is made. Halothane is not a norepinephrine releaser as are cyclopropane and ether.[25] Because of this, hypotension may occur during maintenance. This is a result of a combination of several factors, among which are a decrease in cardiac output caused by myocardial depression and a possible ganglionic blockade, particularly when halothane is used in conjunction with some muscle relaxants.[1, 25] The drug is used in combination with nitrous oxide, which acts both as a carrier gas for the vapor and additively to enhance the anesthetic effect, and a neuromuscular blocking agent.[3]

The blood–gas ratio for halothane is 2:3, a value higher than that of the gases but less than that of ether and chloroform. Induction time is longer than it is with cyclopropane or nitrous oxide, but more rapid than it is with ether and chloroform—5 to 8 minutes. An induction concentration of 1.5 per cent is required, followed by a cutback to 1 per cent or less for maintenance. During prolonged procedures, the maintenance concentration is gradually decreased as the watery tissues become saturated. Fatalities may occur as a result of overconcentration toward the end of the procedure, particularly when the patient is not monitored closely. Recovery occurs within 10 to 15 minutes and depends on the total anesthesia time.[3, 5] Temperature-compensated vernier-type vaporizers are used in a semi-open system to provide unvarying concentrations of the vapor.

Halothane is highly lipophilic. The oil–water ratio is 330, making it second in rank to methoxyflurane. Some accumulation occurs in adipose tissue, but not to the extent that it does with methoxyflurane.[2]

Liver functions, as with other potent inhalation anesthetic agents, are depressed, but less so than with chloroform. They return to normal within several days after anesthesia. These depressions of liver function are unrelated to the hepatotoxic effects of halogenated anesthetic drugs.[3] Unlike chloroform, halothane is not directly hepatotoxic, but hepatitis is associated with its use. The histologic picture of hepatitis associated with halothane administration is difficult to distinguish from that of viral hepatitis.[26, 27] There is much speculation as to its cause. It has been suggested that intermediate metabolites may cause injury of hepatic cells. Anywhere from 10 to 30 per cent of inhaled halothane is metabolized, and metabolites may be detected in the urine for a period of several days after inhaling halothane. Various intermediate metabolites have been isolated; however, trichlorofluoroacetic acid is the principal end-product isolated from the urine. The suggestion is also made that the liver injury may be a hypersensitivity response. Unlike the case with chloroform, halothane-associated hepatitis usually occurs after a second exposure to the drug, although in some cases it has developed after a first use. A history of an unexplained febrile reaction several days after administration of halothane should arouse suspicion, and the drug should be withheld a second time. Unlike hepatitis following chloroform, which appears promptly after exposure (48 hours) and is dose-related, halothane-associated hepatitis may not appear until 7 to 10 or more days after exposure to the drug. No correlation can be made between intensity of the response dose and the duration of exposure. The patient may be discharged from the hospital, only to be readmitted later complaining of malaise and fever, asthenia, loss of appetite, and lassitude. Later, jaundice develops. The severity of the response may be assessed by liver function studies, particularly blood enzyme levels (SGOT, SGPT, and so on), alkaline phosphatase, and other parameters of a liver profile. The mortality rate may be as high as 50 per cent of those affected.

Some halothane enthusiasts do not concede that the clinical entity called "halothane hepatitis" exists; however, the existence of halothane-associated hepatitis cannot be denied. Some clinicians feel impaired liver function is not a contraindication to administration of halothane.[27, 28] From the standpoint of common sense and safety, other drugs that have not been incriminated in causing hepatitis and jaundice should be used, since the etiology of halothane-associated hepatitis is not known. Future exposure should be avoided in all patients who develop jaundice and recover following the administration of halothane.

During the past several decades, halothane was the most popular and widely used of the volatile anesthetics.[5] The agent is now gradually being supplanted by enflurane and isoflurane, with which hepatitis occurs far less frequently.[29]

Methoxyflurane

Methoxyflurane (Penthrane) is a chlorinated and fluorinated nonflammable methyl ethyl ether and not a hydrocarbon. The drug, introduced in 1960, resembles nonhalogenated ethers in many of its pharmacologic properties. Two chlorine atoms are present on the terminal carbon of the ethyl group and two fluorine atoms on the carbon adjacent to the oxygen atom: $HCl_2C\text{-}CF_2\text{-}O\text{-}CH_3$. The vapor is nonpungent and nonirritating, is easily inhaled, and has a fruity odor. Unlike other volatile liquid anesthetic gases, methoxyflurane has an unusually high boiling point (104°C), more than that of water (100°C). Were it not that the agent is potent (MAC, 0.16)—the heat of vaporization (49 cal/gm) is only a fraction of that of water (537 cal/gm)—it would not be suitable for anesthesia. The vapor pressure generated at room temperature ranges between 20 and 25 mm Hg. Since anesthesia is maintained with 0.5 to 1 per cent concentrations (3.5 to 7.5 mm Hg), adequate vapor tensions can be attained at room temperature. As is the case with ethyl ether, concentrations exceeding 1 per cent are required for induction. Subanesthetic concentrations of methoxyflurane are highly analgesic. Muscle relaxation is obtained using it as a sole agent at lower levels of anesthesia. Presumably it acts at the internuncial neurons.[1, 3, 9, 12, 28]

Methoxyflurane combines some of the characteristics of ethyl ether with those of the halogenated hydrocarbons. The drug has a blood–alveolar air ratio of 13.0. This is slightly higher than that of ethyl ether (12.0). Induction and recovery, therefore, are slow, like those of ether. The drug has the highest oil–water ratio of all volatile anesthetics known (400). Uptake by the adipose tissues is exceptional, because the relatively high degree of water solubility allows for better perfusion through the adipose tissues than would a poorly water-soluble drug. Adipose tissues are poorly perfused; therefore, whatever is taken up lingers in the body fat for many days. Prolonged somnolence during the postanesthetic period is common.[3, 5]

Myocardial contractility is decreased, and irritability of conducting tissues is increased. Arrhythmias and hypotension occur frequently at lower levels of anesthesia. Hepatitis has occurred far less frequently with methoxyflurane than it has with halothane.

The drug attained only limited acceptance, however, and is now falling into disuse because of its nephrotoxic potential.[3, 28] Methoxyflurane is metabolized in the liver microsomal reticulum, as are other halogenated lipophilic hydrocarbons and ethers. Oxalic acid is one of the metabolized byproducts. It forms calcium oxalate, which precipitates in the glomeruli and tubules and may cause an acute renal shutdown. Additionally, because it is highly lipophilic, there is a pronounced uptake by adipose tissues, particularly when administered over long periods of time and at deep levels of anesthesia. The drug is slowly released over a period of many days and metabolized by the liver to various fluorinated compounds, among which is the fluoride ion. Fluoride blood levels may become markedly elevated. The concentration of fluoride is so high that it exerts a deleterious effect on the distal renal tubules. A high-output renal failure results, which may be fatal.[3, 28]

Enflurane

Enflurane (CHF_2-O-CF_2-CHClF) is a pleasant-smelling, nonflammable, chlorinated and fluorinated ether that provides rapid induction with little or no excitement.[3, 5] The vapor pressure generated at room temperature is 180 mm Hg. Because it has an MAC of 1.2, and 1 to 2 per cent (7.2 to 14.4 mm Hg) are necessary for induction and maintenance, there is no problem in vaporizing the drug in sufficient quantities for anesthesia. The blood–gas ratio is 1.8, less than that of halothane. Induction and recovery, therefore, are rapid. It provides better muscle relaxation than halothane, but high concentrations may cause cardiovascular depression and seizures.

Enflurane is generally used with nitrous oxide, which not only acts as a carrier gas for the vapor but also augments its anesthetic properties. Neuromuscular agents are used to facilitate muscle relaxation and maintain lighter levels of anesthesia. The cardiovascular system remains relatively stable at upper levels of anesthesia. Enflurane has little effect on the pulse rate and cardiac rhythm at upper levels of anesthesia but depresses the circulatory system at lower levels. The arterial pressure decreases moderately following induction and tends to return to near normal from surgical stimulation and then remain stable. Depression of the cardiovascular system is dose related. As is the case with ethers, enflurane does not significantly sensitize the heart to epinephrine and other catecholamines.[3]

Enflurane is a respiratory depressant. The respiratory rate remains essentially constant or slightly elevated, but the tidal volume is decreased, with a resulting depression of minute volume exchange. Assisted ventilation, therefore, is required. Transient mild abnormalities in liver function tests are observed, similar to those occurring after other anesthetics. There have been a number of isolated cases of hepatic damage but not to the same extent as with halothane.[9] The drug does not appear to be nephrotoxic, as is the case with methoxyflurane.[3, 5]

Enflurane undergoes biotransformation to organic halogenated compounds and fluoride and chloride ions, but to a lesser degree than do halothane and methoxyflurane. It has not caused any significant incidence of renal dysfunction, as has methoxyflurane. Fluoride ion plasma concentration is below the toxic threshold of normal individuals but may be hazardous in those with renal disease.[3]

Central nervous system stimulation, manifested by excitation, tremors, and convulsions, may occur during enflurane anesthesia. Infrequent seizure-like patterns are noted in the electroencephalogram. They occur as anesthesia deepens and develop at the lower levels of anesthesia in the presence of hypercapnia. Seizure activity disappears if administration of the drug is discontinued.[3]

Isoflurane

Isoflurane (Forane) (CHF_2-O-CF_2CHClF) is a highly volatile, nonflammable, halogenated ether that was released for general use in 1980.[30] Although it is an isomer of enflurane, some pharmacologic differences exist between the two drugs and between it and halothane.[3, 30]

Isoflurane is less potent than halothane. The vapor pressure generated at room temperature is 250 mm Hg. The alveolar concentration necessary for surgical anesthesia is 1.5 to 2 per cent (10 to 15 mm Hg). It has an MAC of 1.3, which decreases in patients over 60 years of age. The range of concentrations used for anesthesia is 0.5 to 3 per cent (3.7

to 22 mm Hg). The blood–gas ratio is 1.38, less than that of halothane. Induction and recovery, therefore, are rapid. It is highly lipophilic and poorly water soluble.

Induction is smooth, with little excitement when premedication is given. It is administered with nitrous oxide and oxygen, which act both as carrier gas and additively to augment isoflurane's anesthetic effects. The MAC with 50 per cent nitrous oxide is 0.7 per cent. Satisfactory relaxation can be obtained with the sole agent; however, use of neuromuscular blocking agents allows use of upper levels of anesthesia.

Isoflurane potentiates the effects of nondepolarizing neuromuscular blocking agents. It causes little or no cardiovascular depression, and there is less tendency to develop arrhythmias, even at deeper levels of anesthesia, than with halothane or enflurane. Central nervous system stimulation characterized by seizures does not occur during isoflurane anesthesia, as it does with enflurane. Respiration is depressed, and the respiratory rate should not be used as an index to ventilation in patients breathing spontaneously. Mental alertness may be depressed for 2 or 3 hours after anesthesia depending on duration of administration; however, postoperative nausea, vomiting, and excitation are uncommon.[3, 29]

Isoflurane is minimally metabolized (2.5 to 3.5 per cent). The principal metabolites are trifluoroacetic acid and fluoride ion, which appear in urine in a ratio of about 2:1.

DISCONTINUED VOLATILE AGENTS

A dozen or more effective volatile drugs once widely used as general anesthetics have fallen into disuse because they are flammable, hepatotoxic, or carcinogenic. Some are still available for laboratory or industrial use. Occasionally patients who have access to these and who are inadvertently exposed or deliberately inhale them require emergency treatment for overdosage. Ether and cyclopropane, two mainstays of anesthesiology, are no longer in use as anesthetics. The pharmacologic behavior of currently used volatile anesthetics was elucidated by comparing the pharmacologic actions to these two agents.

Ether

Ethyl ether is used as a solvent in laboratory settings and for industrial purposes. Its pharmacologic action is similar to that of methoxyflurane in many respects. Induction is prolonged; recovery varies usually from 10 or 15 minutes to 30 or 40 minutes, depending on duration of exposure. Emergence is characterized by delirium, confusion, and agitation. Overdosage causes respiratory failure, followed by cardiac arrest. Management of overdosage is basically the same as for other volatile agents.

Cyclopropane

Cyclopropane is a sweet-smelling, flammable gas that has little or no laboratory, commercial, or industrial use. Poisoning is highly unlikely because of its unavailability, but if poison is encountered, management should be the same as for other volatile anesthetics. Recovery is rapid, usually within 10 minutes after inhalation irrespective of the duration of exposure. Overdose causes respiratory arrest, followed by cardiac arrest.

Chloroform

Chloroform never had widespread acceptance as an inhalation anesthetic in the United States and is no longer used for that purpose, because it is both hepatotoxic and cardiotoxic. It is available as a solvent in laboratories and in the chemical industry, but has been banned as a flavorant in toothpastes and other over-the-counter drug products as a result of carcinogenicity in animals after chronic exposure. Acute and chronic poisoning can occur from exposure to the vapors. It produces all stages of anesthesia when inhaled, and has a narrow margin of safety, because it causes cardiac and respiratory failure almost simultaneously.

Phosgene forms when chloroform vapors are exposed to flames and cauteries. Inhaled phosgene is converted to hydrochloric acid and carbon dioxide when it reacts with the water in the alveoli. The acid causes pulmonary edema. Unlike halothane, chloroform is directly hepatotoxic. Jaundice may follow within 2 or 3 days after exposure, and one exposure may precipitate hepatitis. The severity is dose-related.

A spontaneously breathing subject who is overdosed should be removed to a well-ventilated area. Oxygen should be administered if available. Subjects who have ceased breathing should be resuscitated using an effective method of lung inflation and external cardiac compression.

Trichloroethylene

Trichloroethylene ($CHC=CCl_3$) is a slowly volatilizing liquid (boiling point, 87°C) resembling chloroform in odor and physical properties. It was used extensively for analgesia but is not satisfactory for general anesthesia. Oxidation converts it to phosgene which, if inhaled, causes pulmonary edema. Trichloroethylene depresses the myocardium and increases cardiac irritability, resulting in arrhythmias. Most of the inhaled drug is eliminated unchanged by exhalation, but some is metabolized and excreted into the urine as trichloroacetic acid for several days after exposure. Bilateral anesthesia of the face and palsies of the other cranial nerves have occurred after chronic exposure in industrial settings as a result of the presence of an impurity, dichloroacetylene. Trichloroacetylene has the potential for abuse. Trichloroethylene "sniffers" were not uncommon when the drug was readily available as an anesthetic.

Drowsiness, loss of consciousness, and respiratory arrest may occur from exposure to the vapors. Patients breathing spontaneously can be revived by removing them to a well ventilated area. Patients who are apneic require effective intermittent lung inflation and, if asystole is present, external cardiac compression.

Ethyl Chloride

Ethyl chloride is a saturated, chlorinated, flammable liquid hydrocarbon that causes general anesthesia when the vapors are inhaled. It is rapid acting, and the level of anesthesia is difficult to control. It is no longer used as a general anesthetic because it is cardiotoxic; overdosage causes almost simultaneous respiratory and cardiac arrest.

The liquid is highly volatile (boiling point, 15°C). When sprayed on the skin, tissue temperature is reduced to −10°C or lower, causing tissues to freeze. The water vapor in the air condenses, and ice forms at the site of application, producing anesthesia. Painful cutaneous stimuli are obtunded, but frostbite has resulted from overuse. Ethyl chloride was used as a local anesthetic for short procedures such as myringotomy and cutaneous abscess and for introducing large-bore needles. Once widely used in emergency rooms, the drug has gradually disappeared from these areas because of its limited use and flammable vapors.

Acute poisoning is characterized by unconsciousness, which proceeds to respiratory and cardiac failure if inhalation of the vapors persists. The drug is quickly eliminated within 2–3 minutes when a spontaneously breathing subject inhales fresh air or oxygen.

MANAGEMENT OF ACUTE ANESTHETIC DRUG OVERDOSAGE

Overdosage from anesthetic drugs occurring in an operating room setting is managed by trained anesthesia personnel. The inhalor of the anesthetic apparatus (gas machine) may be quickly converted into a ventilator to permit intermittent lung inflation or assisted respiration. Adjunctive and antidotal drugs, airways, suction apparatus, monitoring devices, and other necessary paraphernalia, as well as skilled personnel versed in cardiopulmonary resuscitation, are immediately available. The patient's medical history, the drugs administered, and dosage used are known. Overdosage is anticipated as a possibility, and anesthetists are prepared to immediately cope with it should it occur. The situation is entirely different in areas other than operating rooms. In most instances, neither facilities for diagnosis nor skilled personnel are immediately available. The medical history is fragmentary or unknown, and the nature of the drug or drugs and the quantities ingested are often uncertain.

All CNS depressants, including sedatives, cause semi-coma or comatose states if given in excess. The initial treatment should be the same as that instituted for any comatose state of unknown etiology. The first and immediate steps to undertake are: (1) The establishment of an unobstructed airway with an adequate minute volume exchange, and (2) an assessment of the status and correction of any aberration of the circulatory system. Apneic patients should be ventilated with an Ambu bag or similar inhalor or by mouth-to-mouth breathing if nothing else is available. Steps should be taken to correct hypotension with fluids and vasopressors. Essentially, a general approach to the emergency management of poisoning should be utilized, as outlined in Chapter 1.

Acute overdosage from CNS depressants is far more common with nonvolatile drugs than with volatile drugs and generally results in a comatose state; recovery time depends on the half-life of the ingested drugs and the physiologic state of the patient. Unconsciousness in some cases may be prolonged for hours.

Salts of rapid-acting drugs that are weak acids, such as thiopental, are converted to the nonionized, lipid-soluble acid in the stomach. When taken orally, these and other drugs that are not salts but are lipid soluble are quickly absorbed from the stomach and upper intestinal tract and undergo some metabolic change on their first pass through the liver. A dose given by the oral route is far less effective than the same dose administered parenterally. Patients ingesting such a drug may merely be disoriented, confused, or semi-comatose and not necessarily comatose. Larger oral doses are therefore required to depress the nervous system to the point of inducing coma than would be required by parenteral doses.

Patients who have been exposed to volatile agents, if breathing spontaneously, usually recover quickly and are usually conscious by the time they are transported to the emergency department. When treated at the scene of exposure, they should be removed to an area where they can breathe fresh air. The level of anesthesia may be assessed by noting reflex activity and muscle tone. Usually patients who were still inhaling the offending agent at the time of discovery are in some level of Stage III or Stage IV anesthesia. They begin to recover after breathing fresh air or oxygen and gradually pass into Stage II or I. If the gas or vapor that was inhaled was diluted with air, the level of narcosis may be no deeper than Stage II or I. The patient moves about and shows signs of return of consciousness. Some drowsiness may persist after recovery, particularly after inhaling vapors of drugs such as methoxyflurane.

Some poisonings with volatile anesthetic agents occur in industrial or laboratory settings where these substances are used as reagents, solvents, or ingredients for manufacturing purposes. Industrial settings generally have facilities for rendering first aid to victims who inhale these ingredients. Most volatile agents cause nausea and emesis upon emergence. Precautions to avert aspiration should be taken by suctioning the pharynx and placing the subject in the tilted position, with head down.

Apneic or severely depressed patients who have been resuscitated and who fail to regain consciousness within a reasonable period of time may have sustained hypoxic brain damage. The severity of such damage may be assessed by neurologic examination and use of the electroencephalogram (EEG). The EEG may indicate "brain death" in deeply comatose patients, particularly those who have ingested nonvolatile agents at the time of admission. However, early tracings may be misleading, particularly when excessive doses of nonvolatile drugs have been ingested. The electrical pattern then may simulate that of brain death. Electrical activity returns as the drug is eliminated.

CNS depressants have the propensity for abuse. Repeated exposure results in tolerance, as well as a psychic and physical dependence. Subjects who have developed a tolerance require a larger dose than usual to achieve the usual anticipated pharmacologic effect. Cross-tolerance to other CNS depressants is not unusual. A person tolerant to a non-barbiturate hypnotic may also be tolerant to barbiturates. Dependent persons may become overdosed when they substitute a drug to which they have access for the one they customarily take that is unavailable (i.e., a barbiturate for a chlordiazepoxide). These facts are of significance in CNS-depressant overdosage management. In these days of widespread drug dependence, syringes and needles are available to non-health professionals. Poisoning by the parenteral route, therefore, is not uncommon.

Airway obstruction is invariably present in semi-comatose and comatose patients. This requires immediate relief. Too often correction is undertaken by persons of limited experience attempting tracheal intubation. A reversible situation is converted to one that is irreversible. Intubating a patient in the operating room with the benefits of anesthesia, with total paralysis of neck and jaw muscles induced by neuromuscular blocking agents, and with absent pharyngeal and laryngeal reflexes, is an entirely different procedure than one attempted in a patient with partially obtunded or active reflexes and with partial or full muscle tone in a bed or on a stretcher that does not permit proper positioning. Even anesthesiologists and others expert at intubating experience difficulty in these situations and avoid trying. If they do, they cease trying after one or two attempts if unsuccessful. It is not necessary to routinely intubate to resuscitate. An oral or nasal airway is usually effective in most situations, at least at the outset, until preparations are made to intubate under more optimal conditions. An airway suffices if the patient is breathing spontaneously and ventilating adequately. Airways should be lubricated with benzocaine or lidocaine ointment; otherwise they may not be tolerated, because the pharyngeal reflex is only partially inactivated. Oxygen is supplied at a 3- to 5-liter flow nasally. Intubation should always be attempted with patients on their back; never in the prone, lateral, or sitting position.

Repeated attempts at intubation may precipitate laryngeal spasm, particularly if some degree of glottic edema is present or the laryngeal reflex is hyperactive. This may be the case when volatile agents are inhaled. Laryngeal spasm uncomplicated by glottic edema may be overcome by a single dose (75 to 100 mg) of succinylcholine or other rapid-acting muscle relaxant of short duration in adults. Smaller doses are required for infants and children. Some physicians, after failing to intubate, unwisely attempt to perform a classical midline tracheotomy to overcome laryngeal spasm, which is unwise. Profuse bleeding is always encountered. The result of such an attempt is a severely brain-damaged, profusely bleeding, or dead patient. Cricothyroidotomy is the procedure of choice in urgent situations. It can be quickly performed to re-establish a patent airway. A classical tracheotomy can then be performed under conditions that provide asepsis and adequate hemostasis. Physicians with little or no experience should not attempt intubation, as book instruction alone is not adequate to properly learn the technique.

After initial emergency treatment has been rendered and the patient is "stabilized," further treatment should be continued in an intensive care unit until the drug is eliminated, with modern standards of critical care.

SUMMARY

An overview of the concepts of anesthesia and specific anesthetic agents has been presented. Clinical overdose may result from complications during anesthesia and from abuse of anesthetic agents by either hospital personnel or the public. Clinical management involves monitoring of pertinent clinical parameters and supportive therapy, with particular attention given to the respiratory, cardiovascular, and central nervous systems.

References

1. Adriani J: Pharmacology of Anesthetic Drugs. Springfield, IL, Charles C Thomas, 1970.
2. Adriani J: The Chemistry and Physics of Anesthesia. Springfield, IL, Charles C Thomas, 1962.
3. American Medical Association, Drug Evaluations: General Anesthetics. 6th ed., pp 291–308, Chicago, IL, 1987.
4. Matteo RS, Katz RL, Papper EM: The injection of epinephrine during general anesthesia with halogenated hydrocarbon and cyclopropane in man. Anesthesiology *23*:360, 1962.
5. Dripps R, Eckenhoff JE, Vandam LD: Introduction to Anesthesia. 6th ed. Philadelphia, W. B. Saunders Company, 1982.
6. Miller RD: Anesthesia. 2nd ed. New York, Churchill Livingstone, 1986.
7. American Medical Association: Drug Evaluations: Adjuncts to Anesthesia. Chicago, IL, 1986, pp 309–326.
8. Kaiko RE: Basics of pain; Opioid analgesics. Pain 2:32–26, 1985.
9. O'Sullivan GF, Waldon DM: Flumazenil in management of acute overdose with benzdiazepines. Clin Pharmacol Therap *42*:254–259, 1987.
10. Innovar. Med Lett *23*:74, 1982.
11. Adriani J: Labat's Regional Anesthesia. 4th ed. St. Louis, MO, Warren H Green, Inc., 1985, pp 55–107.
12. American Medical Association: Drug Evaluations: Local Anesthetics. 6th ed. Chicago, IL, 1987, pp 275–290.
13. Cohen EN, Belleville JW, Brown BW: Anesthesia, pregnancy and miscarriage: The study of operating room nurses and anesthetists. Anesthesiology *35*:343, 1971.
14. Cohen EN, Brown BW, Wu ML, et al: Occupational disease in dentistry and chronic exposure to trace anesthetic gases. J Am Dent Assoc *101*:21, 1980.
15. Cohen EN: Toxicity of inhalation anesthetic agents. Br J Anaesth *50*:655, 1978.
16. Guedel AE: Inhalation Anesthesia: A Fundamental Guide. 2nd ed. New York, Macmillan, 1951.
17. Faulconer A Jr, Bickford RG: Electroencephalography in Anesthesiology. Springfield, IL, Charles C Thomas, 1964.

18. Sabin LJ, Eger EI II, Munson ES: Minimum alveolar concentration of methoxyflurane, halothane, ether and cyclopropane in man. Anesthesiology *28*:994, 1967.
19. Adriani J, Naraghi M: Drug abuse in hospitalized patients. *In* National Clearinghouse for Drug Abuse Information: Acute Treatment for Drug Abuse Emergencies Manual. Washington, DC, U.S. Government Printing Office, 1973, pp 125–136.
19a. Bourne P: Chapter 23. *In* Acute Drug Abuse Emergencies. San Francisco, Academic Press, 1978, pp 231–248.
20. Smith RA, Winter PN, Smith M, Eger EI II: Tolerance to and dependence on inhalation anesthetics. Anesthesiology *50*:505, 1979.
21. DAWN, National Institute of Drug Abuse, Public Health Service: Emergency Room Figures. Washington, DC, US Government Printing Office, 1980.
22. Nitrous oxide hazards. FDA Drug Bulletin *10*:13, 1980.
23. Rosenberg H, Orkin FK, Springstead J: Abuse of nitrous oxide. Anesth Analg *58*:104, 1979.
24. Spencer JD, Raasch F, Trefny FA: Halothane abuse in hospital personnel. JAMA *235*:1034, 1976.
25. Price HL: Circulation During Anesthesia and Operation. Springfield, IL, Charles C Thomas, 1967.
26. Aach R: Halothane and liver failure. JAMA *211*:2145, 1970.
27. Carney FMI, Van Dyke RA: Halothane hepatitis—A critical review. Anesth Analg *51*:135, 1972.
28. Adriani J: Toxicity of halogenated anesthetics, hypnotics and sedatives. J Am Assoc Nurse Anesth *40*:95, 1972.
29. Eger EI II: Isoflurane (Forane). Madison, WI, Airco, Inc., 1981.
30. Fineberg HV, Pearlman LA, Gabel RA: The case for abandonment of explosive anesthetic agents. N Engl J Med *303*:613, 1980.
31. Chenoweth MD: Modern Inhalation Anesthetic Agents. New York, Springer-Verlag, 1972.
32. Drug Poisoning. Merck Manual. 15th ed. 1987, Rahway, NJ, Merck & Co., pp 2543–2546.

CHAPTER 76
PETROLEUM DISTILLATES AND TURPENTINE

Michael E. Ervin, M.D.
Michael G. Manske, M.D.

DEFINITIONS OF TERMS

The goal of this chapter is to clarify the treatment of petroleum distillate ingestions. Confusion has resulted from anecdotal opinion and the fact that a number of similar, yet different, petroleum distillates are involved. Petroleum distillates come from diverse crude oil sources throughout the world and are produced by different processes, such as distillation and cracking. Also, they often are mixed with each other or contain additives (e.g., insecticides) that can be more dangerous than the petroleum distillates themselves.

The terms *hydrocarbons* and *petroleum distillates* have been used interchangeably erroneously. Therefore, let us define them. Hydrocarbons are a broad group of organic compounds that contain carbon and hydrogen only. Hydrocarbons are divided into aliphatic (straight-chain) and aromatic (containing a benzene ring). The basic aliphatic hydrocarbons include methane (CH_4), ethane (CH_3CH_3), propane ($CH_3CH_2CH_3$), and butane ($CH_3[CH_2]_2CH_3$), all of which are flammable gases. Natural gas is primarily methane and ethane. Liquefied petroleum gas (LPG, "bottled gas") contains propane and butane.

Hydrocarbons do not necessarily have to be petroleum distillates. Turpentine is a hydrocarbon made from pine oil, not from petroleum. Carbon tetrachloride is a hydrocarbon but not a petroleum distillate. Petroleum distillates are the breakdown products remaining after the processing of crude oil. Some examples are kerosene, gasoline, mineral seal oil (used for red furniture polish), and naphtha (as found in charcoal lighter fluid).

Insecticides, heavy metals, and other toxic

chemicals with a petroleum base must be considered separately, because their treatment differs from that of other petroleum distillates. Therefore, it is important in any petroleum distillate ingestion to know whether the petroleum distillates have any other toxic additives. However, the presentation and management of patients with petroleum distillate and turpentine poisoning are for practical purposes similar, and the following discussion is confined to those agents alone.

EPIDEMIOLOGY

It has been estimated that each year 28,000 children under the age of 5 years ingest petroleum distillates.[1] These ingestions account for 5 per cent to 25 per cent of all poison deaths in this age group. As one study indicated, these figures may underestimate the problem and not show regional differences.[2] Poison centers that gather statistics are more likely to be contacted about unfamiliar poisons, and more commonly ingested substances such as petroleum distillates tend to be under-reported.

The most commonly ingested products in this group in order of frequency are: (1) gasoline, (2) pine oil and turpentine, (3) mineral spirits, (4) kerosene, (5) lubricating oils, and (6) lighter fluid.[3, 4] There may be regional differences and seasonal differences in the ingestion of particular products. One study reported a summer peak for gasoline ingestion but an autumn/winter peak for household cleaning products.[5] Kerosene ingestion is particularly common in the southern United States. Kerosene (called paraffin in the United Kingdom) is often placed in soft drink bottles or other unlabeled containers and left around the house or garage, making it easily accessible to a child. It is also widely used as a starter for wood-burning stoves and as fuel for space heaters. As shown in Table 76–1, many products found in the home or garage contain petroleum distillates.

Mineral seal oil preparations such as red furniture polish are extremely dangerous. Unfortunately they have an attractive color, are pleasantly scented, and are therefore attractive to a child. Patients ingesting mineral seal oil generally have a more severe clinical course and a longer period of hospitalization.

The majority of petroleum distillate poisonings are oral ingestions in infants and toddlers.[3, 4] These substances are usually ingested accidentally, without the intention of suicide. Although rare, intravenous use of a hydrocarbon has been reported in a drug abuser.[6]

Most morbidity from ingestion of petroleum distillates is related to pulmonary complications secondary to aspiration. Deaths resulting from petroleum distillate poisoning almost always are caused by pulmonary complications rather than by central nervous system or other involvement.

PATHOPHYSIOLOGY

The toxicity of petroleum distillates can affect many organ systems in the body, but the majority of serious problems are related to the pulmonary, cardiovascular, and central nervous systems and, to a lesser extent, the gastrointestinal system.[5, 7, 8]

Numerous studies in animals have shown that pulmonary injury after ingestion results from aspiration, not from gastrointestinal absorption.[5, 9–11] Aspiration may occur when the hydrocarbon is initially ingested or during vomiting.[12] A hydrocarbon's aspiration potential is dependent on its viscosity, volatility, and surface tension. The risk of aspiration involving any particular petroleum distillate increases with low surface tension, low viscosity, and high volatility.[12] Low surface tension allows the petroleum distillate to spread rapidly over the surface contacted (i.e., the pulmonary parenchyma). Viscosity, which is the resistance to flow, is the most important physical property that determines the aspiration hazard. Low viscosity enables a substance to seep and spread thinly over a surface, allowing deeper penetration of fluid into the distal airway.[13] Viscosity is expressed as the efflux time in seconds (standard Saybold universal seconds, or SSU) of a particular substance flowing through a Saybold viscometer at 37.8°C. A petroleum distillate with a viscosity below 45 SSU (e.g., petroleum ether, petroleum naphtha, gasoline, mineral spirits, kerosene, lamp oil, and mineral seal oil) is highly toxic by aspiration. However, hydrocarbons with viscosity between 45 SSU and 100 SSU still pose a risk of aspiration.[14] The volume of petroleum distillate ingested is not related to the incidence of aspiration; in fact, many cases of aspiration

Table 76–1. EXAMPLES OF COMMERCIAL PRODUCTS FOUND IN THE HOME OR GARAGE

BRAND NAME	CHEMICAL TYPE
Aviation Form-A-Gasket	Isopropyl alcohol
Blue Max Shield One-Step Polymer Car Coating	Petroleum distillate
Brasso	Petroleum distillate, ammonia
Bruce Cleaning Wax	Petroleum naphtha
Collinite Fleetwax	Petroleum distillate
Collinite Insulator Wax	"
Collinite Metal Wax	"
CRC Marine Formula 6-66	"
CRC Marine Lectra-Clean Motor and Equipment Cleaner	Carbon tetrachloride
CRC Marine Silicone Lubricant	Silicone, petroleum distillate
CRC Marine Zinc-Mate (Rust preventative and touch-up)	95% zinc
Du Pont Acrylic Enamel Reducer	Petroleum naphtha >60%
Du Pont Engine Cleaner and Degreaser	Kerosene 85%
Du Pont Good and Clean Lotion	Mineral spirits
Du Pont Imron Paint Additive	Xylene
Du Pont Plastic Cement	Toluol
Du Pont Rain Dance	Aliphatic hydrocarbons
Du Pont Windshield Washer	Methanol
Du Pont Zerex Anti-Rust Antifreeze	100% ethylene glycol
Du Pont Zerex Gas Line Antifreeze	>90% methanol
Du Pont Zerex Windshield De-Icer	90% methanol
El Pico Marine Paint and Varnish Remover	Methanol, methylene chloride, ethylene dichloride
El Pico Sandeze (Sta-Lube)	Acetone, toluene, methanol
Fixall Enamel	Mineral spirits
Fixall Varnish	"
Formby's Furniture Cleaner	Petroleum distillate
Formby's Furniture Refinisher	Methanol, toluene, methylene chloride
Formby's Furniture Treatment	Petroleum distillate
Fulton Acetone	Acetone
Fulton Lacquer Thinner	Toluol, xylol, methyl isobutyl ketone
Gulf Charcoal Lighter Fluid	Petroleum naphtha
Johnson's Paste Wax	"
Jubilee Kitchen Wax	"
Lamplight Farms Lamp Oil	Petroleum distillate
Lemon Pledge Furniture Polish (Johnson)	Petroleum naphtha
Lighting Starting Fluid	Ether, hydrocarbons
Liquid Wrench	Petroleum distillate
Mac's Brake and Electric Motor Cleaner	Trichloroethane, perchloroethylene, methylene chloride
Mac's Carburetor and Choke Cleaner	Petroleum distillate
Mac's Cleaner Wax	"
Mac's Gas Line Antifreeze	Methanol
Mac's Moisture and Rust Control	Propane, petroleum distillate
Mac's Valve Tune	Petroleum distillate
Mac's Windshield De-Icer	Methanol
Magic Pre-Wash (Armour-Dial)	Petroleum distillate
Mobil Gas Line Antifreeze	Isopropyl alcohol, methyl alcohol
Mobil Oil Cooling System Cleaner	Kerosene
Mobil Oil Fast Flush	Kerosene, orthodichloro-benzene
Mobil Oil Super Solvent	Methanol
Mobil Permazone Antifreeze	Ethylene glycol
Mobil Windshield Washer Concentrate	Methanol
Monochem T-5 Toilet Chemical	Paraformaldehyde
Napa Auto Air Conditioner Recharge Kit	Freon
Napa Balkamp Form-A-Gasket Sealant	Isopropyl alcohol
Napa Balkamp Gasket Remover	Toluene
Napa Balkamp Liquid Solder	Toluene, methyl ethyl ketone
Napa Balkamp Liquid Steel	Toluene
Napa Chain and Cable Lube	"
Napa Concrete Cleaner	Caustic soda
Napa Contact Cement	Toluene, petroleum naphtha, acetone

Table continued on following page

Table 76–1. EXAMPLES OF COMMERCIAL PRODUCTS FOUND IN THE HOME OR GARAGE *Continued*

BRAND NAME	CHEMICAL TYPE
Napa Refrigerant 22	Monochlorodifluoromethane
Napa Spray Lube for Open Gears	Toluene
Old English Furniture Polish	Mineral seal oil
Ospho Metal Primer	Phosphoric acid
Pettit Marine Paint Old Salem Brushing Thinner	Petroleum distillate
Pine Power	Pine oil
Pinesol	Pine oil
Poco Marine Safety Clean	Hydrochloric acid
Quaker State Deluxe Motor Oil	Crude oil
Rustoleum Stops Rust	Petroleum naphtha
Scott's Liquid Gold	Petroleum distillate, trichloroethane
Shell Barbecue and Fireplace Lighter Fuel	Petroleum distillate
Shell Carburetor and Combustion Chamber Cleaner	Aromatic petroleum distillate
Shell Furniture Polish	Mineral spirits
Shell Lighter Fluid and Spot Remover	Petroleum naphtha
Shell Liquid Tire Chain	Methanol
Shell Parts Loosener	Petroleum naphtha
Shell Refrigerant	Freon 12
Shout Laundry Soil and Stain Remover	Petroleum naphtha
Siloo Enginkool	Sodium nitrite
Siloo Octane Treatment Gasoline Additive	Methanol, petroleum distillate
Siloo Trans Kleen Transmission Additive	Petroleum distillate, xylene
Southern Pine Denatured Alcohol	Ethyl alcohol
Southern Pine Paint Remover	Petroleum distillate
Southern Pine Pure Turpentine	Turpentine
STP Gas treatment	Mineral spirits, xylene
3-In-1 Household Oil	Petroleum distillate
Valvoline Outboard Extreme Pressure Gear Oil	"
Valvoline Special Moly EP Grease (Ashland)	Petroleum distillate. Soap base: lithium 12-hydroxystearate, molybdenum disulfide
WD-40	Petroleum distillate

involve ingestion of only small volumes of distillates.[15]

Aspiration of a petroleum distillate results in chemical pneumonitis. Bronchospasm, hyperemia, edema, and atelectasis are noted.[16] Diffuse hemorrhagic alveolitis with granulocytic infiltrates occurs soon after aspiration and peaks at about 3 days.[16] Frank necrosis of bronchial, bronchiolar, and alveolar tissues can occur, along with vascular thrombosis and micro abscess formation.[12] A late proliferative process with alveolar thickening may occur later and peaks at about 10 days.[16] Late complications may include bacterial pneumonia,[12] residual small airway abnormalities,[17, 18] and pneumatoceles.[19] An alteration of surfactant may result in a lung picture resembling hyaline membrane disease. Giammona[20] felt that petroleum distillates cause changes in surface tension leading to instability and collapse of unstable alveoli with resulting atelectasis, edema, and early distal airway closure. This produces ventilation/perfusion abnormalities resulting in hypoxia. Giammona theorizes that the initial pulmonary injury may be caused by the interaction of the petroleum distillate with surfactant instead of by direct parenchymal destruction.[20]

Upper airway pathology may occur with or without aspiration and includes hyperemia, mucosal irritation, and inflammation of the oropharynx.[7, 8] At least one case of epiglottitis has been reported following gasoline ingestion.[21]

Central nervous system effects of petroleum distillates are probably caused by hypoxia secondary to pulmonary injury.[22] In rats fed moderate-to-large volumes of petroleum distillates, no brain pathology was noted.[23]

Although petroleum distillates are poorly absorbed from the gastrointestinal tract, some systemic absorption does occur.[12] The gastrointestinal pathology of petroleum distillate ingestion is generally mild and self limited. Mucosal inflammation and superficial ulceration is common,[12] and although fatty infiltration of the liver may occur, frank necrosis is uncommon.[13]

Petroleum distillate ingestion may cause myocarditis and mild degenerative changes of myofibrils.[24] At least one case of petroleum distillate ingestion resulted in electrocardiographic and vectorcardiographic evidence of myocardial infarction.[25] Petroleum distillates are said to sensitize the myocardium to catecholamines.[7, 8]

Petroleum distillates have also been reported to cause intravascular hemolysis and renal damage, which usually consists of mild degenerative changes of the renal tubules but may rarely result in acute tubular necrosis.[12] At least one case report has associated turpentine ingestion with hemorrhagic cystitis.[26]

CLINICAL PRESENTATION AND COURSE

The clinical presentation of petroleum distillate ingestion does not vary significantly according to the particular petroleum distillate ingested. Nevertheless, a wide range of presentations occurs, from the asymptomatic patient to the patient with significant pulmonary or neurologic manifestations. The vast majority of children are asymptomatic at the time of presentation.[27, 28] Presenting symptoms and signs, however, are usually related to three main organ systems: pulmonary, central nervous, and gastrointestinal. Older children may complain of a burning sensation in their mouths or an unpleasant taste, but gastrointestinal presentation primarily consists of vomiting, and therein lies the danger for aspiration into the lungs. The vomitus has a characteristic odor, except when the ingestion took place some time before or if previous vomiting has cleared the stomach. Diarrhea may occur, and it may be blood-tinged or have a hydrocarbon odor.[13] Perianal excoriation can occur, especially with mineral seal oil. Nausea, belching, and abdominal pain are other common gastrointestinal symptoms. However, gastrointestinal system presentation alone is not a significant problem to the patient.

Complaints relating to pulmonary involvement include coughing paroxysms, choking, or gagging, and these are indicative of a high likelihood of aspiration.[5] Symptoms of central nervous system involvement include light-headedness, headache, visual changes, impaired memory, or unusual behavior.

Physical exam may reveal fever, tachypnea, and tachycardia. Stridor may be present and is an indication to consider upper respiratory obstruction as an immediate concern.[21] The patient may have transient cyanosis as a result of the displacement of alveolar gas by the ingested hydrocarbon.[29] Dyspnea, tachypnea, tachycardia, intercostal retractions, and nasal flaring are often noted within 30 minutes of aspiration,[12] but may not manifest for up to 2 days.[5] Auscultation may reveal rales, wheezes, or coarse or decreased breath sounds, especially in the lower lobes. Normal auscultation, however, does not exclude lower airway involvement.[29]

The usual clinical course is progression during the first 24 hours after aspiration, reaching a plateau and then subsiding between the second and fifth days. With severe injury, pulmonary edema and hemoptysis may occur. Barring complications, the usual hospitalization is 3 to 5 days.

Abnormalities on chest x-ray films may be seen within 30 minutes of aspiration and may occur even with an absence of auscultatory findings. A large percentage of patients with lung involvement show x-ray findings of chemical pneumonitis within 12 hours, but in many patients the first x-ray study will be deceptively clear. Fine, punctate, mottled densities in the perihilar areas may be seen; basal pneumonitis, atelectasis, or both, also may be present. Obstructive emphysema (air-trapping), usually peripheral, is often present, and pleural effusions, pneumatoceles, pneumothorax, pneumomediastinum, pneumopericardium, and subcutaneous emphysema may develop.[19, 29–31]

Lung involvement is often bilateral, reaches its maximum at 72 hours, and usually clears within a few additional days. Occasionally, the radiologic changes shown on x-ray films may persist for several weeks or months. Respiratory signs and symptoms usually disappear before the x-ray picture improves.[29, 31] Treat the patient and not the roentgenogram! If the initial chest x-ray film is normal but the patient is in obvious respiratory distress, hospitalize the patient. Similarly, do not wait for the x-ray film of an admitted patient to improve before discharging that patient; instead, use clinical judgment. In one series, a double gastric fluid level was noted on the upright chest x-ray film in 22 of 52 cases of kerosene ingestion; experiments showed that 5 mL was the minimal amount of kerosene needed to produce this sign. The investigators in this series, Daffner and Jimenez, advocate giving the patient a glass of water prior to the x-ray study to help demonstrate the double fluid level by providing the aqueous layer.[32]

Not enough studies exist for definitive comment on long-term sequelae. In one study, 13 patients ingesting kerosene were followed over a 6-month to 4-year period. None had evidence of persistent injury as shown by physical examination or chest x-ray film. Not all these patients, however, had evidence of pulmonary injury at the time of ingestion.[33] Foley et al. followed 30 of 101 patients who had ingested kerosene. Only one had an abnormal chest roentgenogram suggestive of bronchiectasis. Over half the group of 30 gave histories of repeated respiratory tract infections of long duration. Several had a persistent cough, and three had a subsequent episode of pneumonia.[31]

The indications for a chest roentgenogram and other laboratory testing is a frequently discussed issue. Patients who are symptomatic (coughing, short of breath, etc.) should all have a baseline chest roentgenograms. Additionally, if there are any signs of respiratory distress, baseline arterial blood gas should be determined. Hospitalized patients may need further testing as clinically indicated. (e.g., complete blood count with differential, electrolytes, renal, and liver function tests; urinalysis and electrocardiogram).

Central nervous system symptoms can range from lethargy to coma to seizures. Although such symptoms are somewhat frightening, they rarely are a cause of death. The cardiovascular system may be involved, and arrhythmias may result. These may range from atrial fibrillation or flutter to ventricular fibrillation. There have been several case reports of sudden death in young healthy people after siphoning gasoline.[34] As reported, they siphoned gasoline, ran from the automobile, and then died. Autopsies showed no pathology. It has been postulated that these people perhaps aspirated some of the gasoline into the lungs, resulting in some absorption of gasoline that sensitized the myocardium to arrhythmias. It has been further postulated that some of the gasoline vapors replaced the oxygen in the alveoli, resulting in hypoxia followed by ventricular fibrillation and sudden death.

Although an isolated event, acute renal failure after the use of diesel fuel as shampoo has been reported.[35] Renal failure is also a complication of turpentine and pine oil product ingestions. Also, hemoglobinuria with a fall in hemoglobin secondary to intravascular hemolysis has been seen in one case after ingestion of gasoline.[36] Hepatosplenomegaly has occasionally been observed but generally has not resulted in any major clinical problem. Also, the skin can sustain severe burns after prolonged immersion in gasoline, with fatal results.[37]

Caregivers should not use smell to determine whether to treat a patient. A child may smell strongly of gasoline, but actually have all the petroleum distillate on clothing and have ingested none. Similarly, the breath may reek of volatile liquid but should not be relied on as a certain sign of danger, since only a small amount may have been swallowed without aspiration occurring.

Finally, the clinical presentation will often be described to the physician or poison control center over the phone. If the caller states that someone has ingested a petroleum distillate and is coughing or otherwise symptomatic, the person definitely should be evaluated by a physician in the emergency department or office. For an asymptomatic patient in a stable, responsible, and known home environment, observation at home with instructions to check with the doctor in 4 to 6 hours or to bring the person in if symptoms develop may be appropriate advice. More conservative advice would be to have every person with petroleum distillate ingestion evaluated by a physician.

TREATMENT

Much controversy surrounds different aspects of treatment: the induction of vomiting, nasogastric lavage, administration of oils to thicken the petroleum distillate, administration of prophylactic steroids, and the use of antibiotics. The morbidity and mortality related to petroleum distillate poisoning are primarily from pulmonary complications. For example, it is well documented and not in dispute that aspiration is the cause of pneumonia. The risk of aspiration and lung damage involving any particular petroleum distillate increases with low surface tension, low viscosity, and high volatility. Mineral seal oil with its low viscosity and high volatility is more likely to cause a serious aspiration pneumonia than are diesel oils, petroleum jelly, and other petroleum distillates that are highly viscous and thus pose almost to risk of aspiration.

Clinical and x-ray evidence as well as Giammona's studies of altered surface tensions suggest that collapsing alveoli and distal airways may be a major part of the respiratory problem.[20] Therefore, positive end-expiratory pressure (PEEP) can be an important therapeutic adjunct. However, care must be taken to observe for pneumothorax, since patients with hydrocarbon pneumonitis are prone to develop pneumatoceles and pneumothorax.

When a patient is coughing, is in some respiratory distress, and is wheezing, the physician may consider using epinephrine to correct bronchospasm. However, this is contraindicated. Because petroleum distillates may sensitize the myocardium and aspiration pneumonia can produce hypoxia, the patient is susceptible to arrhythmias. Under these circumstances, epinephrine could precipitate lethal arrhythmias. If a bronchodilating drug must be used, then a beta$_2$-stimulant drug such as terbutaline should be considered.

Induction of Vomiting

The first controversial area is evacuation of the stomach. The question of whether to induce vomiting and clear the stomach is actually the question of whether significant pulmonary pathology can result from gastrointestinal absorption. Also, can central nervous system problems be caused by gastrointestinal absorption? If it can be shown that petroleum distillates in the gastrointestinal tract do not cause serious pulmonary or CNS pathology, then the patient should not be made to vomit. Bratton and Haddow showed that if massive doses of petroleum distillates are placed in the gastrointestinal tract of laboratory animals, no pulmonary pathology results.[9] Petroleum distillates are very poorly absorbed from the gastrointestinal tract; even if they were absorbed, they would be filtered out by the first capillary or sinusoidal bed they reach (i.e., the liver), thus protecting the lungs. This was shown by injecting massive doses of naphtha into the portal veins of laboratory animals, with no resulting damage to the lungs. However, this study documented that small amounts of petroleum distillate injected directly into the trachea caused the chemical pneumonitis typical of petroleum distillate poisoning. It also showed that intravenously administered petroleum distillate caused an almost immediate pneumonitis, as had been reported clinically in a drug abuser.[6] In another study by Foley et al., the esophagi of rabbits were exposed and ligated under anesthesia.[31] Through an esophageal incision distal to the ligature, a tube was introduced, and kerosene was slowly instilled into the stomach in quantities varying between 25 and 50 mL/kg. As the tube was withdrawn, the esophagus was ligated distal to the incision. The lungs were normal when the animals were sacrificed. When small amounts of kerosene were injected into the endotracheal tube, severe pneumonitis ensued.[31] Other investigators have reproduced these results.[11, 38, 39]

Wolfsdorf went a step further.[22] He looked specifically at the effects of kerosene on the central nervous system and showed that this petroleum distillate had very little direct effect on it. It has been postulated that the central nervous system effects that are sometimes seen (such as somnolence and, occasionally, seizure activity) are from hypoxia secondary to pulmonary involvement. The implications here are that therapy of petroleum distillate poisoning should be directed toward the prevention of vomiting, aspiration, and hypoxia. Arena has supported this traditional view of noninduction of emesis.[40]

However, another point of view, the concept of selected emesis, has also been supported.[41] Because petroleum distillates vary widely, they are divided into three groups depending on their viscosity. Group one is composed of thick, viscous petroleum distillates. They need no specific therapy because of their lack of absorption and low potential for spreading. These agents are generally considered nontoxic, although they may cause a low-grade lipoid pneumonia instead of severe, progressive chemical pneumonitis. Examples are asphalt, tar, lubricants, heavy greases, mineral oil, baby oil, suntan oil, and diesel oil. Group two has a medium-range viscosity and includes most of the petroleum distillates seen in poisonings, such as gasoline, kerosene, turpentine, and naphthas. Theoretically, the risk of aspiration is not very great in this category, and if a large amount is ingested (1 mL/kg) the patient should be made to vomit. Rumack has also postulated that if a poison is going to be aspirated, it is more likely to occur when ingesting the poison rather than after or during induced emesis. Group three petroleum distillates have a very low viscosity. They spread very easily over a large surface area and can cause a serious aspiration pneumonia. The classic example is mineral seal oil, found in furniture polishes. No emesis is recommended, because the risk of aspiration is too high as a result of the low viscosity of the agent.

After review of the scientific experimental evidence, no advantage appears in separating these petroleum distillates into three categories and selectively inducing vomiting; an element of unnecessary risk taking is possible. Even if one agrees with the division into three groups, very seldom is it known exactly how much the patient has ingested. Vomiting should not be induced because there appears to be no pulmonary damage from gastrointestinal absorption and no significant central nervous system toxicity. All the scientific evidence supports the traditional view of noninduction of emesis in petroleum distillate poisoning. It must be pointed out, however, that petroleum distillates that also contain heavy metals, pesticides, or other toxic additives (which are potentially far more toxic than the petroleum distillate ingested) should be eliminated from the gastrointestinal tract in accordance with standard practice for the specific agent involved.

Nasogastric Lavage

The second controversy concerns nasogastric lavage. Cautious gastric lavage was previously advocated by some, but this is no longer the case. First, there is no such thing as "cautious gastric lavage" in an awake, screaming child. Also, one study showed the complication rate of pneumonitis to be twice as high for the nasogastric lavage–treated group of children as for the ipecac-treated group.[42] It is thought that the nasogastric tube may allow the petroleum distillate to come up from the stomach through the open esophagogastric junction and then be aspirated. Gastric lavage should never be considered in such a patient. Some clinicians advocate lavage after an endotracheal tube has been inserted in comatose patients.[41]

Administration of Oils

The third area of controversy concerns the use of olive or mineral oil to increase viscosity, thereby decreasing the chance of aspiration if vomiting occurs after the initial ingestion. Such oil also acts as a cathartic to hasten the petroleum distillate from the gastrointestinal tract. However, if aspirated, the oil can cause lipoid pneumonia. A 6-year retrospective study showed an increased incidence of pneumonia in children who were given oils;[15] therefore the use of oils should be avoided.

Administration of Steroids and Antibiotics

Antibiotics should not be used for routine prophylaxis. Their use should be guided by clinical judgment, taking pre-existing underlying disease into account. This is often difficult, since fever and leukocytosis are to be expected in the initial chemical, nonbacterial pneumonitis. Gram stains of sputum should be watched closely. The routine use of steroids and antibiotics for kerosene-induced aspiration pneumonia has been evaluated.[43] Steroids were found to be undesirable, as there was a very significant increase in positive lung cultures with daily steroid administration; an even higher incidence of positive cultures was found when steroids and antibiotics both were used. While steroids are not routinely indicated, they are employed in the management of "shock lung," should this develop as a complication.

Summary of Therapy

For treatment of petroleum distillate ingestion, utilize the usual supportive measures for any type of poisoning or acute illness. Do *not* induce vomiting unless an insecticide or other more toxic poison is ingested along with the petroleum distillate. Do *not* use nasogastric lavage (unless preceded by endotracheal intubation in the unresponsive, comatose patient). Do *not* use mineral oil or olive oil to thicken hydrocarbons. The use of activated charcoal is indicated, especially with pine oil product ingestions. Magnesium or sodium sulfate or citrate may be used as a cathartic. Avoid epinephrine if possible.

Use antibiotics or steroids only if there is a specific indication. As aspiration is always a possibility, a baseline chest x-ray film and arterial blood gas levels should be obtained on all hospitalized patients, coupled with appropriate observation. With turpentine or pine oil ingestions, serial measurements of serum BUN and creatinine and repeated urinalyses are indicated. In the event of renal failure, assessment and management as outlined in Chapters 8 and 9 may be appropriate.

With all these rules, clinical judgment still is needed for the many variations that may occur. For example, what should be done with a child who was initially coughing but is now asymptomatic, has a negative chest x-ray film and normal blood gas levels, and has been observed in the emergency department for 4 to 6 hours without change? This child could be sent home with instructions for follow-up with the pediatrician or to return if symptomatic. If the parents' reliability is questionable, it might be better to hospitalize the child.

Based on these recommendations, the management of petroleum distillate, turpentine, and pine oil ingestions consists of diagnosing any complications, such as aspiration pneumonia or renal failure, and providing appropriate supportive care.

References

1. Press E, Adams WC, Chittenden RF, et al: Cooperative kerosene poisoning study; Evaluation of gastric lavage and other factors in the treatment of accidental ingestion of petroleum distillate products. Pediatrics *29*:648, 1962.
2. Gehlbach SH, Wall JB: Childhood poisoning; A community hospital experience. South Med J *70*:674, 1977.
3. Litovitz TL, Schmitz BF, Matyunas N, et al: 1987 annual report of the American association of poison control centers national data collection system. Am J Emerg Med *6*:479, 1988.
4. Litovitz TL, Martin TG, Schmitz B: 1986 annual report of the American association of poison control centers national data collection system. Am J Emerg Med *5*:405, 1987.
5. Truemper E, Reyes De La Rocha S, Atkinson SK: Clinical characteristics, pathophysiology, and management of hydrocarbon ingestion; Case report and review of the literature. Ped Emerg Care *3*:187, 1987.
6. Neeld EM, Limacher MC: Chemical pneumonitis after the intravenous injection of a hydrocarbon. Radiology *129*:36, 1978.
7. Arena JM: Hydrocarbon poisoning—current management. Pediatric Annals *16*:879, 1987.
8. Tinker TD: Hydrocarbon ingestion in children; Its sequelae and management. J Okla State Med Assoc *79*:95, 1986.
9. Bratton L, Haddow JE: Ingestion of charcoal lighter fluid. J Pediatr *87*:633, 1975.
10. Dice WH, Ward G, Kelly J, et al: Pulmonary toxicity following gastrointestinal ingestion of kerosene. Ann Emerg Med *11*:138, 1982.
11. Wolfe BM, Brodeur AE, Shields JB: The role of gastrointestinal absorption of kerosene in producing pneumonitis in dogs. J Pediatr *76*:867, 1970.
12. Klein BL, Simon JE: Hydrocarbon poisonings. Pediatr Clin N Am *33*:411, 1986.
13. Haddad, LM: Petroleum distillates. *In*: A Study Guide in Emergency Medicine. Dallas, TX, 1980, American College of Emergency Physicians, pp 4–53.
14. Kulig K, Rumack B: Hydrocarbon ingestion. Curr Top Emerg Med *3*:1, 1981.
15. Beamon RF, Siegel CJ, Landers G, et al: Hydrocarbon ingestion in children; A six year retrospective study. JACEP *5*:771, 1976.
16. Gross P, McNerney JM, Babyak MA: Kerosene pneumonitis; An experimental study with small doses. Am Rev Resp Dis *88*:656, 1963.
17. Gurwitz D, Kattan M, Levison H, et al: Pulmonary function abnormalities in asymptomatic children after hydrocarbon pneumonitis. Pediatrics *62*:789, 1978.
18. Tal A, Aviram M, Bar-Ziv J, et al: Residual small airways lesions after kerosene pneumonitis in early childhood. Eur J Pediatr *142*:117, 1984.
19. Bergeson PS, Hales SW, Lustgarten MD, et al: Pneumatoceles following hydrocarbon ingestion. Am J Dis Child *129*:49, 1975.
20. Giammona ST: Effects of furniture polish on pulmonary surfactant. Am J Dis Child *113*:658, 1967.
21. Grufferman S, Walker FW: Supraglottitis following gasoline ingestion. Ann Emerg Med *11*:368, 1982.
22. Wolfsdorf J: Kerosene intoxication: An experimental approach to the etiology of the CNS manifestation in primates. J Pediatr *88*:1037, 1976.
23. Ashkenazi AE, Berman SE: Experimental kerosene poisoning in rats. Pediatrics *28*:642, 1961.
24. Deichmann WB, Kitzmiller KV, Witherup S, et al: Kerosene intoxication. Ann Intern Med *21*:803, 1944.
25. James FW, Kaplan S, Benzing G: Cardiac complications following hydrocarbon ingestion. Am J Dis Child *121*:431, 1971.
26. Klein FA, Hackler RH: Hemorrhagic cystitis associated with turpentine ingestion. Urology *16*:187, 1980.
27. Anas N, Namasonthi V, Ginsburg CM: Criteria for hospitalizing children who have ingested products containing hydrocarbons. JAMA *246*:840, 1981.
28. White LE, Driggers DA, Wardinsky TD: Poisoning in childhood and adolescence; A study of 111 cases admitted to a military hospital. J Fam Pract *11*:27, 1980.
29. Eade NR, Taussig LM, Marks MI: Hydrocarbon pneumonitis. Pediatrics *54*:351, 1974.
30. Brunner S, Rovsing H, Wulf H: Roentgenographic changes in the lungs of children with kerosene poisoning. Am Rev Resp Dis *89*:250, 1964.
31. Foley JC, Dreyer NB, Soule AB, et al: Kerosene poisoning in young children. Radiology *62*:817, 1954.
32. Daffner RH, Jimenex JP: The double gastric fluid level in kerosene poisoning. Pediatr Radiol *106*:383, 1973.

33. Reed ES, Leikin S, Kerman HD: Kerosene intoxication. Am J Dis Child *79*:623, 1950.
34. Bass M: Death from sniffing gasoline. (Letter). N Engl J Med *299*:203, 1978.
35. Barrientos A, Ortuno MT, Morales JM, et al: Acute renal failure after use of diesel fuel as shampoo. Arch Intern Med *137*:1217, 1977.
36. Stockman JA: More on hydrocarbon—induced hemolysis. (Letter) J Pediatr *90*:848, 1977.
37. Walsh WA, Scarpa FJ, Brown RS, et al: Gasoline immersion burn case report. N Engl J Med *291*:830, 1974.
38. Waring JI: Pneumonia in kerosene poisoning. Am J Med Sci *185*:325, 1933.
39. Lesser LI, Weens HS, McKey JD: Pulmonary manifestations following ingestion of kerosene. J Pediatr *23*:352, 1943.
40. Arena JM: Poisoning; Toxicology, Symptoms, Treatment. 2nd ed. Springfield, IL, Charles C Thomas, 1970.
41. Rumack H (ed): Poisindex; Hydrocarbons. Denver, Micromedex, 1982.
42. Ng RC, Darwish H, Steward DA: Emergency treatment of petroleum distillate and turpentine ingestion. Can Med Assoc J *111*:537, 1974.
43. Brown J, Burke B, Danjani AS: Experimental kerosene pneumonia; Evaluation of some therapeutic regimens. J Pediatr *84*:396, 1974.

CHAPTER 77

INDUSTRIAL TOXICOLOGY: General Concepts and The Microcomputer Industry

A. General Concepts

Jeffrey Jones, M.D.
M. Jo McMullen, M.D., FACEP

A hazardous material is any substance that poses any threat to human life or health, either in itself or in accidents such as a fire or explosion. A hazardous material is considered hazardous if it is explosive, flammable, combustible, an oxidizer, poisonous (toxic), corrosive, or radioactive. The most commonly shipped hazardous materials are gasoline, anhydrous ammonia, propane, LPG (liquefied petroleum gas), chlorine, and sulfuric acid.

More than 5 million different chemical substances are known. Chemical companies produce commercially and ship about 35,000 different dangerous chemicals to which industrial workers and others may be exposed. Toxicity data are not available for more than 80 per cent of these agents. It is important to know the general management of certain classes of chemicals and of a few more common, specific compounds. It is equally important to know the sources of information that are routinely available, how to gain access to that information, and what level of help can be expected in an emergency. Incidents of hazardous material spills reported to the US Department of Transportation between 1971 and 1980 numbered 111,293, with 248 deaths and 6873 injuries.[1]

In the seventeenth century, Bernadino Ramazzini, often called the "father of industrial medicine," implored physicians of Italy to ask patients not only about their symptoms but also to go carefully into the nature of their work.[2] Today, few occupations do not involve some contact with a metal, gas, solvent, or unusual chemical that has the potential to poison, irritate, or sensitize.[3] It has been estimated that in the United States 100,000 persons die each year from industrially related disease, and there are about 400,000 new cases of occupational diseases per year.[4] These numbers may be significant underestimates because of inadequate data collection systems and problems with recognition and diagnosis of occupational disease. Table 77–1 lists some of these problems. See Table 77–2 for a useful list of terms and Table 77–3 for abbreviations used in industrial toxicology.

Recognition of industrial poisoning is simplified when the acutely ill person is transported directly from the workplace where an unprotected exposure to a known toxic substance has occurred. However, if there is a latent period between exposure and clinical illness, if potential toxins are multiple or unknown, or if the resultant illness mimics common diseases, recognition and appropriate management of acute industrial poisoning may be delayed.[4–6] Moreover, physicians are often inadequately prepared to diagnose or treat diseases caused by industrial toxins. Formal training in medical schools and postgraduate programs in occupational health issues are minimal.[7]

The diagnosis of industrial poisoning is important, not only for the care of the patient but also because accurate diagnosis makes it possible to identify potential workplace hazards and health risks to the community. Efficient diagnosis and treatment are facilitated when emergency department personnel maintain a high index of suspicion for the possibility of industrial poisoning, familiarize themselves with the industrial processes and toxic substances used locally, maintain an adequate reference library, and obtain occupational histories from their patients.[6]

Table 77–1. OBSTACLES TO THE DIAGNOSIS OF INDUSTRIAL POISONING[4, 5]

1. Most occupational illnesses are clinically and pathologically indistinguishable from common medical disorders.
2. Toxicologic data are not currently available on more than 80% of hazardous chemicals used in industry.
3. For many industrial toxins, there is a latent period (hours to days) between the toxic exposure and the onset of symptoms.
4. Nonoccupational factors (i.e., smoking) may act synergistically with occupational exposure to cause disease.
5. Many toxins occur in mixtures or may be contaminants of other products.
6. Privacy about proprietary formulations and fear of litigation limit the free flow of chemical information from employers and manufacturers.
7. Physicians often are inadequately prepared to diagnose or treat a disease caused by an industrial toxin.

Table 77–2. TERMINOLOGY IN INDUSTRIAL TOXICOLOGY

Absorption: the taking in of any material by direct contact with the skin.
Acid: a chemical compound of electronegative elements or groups plus one or more ionizable hydrogen(s) (H^+). These are very active chemically.
Alkali: a chemical compound that reacts to form the hydroxyl ion (OH^-). Also known as a base, very active chemically.
Asphyxiant: any chemical substance that can cause hypoxia, and potentially death, by displacing the air in a given environment.
Combustible: capable of burning; a substance with a flash point equal to or above 37.8° C (100° F). Combustion (burning) is an exothermic chemical reaction caused by light or heat with a rapid oxidation of fuel, accompanied by flames.
Corrosive: liquid or solid material that causes visible destruction or irreversible alterations in any living tissue (e.g., human skin tissue) by its chemical action. In the case of leakage from its packaging, a liquid that has a severe corrosive rate on steel.
Explosimeter: a mechanical device to check for dangerous concentrations of gases.
Explosive: any material capable of burning or detonating suddenly and violently.
Flammable: capable of burning with a flash point below 37.8° C (100° F).
Flash point: the minimum temperature of a liquid or solid at which it gives off enough vapors to form an ignitable mixture with the air.
Fumes: particulate matter floating in air, an aerosol of solid particles generated by condensation from the gaseous state.
Gas: a state of matter which is a fluid with a vapor pressure under 40 psi at 37.8° C (100° F).
Irritant: a substance that is not classified as a poison but may produce intensely irritating fumes.
Lower explosive limit (LEL): the minimum concentration of gas or vapor in air below which the mixture will not explode.
Oxidant (Oxidizer): a substance that contains oxygen and gives it up readily; will support combustion.
Poison: any substance that can cause injury, illness, or death to living tissues by chemical means. This is synonymous with toxin or toxic material.
Reactive: capable of reacting or tending to react chemically with other substances.
Vapor: a substance that is liquid under ordinary conditions at 25°C.
Vapor pressure: the gas pressure exerted on the sides of a closed container by the collision of molecules.
Water-reactive: the reaction of a substance as it comes into contact with water or humid air such that it produces hazardous vapors or releases energy.

The history of work experience may provide critical information that relates the patient's symptoms and signs to exposure to a specific job hazard. Thus, Ramazzini's advice concerning the occupational history is just as relevant if not more so today than it was in the seventeenth century.

Table 77–3. ABBREVIATIONS IN INDUSTRIAL TOXICOLOGY

LC_{50}: lethal concentration; 50% of test animals (and potentially humans) exposed to this concentration of a gas, vapor, dust, or fume in air will be killed.
LCL_0: lowest published lethal concentration.
LD 100: The dosage of an active ingredient taken by mouth that is expected to cause death.
LD_{50}: lethal dose resulting in 50% kill. This represents an experimentally derived value. This is obtained by a statistical estimate of the dosage necessary to kill 50% of an infinite population of animals. Usually expressed as weight of a substance in mg/kg of body weight.
LDL_0: lowest published toxic dose.
mg/m^3: used to measure fumes, mists, or dusts. Standards defined by the Occupational Safety and Health Act of 1970.
PPM: parts per million. This measures the parts of a gas or vapor per million parts of air. Used in environmental research more than in human studies.
TCL_0: lowest published toxic concentration of an active substance taken by mouth or absorbed by the skin that is expected to cause death in 50% of the test animals. This is reported in mg/kg of body weight.
TDL_0: lowest published toxic dose.
TLV: threshold limit value. Formerly known as the maximum allowable concentration (MAC). This term refers to airborne concentrations and represents conditions under which nearly all workers may be repeatedly exposed for 8 hours a day, 5 days a week, without harmful effects. Defined under the Toxic Substances Control Act of 1977.

CLASSIFICATION OF HAZARDOUS MATERIALS

The US Department of Transportation requires all shipping papers to have classification as well as ID numbers.[8] This classification and numbering system is used by many other regulatory agencies and authorities to identify potentially hazardous substances[9] (Table 77–4).

The National Fire Protection Association (NFPA) Committee on Fire Hazards of Materials developed a Hazard Signal System: NFPA–704 (Fig. 77–1).[10] This includes a numerical rating scale to identify the degree of hazard in the categories of health, fire, and reactivity (Table 77–5). This system is frequently used as a labeling system by chemical manufacturers, although not required by law for chemicals in transit across state lines.

Health hazard refers specifically to the capacity of a material to cause personnel injury from contact with or absorption into the body

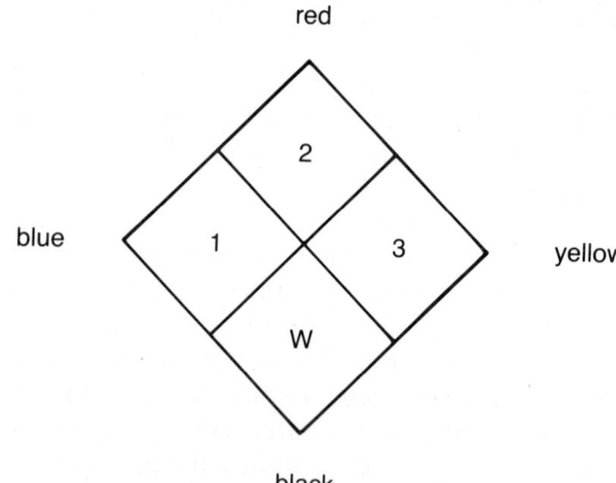

Figure 77–1. Symbol of the National Fire Protection 704 Hazard Signal System. See Table 77–5 for explanation.

of a chemical. In fire fighting or other emergency conditions, health hazard refers to a single exposure, which may vary from a few seconds to an hour. It is not applicable to the situation of an industrial worker being exposed on a routine basis. Table 77–5 of the NFPA-704 system shows the five ratings of

Table 77–4. LABELING AND CLASSIFICATION SYSTEMS[1, 8]

US DEPARTMENT OF TRANSPORTATION
1. class A explosives
2. class B explosives
3. blasting agent
4. poison A
5. flammable gas
6. nonflammable gas
7. nonflammable gas (chlorine)
8. nonflammable gas (oxygen, pressurized liquid)
9. flammable liquid
10. combustible liquid
11. flammable solid
12. flammable solid (dangerous when wet)
13. oxidizer
14. organic peroxide
15. poison B (nonflammable gas—fluorine)
16. radioactive material
17. corrosive material
18. irritating material

UNITED NATIONS CLASSIFICATION NUMBERS
1. explosives
2. gases
3. flammable and combustible liquids
4. flammable solids, spontaneous combustion substances
5. oxidizers and organic peroxides
6. poisonous materials
7. radioactive materials
8. corrosives
9. miscellaneous hazardous materials

Table 77–5. NFPA HAZARD SIGNAL SYSTEM "704"

FLAMMABLE (RED)
- 4—extremely flammable
- 3—ignites at normal temperatures below 37.8° C (100° F)
- 2—ignites at temperatures below 93.3° C (200° F)
- 1—must be preheated to burn
- 0—will not burn

HEALTH HAZARD (BLUE)
- 4—too dangerous to enter vapor or liquid
- 3—extreme danger
- 2—hazardous
- 1—slightly hazardous
- 0—normal material

REACTIVITY (YELLOW)
- 4—may detonate
- 3—shock and heat may detonate
- 2—violent chemical change
- 1—unstable if heated
- 0—stable

SPECIFIC HAZARD (BLACK)
- OXY—oxidizer
- ACID—acid
- ALK—alkali
- COR—corrosive
- -W- —use no water
- 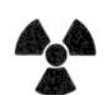 —radiation hazard

the degree of hazard of a specific chemical, as follows:

0—Materials which on exposure under fire conditions would offer no hazard beyond that of ordinary combustible materials.

1—Materials which on exposure would cause irritation but only minor residual injury even if no treatment is given.

2—Materials which on intense or continued exposure could cause temporary incapacitation or possible residual injury unless prompt medical treatment were given.

3—Materials which on short exposure could cause serious temporary or residual injury even though prompt medical treatment were given.

4—Materials which on very short exposure could cause death or major residual injury even though prompt medical treatment were given.

The US Department of Labor (DOL) requires a *Material Safety Data Sheet (MSDS)* for hazardous materials with which shipbuilders work. These data sheets contain detailed information about specific chemicals and their toxicity. Because of their standard format and availability, these sheets have become required by many fire department HAZMAT (Hazardous Material) units and in Right to Know ordinances. A booklet defining the terminology used and giving an example of an MSDS is available from the US DOL Occupational Safety and Health Administration: OSHA publication 2265, 1977.[11]

OCCUPATIONAL HISTORY

The complete occupational history is too cumbersome and time-consuming for use as a screening instrument in all emergency evaluations or office visits. Goldman and Peters[5] developed a systematic approach (Fig. 77–2) for evaluating hazardous exposures. The algorithm begins with a quick survey that can be performed routinely on all patients. The clinician may then proceed to a more detailed line of questioning to follow up any indications of toxic exposure.

Routine Survey. This first step includes three essential questions easily incorporated into routine history taking: current and past job titles; known exposure to fumes, chemicals, dusts or radiation; and any temporal relationship of the chief complaint to work activities or other contributory factors. The work and exposure history acts as a broad screen to elicit potentially hazardous exposures at home or work. When conditions with short latency periods are under evaluation, such as occupational asthma, then the emphasis should be on the current job and exposures. For conditions of longer latency, such as asbestosis, the history must focus on jobs and exposures in the past. Allergic responses to agents may develop even after years of asymptomatic exposure.

A temporal relationship between the onset of symptoms and work or home activities can provide an important clue to recent sources of exposure. In general, symptoms that recede on the weekend or at vacation time and return at the start of the work week indicate some current job-related exposure.[5] For example, acute systemic solvent toxicity, which includes the symptoms of headache, gastrointestinal disturbance, and lightheadedness, will usually occur with a short time of exposure and lessen within hours following removal from exposure. The expression of toxic symptoms is also influenced by the use of medications, pre-existing medical disease, and exposure to other hazardous substances. In addition, some personal habits (e.g., use of tobacco or alcohol) represent significant environmental exposures that may interact with or add to occupational exposures (Table 77–6).

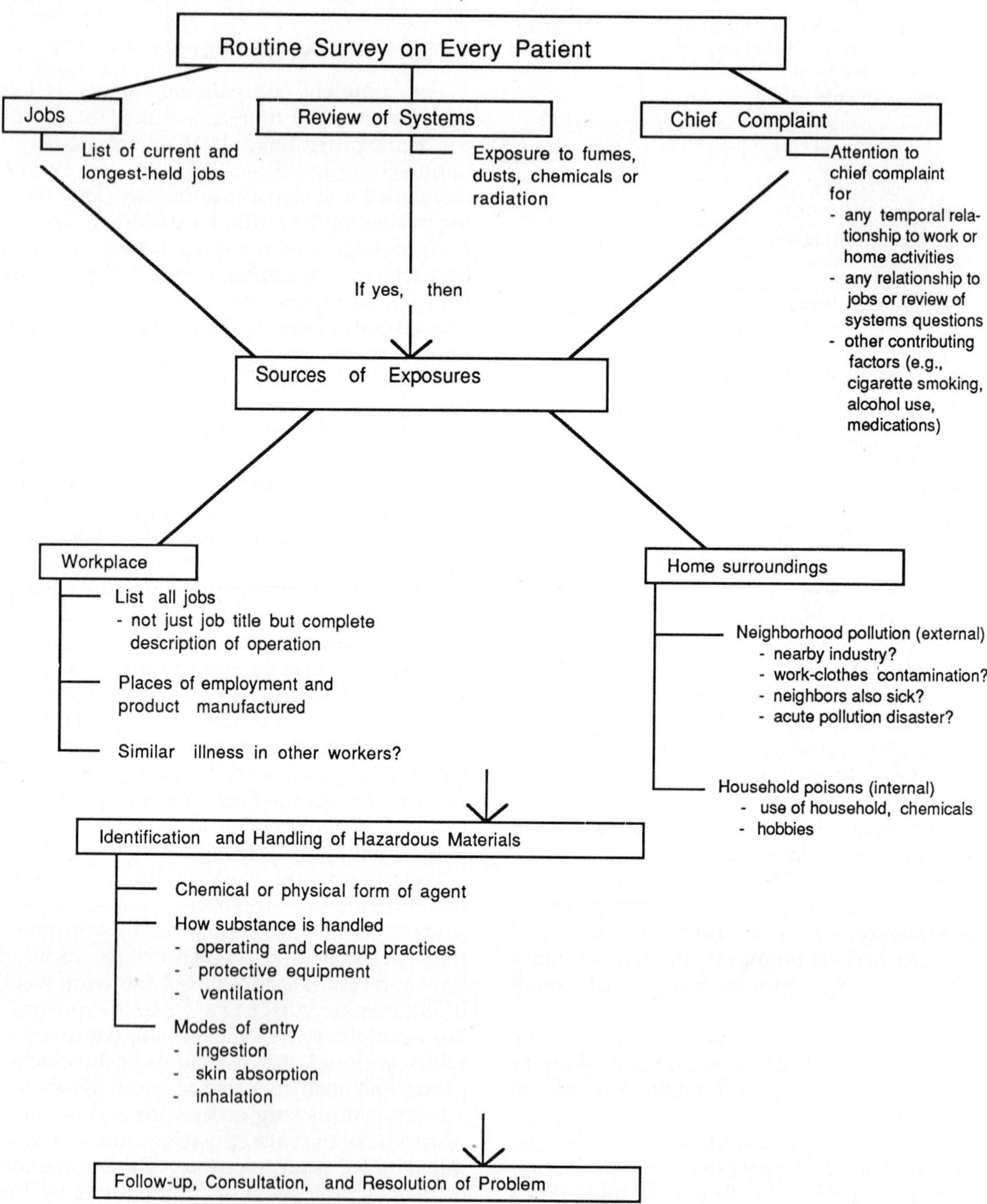

Figure 77–2. Systematic approach to history taking and diagnosis of occupational illness. (From Goldman RH, Peters JM: The occupational and environmental health history. JAMA *246*:2831–2836, 1981.)

Table 77–6. FACTORS THAT MODIFY RISK OF OCCUPATIONALLY RELATED ILLNESS

MODIFYING FACTOR	KNOWN OR PROBABLE EFFECT
General	
Age	Youth—latency for cancer; elderly—more susceptible to toxicity
Sex	Sex differences exist for some toxicity states; reproductive effects
Smoking status	
Current smoker	Confers additive risk in some situations
Smoker at time of exposure	Confers synergistic risk in some situations
Smoking during exposure	Modifies toxic exposure in some situations, such as polymer fume fever
Family history	Hereditary conditions or predispositions may be exacerbated or triggered, such as cancer-prone families
Exercise	
Conditioning	Fitness may reduce susceptibility in some situations
At time of exposure	Generally, increased susceptibility
Metabolic states	Activity of certain enzyme systems involved in activation, detoxification, and adaptation to toxic exposures may modify response although within range of normal
Medical	Generally, any debilitating condition may enhance clinical susceptibility
Atopy	
Asthma	Tendency toward easy sensitization
Eczema	Increased bronchial reactivity
Chronic respiratory disease	
Respiratory insufficiency	Diminished pulmonary reserve
Bronchitis	Increased bronchial reactivity; exacerbated bronchial irritation
Chronic cardiovascular disease	
Cardiac insufficiency	Increased susceptibility
Coronary artery disease	Angina in some situations, such as carbon monoxide, methylene chloride exposure
Infection	
Acute viral illness	Increased susceptibility to bronchial irritation; possibly synergistic effect
Exposure to infectious agents	Certain exposures may depress host defenses
Immune deficiency states	Increased susceptibility to infections
Hereditary	
Immunosuppressive therapy	
Renal disease	Additive or synergistic effects may occur with exposure to nephrotoxic agents
Renal insufficiency	Increased susceptibility to toxic agents excreted via renal route
Chronic renal disease	Immunodeficiency; increased susceptibility to toxic effects
Neurologic conditions	
Diminished mental capacity	May affect judgment and response to exposure situation
Neurologic disease	Toxic effects may be additive; increased clinical susceptibility
Seizure disorder	Certain toxic exposures may alter threshold
Impaired perceptive ability (visual or hearing impairment, anosmia)	Impaired ability to avoid hazard
Dermatologic conditions	Skin rashes may increase dermal absorption; may condition response
Substance abuse	Concomitant alcohol and drug abuse may have additive or synergistic effects in some situations
Hepatic insufficiency	Increased susceptibility to toxic agents detoxified by liver; increased susceptibility to hepatotoxic agent; reduced hepatic reserve
Systemic conditions	
Malnutrition (general)	Increased susceptibility to toxic effects
Vitamin deficiency (selective)	Diminished host defenses against toxic effects
Inborn errors of metabolism	Selective susceptibility (depending on abnormality)
Genetic diseases	Certain genetic diseases associated with increased susceptibility to mutagenic effects
Mental status	Stress may increase susceptibility to some toxic exposures. Stress, affective disorders, neuroses, or psychoses may mask, mimic, or subtly modify the clinical presentation

(From Occupational and Environmental Health Committee of The American Lung Association of San Diego and Imperial Counties: Taking the occupational history. Ann Intern Med *99*:641–651, 1983.)

Sources of Exposure. In assessing the likelihood of the work place as a source of toxic exposure, the physician should obtain a complete description of all jobs, including the products manufactured and the processes involved. Many workers will be well-informed about specific exposures at the work place, and the information they provide will be sufficient for documentation. Often, however, the exposure history will require further detective work to identify specific components of products and documentation of exposure levels.[4]

Patients should be asked whether fellow workers have similar complaints; the clustering of symptoms among employees may be the first clue to an occupational hazard.[4] The plant physician or manager can often provide the most useful information on working conditions and chemicals in use.

In addition to the occupational history, the physician needs to be aware of possible sources of home contamination. The patient should be asked about neighborhood environmental exposure, such as a nearby factory or chemical waste dump. An obvious source of external pollution is dust or chemicals carried into the home on work clothes. For example, children of employees at a lead storage battery facility showed excessive serum lead levels.[12] However, some of the most toxic industrial chemicals are readily available for home use: pesticides, solvents, cleaning fluids, or disinfectants. Dangerous situations may arise when two substances are mixed together in hope of producing a more potent compound (e.g., chloramine fumes produced from the mixture of ammonia and sodium hypochlorite).

The growth and diversification of hobbies have introduced a multitude of hazardous substances into the household. Artists and craftsmen often face daily exposure to toxic substances, including solvents in paints, inks, and thinners; lead, cadmium and other metals in pigments, pottery glazes, copper enamels, and silver solders; and dusts such as silica and asbestos in clays, talcs, and glazes.[13] Further compounding this problem is the inadequate labeling of many art materials. This brings the clinician to the next step in the algorithm—to identify and describe the use of the suspected agents.

Identification. To characterize the health effects of a chemical exposure, it is important to determine not only the generic ingredients of the compound involved but also its physical state and concentration. For example, at high temperatures the chlorinated hydrocarbon trichloroethylene, widely used as an industrial solvent, produces phosgene, which may cause pulmonary edema.[14] Prehospital medical care personnel or fire department HAZMAT team members may be helpful in locating chemical labels, manifest sheets, shipping papers, or knowledgeable personnel to identify the agent involved.

Besides the character of an exposure, history-taking should not neglect the quantity. As in pharmacology, the effect of any substance will be related to the amount that enters the body and how it is eliminated. Key elements of the quantitative exposure history include the nature and use of protective equipment and clothing, ventilation, duration of exposure, and the general level of cleanliness of the work setting.

The final factor in the assessment of industrial poisoning is the mode of entry into the body. Industrial toxins can harm exposed workers by inhalation, skin contact, and ingestion. The most common effects are the dermatoses, consisting mainly of irritant and allergic dermatitis. Inhalation exposures to toxic fumes, vapors, and gases pose the greatest danger because they have the potential to affect many people at the same time, with immediate compromise of the respiratory system. Toxic ingestion is infrequent; however, eating, drinking, or smoking in the work area may increase the body's exposure.

Follow-Up. Despite all best efforts, the clinician is often faced with an incomplete data base on which to begin treatment. If adequate information on the toxic agent is not available on site or from the manufacturer, the nearest poison control center should be contacted once the chemical or a chemical class has been identified. Poison control centers rely on a wide variety of information sources and specialty consultants to assess toxicity and advise treatment personnel.

PATHOPHYSIOLOGY

The pathologic effects that may occur with exposure to a specific hazardous substance include direct injury, sensitization, asphyxiation, systemic toxicity, carcinogenesis, mutagenesis, and teratogenesis. The latter three effects have long latency periods and are not considered in the category of toxicologic emergencies.

Irritant contact dermatitis is a direct injury to the skin, commonly associated with acids, alkalis (caustics), and certain metal compounds, as well as repeated exposures to detergents or solvents.[4] Strong corrosives may coagulate skin proteins or cause extensive tissue dehydration. The net effect is necrosis of the dermal cells, resulting in a vesicular (blistering) or ulcerative injury. Milder irritants, such as soaps and detergents, remove surface lipids and cause dryness and cracking of the skin. Generally, eyes are much more readily damaged by these actions, and ingesting the toxin can cause irritate mucosal surfaces on contact. Such damage leads to vomiting, diarrhea, intestinal cramping, and hemorrhage.

Irritant gases, metal dusts or fumes, and chemicals of extreme pH or reactivity, may produce mucosal damage to the respiratory tract (Table 77–7). The location of injury depends upon the water solubility and particle size of the substance. The highly water-soluble gases—ammonia, hydrogen chloride, and hydrogen fluoride—dissolve readily in the moisture associated with the mucous membranes of the nose and upper respiratory tract. Inflammation, ulceration, edema, and necrosis may acutely obstruct the upper airway. Gases with a low solubility in water—ozone, nitrogen dioxide, and phosgene—will reach the lower airway, producing pneumonitis and pulmonary edema. Potential late effects from the inhalation of these substances include bronchiolitis fibrosa obliterans, bronchiectasis, chronic bronchitis, and varying degrees of pulmonary fibrosis.

Most respiratory irritants are gases or vapors, but they may also exist as particulates (e.g., mist) or be absorbed onto particulates (e.g., sulfur dioxide).[15] The particle size largely determines the extent of their accessibility to small airways. Particles between 1 and 5 μ can diffuse within the alveoli.[16] Pneumoconiosis is the result of chronic exposure to dusts (e.g., asbestos) resulting in the development of fibrorestrictive disease.

Hypersensitivity reactions are caused by repeated exposure to any one of a number of organic and inorganic agents. Exposure does not lead to clinical disease in every individual. The two basic immunologic reactions are the immediate response (Type I), as seen in bronchial asthma, and the cell-mediated response (Type IV), as seen in hypersensitivity pneumonitis and allergic contact dermatitis. The early appearance of hypersensitivity reactions is quite similar if not indistinguishable from that of chemical irritations.[4]

Poisonous gases need not damage the lungs directly to have adverse effects on the body. Interfering with the supply of oxygen to the tissues will cause asphyxiation. When present in sufficient quantities, biologically inert gases, such as hydrogen and methane, will reduce the oxygen content of inspired air. These gases are called "simple asphyxiants." Symptoms are usually evident by the time these gases exceed 20 to 30 vol per cent of inspired air.[18] Chemical or toxic asphyxiants include carbon monoxide, cyanide, and hydrogen sulfide. These gases lead to profound disruptions of cellular metabolism by blocking the delivery or utilization of oxygen. Both types of asphyxiants produce minimal direct injury to the respiratory tract but can cause marked neurologic and metabolic alterations.[19]

Many toxic agents affect other organ systems through secondary systemic spread. Under normal conditions, the skin is remarkably successful in preventing diffusion when

Table 77–7. TOXIC INDUSTRIAL GASES[4, 6, 7]

IRRITANT GASES	METAL FUMES	SIMPLE ASPHYXIANTS	CHEMICAL ASPHYXIANTS
Ammonia	Beryllium	Nitrogen	Carbon monoxide
Chlorine	Cadmium	Methane	Hydrogen sulfide
Nitrogen dioxide	Mercury	Carbon dioxide	Hydrogen cyanide
Ozone	Nickel	Argon	Acetonitrile
Phosgene	Vanadium	Helium	Methylene chloride
Sulfur dioxide	Zinc	Nitrous oxide	
Fluorine	Chromium	Hydrogen	
Bromine	Osmium		
Acetic acid			

exposed to toxic chemicals. The amounts absorbed are usually of little significance. Exceptions include chlorinated hydrocarbons, warfarin, organophosphates, organic mercury, tetraethyl lead, and dimethylsulfoxide.[20]

Inhalation of toxicants presents the most rapid and direct avenue of entry into the body because of the intimate association of air passages in the lung with the circulatory system. Once a hazardous substance has been absorbed, the clinical manifestations depend on many factors, including the inherent toxicity of the chemical, the total dose, and the duration of exposure. Exposure to other agents, like alcohol or drugs, may modify the response (see Table 77–6). The clinical spectrum is accordingly very broad. When managing poisoning cases, the clinician must obtain a thorough history and physical examination with appropriate laboratory studies, and must be observant for injury to target organ systems, especially central nervous, renal, cardiac, and hepatic systems.

Because of its strategic position, both anatomically and biochemically, the liver not only is exposed to direct cytotoxins but also is the major site in the body for biotransformation of chemical substances.[21] Hepatic enzyme systems oxidize lipid-soluble chemicals to their water-soluble metabolites. These metabolites may then be harmlessly excreted in aqueous media such as urine or bile. However, in some instances the oxidation system converts inactive chemicals to highly reactive toxins with resulting hepatocellular necrosis.

Table 77–8 is a guide to clinical manifestations of acute exposure to common industrial

Table 77–8. CLINICAL SIGNS OF INDUSTRIAL POISONING[4, 16, 22, 23]

ORGAN	SYMPTOM/SIGN	EXPOSURE
Eye	Corneal burns	Caustic agents, irritant gases, solvents
	Diplopia	Carbon disulfide, CO, ethylene glycol, lead, methyl bromide, methyl chloride, methyl iodide, triethyl tin
	Miosis	Carbamates, nicotine, organophosphates
	Mydriasis	Barium, benzene, ethyl bromide, ethylene glycol, methanol, methyl chloride
	Nystagmus	Carbon disulfide, CO, ethylene glycol, mercury, methyl bromide, methyl chloride, methyl iodide
	Papilledema	Ethylene glycol, lead, methanol, phosphorus, triethyl tin
	Ptosis	Thallium
	Retinal hemorrhages	Acetylphenylhydrazine, benzene, lead, methyl bromide, triethyl tin, warfarin
	Vision disturbance	Carbon tetrachloride, dinitrobenzene, lead, methanol, naphthalene, thallium, toluene, triethyl tin
Head	Epistaxis	Acrylonitrile, benzene, bromine, chromium, phosphine, tetryl
	Gum discoloration	Arsenic, bismuth, lead, mercury
	Pharyngitis	Acetone, acrolein, antimony, formaldehyde, hydrogen sulfide, iodine, tin
	Rhinitis	Acrolein, ammonia, antimony, chlorobenzenes, epoxy resins, formaldehyde, mercury, hydrochloric acid, ozone, organic dusts, phenylenediamine, thallium
	Salivation	Arsenic, bismuth, lead, mercury, organophosphates
	Tinnitus	Carbon dioxide, heavy metals, methanol, methyl bromide, nitrobenzene, toluene, xylene
Pulmonary	Asthma	Grain dusts, isocyanate, metal fumes, phenylenediamine, polyvinyl chloride, toluene
	Dyspnea	Asphyxiants, beryllium, chloramine-T, dusts, nickel carbonyl, phosphate ester insecticides
	Pulmonary edema	Hydrogen sulfide, irritant gases, metal fumes, methyl bromide, methyl chloride
Cardiovascular	Angina	Arsenic, asphyxiants, carbon disulfide, methylene chloride, nitrates
	Bradycardia	Nitrites, organophosphates
	Dysrhythmias	Arsenic, chlorinated hydrocarbons, fluorocarbons, nitrates, phenol, any agent causing ischemia
	ECG abnormalities	Antimony, arsenic, arsine
	Hypertension	Cadmium, diphenyl oxide, lead, nicotine, vanadium

Table 77–8. CLINICAL SIGNS OF INDUSTRIAL POISONING[4, 16, 22, 23] *Continued*

ORGAN	SYMPTOM/SIGN	EXPOSURE
Cardiovascular Continued	Hypotension	Arsenic, arsine, carbon tetrachloride, fluorides, iron salts, methyl bromide, nickel carbonyl, nitrites, phosphine, phosphorus
	Tachycardia	Arsenic, dinitro-cresol, dinitrophenol, iron salts, nicotine, pentachlorophenol, potassium bromate
Gastrointestinal	Abdominal colic	Arsenic, inorganic lead, organophosphates, thallium
	Constipation	Barium sulfate, lead, thallium
	Diarrhea	Arsenic, barium, carbamates, organophosphates, phosphorus, heavy metals
	Jaundice	Hepatotoxins (carbon tetrachloride), hemolytic agents (arsine, stibine)
	Melena	Corrosives, iron, thallium
	Nausea and vomiting	Chlordane, CNS depressants (acetone, benzene), irritants (epoxy resins, copper, tin), organophosphates, methemoglobin formers
Renal	Anuria	Bismuth, carbon tetrachloride, chlordane, chlorohydrin, ethylene glycol, mercurials, phosphorus, trinitrotoluene, turpentine
	Hematuria	Chlorates, heavy metals, naphthalene, nitrates
	Myoglobinuria	Aniline dyes, aromatic amines, chlorate, ethylene glycol, nitrates, nitrites
	Oliguria	Lead
	Proteinuria	Arsenic, mercury, organic solvents, phosphorus
Hematopoietic	Anemia	Arsine, arsenic, benzene, copper, lead, oxidant chemicals, stibine, trinitrotoluene
	Neutropenia	Arsenic, benzene, organochlorine insecticides
	Thrombocytopenia	Benzene, organochlorine insecticides
Nervous System	Ataxia	Chlordane, heavy metals, hexane, methyl chloride, organophosphates, toluene
	Cranial neuropathy	Carbon disulfide, trichloroethylene
	Delirium	Boric acid, bromides, chlordane, DDT, lead
	Depression	Alcohols, boric acid, carbon monoxide, cationic detergents, cyanide, heavy metals, insecticides, kerosene, naphthalene, phenol, solvents
	Motor neuropathy	Lead
	Myoclonus	Benzene hexachloride, mercury
	Parkinsonism	Carbon disulfide, carbon monoxide, manganese
	Psychosis	Bromides, carbon disulfide, manganese, toluene
	Seizures	Carbon monoxide, cyanide, lead, organic mercurials, organochlorine insecticides, organotin compounds
	Sensorimotor neuropathy	Acrylamide, arsenic, carbon disulfide, carbon monoxide, DDT, hexane, mercury
	Severe headache	Carbon monoxide, carbon tetrachloride, lead, nickel, nitrates, nitrites, organophosphates, trinitrotoluene
	Tremor	Arsenic, carbon disulfide, chlordecone, DDT, manganese, mercury
Endocrine	Decreased libido	Lead, mercury, other heavy metals
	Menstrual irregularities	Bismuth, lead, mercurials
Skin	Acne	Chlorobenzene, coal tar, paraffin
	Alopecia	Arsenic, boric acid, selenium, thallium
	Bullous lesions	Carbon monoxide, caustic agents
	Burns	Acids, formaldehyde, hypochlorite, lye
	Depigmentation	Arsenic, hydroquinone, phenols
	Diaphoresis	Nicotine, organophosphates
	Eczema	Detergents, solvents, soaps
	Flushing	Boric acid, cyanide
	Hyperpigmentation	Arsenic, halogenated aromatics
	Photosensitization	Phenanthrane, tars
	Purpura	Chlorinated biphenyls, dioxins
Musculoskeletal	Arthralgias	Arsenic, dinitrotoluene, lead
	Gout	Lead
	Muscle fasciculations	Manganese, organophosphates
	Muscle weakness/paralysis	Arsenic, chlordane, lead, organophosphates, organic mercurials, thallium
	Osteomalacia	Cadmium, fluoride, phosphorus

poisons. Note that no organ system is spared. The complexity, diversity, and unpredictability of industrial poisonings require a clinical approach that concentrates on effective management of the presenting problems, vital signs, symptom complexes, and ultimately the major organ systems involved.

PREHOSPITAL CARE AND DECONTAMINATION

Prompt and safe removal from exposure is the first consideration in the management of industrial poisoning. If rescue of a disabled victim is required, emergency personnel should wear protective garments and respirators appropriate to the chemical involved. Information about the appropriate gear is readily available if the chemical is known.[24]

If the chemical is unknown, attempts must be made by the initial responders to identify it. The scene of the exposure should be assessed for clues to the nature of the accident and the likelihood of associated medical or traumatic injuries. After the chemical agent has been identified, much information is obtained to assist in rescue and evacuation.

Decontamination is often the most overlooked area in the treatment of the chemically injured patient.[25] The extreme toxicity of many agents (e.g., organophosphates) and the risk of cross-contamination make thorough decontamination essential. The procedure is relatively uncomplicated unless it is compounded by associated injuries. Decontamination for inhaled agents, such as cyanide, may require simply removing the patient from the source of exposure and administering high-flow oxygen.[26]

Toxic chemicals that are absorbed dermally or act on the skin will require aggressive cleansing for removal. Emergency personnel wearing protective clothing (rubber gloves, gown, safety goggles) remove all the victim's clothing and seal it in a plastic bag. Soap and cool water provide adequate initial decontamination for most chemical toxins. A rare exception to this rule is exposure to agents insoluble in water (e.g., phosphorus) or to those that react violently with water (e.g., chlorosulfonic acid, calcium oxide, sodium, and titanium tetrachloride). The best approach for an unknown exposure is first to flush a small area with a stream of water and observe for an adverse reaction.

Tincture of green soap is an alkaline detergent in 30 per cent alcohol that is frequently employed in initial decontamination. The body must be thoroughly and repeatedly washed, with attention paid to the hair and fingernails. The water temperature may be gradually increased as the process continues. Initial use of cool water avoids opening the skin pores and reduces dermal absorption of the chemical.[26] The stable patient should be placed in a portable shower with a self-contained waste water system. A child's plastic wading pool may be used and the wash water saved for proper disposal.[24] Chemicals splashed in the eyes should be flushed out immediately with copious amounts of water or normal saline; this may be continued for up to 30 minutes (alkali burns).

When intoxication is caused by ingestion, an attempt should be made as soon as possible to prevent further absorption by emesis or lavage, depending on the patient's level of consciousness. For a treatment overview, see the algorithm outline in Figure 77–3.

HOSPITAL MANAGEMENT

As with any poisoning victim, initial management first involves assessing the overall severity of illness, determining the systems affected, and preventing further absorption of the toxin. Arterial blood gases should be measured and volume status should be assessed for signs of hypovolemia; baseline liver and renal function tests should be performed. Potentially lethal dysrhythmias must be identified and treated rapidly. Occasionally, CNS depression may be life threatening as well. Patients with thermal burns and traumatic injuries need to be identified and stabilized.[17]

Most patients will have been adequately decontaminated by the time the emergency physician becomes involved with the case, but this should always be ascertained. Specific note of the decontamination procedures should be made when communicating with field personnel. If a patient arrives at the emergency department prior to decontamination, the procedures outlined earlier are followed before the patient actually enters the department. The risk of medical personnel becoming poisoned by contamination from victims should always be kept in mind. Systemic absorption of ingested poisons is

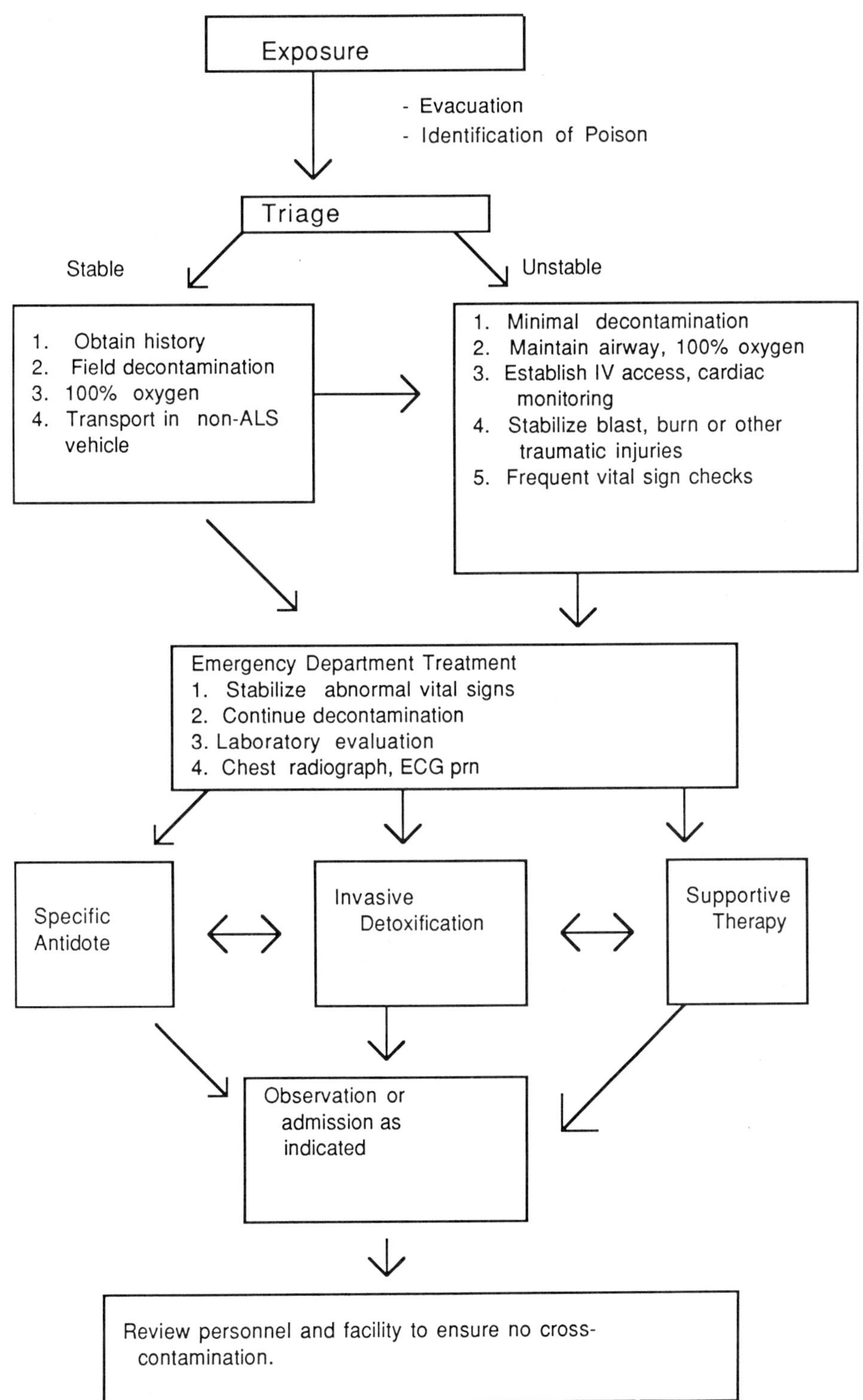

Figure 77–3. The management of industrial poisoning.

reduced by emesis or gastric lavage, administration of activated charcoal, and catharsis.

When initial decontamination is completed, attention is directed to aggressive airway management and supportive pulmonary therapy. Patients exposed to noxious gases should receive humidified 100 per cent oxygen until carbon monoxide poisoning can be ruled out. Immediate transportation to a facility where hyperbaric oxygen therapy is available should be considered for patients who have carboxyhemoglobin levels over 30 to 40 per cent, or for those who do not promptly respond to normobaric oxygen treatment.[17] The management of inhalation injuries may require endotracheal intubation because of oropharyngeal and laryngeal edema. Emergency cricopharyngeal puncture is occasionally needed, especially after ammonia inhalation. Once intubation is accomplished, continuous positive airway pressure (CPAP) and positive end-expiratory pressure (PEEP) are useful for treating noncardiogenic pulmonary edema. Aminophylline and other parenteral bronchodilators may be recommended in patients who have lower respiratory tract injury.[17] Any patient with a history of significant toxic inhalation should be carefully monitored in the hospital for at least 24 hours because of the latency of toxicity of many compounds and the potential for sudden deterioration.

Treatment of minor chemical burns consists of debridement, tetanus immunization, topical antibiotic cream, and occlusive dressing for comfort. Because of the risk of underestimating the extent of chemical burns, close follow-up should be arranged. Extensive burns require aggressive treatment to protect against hypovolemic shock and secondary complications (e.g., infections).[27] Any burn that covers greater than 20 per cent of the body surface area requires immediate transport of the patient to a burn center. If the dermal injury is limited to superficial or localized irritation, wet dressings should be applied for comfort. A short-term course of systemic steroids may be necessary for extensive dermatitis. Additional treatment includes oral antihistamines for sedation and relief of itching.[16]

When a chemical agent has been splashed into the eye, immediate irrigation is imperative; this is best begun during transport to the medical facility and is continued for up to 30 minutes. Extensive irrigation is necessary with alkali burns of the eyes because of the inability of the eye to buffer pH changes of a severely basic nature and the capacity of alkalis to penetrate ocular tissues rapidly.[16] After irrigation, examination of the cornea with fluorescein dye and slit lamp should be performed. A cycloplegic agent, such as 0.2 per cent scopolamine or 2 per cent atropine, may be used for associated iritis. The application of an antibiotic ointment and eye patch will give the victim symptomatic relief. More significant injuries caused by alkalis and strong acids saponify plasma membranes, denature collagen, and cause vascular thrombosis.[28] The application of collagenase inhibitors, such as cysteine and calcium EDTA, during regeneration of corneal epithelium has greatly reduced the incidence of ulceration associated with alkali burns.[29] All these injuries require ophthalmologic consultation.

Intensive supportive care is the mainstay of management of the poisoning victim, with the goal of preservation of vital organ function until the poison has been metabolized. This includes the early symptomatic treatment of complications such as peripheral vascular collapse, hypoxia, dysrhythmias, seizures, fluid and electrolyte disturbances, and pulmonary or cerebral edema. Hepatic, renal, and hematologic failures tend to occur only slightly later. Close expectant management in these patients has reduced the mortality in hospitalized patients to less than 1 per cent.[30] A small group of severely poisoned patients, however, may benefit from the use of artificial organs to enhance elimination of toxins from the blood. Hemodialysis, hemoperfusion, and other modalities are considered state of the art in invasive detoxification (see Chapter 8).

LABORATORY EVALUATION

The current role of the clinical laboratory in the medical management of industrial poisoning is primarily that of providing data on acid-base status, levels of hypoxia, and organ function tests (liver, kidney, and hematologic systems). If suspicion of a specific exposure is raised by the history, additional testing, such as a methemoglobin level, may be necessary. Several types of chemical intoxication may be evaluated further by determining the concentration of the suspected toxin or its metabolites in the blood or urine, or an affected enzyme in the blood. All patients with inhalation exposure should have a carboxyhemoglobin level determination.

Central to evaluating pulmonary problems are the chest radiograph and pulmonary function testing. The radiograph may reveal aspiration pneumonitis, noncardiogenic pulmonary edema, pleural effusions, or interstitial fibrosis. In addition to the routine posteroanterior view, one should consider oblique views if, for example, changes in the pleural surfaces are suspected following asbestos exposure. For diagnosis, it is helpful to be able to characterize pulmonary function abnormalities as obstructive or restrictive.[22] A xenon ventilation-perfusion lung scan may be useful in patients with suspected inhalation injury.

Abnormalities found on the resting electrocardiogram (ECG) are neither very sensitive nor specific for diagnosing occupational exposure. Chemical asphyxiants or arsenic may produce an ECG picture of myocardial ischemia by interfering with cellular respiration. Both arsine and antimony have been associated with abnormalities in the T waves. Overexposure to phosphorus, organic mercury, or arsenic causes QT prolongation and ST-T wave abnormalities.[4]

SUMMARY

Legislative measures, such as the Toxic Substances Control Act of 1976, alone may not be sufficient to reduce occupational disease significantly. Approximately 60,000 chemical substances are in common use, and several hundred new compounds are added by industrial processes each year. Unpredicted health hazards from new processes continue to emerge and "well-known" occupational exposures still escape surveillance and control.[5] As a result, any patient presenting with an unusual symptom or group of symptoms should always raise the suspicion of an occupationally related disease. A systematic approach to the occupational history serves as a guide to discovering a specific toxic exposure that may be the cause of the presenting symptoms. Even when such a history is unavailable, a thoughtful physical examination and initial laboratory analysis often lead the clinician to an early toxicologic diagnosis.

The second part of this chapter will take a look at a specific industry, the microelectronics industry, in order to develop an appreciation for the concepts involved in industrial toxicology.

References

1. Wanke LA: Toxic chemical spills. Topics Emerg Med 7(1):9–19, 1985.
2. Ramazzini B: Diseases of Workers (translated by Wright CW). New York, Hafner, 1964.
3. Kunkel DB: Occupational asthma. Part II: Causes and management. Emerg Med *19*:86–94, 1987.
4. Rosenstock L, Cullen MR (eds): Clinical Occupational Medicine. Philadelphia, WB Saunders, 1986.
5. Goldman RH, Peters JM: The occupational and environmental health history. JAMA *246*:2831–2836, 1981.
6. Linz DH, Barker AF, Morton WE, et al: Occupational toxic inhalations. Topics Emerg Med *7*:21–33, 1985.
7. Levy B: The teaching of occupational health in American medical schools: Five-year follow-up of an initial study (abs). Am J Public Health *75*:79–80, 1985.
8. DOT Hazardous Materials Warning Placards. Washington, DC, US Department of Transportation, Research and Special Programs Administration, Materials Transportation Bureau, Office of Operations and Enforcement, 1981.
9. Stutz DR, Ricks RC, Olsen MF: Hazardous Materials Injuries: A Handbook for Prehospital Care. Greenbelt, MD, Bradford Communications Corp, 1982.
10. NFPA: Fire Protection Guide on Hazardous Materials. Boston, National Fire Protection Association, 1981.
11. Material Safety Data Sheet: Requirements for reporting hazardous materials safety and health regulations for ship repairing, shipbuilding and shipbreaking. Washington, DC, US Department of Labor, OSHA, 1977.
12. Increased lead absorption in children of lead workers—Vermont. MMWR *26*:61–62, 1977.
13. McCann M, Barazani G (eds): Health Hazards in the Arts and Crafts. Washington, DC, Society for Occupation and Environmental Health, 1980.
14. Finkl AJ: Hamilton's and Hardy's Industrial Toxicology. 4th ed. Boston, John Wright–PSG Inc, 1983.
15. Wald PH, Balmes JR: Respiratory effects of short-term, high-intensity toxic inhalants: Smoke, gases, and fumes. J Intens Care Med 2:260–278, 1987.
16. Proctor NH, Hughes JP (eds): Chemical Hazards of the Workplace. Philadelphia, JB Lippincott, 1978.
17. Kizer KW: Toxic inhalations. Emerg Med Clin North Am 2:649–666, 1984.
18. Goldfrank LR, Bresnitz EA: Toxic inhalants. *In* Goldfrank LR, Flomenbaum NE, Lewin NA, et al (eds): Goldfrank's Toxicologic Emergencies. Norwalk, CT, Appleton-Century-Crofts, 1986, pp 651–661.
19. Hedges JR: Acute noxious gas exposure. Curr Topics 2:1–9, 1978.
20. Stokinger HE: Routes of entry and modes of action. *In* Key MM (ed): Occupational Diseases—A Guide to Their Recognition. Washington, DC, US Government Printing Office, 1977, pp 11–21.
21. Tolman KG: Gastrointestinal system. *In* Rom WN

(ed): Environmental and Occupational Medicine. Boston, Little, Brown, 1983, pp 397–402.
22. Frank AL: The occupational history and examination. *In* Rom WN (ed): Environmental and Occupational Medicine. Boston, Little, Brown, 1983, pp 23–32.
23. Block JB: The Signs and Symptoms of Chemical Exposure. Springfield, MA, Bannerstone House, 1980.
24. Doyle CJ, Little NE, Ulin LS: Acute exposure to hazardous materials. *In* Haddad LM, Winchester JF (eds): Clinical Management of Poisoning and Drug Overdose. Philadelphia, WB Saunders, 1983, pp 250–263.
25. US Department of Transportation: Hazardous Materials, 1980; Emergency Response Guide. Publication DOT-P, 5800.2. Washington, DC, Research and Special Projects Administration, Materials Transportation Bureau, 1980.
26. Barr SJ: Chemical warfare agents. Topics Emerg Med *7*:62–70, 1985.
27. Klein DG, O'Malley P: Topical injury from chemical agents: Initial treatment. Heart Lung *16*:49–54, 1987.
28. Pfister RR: Chemical injuries of the eye. Ophthalmology *90*:1246–1250, 1983.
29. Slansky HH, Dohlman CH, Berman MB: Prevention of corneal ulcers. Trans Am Acad Ophthalmol Otolaryngol *75*:1208–1212, 1971.
30. Vale JA: The epidemiology of acute poisoning. Acta Pharmacol Toxicol *41*(Suppl):443–458, 1977.
31. Done AK: Of metals and chelation. Emerg Med *11*:186–214, 1979.
32. Fleisher G, Ludwig S: Textbook of Pediatric Emergency Medicine. Baltimore, Williams and Wilkins, 1983, pp 494–496.
33. Dreisbach RH: Handbook of Poisoning. Los Altos, CA, Lange Medical Publishers, 1983.

General Bibliography

Bureau of Explosives: Emergency Handling of Hazardous Materials in Surface Transportation. Washington, DC, Association of American Railroads, 1977.

Gosselin RE, et al: Clinical Toxicology of Commercial Products: Acute Poisoning. 5th ed. Baltimore, Williams and Wilkins, 1984.

Sax NI: Dangerous Properties of Industrial Materials. New York, Van Nostrand Reinhold, 1979.

Toxic and Hazardous Industrial Chemicals Safety Manual for Handling and Disposal with Toxicity and Hazard Data. Tokyo, The International Technical Information Institute, 1985.

Urez RC: Chemical Emergency Action Manual. Buffalo, NY, American Lung Association of Western New York, 1981.

US Department of Transportation: Emergency Action Guide for Selected Hazardous Materials. Washington, DC, 1978.

B. The Microelectronics Industry

Joseph LaDou, M.D.
Philip A. Edelman, M.D.

The microelectronics industry is major throughout the world. Its explosive growth, stemming from a series of scientific discoveries and rapid developments in manufacturing processes, has created a world market for semiconductor devices alone of more than $19 billion and a work force of more than half a million people. Just a few years ago, we thought of semiconductor manufacture as the activity of a few regions, such as Silicon Valley (Santa Clara County in northern California), Route 128 outside Boston, the area surrounding Texas Instruments near Dallas, and the IBM plant at East Fishkill, New York. Today, the pre-eminence of American technology is being challenged by that of Japan; there are many active Asian and European producers of microelectronic devices. In the United States, semiconductor and related companies are now located in most industrialized areas.

The industry began in 1948 with the development of the transistor, a small, low-power amplifier that replaced the cumbersome, inefficient vacuum tube. The industry grew rapidly, finding large and ready markets in the burgeoning computer industry and other consumer products. Miniaturized electronic circuits are produced for a vast number of devices for the military and space agencies and for an array of data communication industries. The importance of microelectronics to contemporary life is measured in our increasing reliance on information and entertainment derived from home computers, radios, video games, and soon the wristwatch television set. Some analysts speculate that the microelectronics industry will be America's fourth largest by the end of the century. In terms of gross national product, jobs, quality of life, and a number of other yardsticks, all of us share a hope that the industry continues its history of uncomplicated growth and development.

Development of the Industry and Health Considerations

When microelectronics companies began to develop, it was assumed by many urban planners, municipalities, industry organizations, and related groups that the manufacture of microelectronics components would entail much the same processes as those of conventional electronics. They envisioned large numbers of workers seated at workbenches quietly soldering conductive wires to printed circuit boards. For that reason, issues of toxic chemicals, gases, fumes, waste materials, explosion hazards, and the like were not directly considered.

The new technology is largely maintained in secrecy. Most companies, particularly small ones, keep their manufacturing processes to themselves and carefully screen information on manufacturing materials before providing these data to persons or agencies outside the company. This is not a condemnation of company policies, for there are serious problems of industrial theft in this highly competitive industry, but it is mentioned as a reason for the general level of ignorance of possible health hazards in the microelectronics industry.

Initially, microelectronic devices were primarily developed in California, which continues to lead the industry in technologic advances and consumer applications. From the beginning, physicians treating patients from microelectronic companies shared the community acceptance of a clean industry. No ugly smokestacks commonly associated with heavy industries nor contamination of rivers and streams was apparent. Injured patients reported to management and sent to medical facilities reflected the typical industrial experience with back strains and other musculoskeletal problems that represent the majority of patient complaints—as they continue to do to this day.

Early Health Concerns and Problems

From the outset, however, new and somewhat unique problems were associated with semiconductor manufacture. Company health and safety personnel were concerned with exposure to arsenic and other metals, even before it was clear that arsenic was a carcinogen. Screening programs were conducted by the larger companies to monitor the levels of arsenic in the hair, nails, and urine of workers in some areas of the production process. Skin rashes appeared from work with epoxy resins; a number of dermatologists became skilled in recognizing the epoxy-sensitive worker and his or her need to prevent further exposure.

Most apparent of all was the common hydrofluoric acid burn: a slow, often insidious burn of deep tissues as the fluoride ion passed through the skin and moved toward bone. When not immediately attended to with thorough washing and inactivation, the burns often became severe on the hands, arms, face, and other exposed areas. Hydrofluoric acid is used to etch glass (silicon dioxide) from the surface of the silicon wafers so that dopant ions can be deposited into areas of silicon stripped of its protective glass coating. Although the technology was well established, the sheer number of hydrofluoric acid burns that occurred created the first awareness that microelectronics shared with other industries a measurable level of risk to the health and safety of workers. In a typical year, more than a thousand cases of chemical burns and splashes affecting the eyes or skin are reported by electronics workers in California.

Changing Processes and Health Problems

Recently, a spectrum of health and safety problems has emerged, not only in semiconductor manufacture but also in the manufacture of related devices such as light-emitting diodes, microwave-integrated circuits, and liquid crystal displays. The number and severity of hydrofluoric acid burns appears to be declining in larger companies because specific health and safety measures have been developed within the companies.[1] Now, other serious problems have taken their place.

A good example of the dynamic nature of the industry is found in the replacement of "wet etching" with hydrofluoric and other acids by a process called "dry plasma etching," done in a closed system with presumably much greater safety for the workers. The energy source for dry plasma etching devices is radiofrequency (RF) power; the health consequences of exposures to these fields have not been thoroughly investigated. In this particular example, one health hazard may be replaced by yet another, with an outcome more difficult to measure than that of the established process. Radiofrequency power is also commonly used in a variety of other high-technology machines in the semiconductor manufacturing process, such as the epitaxy reactor and metallization equipment. Radiofrequency equipment of this nature, however, is used in many other industries.

The addition of dopant ions to the semiconductor wafers is accomplished by a number of techniques. Initially, dopants were added to melted silicon to form an ingot from which wafers would be cut. The amounts of arsenic, phosphorus, and boron were small, and these substances generally were handled with caution. Now, more advanced technology demands the use of more arsenic (the making of gallium arsenide ingots rather than silicon ingots) and the implantation of ions of arsenic, phosphorus, and boron from sources of the highly toxic gases arsine, phosphine, and diborane. These dopant molecules, imbedded in the silicon crystal lattice, create the electrical potentials and thus circuits in the chip.

Herein may lie the current greatest health concern for workers, at least until the next level of technology replaces these toxic materials with a new set of problems.

Statistical Evidence of Health Hazards

The high-technology manufacturing techniques of the microelectronics industry have produced health statistics in California that have not yet been explained. These statistics are derived from state workers' compensation insurance records (considered the most complete in the country) from information supplied by the many hundreds of companies engaged in electronics and microelectronics manufacture. They tend to support the view that the microelectronics industry deserves the public impression of relative health and safety. The electronics industry traditionally has had a lower combined incidence of occupational injury and illness than that of heavier industries, and the subgroup of workers engaged in semiconductor manufacture demonstrates the same enviable record that is indicative of a safe and healthy work environment.

The reasons for this relatively low rate of combined injury and illness among electronics (and semiconductor) workers are many. Electronics workers are seldom exposed to large machines with dangerous moving parts. The product being made is exceptionally small, requiring absolute cleanliness, and much of the work is done seated at microscopes. Most important, however, is the fact that the composition of the work place is unique among manufacturing industries. Unlike heavy industries, such as automobile manufacture, petrochemical production, and mining, in which the production force constitutes the preponderance of employees, the semiconductor industry is heavily weighted with nonmanufacturing employees—managers, engineers, technicians, and business and clerical workers. An industry study revealed that production workers constitute only 31 per cent of the work force and maintenance workers only 2.5 per cent. Yet, these two groups accounted for almost 60 per cent of injury and illness cases. Thus, a comparison of cases of injury and illness in semiconductor manufacturing versus other industries could result in an undeserved lower incidence figure for the microelectronics industry. Finally, most production workers in the microelectronics industry are women and racial minorities, two groups that tend to change jobs frequently. Consequently, the high turnover of employees may distort statistics on health and safety problems.

Despite the overall record of occupational safety, the semiconductor industry has been troubled by an unusually high incidence of occupational illness. The California survey of the industry's work-related illness records conducted annually by the Division of Labor Statistics and Research indicates that the rate of occupational illness among semiconductor workers is more than three times that among workers in general manufacturing industry—26.4 per cent of workloss cases as compared with 7.0 per cent (Fig. 77–4).

Occupational illness data may reflect the widespread use of toxic materials in the semiconductor industry, which has developed process applications for many metals, chemicals, and toxic gases in a wide variety of combinations and plant settings. An industry considered "clean" 20 years ago is today recognized as a "chemically intensive" manufacturing industry. American semiconductor companies consume 200,000,000 gallons of wet chemicals annually.

The statistical category of occupational ill-

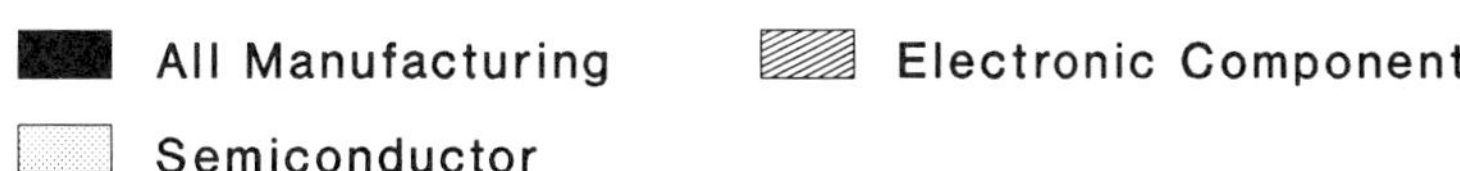

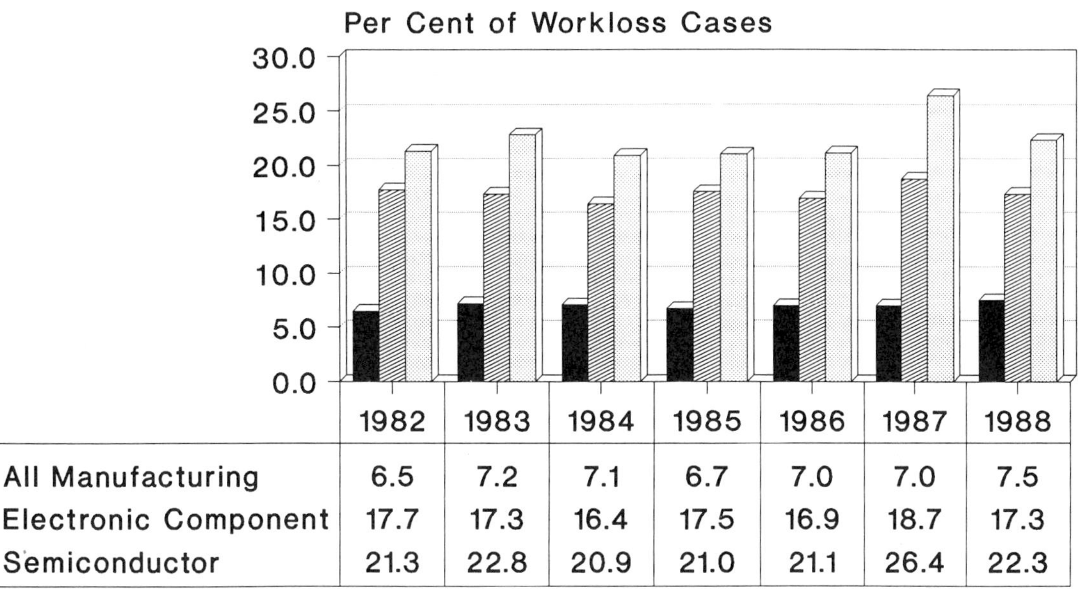

	1982	1983	1984	1985	1986	1987	1988
All Manufacturing	6.5	7.2	7.1	6.7	7.0	7.0	7.5
Electronic Component	17.7	17.3	16.4	17.5	16.9	18.7	17.3
Semiconductor	21.3	22.8	20.9	21.0	21.1	26.4	22.3

Figure 77–4. Occupational illness as per cent of workloss cases.

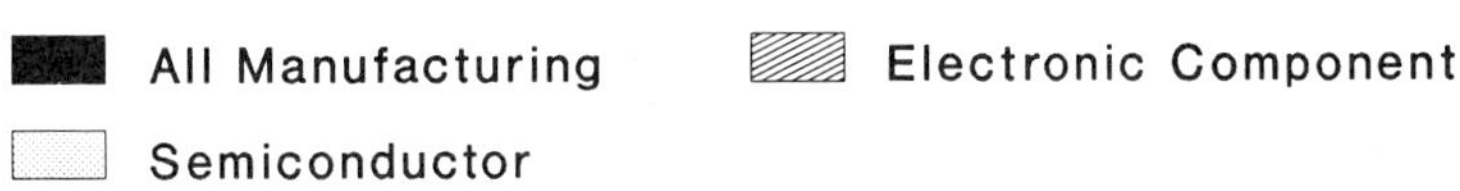

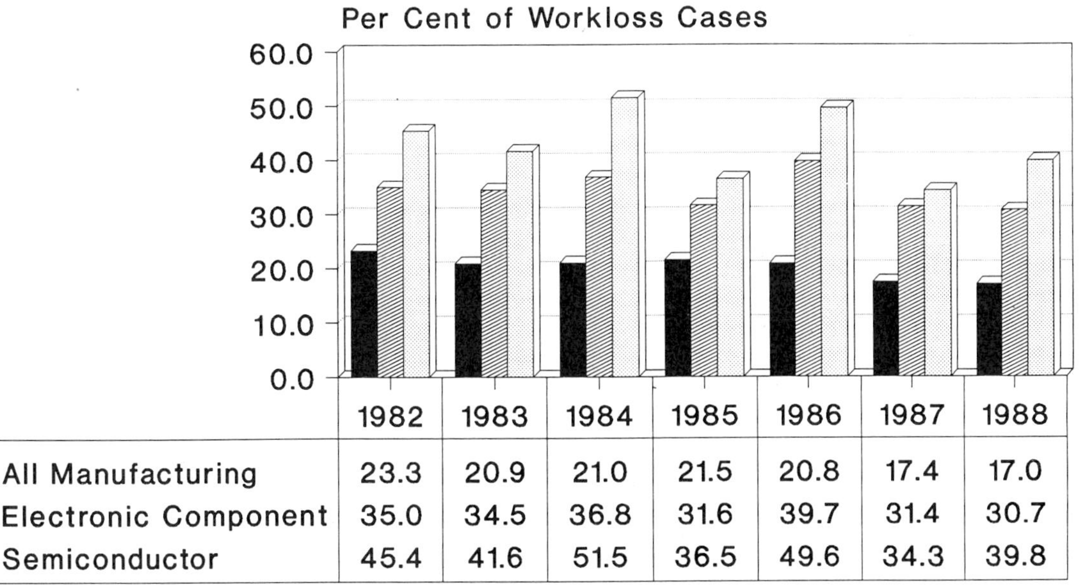

	1982	1983	1984	1985	1986	1987	1988
All Manufacturing	23.3	20.9	21.0	21.5	20.8	17.4	17.0
Electronic Component	35.0	34.5	36.8	31.6	39.7	31.4	30.7
Semiconductor	45.4	41.6	51.5	36.5	49.6	34.3	39.8

Figure 77–5. Systemic poisoning as per cent of occupational illness.

ness termed "systemic poisoning" is elevated each year among electronics workers, primarily because of the high incidence among semiconductor workers. Systemic poisoning data reflect exposure to toxic materials resulting in occupational illness, as shown in Figure 77–5.

We emphasize that systemic poisoning includes a number of disease possibilities in addition to exposure to toxic materials. Many physicians object to a category of occupational illness that includes so wide a variety of diseases as anemias, emphysema, hepatitis, and peptic ulcer, giving the false impression that each of these is the result of toxic exposure. To compound the statistical problem, the data are derived from the "First Report of Injury" compiled by the state Department of Industrial Accidents.[2] These reports seldom contain a confirmed diagnosis, which, in the case of toxic exposure, usually requires a number of diagnostic tests before systemic poisoning is either diagnosed or ruled out.

However, the wide variety of medical problems that can be included in the definition of systemic poisoning does not account for much of the statistical experience in the electronics and semiconductor industries, as shown in Figure 77–6.

The complaints of workers in the semiconductor group are confined to systemic effects caused by toxic agents, upper respiratory conditions, and a wider group of pulmonary complaints including infections, allergic reactions, and emphysema. These complaints are compatible with toxic exposure, although not diagnostic of significant illness. Thus, rather than accurately indicating the incidence of systemic poisoning cases, the data merely indicate an area for concern about the semiconductor working environment.[3]

One distinguishing feature of the semiconductor manufacturing environment is the development and widespread application of the "cleanroom" in which chips are processed with a minimum of exposure to workroom dust. Filters are used to remove dust from the air and to filter replacement air for that which is removed by hoods and vents or is lost in small leaks in the ventilating system. Typically, in an effort to minimize the replacement and maintenance of filters, air is recirculated in cleanrooms. Thus, in a single hour, a total air replacement in the cleanroom is accomplished more than 500 times, with

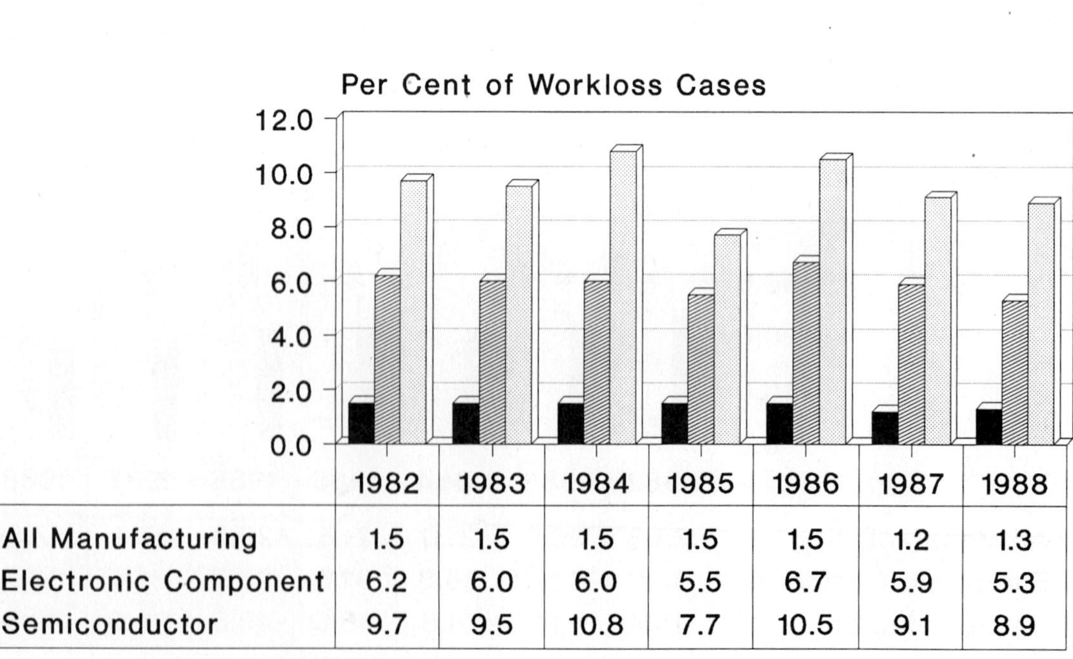

	1982	1983	1984	1985	1986	1987	1988
All Manufacturing	1.5	1.5	1.5	1.5	1.5	1.2	1.3
Electronic Component	6.2	6.0	6.0	5.5	6.7	5.9	5.3
Semiconductor	9.7	9.5	10.8	7.7	10.5	9.1	8.9

Figure 77–6. Systemic poisoning as per cent of workloss cases.

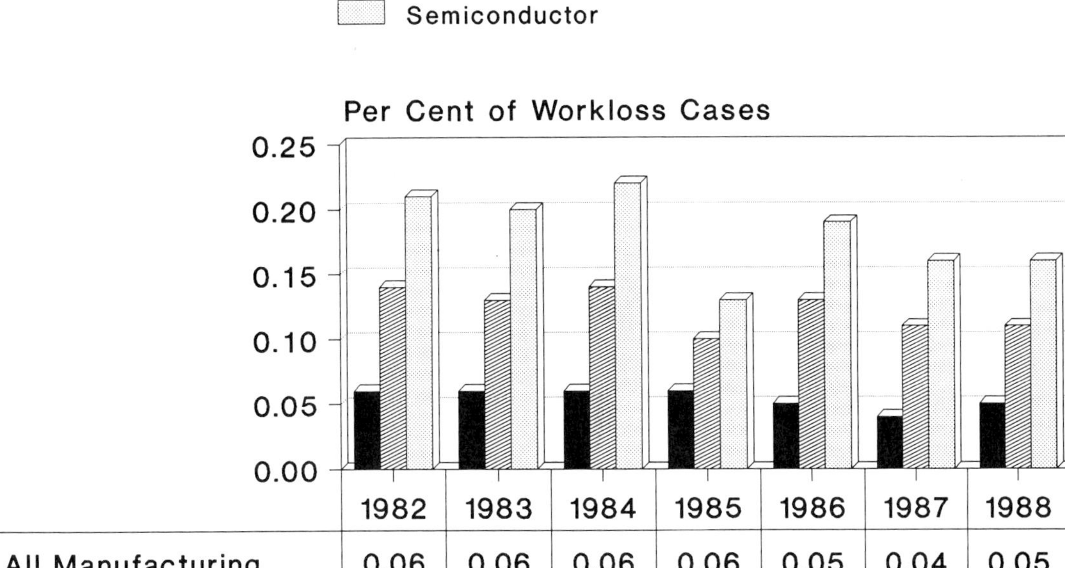

	1982	1983	1984	1985	1986	1987	1988
All Manufacturing	0.06	0.06	0.06	0.06	0.05	0.04	0.05
Electronic Component	0.14	0.13	0.14	0.10	0.13	0.11	0.11
Semiconductor	0.21	0.20	0.22	0.13	0.19	0.16	0.16

Figure 77–7. Systemic poisoning as per cent of total workforce.

more than 80 per cent of the air being recirculated and less than 20 per cent of the air newly introduced after appropriate particle filtering. This recirculation of cleanroom air is suspected of causing at least some of the high incidence of occupational illness in microelectronics workers, since chemicals are recirculated and not filtered out along with the dust. Cleanroom air refers to low dust levels, not to low chemical vapor levels.

In view of the fact that production and maintenance workers constitute only 31 per cent of the workforce yet account for 60 per cent of injuries and illnesses, the argument could easily be sustained that the overall data for the semiconductor industry seen in Figures 77–6 and 77–7 underrepresent the actual incidence of occupational illness in this industry relative to other manufacturing industries.

The technology underlying this industry is continually changing. For example, the space on a chip required for a given electronic function has decreased by a factor of two about every 18 months. New processes and new materials are replacing old ones in rapid succession. This fast-paced change, as well as the stringent security precautions of the industry, has added to the difficulty of instituting proper health and safety measures in the microelectronics industry. Two vitally important questions need to be answered. First, what health hazards do microelectronics workers face in doing their jobs? Second, what health hazards may exist for the communities in which microelectronics companies operate?

The Microelectronic Process

Over the past decade, multiple process techniques and variations have developed. New substrates (wafers) are being used. For the purpose of general discussion, we have typified the following summary of a silicon chip production.

The typical manufacture of semiconductor chips begins with silicon, which is prepared in wafer form, usually by a company that specializes in growing the silicon crystals. In the first step of the process, raw silicon is reduced from its oxide (the main constituent of common sand) and purified by a series of chemical additions. It is then melted in a crucible at 1420°C in an atmosphere of inert gas to prevent oxidation and unwanted impurities. Dopants (typically arsenic, phosphorus, or boron) may be added during this step to enhance electrical conductivity. A perfect single-crystal silicon seed is then inserted into the melted silicon and slowly twisted and withdrawn from the crucible. The resulting silicon ingot can be three to four inches in diameter and several feet long. The uneven surface of the ingot is next polished to standard diameter dimensions. The ingot is then sliced into wafers using a thin, high-speed diamond saw. Finally, the wafers are ground and polished, with one side given a flawless, polished surface.

The wafers are cleaned in acid and solvent baths (sulfuric and nitric acids and a variety of solvents) to remove grease and other unwanted substances. The wafer is then heated at between 1000°C and 1200°C in an atmosphere of oxygen and water vapor to develop a silicon dioxide film on its surface. This film is hard and durable and serves as an excellent insulator. The desired thickness of the silicon dioxide film is achieved by careful control of temperature and timing.

A photoresist pattern is applied to the oxidized wafer; the photoresist is a light-sensitive polymeric material dissolved in a solvent. It is usually applied in an enclosed, exhausted system by a spin-on (centrifugal) or spray system. The resulting film on the wafer is dried thoroughly by heat, which also adheres it firmly to the underlying silicon dioxide. A photomask is applied to allow selective ultraviolet exposure, causing polymerization of precise areas of the photoresist. Polymerization of the photoresist alters its solubility in certain solvents. Thus, the soluble photoresist can be removed with microscopic accuracy.

The wafer, now equipped with its polymerized photoresist pattern and its exposed silicon dioxide, is again hardened by heating and placed in a solution of hydrofluoric acid. The acid dissolves the silicon dioxide layer wherever it is unprotected, but does not affect either the photoresist or the wafer itself. When the acid has removed the exposed silicon dioxide, the wafer is rinsed and dried and the photoresist is removed by a stripping agent (e.g., phenols or acids).

The semiconductor fabrication process is very similar to photolithography in printing. As with lithography, each semiconductor layer is built up one after another until the desired circuitry is completed. Similarly, each pattern (photomask) must be positioned with extreme accuracy with respect to the underlying layers. This requires technicians to use special binocular microscopes to "align" the wafers. When the mask is in the exact position, the wafer is exposed to ultraviolet radiation and the next desired pattern of integrated circuitry is transferred to its photoresist-coated surface. The exposure is then developed as before, after which it is inspected for flaws and, if acceptable, is heated again.

The wafer is next given at least two baths in acid (hydrochloric or hydrofluoric acid) and heated to a temperature higher than boiling water to remove unexposed material from around the desired circuitry. This step is followed by a wash in distilled water. The wafer may be placed in a closed furnace containing a dopant (arsine, phosphine, or diborane gas) and heated to 1000°C. In this step, called diffusion, the dopant penetrates the surface of the wafer to alter the electrical characteristics. Dopants also can be deposited in an ion implantation chamber, with the dopants supplied as either solids or gases. The dopant molecules are ionized, then accelerated into the wafer. Ion implantation has become the prime method of doping wafers. Solid chemical sources have, in some cases, replaced toxic gases such as arsine.

The photoresist, masking, etching, and diffusion steps may be repeated for the same wafer many times, depending on the number of layers of circuitry that is needed to create the three-dimensional circuit. The wafer with its complete circuitry deposited by dopants is again masked with photoresist, exposed, and acid-etched to deposit aluminum contacts for connecting external wiring. It is then heated to remove any unwanted metal, washed with distilled water, and coated with a surface layer of glass at a temperature of 420°C. This step is followed by another acid-etching and rinse.

Each completed wafer has scores of individual integrated circuit chips built up on its surface, and these must be separated. Each chip is inspected by microscopic and computer methods for accuracy. Imperfect chips are marked for disposal. The wafer is then sliced into separate chips using a diamond-blade saw. The individual integrated circuit chips are then bonded to ceramic frames containing a dozen or more conductive metal legs to attach them to the final printed circuit boards. The chips are connected to the legs by soldering ultrathin gold or silver wires to the aluminum contacts on the chips. Finally, the chips are enclosed in a plastic or ceramic capsule which is sealed with epoxy. The capsules are then tested for air-tightness by placing them in radioactive krypton and measuring them for leaks.

The completed chips are sold to electronics manufacturers where they are assembled on circuit boards and installed in a myriad of electronic products. There are, of course, many hundreds of advanced techniques which augment this basic semiconductor process.

Identifying Sources of Work-Related Exposures

Diversified electronics companies will store, use, and often recycle thousands of different materials. To satisfy various laws and regulations, these companies will maintain more than 3000 Material Safety Data Sheets for their employees and staff to utilize, and for physicians studying cases of work exposure. Unfortunately, MSDSs share the common problem of providing useful data on acute spill and leak containment and important information on flammability, but may be of little value to the clinical management of any given case of exposure. The treating physician should obtain the necessary MSDSs and any other available information from the company where the exposure occurred. In most cases, the MSDS does tell the contents of commercial products used, and from there, more traditional sources of information on toxicity can be consulted. The use of the chemical and the waste or byproducts may not be apparent. For example, a halogenated hydrocarbon may be used in a plasma etcher at very high temperature to degrade the chemical to phosgene and acid mists.

If the physician has established rapport with company health and safety personnel before the exposure occurs, she or he is much more likely to receive full disclosure of the event and its seriousness. Visiting the work place is important, not only to learn the nature of the work and the possibilities for injury and illness, but also to meet the other members of the health and safety team and to plan a team approach to the care that may later be rendered to workers.

The major problems resulting from microelectronics manufacture are related to acute exposure to chemicals, toxic gases, and dopant metals. Chronic illnesses resulting from chemical, metal, and gas exposure are not yet studied in this industry, and little is known regarding the widespread exposure of workers to ionizing and non-ionizing radiation. Major health studies are being contemplated by a number of countries, but, to date, only a few preliminary epidemiologic studies are available to assist the clinician in the attempt to diagnose and treat many of the exposure cases presented by the microelectronics industry.

EXPOSURE TO CHEMICALS

Solvents

A large percentage of microelectronics production workers are potentially exposed to solvents.[4] The number of solvents and their various classes present problems of clinical recognition and treatment. Solvents are known to affect every human organ system, but their presenting symptoms and signs are seldom specific to any given solvent or class of solvents. A study of the California semiconductor industry gives some idea of the solvent use of this growing manufacturing process, as shown in Table 77–9.[4]

In general, the common acute effects of solvent exposure are intoxication from depression of the central nervous system, irritation of the eyes and respiratory tract, and a defatting of the skin resulting in dermatoses. Acute exposure to solvents may result in loss of manual dexterity, response speed, coordination, or balance. Neurobehavioral effects of chronic exposure to low

Table 77–9. SOLVENT USAGE BY U.S. SEMICONDUCTOR COMPANIES IN 1988

SOLVENT	GALLONS
Acetone	890,000
Isopropanol (2-propanol)	786,000
Toluene	313,000
Trichloroethylene	273,000
n-Butyl acetate	240,000
Methanol	105,000
Xylene	97,000

Source: Rose Associates, Los Altos, CA.

doses of organic solvents demonstrate what is commonly referred to as the "psycho-organic syndrome." The hallmarks of this syndrome are memory disturbances, difficulties in understanding, and mood changes. Anxiety and depression occur later in the development of the chronic syndrome, along with dysfunction of the autonomic nervous system. The intensity and duration of exposure necessary to cause this problem are still being defined. This syndrome has not been clearly documented in this industry. Polyneuropathy also accompanies long-term exposure to some organic solvents. The growing recognition of the hazards of solvent exposure emphasizes the necessity to institute engineering controls in the workplace to protect workers from exposure to the solvents, to isolate workers from areas of possible solvent exposure, and to provide workers with appropriate protective clothing and respirators when necessary. The principal area of potential exposure in this industry is for chemical handlers and technicians in the photomasking areas.

Aliphatic Hydrocarbons

Alkanes, aliphatic hydrocarbons with single-bonded (saturated) carbons, are generally of low toxicity. An exception is *n*-hexane, capable of causing a severe peripheral neuropathy. The alkenes, with their double (unsaturated) bonds, are also of generally low toxicity.

Alcohols

Alcohols are more potent CNS depressants and irritants than are the aliphatic hydrocarbons. The most commonly used, isopropanol, irritates the eyes and respiratory tract to provide useful warning symptoms. At higher concentrations, CNS depression occurs but is seldom accompanied by neurobehavioral effects, probably because the threshold limit value (TLV) for isopropanol is determined by irritation, which occurs at levels far below those at which CNS effects would be anticipated.

Methanol is used in some microelectronics companies and should be suspected with cases of blurred vision or other visual disturbances.

Aromatic Hydrocarbons

Benzene produces a reversible pancytopenia, an aplastic anemia, and acute nonlymphocytic leukemia. It is the only solvent recognized to be a human carcinogen. For this reason, its use is being markedly curtailed. It is not frequently found in microelectronics formulation.

Toluene and xylene are stronger irritants and anesthetics (CNS depressants) than the aliphatics. Xylene is more acutely toxic in low doses than is toluene. Nonetheless, xylene appears to be a more common replacement for benzene in the microelectronics industry than is toluene. Toluene potentiates the effects of exposure to other solvents, especially benzene and chlorinated hydrocarbons. Persistent cerebellar ataxia has been reported in workers chronically exposed to toluene. Flushing is a prominent sign of xylene exposure. Xylene may cause sudden death by increasing myocardial sensitivity to epinephrine.

Phenols and Substituted Phenols

These compounds are solvents and have had particular application as "strippers." They are used to remove the photoresist materials from the wafers after the photolithographic process. They are irritants but also are strong CNS depressants. They penetrate the skin readily. As they are volatile, they easily create an inhalation hazard. Phenols may cause cardiac conduction disturbances and liver and kidney injury. Some of the substituted phenols may be strong cellular poisons.

Petroleum Distillates

Petroleum distillates are solvents composed of mixtures of aliphatic and aromatic hydrocarbons. Irritation and anesthesia increase as the percentage of aromatic hydrocarbons in the mixture increases. However, as the fraction becomes heavier, the volatility decreases, offsetting the toxicity.

Glycols

Ethylene glycol, a commonly used glycol, is not usually a problem in the work setting. This is because it has a very low vapor pressure and therefore does not present for inhalation; it is poorly absorbed by the skin. If heated to create a vapor, it would present a hazard. It is certainly toxic if accidentally ingested. However, in a fashion similar to most all solvents, it can produce a chronic dermatitis from the defatting of the skin.

Ketones

Ketones have irritant warning properties at levels well below those required to cause CNS depression. Acetone is one of the most commonly used solvents in this industry. Methyl ethyl ketone, widely used in microelectronics, does not cause peripheral neuropathy as does methyl *n*-butyl ketone, but it does potentiate the toxicity of other solvents.

Esters

N-butyl acetate is similar to other esters in having a very low odor threshold. Its distinctive sweet odor is one of the most characteristic smells of microelectronics manufacture. Esters are more potent anesthetics than corresponding alcohols, aldehydes, and ketones. However, they are also strong irritants, whose odor and irritation occur at levels that protect workers from CNS depression.

Glycol Ethers

These glycol ether solvents are frequently found in photoresists and other chemicals in the microelectronics industry. The trade name Cellosolve includes several alkyl-substituted glycol ethers. Encephalopathy in the absence of acute CNS depression has been reported in workers. Bone marrow toxicity resulting in pancytopenia is another acute effect of exposure reported anecdotally in a few cases. 2-Methoxyethanol, 2-ethoxyethanol, and their acetate derivatives result in reproductive toxicity in animals and are teratogenic. The butyl and propyl alkoxy ethanols may have less toxicity, and their substitution is being tested as a control measure.

Chlorinated Hydrocarbons

Chlorinated hydrocarbons represent a significant percentage, perhaps a majority, of the solvents used in the microelectronics industry. They are potent anesthetics, hepatotoxins, and nephrotoxins; many are demonstrated animal carcinogens. Their reproductive toxicity has not been extensively studied. Methylene chloride is converted to carbon monoxide, formaldehyde, and carbon dioxide in the body. Workers with elevated end-of-shift carboxyhemoglobin in the absence of cigarette smoking may reflect methylene chloride exposure, and the work setting should be appraised by an industrial hygienist. The principal chlorinated hydrocarbon exposures in the semiconductor industry appear to be 1,1,1-trichloroethane, trichloroethylene, tetrachloroethylene, and methylene chloride (dichloromethane). Chlorofluorocarbons are increasingly used by this industry and share some of the toxicity outcomes mentioned earlier. They are generally marketed and used under the tradename Freon. The halogenated hydrocarbons can cause respiratory tract irritation and bronchospasm in moderate exposures (above the TLV), and they sensitize the myocardium.

Photoresist Chemicals

The photolithographic processes that transpose circuit patterns to the surface of the silicon wafer do so by coating the wafer with light-sensitive materials known as photoresists. Photoresists may be composed of many different chemicals and characteristically undergo chemical reactions during the manufacturing process.

Adequate toxicology information about resins and polymers is seldom provided for their industrial applications. The toxicity of plastic monomers is greater than that of their respective polymers. For instance, the monomer vinyl chloride, used in the microelectronics industry, is carcinogenic, whereas the polymer of vinyl chloride is not. Likewise, vinyl chloride monomer is much more toxic than polyvinyl chloride. Glycol ethers are common solvent carrier vehicles in commercial photoresists, adding to the reproductive toxicity posed by resins and monomers.

Some of the many chemicals used in the photoresist phase of the manufacturing of microelectronic devices include styrene monomer, polyvinyl alcohol, polyvinyl cinnamate (a commonly used resin with no toxicology information available from the standard sources, the Registry of Toxic Effects of Chemical Substances or others), isoprenes, various butadienes, bisphenol A diglycidyl ether, various metal halides, phenol formaldehyde, and urethanes. The list could be quite formidable.

When exposure is suspected, the number and complexity of these chemicals make it a necessity to search out each component and then to consider the literature regarding most of the chemicals as being far from a complete toxicologic review of the possible biologic effects.

Hydrofluoric Acid

Acids and alkalis are used in great volume by the microelectronics industry. A survey in California found their application in greater volume than that of the organic solvents. This discussion will cover the recognition and treatment of hydrofluoric acid burns, since they represent the most common burn injury and illness and are typically of far more clinical significance than other chemical burns. Some other agents causing chemical burns in the industry include sulfuric acid, peroxides, nitric acid, phenols, methylene chloride, and cryogenics.

Hydrofluoric acid burns occur primarily from splashes onto unprotected areas of skin or through porous leaks in protective gloves. The acid, in dilute concentration, can penetrate the skin without pain and begin a process of tissue damage which is itself the result of fluoride's interference with cellular enzymes and damage to cellular membranes and organelles. Concentrated hydrofluoric acid, as in the case of other strong acids, will result in burning of the skin and thus provide a better indication of the need for lavage.

Blanched tissue results from burns with concentrated acid (greater than 40 per cent). There is a characteristic blanching of the nail bed when dilute acid has been allowed to penetrate the cuticle margin. Erythema, swelling, and pain ensue. Blisters are uncommon with hydrofluoric acid burns. The skin color may darken as the subcutaneous damage progresses to frank necrosis of wide areas and deep ulcerations. Although these findings may vary depending on location and extent of the burn, the symptom of pain is reliable in determining the continuing damage to tissues.

Immediate treatment is important because the patient may be in extreme pain, tissue destruction is taking place, and there is a risk that death may ensue from a sudden cardiac event resulting from the hypocalcemia that accompanies systemic effects of fluoride ion absorption.

Emergency treatment of all suspected and confirmed hydrofluoric acid burns consists of copious water lavage with running water for 15 minutes. In most cases of hydrofluoric acid splash to skin surfaces, no symptoms will result following this simple practice of lavage. When pain occurs, early on in the case of concentrated acid burns and over a period of many hours depending on the level of dilution of the acid, the burn must be considered significant and fluoride inactivation with calcium gluconate undertaken. The patient should keep the affected skin area in magnesium sulfate (25%) or a quaternary ammonium compound (Zephiran) for 15 minutes (other solutions or vehicles may be effective but require available calcium or magnesium). If the pain ceases, no further tissue damage is taking place. If pain persists, it is a reliable indication that further treatment is needed.

Injection of calcium gluconate (5 to 10 per cent concentration) with the smallest needle available (30 gauge) is done directly under the swelling of the skin until the pain is abated. No more calcium gluconate should be injected than is required to reach cessation of pain. It is best to disregard suggestions to mix calcium gluconate with lidocaine (Xylocaine) since this practice may erase the value of the pain end-point. Generally 0.5 ml of 10 per cent calcium gluconate per cm^2 of burned tissue is used. For digits, avoid overinjection as this may cause vascular compromise; use no more than 0.5 ml per phalanx. Never inject calcium chloride.

Nailbed burns do not lend themselves to injection with calcium gluconate. In this very painful burn, removal of the nail is usually necessary. The patient should be followed for pain relief after the digital block has worn off.

Bullae should be debrided, and burn areas can be dressed with calcium gluconate preparations. Healing occurs rapidly once the pain and tissue damage have been reversed.

Calcium gluconate gel has been advanced as a treatment measure for minor burns where injection of small quantities of calcium gluconate would have been necessary. The gel must be applied with lengthy massage and has not been studied sufficiently. In the usual treatment setting, it is more appropriate to attempt the soaking for 15 minutes, followed by injection, to obtain reliable results with treatment. In serious extremity burns, intra-arterial calcium infusions have been used by a limited number of clinicians.

Microelectronics workers can be exposed to hydrofluoric acid mists that may seriously burn respiratory tissues. Hydrofluoric acid burns of the eyes are acute emergencies. Whatever the area of burn, immediate recognition and conservative medical management are warranted.

Toxic Gases

Arsine is the most toxic of the gases used in the microelectronics industry. Exposure to 250 ppm is instantly lethal. Exposure to 25 to 50 ppm is lethal after 30 minutes, and exposure to 10 ppm is lethal after longer exposures. Arsine, the hydride gas used in diffusion furnaces and ion implanters to deposit arsenic on the surface of silicon wafers, is the most toxic form of arsenic. The older literature stresses the delayed hemolysis and ensuing renal failure of arsine exposure cases. However, because of numerous fatalities in recent years in semiconductor plants, further clinical features should be emphasized.

Arsine gas is a pancytotoxin, toxic to every mammalian organ thus far studied. It is almost immediately toxic to the central nervous system, creating confusion in victims of exposure. This will be a serious problem when an event occurs that requires clear heads to formulate an evacuation plan. It is toxic to the lungs, resulting in pulmonary edema with massive exposure. Death occurred promptly following exposure of seven Japanese workers in recent accidents. The deaths may have resulted from a combination of immediate heart, lung, and CNS effects. Arsine is also toxic to the liver, kidney, gastrointestinal tract, bone marrow, and skeletal muscle, in addition to its better-known effect of massive hemolysis.

The common clinical picture of a moderate exposure is that of presenting symptoms of headache, malaise, abdominal pain, nausea, and vomiting. Over the course of 2 to 24 hours, these symptoms are followed by hematuria, which is first recognized by the patient as tea-colored urine and a bronzelike jaundice. Hepatosplenomegaly may be prominent.

Laboratory evaluation of the patient will demonstrate a severe hemolytic anemia. Plasma-free hemoglobin is elevated (>1.5 gm/dl) and, when accompanied by a history of arsine exposure and symptoms, is an indication for exchange transfusions. Acute renal failure will continue to develop if arsenic-impregnated red blood cells are allowed to continue to circulate. Treatment by maintaining the hematocrit with blood loss replacement is inadequate. If renal failure develops, hemodialysis is indicated until renal function returns. Alkaline diuresis will favor solubility and help prevent the precipitation of hemoglobin in the kidney. Exchange transfusions are vital because hemolysis will continue as long as the nondialyzable arsine-hemoglobin-haptoglobulin complex remains in the blood. British antilewisite (BAL) is not effective in the treatment of arsine poisoning. Lower-dose exposures may cause headache, confusion, and lethargy without hemolysis.

Arsine gas represents one of the most serious community hazards posed by the microelectronics industry. The dopant gas is vital to the industry, and no replacement material of less toxicity is soon to be introduced in the many hundreds of locations using the gas. Arsine is conveyed in metal cylinders that require manufacturing, filling, and mixing; transportation by truck or railbed; often refilling and mixing; and delivery to the company before the cylinder is installed in a furnace or implanter and calibrated for use. One cylinder of gas released in a plant could provide sufficient arsine to deliver a lethal dose through the ventilation system to virtually all the production force. The question of evacuation and treatment in this setting is almost academic, with many worst-case scenarios. Most companies provide extensive engineering controls and seldom use 100 per cent gas. However, pure arsine is used in the production of gallium-arsenide devices. Smaller companies often do not have adequate engineering controls as they are costly.

The loss of a cylinder of gas from a delivery truck could provide a lethal level of gas for several square blocks of the community, resulting in hundreds of fatalities. Hospital emergency departments are equipped to provide the life-saving treatment of choice to only a few of the many thousands of residents of an exposed community who would survive with exchange transfusion if such quantities of blood were available. How does a community plan for a disaster that will require hundreds of exchange transfusions?

Phosphine

Phosphine is the hydride of phosphorus, which, like arsenic, is a common dopant in the semiconductor industry. Phosphine gas is highly toxic and has an IDLH (immediately dangerous to life and health) level of 200 ppm. Its toxicity is similar to that of arsine, with pulmonary edema and myocardial and CNS depression as early effects of exposure. Phosphine also affects the kidney, liver, and peripheral muscles and rarely causes a hemolysis of limited extent and significance. Unlike the case with arsenic, there is no single, life-saving treatment for phosphine poisoning. Treatment is nonspecific and supportive. Long-term effects are not known.

As with arsine, phosphine provides considerable concern to the community with its transportation, storage, and utilization in multiple industrial sites. Phosphine is often transported and used in 100 per cent concentration. This is not necessary to any particular manufacturing process. It is merely a convenience in process control not to have to make as many cylinder changes as are required by the use of phosphine in cylinders of lower concentration—a good example of the need for health and safety staff participation in the planning phase of industrial operations, for the increased risk of exposure of workers and the community to phosphine gas may be a consideration overlooked by industrial engineers.

The common use of 100 per cent phosphine makes it a good example of an extremely hazardous gas. It is flammable, pyrophoric, and toxic, with a permissible exposure level (PEL) of 0.3 ppm. The maximum concentration tolerated is 100 to 190 ppm for about 1 hour—death occurs within a few minutes at 2000 ppm. Accidental release of a 20-pound cylinder (the small cylinders are often referred to as lecture bottles, holding about one tenth the quantity of gas as a standard cylinder) of this gas would require a block of air 10 feet high covering 1792 acres of 276 city blocks (21,755,000 cubic meters of air) to dilute to its threshold limit value (TLV) of 0.3 ppm.

Diborane

Diborane is an extremely reactive gas and immediately affects the respiratory tract, resulting in pulmonary edema. Probably because of this response, a clear-cut clinical presentation of diborane toxicity is lacking. The symptoms of mild-to-moderate exposure to diborane are likened to metal fume fever, with tightness and burning in the chest, coughing, shortness of breath, chills, fever, nausea, and shivering. CNS effects include drowsiness, headaches, and vertigo. As with phosphine poisoning, there is no treatment of diborane exposure except that of supportive measures.

Dopant Metals

A wide variety of metals are used in small quantity to change the electrical characteristics of the silicon wafer substrate. The most common are arsenic, phosphorus, and boron. Arsenic is a common trace metal in the diet. As found in fish, particularly shellfish, arsenic is organically bound and not toxic to the mammalian species. Pentavalent arsenic (arsenate) is common in the soil and of low toxicity to humans.

It is trivalent arsenic trioxide (arsenite) that is toxic to humans. This poison of legendary potency is now recognized as a carcinogen as well. Trivalent arsenic is associated with skin cancers in chemical workers and winemakers. It has resulted in angiosarcoma of the liver through consumption of arsenic-contaminated drinking water and wine.

Arsenic trioxide is absorbed primarily by inhalation and ingestion. It is rapidly taken up by red blood cells, then redistributed to a number of organs, primarily the kidney, liver, and muscles. Metabolism results in urinary excretion of 70 per cent of As_2O_3 as methylated arsenous acid and in the less toxic arsenate form. Biomethylation thus results in effective detoxification of a significant portion of arsenite. Within 30 hours, half the arsenite is excreted. After 1 week, only traces are found in the body, principally in the keratin-containing tissues, thus the popularity of measuring long-term arsenic exposure in hair and nails (a poor method for individual diagnosis).

The use of arsenic trioxide for incidental production in the semiconductor industry has caused concern among health and safety professionals because the material is both toxic and carcinogenic. Carcinogenicity is basically preventable by monitoring arsenic exposure. Unfortunately, there is no reliable test of arsenic exposure in low-level exposures. A blood or urine arsenic assay may be helpful in the case of an acute exposure, but periodic surveillance tests for arsenic are seldom of value.

What is needed is an inexpensive laboratory assay for inorganic metabolites rather than the assay for total arsenic (atomic absorption). This test is not available except in a few reference laboratories, and at currently prohibitive costs.

It is also clear that arsine gas, when inhaled in low concentrations, is excreted as trivalent arsenic and may reflect that arsine is a carcinogen requiring further regulation in the workplace.

SOURCES OF EXPOSURE

Arsenic Compounds

Several sources of potential exposure to arsenic compounds exist in the semiconductor industry. Arsine, the hydride of arsenic and distinctly different from other inorganic arsenic compounds, is highly toxic acutely. It also forms small amounts of arsenic trioxide in air, but, more significantly, it forms arsenic trioxide when burned. Many of the semiconductor processes using arsine are done at high temperatures. Arsine cracks at about 260 to 315.5° C (500 to 600° F). Therefore, arsenic or arsenic trioxide is deposited out on many surfaces of reaction vessels. Ion implantation of dopants minimizes this effect; that is, the efficiency of the deposition is much greater.

In gallium arsenide wafer crystal growth, 100 per cent arsine is frequently used; the reaction chamber requires frequent cleaning (as often as after each run). The inside of the chamber is coated with a black arsenic coating, which is usually scraped off by a technician. At many facilities, workers have been observed to accomplish this procedure without any protective clothing or breathing devices, even though large amounts of arsenic dust are produced during this operation.[5]

Likewise, ion implanters require periodic maintenance and cleaning as they have critical parts that may form deposits. Cleaning is usually done by removing the part and bringing it to a maintenance area where bead-blasting is done. The bead material becomes contaminated with the arsenic and must be handled as hazardous waste. Frequently, these maintenance areas are poorly controlled and unmonitored. We have seen some with gross contamination of all surfaces in the room. Poor worker education and the infrequency of the operation have contributed to unacceptable levels of contamination.

Sawing of the gallium arsenide wafers also carries the potential for worker exposure. Recent literature has demonstrated that the arsenic in gallium arsenide may be released in biologic matrices, allowing absorption of arsenic. Therefore, sources of respirable gallium arsenide must be viewed as possible sources of arsenic exposure. Pump oils represent another source of exposure to various contaminants, including heavy metals. The pump oils for furnaces, ion implanters, chemical vapor deposition chambers, and other devices should be considered as contaminated with toxic substrates until consistently proved otherwise.

Hydrogen Fluoride

Hydrogen fluoride is used as an etchant for the wafers; however, it is also used for cleaning the quartz tubes used in the furnaces. These tubes are placed into horizontal or vertical tube washers and concentrated hydrofluoric acid may be used to clean them. Because of poor ergonomic design or ventilation system failures, this operation may allow employees to be exposed to the HF. Dry or plasma etchers are used in the production of the wafers. Various chemicals are used in conjunction with the radiofrequency-generated high temperatures to etch the wafer. Hydrochloric acid, chlorinated hydrocarbons (including chloroform and carbon tetrachloride), or Freons are used for this purpose. They all have the potential to form active free radicals in the chamber and free halogen radicals. If there is a leak, HF and hydrochloric acid will be produced in conjunction with other possible materials, such as carbonyl chloride (phosgene) or carbonyl fluoride. Even when the chemicals do not escape, they may collect in the pump oils. Minor cracks in the housing of the plasma etchers may allow radiofrequency radiation to escape into the operator's work area.[6]

Photoresists

Photoresist compounds consist of a variety of chemicals necessary to produce positive or negative images on the wafers. They are generally UV- or light-reactive. The formulation of these materials is difficult to obtain because they are generally ornate compounds of particular proprietary concern. Various solvents are used in conjunction with them, including xylenes, glycol ethers, and related materials. The stripping agents (used to remove the unpolymerized material after light exposure) are often methylene chloride or phenolic compounds that are corrosive and are often volatile enough to present inhalation hazards. They also frequently have significant dermal penetration. Systemic toxicity must therefore be considered.

Physical Agents

Ionizing radiation at ion implanters, lasers in various equipment, radiofrequency radiation at plasma etchers and other devices, and ultraviolet at align and masking stations should also be considered as sources of worker exposure.

General Problems

The dry atmosphere of the cleanroom and the potential low levels of airborne irritants (acids, solvents, and so on) provide an atmosphere that is not optimal for many workers. Bronchitis or asthma may be exacerbated by these environmental conditions. Most important, for the whole industry there are insufficient baseline industrial hygiene data and medical information. Similarly, medical monitoring programs have not been widely employed in this industry. Methods of biologic monitoring for many of the compounds are not established, and because of legal concerns companies often are loath to experiment and develop needed methodologies. The turnover of employees in this industry is substantial; the workers often find similar jobs at other companies. It is therefore necessary to be able to track such employees from one place of employment to another for any longitudinal studies of health risks. This undertaking would require an industry-wide, standard medical program.

Modern facilities store most of the chemicals in properly segregated block houses with specially designed plumbing to deliver the reagents to the laboratory. However, some small quantities of bulk chemical are brought into the laboratory manually. This is usually done by a designated and specially trained "chemical handler." These individuals will transport and handle the chemicals, such as filling tanks, reservoirs, and related devices, and should have more intensive medical evaluation and surveillance. Maintenance workers are also usually overlooked.

Community Exposures

The effect of these facilities on the community has been addressed only recently. Although in several areas of the country groundwater has been contaminated because of the leakage of solvents from underground storage tanks, the potential for pollution beyond that of the solvents has not been evaluated. In particular, the effluent of arsenic from semiconductor plants has not been quantified at most facilities. Although ion implantation for doping silicon wafers does not present a large amount of arsenic as effluent, those facilities in the manufacture of gallium arsenide and related devices often use 100 per cent arsine for epitaxial growth, and this procedure uses large amounts of arsine with low efficiency of deposition on the wafer. Thus, more than 90 per cent of the arsine used becomes effluent. The amount of fugitive emissions is unknown. Some arsine is contained in solid waste from maintenance operations on the equipment, and if it is recognized and properly contained, it will be disposed of as hazardous waste and require recycling or burial at a Class I landfill. However, the bulk of the material will leave the chamber as gaseous effluent.

Several systems may attempt to recover the arsenic. Charcoal filters may be used to trap the arsine. Alternatively, the arsine is burned to form arsenic trioxide, and the As_2O_3 is then scrubbed to recover the material in a liquid phase. The resultant material then must be treated and solidified and buried in another appropriate manner. Most semiconductor companies, however, have not routinely monitored the exact efficiencies of these systems. Other innovative systems are being implemented to attempt to increase the efficiency of the process and to control emissions. As many smaller facilities are in mixed industrial-residential zoned areas, the impact on the community should be assessed.

New and Future Technology

The development of novel process techniques and variations of existing methods are as diverse as the applications of these devices. Light-emitting diodes (LEDs) of different colors, solar energy panels, infrared circuitry, and many other uses have necessitated that greater electronic acuity, thermal properties, resistance to ionizing radiation and other factors be considered and employed.

This industry has also developed and employs the use of various special metals for packaging the chips, new electrically conductive epoxies, novel ceramics, and compound substrates. The compound substrates consist of more than a single element in the base crystal (e.g., silicon) and may include gallium, indium, arsenic, silicon, germanium, phosphorus, and other elements. Photoactive chemicals, solvents, lasers, ion implanters, etching techniques and other aspects of chip manufacture continue to evolve, making this a dynamic industry and therefore a challenge for the medical community to understand and evaluate the potential exposures.

CONCLUSION

It hardly overstates the case to say that the microelectronics industry provides the complete spectrum of occupational exposures found in most industries: a broad spectrum of chemicals, metals, dusts; physical hazards such as ionizing and non-ionizing radiation; ergonomic and psychologic stressors; and various other hazards such as explosion, fire, and, a major cause of fatalities to date, electrocution.

As this industry establishes diversified companies throughout the world, health and safety professionals will need to become familiar with the spectrum of toxic materials and the need to recognize and suggest remedial measures in the workplace.

References

1. LaDou J (ed): The microelectronics industry. State of the Art Reviews: Occupational Medicine 1(1):Jan-Mar 1986. Hanley & Belfus, Inc., available by writing PO Box 1377, Philadelphia, PA 19105-9990.
2. California Work Injuries and Illnesses, July, 1989. Department of Industrial Relations, Division of Labor Statistics and Research, PO Box 603, San Francisco, CA 94101.
3. Robbins PJ, Butler CR, Mahaffey KR: Occupational Injury and Illness in the Semiconductor Industry for 1980–1985. NIOSH Report. Available from Robert A. Taft Laboratories, 4676 Columbia Parkway, Cincinnati, OH 45226-1998.
4. Wade R, Williams M, Thomas M: Semiconductor Industry Study. California Department of Industrial Relations, Division of Occupational Safety and Health, Taskforce on the Electronics Industry, 1981.
5. Yoshida T, Shimamura T, Kitagawa H, Shigeta S: Enhancement of the proliferative response of peripheral blood lymphocytes of workers in semiconductor plants (translated from Japanese). Indust Health 25:29–33, 1987.
6. Wald PH, Jones J: Semiconductor manufacturing: A review of processes and hazards. Am J Indust Med 11(2):203–221, 1987.

CHAPTER 78

CHLORINATED HYDROCARBONS

Brian F. Keaton, MD, FACEP

Chlorinated hydrocarbons are commonly encountered industrial chemicals. For the most part, they are excellent organic solvents and are relatively inexpensive. Most are liquids at room temperature but are extremely volatile, and fortunately, most are nonflammable. These properties make them valuable as degreasing agents, dry cleaning compounds, paint removers, and as vehicles for paints and varnishes.[1] This group also includes two common household products containing trichloroethane.

Because of the high volatility of chlorinated hydrocarbons, most significant exposures are via the pulmonary route, with gastrointestinal and cutaneous exposures assuming much less significance. An exception to this rule is carbon tetrachloride, which can be absorbed through the skin in toxic amounts. Most of these agents cause dose-related central nervous system (CNS) depression progressing through the stages of general anesthesia. Hepatotoxicity is common, and while skin sensitization is rare, extreme drying and cracking of the skin is seen with some of the degreasing agents in this group. Experimental evidence has suggested that exposure to chemicals in this group can sensitize the myocardium to the effect of endogenous catecholamines.[1]

Diagnosis is usually made based on the history of exposure and the patient's physical presentation. Other than providing baseline information regarding hepatic, pulmonary, hematologic, and renal function, the laboratory is seldom of significant help during the initial evaluation and treatment of these patients as most of these toxins are not screened by standard toxicology techniques. In fact, most of these chemicals are cleared via the lungs, making analysis of the exhaled gasses the preferred screening method: this is not readily available to most emergency care providers.

With few exceptions, treatment is supportive, with removal from the source of exposure and decontamination being most important. Special attention must be paid to airway support and oxygenation. It is also crucial that the rescuer and medical personnel involved in the treatment of the victims be protected from exposure to the toxin. Gloves, gowns, double bagging of all contaminated clothing, adequate ventilation, and careful and repeated hand washing are essential. These victims frequently suffer delayed pulmonary, hepatic, renal, and neurologic dysfunction, making careful follow-up extremely important. Some of the chemicals in this group are also known or suspected carcinogens and teratogens. While all of the short-chain aliphatic chlorinated hydrocarbons are found in the environment in minute quantities, they are fairly rapidly degraded to carbon dioxide, water, and the chloride ion. With few exceptions, there is no evidence of significant bioaccumulation or risk to man via the food chain.[2]

Methyl Chloride

Until several years ago, methyl chloride (chloromethane, CH_3Cl) was used extensively as a refrigerant. However, its significant and sometimes fatal acute CNS depression and reported persistent neurologic and psychiatric sequelae have made it a seldom-used chemical today.[1] It is now used primarily as a methylating agent in the chemical industry, where chronic exposure has been associated with a variety of neurologic symptoms.[3] Acute exposure can cause headache, CNS depression, seizures, anorexia, nausea, vomiting, and conjunctivitis. Methyl chloride is a gas at room temperature but is usually encountered as a liquid under pressure. Exposure to escaping gasses can result in freezing of the exposed tissues. Treatment consists of removal from the contaminating environment, decontamination, general supportive care, and observation for delayed or persistent neurologic sequelae.[4] Most patients experience a complete recovery within 10 to 30 days, although long-term CNS disability has been reported, ranging from depression to peripheral neuropathies. The

Threshold Limit Value (TLV) for methyl chloride is 100 ppm.[5]

Methylene Chloride

Methylene chloride (CH_2Cl_2) is an extremely volatile, colorless, relatively nontoxic liquid that is a very potent solvent and extraction agent. It is a common ingredient in paint removers and strippers. While it has the same potential for direct CNS depression common to all of the chlorinated hydrocarbons, it has the additional toxic potential of being metabolized to carbon monoxide (CO) in humans. This is usually not a problem when used in a well-ventilated environment. Studies have demonstrated that exposures to 100 ppm of methylene chloride for 7.5 hours result in carboxyhemoglobin (COHb) saturations of approximately 3 per cent, which is well within accepted standards.[6] However, if used in a poorly ventilated area, local concentrations can reach dangerously high levels quickly, resulting in severe carbon monoxide poisoning. There is a linear relationship between the COHb level and the methylene chloride exposure concentrations.[6] The signs and symptoms and the management of the methylene chloride–induced carbon monoxide poisoning are the same as for the more common respiratory exposure to carbon monoxide. Because of continued metabolism of methylene chloride to carbon monoxide, the treatment of methylene chloride–induced carbon monoxide poisoning is often prolonged. Increased physical activity tends to increase the metabolism of methylene chloride to carbon monoxide, and patients with underlying coronary artery disease are more sensitive to the toxic effects of the increasing COHb level.[6] A large study has failed to demonstrate any evidence linking chronic low-level methylene chloride exposure to a decreased life span.[7] Another rare though potentially serious hazard associated with methylene chloride is the danger of phosgene gas formation via combustion.[1] The permissible exposure limit for methylene chloride is 100 ppm with a TLV of 250 ppm.[5]

Chloroform

Chloroform (trichloromethane, $CHCl_3$) was initially used as an anesthetic agent, but its use in this capacity was discontinued as a result of severe hepatic and renal toxicity. Its primary use today is as an industrial solvent and chemical intermediary. It is a sweet-smelling and tasting liquid that is colorless, nonflammable, extremely volatile, and highly lipid soluble. It is known to be carcinogenic in laboratory animals, and its use in foods and pharmaceuticals has been essentially eliminated by the Food and Drug Administration (FDA).[8]

Chloroform is a potent anesthetic, and acute toxicity is the result of profound CNS depression. In humans, death has been reported with ingestions of as little as 10 ml orally. Prolonged or repeated exposures can result in severe hepatotoxicity characterized by centrilobular necrosis. Fatty degeneration has been described in kidney, liver, and heart. This damage is felt to be caused by hepatic microsomal oxidation of chloroform via the P_{450} system to phosgene, which then binds to hepatic and renal macromolecules, leading to necrosis (Fig. 78–1).[9] It has been experimentally shown that pretreatment with certain agents (e.g., piperonyl butoxide) that block this enzyme system leads to a reduction of hepatic damage, though treatment with this agent 1 hour after chloroform administration was of no benefit.[10] Pretreatment with

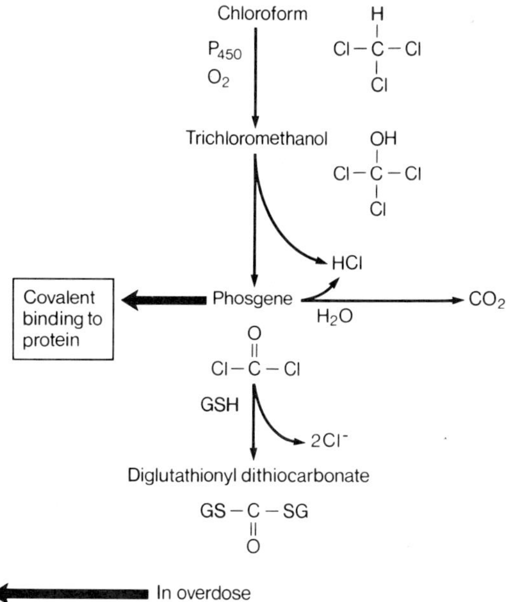

Figure 78–1. Metabolism and mechanism of toxicity of chloroform.

diethyl maleate, an agent that depletes glutathione stores, or P_{450} induction with an agent such as phenobarbital has been shown to significantly increase hepatotoxicity.[10, 11]

Symptoms resulting from acute exposure via pulmonary, gastrointestinal, or dermal routes are dose related. Chloroform cannot be detected by the human nose until concentrations exceed 400 ppm. Exposures of 1000 ppm for 10 minutes can result in nausea, vomiting, headache, and vertigo. Exposures of 1000 to 4000 ppm cause disorientation, and concentrations of 10,000 to 20,000 ppm result in loss of consciousness and may be fatal. Contact with the skin results in a local dermatitis caused by defatting of the tissues, and eye contact results in corneal irritation via the same mechanism.[9] Chronic low-level exposures can cause lassitude, marked mental dullness, and gastrointestinal disturbances, though no changes in liver function tests are seen.[8]

Management of acute exposures is entirely supportive and includes removal from the contaminating environment and decontamination. Special attention must be paid to liver and renal function.

The recommended National Institute for Occupational Safety and Health (NIOSH) standards for industrial exposures is 10 ppm as a time-weighted average for a 10-hour work day and 40-hour work week, and 50 ppm for any 10 minute period.[12]

Carbon Tetrachloride

Carbon tetrachloride (tetrachloromethane, CCl_4) is a clear, colorless, nonflammable liquid with a sweet odor similar to that of chloroform. Historically, it has been used as an anesthetic agent, a dry cleaning agent, an antihelminthic, a dry shampoo, a degreaser, a grain fumigant, and a fire retardant. Because of its excessive toxicity, its use has been severely restricted by the FDA, and now it is used primarily as an intermediary in the synthesis of refrigerants, solvents, and propellants; as a solvent in chromatography; and to extract tin from scrap metal.[1] Major spills of carbon tetrachloride have resulted in the contamination of drinking water; however, no serious sequelae have been reported.[13]

Carbon tetrachloride is a potent anesthetic and is capable of causing death from its CNS depression alone. However, it is also an extremely potent hepatic and renal toxin. In the liver, carbon tetrachloride has been shown to cause its toxic effect via two different mechanisms. The first involves disruption of the hepatocyte's ability to bind triglycerides to lipoprotein carriers, resulting in intracellular accumulation of lipids and fatty degeneration of the liver. The second mechanism of toxicity involves the formation of an extremely toxic metabolite, which causes cell death and centrilobular hepatic necrosis.[14] This metabolic process is mediated via the P_{450} microsomal enzyme system, and prior induction of this sytem by agents such as ethanol enhance the hepatotoxicity of carbon tetrachloride. Renal damage occurs as a result of the direct effects of carbon tetrachloride on the proximal tubule and the loop of Henle.[1] A variety of other problems have been attributed to chronic carbon tetrachloride exposure. These include dermatitis secondary to skin defatting, polyneuritis, visual deficits, parkinsonism, bone marrow depression, hepatic and renal dysfunction, and cirrhosis. There is no evidence that carbon tetrachloride is carcinogenic.[1] Carbon tetrachloride has a prolonged half-life in the body and is still detectable in exhaled gasses as long as a month after exposure.[8]

Following acute exposure, the patient experiences nausea, vomiting, abdominal pain, and CNS depression proportionate to the severity of the exposure. Patients who survive the acute CNS depressant effects and regain consciousness may become asymptomatic or have persistent nausea and anorexia.

A latent period often ensues. Patients have been discharged or transferred to a psychiatric unit because of apparent recovery, only to have them develop hepatic and/or renal shutdown during the following 24 to 72 hours.

Liver enzymes are usually significantly elevated by 48 hours post exposure, with the clinical signs of hepatitis developing in the next several days. Acute renal failure caused by acute tubular necrosis becomes clinically evident at 1 to 7 days post exposure. Renal failure in the absence of hepatitis is occasionally seen. There is marked individual variation as to susceptibility to the toxic effect of carbon tetrachloride, though pre-existing hepatic and/or renal disease and alcohol abuse tend to predispose the patient to increased severity.[8]

Treatment is, for the most part, supportive, with removal from the contaminating environment and decontamination being of highest initial priority. Prolonged in-hospital observation is necessary to avoid missing the delayed hepatorenal complications. Hemodialysis may be necessary if the acute renal failure is severe. If the patient survives the acute exposure and the initial hepatorenal failure with its attendant host of complications, recovery can be complete over a period of months.[1] Several theoretically sound suggestions have been made in the literature regarding possible specific treatments for carbon tetrachloride poisoning. These include the use of *N*-acetylcysteine to bind the toxic metabolite phosgene and to supply a source for the formation of glutathione (similar to the way it is currently used for acetaminophen poisoning), use of 16, 16-dimethyl prostaglandin E_2 to block the accumulation of intracellular lipids, and hyperbaric oxygen. All have promise theoretically and a few limited animal studies have been encouraging; however, at this time, there is no indication for use of these treatments in humans.[8, 15]

The recommended TLV for carbon tetrachloride is 10 ppm, and the NIOSH standard is 2 ppm as a time-weighted average for a 10-hour day and a 40-hour work week.[16]

Ethyl Chloride

Ethyl chloride (chloroethane, monochloroethane, chloroethyl, CH_3CH_2Cl) is a gas at room temperature that is easily liquefied under pressure. It is used primarily as a chemical intermediary in the production of tetraethyl lead and other ethyl compounds, as a solvent in perfumes, and as a topical anesthetic, where it is sprayed on the skin to "freeze" a local area.[1] It is mildly anesthetic in high concentrations and can be irritating to mucous membranes. Contact with the liquefied gas can cause frostbite. Its systemic toxicity is limited, with a TLV of 1000 ppm.[4] Treatment is symptomatic and supportive.

1,1-Dichloroethane and 1,2-Dichloroethane

Though both 1,1-dichloroethane (ethylidene dichloride, CH_3CHCl_2) and 1,2-dichloroethane (ethylene dichloride, CH_2ClCH_2Cl) are isomers that have similar properties and industrial uses, the bulk of medical experience has been with 1,2-dichloroethane. Both are used as solvents and degreasers and as chemical intermediaries. 1,2-dichloroethane is used primarily as a lead scavenger in leaded gasolines and in the synthesis of vinyl chlorides. Toxic exposures result in dose-related anesthesia, headaches, dizziness, nausea, vomiting, and abdominal pain. Severe exposures can lead to hepatic and renal injury. Following removal from the contaminating environment and decontamination, treatment is entirely supportive. Recent animal studies suggesting that 1,2-dichloroethane might be carcinogenic have resulted in a reduction in the NIOSH limits to 1 ppm determined as a time-weighted average over a 10-hour work day, with a ceiling limit of 2 ppm for any 15-minute period. The standard for the 1,1-dichloroethane isomer is 100 ppm.[1]

1,1,1-Trichloroethane

1,1,1-Trichloroethane (methyl chloroform, CH_3CCl_3) is one of the most widely encountered halogenated hydrocarbons. Two common household products containing this chemical include Liquid Paper (52% methyl chloroform) and Scott's Liquid Gold. Liquid Paper overdose by inhalation and particularly by ingestion is not an uncommon cause of emergency department visits, particularly in the teen-age population. It is used in industry as a metal cleaner and degreaser, as a solvent, an aerosol propellant, a dry cleaning agent, and a pesticide.[17] A colorless and nonflammable liquid, it has an odor similar to chloroform and, for the most part, is of very low toxicity.[18] Only a handful of fatal cases have been reported, and all of these have been a result of prolonged closed-space respiratory exposures. Such fatalities are felt to be caused by respiratory depression secondary to the general CNS depressant effects of this agent. Some researchers also suggest that this agent sensitizes the myocardium to the effects of endogenous epinephrine, leading to increased risk of fatal dysrhythmias.[1] There is no evidence that chronic exposure to this agent causes significant hepatic, renal, or cardiovascular damage.[18] Diagnosis is usually based on clinical and historical information, with the laboratory offering little assistance. If available, gas chromatography of the patient's expired gases can be used to confirm diagnosis.

Treatment is supportive. With environmental exposure, symptoms resolve rapidly after the patient is removed from the contaminating environment and the general anesthetic effects of the agent are allowed to run their course.[17] Contaminated clothing should be removed, and the patient should be washed with soap and water. Health care workers should wear rubber gloves while cleaning these patients. With overdose, emergency management and in-hospital observation and supportive care may be indicated.

The recommended TLV for exposure is 350 ppm. There have been no reported teratogenic or carcinogenic properties.[19]

1,1,2-Trichloroethane

1,1,2-Trichloroethane (vinyl trichloride, $CH_2ClCHCl_2$) is an isomer of methyl chloroform that is a stronger anesthetic than methyl chloroform. It is also an irritant to mucous membranes and significantly toxic to the liver and kidneys. It is suspected as a human carcinogen, which has led to a strict NIOSH exposure standard of 10 ppm. Treatment is entirely supportive.[1]

1,1,2,2-Tetrachloroethane

1,1,2,2-Tetrachloroethane (acetylene tetrachloride, $CHCl_2CHCl_2$) is one of the best solvents among the chlorinated hydrocarbons. However, it is also among the most toxic. Its toxicity is similar to but much more severe than that seen with carbon tetrachloride. For this reason, it has been almost completely eliminated from industrial use in the United States. Early signs of toxicity include fine hand tremor, vertigo, headache, abdominal pain, anorexia, nausea, constipation, lethargy, and paresthesias. Hepatic toxicity results in acute or subacute zonal necrosis and steatosis with hepatomegaly and jaundice. The NIOSH standard is 1 ppm as a time-weighted average for a 10-hour work day and 40-hour work week.[1, 20]

1,2-Dichloroethylene

1,2-Dichloroethylene (1,2-dichloroethane, acetylene dichloride, CHCl=CHCl) is used as a low-temperature extracting agent for heat-sensitive materials such as perfumes and for decaffeinated coffee. It is a mild CNS depressant and is otherwise without significant toxicity.[1] Treatment is symptomatic.

1,1-Dichloroethene

1,1-Dichloroethene (vinylidene chloride, $CH_2{=}CCl_2$) is used as a reagent in the formation of copolymeric plastics and has hepatic and nephrotoxicity similar to that seen with carbon tetrachloride. Laboratory studies have shown it to be associated with hepatic hemangiosarcomas and bronchoalveolar adenomas. Treatment is supportive, with special attention paid to hepatic and renal function.[1]

Trichloroethylene

Trichloroethylene (acetylene trichloride, trichloroethene, $CHCl{=}CCl_2$) is a solvent used most commonly in vapor degreasing operations as well as in the dry cleaning of fabrics, in selective extraction of medicines and foods, and as a chemical intermediate. Prior to the mid 1970s, trichloroethylene was used as a general anesthetic agent for minor surgeries and obstetrics. It is estimated that as many as 200,000 workers in the United States are exposed to this agent on a regular basis.[21] Trichloroethylene is a clear, colorless, nonflammable liquid with an odor similar to carbon tetrachloride. It is frequently used as a substitute for carbon tetrachloride, because it has much lower toxic potential. It is readily absorbed from the lungs and gastrointestinal tract and minimally via the skin. Most severe toxic effects are caused by respiratory depression, which is part of its generalized CNS depressant effect. It has also been reported to sensitize the myocardium to the effects of epinephrine, leading to deaths from primary venticular fibrillation.[1] Acute respiratory exposure usually results in CNS depression with associated prolonged severe nausea and vomiting. Some victims experience a "high" during the early stages of exposure. Most workers experience a dose-related decline in their psychomotor skills, which resolves after removal from the contaminating environment. Transient renal and hepatic toxicity have been described.[22] A single case of trichloroethylene-associated cirrhosis has been reported.[23] Dermatitis resulting from defatting of the skin and irritation of the nose and eyes have been noted in some individuals. Several unusual syndromes have been described following repeated and chronic exposures. "Degreasers' flush" has been described in workers exposed to trichloroethylene who then consume ethanol-containing beverages. These workers develop a characteristic blotching or flushing of the face and neck beginning within an hour of ethanol consumption. The flush begins around the nose and malar regions and quickly spreads to the entire face and neck, with a sharp line of demarcation separating the involved and noninvolved areas. The flush begins to clear within a couple of hours, leading to complete resolution without sequelae. There are no associated changes in vital signs, nor are there any physical complaints such as pain or itching. The exact mechanism is unknown, though trichloroethylene blood levels in these subjects are elevated above those of controls during the "flushing," possibly a result of ethanol inhibition of trichloroethylene's normal metabolic pathway.[24] Isolated trigeminal peripheral neuralgia secondary to trichloroethylene exposure has been described following acute exposures. Though the exact mechanism is unclear, demyelination of the trigeminal nerves has been seen on autopsy. All demyelination survivors have recovered fully, though symptoms have lasted for a year or more.[25] There is no evidence that this agent is carcinogenic or teratogenic in humans. Diagnosis is based on history and clinical findings and can be confirmed by sampling expired gasses for trichloroethylene levels. Treatment is entirely supportive.

Tetrachloroethylene

Tetrachloroethylene (perchloroethylene, $CCl_2{=}CCl_2$) is a colorless, nonflammable liquid that is used primarily as a dry cleaning and degreasing agent. Absorption is primarily pulmonary, with limited exposure through the skin. It has toxic properties similar to those described for trichloroethylene, including CNS depression, skin rashes, and mucous membrane irritation. Nausea, vomiting, and hepatorenal dysfunction are also seen in some cases. Treatment is entirely supportive. The NIOSH standard is 50 ppm.[1, 8]

Dichloropropane

Dichloropropane ($CH_2ClCHClCH_3$) is used as a soil fumigant prior to crop planting. Toxicity is the result of CNS depression and pulmonary irritation. Treatment is entirely supportive.[8]

Ethylene Chlorohydrin

Ethylene chlorohydrin (2-chloroethanol, $ClCH_2CH_2OH$) is used as a solvent in the manufacturing of paper products and textiles and is also used to speed the germination of seeds and potatoes. It is used in the manufacturing of ethylene glycol, ethylene oxide, and some insecticides.[4, 8] Ethylene chlorohydrin has been reported as an occasional by-product of ethylene oxide sterilization of some plastic products, though no toxic effects have been attributed to this type of exposure.[26] It is a colorless liquid at room temperature, with a mild ether-like odor and a flash point of 60°C.[4] Ethylene chlorohydrin is extremely toxic, with exposure limits of 1 ppm and an estimated fatal adult inhalation dose of 1 to 2 mL. Even in dangerous concentrations, there is no characteristic warning odor and no significant irritation of the nose or throat. Ethylene chlorohydrin is toxic to the lungs, liver, and kidneys, but the exact mechanism of toxicity is unknown. Though initial symptoms are usually minimal, respiratory exposure can cause minor irritation of mucous membranes, followed by sleepiness, drowsiness, giddiness, nausea, and vomiting. After a latent period that can be as long as 72 hours, headache, thirst, and delirium are seen, followed by pulmonary edema, hypotension, stupor, and coma. Fatty infiltration of the liver and kidneys and cerebral and pulmonary edema are seen on autopsy. Treatment is primarily supportive and includes removing the patient from the offending environment and thorough decontamination. The patient must be followed closely, looking for the delayed development of pulmonary, renal, hepatic, and neurologic complications. For the most part, survival is expected if a victim survives the first 18 hours following exposure.[8]

References

1. Chlorinated hydrocarbons. *In* Hamilton and Hardy's Industrial Toxicology. 4th ed. Boston, John Wright-PSG Inc., 1983, p 255-234.

2. McConnell G: Chlorinated hydrocarbons and the environment. Endeavors *34*:13-18, 1975.
3. Scharnweber HC, Spears GN, Cowles SR: Chronic methyl chloride intoxication in six industrial workers. J Occup Med *16*:112-113, 1974.
4. International Technical Information Institute: Toxic and Hazardous Industrial Chemicals Safety Manual. Tokyo, Japan, 1975.
5. Plunkett ER: Handbook of Industrial Toxicology. New York, Chemical Publishing Company, 1978.
6. DiVincenzo GD, Kaplan CJ: Uptake, metabolism, and elimination of methylene chloride vapors. Hum Toxicol Appl Pharmacol *59*:130-140, 1981.
7. Friedlander BR, Hearne T, Hall S: Epidemiologic investigation of employees chronically exposed to methylene chloride; Mortality analysis. J Occup Med *20*:657-666, 1978.
8. Meredith TJ, Vale JA: The halogenated hydrocarbons. *In* Haddad LM, Winchester JF (eds): Clinical Management of Poisoning and Drug Overdose. Philadelphia, WB Saunders, 1983, p 779-785.
9. Hygenic guide series; Chloroform, Am Hyg Assoc J *26*:636, 1965.
10. Kluwe WM, Hook JB: Potentiation of acute chloroform nephrotoxicity by the glutathione depletor diethyl maleate and protection by the microsomal enzyme inhibitor piperonyl butoxide. Toxicol Appl Pharmacol *59*:457-466, 1981.
11. Pohl LR, Bhooshan B, Krishna G: Mechanism of the metabolic activation of chloroform. Toxicol Appl Pharmacol *45*:238, 1978.
12. NIOSH: Criteria for a Recommended Standard . . . Occupational Exposure to Chloroform. Washington, DC, National Institute for Occupational Safety and Health (NIOSH 75-114), 1974.
13. Marx JL: Drinking water; Getting rid of carbon tetrachloride. Science *196*:632-636, 1977.
14. Recknagel RO: Carbon tetrachloride hepatotoxicity. Pharmacolog Rev *19*:145-208, 1967.
15. Burk RF, Reiter R, Lane JM: Hyperbaric oxygen protection against carbon tetrachloride hepatotoxicity in the rat. Gastroenterology *90*:812-818, 1986.
16. NOISH: Criteria for a Recommended Standard . . . Occupational Exposure to Carbon Tetrachloride. Washington, DC, National Institute for Occupational Safety and Health (NIOSH 76-133), 1975.
17. Stewart, RD: Methyl chloroform intoxication. JAMA *215*:1789, 1971.
18. Meredith TJ, Vale JA: The halogenated hydrocarbons. *In* Clinical Management of Poisoning and Drug Overdose. Philadelphia, WB Saunders, 1983 p 779-785.
19. NIOSH: Criteria for a Recommended Standard . . . Occupational Exposure to 1,1,1-Trichloraoethane (Methyl Chloroform). Washington, DC, National Institute for Occupational Safety and Health (NIOSH 76-184), 1976.
20. NIOSH: Criteria for a Recommended Standard . . . Occupational Exposure to 1,1,2,2-Tetrachloroethane. Washington, DC, National Institute for Occupational Safety and Health (NIOSH 77-121), 1976.
21. Messite, J: Commentary; Trichloroethylene standards. J Occup Med *16*:194, 1974.
22. NIOSH: Criteria for a Recommended Standard . . . Occupational Exposure to Trichloroethylene. Washington, DC, National Institute for Occupational Safety and Health (NIOSH 73-11025), 1973.
23. Thiele, DL, Eigenbrodt, EH, Ware, AJ: Cirrhosis after repeated trichloroethylene and 1,1,1-trichloroethane exposure. Gastroenterology *83*:926, 1982.
24. Stewart, RD, Hake, CL, Peterson, JE: "Degreasers' Flush." Arch Environment Health *29*:1, 1974.
25. Feldman, RG, Mayer, RM, Taub, A: Evidence for peripheral neurotoxic effect of trichloroethylene. Neurology *20*:599, 1970.
26. Lawrence, WH, Turner, JE, Autian, J: Toxicity of ethylene chlorohydrin I; Acute toxicity studies. J Pharmaceut Sci *60*:568, 1971.

CHAPTER 79

BENZENE AND THE AROMATIC HYDROCARBONS

Darell E. Heiselman, D.O., FACC, FCCP
Louis A. Cannon, M.D.

BENZENE

Aromatic hydrocarbons are hydrocarbons that contain a benzene ring. The primary aromatic hydrocarbons are benzene, toluene, xylene, styrene, and vinyl chloride.

There are many synonyms for benzene, including cyclohexatriene, benzol, coal tar naphtha, and phenyl hydride. Benzene is a clear, highly flammable liquid with a sweet, pleasant, aromatic odor. It is incompatible with chlorine, bromine, and iron. Common commercial grades contain various percentages of benzene, usually between 50 per cent and 100 per cent, with the remaining constituents containing other aromatic compounds such as toluene and xylene.

Benzene is often used as an industrial intermediate in the production of other chemicals such as styrene and phenol. It is involved in the distillation of coal and coal tar and is also used in the manufacturing of dyes, detergents, explosives, paints, varnishes, plastics and rubbers.

Benzene is also a constituent in motor fuels. As the production of unleaded gasoline increases for automobiles equipped with catalytic converters, greater potential for exposure to benzene arises, as the content of benzene is higher in unleaded gasoline.

Benzene's toxicity to bone marrow was recognized in the 1800s, when four fatal cases of benzene poisoning were reported in factory workers in Stockholm.[1] It was not until 1910 that Selling elucidated the important characteristic of benzene poisoning to be leukopenia with aplasia, an extreme reduction in cells produced by the bone marrow.[2]

Benzene's leukocytotoxic action was once used therapeutically in the treatment of leukemias in the early 1900s, but its toxicity limited its use, with cases of severe purpura and drastic reductions in red as well as white blood cell lines.

In the 1920s and 1930s, the Chemical and Rubber Sections of the U. S. National Safety Council encouraged U.S. industry to limit the concentration of benzene to less than 100 ppm.[3] As these safety proposals slowly became adopted, industry began to turn to safer substitutes for benzene such as toluene and liquid rubber latex.

As early as 1928, evidence that benzene may be an etiologic agent in several types of leukemias began to accumulate when Penati and Vigliani collected 10 cases of leukemia in patients exposed to benzene.[4] Since that time, excessive chromosome aberrations in the nuclei of lymphocytes have been well documented as well as a strong association between benzene exposure and leukemia.[5–8] Greenlee et al. have proposed a mechanism for benzene's toxicity, which may involve conversion of benzene metabolites to cytotoxic quinone and superoxide radicals.[9]

Despite the accumulated evidence, benzene's potential for carcinogenicity has been a hotly debated issue, with strong proponents on both sides. In 1987, Rinsky et al. reported a large case control study showing a strongly positive correlation between exposure to benzene and leukemia as well as multiple myeloma.[10] This was not taken without issue, however, for 2 months later, four pages of editorial comments took issue with their findings.[11, 12]

A similar cohort study published in the same year involving over 28,000 Chinese workers exposed to benzene showed similar results.[13] Rinsky estimated that the risk of cancer over a 40-year period of exposure to benzene would be lowered from 154.5 to 1.7 by lowering the permissible exposure limit (PEL) from 10 ppm to 1 ppm. The National Institute for Occupational Safety and Health (NIOSH) responded by lowering the PEL from 10 ppm to 1 ppm in September of 1987, less than 6 months after the data were published.

It is hard to deny that there is a very strong if not proven association between benzene and cancer, particularly leukemia. In order to monitor benzene exposure, NIOSH recommends measuring phenol excretion in the urine. If more than 75 mg of phenol per liter of urine are found, monthly monitoring of complete blood counts by serial examinations should be performed for 2 to 3 months to monitor thrombocyte, leukocyte, and erythrocyte counts.[14, 15]

Pre-employment evaluation of personnel with potential benzene exposure should be comprehensive. A history should include a detailed work history to evaluate previous exposure to marrow toxins; a family and personal history of blood dyscrasias, cancer, liver, and renal function; and a history of alcohol intake and the ingestion of medications and other drugs. Laboratory tests should include a baseline complete blood count with indices and platelet count as well as evaluation of kidney and liver function.

Treatment of Acute Exposure

The treatment of acute exposure to benzene and the other aromatic hydrocarbons is shown in Table 79–1. The clinical signs and symptoms of acute exposure largely depend on the organ involved and the duration of contact. Benzene is a direct irritant to eyes and skin, causing erythema and blistering, and a scaly dermatitis may develop from defatting of the subcutaneous tissues.

Table 79–1. TREATMENT PROTOCOL FOR ACUTE EXPOSURE TO AROMATIC HYDROCARBONS

1. Remove worker from area of exposure.
2. Irrigate eyes copiously with normal saline or other irrigant if there has been exposure to the eyes for 30 minutes.
3. Wash contaminated areas of the body with soap and water.
4. Perform gastric lavage if indicated, but only under experienced medical supervision. Do not induce emesis.
5. Provide oxygen for inhalation.
6. Perform CPR and supportive care as indicated. Be wary of isoproterenol, epinephrine, or other sympathomimetic drugs, as the myocardium may be sensitized to these medications.
7. Treat any neurologic deficits or emotional lability supportively.
8. Perform chest roentgenogram, liver profile, urinalysis, and complete blood counts as necessary. Monitor as needed.
9. Perform pregnancy testing.
10. Monitor urine for degradation products of each aromatic hydrocarbon involved.

Lung aspiration may cause pulmonary edema and hemorrhage; therefore, emesis should not be artificially induced without adequate airway protection. Ventricular fibrillation has been reported and may be produced by aromatic hydrocarbon–produced myocardial sensitization to circulating catecholamines. This may be aggravated by the use of isoproterenol and epinephrine, so these should be reserved for patients not responding to other therapeutic maneuvers.

The gastrointestinal and nervous systems may also be affected in a significant acute exposure to benzene. Nausea, vomiting, and colic are often produced from exposure, and liver damage may result. Acute exposure to benzene may also produce nervous system toxicity with severe headache. Euphoria, ataxia, dizziness, nausea, convulsions, coma, and death may also result if central nervous system depression occurs.

Concerns related to chronic exposures to benzene at higher-than-permissible levels center around its potential for hematologic and myelotoxicity. Its initial effects may actually produce a nonspecific stimulation of the marrow, followed by anemia, leukopenia, thrombocytopenia, and myeloid metaplasia. Aplastic anemia may develop, and peripheral blood counts may not necessarily reflect marrow changes.

Benzene is considered by NIOSH to be leukemogenic. Evidence is substantial for benzene's induction of acute myelogenous leukemia, acute erythroleukemia, and possibly multiple myeloma; however, correlation with chronic leukemias is less substantiated.[16]

TOLUENE

Toluene is a colorless, volatile liquid with an aromatic odor. Common synonyms for toluene include toluol, methyl benzene, and phenyl methane. Although poorly soluble in water, it is rapidly absorbed, with an onset of action in minutes. Toluene is extensively metabolized via oxidation to benzyl alcohol then to benzaldehyde by alcohol dehydrogenase. Further oxidation then forms benzoic acid. Conjugation with glycine produces the major metabolite, hippuric acid, which is excreted in the urine. Benzyl glucuronide is formed in smaller amounts by conjugation with glucuronic acid.

Toluene is an organic solvent for paints and coatings. It is used in the manufacture of benzene and of products such as detergents, dyes, adhesives, lighter fluid, and explosives. Toluene is the major ingredient of airplane model glue. Unleaded gasoline may contain toluene as an additive. Printers, spray painters, shoemakers, cabinetmakers, and those involved in the manufacture or refinement of petroleum products appear to have a significant risk of constant exposure.[17–21] Commercial preparations may contain various amounts of benzene.

In comparison to other organic solvents, toluene appears to have more severe acute effects in vapor exposure than benzene. Bone marrow depression and hematologic side effects from toluene reported previously in the literature are now felt to have been secondary to contamination with benzene and not caused by toluene itself.[22] Bone marrow depression has not been described from either chronic or acute exposure to pure toluene. Children with microcephaly, central nervous system dysfunction, minor craniofacial and limb anomalies, and variable growth deficiency were born to women who inhaled large amounts of pure toluene throughout pregnancy.[23]

In the early 1960s, toluene was used as an industrial solvent in place of benzene, which had known hematologic toxicity. Because of the euphoria and central nervous system depression seen with exposure to toluene, it has become an abused substance by "sniffers."[24] The abuse seen with toluene involves inhaling paint thinners, glue, fingernail polish removers, and others. Several deaths have been reported from model airplane glue being placed in plastic bags that were then placed over an individual's head.[25] The cause of death most likely relates to narcosis and anesthesia from the toluene, followed by asphyxia in the plastic bag.

During acute exposure, toluene is an irritant to eyes, lungs, skin, and other areas of direct exposure. Erythema, defatting dermatitis, skin paresthesias, conjunctivitis, and keratitis occur from direct contact. Dilated pupils and lacrimation may be observed following exposure to toluene vapors. Arrhythmias, sudden death, respiratory arrest, and chemical pneumonitis have been reported with acute inhalation.[26–28] Nausea, vomiting, and anorexia are frequently present with acute toluene poisoning. Electrolyte and acid-base disturbances may present as Type I (distal) renal tubular acidosis, hypokalemia, hypophosphatemia, and anion gap acidosis.[29] Rhabdomyolysis with elevated CPK has been described.[30] Toluene may cause headache, dizziness, mental confusion, euphoria, hallucinations, status epilepticus, incoordination, ataxia, nervousness, insomnia, muscle fatigue, and eventual narcosis.[31]

For the treatment of acute exposure of toluene, follow the recommendations given in Table 79–1. In addition, if exposure is massive, perform chest roentgenograms, hepatic and renal profiles, and urinalysis. Bicarbonate therapy should not be given until potassium and calcium are replaced adequately. Potassium replacement should be in the form of potassium phosphate, since both potassium and phosphate are usually low. Serial measurements of potassium, calcium, magnesium, and phosphate should be performed.

The recommendation for occupational safety and health hazards is 200 ppm at an 8-hour time-weighted average (TWA), with a 300 ppm acceptable ceiling, and a 500 ppm maximum ceiling at 10 minutes.[32] Levels of exposure greater than 600 ppm cause confusion and delirium. Toluene abusers may be exposed to over 1000 ppm for excessive periods of time. The various components in abused solvent mixtures may be additive in their toxic effects.

Occupational exposure to toluene requires a comprehensive preplacement and annual medical examination, with emphasis on liver, kidney, and central nervous systems. Laboratory tests should include complete blood counts, hepatic and renal profiles, and urinalysis.

Pulmonary hypertension, hemorrhagic alveolitis, sensitization of the myocardium to catecholamines, atrioventricular block, sudden death, and bradyarrhythmias have been reported during chronic exposure.[33–35] Nausea, vomiting, and anorexia are not infrequent symptoms. Hepatomegaly and centrilobular necrosis have been described with chronic exposure as well.[36, 37] Hypokalemic periodic paralysis may be seen as a result of Type I renal tubular acidosis.[38, 39] Urinalysis abnormalities include hematuria, pyuria, myoglobinuria, and proteinuria. Chronic exposure to toluene may carry the attendant risk of urinary calculi and reversible renal failure.[40, 41] Toluene exposure may produce elevated CPK with rhabdomyolysis.

Toluene exposure may cause dementia, cerebellar degeneration, cranial nerve abnormalities, spasticity, hyperactive tendon reflexes, corticobulbar and corticospinal damage, encephalopathy, postural tremor, and sensorineural hearing loss. In addition, peripheral and optic neuropathies, brain stem atrophy, status epilepticus, psychosis, myopathy, myoclonus, choreoathetotic movement disorders, insomnia, irritability, personality changes, and memory impairment have all been reported with toluene exposure.[42–50]

In addition to the treatment recommendations in Table 79–1, biologic monitoring can be of serum toxicology or urinary hippuric acid levels can be performed on all workers at risk for excessive exposure.[51] Hippuric acid levels may be inaccurate as a result of the ingestion of benzoates in food.[52]

XYLENE

Xylene is a clear, flammable liquid with an aromatic odor. Common synonyms for xylene include dimethyl benzene, xylol, and the three isomers, *o*-, *m*-, and *p*-xylene. It is produced from both petroleum and coal tar, and is an organic solvent for some resins, gums, and oils. Commercial preparations usually contain 85 per cent of the *m*- isomer and only about 5 per cent of the *p*- isomer. Other preparations may contain benzene in various amounts.

Aromatic hydrocarbons such as xylene and benzene may be found in unleaded gasoline. Therefore, the use of unleaded gasoline increases the general population's possible exposure to these hydrocarbons.

Xylene may be found in paints, lacquers, adhesives, and cements. Cleaning fluids, degreasers, dyes, inks, insect repellants, and perfumes are other sources of xylene exposure.

Temporary hepatorenal impairment and death from pulmonary edema have been described from xylene inhalation.[53] There have also been reports of reversible corneal vacuolization during xylene exposure.

Mild toxic effects to the hematopoietic system consisting of a reversible decrease in red and white cell counts and a concomitant increase in platelet count have been demonstrated in animal studies. Nevertheless, evidence in humans is lacking for blood or blood-forming organ toxicity.[54–56] Rodent studies demonstrate the association of prenatal toxicity and developmental defects with mixed and individual isomers of xylene.[57, 58]

NIOSH's recommended PEL is 100 ppm (435 mg/m^3) for an 8-hour TWA.[59] After exposure, xylene can be measured in expired air and blood. The presence of methyl hippuric acid in the urine has been used as a diagnostic test for exposure.[60–62]

Xylene in liquid form is a direct irritant to skin, causing erythema, dryness, and defatting. Vesicles may form with prolonged contact, and facial flushing has been described with acute exposure. Vapors may be irritating to the nose and throat. Ocular complications include conjunctivitis, corneal vacuolization, and keratitis.

Cardiopulmonary complications include catecholamine-induced ventricular arrhythmias, acute pulmonary edema, and respiratory depression from acute exposure. Nausea, vomiting, anorexia, and abdominal pain are often observed; less frequently, reversible hepatic impairment occurs. High concentrations of xylene may cause dizziness, ataxia, drowsiness, excitement, incoordination, headache, confusion, vertigo, tremor, and coma.[63, 64]

Treatment of acute and chronic exposure to xylene is the same as that for exposure to other aromatic hydrocarbons (Table 79–1). Additionally, patients with severe exposure should be hospitalized and observed for possible pulmonary edema that may be delayed as much as 72 hours. A chest roentgenogram, ECG, complete blood count, determination of arterial blood gas levels, and liver and renal profiles should also be performed.

Occupational exposure to xylene requires a comprehensive preplacement medical examination. This should include special attention to symptoms of headache, dizziness, nausea, other gastrointestinal symptoms, and alcohol consumption.[65–67] Detailed examination of eyes, lungs, mucous membranes, and skin should be performed. These medical examinations should be repeated every 2 years and should include complete blood count, routine urinalysis, and liver function tests.[68] Biologic monitoring can be performed on all workers at risk for excessive exposure by following urinary methyl hippuric acid levels.[69–71]

At present, there is no evidence to indicate that xylene is toxic to blood and blood-forming organs.[72] However, xylene is often found in combination with other hydrocarbons (e.g., benzene). In these situations, the standards for any additive chemicals should be applied.

STYRENE

Commonly encountered synonyms used for styrene include styrol, styrolene, vinylbenzene, cinnamene, cinnamol, and phenylethylene. Styrene is a flammable, colorless-to-yellowish liquid that has an attractive, sweet odor at low concentrations, which becomes unpleasantly penetrating at higher levels. It is a very refractive, oily liquid that boils at 145°C and polymerizes to form a plastic (polystyrene) at approximately 200°C.

Styrene is used as an industrial intermediate in combination with acrylonitrile and butadiene to form copolymer and rubber products. Styrene is also used in the synthesis of resins, as a dental filling component, as a chemical in agricultural products, in the production of insulators and polyesters, and in drug manufacturing. It is commonly used in boat and yacht manufacturing, in the reinforced plastics industry, and in photostat copying systems.

Styrene is often stabilized by the addition of tertbutylcatechol or another polymerization inhibitor. Spontaneous polymerization may take place at higher temperatures or if a polymerization inhibitor is not present in sufficient levels. This may result in spontaneous rupture of containers storing this chemical. Styrene will corrode copper alloys and dissolve rubber. Contact with oxidizing agents, strong acids, or aluminum chloride should be avoided.

A fire involving styrene may release harmful by-products, including carbon monoxide. Fumes are acrid, and the odor threshold is considerably lower than the PEL and should therefore provide adequate warning to a potential toxic exposure.

Current Occupational Safety and Health (OSHA) standards for styrene are 100 ppm for an 8-hour TWA, with a 200 ppm ceiling. The level defined as immediately dangerous to life or health (IDLH) is 5000 ppm. Workers exposed to levels above 500 ppm should have a self-contained breathing apparatus with a chemical cartridge respirator with organic vapor cartridges.[73]

Styrene in both liquid and vapor forms is irritating to the skin and mucous membranes. Humans exposed at 376 ppm experienced rapid onset of eye and nasal irritation.[74] Corneal burns have also been reported with direct contact to the eyes. Skin contact may produce acute as well as chronic dermatitis. Chest burning, wheezing, dyspnea, and angina have been reported with some acute exposures; however, objective changes in pulmonary function occurred only in workers who also smoked.[75, 76]

Styrene is a CNS depressant. After approximately 1 hour of exposure to styrene, headache, nausea, incoordination, impaired dexterity, and other signs of transient neurologic impairment develop. Studies have also shown impaired cognition, slower reaction times, and subjective feelings of tiredness following styrene exposure. Abnormal EEGs have also been noted. These reports have been largely inconclusive observational studies, which are often subjective and difficult to interpret.[77, 78]

Studies to date have been conflicting and inconclusive regarding embryotoxicity, fetotoxicity, or teratogenicity.[79, 80] However, because birth defects have been noted, pregnant workers exposed to styrene may desire an amniocentesis during pregnancy to help detect potential fetal abnormalities.

Recommendations for treating acute and chronic exposures to styrene are shown in Table 79–1. Chronic exposure to styrene may produce alterations in liver enzymes and liver function tests. Alterations in glucose metabolism have been noted, but well-defined alterations have not clearly been shown.[81]

Objective changes in pulmonary function have also been poorly documented. One study of workers exposed to styrene found that only 20 per cent of cases showed any significant change in FEV_1. The study was poorly controlled, and other factors may have had a primary impact on the changes observed.[75, 76]

In addition to the neurologic effects noted in acute exposure, an association with peripheral neuropathy has also been shown. Long-term exposures may result in persistent and premature dementia in some workers.[82, 83]

Recent literature suggests a potential for nephrotoxicity localized to the proximal tubule in rats exposed at chronic, low, nontoxic doses of styrene. Human studies are lacking.[84] Congenital defects and increases in spontaneous abortions have been reported but not supported by recent investigations.[79, 80]

Although studies to date have not shown conclusively that styrene directly causes cancer, numerous studies implicate styrene and styrene oxide as possible carcinogens. Lymphomas and leukemias have largely been associated with styrene, and Hodgson and Jones also found an increased incidence of laryngeal carcinoma.[85] To help in assessing the significance of an exposure to possible toxic quantities of styrene, biologic monitoring should be performed on all workers by following urinary mandelic or hippuric acid excretion.[86, 87]

VINYL CHLORIDE

Vinyl chloride is a colorless, sweet-smelling gas that is highly explosive and flammable. Other common synonyms for vinyl chloride include ethylene monochloride, monochloroethene, monochloroethylene, chloroethene, and chloroethylene. It has a lower and upper explosive limit of 4 per cent and 26 per cent, respectively. At normal temperatures it is noncorrosive, but in contact with water and at elevated temperatures, it increases the corrosion of iron and steel. Vinyl chloride is usually handled as a liquid under pressure. The half-life in air ranges from 3 to 20 hours. Easy absorption occurs across cell membranes because of its low molecular weight, even though its low solubility impedes the process. Approximately 80 per cent of vinyl chloride is cleared from the blood in 10 minutes after cessation of exposure.

Vinyl chloride is used as an intermediate in the production of plastics, methyl chloroform, and aerosol propellants. Vinyl chloride has been detected in small amounts in cigarette smoke (16 ng per cigarette, 27 ng per cigar).

Vinyl chloride was originally used in the early 1930s for its anesthetic action. Its use was later discontinued because of the significant cardiac arrhythmias induced during anesthesia.[88] In 1949, reports of Russian workers with liver changes consistent with hepatitis from exposure were observed. A severe neurologic disorder was described in Minamata, Japan, associated with the production of vinyl chloride in 1960.[89] Later, in 1966, acro-osteolysis was described in vinyl chloride autoclave cleaners in Belgium.[90] Viola et al. attempted to reproduce this in animal experiments, which incidentally revealed vinyl chloride–induced cancer.[91] Maltoni and Lefemine continued studies with vinyl chloride and demonstrated angiosarcoma of the liver in rodents.[92, 93]

Creech and Johnson reported two cases of hepatic angiosarcoma in employees at a chemical plant.[94] Retrospective studies of vinyl chloride workers confirmed a significant risk of 400:1 and a latency period of 12 to 30 years for liver cancer. These and other studies caused American and European industry to change acceptable exposure levels of vinyl chloride to levels of 10 ppm or less for an 8-hour TWA.

Additional evidence for the mutagenicity of vinyl chloride is demonstrated by increased chromosomal aberrations in lymphocytes of workers exposed to vinyl chloride.[95–98] Of significance is the abnormally high rate of fetal wastage found in wives of male workers with occupational exposure to vinyl chloride.[99, 100]

Exposure to vinyl chloride is usually through the lungs. Metabolic activation through a three-step process is required for vinyl chloride to become mutagenic, carcinogenic, or cytotoxic. The alcohol dehydrogenase system metabolizes vinyl chloride at low concentrations (< 50 ppm) into chloroacetaldehyde and monochloroacetic acid.[101] At moderate levels (> 50 ppm), oxidation by the peroxidase-catalase system produces chloroacetaldehyde. At very high levels (> 250 ppm), oxidation occurs mainly via the hepatic microsomal mixed-function oxidase system (cytochrome P_{450}-dependent) to the end product, chloroethylene oxide. When the oxidative systems become saturated, vinyl chloride is excreted unchanged via the lungs.

Chloroethylene oxide and chloroacetaldehyde may be further oxidized or conjugated with glutathione via glutathione transferases or epoxide hydrase. The remaining nondegraded electrophilic intermediates may cause cytotoxicity by interfering with protein synthesis or forming DNA adducts (chemicals that bind to DNA). DNA adducts may cause distortion of the symmetrical helical structure, resulting in mutagenic or carcinogenic interference in DNA replication.

Skin contact with vinyl chloride in liquid form can cause redness, irritation, and frostbite. Acute exposure to vapors or direct contact may cause irritation and erythema to the eyes, throat, and nose. In severe exposures, cardiac arrhythmias have been reported. Nausea, vomiting, and abdominal pain are frequently present and may be associated with hepatic cell necrosis and hepatitis. Dose-related effects observed with acute vinyl chloride exposure include lightheadedness, dizziness, decreased auditory and visual responses, and disorientation.[102, 103]

Treatment of acute exposure to vinyl chloride follows the protocol given in Table 79–1. In addition, the patient should have close observation after significant exposure for hepatic damage. Serial SGOT, SGPT, alkaline phosphatase, bilirubin, and albumin levels and prothrombin time should be obtained on admission and repeated every 24 hours for a 72-hour period.

Because of the long-term implications for increased incidence of tumors,[104–106] acro-osteolysis, and liver abnormalities, an extensive monitoring policy for exposed workers is recommended.[107, 108]

Occupational exposure to vinyl chloride requires a comprehensive preplacement history and physical examination, with special attention to liver and spleen enlargement. At the initial time of employment and annually thereafter, recording of alcohol intake and history of hepatitis, drugs, and chemical exposure, blood transfusions, and hospitalizations should be made. Prior to employment and annually thereafter, laboratory studies should be performed, including measures of SGOT, SGPT, bilirubin, GGTP, and alkaline phosphatase. If the person being screened has been exposed for 10 years or more to vinyl chloride monomer production or polymerization, screening should be performed every 6 months. It is recommended that no woman who is pregnant or expects to become pregnant be directly exposed to vinyl chloride monomer operations. Vinyl chloride is a demonstrated carcinogen, and NIOSH's recommended PEL is 1 ppm for an 8-hour TWA, with a 5 ppm ceiling at 15 minutes.

Although no definitive and reliable sign, symptom, or laboratory test has been found to be specific for the early diagnosis of angiosarcoma of the liver,[93] special attention should be made to complaints of fatigue, lassitude, epigastric pain, pleuritis, chest pain, dyspnea, or gastrointestinal hemorrhage.

Chronic exposure to vinyl chloride may present with a variety of clinical manifestations. Sclerodermatous (or scleroedema) skin changes[109] and Raynaud's phenomenon[110] may present either together with acro-osteolysis as a triad or separately. A genetic predisposition may play a role in the development of scleroderma-like skin changes with vinyl chloride exposure.[111] Acro-osteolysis has been reported in approximately 3 per cent of workers (usually reactor cleaners) exposed to vinyl chloride.[90, 112, 113] It does not necessarily improve with removal of exposure, but radiographic improvement of phalangeal lesions has been reported. Recent reports suggest a possible association with malignant melanoma,[114] and a case report has been published of vasculitic purpura.[115]

Chronic exposure can cause pneumoconiosis with dyspnea and impaired pulmonary function (restrictive and/or obstructive insufficiency).[116–118] Biopsy abnormalities consist of desquamation of macrophages, minor interstitial and alveolar inflammatory changes, or pulmonary fibrosis.[119] An increased incidence of large cell or adenocarcinoma of the lung has been reported in several retrospective, epidemiologic studies.[120–123]

Hepatic angiosarcoma, hepatocellular carcinoma, portal hypertension, splenomegaly, and hepatic fibrosis have all been reported with exposure to vinyl chloride.[94, 124–130] A retrospective study of 1294 workers exposed to vinyl chloride revealed an increased incidence of brain cancer (glioblastoma multiforme).[131] A polyneuropathy may be associated with vinyl chloride exposure.[132] Evidence is substantial for vinyl chloride's induction of anemia, reticulocytosis, thrombocytopenia, leukopenia, and lymphatic malignancies.

References

1. Santesson CG: Arch Hyg *31*:336, 1897.
2. Selling L: Bulletin of Johns Hopkins Hospital. Johns Hopk Hosp Rep *17*:83, 1910.
3. Hamilton A: J Ind Hyg *10*:227, 1928.
4. Penati F, Vigliani EC: Rass Med Ind *9*:345, 1938.
5. Vigliani EC: Leukemia associated with benzene exposure. Ann NY Acad Sci *271*:143, 1976.
6. Clare MG, Yardley JA, Maclean AC, Dean BJ: Chromosome analysis from peripheral blood lymphocytes of workers after an acute exposure to benzene. Br J Ind Med *41*(2):249-253, 1984.
7. Eikmann, T, Stinner D, Prajsnar D: Haematological data relating to phenol excretion in urine with chronic benzene exposure; I; Epidemiological studies of adults (from author's translation). Zentralbl Bakteriol Mikrobiol Hyg *174*(1-2):57-76, 1981.
8. Mehlman, MA: Carcinogenicity and Toxicity of Benzene. Princeton, NJ, Princeton Scientific Publishers, 1983.
9. Greenlee WF, Sun JD, Bus JS: A proposed mechanism of benzene toxicity; Formation of reactive intermediates from polyphenol metabolites. Toxicol Appl Pharmacol *59*:187, 1981.
10. Rinsky RA, Smith AB, Hornung R, Filloon TG: Benzene and leukemia; An epidemiologic risk assessment. N Engl J Med *316*:1044-1050, 1987.
11. Bader M: Benzene and leukemia (editorial). N Engl J Med *317*:1027, 1987.
12. Hu H: Benzene associated myelofibrosis (editorial). Ann Intern Med *106*:172-173, 1987.
13. Yin SN, Li GL, Tain FD, Jin C: Leukemia in benzene workers: a retrospective cohort study. Br J Ind Med *44*:124-148, 1987.
14. National Institute for Occupational Safety and Health, US Department of Health, Education and Welfare: Revised Recommendation for an Occupational Exposure Standard for Benzene (NIOSH) 657-012/325. Washington, DC, US Government Printing Office, 1979.
15. National Institute for Occupational Health, US Department of Health, Education and Welfare: NIOSH Pocket Guide to Chemical Hazards. DHHS (NIOSH) publ 85-114. Washington, DC, September, 1985.
16. Irons RD: Toxicology updates; Benzene. J Appl Toxicol *2*:57, 1982.
17. Anshelm Olson B, Gamberale F, Gronqvist B: Reaction time among steel workers exposed to solvent vapors; A longitudinal study. Int Arch Occup Environ Health *48*:211-218, 1981.
18. Anshelm Olson B: Effects of organic solvents on behavior performance of workers in the paint industry. Neurobehav Toxicol Teratol *4*:703-708, 1982.

19. Baelum J, Anderson IB, Lundqvist GR, Mlhave L, Pedersen OF, Vaeth M, Wyon DP: Response of solvent-exposed printers and unexposed controls to six-hour toluene exposure. Scand J Work Environ Health *11*:271-280, 1985.
20. Cherry H, Hutchins H, Pace T, Waldron HA: Neurobehavioral effects of repeated occupational exposure to toluene and paint solvents. Br J Ind Med *42*:291-300, 1985.
21. Takeichi S, Yamade T, Shikata I: Acute toluene poisoning during painting. Forensic Sci Int *32*:109-115, 1986.
22. Powars D: Aplastic anemia secondary to glue sniffing. N Engl J Med *273*:700-702, 1965.
23. Hersh JH, Podruch PE, Rogers G, Weisskopf B: Toluene embryopathy. J Pediatr *106*:922-927, 1985.
24. Streicher HZ, Gabow PQ, Moss AH, et al: Syndromes of toluene sniffing in adults. Ann Intern Med *94*:758-762, 1981.
25. Paterson SC, Sarvesvaran R: Plastic bag death—a toluene fatality. Med Sci Law *23*:64-66, 1983.
26. Bass M: Sudden sniffing death. JAMA *212*:2075-2079, 1970.
27. Reinhardt CF, Azar A, Maxfield ME, et al: Cardiac arrhythmias and aerosol "sniffing." Arch Environ Health *22*:265-279, 1971.
28. Cronk SL, Barkley DE, Farrell MF: Respiratory arrest after solvent abuse. Br Med J *290*:897-898, 1985.
29. Fischman CM, Oster JR: Toxic effects of toluene: a new cause of high anion gap metabolic acidosis. JAMA *241*:1713-1715, 1979.
30. Reisin E, Teicher A, Jaffe R, et al: Myoglobinuria and renal failure in toluene poisoning. Br J Ind Med *32*:163-168, 1975.
31. Glowa JR, DeWeese J, Natale ME, Holland JJ, Dews PB: Behaviorial toxicology of volatile organic solvents; I; Methods; Acute effects of toluene. J Environ Pathol Toxicol Oncol *6*:153-168, 1986.
32. National Institute for Occupational Safety and Health, US Department of Health, Education, and Welfare: Criteria for a Recommended Standard; Occupational Exposure to Toluene. (HSM) 73-11023. Washington, DC: US Government Printing Office, 1973, pp 14-45.
33. Garriott J, Petty CS: Death from inhalant abuse; Toxicological and pathological evaluation of 34 cases. Clin Toxicol *16*:305-315, 1980.
34. Zee-Cheng C, Mueller CE, Gibbs HR: Toluene sniffing and severe sinus bradycardia. Ann Intern Med *103*:482, 1985.
35. Engstrand DA, England DM, Huntington RW: Pathology of paint sniffers' lung. Am J Forensic Med Pathol *7*:232-236, 1986.
36. Howell SR, Christian JE, Isom GE: The hepatotoxic potential of combined toluene-chronic ethanol exposure. Arch Toxicol *59*:45-50, 1986.
37. O'Brien ET, Yeoman WB, Hobby JA: Hepatorenal damage from toluene in a glue sniffer. Br Med J *2*:29-30, 1971.
38. Bennet RH, Forman HR: Hypokalaemic periodic paralysis in chronic toluene exposure. Arch Neurol *37*:673, 1980.
39. Taher SM, Anderson RK, McCartney R, et al: Renal tubular acidosis associated with toluene "sniffing." N Engl J Med *290*:765-768, 1974.
40. Kroeger RM, Moore RJ, Lehman TH, et al: Recurrent urinary calculi associated with toluene sniffing. J Urol *123*:89-91, 1980.
41. Will AM, McLaren EH: Reversible renal damage due to glue sniffing. Br Med J *283*:525-526, 1981.
42. Boor JW, Hurtig HI: Persistent cerebellar ataxia after exposure to toluene. Ann Neurol *2*:440-442, 1977.
43. Channer KS, Stanley S: Persistent visual hallicinations, secondary to chronic solvent encephalopathy; Case report and review of the literature. J Neurol Neurosurg Psychiatr *46*:83-86, 1983.
44. Ehyai A, Freemon FR: Progressive optic neuropathy and sensorineural hearing loss due to chronic glue sniffing. J Neuro Neurosurg Psychiatr *46*:349-351, 1983.
45. Fornazzari L, Wilkinson DA, Kapur BM, Carlen PL: Cerebellar, cortical and functional impairment in toluene abusers. Acta Neurol Scand *67*:319-329, 1983.
46. Hormes JT, Filley CM, Rosenberg NL: Neurologic sequelae of chronic solvent vapor abuse. Neurology *36*:698-702, 1986.
47. King MD: Neurological sequelae of toluene abuse. Human Toxicol *1*:281-287, 1982.
48. Juntunen J, Matikainen E, Antti-Poika M, Suoranta H, Valle M: Nervous system effects of long-term occupational exposure to toluene. Acta Neurol Scand *72*:512-517, 1985.
49. Prockop L: Neurotoxic volatile substances. Neurology *29*:862-864, 1979.
50. Lazar RB, Ho SU, Melen O, Daghestani AN: Multifocal central nervous system damage caused by toluene abuse. Neurology *33*:1337-1340, 1983.
51. De-Rosa E, Bartolucci GB, Sigon M, Callegaro R, Perbellini L, Brugnone F: Hippuric acid and ortho-cresol as biological indicators of occupational exposure to toluene. Am J Ind Med *11*:529-537, 1987.
52. De-Rosa E, Brugnone F, Bartolucci GB, Perbellini L, Bellomo ML, Gori BP, Sigon M, Chiesura Corona P: The validity of urinary metabolites as indicators of low exposures to toluene. Int Arch Occup Environ Health *56*:135-145, 1985.
53. Morley R, Eccleston DW, Douglas CP, Greville WET, Scott DJ, Anderson J: Xylene poisoning; A report on one fatal case and two cases of recovery after prolonged unconsciousness. Br Med J *3*:442, 1970.
54. Moszczynski P, Lisiewicz J: Enzymes of neutrophils in workers occupationally exposed to benzene, toluene, and xylene. Rev Esp Oncol *31*:435-441, 1984.
55. Pap M, Varga C: Sister-chromatid exchanges in peripheral lymphocytes of workers occupationally exposed to xylenes. Mutat Res *187*:223-225, 1987.
56. Dean BJ: Recent findings on the genetic toxicology of benzene, toluene, xylenes, and phenols. Mutat Res Nov *254*:153-181, 1985.
57. Hood RD, Ottley MS: Developmental effects associated with exposure to xylene; A review. Drug Chem Toxicol *8*:281-297, 1985.
58. Mirkova E, Zaikov C, Antov G, Mikhailova A, Khinkova L, Benchev I: Prenatal toxicity of xylene. J Hyg Epidemiol Microbiol Immunol *27*:337-343, 1983.
59. National Institute for Occupational Safety and Health, US Department of Health, Education, and Welfare: Criteria for a Recommended Standard for Occupational Exposure to Xylene (NIOSH) 75-168. Washington, DC, US Government Printing Office, 1975.
60. Lundberg I, Sollenberg J: Correlation of xylene

exposure and methyl hippuric acid excretion in urine among paint industry workers. Scand J Work Environ Health *2*:140-153, 1986.

61. Ogata M, Taguchi T: Quantitation of urinary metabolites of toluene, xylene, sytrene, ethylbenzene, benzene, and phenol by automated high performance liquid chromatography. Int Arch Occup Environ Health *59*:263-272, 1987.
62. Ogata M, Taguchi T: Quantitative analysis of urinary glycine conjugates by high performance liquid chromatograph; Excretion of hippuric acid and methylhippuric acids in the urine of subjects exposed to vapours of toluene and xylenes. Int Arch Occup Environ Health *58*:121-129, 1986.
63. Savolainen K, Riihimaki V, Linnoila M: Effects of short-term xylene exposure on psychophysiological functions in man. Int Arch Occup Environ Health *44*:201-211, 1979.
64. Savolainen K, Riihimaki V, Seppalainen AM, Linnoila M: Effects of short-term xylene exposure and physical exercise on the central nervous system. Int Arch Occup Environ Health *45*:105-121, 1980.
65. Riihimaki V, Savolainen K, Pfaffli P, Pekari K, Sippel HW, Laine A: Metabolic interaction between m-xylene and ethanol. Arch Toxicol *49*:253-263, 1982.
66. Savolainen K, Riihimaki V, Luukkonen R, Muona D: Changes in the sense of balance correlate with concentrations of m-xylene in venous blood. Br J Ind Med *42*:765-769, 1985.
67. Savolainen K: Combined effects of xylene and alcohol on the central nervous system. Acta Pharmacol Toxicol *46*:366-372, 1980.
68. Engelmeier RL: Effective measures to reduce xylene exposure. J Prosthet Dent *53*:564-565, 1985.
69. Riihimaki V: Conjugation and urinary excretion of toluene and m-xylene metabolites in a man. Scand J Work Environ Health *5*:135-142, 1979.
70. Engstrom K, Husman K, Pfaffli P, Riihimaki V: Evaluation of occupational exposure to xylene by blood, exhaled air, and urine analysis. Scand J Work Environ Health *4*:114-121, 1978.
71. Sedivec V, Flek J: The absorption, metabolism and excretion of xylenes in man. Int Arch Occup Environ Health *37*:205-217, 1976.
72. Sollenberg J, Baldesten A: Isotachophoretic analysis of mandelic acid, phenylglyoxylic acid, hippuric acid and methylhippuric acid in urine after occupational exposure to styrene, toluene, and/or xylene. J Chromatogr *132*:469-476, 1979.
73. National Institutes for Occupational Safety and Health, US Department of Health, Education and Welfare: Criteria for a Recommended Standard. Occupational Exposure to Styrene. (NIOSH) Publication 83-119. Cincinnati, OH, 1983, pp 1-250.
74. McLaughlin RS: Chemical burns of the human cornea. Am J Ophthamol *29*(11):1353-1362, 1946.
75. Chmielewski J, Renke W: Clinical and experimental studies on the pathogenesis of toxic effects of styrene—Part II; The effect of styrene on the respiratory system. Bull Inst Marit Trop Med Gdynia *26*:299-302, 1975.
76. Stewart RD, Dodd HC, Baretta ED, Schaffer AW: Human exposure to styrene vapor. Arch Environ Health *16*:656-662, 1968.
77. Lorimer WV, Lillis R, Nicholson WJ, Anderson H, et al: Clinical studies of styrene workers—initial findings. Environ Health Perspect *17*:171-181, 1976.
78. Axelson O, Gustavson J: Some hygienic and clinical observations on styrene exposure. Scand J Work Environ Health *4* (Suppl 2):215-219, 1978.
79. Hemminki K, Franssila E, Vainto H: Spontaneous abortions among female workers in Finland. Int Arch Occup Environ Health *45*:123-126, 1980.
80. Harkonen H, Holmberg PC: Obstetric histories of women occupationally exposed to styrene. Scand J Work Environ Health *8*:74-77, 1982.
81. Chmielewski J: Clinical and experimental research into the pathogenesis of the toxic effect of styrene—Part V; Impact of styrene on carbohydrate balance in people in the course of their work. Bull Inst Marit Trop Med Gdynia *27*:177-184, 1976.
82. Baker EL, Smith TJ, Landrigan PJ: The neurotoxicity of industrial solvents; A review of the literature. Am J Ind Med *8*:207-217, 1985.
83. Behari M, Choudhary C, Roy S, Maheshwari MC: Styrene-induced peripheral neuropathy; A case report. Eur Neurol *25*:424-427, 1986.
84. Chakrabarti SK, Labelle L, Tuchweber B: Studies on the subchronic nephrotoxic potential of styrene in Sprague-Dawley rats. Toxicology *44*:355-365, 1987.
85. Hodgson JT, Jones RD: Mortality of styrene production, polymerization and processing workers at a site in northwest England. Scand J Work Environ Health *11*:347-352, 1985.
86. National Institute for Occupational Safety and Health, US Department for Health and Human Services: NIOSH Recommendations for Occupational Safety and Health Standards. Morbidity and Mortality Weekly Report Supplement, Vol 35, No 1s, September 1986.
87. National Institute for Occupational Safety and Health, US Department of Health, Education and Welfare: NIOSH Pocket Guide to Chemical Hazards. DHHS NIOSH 85-114. Washington, DC, September 1985.
88. Oster RH, Carr CJ, Krantz JC: Anesthesia; Narcosis with vinyl chloride. Anesthesiology *8*:359, 1947.
89. Kurland LT, Faro SN, Siedler H: Minamata disease. World Neurology *1*:370, 1960.
90. Cordier JM, Fievez C, Lefevre MJ, Sevrin A: Acroosteolysis and related cutaneous lesions in two workers engaged in cleaning autoclaves. Cahiers Med Travail *4*:14, 1966.
91. Viola PL, Bigotti A, Caputo A: Oncogenic response of rat skin, lungs, and bones to vinyl chloride. Cancer Res *31*:516-552, 1971.
92. Maltoni C, Lefemine GL: Carcinogenicity bioassays of vinyl chloride 1; Research plan and early results. Environ Res *7*:387-405, 1974.
93. Maltoni C, Lefemine GL: Carcinogenicity bioassay of vinyl chloride: current results. Ann NY Acad Sci *246*:195-218, 1975.
94. Creech JL Jr, Johnson MN: Angiosarcoma of the liver in the manufacture of polyvinyl chloride. J Occup Med *16*:150-151, 1974.
95. Ducatman A, Hirschhorn K, Selikoff IJ: Vinyl chloride exposure and human chromosome aberrations. Mutat Res *31*:163, 1975.
96. Heath CW Jr, Dumont CR, Gamble J, Waxweiller RJ: Chromosomal damage in men occupationally exposed to vinyl chloride monomer and other chemicals. Environ Res *14*:68-72, 1977.
97. Leonard A, Decat G, Leonard D, et al: Cytogenetic investigations on lymphocytes from workers exposed to vinyl chloride. J Toxicol Environ Health 2:1135-1141, 1977.

98. Purchase IF, Richardson CR, Anderson D, Paddle GM, Adams WG: Chromosomal analyses in vinyl chloride-exposed workers. Mutat Res *57*:325-334, 1978.
99. Infante PF, Wagoner JK, Waxweiller RJ: Carcinogenic, mutagenic, and teratogenic risks associated with vinyl chloride. Mutat Res *41*:131-142, 1976.
100. Theriault G, Iturra H, Gingras S: Evaluation of the association between birth defects and exposure to ambient vinyl chloride. Teratology *27*:359-370, 1983.
101. Bolt HM, Kappus H, Buchter A, Bolt W: Metabolism of vinyl chloride. Lancet *1*:425, 1975.
102. Langauer-Lewowicka H, Kurzbauer H, Byczkowska Z, Wocka-Marek T: Vinyl chloride disease-neurological disturbances. Int Arch Occupat Environ Health *52*:151-157, 1983.
103. Styblova V, Lambl V, Chumcal O, Kellerova V, Paskova V, Vitovcova J, Zlab L: Neurological changes in vinyl chloride-exposed workers. J Hyg Epidemiol Microbiol Immunol *25*:233-243, 1981.
104. Emmerich KH, Norpoth K: Malignant tumors after chronic exposure to vinyl chloride. J Cancer Res Clin Oncol *102*:1-11, 1981.
105. Nicholson WJ, Hammond EC, Seidman H, Selikoff IJ: Mortality experience of a cohort of vinyl chloride-polyvinyl chloride workers. Ann NY Acad Sci *246*:225-230, 1975.
106. Tabershaw IR, Gaffey WR: Mortality study of workers in the manufacture of vinyl chloride and its polymers. J Occup Med *16*:509-518, 1974.
107. National Institute for Occupational Safety and Health, US Department of Health, Education, and Welfare: Criteria for a Recommended Standard for Occupational Exposure to Vinyl Chloride (NIOSH) 657-012/302. Washington, DC, Government Printing Office, 1979.
108. National Health Council of the Netherlands, Committee on the Evaluation of Carcinogenic Substances: A scientific basis for the risk assessment of vinyl chloride. Regul Toxicol Pharmacol *7*:120-127, 1987.
109. Rush PJ, Bell MJ, Fam AG: Toxic oil syndrome and chemically induced scleroderma-like conditions. J Rheumatol *11*:262-264, 1984.
110. Falappa P, Magnavita N, Bergamaschi A, Colavita N: Angiographic study of digital arteries in workers exposed to vinyl chloride. Br J Ind Med *39*:169-172, 1982.
111. Black C, Periera S, McWhirter A, Welsh K, Laurent R: Genetic susceptibility to scleroderma-like syndrome in symptomatic and asymptomatic workers exposed to vinyl chloride. J Rheumatol *13*:1059-1062, 1986.
112. Cook WA, Giever PM, Dinman BD, Magnuson HJ: Occupational acro-osteolysis. Arch Environ Health *22*:74, 1971.
113. Harris DK, Adams WGF: Acro-osteolysis occurring in men engaged in the polymerization of vinyl chloride. Br Med J *3*:712-714, 1967.
114. Storetvedt Heldass S, Andersen AA, Langard S: Incidence of cancer among vinyl chloride and polyvinyl chloride workers; Further evidence for an association with malignant melanoma. Br J Ind Med *44*:278-280, 1987.
115. Magnavita N, Bergamaschi A, Garcovich A, Giuliano G: Vasculitic purpura in vinyl chloride disease: a case report. Angiology *37*:382-388, 1986.
116. Arnaud A, Pommier de Santi P, Garbe L, Payan H, Charpin J: Polyvinyl chloride pneumoconiosis. Thorax *33*:19, 1978.
117. Lilis R: Review of pulmonary effects of poly(vinyl chloride) and vinyl chloride exposure. Environ Health Perspect *41*:167-169, 1981.
118. Miller A, Tierstein AS, Chuang M, Selikoff IJ, Warshaw R: Changes in pulmonary function in workers exposed to vinyl chloride and polyvinyl chloride. Ann NY Acad Sci *246*:42-52, 1975.
119. Cordasco EM, Demeter SL, Kerkay J, Van Ordstrand HS, Lucas EV, Chen T, Golish JA: Pulmonary manifestations of vinyl and polyvinyl chloride; Newer aspects. Chest *78*:828, 1980.
120. Buffler PA, Wood S, Eifler C, Saurez L, Kilian DJ: Mortality experience of workers in a vinyl chloride monomer production plant. J Occup Med *21*:195-203, 1979.
121. Wagoner JK: Vinyl chloride and pulmonary cancer. J Environ Pathol Toxicol *1*:361-362, 1978.
122. Waxweiler RJ, Stringer W, Wagoner JK, Jones J, Falk H, Carter C: Neoplastic risk among workers exposed to vinyl chloride. Ann NY Acad Sci *271*:40-48, 1976.
123. Belli S, Bertazzi PA, Comba P, Foa V, Maltoni C, Masina A, Pirastu R, Reggiani A, Vigotti MA: A cohort study on vinyl chloride manufacturers in Italy; Study design and preliminary results. Cancer Lett *35*:253-261, 1987.
124. Blendis LM, Smith PM, Lawrie BW, Stephens MR, Evans WD: Portal hypertension in vinyl chloride monomer workers; A hemodynamic study. Gastroenterology *75*:206-211, 1978.
125. Block J: Angiosarcoma of the liver following vinyl chloride exposure. JAMA *229*:53, 1974.
126. Brady JS, Liberatore F, Harper P, Greenwald P, Burnett W, Davies JNP, Bishop M, Polan A, Vianna N: Angiosarcoma of the liver; An epidemiologic survey. J Natl Cancer Inst *59*:1383, 1977.
127. Forman D, Bennett B, Stafford J, Doll R: Exposure to vinyl chloride and angiosarcoma of the liver; A report of the register of cases. Br J Ind Med *42*:750-753, 1985.
128. Louagie YA, Gianello P, Kestens PJ, Bonbled F, Haot JG: Vinyl chloride induced hepatic angiosarcoma. Br J Surg *71*:322-323, 1984.
129. Sugita M, Masuda Y, Tsuchiya K: Early detection and signs of hepatoangiosarcoma among vinyl chloride workers. Am J Ind Med *10*:411-417, 1986.
130. Tamburro CH: Relationship of vinyl monomers and liver cancers; Angiosarcoma and hepatocellular carcinoma. Semin Liver Dis *4*:158-169, 1984.
131. Moss AR: Occupational exposure and brain tumors. J Toxicol Environ Health *16*:703-711, 1985.
132. Perticoni GF, Abbritti G, Cantisani TA, Bondi L, Mauro L: Polyneuropathy in workers with long exposure to vinyl chloride; Electrophysiological study. Electromyogr Clin Neurophysiol *26*:41-47, 1986.

CHAPTER 80
CHLORINE

Thomas Stair, M.D.

The odor of chlorine gas (Cl_2) is familiar from household bleach and chlorinated swimming pool and tap water. Chlorine is a potent oxidizing and bleaching agent that is widely used in the manufacture of chemicals, plastic, cloth, and paper. Although chlorine gas has not been used regularly for chemical warfare since World War I, industrial accidents and leaks from storage and transport tanks can produce casualties of comparable number and severity.[1–7] Other exposures may occur in chemistry laboratories,[8] in large swimming pools chlorinated with gas (smaller pools usually use hypochlorite),[9–11] when household bleach is mixed with a strong acid,[12] and even voluntarily.[13]

Chlorine gas combines with tissue water to form hydrochloric and hypochlorous acids,

$$Cl_2 + H_2O \rightarrow HCl + HOCl$$

and hypochlorous acid further breaks down into HCl and oxygen. Chlorine gas, hydrochloric and hypochlorous acids, and oxygen-free radicals all react with sulfhydryl bonds in proteins to form chloramine and thiol radicals.

Chlorine is toxic to surfaces with which it comes in contact, which can be skin, eyes, pulmonary epithelium, or the gastrointestinal tract. Injury is proportional to concentration of gas, duration of contact, and water content of the exposed tissue. Chlorine gas is 10 to 30 times more irritating to the respiratory mucosa than hydrochloric acid. A few seconds of exposure to chlorine gas can be fatal, probably because the heavier-than-air chlorine produces anoxia and cardiac arrest.[1, 14, 15]

Because of its intermediate water solubility and multiple reactive products, chlorine irritates the entire respiratory tree, from nose to alveoli. Within seconds to minutes of exposure, there are symptoms of irritation of the exposed mucosa of eyes, nose, and throat, followed by symptoms of stepwise irritation of the respiratory mucosa, including coughing, dyspnea, wheezing, sputum production, and chest pain.[14] Pulmonary function tests show large and small airway restriction, which may resolve completely over time.[2–4, 10, 16, 17] Loss of pulmonary surfactant can decrease compliance and produce a respiratory distress syndrome early on, but pulmonary edema peaks at 12 to 24 hours. Enough HCl may be absorbed in a nonfatal injury to produce a hyperchloremic metabolic acidosis.[18]

At autopsy, chlorine fatalities can show sloughing of the bronchial columnar epithelium, purulent intraluminal exudate, hyaline membranes in the alveolar spaces, thrombi in the pulmonary vessels, and interstitial and alveolar pulmonary edema.[19]

Treatment begins at the site of exposure with extrication of the victim. Chemical workers may be trained not to hyperventilate or flee downwind. The odor of chlorine on the patient may correlate roughly with the exposure. Victims with no immediate symptoms require no treatment. Because skin exposure may result in partial or full-thickness burns, exposed skin, corneas, or mucosa should be flushed with water, after which standard burn therapy may be initiated.[1]

Tracheobronchitis is treated with cool mist inhalation. Bronchospasm should respond to systemic or inhaled bronchodilators. Oxygen should be provided for dyspnea, but its concentration should eventually be reduced to avoid toxicity. Respiratory distress may require mechanical ventilation with positive end-expiratory pressure. Pulmonary edema therapy may require Swan-Ganz catheter pressure measurements. Corticosteroids are recommended to inhibit inflammation of the respiratory tree, although their benefit remains unproven. Prophylactic antibiotics only promote resistant infection. Bronchoscopy may help clear mucosal plugs.[1]

Although household bleach (5.25 per cent sodium hypochlorite) is not by itself very caustic, it can, after mixing with a strong acid, liberate a toxic dose of chlorine gas.[12, 18, 20] Another hazard, the mixing of two household cleansers, bleach and ammonia,

$$NaOCl + NH_3 \rightarrow NaOH + NH_2Cl$$

liberates chloramine gas, which, being less soluble in water, is better delivered to the distal airways, where it reacts with tissue water to revert to ammonia and hypochlorous acid,

$$NH_2Cl + H_2O \rightarrow NH_3 + HOCl$$

resulting in a toxic pneumonitis.[20, 21] Intravenous drug users are learning to use bleach to sterilize their utensils in an effort to avoid spreading AIDS, and inadvertent injection has been reported with little toxicity.[22]

References

1. Hedges JR, Morrissey WL: Acute chlorine gas exposure. Ann Emerg Med *8*:59-63, 1979.
2. Kaufman J, Burkons D: Clinical, roentgenologic and physiologic effects of acute chlorine exposure. Arch Environ Health *23*:29-34, 1971.
3. Charan NB, Lakshminarayan S, Myers GC, et al: Effects of accidental chlorine inhalation on pulmonary function. West J Med *143*:333-336, 1985.
4. Hasan FM, Gehshan A, Fuleihan FJD: Resolution of pulmonary dysfunction following acute chlorine exposure. Arch Environ Health *38*:76-80, 1983.
5. Fleta J, Calvo C, Zuniga J, et al: Intoxication of 76 children by chlorine gas. Human Toxicol *5*:99-100, 1986.
6. Dixon WM, Drew D: Fatal chlorine poisoning. J Occup Med *10*:249-251, 1968.
7. Joyner RE, Durel EG: Accidental liquid chlorine spill in a rural community. J Occup Med *4*:152-154, 1962.
8. Edwards IR, Temple WA, Dobbinson TL: Acute chlorine poisoning from a high school experiment. New Zealand Med J *96*:720-721, 1983.
9. Decker WJ, Koch HF: Chlorine poisoning at the swimming pool; An overlooked hazard. Clin Toxicol *13*:377-381, 1978.
10. Ploysongsang Y, Beach BC, DiLisio RE: Pulmonary function changes after acute inhalation of chlorine gas. South Med J 75:23-26, 1982.
11. Wood BR, Colombo JL, Benson BE: Chlorine inhalation toxicity from vapors generated by swimming pool chlorinator tablets. Pediatrics *79*:427-430, 1987.
12. Jones FL: Chlorine poisoning from mixing household cleaners. JAMA *222*:1312, 1972.
13. Rafferty P: Voluntary chlorine inhalation. Br Med J *281*:1178-1179, 1980.
14. Chlorine poisoning (editorial). Lancet *1*:321-322, 1984.
15. Barrow CS, Plarie Y, Warrick JC, et al: Comparison of the sensory irritation response of mice to chlorine and hydrogen chloride. Arch Environ Health *32*:68-76, 1977.
16. Rotman HH, Fleigelman MJ, Moore T, et al: Effects of low concentrations of chlorine on pulmonary function in humans. J Appl Physiol *54*:1120-1124, 1983.
17. Jones RN, Hughes JM, Glindmeyer H, et al: Lung function after acute chlorine exposure. Am Rev Respir Dis *134*:1190-1195, 1986.
18. Szerlip HM, Singer I: Hyperchloremic metabolic acidosis after chlorine inhalation. Am J Med *77*:581-582, 1984.
19. Adelson L, Kaufman J: Fatal chlorine poisoning; Report of two cases with clinicopathologic correlation. Am J Clin Path *56*:430-442, 1971.
20. Reisz GR, Gammon RS: Toxic pneumonitis from mixing household cleaners. Chest *89*:49-52, 1986.
21. Gapanay-Gapanavicius M, Molho M, Tirosh M: Chloramine-induced pneumonitis from mixing household cleaning agents. Br Med J *285*:1086, 1982.
22. Froner GA, Rutherford GW, Rokeach M: Injection of sodium hypochlorite by intravenous drug users. JAMA *258*:325, 1987.

CHAPTER 81
PHOSPHINE AND PHOSGENE

Daniel T. Schelble, M.D., FACEP

PHOSPHINE

Phosphine is a colorless flammable gas with an odor of garlic or rotten decaying fish. Synonyms include *hydrogen phosphide, phosphoretted hydrogen,* and *phosphorus trihydride.* Its chemical identification number is 2199. It has a chemical formula of PH_3 and the following structure:

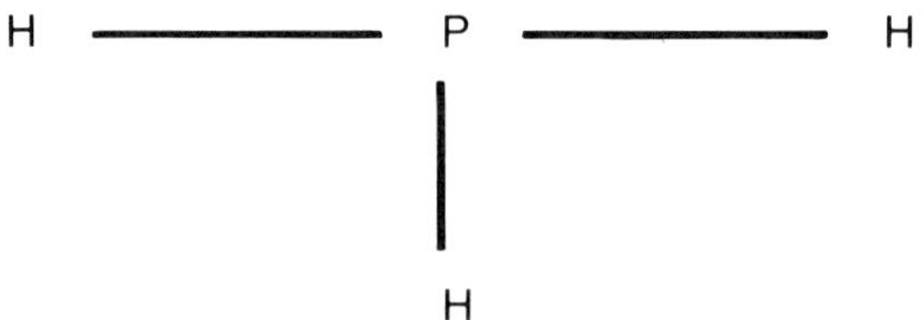

Phosphine gas is used in silicon crystal treatment in the semiconductor industry, in the "pickling" of metals, and in the preparation of phosphonium halides. It is a contaminant in acetylene. Significant phosphine gas exposure is relatively rare, and from 1900 to 1958 only 59 cases of phosphine gas exposure with 26 deaths were reported in the literature.[1–4]

During the past 30 years, cases of significant exposures with a high mortality have been reported secondary to the hydrolysis of aluminum phosphide and zinc phosphide. Aluminum phosphide (ALP—Celphos, Phostoxin, Quick Phos) is used as a grain preservative in silos and elevators and aboard ships. ALP is effective against rodents and insects and is used in tablet form. Zinc phosphide (ZNP—Field Rat Powder) is a gray crystalline powder that, like ALP, is used as a rodenticide in agricultural regions. It is often mixed with bait foods like cornmeal and, when used indiscriminantly, represents a definite risk to pets and children. Although there have been rare reports of accidental exposure secondary to grain fumigation and professional exterminating, the majority of cases reported are intentional suicide acts. In some parts of India, ALP and ZNP became so popular as suicide agents that their production and sale were banned. Half a tablet (1.5 gm) of ALP ingested by mouth has been reported successful in causing suicide.[5] Both ALP and ZNP, when exposed to moisture, release phosphine.[6–8]

The threshold limit value (TLV) of phosphine is 0.3 ppm (gas) or 0.4 mg/m^3 (liquid). One 3-gm tablet of ALP, when brought into contact with water, slowly produces 1 gm of phosphine gas. It is monitored in the workplace or ambient air by gas chromatographic techniques. The gas is detectable by odor at 2 ppm, and even brief exposure is fatal in the range of 400 ppm.

Pathophysiology

In general, phosphine is a protoplasmic poison that interferes with enzymes and protein synthesis and primarily attacks the cardiovascular and respiratory systems. This poison ultimately results in peripheral vascular collapse, cardiac arrest, and pulmonary edema. Singh has shown in animals that phosphine causes noncompetitive inhibition of cytochrome oxidase of the myocardial mitochondria.[8] Similarly, other authors have shown that phosphine inhibits the incorporation of amino acids into myocardial protein.[5] This conclusion is consistent with autopsy studies that have demonstrated fatty degeneration with myofibril necrosis. It has been suggested that these alterations in myocardial mitochondria and protein produce permeability disturbances to sodium, potassium, magnesium, calcium, and other ions giving rise to changes in transmembrane action potentials.[6] For still unknown reasons, these changes are much more prevalent in the myocardium, small peripheral vessels, and pulmonary cells while sparing the large vessels and major coronary arteries.

Pulmonary edema and pneumonitis are felt to result from direct cytotoxicity to the pulmonary cells. Autopsy studies have also shown fatty infiltrates, central necrosis with hemorrhage, and lymphocytic granulomas in the liver and medullary congestion and tubular epithelial degeneration in the kidneys.[9] The propensity for phosphine to attack the small peripheral vessels can cause a profound decrease in systemic vascular resistance leading to marked hypotension that is sometimes unresponsive to pressor agents.

The majority of deaths occur within the first 12 to 24 hours and are usually cardiovascular in origin. Deaths after 24 hours are usually due to liver failure.[10]

Signs and Symptoms

Symptoms are primarily related to the cardiovascular and pulmonary systems and, if oral ingestion has taken place, the gastrointestinal system. Symptoms may include restlessness, irritability, drowsiness, tremors, paresthesias, vertigo, diplopia, ataxia, cough, dyspnea, retrosternal discomfort, abdominal pain, and vomiting.

Signs, like symptoms, are multiple and represent various stages of cardiovascular collapse. Signs may include hypotension, tachycardia, oliguria, anuria, cyanosis, pulmonary edema, tachypnea, jaundice, hepatosplenomegaly, ileus, seizures, and diminished reflexes. Electrocardiographic (ECG) findings include ST-segment elevation or depression, T-wave inversion, sinus tachycardia, SVT, atrial fibrillation, and atrioventricular (AV) conduction problems, especially right bundle branch block (RBBB) and complete AV dissociation. Of interest is the fact that if the patient survives the initial 24 hours, the ECG returns to normal in 10 to 25 days, indicating that the myocardial damage is reversible. Potentially life-threatening ECG abnormalities are found in more than 50 per cent of these patients.[10, 11]

Chest x-ray usually reveals pulmonary edema. Laboratory studies reveal abnormalities in myocardial enzymes and liver function tests. Blood urea nitrogen (BUN) and creatinine levels are usually elevated. Blood gas measurements demonstrate a combined respiratory and metabolic acidosis. Complete blood count (CBC) may reveal a leukopenia and low red blood cell count. Chronic skin exposure to phosphine 0.6 ppm has caused hyperemia and hypersensitivity to touch.[10]

Of interest, workers exposed intermittently to phosphine levels of up to 35 ppm but averaging less than 10 ppm complained of mild symptoms that resolved, and no cumulative effects were noted. Chronic, low-level exposure led to toothache and mandibular swelling and ultimately jaw necrosis, the so-called phossy jaw.[9]

Signs and symptoms may mimic, in mild form, the symptoms of viral upper respiratory infections. More severe forms of phosphine exposure may be confused with cardiogenic pulmonary edema, viral or bacterial pneumonias, or full-blown adult respiratory distress syndrome (ARDS) from any cause.

Treatment

Initially, the patient must be removed as quickly and safely as possible from the environment. All clothing should be removed and the skin washed. Oxygenation, IV administration of fluids, vasopressors, plasma expanders, fresh blood transfusion, bronchodilators, and digoxin or calcium channel blockers must be considered based on the clinical picture. Persistent hypotension that is unresponsive to vasopressors (e.g., dopamine) is much more prevalent in the setting of oral phosphide ingestion than in situations of phophine gas exposure. Diuretics, if the patient is not hypotensive, should be considered for pulmonary edema. Seizures are controlled by the usual therapeutic modalities.

Calcium gluconate and 25 per cent magnesium sulfate, because of their membrane stabilizing effects, have been advocated and utilized with good results. If ingestion of phosphine has occurred, gastric lavage with a potassium permanganate solution (in a 1:10,000 dilution) is recommended. Permanganate oxidizes phosphine in the stomach to form phosphate, thereby reducing the available amount of toxic phosphine. The results of potassium permanganate lavage are much better if this treatment is instituted within 60 minutes of ingestion.[11, 12] Singh reported the survival of one patient with massive renal failure due to phosphine toxicity by utilizing hemodialysis.[8] The value of steroids has not been proved but is thought to be helpful in reducing inflammation, especially in the pulmonary system.[2]

Prevention, the ultimate treatment, consists primarily of adequate ventilation and respiratory protection from phosphine gas. The accidental ingestion of phosphide is best avoided by controlling its production and distribution and by adequate warnings and education in areas where it is used. Pediatric exposure is best prevented by continued adult vigilance. Any person with underlying cardiac, pulmonary, liver, or renal disease should be precluded from possible exposure.

Annual physical examinations and chest x-rays should be conducted on workers with potential exposure. In the workplace frequent clothing changes and appropriately located showers and eye fountains should be utilized.

Long-Term Implications

The great majority of deaths occur within the first 24 hours and depend on the concentration and duration of exposure as well as its prompt recognition and treatment. In those fortunate individuals who survive the initial 24 hours, most show no permanent disabilities within 30 days, and all return to their normal baseline values within 4 months.[11, 12, 14] All liver, pulmonary, and renal function studies as well as ECG changes return to normal within this time frame. In summary, full recovery is anticipated if the patient survives the initial insult.

PHOSGENE

Phosgene is a colorless gas, heavier than air, and has a musty odor resembling fresh-mown hay or green corn. In high concentrations it is reported to be rather pungent and mildly irritating. Smokers have reported a flat, metallic taste when smoking in the presence of phosgene. Synonyms include carbonic dichloride, carbonyl chloride, carbon oxychloride, and chloroformyl chloride. Its chemical identification number is 1076, a potentially useful fact in identifying spills in railway or truck accidents. Phosgene is an acidic chloride with a chemical formula of $COCl_2$ and the following structure:[15–18]

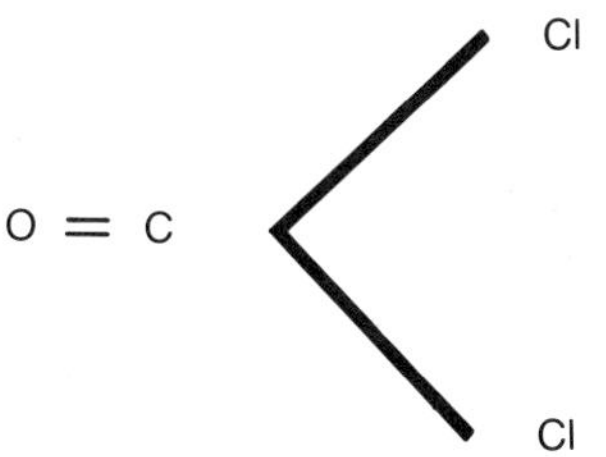

Phosgene does not occur naturally and was first synthesized by Sir Humphry Davy in 1812 by means of passing carbon monoxide and chlorine through charcoal. During the Industrial Revolution, the use of phosgene in manufacturing gradually increased; however, morbidity and mortality attributable to phosgene largely went unrecognized and unreported. Because of its properties (colorless, heavier than air), phosgene was used extensively in gas warfare in World War I, and numerous authors have reported that it caused 80 per cent of the deaths by gas in that conflict.[19–21]

Because of its devastating effects in World War I and follow-up studies on veterans from that war, the industrial nations recognized the need for personnel protection, and by 1940 occupational exposure standards were widely recognized in the United States and other nations. A maximum allowable concentration (MAC) of 1.0 ppm (gas) or 0.4 mg per m^3 (liquid) and a threshold limit value (TLV) of 0.1 ppm of continuous exposure during a 10-hour day were established and were widely accepted.[17, 19] Fortunately, gas warfare was sparingly used in World War II, and exposure now is primarily industrial and occurs relatively rarely and in isolated instances.

Phosgene is used in the synthesis or manufacture of isocyanates, polyurethane, polycarbonate resins, aniline dyes, pharmaceuticals, plastics, and insecticides and in the "uranium enrichment" process. Phosgene is also a combustion or decomposition byproduct of most volatile chlorine compounds (e.g., carbon tetrachloride, chloroform, and methylene chloride). These substances are widely found in common household substances such as solvents, paint removers, and dry cleaning fluids, which, when exposed to heat or fire, can produce phosgene gas. In December, 1987, in Tampa, Florida, an individual was filling an air mattress with a hair dryer when the mattress exploded, burned, and released phosgene into the apartment.[22] This gas represents one of the many hazards to firefighting personnel and fire victims. Welding in a poorly ventilated, confined space in the presence of chlorinated solvents or other halides can cause phosgene to form rapidly in lethal concentrations. The Occupational Safety and Health Administration (OSHA) placed the yearly production of phosgene in the United States at two million pounds and estimated that 10,000 workers are at risk of phosgene exposure.[23]

Phosgene was implicated in the Bhopal, India, tragedy that occurred in December, 1984. Approximately 150,000 to 200,000 people were affected, significant morbidity occurred in more than 10,000, and mortality was approximately 3,300. This industrial accident was the worst of its kind in civilian history. Nearly 50,000 pounds of stored methylisocyanate (MIC) were released in vapor and liquid forms over a period of 2 hours. MIC is made from phosgene and methylamine and is used as an intermediate product in the manufacture of the carbamate insecticide Carbaryl, or Sevin (Union Carbide Corp. trade name). Because of the hypothesized reactions that took place within the storage tank and in the surrounding atmosphere, it is thought that MIC, phosgene, and hydrogen cyanide all played a significant role in this well-known disaster.[24]

Prevention of exposure to phosgene is the key to success in the workplace and home. At work, appropriate ventilation, exhaust fans, frequent checks of tank apparatus and piping seals, respiratory protection, chemical goggles, frequent changing and washing of work clothes, regular scheduled use of phosgene dosimeters or chemically impregnated strips, and physical examinations at regular intervals all have made significant phosgene exposure a rare occurrence. In the home, strict adherence to label precautions regarding both the use and storage of chemicals and solvents should be employed and encouraged.

Pathophysiology

As in most exposures to toxic substances, the concentration, duration, and water solubility of phosgene are the three key factors in the individual's response to phosgene. Phosgene slowly hydrolyzes in mucous membrane water to produce carbon dioxide and hydrochloric acids. This reaction may take place in minutes to several hours, rarely exceeding 24 hours, depending on concentration and duration of exposure. Because this hydrolysis tends to occur slowly, phosgene is less irritating to the mucous membrane of the upper airway and eyes and therefore penetrates more deeply into the lungs. This initial formation of hydrochloric acid causes epithelial damage and necrosis in the bronchi and small bronchioles, leading to an increase in permeability and edema. Tobias et al (1949)[25] demonstrated in the animal model the direct action of low concentrations of phosgene causing bronchial and bronchiolar necrosis and severe pulmonary edema. The same group also demonstrated massive red blood cell hemolysis at high concentrations of phosgene with resultant capillary plugging. Following the epithelial damage, focal disruption of type I pneumatocytes occurs, causing further alveolar and interstitial edema. This result is later followed by derangements in type II pneumatocytes, interstitial cell necrosis, and alveolar collapse.[25]

If the initial concentration of phosgene was high, there may be a rapid onset of direct cytotoxicity and enzymatic poisoning. Since phosgene is an acidic chloride, it reacts readily with NH_2^-, OH^- and SH^- groups. These radicals are found in essentially all living tissue as components of albumin, amino acids, intermediary metabolites, enzymes, and vitamins. For example, phosgene reacts with glutathione in renal and hepatic tissue to form diglucathionyl dithiocarbamate. As soon as glutathione stores are depleted, phosgene covalently binds with proteins in cellular enzymes in macromolecules, leading to hepatic and renal necrosis.[26] Ivanhoe and Meyers (1964) demonstrated in rabbits that phosgene also causes neuroparalysis of the sympathetic system, resulting in marked pulmonary vasoconstriction and further contributing to pulmonary edema.[27]

The end result of phosgene toxicity clinically is hypovolemia, hemoconcentration, hypotension, progressive respiratory distress with pulmonary edema and oxygenation abnormalities, and pulmonary, hepatic, and renal cellular necrosis. If phosgene toxicity is unrecognized or irreversible with treatment, full-blown ARDS develops, leading to death.

Clinical Signs and Symptoms

Eye irritation with conjunctivitis, excessive lacrimation, or corneal damage has been reported secondary to phosgene exposure in gas or liquid states. Dryness and burning of the throat, thirst, cough with thick sputum or hemoptysis, headache, nausea, vomiting, weakness, cyanosis, and chest discomfort all may be present in varying degrees. Skin irritation, especially if the victim is hot and sweaty, has been reported secondary to both gas and liquid exposure. The initial constellation of signs and symptoms is proportional to the duration and concentration of the substance.[28] In terms of specific exposure levels, 3 ppm can cause immediate throat irritation; 4 ppm will affect the eyes; and 5 to 10 ppm will cause an immediate cough. Exposure to 25 ppm for 30 minutes is very dangerous, and even brief exposure to 50 ppm or greater may be rapidly fatal. Rat studies have shown that 2 days of continuous exposure to 0.5 ppm was lethal, and 1 hour of continuous exposure to 2 ppm caused permanent lung damage.[16, 18, 19]

In most cases, a relatively asymptomatic latent period follows the initial symptoms; this may last for a few minutes to 72 hours. The duration of the latent period is inversely proportional to the severity of the initial exposure. Most cases of significant exposure have a latent period of less than 24 hours, and 80 per cent of mortalities occur within 48 hours of the initial exposure.[21]

Other than a high index of suspicion and a very careful, detailed history that pays attention to possible exposure, there are no specific diagnostic tests for phosgene. Chest x-ray findings of pulmonary edema, hilar enlargement, and ill-defined central, patchy infiltrates are rather late findings that occur within 6 to 8 hours of exposure. Entities that may mimic phosgene exposure include exposure to other noxious gases (e.g., oxides of nitrogen, chlorine, ammonia, and sulfur dioxide), upper respiratory infections (viral or bacterial), cardiogenic pulmonary edema, pneumonia, or ARDS from other causes.

General and Specific Treatment

Due to the latent period, high mortality rate, and permanent morbidity, essentially all victims with known phosgene exposure should be admitted and closely observed. Obviously, the victim must be immediately removed from the contaminated environment, and all contaminated clothing must also be removed.

Exposure of the eye or skin, whether to liquid or gas, should be treated with copious lavage. Treatment is aimed primarily at the pulmonary system and includes supplemental oxygen delivered by the most appropriate route, pulmonary arterial catheter monitoring for fluid and oxygenation management, and bronchodilators. Continuous oximeter monitoring, serial blood gas analysis, and pulmonary function testing should be employed. Prophylactic antibiotics are recommended because autopsy studies have uniformly found evidence of pneumonia and bronchitis. Dopamine may be necessary for treatment of hypotension, bradycardia, or renal failure. The benefits of sedation should be weighed against the sedative effect on the respiratory center. Diuretics are contraindicated because pulmonary edema is not hypervolemic in origin, and phosgene victims tend to be hypovolemic and hypotensive.

Specific therapeutic regimens for phosgene have been controversial. Russian and German scientists during both World Wars felt that hexamethylene tetramine (HMT; methenamine; Urotropin) was a specific antidote, and both countries utilized the substance in their gas masks. This subject was extensively studied during and after both World Wars, and the controversy raged in the literature. Diller (1980) undertook an extensive review of the world literature plus experimentation and concluded that there was a limited prophylactic effect of HMT if it were administered *before* phosgene exposure, but there was no convincing proof of a therapeutic effect of HMT administered *after* phosgene exposure.[26]

Cysteine in vitro traps phosgene and converts it to a less harmful metabolite. It has, therefore, been suggested that the administration of *N*-acetyl cysteine (Mucomyst) may afford some protection. To date, no controlled in vivo studies have been reported.[29, 30] Plunkett (1980) suggests the use of aminocaproic acid (Amicar) to prevent fibrinolysis and to enhance hemostasis in the presence of a phosgene-induced bleeding diathesis.[17]

Administration of steroids is suggested throughout the phosgene literature and seems reasonable in light of the intense inflammation, especially in the respiratory epithelium. The Bhopal experience clearly demonstrated the efficacy of steroid use throughout the acute treatment phase.[24]

Long-Term Implications

Studies performed during the 1920s and 1930s on veterans implied that phosgene exposure caused chronic and recurrent morbidity and increased mortality from bronchitis, emphysema, and reactivation of tuberculosis. However, these studies were limited by the fact that the duration and concentration of the exposure in the battlefield setting were unknown.

Polednak (1980)[31] did an extensive 30-year outcome review of over 800 uranium processing plant workers with known levels and duration of exposure. Utilizing standardized mortality ratios (SMRs), he concluded that in the group of workers with low levels of daily exposure (699 men) there was no evidence of excessive overall mortality, or mortality from diseases of the respiratory system. However, in the group with known high levels of exposure (106 men) there did appear to be an increase in mortality and morbidity (pneumonitis, chronic bronchitis, emphysema, impaired pulmonary function studies), although the sample size was such that no definitive conclusions could be reached. Similarly, the same author concluded, with the same caveat regarding sample size, that there was no evidence of increased lung cancer mortality after exposure to phosgene.

References

1. Plunkett ER: Handbook of Industrial Toxicology. 3rd ed. New York, Chemical Publishing Co, 1987, pp 430–432.
2. Haddad LM, Winchester JF: Clinical Management of Poisoning and Drug Overdose. Philadelphia, WB Saunders Co, 1983, Chap. 84.
3. Stutz DR, Ricks RC, Olsen MF: Hazardous Materials Injuries: A Handbook for Pre-Hospital Care (Protocol 67). Greenbelt, MD, Bradford Communications Corp, 1982.
4. Morgan DP: Recognition and Management of Pesticide Poisonings. 3rd ed. Washington DC, US Environmental Protection Agency, 1982, Chap. 12.
5. Chan LTF, Crowley RJ, Dellion D, et al: Phosphine analysis in post mortem specimens following ingestion of aluminum phosphide. J Anal Toxicol *7*:165–167, 1983.
6. Jain SM, Bharani A, Sepaha GC, et al: Electrocardiographic changes in aluminum phosphide (ALP) poisoning. J Assoc Phys India *33*:406–409, 1985.
7. DiPalma JR: Human toxicity from rat poisons. Clin Pharm *24*:186–189, 1981.
8. Singh S, Dilawari JB, Vashist R, et al: Aluminum phosphide ingestion. Br Med J *290*:1110–1111, 1985.
9. Dreisbach RH, Robertson WO: Handbook of Poisoning: Prevention, Diagnosis, and Treatment. Norwalk, CT, Appleton and Lange, 1987, Chap. 15.
10. Raman R, Dubey M: The electrocardiographic changes in quick phos poisoning. Indian Heart J *37*:193–195, 1985.
11. Khosla SN, Chugh SN, Nand N, Saini RS: Systemic involvement in aluminium phosphide poisoning. J Assoc Physicians India *34*:227–230, 1986.
12. Sepaha GC, Bharani AK, Jain SM, Raman PG: Acute aluminium phosphide poisoning. J Indian Med Assoc *83*:378–379, 1985.
13. Proctor NH, Hughes JP: Chemical Hazards of the Workplace. Philadelphia, JB Lippincott Co, 1978, pp 415–416.
14. Shusterman D: Problem-solving techniques in occupational medicine. J Fam Prac *21*:195–199, 1985.
15. Misra NP, Manoria PC, Saxena K: Fatal pulmonary oedema with phosgene poisoning. J Assoc Phys India *33*:430–431, 1985.
16. Stutz DR, Ricks RC, Olsen MF: Hazardous Materials Injuries: A Handbook for Pre-Hospital Care (Protocol 12). Greenbelt, MD, Bradford Communications Corp, 1982.
17. Plunkett ER: Handbook of Industrial Toxicology. 3rd ed. New York, Chemical Publishing Co, 1987, pp 428–430.
18. Proctor NH, Hughes JP: Chemical Hazards of the Workplace. Philadelphia, JB Lippincott Co, 1978, pp 414–415.
19. Bradley BL, Unger KM: Phosgene inhalation: a case report. Texas Med *78*:51–53, 1982.
20. Goldfrank LR: Toxicologic Emergencies: A Comprehensive Handbook in Problem Solving. New York, Appleton-Century-Crofts, 1982, Chap. 25.
21. Haddad LM, Winchester JF: Clinical Management of Poisoning and Drug Overdose. Philadelphia, WB Saunders Co, 1983, Chap. 84.
22. Akron Beacon Journal: Thrifty Couple Gets Big Bang from Mattress. December 13, 1987, p. A–13.
23. Occupational Exposure to Phosgene: Criteria for a Recommended Standard. Washington, DC, National Institute for Occupational Safety and Health, 1976.
24. Lorin HG, Kulling PEJ: The Bhopal tragedy—What has Swedish disaster medicine planning learned from it? J Emerg Med *4*:311–316, 1986.
25. Tobias JM, et al: Localization of the site of action of a pulmonary irritant, diphosgene. Am J Physiol *158*:173–183, 1949.
26. Diller WF: The methenamine misunderstanding in the therapy of phosgene poisoning. Arch Toxicol *46*:199–206, 1980.
27. Ivanhoe F, Meyers PH: Phosgene poisoning, as an example of neuroparalytic acute pulmonary oedema. The sympathetic vasometer reflex involved. Dis Chest *46*:211–218, 1964.
28. Dreisbach RH, Robertson WO: Handbook of Poisoning: Prevention, Diagnosis, and Treatment. Norwalk, CT, Appleton and Lange, 1987, Chap. 10.
29. Kubic VL, Anders MW: Metabolism of carbon tetrachloride to phosgene. Life Sci *26*:2151, 1980.
30. Pohl LR, Bhooshan B, Krishna G: Mechanism of activation of chloroform. Toxicol Appl Pharmacol *45*:238, 1978.
31. Polednak AP: Mortality among men occupationally exposed to phosgene in 1943–1945. Environ Research *22*:357–367, 1980.

CHAPTER 82

METHYL BROMIDE AND RELATED COMPOUNDS

John C. Bradford, D.O., FACEP

METHYL BROMIDE

Methyl bromide (CH_3Br) is in relatively widespread industrial use as a fumigant and insecticide because of its effective penetrating power and absence of fire or explosion hazard. It is estimated that 75,000 American workers are occupationally exposed to methyl bromide annually.[14] Its toxicity is severe, and despite safeguards, cases of acute and chronic intoxication occur, chiefly in the fruit and tobacco industries.[1, 2] It has also been used as a refrigerant, solvent, methylating agent, and in dyes and fire extinguishers. Methyl bromide is also known as bromomethane, monobromomethane, Embafume, or iscobrome.[3]

Pathophysiology

Pure methyl bromide is a colorless gas that is heavier than air. Odorless and tasteless in low concentrations, it has a musty, acrid smell in high concentrations.[4] Toxic exposure can occur by inhalation or by skin absorption. Excretion takes place mainly through the lungs. The remainder is metabolized in the body, and inorganic bromine is excreted in the urine.[5]

The mechanism of action of methyl bromide is incompletely understood. Neither inorganic bromide nor methyl alcohol are primarily responsible for the common clinical presentations. An intracellular site of action has been postulated, possibly by methylation of sulhydryl groups of complex enzyme systems.[3, 5–8] This cellular disruption seems to have an affinity for the central nervous system, resulting in progressive dysfunction. At autopsy, cerebral edema, hyperemia of the meninges, subarachnoid and cerebral hemorrhages, demyelination, and loss of neurons have been described. Cardiac, hepatic, pulmonary, and renal damage may also occur.[4, 9, 10]

In methyl bromide poisoning, symptoms can occur at a bromide level of 3 mg per dL, and levels of 8 or 9 mg per dL may be fatal.[1, 4, 12] In contrast, bromism resulting from poisoning by inorganic bromides does not appear until levels of 50 to 100 mg per dL are reached.[11]

Clinical Features

While very high concentrations (>250 ppm) can cause pulmonary edema and death from respiratory collapse, lower level exposure frequently results in central and peripheral nervous system toxicity.[9, 12, 13]

The onset of symptoms is usually delayed from 30 minutes to several hours or longer, depending on the concentration of the gas and length of exposure. Chemosis, conjunctivitis, and vesicular skin eruptions can occur locally.[2, 3, 4, 16]

Neurologic manifestations include vomiting, headache, vertigo, gait disturbances, diplopia, delirium, mania, seizures, and a Reye-like syndrome. Hallucinations, paresthesias, amnesia, aphasia, and depression may also occur.[2, 4, 10, 14, 15] In some cases, mental disturbances may predominate with only mild neurologic signs and no seizures. In others, severe status epilepticus may be present, which is often refractory to therapy.[9, 15]

Proteinuria and oliguria may occur because of renal cortical necrosis. With liver involvement, a hepatitis-like picture may be present.[9, 10, 15]

Treatment

Initial decontamination is vitally important. The patient should be immediately evacuated from the scene and the clothing removed, as methyl bromide can penetrate cloth, leather, or rubber.[17–19] Exposed skin should be washed with water, and the eyes should be flushed. Symptomatic care should be provided as soon as possible with oxygen, diazepam, and/or phenytoin for seizures, aggressive pulmonary toilet, and standard burn care for skin exposure. Pulmonary edema should respond to diuretics and bronchodilators. Mechanical ventilatory support may be necessary.[1, 3, 9, 13]

In an attempt to improve the elimination of bromide, dimercaprol (BAL) has been recommended as a chelating agent because of methyl bromide's postulated combination with sulfhydryl groups.[1, 5, 20] Reduced glutathione levels have been demonstrated with methyl bromide toxicity in animal models, and elevated glutathione levels are thought to be potentially protective. *N*-Acetylcysteine has been shown to serve as a precursor to glutathione and has also been recommended as an adjunct to treatment.[5, 21]

Long-term Implications

Psychiatric and neurologic recovery may take months to years, and in severe cases, permanent defects, including vertigo, hallucinations, anxiety, depression, myoclonus, and optic atrophy may occur.[5, 13–15, 22]

In chronic, low-level exposures, slight EEG and serum transaminase changes have been noted, but no relationship has been found with clinical signs or symptoms.[23]

METHYL IODIDE

Methyl iodide (CH_3I), also known as iodomethane, is a colorless, transparent liquid with a pungent odor. It is produced by the reaction of methanol, iodine and phosphorus and is used primarily as a methylating agent in pharmaceutical and chemical synthesis. Methyl iodide formerly was used as a grain and tobacco fumigant but is reported to be no longer used in agricultural applications.[24]

Methyl iodide intoxication has been infrequently reported in the medical literature, with exposures occurring in much smaller numbers than with methyl bromide.[25] This most likely reflects methyl iodide's more limited use and potential for worker exposure, as it remains a liquid at room temperature.

Pathophysiology

While the exact mechanism of action of methyl iodide remains unclear, methylation of intracellular sulfhydryl groups is postulated.[7, 25]

Clinical Features

As in methyl bromide exposure, neurologic dysfunction is the predominant clinical presentation. Pulmonary edema, renal failure, and cardiovascular collapse have all been reported. Prolonged or repeated exposure markedly increases the chance for toxicity.[7]

Neurologic and psychologic manifestations are similar to those found in methyl bromide toxicity. The dysfunction may progress rapidly to seizures, coma, and death or may be chronic, with persistent cerebellar and psychologic disturbances present indefinitely after exposure.[25]

Direct, long-term skin exposure to methyl iodide can cause burns or blistering. The latency period between exposure and the presentation of clinical symptoms ranges from hours to days.[25, 27]

Treatment

The treatment of methyl iodide exposure is essentially the same as for methyl bromide, with elimination of the toxin, supportive care, and the possible use of BAL or *N*-acetylcysteine.[1, 5, 21, 26]

Long-term Implications

Psychiatric disturbances similar to those noted in methyl bromide toxicity may persist indefinitely.[23]

ETHYLENE DIBROMIDE

Ethylene dibromide (EDB,1,2-dibromomethane) has been widely used for some 40 years as a soil fumigant for nematodes, and as an insect control for citrus fruits and grains. It is also used as a lead scavenger in gasoline refinement. Its toxicity to humans comes from its potential carcinogenicity from long-term, low-level exposure, with direct high-level exposure producing acute symptoms.[28] In 1984, the Environmental Protection Agency severely restricted the use of ethylene dibromide when it was detected in commercial products such as baking mixes.

Pathophysiology

Pure ethylene dibromide is a clear, colorless liquid with a distinctive odor usually described as sweet. It is considered an alkylating agent that effects DNA replication and ultimately cell division. It alters intracellular functions and can disrupt biologic systems.[29]

Clinical Features

Direct exposure can cause skin ulcerations, conjunctivitis, gastrointestinal and respiratory mucosal irritation, central nervous system irritation, and depression.[29] Two fatalities have been reported after extensive dermal and respiratory exposure. These individuals experienced respiratory irritation, vomiting, diarrhea, confusion, and obtundation. Severe metabolic acidosis and hepatic and renal failure developed, and both succumbed to multiple organ system failure.[30] One reported case of oral ingestion of 140 mg per kg of EDB resulted in massive liver necrosis and renal damage.[29]

Laboratory values after an acute exposure may reflect a severe metabolic acidosis, renal failure, and hepatic necrosis. Serum bromide levels will be elevated.[30]

Hepatotoxicity and squamous cell carcinoma of the stomach have been implicated in EDB exposure in animal studies.[28, 30, 31]

References

1. Rathus EM, Landy PJ: Methyl bromide poisoning. Br J Ind Med *18*:53-57, 1961.
2. MacDonald AC, Monro IC, Scott GI: Fatal case of poisoning due to inhalation of methyl bromide. Br Med J *2*:112-116, 1965.
3. Proctor NH, Hughes JP: Chemical Hazards of the Workplace. Philadelphia, JB Lippincott, 1978, pp 332-333.
4. Clarke CA, Roworth CG, Holling HE: Methyl bromide poisoning; An account of four recent cases met with in one of HM ships. Br J Ind Med *2*:17-23, 1945.
5. Zatuchni J, Hong K: Methyl bromide poisoning seen initially as psychosis. Arch Neurol *38*:529-530, 1981.
6. Miller DP, Haggard HW: Intracellular penetration of bromide as a feature in the toxicity of alkyl bromides. J Ind Hyg Tox *25*:423-433, 1943.
7. Lewis SE: Inhibition of SH proteins by methyl bromide. Nature *161*:692-693, 1948.
8. Nishimura M, Umeda M, Ishizu S, et al: Effects of methyl bromide on cultured mammalian cells. J Toxicol Sci *5*:321-330, 1980.
9. Hine CH: Methyl bromide poisoning; A review of ten cases. J Occup Med *11*:1-10, 1969.
10. Prain JH, Smith GH: A clinical-pathological report of eight cases of methyl bromide poisoning. Br J Ind Med *9*:44-49, 1952.
11. Hoffman WS: The Biochemistry of Clinical Medicine. 2nd ed. Chicago, Year Book Medical Publishers, 1959, pp 223-225.
12. Collins RR: Methyl bromide poisoning; A bizarre neurological disorder. Calif Med *103*:112-116, 1965.
13. Behrens RH, Dukes DC: Fatal methyl bromide poisoning. Br J Ind Med *43*:561-562, 1986.
14. Chavez CT, Hepler RS, Straatsma BR: Methyl bromide optic atrophy. Am J Ophthalmol *99*:715-719, 1985.
15. Shield LK, Coleman TL, Markesberg WR: Methyl bromide intoxication; Neurologic features, including simulation of Reye Syndrome. Neurology *27*:959-962, 1977.
16. Irish DD: Halogenated hydrocarbons; I; Aliphatic. *In* Patty FA, Fassett DW, Irish DD (eds): Industrial Hygiene and Toxicology, Vol. II. Toxicology. New York, John Wiley and Sons, 1963, pp 1243-1332.
17. Plukett ER: Handbook of Industrial Toxicology. 3rd ed. New York, Chemical Publishing Company, Inc., 1987, pp 347-349.
18. Stutz DR, Ricks RC, Olsen MF: Hazardous Materials Injuries. Greenbelt, MD, Bradford Communications Corp., 1982.
19. O'Neal L: Acute methyl bromide toxicity. J Emerg Nurs *13*:96-98, 1987, pp 216-217.
20. Marraccini J, Thomas G, Ongley J: Death and injury caused by methyl bromide. J Forensic Sci *28*:601-607, 1983.
21. Alexeef GV, Munoz P, Watt D: Determination of acute toxic effects in mice following exposure to methyl bromide. J Toxicol Environ Health *15*:109-123, 1985.
22. Prockop LD, Smith AO: Seizures and action myoclonus after occupational exposure to methyl bromide. J Flor Med Assoc *73*:690-692, 1986.
23. Verberk MM, Rooyakkers-Beemster T, DeVireger M, et al: Bromide in blood, EEG and transaminases in methyl bromide workers. Br J Ind Med *36*:59-62, 1979.
24. IARC Manographs: Methyl iodide. *41*:213, 1986.
25. Appel GB, Galen R, O'Brien J, Schoenfeldt R: Methyl iodide intoxication. A case report. Ann Intern Med *82*:534-536, 1975.
26. Buckell M: 2:3 Dimercaptopropanol (BAL) and methyl iodide intoxication. Nature (Lond) *163*:330, 1949.
27. Hartman TL, Wacker W, Roll R: Methyl chloride intoxication. N Engl J Med *253*:552-554, 1955.
28. Sun M: EBD contamination kindles federal action. Science *223*:464-466, 1984.
29. Alexiou NG: Ethylene dibromide, a diagnostic and therapeutic problem for the practitioner. J Flor Med Assoc *71*:151-174, 1984.
30. Letz GA, Pond SM, et al: Two fatalities after acute occupational exposure to ethylene dibromide. JAMA *252*:2428-2431, 1984.
31. Goldman L, Smith RF: Behavioral effects of prenatal exposure to ethylene dibromide. Neurobehav Toxicol Teratol *5*:579-585, 1983.

CHAPTER 83
HYDROGEN SULFIDE AND CARBON DISULFIDE

Ingrid M. O. Vicas, M.D., C.M.
Daniel D. Whitcraft III, M.D.

HYDROGEN SULFIDE

Hydrogen sulfide (H_2S) is a highly toxic, malodorous, intensely irritating gas. It results in significant numbers of fatalities, often multiple, due to inadequately protected coworkers who succumb during rescue procedures.

Sources

H_2S is released from a variety of natural sources, including decaying organic material, natural gas, volcanic gases, and sulfur springs. H_2S is routinely generated in agriculture and in the course of oil and gas exploration. More than 70 occupations involve some risk of hydrogen sulfide toxicity, including workers in viscose rayon manufacture, paper mills, petrochemical plants, natural gas plants, petroleum refineries, heavy water production, coke oven plants, iron smelters, food processing plants, sugar beet processing, tanneries, and pesticide and sulfur production.[1] The petroleum industry, however, is the single highest source of H_2S exposure to workers.[2]

H_2S toxicity is invariably the result of occupational exposure. There have been no reports in the English language literature of deliberate suicidal exposure to H_2S.

Mechanism of Action

By inhibiting mitochondrial cytochrome oxidase aa3, H_2S paralyzes the electron transport system, resulting in inhibition of cellular utilization of oxygen, metabolic acidosis secondary to anaerobic metabolism, and cytotoxic anoxia.[3] In body fluids at physiologic pH, undissociated and dissociated hydrogen sulfide exist in equal proportions. The undissociated acid, H_2S, is thought to be more inhibitory than its dissociated form, HS^-.[4]

Although the mechanism of toxicity of H_2S resembles that of cyanide, sulfide is a more potent cytochrome oxidase inhibitor than cyanide.[3]

Single sublethal doses of H_2S directly stimulate the carotid body, resulting in a brief but dramatic hyperpnea.[5] However, in persons with lethal doses the primary cause of death has been attributed to respiratory paralysis due to the toxic effect of sulfides on the respiratory centers of the brain.[6,7] Experimental evidence showing selective uptake of sulfide by the brain stem seems to support this observation.[8,9]

Pharmacokinetics

Absorption. H_2S is rapidly absorbed almost exclusively through the inhalational route. Percutaneous absorption is minimal, although toxicity and even fatalities have been reported following cutaneous application of sulfur-containing dermatologic preparations or ammonium sulfide permanent-wave solutions.[10]

Distribution. H_2S is distributed to the brain, liver, kidney, pancreas, and small intestine.[11]

Metabolism. The metabolism of H_2S involves three different pathways: (1) oxidation to sulfate (considered to be the major metabolic pathway), (2) methylation, and (3) reaction with metallic ion or disulfide-containing proteins. Oxidation and methylation represent detoxification routes, whereas interaction with essential proteins is responsible for the toxic action of H_2S.[6]

Sulfides undergo spontaneous oxidation through both enzymatic and nonenzymatic mechanisms to nontoxic products such as thiosulfate, polysulfides, or sulfate. The major site of this conversion appears to be the liver, although other tissues such as the kidneys, lungs, and plasma may function as secondary sites. The process of sulfide autooxidation consumes oxygen.[7]

The reaction of H_2S with nonessential proteins containing disulfide bonds (e.g., glutathione) may represent yet another detoxification pathway with interesting therapeutic implications.[10]

H_2S, produced endogenously by anaerobic bacteria in the gut, is detoxified through sequential methylation by intestinal tract cells.[12] The importance, if any, of this metabolic route for the detoxification of exogenously administered hydrogen sulfide remains to be determined.[6]

Excretion. Nontoxic oxidation products are excreted primarily by the kidneys.[13] Neither hydrogen sulfide nor its metabolites have been shown to be excreted by the lungs.[14]

H_2S is not a cumulative poison because it is metabolized and excreted.

Table 83–1. PHYSIOLOGIC EFFECTS OF HUMAN EXPOSURE TO H_2S

H_2S CONCENTRATION (ppm)	EFFECT
0.02	Odor threshold
100–150	Nose/eye irritation
250–500	Sore throat, cough
	Keratoconjunctivitis
	Chest tightness
	Pulmonary edema
500–1000	Headache
	Disorientation
	Loss of reasoning
	Cyanosis
	Coma, convulsions
> 1000	Death

(Adapted from Beauchamp RO, Bus JS, Popp JA, Boreiko CJ, Andjelkovich DA: A critical review of the literature on hydrogen sulfide toxicity. CRC Crit Rev Toxicol *13*:25–49, 1984.)

Clinical Presentation

Epidemiology. Because this condition is predominantly an occupational exposure, men tend to be more commonly affected.[2] However, a number of reports describe spouses[15] or children[15, 16] who have accidentally been exposed to H_2S.

Acute Exposure

Two major effects of hydrogen sulfide on the human system can be identified: a local irritative effect that develops after prolonged exposure and a rapidly fatal systemic effect of the inhalation of high concentrations of H_2S.[6] The primary targets of systemic H_2S toxicity appear to be the central nervous system and the respiratory system. The mucous membranes of the eyes and the respiratory tract are the targets of local irritative and inflammatory effects. Severity of clinical effects is related both to the concentration of H_2S (Table 83–1) and the duration of exposure.

Symptoms in seriously affected patients, not surprisingly, include unconsciousness, cyanosis, dilated pupils, decreased respirations or apnea, and generalized tremors or convulsions and agitation.

Neurologic Manifestations. Transient loss of consciousness, prolonged coma, lateralizing motor signs, headache, agitation, somnolence, tremulousness, convulsions, opisthotonus, and vertigo have been described as central nervous system manifestations of toxicity.[15, 17–29] In a large series of workers exposed to H_2S, even though 75 per cent demonstrated a period of loss of consciousness at the site of exposure, only 13 per cent were still comatose on arrival at the hospital.[2] Table 83–1 summarizes the clinical effects seen in three series with a total of 523 patients.[2, 30, 31] Neurologic complaints consisting of altered behavior patterns, confusion, vertigo, agitation, and somnolence were common in all three series. Although headache may not necessarily occur immediately after exposure, it is usually present in 16 to 25 per cent of patients by the time they arrive at the hospital.[2]

Sudden loss of consciousness on exposure to toxic concentrations, commonly referred to as "knockdown" by workers, is usually associated with spontaneous recovery. Workers may continue at their jobs without seeking medical attention until the end of the workday, at which point they are essentially asymptomatic.

Pulmonary Manifestations. Minor pulmonary manifestations include cough, dyspnea, and hemoptysis (Table 83–2). Clinical and radiologic evidence of pulmonary edema[2, 17, 20, 23, 24, 25, 30, 42] and apnea[17, 18, 19, 21, 22, 30, 32] represent life-threatening pulmonary symptoms. Once respirations cease, they do not resume spontaneously if the patient is removed from the toxic source.[33] Apnea is often followed by convulsions, cardiovascular collapse, and death.

Table 83–2. CLINICAL FEATURES OF H_2S TOXICITY

	REFERENCE			
SYMPTOM	*Kleinfeld (ref 30) n=52*	*Burnett (ref 2) n=221*	*Arnold (ref 31) n=250*	*Total n=523*
Unconsciousness	11	163	135	309
Dizziness, vertigo, agitation, confusion	39	50	54	143
Headache	11	27	65	103
Nausea or vomiting	12	38	62	112
Dyspnea	5	6	57	68
Convulsions	1	16	5	22
Pulmonary edema	2	34	14	50
Cyanosis	5	19	3	27
Conjunctivitis	2	19	46	67
Sore throat, cough	5	24	41	70
Weakness	13	8	19	40
Hemoptysis		2	1	3
Miscellaneous	34*		79†	113
Death	4	10	7	21

*Includes hoarseness, tachycardia, numbness, chest burning, tremors, hyperreflexia.
†Includes malaise, chest pain, bradycardia, neuropsychologic symptoms.

Up to 20 per cent of patients exposed to H_2S arriving in an emergency department demonstrated pulmonary edema.[2] This pulmonary edema can be very extensive in nature with copious frothy, bloody secretions. Experimentally, a similar massive pulmonary edema can be demonstrated after acute inhalational exposure to H_2S.[34]

Marked cyanosis is a common phenomenon described in both survivors and fatalities.[17, 19, 20, 21, 22, 25, 27] Although the reason for this cyanosis is unclear, several explanations can be considered: (1) inadequate oxygenation due to marked pulmonary edema, (2) poor tissue perfusion due to hypotension, and (3) formation of a pigmented sulfhemoglobin. This third theory is controversial, some authors contending that H_2S toxicity does not induce sulfhemoglobin formation.[38]

Cardiologic Manifestations. Myocardial infarction and electrocardiographic (ECG) changes may occur. However, these effects may be secondary to prolonged hypoxia rather than to a direct cardiotoxic or arrhythmogenic effect of H_2S.

Other Manifestations. Local irritating effects such as sore throat and gastrointestinal symptoms such as nausea and vomiting have been described.[2] Ocular effects include keratoconjunctivitis and subjective symptoms such as blurring of vision, "haloes around lights" ("gas eye"), photophobia, and blepharospasm. These ocular symptoms occur early in a patient with subacute exposure to H_2S, even before the manifestation of any respiratory symptoms.[6]

At concentrations of up to 30 ppm, H_2S has a rotten egg odor, whereas at 30 ppm the odor is described as sickeningly sweet. The pungent odor of H_2S provides inadequate warning at low levels of exposure. At higher concentrations, olfactory nerve fatigue and later paralysis of the nerve results in an inability to detect the odor. The assumption that odor will warn of levels of H_2S that are life-threatening is erroneous because instantaneously introduced doses (>150 ppm) may not be perceived at all.[33] Workers who recover from H_2S exposure either have no recollection of any odor or may describe a sickeningly sweet odor prior to losing consciousness.

Disposition

In a series of 221 victims, 21 per cent were seen in a physician's office and discharged. Of the 78 per cent seen in hospital, 65 per cent were admitted, 6 per cent were dead on arrival, and the remainder (29 per cent) were discharged. Ultimately, 10 per cent of all admitted patients required transfer to a tertiary care facility.[2] In another series of 250 workers with H_2S exposure, 22 per cent required hospitalization for overnight observation.[31]

Outcome

The overall mortality in three series of H_2S victims is 4 per cent (range 2.8 to 6 per cent) (Table 83–2). Ultimate survival despite complete cardiopulmonary arrest has been described.[8, 23]

Most exposures result in 2 days or less of lost work time.[31] The majority of case reports describe no long-term sequelae even in patients who were in critical condition at presentation. However, most studies make no specific mention of the nature of long-term follow-up. Permanent neurologic sequelae include prolonged coma, convulsions, increased tone with extensor spasms,[35] chronic vegetative state,[16, 18] intention tremor, and pseudobulbar impairment.[19]

The potential for increased H_2S sensitivity from repeated exposures has been considered. No good evidence supports increased or decreased sensitivity to H_2S with multiple overexposures. Although H_2S is said not to be a cumulative poison,[5] it is possible that repeated knockdown episodes may result in long-term effects, or a knockdown experience may render the individual more susceptible to a lower concentration of H_2S on reexposure.

Chronic Exposure

Whether chronic poisoning exists as an entity or whether it is a subjective response to an obnoxious agent remains unresolved.[6] Although the majority of serious exposures are acute in nature, there is continued concern about the effects of long-term exposure on an individual's general health, particularly the development of the fetus and the immature central nervous system. However, data are incomplete on the teratogenic, carcinogenic, and long-term effects of chronic low-dose exposure.[1]

Laboratory Features

Arterial Blood Gases. Arterial PO_2 is usually normal. However, because of its action of binding to cytochrome oxidase, H_2S results in cellular impairment of oxygen extraction, leaving an expected elevated venous PO_2. Although it has not been documented specifically for H_2S, one would expect to find a decrease in the arterial-venous PO_2 difference.

An oxygen saturation gap (calculated oxygen saturation minus measured oxygen saturation) has been reported in a patient exposed to H_2S.[18] After accounting for methemoglobin and carboxyhemoglobin concentrations, it was implied that the O_2 saturation gap was due to an abnormal hemoglobin, in this case thought to be sulfhemoglobin.

Sulfhemoglobin Controversy. The presence of sulfmethemoglobin as a consequence of H_2S poisoning has been disputed. Although the formation of sulfhemoglobin has been reported or suggested after a variety of drug ingestions[36] or after H_2S exposure,[18, 21] sulfhemoglobin is thought not to occur in H_2S poisoning.[33, 37]

Radiologic Investigations. A chest radiograph may show evidence of pulmonary edema. CT scan of the brain has been reported to show evidence of basal ganglial lesions.[35, 38]

Sulfide Measurements. Techniques developed to measure either plasma or brain sulfide levels[8, 39] have been applied either after acute exposure to H_2S in workers[39] or in postmortem samples.[8, 40]

The brain sulfide technique involves gas dialysis and ion chromatography coupled to electrochemical detection. Endogenous brain sulfide levels have been measured experimentally in rats poisoned with H_2S or sodium sulfide,[9] in normal human postmortem brain stem,[8] and in brain stem specimens of H_2S fatalities.[40] Endogenous brain sulfide levels in normal human postmortem brain stem have been measured at 0.67 ± 0.05 μg per gram. This technique may be useful in confirming death due to acute H_2S poisoning by inhalation.

Brain stem selectively accumulates H_2S,[16] specifically in the myelin and mitochondrial fractions.[8] It is known that H_2S is more soluble in lipophilic solvent than water. Since the brain stem has a higher concentration of white matter, and white matter contains more lipid than gray matter, it is not surprising that H_2S is preferentially concentrated in the brain stem.

Treatment

Supportive Measures. Because many victims of H_2S exposure may be apneic at the scene, immediate resuscitation measures are imperative (Table 83–3). There is no evidence that performing mouth-to-mouth resuscitation on a victim of H_2S inhalation poses any danger to the rescuer. However, rescuers should first ensure that the environment is

Table 83–3. PRINCIPLES OF MANAGEMENT OF H_2S EXPOSURE

Rescuer protection
Basic life support
Aggressive supportive care
Sodium nitrite (3 per cent)
Adult: 10 ml at 2.5 to 5 ml/min
Child: 0.2 ml/kg
Hyperbaric oxygen therapy
may be considered under select circumstances

safe and wear a self-contained breathing apparatus before attempting rescue procedures. Numerous reports[21, 24, 41–47] describe rescuer exposure to the toxic environment, often with fatal outcomes.[16, 41, 43–46]

In hospital, early and aggressive management of convulsions, pulmonary edema, and acidosis may result in ultimate survival with no long-term sequelae.[5, 17, 19, 25, 26, 28, 30, 44, 45]

Oxygen. Experimentally, oxygen alone does not affect the course of acute sulfide poisoning.[47]

Hyperbaric Oxygen. Anecdotal evidence suggests an apparent benefit of hyperbaric oxygen (HBO) therapy in victims of H_2S poisoning.[23, 24] In both cases, the patients did not seem to demonstrate significant improvement after standard nitrite therapy. HBO therapy, instituted even after a 10-hour delay, resulted in marked improvement in mental status as early as the first treatment.[23] In the second report, nitrite therapy, administered within 30 to 60 minutes after exposure, resulted in minimal improvement in mental status. Three treatments of HBO therapy at 2.5 atmospheres for 90 minutes resulted in complete recovery.[24] Another patient demonstrated an initial improvement in mental status after HBO therapy but was left with a persistent memory deficit.[61] In only one case report was HBO therapy ineffective.[62]

HBO therapy is postulated to be effective by one of several mechanisms: (1) increased O_2 concentration results in increased O_2 competition for binding sites on cytochrome oxidase; (2) since oxyhemoglobin is a natural catalyst of sulfide oxidation, increased oxyhemoglobin concentration favors auto-oxidation of sulfide; (3) increased O_2 plasma diffusion results in improved oxygenation of marginally perfused tissue.[24]

Although an interesting therapeutic modality, use of HBO therapy in H_2S exposure has not been sufficiently proved to be recommended indiscriminately. However, it is of sufficient interest to warrant further research. It is possible that it may be of significant benefit in patients in whom CNS symptoms do not resolve either spontaneously or after prompt institution of nitrite therapy. The effect of HBO therapy in patients with marked pulmonary edema remains to be demonstrated.

Antidotes

Nitrites

The similarity between the mechanism of toxicity of hydrogen sulfide and cyanide has led to the suggestion that nitrite therapy be used in H_2S poisoning.[47, 48] Nitrites are thought to be effective by inducing methemoglobinemia. The resulting large available pool of ferric heme has a greater affinity for hydrogen sulfide than cytochrome oxidase, thereby sequestering sulfide ion and freeing cytochrome oxidase. With removal of hydrogen sulfide from cytochrome oxidase, aerobic metabolism resumes. The sulfmethemoglobin complex is then detoxified through endogenous routes.[4, 49]

The application of this theory remains unclear. An understanding of the experimental and clinical evidence for and against nitrite therapy will help the clinician make an informed and independent decision.

Experimental Evidence. A number of animal and in vitro studies support the use of nitrite therapy. Under experimental conditions, when cytochrome oxidase is completely inhibited by sulfide, the addition of methemoglobin results in increased oxidation of cytochrome oxidase.[4]

Pretreatment of several animal species with sodium nitrite improved both mortality and survival time after exposure to either parenteral sodium sulfide or to H_2S gas by inhalation.[48, 49] However, pretreatment with sodium nitrite was ineffective with high concentrations of H_2S (1872 ppm). Pretreatment with parenteral administration of human methemoglobin protected mice from lethal doses of sodium sulfide.[50]

In one of the few studies reported in which nitrite therapy was administered after sulfide poisoning, nitrite decreased mortality.[48] However, the dose of nitrite used was 20-fold that recommended for cyanide poisoning; it was administered 2 minutes after sulfide injection and produced up to an 82 per cent methemoglobinemia in the animals.[51]

However, the effectiveness of the sulfmethemoglobin complex in sulfide detoxification is questionable in light of two observations: (1) sulfide is not bound as strongly to methemoglobin as cyanide,[50] and (2) sulfmethemoglobin undergoes gradual auto-oxidation-reduction to ferrohemoglobin and possibly to some oxided form of sulfur.[4] Animal experiments with cyanide poisoning have demonstrated the efficacy of nitrites even in the presence of methylene blue, which blocks methemoglobin formation.[52] Alternative explanations for the efficacy of nitrite therapy in cyanide and H_2S poisoning have been suggested as follows; (1) vasoactive changes in microcirculation; (2) a direct cytochrome oxidase–stimulating effect; (3) a direct effect on hydrogen sulfide–cytochrome oxidase binding that is not mediated by methemoglobin induction.[18]

Recently, this mechanism has been called into question in the case of cyanide poisoning.[52] The clinical response to nitrites occurs more rapidly than can be explained by the rate of methemoglobin formation. Some experimental evidence points to the importance of the vasodilatory effects of nitrites. Alpha-blocking agents such as chlorpromazine and phenoxybenzamine in combination with thiosulfate have been shown to be as effective in treating cyanide poisoning as the nitrite-thiosulfate combination.[52] No parallel experiments have been conducted questioning the traditional explanation of the effectiveness of nitrites in H_2S poisoning.

Alternatively, it may be that nitrite-induced methemoglobinemia is a more effective oxidation catalyst for sulfide than is oxyhemoglobin.[51] In vitro evidence shows that both oxyhemoglobin and methemoglobin are effective catalytic agents for sulfide, with methemoglobin being somewhat more efficacious.[31] On this basis it is not surprising that animals pretreated with nitrite show a reduced sensitivity to sulfide because the faster reaction catalyzed by the methemoglobin permits a faster turnover of sulfide. However, the oxyhemoglobin-catalyzed reaction is also rapid, resulting in elimination of more than 90 per cent of sulfide within 20 minutes. Additionally, nitrite produces methemoglobin slowly under air or oxygen but acts more rapidly under oxygen-depleted conditions. Furthermore, nitrite inhibits sulfide detoxification catalyzed by oxyhemoglobin. From this study, the authors inferred that the lifetime of sulfide in an oxygenated blood stream is in the order of minutes. Their final conclusions, based on these in vitro data, were that (1) nitrites are effective only if they are given very early in the course of management; and (2) the methemoglobinemia so produced is relatively slow in light of the rapid catalytic effect of oxyhemoglobin. Their final conclusion was that the induction of methemoglobinemia about 10 minutes after exposure confers no added benefit. These data have not been confirmed in vivo by either animal experimentation or human observation.

Other Antidotes

A number of alternative antidotes are being investigated. All the data to date are still experimental in nature. It remains to be determined whether any of these therapeutic agents will prove clinically efficacious.

Thiosulfate. Experimental evidence indicates that thiosulfate has no significant protective effect on the mortality of mice.[47] Unlike cyanide poisoning, in which sodium thiosulfate is known to serve as a substrate for the enzyme rhodanese, which catalyzes the conversion of cyanide to the nontoxic thiocyanate, no parallel rationale is known for the use of thiosulfate as an antidote to sulfide poisoning.

Pyruvate. Pretreatment with 1 gm per kg of pyruvic acid offers mice approximately the same protection from the lethal effects of parenteral sodium sulfide as that afforded by nitrites.[53, 54] Additionally, pyruvic acid increases the effectiveness of sodium nitrite.[53] Pyruvic acid treatment after exposure to parenteral administration of sodium sulfide reduced the lethality of parenterally administered sulfide.[53]

α-Ketoglutarate. Prophylactic administration of a combination of α-ketoglutaric acid and pyruvic acid reduced the lethality of sodium sulfide when given either parenterally or orally.[55] Additionally, the protective effect of this combination was further enhanced by administration of amyl nitrite after exposure to sodium sulfide.[55]

Dithiothreotol. Dithiothreotol (DTT) reduces disulfide bridges to maintain sulfhydryl groups in their reduced states. Experimental data indicate that DTT increases brain sulfide concentrations in both control and sulfide-poisoned brain homogenates.[56] This fact leads to interesting speculation about the application of such a therapeutic agent after exposure, resulting in detoxification of sites that have been inactivated by sulfide.

Summary

Despite some uncertainty, available experimental and clinical data indicate that sodium nitrite therapy (10 ml of a 3 per cent solution at the rate of 2.5 to 5 ml per minute) may be beneficial after basic life support measures have been instituted. Based on in vitro evidence, greater benefit may be realized if the nitrite therapy is instituted early in the clinical course. Further investigation of the clinical effectiveness of nitrites administered at varying times after exposure may determine the usefulness of nitrite therapy beyond the first few minutes after exposure.

Clinical use of nitrite therapy in cases of H_2S poisoning is limited to a handful of anecdotal reports. Recovery after nitrite treatment may not necessarily indicate therapeutic efficacy. Victims of H_2S poisoning have survived equally well without sequelae after supportive care alone. Pulmonary edema, a cause of early death from H_2S toxicity, should be treated promptly and aggressively.

The use of hyperbaric oxygen is controversial but may be of some benefit in patients who do not respond to nitrite therapy or who demonstrate persistent neurologic abnormalities. Its role in management warrants further investigation.

A number of alternative therapeutic agents show some promise experimentally, but further research is required to determine their application in a clinical setting.

Prevention

A significant number of potentially preventable deaths have occurred when rescuers did not protect themselves prior to attempting rescue procedures. Companies and workers at risk should be aware of the dangers of exposure to H_2S and should take appropriate precautions including wearing protective equipment and following precautionary protocols that include a "buddy system" approach. A number of symptomatic exposures have resulted from equipment failure (mask knocked off, hose pinched off, valve frozen).[31] All workers at a facility where H_2S exposure is a risk should be trained in basic life-support rescue methods. An overall improvement in worker awareness as well as improvement in on-site first-aid procedures may contribute significantly to an observed decrease in overall mortality (Table 83–2).[31]

CARBON DISULFIDE

Carbon disulfide (CS_2) is a synthetic toxin with a sweet aromatic odor that resembles that of decaying cabbage. It is used as a fumigant for grains and as a solvent, particularly in the rayon industry. It has been used in the production of cellophane and viscose rayon and as a solvent for waxes, resins, gums, and rubber.[57]

Primarily absorbed by inhalation, CS_2 is highly tissue bound and is rapidly distributed to the liver, kidney, and brain.[58] Metabolism of CS_2 involves two distinct pathways: direct reaction with amine or thiol components of cells and microsomal oxidation to reactive intermediates that covalently bind to cellular macromolecules. These dithiocarbamate derivatives inactivate enzymes by chelating metal ions like copper or zinc. Alternatively, these derivatives can bind directly to active components of proteins. These mechanisms may play an important role in CS_2 neurotoxicity. Reactive intermediates formed through the P-450 system are felt to play a role in CS_2-induced hepatotoxicity. One per cent of CS_2 is excreted in urine, whereas 5 per cent is eliminated unchanged through the lungs.

Clinical Effects

Acute exposure is uncommon. Acute dermatologic exposure causes burning, erythema, and peeling of the skin. Ocular exposure results in immediate severe irritation. Acute inhalation also results in a significant irritative effect.

Chronic exposure results in by far the most significant expression of toxicity of this compound. The central and peripheral nervous systems are the major target organs for toxicity, of which psychosis, tremor, and polyneuritis are common manifestations. Polyneuritis, seen in up to 88 per cent of toxic patients, includes lower extremity weakness and paresthesias. The peripheral neuritis frequently involves the radial, ulnar, sciatic, and external peroneal nerves.[59] Extrapyramidal signs, chorea, and athetosis may also occur.

The behavioral changes are the most striking aspect of CS_2 toxicity. These consist primarily of manic-depressive type psychoses with psychomotor excitation, delirium, and hallucinations. In milder forms of toxicity, personality changes are evident, with emotional lability, depression, memory impairment, and irritability.[57]

Other systemic manifestations include gastric disturbances and visual disturbances. CS_2 is felt to be atherogenic and diabetogenic. The death rate from coronary artery disease in workers in the viscose rayon manufacturing industry was found to be 2.5 times that of nonexposed men.[60]

Treatment

Removal from the environment and decontamination along with supportive care form the mainstay of therapy. Prevention of toxicity is preferable.

References

1. Tabacova J: Maternal exposure to environmental chemicals. Neurotoxicology *7*:421–440, 1986.
2. Burnett WW, King EG, Grace M, Hall WF: Hydrogen sulfide poisoning: Review of 5 year's experience. Can Med Assoc J *117*:1277–1280, 1977.
3. Nichols P: The effect of sulfide on cytochrome aa3, isosteric and allosteric shifts of the reduced a1-peak. Biochim Biophys Acta *396*:24–35, 1975.
4. Smith L, Kruszyna H, Smith RP: The effect of methemoglobin on the inhibition of cytochrome c oxidase by cyanide, sulfide or azide. Biochem Pharmacol *26*:2247–2250, 1977.
5. Amman H: A new look at physiologic respiratory response to H_2S poisoning. J Haz Materials *13*:369–374, 1986.
6. Beauchamp RO, Bus JS, Popp JA, Boreiko CJ, Andjelkovich DA: A critical review of the literature on hydrogen sulfide toxicity. CRC Crit Rev Toxicol *13*:25–49, 1984.
7. Evans CL: The toxicity of hydrogen sulphide and other sulphides. Q J Exp Physiol *52*:231–248, 1967.
8. Warencyia MW, Goodwin LR, Benishin CG, Reiffenstien RJ, Francom DM, Taylor JD, Dieken FP: Acute hydrogen sulfide poisoning. Demonstration of selective uptake of sulfide by the brainstem by measurement of brain sulfide levels. Biochem Pharmacol *38*:973–981, 1989.
9. Warencyia MW, Goodwin LR, Francom DM, Reiffenstien RJ, Dieken FP, Taylor JD: Regional brain distribution of sulfide after H_2S poisoning. In Jones GR, Singer PP (eds): Proceedings of the 24th International Meeting of the International Association for Toxicology. University of Alberta Press, 1988.
10. Gosselin RE, Smith RP, Hodge HC: Clinical Toxicology of Commercial Products. 5th ed. Baltimore, Williams & Wilkins, 1984.
11. Voight GE, Mueller P: Versuche zum histochemischen Nachweis der Schwefelwasserstoff-Vergiftung [The histochemical effect of hydrogen sulfide poisoning]. Acta Histochem *1*:223–239, 1955.
12. Weisiger RA, Pinkus LM, Jakoby WB: Thiol S-methyltransferase: Suggested role in detoxification of intestinal sulfide. Biochem Pharmacol *29*:2885–2887, 1980.
13. Marcus SM: Hydrogen sulfide. Clin Toxicol Rev *5*(4), 1983.
14. Susman JL, Hornig JF, Thomae SC, Smith RP: Pulmonary excretion of hydrogen sulfide, mathanethiol, dimethyl sulfide, and dimethyl disulfide in mice. Drug Chem Toxicol *1*:327–388, 1978.
15. Thoman M: Sewer gas: hydrogen sulfide intoxication. Clin Toxicol *2*:383–386, 1969.
16. Berlin CM: Death from anoxia in an abandoned cesspool (letter). Ann Intern Med *95*:387, 1981.
17. Kemper FD: A near-fatal case of hydrogen sulfide poisoning. CMAJ *94*:1130–1131, 1966.
18. Hoidal CR, Hall AH, Robinson MD, Kulig K, Rumack BH: Hydrogen sulfide poisoning from toxic inhalations of roofing asphalt fumes. Ann Emerg Med *15*:826–830, 1986.
19. Hurwitz LJ, Taylor GI: Poisoning by sewer gas. Lancet *1*:1110–1112, 1954.
20. Stine RJ, Slosberg B, Beacham BE: Hydrogen sulfide intoxication: A case report and discussion of therapy. Ann Intern Med *85*:756–758, 1976.
21. Peters JW: Hydrogen sulfide poisoning in a hospital setting. JAMA *246*:1588–1589, 1981.
22. Huang CC, Chu NS: A case of acute hydrogen sulfide (H_2S) intoxication successfully treated with nitrites. J Formosan Med Assoc *86*:1018–1020, 1987.
23. Smilkstein MJ, Bronstein AC, Pickett HM, Rumack BH: Hyperbaric oxygen therapy for severe hydrogen sulfide poisoning. J Emerg Med *3*:27–30, 1985.
24. Whitcraft DD, Bailey TD, Hart GB: Hydrogen sulfide poisoning treated with hyperbaric oxygen. J Emerg Med *3*:23–25, 1985.
25. Ravizza AG, Carugo D, Cerchiari EL, Cantadore R, Bianchi GE: The treatment of hydrogen sulfide intoxication: Oxygen versus nitrites. Vet Hum Toxicol *24*:4–5, 1982.
26. Milby TH: Hydrogen sulfide intoxication. Review of the literature and report of unusual accident resulting in two cases of nonfatal poisoning. J Occup Med *4*:431–437, 1962.
27. Simson RE, Simpson GR: Fatal hydrogen sulphide poisoning associated with industrial waste exposure. Med J Aust *1*:3310–334, 1971.
28. Deng JF, Chang SC: Hydrogen sulfide poisonings in hot-spring reservoir cleaning: Two case reports. Am J Ind Med *11*:447–451, 1987.
29. Audeau FM, Gnanaharan C, Davey K: Hydrogen sulphide poisoning: Associated with pelt processing. NZ Med J *98*:145–147, 1985.
30. Kleinfeld M, Giel C, Rosso A: Acute hydrogen sulfide intoxication: An unusual source of exposure. Ind Med Surg *33*:656–660, 1964.
31. Arnold IMF, Dufresne RM, Alleyne BC, Stuart PJW: Health implication of occupational exposures to hydrogen sulfide. J Occup Med *27*:373–376, 1985.
32. Hagley SR, South DL: Fatal inhalation of liquid manure gas. Med J Aust *2*:459–460, 1983.

33. Smith RP, Gosselin RE: Hydrogen sulfide poisoning. J Occup Med *21*:93–97, 1979.
34. Lopez A, Prior M, Reiffenstien RJ, Goodwin LR: Peracute toxic effects of inhaled hydrogen sulfide and injected sodium hydrosulfide on the lungs of rats. Fund Appl Toxicol *12*:367–373, 1989.
35. Matsuo M, Cummins JW, Anderson RE: Neurological sequelae of massive hydrogen sulfide inhalation. Arch Neurol *36*:451–452, 1979.
36. Park CM, Nagel RL: Sulfhemoglobinemia. Clinical and molecular aspects. N Engl J Med *310*:1579–1584, 1984.
37. Curry SC, Gerkin RD: A patient with sulhemoglobin? (letter) Ann Emerg Med *16*:828–829, 1987.
38. Gaitonde UB, Sellar RJ, O'Hare AE: Long-term exposure to hydrogen sulphide producing subacute encephalopathy in a child. Br Med J *294*:614, 1987.
39. Lindell H, Jappinen P, Savolainen H: Determination of sulphide in blood with an ion selective electrode by pre-concentration of trapped sulphide in sodium hydroxide solution. Analyst *113*:839–840, 1988.
40. Goodwin LR, Francom DM, Dieken FP, Taylor JD, Warencyia MW, Reiffenstien RJ, Dowling G: Determination of brain sulfide in brain tissue by gas dialysis/ion chromatography: Postmortem studies and two case reports. J Anal Toxicol *13*:105–109, 1989.
41. Deaths at a rendering plant. Morbid Mortal Weekly Rep, pp 435–436, 1975.
42. Occupational fatality following exposure to hydrogen sulfide—Nebraska. Morbid Mortal Weekly Rep *35*:533–535, 1986.
43. Adelson L. Sunshine I: Fatal hydrogen sulfide intoxication. Arch Pathol *81*:375–380, 1966.
44. Osbern LN, Crapo RO: Dung lung: A report of toxic exposure to liquid manure. Ann Intern Med *95*:312–314, 1981.
45. Oderda GM: Fatality produced by accidental inhalation of drain cleaner fumes. Clin Toxicol *8*:547–551, 1975.
46. Donham KJ, Knapp LW, Monson R, Gustafson K: Acute toxic exposure to gases from liquid manure. J Occup Med *24*:142–145, 1982.
47. Smith RP, Kruszyna R, Kruszyna H: Management of acute sulfide poisoning: Effects of oxygen, thiosulfate, and nitrite. Arch Environ Health *31*:166–169, 1976.
48. Smith RP, Gosselin RE: Current concepts about the treatment of selected poisonings: Nitrite, sulfide, barium, and quinidine. Annu Rev Pharmacol Toxicol *16*:189–199, 1976.
49. Smith RP, Gosselin RE: The influence of methemoglobinemia on the lethality of some toxic anions: II. Sulfide. Toxicol Appl Pharmacol *6*:584–592, 1964.
50. Smith RP, Gosselin RE: On the mechanism of sulfide inactivation by methemoglobin. Toxicol Appl Pharmacol *8*:159–172, 1966.
51. Beck JF, Bradbury CM, Connors AJ, Donini JC: Nitrite as an antidote for acute sulfide intoxication? Am Ind Hyg Assoc J *42*:805–809, 1981.
52. Way J, Sylvester D, Morgan RL, et al: Recent perspectives on the toxico-dynamic basis of cyanide antagonism. Fund Appl Toxicol *4*:S231–S239, 1984.
53. Dulaney M Jr, Hume AS: Pyruvic acid protects against the lethality of sulfide. Res Commun Chem Pathol Pharmacol *59*:133, 1988.
54. Hume AS, Dulaney MD: The effectiveness of various α-ketocarboxylic acids in preventing sulfide-induced lethality. Toxicologist *8*:28, 1988.
55. Dulaney MD, Hume AS: The effectiveness of the combination of pyruvate (PYR) and alpha-ketoglutarate (AKG) as prophylactic antidotes against sulphide lethality. Proceedings of the International Conference on Hydrogen Sulfide Toxicity, Banff, Canada, 1989.
56. Warencyia MW, Reiffenstien RJ, Goodwin LR, Dieken FP: Dithiothreitol liberates additional brain sulphide. Proc West Pharmacol Soc *32*:333, 1989.
57. Finkel AJ: Hamilton and Hardy's Industrial Toxicology. 4th ed. Littleton, MA, PSG Publishing Co, 1983.
58. Bus JS: The relationship of carbon disulfide metabolism to development of toxicity. Neurotoxicology *6*:73–80, 1985.
59. Beauchamp RO, Bus JS, Popp JA, Boreiko CJ, Goldberg L: A critical review of the literature on carbon disulfide toxicity. Crit Rev Toxicol *11*:169–278, 1983.
60. Tiller JR, Schilling RSF, Morris JN: Occupational toxic factors in mortality from coronary heart disease. Br Med J *4*:407, 1968.
61. Vicas, IMO: Hydrogen sulfide exposure treated with hyperbaric oxygen. Vet Hum Toxicol *31*:353, 1989.
62. Al-Mahasneh OM, Cohle SD, Haas E: Lack of response to hyperbaric oxygen in a fatal case of hydrogen sulfide poisoning. Vet Hum Toxicol *31*:353, 1989.

CHAPTER 84
TEAR GAS AND RIOT CONTROL AGENTS

David R. Graham, M.D.

The chemical agents used in riot control differ from those used in warfare in that they are chosen to produce immediate, disabling, but above all transient effects. Systemic toxicity due to the chemical agents used is minimal, yet they are so highly irritant to the eyes, skin, and upper respiratory tract that persons in contact with them are forced to seek immediate escape.

It is thought that the Paris police in 1912 were the first to use chemical agents to control a civic disturbance when they used "hand bombs" of an optic irritant, ethylbromacetate against "lawless gangs."[1, 2] In the United States during the crime wave of the 1920s chemicals were used to combat urban gangsters. Dispersal systems were refined, resulting in the development of antiriot guns, which were capable of firing chemical agents into crowds or buildings from a distance, thereby avoiding direct confrontation.[1]

EFFECTS

Riot control agents (also termed "short term incapacitants" or "harassing agents") act locally on peripheral sensory receptors at the site of contamination, producing uncomfortable sensations with reflex effects that interfere with co-ordinated motor activity.[1, 2] The effects at various sites are shown in Table 84–1. Although up to 15 sensory irritants have been used worldwide in riot control, only three agents are commonly used today.

1. 1-Chloroacetophenone (CN or Mace)
2. 2-Chlorobenzylidene malononitrile (CS)
3. Dibenzoxapine (CR)

METHODS OF DISPERSAL

The way in which chemical agents are dispersed depends on the situation in which they are used. If these agents are used to control large-scale riots or violent demonstrations, irritant smokes can be produced by combining the agent with a pyrotechnic mixture such as chlorate and lactose, which on ignition causes the irritant to vaporize and then condense to a cloud of solid or liquid particles of a respirable size (1 to 2 μ). Riot control agents can also be delivered by grenades or by cartridges fired from a gun; and devices such as the "rubber bursting grenade," which disperses many sources over a wide area on explosion, can be used to produce a multifocal smoke.[3]

Chemical agents can also be deployed as powders or aerosols. Powders have been used by the police against smaller numbers of violent criminals and are dispersed by explosion from tear gas pistols. CS powders have been reported to cause eye damage, particularly when fired at close range.[4, 5, 6] Aerosols are safer and are used as personal protection devices. These are available commercially in some countries. Chemical Mace and Federal Streamer contain CN or Mace, the Paralyser contains CS, and Guardian contains capsicum.[1, 7] The aerosol cans containing the sensory irritants are fired at would-be attackers and produce immediate eye pain, blepharospasm, and severe stinging of the skin, rendering the attacker disabled.

Table 84–1. LOCAL EFFECTS OF RIOT CONTROL AGENTS

SITE	EFFECT
Eye	Discomfort or pain with blepharospasm and lacrimation
Mouth	Stinging or burning of palate and tongue with excess salivation
Nose	Discomfort and rhinorrhea
Respiratory tract	Tightness or burning sensation in the chest with coughing, sneezing, and increased tracheobronchial secretions
Skin	Stinging and burning with erythema

(Modified from Ballantyne B: Biomedical and health aspects of the use of chemicals in civil disturbances. In Scott RB, Frazer J (eds): Medical Annual. Bristol, Wright and Sons, 1977, pp 7–41.)

SPECIFIC IRRITANTS

Chloroacetophenone

Chloroacetophenone (CN, tear gas Mace), which was prepared by Graebe in 1871, was first used in World War I as a "tear gas." It has been used as a smoke and a powder but is usually discharged as an aerosol.

The effects are immediate and include an intense stinging and burning sensation in the nose, throat, and eyes. This sensation is accompanied by lacrimation, blepharospasm, salivation, and rhinorrhea. The exposed individual experiences constriction in the chest with dyspnea, gagging, and stinging of the skin. Although some effects may disappear within 20 minutes, there is usually prolonged conjunctivitis with blurred vision.[8] CN is more toxic than CS or CR and if inhaled in any quantity, as may occur in an enclosed space, lung damage can lead to asphyxia. Deaths have been reported following the use of CN grenades.[1, 9, 10, 11] In high concentrations, CN can cause corneal damage and contact dermatitis.[12–16]

Treatment

Treatment consists of decontamination. Exposed areas should be thoroughly washed with water, and contaminated clothes should be removed and placed in polyethylene bags by persons wearing gloves.[17] Eyes should be irrigated for at least 30 minutes, especially in patients who complain of blurred vision or have conjunctivitis. Examination with a slit lamp and follow-up ophthalmology consultation are required. Contact dermatitis may require topical steroids if it is severe. Respiratory effects usually disappear within 15 minutes; however, if symptoms persist, injury to the respiratory tract should be suspected, and the subject should be x-rayed and admitted to the hospital for observation.

Chlorobenzylidene Malononitrile

Chlorobenzylidene malononitrile (CS), which was first developed in 1958 by Corson and Stoughton,[18] is the most frequently used riot control agent. It is more effective and safer than CN because it is 10 times more potent as an irritant yet is significantly less lethal.[1, 9] The comparative effects and toxicity of the riot control agents are shown in Table 84–2.[19]

CS is dispersed by grenade or fixed cartridge or as an aerosol. The active chemical rapidly breaks down to nonirritating substances, and the symptoms persist only as long as exposure occurs. At concentrations of 4 mg per m^3 the symptoms are severe, with a burning sensation in the eyes accompanied by lacrimation, blepharospasm, and conjunctival injection.[1, 20, 21] A minority of subjects have photophobia for up to 1 hour. The severity of these ocular symptoms has been reduced in exposed policemen by the wearing of soft contact lenses.[22]

The effects on the respiratory tract include sneezing, cough, chest tightness, and rhinobronchorrhea. Within minutes of exposure there is stinging of the exposed skin, particularly in moist areas, followed by erythema. Occasionally these symptoms are accompanied by nausea and vomiting. Recovery is complete within 30 minutes, although most symptoms have subsided after 15 minutes. Exposure to CS gas under controlled conditions has not been associated with any serious systemic upset.[1, 20, 23] Indeed, the concentrations required to cause death are thought to be several hundred times greater than the dose required to produce acute harassment.[23–25] The Himsworth report further states that with pyrotechnically produced CS smoke the likelihood of death is virtually negligible.[23] No deaths have been reported in riot control situations, although in confined areas high concentrations could lead to inflammatory changes within the lungs.

Table 84–2. RIOT CONTROL AGENTS: COMPARISON OF POTENCY AND TOXICITY

	CN	CS	CR
Eye irritation threshold (mg/m^3)	0.3	0.004	0.002
LD_{50} (mg/kg) intraperitoneal (guinea pig)	17	73	390
Oral (rabbit)	118	230	1760
Estimated lethal dose (mg/min/m^3)	10×10^3	60×10^3	$>100 \times 10^3$

(Modified from Beeswick FW: Chemical agents used in riot control and warfare. Human Toxicol 2:247–256, 1983.)

Treatment

Because the effects are transient, exposed persons rarely require hospitalization; however, care should be exercised in the assessment of asthmatics and persons with bronchitis. First aid treatment includes moving to fresh air and facing into the wind with the eyes open (the Medical Manual on Defence).[21] The skin should be decontaminated with soap and water and the eyes irrigated with saline if symptoms persist. Skin erythema settles within 24 hours and does not require treatment.

Dibenzoxapine

Dibenzoxapine (CR) was first synthesized in 1962.[26] Its potency as a peripheral sensory irritant is about 10 times that of CS, and it has a low toxicity in man.[1, 27] Because it is chemically more stable, CR can be dispersed in aerosol or solution form. The symptoms of CR exposure are similar to those of CS, but the concentrations required are significantly lower (Table 84–2). Because CR is delivered in solution the effects tend to be localized to the skin and eyes, and the low vapor pressure of CR in solution means that it has little effect on the respiratory tract. Eye pain, lacrimation, and blepharospasm last for 15 minutes after exposure, although conjunctival injection and lid edema may last up to 6 hours. If the solution enters the mouth or nose, pain is accompanied by salivation and rhinorrhea, which last for 15 minutes. If CS is dissolved in saliva and swallowed, the symptoms are accompanied by nausea and abdominal pain. The burning sensation of exposed skin appears within minutes and lasts for up to a half hour, leaving a well-demarcated erythema that lasts for 1 to 2 hours. Biomedical studies have shown that the effects of CR are significantly less toxic than those of either CN or CS,[1, 19] although CR has been shown to raise the blood pressure,[1] an effect that could also be explained by stress or pain. CR exposure has also been reported to cause a rise in intraocular pressure.[28]

Summary

In general, the morbidity and mortality associated with riots are related to physical injury rather than to effects due to riot control agents. The use of chemicals is intended to save life, reduce casualties, and protect property. The most effective agents are peripheral sensory irritants, and the best agents are those that produce a rapid onset of distressing symptoms that resolve quickly after exposure ceases without any long-term effects. The ideal agent should cause maximal harassment with low toxicity. The uncomfortable nature of the symptoms with associated reflexes, blepharospasm, lacrimation, rhinorrhea, and salivation make further activity impossible and cause the individual to attempt to escape from the exposure. Smoke affects the eyes and respiratory tract and has a lesser effect on the skin, whereas liquid sprays and aerosols have less effect on the respiratory tract but produce more marked effects on the skin and eyes. If the mouth is affected, the agent may be swallowed, producing abdominal pain.

Recovery is rapid when exposure ceases. Treatment consists of decontamination by washing or saline lavage of affected areas. Medical attendants should take precautions to avoid self-contamination from casualties. In the usual circumstances specific therapy is not required. Only if exposure occurs in a confined space when escape is impossible is there likely to be any serious systemic upset, the most profound effects in such a case being on the respiratory tract. Patients with prolonged symptoms or signs require appropriate subspecialty follow-up.

References

1. Ballantyne B: Biomedical and health aspects of the use of chemicals in civil disturbances. In Scott RB, Frazer J (eds): Medical Annual. Bristol, Wright and Sons, 1977, pp 7–41.
2. Swearengen TF: Tear Gas Munitions. Springfield, IL, Charles C Thomas, 1966.
3. Ballantyne B, Johnson WG: Chlorobenzylidene malononitrile (CS) and the healing of cutaneous injuries. Med Sci Law *14*:93–97, 1974.
4. Oaks LW, Dorman JE, Petty R: Tear gas burns of the eye. Arch Ophthalmol *63*:698–706, 1960.
5. Hoffman DH: Eye burns caused by tear gas. Br J Ophthalmol *51*:265–268, 1967.
6. Grant WM: Toxicology of the Eye. Springfield, IL, Charles C Thomas, 1974.
7. Sreenivasan VR, Boese RA: Identification of lacrimators. J Forensic Sci *15*:433–442, 1970.
8. Punte CL, Gutentag PJ, Owens EJ, et al: Inhalation studies with chloroacetophenone, diphenylaminochlorasine and pelargonic morpholide. 11 human exposures. Am Industr Hyg Assoc J *23*:199–202, 1962.

9. Gonzales TA, Vance M, Helpern M, et al: Legal Medicine. New York, Appleton-Century-Crofts, 1954.
10. Stein AA, Kirwan WE: Chloroacetophenone (tear gas) poisoning—a clinico-pathological report. J Forensic Sci *9*:374–382, 1964.
11. Ballantyne B, Gazzard MF, Swanston DW, et al: The comparative ophthalmic toxicology of 1-chloroacetophenone (CN) and dibenz (b.f)1:4-oxapine (CR). Arch Toxicol *34*:183–201, 1975.
12. Macrae WG, Willinsky MD, Basu PK: Corneal injury caused by aerosol irritant projectors. Can J Ophthalmol *5*:3–11, 1970.
13. Leopold IH, Lieberman TW: Chemical injuries to the cornea. Fed Proc *30*:92–95, 1971.
14. Schwartz L, Tulipan L, Birmingham DJ: Occupational Diseases of the Skin. Philadelphia, Lea & Febiger, 1957.
15. Jolly HW, Carpenter CL: Tear gas dermatitis. JAMA *203*:808, 1968.
16. Holland P, White RG: The cutaneous reactions produced by *o*-chlorobenzylidene malononitrile and ω-chloroacetophenone when applied directly to the skin of human subjects. Br J Dermatol *86*:150–154, 1972.
17. Fine K, Bassin RH, Stewart MM: Emergency care for tear gas victims. J Am Coll Emerg Phys *6*:144, 1977.
18. Corson BB, Stoughton RW: Reactions of alpha, beta unsaturated dinitriles. J Am Chem Soc *50*:2825–2837, 1928.
19. Beswick FW: Chemical agents used in riot control and warfare. Hum Toxicol *2*:247–256, 1983.
20. Beswick FW, Holland P, Kemp KH: Acute effects and exposure to ortho chlorobenzylidene malononitrile (CS) and the development of tolerance. Br J Ind Med *29*:298–306, 1972.
21. Ministry of Defence. The Medical Manual of Defence Against Chemical Agents. London, Her Majesty's Stationery Office, 1972.
22. Kok-Van Aalphen CC, vander Linden JW, Vissar R, et al: Protection of police against tear gas with soft contact lenses. Military Med *150*(8):451–454, 1985.
23. Himsworth Report. Report of the Enquiry into the Medical and Toxicological Aspects of CS (Orthochlorobenzylidene Malononitrile). Part I. Enquiry into the Medical Situation Following the Use of CS in Londonderry on 13th and 14th August 1969. Command 4173. London, Her Majesty's Stationery Office, 1969.
24. Punte CL, Weimer JT, Ballard TA, et al: Toxicological studies on o-chlorobenzylidene malononitrile. Toxicol Appl Pharmacol *4*:656–662, 1962.
25. WHO Health Aspects of Chemical and Biological Weapons. Report of a World Health Organization Group of Consultants. Geneva, WHO, 1974.
26. Higginbottom R, Suschitzsky H: Synthesis of heterocyclic compounds. Part II. Cyclisation of o-nitrophenyl oxygen ether. J Chem Soc *2*:2367–2370, 1962.
27. Riot control agents. Br Med J *3*:5, 1973.
28. Ballantyne B, Swanston DW: The scope and limitations of acute eye irrigation tests. *In* Ballantyne B (ed): Current Approaches in Toxicology. Bristol, Wright, 1977, pp 139–157.

CHAPTER 85

SOLVENT ABUSE

David R. Graham, M.D.

Solvent abuse is the deliberate inhalation of volatile organic substances to produce alterations in the state of consciousness and perception for recreational purposes. A wide variety of substances can be employed for this purpose including solvents, glues, gasoline (petrol), lighter fuel, paints, antifreeze, and aerosol sprays.

Despite its more recent popularity, particularly among adolescents, solvent abuse is not, as has been suggested,[1] a new phenomenon. It remains supposition that the Oracle at Delphi gained her powers from the inhalation of vapors, but it is well known that the inhalation of gases and vapors[2] was popular in the nineteenth century.[2] Chloroform and ether were used to produce intoxication, and nitrous oxide (laughing gas) was considered a genteel way of becoming drunk.

In recent times the practice of solvent abuse appears to have begun with gasoline (petrol) sniffing, which is thought to have originated in California.[2, 3] The first reports of glue sniffing came in 1962 from Glaser and Massengale in the US and from Merry and Zaccariadis in the UK.[4, 5] Gasoline sniffing was later identified in Australia[6] and in New Mexico.[7] Denver, Colorado, was the first city with a serious glue sniffing problem, but by the mid-1960s the problem of solvent abuse was thought to be present in every state in America.[8] It is not clear whether the practice started "de novo" in many different places or spread from state to state.

Following awareness of the abuse of gasoline and glue there were reports of inhalation of a variety of volatile organic substances, including nail polish remover, antifreeze, marker pens, cleaning fluids, paint thinners, chloroform, lighter fuels, and aerosol products.[8–11] The problem of solvent abuse was no longer confined to the US but was encountered worldwide.[12–16]

CURRENT PROBLEM

The prevalence of solvent abuse is uncertain. It is most often carried out as a group activity, usually involving teenage boys, the peak age being 13 to 15 years.[17–19] Most young abusers grow out of the habit, although some become chronic dependent users, and others progress to heavy drinking.[17, 19, 20] Although most commonly recognized in adolescence, solvent misuse does occur in adults,[21] when, interestingly, the numbers of male and female abusers are reported to be similar.[22]

Solvent abuse bears no particular relationship to socioeconomic factors.[23] However, some studies have shown a greater incidence in single parent families and in children whose parents were unemployed,[2, 17, 19] whereas others found no such relationship.[1, 7] Many solvent abusers appear to be otherwise normal children from normal homes and become involved only transiently because of curiosity, chance encounters, or peer group pressure.[2]

The method of inhaling the solvent varies depending on the particular substance abused. Gasoline (petrol sniffing) occurs directly from a tank or container, adhesives are most often inhaled from a bag, typically a potato chip bag (known as bagging), and solvents are poured or sprayed onto a cloth and held against the nose and mouth (huffing). Aerosol sprays can be inhaled directly, bagged, or huffed.

The constituents of the various inhaled substances are shown in Table 85–1.[25]

Metabolism and Effects. Solvent vapors are readily absorbed through the lungs, cross cell membranes with great ease, and, because of their fat-soluble properties, reach highest concentrations in the central nervous system. Solvents are excreted in the breath, and those that are metabolized in the body undergo oxidation in the liver to form water-soluble compounds that can be excreted in the urine.[1, 2, 24] Several of these metabolites can be detected and provide a means of monitoring solvent abuse (Table 85–2).[25]

As well as being central nervous system depressants, solvents produce subjective effects that are reported to be similar to those of marijuana, although vivid visual hallucinations are more evident. Further symptoms include euphoria, excitement, and a feeling of omnipotence. There may be accompanying blurred vision, tinnitus ("buzzed up on glue"), slurred speech, headache, abdominal pain, chest pain, or bronchospasm.

Clinically, patients appear drunk, but their breath, hair, or clothing may smell of solvent. There may be clouding of consciousness with progression to convulsions, status epilepticus, and coma. If the method used to inhale

Table 85–1. CHEMICAL COMPOSITION OF ABUSED SOLVENTS

INHALED SUBSTANCE	CHEMICAL
Aerosol	Fluorocarbons
Airplane glue (polystyrene cement)	Toluene
Dry cleaning fluid	Methylene chloride Trichloroethylene Carbon tetrachloride
Dyes	Acetone Methylene chloride
Gasoline	Petroleum distillates Benzene
Glues and adhesives	Toluene, benzene, xylene Acetone Trichloroethylene Trichloroethane
Lighter fluid	Butane
Liquid "white-out" products	Trichloroethane
Nail polish remover	Acetone, amyl acetate

Table 85–2. METABOLITES OF SOLVENTS

SOLVENT	METABOLITE
Benzene	Phenol
Toluene	Hippuric acid
Trichloroethylene	Trichloroacetic acid and trichloroethanol
Xylene	Methylhippuric acid

is bagging or huffing, a characteristic rash may be present around the nose and mouth—"glue sniffers rash." Sudden death is now a well-recognized risk of solvent abuse and is thought to be due to cardiac dysrhythmias.[2, 3, 25, 26]

Long-Term Effects. The long-term effects of solvent abuse are due to damage to the liver, kidneys, nervous system, and bone marrow. Hepatorenal damage is well recognized with toluene, trichloroethylene, chloroform, and carbon tetrachloride. Bone marrow depression and aplastic anemia have been associated with the sniffing of benzene-containing glues.[27] Long-term effects on the central nervous system are observed in abusers of toluene and include encephalopathy, optic atrophy, cerebellar degeneration, and disorders of equilibrium.[28–31] Peripheral neuropathy has been particularly associated with glues that contain toluene in combination with *N*-hexane.[32] Solvent abuse also produces nonspecific symptoms and should be suspected if adolescents suffer from unexplained anorexia, listlessness, or marked moodiness. Toluene has been shown to have adverse effects on the fetus,[22] gasoline may be teratogenic,[33] and several solvents have been shown to be carcinogenic in animals, although this has never been proved in humans.[2, 25, 34]

Glue Sniffing

It is only those glues that use aromatic hydrocarbons as a vehicle that are abused. The most important solvent to consider is toluene. This can cause neurologic damage after being sniffed for less than 1 year, and the symptoms may progress after abuse is stopped.[25, 35] Problems have been noted particularly when *N*-hexane is combined with toluene.[32, 36] This combination seems to be associated with muscle weakness and a peripheral neuropathy that may be either glove and stocking or sensory-motor in type.[2, 25] The symptoms can be so severe that at presentation affected abusers may be thought to have Guillain-Barré syndrome.[22]

The renal abnormalities found in glue sniffers include proteinuria, hematuria, distal renal tubular acidosis, and renal calculi.[25, 37–39] A review of adult sniffers[22] reported three major presentations including neuropsychiatric disorders, gastrointestinal complaints, and muscle weakness. The study revealed some interesting biochemical changes with hypokalemia, hypophosphatemia, hypochloremia, and a low serum bicarbonate level in many subjects and evidence of rhabdomyolysis (elevated levels of creatinine phosphokinase) in patients with muscle weakness.[22] Therefore, in addition to the clinical picture already outlined, the above biochemical abnormalities should alert one to the possibility of solvent abuse. In cases of glue sniffing the diagnosis can be confirmed by recovering hippuric acid in the urine or toluene in the blood. In the latter case, toluene blood levels have been shown to correlate with clinical severity. At a level of 0.4 μg per gm solvent can be detected on the breath, a level of 5 μg per gm causes severe symptoms, and a level of greater than 10 μg per gm is likely to prove fatal.[2, 40]

Gasoline

Gasoline (petrol) is not a single substance but a complex mixture of hydrocarbons with various additives such as lead, antioxidants, dyes, and rust inhibitors. Certain saturated hydrocarbons have powerful narcotic properties and also cause nausea, ataxia, and loss of consciousness. The saturated hydrocarbons are mild anesthetic agents.

Gasoline is inhaled directly, and intoxication occurs after 10 to 20 breaths and lasts for 3 to 5 hours.[25] Intoxication is often accompanied by nausea and vomiting, and if inhalation is intense the sniffer may experience intense excitement followed by coma. Clinical examination at this time may reveal convulsive movements, and the pupils can be dilated, fixed, or unequal. Nystagmus and conjugate deviation may also be present. Deep intoxication may cause respiratory depression or cardiac sensitization and on occasion has caused death.[25, 40] Persons who have died from gasoline inhalation may display cerebral and pulmonary edema as well as hepatic and renal damage. Chronic abusers may inhale daily and develop anorexia, weight loss, and muscle weakness. Neuropsychologic damage also occurs, and ECG abnormalities have been demonstrated. If gasoline contains lead as an antiknock agent the abuser can also develop lead poisoning.[41, 42]

Chlorinated Hydrocarbons

Inhalation of the chlorinated hydrocarbons such as carbon tetrachloride, trichloroethylene, and trichloroethane cause euphoria or excitement often associated with headache, dizziness, nausea, vomiting, stupor, coma, and convulsions. Specific adverse effects noted with the chlorinated hydrocarbons include centrilobular hepatic necrosis and acute renal failure.[43, 44] Chlorinated hydrocarbons also sensitize the myocardium, and deaths have been presumed to be due to cardiac dysrhythmias. Trichloroethylene has also been reported to cause optic atrophy and cranial nerve damage.[25] One of the worst abused substances in US teenagers today is "Liquid Paper," which is 52 per cent methyl chloroform (trichloroethane). Overdose is a not uncommon event. See Chapter 78.

Aerosols

Fluorinated hydrocarbons (Freons) are used as aerosol propellants. Aerosols can be inhaled directly or from a bag or cloth into which they are first sprayed. The most important and sinister sequel to abuse of the fluorinated hydrocarbons is sudden death. Initially, the deaths were thought to be due to asphyxia from plastic bags, but many deaths have since been reported without any evidence of asphyxia.[3] Classically, after inhalation there is a period of intense excitement often involving physical exertion such as running, which is followed by collapse and death.[3, 25] At autopsy no specific features are identified, and it is thought that deaths are due to cardiac dysrhythmias.[25] Further evidence that supports this thesis is the fact that volatile hydrocarbons have been shown in animals to be capable of producing both asystole (in the presence of hypoxia) and ventricular fibrillation (due to sensitization of the myocardium by circulating catecholamines).[25, 45-47]

MANAGEMENT

Given any or some of the clinical or biochemical features mentioned above it is important to suspect solvent abuse. If the diagnosis of solvent abuse is suspected it can be confirmed by biochemical examination of the blood or urine (Table 85–1). Emergency treatment is supportive and includes decontamination, oxygen, and any specific therapy required in a particular case such as antiarrhythmics or anticonvulsants. A few patients may require intermittent positive-pressure ventilation, dialysis, or treatment for hepatic failure.

For the future, prevention of solvent abuse relies first on recognition of the problem, followed by education, in particular, alerting young people to the serious long- and short-term hazards of sniffing.

References

1. Sourindhrin I: Solvent abuse. Br Med J *290*:94–95, 1985.
2. Watson JM: Solvent Abuse. The Adolescent Epidemic. London, Croom Helm, 1986.
3. Bass M: Sudden sniffing death. JAMA *212*:2075–2079, 1970.
4. Glaser HH, Massengale ON: Glue sniffing in children. Deliberate inhalation of vapourised plastic cements. JAMA *181*:300–303, 1962.
5. Merry J, Zaccariadis N: Addiction to glue sniffing. Br Med J *2*:1448, 1962.
6. Nurcombe B, Bianchi GN, Money J, et al. A hunger for stimuli: The psychosocial background of petrol inhalation. Br J Med Psychol *43*:367–374, 1970.
7. Kaufman A: Gasoline sniffing among children in a Pueblo Indian village. Pediatrics *51*:1060–1064, 1973.
8. Corliss LM: A review of evidence on glue sniffing—a persistent problem. J School Health *35*:442–449, 1965.
9. Gellman V: Glue sniffing among Winnipeg school children. Can Med Assoc J *98*:411–413, 1968.
10. Weinraub M, Groce P, Karno M: Chloroformism—a new case of a bad old habit. Calif Med *117*:63–65, 1972.
11. Guaraldi GP, Bonasegla P: Su di un caso di tossicomania da tricloroetilene. Riv Sper Freniatria *92*:913–920, 1968.
12. Blatherwich CE: Understanding glue sniffing. Can J Publ Health *63*:272–275, 1968.
13. Cohen S: The volatile solvents. Publ Health Rev *2*:185–214, 1973.
14. Alha A, Korte T, Tenhu M: Solvent sniffing death. Rechtsmed *72*:299–305, 1973.
15. Goto I, Matsumura M, Inoui N. et al: Toxic polyneuropathy due to glue sniffing. J Neurol, Neurosurg Psychiatr *37*:843–853, 1976.
16. Shirabe T, Tsudo T, Terao A, et al: Toxic polyneuropathy due to glue sniffing. J Neurol Sci *21*:101–113, 1974.
17. Masterson G, Sclare AB: Solvent abuse. Health Bull (Edinb) *36*:305–309, 1978.
18. Watson JM: Solvent abuse: Presentation and clinical diagnosis. Hum Toxicol *1*:249–256, 1982.
19. Sourindhrin I, Baird JA: Management of solvent abuse: A Glasgow community approach. Br J Addict *79*:227–232, 1979.
20. Cohen S: Glue sniffing. JAMA *231*:653–654, 1975.
21. Hershey CO, Miller S: Solvent abuse: A shift to adults. Int J Addict *6*:1085–1089, 1982.
22. Streicher HZ, Gabow PA, Moss A: Syndromes of toluene sniffing in adults. Ann Intern Med *94*:758–762, 1981.
23. Press E, Done AK: Solvent sniffing—physiological

effects and community control measures for intoxification from the intentional inhalation of organic solvents. Pediatrics *39*:51–61, 1967.
24. Waldron HA: Effects of organic solvents. Br J Hosp Med *26*:645–649, 1981.
25. Vale JA, Meredith TJ: Solvent abuse. In Haddad LM, Winchester JR (eds): Clinical Management of Poisoning and Drug Overdose. Philadelphia, WB Saunders, 1983, pp 801–804.
26. Anderson HR, MacNair RS, Ramsey JD: Deaths from abuse of volatile substances: A national epidemiological survey. Br Med J *290*:304–307, 1985.
27. Powars D: Aplastic anemia secondary to glue sniffing. N Engl J Med *273*:700–702, 1965.
28. Keane JR: Toluene optic atrophy. Ann Neurol *4*:390, 1978.
29. Knox JW, Nelson JR: Permanent encephalopathy from toluene inhalation. N Engl J Med *275*:1494–1496, 1966.
30. Grabaski DA: Toluene sniffing producing cerebellar degeneration. Am J Psychiatr *118*:401–462, 1961.
31. Sasa M: Equilibrium disorders with diffuse brain atrophy in long term toluene sniffing. Arch Otorhinolaryngol *221*:163–169, 1978.
32. Korobkin R, Asbury AK. Saumner AJ et al: Glue sniffing neuropathy. Arch Neurol *32*:158–162, 1975.
33. Hunter AGW, Thompson D, Evans JA: Is there a fetal gasolene syndrome. Teratology *20*:75, 1979.
34. National Cancer Institute: Technical report services No 2. Bethesda, United States Department of Health, Education, and Welfare, 1976.
35. King MD, Day RE, Oliver JS et al: Solvent encephalopathy. Br Med J *283*:663–665, 1981.
36. Yamamura Y: n-Hexane polyneuropathy. Folia Psychiatr Neurol Japonica *23*:45–57, 1969.
37. Moss AH, Gabow PA, Kaehny WD, et al: Fanconi's syndrome and distal renal tubular acidosis after glue sniffing. Ann Intern Med *92*:69–70, 1980.
38. Taher SM, Anderson RJ, McCartney R, et al. Renal tubular acidosis associated with toluene sniffing. N Engl J Med *290*:765–768, 1974.
39. Kroeger RM, Moore RJ, Lehman TH, et al. Recurrent urinary calculi associated with toluene. J Urol *123*:89, 1980.
40. Poklis A, Burkitt CD: Gasoline sniffing: A review. Clin Toxicol *11*:35, 1977.
41. Robinson RO: Tetraethyl lead poisoning from gasoline sniffing. JAMA *240*:1373, 1978.
42. Hansen KS, Sharp FR: Gasoline sniffing, lead poisoning and myoclonus. JAMA *240*:1375, 1978.
43. Litt IF, Cohen MI: "Danger . . . vapour harmful." Spot remover sniffing. N Engl J Med *281*:543, 1969.
44. Baerg RD, Kimberg DV: Centrilobular hepatic necrosis and acute renal failure in solvent sniffers. Ann Intern Med *73*:713–720, 1970.
45. Price HL, Laurie AA, Jones RE: Cyclopropane anaesthesia II. Epinephrine and norepinephrine in initiation of ventricular arrhythmia by carbon dioxide inhalation. Anaesthesiology *19*:288–294, 1958.
46. Lord CO, Katz RL, Ealings KE: Antiarrhythmic properties of stereoisomer of beta adrenogenic blocking agent (H56/28). Anaesthesiology *29*:288–294, 1968.
47. Orth OS, Letgh MB, Mellish CHM, et al: Action of sympathomimetic amines in cyclopropane ether and chloroform anaesthesia. J Pharmacol Exp Ther *67*:1–16, 1939.

CHAPTER 86
SMOKE INHALATION

Mark A. Eilers, M.D.

Eight to ten thousand persons die annually from injuries related to fires. Approximately 2 million patients seek medical care for cutaneous burns in the United States per year, of which 130,000 must be hospitalized. More than 50 per cent of these patients require intensive care. Of these patients, as many as 70 per cent have significant smoke inhalation as a factor complicating their injury. The vast majority of deaths are not caused by cutaneous burns or wound sepsis but are secondary to inhalation of toxic products of combustion.

Seventy per cent of all fire-related fatalities occur as a result of residential fires. The cost in property loss alone is 3 to 4 billion dollars per year. Dayton, Ohio, population 202,000, lost approximately 47 million dollars to fires in the past calendar year.[1–3]

The vast majority of patients who sustain cutaneous burns die as a result of complications of smoke inhalation. The most common cause of immediate death in fires is smoke inhalation injury. The most common toxin inhaled is carbon monoxide.[1, 4–16]

Few data on smoke inhalation existed in the medical literature prior to the 1942 Coconut Grove (Boston) Nightclub fire. In that fire 491 people were killed. Of the 114 victims transported to Massachusetts General Hospital, 75 were dead on arrival. Thirty-five of 36 who survived initial burn therapy died as a direct result of pulmonary injuries, not cutaneous burns.[17]

The MGM Grand Hotel fire (1980, 85 deaths), the Stouffer's White Plains fire (1980, 26 deaths), and the Las Vegas Hilton fire (1982, 12 deaths) have recently focused attention on the role inhalation injury plays in fire-related deaths.[1] In each instance, the majority of deaths occurred in guests found on higher floors where no soot or direct combustion was found. Autopsy evidence indicated that people died immediately, presumably owing to toxic gas inhalation.[1, 4–16]

Inhalation injury occurs as a result of carbon monoxide toxicity, direct thermal injury, and chemical insult.

Thus, because of the potential lethality of inhalation injury, the subject warrants an emergency physician's keen awareness whenever a history of fire or combustion is present.

ENVIRONMENT

The components of a fire include visible flame, luminous gas, heat, and smoke. The gaseous fraction is primarily carbon monoxide, carbon dioxide, and a variety of mixtures of other potentially lethal gases. Smoke is a suspension of small particles in hot gas that yields intense irritation of the eyes and upper airways. Visual obscuration is also prominent.

In a Center for Fire Research paper published in 1981, Birky and Clarke reported on the inhalation of toxic products from fires.[5] Their report reviewed the types of materials burned as well as who gets burned and how those factors interrelate to cause death and disability. The findings suggested that carbon monoxide and cyanide each alone could easily account for more than 50 per cent of the immediate deaths involved in inhalation injuries.

As combustion proceeds, available oxygen is consumed. It is not infrequent that even very early in a fire the ambient oxygen content drops to 15 per cent or lower. The resulting hypoxic environment is further exacerbated by oxygen displacement by gaseous products produced during combustion. Carbon monoxide and carbon dioxide mechanically and chemically displace oxygen, leading to further hypoxia and asphyxiation. In addition, many gases produced during combustion are themselves highly toxic and may alone be rapidly fatal. Pitt and colleagues in 1979 in a laboratory study,[18] Burns and associates in a 1985 autopsy study,[19] Jones and coworkers in a 1987 clinical study,[20] and Gold and colleagues in a 1978 field study[21] have all demonstrated the presence of potentially lethal amounts of carbon monoxide and/or cyanide in either the fire itself or the body tissues of those killed.

A synergism is postulated between the toxic effects of alcohol, carbon dioxide, and cyanide in producing deaths.[18–26] An international symposium sponsored by the Committee on Fire Research and the National Research Council[27] and a number of other studies[18–26] site factors such as ethanol ingestion, carbon monoxide, and cyanide as major contributors to inhalation injury deaths. Factors such as carbon monoxide, carbon dioxide, ethanol, and cyanide create an incapacitation. Intoxication due to individual agents or combinations noted previously plus others create a physical immobilization or altered mental capability, hindering the escape response. This yields prolonged exposure to toxic chemicals as well as prolonged thermal injury and is markedly contributory to death. Smith and coworkers[27] and Barillo and coworkers[25] represent an increasing body of evidence that suggests that sublethal amounts of various toxins are synergistic in creating morbidity. Elevated blood and ethanol levels have been strongly correlated with death from toxic gas exposure in fires.[22, 25] Smith and coworkers[27] have demonstrated that the combination of carbon monoxide and cyanide produced substantially more morbidity and mortality than either agent alone. Watanabe and Makino[23] have demonstrated in a laboratory model that carbon dioxide produces significantly greater pulmonary injury than heated air alone. The weight of this evidence would lend credence to the number of deaths and victims not consumed by flames.

It cannot be too strongly stressed that this exposure may create incapacitation in only 2 to 3 breaths. It is important to bear in mind that in the stress, both mental and physical, of fighting or escaping a fire, hyperventilation, toxic exposure, incapacitation, and death are very immediate threats.

Toxic Components

Since the late 1960s, there has been a progressive increase in the use of plastics and synthetic materials in furniture, carpets, wall coverings, and electrical materials that has radically changed the composition of the toxic products of fire and combustion. Today, the potentially toxic load of combustible materials in a residential structure has become overwhelming. Lethal risk to people within the first few moments of fire from inhalation products has become a much greater hazard than that from fatal burns or any other attendant hazards. Inhalation of toxic products combined with asphyxia and an exacerbation of underlying disabilities has been demonstrated to cause rapid physical and/or mental incapacitation. This incapacitation leads to sustained toxic exposure and/or cutaneous thermal burns and may contribute to death.[28–34]

The burning of products containing polyurethanes, silk, nylon, cyanide, and nitrogen yields two highly toxic compounds: cyanide and acrolein. Acrolein is an aldehyde produced by the burning of cotton or wood. It is very irritating, especially to the mucous membranes of the upper airways and eyes. It rapidly denatures protein. In a concentration of 10 parts per million (ppm) (a commonly achieved level of concentration in residential fires), it produces pulmonary edema and death within minutes.[35]

When plastics burn a number of factors affect the toxins produced, including temperature, fuel load, rate of burning, and other intangibles. Each individual plastic or substance will produce different toxic products. Polyvinylchloride (PVC) is an example.[28–31] Hydrochloric acid gas is produced during PVC combustion along with at least 72 other known products. The exact toxicities of these products have yet to be established.[35] Thus, when considering what potential hazards may have been encountered in a toxic inhalation, it becomes evident that there are immediate killers, such as hypoxia, cyanide, and carbon monoxide, along with literally thousands of other potential complicating substances.

Resources outlining toxic combustion products are numerous.[1, 6, 27–30, 35] Many different combinations and factors exist, making prediction or analysis essentially impossible. A variety of animal studies, laboratory fire models, autopsy studies, clinical studies, and field studies have confirmed the wide variability of the presence and concentrations of multiple toxic substances within the same blaze.[5, 6, 8, 9, 18–23]

Although precise prediction or analysis of toxic inhalation products may be highly impractical at this juncture, the evidence points toward the cause of death from direct thermal injury, carbon monoxide, cyanide, and other substances. Maintaining one's index of suspicion for thermal, cyanide, and carbon monoxide injury will serve as an excellent starting point. Table 86–1 outlines the more common toxic products of combustion, their sources, and associated clinical syndromes. A history of the fire location and its content as well as the duration and extent of exposure is key to proper emergency management. Assistance from an occupational medicine, toxicology, or certified regional poison control center will often prove valuable.

PATHOPHYSIOLOGY

Thermal Burns. Clinical and animal studies have documented the highly efficient cooling capacity of the upper airway. This is usually sufficient to prevent burns distal to the glottis. Hot dry air, even when forced past the upper airways directly into the trachea, will only produce burns in the proximal portion of the trachea. When steam is the agent of injury, massive and direct deep pulmonary parenchymal injury is possible. Steam has a 4000 times greater heat-carrying capacity than hot air. Thus, eliciting the history of a steam component to a burn should alert one to the possibility of a severe direct pulmonary injury.[1, 6, 10–16]

Chemical Injury. Soluble gases such as sulfur dioxide, ammonia, chlorine, and hydrochloric acid produce burns of the respiratory mucosa with resultant edema and potentially life-threatening upper airway obstruction.

Hydrochloric acid is noted to be absorbed on soot particles ranging in size from 0.1 to 2.5 μm in diameter. This size particle could be inhaled as far distally as the alveoli. When these contaminated soot particles reach the alveoli, the hydrochloric acid produces an immediate inflammatory reaction. Alveolar surfactant is destroyed, and the alveoli collapse. This combination of microatelectasis and inflammatory response produces hypoxia, distal airway collapse, and interstitial and alveolar pulmonary edema. The clinical appearance is almost immediate and rapidly fatal.[1, 6, 10–16, 19, 23, 28, 35–45]

Volatile, insoluble gases such as acrolein and phosgene absorbed on carbon particles can and do reach the lower respiratory tract and lung parenchyma. As a result, cilia of the mucociliary blanket cease to function, and the removal of debris is impaired. In addition, these toxic gases produce congestion, edema, necrosis, and sloughing of the bronchi, small airways, and pulmonary alveoli, leading to both immediate and delayed lower airway obstruction. Bronchospasm, either from direct irritation or neural reflexes, further decreases air flow. Peribronchial edema and premature small airway closures further exacerbate bronchospasm. After the initial injury, necrosis, ulceration, and sloughing lead to segmental, lobular, or total airway obstruction.[1, 6, 10–14, 19, 28, 29, 36–46]

Bacterial invasion with frank bacterial pneumonitis is a rare finding on initial presentation. Bacterial pneumonia is more common 3 to 5 days after initial injury.[1, 6, 10–16]

CLINICAL MANIFESTATIONS

History of Exposure. The 12 points listed hereafter are the most important factors in the fire environment that may be crucial in establishing a high index of suspicion for the presence of smoke inhalation injury.[1]

1. Open versus closed space,
2. Estimated duration of exposure,
3. Presence of steam,
4. Explosion,
5. Nature of burning material,
6. Presence of other injured or dead victims,
7. Amount, color, unique odor of smoke,
8. History of a fall or jump,
9. For fire fighters, nature of mask used (intermittent, demand, or continuous) and mask function,
10. Suicide note,
11. Suspicion of arson, and
12. Involvement of plastics.

Past History. Whenever possible, a careful evaluation of a patient's past history may yield significant information. Patients with underlying chronic obstructive pulmonary disease and/or cardiovascular disease will be at increased risk. It is particularly helpful and important to elicit any occupational or hobby exposures. A history of any other chronic illnesses and, especially, depression with suicidal ideation and/or drug or alcohol dependence may be elicited.

Symptoms and Signs. The classic signs and symptoms of inhalation injury include primary respiratory findings, but any organ system can be affected. Singed nasal hairs, soot in the upper airways, stridor, hoarseness, cough, carbonaceous sputum, tachypnea, dyspnea, cyanosis, wheezing, rales, rib fractures, pneumothorax, neck pain, and sore throat are all considered suggestive of respiratory injuries.[1, 6, 10–16]

Classic physical findings of smoke inhalation have been seriously questioned by Moylan,[47] who found the criteria of limited usefulness. He found that only two-thirds of patients with facial burns had inhalation injuries. Furthermore, up to 86 per cent of patients with upper respiratory tract burns had no associated facial burns. He found that patients with inhalation injuries usually had no carbonaceous sputum at initial presentation, and 50 per cent never produced any. Singed nasal hairs proved to be only 13 per cent predictive of inhalation injuries. Less than 25 per cent of patients with upper respiratory tract burns requiring intubation developed hoarseness. Moylan also noted that lethal upper airway obstruction may occur acutely and without any signs of facial burns.

Any number of central nervous system expressions of respiratory tract injury may be present. Patients found unconscious in a fire probably have the most likelihood of sustaining serious inhalation injuries. Fire fighters removing their masks during any portion of the extinguishing or cleanup phases of fire fighting may be subject to very high risk of smoke inhalation injury.[1, 6, 21] Seizures, hallucinations, confusion, headache, and dizziness exacerbated by behavioral dysfunction (confusion, anxiety, or compromised judgement) should lead one to be particularly suspicious of a toxic inhalation. Hyperthermia or hypothermia as well as orthopedic, gastrointestinal, and/or ophthalmologic manifestations should be anticipated.[1, 6, 10–16]

LABORATORY AND DIAGNOSTIC SUPPORT

After the basics of initial evaluation, resuscitation, and stabilization have taken place,

Table 86–1. TOXIC PRODUCTS OF COMBUSTION

Hydrogen Cyanide (HCN)
Source: Wool, silk, polyacrylnitrile, nylon, polyurethane, paper.
Toxicity: Systemic (cellular poison). This is a rapidly fatal asphyxiant that induces cellular hypoxia by formation of a stable complex with cytochrome oxidase.
Clinical aspects: HCN may be inhaled or absorbed through the skin. The characteristic odor of bitter almonds cannot be smelled by 30 to 50% of the population. Usually seen are emesis, palpitations, confusion, anxiety, and vertigo. Initially the blood pressure may be elevated, with a slow pulse, followed by a diminution of the blood pressure and a rise in pulse rate. Rapid respirations give way to slow and labored respiratory patterns, with coma and convulsions following. The ECG may show S-T elevation or depression. Acute pulmonary edema and lactic acidosis may be seen.
Treatment: Cyanide Antidote Kit by Lilly. Basic goal is to produce methemoglobin, then thiocyanate. Rapid treatment at the scene, if possible, is required for life salvage.

Hydrogen Chloride (HCl)
Source: Polyvinylchloride, chlorinated acrylics, and retardant-treated materials.
Toxicity: Direct pulmonary irritant; it inflames conjunctiva of eyes. At concentrations of 15 ppm, localized irritation of throat is noted. A concentration greater than 100 ppm may result in pulmonary edema and laryngeal spasm. Mists of HCl are less harmful than anhydrous HCl because the mist droplets have no desiccant action. The HCl gas reacts with moisture in the lungs to produce the acid destruction manifest by violent inflammation.
Clinical aspects: May be insidious and frequently delayed in onset, as much as 1 to 2 days, but 1 to 6 hours is usually noted. Skin irritation with frank burns may be noted. Pain and swelling of the conjunctiva may be noted as well as corneal erosions. Pulmonary damage manifests as dyspnea, chest pain and tightness, and pulmonary edema.
Treatment: Prompt evacuation of the victim, irrigation (decontamination) of the skin and eye, and administration of 100% oxygen. These patients should be observed for at least 24 hours for delayed toxicity.

Ammonia
Source: Wool, silk, nylon, melamine.
Toxicity: Direct irritant to respiratory structures and skin. It is capable of exerting a profoundly caustic action. Coma and convulsions are noted as systemic aspects of toxicity.
Clinical aspects: Readily identifiable by its pungent odor, conjunctivitis and lacrimation are noted early, producing temporary blindness. Restlessness, chest tightness, a frothy sputum, and cyanosis with collapse may be noted. These appear at concentrations greater than 1000 ppm. At greater than 1500 ppm, laryngospasm and immediate death may occur. Victims usually complain of intense pain in eyes, mouth, and throat and manifest a feeling of suffocation. There may be an inability to speak secondary to laryngeal edema, with stridor noted. Ammonia increases respiratory secretions. Skin contact will produce local irritation or burns.
Treatment: Predicated on decontamination and dilution. Airway control to overcome laryngeal edema and glottic spasm is of fundamental importance, as is respiratory care for pulmonary edema.

Sulfur Dioxide
Source: From all sulfur sources, this represents the common oxidation product of same.
Toxicity: Direct irritant on contact with moistened mucous membrane surfaces and the lung by virtue of the formation of sulfurous acid.
Clinical aspects: Patients often have dyspnea, cough, chest tightness, and chest "burning." Pulmonary edema with respiratory distress and failure is noted. Vomiting, difficulty swallowing, fever, pharyngeal and glossal erythema, headache, vertigo, agitation, memory loss, abdominal pain, diarrhea, tremor, convulsions, pneumonia, and peripheral neuritis may be noted.
Treatment: Decontamination with irrigation and dilution. Meticulous pulmonary care is mandatory.

Table 86–1. TOXIC PRODUCTS OF COMBUSTION *Continued*

Hydrogen Fluoride
Source: Fluorinated resins or films.
Toxicity: Direct irritant to mucosal surfaces, skin, and pulmonary tract. The fluoride ion is a direct cellular poison and interferes with calcium metabolism. It reacts with tissue proteins.
Clinical aspects: On the skin, it will produce irritation and deep penetrating necrotic lesions. Inhalation results in a severe pneumonitis with shortness of breath, chest tightness, and coughing.
Treatment: Termination of exposure followed by decontamination with irrigation. Meticulous pulmonary care may be required for treatment of the lung damage produced.

Acrolein
Source: From polyolefins and cellulosics.
Toxicity: Direct irritant.
Clinical aspects: Causes lacrimation with intense irritation of the upper respiratory passages.
Treatment: Meticulous respiratory care. Usually minor irritation will resolve with cessation of exposure.

Hydrogen Sulfide
Source: Hair, wools, meats, and hides, from decomposition of sulfur-containing organic materials.
Toxicity: With moisture, forms a caustic, sodium sulfide, that is a direct irritant to eyes, wet skin, and respiratory passages. Rotten egg odor is unmistakable, but low concentrations will fatigue the sense of smell rapidly. Capable of producing respiratory paralysis and death.
Clinical aspects: Consistent with respiratory tract irritation, manifested by cough, chest tightness, and dyspnea.

Nitrogen Oxides
Source: Fabrics, cellulose nitrate, and celluloid.
Toxicity: Converted to nitric acid with hydration. Because the oxides are poorly soluble in water, delayed effects are common, with a latent period of 5 to 24 hours as hydration takes place in the lungs.

Isocyanate (Toluene di-isocyanate)
Source: Urethane isocyanate polymers.
Toxicity: Exerts a pharmacodynamic reaction (universally experienced) with severe irritation being noted, especially of the eyes, GI tract, and lungs. An allergic reaction will also be noted in selected individuals manifested by an acute pneumonitis with edema.
Clinical aspects: Skin—irritation and inflammation. Eyes—conjunctival irritation and inflammation. GI tract—nausea, vomiting, and abdominal pain (from inhalation). Lungs—severe coughing, burning, and irritation of the upper tract with a choking sensation. There is sputum production with laryngitis, retrosternal soreness, chest pain, and asthma (a chemical bronchitis with bronchospasm). Chronic bronchitis may result. CNS—headache, insominia, euphoria, ataxia, and anxiety neurosis, depression, and paranoia.
Treatment: Irrigation and decontamination are the mainstays of early treatment. The asthmatic component may require theophylline treatment.
Clinical aspects: In high concentrations, there is immediate cough and chest pain. At low concentrations, there may be no warning, and the appearance of red-brown, orange, or copper-colored gases at the fireground is indication for immediate use of breathing apparatus. Insidious symptoms include chest tightness, dyspnea, shortness of breath, coma, and death.
Treatment: Meticulous pulmonary care in addition to decontamination and irrigation.

Phosgene
Source: From decomposition of heated organic compounds with chlorine, such as when carbon tetrachloride fire extinguishers are used. Chlorinated hydrocarbons and a number of plastics will produce same. Phosgene will decompose to HCl and CO.
Toxicity: Poor water solubility leads to delayed appearance of clinical toxicity. Direct irritant of pulmonary tract.
Clinical aspects: Choking, cough, chest pain, and hemoptysis.
Treatment: Irrigation after decontamination. Meticulous pulmonary care.

TERMINOLOGY USED IN COMBUSTION TOXICITY

Escape impairment—the inability of an individual or test animal to *escape* from a fire environment or simulation thereof. Strictly speaking, this term must be distinguished from "incapacitation," with which it is commonly confused. Incapacitation refers to the inability of a test animal to perform a *normal* or *trained* activity or task. Escape impairment may result from the toxic effects of fire effluents, including impaired vision, diminished motor coordination, and altered mental status.

Incapacitation—the inability of the subject animal to perform a normal activity or trained task. Synonyms used in the literature include intoxication and sublethal end-point. Incapacitation may be measured by observing the decrement in animal performance of a variety of mechanical tasks or by observing staggering, collapse, or convulsions.

Fire risk—the probability that a fire will occur and the potential for harm to life and property resulting from such an occurrence. Fire risk is a quantitative description for injury or property loss. As such it is a mathematically knowable value without the implication of acceptance of the value by an individual or society.

Fire hazard—a fire risk that is unacceptable. The declaration of a given risk as a hazard by an individual or community is arrived at by the less scientific, more cumbersome, but behaviorally more relevant process of consensus and is rooted in human perception.

(Reprinted with permission from Dinerman N, Huber JA: Inhalation Injuries. *In* Rosen P (ed): Emergency Medicine: Concepts and Clinical Practice. Vol. 1, 2nd ed. St. Louis, CV Mosby, 1988.)

some ancillary support may be of considerable benefit.

Arterial Blood Gases. Determination of PO_2, PCO_2, pH, and carboxyhemoglobin saturation should be undertaken on anyone with suspected pulmonary injury. When carbon monoxide exposure is suspected, obtain a measured oxygen saturation determination, as a calculated level will be artificially high. Carboxyhemoglobin levels should be obtained in anyone involved in a fire or suspected of exposure to toxic products of combustion. Carboxyhemoglobin levels, when measured, are usually lower than actually experienced at the time of exposure, universally as a result of prehospital oxygen therapy.

Hyperbaric oxygen therapy should be considered for any patient who may have sustained significant carbon monoxide levels. A body of literature supports the use of hyperbaric oxygen therapy for any patients suspected or having actual measured levels of 40 per cent or greater.[1, 6, 10–16, 18, 21, 23, 26, 27]

Cyanide Level. Cyanide levels in the emergency department are fundamentally an academic folly. Levels may, however, be of some retrospective value. Anyone suspected of cyanide exposure must be treated presumptively and urgently.[1, 6, 9–16, 18, 20, 21, 26]

Electrocardiogram and Cardiac Monitor. Any suspected serious inhalation exposure, especially in older patients with chronic obstructive pulmonary disease (COPD) or underlying cardiovascular disorders, indicates the need for continuous cardiac monitoring. The presence of a myocardial infarct may be the first suggestion that a patient has been seriously intoxicated or asphyxiated from toxic products of combustion.

Chest X-Rays. Much has been written about the usefulness or uselessness of chest radiology in this setting. Reason can suggest that a baseline chest x-ray may be of benefit even in patients with little suspicion of injury. Most studies confirm this reasoning.[1, 6, 10–16, 29, 36, 48] A normal chest radiograph does not rule out severe pulmonary injury. Indeed, patients with severe pulmonary injury, hypoxia, and respiratory failure may have a completely normal chest x-ray. Similarly, seemingly asymptomatic patients may present with severe chest radiographic findings.

Several studies have suggested that up to 40 per cent of patients with serious pulmonary injuries may manifest essentially normal chest x-rays.[1, 6, 10–16, 48]

Other chest x-ray findings include local, patchy, or diffuse infiltrates, although they may not become evident until 24 to 36 hours after exposure. A diffuse alveolar filling pattern may develop as late as 96 hours after admission. As a rule, resolution without residua generally follows.

Pulmonary Function Tests. Spirometry continues to be of great usefulness in the emergency department. Although somewhat effort dependent, spirometry is inexpensive, easy to reproduce, and useful as an evaluative and prognostic tool. Altered peak expiratory flow rate, forced expiratory volume in 1 second or in the more sophisticated tools, and flow volume loops can help identify subtle respiratory injury. Normal spirometry probably excludes significant injury to the lower respiratory track. No specific parameters have been firmly established for diagnostics.[1, 6, 10–16, 45, 49]

Xenon^{133} Perfusion-Ventilation Scanning. Ventilation-perfusion scanning using xenon is considered diagnostic of ventilation injury if abnormal retention after 90 seconds occurs. Any pre-existing chronic obstructive airway disease will yield false-positive results. This may be a very useful test in patients who have more minimal injuries.[1, 6, 10–16]

Xenon scanning requires considerable patient cooperation, removal of the patient from the emergency department and its attendant monitoring, and approximately 45 minutes. A technician with the expertise to perform this examination must be available. These factors may conspire to limit the practicality of xenon scanning in this setting.

Fiberoptic Bronchoscopy. Bronchoscopy can be used to directly and rapidly assess the upper airway for pulmonary injury. This procedure may unveil the need for early or even prophylactic intubation. The finding of soot, burns, edema, ulceration, necrotic tissue, or debris strongly argues for intubation. Patients with marginal or borderline clinical suspicion of pulmonary injury may have fiberoptic bronchoscopy done. If it is normal (and they have normal spirometry) they can be discharged after 6 to 10 hours of observation with relative safety.[1, 6, 10–16, 50, 51]

THERAPY AND MANAGEMENT

Some of these patients may present as traumatic, hypoxic, and comatose in extremis, and others may present as the merely walking worried. Appropriate and timely prehospital and emergency department evaluations will be the pivot upon which a good outcome turns.

Prehospital Care. When dealing with the prehospital care phase, as much information as possible should be gathered from the paramedics, fire fighters, and others on the scene. The nature of the explosion, the type of chemicals or structure involved, the length of exposure, the presence of unconsciousness, open versus closed space, how patients were rescued, and any trauma are critical factors in determining patient outcome.

Decontamination of toxic or radioactive materials, oxygen therapy, and relief of airway obstruction should be begun at the fire scene. Burns should be treated in the usual fashion; i.e., removing the patient's clothing and covering him or her with a sterile sheet.

Emergency Department. Immediate threats to life, such as airway obstruction or hypoventilation, must be urgently assessed and corrected. Frank asphyxia or cyanide or carbon monoxide exposure will kill the vast majority of these patients. One-hundred per cent oxygen must be administered to patients with even a slight suspicion of carbon monoxide or cyanide intoxication and may prove to be life-saving. Careful attention to providing a secure airway and an assessment of breathing, circulation, neurologic disability, and other injuries are the initial priorities. Head to toe primary assessment, resuscitation, and a secondary survey to assess any and all concomitant system injuries must be completed.

Aggressive pulmonary toilet with bronchodilator therapy using either intravenous or oral aminophylline and/or beta agonist agents and fiberoptic bronchoscopy are the primary therapeutic tools. Evaluation of the extent and degree of injury; removal of debris via bronchoscopy; pulmonary toilet including humidified oxygen, coughing, deep breathing, and postural drainage; and careful gentle suctioning to maintain airway patency are critical for survival. Arterial blood gases, chest radiography, and other measurements may be taken at this time.

Pulmonary edema may be mild and very responsive to simple diuretic therapy. Other pulmonary edema presentations may be much more fulminating and refractory, requiring aggressive intubation, positive end-expiratory pressure, and multiple pharmacologic manipulations.

Prophylactic antibiotics are not recommended. Antibiotics are only useful when cultures, temperature elevation, leukocytosis, or infiltrates on the chest x-ray have firmly suggested the diagnosis.[1, 6, 10–15, 36]

Steroids should not be administered. Many studies have demonstrated either equivocal or frankly morbid results from the use of steroids in the management of patients with pulmonary injuries.[1, 6, 10–16, 29, 36, 52, 53]

Any other injuries should be managed knowing that the pulmonary injury alone will increase the morbidity from the burn by 30 to 70 per cent.[54, 55]

In the comatose patient with a carboxyhemoglobin value of greater than 40 per cent, hyperbaric oxygen may be indicated.[1, 6, 10–16, 18, 21, 23, 26, 27]

Antidotal therapy for cyanide poisoning may be indicated, especially in patients found unconscious at the scene of the fire, exposed to plastics burning, or involved in a fire where production of cyanide gas has been suspected.[1, 6, 10–16, 18, 20, 21, 26–46, 56]

ADMISSION CRITERIA

Patients with suspected smoke inhalation who are asymptomatic and without indications of prolonged concentrated exposure may be discharged after 4 to 6 hours of observation. These patients include those with no history of loss of consciousness or mental dysfunction at the scene and those with a documented carbon monoxide level of less than 10 per cent before oxygen therapy.

Patients who are asymptomatic with normal laboratory data but who have a high probability of a significant smoke exposure are best observed in a regular hospital bed for 24 hours.

Patients who are candidates for intensive care include the following:

1. Those with multiple system trauma or significant cutaneous burns;
2. Those with symptoms, signs, or laboratory evidence of cardiac or central nervous system dysfunction;
3. Those with respiratory symptoms such as wheezing, rales, rhonchi, hoarseness, tachypnea, or stridor;
4. Those with carboxyhemoglobin determinations of 15 per cent or greater; and
5. Those with abnormal chest x-rays, pulmonary function tests, arterial blood

gases, xenon scans, or fiberoptic bronchoscopy or any deterioration in clinical or laboratory data.

Treatment of these patients in the intensive care unit continues with vigorous pulmonary toilet, maintenance of oxygenation with mechanical ventilation or assistance as indicated, antibiotic therapy (when clinically indicated), hemodynamic monitoring, and routine nursing care.

LONG-TERM EFFECTS

Long-term sequelae of smoke inhalation are actually quite rare. Tracheal stenosis when upper airways have been burned is a common finding. Bronchiolitis obliterans, saccular bronchiectasis, and repeated pulmonary infections have been observed. Severe persistent obstructive airway disease has also been identified. These factors argue for long-term follow-up with appropriate specialists.[57–60]

References

1. Dinerman N, Huber JA: Inhalation injury. *In* Rosen P (ed): Emergency Medicine: Concepts and Clinical Practice. Vol 1, 2nd ed. St. Louis, CV Mosby, 1988, pp 585–608.
2. Hoffman MS (ed): The World Almanac and Book of Facts. New York, Scripps-Howard Company, 1988.
3. Blackburn GW, Hatchl BL, Braley GE, et al: Statistical Abstract of the United States. 107th ed. 1987.
4. Autian J: Medical aspects of toxicity resulting from fire exposure, physiological and toxicological aspects of combustion products. International Symposium, Salt Lake City, March 18–20, 1974, pp 47–56.
5. Birky MM, Clarke FB: Inhalation of toxic products from fires. Toxicity of Organic Compounds *57*(10):997–1013, 1981.
6. Johnston BD: Inhalation injuries. *In* Auerbach PS, Geehr EC (eds): Management of Wilderness and Environmental Emergencies. 1st ed. New York, Macmillan, 1983, pp 585–605.
7. Zikria BA, Budd DC, Floch HF, et al: A clinical view of "smoke poisoning," physiological and toxicological aspects of combustion products. International Symposium, Salt Lake City, March 18–20, 1974, pp 36–43.
8. DeKorver L: Smoke problems in urban fire control, physiological and toxicological aspects of combustion products. International Symposium, Salt Lake City, March 18–20, 1974, pp 4–10.
9. Radford EP, Pitt B: Study of fire deaths in Maryland Sept. 1971–Jan. 1974, physiological and toxicological aspects of combustion products. International Symposium, Salt Lake City, March 18–20, 1974, pp 26–35.
10. Robinson L, Miller RH: Smoke inhalation injuries. Am J Otolaryngol *7*(5):375–380, 1986.
11. Crapo RO: Smoke-inhalation injuries. JAMA *246*(15):1694–1696, 1981.
12. Coleman DL: Smoke inhalation. West J Med *135*(4):300–309, 1981.
13. Ellenhorn MJ, Barceloux DG: Smoke inhalation. *In* Ellenhorn MJ, Barceloux DG: Medical Toxicology, Diagnosis and Treatment of Human Poisoning. 1st ed. New York, Elsevier, 1988, p 888.
14. Parish RA: Smoke inhalation and carbon monoxide poisoning in children. Pediatr Emerg Care *2*(1):36–39, 1986.
15. Peters WJ: Inhalation injury caused by the products of combustion. CMAJ *125*:249–252, 1981.
16. Rubenstein E: Smoke inhalation. *In* Rubenstein E, Federman DD: Scientific American Medicine. New York, Scientific American, Inc, 1984, p 1.
17. Pittman JC: The pulmonary complications: A clinical description. Ann Surg *117*:834–840, 1943.
18. Pitt BR, Radford EP, Gurtner GH, et al: Interaction of carbon monoxide and cyanide on cerebral circulation and metabolism. Arch Environ Health *34*(5):354–359, 1979.
19. Burns TR, Greenberg SD, Cartwright J, et al: Smoke inhalation: An ultrastructural study of reaction to injury in the human alveolar wall. Environ Res *41*:447–457, 1986.
20. Jones J, McMullen J, Dougherty J: Toxic smoke inhalation: Cyanide poisoning in fire victims. Am J Emerg Med *5*(4):317–321, 1987.
21. Gold A, Burgess WA, Clougherty EV: Exposure of firefighters to toxic air contaminants. Am Indust Hygiene Ass J *39*:534–539, 1978.
22. Mierley MC, Baker SP: Fatal house fires in an urban population. JAMA *249*(11):1466–1468, 1983.
23. Watanabe K, Makino K: The role of carbon monoxide poisoning in the production of inhalation burns. Ann Plastic Surg *15*(3):284–295, 1985.
24. Barillo DJ, Goode R, Rush BF Jr, et al: Lack of correlation between carboxyhemoglobin and cyanide in smoke inhalation injury. Curr Surg: Sept/Oct:421–425, 1986.
25. Barillo DJ, Rush BF Jr, Goode R: Is ethanol the unknown toxin in smoke inhalation injury? Am Surg *52*:641–645, 1986.
26. Hart GB, Strauss MB, Lennon PA, et al: Treatment of smoke inhalation by hyperbaric oxygen. J Emerg Med *3*:211–215, 1985.
27. Smith PW, Crane CR, Sanders DC, et al: Effects of exposure to carbon monoxide and hydrogen cyanide, physiological and toxicological aspects of combustion products. International Symposium, Salt Lake City, March 18–20, 1974, pp 75–88.
28. Einhorn IN: Physiological and toxicological aspects of smoke produced during the combustion of polymeric materials. Environ Health Per *11*:163–189, 1975.
29. Cohen MA, Guzzardi LJ: Inhalation of products of combustion. Ann Emerg Med *12*(10):628–632, 1983.
30. Purser DA, Buckley P: Lung irritance and inflammation during and after exposures to thermal decomposition products from polymeric materials. Med Sci Law *23*(2):142–150, 1983.
31. Carter VL, Bafus DA, Harris ES: Toxicity associated with flame-retarded plastics, physiological and toxicological aspects of combustion products. International Symposium, Salt Lake City, March 18–20, 1974, pp 96–104.

32. Seader JD, Chien WP: Factors affecting smoke development and measurement, physiological and toxicological aspects of combustion products. International Symposium, Salt Lake City, March 18–20, 1974, pp 166–180.
33. Hileman FD, Voorhees KJ: Pyrolysis of a flexible-urethane foam, physiological and toxicological aspects of combustion products. International Symposium, Salt Lake City, March 18–20, 1974, pp 226–244.
34. Zapp JA Jr: Fires, toxicity and plastics, physiological and toxicological aspects of combustion products. International Symposium, Salt Lake City, March 18–20, 1974, pp 58–74.
35. Ellenhorn MJ, Barceloux DG: Inhalant abuse. *In* Ellenhorn MJ, Barceloux DG: Medical Toxicology Diagnosis and Treatment of Human Poisoning. New York, Elsevier, 1988, pp 840–887.
36. Herndon DN, Langner F, Thompson P, et al: Pulmonary injury in burned patients. Surg Clin North Am *67*:31–46, 1987.
37. Herndon DN, Traber LD, Linares H, et al: Etiology of the pulmonary pathophysiology associated with inhalation injury. Resuscitation *14*:43–59, 1986.
38. Madden MR, Finkelstein JL, Goodwin CW: Respiratory care of the burn patient. Clin Plastic Surg *13*(1):29–38, 1986.
39. Stewart RJ, Yamaguchi KT, Rowland RRR, et al: Early detection of extravascular lung water in an inhalation injury animal model. Burns *12*(7):457–460, 1986.
40. Walker HL, McLeod CF Jr, McManus WF: Experimental inhalation injury in the goat. J Trauma *21*(11):962–964, 1981.
41. Traber DL, Herndon DN, Stein MD, et al: The pulmonary lesion of smoke inhalation in an ovine model. Circ Shock *18*:311–323, 1986.
42. Thorning DR, Howard ML, Hudson LD, et al: Pulmonary responses to smoke inhalation: Morphologic changes in rabbits exposed to pine wood smoke. Hum Pathol *13*(4):355–364, 1982.
43. Herndon DN, Traber DL, Niehaus GD, et al: The pathophysiology of smoke inhalation injury in a sheep model. J Trauma *24*(12):1044–1051, 1984.
44. Loke J, Paul E, Virgulto A, et al: Rabbit lung after acute smoke inhalation. Arch Surg *119*:956–959, 1984.
45. Haponik EF, Meyers DA, Munster AM, et al: Acute upper airway injury in burn patients. Am Rev Respir Dis *135*:360–366, 1987.
46. Cahalane M, Demling RH: Early respiratory abnormalities from smoke inhalation. JAMA *251*(6):771–773, 1984.
47. Moylan JA: Inhalation injury—a primary determination of survival. JBCR *3*:78–84, 1981.
48. Teixidor HS, Rubin E, Novick GS, et al: Smoke inhalation: Radiologic manifestations. Radiology *149*:383–387, 1983.
49. Cooke NT, Cobley AJ, Armstrong RF: Airflow obstruction after smoke inhalation. Anesthesia *37*(8):830–832, 1982.
50. Clark CJ, Reid WH, Telfer ABM, et al: Respiratory injury in the burned patient. Anesthesia *38*(1):35–39, 1983.
51. Tan WC, Lee ST, Lee CN, et al: The role of fiberoptic bronchoscopy in the management of respiratory burns. Ann Acad Med Singapore *14*(3):430–434, 1985.
52. Robinson NB, Hudson LD, Riem M, et al: Steroid therapy following isolated smoke inhalation injury. J Trauma *22*(10):876–879, 1982.
53. Beeley MJ, Crow J, Jones JG, et al: Mortality and lung histopathology after inhalation lung injury. Am Rev Respir Dis *133*(2):191–196, 1986.
54. Shirani KZ, Pruitt BA Jr, Mason AD: The influence of inhalation injury and pneumonia on burn mortality. Ann Surg *205*(1):82–87, 1987.
55. Thompson PB, Herndon DN, Traber DL, et al: Effect on mortality of inhalation injury. J Trauma *26*(2):163–165, 1986.
56. Moritz AR, Henriques FC, McLean R: The effect of inhaled heat on the air passages and lungs: An experimental investigation. Am J Pathol *21*:311–331, 1945.
57. Williams DO, Vanecko RM, Glassroth J: Endobronchial polyposis following smoke inhalation. Chest *84*(6):774–776, 1983.
58. Kato M: Chronic effects of fire casualty on pulmonary function. 15(1,2):77–85, 1982.
59. Jaspar N, Bracamonte M, Sergysels R: Severe peripheral airway obstruction after inhalation burn. Intensive Care Med *8*:105–106, 1982.
60. Minty BD, Royston D, Jones JG, et al: Changes in permeability of the alveolar-capillary barrier in firefighters. Br J Indust Med *42*:631–634, 1985.

CHAPTER 87

AMMONIA, NITROGEN, NITROUS OXIDES, AND RELATED COMPOUNDS

M. Jo McMullen, M.D., FACEP
Thomas J. Hetrick, M.D., FACEP
Louis A. Cannon, M.D.

AMMONIA

The usual setting of patient exposure to ammonia is an industrial accident. Industrial-strength ammonia at concentrations of 27 to 30 per cent is considered a caustic or alkali. It is used as a chemical in the manufacture of fertilizer; because of its high nitrogen concentration (82 per cent), it is one of the best fertilizers available commercially. Ammonia is also used as a solvent in the manufacture of textiles, leather, and pulp and paper processing and as a stabilizer in rubber manufacturing. It is also used in the synthesis of nitrous oxide, plastics, pharmaceuticals, pesticides, cyanide, explosives, rocket fuels, and flame retardants. Ammonia is also used in petroleum refining processes and in the treatment of metals. In the past ammonia was a common refrigerant and may still be found in some food processing installations and in ice production and cold storage facilities.[1–6]

Commonly used as a household cleaner or bleaching agent, ammonia is found in 5 to 10 per cent concentrations with a pH of less than 12. If an ammonia-containing cleaner is mixed with a chlorine-containing bleach, fumes of both ammonia and chlorine are released. In this concentration, it is generally considered an irritant and is rarely reported to cause burns.[5] However, three patients who attempted suicide by ingesting household ammonia were reported to have esophageal burns; there was one fatality.[7] Ammonia may also be found around the home as a liniment and in spirits of ammonia.[8]

Anhydrous ammonia (NH_3) at atmospheric pressure is a colorless gas with an extremely pungent odor. This gas may burn but does not ignite readily; however, the container may explode in heat or fire. The explosive limit in air is 16 to 25 per cent. Usual shipping containers include tank cars, tank trucks, barges, and steel cylinders.[1, 3, 5, 9]

Pathophysiology

The extent of injury from ammonia depends on the duration of the exposure, the concentration of the gas or liquid, and the depth of inhalation (see Table 87–1). Ammonia vapor per se is not poisonous, but its high solubility in water is responsible for its irritant and corrosive actions. The anhydrous gas ammonia is absorbed on mucosal membranes such as the eyes, oral cavity, pharynx, and lungs and mixes with moisture found there to convert to ammonium hydroxide (NH_4OH), which is both irritant and caustic to these areas. This conversion is an exothermic reaction and will cause a thermal injury as well as a chemical injury. This type of burn results in the liquefaction of the tissues and a deeper penetration of the chemical burn with subsequent scarring. Burns will feel soapy due to the saponification of the tissues. Edema of all involved tissues is common.[1–3, 5, 8–10, 12]

Desquamation of the epithelial layer of the upper tracheobronchial tree (tracheobronchitis) with membrane formation is the usual pathology found. There tends to be relatively little effect on the lower airways because of the agent's high solubility. With very high

Table 87–1. EFFECTS OF AMMONIA AT DIFFERENT CONCENTRATIONS

25–50 ppm	Odor threshold; tolerance may develop to the odor
25 ppm	TLV
50 ppm	OSHA and NIOSH exposure limits TWA
100 ppm	Eye irritant
500 ppm	Immediate danger to life or health
1000 ppm	Direct caustic effects on respiratory tract
2500 ppm	Death has been reported after ½ hour of exposure
30,000 ppm	LCLD after 5 minute exposure in human references[1, 3, 5, 10 11]

concentrations of the vapors, terminal bronchiolitis and alveolar injury leading to pulmonary edema can occur. Noncardiogenic pulmonary edema is secondary to damage to the alveolar-capillary membrane with resultant increased permeability and the exudation of fluid into the alveolae.[2, 4, 12–14]

Intra-alveolar fibroblastic proliferation has been reported. Bronchial mucosa is replaced by granulation tissue. Cystic bronchiectasis—thinning of the walls with cystic dilatation—follows destruction of mucous glands, smooth muscle, and cartilage. The small airways become filled with collagenous tissue, and inflammatory cells.[3, 15, 16]

Skin exposure to the liquid (−33°C) causes frostbite-type injuries with first- to third-degree burns. Extensive systemic absorption with death has been reported. Also, deaths have resulted from extensive skin burns.[3, 10]

Oral ingestion causes burns, ulcer formation, and esophageal or stomach perforation by the same mechanism that causes skin burns.[9]

Clinical Signs and Symptoms

Facial Signs. Exposure of the head and neck region to fumes commonly causes headache, salivation, swelling around the eyes and lips, and restlessness. Concentrated ammonia fumes cause a burning sensation in the eyes, followed by lacrimation, swelling, blurred vision, and severe pain. Corneal opacification with scarring and neovascularization, iritis, lens damage, and cataract formation are all common complications of severe exposure, particularly if the patient is not treated promptly. Increased intraocular pressure will mimic acute narrow-angle closure glaucoma. Ammonia has a greater tendency than any other alkali to penetrate and damage the eye.[1, 3, 4, 5, 9, 10, 12, 15, 16]

Lungs. Injury due to ammonia inhalation is often classified as mild, moderate, or severe, depending on the extent of pulmonary injury. There may be initial primary respiratory failure on the basis of severe local edema with acute obstruction of the airway. If this does not occur immediately, the patient will present with cough, dyspnea, or tightness in the chest, laryngitis, bronchospasm manifest by wheezing and tracheitis, and hypoxia. Occasionally these patients will be unable to speak. Respiratory irritation may occasionally be delayed in onset. Eventually, pulmonary edema may present with rales and rhonchi if the concentration was sufficiently high to have penetrated the lower airways. Copious amounts of tracheal secretions are usually reported. Hemoptysis and fever are not uncommon. Consolidation and pneumonia can occur.[1, 3–6, 9, 10, 12, 15, 16]

Inhalation injury may follow a biphasic course with an initial chemical pneumonitis, edema, congestion, hemorrhage, and atelectasis. This phase is followed by some improvement during the next 48 to 72 hours. Then the gradual onset of airway obstruction and respiratory failure develops with sloughing of tissue; a persistent obstructive pattern may then develop. Most patients who survive the first 24 hours will recover.[3, 17]

The initial chest x-ray is usually clear but may eventually suggest tracheobronchitis and mild pulmonary edema. Xenon-133 scanning or direct examination of the airway by fiberoptic bronchoscopy will help to determine the extent of injury.[4, 18]

Gastrointestinal Signs. Ingestion causes severe pain in the mouth, chest, and abdomen and cough, nausea, and vomiting. Shock frequently occurs early. Severe local edema of the lips and mouth will be present. Burns of the soft palate may occur. The airway must be examined for edema, which may lead to primary respiratory obstruction. Early endoscopy will be helpful in determining the extent of injury. Twenty-four to 72 hours later, esophageal and gastric perforation with mediastinitis may occur. These patients will have severe abdominal pain and rigidity and may have associated respiratory complications including pulmonary edema. Late complications from ulcerative esophagitis include stricture formation.[1, 5, 10, 12]

Skin Signs. Initially, the patient will notice sweating and a burning sensation, followed rapidly by blister or vesicle formation. Injuries may include mild erythema and edema following exposure to a low concentration of ammonia or severe edema with liquefaction necrosis and deep penetrating burns following a more concentrated vapor exposure. Exposure to the liquid form of ammonia will produce deep frostbite injuries.[1, 5, 10, 16, 19]

Laboratory Features. The laboratory generally yields nonspecific results and is not helpful. It is important to obtain serial arterial blood gases, both to follow the progress of respiratory failure and because these patients have a propensity to develop a metabolic acidosis. The serum ammonia level does not correlate with the degree of injury.[10, 15]

Treatment

Prehospital management must be started early and aggressively. It is necessary to remove the patient from the exposure situation to fresh air and to remove all clothing, even the shoes. For a skin exposure, the emergency medical service (EMS) personnel should wash the affected area twice with soap and copious amounts of water for at least 15 to 20 minutes; then the area can be covered with a dry, clean dressing. After cleaning as noted, skin burns should be dressed with Silvadine. Fluid resuscitation by the standard burn protocol is recommended, but it is important to remember that noncardiogenic pulmonary edema may occur. Pulmonary capillary wedge pressure monitoring may be required in the seriously burned patient. Tetanus prophylaxis is indicated.[3, 9, 15]

It is important for EMS personnel to wash out the eyes continuously until a physician can examine them and check the pH.[1, 5, 7, 9] After the eyes have been adequately irrigated to a normal pH, slit-lamp evaluation with fluorescein stain should be done and the pressure levels should be checked. Ophthalmic antibiotics and atropine are recommended. Steroids are also frequently recommended, but no controlled trials are available to support these recommendations.[3]

If ammonia has been ingested it is generally recommended that the patient be given 4 to 8 ounces of water or milk to dilute the ammonia. It is important that the prehospital personnel do nothing to induce emesis.[1, 5] After dilution and endoscopy, some authors recommend steroids as treatment for esophageal burns. Antibiotics will be needed if mediastinitis develops.[5, 10]

In any case of exposure to ammonia by inhalation, support of respirations with high-flow oxygen is important in the prehospital setting, although early intubation, if feasible, is the treatment of choice.[1, 7]

In the hospital, early aggressive control of the airway is essential. Earlier authors recommended immediate tracheostomy for all patients exposed to ammonia fumes who had any clinical signs at presentation. More recently, early intubation, before edema makes it impossible, is usually suggested. However, emergency tracheostomy may be needed if upper airway obstruction is present. Humidified oxygen and bronchodilators are essential components of therapy, as is frequent suctioning. Positive end-expiratory pressure (PEEP) ventilation may be necessary to maintain adequate oxygen levels.[2–5, 7, 8, 17]

Fiberoptic bronchoscopy can be both a diagnostic aid and a therapeutic benefit in assisting with the removal of sloughed tissue and secretions. In addition to serial arterial blood gas measurements and radiographs, serial pulmonary function testing may also be useful.[3, 5, 8, 10] Use of systemic steroids for inhalation injury is controversial, although most case reports include their use. Prophylactic systemic antibiotics are generally no longer recommended.[2, 4, 8, 17, 19]

Long-Term Implications

Patients who survive for more than 24 hours are likely to recover. Although complete pulmonary recovery is the usual outcome, residual bronchoconstriction, bronchiectasis, and small airway disease have been reported. Fibrous obliteration of the small airways, thought to be a late stage of bronchiolitis obliterans, is felt to be the cause of the chronic obstructive pulmonary disease that occasionally develops.[5, 8, 10, 13, 16, 17, 20]

Eye damage varying in degree to total blindness may be the permanent residual effect of an exposure to ammonia. Cataract formation, permanent corneal ulceration, and lenticular opacification have been reported.[1, 17]

Follow-up barium swallow at 10 to 21 days is recommended in patients who have ingested ammonia because stricture formation may present at this time.[5]

Repeated exposure may cause chronic irritation of the conjunctiva and upper respiratory tract. Chronic bronchitis has been reported after repeated inhalation exposures. However, chronic exposure to low concentrations of ammonia vapor rarely causes serious injury to the lung parenchyma.[1, 11, 15]

NITROUS OXIDE

Toxic gas inhalations involving nitrogen oxides have been reported in both single victims and large groups for the last 200 years. The earliest recorded case of toxic inhalation of fumes involved a French merchant who died after breathing concentrated nitric acid fumes in 1804.[21] Nitrous oxides were not recognized as the cause of silo filler's disease until 1956,[22] although the clinical entity had been recognized as early as 1914.[23] The mortality for silo filler's disease, based on a review of the literature, is about 30 per cent. In one Wisconsin study, 4.2 per cent of all farmers have become symptomatic working around silos.[24]

Membrane irritation is noted with exposure to 13 ppm of nitrogen dioxide (NO_2),[25] but most people can note the odor on exposure to 1 to 3 ppm. The maximum allowable exposure is 3 ppm (threshold limit value, TLV) for NO_2 and 25 ppm for nitric oxide (NO).[26] At 50 to 150 ppm NO_2 is only a mild to moderate irritant of the eyes and upper airways,[24] so patients tend to stay in the toxic environment longer. The LD_{50} is 174 ppm at 1 hour.[27] Using the level found in environmental research, 50 to 150 mg per m^3 is needed to produce bronchitis or pneumonia, whereas 560 to 940 mg per m^3 is considered lethal.[28] Table 87–2 lists the chemical composition of the nitrogen compounds.

Sources of Exposure

The most common toxic effect of exposure to nitrogen oxide fumes is pulmonary disease following exposure to silage gas, or silo filler's disease.[24, 29, 30] Another common occupation that involves exposure to these fumes is firefighting. Fumes may come from slow-burning nitrocellulose in x-ray film such as in the Cleveland Clinic disaster of 1929.[21, 29] Firefighters may be exposed because of other burning materials such as bed mattresses or fires at chemical plants.[25]

Other common sources of exposure include acetylene welding in confined spaces, detonation of explosives, especially shot firing in coal mines and dynamite blasting, and accidents involving nitric acid. Diesel fumes or fumes from any internal combustion engine, furnace gases, and smoking cigarettes, cigars, and pipes can cause low-level exposure. Many chemical processes such as the manufacture of dyes and lacquers are associated with the release of nitrous oxide fumes,[21, 29–31] as is cleaning coins.[32]

Missile silos, where nitrogen tetroxide is used as a fuel oxidizer, have been the site of accidental exposures; there is one report of 24 workers exposed at one time; three Apollo astronauts were also exposed.[24, 33]

Table 87–2. NO_x

Nitrogen oxide	NO (nitric oxide)
Nitrous oxide	N_2O
Nitrogen dioxide	NO_2 (red-brown or copper)
Nitrogen peroxide	N_2O_2
Dinitrogen trioxide	N_2O_3
Dinitrogen tetroxide	N_2O_4 (nitrogen tetroxide, yellow)
Dinitrogen pentoxide	N_2O_5

Silo Filler's Disease

Death occurring on entering a silo was first described in 1914 but was incorrectly attributed to asphyxiation. The study of this case involved returning to the silo the next day and dropping in a guinea pig, a rabbit, and a "large slender collie dog." After all three had dropped dead, one of the investigators went in. He described the odor we now know as nitrogen dioxide; however, this compound was not appreciated on gas analysis, and the deaths were mistakenly attributed to carbon dioxide.[23] The first reports that correctly attributed silo filler's disease to nitrogen dioxide appeared in 1956.[22, 34, 35]

High concentrations of nitrogen oxides can be found when silage, usually corn, is grown under conditions of drought, heavy sunlight, or premature harvest. The oxides of nitrogen are derived from nitrates in the silage, which are fermented into nitrites that combine with organic acids to form nitrous acid. This then decomposes into water and a mixture of nitrogen oxides. Nitrogen dioxide, which is reddish brown and has a pungent odor, and nitrogen tetroxide, which is yellow, are thought to be the principal agents responsible for the pulmonary injury. The decomposing process begins very shortly after putting crops into a silo (within 4 hours of filling) and continues for at least 10 days. Dangerous amounts of gas may remain in the silo for a month if it is not opened. One case report involved a man exposed 6 weeks after silage was stored.[29, 31, 36–39]

Pathophysiology

Because nitrogen oxides are less soluble (hydrolyze more slowly) than most irritant gases, they reach the bronchioles and alveoli, whereas most irritant gases do not. Within the lungs, nitrogen oxides react with water to form nitrous and nitric acids, which cause extensive local damage that results in a profound chemical pneumonitis and pulmonary edema. Pulmonary edema occurs when high concentrations of the gases are inhaled. At lower concentrations, an inflammatory exudate and bronchoconstriction occur.[24, 29, 30, 40] There is both increased airway resistance and decreased diffusion capacity. The acute increase in airway resistance that occurs following NO_2 exposure, even at low doses, appears to be mediated by histamine release.[21] Inhalation of as little as 0.3 ppm of nitrogen dioxide has been shown to potentiate induced bronchospasm in asthmatics.[31]

There appears to be an increased susceptibility to both bacterial and viral respiratory infections and interference with the ability of the lungs to remove inhaled deposited particles after exposure to NO_2.[25, 28] In addition, the nitrogen oxides participate in several reactions that interfere with other biologic systems. In addition to direct alveolar epithelial injury from NO_2 combined with water to form acid, NO_2 oxidizes lecithin in membranes and pulmonary surfactant, forming stable free radicals. It is involved in direct oxidation of unsaturated fatty acids and *N*-nitrosation to nitrosamines, which play a significant role in gastrointestinal cancers. There may also be a poisoning of the cytochrome electron transfer reaction.[21]

Clinical Signs and Symptoms

Clinical presentation is generally divided into three clinical stages, acute, delayed, and subacute.[21]

Acute Phase. In this group of patients mucosal irritation results in immediate weakness and choking followed by dyspnea and bronchospasm, cough, nausea, vomiting, headache, conjunctivitis, vertigo, tachycardia, and chest pain (which may be pleuritic). There may also be eye irritation and vertigo. Skin burns from the mixture of fumes with sweat producing nitric acid have been reported. Many effects terminate at this point if there has been only a mild, brief exposure. Symptoms may persist for 1 to 2 weeks, although clinically obvious pulmonary pathology does not occur, and these patients usually recover completely. A leukocytosis and fever may be present at this stage.[24, 25, 37, 42, 43] Following the acute phase, there is a symptom-free interval of 3 to 36 hours (may be as long as 10 days).

Delayed Phase. This phase is characterized by noncardiogenic pulmonary edema, which may occur even with only minimal initial symptoms. In one study, this phase occurred in 5 of 23 patients initially presenting with acute symptoms.[24] Symptoms commonly include tachypnea, dyspnea, tachycardia, fever, cyanosis, rales, both restrictive and obstructive ventilatory defects with decreased diffusion capacity, and hypoxia. X-ray findings generally start with perihilar infiltrates and progress to fulminant pulmonary edema. Fibrinous bronchiectasis may be found on biopsy. In one study of 34 patients,[21] 40 per cent of the patients who developed pulmonary edema died.[21, 24–26, 30, 32] Those that survived either developed long-term complications, experienced a subacute phase, or recovered completely.

A further asymptomatic phase may then occur during which the chest x-ray clears, although the patient may still have a mild cough, dyspnea, and malaise.[30] This phase lasts anywhere from 2 to 6 weeks.

Subacute Phase. This phase usually occurs 2 to 4 weeks later. The patient again becomes acutely ill with cough, dyspnea, chest tightness, hypoxia, confusion, hypotension, fever and chills, rales, and wheezing. The chest x-ray at this point may again resemble that characteristic of pulmonary edema, or it may show multiple discrete nodules (miliary pattern). Pulmonary function testing will show both obstructive and restrictive defects. The pathologic picture may be that of a bronchitis and bronchiolitis with persistent cough or that of bronchiolitis obliterans. Bronchiolitis obliterans will appear on biopsy as a proliferation of granulation tissue with eosinophils and plasma cells in the lumen of the bronchioles and alveolae, and fibrosis with preservation of the background architecture of the lung. There may be progressive deterioration with developing pneumonia. This stage may prove fatal.[21, 30, 33, 37]

The clinical presentation and progression of disease will depend on the concentration and duration of exposure, and perhaps on the patient's predisposition to lung disease. Hypotension (direct effects of nitrates on blood vessels), metabolic acidosis (nitrous acid and lactic acidosis), and methemoglobinemia are frequently reported.[34, 35]

Diagnosis is based on the history of exposure to inhaled organic dust such as entering a freshly filled silo in the summer or early fall, or an industrial exposure. The latency period of several hours followed by the symptoms of cough, fever and chills, chest pain, dyspnea, headache, myalgias, and nausea and vomiting is very suggestive of this exposure. Differential diagnosis should include allergic lung disease due to molds (farmer's lung due to a hypersensitivity reaction), pneumonia, miliary tuberculosis, viral influenza, carbon monoxide, myocardial infarction, or pulmonary edema following exposure to a fire.[21, 36]

Treatment

Treatment will depend on the patient's phase of clinical illness and the symptomatic presentation. High-flow oxygen and intubation with positive pressure ventilation as needed are considered the mainstays of treatment.[21, 26, 29, 47] Aminophylline and inhaled bronchodilators are recommended for symptomatic bronchoconstriction. Albumin to raise the plasma oncotic pressure has been suggested, but its use is not well documented. Diuretics, digitalis, and volume reduction are not considered helpful. Hyperbaric oxygen is contraindicated.[21]

Steroids are felt to be beneficial both in prevention of the delayed and subacute phases and in treatment. High-dose corticosteroids should be continued for 8 weeks and tapered gradually to prevent relapses. Steroids may assist in suppressing the diffuse alveolar damage that is induced by toxic inhalation. Many authors report dramatic improvement in symptoms following use of steroids and the recurrence of symptoms when the steroids are abruptly stopped; the symptoms then respond to reinstitution of the steroids.[21, 24, 29, 31, 33, 37, 44] Steroids are the treatment of choice for the phase of bronchiolitis obliterans.

Correction of acid-base abnormalities, standard therapy for methemoglobinemia, and, because these patients are prone to infection, frequent sputum cultures and antibiotics when appropriate are indicated.

In-hospital observation for 6 hours is recommended for all persons with potential exposure. If the patient is asymptomatic at that time and has relatively rapid access to medical care, he or she may be discharged for close follow-up. Repeat examinations for 6 weeks are recommended.

Long-Term Implications

In animals, chronic exposure has caused a pattern of emphysema, decreased body weight, and increased incidence of spontaneous tumors. The development of emphysema with chronic exposure occurs in coal miners. Studies have also shown an increased incidence of bronchitis in children who have had chronic low-dose exposure.[24, 25, 28, 50, 51]

Six of twenty-four cases from a missile silo accident had neurologic sequelae that have remained unexplained. In one study of 23 cases, of the five cases that progressed beyond the acute phase, all had some persistent pulmonary dysfunction on follow-up of several years.[24, 43] The ability to predict who will have long-term complications from a single acute exposure is poor, and meaningful numbers from studies are essentially nonexistent. Generally, a patient who does not progress beyond the acute phase will not have subsequent problems, and patients who have pulmonary edema or progress to bronchiolitis obliterans seem to have a high chance of developing long-term complications.

LIQUID NITROGEN

Nitrogen gas comprises 78 per cent of the atmospheric air. It is a colorless, nonflammable elemental compound that is odorless and is liquid between −210°C and −195°C. Liquid nitrogen is used in industry as a refrigerant and storage medium for nitrogen gas. It is utilized in cryogenic therapy in numerous medical specialties.[52]

Pathophysiology

Liquid nitrogen has two toxic mechanisms. In the gaseous phase, it can act as an asphyxiant by displacing ambient atmospheric oxygen. In the liquid or supercool gaseous phases, it acts as a rapid freezing agent on exposed tissues.

Clinical Signs and Symptoms

Inert gaseous nitrogen in sufficient quantities will displace ambient oxygen, causing asphyxia. Oxygen concentrations of 15 to 16 per cent will produce symptoms.[53] Initially, the respiratory rate and pulse will increase, and psychomotor coordination will decrease. At an oxygen concentration of 10 to 12 per cent, poor judgment, giddiness, Cheyne-Stokes respiration, and cyanosis occur; unconsciousness occurs at an oxygen concentration of 8 to 10 per cent;[53, 54] and rapid onset of convulsions, coma, and death occurs at levels of 6 per cent oxygen or less.[54]

Liquid or supercooled pressurized gaseous nitrogen produces rapid freezing of exposed tissues. Mild dermal exposure causes pain on freezing and thawing[55] with localized erythema.[56] Transient urticarial lesions occur secondary to mast cell degranulation.[57] Bullae separating the dermal-epidermal layer generally result, with later sloughing and healing without scarring. Injury to the deeper tissues from liquid nitrogen is typical of a classic frostbite injury. The dermis can be anesthetic and pale. Bullae will not form. Red cell thrombi occlude the local vascular supply with subsequent necrosis and gangrene.[57] Rockswold[52] described the intraoral lesions caused by an accidental inhalation of liquid nitrogen. Frank charring, inflammation, and edema of the lips were present. The patient had inspiratory stridor secondary to a pale, edematous, swollen epiglottis. Bullae of the palate subsequently developed and later sloughed, leaving an ulcerated base.

Local complications from therapeutic exposure to liquid nitrogen have included digital and ulnar nerve neuropathies,[58, 59] onchodystrophy,[60] and pyogenic granuloma.[61, 62] Patients have also suffered syncope[63] and cardiac arrest[64] during liquid nitrogen application, probably due to vasomotor reactions from the stress and pain of the procedure.[63]

Treatment

Asphyxiated patients should be removed from the offending environment and given 100 per cent oxygen supplementation. Cardiac monitoring and supportive care for CNS complications are indicated.

For external dermal exposure, rapid rewarming in a water bath at 40 to 42°C is indicated until vascular flush has returned. Standard frostbite management including elevation of the limb, protective dressings, and late surgical debridement of necrotic tissue should be initiated. Whether or not pharmacologic agents should be used to enhance circulation is an unresolved issue.

For intraoral injuries, acute evaluation for impending or actual upper airway obstruction is mandatory. Aggressive airway management including tracheostomy may be necessary. Use of parenteral steroids is felt to be of benefit.[52]

Long-Term Implications

There is nothing uniquely peculiar about the long-term effects of liquid nitrogen. Sequelae of tissue injury may be seen: tissue loss through gangrene, scarring, neuropathy, or changes in pigmentation. The chronic stigmata of CNS hypoxia may occur. As the predominant component of the atmosphere, nitrogen has no adverse environmental implications.

DIMETHYLNITROSAMINE

Dimethylnitrosamine (DMN, *N*-nitrosodimethylamine, DMNA, NDMA, *N*-methyl-*N*-nitrosomethanamine) is a yellow liquid that is soluble in water, ether, or alcohol. It is of low viscosity and has a boiling point of 152°C. It has no appreciable odor and is incompatible with strong oxidizing agents.

DMN is used commonly as an industrial solvent in the production of dimethylhydrazine. It is used in the production of hypergolic rocket fuels and thiocarbonyl fluoride polymers and as a soluble cutting oil. Other potential sources of exposure include its use as a gasoline additive, lubricant additive, plasticizer for acrylonitrile polymers, and component in high-energy battery systems with active metal anode-electrolyte systems. DMN has also been found in multiple cosmetic products, hand and body lotions, and shampoos. Various nitrosamines have also been patented for use in pesticides and nematocides. High levels of DMN have been found in soil, postulated to be from the use of triazine herbicide, which can react with ubiquitously used nitrogenous fertilizers.[65]

DMN is currently classified as a potential occupational carcinogen by The National Institute for Occupational Safety and Health (NIOSH) and the American Conference of Governmental Industrial Hygienists (ACGIH) and has no acceptable PEL (permissible exposure limit).

Pathophysiology

DMN was discovered to be a powerful carcinogen almost 30 years ago when investigators found hepatotoxicity, jaundice, and liver damage in workmen exposed to this chemical. Since that time, research has shown that DMN is one of the most powerful carcinogenic materials recognized, its pathologic effects stemming from the alkylation of DNA. DMN's pathologic effects appear to be both dose and time related. In rodents, a single large dose of DMN will result in renal cancer, whereas exposure to low doses over long periods of time causes hepatic cancer.[66, 67, 68, 69]

It is interesting that this dose- and time-related organotropism has been used in cancer chemotherapy with the drug streptozotocin, an *N*-methylnitrosamine. This agent is currently being used to treat metastatic insulin-secreting tumors of the pancreas because of its high affinity and cytotoxicity to this specific cell type located in the human pancreas.[70]

Pre-employment screening of workers who may be exposed to DMN should include attention to a family history of cancer and liver disease, smoking, the potential for pregnancy during periods of exposure, steroid use, and immunocompetence.

Clinical Signs and Symptoms

Local direct exposure to DMN produces minimal direct irritation to the skin and mucous membranes. Therefore, the warning signs of potential exposure by contact are poor. In persons with acute poisoning due to systemic exposure, headaches, a feeling of generalized malaise, fever, and weakness often occur. Gastrointestinal effects are frequent and include abdominal cramping and nausea. Vomiting and diarrhea occur within hours of absorption. Liver enlargement and jaundice may follow.[71, 72]

Treatment

The worker should be removed from the area of exposure. The eyes should be irrigated with water if there has been a potential exposure of the conjunctival membranes. Contaminated parts of the body are washed with soap and water. It is necessary to evaluate liver size and function by monitoring serum albumin, prothrombin time, conjugated bilirubin, or other indices of hepatic function.

It is also necessary to monitor changes in the patient's chest x-ray and renal function parameters. The patient should be followed for other possible malignant changes as dictated by the family history or other factors, i.e., breast cancer screening in female patients or sputum cytology in an employee who smokes or has a family history of lung cancer.

Chronic Poisoning or Long-Term Implications

Clinical manifestations of chronic exposure to DMN may include severe liver damage, with acute centrilobular necrosis, jaundice, and ascites. Inhalation and ingestion of DMN have produced malignant tumors in rodents involving the liver, kidney, and lung. Such tumors have not been conclusively reported in humans, but in light of the potent carcinogenicity found in experimental animals, every precaution to avoid chronic exposure should be taken. Evaluation of a patient with a history of chronic exposure should make optimum use of cancer screening tools such as sputum cytology, chest x-ray, liver function tests, pelvic examination, and breast cancer screening in appropriate individuals as dictated by exposure and family history.[73, 74, 75]

DIETHYLAMINE AND TRIETHYLAMINE

Diethylamine (diethamine, *N*-ethylethanamine) and triethylamine (*N,N*-diethylethanamine) are alkaline colorless liquids with a strongly ammoniac or fishy odor. This odor often gives warning of their presence because the odor threshold is as low as 0.14 ppm, and the permissible exposure limit (PEL) is more than 100 times greater. Diethylamine has a boiling point of 56°C; that of triethylamine is 90°C. These compounds are incompatible with strong oxidizers and acids. Both compounds are unstable when exposed to heat, and hazardous decomposition products such as carbon monoxide and oxides of nitrogen may be released in a fire involving these compounds. Extinguishants should be dry chemicals, alcohol foam, or carbon dioxide.

The sources of exposure are varied. Diethylamine is often used in the petroleum and rubber industries. It is also utilized in the manufacturing of pharmaceutical products, resins, and dyes. Triethylamine is used as an antilivering agent for urea and melamine-based enamels and as a corrosion inhibitor in paint remover formulations based on methylene chloride. It is used as a rubber accelerator and propellant.

Diethylamine and triethylamine have permissible exposure limits of 25 ppm by the Occupational Safety and Health Administration (OSHA) and 10 ppm by the ACGIH. The immediately dangerous to life or health (IDLH) levels are set at 2000 ppm and 1000 ppm, respectively.[76–78]

Clinical Signs and Symptoms

In the setting of an acute local exposure, both of these compounds are direct irritants to the mucous membranes and the eyes. Acute dermatitis with dermal burns as well as a nonspecific irritation can result from exposure. As with all alkaline products, these compounds can significantly damage the eyes by direct contact. Exposure may cause keratitis or conjunctivitis with severe photophobia, corneal edema, coagulation necrosis of tissues, and severe eye damage.[79]

Systemic symptoms involve the respiratory tract with cough, dyspnea, chest pain, and pulmonary edema. Pulmonary edema may be delayed up to 72 hours after the initial exposure, and patients who have had significant tracheobronchial exposure should be monitored closely. Exposure to a fire involving these chemicals may mean exposure to the breakdown products of carbon monoxide and oxides of nitrogen. Laboratory evaluation and treatment should be performed accordingly.

Treatment

The worker should be removed from the scene of the exposure, and affected clothing should be removed promply. Soap and water should be used to wash the contaminated areas of the body.

Copious irrigation with normal saline or water should be begun as soon as possible following ocular exposure. Apply a local anesthetic and irrigate continuously, preferably with a contact lens irrigation set-up, for at least 20 minutes. pH measurements should be taken to ensure satisfactory irrigation. If the pH of the eye is still alkaline, continued irrigation must be performed to terminate coagulation necrosis. A cycloplegic may be used for the pain associated with ciliary spasm. An antibiotic in either drop or ointment form should be used along with an eye patch. Ophthalmologic referral for all alkaline injuries to the eye is standard. Collagenase inhibitors and steroids should be used only following ophthalmology referral.

Ingestion of either of these agents should be treated initially with milk to counteract the alkaline pH damage to the stomach and esophageal mucosa. Lavage and induced emesis are not recommended. Endoscopy may be needed.

Oxygen should be given for all patients with inhalation exposure, and chest x-rays and arterial blood gas measurements are recommended for symptomatic patients. A high index of suspicion for delayed onset of pulmonary edema is warranted.[80]

Long-Term Implications

The condition of workers subjected to chronic exposure should be followed with the use of liver function profile tests, renal function tests, blood counts, electrocardiography and chest x-rays.

References

1. Occupational Health Services: Material Safety Data Sheet (MSDS). Secaucus, NJ, Occupational Health Services; 1985.
2. Flury KE, Dines DE, et al: Airway obstruction due to inhalation of ammonia. Mayo Clinic Proc *58*:389–393, 1983.
3. Arwood R, Hammond J, Ward GG: Ammonia inhalation. J Trauma *25*:444–447, 1985.
4. Montague TJ, Macneil AR: Mass ammonia inhalation. Chest *77*:496–498, 1980.
5. Decker WJ: Ammonia. Micromedex *52*, 1987.
6. Dalton ML, Bricker DL: Anhydrous ammonia burns of the respiratory tract. Texas Med *74*:51–54, 1978.
7. Klein J, Olsen KR, McKinney HE: Caustic injury from household ammonia. Am J Emerg Med *3*:320, 1985.
8. Hockberter RS: Toxic gas inhalation. Digest Emerg Med Care *3(1)*:1–8, 1983.
9. Levy DM, et al: Ammonia burns of the face and respiratory tract. JAMA *190(10)*:95–98, 1964.
10. Proctor NH, Hughes JP: Chemical Hazards of the Workplace. Philadelphia, J. B. Lippincott, 1978.
11. Proctor NH, Hughes JP: Exposure to ammonia during removal of paint from artificial turf—Ohio. Morbid Mortal Wkly Rep *33*(40):567–568, 1984.

12. Kass J, et al: Bronchiectasis following ammonia burns of the respiratory tract: A review of two cases. Chest *62*(3):282–285, 1972.
13. Murphy DMP, et al: Severe airway disease due to inhalation of fumes from cleaning agents. Chest *69*:372–376, 1976.
14. Sternbach GL: Noncardiogenic pulmonary edema. TEM *2*:35–44, 1980.
15. Birken GS, Fabri PJ, Carey LC: Acute ammonia intoxication complicating multiple trauma. J Trauma *21*:820–822, 1981.
16. Sobonya R: Fatal anhydrous ammonia inhalation. Hum Pathol *8(3)*:293–299, 1977.
17. Plunkett ER (ed): Handbook of Industrial Toxicology. New York, Chemical Publishing Co, 1987.
18. Chu CS: New concepts of pulmonary burn injury. J Trauma *21*:958–961, 1981.
19. Welch GW, Lull RJ, Petroff PA, et al: The use of steroids in inhalation injury. Surg Gynecol Obstet *145*:539–544, 1977.
20. Vale JA, Meredith TJ: Ammonia, nitrogen oxide, silo-filler's disease and chlorine. In Haddad LM, Winchester JF (eds): Clinical Management of Poisoning and Drug Overdose. Philadelphia, W. B. Saunders, 1983.
21. Guidotti TL: The higher oxides of nitrogen: Inhalation toxicology. Environ Res *15*:443–472, 1978.
22. Grayson RR: Silage gas poisoning: Nitrogen dioxide pneumonia, a new disease in agricultural workers. Ann Intern Med *45*:393–396, 1956.
23. Hayhurst ER, Scott E: Four cases of sudden death in a silo. JAMA *63*:1570, 1914.
24. Horvath EP, doPico GA, Barbee RA, Dickie HA: Nitrogen dioxide-induced pulmonary disease. J Occup Med *20(2)*:103–110, 1978.
25. Tse RL, Bockman AA: Nitrogen dioxide toxicity—Report of four cases in firemen. JAMA *212(8)*:1341–1344, 1970.
26. Olson KR, Insley, BM: Nitrogen oxides. Micromedex 53, 1987.
27. Morrow PE: Toxicology data on NO_x: An overview. J Toxicol Environ Health *13(2–3)*:205–227, 1984.
28. Morrow PE: Oxides of nitrogen and health. Lancet *1*:81–82, 1981.
29. Fleetham JA, Munt PW, Tunnicliffe BW: Silo-fillers' disease. Can Med Assoc J *119*:482–484, 1978.
30. Haggerty MA, Soto-Green M, Reichan LB: Caring for victims of toxic gas inhalation. J Crit Illness *2(7)*:77–87, 1987.
31. Haggerty MA, Soto-Green M, Reichan LB: Silo-filler's disease in rural New York. Morbid Mortal Wkly Rep *31(28)*:389–391, 1982.
32. Sriskandan K, Pettingale KW: "Numismatist's pneumonitis": A case of acute nitrogen dioxide poisoning. Postgrad Med J *61*:819–821, 1985.
33. Jonas DO: Case for diagnosis. Mil Med *149*:481–485, 1984.
34. Lowery T, Schuman LM: Silo-filler's disease—a syndrome caused by nitrogen dioxide. JAMA *162*:153–160, 1956.
35. Delaney LT, Schmidt HW, Stroebel CF: Silo-filler's disease. Proc Mayo Clinic *31*:189–200, 1956.
36. Cockcroft DW, Dosman JA: Respiratory health risks in farmers. Ann Intern Med *95*:380–382, 1981.
37. Maurer WJ: Silo-filler's disease: A historical perspective and report of a case. Wisc Med J *84*:13–16, 1985.
38. Moskowitz RL, Lyons HA, Cottle HR: Silo-filler's disease. Clinical, physiological and pathologic study of a patient. Am J Med *36*:457–462, 1964.
39. Scott EG, Hunt WB: Silo-filler's disease. Chest *63*:701–702, 1973.
40. Fleming GM, Chester EH, Montenegro HD: Dysfunction of small airways following pulmonary injury due to nitrogen dioxide. Chest *75*:720, 1979.
41. Bauer MA, et al: Inhalation of 0.30 ppm nitrogen dioxide potentiates exercise-induced bronchospasm in asthmatics. Am Rev Resp Dis *134*:1203–1208, 1986.
42. Ramirez RJ, Dowell AC: Silo-filler's disease. Nitrogen dioxide-induced lung injury. Long-term follow-up and review of the literature. Ann Intern Med *74*:569–576, 1971.
43. Yockey CC, Eden BM, Byrd RB: The McConnell missile accident. Clinical spectrum of nitrogen dioxide exposure. JAMA *244*:1221–1223, 1980.
44. Brey RL, Seidenfeld JJ: Lung toxicity resulting from exposure to nitrogen dioxide: A possible occurrence due to Titan missile accidents. Ariz Med *38(5)*:344–348, 1981.
45. Fleetham JA, Tunnicliffe BW, Munt PW: Methemoglobinemia and the oxides of nitrogen (letter). N Engl J Med *298*:1150, 1978.
46. Pratt DS, May JJ: Feed-associated respiratory illness in farmers. Arch Environ Health *39(1)*:43–48, 1984.
47. Welch HW, Lull RJ, Petroff PA: The use of steroids in inhalation injury. Surg Gynecol Obstet *145*:539–544, 1977.
48. Jones GR, Proudfoot AT, Hall JI: Pulmonary effects of acute exposure to nitrous fumes. Thorax *28*:61–65, 1973.
49. Jakab GJ: Modulation of pulmonary defense mechanisms by acute exposures to nitrogen dioxide. Environ Res *42*:215–226, 1987.
50. Fishbein L: Atmospheric mutagens I: Sulfur oxide and nitrogen oxides. Mutation Res *32*:309–330, 1976.
51. Kennedy MCS: Nitrous fume poisoning in coal-miners. Rev Instit Hyg Mines *29(1)*:167–174, 1974.
52. Rockswold G: Inhalation of liquid nitrogen vapor. Ann Emerg Med *11*:553–555, 1982.
53. Kizer KW: Toxic inhalation. Emerg Med Clin North Am *2*:649–666, 1984.
54. Freon compounds and safety. Freon Products Information S-16. Wilminton, DE, E. I. Dupont DeNemours & Co., Freon Products Division, 1969, p 6.
55. Moschella SL, Heuley HJ: Dermatology. Philadelphia, W. B. Saunders, 1985, pp 1996–2000.
56. Domonkos AN: Andrew's Diseases of Skin: Clinical Dermatology. Philadelphia, W. B. Saunders, 1971, pp 966–967.
57. Fitzpatrick TB, Eisen AZ, Wolff K, Freedburg IM, Austen KF: Dermatology in General Medicine. New York, McGraw Hill Book Co., 1979, pp 925–927.
58. Nix E: Liquid-nitrogen neuropathy. Arch Dermatol *92*:185–187, 1965.
59. Finelli PF: Ulnar neuropathy after liquid nitrogen therapy. Arch Dermatol *111*:1340–1342, 1975.
60. Caravati CM Jr, Wood BT, Richardson DR: Onychodystrophies secondary to liquid nitrogen cryotherapy. Arch Dermatol *100*:441–442, 1969.
61. Greer KE, Bishop GF: Pyogenic granuloma as a complication of cryosurgery. Arch Dermatol *111*:1536–1537, 1975.
62. McKeekin TO, Moschella SL: Iatrogenic complications of dermatologic therapy. Primum non nocere. Med Clin North Am *63(2)*:442, 1979.
63. Epstein AM: Syncope associated with liquid nitrogen therapy. Arch Dermatol *100*:847, 1977.

64. Goldstein N: Cardiac arrest following application of liquid nitrogen. J Dermatol Surg Oncol *5*:602, 1979.
65. Cassarett and Doull: *N*-Nitrosodimethylamine. *In* The Basic Science of Poisons. New York, Macmillan, 1986, pp 668–670.
66. Magee P (ed): Nitrosamines and human cancer. Banbury Report 12. Cold Spring Harbor, NY, Cold Spring Harbor Laboratory, 1982.
67. O'Neill IK, Von Borstel RC, Miller CT, et al: *N*-Nitroso Compounds: Occurrence, Biological Effects and Relevance to Human Cancer. IARC Sci Publ 57. Lyon, International Agency for Research on Cancer, 1984.
68. Searle CE (ed): Chemical Carcinogens, 2nd ed. ACS Monograph 173. Washington DC, American Chemical Society, 1984.
69. Shimkin MB: Some Classics of Experimental Oncology. NIH Publ No. 80-2150. Washington DC, U.S. Government Printing Office, 1980.
70. American Medical Association, Department of Drugs: AMA Drug Evaluations, 5th ed. Chicago, American Medical Association, 1983.
71. U.S. Environmental Protection Agency: Dimethylnitrosamine: Health and Environmental Effects, No. 86. Washington DC, Office of Solid Waste, 1980.
72. Sax NI (ed): Dangerous Properties of Industrial Materials, No. 6 (*N*-Nitrosodimethylamine). New York, Van Nostrand Reinhold, 1982, pp 65–69.
73. National Institute for Occupational Safety and Health, U.S. Department of Health Education and Welfare: NIOSH Pocket Guide to Chemical Hazards. Washington DC, Department of Health and Human Services (NIOSH), 1985, pp 85–114.
74. NASA Occupational Health Office: OSHA Medical Surveillance Requirements and NIOSH Recommendations: For Employees Exposed to Toxic Substances and Other Work Hazards. Washington, DC, Bio Technology Inc., 1980.
75. National Institute for Occupational Safety and Health, U.S. Department of Health and Human Services: NIOSH recommendations for occupational safety and health standards. Morbid Mortal Weekly Rep Suppl *35*:1s, 1986.
76. National Institute for Occupational Safety and Health, U.S. Department of Health and Human Services and U.S. Department of Labor: Occupational Health Guidelines for Chemical Hazards. Washington DC, Department of Health and Human Services (NIOSH), 1981, pp 81–123.
77. American Conference of Governmental Industrial Hygienists: Diethylamine: Documentation of the Threshold Limit Values for Substances in the Workroom Air, 3rd ed. Cincinnati, ACGIH, 1974.
78. American Conference of Governmental Industrial Hygienists: Triethylamine: Documentation of the Threshold Limit Values for Substances in the Workroom Air, 3rd ed. Cincinnati, ACGIH, 1974.
79. Akesson B, et al: Visual disturbances after experimental human exposure to triethylamine. Br J Indus Med *42*:848, 1985.
80. National Institute for Occupational Safety and Health, U.S. Department of Health, Education and Welfare: NIOSH Pocket Guide to Chemical Hazards. Washington DC, Department of Health and Human Services (NIOSH), 1985, pp 85–114.

CHAPTER 88

FREON AND OTHER INHALANTS

James M. Dougherty, M.D., FACEP
Richard E. Gradisek, M.D., FACEP
Thomas J. Hetrick, M.D., FACEP

FREONS

Fluorocarbons are organic compounds containing atoms of fluorine. In addition, certain fluorocarbons contain atoms of chlorine or bromine. Collectively, a group of nonflammable, nonexplosive fluorocarbons are frequently identified by the trademarked name Freons (E.I. Dupont De Nemours & Co., Inc.). Freon compounds have a varied range of boiling points and exist as liquids and gases at room temperature.

Freons, initially introduced for use in the 1930s, now have widespread applications in refrigeration systems and fire extinguishers, and as propellants in millions of aerosol products. Freon 12 (dichlorodifluoromethane), Freon 11 (trichloromonofluoromethane), and Freon 114 (dichlorotetrafluoroethane) are the most commonly used aerosol propellants.[1] Freon 12, Freon 113 (trichlorotrifluoroethane), and Freon 22 (chlorodifluoromethane) are commonly used in refrigeration systems.

Freons are toxic to humans by several mechanisms. Inhaled fluorocarbons sensitize the myocardium to catecholamines, frequently resulting in lethal ventricular arrhythmias. Because they are gases heavier than air, fluorocarbons can displace atmospheric oxygen, thus resulting in asphyxiation. These compounds also have a central nervous system (CNS) anesthetic effect analogous to a structurally similar general anesthetic, halothane. Pressurized refrigerant or liquid fluorocarbons with a low boiling point have a cryogenic effect on exposed tissues, causing frostbite, laryngeal or pulmonary edema, and gastrointestinal perforation.[2] Certain fluorocarbons degrade at high temperatures into toxic products of chlorine, hydrofluoric acid, or phosgene gases.

Pathophysiology

Fluorocarbons were initially believed to be compounds low in toxicity. In the late 1960s there were early reports of deaths caused by intentional inhalation abuse of various aerosols.[3] Victims frequently discharged the aerosol contents into a plastic bag and then inhaled the gaseous contents. Suffocation was initially considered to be the cause of death. In 1970, Bass[4] reviewed 110 cases of "sudden sniffing death" without finding evidence of suffocation. The majority of those deaths (59) involved fluorocarbon propellants. He noted that in several cases sudden death followed a burst of emotional stress or exercise. No significant findings were noted at autopsy. Taylor and Harris[5] found a relationship in mice between fluorocarbon inhalation, asphyxia, and cardiac dysrhythmias. Flowers and Horan[6, 7] found that fluorocarbon inhalation alone caused dysrhythmias in dogs, in which normal blood gas parameters were maintained. The dysrhythmic pattern was sinoatrial slowing with junctional or ventricular escape rhythms and finally ventricular fibrillation or asystole. Reinhardt et al[8] also found that fluorocarbon inhalation in dogs resulted in dysrhythmias that were enhanced by anoxia, injected epinephrine, and noise stress. He found that fatal responses resulted from inhaled concentrations of 0.35 to 0.61 per cent of Freon 11 and of 5 per cent of Freon 12 and 114. These concentrations are well above the current human threshold limit value (TLV) for these fluorocarbons of 1000 ppm (0.1 per cent).[9]

The above authors and others[1, 10] concluded that fluorocarbon inhalation caused myocardial sensitization to catecholamines. The dysrhythmia potential of circulating adrenergics, which are increased with the victim's stress, is greatly enhanced. Harris[1] found that this effect lasted 15 minutes in mice and 1.5 to 3 minutes in dogs and monkeys. It is controversial whether bronchodilator aerosols utilizing fluorocarbon propellants cause cardiac sensitization. They may produce concentrations of 1000 ppm only at excessive doses of 12 to 24 inhalations in 2 minutes.[11]

The mechanisms of the cardiac effects of fluorocarbons are not clearly delineated. Abolition of ventricular arrhythmias by propranolol pretreatment suggested that they may have an effect on beta-adrenergic receptor pathways.[1] Thyrum[12] suggested that alteration of calcium binding on cell membranes may be a possible mechanism. Lessard et al[13] concluded that Freon 12 mainly decreased membrane ionic permeability in rats and found no significant inhibition of cellular metabolism.

Fluorocarbons in high concentrations can displace atmospheric oxygen and result in victim asphyxia. Morita et al[14] attributed the deaths of four sailors exposed to a fluorocarbon 22 refrigerant leak to asphyxia at autopsy. The deceased sailors were asleep in the mid or lower level bunks. Sailors from high bunks were able to escape and survive. The CNS signs of hypoxia may also be additive to the anesthetic CNS effects of fluorocarbons. Early giddiness, psychomotor incoordination, slurred speech, and later decreasing consciousness are common to both. CNS effects of Freon 113 in man were found at a concentration of 2,500 ppm (0.25 per cent).[15] Although above the TLV of 1000 ppm, this concentration is below the 5000 ppm (0.5 per cent) level associated with cardiac sensitization in animals. Exposed victims should experience CNS alterations before cardiac sensitization.[16] These alterations, however, may blunt or eradicate a victim's withdrawal response from fluorocarbon exposure.

Clinical Signs and Symptoms

Inhalation of Freon compounds at moderate concentrations initially produces CNS anesthetic effects of intoxication and loss of psychomotor coordination. In humans, this effect occurred at levels of 2,500 ppm for Freon 113[15] and 10,000 ppm for Freon 12.[17] Higher concentrations produce marked incoordination, slurring of speech, apprehension, and finally decreasing levels of consciousness.[17] Attendant hypoxia at high concentrations may also produce tremors, convulsions, and cerebral edema.

Cardiac sensitization occurs at higher concentrations than initial CNS intoxication. Onset of lethal cardiac arrhythmias is frequently preceded by a burst of emotional or physical exertion followed by collapse.[4] Sinoatrial bradycardia with junctional escape rhythm and ventricular fibrillation or asystole are frequently the terminal rhythms.[6, 7]

Exposure to low-boiling-point Freons or release of pressurized Freons has a cryogenic effect on the soft tissues. The classic findings of frostbite occur with erythema, pain, bullae, and, in severe cases, tissue necrosis. Although these signs usually occur on the extremities, Haj et al[2] reported a case of gastric perforation that occurred one-half hour after accidental ingestion of refrigerated Freon 11; transient jaundice and liver enzyme elevation postoperatively was reported in this patient. Serious cardiac complications are not seen with ingested fluorocarbons because their absorption by this route is 35 to 48 times lower than after inhalation.[11] A patient who ingested 1 liter of Freon 113 experienced transient cyanosis and suffered rectal irritation and diarrhea only.[16]

Higher-boiling-point Freons can cause dermal dryness or irritation owing to their ability to dissolve or necrose soft tissue fat. Ocular contact results in transient irritation.

Mild respiratory tract irritation and bronchoconstriction may occur with inhaled gaseous Freons.[18] Aspiration of liquid Freons may cause pulmonary edema or pneumonia. Certain Freons, when exposed to high temperatures, decompose into phosgene, chlorine, and hydrofluoronic acid, which produce significant respiratory tract injury and pulmonary edema.

Specific Treatment

Victims of Freon inhalation require management for hypoxic, CNS anesthetic, and cardiac symptoms. Patients must be removed from the exposure environment, and high-flow supplemental oxygen should be utilized. The respiratory system should be evaluated for injury, aspiration, or pulmonary edema and treated appropriately. CNS findings should be treated supportively. A calm environment with no physical exertion is imperative to avoid increasing endogenous adrenergic levels. Exogenous adrenergic drugs must not be used to avoid inducing sensitized myocardial dysrhythmias.[16, 18] Atropine is ineffective in treating bradyarrhythmias. For ventricular dysrhythmias, diphenylhydantoin and countershock may be effective.[18]

Cryogenic dermal injuries should be treated by water bath rewarming at 40 to 42°C until vasodilatory flush has returned. Elevation of the limb and standard frostbite management with late surgical debridement should be utilized.[18] Ocular exposure requires irrigation and slit-lamp evaluation for injury.

Long-Term Implications

Long-term effects of exposure to Freons are primarily limited to the sequelae of the CNS, cardiac, and dermal injuries described. Chronic low-level inhalation exposure to Freons is generally considered low in toxicity. No evidence of carcinogenicity of Freon 11 or 12 has appeared,[19] and there is inadequate evidence for Freon 22.[20]

Freons have been implicated environmentally in the depletion of the stratospheric ozone layer. This depletion theoretically results in increased levels of ultraviolet B radiation and an increased incidence of skin cancers. Consequently, fluorocarbon propellants in nonessential aerosols were banned in the United States in 1979.[21] Recent convincing evidence of ozone depletion prompted the Dupont Company to announce a phased termination of their chlorofluorocarbon production in March, 1988.

THE ISOCYANATES

Isocyanates (ICs) are widely used in the manufacture of flexible and rigid forms, fibers, coatings, and elastomers. They are currently finding increasing use in the automobile industry because of the need to develop rigid replacement materials that are lighter than steel to produce more energy-efficient vehicles.[22]

The worldwide production of ICs now exceeds 1 billion pounds annually; of this, at least 400 million pounds are of toluene diisocyanate (TDI), the most intensely studied of the isocyanates. Isocyanates are also being increasingly used in the replacement of building insulation following recognition of the cancer-causing potential of asbestos.

It is estimated that in the United States approximately 250,000 persons are exposed occupationally each year to isocyanates.[22] The most notorious of the isocyanates, methyl isocyanate (MIC) was responsible for the Bhopal, India tragedy of December, 1984. This accidental release of methyl isocyanate now ranks as the worst industrial catastrophe in world history.

Chemical Structures and Properties

All isocyanates contain the –N=C=O group, which reacts readily with compounds containing reactive hydrogen ions to form urethanes (Fig. 88–1). The di- and polyisocyanates contain, respectively, two and three or more of these groups. The chemical reactivity of the ICs makes them ideal for polymer formation; hence their widespread use in the manufacture of polyurethane foams, paints, adhesives, fibers, resins, and sealants.[23]

The low-molecular-weight ICs tend to be more readily volatilized into the workplace atmosphere than the higher molecular weight diisocyanates (DICs). Although the vapor pressures of the higher molecular weight DICs are relatively low, they may generate vapor concentrations sufficient to cause respiratory and mucous membrane irritation if they are handled in poorly ventilated areas.[23] Also, the potential for skin irritation is generally higher for the lower molecular weight DICs, and the severity of these irritant responses is reduced with increasing molecular weight.[23]

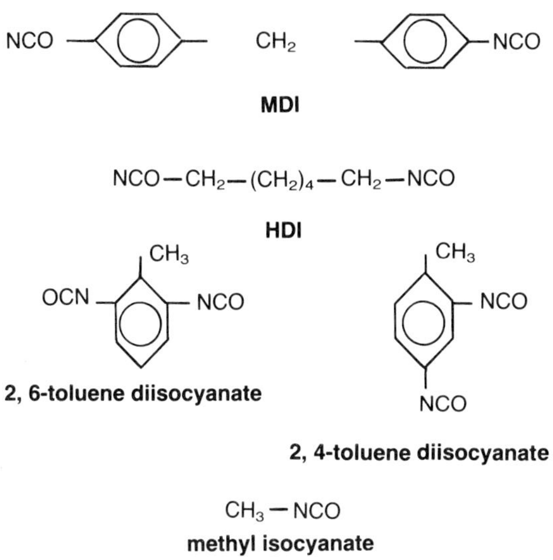

NCO — C6H4 — CH2 — C6H4 — NCO

MDI

$NCO—CH_2—(CH_2)_4—CH_2—NCO$

HDI

2, 6-toluene diisocyanate

2, 4-toluene diisocyanate

$CH_3—NCO$

methyl isocyanate

Figure 88–1. Chemical structures of isocyanates.

Pathophysiology

ICs probably cause nonspecific inhibition of a variety of membrane receptors and enzyme systems, effects that are consistent with the highly reactive properties of these substances.[24]

TDI was found to compete with isoproterenol-induced production of intracellular cyclic-AMP in peripheral blood lymphocytes. This effect appears to be dose dependent. This antagonistic property of TDI differs from classic beta-adrenergic blockade because it also affects prostaglandin E_1 and glucagon receptors. These effects occurred only with relatively high concentrations of TDI.[25]

Two main types of reactions (using TDI as the prototype) have been observed. The first is a *toxic reaction*. This reaction is usually seen at high concentrations (>5 ppm), affects nearly all individuals, and is usually secondary to accidental exposure. The pulmonary, ocular, and dermatologic systems are usually affected, although the symptomatology is usually reversible, especially if treatment is started early.[22, 26]

The second reaction, *occupationally induced asthma*, is of far greater importance clinically. Approximately 5 per cent of those exposed to TDI will develop asthma. Sensitization occurs within the first 6 months of exposure, and once a worker has been "sensitized," he will react to as little as 0.005 ppm during a 15-minute exposure. Symptoms include dyspnea, chest tightness, wheezing, headaches, and vomiting.[22]

There is still a great amount of confusion about the nature of the mechanism of TDI sensitivity. At present, no definitive diagnostic test is available to determine who will develop sensitivity. Another important problem that needs to be addressed involves the mechanism of cross reactivity between different isocyanate compounds.[22, 28]

Clinical Signs and Symptoms

Exposure to ICs can cause skin and mucous membrane irritation, nausea, vomiting, and abdominal pain. In high concentrations, ICs have a primary irritant effect on the respiratory tract. In one study, all volunteers exposed to 0.5 ppm of TDI experienced irritation of the eyes, nose, and throat.[28]

Once sensitization has occurred at the workplace and asthma has developed in workers exposed to TDI, asthma may be prolonged or even permanent, even when the workers are removed from isocyanate exposure.[29] Moller and coworkers reported that 7 of 12 patients with TDI asthma had persistent asthma even though they had been removed from exposure for a mean period of 1.9 years. These patients retained their TDI "sensitivity," as shown by bronchial challenge tests.[30]

The most infamous of the isocyanates, methyl isocyanate, was responsible for the estimated 6000 to 20,000 deaths, 15,000 injuries, and toxic chemical exposure to between 100,000 and 200,000 people in Bhopal, India.[31–33] It is hypothesized that a substantial amount of water was introduced into a storage tank containing 45 tons of the chemical together with a higher than normal amount of chloroform and an iron catalyst at a high reaction temperature. This caused a rupture of the storage tank and release of a toxic plume of MIC that extended as far as 8 kilometers from the factory and covered an area of 40 square kilometers.[32, 33]

As with all low-molecular-weight ICs, MIC is a strong irritant. Its irritant action is nonspecific and resembles that of other irritant gases such as chlorine, ammonia, and sulfur dioxide. MIC breaks down rapidly in the presence of water (on mucous membranes) to dimethylurea, which is relatively nontoxic. Because of this property, MIC is not hazardous for a prolonged period of time.[32, 34]

Survivors from Bhopal described an acute clinical picture of irritation and redness of the skin and intense irritation of the eyes including photophobia, blepharospasm, profuse eyelid edema, and superficial corneal abrasions. Respiratory findings included rhinitis, pharyngitis, coughing, respiratory distress, bronchoconstriction, dyspnea, choking, pulmonary edema, and adult respiratory distress syndrome (ARDS).[32, 34]

Upper gastrointestinal symptoms were common in the initial stages of exposure. These were probably secondary to swallowed dimethylurea produced by a combination of MIC and water from mucous membranes in the mouth and nose.

Selected autopsies revealed the following bronchiolar pathologic lesions: bronchiolitis, pneumonitis, pulmonary edema, and ARDS.[34] Edema, substantial destruction or necrosis of alveolar walls, desquamative or ulcerative bronchitis, bronchiolitis, and macrophage invasion were all seen. It was felt that the gas did not penetrate deeply into the lungs, thus producing the large amount of bronchial pathology that was seen.[34]

Only a handful of patients had severe visual impairment, and no cases of blindness were identified. The injuries seen were similar to those resulting from a mild chemical burn, and the water content in the tears may have helped break down the gas and modify the damage.[34]

No direct effects of MIC involving the CNS, circulation, liver, or other organs were identified. Possible secondary effects (acute tubular necrosis, miscarriages) were noted but were felt to be secondary to hypoxia.[31, 34]

Specific Treatment

For acute exposure:

1. Remove patient immediately from the source of exposure.
2. Treat symptomatically.
3. Main problems will be *ophthalmic* and *respiratory*. For these, provide the following:
   - High-flow humidified oxygen.
   - Airway support, including suctioning as required.
   - Bronchodilators for bronchospasm.
   - Monitoring for hypoxia.
   - Consideration of arrhythmias secondary to hypoxia.
   - Copious irrigation of the eyes with water.

For chronic exposure:[35]

1. Ideally, transfer the worker from source of exposure.
2. If worker is unable to change jobs:
   - Use protective devices to minimize exposure (dust masks, respirators).
   - Recognize that dust masks are often ineffective due to poor fit.
   - Realize that compliance is low for respirators (hot, heavy).

- Emphasize that the use of respirators is for temporary protection only and should not be regarded as a method of controlling occupational asthma.

Workers should be followed regularly with serial lung function tests and nonspecific bronchial reactivity testing.[25]

Recommendations and Long-Term Implications

In the United States, the exposure standards of the federal Occupational Safety and Health Administration (OSHA) for diisocyanates have been established only for toluene diisocyanate and methylene bisphenyl isocyanate. The current federal OSHA standard for TDI is a ceiling limit of 0.02 parts per million parts of air (ppm), or 0.14 mg per m^3. The OSHA standard for MDI is a ceiling limit of 0.02 ppm (0.2 mg per m^3).[23]

The current National Institute of Occupational Safety and Health (NIOSH) recommended exposure limit (REL) for occupational exposure to hexamethylene diisocyanate (HDI) and TDI is 0.035 mg per m^3 for up to a 10-hour work shift and 40-hour work week, and 0.14 mg per m^3 as a ceiling concentration for any 10-minute sampling period.[23] The NIOSH REL for MDI is 0.005 ppm (0.05 mg per m^3) for up to a 10-hour work period and a ceiling concentration of 0.02 ppm (0.2 mg per m^3) for a 10-minute period. The NIOSH REL for diisocyanates was based on three types of effects of exposure: direct irritation, sensitization, and chronic decrease in pulmonary function. These REL apply to diisocyanate monomers only and not to higher polymers of these compounds.[23]

Little is known about the toxic effects of polymeric isocyanates. No long-term studies have been conducted on polymeric isocyanates, and further, their potential for inducing pulmonary hypersensitivity, as shown for monomeric isocyanates, has not been investigated.

BORON HYDRIDES

The boron hydrides exist as highly toxic crystals, colorless gases, and colorless liquids.[36] Their repulsive odor has been described as similar to that of rotten eggs.[37] Collectively, the boron hydrides are used in welding, fuel synthesis, chemical synthesis, and rubber synthesis, as fluxing agents, reducing agents, and rocket propellants, and in polymerization of ethylene, vinyl, and styrene.[36, 37] They are highly toxic as inhalants and ingested substances and in percutaneous exposures. They are not readily degraded and may remain unchanged in sealed containers well in excess of 20 years.[38]

Pathophysiology

Diborane exhibits primarily bronchopulmonary toxicity at 0.1 ppm.[36, 37] Decaborane and pentaborane act as central nervous system depressants and produce significant gastrointestinal toxicity at levels of 0.5 ppm and 0.005 ppm, respectively.[36, 37]

It is postulated that early central nervous system toxicity results from the direct actions of the boron hydrides or their metabolites rather than from hypoxia. CNS norepinephrine depletion has been demonstrated after exposure to pentaborane and decaborane.[39] Intracranial hypertension and eventual cortical atrophy have been reported.[38]

In addition, severe anion gap lactic acidosis has been demonstrated due to myoclonus, seizures, circulatory collapse, and shock in some cases. The direct effect of the boron hydrides on cellular oxidative metabolism is a possible contributing factor. Despite the severe metabolic acidosis, there is no respiratory compensation. In fact, a superimposed respiratory acidosis due to CNS depression and seizures has been demonstrated.[38]

There is also evidence of fatty necrosis of the liver with consequent mild elevation of alkaline phosphatase level. After severe exposure impressive elevation of transaminase levels to four to six times normal has been reported.[38]

Rhabdomyolysis and resultant myoglobinuria occur owing to myoclonus, seizures, dehydration, and direct myotoxic effects of the boron hydrides. Peak creatine phosphokinase levels occur several days after initial exposure. Patients do not develop hypokalemia.[38]

Signs and Symptoms

Prolonged low-level exposure may result in vague neurologic symptoms including headache, lightheadedness, vertigo, dizziness, drowsiness, personality changes,[40] muscular weakness, cramps, and spasm.[37] Chest tightness, shortness of breath, nonproductive cough, and precordial pain may also be experienced. More serious exposures may result in lethargy, slurred speech, nystagmus, confusion, incoordination, convulsions, coma, and frank pulmonary edema.[36–38] Atrial fibrillation, ventricular tachycardia, and asystole have been reported after severe acute exposure to pentaborane.[38] On rare occasions after severe exposures, symptoms may present within 60 minutes. More likely, severe symptoms will be delayed up to 40 hours.[38] Signs and symptoms must be differentiated from those characteristic of acute hypoglycemia, cerebral vascular accidents, acute pneumonia, and acute congestive heart failure.

Treatment

There is no known antidote for boron hydride poisoning. Specific treatment for exposure consists of thorough washing of skin areas with a 3 per cent aqueous ammonia solution, irrigation of the eyes, and prompt removal from the source of exposure. If ingestion has occurred gastric lavage should be followed by administration of activated charcoal and catharsis. If high-level inhalation has occurred, hospitalization for observation for 48 to 72 hours is recommended. Chest x-ray and arterial blood gases should be monitored. Metabolic acidosis should be aggressively normalized. Administration of oxygen, intubation, positive end-expiratory pressure (PEEP), and mechanical ventilation may be necessary. A norepinephrine drip is indicated for hypotension below 90 mm Hg systolic blood pressure. Use of steroids to decrease inflammatory response is controversial. Treatment is otherwise symptomatic and supportive after all other causes have been ruled out.

Long-Term Implications

Symptoms of acute exposure may last for several days. Chronic liver and renal failure as well as cerebral atrophy may result from prolonged high-level exposure.[38] Low-level prolonged exposure may result in chronic mentation changes including poor emotional control, difficulty in decision making, poor concentration, and personality changes.[41]

HYDRAZINES

Hydrazine is a colorless, oily or crystalline solid with an ammoniac odor. It is used most commonly as a solder fluxing agent, in metallurgy, and in agricultural chemicals. It is also used as a silvering agent for mirrors, as a rocket fuel, in chemical synthesis and photographic developing, and in the manufacture of drugs, dyes, textile treatments, explosives, and plastics.[41] Monomethylhydrazine is also found in the group III mushrooms *Gyrometra* spp., or false morels.

Hydrazines are extreme local irritants, convulsants, hepatotoxins, and hemolytic agents. Primary exposure occurs through skin absorption and inhalation. Delayed death has been reported after acute exposure to low concentrations.

Pathophysiology

Hydrazines are absorbed well by all routes of administration including the lungs, gastrointestinal tract, and skin. None of the hydrazines are concentrated in any specific organ.[42] Acetylation is a major pathway of metabolism. Persons who are slow acetylators may be more susceptible to toxic effects.[43] The hepatotoxicity and general toxicity of the hydrazines depend on the competing rates of conversion to hydrazine and monoacylhydrazine, which are hepatotoxic, versus conversion to diacylhydrazine, which is not hepatotoxic. Liver damage results from nuclear and nucleolar enlargement, mitochondrial swelling and increased formation of antibodies.[44] Fatty degeneration, fatty infiltration, and cellular damage have also been reported.[41]

Clark et al have demonstrated that hydrazines produce a functional pyridoxine deficiency through inhibition of coenzyme synthesis or deactivation of coenzymes.[45] Central nervous system toxicity is due to direct toxicity of the brain stem and spinal cord.[46] Hydrazine is a moderate hemolytic agent that may result directly in renal damage or indirectly in acute tubular necrosis or nephritis.[42]

Additional effects include generalized severe mucous membrane irritation and cardiovascular depression. Hypotension results from a direct negative inotropic effect on the myocardium. Both direct and indirect effects on vascular smooth muscle also contribute to the hypotensive effects.[47]

A milligram-per-kilogram oral toxic dose has not yet been developed for humans. The threshold limit value (TLV) is in the range of 0.1 to 0.5 ppm.[36]

Clinical Signs and Symptoms

The most prominent early symptom is extreme mucous membrane irritation, which produces coryza, rhinorrhea, salivation, chemical conjunctivitis, and even severe facial edema.[43] Respiratory compromise is common and may progress to noncardiac pulmonary edema. Other vague nonspecific symptoms include dizziness, nausea, generalized myalgias, generalized excitation, convulsions, and coma.[37]

Several different organ systems are targeted in delayed toxicity. Hydrazines cause kidney damage by red blood cell hemolysis resulting in severe tubular necrosis and nephritis. Intravascular hemolysis has been reported after a single 4-hour exposure.[42] Consequent hemolytic anemia may cause dyspnea and generalized weakness or may exacerbate pre-existing cardiovasular symptomatology. Methemoglobinemia has been demonstrated to varying degrees in animals.[45]

As a hepatotoxin, hydrazine may cause varying degrees of acute or delayed liver failure. Hyperglycemia and hypoglycemia have been reported depending on liver glycogen stores at the time of exposure and the amount of liver damage that develops.[41] Lupuslike syndromes have been reported after exposure to hydrazine sulfate.[43]

Treatment

Specific treatment for exposure consists of thorough washing of all exposed skin areas with soap and water, copious irrigation of the eyes, and prompt removal of the patient from the source of exposure.

After inhalation, observation for progressive respiratory distress is necessary. Chest x-ray and arterial blood gases should be monitored. Administration of oxygen, intubation, and assisted ventilation may become necessary. Pneumonia and bronchitis need to be excluded.

If ingestion has occurred, gastric lavage or emesis should be followed by administration of activated charcoal and catharsis. Emesis is most effective if it is initiated within 30 minutes of ingestion.

Pyridoxine may be antidotal. The suggested dose is 25 mg per kg with half of this dose given intramuscularly and two-thirds given IV over 3 hours.[41] Seizures should be controlled with diazepam, phenytoin, or phenobarbital. Blood sugar levels should be monitored for severe hypoglycemia, which may appear with or without preceding significant hyperglycemia. The patient should be observed for evidence of intravascular hemolysis, methemoglobinemia, and consequent deterioration of renal function. Patients who are symptomatic or who demonstrate a methemoglobin level greater than 30 per cent should be treated with methylene blue 1 to 2 mg per kg slowly IV every 4 hours as needed.[41] Improvement is dramatic if diagnosis is correct. Liver function should be monitored because hydrazines are known hepatotoxins.

Elimination is enhanced by forced diuresis and acidification of the urine.[45] Hemodialysis and peritoneal dialysis should be effective, but insufficient human data exist on the use of these modalities.[41] Treatment is otherwise symptomatic and supportive.

Long-Term Implications

A lupuslike syndrome has been reported after chronic exposure in predisposed slow acetylators.[48] Hydrazine has been shown to cause cancer in animals and is suspected of being carcinogenic in humans.[49–51] Animal models demonstrate an increased incidence of pulmonary adenocarcinoma and hepatocarcinoma.[37]

ACROLEIN

Acrolein is a yellow liquid with a pungent odor that is used in the manufacture of pharmaceuticals, resins, food supplements, herbicides, perfumes, plastics, sewage treatment, and textiles and as an odor-warning agent in methylchloride refrigeration units.[36] Exposure occurs primarily through inhalation, although ingestion and percutaneous contact does occur.

Pathophysiology

Acrolein is a direct irritant of the mucous membranes and pulmonary parenchyma and causes severe lacrimation.[37] It appears to act on glyceraldehyde-3-phosphate dehydrogenase to suppress glycolysis.[36, 41] As little as 0.25 ppm has been reported to cause severe lacrimation and upper respiratory tract irritation.[37, 41] Exposure to 1 ppm for 5 minutes is not acceptable to workers and rapidly becomes intolerable.[52] Pulmonary edema and death have been reported after exposure to 10 ppm for 10 minutes.[52] The severe irritant properties and pungent odor usually prevent more serious exposure.[37, 41] No OSHA standards currently exist for acrolein.[53]

Signs and Symptoms

Percutaneous exposure causes severe dermatitis with erythema, skin burns, edema, and induration.[36, 41] Splashes in the eye result in conjunctivitis, edema, corneal damage, and severe lacrimation.[54] After inhalation, symptoms may mimic those of a viral upper respiratory infection with rhinitis, pharyngitis, dyspnea, bronchitis, and shortness of breath.[55] As symptoms progress, pain in the chest may develop along with cyanosis and pulmonary edema. Care must be taken to differentiate between infection and cardiogenic etiologies. Nausea, vomiting, diarrhea, and progressive decreased level of consciousness may also occur.[36]

Treatment

Specific treatment for exposure to acrolein consists of thorough cleansing of skin areas, eye irrigation if indicated, and prompt removal from the source of exposure. If ingestion has occurred, gastric lavage should be followed by activated charcoal and catharsis. Following high-level inhalation, hospitalization for 48 to 72 hours of observation for delayed-onset noncardiogenic pulmonary edema is recommended. Chest x-ray and arterial blood gas measurements are recommended. Administration of oxygen, intubation, and mechanical ventilation may be necessary. Adquate hydration must be maintained. Use of steroids to decrease the inflammatory response of the lung is controversial. Dermatitis and burns should be treated in the usual manner. All other treatment is symptomatic and supportive. Antibiotics are tailored to specific infections and are not routinely used prophylactically.

Long-Term Implications

No permanent effects have been reported. Respiratory insufficiency may exist for at least 18 months after significant exposure.[36]

References

1. Harris WS: Toxic effects of aerosol propellants on the heart. Arch Intern Med *131*:162–166, 1973.
2. Haj M, et al: Perforation of the stomach due to trichlorofluoromethane (Freon 11) ingestion. Israel J Med Sci *16*:392–394, 1980.
3. Baselt RC, Cravey RH: A fatal case involving trichloromonofluoromethane and dichlorodifluoromethane. J Forensic Sci *13*:407–410, 1968.
4. Bass M: Sudden sniffing death. JAMA *212*:2075–2079, 1970.
5. Taylor G, Harris WS: Cardiac toxicity of aerosol propellants. JAMA *214*:81–85, 1970.
6. Flowers NC, Horan LG: Nonanoxic aerosol arrhythmias. JAMA *219*:33–37, 1972.
7. Flowers NC, Horan LG: The electrical sequelae of aerosol inhalation. Am Heart J *83*:644–651, 1972.
8. Reinhardt CF, Azar A, Maxfield MG: Cardiac arrhythmias and aerosol "sniffing." Arch Environ Health *22*:265–279, 1971.
9. American Conference of Governmental Industrial Hygienists, 1985: TLV's Threshold Limit Values of Biological Exposures Indices for 1985–86. Appendix of Clinical Guide to the OHSA Hazard Communication Standard, 1st ed. Bethesda, Raytech Publications, 1986.
10. Aviado DM: Toxicity of aerosols. J Clin Pharmacol *15*:86–104, 1975.
11. Charlesworth FA: The fate of fluorocarbons, inhaled or ingested. Food Cosmet Toxicol *13*:572–574, 1975.
12. Thyrum PT: Fluorinated hydrocarbons and the heart. Anesthesiology *36*:103–104, 1972
13. Lessard Y, Begue JM, Paulet G: Fluorocarbons and cardiac arrhythmia: Does difluorodichloromethane (FC 12) inhibit cardiac metabolism? Acta Pharmacol Toxicol *58*:71–73, 1986.
14. Morita M, Miki A, Kazama H, Sakata M: Case report of deaths caused by Freon gas. Forensic Sci *10*:253–260, 1977.
15. Stoops GJ, McLaughlin M: Psychophysiological testing of human subjects exposed to solvent vapor. Am Ind Hyg Assoc J *28*:43–50, 1967.
16. Toxicity Studies with 1, 1,2-Trichloro-1,2,2-Trifluoroethane. Freon Product Information S-24. Wilmington, DE, E. I. Dupont De Nemours & Co. Freon Products Division, 1979.
17. Azar A, Reinhardt CF, Maxfield MG: Experimental human exposures to fluorocarbon 12 (dichlorodifluoromethane). Am Ind Hyg Assoc J *33*:207–216, 1972.
18. Rumack BH (ed): Fluorinated hydrocarbons. Poisindex, Micromedex, Denver, 1990.
19. Sittig M: Priority Toxic Pollutants: Health Impacts and Allowable Limits. Park Ridge, NJ, Moyes Data Corp, 1980, p 235.
20. International Agency for Research on Cancer: Chlorodifluoromethane. Monograph 41. Lyon, France. 1986, pp 237–252.
21. Kruus P, Valeriote IM, et al: Controversial Chemi-

cals—A Citizens Guide. 2nd ed. Montreal, Multiscience Publications, 1984, pp 102–113.
22. Butcher BT: Isocyanate induced asthma. Eur J Resp Dis 63:Suppl. *123*, 78–81, 1982.
23. Stephenson RL: Personal communication.
24. Bernstein IL. Isocyanate-induced pulmonary disease: A current perspective. J Allergy Clin Immunol Suppl *24–31*:70, 1982.
25. Chan-Yeung M, Lam S: Occupational asthma. Am Rev Resp Dis, *133*:686–703, 1986.
26. Kalra S, Malik SK, Behera D: Acute exposure to toluene diisocyanate (TDI): Report of a case and review of literature. Indian J Chest Dis Allergy Sci *26(4)*:269–271, 1984.
27. Mapp CE, Vecchio LD, Boschetto P, Fabbri LM: Combined asthma and alveolitis due to diphenylmethane diisocyanate (MDI) with demonstration of no crossed respiratory reactivity to toluene diisocyanate (TDI). Ann Allergy *54*:424–429, 1985.
28. Henschler D, Assman W, Meyer KO: The toxicology of the toluene diisocyanates. Arch Toxicol *19*:364–387, 1962.
29. Axford AT, McKerrow CB, Jones A, Parry J, Le Quesne, PM: Accidental exposure to isocyanate fumes in a group of firemen. Br J Ind Med *33*:65–71, 1976.
30. Moller DR, McKay RTK, Bernstein IL, Brooks S: Long term follow-up of workers with TDI asthma (abstract). Am Rev Resp Dis *129d*:A159, 1984.
31. Kamat SR, Mahashur AA, Tiwaris AKB, et al: Early observations on pulmonary changes and clinical morbidity due to the isocyanate gas leak at Bhopal. J Postgrad Med *31*:63–72, 1985.
32. Lorin HG, and Kulling PEJ: The Bhopal tragedy—What has Swedish disaster medicine planning learned from it? J Emerg Med *4*:311–316, 1986.
33. Bhopal Working Group: The public health implications of the Bhopal disaster. Am J Public Hlth *77*:230–236, 1987.
34. Medical News. JAMA *253*:2001–2014, 1985.
35. Gazaleh S: Toluene di-isocyanate. In Haddad LM, Winchester JF (eds): Clinical Management of Poisoning and Drug Overdose. Philadelphia, W. B. Saunders, 1983, pp 797–799.
36. Plunkett ER: Handbook of Industrial Toxicology. New York, Chemical Publishing Co, 1976.
37. Proctor NH, Hughes JP: Chemical Hazards of the Workplace. Philadelphia, JB Lippincott, 1978.
38. Yarbrough BE, Garrettson LK, Zolet DI: Severe central nervous system damage and profound acidosis in persons exposed to pentaborane. J Toxicol Clin Toxicol *23*:519–536, 1985-1986.
39. Merrit JH, Schultz EJ: The effect of decaborane on the biosynthesis and metabolism of norepinephrine in the rat brain. Life Sci *5*:26–32, 1966.
40. Silverman JJ, Hart RP, Garrettson LK, et al: Posttraumatic stress disorder from pentaborane intoxication. JAMA *254*:2603, 1985.
41. Rumack BH (ed): Acrolein. Poisindex, Micromedex, Denver, 1990.
42. Clayton GD, Clayton FE: Patty's Industrial Hygiene and Toxicology, 3rd ed. New York, John Wiley and Sons, 1981.
43. Durrant PJ, Harris RA: Hydrazine and lupus. N Engl J Med *303*:584–585, 1980.
44. Ganote CE, Rosenthal AS: Characteristic lesions of methylazoxymethanol-induced liver damage. Lab Invest *19*:382–398, 1968.
45. Clark DA, Bairrington JD, Bitter HL, et al: Pharmacology and toxicology of propellant hydrazines. Aeromedical Rev *11*:68, 1968.
46. Fine EA, Kunkel AM, Wills JH: Pharmacologic action of hydrazine. Fed Proc *9*:272, 1950.
47. Murtha EF, Wills JH: Effect of hydrazine on cat papillary muscle. Fed Proc *12*:354, 1953.
48. Reidenberg MM, Durant PJ, Harris RA: Lupus erythematosus-like disease due to hydrazine. Am J Med *75*:365, 1983.
49. Albert DM, Puliafito CA: Choroidal melanoma: Possible exposure to industrial toxins. N Engl J Med *296*:634, 1977.
50. Wald NJ: Hydrazine: Epidemiological evidence. IARC Sci Publ *65*:75–80, 1985.
51. International Agency for Research on Cancer: Monographs on the Evaluations of Carcinogenic Risk of Chemicals to Humans. Suppl 4. Chemicals, Industrial Processes, and Industries Associated with Cancer in Humans (IARC Monographs, Vol. 1–29). Lyon, IARC, 1982, pp 136–138.
52. American Conference of Government Industrial Hygiene: Documentation of the Threshold Limit Values, 4th ed. Cincinnati, American Conference of Government Industrial Hygiene, 1980.
53. International Agency for Research on Cancer: Acrolein. IARC Monograph 36 on the Evaluation of the Carcinogenic Risks of Chemicals to Humans, 1985.
54. Corant WM: Toxicology of the Eye, 2nd ed. Springfield, IL, Charles C Thomas, 1974.
55. Nielsen GD: Sensory irritation and pulmonary irritation caused by airborne allyl acetate, allyl alcohol, and allyl ether, compared to acrolein. Acta Pharmacol Toxicol *54*:292–298, 1984.

CHAPTER 89
PHENOL AND RELATED AGENTS

Lester M. Haddad, M.D., FACEP

This chapter will review the effects of phenol, dinitrophenol, and pentachlorophenol. Phenol and dinitrophenol, although chemically related, have distinct clinical syndromes. Pentachlorophenol shares the clinical effects of both phenol and dinitrophenol. Propofol is a derivative of isopropylphenol and is a new, rapidly acting, intravenous anesthetic; it is briefly discussed in Chapter 76, General Anesthetics.

PHENOL

Phenol is carbolic acid and was originally introduced as an antiseptic. It was used preoperatively as a skin disinfectant and employed in wound dressings. It was used recently to cauterize the appendiceal stump after appendectomy and in a few places is still employed in modern surgical procedures. Phenol is still used today in disinfectants, in insecticides, and in outpatient surgery by podiatrists. Chemical peeling of skin lesions and wrinkles with phenol is an increasingly common practice in plastic surgery, dermatology, and otolaryngology. Mallinckrodt, Inc. produces a product containing 89 per cent phenol for medical use. An over-the-counter product, Campho-Phenique, contains 2 to 5 per cent phenol. Table 89–1 lists compounds related to phenol that produce similar clinical syndromes.

Toxicology. Phenol denatures proteins; otherwise, little is known about its cellular effects except that it is poisonous. It is readily absorbed from all surfaces of the body. It is caustic and, if spilled on the skin or ingested, causes intense pain and blanching of the area. The skin will have a brown stain following exposure and healing.

Phenol is rapidly secreted through the kidney, primarily conjugated with glucuronide but also as free phenol. A fraction of phenol may be excreted by the lungs and may impart an aromatic odor to the breath.

Clinical Presentation. Phenol today is an uncommon but definite cause of clinical poisoning. Ingestion of tar shampoos and some over-the-counter antiseptics that have very low concentrations of phenol usually result only in gastrointestinal symptoms, if any.

Ingestion of germicidal or fungicidal agents or the medicinal 89 per cent phenol preparation can be life-threatening and usually constitutes a major medical emergency. The lethal dose is generally given as 3 to 6 grams.

A 1979 report described an unusual case in which 1 ounce of 89 per cent phenol was mistakenly given in a measured container to an outpatient. The patient survived following a stormy, 15-day hospital course. The report describes the classic presentation of phenol poisoning.[1] The patient immediately clutched her throat on drinking the "medicine" and collapsed. Within 30 minutes she had an unrecordable blood pressure and sustained a respiratory arrest. During endotracheal intubation in the emergency department, the mouth and hypopharynx were noted to be white. A "lamp oil" odor was noted while

Table 89–1. EXAMPLES OF PHENOL-RELATED COMPOUNDS

CHEMICAL	USE
Amyl phenol	Germicide
Creosol	Antiseptic
Creosote	Wood preservative
Cresol*	Germicide
Guaiacol	Antiseptic
Hexachlorophene	Antiseptic
Medicinal tar†	Treatment of dermatologic conditions
Phenol	Outpatient podiatric surgery
Phenylphenol	Disinfectant
Resorcinol	Bactericidal ointment
Tetrachlorophenol	Fungicide
Thymol	Fungicide and anthelmintic

*Cresol and Soap Solution (B.P.) is part of the British Pharmacopoeia and is known as Lysol (not to be confused with the American brand name "Lysol Disinfectant," some products of which may contain phenol but not cresol).

†Medicinal tars include coal tar, pine tar, and juniper tar preparations; the term "tar acids" refers specfically to the phenolic constituents of tar.

(Adapted from Gosselin RE, Hodge HC, Gleason MN, Smith RP: Clinical Toxicology of Commercial Products. 4th ed. Baltimore, Williams & Wilkins, 1976.)

the patient was ventilated with bag and mask.

The patient experienced ventricular tachycardia 1 hour post ingestion, and resuscitation was effected with cardioversion. During the first 24 hours, she exhibited ventricular arrhythmias, seizures, and metabolic acidosis. Hepatic failure and renal failure with anuria have also been described with phenol poisoning[2] but were not observed in this patient. Selective elevation of uric acid levels and subsequent esophagitis and gastrointestinal bleeding occurred also in this patient.[1]

Cardiac dysrhythmias[3, 4] have been noted as well as laryngeal edema[5] secondary to chemical peeling with phenol.

Management. Management of phenol poisoning includes decontamination of the skin with extensive irrigation, using first water and then olive oil; removal of ingested phenol; and supportive therapy. Removal of ingested phenol should be accomplished by gastric lavage. Olive oil is the best medium because it dissolves phenol but does not hasten absorption.[6, 7] Alcohol increases gastric absorption of phenol, and mineral oil is ineffective in dissolving phenol. Following lavage, olive oil should be left in the stomach to retard subsequent absorption of any remaining phenol. Activated charcoal, which also retards phenol absorption, is also indicated.

Treatment of persons with systemically absorbed phenol is strictly supportive because dialysis is not thought to benefit those with phenol intoxication. Management of esophagitis with steroids may be indicated, and long-term follow-up of patients with esophageal stricture is appropriate.

DINITROPHENOL

Dinitrophenol and related products are phenol derivatives that are used principally as herbicides and also for control of mites and aphids. Table 89–2 lists some chemicals and products in this group.

Table 89–2. DINITROPHENOL AND RELATED PRODUCTS

CHEMICAL	PRODUCT
Dinitrophenol	Dowicide F
Dinitro-O-sec-butyl phenol	Sinox PE Herbicide (50%)
Di-isophenol	Vet. anthelminthic

A characteristic of dinitrophenols is that they uncouple oxidative phosphorylation in cell mitochondria. The increase in oxidative metabolism rapidly depletes body fat stores, and for this reason these compounds were once used for weight reduction. Weight loss is the usual sign exhibited in patients with chronic poisoning from these agents. Dinitrophenol has recently found a role in the study of calcium metabolism and muscle physiology.[8, 9] It is absorbed by all routes, including inhalation.

Clinical Presentation. The dinitrophenols are highly toxic and can rapidly produce death. As a result of increased metabolism of body cells, patients have profuse diaphoresis, fever, thirst, tachycardia, and respiratory distress. Because normal cardiorespiratory function cannot keep up with metabolic demand, anoxia and metabolic acidosis rapidly ensue. Coma, convulsions, pulmonary edema, and severe hyperpyrexia are usually preterminal events. Methemoglobinemia also occurs.

As with other phenols, renal and hepatic failure can occur. Delayed cataract formation and agranulocytosis have also been described.[6]

Trinitrophenol (picric acid), used in the explosives industry, has effects similar to those of dinitrophenol but can also cause intravascular hemolysis. Picric acid is also highly irritant to the eyes and skin.

The major differential in the diagnosis of dinitrophenol poisoning is salicylate poisoning, which also uncouples oxidative phosphorylation. Other causes of hyperpyrexia, such as anticholinergic agents, also should be included in the differential diagnosis.

Management. Management of dinitrophenol poisoning follows the general principles of management of all poisoning patients. Eyes should be flushed with copious amounts of water; skin and hair should be washed with soap and water. Yellow staining of the skin usually occurs following contact with dinitrophenol. Care must be taken to avoid contamination of hospital personnel.

Gastric lavage followed by activated charcoal and a cathartic is usually necessary to manage a patient who has ingested this substance. Salicylates and anticholinergics are obviously contraindicated in management of these patients.

Table 89–3. EXAMPLES OF PRODUCTS[6] CONTAINING PENTACHLOROPHENOL

Dowicide 7 Antimicrobial
Forpen-50 Wood Preservative (Forshaw)
Ontrack WE Herbicide (Ciba-Geigy)
Ortho Triox Liquid Vegetation Killer
Osmose Wood Preserving Compound
Watershed Wood Preservative (Forshaw)
Weed and Brush Killer (State Chemicals)

Supportive therapy is the mainstay of treatment. Oxygen, intravenous fluids, maintenance of acid-base and electrolyte balance, and control of hyperpyrexia with a hypothermia blanket are indicated. Diazepam may be necessary to control seizures. Significant methemoglobinemia may require treatment.

PENTACHLOROPHENOL

Pentachlorophenol has considerable use as a herbicide, fungicide, weed killer, molluscicide, and wood preservative. Table 89–3 lists several products that contain pentachlorophenol.

Pentachlorophenol resembles both phenol and dinitrophenol in its toxic aspects. Like phenol, it is toxic to the liver, kidney, and central nervous system. It resembles dinitrophenol in that it stimulates oxidative metabolism by uncoupling oxidative phosphorylation in the mitochondria.

The clinical syndromes of pentachlorophenol toxicity likewise resemble those of both phenol and dinitrophenol poisoning. Armstrong and Robson described 20 newborn infants in a small hospital who developed an unusual illness characterized by profuse, generalized diaphoresis, fever, tachycardia, tachypnea, hepatomegaly, and acidosis. Two infants died. Pentachlorophenol was used in the terminal rinse of the diapers and nursery linens and was implicated as the causative agent.[10]

Treatment follows the general principles of management and is supportive in nature. Armstrong and Robson were successful in saving six of seven patients in the above group with the use of exchange transfusion. Eye exposure requires irrigation and ophthalmologic consultation.

References

1. Haddad LM, Dimond KA, Schweistris JE: Case report: Phenol poisoning. J Am Coll Emerg Phys 8:267, 1979.
2. Baker EL, Landrigan PJ, Bertozzi PE, Field PH, Basteyns BJ, Skinner HG: Phenol poisoning due to contaminated drinking water. Arch Environ Health 33:89, 1978.
3. Warner MA, Harper JV: Cardiac dysrhythmias associated with chemical peeling with phenol. Anesthesiology 62:366, 1985.
4. Truppman ES, Ellenby JD: Major electrocardiographic changes during chemical face peeling. Plast Reconstr Surg 63:44, 1979.
5. Klein DR, Little JH: Laryngeal edema as a complication of chemical peel. Plast Reconstr Surg 71:419, 1983.
6. Gosselin RE, Hodge HC, Gleason MN, Smith RP: Clinical Toxicology of Commercial Products, 4th ed. Baltimore, Williams & Wilkins, 1976.
7. Gilman AG, Goodman LS, Gilman A: The Pharmacological Basis of Therapeutics, 6th ed. New York, Macmillan, 1980.
8. Heller SL, Brooke MH, Kaiser KK, Choski R: 2,4-Dinitrophenol, muscle biopsy, and McArdle's disease. Neurology 38:15, 1988.
9. Elz JS, Nayler WG: Calcium gain during postischemic reperfusion—the effect of 2,4-dinitrophenol. Am J Pathol 131:137, 1988.
10. Armstrong RW, Robson AM: Pentachlorophenol poisoning, I and II. J Pediatr 75:309, 1969.

SECTION H

Cardiovascular and Hematologic Agents

CHAPTER 90
DIGITALIS

Lloyd S. Goodman, M.D., FACC

Digitalis was introduced into clinical medicine by William Withering in 1785 after his investigation of a home remedy used by herbalists in the English countryside. He reported on 10 years of observation of 163 patients and recommended that

> . . . it be continued until it acts either on the kidneys, the stomach, the pulse, or the bowel . . . Let it be stopped upon the first appearance of any of these effects and I will maintain that the patient will not suffer from its exhibition, nor the practitioner be disappointed in any reasonable effects.

He further gave a most accurate account of digitalis intoxications:

> The foxglove when given in very large and repeated doses, occasions sickness, vomiting, purging, giddiness, confused vision, objects appearing green and yellow; increased secretion of urine, with frequent motions to part with it, and sometimes inability to retain it; slow pulse, even as slow as 36 in a minute, cold sweats, convulsions, syncope, death.

Scope of Problem

Digitalis preparations continue to be among the top ten drugs prescribed in the United States. Prior to our present understanding of digitalis pharmacology, up to 15 per cent of all medical admissions were taking digitalis, and 20 to 30 per cent of these patients showed signs of toxicity. The mortality of patients with toxicity varied from 3 to 25 per cent and was especially common in the elderly.[1, 2] However, recent advances have considerably altered this incidence for the following reasons: (1) Our understanding of digitalis pharmacodynamics is much better, and we use it to determine the more appropriate maintenance dose; (2) serum digoxin levels are now easily and rapidly available to almost every physician, thus identifying many unexpected responses; (3) drug bioavailability is more standardized; and (4) the available drug therapy for congestive heart failure has expanded rapidly and has eliminated the need to push digitalis to higher and more potentially toxic levels.[3] Nevertheless, the number of patients on maintenance digitalis therapy remains high, and the numerous common untoward effects still demand attention and understanding, especially because the margin between therapeutic and toxic doses is very small, and many of the abnormal rhythms are found in patients with advanced heart disease who are being treated without digitalis, making determination of toxicity all the more difficult. Because toxic effects are a consequence of excessive therapeutic effects, one must first understand the basic pharmacology of digitalis in order to manage the intoxicated patient.

PHARMACOLOGY

Basic Mechanism

Digitalis acts at the subcellular level by altering the Na^+-K^+-ATPase transport system. The net effect is intracellular loss of K^+ and gain of Na^+ and Ca^{++}. In short, digitalis acts to increase the Ca^{++} available to the contractile elements of the myocardium after excitation.[4] The increased Ca^{++} augments myofibrillar interaction in cardiac muscle and leads to positive inotropic action.[5] Any drug affecting Na^{+}, K^{+}, or Ca^{++} fluxes across cell membranes can exert a significant effect on conduction (Fig. 90–1).

In the intact heart, the effects of digitalis can be separated into mechanical and electrophysiologic actions, and toxicity can be related to its excessive therapeutic effects and the status of the patient at the time of drug administration.

Pharmacodynamics and Preparations

Several preparations of digitalis are available. However, because of ease of oral administration and duration of action, only two preparations are used in most clinical practices today—digoxin (half-life, 33 to 34 hours) and digitoxin (half-life, 6 to 7 days). Digoxin and digitoxin are passively absorbed from the small intestine, with an effective absorption of 55 to 75 per cent for digoxin tablets, 90 to 100 per cent for digitoxin tablets, and 90 to 100 per cent for the liquid or encapsulated liquid form of digoxin.[4] Figure 90–2 illustrates the average values for absorption and the half-lives of digoxin and digitoxin.[6] Detailed pharmacodynamic studies have shown that the drug action depends on the tissue concentration, which is relatively constant in relation to serum levels, and that the major depot in man is skeletal muscle.[7] These findings lead to two conclusions: First, the constant relationship of the myocardial digoxin concentration to the serum concentration supports measuring serum levels to monitor patient compliance, and second, dosage requirements and the likelihood of toxicity can be anticipated on the basis of muscle mass rather than overall body weight.

Digoxin and digitoxin are eliminated in different ways. Digoxin is excreted primarily through the renal route, whereas digitoxin is eliminated primarily through metabolic change to inactive breakdown products. Since enterohepatic circulation plays a role in the metabolism of both drugs, biliary production will affect digitalis elimination. Bioavailability of the drug may vary owing to different manufacturing processes, malabsorption syndromes, and inactivation by gut flora, which can be altered by antibiotics.[8] Furthermore, digoxin is one of the breakdown products of digitoxin metabolism (about 8 per cent) (see Figs. 90–2 and 90–3). Other important factors in patient handling and response to digitalis include disease state, patient's age, and drug interactions.

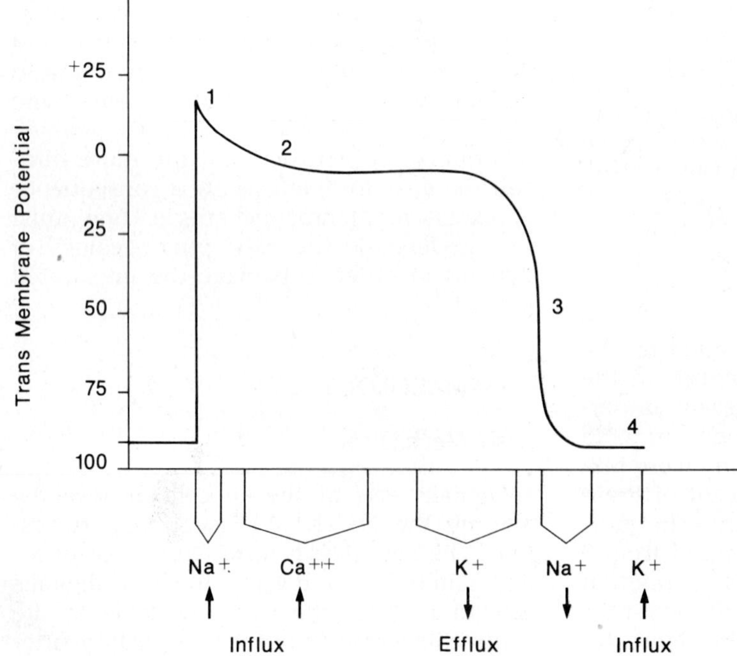

Figure 90–1. Ion (Na^{+}, K^{+}, Ca^{++}) fluxes associated with myocardial action potential. Any drug altering these ion fluxes will alter the action potential and thereby affect myocardial conduction.

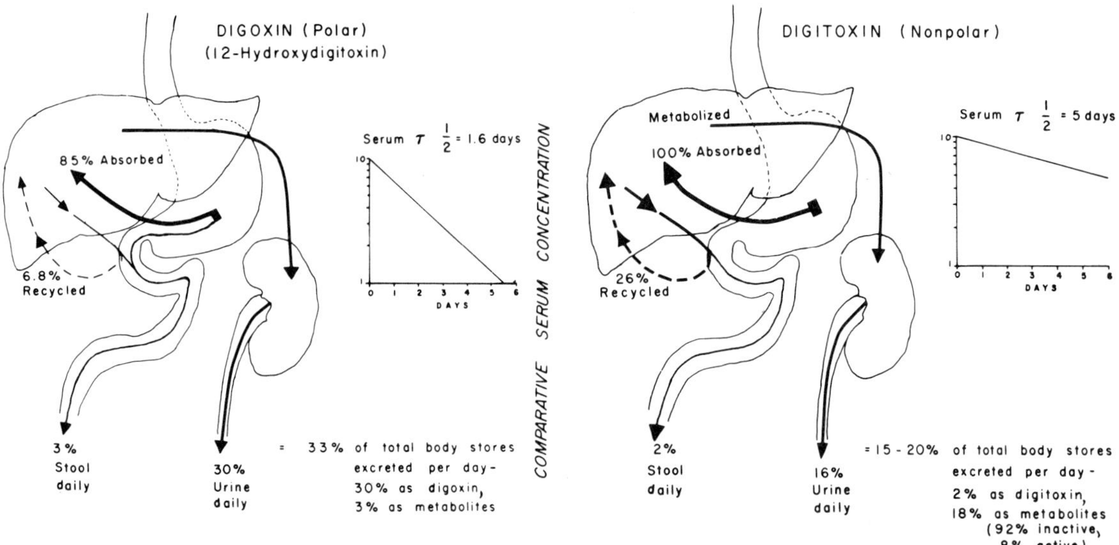

Figure 90–2. Digoxin and digitoxin pharmacokinetics, showing average values for absorption, excretion, enterohepatic circulation, and half-life. (Reproduced with permission from Doherty JE: Digitalis glycosides; Pharmacokinetics and their clinical implications. Ann Intern Med *79*:229, 1973.)

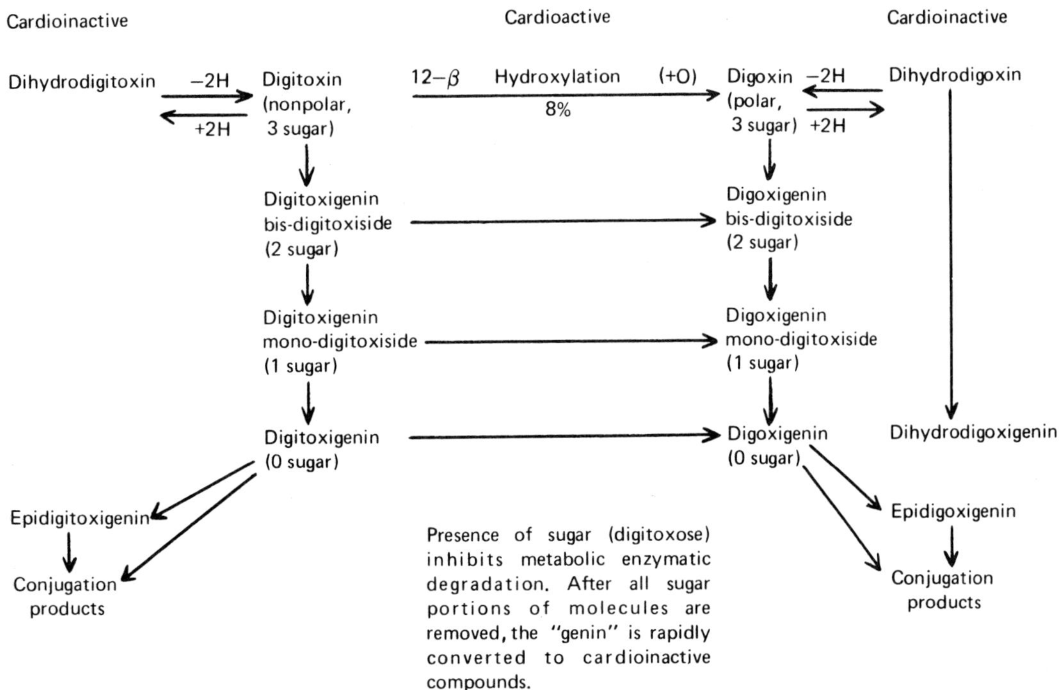

Figure 90–3. Metabolic pathways of digoxin and digitoxin. Note that digoxin is part of the metabolic pathway of digitoxin. (Reproduced with permission from Doherty JE: Digitalis glycosides; Pharmacokinetics and their clinical implications. Ann Intern Med *79*:229, 1973.)

Normal Therapeutic Effects on Intact Heart (Summary of Actions)

The most important therapeutic use for digitalis is its inotropic effect. Digitalis augments the force of myocardial contractions by increasing the velocity of shortening and the velocity of developed tension of the cardiac muscle.[9] Therefore, there is less encroachment on compensatory mechanisms, allowing greater cardiac reserve. In patients with heart failure, digitalis causes a decrease in end-diastolic pressure and volume, increasing cardiac output and stroke work. The usefulness of digoxin for congestive heart failure in patients in sinus rhythm has been the subject of some controversy. However, most authors conclude that digoxin is a weak inotrope.[10–14] In the nonfailing heart, the effects of digitalis are more controversial. Positive inotropic action may occur, but it is not manifested by a measurable change in cardiac output or by a decrease in left ventricular filling pressure.[15]

The chronotropic effect of digitalis is primarily central and is mediated through increases in vagal tone, which decreases the rate of sinoatrial node depolarization. Other effects of digitalis may vary depending on the interaction of drug concentration and autonomic tone. Digitalis decreases the refractory period of both atrial and ventricular cells and tends to increase action potential amplitude and V_{max}. This improves conduction within the muscle, as reflected in a shortened Q-T interval. The same mechanism accounts for the increased atrial rate seen in atrial flutter or atrial flutter-fibrillation.[16]

Digitalis increases the refractory period of the A-V node and the bundle of His. It prolongs phase 3 of the action potential, accounting for the decreased ventricular response seen in atrial fibrillation. Some A-V nodal effects are independent of vagal tone and affect phase 0, thus decreasing conduction velocity.[9] Most, if not all, of the effects of digitalis on the Purkinje system and ventricular muscle are direct effects and do not depend on autonomic interaction.[4]

Digitalis causes significant effects on myocardial automaticity (ability of tissue to undergo spontaneous depolarization) and excitability (ability of tissue to respond to a given stimulus). Inhibition of the Na^+ pump leads to an influx of Na^+ into the cell. This Na^+ influx increases phase 4 depolarization in all cardiac tissue except the sinoatrial node and leads to the appearance of new or latent pacemakers, thus increasing automaticity. It also lowers the resting membrane potential threshold, thus increasing excitability.[17] A number of investigators have recently described another and possibly more important effect of this Na^+ influx. According to Rosen et al, this inward current causes delayed afterpotentials (oscillations in transmembrane potentials that follow full repolarization of the membrane) that "provide a more logical basis" for understanding digitalis-induced arrhythmias.[18]

Digitalis possesses a relatively narrow therapeutic index, 40 to 60 per cent of the lethal dose being required to achieve the maximal therapeutic effect. The toxic effects that occur when levels exceed the therapeutic range are almost uniformly a consequence of excessive normal physiologic responses.

Use and Abuse of Serum Levels

The concentration of digitalis in the serum is the net result of whole body absorption, distribution, and excretion. Attempts to predict serum levels based on age, sex, and renal function have not been successful, even with computer assistance, and such attempts cannot replace actual measurement of serum levels. However, the serum level does not necessarily indicate toxicity.[19–22] Three major problems arise in the diagnosis of toxicity.

First, the accuracy and reproducibility of the test may be questionable. Testing methods vary with the sophistication of the laboratory, and commercial kits may give inconsistent measurements of serum levels. Assays of different digitalis preparations often overlap, and accurate interpretation of results is possible only if the exact preparation is known. In addition, the correlations between clinical effects and therapeutic and toxic levels have been made at steady-state levels. These levels are reached 6 to 8 hours after administration, and any measurements made prior to this time may give values two to three times greater than those seen at steady state. False-positive drug elevations may occur for several reasons. For example, spironolactone and hyperbilirubinemia will interfere with the test. Far more frequent is a false-positive assay in patients with chronic

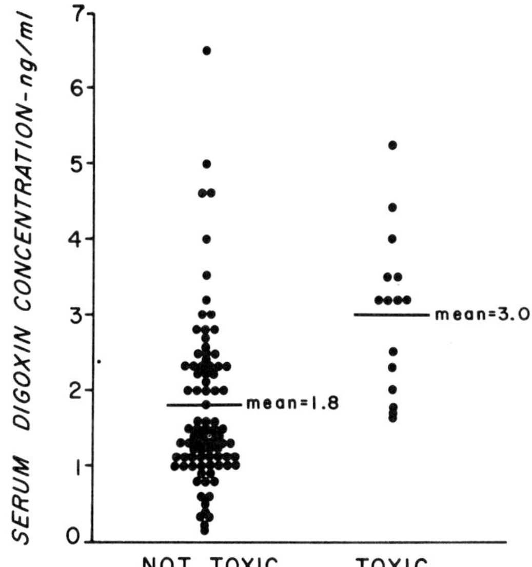

Figure 90–4. Results of 100 serum digoxin radioimmunoassay measurements. Sixteen patients were believed to be clinically toxic; their mean serum level was 3.0 ng/ml. Seven patients thought to be nontoxic also had serum levels of more than 3.0 ng/ml. Overlap of normal and toxic values does occur; therefore judgment must be used when evaluating results. (From Doherty JE: Digitalis glycosides; Pharmacokinetics and their clinical implications. Ann Intern Med 79:229, 1973.)

renal failure. This result is thought to be due to an endogenous circulating digoxinlike substance that has been reported in more than 60 per cent of patients with chronic renal insufficiency.[23]

A second problem in diagnosing toxicity arises because serum levels of patients demonstrating clinical toxicity overlap considerably. Specific and sensitive laboratory criteria are not available as alternatives to clinical assessment. The inability to define toxicity levels accurately has been a major defect in the analysis of most studies (Fig. 90–4).

A third problem is that several factors predispose patients to toxicity at levels well below the 2 ng per ml level, which is usually considered the upper limit of normal. Hypokalemia is the most important of these factors. Anoxia due to chronic pulmonary disease or advanced forms of heart disease is also important. In addition, enhanced sympathetic activity for any reason seems to sensitize the patient to digitalis-induced arrhythmias.[24]

Therefore, serum levels should be used only as a guide to appropriate therapeutic doses and as an indication of toxicity. Serum levels also may verify drug compliance and aid dose regulation in patients with changing renal function, those who have undergone cardiac surgery, or those with severe congestive heart failure.[25] However, serum levels alone do *not* diagnose those who have toxicity.

DIGITALIS TOXICITY

Toxicity from digitalis can produce cardiac and extracardiac symptoms. Drug interactions may increase the effective drug level, and other factors, such as ischemia or inflammation, affect sensitivity to digitalis. The cardiac mechanism of digitalis toxicity is usually ascribed to depression of conduction and alterations of impulse formation; noncardiac symptoms are listed in Table 90–1.

Interaction with Other Drugs

The importance of drug interactions in the development of digitalis toxicity was not truly appreciated until reliable assays of digoxin levels became widespread. Several drugs such as cholestyramine, antacids, kaolin-pectin, bran, and some antibiotics such as neomycin, sulfasalazine, and para-aminosalicylic acid, alter absorption and effectively decrease the bioavailability of digoxin.[26, 27] This fact is important because discontinuing these drugs without changing the digoxin

Table 90–1. SIGNS AND SYMPTOMS OF DIGITALIS TOXICITY

MANIFESTATION	PREVALENCE (PER CENT)
Fatigue	95
Visual symptoms	95
Weakness	82
Nausea	81
Anorexia	80
Psychic complaints	65
Abdominal pain	65
Dizziness	59
Abnormal dreams	54
Headache	45
Diarrhea	41
Vomiting	40

(From Smith TW, Antman EM, Friedman PL, Blatt CM, Marsh JD: Digitalis glycosides: Mechanisms and manifestations of toxicity. Part III. Prog Cardiovasc Dis *27(1)*:26, 1984.)

dose may lead to a digitoxic state. Other antibiotics, such as erythromycin and tetracycline, may significantly increase digoxin levels by altering the gut flora, which is important in metabolizing digoxin.[8] This is less of a problem when the capsule form is used. By far the most important drugs interacting with digoxin are the antiarrhythmics. Quinidine causes an increase in serum digoxin in up to 90 per cent of patients. The magnitude of the increase varies but is often twofold. The serum digoxin level begins to increase with the onset of quinidine therapy and remains elevated as long as both drugs are continued. The exact mechanism that causes this interaction is still being investigated. It is known that the half-life of digoxin is not prolonged and that total body clearance is reduced. The findings so far are best explained by the fact that digoxin is displaced from tissue-binding sites.[29, 31] Some evidence has suggested that there may be paradoxical increased concentrations in areas of the brain and has prompted speculation that some of the toxic effects may be the result of central nervous system stimulation.[4] The adverse effects of elevated digoxin levels due to quinidine are similar to those experienced with an overdose of digoxin, though the mechanism that causes this elevation is still not settled.

Another major antiarrhythmic drug that interacts with digoxin is amiodarone. Digoxin levels increase by 25 to 70 per cent within 24 hours after amiodarone is added.[27] The effect is mediated through a decrease in renal and nonrenal clearance.[32] The result is more frequently a bradyarrhythmia or heart block than a tachyarrhythmia.[33]

There is no evidence to date that other antiarrhythmics similar to quinidine in action (type I) interact with digoxin. Procainamide, disopyramide, lidocaine, mexiletine, tocainide, flecainide, and encainide do not increase serum digoxin levels. Likewise, other antiarrhythmics such as aprindine, ajmaline, and ethmozine (some still in clinical trials) do not affect digoxin levels.[27, 34]

The interaction of Ca^{++} channel-blocking drugs with digoxin varies greatly. Nifedipine has no effect,[35] whereas diltiazem has such a small effect that toxicity is unlikely.[27] On the other hand, verapamil increases serum digoxin levels by up to 70 per cent by altering renal and extrarenal clearance, which can lead to lethal cardiac toxicity.[36, 37] Potentially toxic interaction may also occur with potassium-sparing diuretics (such as spironolactone), which inhibit tubular secretion of digoxin; with antihypertensive agents, which can significantly alter renal reperfusion and glomerular filtration rate; and with anti-inflammatory drugs, especially indomethacin, in neonates or in the presence of renal dysfunction.[27, 38] Some antiadrenergic agents, such as clonidine, methyldopa, reserpine, and beta-blockers, in combination with digitalis may lead to severe bradyarrhythmias, especially in patients with sinus node disease.[27]

Altering Sensitivity to Digitalis

Digitalis toxicity can occur in a patient with any condition that increases total body digitalis or modifies the cardiac sensitivity to digitalis. Aside from the drug interactions discussed above, renal dysfunction leading to decreased renal excretion of digitalis is the major factor leading to increased total body digitalis. Neither dialysis nor cardiopulmonary bypass cause much body loss of digitalis, although hemoperfusion may increase its removal (see Chapter 8). Cardiac factors that increase sensitivity to digitalis and may lead to toxicity include myocardial infarction or ischemia, myocarditis, cardiomyopathy, amyloidosis, and other trauma including surgery.[39] A healthy heart tolerates large amounts of digitalis, whereas diseased myocardium appears to manifest arrhythmias at lower serum levels.[40] Myocardial disease leads to local areas of altered electrophysiology, which in turn can cause variation in digitalis uptake by cardiac tissue. The concentration differences and local ischemia lead to variations in cellular recovery times and set the stage once again for re-entry phenomena (Fig. 90–5). Intrinsic cardiac disease alone may produce similar rhythm disturbances, of which several are common in acute myocardial infarction. There are no specific distinguishing features of these rhythm disturbances. However, digitalis toxicity may be implicated in most instances when withdrawal of the drug is followed by resolution of the arrhythmia. This increased sensitivity does not preclude careful use of digitalis when it is clinically indicated.[41]

Metabolic factors are important in enhancing myocardial sensitivity to digitalis. Electro-

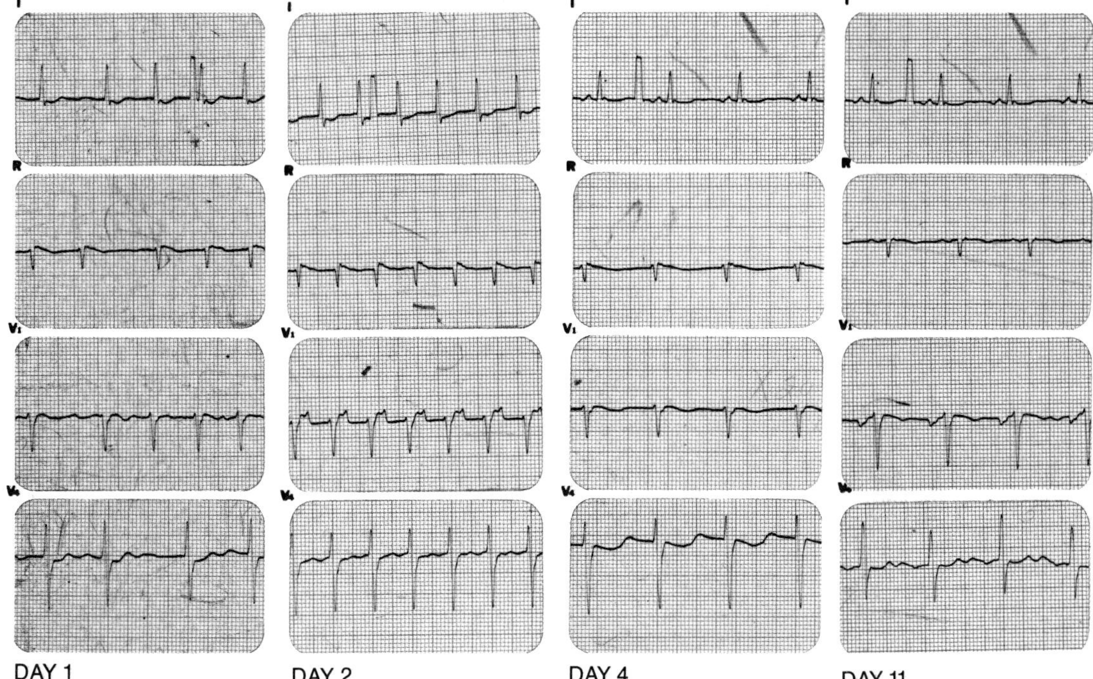

Figure 90–5. Electrocardiograms of a 67 year old man with coronary disease and previous myocardial infarction, who was admitted to the hospital with congestive heart failure. He was on maintenance digoxin therapy.

Day 1. The patient developed atrial fibrillation and was given an extra dose of digoxin and Lasix. *Day 2*. Accelerated junctional rhythm with retrograde P waves (seen clearly in V_1). *Day 4*. Junctional rate slowed with marked ST-T changes (K^+ noted to be 2.3). *Day 11*. After fluid restriction and withholding digoxin and diuretics, sinus rhythm was re-established. This sequence demonstrates problems of digoxin toxicity worsened by ischemia.

lyte abnormalities, especially hypokalemia, are well known, but aberrations of magnesium and calcium may play a role and are important considerations.[42, 43] Other metabolic abnormalities, including acidosis, alkalosis, hypoxemia, and hyperthermia, may play a role but are probably not independent risk factors. Diseases of other organ systems, especially chronic lung disease and hypothyroidism, predispose a patient to digitalis toxicity. Acute cerebral vascular events may lead to toxicity by a large sympathetic discharge, which may lower the arrhythmia threshold[39] (Table 90–2).

Cardiac Mechanisms

The diagnosis of digitalis cardiotoxicity is often difficult, because arrhythmias similar to those characteristic of digitalis toxicity, are frequently manifestations of underlying cardiac disease. A change in the rhythm may be the most important clue. Rhythm distur-

Table 90–2. PREDISPOSING FACTORS TO DIGITALIS INTOXICATION

Patient abnormalities
Old age
Severe heart disease
Myocardial infarction
Myocarditis
Recent cardiac surgery
Cor pulmonale
Renal failure
Hemodialysis
Hypothyroidism
Anoxia
Amyloidosis
Electrolyte abnormalities
Hypokalemia
Hypernatremia
Hypercalcemia
Hypomagnesemia
Alkalosis
Drugs
Diuretics
Steroids
Reserpine
Catecholamines
Quinidine
Verapamil
Amiodarone

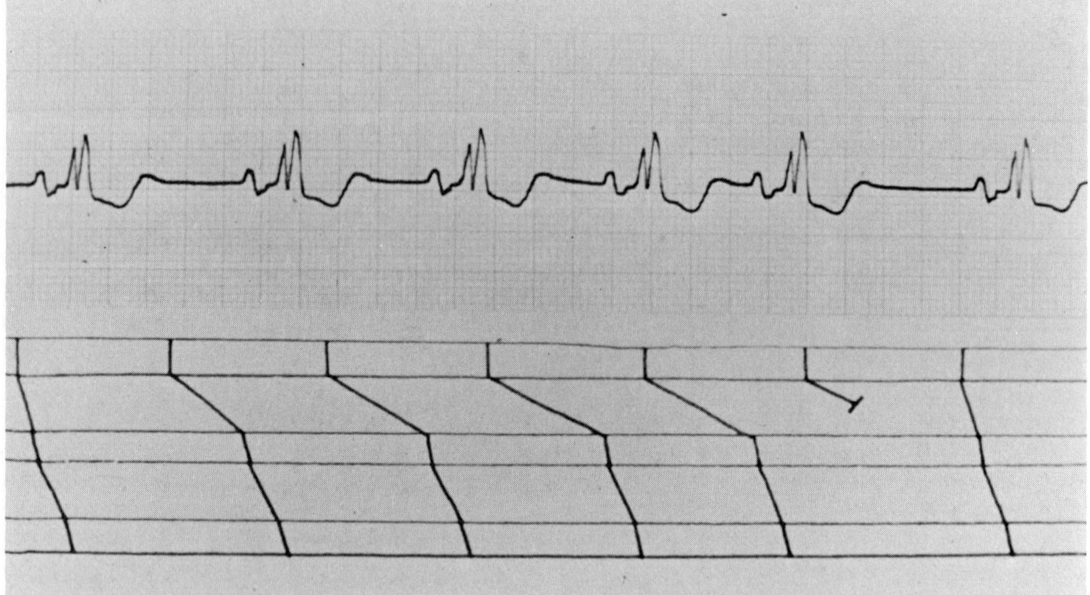

Figure 90–6. SA nodal Wenckebach. P to P interval increases by decreasing increments until P wave is dropped.

bances can now be evaluated by detailed and complex electrophysiologic studies. Most authorities attribute digitalis cardiotoxic rhythms to *depression of conduction* or *alteration of impulse formation* with increased heterogeneity of refractory periods. Fisch and Knoebel offer a somewhat more detailed classification "based on probable physiologic mechanisms,"[44] but for clarity, the standard mechanisms are discussed below.

Depression of Conduction

Depression of conduction results in heart block at the sinoatrial (SA) and atrioventricular (A-V) nodes. Sinoatrial nodal block is relatively common and may range from sinus pauses to the SA nodal Wenckebach phenomenon, or to total sinoatrial nodal exit block (Figs. 90–6 and 90–7). A-V block is usually type I A-V nodal block. The designation of type I or type II block is a relatively new approach in describing A-V block based on His bundle recordings. In this scheme, block above the bundle of His is considered type I and block below the bundle of His is considered type II. On the scalar electrocardiogram both types consistently manifest as first-degree block (prolonged P-R interval), second-degree A-V block (intermittent dropped beats), or third-degree block (complete A-V dissociation).[45]

Digitalis is usually associated with type I block in its many forms. First-degree block from digitalis is indistinguishable from other causes and is seen as a prolonged P-R interval. Second-degree block is usually A-V nodal Wenckebach (Mobitz type I) (Fig. 90–8). The resultant heart rate may be complicated

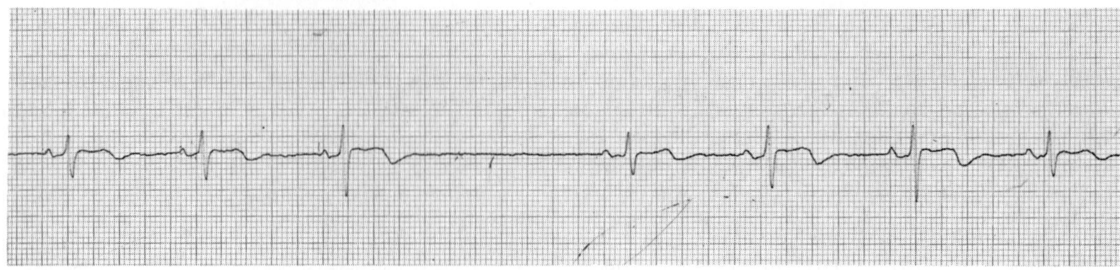

Figure 90–7. Sinus node exit block: Long pause between beat 3 and beat 4 is twice the normal sinus interval.

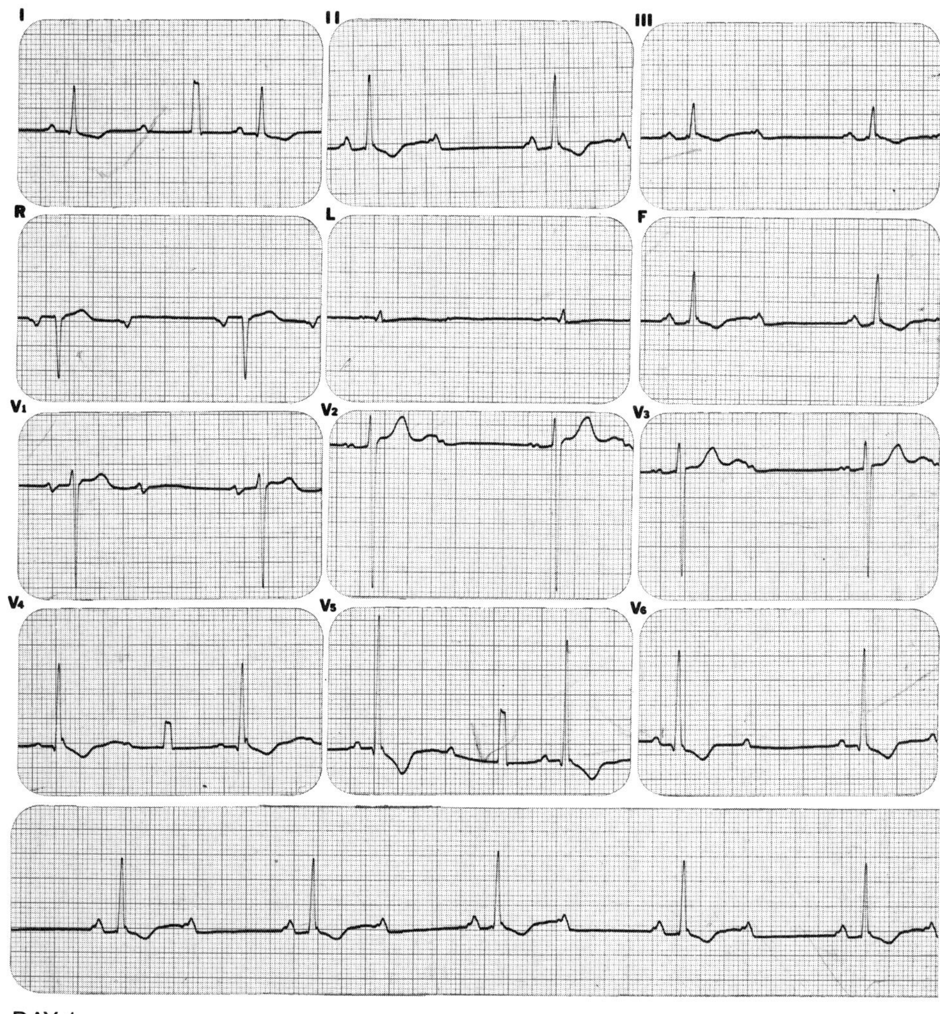

DAY 1

Figure 90–8. Electrocardiograms of a 52 year old woman with hypertension and congestive failure, seen in the emergency room for weakness. She was taking 0.25 mg of digoxin daily. Digoxin was withheld, and the patient was observed.

Admission ECG shows 2:1 A-V block, narrow QRS, increased voltage, and short Q-T and S-T changes compatible with digitalis and/or left ventricular hypertrophy.

Illustration continued on following page

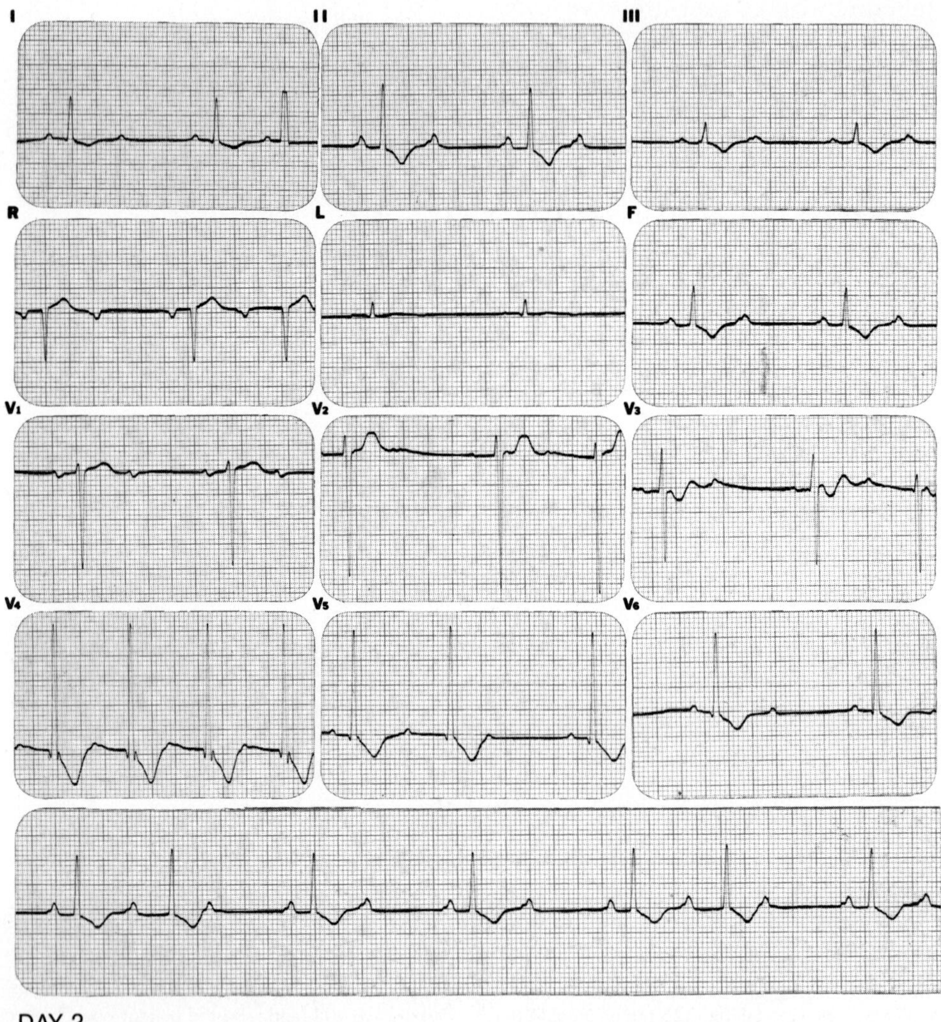

Figure 90–8 *Continued.* Day 2 ECG showed some areas of 2:1 conduction but also 3:2 Wenckebach and periods of first-degree A-V block (lead V_4). By day 6, the ECG showed sinus rhythm, first-degree A-V block, and the typical "scooped-out" S-T changes of digitalis.

This sequence demonstrated first- and second-degree block associated with digitalis toxicity and 2:1 block with a narrow QRS (as a manifestation of Mobitz I block).

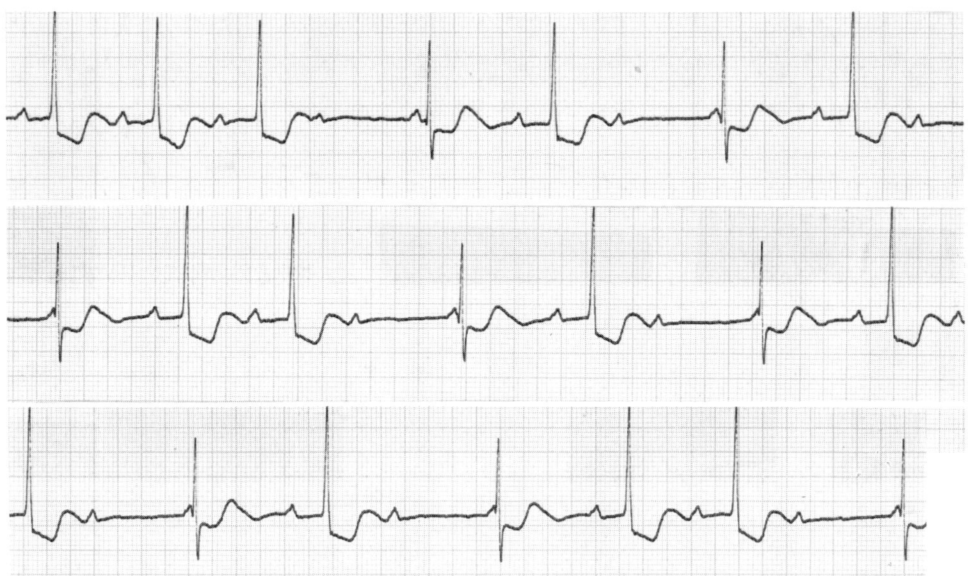

Figure 90–9. A-V nodal Wenckebach with 2:1, 3:1, and 4:1 conduction. After each dropped beat there is a junctional escape beat prior to re-establishment of SA conduction. The ECG strips are continuous.

because of accelerated junctional escape beats (Fig. 90–9). Third-degree block, or A-V dissociation, is usually associated with a narrow QRS escape focus at adequate rates, but hemodynamic alterations are rare in the absence of other cardiac abnormalities (Figs. 90–10 and 90–11). Type II (infra-His) block and bilateral bundle branch block are rare consequences of digitalis toxicity but may be seen if there is underlying heart disease.

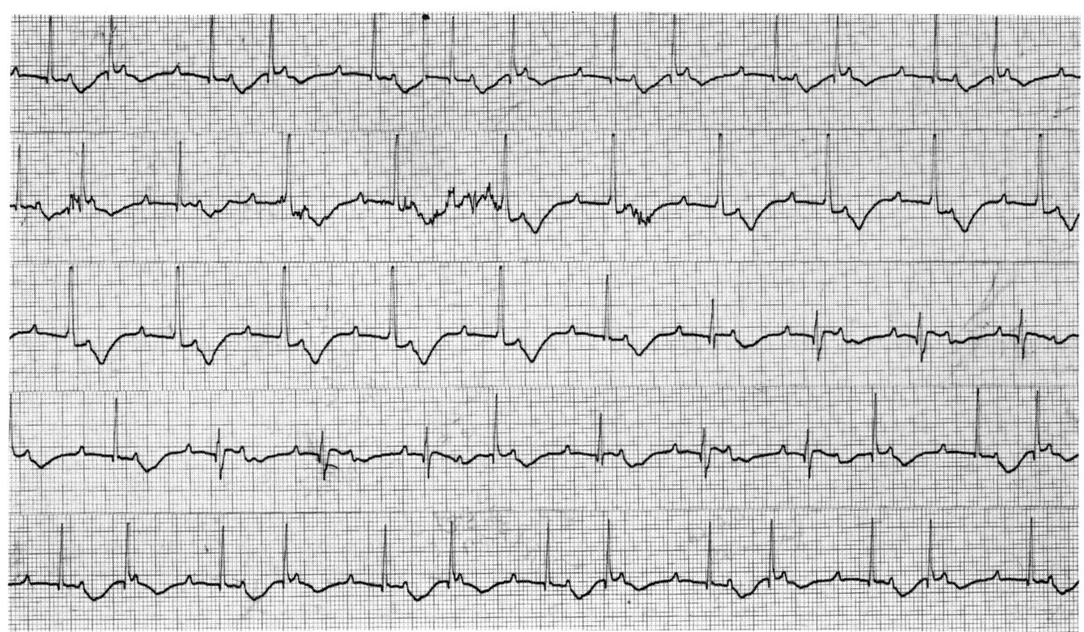

Figure 90–10. Electrocardiogram of an elderly man on maintenance digoxin for congestive heart failure. He was admitted to hospital for an irregular heartbeat and showed no other symptoms. Heart rhythm resolved to regular sinus rhythm 3 days after digoxin was discontinued.

Admission ECG: Strip 1, 3:2 Wenckebach; Strip 2, 3:2 → 2:1 block; Strips 3, 4, and 5 exhibit 2:1 block changing to A-V dissociation related to high-grade block. Note the slight variation in QRS configuration, the change in rate, and fusion beats (Strip 3, fourth beat from right and Strip 4, seventh beat). (ECG strips are continuous.)

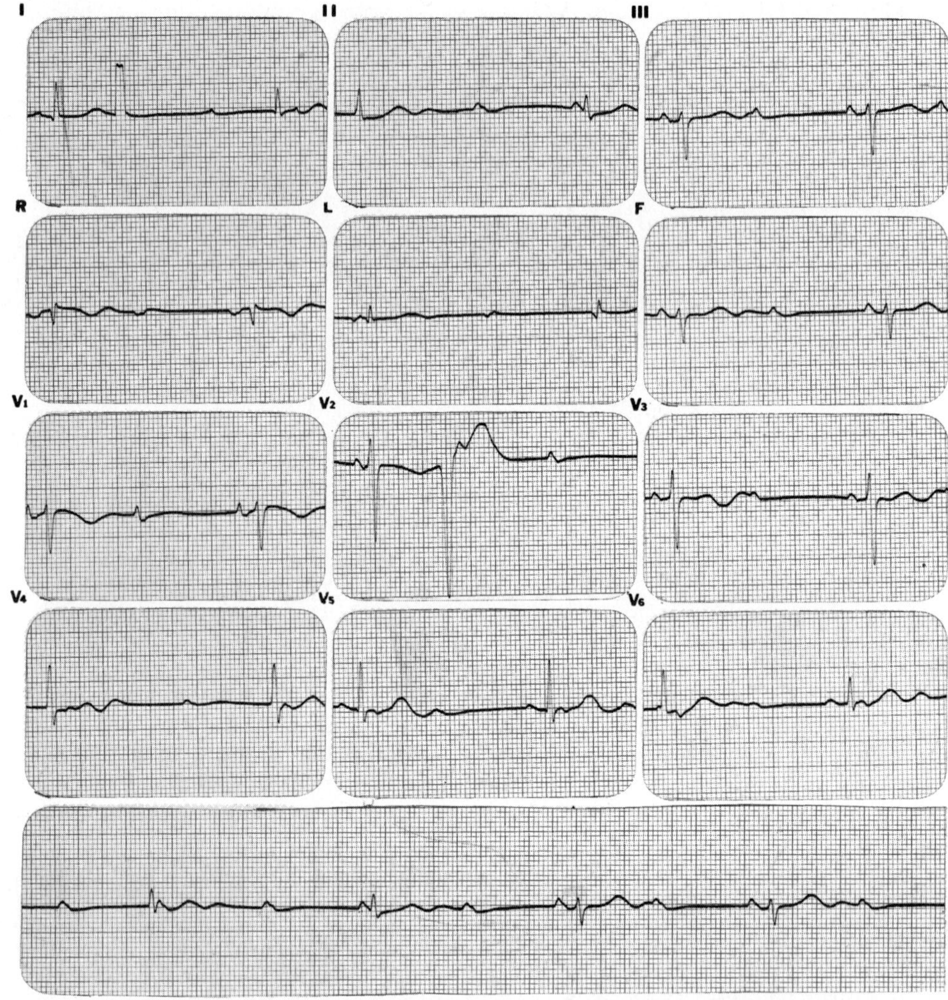

Figure 90–11. Electrocardiogram of a 79 year old woman admitted with shortness of breath and weight loss. She was on maintenance digoxin therapy. The ECG shows A-V dissociation secondary to a high-grade A-V block with narrow QRS.

Alteration of Impulse Formation

Alterations of impulse formation may be divided into those that suppress higher pacemakers and those that excite lower pacemakers. Suppression of higher pacemakers is limited primarily to sinus bradycardia (Fig. 90–12). The extent of the bradycardia may be quite severe, especially in elderly patients and in those with sinus node disease (Fig. 90–13). Excitation may take the form of accelerated junctional (Fig. 90–14) or accelerated ventricular tachycardias (Fig. 90–15) to every known extrasystolic mechanism, such as premature ventricular contractions (PVCs) (Fig. 90–16), ventricular parasystole, and ventricular or bidirectional tachycardia. The PVCs may be multifocal, bigeminal, paired, or in couplets. The ventricular tachycardia related to digitalis toxicity carries a 50 per cent mortality. Bidirectional tachycardia is almost always fatal.

The combination of suppressant and excitant effects is almost always diagnostic of digitalis toxicity and is manifested usually by an increased sinus rate with block or second-degree A-V block with accelerated lower pacer. Examples are atrial tachycardia with block (Fig. 90–17) or Wenckebach block with accelerated junctional escape beats (Fig. 90–10).

Digitalis toxicity is an exacerbation of the drug's normal effects on refractory periods of the conduction system and myocardial cells. There is an increased heterogeneity of refractory periods, allowing the development

Text continued on page 1309

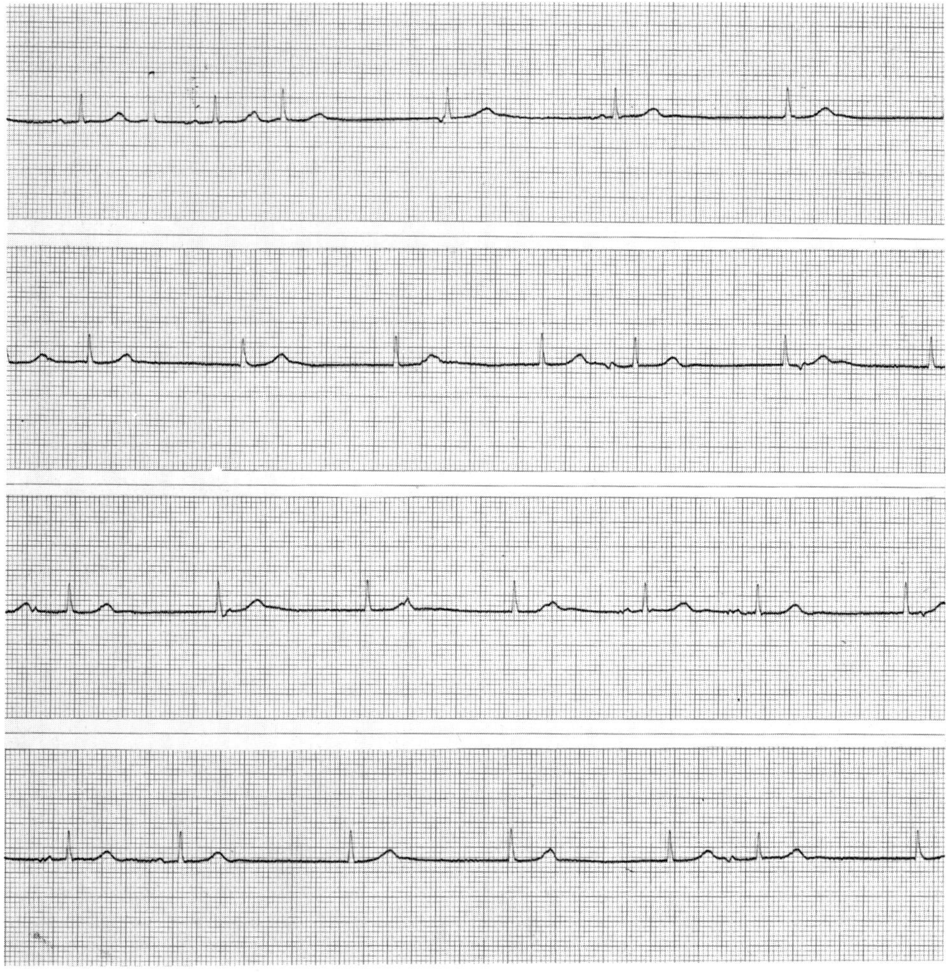

Figure 90–12. The electrocardiogram of an 82 year old woman recently begun on digitalis shows sinus rhythm with sinus arrest and A-V dissociation with slow atrial escape and faster junctional escape rhythm.

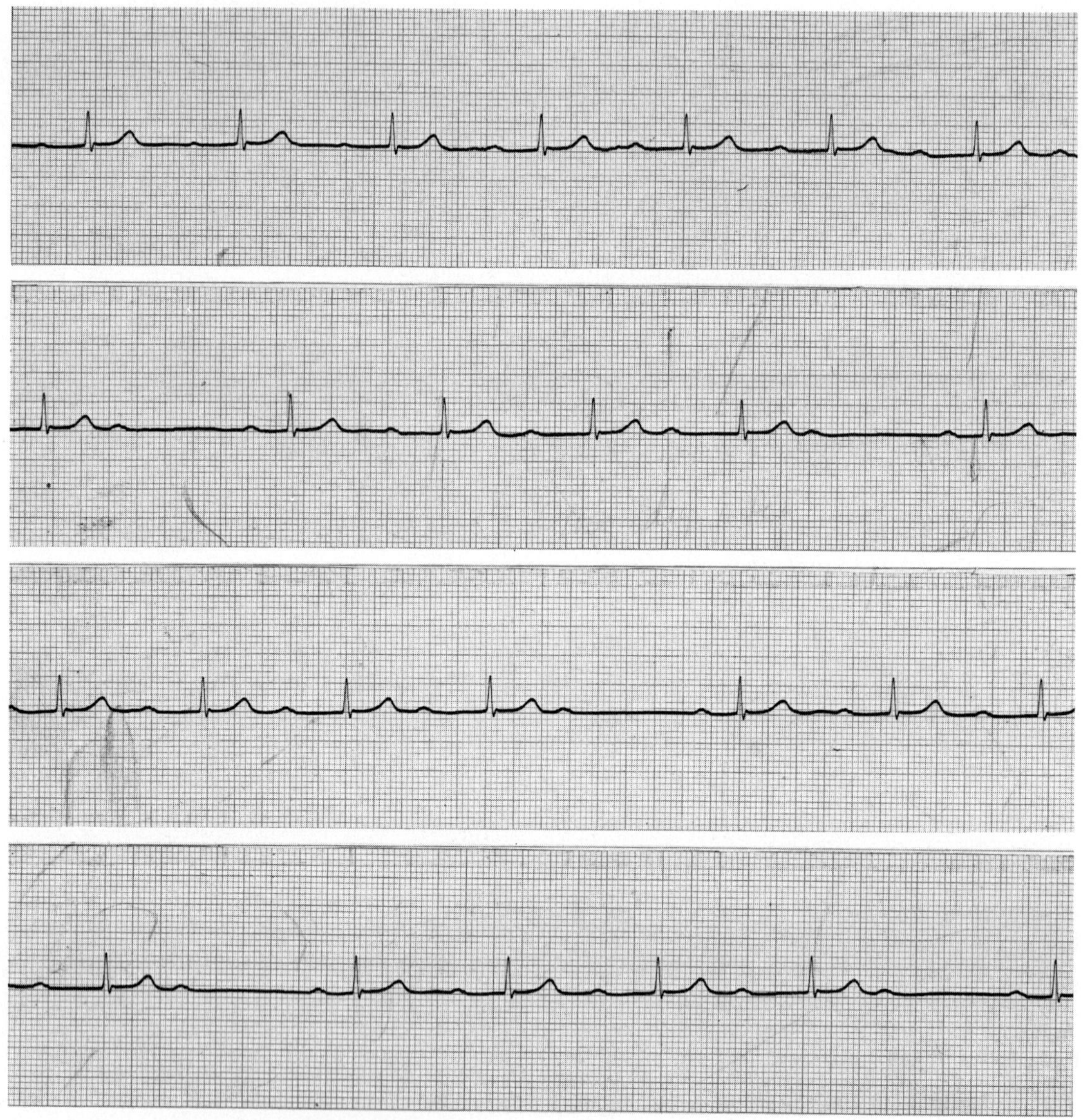

Figure 90–13. An 82 year old man was referred for slow pulse. An ECG one day prior to the present ECG showed 2:1 heart block. The patient was taking digoxin, 0.25 mg/day. Strips show 5:4 A-V nodal block with narrow QRS.

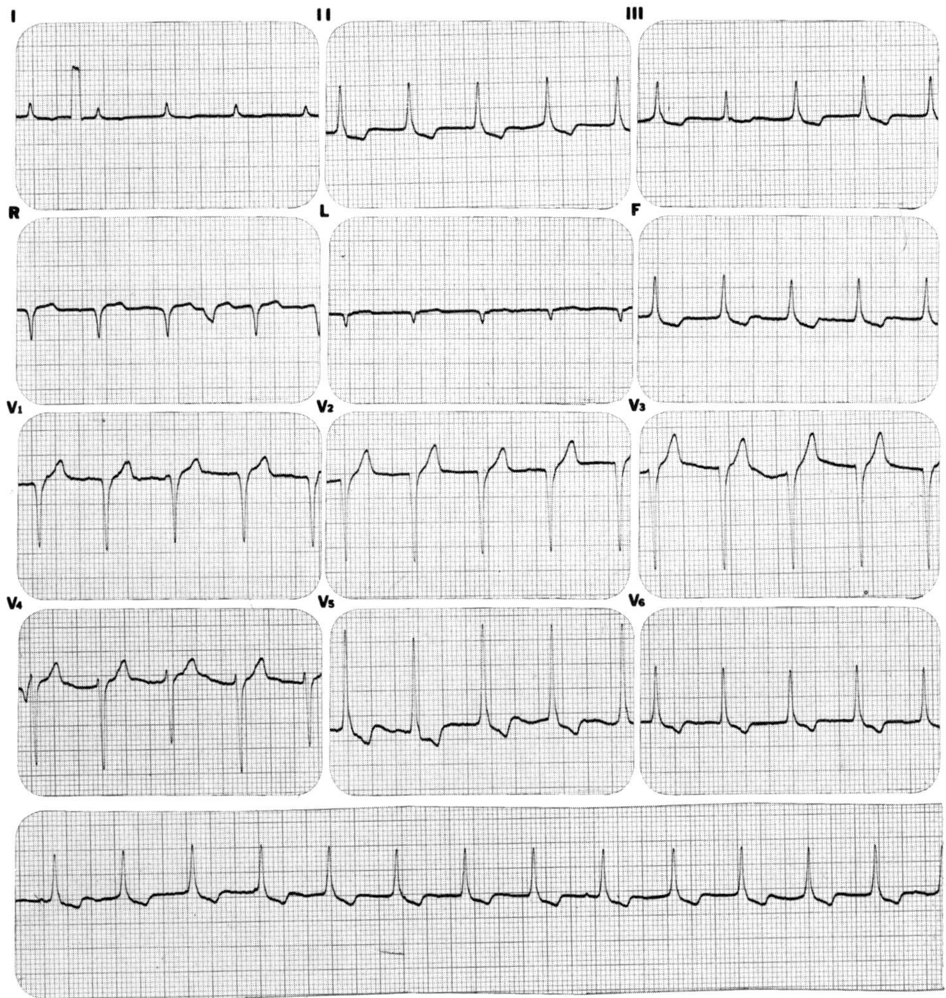

Figure 90–14. Electrocardiogram of a patient admitted to the cardiac care unit because of nausea and palpitations. Findings were an A-V dissociation secondary to accelerated junctional rhythm.

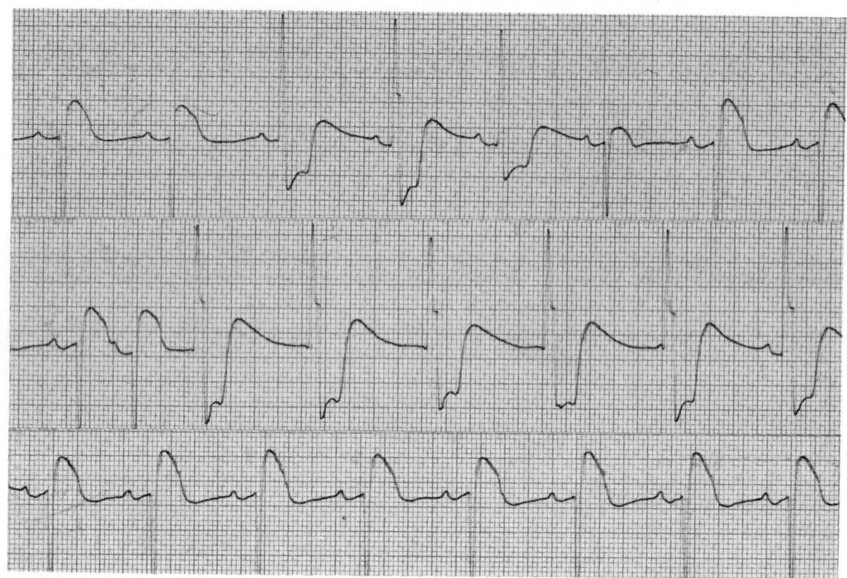

Figure 90–15. Sinus rhythm, A-V dissociation related to accelerated ventricular rhythm, and occasional premature atrial contractions (second beat of middle strip) in an elderly woman admitted to the coronary care unit with a digoxin level of 9.2 ng/ml.

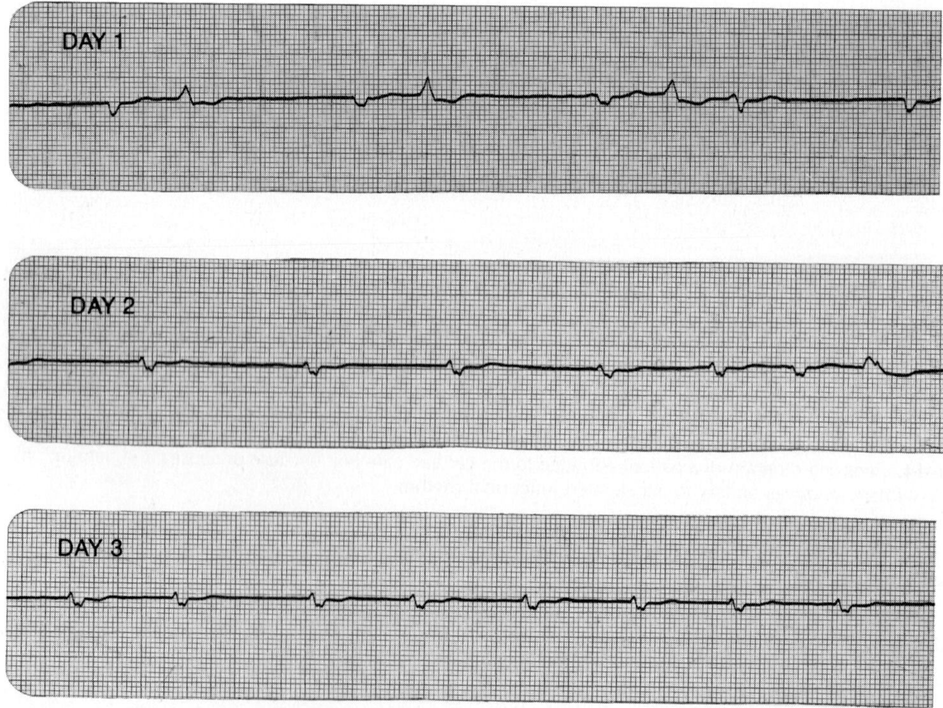

Figure 90–16. Electrocardiograms of a 73 year old man with known atrial fibrillation, admitted for weakness. Day 1: Atrial fibrillation. Periods of regularization compatible with high-grade block and PVCs. Digoxin level 5.0 ng/ml. Day 2: Rate is slightly faster. PVCs are less. Day 3: Rate is faster. Ectopy is resolved.

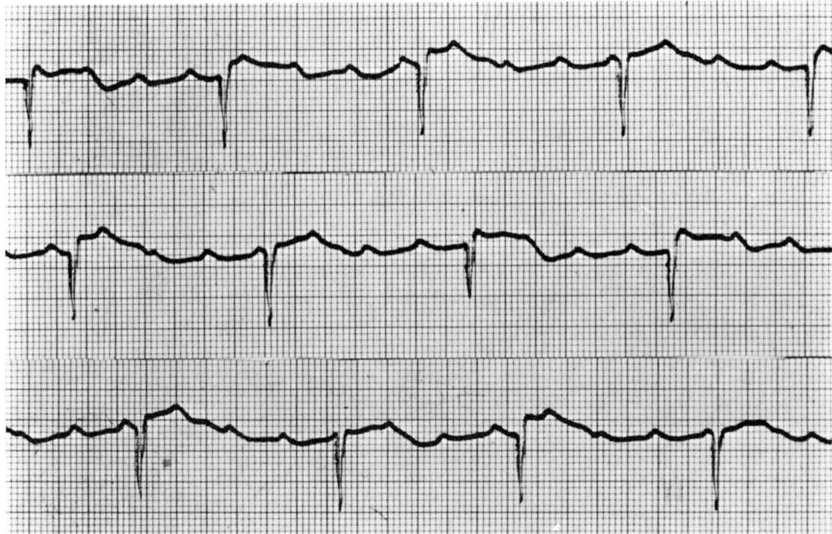

Figure 90–17. This rhythm strip shows atrial tachycardia with block. There is an atrial rate of approximately 150 per minute with a 3:1 block.

of re-entry phenomena, which probably account for the tachyarrhythmias (Table 90–3).

THERAPY OF DIGITALIS INTOXICATION

Conventional Therapy

Successful therapy of digitalis intoxication depends on early recognition (see Table 90–4). Physicians must maintain a high index of suspicion if they are to make this diagnosis, especially in patients with predisposing factors, such as old age, renal disease, chronic lung disease, or quinidine use. Most patients suffer from chronic overdose as opposed to severe acute ingestion, which is usually suicidal or accidental. Two recent reports vividly illustrate this point. Webster et al reported a patient who developed digitalis toxicity from drinking herbal tea made with foxglove leaves mistaken for comfrey.[46] Wamboldt et al reported three patients in whom digitalis intoxication was misdiagnosed as depression.[47] In cases such as these, gastrointestional manifestations, such as anorexia, nausea, or vomiting, are often the first clinical signs. The earliest electrocardiographic manifestations of digitalis effect include a prolonged P-R interval and a sagging ("scooped-out") S-T depression with a relatively short Q-T interval (Fig. 90–18). Neither the S-T changes nor the prolonged P-R interval indicate intoxication, but they do increase suspicion.

On the other hand, arrhythmias are the hallmark of toxicity. As previously noted, the arrhythmias may take every possible form; the most common of these, PVCs, first-degree A-V block, and atrial fibrillation with a

Table 90–3. RHYTHM AND CONDUCTION DISTURBANCES IN DIGITALIS INTOXICATION

Excitant
Atrial premature beats
Atrial tachycardia
Atrial flutter (rare)
Atrial fibrillation (rare)
Junctional premature beats
Accelerated junctional rhythms
Ventricular premature beats, bigeminy and multiformed
Ventricular tachycardia
Bidirectional tachycardia
Ventricular fibrillation
Suppressant
Sinus bradycardia
Sinoatrial block
Type I second degree A-V block (Wenckebach)
Bundle branch block
Complete A-V block
Type II second degree A-V block (?)
Combination excitant and suppressant
Atrial tachycardia with A-V block
Sinus bradycardia with junctional tachycardia
Wenckebach with junctional premature beats
Regularization of ventricular rhythm with atrial fibrillation

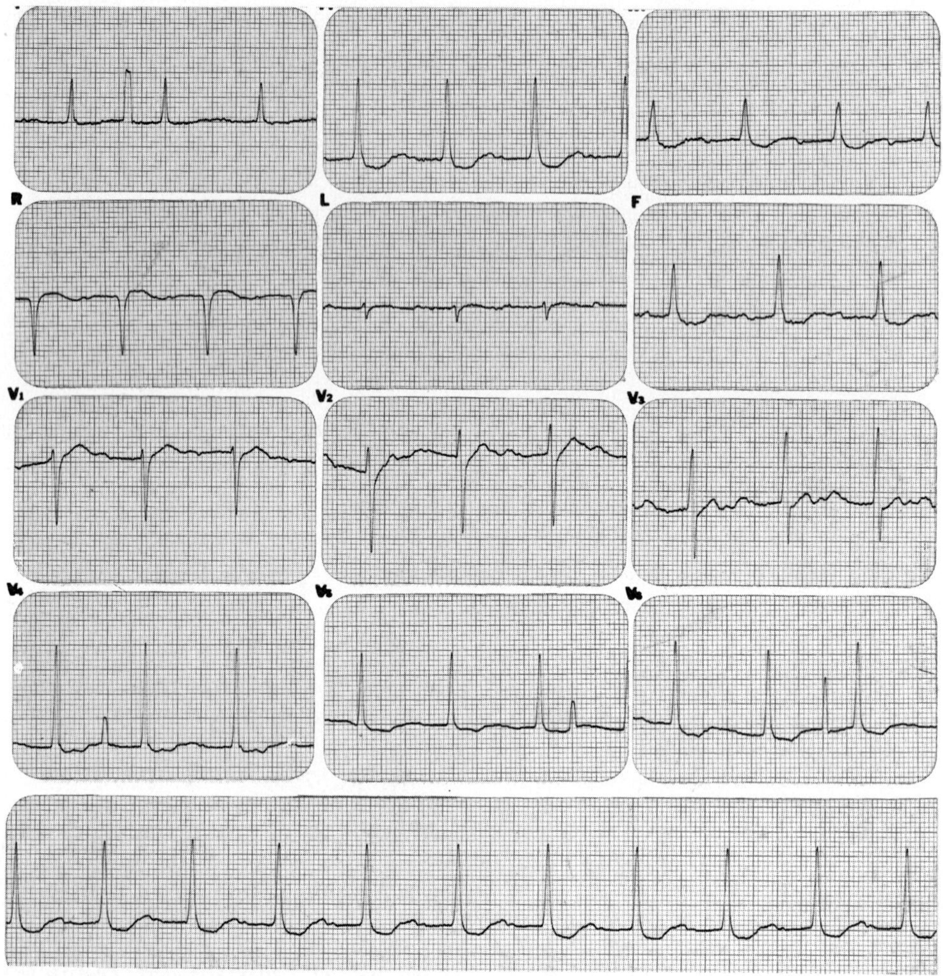

Figure 90–18. Electrocardiogram showing sinus rhythm, first-degree A-V block, and marked S-T changes compatible with digoxin effect. The patient was asymptomatic with a normal digoxin level.

very slow rate, require no special therapy except drug withdrawal. Any disturbance that affects the patient's hemodynamic status, whether it be tachycardia or bradycardia, should be treated more aggressively.

Treating Bradyarrhythmia

Severe bradyarrhythmias are often related to increased vagal tone. If the patient is symptomatic, a trial of atropine intravenously at a dose of 0.5 to 2.0 mg is useful. If the arrhythmia does not respond and hemodynamic status is unstable, a temporary transvenous pacing catheter should be used. Beta-agonists, such as isoproterenol, should be avoided because the risk of precipitating more severe arrhythmias is too high.

Treating Ectopy

Ectopy is a greater problem, especially because half to three-fourths of patients developing high-grade ventricular tachyarrhythmias from digitalis toxicity will die. Therapy should include:

1. Potassium. IV potassium must be administered carefully because the potential is high for worsening arrhythmias, especially bradyarrhythmias. Intravenous potassium solutions should not exceed 120 to 160 mEq per liter and infusion rates of 0.5 to 1.0 mEq per minute are maximal.
2. Lidocaine and phenytoin. Lidocaine (and its congeners, mexiletine and tocainide) and phenytoin (Dilantin) may also be useful because they have the least effect on

Table 90–4. SUMMARY OF TREATMENT FOR DIGITALIS TOXICITY

I. Initial approach
   A. Withdraw drug and obtain serum drug level if possible.
   B. Maintain close observation in monitored setting.
   C. Reserve therapy for hemodynamically significant arrhythmias.
II. Conventional or chronic overdose
   A. Bradycardia. There is no absolute critical rate, and no therapy is needed unless patient is symptomatic.
      1. Initiate trial of atropine first.
      2. Temporary demand pacemaker may be needed if symptomatic bradycardia persists.
      3. Avoid beta-agonists if possible. These often precipitate more serious arrhythmias.
   B. Ectopy. Reserve therapy for more complex forms.
      1. Begin with normalization of K^+ unless K^+ is greater than 5.0 mEq per liter or severe renal failure exists.
      2. Lidocaine and phenytoin are antiarrhythmic drugs of first choice if K^+ replacement is unsuccessful.
      3. Other class I antiarrhythmics, such as quinidine or pronestyl, are not useful as initial agents.
      4. Consider $MgSO_4$ if K^+ is elevated or serum magnesium is low.
      5. Verapamil is useful only if supraventricular tachycardia is present.
      6. Beta-blockers have limited usefulness but may decrease automaticity.
      7. Cardioversion should be limited to patients with life-threatening arrhythmias and used at lowest effective energy level.
III. Resistant or massive overdose
   A. Digoxin-specific antibodies should be considered when:
      1. There has been ingestion of more than 10 mg of digoxin (adult) or 4 mg (children).
      2. The serum digoxin concentration is greater than 10 ng/ml.
      3. Serum K^+ is greater than 5.0 mEq per liter in this setting.

atrial tissue and the A-V node. In fact, phenytoin is more effective for digitalis-induced ectopy than for most other causes of ectopy. Lidocaine dosage regimens are well outlined.[48] The phenytoin dosage recommendation is 50 to 100 mg given slowly every 5 minutes to a dose not exceeding 600 mg while blood pressures are monitored until toxicity is reached or arrhythmia is controlled.

3. Quinidine, procainamide, and disopyramide. These drugs are less effective for digitalis-induced ventricular ectopy. Their potential for toxicity is too high to make them initial agents. The usefulness of type Ic antiarrhythmics, flecainide and encainide, is presently unknown.
4. Verapamil. Verapamil can alter triggered automaticity and may be useful in supraventricular arrhythmias, but it is ineffective in ventricular ectopy.
5. Beta-blockers. Beta-blockers may be useful in inducing decreased automaticity. They decrease the refractory period in cardiac muscle and conduction tissue and slow conduction velocity. However, bradycardia and hypotension limit their usefulness.
6. Others. Bretylium tosylate and other newer antiarrhythmics are still unproven and their use should be reserved.[4, 49] However, magnesium sulfate has some theoretical indications, especially if the serum magnesium is low or the serum potassium is elevated.[43]
7. Cardioversion. Direct current (DC) countershock should be the last resort in life-threatening arrhythmias; if used, the lowest effective energy level for cardioversion is suggested. Even at low energy levels, the highest mortality for DC cardioversion occurs in patients with digitalis toxicity. A recent report emphasized the safe use of cardioversion for atrial arrhythmias in patients taking digoxin who are not toxic.[50] However, the danger remains high when the abnormal rhythm is induced by toxic digitalis levels.[50]

Resistant or Massive Overdose

Digitalis in massive doses may be lethal; suicidal or accidental overdoses are not uncommon. Massive doses poison membrane-bound Na^+-K^+-ATPase in the heart and all body tissues that contain this enzyme. The poisoned membranes can no longer maintain electrolyte gradients, and extremely high serum levels of potassium result. In the absence of Na^+ and K^+ gradients, resting membrane potentials are reduced, and the cells of the conduction system cannot function as pacemakers. The result is asystole and finally a complete loss of any cardiac electrical activity.[51]

Treating massive digitalis overdose presents some difficult problems. The most immediate lethal problem is the mounting hyperkalemia. Hemodialysis, the treatment of choice for refractory hyperkalemia, may temporarily reduce excess serum potassium but will not eliminate digitalis because of its high tissue binding. Charcoal or resin hemoperfusion coupled with dialysis has been attempted but with minimal effect.[52]

The most promising method for treating very high levels of digitalis poisoning is the use of digoxin-specific antibodies.[53] This method is now generally available and has been well accepted since Smith et al reported its successful use in 26 patients from 20 centers in 1982.[54] These studies were updated to 63 patients by Wenger and associates in 1985.[55] Study reports have shown that Fab fragments of the antibody can be used successfully. These molecules (50,000 daltons) neutralize digoxin toxicity and increase its speed of excretion. The fragments bind free digoxin and reverse tissue binding of digitalis. The serum concentrations reach very high levels, but the small molecular size allows glomerular filtration and relatively rapid excretion of digoxin (Fig. 90–19) in the presence of near-normal renal function.

The method of using digoxin-specific antibodies is well described by Smith and associates. Skin testing is performed to exclude immediate hypersensitivity. The digoxin-specific Fab fragments are given intravenously over 15 to 30 minutes. The dose is calculated to be equimolar to the estimated total body digoxin. This estimate is derived from the history or from serum levels (1 mg of digoxin for each nanogram of digoxin per milliliter of serum). The results are usually rapid and are uniformly successful when the diagnosis is correct, the dose adequate, and the patient not already agonal. Significant adverse effects have not been noted.[53, 55]

Digoxin-immune Fab (ovine) is marketed

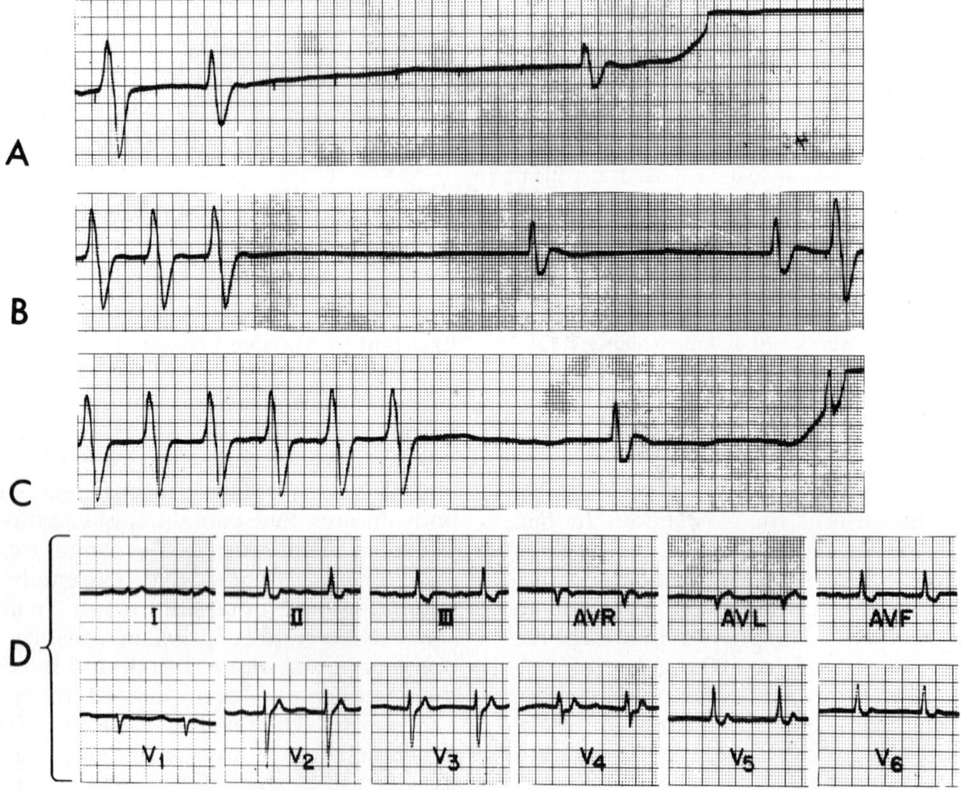

Figure 90–19. Sequential electrocardiograms recorded above, during, and after treatment with digoxin-specific Fab fragments. In *A*, the tracing recorded immediately before the start of Fab infusion, serum potassium is 8.7 mEq per liter; the escape interval when pacer stimulus is reduced below threshold is 4.60 seconds. In *B*, the tracing recorded 15 minutes after the start of Fab infusion, serum potassium is 8.0 mEq per liter; the escape interval is 3.96 seconds. In *C*, the tracing recorded 30 minutes after the start of Fab infusion, the escape interval is 2.76 seconds. In *D*, the tracing recorded 2 hours after the start of Fab infusion, serum potassium is 7.4 mEq per liter; a sinus mechanism is present at a rate of 75 per minute, with first-degree atrioventricular block (P-R interval of 0.24 second). (From Smith TW, Haber E, Yeatman L, Butler VP Jr: Reversal of advanced digoxin intoxication with Fab fragments of digoxin-specific antibodies. N Engl J Med *294*:797, 1976. Reprinted by permission.)

as Digibind by Burroughs Wellcome. At present, indications for this therapy are limited to patients with severe digitalis overdose in whom there is actual or potential life-threatening toxicity. Manifestations of life-threatening toxicity include life-threatening rhythm disturbances (whether tachyarrhythmias, bradyarrhythmias, or heart block) that do not respond to conventional measures, or hyperkalemia that is unresponsive to the usual therapies. In addition, immunotherapy is considered appropriate in patients in whom toxic exposure is so great that a satisfactory outcome with conventional therapy is unlikely. According to the package insert included with Digibind, this situation should be considered when there has been ingestion of more than 10 mg of digoxin in previously healthy adults or 4 mg in children. In addition, a steady-state serum concentration of greater than 10 ng per milliliter or a serum potassium level of greater than 5 mEq per liter in the setting of severe digoxin intoxication often presages cardiac arrest and satisfies this condition. It is hoped that continued experience will confirm the safety of the method, and its use may be extended to diagnostic testing as well as to first-line therapy for digitalis toxicity when the diagnosis has not been confirmed.[55, 56]

The majority of these expensive, time-consuming, complicated therapies for digitalis toxicity can be avoided by allocating adequate time and effort to educating the patient. Many early signs and symptoms can be easily recognized by patients. Stressing the potential for toxicity may prevent the self-administration by patients of higher doses.

Summary

Digitalis intoxication is common. Toxicity is manifest by multiple systemic symptoms, the most important of which clinically are cardiac arrhythmias. Virtually every arrhythmia has been reported from digitalis excess. However, each disturbance also occurs in the presence of intrinsic cardiac disease, and distinguishing one from the other is not always easy, even with measurement of serum levels of digitalis. Management of arrhythmias often requires little more than drug withdrawal, but more sophisticated techniques, including the use of digoxin-specific antibodies for severe overdose, are available and should become familiar to physicians using digitalis. Hemodialysis or hemoperfusion may not be useful because the drug has a large volume of distribution and is highly tissue bound. Direct-current countershock should be either avoided or used at the lowest possible energy levels.

Finally, the most important aid in the successful treatment of digitalis intoxication is prevention through patient education. This method allows the earliest recognition of potential problems and is especially important in view of the duration of digitalis use.

References

1. Beller GA, Smith TW, Abermann WH, Haber E, Hood WB Jr: Digitalis intoxication: A prospective clinical study with serum level correlations. N Engl J Med *284*:989, 1971.
2. National Center for Health Statistics: Yearly Report. Washington DC, US Government Printing Office, 1977.
3. Smith TW: Digitalis—A bicentennial progress report. West J Med *145*(1):92, 1986.
4. Smith TW, Antman EM, Friedman PL, Blatt CM, Marsh JD: Digitalis glycosides: Mechanisms and manifestations of toxicity (in three parts). Prog Cardiovasc Dis, Part I *26*:413, 1984; Part II *26*:495, 1984; Part III *27*:26, 1984.
5. Schwartz A: Is the cell membrane Na^+-K^+-ATPase enzyme system the pharmacological receptor for digitalis? Circ Res *39*:1, 1976.
6. Doherty JE: Digitalis glycosides: Pharmacokinetics and their clinical implications. Ann Intern Med *79*:229, 1973.
7. Doherty JE, deSoyza N, Kane JJ, Bissett JK, Murphy ML: Clinical pharmacokinetics of digitalis glycosides. Prog Cardiovasc Dis *21*:141, 1978.
8. Lindenbaum J, Rund DG, Butler VP Jr, Tse-Eng D, Saha JR: Inactivation of digoxin by the gut flora: Reversal by antibiotic therapy. N Engl J Med *305*:789, 1981.
9. Smith TW, Haber E: Digitalis. N Engl J Med *289*:945, 1973.
10. Arnold SB, Byrd RC, Meister W, et al: Long-term digitalis therapy improves left ventricular function in heart failure. N Engl J Med *303*:1443, 1980.
11. Lee DCS, Johnson RA, Bingham JB, et al: Heart failure in outpatients: A randomized trial of digoxin versus placebo. N Engl J Med *306*:699, 1982.
12. Fleg JL, Gottlieb SH, Lakatta EG: Is digoxin really important in treatment of compensated heart failure? A placebo-controlled crossover study in patients with sinus rhythm. Am J Med *73*:244, 1982.
13. Ware JA, Snow E, Luchi JM, Luchi RJ: Effect of digoxin on elderly patients with congestive heart failure. J Am Geriatrics Soc *32*:631, 1984.
14. Mulrow CD, Feussner JR, Velez R: Reevaluation of digitalis efficacy: New light on an old leaf. Ann Intern Med *101*:113, 1984.
15. Braunwald E: Effects of digitalis on the normal and the failing heart. J Am Coll Cardiol *5*:51A, 1985.

16. Smith TW: Drug therapy: Digitalis glycosides. N Engl J Med *288*:719, 1973.
17. Rosen MR, Wit AL, Hoffman B: Electrophysiology and pharmacology of cardiac arrhythmias. IV. Cardiac antiarrhythmic and toxic effects of digitalis. Am Heart J *89*:391, 1975.
18. Rosen MR: Cellular electrophysiology of digitalis toxicity. J Am Coll Cardiol *5*:22A, 1975.
19. Marcus FI: Current concepts of digoxin therapy. Mod Concepts Cardiovasc Dis *45*:77, 1976.
20. Inglefinger JA, Goldman P: The serum digitalis concentration—Does it diagnose digitalis toxicity? N Engl J Med *294*:867, 1976.
21. Lasagna L: How useful are serum digitalis measurements? (editorial). N Engl J Med *294*:898, 1976.
22. Sarangi A, Tripathy N, Lal D, Patnaik BC, Swain AK: Study of serum digoxin status in digitoxicity by radioimmunoassay. Am Heart J *99*:289, 1980.
23. Graves SW, Brown B, Valdes RJ: An endogenous digoxin-like substance in patients with renal impairment. Ann Intern Med *99*:604, 1983.
24. Marcus FI: Use of digitalis in acute myocardial infarction (editorial). Circulation *62*:17, 1980.
25. Duhme DW, Greenblatt DJ, Koch-Weser J: Reduction of digoxin toxicity associated with measurement of serum levels. Ann Intern Med *80*:516, 1974.
26. Brown DD, Juhl RP: Decreased bioavailability of digoxin due to antacids and kaolin-pectin. N Engl J Med *295*:1034, 1976.
27. Marcus FI: Pharmacokinetic interactions between digoxin and other drugs. J Am Coll Cardiol *5*:82A, 1985.
28. Hager WD, Fenster P, Mayersohn M, Perrier D, Graves P, Marcus FI, Goldman S: Digoxin-quinidine interaction: Pharmacokinetic evaluation. N Engl J Med *300*:1238, 1979.
29. Bigger JT Jr: The quinidine-digoxin interaction—What do we know about it? N Engl J Med *301*:779, 1979.
30. Ochs HR, Pabst J, Greenblatt DJ, Dengler HJ: Noninteraction of digitoxin and quinidine. N Engl J Med *303*:672, 1980.
31. Hirsh PD, Weiner JH, North RL: Further insights into digoxin-quinidine interaction: Lack of correlation between serum digoxin concentration and inotropic state of the heart. Am J Cardiol *46*:863, 1980.
32. Fenster PE, White NW Jr, Hanson CD: Pharmacokinetic evaluation of the digoxin-amiodarone interaction. J Am Coll Cardiol *5*:108, 1985.
33. Nademanee K, Kannan R, et al: Amiodarone-digoxin interaction: Clinical significance, time course of development, potential pharmacokinetic mechanisms and therapeutic implications. J Am Coll Cardiol *4*:111, 1984.
34. Leahey EB, Reiffel JA, Giardina E-GV, Bigger JT Jr: The effect of quinidine and other oral antiarrhythmic drugs on serum digoxin. Ann Intern Med *92*:605, 1980.
35. Schwartz JB, Raizner A, Akers S: The effect of nifedipine on serum digoxin concentrations in patients. Am Heart J *107*:669, 1984.
36. Klein HO, Land R, Segni ED, Kapinsky E: Verapamil-digoxin interaction. N Engl J Med *302*:160, 1980.
37. Zatuchni J: Verapamil-digoxin interaction. Am Heart J *108*:412, 1984.
38. Wilkerson RD, Mockridge PB, Massing GK: Effects of selected drugs on serum digoxin concentration in dogs. Am J Cardiol *45*:1201, 1980.
39. Surawicz B: Factors affecting tolerance to digitalis. J Am Coll Cardiol *5*:69A, 1985.
40. Iesaka Y, Aonuma K, Gosselin AJ, et al: Susceptibility of infarcted canine hearts to digitalis—toxic ventricular tachycardia. J Am Coll Cardiol *2*:45, 1983.
41. Muller JE, Turi ZG, Stone PH, et al: Digoxin therapy and mortality after myocardial infarction: Experience in the MILIS study. N Engl J Med *314*:265, 1986.
42. Sonnenblick M, Abraham AS, Meshulam Z, Eylath U: Correlation between manifestations of digoxin toxicity and serum digoxin, calcium, potassium, and magnesium concentrations and arterial pH. Br Med J *286*:1089, 1983.
43. Reisdorff EJ, Clark MR, Walters BL: Acute digitalis poisoning: The role of intravenous magnesium sulfate. J Emerg Med *4*:463, 1986.
44. Fisch C, Knoebel SB: Digitalis cardiotoxicity. J Am Coll Cardiol *5*:91A, 1985.
45. Kastor JA: Atrioventricular block. N Engl J Med *292*:462, 1975.
46. Webster J, Newnham DM, Petrie JC: Accidental digitalis poisoning due to drinking herbal tea. Br Med J *290*:1624, 1985.
47. Wamboldt FS, Jefferson JW, Wamboldt MZ: Digitalis intoxication misdiagnosed as depression by primary care physicians. Am J Psychiatr *143*:219, 1986.
48. Greenblatt DJ, Bolognini V, Koch-Weser J, Harmatz JS: Pharmacokinetic approach to the clinical use of lidocaine intravenously. JAMA *236*:273, 1976.
49. Koch-Weser J: Drug therapy—bretylium. N Engl J Med *300*:473, 1979.
50. Ditchey RV, Karliner JS: Safety of electrical cardioversion in patients without digitalis toxicity. Ann Intern Med *95*:676, 1981.
51. Reza MJ, Kovick RB, Shine KI, Pearce ML: Massive intravenous digoxin overdosage. N Engl J Med *291*:777, 1974.
52. Warren SE, Fanestil DD: Digoxin overdose—Limitations of hemoperfusion-hemodialysis treatment. JAMA *242*:2100, 1979.
53. Smith TW, Haber E, Yeatman L, Butler VP Jr: Reversal of advanced digoxin intoxication with Fab fragments of digoxin-specific antibodies. N Engl J Med *294*:797, 1976.
54. Smith TW, Butler VP Jr, Haber E, et al: Treatment of life-threatening digitalis intoxication with digoxin-specific Fab antibody fragments. N Engl J Med *307*:1357, 1982.
55. Wenger TL, Butler VP Jr, Haber E, Smith TW: Treatment of 63 severely digitalis-toxic patients with digoxin-specific antibody fragments. J Am Coll Cardiol *5*:118A, 1985.
56. Burroughs-Wellcome: Digoxin-immune Fab (ovine), Digibind (package insert).

CHAPTER 91
BETA-ADRENOCEPTOR BLOCKER POISONING

Neal L. Benowitz, M.D.

Beta-adrenergic receptor blocking drugs are widely used in medicine for the treatment of hypertension, arrhythmias, angina pectoris, open-angle glaucoma, migraine headaches, and various other disorders, and for prophylaxis against sudden death after myocardial infarction. Beta-adrenergic receptor blocking drugs are among the top-selling drugs in the world, and among cardiovascular drug overdoses β-blockers overdoses are relatively common. Although most patients with β-blocker poisoning or toxicity during therapeutic dosing respond well to treatment and recover fully, a significant number of cases are life-threatening and present a therapeutic challenge to the clinician, and many fatalities have been reported.[1]

PATHOPHYSIOLOGY OF β-BLOCKER POISONING

Pharmacology of β-Adrenergic Receptor Blockers

Actions of β-blockers can best be understood by considering the distribution and function of β-adrenergic receptors in the body (Table 91–1). Receptors have been classified as β_1 or β_2 on the basis of relatively selective effects of particular agonists and antagonists on groups of organ systems. It should be recognized that β_1, or cardioselective antagonists such as metoprolol and atenolol, are relatively selective only in therapeutic doses; with increasing doses and after overdose in particular, generalized β-blockade occurs.

The normal physiologic functions mediated by β-adrenergic receptors are as follows: Beta-1 stimulation increases sinoatrial rate; myocardial contractility; conduction velocity in atrial tissue, atrioventricular node, and ventricular tissue; and nonsinus node pacemaker automaticity. Renin is released from the kidney.

Beta-2 stimulation dilates bronchial smooth muscle and arterioles in skeletal muscle; relaxes the gravid uterus; stimulates insulin secretion; and increases lactic acid production, lipolysis, and glycogenolysis. As a consequence of β_2 effects, blood glucose and free fatty acid concentrations rise. Recent evidence also indicates that β_2 stimulation affects body distribution of potassium, moving potassium into cells and decreasing the blood potassium concentration.[2]

Adverse Consequences of β-Blockade

Beta-adrenergic receptor blockers reverse the actions of β stimulation. Most patients tolerate therapeutic doses of β-blockers quite well; serious adverse reactions (Table 91–2) usually result from the interaction of β-blockade and underlying medical illness or other drugs.[3] For example, cardiac failure, including pulmonary edema, and hypotension occur primarily in patients who have poor ventricular function and who are dependent on sympathetic drive to maintain adequate cardiac output. Atrioventricular conduction disturbances and sinus node dysfunction resulting in bradyarrhythmias occur most often in persons who have underlying intraventricular conduction or sinus node disease or who are taking other drugs (such as calcium block-

Table 91–1. DISTRIBUTION AND FUNCTION OF β-ADRENERGIC RECEPTORS

β_1	β_2
Heart (rate and contractility; conduction velocity)	Bronchus (dilation)
Kidney (plasma renin release)	Blood vessels (arteriolar dilation)
Eye (aqueous humor production)	Intestinal smooth muscle (relaxation)
	Uterus (relaxation)
	Pancreas (insulin release)
	Adipose tissue (lipolysis)
	Liver (glycogenolysis; lactic acid production)
	Potassium distribution (into cells)

Table 91–2. ADVERSE REACTIONS RESULTING FROM β-ADRENERGIC RECEPTOR BLOCKADE

Hypotension, circulatory collapse
Cardiac failure, acute pulmonary edema
Sinus bradycardia
Atrioventricular nodal conduction delay, heart block
Bronchospasm
Raynaud's phenomenon, intermittent claudication
Hypoglycemia
Depression, somnolence, insomnia, vivid dreams, delirium
Fatigue, weakness, impotence*

*May reflect depression rather than consequence of β-blockade.

ers) that also depress conduction. Bronchospasm usually occurs in persons with asthma or chronic obstructive pulmonary disease (although the history of such a disorder may be in the distant past or may be atypical).[4] Cold extremities and Raynaud's phenomenon occasionally occur in persons with no apparent vascular disease, but the development of intermittent claudication suggests peripheral arterial obstructive disease. The mechanism of vascular insufficiency is believed to be antagonism of β_2-mediated arteriolar dilation with persisting α-mediated arteriolar constriction.

Hypoglycemia has been described during therapeutic use of β-blockers in children after a period of reduced oral intake, in diabetic patients concomitantly receiving insulin or other hypoglycemic drugs, and in uremic patients. In humans receiving therapeutic doses of β-blockers, the magnitude of hypoglycemia induced by insulin is unaffected, but the time course of recovery and hence the duration of hypoglycemia is prolonged by β_2-blockers, presumably by blocking glycogenolysis. Insulin-induced hypoglycemia in the presence of nonselective β-blockade may be associated with severe hypertension due to epinephrine release with unopposed α-adrenergic vasoconstriction.

Differences Among β-Adrenergic Blocking Drugs

Manifestations of overdose with a β-blocking drug include the consequences of β-blockade, common to all drugs in this class, and other pharmacologic effects, which differ among different preparations. Table 91–3 shows the β-blockers currently in use in the United States and the differences in pharmacologic properties that can influence the effects of poisoning.[5] For example, an overdose with a β-blocker such as propranolol, which has membrane-depressant effects, may result in depressed myocardial contractility and intraventricular conduction, hypotension, and heart block. Membrane-active drugs also are more likely to affect the central nervous system and cause sedation, coma, and convulsions. An overdose of a β-blocker such as pindolol, which has partial receptor agonist activity, can cause tachycardia and hypertension. Sotalol, which has type III antiarrhythmic activity and prolongs the Q-T interval in a dose-dependent manner, may

Table 91–3. PHARMACOLOGIC AND PHARMACOKINETIC DIFFERENCES AMONG β-BLOCKERS

DRUG	CARDIO-SELECTIVE	MEMBRANE DEPRESSION	PARTIAL AGONIST	HALF-LIFE (hr)	Cl (m/min)	Vd (L/kg)	PER CENT PROTEIN BOUND
Acebutolol*	+	+	+	7	300	1.2	20
Alprenolol*	0	+	+ +	2–3	450	1.1	76
Atenolol	+	0	0	6–9	180 (R)	1.1	3
Esmolol†	+	0	0	7 min	18000	2.5	56
Labetolol‡	0	+	0	3–5	1500	5.6	50
Metoprolol*	+	+	0	3–4	1100	5.5	8
Nadolol	0	0	0	14–24	200 (R)	1.9	28
Oxyprenolol	0	+	+ +	2	200	1.3	92
Pindolol	0	+	+ + +	3–4	500	1.2	50
Propranolol*	0	+ +	0	2–6	1000	2.8	93
Sotalol	0	0	0	7–15	160 (R)	1.3	1
Timolol	0	0	0	4–5	500	1.7	60

*Active metabolites.
†For intravenous use only.
‡Additional α-blocking activity.
R = primary renal excretion.

produce ventricular tachycardia (often of the torsades de pointes type) or ventricular fibrillation.[6]

Depression, insomnia, and vivid dreams are relatively common adverse effects and are probably due to neural membrane effects rather than to effects on the β-adrenergic receptor. The lipophilic and less membrane-active drugs, such as nadolol and atenolol, may have fewer effects on the central nervous system.

CLINICAL PRESENTATION OF β-ADRENERGIC RECEPTOR BLOCKER OVERDOSE

Cardiopulmonary Effects

Both β-adrenergic receptor blockade and nonadrenergic actions contribute to the cardiovascular manifestations of a massive overdose (Fig. 91–1, Table 91–4). The main features are bradycardia and hypotension. As discussed earlier, pulmonary edema and bronchospasm may also occur, but usually in persons with underlying myocardial disease and obstructive airways disease, respectively.

Arrhythmias result as a consequence of β-blockade and membrane depression. In therapeutic doses, PR internal prolongation and slowing of the sinus rate are observed. At higher doses, sinus bradycardia, atrioventricular block, A-V junctional rhythm, loss of atrial activity, widening of the QRS complex, idioventricular rhythm, and asystole have

Table 91–4. CLINICAL MANIFESTATIONS OF β-BLOCKER OVERDOSE

Cardiovascular
Arrhythmias and electrocardiographic abnormalities
Sinus, atrioventricular nodal, ventricular bradycardia
Atrioventricular block (all degrees)
Loss of atrial activity
Widened QRS
Q–T prolongation (sotalol)
Bundle branch block
Ventricular arrhythmias (usually bradycardia-dependent escape rhythms; ventricular tachycardia, often torsades de pointes, with sotalol)
Asystole
Hypotension, cardiogenic shock
Tachycardia and hypertension (pindolol)
Central nervous system
Depressed consciousness, delirium, coma
Convulsions
Respiratory depression
Other
Bronchospasm
Pulmonary edema
Hyperkalemia
Hypoglycemia

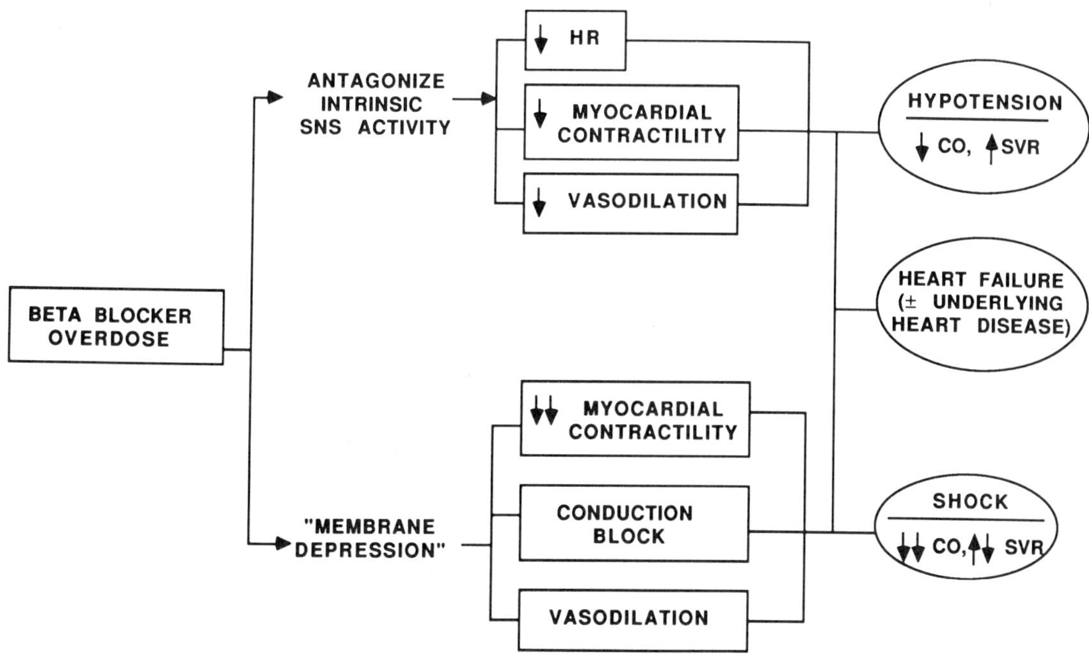

Figure 91–1. Pathophysiology of β-blocker overdose.

been observed. Sotalol in particular may produce Q-T prolongation, both in therapeutic doses and in overdose. Ventricular tachycardia of the torsades de pointes type has been reported during therapy with this drug. Because of its intrinsic sympathomimetic activity, pindolol produces less heart rate slowing than other β-blockers and may even cause tachycardia.

Arrhythmias due to β-blockers may be observed with therapeutic doses in patients with intrinsic conduction disease or those who are taking other drugs that depress cardiac conduction. For example, complete heart block may develop in patients with atrioventricular nodal disease. Because the lower conduction system is not affected by β-blockers, a narrow complex junctional escape rhythm is expected. Bradyarrhythmias including asystole have been observed in patients receiving β-blockers and intravenous verapamil. Details of this and other drug interactions involving β-blockers are described in a later section.

Hypotension most often results from bradycardia and reduced myocardial contractility, which combine to reduce cardiac output. In anesthetized dogs intoxicated with metoprolol, the fall in cardiac output was associated with increases in pulmonary capillary wedge pressure and central venous pressure, findings consistent with impairment of myocardial contractility.[7] Of note is that the greatest decline in heart rate occurred early in the course of metoprolol intoxication, whereas blood pressure did not decrease until much later when the concentration of metoprolol in the blood was much higher. This observation suggests that hypotension is primarily related to depressed contractility and shows that the magnitude of heart rate slowing is not a useful indicator of the severity of poisoning. Thus, high doses of β-blockers, presumably owing to membrane-depressant actions, may result in profound myocardial depression and cardiogenic shock.

In dogs, peripheral vascular resistance increased shortly after initial dosing with metoprolol, but as intoxication became more severe, resistance fell toward the baseline value.[7] The initial vasoconstriction presumably resulted from β_2-blockade or as a reflex response to hypotension, but with higher doses membrane effects resulted in vasodilation, which contributed to hypotension.

Occasionally, severe or fatal reactions to β-blockers occur after only small doses. For example, cases of profound shock, often with severe bradycardia, or pulmonary edema have occurred with doses of propranolol as low as 10 mg orally.[8] Likewise, severe or even fatal asthma has been noted after small doses of propranolol in people, usually with a history of asthma (sometimes remotely in the past) or with chronic obstructive lung disease.[4, 9] Most patients with β-blocker overdose continue to breathe despite cardiovascular toxicity; however, respiratory arrest can occur following an overdose. A study of experimental β-blocker poisoning in anesthetized but spontaneously breathing rats showed that with progressively severe intoxication respiratory arrest appeared before cardiac failure.[10] Rats who were artificially ventilated tolerated larger doses of β-blockers before death, which was due to circulatory failure.

Central Nervous System Manifestations

Mild or moderate overdoses are typically associated with lethargy. Severe overdoses may result in delirium, coma, convulsions, and respiratory arrest. Coma due to β-blocker overdose is preceded by evidence of cardiovascular toxicity. In the absence of such toxicity other causes for coma should be sought. A recent case report describes convulsions related to a therapeutic infusion of esmolol.[11]

Gastrointestinal Disturbances

Gastrointestinal disturbances, such as indigestion or diarrhea, are occasionally experienced by patients receiving therapeutic doses of β-blockers. An interesting complication of propranolol overdose is esophageal spasm that obstructs insertion or withdrawal of an orogastric or nasogastric tube.[12] The presumed mechanism is inhibition of β-adrenoceptor-mediated smooth muscle relaxation with unopposed α-mediated muscle contraction.

Metabolic Disturbances

Hypoglycemia is not common but has been reported after β-blocker intoxication in children. Hypoglycemia should be considered a potential cause of coma and convulsions.

Hyperkalemia is of theoretical concern because of the inhibition of potassium movement into cells by β_2-blockade. In patients taking propranolol, muscular activity, such as intense physical exercise, can produce hyperkalemia. Presumably the same effect would occur in patients with convulsions in the presence of β-blockers.

RELEVANT PHARMACOKINETICS

Understanding the pharmacokinetics (Table 91–3) of β-blockers is useful in anticipating the time course of poisoning and in designing therapy for patients overdosed with various β-blocking drugs. (For a recent review of the pharmacokinetics of β-blockers the reader is referred to reference 13.) Lipophilicity is a useful way to classify β-blocking drugs. More lipophilic drugs tend to be distributed extensively in body tissues and to be extensively and rapidly metabolized by the liver. Less lipophilic drugs are distributed less extensively to tissues and are excreted largely unmetabolized by the kidneys.

Propranolol is the most lipophilic of the currently available β-blockers. Metoprolol, timolol, and pindolol are moderately lipophilic, whereas nadolol and atenolol are the least lipophilic.

The more highly lipophilic drugs are well absorbed but undergo extensive first-pass metabolism. For example, propranolol is completely absorbed but has an average of 30 per cent bioavailability. The bioavailability of drugs with high first-pass metabolism is quite variable among people and is susceptible to changes in hepatic and splanchnic hemodynamics. In contrast, nadolol is only about 30 per cent absorbed, but all of it is bioavailable. Timolol is marketed both as a tablet and as an ophthalmic solution for treatment of glaucoma. It should be noted that even after ophthalmic application, significant systemic absorption with toxicity typical of β-blockade (bradycardia, hypotension, and bronchospasm) can occur.

Propranolol and metoprolol are eliminated almost entirely through metabolism by the liver, whereas nadolol and atenolol are eliminated by the kidney. Acebutolol and pindolol are eliminated by both metabolism and renal excretion. Half-lives of the metabolized drugs tend to be shorter (i.e., propranolol half-life is 3 to 6 hours) than those of drugs excreted by the kidney (nadolol half-life is 14 to 24 hours).

Protein binding does not correlate well with lipophilicity. Propranolol and oxyprenolol are extensively bound (93 per cent); the others are more weakly bound.

Pharmacokinetic differences have therapeutic implications. For example, drugs with relatively short half-lives, such as propranolol, assuming normal metabolism, are eliminated nearly completely within 24 hours. Thus most patients are substantially recovered within 1 to 2 days of an overdose of propranolol. In contrast, drugs such as nadolol, which have long half-lives, can be expected to persist in the body with attendant toxicity for several days.

Hemodynamic complications of an overdose with β-blockers can affect disposition kinetics. For example, propranolol reduces hepatic blood flow and the metabolism of some other rapidly metabolized drugs such as lidocaine. With severely depressed circulatory function, reduced hepatic blood flow as well as hepatocellular damage might result in delayed metabolism of propranolol itself or of coingested drugs. Hypotension is also associated with reduced renal blood flow and reduced glomerular filtration rate, which might retard excretion of nadolol or atenolol and prolong the course of intoxication with these drugs.

Pharmacokinetic considerations may be useful in predicting the usefulness of accelerated drug removal techniques. Lipophilic drugs, such as propranolol, which have large volumes of distribution, rapid intrinsic metabolism, and extensive protein binding, are not appreciably removed by either hemodialysis or hemoperfusion. However, less lipophilic drugs such as nadolol, which have a smaller volume of distribution, a relatively low intrinsic clearance, and low protein binding, are good candidates for hemodialysis or hemoperfusion.

Laboratory Toxicology

There is no clear relationship between blood or plasma levels of β-blockers and the outcome of poisoning. A summary of toxic and fatal plasma concentrations is found in Table 91–5.

Table 91–5. LABORATORY TOXICOLOGY OF β-BLOCKERS

	PLASMA CONCENTRATIONS (mg/L)	
	Severe Poisoning with Survival	*Fatality*
Acebutalol	17.0	21.5
Alprenolol	1.3	1.3
Atenolol	2.1	—
Labetalol	11.1	—
Metoprolol	18.0	50.0–56.6
Nadolol	—	—
Oxyprenolol	3.1	10.0
Pindolol	1.5	—
Propranolol	4.7	0.4–28.0
Sotalol	17.2	40.0
Timolol	—	—

(Adapted from Heath A: β-adrenoceptor blocker toxicity: Clinical features and therapy. Am J Emerg Med 2:518–525, 1984; and Weinstein RS: Recognition and management of poisoning with beta-adrenergic blocking agents. Ann Emerg Med *13*:1123–1131, 1984.)

DRUG INTERACTIONS INVOLVING BETA BLOCKERS

Pharmacokinetic Interactions

Although many pharmacokinetic interactions involving β-blockers have been described (Table 91–6), they are not perceived as creating a substantial therapeutic problem. This perception results from the difficulty of appreciating inadequate dosing in patients with dynamic diseases such as angina or hypertension, because of the high toxic-therapeutic ratio, and because of the intrinsic wide individual variability in the pharmacokinetics of many of the β-blockers. However, pharmacokinetic interactions can be of substantial magnitude and should be considered when there is unexpected toxicity.

For β-blockers with a high presystemic (first-pass) metabolism, interacting drugs that affect the rate of metabolism will influence both bioavailability and systemic clearance. When bioavailability is low owing to extensive first-pass metabolism, small changes in clearance may have large effects on bioavailability. For example, phenytoin, phenobarbital, and rifampin accelerate the metabolism of propranolol and metoprolol, resulting in reduced bioavailability of the latter β-blockers. Half-life after absorption may or may not be shortened owing to the concomitant increase in systemic clearance. Conversely, cimetidine decreases the metabolism and increases the bioavailability of propranolol and metoprolol. As a consequence, excessive bradycardia associated with high levels of propranolol may result when cimetidine is added to propranolol therapy.[14]

Hydralazine has unusual effects on propranolol kinetics. Both systemic clearance and bioavailability increase.[15] Extraction of propranolol by the liver is high, so that propranolol clearance is regarded as being dependent on hepatic blood flow. Hydralazine increases systemic clearance of propranolol by increasing cardiac output and hepatic blood flow. However, hydralazine may also increase bioavailability owing to rapid delivery of the drug to the liver and saturation of metabolic pathways. The magnitude of the increased bioavailability far exceeds the change in systemic clearance. As a result, propranolol levels increase in the presence of hydralazine (and presumably other vasodilators).

The β-blockers that are eliminated by renal excretion are not subject to metabolic interactions but are sensitive to changes in renal function. Drugs that might affect renal function, such as nonsteroidal anti-inflammatory drugs, could, therefore, influence the elimination rate of renally excreted β-blockers.

Pharmacodynamic Interactions

Adverse drug interactions most commonly occur in people who are taking other myocardial depressant drugs. Among these are the calcium entry blockers and type I antiarrhythmic drugs, particularly disopyramide. Of the calcium entry blockers, verapamil has been implicated in adverse interactions with β-blockers most often, presumably because among the calcium blockers verapamil has the greatest myocardial depressant activity at the usual therapeutic doses. Most instances of hypotension or asystole have occurred in patients taking β-blockers following intravenous verapamil, possibly related to high circulating levels of verapamil after rapid administration.[16, 17] Nifedipine or diltiazem combined with β-blockers are usually well tolerated. However, in patients with depressed cardiac function, hypotension or cardiac failure may occur with these combinations as well.[18, 19] In high-risk patients on β-blockers, verapamil is best avoided; other

Table 91–6. DRUG INTERACTIONS INVOLVING β-BLOCKERS

DRUG	INTERACTING DRUG	EFFECTS	PROBABLE MECHANISM	COMMENTS
All β-blockers	Verapamil and possibly other calcium entry blockers	Excessive bradycardia, complete heart block, asystole,* cardiac failure	Additive depression of myocardial conduction and contractility	Primarily seen in patients with pre-existing left ventricular dysfunction or conduction disturbance
	Amiodarone	Same as calcium entry blockers	Additive myocardial depressant and sympathetic blocking actions	
	Epinephrine, insulin, or oral hypoglycemic agents (hypoglycemia, epinephrine release)	Hypertension (stroke)	Unopposed α-adrenergic vasoconstriction	Primarily seen with nonselective β-blockers; possibly also with high doses of selective blockers
	Antacids, cholestyramine, colestipol	Reduced absorption	Binding in gut	Separate dosing by at least 1 hour
Propranolol and metoprolol	Phenytoin, phenobarbital, rifampin	Reduced bioavailability	Accelerated metabolism, increased first-pass metabolism	May need higher doses of propranolol
	Cimetidine	Increased bioavailability	Decreased first-pass metabolism	May need to decrease propranolol dose
	Hydralazine	Increased bioavailability, increased systemic clearance; variable effect on propranolol blood levels	Accelerated systemic metabolism; saturation of presystemic metabolism	Interaction is probably of hemodynamic nature; fixed relationship between propranolol and hydralazine dosing desirable
	Lidocaine	Propranolol may reduce lidocaine clearance, resulting in higher than expected levels; may occur with other β-blockers as well	Reduced liver blood flow; direct inhibition of metabolism	Reduce lidocaine infusion rate
Propranolol and pindolol	Indomethacin, possibly other NSAIDs	Reduced antihypertensive action of β-blockers	Inhibition of prostaglandin synthesis	Avoid combination if possible; if NSAIDs are necessary, monitor BP closely

*After IV verapamil

calcium entry blockers should be administered initially in low doses and under careful observation. Amiodarone has sympathetic blocking activity and may also have additive myocardial depressant effects with β-blockers.[20]

All β-blockers inhibit reflex tachycardia. This property is used therapeutically in combining β-blockers with vasodilators in the therapy of hypertension. However, instances of profound hypotension in patients receiving β-blockers followed by parenteral vasodilators such as intravenous hydralazine or diazoxide, and potentiation of postural hypotension due to prazosin have been reported.

A consequence of nonselective β-blockade is the epinephrine reversal phenomenon. In the absence of β-blockers, epinephrine increases systolic blood pressure slightly and decreases diastolic blood pressure. After pretreatment with propranolol, epinephrine produces marked systolic and diastolic hypertension.[21] Epinephrine alone constricts and dilates resistance blood vessels by stimulating α_1- and β_2-receptors, respectively. These actions counterbalance one another. Blocking β_2-receptors, as occurs with nonselective β-blockade, results in unopposed α_1 stimulation and therefore hypertension. In patients receiving nonselective β-blockers, epinephrine administered therapeutically or released endogenously (as in association with insulin-induced hypoglycemia or an epinephrine-secreting pheochromocytoma) may result in severe hypertension with cerebral vascular accident or myocardial injury or infarction.

MANAGEMENT OF β-BLOCKER OVERDOSE

General Considerations

Respiratory support, emesis or lavage, and administration of charcoal are indicated as for other drug ingestions (Table 91–7). Intensive monitoring of intoxicated patients must continue until it is clear that absorption of the toxicant from the gastrointestinal tract is

Table 91–7. MANAGEMENT OF BETA-BLOCKER OVERDOSE*

GENERAL MANAGEMENT
Support respiration
Emesis or lavage and charcoal
Glucose (hypoglycemia particularly prominent in children)
Correct hyperkalemia
Treat convulsions (diazepam, 5–10 mg in adults or 0.1–0.3 mg/kg/min in children, IV; if necessary, add phenobarbital or phenytoin.

ARRHYTHMIAS
Sinus bradycardia
- If hemodynamically stable, no specific therapy
- If hypotensive:
  - (1) atropine: 0.6 mg IV; if inadequate response, repeat every 3 min to total of 2–3 mg
  - (2) isoproterenol: begin 4 μg/min; may need very large doses (dose may be limited by peripheral vasodilation and hypotension)
  - (3) glucagon: 5–10 mg IV over 1 min, then 1–5 mg/hr infusion
  - (4) If unresponsive to above, pacemaker

Atrioventricular block with junctional or ventricular bradycardia:
- Pacemaker
- Atropine, isoproterenol, glucagon as above

Ventricular premature beats or tachycardia:
- If rhythm is related to bradyarrhythmias (i.e., escape rhythm), treat as discussed above.
- Lidocaine, phenytoin, bretylium, overdrive pacing
- Potassium (if hypokalemic, particularly with sotalol intoxication)
- Avoid type 1A or 1C antiarrhythmic drugs

HYPOTENSION
Normal saline: 200 ml every 10 min until 1000–2000 ml or evidence of pulmonary edema
Treat bradyarrhythmias as discussed above
If unresponsive to fluids (± dopamine or norepinephrine), administer glucagon (dose as for arrhythmia)
If still hypotensive:
1. Consider hemodynamic monitoring to guide further fluid therapy and measure SVR
2. Pressor drugs:
   - Normal or high SVR:
     - Isoproterenol
     - Dobutamine
     - Prenalteral
   - Low SVR:
     - Epinephrine
     - Dopamine
     - Norepinephrine

(*Note*: Combination of isoproterenol to increase heart rate and myocardial contractility and dopamine or norepinephrine to maintain vascular resistance is often necessary)
If intractable cardiogenic shock, insert intra-aortic balloon or cardiopulmonary bypass

ACCELERATED DRUG REMOVAL
Consider hemoperfusion or hemodialysis for acebutolol, atenolol, nadolol, or sotalol, particularly if there is evidence of renal insufficiency

*Drug doses for adults; for children reduce dose according to body weight.

complete and cardiovascular manifestations have resolved. It is particularly important to observe patients for an adequate period of time after ingestion of slow-release formulations that are available for some β-blockers. Intravenous glucose should be administered because hypoglycemia may complicate the overdose, particularly in children and diabetics. Serum potassium should be measured and, if necessary, hyperkalemia should be corrected. Convulsions usually respond to intravenous diazepam; phenytoin or phenobarbital should be added if seizures are unresponsive to diazepam.

Experimental Studies

Few studies have systematically evaluated therapy for β-blocker poisoning. One study in anesthetized dogs showed that prenalterol, a β_1-adrenoceptor agonist, reversed the depression of cardiac output and the elevation of pulmonary capillary wedge and central venous pressures induced by high doses of metoprolol.[7] Prenalterol-treated dogs survived, whereas control dogs died. Thus it appears that effective therapy of severe β-blocker poisoning rests with the ability to reverse myocardial depression. Another study compared a number of therapies in anesthetized, ventilated rats intoxicated with a continuous infusion of propranolol.[22] With this preparation heart rate declined and blood pressure fell, resulting in a decline in both cardiac output and peripheral vascular resistance. Isoproterenol was most effective in reversing both hypotension and bradycardia. Dopamine, norepinephrine, and epinephrine reversed the hypotension but did not affect heart rate. Glucagon and theophylline increased heart rate but did not raise blood pressure. Atropine was ineffective.

Glucagon

Glucagon is a pancreatic polypeptide that, acting at a site distinct from the β-receptor, activates myocardial adenyl cyclase, thereby stimulating cyclic AMP synthesis and producing effects in the heart similar to those of β-agonists. Glucagon increases myocardial contractility and heart rate, even in the presence of β-blockers (Fig. 91–2).[23] In addition, glucagon decreases vascular resistance, which may help to improve cardiac output if vascular resistance (afterload) is high. Glucagon has been used successfully in many cases of β-blocker poisoning.[24–26] The response to glucagon is sometimes dramatic, and the drug should be given early in the course of severe β-blocker overdose. Effects of a single 5-mg dose of glucagon are generally observed within 5 to 10 minutes and last for 15 to 30 minutes. If no response is seen in 10 minutes a larger dose (up to 10 mg) should be administered. Once a beneficial response is observed, a constant infusion (1 to 5 mg/hr) may be necessary to sustain the benefit. Major side effects of glucagon are vomiting and hyperglycemia.

Management of Arrhythmias

Treatment of β-blocker-induced arrhythmias is summarized in Table 91–7. Sinus bradycardia without hypotension requires no specific treatment; with hypotension, administration of atropine followed by isoproterenol or intracardiac pacing is indicated. Because excessive parasympathetic tone is not a major factor in the pathophysiology of β-blocker-induced bradycardia, atropine is not usually successful or adequate. Because of competitive blockade with β-blockers, enormously high doses of isoproterenol may be required to increase the heart rate. Doses as high as 1600 μg per minute have been administered to β-blocker-poisoned patients.[27] The maximum tolerable dose of isoproterenol may be limited by peripheral vasodilation and worsening hypotension before adequate heart rate acceleration is achieved. Glucagon may increase heart rate even when large doses of atropine and isoproterenol have failed.[28, 29] Advanced atrioventricular block is an indication for intracardiac pacing, which is usually successful. Of note are two recent reports of external cardiac pacing used to manage bradyarrhythmias induced by propranolol overdose.[30, 31] A slow atrioventricular rhythm, if hemodynamically compromising, should be treated with intravenous isoproterenol or glucagon or both, pending pacemaker insertion.

Ventricular premature beats, when frequent or occurring in runs, are best treated with lidocaine or, if unsuccessful, phenytoin. Type 1A and IC antiarrhythmic drugs may further depress myocardial function and

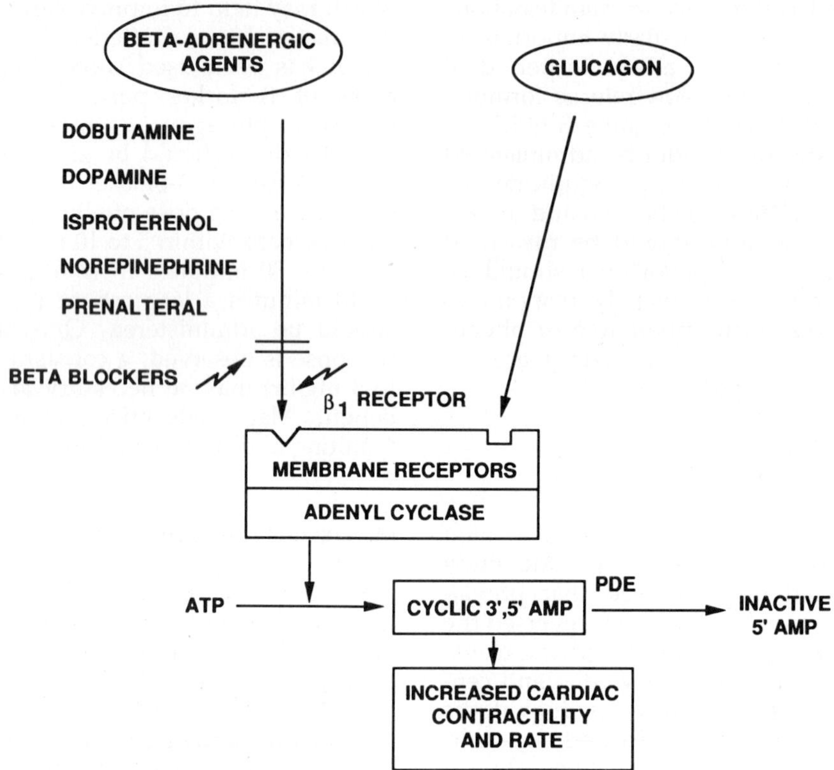

Figure 91–2. Interactions of β-adrenergic agonists and blockers, glucagon, and theophylline on myocardial cyclic 3′,5′-AMP concentrations and resultant cardiac inotropic and chronotropic effects. *AMP*, adenosine monophosphate; *ATP*, adenosine triphosphate; *PDE*, phosphodiesterase.

should be avoided. Polymorphous ventricular tachycardia in a patient with Q–T interval prolongation due to sotalol can be treated with an isoproterenol infusion or overdrive ventricular pacing.[32] Some cases of torsades de pointes related to sotalol occur in patients who are hypokalemic, in which case replacement of potassium is necessary.[33] Electrical cardioversion is indicated for ventricular tachycardia that is unresponsive to drug therapy or pacing, and for ventricular fibrillation.

Management of Hypotension

As discussed previously, hypotension due to β-blocker poisoning results in most cases from reduced cardiac output due to myocardial depression and bradycardia. Hypotension due to bradycardia or mild cardiac depression usually responds to intravenous fluids. Bradyarrhthmias should be corrected as described above. Management of hypotension in the presence of severe myocardial depression requires therapy with inotropic agents or extracorporeal circulatory assistance. A number of inotropic agents including isoproterenol, glucagon, dopamine, norepinephrine, epinephrine, dobutamine, and prenalterol have been administered to β-blocker-poisoned patients.[24, 26] Although no systematic comparisons have been conducted, a review of clinical reports suggests that glucagon and epinephrine are most effective at increasing blood pressure[24] (note: prenalterol was not evaluated in this review).

It is likely that combinations of pressor drugs will be needed to treat many patients. A β-adrenoceptor agonist such as isoproterenol or prenalterol may be needed to reverse myocardial depression, whereas a vasoconstrictor such as dopamine or norepinephrine may be needed to reverse vasodilation (due to actions of the ingested β-blocker or the therapy with β-agonists). It is logical to titrate β-agonists and vasoconstrictors separately to optimize hemodynamics. The success of epinephrine as a single agent is probably due to its combination of β- and α-agonist actions, which resemble a combination of isoproterenol and norepinephrine. Because of the competitive nature of the β-blockade, extremely high doses of catecholamines or other β-agonists are usually required for therapeutic benefit.

In the presence of pulmonary edema or after administration of large volumes of fluid, monitoring of intracardiac pressures and cardiac output is useful. Such monitoring will help to optimize fluid therapy and help in the selection of pressor drugs needed to optimize systemic vascular resistance. For example, if vascular resistance is high, isoproterenol or glucagon, which lower vascular resistance, would be logical choices. If vascular resistance is low, norepinephrine, epinephrine, or dopamine, all of which increase vascular resistance, might logically be selected.

A patient with cardiogenic shock who is unresponsive to pharmacologic therapy due to propranolol overdose was successfully resuscitated using an intraaortic balloon pump.[30] Mechanical circulatory assistance devices may be the only way to resuscitate the most severely intoxicated patients.

Accelerated Drug Removal

Hemodialysis or hemoperfusion is likely to be ineffective in accelerating the removal of many β-blockers because of their high lipid solubility, large volumes of distribution, or high endogenous clearance. Those β-blockers with reasonably small volumes of distribution (less than 2 liters/kg), low endogenous clearance (300 ml/min or less), and half-lives that are long enough to warrant consideration of accelerated drug removal include acebutolol, atenolol, nadolol, and sotalol. Absorption of some β-blockers to amberlite resin has been studied in vivo.[34] Atenolol (the only one of the group that is a good candidate for hemoperfusion) demonstrated an extraction ratio of 0.49. No data are available on adsorption to charcoal, nor have clinical reports of hemodialysis or hemoperfusion been published at this time.

References

1. Kulling P, Eleborg L, Persson H: β-adrenoceptor blocker intoxication: Epidemiological data. Prenalterol as an alternative in the treatment of cardiac dysfunction. Hum Toxicol 2:175–181, 1983.
2. Brown MJ, Brown DC, Murphy MB: Hypokalemia from beta$_2$-receptor stimulation by circulating epinephrine. N Engl J Med *309*:1414–1419, 1983.
3. Frishman W, Silverman R, Strom J, Elkayam U, Sonnenblock E: Clinical pharmacology of the new beta-adrenergic blocking drugs. Part 4. Adverse effects. Choosing a β-adrenoreceptor blocker. Am Heart J *98*:256, 1979.
4. Vedal S, Anantharaman A, Israel RH: Hidden asthmatic. NY State J Med 80:648–649, 1980.
5. Frishman WH: Clinical differences between beta-adrenergic blocking agents: Implications for therapeutic substitution. Am Heart J *113*:1190–1198, 1987.
6. Neuvonen PJ, Elonen E, Vuorenmaa T, Laakso M: Prolonged QT-interval and severe tachyarrhythmias, common features of sotalol intoxication. Int J Clin Pharmacol *20*:85–89, 1981.
7. Andersson T, Heath A, Mattsson H: Prenalterol as an antidote to massive doses of metoprolol—a cardiovascular study in the dog. Acta Med Scand Suppl *659*:71–88, 1982.
8. Beutler E, Fairbanks V, Fahey J: Hypotension after oral propranolol. Lancet 2:100, 1963.
9. Raine JM, Palazzo MG, Kerr JH, Sleight P: Near-fatal bronchospasm after oral nadolol in a young asthmatic and response to ventilation with halothane. Br Med J *282*:548–549, 1981.
10. Langemeijer J, de Wildt D, de Groot G, Sangster B: Respiratory arrest as main determinant of toxicity due to overdose with different β-blockers in rats. Acta Pharmacol Toxicol *57*:352–356, 1985.
11. Das G, Ferris JC: Generalized convulsions in a patient receiving ultrashort-acting beta-blocker infusion. Drug Intell Clin Pharm *22*:484–485, 1988.
12. Panos RJ, Tso E, Barish RA, Browne BJ: Esophageal spasm following propranolol overdose relieved by glucagon. Am J Emerg Med *4*:227–228, 1986.
13. Riddell JG, Harron DWG, Shanks RG: Clinical pharmacokinetics of β-adrenoceptor antagonists; An update. Clin Pharmacokinet *12*:305–320, 1987.
14. Donavan MA, Heagerty AM, Patel L, et al: Cimetidine and bioavailability of propranolol. Lancet *1*:164, 1981.
15. McLean AJ, Skews H, Bobik A, et al: Interaction between oral propranolol and hydralazine. Clin Pharmacol Ther *27*:726, 1980.
16. Benaim ME: Asystole after verapamil. Br Med J *15*:169, 1972.
17. Wayne VS, Harper RW, Laufer E, et al: Adverse interaction between beta-adrenergic blocking drugs and verapamil: Report of three cases. Aust NZ J Med *12*:285, 1982.
18. Anastassiades CJ: Nifedipine and beta-blocker drugs. Br Med J *281*:1251, 1980.
19. Opie LH, White DA: Adverse interaction between nifedipine and beta-blockade. Br Med J *281*:1462, 1980.
20. Derrida JP, Ollagnier J, Benaim R, et al: Amiodarone et propranolol: une association dangereus? Nouv Presse Med *8*:1429, 1979.
21. van Herwaarden CLA, Fennis JFM, Binkhort RA, et al: Haemodynamic effects of adrenaline during treatment of hypertensive patients with propranolol and metoprolol. Eur J Clin Pharmacol *12*:397, 1977.
22. Strubelt O: Evaluation of antidotes against the acute cardiovascular toxicity of propranolol. Toxicology 31:261–270, 1984.
23. Parmley WW, Glick G, Sonnenblick EH: Cardiovascular effects of glucagon in man. N Engl J Med *279*:12, 1968.

24. Weinstein RS: Recognition and management of poisoning with beta-adrenergic blocking agents. Ann Emerg Med *13*:1123–1131, 1984.
25. Peterson CD, Leeder JS, Sterner S: Glucagon therapy for β-blocker overdose. Drug Intell Clin Pharm *18*:394–398, 1984.
26. Heath A: β-Adrenoceptor blocker toxicity: Clinical features and therapy. Am J Emerg Med 2:518–525, 1984.
27. Lewis M, Kallenbach J, Germond C, Zaltzman M, Muller F, Steyn J, Zwi S: Survival following massive overdose of adrenergic blocking agents (acebutolol and labetalol). Eur Heart J *4*:328–332, 1983.
28. Salzberg MR, Gallagher EJ: Propranolol overdose. Ann Emerg Med *9*:26, 1980.
29. Agura ED, Wexler LF, Witzburg RA: Massive propranolol overdose. Am J Med *80*:755–757, 1986.
30. Lane AS, Woodward AC, Goldman MR: Massive propranolol overdose poorly responsive to pharmacologic therapy: Use of the intra-aortic balloon pump. Ann Emerg Med *16*:1381–1383, 1987.
31. Kenyon CJ, Aldinger GE, Joshipura P, Ziad GJ: Successful resuscitation using external cardiac pacing in beta adrenergic antagonist-induced bradyasystolic arrest. Ann Emerg Med *17*:711–713, 1988.
32. Totterman KJ, Turto H, Pellinen T: Overdrive pacing as treatment of sotalol-induced ventricular tachyarrhythmias (torsade de pointes). Acta Med Scand (Suppl) *663*:28–33, 1982.
33. McKibbin JK, Pocock WA, Barlow JB, Millar S, Obel IW: Sotalol, hypokalemia, syncope and torsade de pointes. Br Heart J *51*:157–162, 1984.
34. Heath A, Gabrielsson M, Redgardh G: Absorption of β-adrenoceptor antagonists to amberlite resin. Br J Clin Pharmacol *15*:290–492, 1983.

CHAPTER 92

CALCIUM ENTRY BLOCKER POISONING

Neal L. Benowitz, M.D.
Janice B. Schwartz, M.D.

Calcium entry blockers increasingly are being more widely used for treatment of angina pectoris, coronary spasm, supraventricular arrhythmias, hypertension, hypertrophic cardiomyopathy and migraine headache and are being evaluated for a number of other applications. Now, three calcium entry blockers are available in the United States: verapamil, diltiazem and nifedipine. Since worldwide the most information is available on these drugs, this chapter will focus on them. Several other calcium entry blockers are available elsewhere in the world and will eventually become available in the United States. Because calcium entry blockers can affect cardiovascular function profoundly, intoxication should always be considered potentially life-threatening.

PHARMACOLOGY AND PATHOPHYSIOLOGY
(Fig. 92–1)

Cardiac Electrophysiologic Actions

Calcium entry blockers inhibit the movement of calcium ions across cell membranes through calcium channels. Calcium entry into sinoatrial (SA) and atrioventricular (AV) nodal cells provides the slow inward current that results in depolarization. Calcium-mediated depolarization determines conduction time through the AV node. Calcium entry blockers, such as verapamil, are able to inhibit markedly the slow inward calcium current into myocardial cells.

In therapeutic doses, verapamil slows heart rate and prolongs AV conduction. The prolongation of AV conduction can be used to therapeutic benefit to interrupt AV nodal re-entry supraventricular tachyarrhythmias, and to slow the ventricular response rate to atrial fibrillation or atrial flutter. Excess verapamil may also depress phase 4 depolarization to the extent that sinus bradycardia or even sinus arrest may occur. Even at lower concentrations, verapamil may impair sinus node function in patients with underlying sinus node dysfunction. Excess verapamil also may cause marked prolongation of AV nodal conduction, which may result in advanced heart block, often with a narrow QRS escape rhythm, most likely of His-Purkinje cell origin. In this setting, beta-adrenergic

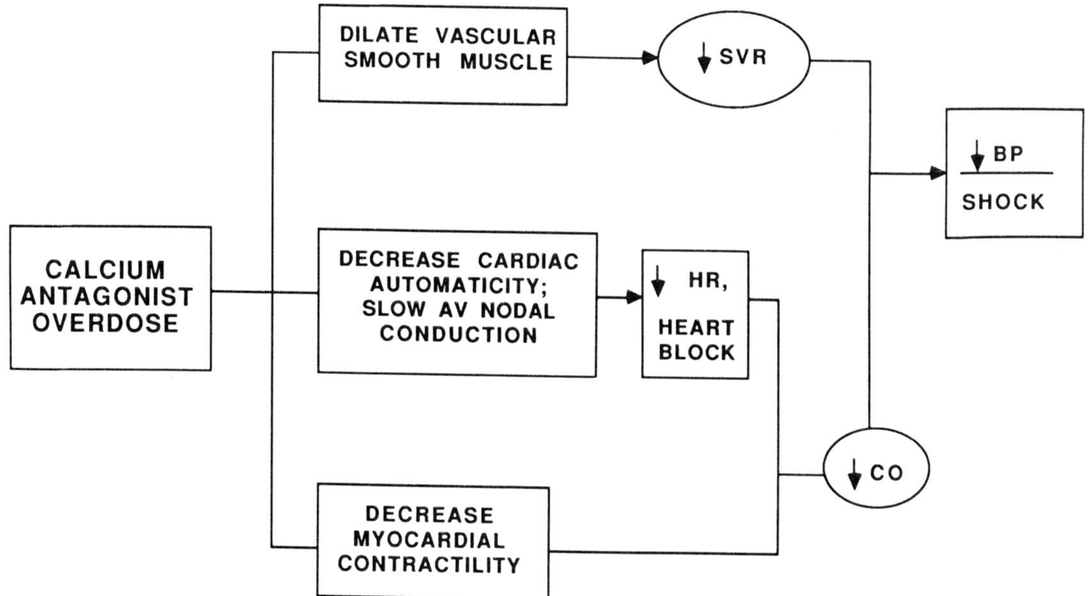

Figure 92–1. Pathophysiology of cardiovascular consequences of calcium antagonist overdose.

blocking drugs produce additional decreases in sinus and AV nodal activity and may also suppress the junctional escape rhythm, leading to failure of impulse generation and to asystole.

Myocardial Contractility

Calcium entry during phase 2 of cardiac depolarization triggers release of calcium bound to the sarcoplasmic reticulum, which in turn results in attachment of actin and myosin and to muscular contraction (Fig. 92–2). Calcium entry blockers impede the inward calcium current responsible for triggering contraction and may also affect binding of calcium within the cardiac cell. In therapeutic doses, calcium entry blockers depress contractility to some degree, but this depression is often counterbalanced by reflex sympathetic nervous activation, occurring in response to lowering of the blood pressure.

In toxic doses, or in therapeutic doses in subjects with depressed myocardial function or receiving additional myocardial depressant drugs, calcium entry blockers may result in significant depression of contractility with worsening of heart failure, acute pulmonary edema, or hypotension.

Vascular Smooth Muscle

Calcium entry blockers inhibit calcium-mediated contraction of vascular smooth muscle, similar to their effects on cardiac muscle. Calcium entry blockers also appear to inhibit calcium influx stimulated by alpha-adrenergic receptors and to interfere with intracellular binding and release of calcium. As a result, calcium entry blockers reduce arterial resistance and blood pressure. Reflex sympathetic neural activation with increased circulating catecholamines may lessen the degree of blood pressure lowering, especially during initial treatment. This has been noted most frequently with nifedipine.

Pharmacologic Differences Among Calcium Entry Blockers

Individual calcium entry blockers have different profiles of effect on the cardiovascular system—presumably because of different membrane sites of actions and different tissue affinities. These differences are summarized in Table 92–1. In brief, all calcium entry blockers can reduce blood pressure and are equally efficacious in treating hypertension. Nifedipine is the most potent vasodilator and has little appreciable in vivo effect on cardiac contractility or conduction. Verapamil and diltiazem depress cardiac contractility and cardiac output to a similar degree. Verapamil and diltiazem have the greatest effect on sinus node automaticity and AV nodal conduction. Nifedipine and other dihydropyridines have no appreciable negative chronotropic effects in vivo.

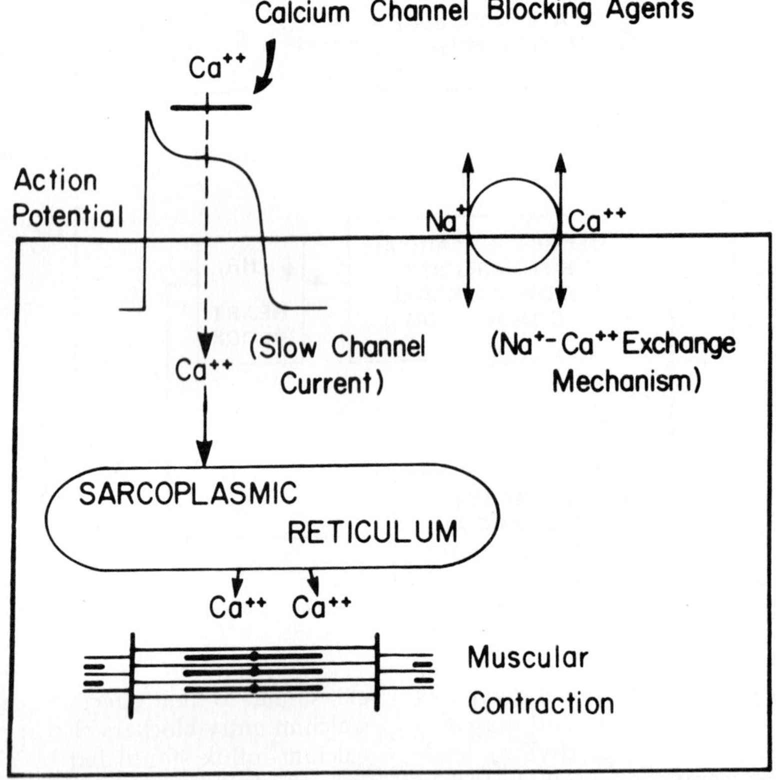

Figure 92–2. Role of calcium in excitation and contraction of myocardial cells. Calcium entry blockers inhibit these processes. (From Antman EM, Stone PH, Muller JE, et al: Calcium channel blocking agents in the treatment of cardiovascular disorders. Part I: Basic and clinical electrophysiologic effects. Ann Intern Med 93:875, 1980.)

In addition to calcium-blocking actions, verapamil also has postsynaptic alpha-adrenergic blocking activity, which may also contribute to vasodilatation.

Dose Response Considerations

Dose response studies performed in anesthetized dogs aid in understanding the time course of progression and resolution of calcium entry blocker overdose.[1] At low concentrations (about 50 ng/ml), verapamil increased the atrium-to-His bundle (A-H) conduction time, a measure of AV nodal refractoriness, and was associated with P-R prolongation. At high concentrations (about 200 ng/ml), second or third degree heart block occurred, and at somewhat higher concentrations (400 ng/ml), sinus arrest occurred. The threshold concentration for reduced contractility in dogs was about 150 ng/ml, and significant depression of cardiac output was seen at 300 to 400 ng/ml. The dose response curve may vary according to the anesthetic and autonomic state of the animal, but the sequence of progression of AV nodal blockade with increasing doses seems to be consistent.

Table 92–1. CLINICAL PHARMACOLOGIC DIFFERENCES AMONG CALCIUM ENTRY BLOCKERS

	RESTING HEART RATE	BLOOD PRESSURE	SYSTEMIC VASCULAR RESISTANCE	CARDIAC CONTRACTILITY	AV NODAL CONDUCTION
verapamil	↓	↓	↓	↓↓	↓↓↓
diltiazem	↓	↓	↓↓	↓	↓↓
nifedipine	↔ or ↑	↓↓	↓↓↓	±	±

For perspective, in humans the therapeutic concentration of verapamil is 15 to 100 ng/ml, and severe poisoning results from concentrations of several thousand nanograms per milliliter.[2–4] In the presence of beta-blockers, the cardiac dose response for verapamil and diltiazem may be shifted, so that calcium blockers have enhanced effects at low concentrations.[5, 6] Although concentration-response relationships may be well defined in experimental preparations, the individual response is highly variable.

Pathophysiology of Calcium Entry Blocker Toxicity in Specific Disease States

Severe toxicity may follow therapy with calcium entry blockers in conventional doses in certain disease states or in patients taking other drugs. Drug interactions are discussed later. Patients with sick sinus syndrome or AV nodal conduction disease may develop sinus arrest or high-grade atrioventricular block after small doses of verapamil or diltiazem. In patients with supraventricular tachycardia from Wolff-Parkinson-White syndrome, intravenous verapamil indirectly may enhance antegrade conduction down accessory AV pathways, resulting in an increased ventricular rate and potentially ventricular fibrillation and cardiac arrest.[7] Verapamil should be avoided in the presence of supraventricular tachycardia with pre-excited ventricular complexes. Neonates with supraventricular tachycardia and cardiac failure appear to be at high risk of complications from intravenous verapamil. Two reports describe eight infants, 2 to 6 weeks of age, who developed severe bradycardia and hypotension after 0.1 to 0.3 mg/kg of verapamil intravenously.[8, 9] Two of these children died. The authors of this report conclude that verapamil therapy should not be employed in treating supraventricular tachycardia in neonates.

Calcium entry blockers may produce life-threatening toxicity in patients with obstructive valvular disease or hypertrophic cardiomyopathy. Nifedipine administration was reported to cause acute pulmonary edema in patients with valvular aortic stenosis, presumably due to vasodilatation with the inability to appropriately increase cardiac output.[10]

Several patients have developed hypotension or pulmonary edema after verapamil or nifedipine treatment of hypertrophic cardiomyopathy.[11–14] Nifedipine, owing to vasodilatation and reflex sympathetic stimulation may increase left ventricular outflow obstruction and left ventricular filling pressures.[11] Verapamil may produce adverse affects by several mechanisms (Fig. 92–3). Vasodilatation resulting in increased outflow obstruction, hypotension, or pulmonary edema occurs as described for nifedipine. In addition, verapamil can produce hypotension by sinus node depression with decreased heart rate, AV block resulting in impaired ventricular filling and increased outflow obstruction, and direct myocardial depression. In a series of 233 patients receiving verapamil for long-term treatment of obstructive cardiomyopathy, 24 experienced AV dissociation (with junctional escape rhythm in 23 and ventricular rhythm in 1); 5 developed sinus arrest; 6 developed Wenckebach heart block; 17, pulmonary congestion; and 12, hypotension.[12] Four deaths in these patients (resulting from pulmonary edema, hypotension, and probable arrhythmias) were considered to be related to verapamil therapy. Most adverse effects in this population occur early in the course of treatment. It has been recommended to avoid verapamil in patients with hypertrophic cardiomyopathy and increased pulmonary capillary wedge pressure, a history of orthopnea, or paroxysmal nocturnal dyspnea (with or without obstruction); or low systolic blood pressure in the presence of outflow obstruction.

Reversal of Drug Effects by Calcium

It is logical that increasing extracellular calcium concentrations should reverse the effects of calcium entry blockers. However, as shown by animal studies, this is not always the case. In dogs intoxicated with verapamil, calcium fully reversed the depressed cardiac contractility.[15] Reversal was seen with an increase in serum calcium of about 2 mEq/L (equivalent to 4 mg/dl), which requires fairly large doses of calcium.

Calcium chloride only partially reversed effects of verapamil on AV nodal conduction, and required an even greater increment in serum calcium (4 mEq/L or 8 mg/dl). Calcium was totally ineffective in reversing reduced vascular resistance. Thus the antidotal actions of calcium must be considered to be limited to selected hemodynamic actions of

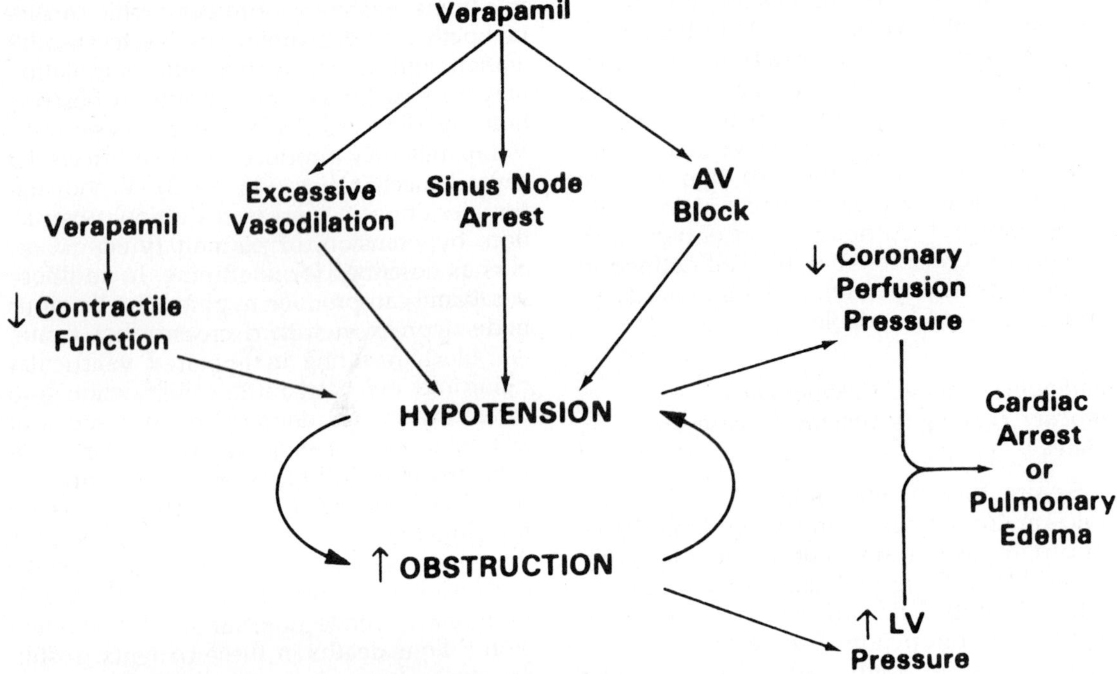

Figure 92–3. Mechanisms by which verapamil can produce hypotension, pulmonary edema, or sudden death in patients with hypertrophic cardiomyopathy. (From Epstein JE, Rosing DR: Verapamil: Its potential for causing serious complications in patients with hypertrophic cardiomyopathy. Circulation *64*:437, 1981.)

calcium entry blockers. Certain toxic manifestations may require other treatments, in addition to calcium, as discussed later.

CLINICAL PRESENTATION OF THE OVERDOSE

(Table 92–2)

Cardiovascular

The most serious complications of calcium entry blocker overdose are those involving the cardiovascular system. *The typical features include hypotension, bradycardia and AV block, or an accelerated junctional rhythm.*[2–4, 16–30]

Typical electrocardiographic findings and arrhythmias caused by calcium entry blockers are shown in Figures 92–4 to 92–10. With therapeutic doses of verapamil, P-R interval prolongation is seen. With higher doses, sinus bradycardia, AV nodal block (often of a Wenckebach type), or AV dissociation with an accelerated junctional rhythm occurs. In overdose, sinus arrest with a junctional rhythm is most common. QRS complexes are usually narrow; however, occasionally wide complexes with bundle branch block patterns have been observed. Asystole may occur after massive overdose or, occasionally, after IV verapamil in patients taking beta-blockers.[31] Diltiazem has the same spectrum of electrophysiologic actions as verapamil, although this does not seem to be as well

Table 92–2. CLINICAL FEATURES OF CALCIUM ENTRY BLOCKER OVERDOSE

CENTRAL NERVOUS SYSTEM
Lethargy, slurred speech, confusion, coma
Respiratory arrest
Seizures
GASTROINTESTINAL
Nausea, vomiting
CARDIOVASCULAR
Hypotension
Bradycardia and other arrhythmias
Sinus bradycardia
Accelerated AV nodal rhythm
2° AV block (Wenckebach)
3° AV block with junctional or ventricular escape rhythm
Sinus arrest with junctional rhythm
Asystole
METABOLIC DISTURBANCES
Hyperglycemia
Lactic acidosis

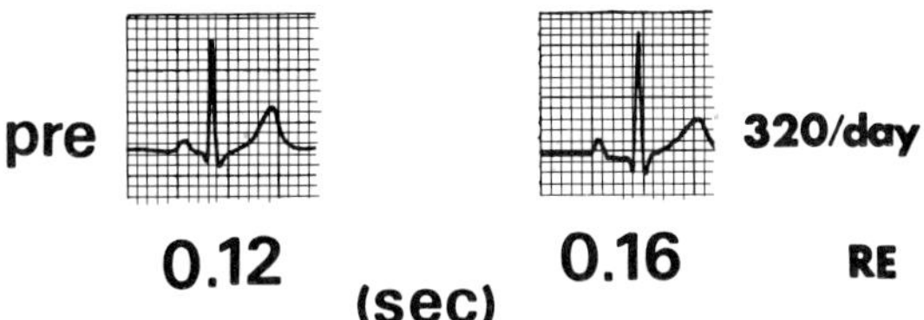

Figure 92–4. The initial ECG manifestation of calcium entry blocker effect with verapamil or diltiazem is usually prolongation of the P-R interval AV nodal re-entry tachycardias. Before verapamil (pre), this patient's P-R interval measured in lead II was 0.12 sec. After one week of verapamil, 320 mg/day, the P-R interval increased to 0.16 sec. At electrophysiologic study, this correlated with an increased A-H interval and noninducible supraventricular tachycardia.

recognized (Figs. 92–9 and 92–10). The current practice of co-administration of diltiazem with beta-blockers frequently leads to sinus or AV nodal dysfunction. Nifedipine, in massive intoxications, may or may not produce adverse cardiac electrophysiologic effects.[25, 26]

Hypotension or shock from calcium entry blockers may result from either reduced cardiac output or vasodilatation or a combination of the two. With nifedipine, hypotension is primarily due to vasodilatation. With verapamil or diltiazem, both impaired contractility and vasodilatation contribute. Hypotension is relatively common when verapamil is given by rapid intravenous infusion for treatment of supraventricular arrhythmias, presumably as a result of transiently high blood and myocardial concentrations. Recent studies suggest that calcium chloride pretreatment can reduce the degree of hypotension without impairing the antiarrhythmic efficacy of verapamil.[32] Hypotension and cardiac failure caused by the interaction between calcium entry blockers and other drugs is discussed in a later section.

Aggravation of chronic cardiac failure or precipitation of pulmonary edema is well described with therapeutic use of calcium entry blockers. Usually this occurs in patients with severe underlying myocardial dysfunction, obstructive valvular disease, or hypertrophic cardiomyopathy or in those patients taking other myocardial depressant drugs. Pulmonary edema is uncommon in people with normal cardiac function, even after overdose of calcium entry blockers.

Central Nervous System Manifestations

Calcium entry blocker overdoses have been associated with variable degrees of central

Text continued on page 1336

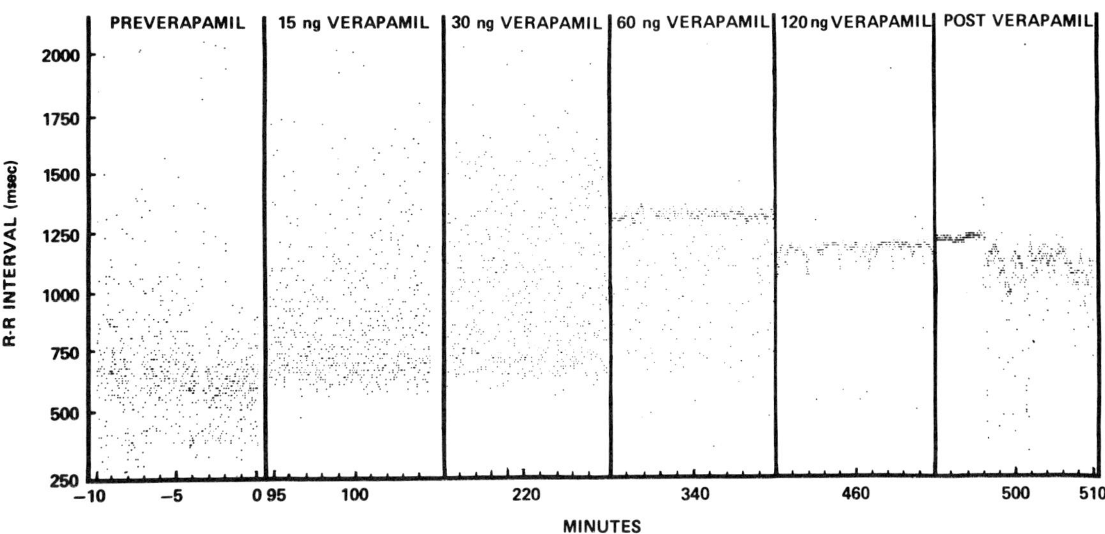

Figure 92–5. Regularization of the ventricular response rate to atrial fibrillation is frequently seen during verapamil or diltiazem administration. This may be seen in the absence of digitalis therapy and does not necessarily represent toxicity. Continuous R-R interval data were collected during steady state infusions of verapamil in a patient with chronic atrial fibrillation and a mitral valve replacement. In the pre-verapamil panel of the figure, representing 10 minutes of continous ECG data, atrial fibrillation is manifested by the tremendous scatter of the R-R intervals. Verapamil at concentrations of 15 to 30 ng/ml lead to a decrease in the ventricular response rate to atrial fibrillation (note the drop out of shorter R-R intervals). At 60 ng/ml, the longer R-R intervals also drop out, and a dominant rate with an R-R interval of about 1260 msec appears. At 120 ng/ml of verapamil and immediately after ending the infusion, a "regular" rate with an R-R interval of about 1200 msec is seen. Interval data after termination of verapamil show a return to widely scattered R-R intervals.

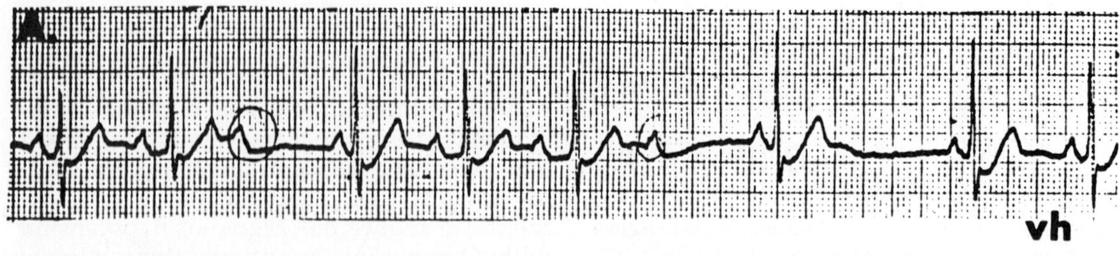

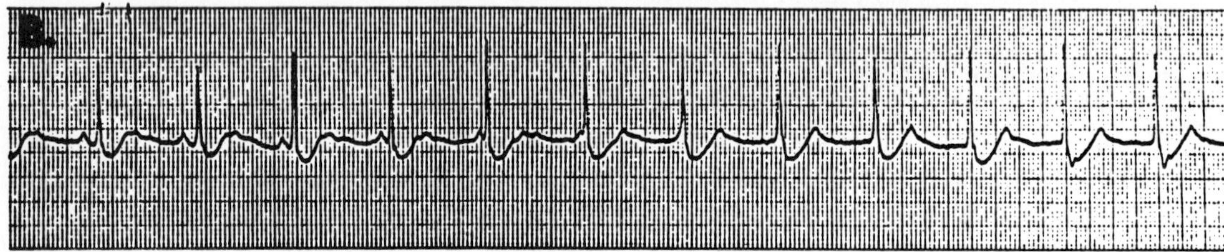

Figure 92–6. A, Increasing pharmacologic effect of calcium blocker therapy is manifested as AV block. This ECG shows second-degree AV block of the Wenckebach type that developed in a previously digitalized (serum digoxin level = 1.7 ng/ml) middle-aged woman immediately after receiving IV verapamil for paroxysmal atrial tachycardia. B, Continued therapy with verapamil (in combination with digoxin) in this patient led to the appearance of an accelerated junctional rhythm. Note the narrow regular rhythm with an R-R interval of about 800 msec. Dissociated atrial (sinus) activity is seen at a P-P interval of 840 msec. Thus, there is isorhythmic dissociation. Atropine administration did not restore sinus rhythm.

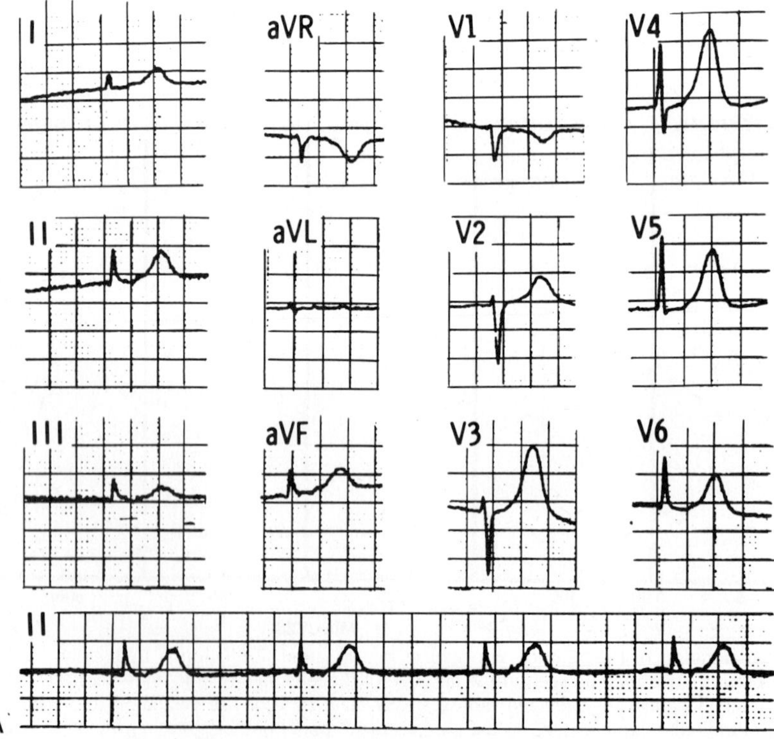

Figure 92–7. A, A 42 year old man with a history of alcohol abuse and without known cardiac disease presented to the emergency department 1 hour after ingestion of approximately 2400 mg of verapamil, 5 mg of lorazepam, and 1 liter of vodka. His blood pressure was 60/40 mm Hg. Initial electrocardiogram reveals a narrow junctional escape rhythm and a rate of 45 beats per minute, without obvious P waves. The T waves are broad and peaked with a QT interval of 520 msec.

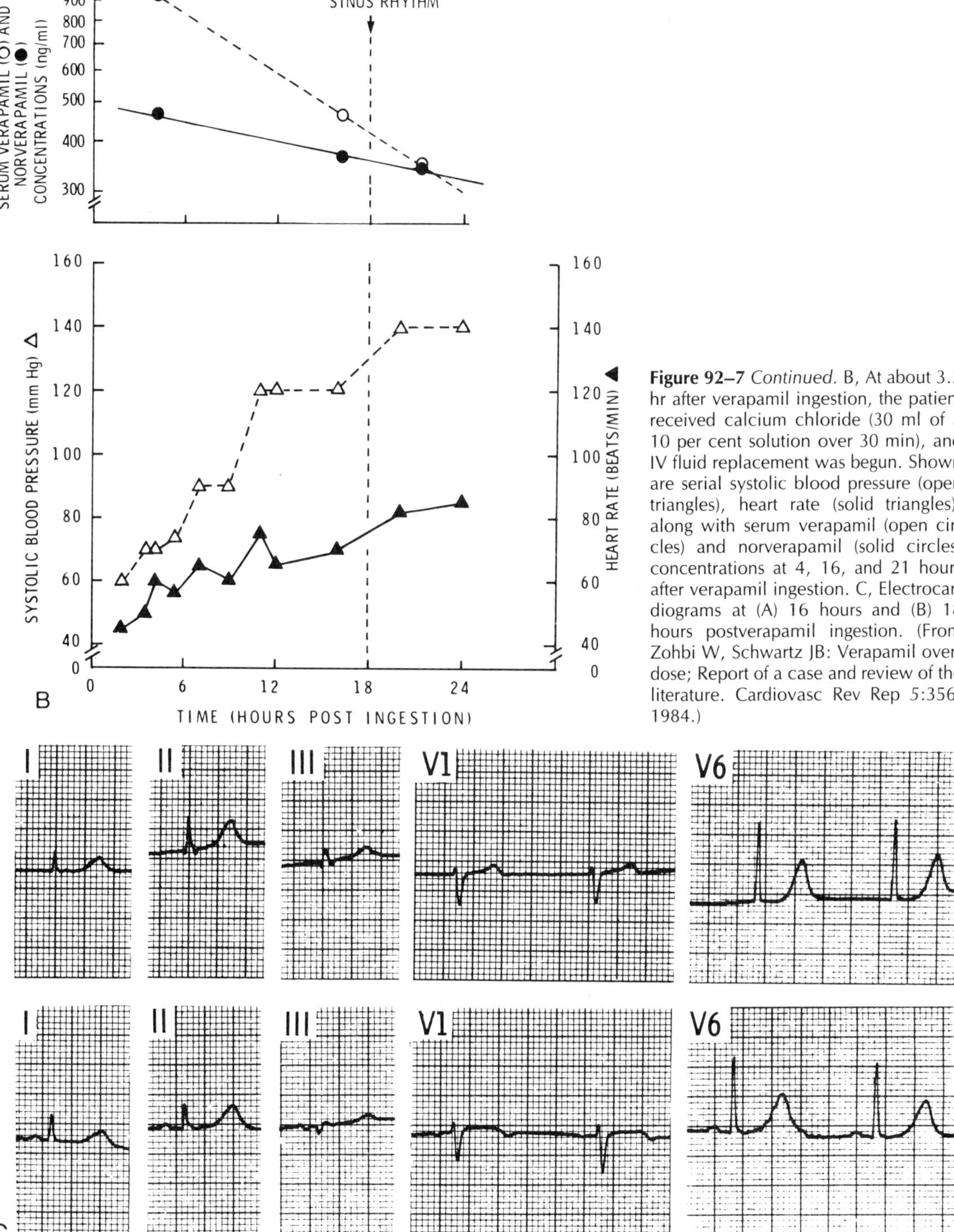

Figure 92–7 *Continued.* B, At about 3.5 hr after verapamil ingestion, the patient received calcium chloride (30 ml of a 10 per cent solution over 30 min), and IV fluid replacement was begun. Shown are serial systolic blood pressure (open triangles), heart rate (solid triangles), along with serum verapamil (open circles) and norverapamil (solid circles) concentrations at 4, 16, and 21 hours after verapamil ingestion. C, Electrocardiograms at (A) 16 hours and (B) 18 hours postverapamil ingestion. (From Zohbi W, Schwartz JB: Verapamil overdose; Report of a case and review of the literature. Cardiovasc Rev Rep 5:356, 1984.)

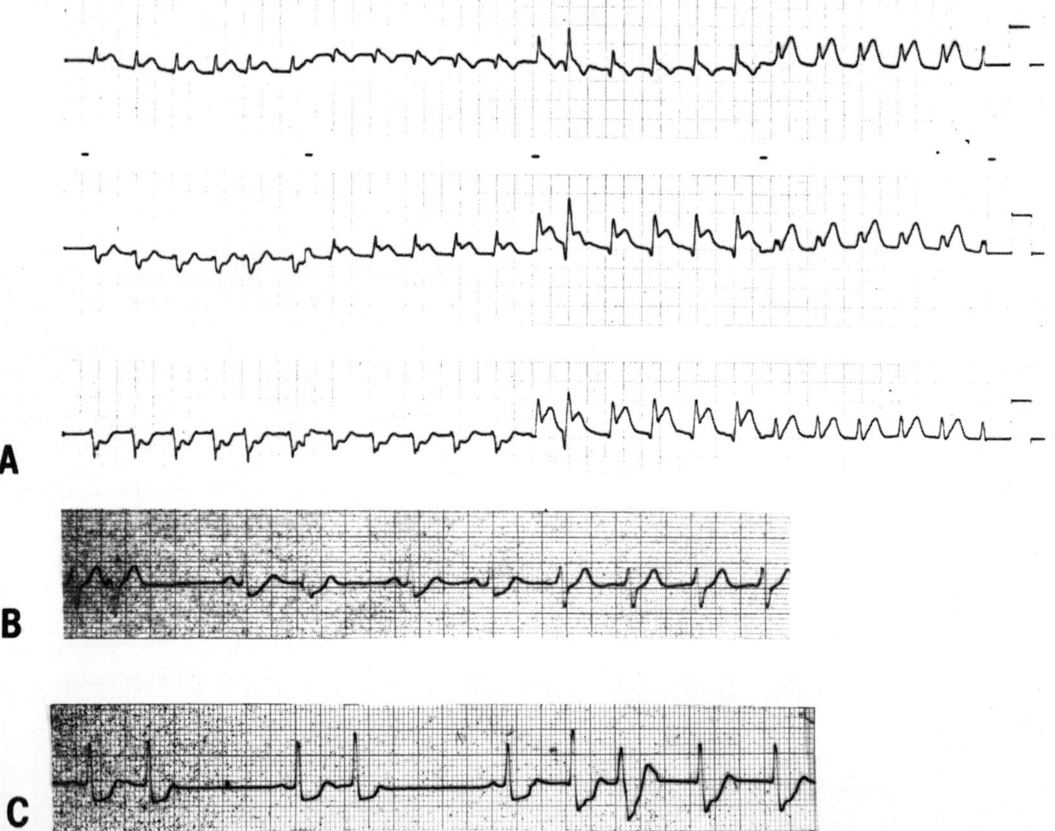

Figure 92–8. This 12-lead ECG *(A)* and rhythm strip *(B)* is from a 69 year old man admitted to the CCU with chest pain. Because of the paroxysmal tachycardia that was thought to be a "narrow QRS tachycardia" on the monitor, he received IV verapamil. Close examination of the ECG, however, shows a slightly irregular wide QRS tachycardia with a rate of about 135 per min and an acute anterior MI. Retrograde P waves can be appreciated in several leads.

C, Following verapamil, the patient became hypotensive. The rhythm strip from the monitor shows an irregular bradycardia most likely resulting from second degree Wenckebach AV block, prolonged sinus node recovery time, and the emergence of an escape rhythm (probably junctional) at a rate of about 100 per min.

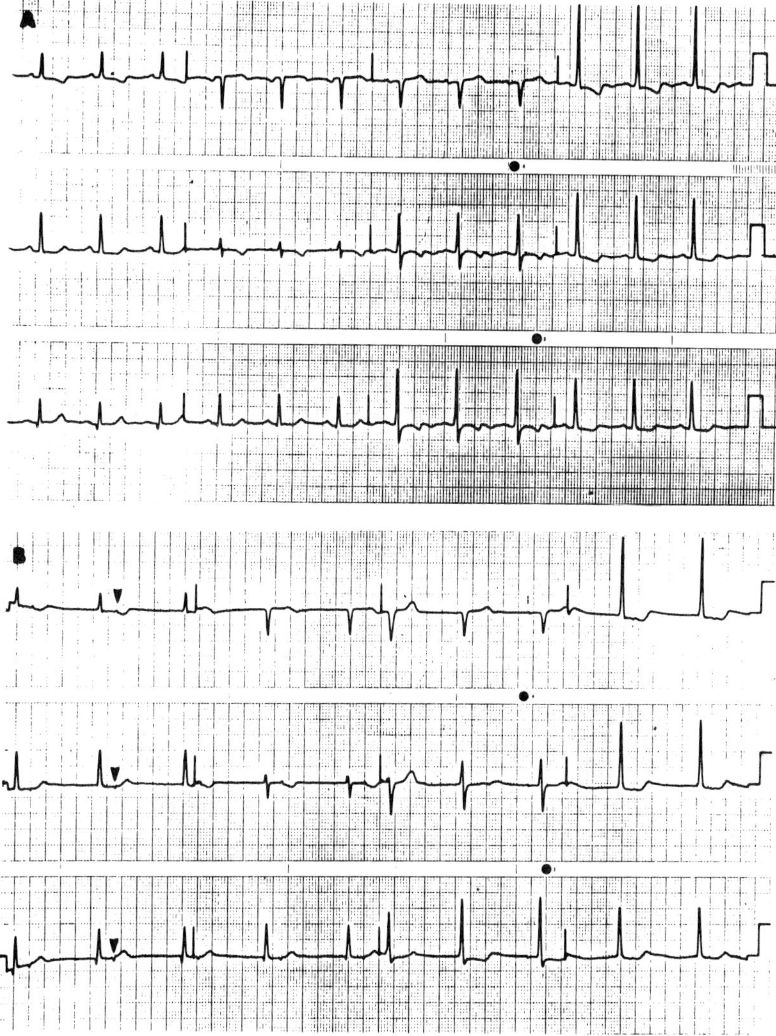

Figure 92–9. These electrocardiograms were taken from a 71 year old insulin-requiring diabetic woman with known coronary artery disease (previous inferoposterior MI and coronary bypass surgery). *A*, ECG was taken when she was seen in clinic reporting increasing angina. The inferoposterior MI seen on ECG was previously present but the anterior T wave inversion was new. The P-R interval was 180 msec. She was receiving isosorbide dinitrate, 20 mg every 4 hours; procainamide SR, 500 mg qid; furosemide, 80 mg/day; one ASA/day, in addition to varying insulin doses and pilocarpine eyedrops. Diltiazem, 60 mg bid, was begun without problems, and the dose was then increased to 60 mg qid.

B, On the second day of qid dosing, the patient developed paroxysmal nocturnal dyspnea, indigestion, and lightheadedness and returned to the clinic where this ECG was made. This shows a junctional rhythm of 60 bpm with retrograde P waves (arrows). Clinical examination demonstrated congestive heart failure that responded to IV furosemide and nitropaste administration. Diltiazem was withheld for 24 hours, with return of sinus rhythm. Serial enzyme determinations and ECG ruled out myocardial infarction. She was restarted on diltiazem, 30 mg tid, for angina control; subsequent 24-hour ambulatory ECG recordings showed no AV block, bradycardia, or junctional rhythms.

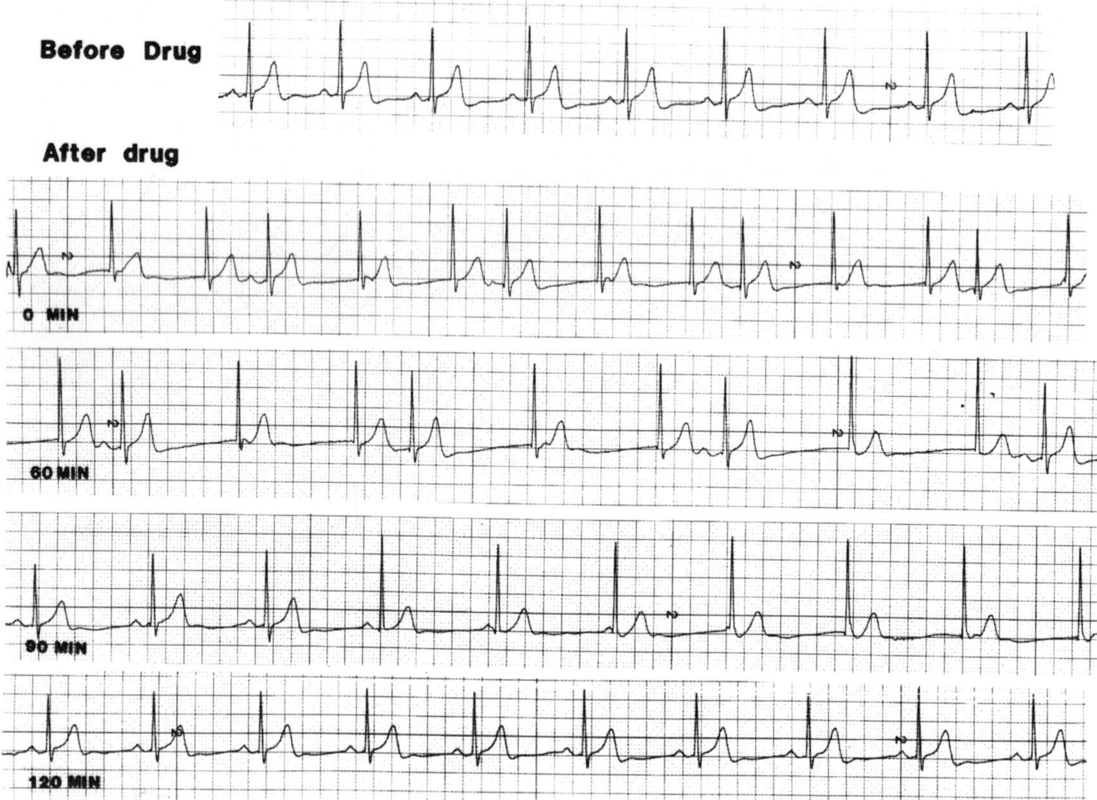

Figure 92–10. This series of electrocardiograms (surface lead 2) shows the changes in AV conduction seen in a 72 year old hypertensive man following a 10-minute infusion of 50 mg of diltiazem. Before the drug, the rhythm is normal sinus at a rate of 58/min, and a P-R interval is 190 msec. At the end of drug infusion (0 min), sinus bradycardia with a cycle length of 1260 msec is seen, and a junctional escape rhythm at 48/min appears (beats 2, 3, 5–6, 8–9, and so on). The P-R interval of conducted beats is 240 msec. Blood pressure was markedly reduced. Sixty minutes after the drug, sinus bradycardia (CL = 1700) persists, and the junctional escape rate has slowed. Sinus bradycardia with AV dissociation is present 90 minutes after the drug. At 2 hours postdrug, sinus rhythm at a rate of 52/min (P-R 200 msec) is seen.

nervous system depression, ranging from drowsiness or confusion to coma. Headache, flushing, weakness and vertigo have been reported. Respiratory arrest generally does not occur as a primary effect but may complicate profound shock. Seizures have been reported after overdose but are not common. Acute respiratory failure has followed intravenous verapamil in a patient with Duchenne's muscular dystrophy.[33]

Gastrointestinal Manifestations

Nausea and vomiting have been reported. Verapamil therapy has been associated with hepatitis,[34, 35] presumably due to allergic mechanisms; this has not been reported during acute intoxication. Obstipation with fecal impaction due to verapamil therapy has been observed.[36]

Metabolic Manifestations

Hyperglycemia is frequently observed in patients after overdose. Calcium is a trigger for insulin release from the pancreas, and calcium entry blockers theoretically could block such release. Impairment of glucose tolerance has been observed in dogs after verapamil and in humans after nifedipine treatment; however, recent controlled studies have not confirmed that such an effect is uniform, even in diabetic patients.[37–39] Metabolic acidosis is common after overdose, presumably due to hypotension and hypoperfusion.

RELEVANT PHARMACOKINETICS
(Table 92–3)

All currently available calcium entry blockers are rapidly and completely absorbed, but bioavailability is incomplete due to first-pass metabolism. Bioavailability is highest for nifedipine (about 70 per cent) and quite low for verapamil and diltiazem. Calcium entry blockers are extensively metabolized, with very little excreted unchanged in the urine. Verapamil and diltiazem have vasoactive metabolites: norverapamil and desacetyldiltiazem, respectively. Calcium entry blockers are extensively protein bound in the plasma and have large volumes of distribution. Terminal elimination half-lives range from 3 to 8 hours. The half-life of verapamil may be prolonged after overdose.[27] The half-life of diltiazem was 7.9 and 5.5 hours in two overdosed patients.[30, 40] The pharmacokinetics of nifedipine after overdose has not been characterized. The calcium entry blockers as a group are expected to be eliminated more slowly in states of circulatory insufficiency.[41]

The half-lives of the calcium entry blockers are such that the duration of intoxication, even with massive poisoning, is usually less than 24 to 36 hours. An exception may be seen with ingestion of slow-release preparations; however, cases describing such poisonings have not yet been published. Because of extensive protein binding, large volumes of distribution, and high endogenous clearance, neither hemodialysis nor hemoperfusion is expected to accelerate meaningfully the removal of calcium entry blockers from the poisoned patient. The fact that hemodialysis is ineffective in removing verapamil has been demonstrated in an intoxicated patient.[42]

DRUG INTERACTIONS INVOLVING CALCIUM ENTRY BLOCKING DRUGS
(Table 92–4)

A number of interactions involving calcium entry blockers have been reported: these may result in severe calcium blocker toxicity, therefore interactions will be examined in some detail. Drug interactions are most likely to occur in patients with underlying cardiac disease or in patients receiving calcium entry blockers by rapid intravenous injection. Most important are the pharmacodynamic interactions involving calcium entry blockers and other drugs that affect the cardiovascular system. For example, bradyarrhythmias, hypotension, or asystole following intravenous administration of verapamil has been seen in patients taking beta-blockers or digitalis.[31, 43–49] Excessive hypotension or cardiac failure following administration of nifedipine has been observed in patients receiving beta-blockers.[50–52] Worsening angina pectoris, resulting from hypotension, may follow addition of nifedipine to a regimen of beta-blockers, nitrates, or diuretics.[53] Calcium entry blockers should be administered cautiously, beginning at low doses and with careful monitoring, to patients who are hypovolemic due to diuretic use or who are taking other hypotensive medications. Laboratory studies indicate that verapamil decreases cardiac performance in patients on beta-blockers, but if left ventricular function is normal or only moderately depressed, and if there are no conduction abnormalities, myocardial depression due to verapamil is well tolerated.[54, 55]

In addition to direct effects on myocardial function and vascular tone, verapamil has alpha-adrenergic blocking activity. Case reports describe hypotension following combination therapy with quinidine and verapamil, presumably due to additive alpha-blocking effects.[56] Hypotension also might be anticipated after rapid injection of verapamil in any patient whose blood pressure depends on increased adrenergic tone or who is receiving other drugs with alpha-blocking activity. In dogs, infusion of verapamil into the AV nodal artery produced complete heart block, but asystole was seen only after pretreatment with propranolol or reserpine.[57] Presumably, blockade of AV nodal conduction by verapamil, combined with sympatholytic inhibition of AV nodal, His-Purkinje, and ventricular pacemakers, accounts for asystole in such cases.[58]

Many pharmacokinetic interactions have been described and are summarized in Table 92–4. The verapamil-digoxin interaction warrants specific discussion. Verapamil and digitalis are frequently used together. The combination is tolerated well by most patients. However, verapamil substantially slows the metabolism and renal excretion of digoxin, resulting in higher serum digoxin concentrations[59] (Fig. 92–11). There is concern about serious adverse interactions if digitalis toxic-

Table 92–3. PHARMACOKINETICS OF CALCIUM ENTRY BLOCKERS

Drug	*Oral Bioavailability (%)*	*Plasma Protein Binding (%)*	*Steady State Volume of Distribution (L/kg)*	*Clearance (ml/min)*	*Half-Life (hr)*	*"Therapeutic" Plasma Concentration (ng/ml)*
Verapamil*	10–20	90	5	1000	3–7	15–100
Diltiazem†	25–90	80	5	900	4–6	30–130
Nifedipine	65–70	90	1–3	700	5–10	25–100

*Vasoactive metabolite—norverapamil.
†Vasoactive metabolite—desacetyldiltiazem.

Table 92–4. DRUG INTERACTIONS INVOLVING CALCIUM ENTRY BLOCKERS

DRUG	INTERACTING DRUG	EFFECT	PROBABLE MECHANISM	COMMENTS
verapamil (other calcium entry blockers possible but less likely)	β-blocker	Heart block, cardiac failure, asystole (after IV verapamil)	Additive depression of AV conduction, myocardial contractility	Primarily seen with verapamil, should be used with caution in patients on β-blockers
verapamil	digitalis	Aggravates heart block	Additive depression of AV nodal conduction	Avoid use of calcium blockers in patients with digitalis toxicity
verapamil	digoxin	Reduced digoxin clearance, increased digoxin levels	Inhibition of metabolism and renal excretion of digoxin	Reduce digoxin dose after starting verapamil; monitor SDC
verapamil	quinidine	Hypotension (after IV)	Additive α-adrenergic blockade; inhibition of metabolism	Use IV verapamil cautiously in patients taking quinidine or other drugs with α-blocking activity
all calcium entry blockers	oral hypoglycemic agents	Hyperglycemia	Inhibition of insulin release by sulfonylurea drugs	May need to increase oral hypoglycemic or insulin doses to maintain control; caution about hypoglycemia when calcium blockers are stopped
verapamil	halothane	Bradycardia, hypotension	Additive depression of sinus node function and myocardial contractility	Avoid co-administration
verapamil diltiazem	disopyramide flecainide	Cardiac failure	Additive depression of myocardial contractility	Avoid use if possible, particularly in patients with impaired function
verapamil diltiazem	amiodarone flecainide	Sinus arrest Heart block	Additive depression of sinus node function and AV nodal conduction	Use combination with extreme caution
all calcium blockers	cimetidine	Increased oral bioavailability of calcium blockers	Inhibition of metabolism; reduced presystemic metabolism	Reduce calcium entry blocker dose by 30–40%
verapamil	rifampin sulfinpyrazone	Reduced oral bioavailability of verapamil	Accelerated metabolism; increased presystemic metabolism	Increase verapamil dose; use alternative calcium blocker with less presystemic metabolism

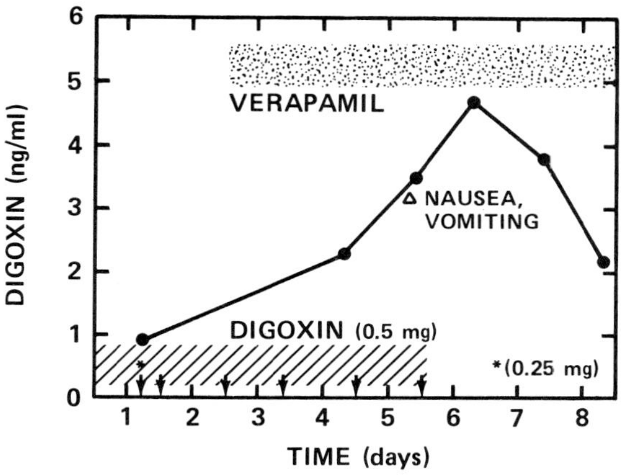

Figure 92–11. Verapamil was added to digitalis therapy for management of paroxysmal atrial tachycardias in an elderly woman with sick sinus syndrome and an implanted dual-chambered pacemaker. Verapamil administration markedly increased the serum digoxin level. Bradyarrhythmias were prevented by her permanent pacemaker, but she developed significant nausea and vomiting. Ventricular arrhythmias were not seen despite the digoxin level of 4.9 ng/ml.

ity develops. Patients receiving verapamil with coexisting digitalis toxicity have developed high-degree heart block or asystole.[48, 49] Ventricular tachyarrhythmias from digitalis toxicity do not seem to be common in the presence of verapamil, possibly owing to a protective effect of calcium entry blockade. Caution and possibly adjustment of the digoxin dose are necessary when adding verapamil to a stable digoxin regimen.

MANAGEMENT OF OVERDOSE
(Table 92–5)

General Considerations

Overall management is similar to that described for other drug overdoses. Evaluation and monitoring of intoxicated patients must continue until it is clear that absorption from the gastrointestinal tract is complete. If a slow-release preparation has been ingested, patients should be hospitalized and monitored for at least 24 hours. Seizures should be treated with intravenous administration of diazepam initially and then phenytoin or phenobarbital.

Experimental Studies

Several studies of treatment of verapamil toxicity have been published. The reversal of cardiovascular effects of verapamil by calcium in dogs has been discussed previously.[15] In another recent study of verapamil toxicity in dogs, a variety of interventions were evaluated. Calcium chloride, isoproterenol, norepinephrine, epinephrine, dopamine, high doses of phenylephrine, and 4-aminopyridine were able to increase myocardial contractility, while dopamine, isoproterenol, 4-aminopyridine, and ventricular pacing increased heart rate.[60] Ventricular pacing was successful in all animals, which is in contrast to poisoning with quinidine-like drugs, in which the myocardium may become unresponsive to electrical stimulation. Similar results were reported in a study of treatment of verapamil intoxication in anesthetized rats.[61] Of note in the latter study is the fact that no pharmacologic treatment was effective in increasing total peripheral resistance, and resistance was significantly further reduced by calcium, dopamine, and isoproterenol.

Calcium

Calcium reverses hypotension due to myocardial depression and, in some patients, increases sinus heart rate and improves AV nodal conduction. Many reports of beneficial

Table 92–5. MANAGEMENT OF CALCIUM ENTRY BLOCKER OVERDOSE

GENERAL MANAGEMENT
Lavage and charcoal
Seizures: diazepam, 5–10 mg IV; phenytoin, 15 mg/kg IV (rate, ≤ 50 mg/min)

ARRHYTHMIAS
Sinus or junctional bradycardia:
- if asymptomatic, general supportive measures
- if symptomatic, atropine, isoproterenol, cardiac pacemaker

Idioventricular rhythm, asystole: isoproterenol, cardiac pacemaker

HYPOTENSION
Treat bradyarrhythmias:
- calcium chloride, 1 gm (10 ml of a 10% solution)
- **OR**
- calcium gluconate, 2–3 gm (30 ml of a 10% solution) IV over 5 min

Normal saline: 200 ml every 10 minutes until 1000–2000 ml or evidence of pulmonary edema

Isoproterenol, epinephrine, norepinephrine, or dopamine infusion (low-to-moderate dose):
- if still hypotensive, insert pulmonary arterial catheter
- if low systemic vascular resistance, dopamine or norepinephrine
- if low cardiac output, amrinone, isoproterenol, dobutamine

NOTE: 4-Aminopyridine, an experimental calcium agonist, may reverse many manifestations of intoxication.

response to calcium administration in patients poisoned with verapamil, and a lesser number with nifedipine or diltiazem, have been published.[2–4, 14, 20, 62–64] The mechanisms, nature of benefit, and limitation of calcium entry block poisoning have been discussed previously. Some patients with severe intoxications do not respond to calcium.[21, 22] Despite its limitations, however, calcium should be administered as first line pharmacologic treatment for all patients with cardiovascular manifestations of calcium entry blocker poisoning.

The optimal dose or formulation of calcium in humans is not known. Animal studies suggest high doses of calcium are needed.[15] Calcium chloride (27 per cent calcium) is generally given in a 10 per cent solution, and 1 gram (10 ml) is infused over 5 minutes; this is repeated every 10 to 20 minutes for two or three additional doses until a response is seen. Doses may be repeated when the beneficial effects dissipate. After repeated doses it is advisable to measure serum calcium to avoid severe hypercalcemia, which itself can be detrimental to cardiovascular function. Calcium gluconate contains only 9 per cent calcium, so doses of 3 grams are required to deliver the same dose of calcium as 1 gram calcium chloride. High-dosage calcium replacement should be given through central venous access, if possible, since extravasation may result in tissue necrosis.

Arrhythmias

Calcium alone may be unsuccessful in correcting bradyarrhythmias. Accelerated junctional rhythms or AV nodal block with escape junctional rhythms do not require treatment per se. Bradyarrhythmias producing symptomatic hypotension may be controlled temporarily by atropine or by infusion of isoproterenol; however, temporary transvenous pacing is the definitive treatment. Ventricular tachyarrhythmias have not been seen in overdoses with calcium entry blocker drugs alone. The presence of ventricular arrhythmias should suggest additional drug toxicity or cardiac disease.

Hypotension

As discussed previously, hypotension may be due to decreased cardic output resulting from bradycardia or myocardial depression or to decreased systemic vascular resistance. Hypotension caused by myocardial depression usually responds to calcium. Bradyarrhythmias should be corrected as described earlier. Based on experimental studies in animals, patients who do not respond adequately to calcium and increasing the ventricular rate should be treated with isoproterenol, epinephrine, or norepinephrine to try to increase cardiac contractility. A case report describes treatment of a patient with verapamil poisoning unresponsive to calcium with a combination of isoproterenol and amrinone with apparent benefit.[65] Hypotension due to vasodilatation should be treated with fluids and, if necessary, vasoconstrictor drugs such as norepinephrine or dopamine. High doses of pressor drugs may be needed in light of the alpha-adrenergic blocking actions of verapamil.

4-Aminopyridine

New drugs that facilitate calcium entry, such as 4-aminopyridine, are currently being developed. 4-Aminopyridine acts by blocking voltage-dependent potassium channels, which in turn increases calcium influx. This drug has been used for many years in eastern Europe as an antagonist of non-depolarizing neuromuscular blocking drugs. In anesthetized, ventilated cats, 4-aminopyridine rapidly reversed hypotension and bradycardia and prevented death from verapamil intoxication.[66] In sedated, spontaneously breathing dogs, 4-aminopyridine reversed the hemodynamic consequences of verapamil poisoning.[60] However, in spontaneously breathing rabbits, 4-aminopyridine actually decreased the dose of verapamil that caused death.[67] In one case report, a 67 year old man with accidental verapamil intoxication resulting in hypotension, complete heart block with bradycardia, and cardiac failure received calcium, isoproterenol and 10 mg of 4-aminopyridine twice at 5 minute intervals, and recovery ensued over 90 minutes.[42] However, it was difficult to determine which of the treatments was primarily responsible for the improvement. It is likely that 4-aminopyridine or similar drugs will be evaluated further for treatment of calcium entry blocker intoxication.

References

1. Mangiardi LM, Hariman RJ, McAllister RG, Bhargava V, Surawicz B, Shabetai R: Electrophysiologic

and hemodynamic effects of verapamil—correlation with plasma drug concentrations. Circulation *57*:366, 1978.
2. Perkins CM: Serious verapamil poisoning: Treatment with intravenous calcium gluconate. Br Med J *2*:1127, 1978.
3. Woie L, Storstein L: Successful treatment of suicidal verapamil poisoning with calcium gluconate. Eur Heart J *2*:239, 1981.
4. Orr GM, Bodansky HJ, Dymond DS, Taylor M: Verapamil overdose. Lancet *1*:218, 1982.
5. Hamann SR, Kaltenborn KE, Vore M, Tan TG, McAllister RG: Cardiovascular and pharmacokinetic consequences of combined administration of verapamil and propranolol in dogs. Am J Cardiol *56*:147, 1985.
6. Qi A, Tuna IC, Gornick CC, Barragry TP, Blatchford JW, Ring WS, Bolman RM III, Walker MJ, Benditt DG: Potentiation of cardiac electrophysiologic effects of verapamil after autonomic blockade or cardiac transplantation. Circulation *75*:888, 1987.
7. McGovern B, Garan H, Ruskin JN: Precipitation of cardiac arrest by verapamil in patients with Wolff-Parkinson-White syndrome. Ann Intern Med *104*:791, 1986.
8. Kirk CR, Gibbs JL, Thomas R, Radley-Smith R, Qureshi SA: Cardiovascular collapse after verapamil in supraventricular tachycardia. Arch Dis Child *62*:1265, 1987.
9. Epstein ML, Kiel EA, Victoria BE: Cardiac decompensation following verapamil therapy in infants with supraventricular tachycardia. Pediatrics *75*:737, 1985.
10. Gillmer WJ, Kark P: Pulmonary oedema precipitated by nifedipine. Br J Med 281:1420, 1980.
11. Fedor JM, Stack RS, Pryor DB, Phillips HR: Adverse effects of nifedipine therapy on hypertrophic obstructive cardiomyopathy. Chest *4*:704, 1983.
12. Rosing DR, Idanpaan-Heikkila U, Maron BJ, Bonow RO, Epstein SE: Use of calcium-channel blocking drugs in hypertrophic cardiomyopathy. Am J Cardiol *55*:185B, 1985.
13. Epstein SE, Rosing DR: Verapamil: Its potential for causing serious complications in patients with hypertrophic cardiomyopathy. Circulation *64*:437, 1981.
14. Morris DL, Goldschlager N: Calcium infusion for reversal of adverse effects of intravenous verapamil. JAMA *249*:3212, 1983.
15. Hariman RJ, Mangiardi LM, McAllister RG, Surawicz B, Shabatai R, Kishida H: Reversal of the cardiovascular effects of verapamil by calcium and sodium: Differences between electrophysiologic and hemodynamic responses. Circulation *59*:797, 1979.
16. de Faire U, Lundman T: Attempted suicide with verapamil. Eur J Cardiol *6*:195, 1977.
17. Candell J, Valle V, Soler M, Rius J: Acute intoxication with verapamil. Chest *75*:200, 1979.
18. Da Silva OA, De Melo RA, Filho JPJ: Verapamil acute self-poisoning. Clin Toxicol *14*:361, 1979.
19. Moroni F, Mannaioni PF, Dolara A, Ciaccheri M: Calcium gluconate and hypertonic sodium chloride in a case of massive verapamil poisoning. Clin Toxicol *17*:395, 1980.
20. Immonen P, Linkola A, Waris E: Three cases of severe verapamil poisoning. Int J Cardiol *1*:101, 1981.
21. Crump BJ, Holt DW, Vale JA: Lack of response to intravenous calcium in severe verapamil poisoning. Lancet *2*:939, 1982.
22. Van Der Meer J, Van Der Wall E: Fatal acute intoxication with verapamil. Neth J Med *26*:130, 1983.
23. Enyeart JJ, Price WA, Hoffman DA, Woods L: Profound hyperglycemia and metabolic acidosis after verapamil overdose. J Am Coll Cardiol 2:1228, 1983.
24. Passal DB, Crespin FH Jr: Verapamil poisoning in an infant. Pediatrics *73*:543, 1984.
25. Schiffl H, Ziupa J, Schollmeyer P: Clinical features and management of nifedipine overdosage in a patient with renal insufficiency. Clin Toxicol *22*:387, 1984.
26. Herrington DM, Insley BM, Weinmann GG: Nifedipine overdose. Am J Med *81*:344, 1986.
27. Zohbi W, Schwartz JB: Verapamil overdose: Report of a case and review of the literature. Cardiovasc Rev Rep *5*:356, 1984.
28. Jakubowski AT, Mizgala HF: Effect of diltiazem overdose. Am J Cardiol *60*:932, 1987.
29. Snover SW, Bocchino V: Massive diltiazem overdose. Ann Intern Med *15*:1221, 1986.
30. Malcolm N, Callegari P, Goldberg J, Strauss H: Massive diltiazem overdosage: Clinical and pharmacokinetic observations. Drug Intell Clin Pharmacol *20*:888, 1986.
31. Benaim ME: Asystole after verapamil. Br Med J *264*:169, 1972.
32. Haft JI, Habbab MA: Treatment of atrial arrhythmias. Effectiveness of verapamil when preceded by calcium infusion. Arch Intern Med *146*:1085, 1986.
33. Zalman F, Perloff JK, Durant NW, Campion DS: Acute respiratory failure following I.V. verapamil in Duchenne's muscular dystrophy. Am Heart J *105*:510, 1983.
34. Nash DT, Feer TD: Heptatic injury possibly induced by verapamil. JAMA *249*:395, 1983.
35. Brodsky SG, Cutler SS, Weiner DA, Klein MD: Hepatotoxicity due to treatment with verapamil. Ann Intern Med *94*:490, 1981.
36. Warel DJ, Ward JW, Griffo W, Rochwasger A: I.V. calcium for fecal impaction secondary to verapamil. N Engl J Med *307*:1709, 1982.
37. Giugliano J, Torella R, Cacciapuoti F, Gentile S, Verza M, Varricchio M: Impairment of insulin secretion in man by nifedipine. Eur J Clin Pharmacol *18*:395, 1980.
38. Collins WCJ, Cullen MJ, Feely J: Calcium channel blocker drugs and diabetic control. Clin Pharmacol Ther *42*:420, 1987.
39. Dominic JA, Miller RB, Anderson J, McAllister RG: Pharmacology of verapamil. II. Impairment of glucose tolerance by verapamil in the conscious dog. Pharmacology *20*:196, 1980.
40. Buffet M, Ostermann G, Raclot P, Bertault R, Rambourg MO, Jassard M, Journe B, Seys GA: Cinétique du diltiazam au cours d'un surdosage volontaire. Presse Méd *12*:1338, 1984.
41. Hamann SR, Blouin RA, Chang SL, Kaltenborn KE, Tan TG, McAllister RG Jr: Effects of hemodynamic changes on the elimination kinetics of verapamil and nifedipine. J Pharmacol Exp Ther *231*:301, 1984.
42. ter Wee PM, Hovinga TKK, Uges DRA, van der Geest S: 4-Aminopyridine and haemodialysis in the treatment of verapamil intoxication. Hum Toxicol *4*:327, 1985.
43. Wayne VS, Harper RW, Laufer E, Federman J, Anderson ST, Pitt A: Adverse interaction between beta-adrenergic blocking drugs and verapamil—report of three cases. Aust NZ J Med *12*:285, 1982.

44. Sinche NJ, Brown JI, Hospta CG: Timolol eye drops and verapamil—a dangerous combination. Med J Aust 548, 1983.
45. Hutchison SJ, Lorimer AR, Lakhdar A, McAlpine SG: β-Blockers and verapamil: A cautionary tale. Br Med J *289*:659, 1984.
46. Zatuchni J: Bradycardia and hypotension after propranolol HCl and verapamil. Heart Lung *14*:94, 1985.
47. Winniford MD, Fulton KL, Hillis LD: Symptomatic sinus bradycardia during concomitant propranolol-verapamil administration. Am Heart J *110*:498, 1985.
48. Kounis NG: Asystole after verapamil and digoxin. Br J Clin Pract *34*:57, 1980.
49. Zatuchni J: Verapamil-digoxin interaction. Am Heart J *108*:412, 1984.
50. Anastassiades CJ: Nifedipine and beta-blocker drugs. Br Med J *281*:1251, 1980.
51. White DA: Adverse interaction between nifedipine and β-blockade. Br Med J *281*:1462, 1980.
52. Robson RH, Vishwanath MC: Nifedipine and beta-blockade as a cause of cardiac failure. Br Med J *284*:104, 1982.
53. Boden WE, Korr KS, Bough EW: Nifedipine-induced hypotension and myocardial ischemia in refractory angina pectoris. JAMA *253*:1131, 1985.
54. Packer M, Meller J, Medina N, Yushak M, Smith H, Holt J, Guererro J, Todd GD, Russell BS, McAllister G Jr, Forlin R: Hemodynamic consequences of combined beta-adrenergic and slow calcium channel blockade in man. Circulation *65*:660, 1982.
55. Reddy PS, Uretsky BF, Steinfeld M: The hemodynamic effects of intravenous verapamil in patients on chronic propranolol therapy. Am Heart J *107*:97, 1984.
56. Maisel AS, Motulsky HJ, Insel PA: Hypotension after quinidine plus verapamil. N Engl J Med *312*:167, 1985.
57. Urthaler F, James T: Experimental studies on the pathogenesis of asystole after verapamil in the dog. Am J Cardiol *44*:651, 1979.
58. Vassalle M: On the mechanisms underlying cardiac standstill: Factors determining success or failure of escape pacemakers in the heart. J Am Coll Cardiol *5*:35B, 1985.
59. Klein HO, Lang R, Weiss E, Di Segni E, Libhaber C, Guerrero J, Kaplinsky E: The influence of verapamil on serum digoxin concentration. Circulation *65*:998, 1982.
60. Gay R, Algeo S, Lee R, Olajos M, Morkin E, Goldman S: Treatment of verapamil toxicity in intact dogs. J Clin Invest *77*:1805, 1986.
61. Strubelt O: Antidotal treatment of the acute cardiovascular toxicity of verapamil. Acta Pharmacol Toxicol *55*:231, 1984.
62. Lipman J, Jardine I, Roos C, Dreosti L: Intravenous calcium chloride as an antidote to verapamil-induced hypotension. Intens Care Med *8*:55, 1982.
63. Hattori VT, Mandel WJ, Peter T: Calcium for myocardial depression from verapamil. N Engl J Med *307*:238, 1982.
64. Henry M, Kay MM, Viccellio P: Cardiogenic shock associated with calcium-channel and beta blockers: Reversal with intravenous calcium chloride. Am J Emerg Med *3*:334, 1985.
65. Goenen M, Col J, Compere A, Bonte J: Treatment of severe verapamil poisoning with combined amrinone-isoproterenol therapy. Am J Cardiol *58*:1142, 1986.
66. Agoston S, Maestrone E, van Hezik EJ, Ket JM, Houwertjes, Upes DRA: Effective treatment of verapamil intoxication with 4-aminopyridine in the cat. J Clin Invest *73*:1291, 1984.
67. Wesseling H, Houwertjes MC, de Langen CD, Kingma HJ: Hemodynamic effects of high dosages of verapamil and the lack of protection by 4-aminopyridine in the rabbit. Arch Int Pharmacodyn Ther *266*:106, 1983.

CHAPTER 93

NITROPRUSSIDE AND SELECTED ANTIHYPERTENSIVES

James F. Winchester, M.D.

Table 93–1 presents a market survey of commonly used antihypertensive drugs in 1987; the pattern has considerably changed in the last few years with the introduction of angiotensin-converting enzyme (ACE) inhibitors and calcium channel blockers [Chapter 92]). Overdosage of many of these compounds has not been reported, but an overdosage can be considered an extension of the desired pharmacologic action (that is, profound hypotension) or a physiologic accompaniment of the basic pharmacologic activity (for example, hypoglycemia or cardiac failure with beta-blocker overdosage [Chapter 91]) with certain drugs. Drug interactions, e.g., the hypertensive response to combined clo-

Table 93–1. TOTAL ANTIHYPERTENSIVE DRUG PRESCRIPTIONS—U.S.A., 1987

	CONSTANT 1988 DOLLARS (MILLIONS)	PER CENT OF MARKET
Traditional agents*	510	23
Diuretics	410	18
Beta-blockers	680	30
ACE inhibitors	400	18
Calcium channel blockers	260	11
Total	2,260	100

*Includes methyldopa, clonidine, reserpine, and so on.

nidine (Chapter 94) and desipramine, or phenylpropanolamine with antihypertensive drugs, will not be discussed. Similarly, hypersensitivity reactions, minor side effects, and possible carcinogenic properties of certain compounds (reserpine) will not be discussed. Often the type (class) of drug will determine (or suggest for individual drugs) the toxicity of drugs in the group. When there are differences between the toxicity of the compounds in a single class, this will be emphasized.

DRUGS ACTIVE ON THE PERIPHERAL VASCULATURE

Nitroprusside

Sodium nitroprusside (sodium nitroferricyanide) is a potent, directly acting vasodilator, used in the management of accelerated hypertension because of its rapid onset of action and rapid dissipation of action following cessation of intravenous therapy.[1] Nitroprusside relaxes arterial and venous smooth muscle but has little effect on other smooth muscle organs. A consequence of reduction in venous smooth muscle is the reduction in cardiac preload, such that in the heart failure patient cardiac output will increase. In the normal patient, however, cardiac output either falls or does not change.[2, 3] Renal blood flow and glomerular filtration are maintained, and renin secretion is increased. Angina, on the other hand, often improves, quite the opposite to what is seen with other vasodilators such as hydralazine.

Acute toxicity from nitroprusside is manifested by vasodilatation and hypotension; the latter may be complicated by nausea, vomiting, sweating, headache, palpitation, and substernal distress. But since the half-life of the drug is approximately 2 minutes, stopping the intravenous infusion completely reverses the symptomatology. The other side effects of nitroprusside are methemoglobinemia after prolonged infusion[4] and symptoms related to cyanide toxicity. Fatalities have been reported.[5–7]

Cyanide radical (cyanogen) is an intermediate of nitroprusside metabolism, the final metabolite being thiocyanate; however, although significant cyanide concentrations are often observed, cyanide toxicity is usually uncommon.[8] Thiocyanate is cleared slowly by the kidney, with a half-life of elimination of 4 days, which is prolonged in renal failure.[1] The thiocyanate toxicity (plasma concentration greater than 10 mg/dl) results in weakness, hypoxia, nausea, tinnitus, muscle spasm, disorientation, and psychosis. Bone marrow toxicity in the form of macrocytic megaloblastic anemia has been observed, and this can be prevented with the administration of hydroxocobalamin.[9] If the drug is continued for prolonged periods of time, hypothyroidism may result, since thiocyanate interferes with transport of iodine by the thyroid.[10] In addition, brain cytochrome oxidase is inhibited by cyanogen.[11]

Lactic acidosis[12] developed in a 66 year old woman during the 28th hour of sodium nitroprusside infusion, after a total dose of 490 mg. The serum lactate level was 338 mg/dl; pyruvate, 2.3 mg/dl; and thiocyanate, 2.1 mg/dl (toxic level greater than 8 mg/dl). Lactic acidosis had been reported previously in a patient[13] and in animal studies.[14, 15] Acidosis is the most reliable indicator of toxicity, leading Vesey and Cole[16] to recommend acidosis as one criterion (in addition to greater than 1.5 mg/kg short-term or greater than 4 μg/kg/min long-term nitroprusside infusion) for bolus infusion of 25 ml of a 50 per cent solution of sodium thiosulfate, to reduce plasma and red cell cyanide concentrations.

Treatment of nitroprusside toxicity consists of stopping the infusion and administering fluids, if necessary, and pressor agents. The regimen of a 25-ml bolus of 50 per cent sodium thiosulfate over 10 minutes can be repeated at half the dosage, and patients should be observed over several hours, since toxicity may recur. Massive poisoning may be treated with amyl nitrite inhalations prior to infusion of thiosulfate. It has been pointed out that adherence to correct doses of nitroprusside abolishes any toxicity.[17] In addition, bone marrow toxicity may be obviated by the use of hydroxocobalamin (1000 μg/dl intramuscularly, not available in the United States), the preferred metabolite of vitamin B_{12}, or cyanocobalamin (1000 μg/dl IM). In very severe poisoning, hemodialysis might be considered, since thiocyanate is dialyzable. Management of acidosis is outlined in Chapter 7.

Adrenergic Neuron Blockers

The mixed compounds in this class are guanethidine, guanadrel, debrisoquine, bethanidine, and bretylium. These drugs are postganglionic adrenergic neuron blockers that produce sympathetic blockade. The drugs are fairly equal in their effects, but bretylium is used also for cardiac arrhythmias (see Chapter 4). Overdose of these compounds is extremely rare, but, when it occurs, the drugs do produce extensions of their desired pharmacologic effects, the most important complication of overdose being profound hypotension (usually orthostatic).

Treatment is along the usual lines, with emesis, gastric lavage, and oral charcoal with or without cathartics. Hypotension should be treated by use of the Trendelenburg position, and intravenous fluids should be administered when necessary. Since guanethidine in animals may be associated with an initial episode of hypertension before hypotension develops, this may occur in human beings. For hypotension, the vasopressor of choice is dopamine, since arrhythmias have been observed with other pressor agents. The kinetics of elimination of guanethidine, which follows a triphasic pattern, exhibits a 5.2-day terminal half-life;[18] for this reason, hypotension may be present for many days.

Nonspecific Vasodilators

Examples of drugs in this class are hydralazine and minoxidil.

Hydralazine

Hydralazine produces direct relaxation of vascular arteriolar smooth muscle, with reflex tachycardia following peripheral vasodilatation. A decrease in afterload and preload also occurs, with improvement in cardiac function in those patients with cardiac failure. Consequently, in contrast to the ganglion blockers and adrenergic neuron blockers, postural hypotension is reduced to a minimum. Blood flow in splenic, coronary, cerebral, and renal circulation increases, although renal sodium, water retention, and reduced urine volume also occur. Following oral administration, peak plasma levels are reached within 1 hour; the plasma half-life ranges from 2 to 8 hours, with an average of 3 hours. The major route of elimination appears to be acetylation in the liver,[19] with slow acetylators being placed at a higher risk of developing a lupus erythematosus–like syndrome,[20] in contrast to fast acetylators, who rapidly reduce circulating plasma concentrations of hydralazine.

Acute overdose is usually manifested by profound hypotension. One adult is reported to have survived after taking approximately a hundred 100-mg tablets. Management, therefore, should be directed to control of blood pressure by placing the patient in the Trendelenburg position, administering intravenous fluids, and using dopamine or dobutamine as vasopressors. Since myocardial ischemia and arrhythmias may develop, it is best to avoid drugs that might aggravate cardiac arrhythmias (e.g., phenylephrine and methoxamine).

Minoxidil

Minoxidil results in direct relaxation of artériolar smooth muscle and a decrease in renal vascular resistance unassociated with reduction in glomerular filtration rate.[1] It is metabolized mainly in the liver, with 97 per cent of the drug being recovered in the urine but less than 10 per cent being unchanged; the elimination half-life of minoxidil in plasma is greater than 4 hours.[21] The major adverse effects of minoxidil are related to fluid retention, particularly in patients with renal failure,[22] as well as reflex tachycardia, pericardial effusion,[23] and hirsutism. In addition, minoxidil in high doses produces atrial hemorrhages in dogs, and creatine phosphokinase elevations in human beings also have been reported.

Accidental overdosage of minoxidil in a child revealed that blood pressure was unchanged (120/80 mm Hg) and the pulse rate was 160/min after the ingestion of 100 mg of minoxidil 1 hour before the child was seen.[24] Over a period of 40 hours, the pulse rate fell to 120/min, and the patient was discharged. Serum minoxidil concentrations at 3 and 13 hours after ingestion were 150 ng/ml and less than 0.5 ng/ml, respectively. Electrocardiograms were normal throughout the hospital stay, although flattening and inversion of T waves have been observed after starting minoxidil.[25] The absence of hypotension in the child after 100 mg of minoxidil supports one view that minoxidil was active only in patients with hypertension and was unable to reduce a normal blood pressure.[26] The observed level of 150 ng/ml should be compared with a standard level of 40 ng/ml measured 1 hour after a 30-mg minoxidil dose in an adult.[27] Based on these observations, it appears that minoxidil does not cause hypotension, commonly seen with other vasodilators in patients with normal blood pressure, and that if a hypertensive patient has taken an overdose, treatment should be directed to control of the blood pressure with the patient in the Trendelenburg position and administration of fluids and dopamine or dobutamine.

CENTRAL ACTING AGENTS

This class includes methyldopa, clonidine, guanabenz, and guanfacine.

Methyldopa

Methyldopa inhibits dihydroxyphenylalanine decarboxylase,[1] and it is no longer classified as a peripheral adrenergic neuronal blocking agent.[28] The central antihypertensive action of methyldopa is via stimulation of central alpha-adrenergic receptors as a result of formation of alpha-methyl norepinephrine,[29, 30] with some peripheral activity.[31] Twenty-five per cent of unchanged methyldopa is excreted in the urine within 24 hours, and the plasma elimination half-time of the drug from plasma by hepatic biotransformation is approximately 2 hours.[32, 33] In renal failure, delayed excretion accounts for some accumulation of methyldopa, but there is no evidence that reduction of dosage is necessary in patients with hepatic or renal disease.[34]

The most common accompaniments of methyldopa overdosage are sedation, coma, and postural hypotension. Delayed absorption from the gut and delayed onset of maximal hypotension should be remembered and the patient properly monitored.[35] Other adverse effects commonly associated with methyldopa therapy[1] may accompany the poisoning, such as Coombs' positive hemolytic anemia and Coombs' positive test, impotence, depression, involuntary movement disorders (parkinsonian-like effects),[36] and paradoxic hypertension,[37–40] as well as drug-associated hepatitis.[41]

Only one fatal case of definite methyldopa poisoning has been reported.[42] The autopsy study was in a 44 year old woman who took approximately 25 gm of methyldopa; the blood level was 0.9 mg/dl, with a urinary concentration of 140 mg/dl. In addition, fatty degeneration of liver cells was observed and accompanying changes of hypertension in heart and kidney. Two other suspected overdose cases were reported;[43] serum levels were 0.72 mg/dl and 0.94 mg/dl, while urine levels were 12.6 mg/dl and 12.9 mg/dl, respectively. Chronic methyldopa poisoning also has been observed.[44] The oral LD_{50} in mice is 5.3 to 15 gm/kg,[42] indicating that methyldopa is relatively nontoxic, which may account for the paucity of overdose cases in the world literature. The best-confirmed features of overdose are hypotension and central nervous system depression. Although not reported in overdose, it should be remembered that atrioventricular conduction may be impaired,[45] and that myocarditis[46] also may accompany its administration. The drug may interact with tricyclic antidepressants.[47]

Treatment consists of removing any remaining methyldopa from the stomach by lavage or emesis, administering activated charcoal and cathartics, and establishing respiration. In addition, as Sternbach and Rosen[35] have emphasized, the patient should be put into the Trendelenburg position, and hypotension should be treated initially with infusion of isotonic fluids. Blood pressure should be monitored regularly, and, if there is no response to fluid infusion, dopamine or dobutamine should be initiated (see Chapter 4). Norepinephrine is also useful in treating hypotension, but the use of alpha-blockers is no longer recommended.[35] Hemodialysis has been reported to remove 60 per cent of methyldopa after therapeutic administration in dialysis patients.[48] In severe cases of methyldopa poisoning, hemodialysis may be considered, but the physician should direct attention primarily to the maintenance of good fluid balance and control of hypotension. In the recovery phase from methyldopa withdrawal, it should be remembered that rebound hypertension may occur; however, it is much less common and less severe than that seen with clonidine withdrawal.[1]

Reserpine

Reserpine, a crystalline alkaloid, is derived from *Rauwolfia serpentina,* a tropical shrub. It was introduced for treatment of hypertension in the late 1950s, and several cases of toxicity were reported soon after. The drug in high dosage caused severe mental depression.[49] Reserpine is a centrally active drug that produces reduction in brain concentrations of norepinephrine and dopamine, as well as serotonin.[50, 51] The unwanted side effects of reserpine (drowsiness, fatigue, hallucinations and nightmares, depression, and agitation) are due to the central depletion of norepinephrine and dopamine.[49] Other central manifestations of reserpine in animals are related to the development of spontaneous electrical seizure activity. Convulsions are not commonly described in patients who take large overdoses, although reserpine increases the sensitivity to electroconvulsive therapy and insulin shock therapy.[52, 53] Reserpine can induce extrapyramidal disturbances, with muscle spasm, dystonia, and so on, common to parkinsonism.

The lethal dose of reserpine is unknown, but the LD_{50} for the rabbit and rat is approximately 10 mg/kg of body weight.[49] A 20-month old boy ingested 260 mg of reserpine, and, although drowsy but arousable for 3 days, he eventually recovered completely.[54] Three children, ranging in age from 2 to 4 years—in two of whom the ingested dose was less than 25 mg—experienced coma, bradycardia, and hypothermia; it is interesting that hypertension and sinus tachycardia were observed in the youngest child.[55] Poisoning with reserpine was common in the past; McKown and associates, reporting on 151 cases of reserpine poisoning, demonstrated that about one third of the patients exhibited flushing of the skin and central nervous system depression.[56] Only one patient, however, was reported to be in coma, and two patients had hypotension. Manifestations of the toxicity may persist as long as 1 week after ingestion. Other symptoms of the toxic syndrome of reserpine include peripheral vasodilatation with flushing of the face, hyperchlorhydria,[57] and occasionally gastrointestinal hemorrhage.[58] Severe cardiovascular collapse sometimes may be seen; it was suggested at one time that reserpine and digitalis in combination might lead to a high incidence of cardiac arrhythmias.

Treatment follows the protocol for other drug poisoning, with initial management consisting of eliminating the drug via gastric lavage, emesis, or oral charcoal. Because of the effects of reserpine on hydrochloric acid production, antacid therapy with such compounds as aluminum hydroxide is particularly useful. In general, management should be directed to maintenance of blood pressure; the more common manifestation is hypotension, but monitoring for a hypertensive crisis, as has been reported in one child,[55] is important. Vasopressor drugs may be required, as well as intravenous solutions. The overriding principle of management, however, is one of masterly inactivity, since all patients have recovered from poisoning with reserpine.

GANGLION-BLOCKING AGENTS

These drugs are little used in modern medical practice; they are hexamethonium, mecamylamine, pempidine, pentolinium, and trimethaphan.[59] The latter two drugs are used in the management of accelerated hypertension and for this purpose are given intravenously. Management of poisoning with these drugs essentially is directed to hypotension and to hastening the elimination of the drugs from the blood. Forced acid diuresis may be useful in mecamylamine and pempidine poisoning,[60] in which it has been demonstrated that excretion of these compounds is diminished in alkaline urine. Since the agents produce antagonism of acetylcholine neurotransmission, it has been suggested that cholinesterase inhibitors, such as physostigmine or neostigmine, may help reverse many of the effects of ganglion-blocking drugs.[61, 62]

BENZOTHIADIAZINE AND OTHER DIURETICS

The benzothiadiazine drugs are thiazide diuretics and their derivatives diazoxide and metolazone, all of which are derived from sulfonamide preparations. All these drugs have similar qualitative effects on peripheral blood vessels; however, diazoxide is quantitatively the most potent vasodilator, yet it does not possess any diuretic activity and, in fact, acts as a potent sodium retainer. Diuretics in prolonged high dosage may produce acute renal failure (see Chapter 9*A*).

Diazoxide

Diazoxide is used for treatment of severe hypertension and accelerated hypertension (when it is given intravenously in a dosage of 300 mg or less). Oral diazoxide is used also to treat hypoglycemia, since it blocks insulin release from the pancreas. Whereas diazoxide is commonly used in the United States in the intravenous form for the treatment of accelerated hypertension, in the United Kingdom and in Europe the drug is available in the oral form for the treatment of refractory hypertension.[63] Continued daily use of intravenous or oral diazoxide for the control of severe hypertension may be associated with hirsutism, but the more important side effects are sodium retention and the production of hyperglycemia with nonketotic hyperosmolar coma,[64] as well as ketoacidosis.[65] Pancreatitis also has been reported. The clearance from plasma of diazoxide is approximately 7 ml/min, and 30 per cent of the excretion is through the kidney.[1] The drug is 90 per cent bound to serum albumin, and more free drug is available for smooth muscle blocking activities in the uremic patient as a result of acid moieties blocking the albumin-binding sites, when a greater hypotensive response is seen.[66] The toxicity of diazoxide should be managed by control of blood pressure (with intravenous fluids and the Trendelenburg position), hyperglycemia, and associated acidosis and hyperosmolar coma. The latter is managed with the use of half-normal saline intravenously and small doses of insulin. Prolonged monitoring may be necessary in view of the prolonged elimination half-time of the drug.

The Thiazide Diuretics

Acute intoxication from thiazide diuretics is extremely rare; toxicity more often results from prolonged usage. The most frequent adverse effects are hypokalemia and complications resulting from this. The incidence of hypokalemia varies with the disease state being treated and many other factors, giving rise to considerable controversy on the appropriateness of routine potassium supplementation in diuretic-treated patients.[67] In addition, other common complications are hyperglycemia, hyperuricemia, and hyperlipidemia. Since the duration of activity of the thiazides is greater than that seen with the loop diuretics, alkalosis and hypokalemia are more common. In common with diazoxide, the thiazide diuretics also can produce pancreatitis. In sulfonamide-sensitive patients, they can produce hypersensitivity reactions.

Potassium-Retaining Compounds

These compounds are spironolactone, triamterene, and amiloride. Side effects seen with these compounds are hypokalemia in a small percentage, but more commonly hyperkalemia, especially in renal failure patients or those with diabetes mellitus. Spironolactone also produces gynecomastia and amenorrhea.

Loop Diuretics

These are ethacrynic acid, furosemide, bumetanide, and tienilic acid (ticrynafen); the latter compound is derived from ethacrynic acid, but its renal action is more like that of a thiazide. The major side effects of these compounds are ototoxicity following large intravenous doses and hypokalemia, hypoglycemia, and hyperuricemia. Tienilic acid is no longer available in the United States. It possessed uricosuric activity;[68] however, 5 deaths and 52 cases of hepatotoxicity were seen, after which the compound was withdrawn from the market.[69]

Carbonic Anhydrase Inhibitors

Acetazolamide is the major compound in this group, and it may be associated with metabolic acidosis, the management of which is outlined in Chapter 7.

Mercurial Diuretics

These compounds are unavailable for use in modern therapeutics; they were mersalyl, mercaptomerin, and meralluride; the major toxicity from these compounds in chronic use is nephrotoxicity (see Chapter 9*B*).

Osmotic Diuretics

The compounds in this group are mannitol and glycerol, which may be given intravenously, by mouth, or by enema. The major associated toxicity is the production of intense diuresis, with dehydration, pulmonary edema, or, in chronic use, cerebral edema. Mannitol intoxication is well recognized, usually in patients being treated for barbiturate or salicylate overdose. Although pulmonary edema is stressed, only four cases have been reported.[70, 71] Mannitol intoxication is usually accompanied by hypotension, polyuria that rapidly converts to oliguria, stupor, and convulsions. Aviram and associates reported three patients who had received inappropriately large amounts of mannitol and who developed severe vascular overfilling, thirst, clouded sensorium, hyperosmolality, and hyponatremia.[71] In this situation, hemodialysis may be of some benefit to reduce the serum osmolality.[71, 72]

Management of Diuretic Intoxication

The clinician should attend to the management of dehydration, electrolyte imbalance (hypokalemia and hyponatremia), hyperglycemia, and acidosis or alkalosis. In addition, if the diuretics have been ingested, gastric lavage or emesis should be performed, followed by administration of activated charcoal. Hyperkalemia associated with potassium-retaining diuretics should be managed with insulin and glucose, followed by administration of a potassium-retaining ion exchange resin (Kayexalate). Hemodialysis for the management of diuretic poisoning has been reported for mannitol intoxication[71, 72] and for acetazolamide; the latter is somewhat dialyzable (a 4-hour hemodialysis achieved removal of approximately 30 per cent of the intravenously administered dose in a patient with renal failure, and the drug clearance was found to be 22 ml/min through the dialyzer).[73] Dialysis for acetazolamide was suggested for the management of its life-threatening complications,[73] which include severe renal impairment[74] and liver disease.[75]

ANTIANGIOTENSIN DRUGS

The four available compounds in this category are saralasin (sarcosine-alanine-angiotensin II) captopril, enalapril, and lisinopril. Saralasin is available only for intravenous use, and the immediate problem associated with it is the transient production of hypertension due to its partial agonist activity.[76] On the other hand, captopril, enalapril, and lisinopril are angiotensin-converting enzyme inhibitors that block the conversion of angiotensin I to angiotensin II.[1]

Poisoning with enalapril has been reported; a 46 year old man ingested 300 mg of enalapril in addition to 225 mg of oxazepam and presented with stupor and a blood pressure of 100/60 mm Hg, in addition to complete suppression of angiotensin II. The patient recovered fully after saline infusion increased blood pressure.[77] Although dialysis is unlikely to be necessary, captopril is dialyzable at a rate approximately half that of blood urea nitrogen (BUN),[78] and enalaprilat (the active form of enalapril) is also dialyzable.

ALPHA-ADRENERGIC BLOCKERS

Alpha$_1$-receptors are situated in the postsynaptic region of the neuron, whereas alpha$_2$-receptors are situated in the neuron's presynaptic region. Alpha-receptors are present in blood vessels, eye, and gastrointestinal tract; stimulation of these with alpha-stimulating drugs (for example, norepinephrine) brings about vasoconstriction, dilatation of the pupil, and reduction in gastrointestinal motility. On the other hand, alpha-blockade brings about pupillary dilatation, vasodilatation, and increased gastrointestinal motility. The main alpha-blockers[79] are phenoxybenzamine, phentolamine, and tolazoline (alpha$_1$ and alpha$_2$), dibenamine (alpha$_1$), prazosin (alpha$_1$), terazosin (alpha$_1$), yohimbine (alpha$_2$), and indoramin (not available in the United States).

Prazosin

Prazosin is both an arterial and a renal dilator, with its predominant action being through alpha-adrenergic blocking activity of smooth muscle.[79] The drug is a postsynaptic alpha$_1$-adrenergic receptor blocker and accomplishes a reduction in peripheral vascular resistance without secondary reflex tachycardia or increased renin activity, as occurs with hydralazine, diazoxide, or minoxidil. Like hydralazine, however, with chronic administration the cardiac index is increased, peripheral vascular resistance is reduced, and heart rate increases.[80] Similarly, fluid retention occurs, and postural hypotension may occur. In addition, tachyphylaxis, which may be due to the fluid retention, also may be observed. More than 99 per cent of the drug is metabolized in the liver, and the mean elimination half-time is approximately 3 hours.[81] The major toxicity with prazosin is related to sudden hypotension, or the "first-dose" phenomenon commonly seen after initiation of therapy. Overdosage should be treated expectantly, with management in the Trendelenburg position, with or without fluids, and with or without dopamine or dobutamine.

Overdose of these drugs is extremely rare, since phentolamine and phenoxybenzamine are used mainly for the control of hypertension in pheochromocytoma, and, as would be expected, profound hypotension is the result. Phenoxybenzamine and dibenamine inhibit uptake of catecholamines in adrenergic nerve terminals in the postsynaptic ($alpha_1$) region in an almost irreversible blockade, whereas phentolamine ($alpha_1$ and $alpha_2$), tolazoline ($alpha_1$), prazosin ($alpha_1$), terazosin ($alpha_1$), and yohimbine ($alpha_2$) are reversibly bound, competitive catecholamine inhibitors. It follows that hypotension and reflex tachycardia (except for prazosin, which is a selective alpha-blocker), especially in hypovolemic patients, are the major results, and that alpha-blockade with phenoxybenzamine and dibenamine may be more protracted. Profound reflex tachycardia may result in angina. Phentolamine and tolazoline both stimulate gastric hydrochloric acid and pepsin secretion, which may result in gastritis or peptic ulcer disease. Management of intoxication with these drugs follows standard therapy, with particular attention being paid to gastric lavage if the drug was ingested. Therapy should be directed to control of blood pressure, adoption of the Trendelenburg position, and administration of intravenous fluids and antacids (in the case of phentolamine or tolazoline). Pressor agents usually are not required.

References

1. Rudd P, Blaschke TF: Antihypertensive drugs and the drug therapy of hypertension. *In* Gilman AG, Goodman L, Rall TW, Murad F (eds): The Pharmacological Basis of Therapeutics. 7th ed. New York, Macmillan, 1985, p 784.
2. Schlant RC, Tsagaris TS, Robertson RJ: Studies on the acute cardiovascular effects of intravenous sodium nitroprusside. Am J Cardiol *9*:51, 1962.
3. Bhatia SK, Frohlich ED: Hemodynamic comparison of agents useful in hypertensive emergencies. Am Heart J *55*:365, 1973.
4. Bower PJ, Peterson JN: Methemoglobinemia after sodium nitroprusside therapy. N Engl J Med *293*:865, 1975.
5. Jack RD: Toxicology of sodium nitroprusside. Br J Anaesth *46*:952, 1974.
6. Merrifield AJ, Blundell MD: Toxicology of sodium nitroprusside. Br J Anaesth *46*:324, 1974.
7. Davies DW, Kadar D, Steward DJ, Munro IR: A sudden death associated with use of sodium nitroprusside for induction of hypotension during anaesthesia. Can Anaesth Soc J *22*:547, 1975.
8. Vesey CJ, Cole PV, Simpson PJ: Cyanide and thiocyanate concentrations following sodium nitroprusside infusion in man. Br J Anaesth *48*:651, 1976.
9. Cottrell JE, Casthely P, Brodie JD, Patel K, Klein A, Turndorf H: Prevention of nitroprusside-induced cyanide toxicity with hydroxocobalamin. N Engl J Med *298*:809, 1978.
10. Nourok DG, Glassock RJ, Solomon DH, Maxwell MH: Hypothyroidism following prolonged sodium nitroprusside therapy. Am J Med Sci *248*:129, 1964.
11. Norris JC, Huma AS: In vivo release of cyanide from sodium nitroprusside. Br J Anaesth *59*:236, 1987.
12. Humphrey SH, Nash DA: Lactic acidosis complicating sodium nitroprusside therapy. Ann Intern Med *88*:58, 1978.
13. Greiss L, Tremblay NAG, Davies DW: The toxicity of sodium nitroprusside. Can Anaesth Soc J *23*:480, 1976.
14. McDowall DG, Keaney NP, Turner JM, Lane JR, Okuda Y: The toxicity of sodium nitroprusside. Br J Anaesth *46*:327, 1974.
15. Simpson PJ, Adams L, Vesey CJ, Cole PV: Some physiological and metabolic effects of sodium nitroprusside and cyanide in the dog. Br J Anaesth *51*:81, 1979.
16. Vesey PV, Cole CJ: Sodium thiosulphate decreases blood cyanide concentrations after the infusion of sodium nitroprusside. Br J Anaesth *59*:531, 1987.
17. Verner IR: Direct acting vasodilators (sodium nitroprusside; glyceryl trinitrate; the adenyl nucleotides). *In* Enderby GEH (ed): Hypotensive Anaesthesia. 3rd ed. Edinburgh, Churchill Livingstone, 1985, p 37.
18. Shand DG, Nies AS, McAllister RG, Oates JA: A loading dose regimen for more rapid initiation of the effect of guanethidine. Clin Pharmacol Ther *18*:139, 1975.
19. Reidenberg MM, Drayer D, DeMarco A, Bello CT: Hydralazine elimination in man. Clin Pharmacol Ther *14*:970, 1973.
20. Alarcon-Segovia D: Drug-induced antinuclear antibodies and lupus syndromes. Drugs *12*:69, 1976.
21. Gottlieb TB, Thomas RC, Chindsey CA: Pharmacokinetic studies of minoxidil. Clin Pharmacol Ther *13*:436,1972.
22. Dormois JC, Young JL, Nies AS: Minoxidil in severe hypertension: Value when conventional drugs have failed. Am Heart J *90*:365, 1975.
23. Zarate A, Gelfand MC, Horton JD, Winchester JF,

Gottlieb MJ, Lazarus JM, Schreiner GE: Pericardial effusion associated with minoxidil therapy in dialyzed patients. Int J Artif Organs *3*:15, 1980.
24. Isles C, Mackay A, Barton PJM, Mitchell I: Accidental overdosage of minoxidil in a child. Lancet *1*:97, 1981.
25. Hall D, Charcolos F, Froer KL, Rudolph W: ECG changes during long-term minoxidil therapy for severe hypertension. Arch Intern Med *139*:790, 1979.
26. Zins GR, Martin WB: The clinical pharmacology of minoxidil. *In* Velasco M (ed): Proceedings, Second International Symposium on Arterial Hypertension. Amsterdam, Excerpta Medica, 1979, p 72.
27. Royer ME, Ko H, Goldbertson TJ, McCall JM, Johnston KT, Stryd R: Radioimmunoassay of minoxidil in human serum. J Pharm Sci *66*:1266, 1977.
28. Weber MA: Discontinuation syndrome following cessation of treatment with clonidine and other antihypertensive agents. J Cardiovasc Pharmacol 2 (Suppl 1):S73, 1980.
29. Chaydarian CG, Karashima D, Castagnoli N: Oxidative and cardiovascular studies on natural and synthetic catecholamines. J Med Chem *21*:548, 1978.
30. Freed CR, Quintero E, Murphy C: Hypotension and hypothalamic amine metabolism after long-term α-methyldopa infusions. Life Sci *23*:313, 1978.
31. Ayiteh-Smith E, Varma DR: Mechanism of the hypotensive action of methyldopa in normal and immunosympathectomized rats. Br J Pharmacol *40*:186, 1970.
32. Kwan KC, Foltz EL, Breault GO, Baer JE, Totaro JA: Pharmacokinetics of methyldopa in man. J Pharmacol Exp Ther *198*:264, 1976.
33. Barnett AJ, Bobok A, Carson V, Korman JS, McLean AJ: Pharmacokinetics of methyldopa. Clin Exp Pharmacol Physiol *4*:331, 1977.
34. Myhre E, Brodwall EK, Stenbaek O, Hansen T: Plasma turnover of methyldopa in advanced renal failure. Acta Med Scand *191*:343, 1972.
35. Sternbach GL, Rosen P: Methyldopa overdose. J Am Coll Emerg Phys *4*:325, 1975.
36. Yamadori A, Albert ML: Involuntary movement disorder caused by methyldopa. N Engl J Med *286*:610, 1972.
37. Westervelt FB, Atuk NO: Methyldopa-induced hypertension. JAMA 227:557, 1974
38. Zehnle CG: Paradoxical hypertension experienced during methyldopa therapy. Am J Hosp Pharm *38*:1774, 1981.
39. Nies AS, Shand DG: Hypertensive response to propranolol in a patient treated with methyldopa: A proposed mechanism. Clin Pharmacol Ther *14*:823, 1973.
40. Levine RJ, Strauch BS: Hypertensive responses to methyldopa. N Engl J Med *27*:946, 1966.
41. Elkington SG, Schreiber W, Conn HO: Hepatic injury caused by L-alpha-methyldopa. Circulation *40*:589, 1969.
42. Alha A, Korte T, Lukkari I, Raekallio J, Tamminmen V: Methyldopa poisoning. Report of the first published fatal case. Zacchia *7*:415, 1971.
43. Tompsett SL: Aldomet (methyldopa) in blood, serum and urine. Bull Int Assoc Forensic Toxicol *4*:3, 1967.
44. Guardasole F, De Vivo R: Case of chronic alpha-methyldopa poisoning in a female patient with biliary-digestive fistula. Rass Int Clin Ter *50*:1316, 1970.
45. Cokkinos DV, Vorides EM: Impairment of atrioventricular conduction by methyldopa. Chest *74*:697, 1978.
46. Ferris JA: Drug-induced myocarditis: A report of two cases. Forensic Sci *13*:261, 1979.
47. Van Spanning HW, van Zwieten PA: The interaction between alpha-methyldopa and tricyclic antidepressants. Int J Clin Pharmacol Biopharm *11*:65, 1975.
48. Yeh BK, Dayton PG, Waters WC: Removal of alpha-methyldopa (Aldomet) in man by dialysis. Proc Soc Exp Biol Med *135*:840, 1970.
49. Gosselin RE, Hodge HC, Smith RP, Gleason MN (eds): Reserpine. *In* Clinical Toxicology of Commercial Products. 4th ed. Baltimore, Williams & Wilkins, 1976, p 289.
50. Holzbauer M, Vogt M: Depression by reserpine of the noradrenaline concentration in the hypothalamus of the cat. J Neurochem *1*:8, 1956.
51. Brodie BB, Spector S, Shore PA: Interaction of drugs with norepinephrine in the brain. Pharmacol Rev *11*:548, 1959.
52. Bracha S, Hess JP: Death occurring during combined reserpine–electroshock treatment. Am J Psychiatr *113*:257, 1956.
53. Foster MN, Gayle RF: Chlorpromazine and reserpine as adjuncts in electroshock treatment. South Med J *49*:731, 1956.
54. Hubbard BA: Reserpine. JAMA *157*:468, 1955.
55. Loggie JMH, Saito H, Kahn I, Fenner A, Gaffney TE: Accidental reserpine poisoning: Clinical and metabolic effect. Clin Pharmacol Ther *8*:692, 1967.
56. McKown CH, Verlhurst HL, Crotty JL: Overdosage effects and danger from tranquilizing drugs. JAMA *185*:425, 1963.
57. Schneider EM, Clark ML: Hyperchlorhydria induced by intravenous reserpine. Response to various therapeutic agents. Am J Digest Dis *1*:22, 1956.
58. Duncan DA, Fleeson W: Reserpine-induced gastrointestinal hemorrhage. JAMA *170*:661, 1959.
59. Taylor P: Ganglion stimulating and blocking drugs. *In* Gilman AG, Goodman LS, Rall TW, Murad F (eds): The Pharmacological Basis of Therapeutics. 7th ed. New York, Macmillan, 1985, p 215.
60. Rumack BH (ed): Ganglionic blocking agents—antihypertension. *In* Poisindex. Denver, Micromedix Systems Inc., 1982.
61. Shanor SP, Kinnard WJ, Buckley JP: Cardiovascular activity of mecamyulamine, pempidine and several pempidine analogs. J Pharm Sci *54*:859, 1965.
62. Beani L, Bianchi C, Bieber G, Ledda F: The effect of some ganglionic stimulants and blocking agents on acetylcholine release from the mammalian neuromuscular function. J Pharm Pharmacol *16*:557, 1964.
63. Pohl JEF, Thurston H: Use of diazoxide in hypertension with renal failure. Br Med J *4*:142, 1971.
64. Harrison BDW, Rutter TW, Taylor RT: Severe non-ketotic hyperglycaemic pre-coma in a hypertensive patient receiving diazoxide. Lancet *2*:599, 1972.
65. Updike ST, Harrington AR: Acute diabetic ketoacidosis—a complication of intravenous diazoxide treatment for refractory hypertension. N Engl J Med *280*:768, 1969.
66. Pearson RM, Breckenridge AM: Renal function protein binding and pharmacological response to diazoxide. Br J Clin Pharmacol *3*:169, 1976.
67. Cirksena WJ, Winchester JF: K or no K? That is the question. *In* Schreiner GE, Winchester JR (eds): Controversies in Nephrology. Vol II. Washington, DC, Nephrology Division, Georgetown University, 1980, p 138.
68. Frohlich ED: Ticrynafen: A new thiazide-like uricosuric antihypertensive diuretic. N Engl J Med *301*:1378, 1979.

69. Barclay WR: Ticrynafen's withdrawal from the market. JAMA *243*:771, 1980.
70. Morgan AG, Bennett JM, Pollack A: Mannitol retention during diuretic treatment of barbiturate and salicylate overdosage. Q J Med *37*:589, 1968.
71. Aviram A, Pfau A, Czaczkes JW, Ullman TD: Hyperosmolality with hyponatremia caused by inappropriate administration of mannitol. Am J Med *42*:648, 1967.
72. Feldman DH, Kjellstrand CM, Fraley EE: Mannitol intoxication. J Urol *106*:622, 1971.
73. Vaziri ND, Saiki J, Barton CH, Rajudin M, Ness RL: Hemodialyzability of acetazolamide. South Med J *73*:422, 1980.
74. Orcharad RT, Taylor DJE, Parkins RA: Sulphonamide crystalluria with acetazolamide. Br Med J *3*:646, 1972.
75. Kristinsson A: Fatal reaction to acetazolamide. Br J Ophthalmol *51*:348, 1967.
76. Wallace JM, Case DB, Laragh JH, Sealey JE, Keim HJ, Drayer JI: The immediate pressor response to saralasin: A measure of the degree of angiotensin II vascular receptor vacancy. Trans Assoc Am Phys *40*:300, 1977.
77. Waeber B, Nussberger J, Brunner HR: Self-poisoning with enalapril. Br Med J *288*:287, 1984.
78. Hirakata H, Onoyama K, Omae T, Fujimi S, Kawahara Y: Captopril (SQ 14225) clearance during hemodialysis treatment. Clin Nephrol *16*:321, 1981.
79. Weiner N: Drugs that inhibit adrenergic nerves and block adrenergic receptors. *In* Gilman AG, Goodman LS, Rall TW, Murad F (eds): The Pharmalogical Basis of Therapeutics. 7th ed. New York, Macmillan, 1985, p 181.
80. Lund-Johansen P: Hemodynamic changes at rest and during exercise in long-term prazosin therapy for essential hypertension. Postgrad Med J *58* (Suppl):45, 1975.
81. Bateman DN, Hobbs DC, Twomey TM, Stevens EA, Rawlins MD: Prazosin pharmacokinetics and concentration effect. Eur J Clin Pharmacol *16*:177, 1979.

CHAPTER 94
CLONIDINE

James R. Roberts, M.D.
Brian J. Zink, M.D.

Clonidine hydrochloride, an imidazoline compound structurally related to the alpha-blocking agent phentolamine, was developed in the 1960s as a nasal decongestant. Its potent antihypertensive action was soon appreciated, and it became a commonly prescribed drug for the treatment of essential hypertension. Clonidine produces its antihypertensive effect via complex interactions with adrenergic, endogenous opioid, and other neuroendocrine pathways in the brain stem and higher brain centers. The precise mechanism and location of action have not been fully elucidated, but the hypotensive effect is secondary to a reduction in sympathetic tone that is mediated through central alpha-adrenergic pathways. Although it is used mainly as a primary or secondary oral antihypertensive, the compound recently has been used to ameliorate alcohol, narcotic, and nicotine withdrawal, and for the control of postmenopausal flushing and migraine headaches. Clonidine is a widely prescribed drug with potential for serious overdose toxicity. In addition, a significant withdrawal syndrome may occur following the abrupt discontinuation of clonidine therapy.

SITE AND MECHANISM OF ACTION

Although it is clear that clonidine exerts its hypotensive action via complex alpha-adrenergic pathways in the central nervous system, the specific site of action is unknown.[1, 2] The drug probably has effects in both the hypothalamus and medulla oblongata. The primary control of systemic blood pressure is thought to occur by means of inhibitory reflex loops in the pontomedullary area, specifically in the nucleus tractus solitarius (NTS) and the vasomotor center (VMC). The NTS receives afferent impulses from baroreceptors in the carotid body (9th cranial nerve) and aortic arch (vagus nerve). When blood pressure is elevated, the impulse traffic through the NTS is increased. Subsequently, the VMC receives inhibitory input from the NTS. This causes decreased efferent output in sympathetic neurons, thus completing a negative feedback loop.[2]

Clonidine is primarily an *alpha-2* adrenergic receptor agonist resembling methyldopa, but to some extent it is an *alpha-1* receptor agonist. Clonidine also possesses some alpha-receptor *antagonist* properties.[2–4] Its specific action in the central nervous system probably depends upon the endogenous concentration of norepinephrine. The hypotensive action of clonidine occurs through central rather than peripheral alpha-adrenergic receptors, confirmed by the observation that central alpha-2 receptor blockers, such as yohimbine, also block the hypotensive action of clonidine.[3] Clonidine may act primarily as a *presynaptic* alpha-2 agonist, effecting a decrease of norepinephrine release, leading to decreased sympathetic outflow from the central nervous system. Clonidine also may be an agonist at *postsynaptic* alpha-2 receptors, activating an inhibitory neuron that suppresses CNS sympathetic outflow.[4] Another theory is that clonidine acts as an alpha-2 receptor *antagonist*, thereby decreasing activity in excitatory cardiovascular neurons in the bulbar area and making the activity of inhibitory neurons more effective in decreasing sympathetic outflow. Regardless of the precise mechanism of action, clonidine's stimulation of central alpha-adrenoreceptors results in a reduction of sympathetic outflow to the cardiovascular system, manifested as a decrease in peripheral vascular resistance and a reduction in heart rate and stroke volume.

The initial hypotensive effect of clonidine is attributed primarily to a reduction in cardiac output rather than by a significant reduction in total peripheral vascular resistance. With continued therapy, peripheral resistance may be lowered. Clinically, both bradycardia and decreased stroke volume are noted. Clonidine induces bradycardia by a combination of three mechanisms.[5] The first is by a central reduction in sympathetic outflow, which reduces adrenergic stimulation to the heart. The second is a central alpha-2 or alpha-1 receptor stimulation, which activates the motor nucleus of the vagus nerve, causing vagal reflex bradycardia. The third mechanism is peripheral. It has been proposed that clonidine acts as an agonist at cardiac presynaptic alpha-2 receptors, causing decreased norepinephrine release in cardiac tissues. It has been demonstrated that clonidine does not change electrophysiologic parameters in the heart, such as sinus cycle length, sinus node recovery time, or intraventricular conduction time.[6] Cardiac response to exercise is not altered by clonidine.

There is no appreciable reflex tachycardia or orthostatic hypotension in patients taking clonidine. The lack of reflex tachycardia is due to clonidine's bradycardic effect. The lack of orthostatic hypotension (in the absence of concomitant hypovolemia) is related to the site of action of clonidine in the brain. Clonidine, unlike reserpine, does not affect final sympathetic outflow from the medulla. It acts upon neurons that feed into the vasomotor center (VMC) exerting its effects in conjunction with input from reflex afferent pathways rather than nullifying these reflex pathways by blocking output from the VMC. This allows existing baroreceptor pathways to continue normal functioning in the presence of clonidine.[7]

The CNS-renal axis plays a major role in blood pressure regulation. Chronic clonidine administration affects the axis by reducing renin secretion. This probably occurs by a peripheral stimulation of alpha-receptors rather than by a central mechanism. No acute change in blood pressure results from this in humans.

Clonidine reduces catecholamine levels in the plasma; the effect is more pronounced for norepinephrine (NE) than for epinephrine (E). This further supports the theory that clonidine reduces sympathetic neuron activity centrally and not through suppression of the adrenal medulla.[8] It also has been demonstrated that clonidine decreases NE and its major metabolite 3-methoxy-4-hydroxyphenylglycol (MHPG) in the cerebrospinal fluid. During insulin-induced hypoglycemia in humans, clonidine inhibits the expected rise in norepinephrine and epinephrine levels.[9] The effects of clonidine appear to persist even with stresses that might be expected to override the suppression of catecholamine release.

Through clinical observations that clonidine can be used to treat opiate withdrawal, it became apparent that clonidine interacts with the endogenous opioid system. Opiate receptors are numerous in the major adrenergic nucleus of the brain, the locus ceruleus.

At low doses, clonidine can block firing of locus ceruleus neurons, with resultant decreased norepinephrine outflow.[10] It has not been established whether clonidine influences endogenous opiate receptors by its action on alpha-adrenergic receptors, or whether other systems are involved. Clonidine has been shown in humans to increase central dopamine turnover.[8]

Clonidine produces a number of other effects that are thought to be related to its action on central alpha-adrenoceptors. In human overdoses, clonidine frequently has been noted to produce *hypothermia.* The mechanism is thought to be alpha-adrenoceptor stimulation in serotonin-acetylcholine pathways, which leads to decreased metabolic heat production and increased dry heat loss. Other biochemical activities of clonidine include a significant reduction in serum cortisol and ACTH levels, an increase in growth hormone levels, and an augmentation of antidiuretic hormone (ADH) secretion.[11] Clonidine also decreases gut motility (antidiarrheal effect) and causes some increase in the rate of absorption of fluid from the gut mucosa.

The psychiatric implications of clonidine are tied to its central effects. In depressed patients there is less response to clonidine in terms of growth hormone release, plasma MHPG increase, and heart rate decline. This may indicate that there is reduced activity of alpha-2 adrenergic receptors in depression. Depressed patients have elevated cortisol levels, which can be reduced by clonidine. Clonidine can reduce anxiety in some depressed patients.[12]

The central mechanism of action of clonidine produces a wide variety of pharmacologic effects, most of which are not yet completely understood.

ABSORPTION, DISTRIBUTION, AND METABOLISM

Clonidine is well absorbed from the gastrointestinal tract within 30 minutes after an oral dose. Serum levels peak in 2 to 3 hours. The bioavailability of the tablet is approximately 75 per cent, indicating no appreciable first-pass effect. The drug is 20 to 40 per cent protein bound and is highly lipid soluble, with excellent CNS penetration. Clonidine is excreted primarily by the kidney, and 40 to 50 per cent of an oral dose is excreted unchanged in the urine. Hepatic metabolism occurs by splitting of the imidazoline ring, but none of the metabolites are known to be pharmacologically active.

The volume of distribution is 3.2 to 5.6 liters per kg. Clonidine exhibits first-order kinetics, and a two-compartment model has been proposed: a rapidly equilibrating compartment consisting of the vascular system and organs of high blood flow, and a slower equilibration in a second compartment. There is no accumulation of the drug with chronic dosing. The elimination half-life is 5 to 13 hours. In chronic renal failure, the dose of clonidine may have to be adjusted downward, but no replacement is necessary after dialysis.

CLINICAL USE

Clonidine is marketed in 0.1-, 0.2-, and 0.3-mg tablets (Catapres). It is also combined in similar doses with the diuretic chlorthalidone (Combipres). The drug is available in Europe as a 0.025-mg tablet (Dixaret). The usual recommended therapeutic dose is 0.2 to 0.8 mg per day (divided in two or three doses). For the rapid control of serious hypertension, an oral regimen has been suggested, consisting of an initial dose of 0.2 mg, followed by 0.1 mg per hour until the desired effect is obtained. Clonidine is also available in transdermal patches (Catapres-TTS) that are applied weekly. Patches are designed to slowly release 0.1, 0.2, or 0.3 mg per day and are impregnated with 2.5, 5.0, and 7.5 mg of clonidine, respectively. The transdermal route is as effective as the oral route with fewer side effects. An intravenous preparation is not available.

Clonidine has been used as a first- or second-line antihypertensive agent, either alone or in combination with other medications. It is synergistic with diuretics but not with methyldopa or prazocin. Tricyclic antidepressants may interfere with clonidine's antihypertensive activity. It appears to be safe and effective in pregnant women,[13] in elderly patients, and in patients with renal failure or undergoing chronic hemodialysis. Clonidine has no antihypertensive effect in individuals with complete spinal cord transection.

The major side effects of therapeutic use are dry mouth, sedation, and dizziness. In the absence of volume depletion (such as is seen with the concomitant use of diuretics), orthostatic hypotension is rare. Hallucinations, nightmares, paranoia, and delirium have been reported with therapeutic use.[14, 15]

There is a linear relationship between the plasma concentration of clonidine and its pharmacologic effect. The hypotensive effect occurs in a relatively narrow concentration range of 1.5 to 2.0 ng per ml. At higher plasma levels, the hypotensive effect is diminished, and once levels of greater than 4 ng per ml are reached, hypertension may occur, probably as a result of vasoconstriction secondary to peripheral alpha-receptor stimulation. This therapeutic window has strong implications both for maintenance dosing and in the overdose setting.

OVERDOSE

Epidemiology. Clonidine overdose is a potentially life-threatening condition. Accidental overdose is most commonly reported in children, who seem to be particularly sensitive to even small amounts of the drug.[16, 17] In a common scenario the child is visiting the grandparents' home and ingests a grandparent's unsecured clonidine tablets. Even 1 or 2 of the small and easily swallowed pills can lead to serious toxicity in a small child. Severe symptoms (coma, hypotension, bradycardia) have been described following ingestion of a single adult therapeutic dose (0.1 and 0.3 mg) by a small child.[18, 19]

Significant clonidine poisoning has been described in children who have sucked or chewed on a discarded clonidine transdermal patch.[20, 21] Considering that a patch designed to release 0.3 mg of clonidine per day is impregnated with a total of 7.5 mg of clonidine, the residual drug in a used patch has the potential to cause significant toxicity in a small child. Theoretically, transdermal poisoning is also possible in a small child who applies a patch to the skin.

In adults, significant clonidine toxicity occurs with ingestion of greater than 2 or 3 mg (ten times the therapeutic dose). Unintentional overmedication can occur if there is confusion with dosing (as is often seen in the elderly) or if the patient increases the maintenance dose. Clonidine has been ingested in suicide attempts. The drug may also be intentionally abused, either for its euphoric effect (particularly when combined with diazepam), or if overused when prescribed for narcotic withdrawal.[22] Narcotic addicts may inadvertently overtreat themselves in an attempt to lessen their need for street narcotics during times of short supply.

Clinical Presentation. Signs and symptoms of overdose occur within 30 to 60 minutes following an acute ingestion. The presentation is remarkably similar to that of a narcotic overdose, with the triad of *miosis, coma,* and *respiratory depression.* Most patients with a significant ingestion will present with decreased mental status or in coma, with varying degrees of hypotension, respiratory depression, bradycardia, miosis, hypotonia, hyporeflexia, pallor, and hypothermia.[23, 24] Clonidine will intensify the depressant effect on the central nervous system of alcohol, barbiturates, and other sedative hypnotics. Seizures may rarely occur. The relative frequency of these features differs between adults and children (Table 94–1). Children are more prone to develop deep coma, respiratory depression, and hypothermia. Intermittent apnea responsive to physical stimuli and a peculiar gasping or sighing have been noted in children. Hypothermia is a curious but frequently reported finding in children with clonidine overdose. It is probably related to a combination of hypotension and bradycardia and a central effect of the drug. Theoretically, hypoglycemia may occur in overdose since clonidine blocks the catecholamine inhibition of insulin release.

Hypertension is seen in 25 per cent of adults and about 10 per cent of children with clonidine overdose. It is more common during

Table 94–1. CLONIDINE OVERDOSE IN CHILDREN AND ADULTS

SIGN OR SYMPTOM	CHILDREN (%)	ADULT (%)
Coma or depressed mental status	80–85	75–80
Respiratory depression/ apnea	50–60	20–30
Bradycardia	30–40	50–60
Hypotension	50	40–50
Hypertension	5–10	15–25
Miosis	30–40	30–40
Hyporeflexia/hypotonia	30–40	30–40
Hypothermia	50	10–20
Seizures	≤ 5	≤ 5

Compiled from various references cited in bibliography.

the early stages of massive overdoses. Hypertension is associated with plasma clonidine levels of greater than 10 to 15 ng per ml, whereas hypotension or normal blood pressure is seen with levels below 10 ng per ml.[25] At higher plasma levels, the peripheral alpha-1 agonist properties of clonidine theoretically cause vasoconstriction, leading to hypertension.[26] In patients who present with hypertension, it is likely that a hypotensive phase occurred first, as the clonidine level was rising. The magnitude and time course of the hypertensive phase is unpredictable, but hypertension can be severe (a diastolic pressure to 140 to 150 mm Hg may be encountered) and may persist for minutes or hours. This phase can be followed precipitously by significant hypotension. Rebound hypertension subsequently may be seen in 2 to 4 days during the "withdrawal" period, particularly if the patient has been on chronic therapy. It is not known whether prior use of clonidine or underlying hypertension alters the initial blood pressure response in clonidine overdose.

Diagnosis. The diagnosis of clonidine overdose is usually based on the clinical history and a physical examination. No laboratory tests are of specific clinical value in the diagnosis. Clonopin (clonazepam) may be confused with clonidine because of similar sounding names. Since the overdose may resemble narcotic ingestion, beta-blocker or calcium antagonist toxicity, hypoglycemia, or sepsis, appropriate screening tests are warranted if the diagnosis is uncertain. As with any overdose, concomitant trauma should be investigated. Quantitative plasma levels are generally unavailable and of no therapeutic value, but a complete toxicology screen may be indicated to confirm or rule out concomitant ingestions. Clonidine can be identified in the serum by high-pressure liquid chromatography (HPLC) or mass spectroscopy for academic or investigative purposes, but the drug likely would be *unidentified* by standard drug screens.

MORTALITY AND MORBIDITY

There are no documented cases of death from clonidine alone in overdose. The lethal dose has not been established, but survival has been documented in children after a 10-mg dose[27] and in an adult following a 100-mg ingestion.[28] Serum levels as high as 230 ng per ml have been reported with survival.[28] Rare deaths have occurred in mixed overdose (personal communication with Boehringer Ingelheim, Ridgefield, CT). Concomitant ingestions, underlying medical conditions, and trauma and sequelae such as pulmonary aspiration may be contributory to a fatal outcome.

Hypotension and bradycardia may be severe but are usually responsive to therapy and not associated with lasting morbidity. Respiratory depression may be the most serious element of clonidine overdose. In children and adults there are reports of apnea and respiratory arrest.[23, 29, 30] In most cases there is gradual improvement in level of consciousness, respiratory effort, and hemodynamic parameters within the first 12 to 24 hours. Total recovery is usually seen after 48 to 72 hours. In patients with underlying renal disease, recovery may be delayed owing to decreased clearance. A unique characteristicof clonidine is its ability to produce a with drawal syndrome, with hypertension, tachycardia, and subjective symptoms of adrenergic hyperactivity. This syndrome theoretically can occur in patients with a single acute overdose as clonidine levels fall to zero. The withdrawal syndrome will be discussed later.

TREATMENT

The treatment of clonidine overdose should be conservative. Since there is little threat of death or lasting morbidity, treatment protocols must be designed to provide standard supportive and symptomatic treatment without subjecting the patient to the risks of overaggressive or unproved therapies.

Following recent significant ingestions, gastric emptying procedures are probably warranted. Gastric lavage is preferred to ipecac-induced emesis if coma or an impending decrease in mental status is present. Oral activated charcoal and a cathartic are recommended. No studies validate the efficacy of these commonly recommended toxicologic therapies, but this standard approach is recommended by most investigators. If the patient is stable and ingestion was longer than 2 hours prior to admission, cautious observation may be all that is required. As a general precaution, the patient should be observed in an area with electrocardiographic monitoring capabilities. Vital signs, including temperature, should be recorded frequently.

Specific interventional therapy is aimed toward respiratory support and the treatment of hypotension and bradycardia. The initial management of clonidine overdose involves assessment of the airway and respiratory exchange. In the comatose state, the inability to maintain a patent upper airway and the risk of aspiration or hypoxemia are major concerns. Supplemental oxygen and tracheal intubation with assisted ventilation may be required. Children seem particularly prone to develop respiratory failure with clonidine overdose. Seizures are usually transient but may be treated with diazepam or lorazepam.

Hemodynamic changes can be pronounced. Bradycardia is a hallmark of significant toxicity, but the decision to treat should not be based solely upon the heart rate. Hypothermia is common, particularly in children, and may contribute to the bradycardia. Bradycardia usually responds to atropine, although repeated doses may be required. Hypotension may be managed with crystalloid infusion; occasionally the use of vasopressors, such as dopamine, is required.

Hypertension is less common than hypotension but may be significant following massive ingestions. Hypertension is usually a transient phase in the hemodynamic response to clonidine toxicity, which may be followed immediately by significant hypotension. Observation is usually all that is required during the hypertensive stage,[30] but, on occasion, the use of a short-acting, easily titratable antihypertensive agent, such as phentolamine, nitroprusside, or nifedipine, may be warranted. It is essential to avoid overtreating mild, transient hypertension with an agent that may compound subsequent hypotension. Forced diuresis, charcoal hemoperfusion, and hemodialysis are of no proven value in the treatment of clonidine overdose.

Naloxone

Naloxone has become popular as a possible antidote for clonidine toxicity; its exact role as a classic antidote is not yet established. Based on the similarity between clonidine and narcotic overdose and studies linking clonidine with endogenous opiate receptors, investigators have examined the effects of the opiate receptor antagonist naloxone in reversing the effects of clonidine.[31] Scattered case reports have documented an abrupt improvement in mental status and hemodynamic parameters in both children and adults with clonidine overdose who were given naloxone. However, this antidote effect is inconsistent, and some reports show no benefit. For example, Banner and associates were unable to demonstrate a reversal of clonidine toxicity in children when up to 0.1 mg per kg of naloxone was administered,[32] whereas Niemann and associates[33] and Kulig and colleagues[34] report striking reversal of clonidine toxicity in adults with 2 mg and 0.8 mg of naloxone, respectively.

It is difficult to separate the effects of naloxone from those of concomitant therapy (fluids, vasopressors, atropine) in the available case reports. Although there may be a subset of naloxone-sensitive patients, the specific characteristics of those patients who will respond to the narcotic antagonist have not been identified. There is a theoretic risk of rebound hypertension in patients with clonidine overdose who are given naloxone, but the case reports of this have not established a definite direct temporal effect.[35] Given the clinical similarity between narcotics and clonidine, and the proven safety and possible benefit of naloxone, *the use of naloxone in patients presenting with clonidine overdose is warranted*. The correct dose of naloxone is unknown, but it should be given with the same caveats that apply to the treatment of narcotic overdose. The exact role of naloxone in clonidine poisoning remains to be elucidated.

Tolazoline

Tolazoline, a central and peripheral alpha-adrenergic blocking agent (and partial agonist), which produces peripheral vasodilatation and cardiac stimulation, is another agent that has been touted as an antidote for clonidine toxicity.[23, 24, 36, 37] In theory, tolazoline should block the central alpha-2 agonist properties of clonidine, but no controlled trials have been reported. Its use has been advocated solely on the basis of sporadic case reports, in which it appears to have antidotal properties. However, as with naloxone, tolazoline has been used in conjunction with other therapeutic measures that also could have accounted for the reversal of toxicity. *Tolazoline is not a proven antidote for clonidine overdose.* Potential side effects are unpredictable and include hypertension or hypotension, tachycardia, and arrhythmias. Tolazoline should be cautiously reserved for those unusual cases unresponsive to standard therapy. The correct dose of tolazoline is not known, but most investigators administer the drug intravenously by slow push in 5- to 10-mg bolus doses, with a maximum of 30 to 40 mg in an adult.[38, 39]

CLONIDINE WITHDRAWAL SYNDROME

Adrenergic hyperactivity may occur 24 to 72 hours after the abrupt cessation of long-term clonidine therapy.[40, 41] It is not known exactly how long patients must be on maintenance therapy before withdrawal of the drug will precipitate symptoms, but withdrawal has not been a significant problem following acute overdose or after treatment for a few days. The clinical symptoms are similar to the withdrawal patterns seen with other antihypertensive agents (beta-blockers, methyldopa), alcohol, and sedative-hypnotic agents.[42] The major concern is that an "overshoot" hypertensive crisis may ensue. Numerous prospective human trials have demonstrated a rapid rise in blood pressure to pretreatment levels when clonidine has been withdrawn following maintenance therapy. Although serious hypertension is very rare, hypertensive encepalopathy and death have occurred.

Clinically, the clonidine withdrawal syndrome consists of tachycardia and hypertension accompanied by subjective symptoms of anxiety, nervousness, insomnia, sweating, abdominal pain, headache, nausea, and palpitations. Approximately 50 per cent of patients withdrawn from the drug will have mild symptoms, but most patients have therapy abruptly terminated without any clinically significant adverse effects. Patients who stop clonidine but are continued on concomitant beta-blocker therapy appear to be at greater risk. There is minimal direct correlation between drug dose and the development of a withdrawal syndrome, and individuals taking 1.2 mg a day or more for more than a few months are more likely to have significant symptomatology. Clonidine withdrawal has been associated with an increased incidence of ventricular arrhythmias, including ventricular tachycardia in a patient with underlying cardiac pathology.[43, 44]

The withdrawal syndrome is the result of excessive central adrenergic overactivity. Plasma and urine catecholamine levels increase during withdrawal.[45] Similarities have been drawn to manic-depressive illnesses, in which norepinephrine metabolites are increased during manic phases. Hypomania and psychosis also have been associated with clonidine withdrawal.[46]

Patients given clonidine must be advised of the risk of stopping therapy. When discontinued, the drug should be gradually tapered over 3 to 5 days. Alternative medications or the transdermal patch should be considered in poorly compliant individuals. The withdrawal syndrome is most effectively treated by reinstituting clonidine therapy, but prazocin, phentolamine, captopril, and phenoxybenzamine may be used.[44, 47] Theoretically, beta-blocker therapy may result in unopposed alpha-agonist activity and worsen withdrawal hypertension. Chlordiazepoxide or other benzodiazepines can help control the subjective symptoms of withdrawal. Serious hypertension may require nitroprusside or diazoxide.[47] The treatment of clonidine withdrawal must be tempered by the fact that the syndrome is self-limiting (5 to 7 days), and most patients can be managed with minimal medical intervention.

CLONIDINE IN THE TREATMENT OF WITHDRAWAL SYNDROMES

Narcotic Withdrawal. Clonidine has been demonstrated to be a useful adjunct to ameliorate the signs and symptoms of narcotic (including propoxyphene) withdrawal.[48, 49] The exact mechanism of action is unclear, but clonidine may decrease norepinephrine turnover or release in the locus ceruleus. Opiate withdrawal has been linked to adrenergic hyperactivity in the locus ceruleus, and the central alpha-agonist properties of clonidine may produce an inhibitory effect on this center.[50]

Both inpatient and outpatient therapy are acceptable. The dose of clonidine required to control symptoms is quite variable, but initial doses of 5 to 8 μg per kg per day (in divided doses) are suggested. The specific dose is titrated to control symptoms, and up to 25 μg per kg per day have been necessary. The clinically effective dose is determined and then gradually tapered over 2 to 3 weeks. An alternative to oral clonidine is the use of 2 or 3 transdermal patches (such as Catapres TTS-2) for 1 to 3 weeks, but this may require oral supplementation for the first few days. Sedation and orthostatic hypotension are the main side effects limiting clinical use. Note that the combination of narcotics plus clonidine can produce a significant decrease in mental status, and there is potential for overdose in the unreliable outpatient.[51] Clonidine also has been used to treat the neonatal abstinence syndrome.

Alcohol Withdrawal. Clonidine may also be very effective adjunctive therapy in the treatment of alcohol withdrawal. Several controlled trials have demonstrated that clonidine produces a significant reduction of both subjective symptoms and tachycardia and hypertension in patients experiencing alcohol withdrawal.[52–54] In a comparison of clonidine with chlordiazepoxide, clonidine was superior in reducing heart rate and systolic hypertension during alcohol withdrawal and equally effective in alleviating subjective symptoms.[52] The usual dose of clonidine used for alcohol withdrawal is 0.2 to 0.3 mg, given up to four times per day. Smaller doses can be used in conjunction with benzodiazepines. Side effects such as orthostatic hypotension may limit therapy to closely supervised inpatients, but motivated outpatients may also benefit.

The value of clonidine to ameliorate other drug withdrawal states, such as benzodiazepine withdrawal, is not yet known, but several experimental studies are presently underway. Recently, clonidine has been touted as a useful adjunct for nicotine withdrawal; although further studies are required, there is initial optimism that the drug may help individuals stop smoking.

References

1. Reid JL: The clinical pharmacology of clonidine and related central antihypertensive agents. Br J Clin Pharmacol *12*:295–302, 1981.
2. Isaac L: Clonidine in the central nervous system: Site and mechanism of hypotensive action. J Cardiovasc Pharmacol 2(Suppl 1):S5–S19, 1980.
3. Birkenhager W, Villarreal H, Sambhi M: Central alpha-adrenoceptors in cardiovascular regulation. Chest *83*(2) Suppl, Feb 1983.
4. Van Zwieten PA, Thoolen MJMC, Timmermans BMWM: The hypotensive activity and side effects of methyldopa, clonidine, and guanfacine. Hypertension *6*(5) Suppl 2, Sept-Oct, 1984.
5. Lisander B, Wennergren G: The role of cardiac receptors in clonidine-induced vagal bradycardia. Eur J Pharmacol *54*:109–118, 1979.
6. Toussaint C, Cave D, Saoudi N, et al: Electrophysiological effects of intravenous clonidine on sinus node function and conduction in man. J Cardiovasc Pharmacol *6*:56–60, 1984.
7. Mancia G, Ferrari A, Gregorini L, et al: Clonidine and carotid baroreflex in essential hypertension. Hypertension *1*, No 4, July-Aug, 1979.
8. Martin PR, Ebert MH, Gordon EK, et al: Effects of clonidine on central and peripheral catecholamine metabolism. Clin Pharmacol Ther *35*:322–327, 1984.
9. Metz SA, Halter JB: Effects of clonidine on hormone and substrate responses to hypoglycemia. Clin Pharmacol Ther *28*:441–448, 1980.
10. Gold MS, Pottash AC: The neurobiological implications of clonidine HCl. Ann NY Acad Sci *362*:191–202, 1981.
11. Smythe GA, Bradshaw JE, Gleeson RM, et al: The central vs. peripheral effects of clonidine on ACTH, corticosterone and glucose release. Eur J Pharmacol *111*:401–403, 1985.
12. Siever LJ, Uhde TW, Jimerson DC, et al: Differential inhibitory noradrenergic responses to clonidine in 25 depressed patients and 25 normal control subjects. Am J Psychiatr *141*:6, 1984.
13. Horvath S: Clonidine hydrochloride—A safe and effective antihypertensive agent in pregnancy. Obstet Gynecol *66*:634, 1985.
14. Brown MJ, Salmon D, Rendell M: Clonidine hallucinations. Ann Intern Med *93*:456, 1980.
15. Hoffman WF, Ladogana L: Delirium secondary to clonidine therapy. NY State Med J 382–383, Mar 1981.
16. Mack RB: Toxic encounters of the dangerous kind. NCMJ Vol 44, February 1983.
17. Stein and Volans. Dixarit overdose: The problem of attractive tablets. Br Med J *2*:667–668, 1978.
18. Neuvonen PJ, Vilska J, Keranen A: Severe poisoning in a child caused by a small dose of clonidine. Clin Toxicol *14*:369–374, 1979.
19. Mathew PM, Addy DP, Wright N: Clonidine overdose in children. Clin Toxicol *18*:169–173, 1981.
20. Hamblin JE: Transdermal patch poisoning. Pediatrics *79*:161, 1987.
21. Caravati EM, Bennett DL: Clonidine transdermal patch poisoning. Ann Emerg Med *17*:175, 1988.
22. Schaut J, Schnoll SH: Four cases of clonidine abuse. Am J Psychiatr *140*:1625–1627, 1983.
23. Conner CS, Watanabe AS: Clonidine overdose: A review. Am J Hosp Pharm *36*:906–911, 1979.
24. Artman M, Boerth RC: Clonidine poisoning. Am J Dis Child 137, February 1983.
25. Domino LE, Domino SE, Stockstill MS: Relationship between plasma concentrations of clonidine and mean arterial pressure during an accidental clonidine overdose. Br J Clin Pharmacol *21*:71–74, 1986.
26. Reid JL, Barber ND, Davies DS: The clinical pharmacology of clonidine: Relationship between plasma concentration and pharmacological effect in animals and man. Arch Intern Pharmacodyn Ther (Suppl), 11–16, 1980.
27. Maggi JC, Iskra MK, Nussbaum E: Severe clonidine overdose in children requiring critical care. Clin Pediatr 455, September 1986.

28. Rotellar JAO, Monasterio ES, De La Cruz JS, et al: Clonidine in thousand-fold overdose. Lancet *1*:1312, 1981.
29. Olsson JM, Pruitt AW: Management of clonidine ingestion in children. J Pediatr *103*:646, 1983.
30. Yagupsky P, Gorodischer R: Massive clonidine ingestion with hypertension in a 9-month-old infant. Pediatrics *72*:500–502, 1983.
31. Farsang C, Kapocsi J, Vajda L, et al: Reversal by naloxone of the antihypertensive action of clonidine: Involvement of the sympathetic nervous system. Circulation *69*:461–467, 1984.
32. Banner W, Lund ME, Clawson L: Failure of naloxone to reverse clonidine's toxic effect. Am J Dis Child *137*:1170–1171, 1983.
33. Niemann JT, Getzug T, Murphy W: Reversal of clonidine toxicity by naloxone. Ann Emerg Med *15*:1229–1231, 1986.
34. Kulig K, Duffy J, Rumack BH, et al: Naloxone for treatment of clonidine overdose. JAMA *247*:12, March 26, 1982.
35. Gremse DA, Artman M, Boerth RC: Hypertension associated with naloxone treatment for clonidine poisoning. J Pediatr *109*:776–778, 1986.
36. Mendoza JE, Medalie M: Clonidine poisoning with marked hypotension in a 2 1/2 year old child. Clin Pediatr 123–127, February 1979.
37. Mofenson HC, Greensher J, Weiss TE: Clonidine poisoning: Is there a single antidote? Clin Toxicol *14*:271–275, 1979.
38. Schieber RA, Kaufman ND: Use of tolazoline in massive clonidine poisoning. Am J Dis Child *135*:77–78, 1981.
39. Anderson RJ, Hart GR, Crumpler CP, et al: Clonidine overdose: Report of six cases and review of the literature. Ann Emerg Med *10*:107–112, 1981.
40. Geyskes GG, Boer P, Mees EJD: Clonidine withdrawal. Mechanism and frequency of rebound hypertension. Br J Clin Pharmacol *7*:55–62, 1979.
41. Ram CVS, Engelman K: Abrupt discontinuation of clonidine therapy. JAMA *242*:2104–2105, 1979.
42. Weber MA: Discontinuation syndrome following cessation of treatment with clonidine and other antihypertensive agents. J Cardiovasc Pharmacol 2(Suppl 1):S73–S89, 1980.
43. Peters RW, Hamilton BP, Hamilton J: Cardiac arrhythmias after abrupt clonidine withdrawal. Clin Pharmacol Ther 435–439, October 1983.
44. Nakagawa S, Yamamoto Y, Koiwaya Y: Ventricular tachycardia induced by clonidine withdrawal. Br Heart J *53*:654–658, 1985.
45. Planz G, Beckenbauer U, Bundschu HD: Response of plasma catecholamines and blood pressure to clonidine and to sudden withdrawal of the drug in subjects with essential hypertension. Int J Clin Pharmacol Ther Toxicol *20*:474–478, 1982.
46. Lewis SJ, Fennessy MR, Taylor DA: Central aminergic mechanisms associated with the clonidine withdrawal syndrome. Clin Exp Pharmacol Phys *8*:489–495, 1981.
47. Campbell BC, Reid JL: Regimen for the control of blood pressure and symptoms during clonidine withdrawal. Int J Clin Pharm Res *5*:215–222, 1985.
48. Gold MS, Pottash AL, Sweeney DR, et al: Efficacy of clonidine in opiate withdrawal. Drug Alcohol Depend *6*:201–208, 1980.
49. Agren H: Clonidine treatment of the opiate withdrawal syndrome. A review of clinical trials of a theory. National Institute of Mental Health, Laboratory of Clinical Science, Section on Pharmacology, Bethesda, MD, NIH, 1985.
50. DiStefano PS, Brown OM: Biochemical correlates of morphine withdrawal. 2. Effects of clonidine. J Pharmacol Exp Ther *233*:339–344, 1985.
51. Weigel J, Schlund J, Derlet R: Clonidine overdose and opiate withdrawal. Ann Emerg Med *17*:387, 1988.
52. Baumgartner GR, Rower RC: Clonidine vs. chlordiazepoxide in the management of acute alcohol withdrawal syndrome. Arch Intern Med *147*:1223–1226, 1987.
53. Balldin J, Bokstrom K: Treatment of alcohol abstinence symptoms with the alpha$_2$-agonist clonidine. Clinical Psychologists, Department of Psychiatry and Neurochemistry, St. Jorgen's Hospital, University of Gothenburg, Sweden.
54. Wilkins AJ, Jenkins WJ, Steiner JA: Efficacy of clonidine in treatment of alcohol withdrawal state. Psychopharmacology *81*:78–80, 1983.

CHAPTER 95
QUINIDINE, PROCAINAMIDE, AND DISOPYRAMIDE

Neal L. Benowitz, M.D.

Quinidine, procainamide, and disopyramide are classified as type IA antiarrhythmic drugs and are widely prescribed for long-term management of supraventricular and ventricular arrhythmias. Cases of serious toxicity and poisoning with these drugs are not as commonly encountered as are those with psychoactive drugs, but when they do occur, poisoning is often life-threatening.

PHARMACOLOGY AND PATHOPHYSIOLOGY OF OVERDOSE

The pharmacology of quinidine, the prototype drug, will be discussed. Differences in pharmacologic action of quinidine, procainamide, and disopyramide will be mentioned where relevant. Although not specifically reviewed, quinine, the optical isomer of quinidine, has toxic effects similar to those of quinidine.

The major electrophysiologic action of quinidine is to decrease the rate of inward sodium current through the sodium channel of the cardiac membrane during depolarization (phase 0, Fig. 95–1).[1, 2] The upstroke velocity of the action potential depends on the inward sodium current, so that upstroke velocity is decreased after quinidine treatment. Depression of slow inward calcium and outward potassium currents may explain the reduced action potential plateau (phase 2) and the prolonged terminal repolarization (phase 3) observed after quinidine use. The rate of spontaneous diastolic depolarization of myocardial cells is also decreased by quinidine, as it is by most classes of antiarrhythmic drugs. The net effects of the various electrophysiologic actions of quinidine are decreased automaticity and conduction velocity and prolongation of the effective refractory period, which are critical to the antiarrhythmic actions of quinidine.

Electrocardiographic correlates of slow conduction velocity are prolonged QRS and Q-T intervals. His bundle electrograms in patients receiving therapeutic doses of quinidine show accelerated atrioventricular conduction, related to autonomic neural effects (discussed subsequently), and prolonged His-Purkinje and intraventricular conduction times,[3] owing to direct depressant effects of quinidine. In severe cases of intoxication, quinidine depresses conduction in all parts of the cardiac conduction system, which results in widening of the QRS complex and complete atrioventricular block. Delayed repolarization of the His-Purkinje system results in the electrocardiographic finding of prolonged Q-T interval, which occurs commonly after therapeutic doses of quinidine and less commonly after procainamide or disopyramide.

Depressed automaticity is usually not manifest with therapeutic dosing because of counteracting autonomic effects. Quinidine produces arteriolar dilation and venodilation by both direct action on vascular smooth muscle and alpha-adrenergic blockade.[4] Procainamide causes vasodilation by ganglionic blockade.[5] Vasodilation elicits baroreceptor-mediated reflex sympathetic stimulation and withdrawal of parasympathetic tone. In addition, disopyramide and, to a lesser extent, quinidine and procainamide have significant direct anticholinergic effects. The sum of autonomic effects masks the depressed sinoatrial automaticity that would be expected from therapeutic concentrations of these drugs. But in the overdose situation, depressed automaticity predominates. Thus severe toxicity manifests clinically by sinus bradycardia, sinus arrest, junctional or ventricular rhythms often with extremely low rates, and asystole. Quinidine, even in therapeutic doses, has been reported to depress sinus node automaticity in persons with sinus node disease, resulting in sinus arrest and significant bradyarrhythmias.

Quinidine depresses myocardial contractility in a dose-related fashion in isolated papillary muscle preparations.[2] The ionic mechanisms for this effect are not clearly defined

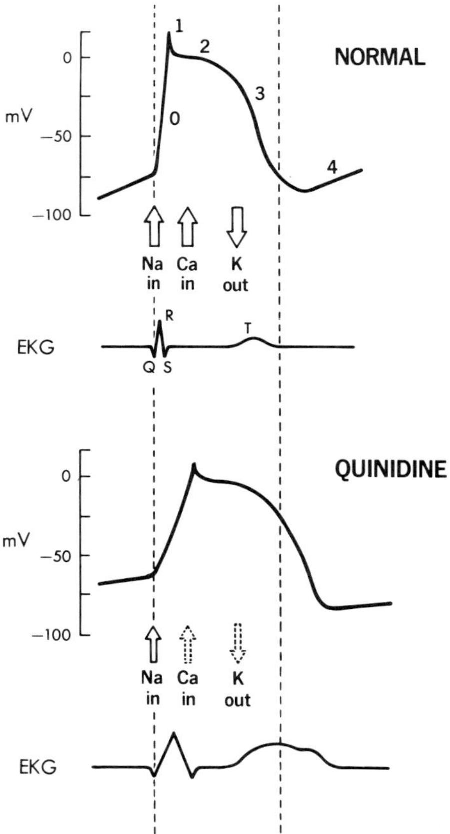

Figure 95–1. Effects of quinidine on action potential characteristics of Purkinje cell (with spontaneous diastolic depolarization). The upper panel shows the normal action potential with its phases: rapid depolarization (0), early repolarization (1), plateau (2), rapid repolarization (3), and diastole (4). Corresponding transmembrane ionic currents are indicated by arrows. The relationship between action potential phase and surface electrocardiogram is also shown.

The lower panel shows (in exaggerated fashion) effects of quinidine. The slope of phase 4 is decreased, the threshold for depolarization is less negative, the rate of phase 0 depolarization is slowed, and the action potential duration is prolonged. The decreased rate of phase 0 depolarization, which results in slowed His-Purkinje conduction velocity, is a consequence of quinidine decreasing the sodium-dependent fast inward current. Effects on action potential duration may be related to quinidine decreasing the calcium-dependent slow inward and potassium-dependent outward currents (this is still controversial). Effects on the surface electrocardiogram include widening of QRS and prolongation of Q-T interval.

but may include inhibition of calcium entry, either by direct inhibition of inward calcium current or secondary to reduced intracellular sodium and consequent reduced calcium-sodium exchange, or by effects of quinidine on calcium binding or release within the sarcolemma. In humans, therapeutic effects of quinidine have little effect on contractility, probably because of the opposing sympathetic neural stimulation, as discussed earlier. However, an overdose can be associated with severe myocardial depression and cardiogenic shock. The hemodynamics of disopyramide poisoning have been studied in anesthetized dogs.[6] With rising concentrations of disopyramide cardiac contractility, heart rate, cardiac output, and blood pressure declined, followed by hypoventilation and cardiac arrhythmias. Cardiovascular collapse was precipitous in many of the animals.[6]

CLINICAL PRESENTATION OF OVERDOSE
(Table 95–1)

Central Nervous System Manifestations

Severe quinidine intoxication may be associated with depressed mental function

Table 95–1. CLINICAL FEATURES OF QUINIDINE, PROCAINAMIDE, AND DISOPYRAMIDE OVERDOSE

I. CENTRAL NERVOUS SYSTEM
   Lethargy, confusion, coma
   Respiratory arrest
   Seizures*
II. GASTROINTESTINAL*
   Vomiting
   Abdominal pain
   Diarrhea
III. CARDIOVASCULAR
   Tachyarrhythmias
   1. Sinus tachycardia (mild poisoning)
   2. Ventricular tachycardia (often polymorphous)
   3. Ventricular fibrillation
   Depressed automaticity and conduction
   1. QRS and Q-T interval prolongation
   2. Bundle branch block
   3. Sinus bradycardia
   4. Sinoatrial block, sinus pauses and arrest
   5. Atrioventricular block
   6. Atrioventricular junctional or ventricular bradycardia
   7. Asystole
   Hypotension
   1. Vasodilation
   2. Depressed myocardial contractility and low cardiac output
IV. METABOLIC AND OTHER FEATURES
   Hypokalemia
   Metabolic acidosis
   Cinchonism†
   Anticholinergic signs and symptoms (urinary retention, mydriasis, dry mucous membranes)‡

*Reported for quinidine only.
†Primarily quinidine.
‡Primarily disopyramide.

even in patients who are hemodynamically stable.[7] Typically, the patient progresses from lethargy to coma, including respiratory arrest. Recurrent generalized motor seizures are also characteristic of severe intoxication. The onset of central nervous system manifestations may be substantially delayed beyond the onset of cardiovascular toxicity, and, conversely, recovery from coma is often delayed, following recovery from cardiac toxicity by hours or days. Presumably penetration and exit of quinidine into and from the brain are slower than those into and out of the heart.

In less severe cases of intoxication with quinidine (and to a greater extent its optical isomer quinine), symptoms and signs of cinchonism may occur. These include (1) disturbed hearing—tinnitus, decreased auditory acuity, and vertigo, (2) disturbed vision or blurred vision, disturbed color perception (yellow vision), photophobia, diplopia, scotomata, and contracted visual fields, and (3) other central nervous system manifestations—headache, fever, apprehension, excitement, confusion, and delirium.

Gastrointestinal Manifestations

Quinidine is extremely irritating to the gastrointestinal tract. Nausea, vomiting, abdominal pain, and diarrhea are common with therapeutic doses as well as with overdose. These problems are much less common with procainamide and disopyramide.

Cardiovascular Manifestations

The most serious complications and usual causes of death with quinidine overdose involve cardiovascular toxicity. Manifestations of cardiovascular toxicity will be discussed as three syndromes (which may occur concurrently): (1) ventricular tachyarrhythmias, (2) depressed automaticity and intracardiac conduction with bradyarrhythmias, and (3) myocardial depression with hypotension.

Ventricular tachyarrhythmias from quinidine have been recognized for many years.[8] These occur infrequently during therapeutic dosing and more commonly after an overdose. Typically, short bursts of polymorphous ventricular tachycardia ("torsades de pointes") and occasionally ventricular fibrillation are observed[9] (see Chapter 5, Figs. 5–3 and 5–13). Generally, but not always, there is evidence of delayed repolarization on the electrocardiogram, that is, Q-T prolongation and/or the presence of a large U wave. Nonhomogeneous ventricular conduction and repolarization are thought to predispose to ventricular re-entry and to ventricular tachycardia (see Chapter 5, Fig. 5–1). There is no direct relationship between blood concentrations of quinidine and the occurrence of ventricular tachycardia.[10] However, quinidine syncope (brief loss of consciousness due to ventricular tachycardia) has been observed, primarily in patients receiving relatively large doses of quinidine for treatment of atrial fibrillation or flutter and, as discussed earlier, may be observed after an overdose of the drug. Among patients who develop ventricular tachycardia during routine therapy, many are taking digitalis and many have prolonged Q-T intervals prior to quinidine treatment.[11]

Depressed automaticity and intracardiac conduction with resultant bradyarrhythmias are clearly dose-related toxic effects of quinidine. Early evidence of impaired conduction is prolongation of the Q-T and QRS intervals. More severe toxicity results in wide, bizarre QRS complexes, bundle branch block, and sinoatrial and atrioventricular block (see Chapter 5, Fig. 5–6). Because of vagolytic effects and perhaps reflex sympathetic stimulation, as discussed previously, sinus or atrial tachycardia can be the presenting arrhythmias in cases of quinidine overdose. However, in more severe cases of intoxication, depressed automaticity is predominant.[12] Sinus bradycardia, sinus pauses or sinus arrest, and, in the presence of atrioventricular block, junctional or ventricular bradycardia and even asystole can occur. Associated with depressed automaticity and conduction is relative or absolute refractoriness of the myocardium to electrical stimulation. Thus higher than usual voltages may be necessary for successful intracardiac pacing, or the pacemaker may not capture at all.[7, 13]

Hypotension can occur after intravenous administration of quinidine, particularly when the administration is rapid, occasionally after therapeutic oral dosing, and commonly after an overdose of the drug. As noted, hypotension from lower doses of quinidine results from a fall in vascular resistance, owing to direct vasodilation and alpha-adrenergic antagonism. Consistent with this action is that some (but not all) poisoned patients have warm, pink skin despite significant hypotension. With higher doses, depressed myocardial contractility becomes the most important cause of hypotension. Pulmonary edema may be associated with myocardial depression, particularly in the context of vigorous fluid therapy. Pulmonary edema was a nearly universal finding in autopsied patients who died of disopyramide overdose.[14] Pulmonary edema with normal cardiac filling pressures has been reported, suggesting that in some patients there is also damage to pulmonary capillaries. The latter is likely a consequence of prolonged hypotension or hypoxia rather than a direct effect of the drug.

Metabolic Effects

Hypokalemia (serum potassium concentrations of 3.0 to 3.5 mEq per liter) has been reported after overdoses in humans and in experimental cases of quinidine intoxication in dogs.[7, 15] It should be remembered that the electrophysiologic effects of toxicity with quinidine resemble hyperkalemia. Extracellular hypokalemia and intracellular hyperkalemia are thought to result from effects of quinidine on the outward potassium current. Management of potassium-related metabolic disturbances is discussed in a later section.

Metabolic acidosis occurs commonly and is most likely due to hypoperfusion related to cardiac toxicity. Hypocalcemia, but not tetany, was reported in one patient.[16]

Procainamide and Disopyramide

Procainamide typically causes lethargy and confusion, hypotension, and impairment of intraventricular conduction (wide, bizarre QRS complexes).[13, 17, 18] The clinical presentation in one series of disopyramide-intoxicated patients differed slightly from that of quinidine or procainamide—a common finding in disopyramide cases was early loss of consciousness with apnea.[14] Cardiac resuscitation was successful initially in four cases, but during the subsequent hospital course malignant arrhythmias occurred and caused death. Four other patients had postmortem evidence of pulmonary edema. A series of 106 disopyramide-poisoned patients collected from French Poison Center reported the full spectrum of cardiovascular complications as described for quinidine, with an overall case mortality of 12.2 per cent.[19]

Severe myocardial depression can occur not only during overdose but also during therapeutic administration of disopyramide and has been associated with aggravation of congestive heart failure, cardiovascular collapse, and death.[20] Usually, patients have severe underlying myocardial disease. In this population, even single doses of disopyramide have been shown to depress myocardial function significantly. It is not known why cardiogenic shock occurs, persists, and is unresponsive to medical intervention in the presence (at least in some patients) of relatively low blood concentrations of disopyramide. Disopyramide may suppress sinus node function and produce bradyarrhythmias in patients with sinus node disease.

Anticholinergic side effects are most common with disopyramide but also can occur with quinidine or procainamide. These may include acute urinary retention (particularly in patients with prostatic hypertrophy), dry mouth and other mucous membranes, mydriasis, and blurred vision. Several cases of hypoglycemia during therapy with disopyramide have been reported, the mechanism of which is unknown.[21, 22] Some cases have been severe, with serum glucose levels of less than 10 mg per dl, associated with hypotension and lactic acidosis.

TOXIC EFFECTS DURING THERAPEUTIC DOSING

Quinidine

Toxicity from type IA antiarrhythmic drugs is not uncommon during therapeutic use. In addition to the toxicity described in the preceding section, other types may occur.

Quinidine has been associated with a variety of hypersensitivity reactions, including drug fever, skin rashes, and hepatitis, and with hematologic reactions, including thrombocytopenia, neutropenia, and agranulocytosis.[23] Hemolytic anemia may occur in patients with glucose-6-phosphate dehydrogenase deficiency. Quinidine hepatitis characteristically develops within one month of initiation of therapy; it is associated with fever and recurs promptly after rechallenge.[24] Histologic examination of the liver may reveal focal necrosis, centrizonal necrosis, or noncaseating granulomatous hepatitis.[24, 25]

Quinidine has been associated with rheumatic syndromes that appear to be of two types.[26, 27] In some patients, polyarthropathy with positive antinuclear and antihistone antibodies developed after 5 to 44 months of therapy. The picture is consistent with that of drug-induced systemic lupus erythematosus (SLE), except that rashes and serositis are uncommon. Other patients develop polyarthritis with a short latency (within 3 months of therapy) without positive antibodies, suggesting a different pathophysiology. In both groups of patients, full recovery followed cessation of quinidine therapy.

Procainamide

The most common adverse reaction limiting the chronic use of procainamide is the systemic lupus erythematosus–like syndrome.[28] This syndrome, developing in 5 to 30 per cent of patients on long-term therapy, is most often manifested by fever, arthritis or arthralgias, myalgia, pleurisy, and/or pericarditis. Skin rash and central nervous system and renal involvement are uncommon in patients with drug-induced SLE. Positive antinuclear antibody tests are seen in up to 80 per cent of patients on long-term therapy. Although these positive tests are usually present in symptomatic patients, they do not strongly predict the development of symptomatic SLE in general. Slow acetylators have been reported to be of greater risk than fast acetylators for development of drug-induced SLE, although this has been questioned recently. Antibodies to histone 2A and guanosine are relatively sensitive and specific for procainamide-induced SLE,[29] whereas antibodies to smooth muscle and native DNA are more suggestive of idiopathic SLE.

In addition to central nervous system symptoms, fever and rash, neutropenia, or agranulocytosis occasionally accompanies procainamide treatment.[30, 31] The latter has an estimated incidence of about 0.5 per cent and may be fatal. Periodic monitoring of the white blood cell count in patients on chronic procainamide therapy has been advocated.

Disopyramide

Aside from its cardiac depressant action, the primary side effects of disopyramide are caused by its anticholinergic actions. Urinary tract obstruction in patients with prostatism is a particularly troublesome problem that often results in cessation of therapy. Pyridostigmine, a cholinesterase inhibitor, has been used along with disopyramide during routine therapy to reverse the anticholinergic effects of disopyramide.[32] Severe fasting hypoglycemia has been reported in patients receiving therapeutic doses of disopyramide.[21, 22]

RELEVANT PHARMACOKINETICS: IMPLICATIONS FOR ACCELERATED DRUG REMOVAL

Although the clinical manifestations of quinidine, procainamide, and disopyramide intoxication are similar, pharmacokinetic differences among the drugs lead to different time courses of toxicity and different approaches to therapy, particularly concerning acceleration of drug removal (Table 95–2).

Table 95–2. PHARMACOKINETICS OF QUINIDINE, PROCAINAMIDE, AND DISOPYRAMIDE (Average Values in Healthy Persons)

	% URINARY EXCRETION *(Unchanged)*	PLASMA PROTEIN BINDING *(%)*	VOLUME OF DISTRIBUTION *(L/kg)*	CLEARANCE *(ml/min/kg)*	HALF-LIFE *(Hr)*	CLEARANCE BY DIALYSIS OR HEMOPERFUSION* *(Ml/min)*
Quinidine[33, 37, 61, 62]	20	71	3.0	4.8	7.8	21(HD), 1.2(PD), 24(HP)
3-OH-Quinidine[34]	26	NA	NA	4.0⁺⁺	12.4	NA
Procainamide[17, 18, 41, 43]	65	16	1.9	9.2	3.0	68(HD), 6.4(PD), 75(HP)
N-Acetylprocainamide[42, 43, 63]	81	10	1.4	3.1	6.0	48(HD), 73(HP), 107(HD & HP)
Disopyramide[44, 47]	55	28⁺	0.8	1.3	7.8	183(HP)

*Data from overdose cases.
†Higher for fast and lower for slow acetylators.
⁺⁺Renal clearance.

HD, Hemodialysis; HP, resin hemoperfusion; PD, peritoneal dialysis.
NA, data not available.

Quinidine

Quinidine is available as a sulfate, a gluconate, and a polygalacturonate. Bioavailability is high (70 to 80 per cent) but is variable among individuals.[33] The sulfate form is usually rapidly absorbed, with peak concentrations at 1.5 hours. The gluconate and the sustained-release sulfate preparations are absorbed more slowly, peaking at about 4 hours. The polygalacturonate form is the most slowly absorbed, peaking at about 6 hours. Of additional importance in overdose is that anticholinergic or direct gastric effects of quinidine may delay absorption so that maximal manifestations of poisoning do not become evident for many hours after ingestion.

Quinidine is metabolized primarily by hydroxylation in the liver. Some of its metabolites are pharmacologically active and could contribute to toxicity. In particular, in humans 3-OH-quinidine has effects similar to those of quinidine.[34] This metabolite has a half-life averaging 12.4 hours, longer that that of quinidine; about 25 per cent of an oral dose of 3-OH-quinidine is excreted unchanged in the urine. A pregnant patient receiving high doses of quinidine for treatment of fetal supraventricular tachycardia developed gastrointestinal toxicity with low therapeutic levels of quinidine but elevated levels of 3-OH-quinidine.[35] It should be recognized that blood concentrations of quinidine in many of the older reported cases of quinidine toxicity were measured by a spectrophotometric assay that is nonspecific and measures both quinidine and its metabolites. About 20 per cent of quinidine is eliminated unchanged in the urine.[33] Urinary excretion has been reported to be increased in acid urine,[36] but the assay used in this study was nonspecific and measured metabolites as well as quinidine.

Quinidine is distributed extensively to body tissues and is substantially bound to plasma proteins (70 per cent). Relatively little quinidine is within the vascular space, making accelerated drug removal difficult.

The average half-life of quinidine at therapeutic doses is 6 to 8 hours, but it may vary from 3 to 19 hours among individuals.[33, 36] Half-lives in poisoned patients are unknown. Because of associated circulatory disturbances, quinidine metabolism would be expected to be slower than normal and the half-life prolonged. The observation that the course of severe quinidine intoxication often lasts 48 or more hours may be related to continued absorption or delayed elimination.

It is difficult to use blood concentrations of quinidine to predict outcome because of individual differences in responses to quinidine, the use of nonspecific assays in the past, and difficulties in determining from case reports when the blood concentrations of drug were measured with respect to the time course of absorption. The range of quinidine concentrations reported in cases of significant intoxications is from 5.1 to 28.4 μg/ml.[7, 16, 37–40] Ratios of serum concentration of 3-OH-quinidine/quinidine average about 0.4, with only occasional patients, presumably fast metabolizers of quinidine, having ratios greater than 1.0.[34, 35] Serum 3-OH-quinidine was 9.7 μg/ml in the pregnant patient with gastrointestinal toxicity previously described.[35]

Procainamide

Procainamide is well absorbed (85 per cent bioavailability) in healthy persons, although there are reports of incomplete or erratic absorption in patients with cardiac failure and slow absorption after an overdose[18] (Fig. 95–2). Procainamide is primarily excreted unchanged in the urine (about 60 per cent), and clearance is significantly decreased in patients with renal insufficiency.[41] Procainamide is also metabolized by the liver and is primarily acetylated to *N*-acetylprocainamide (NAPA), which is in itself pharmacologically active and is undergoing trials as an antiarrhythmic drug. The presence of NAPA, the electrophysiologic effects of which appear to be different from its parent, certainly could influence the toxicity produced by procainamide ingestion, although the interaction between these compounds has not been well defined. The generation of NAPA is faster in persons who are genetically rapid acetylators, and potential effects from NAPA would be of most concern in that population.

Procainamide is extensively distributed to body tissues and is only slightly (15 per cent) protein bound. Like quinidine, a relatively small fraction of the total amount of procainamide in the body is in the vascular compartment, so that extracorporeal removal of the drug is not very effective in removing procainamide. In contrast, NAPA has a

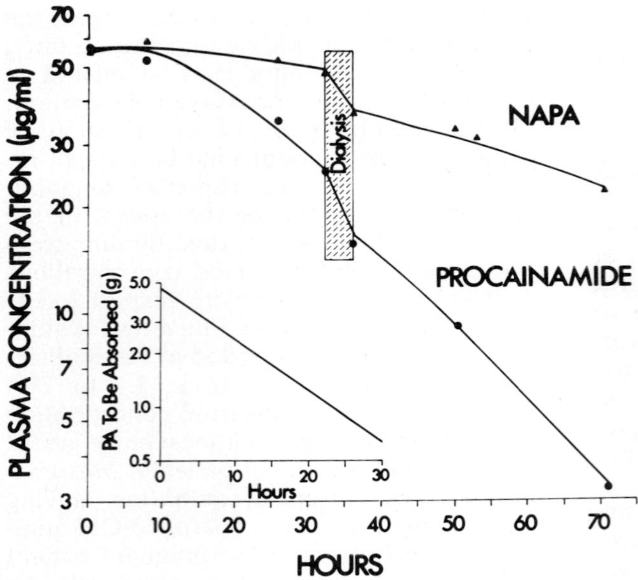

Figure 95–2. Plasma concentrations of procainamide and *N*-acetylprocainamide (NAPA) in a 67 year old woman after intentional overdose of procainamide. Note the apparent continued absorption of procainamide for 30 hours (see inset) during which time the patient was hypotensive and oliguric. The bar indicates a 4-hour period of hemodialysis. After dialysis, procainamide disappeared, with a half-life of 10.5 hours (normal about 3 hours). Computer-estimated NAPA half-life was 35.9 hours, due at least in part to continued conversion of procainamide to NAPA. Levels of the latter remained high for the duration of the observation period. (From Atkinson AJ Jr, Krumlovsky FA, Huang CM, et al: Hemodialysis for severe procainamide toxicity: Clinical and pharmacokinetic observations. Clin Pharmacol Ther *20*:585, 1976.)

smaller volume of distribution and a lower endogenous clearance, so that accelerated drug removal techniques are more useful.[18, 42, 43]

The half-life of procainamide averages 3 hours and the half-life of NAPA approximates 6 hours in healthy persons. Half-lives are longer in patients with renal or cardiac failure. In overdoses, half-lives of 8.8 and 10.5 hours for procainamide and 35.9 hours for NAPA have been reported[18] (Fig. 95–2). Concentrations of procainamide in serious poisonings have ranged from 36 to 77 μg/ml; NAPA in one case was 55 μg/ml.[13, 17, 18] It has been suggested that a combined serum concentration of procainamide and NAPA greater than 60 μg/ml predicts serious toxicity.[18]

Peritoneal and hemodialysis have been studied in two procainamide-intoxicated patients. In one patient, peritoneal dialysis resulted in clearance of 6.4 ml/min, compared with a 27 ml/min clearance via the kidney in the same patient, who had markedly reduced renal function.[17] In another patient, hemodialysis resulted in clearances of 67.5 and 47.7 ml/min for procainamide and NAPA, respectively, compared with estimated total nondialytic clearances of 66.7 and 16.1 ml/min.[18] Again, the nondialytic clearances were lower than in healthy people because the patient had severely compromised renal function. Thus in the poisoned patient with renal insufficiency, hemodialysis may double the clearance of procainamide and quadruple that of NAPA; however, because of the large volume of distribution, hemodialysis for 4 hours removes only a small fraction of total body drug. Longer or repeat dialysis may be necessary to treat severely intoxicated patients.

Hemodialysis, charcoal hemoperfusion, and combined hemodialysis-hemoperfusion were performed in a patient with severe toxicity.[43] Hemoperfusion resulted in clearances of 75.3 and 73.3 ml/min for procainamide and NAPA, respectively; combined hemodialysis-hemoperfusion resulted in a clearance of 107 ml/min for NAPA. Continuous arteriovenous hemofiltration has been used with or without hemodialysis in two patients.[42] Clearances were not calculated, but estimated half-lives for NAPA were 1.5 days for continuous arteriovenous hemodiafiltration and 3.1 days for hemofiltration, compared with 4.1 to 7 days for hemodialysis in the presence of renal failure.

Disopyramide

Disopyramide is highly bioavailable (85 per cent) but is absorbed relatively slowly, probably because of anticholinergic effects, with peak blood concentrations occurring at 2 to 3 hours after ingestion in healthy persons.[44] Even more delayed absorption might be expected in overdose situations. Disopyramide is both excreted in the urine (55 per cent) and metabolized (45 per cent).[44, 45] The monodealkylated metabolite is pharmacologically active and may accumulate in the body in persons with renal insufficiency.

Endogenous clearance and the extent of

distribution of disopyramide to body tissues are much less than those of quinidine or procainamide. Protein binding of disopyramide is concentration dependent, with less than 30 per cent bound when concentrations exceed the therapeutic range (greater than 6 μg/ml). Because of a relatively small volume of distribution with little protein binding (at toxic levels) and low intrinsic clearance, disopyramide is a suitable candidate for removal by hemodialysis or hemoperfusion. In one report of patients on chronic hemodialysis, the half-life of disopyramide was considerably shorter (40 per cent) during hemodialysis compared with patients who were not dialyzed.[46] Studies of experimental disopyramide poisoning in dogs confirm the efficacy of hemoperfusion with columns containing either uncoated charcoal or Amberlite XAD-2 resin.[6] Resin hemoperfusion was reported to remove disopyramide effectively and sharply reduce blood concentrations and toxic effects in one patient.[47] The half-life of disopyramide averages 8 hours in healthy persons. In patients with renal failure, the half-life is prolonged as it might well be in the poisoning circumstance. Blood concentrations of 4.3 to 146 μg of disopyramide/ml (therapeutic range, 2.8 to 7.5) have been reported during serious poisonings or in fatalities.[14, 47, 48] These were measured at various times after overdoses and cannot be interpreted as peak levels.

MANAGEMENT OF OVERDOSE
(Table 95–3)

Table 95–3. MANAGEMENT OF QUINIDINE, PROCAINAMIDE, AND DISOPYRAMIDE OVERDOSE

I. GENERAL MANAGEMENT
- Emesis or lavage and charcoal—even many hours after ingestion
- Seizures—diazepam, 5–10 mg intravenously; phenytoin, 15 mg/kg intravenously (rate ≤ 50 mg/min)
- Sodium bicarbonate—50 mEq intravenously, rapid injection, every 5–10 min to arterial pH of 7.4–7.5

II. ARRHYTHMIAS
- Sinus tachycardia
  - —if hemodynamically stable, no specific therapy
  - —if hypotension or ischemic but not depressed conduction, propranolol
- Ventricular premature beats and tachycardia
  1. Lidocaine, phenytoin, isoproterenol, bretylium
  2. Overdrive pacing
- Bradyarrhythmias
  1. Isoproterenol
  2. Cardiac pacemaker (may require higher than usual pacing voltage)

III. HYPOTENSION
- Normal saline (may be 25–50% bicarbonate)—200 ml every 10 min until 1000–2000 ml or evidence of pulmonary edema
- If still hypotensive, insert pulmonary arterial catheter
- If low cardiac output and low pulmonary arterial wedge pressure, more crystalloid fluid
- If low systemic vascular resistance, dopamine or norepinephrine
- If low cardiac output with slow heart rate, isoproterenol or epinephrine
- If low cardiac output and normal or high pulmonary arterial wedge pressure, isoproterenol, dobutamine
- If intractable cardiogenic shock—intra-aortic balloon pump assistance or cardiopulmonary bypass

IV. ACCELERATED DRUG REMOVAL
- Quinidine—if hepatic failure or extracorporeal circulation, consider hemoperfusion
- Procainamide—if renal insufficiency or extracorporeal circulation, consider hemoperfusion or hemodialysis
- Disopyramide—consider hemoperfusion or hemodialysis for all life-threatening cases of overdose, particularly if there is evidence of renal insufficiency

General Considerations

General management is similar to that described for other drug overdoses. Because of potentially slow absorption, emesis or lavage and charcoal should be used even many hours after ingestion. Similarly, evaluation of intoxicated patients must continue until it is clear that the patient is stable and absorption is complete. Seizures should be treated with intravenous administration of diazepam initially and then phenytoin.

Bicarbonate and Potassium

The approach to management of cardiac toxicity from quinidine has been somewhat controversial. Before specific management is discussed, the role of sodium bicarbonate and sodium lactate should be considered. Sodium lactate has been recommended for treatment of quinidine-induced arrhythmias and hypotension for many years and is supported by some animal data and several anecdotal reports describing dramatic clinical responses.[15, 38, 39, 49] Consideration of the use of sodium lactate for quinidine toxicity began with the observation of its effectiveness in the treatment of cardiac manifestations of hyperkalemia. Because the electrocardiographic changes of quinidine toxicity resemble those of hyperkalemia, sodium lactate was proposed as therapy for quinidine poisoning. Extracellur potassium concentrations modulate the magnitude of the inward sodium currents and rate of rise of action potential and are known to influence the electrophysiologic effects of quinidine.[50, 51] In vivo quinidine effects and toxicity are exaggerated by high concentrations and diminished by low concentrations of potassium.[52] The effectiveness of sodium lactate or sodium bicarbonate may be related in part to lowering extracellular potassium concentrations. Increased extracellular sodium has been shown to reverse toxic electrophysiologic effects of quinidine in vitro.[53] Animal studies suggest that potassium depletion affects the disposition kinetics of quinidine, resulting in lower plasma concentrations for a given quinidine dose compared with controls.[52] Although definitive experimental data are lacking, it seems reasonable to treat serious quinidine or quinidine-like drug overdose with sodium bicarbonate. Repeated bolus injections of sodium bicarbonate until an arterial pH of 7.45 to 7.50 is reached is the usual end point.

Because hypokalemia has been shown to be protective against quinidine toxicity in experimental animals, potassium probably should not be administered to quinidine-poisoned patients even in the presence of moderate hypokalemia (3 to 3.5 mEq/liter), unless it is believed that the hypokalemia is life threatening. One investigator hemodialyzed a quinidine-intoxicated patient against a dialysate containing reduced potassium concentrations (1.5 mEq/liter) and reported substantial clinical improvement in the patient despite relatively little removal of quinidine.[40] It must be recognized that recommendations not to treat or to induce hypokalemia are based on theoretic considerations and have not been evaluated in humans.

Arrhythmias

With respect to specific arrhythmias, sinus tachycardia usually occurs in mild cases of poisoning, is not usually compromising, and requires no specific therapy.

In the presence of sinoatrial or atrioventricular block or significant bradyarrhythmias, insertion of a cardiac pacemaker is warranted. A pacemaker might be useful both in maintaining heart rate and cardiac output in the presence of bradyarrhythmias and in overdrive of escape tachyarrhythmias. As discussed in Chapter 5, however, the pacing threshold is often elevated,[7, 13] and the myocardium sometimes does not respond at all in severe intoxications. Isoproterenol reverses the adverse effects of quinidine on both automaticity and conduction in vitro and in animals[2, 54] and has been shown to be useful in managing quinidine-induced bradyarrhythmias in poisoned patients.

Ventricular ectopy and ventricular arrhythmias are common in cases of quinidine overdose and may be difficult to control. Lidocaine, phenytoin, isoproterenol, bretylium, and overdrive pacing have been successfully used in treating quinidine-induced ventricular arrhythmias.[55–60] Some investigators have questioned using one antiarrhythmic drug to treat the toxicity of another. Lidocaine and phenytoin in therapeutic doses do not usually depress conduction or automaticity. Lidocaine decreases the action potential duration and the refractory period of nonischemic Purkinje cells, effects that are the opposite of those of the quinidine-like drugs. Both lidocaine and phenytoin may shorten the Q-T interval, and phenytoin may shorten the QRS duration as well. Isoproterenol increases automaticity of cardiac pacemakers, accelerates conduction and repolarization, tends to interfere with the re-entry mechanism responsible for many tachyarrhythmias, and reestablishes supraventricular inhibition of junctional or ventricular pacemakers. Isoproterenol has been used successfully to treat recurrent ventricular tachycardia caused by quinidine.[56] Bretylium antagonizes the electrophysiologic effects of quinidine in vitro[57] and has been used to treat quinidine-induced ventricular tachycardia in humans.[50, 59] Overdrive suppression via intracardiac pacemaker has been used successfully for ventricular tachycardia during therapeutic quinidine dosing,[60] but whether it is effective in the case of an overdose is unclear. For polymorphous ventricular tachycardia (torsades de pointes), overdrive pacing, isoproterenol, and bretylium are considered to be the treatments of choice.[9]

Hypotension

As discussed, hypotension may be due to decreased systemic vascular resistance (particularly with quinidine) or to decreased cardiac output secondary to myocardial depression. The latter is most significant in cases of severe intoxication, in which cardiogenic shock may be a cause of death. Cautious use of fluids (as discussed in Chapter 5) is usually effective in managing hypotension due to vasodilating or adrenergic blocking effects. If blood pressure does not respond to fluids, vasoconstrictor drugs such as norepinephrine or dopamine should be used. The doses of pressor drugs required may be unusually high in light of the alpha-adrenergic blocking actions of quinidine.

Differentiating hypotension caused by vasodilation from that caused by myocardial depression and selecting appropriate therapy require measurement of cardiac output. Thus placement of a pulmonary arterial catheter is desirable. If cardiac output is low and cardiac filling pressure is also low, more fluids are necessary. If cardiac output is low despite adequate filling pressures, inotropic agents should be administered. Animal studies have shown isoproterenol to be most effective in reversing disopyramide-induced myocardial depression.[6] Dobutamine should also be considered. If cardiac output is adequate but vascular resistance is low, vasopressors should be administered as discussed earlier.

In severe cases of quinidine poisoning with low-output shock due to myocardial depression, inotropic drugs may not improve contractility. Yet, in contrast to the situation of cardiogenic shock due to myocardial infarction, if the patient can be supported for several hours until the intoxicating drug can be eliminated, myocardial function will return to normal. Thus, drug-induced cardiogenic shock is an ideal situation for use of extracorporeal circulatory assistance techniques. One case of successful use of intra-aortic balloon pump assistance in the treatment of quinidine overdose has been reported.[16]

Accelerated Drug Removal

Techniques for accelerating drug removal are not very effective for quinidine but may be useful for procainamide, NAPA, and disopyramide intoxications. Acidification of the urine can accelerate renal elimination of quinidine. But the increase in drug removal rate is small, and therapy with alkali is probably more important in the management of cardiotoxicity, as discussed earlier. Renal elimination of procainamide appears not to be affected by urinary pH or by urinary flow rate. However, because procainamide, NAPA, and disopyramide are substantially eliminated by the kidney, it is important to maintain adequate renal function in patients intoxicated with these drugs.

Hemodialysis and hemoperfusion remove relatively little quinidine or procainamide because of extensive tissue distribution of the drugs. But when the usual routes of drug elimination are depressed or absent, such as when renal or hepatic failure complicates procainamide or quinidine overdose, respectively, or when extracorporeal circulation is used to support a failing circulation due to either drug, hemoperfusion should be strongly considered, because, even though not terribly effective, it may offer the only route of drug elimination.

Patients with disopyramide poisoning, as discussed earlier, are excellent candidates for hemodialysis or hemoperfusion. Because disopyramide clearance rates are usually higher with hemoperfusion, this method is preferred over hemodialysis, but hemodialysis should be employed if only it is available.

References

1. Hoffman BF, Rosen MR, Wit AL: Electrophysiology and pharmacology of cardiac arrhythmias. VII. Cardiac effects of quinidine and procaine amide. B. Am Heart J *90*:117–122, 1975.
2. Nawrath H: Action potential, membrane currents and force of contraction in mammalian heart muscle fibers treated with quinidine. J Pharmacol Exp Ther *216*:176–182, 1981.
3. Josephson ME, Seides SF, Batsford WP, Weisfogel GM, Akhtar M, Caracta AR, Lau SH, Damato AN: The electrophysiological effects of intramuscular quinidine on the atrioventricular conducting system in man. Am Heart J *87*:55–64, 1974.
4. Schmid PG, Nelson LD, Mark AL, Heistad DD, Abboud FM: Inhibition of adrenergic vasoconstriction by quinidine. J Pharmacol Exp Ther *188*:124–134, 1974.
5. Schmid PG, Nelson LD, Heistad DD, Mark AL, Abboud FM: Vascular effects of procaine amide in the dog. Predominance of the inhibitory effect on ganglionic transmission. Circ Res *35*:948–960, 1974.
6. Hayler AM, Medd RK, Holt DW, O'Keefe BD: Experimental disopyramide poisoning: Treatment by cardiovascular support and with charcoal hemoperfusion. J Pharmacol Exp Ther *211*:491–495, 1979.
7. Kerr F, Kenoyer G, Bilitch M: Quinidine overdose. Neurological and cardiovascular toxicity in a normal person. Br Heart J *33*:629–631, 1971.
8. Reynolds EW, Vander Ark CR: Quinidine syncope

and the delayed repolarization syndromes. Mod Concepts Cardiovasc Dis *45*:117–122, 1976.

9. Smith WM, Gallagher JJ: "Les torsades de pointes": An unusual ventricular arrhythmia. Ann Intern Med *93*:578–584, 1980.
10. Thompson KA, Murray JJ, Blair IA, Woosley RL, Roden DM: Plasma concentrations of quinidine, its major metabolites, and dihydroquinidine in patients with torsades de pointes. Clin Pharmacol Ther *43*:636–642, 1988.
11. Bauman JL, Bavernfeind RA, Hoff JV, et al: Torsades de pointes due to quinidine: Observations in 31 patients. Am Heart J *107*:425–430, 1984.
12. Finnegan TRL, Trounce JR: Depression of the heart by quinidine and its treatment. Br Heart J *16*:341–350, 1954.
13. Gay RJ, Brown DF: Pacemaker failure due to procainamide toxicity. Am J Cardiol *34*:728–732, 1974.
14. Hayler AM, Hold DW, Volans GN: Fatal overdosage with disopyramide. Lancet *1*:968–969, 1978.
15. Luchi RJ, Helwig J Jr, Conn HL Jr: Quinidine toxicity and its treatment. An experimental study. Am Heart J *65*:340–348, 1963.
16. Shub C, Gau GT, Sidell PM, Brennan LA Jr: The management of acute quinidine intoxication. Chest *73*:173–178, 1978.
17. Villalba-Pimentel L, Epstein LM, Sellers EM, Foster JR, Bennion LJ, Nadler LM, Bough EW, Koch-Weser J: Survival after massive procainamide ingestion. Am J Cardiol *32*:727–730, 1973.
18. Atkinson AJ Jr, Krumlovsky FA, Huang CM, del Greco F: Hemodialysis for severe procainamide toxicity: Clinical and pharmacokinetic observations. Clin Pharmacol Ther *20*:585–592, 1976.
19. Jaeger A, Sauder PH, Tempe JD, Mantz JM: Intoxications aigués par le disopyramide. Nouv Presse Med *10*:2883–2887, 1981.
20. Desai JM, Scheinman MM, Hirschfeld D, Gonzalez R, Peters RW: Cardiovascular collapse associated with disopyramide therapy. Chest *79*:545–551, 1981.
21. Nappi JM, Dhanani S, Lovejoy JR, Vander Ark C: Severe hypoglycemia associated with disopyramide. West J Med *138*:95–97, 1983.
22. Goldberg IJ, Brown LK, Rayfield EJ: Disopyramide (Norpace[R])-induced hypoglycemia. Am J Med *69*:463–466, 1980.
23. Cohen IS, Jick H, Cohen SI: Adverse reactions to quinidine in hospitalized patients: Findings based on data from the Boston Collaborative Drug Surveillance Program. Prog Cardiovasc Dis *20*:151–163, 1977.
24. Koch MJ, Seeff LB, Crumley CE, Rabin L, Burns WA: Quinidine hepatotoxicity. A report of a case and review of the literature. Gastroenterology *70*:1136–1140, 1976.
25. Bramlet DA, Posalaky Z, Olson R: Granulomatous hepatitis as a manifestation of quinidine hypersensitivity. Arch Intern Med *140*:395–397, 1980.
26. Cohen MG, Kevat S, Prowse MV, Ahern MJ: Two distinct quinidine-induced rheumatic syndromes. Ann Intern Med *108*:369–371, 1988.
27. West SG, McMahon M, Portanova JP: Quinidine-induced lupus erythematosus. Ann Intern Med *100*:840–842, 1984.
28. Hess E: Drug-related lupus. N Engl J Med *318*:1460–1461, 1988.
29. Weisbart RH, Yee WS, Colburn KK, Whang SH, Heng MK, Boucek RJ: Antiguanosine antibodies: A new marker for procainamide-induced systemic lupus erythematosus. Ann Intern Med *104*:310–313, 1986.
30. Ellrodt AG, Murata GH, Riedinger MS, Stewart ME, Mochizuki C, Gray R: Severe neutropenia associated with sustained-release procainamide. Ann Intern Med *100*:197–201, 1984.
31. Meyers DG, Gonzalez ER, Peters LL, David RB, Feagler JR, Egan JD, Nair CK: Severe neutropenia associated with procainamide: Comparison of sustained release and conventional preparations. Am Heart J *109*:1393–1395, 1985.
32. Teichman SL, Ferrick A, Kim SG, Matos JA, Waspe LE, Fisher JD: Disopyramide-pyridostigmine interaction: Selective reversal of anticholinergic symptoms with preservation of antiarrhythmic effect. J Am Coll Cardiol *10*:633–641, 1987.
33. Ochs HR, Greenblatt DJ, Wood E: Clinical pharmacokinetics of quinidine. Clin Pharmacokinet *5*:150–168, 1980.
34. Vozeh S, Toshihiko U, Guentert TW, Ha HR, Follath F: Kinetics and electrocardiographic changes after oral 3-OH-quinidine in healthy subjects. Clin Pharmacol Ther *37*:575–580, 1985.
35. Killeen AA, Bowers LD: Fetal supraventricular tachycardia treated with high-dose quinidine: Toxicity associated with marked elevation of the metabolite 3(S)-3-hydroxyquinidine. Obstet Gynecol *70*:445–449, 1987.
36. Gerhardt RE, Knouss RF, Thyrum PT, Luchi RJ, Morris JJ Jr: Quinidine excretion in aciduria and alkaluria. Ann Intern Med *81*:927–933, 1969.
37. Reimold EW, Reynolds WJ, Fixler DE, McElroy L: Use of hemodialysis in the treatment of quinidine poisoning. Pediatrics *52*:95–99, 1973.
38. Wasserman F, Brodsky L, Dick MM, Kathe JH, Rodensky PL: Successful treatment of quinidine and procaine amide intoxication. Report of three cases. N Engl J Med *259*:797–802, 1958.
39. Bailey DJ Jr: Cardiotoxic effects of quinidine and their treatment. Review and case reports. Arch Intern Med *105*:13–22, 1960.
40. Woie L, Oyri A: Quinidine intoxication treated with hemodialysis. Acta Med Scand *195*:237–239, 1974.
41. Karlsson E: Clinical pharmacokinetics of procainamide. Clin Pharmacokinet *3*:97–107, 1978.
42. Domoto DT, Brown WW, Bruggensmith P: Removal of toxic levels of *N*-acetylprocainamide with continuous arteriovenous hemofiltration or continuous arteriovenous hemodiafiltration. Ann Intern Med *106*:550–552, 1987.
43. Rosansky SJ, Brady ME: Procainamide toxicity in a patient with acute renal failure. Am J Kidney Dis *VII*:502–506, 1986.
44. Bryson SM, Whiting B, Lawrence JR: Disopyramide serum and pharmacologic effect kinetics applied to the assessment of bioavailability. Br J Clin Pharmacol *6*:409–419, 1978.
45. Hiderling PH, Garrett ER: Pharmacokinetics of the antiarrhythmic disopyramide in healthy humans. J Pharmacokinet Biopharm *4*:199–230, 1976.
46. Horn JR, Hughes ML: Disopyramide dialysability. Lancet *2*:214, 1978.
47. Gosselin B, Mathieu D, Chopin C, Wattel F, Dupuis B, Haguenoer J-M, Despres M: Acute intoxication with disopyramide: Clinical and experimental study by hemoperfusion on amberlite XAD 4 resin. Clin Toxicol *17*:439–449, 1980.

48. Sathyavagiswaran L: Fatal disopyramide intoxication from suicidal/accidental overdose. J Forensic Sci *32*:1813–1818, 1987.
49. Bellet S, Hamdan G, Somlyo A, Lara R: The reversal of cardiotoxic effects of quinidine by molar sodium lactate: An experimental study. Am J Med Sci *237*:165–176, 1959.
50. Watanabe Y, Dreifus LS, Likoff W: Electrophysiologic antagonism and synergism of potassium and antiarrhythmic agents. Am J Cardiol *12*:702–710, 1963.
51. Dreifus LS, de Azevedo IM, Watanabe Y: Electrolyte and antiarrhythmic drug interaction. Am Heart J *88*:95–107, 1974.
52. Brandfonbrener M, Kronholm J, Jones HR: The effect of serum potassium concentration on quinidine toxicity. J Pharmacol Exp Ther *154*:250–254, 1966.
53. Cox AR, West TC: Sodium lactate reversal of quinidine effect studied in rabbit atria by the microelectrode technique. J Pharmacol Exp Ther *131*:212–222, 1961.
54. Gottsegen G, Ostor E: Prevention of the cardiotoxic effect of quinidine by isoproterenol. Am Heart J *65*:102–109, 1963.
55. Kaplinsky E, Yahini JH, Barzilai J, Neufeld HN: Quinidine syncope; Report of a case successfully treated with lidocaine. Chest *62*:764–766, 1972.
56. Nickel SN, Thibaudeau Y: Quinidine intoxication treated by isoproterenol (Isuprel). Can Med Assoc J *85*:81–83, 1961.
57. de Azevedo IM, Watanabe Y, Dreifus LS: Electrophysiologic antagonism of quinidine and bretylium tosylate. Am J Cardiol *33*:633–638, 1974.
58. Vander Ark CR, Reynolds EW, Kahn DR, Tullett G: Quinidine syncope. A report of successful treatment with bretylium tosylate. J Thorac Cardiovasc Surg *72*:464–467, 1976.
59. Koster RW, Wellens HJJ: Quinidine-induced ventricular flutter and fibrillation without digitalis therapy. Am J Cardiol *38*:519–523, 1976.
60. Anderson JL, Mason JW: Successful treatment by overdrive pacing of recurrent quinidine syncope due to ventricular tachycardia. Am J Med *64*:715–718, 1978.
61. Hall K, Meatherall B, Krahn J, Penner B, Rabson JL: Clearance of quinidine during peritoneal dialysis. Am Heart J *104*:646–647, 1982.
62. Haapanen EJ, Pellinen TJ: Hemoperfusion in quinidine intoxication. Acta Med Scand *210*:515–516, 1981.
63. Strong JM, Dutcher JS, Lee W-K, Atkinson AJ Jr: Absolute bioavailability in man of *N*-acetylprocainamide determined by a novel stable isotope method. Clin Pharmacol Ther *18*:613–622, 1975.

CHAPTER 96

LIDOCAINE, MEXILETINE, AND TOCAINIDE

Neal L. Benowitz, M.D.

Lidocaine is widely used as a local anesthetic and parenterally administered antiarrhythmic drug. The actions of mexiletine and tocainide are similar to those of lidocaine, but they have higher oral bioavailability and hence are useful as oral antiarrhythmic agents.

Intoxication with lidocaine is relatively common, occurring as a result of acute massive overdoses, such as after inadvertent acceleration of maintenance IV infusions or with accidental injection of doses meant for dilution (20 per cent solutions) rather than those intended for direct administration (2 per cent solutions).[1] Acute injection of lidocaine has been reported as a method of homicide.[2] More commonly, intoxications result from rapid injections of therapeutic doses of lidocaine in patients with circulatory insufficiency; during maintenance infusions, particularly when clearance is abnormally low due to heart failure, liver disease, advanced age or interactions with drugs that slow the metabolism of lidocaine;[3, 4] or after use of excessive doses or with inadvertent intravenous administration during local anesthesia, including epidural and paracervical blocks.[5, 6] Occasionally, poisoning occurs with inadvertent intramuscular injection during local anesthesia or after swallowing viscous lidocaine prescribed for sore throat; the latter occurs primarily in children.[7] Lidocaine has been one of the drugs most frequently implicated in causing seizures on a general medical service.[8]

Fatal reactions after injection of small doses

of local anesthetics, including lidocaine, into the maxillofacial area or into joint spaces have been attributed to inadvertent arterial injection with retrograde flow into the cerebral circulation.[9, 10] However, a recent experimental study in rats indicates that lidocaine is more toxic when given intravenously as compared with injection into the carotid artery.[11] These results suggest that the toxicity of intra-arterial injection is due to systemic effects that ensue after the drug enters the venous circulation, rather than to retrograde arterial flow.

Intoxications with mexiletine and tocainide are uncommon, owing to their recent introduction into the market. A death has been reported in an adult after ingestion of 16 grams of tocainide.[12] Toxicity from any of the three agents is potentially life-threatening and requires immediate evaluation and intensive care.

PHARMACOLOGY AND PATHOPHYSIOLOGY OF OVERDOSE

Lidocaine acts primarily to inhibit sodium movement across cell membranes. In peripheral nerves, this action results in a decreased rate and degree of depolarization of nerve cells and failure to achieve the threshold potential necessary to propagate action potentials, resulting in conduction blockade and anesthesia. In the heart, lidocaine also inhibits sodium conductance, decreasing the maximal rate of depolarization of myocardial conducting cells. This effect is more prominent in cells that are ischemic and at rapid heart rates. For this reason lidocaine is most effective in the termination of rapid ventricular tachycardia, especially during acute ischemia or after myocardial infarction. Lidocaine may also increase the ventricular fibrillation threshold. At therapeutic doses, lidocaine has minimal electrophysiologic effects on normal cells.

Lidocaine, mexiletine and tocainide, along with phenytoin, are classified as type Ib antiarrhythmic drugs. (See Chapter 97 for discussion of classification.) At therapeutic concentrations, drugs in this class do not affect the QRS interval and have no effect or slightly shorten the Q-T (J-T) interval on the surface electrocardiogram. They have minimal depressant action on the myocardium and are well tolerated by most patients with myocardial disease. The major differences among these three drugs are in their pharmacokinetic properties.

Although relatively little is known of mexiletine and tocainide in overdose, the effects appear to resemble those of lidocaine. In excessive doses, lidocaine can inhibit the sodium channel even in normal tissues. The result may be a clinical picture similar to that seen in quinidine poisoning—marked slowing of cardiac conduction, with development of a wide QRS complex on the electrocardiogram and progressive heart block; depressed myocardial contractility resulting in low output shock; depressed automaticity, resulting ultimately in a slow ventricular rhythm or asystole; and vasodilation.

Central nervous system toxicity, particularly seizures and respiratory arrest, is commonly observed in intoxications and presumably results from disturbances in ion transport across brain cell membranes. Inhibitory neurons are blocked first, producing excitatory stimulation and convulsions; at higher concentrations, both inhibitory and excitatory neurons are inhibited, resulting in generalized central nervous system depression.

CLINICAL PRESENTATION OF THE OVERDOSE AND OTHER TOXIC EFFECTS
(Table 96–1)

Central Nervous System

The most common toxicity of lidocaine and related drugs involves the central nervous system. Even with therapeutic doses of lidocaine, patients may describe dizziness, drowsiness, paresthesias, or euphoria. Typically, with progressive levels of intoxication, lidocaine produces lightheadedness or dizziness, visual disturbances, such as difficulty in focusing the eyes, tinnitus, drowsiness, confusion, agitation and/or disorientation, and even psychosis.

Signs of central nervous system toxicity include shivering, muscle twitching, and tremors. With massive overdoses, seizures, coma, and respiratory arrest may occur. If intoxication develops gradually, as when lidocaine is absorbed from subcutaneous or intramuscular sites or during a constant intravenous infusion, a progression of symp-

Table 96–1. CLINICAL FEATURES OF LIDOCAINE, MEXILETINE, AND TOCAINIDE INTOXICATION

CENTRAL NERVOUS SYSTEM
- Lightheadedness, visual disturbance
- Paresthesias, dysarthria, ataxia, memory loss
- Euphoria, agitation, drowsiness
- Confusion, disorientation, psychosis, coma
- Shivering, muscle twitching, tremor
- Hypotonia (neonates)
- Seizures
- Respiratory arrest

CARDIOVASCULAR
- *Arrhythmias*
  - Sinus arrest
  - Sinus bradycardia
  - AV junctional or ventricular bradycardia
  - Second and third degree heart block
  - Asystole
  - (QRS interval prolongation)*
  - (Ventricular tachycardia or fibrillation)†
- *Hypotension*
  - Vasodilation
  - Depressed myocardial contractility and low cardiac output

GASTROINTESTINAL
- Nausea, vomiting

*Massive poisoning.
†Proarrhythmic effects of mexiletine and tocainide; may occur at therapeutic doses.

toms and signs is often observed. However, with rapid dosing of lidocaine or in the presence of other central nervous system depressant drugs, one may see seizures or coma or both as the first sign of intoxication.

Lidocaine intoxication in the neonate, occurring as a result of inadvertent injection into the fetal scalp or cranium during local anesthesia (caudal or paracervical block or episiotomy), produces apnea, hypotonia, and seizures.[13] Dilated pupils and loss of the oculocephalic reflex may be observed.

Lidocaine-induced respiratory depression may be augmented by general anesthesia or other respiratory depressant drugs.[14] The threshold for lidocaine to induce seizures may be lowered by other drugs, such as the methylxanthines, or by metabolic disturbances.[15, 16]

Central nervous system side effects are common with mexiletine and tocainide even at therapeutic doses; these include paresthesias, ataxia, and loss of memory.[17, 18] Such side effects require termination of therapy in a significant number of patients. Seizures have been observed with overdoses of both these drugs.

Cardiovascular Toxicity

The effects of lidocaine on the cardiovascular system are biphasic. With mild intoxication, blood pressure, heart rate, and cardiac output may be initially elevated due to catecholamine release and peripheral vasoconstriction. At higher doses, heart rate, conduction velocity, and contraction of the heart may be depressed and blood vessels dilated. This may result in arrhythmias, shock, or circulatory collapse. Arrhythmias include sinus bradycardia, sinus arrest, AV nodal or ventricular rhythms, second and third degree heart block, and asystole.[19–26] Other electrocardiographic changes after massive overdose include prolongation of the P-R and QRS intervals.

Arrhythmias also may occur at therapeutic doses. In patients with underlying conduction disease, sinus arrest and AV block have been reported.[19, 20] Lidocaine may increase ventricular ectopy, particularly in the early stages immediately following acute myocardial infarction. Proarrhythmic actions of mexiletine and tocainide, including ventricular tachycardia (sometimes torsades de pointes) or ventricular fibrillation, occur in 5 to 10 per cent of treated patients.[17, 18, 27, 28]

Patients with severe myocardial dysfunction occasionally suffer aggravation of cardiac failure during therapy or poisoning with type Ib antiarrhythmic drugs.

Gastrointestinal

Nausea and vomiting are common, both in therapeutic doses and overdoses with these drugs. Increases in serum concentrations of liver transaminases have been observed during mexiletine therapy. Granulomatous hepatitis has been reported with tocainide treatment.[18]

Hematologic

Tocainide has been associated rarely (0.18 per cent) with hematologic problems, including leukopenia, agranulocytosis, aplastic anemia, and thrombocytopenia.[18] Some experts recommend monitoring of the white blood cell count during the first few months of tocainide therapy. Thrombocytopenia has been reported with use of mexiletine.[17]

Other Toxicity

Topical therapeutic use of lidocaine as a local anesthetic has been associated in case reports with noncardiogenic pulmonary edema (believed to be a manifestation of anaphylaxis) and methemoglobinemia.[29, 30] Therapeutic use of tocainide has been associated in case reports with interstitial pneumonitis, pulmonary fibrosis, a lupus erythematosus syndrome with antinuclear antibodies, and a relatively high incidence of skin rashes.[18]

RELEVANT PHARMACOKINETICS
(Table 96–2)

Absorption

Lidocaine is rapidly metabolized and as a consequence undergoes extensive first-pass metabolism.[31] Oral bioavailability is relatively low (about 35 per cent), so when systemic therapeutic levels are sought, lidocaine is administered by the parenteral route. Because of first-pass metabolism, blood levels of lidocaine remain relatively low, even after repeated oral doses of 300 mg (2 per cent) viscous lidocaine.[32] Although the bioavailability is low, it may be sufficient to result in significant toxicity when oral doses are swallowed, such as has been reported with the use of viscous lidocaine as an oropharyngeal anesthetic primarily in children, but even occasionally after very large doses in adults.[7, 33]

The profile of absorption with the use of lidocaine as a local anesthetic depends on the site of injection and whether a vasoconstrictor like epinephrine has been added.[31] The rate of absorption after a given dose is faster from more vascular sites—from fastest to slowest: intercostal, epidural, brachial plexus, and subcutaneous. The presence of epinephrine decreases the rate of absorption and, therefore, the peak levels of lidocaine. Since the peak level is roughly proportional to the dose administered, it is imperative to keep track of the total dose of lidocaine when multiple doses are given, such as during intercostal nerve blocks. On the other hand, the presence of epinephrine appears to enhance the toxicity of lidocaine after inadvertent intravascular administration.[11] The oral bioavailability of mexiletine and tocainide approaches 100 per cent.[17, 18] Peak concentrations of these drugs are generally seen 1 to 4 hours after an oral dose.

Distribution

After intravenous injection, lidocaine rapidly enters the heart and the brain, producing effects within minutes (Fig. 96–1). Subsequently, concentrations in the blood and highly perfused tissues (such as the brain and the heart) fall, because of distribution to slowly perfused tissues, primarily skeletal muscle and fat. The initial distributional decline in blood concentrations follows a half-life of about 10 minutes (Fig. 96–2) and explains why in some cases the antiarrhythmic action of lidocaine disappears in 10 or 20 minutes after the initial bolus dose. The peak concentration achieved in the blood prior to tissue distribution of the lidocaine depends on the rate of administration. For this reason, a patient can experience a seizure or other transient central nervous system toxicity shortly after a rapid bolus injection, but concentrations of lidocaine may be subtherapeutic when measured a few minutes later. Distribution kinetics are not so important in understanding the course of effects or toxicity of lidocaine when it is used for local anes-

Table 96–2. PHARMACOKINETICS OF LIDOCAINE, MEXILETINE, AND TOCAINIDE (AVERAGE VALUES IN HEALTHY PERSONS)

	LIDOCAINE	MEXILETINE	TOCAINIDE
Oral availability (%)	35	80–90	100
Usual dose	1–4 mg/min IV	600–1200 mg/day PO	800–2400 mg/day PO
Per cent urinary excretion* (unchanged)	2	10	40
Plasma protein binding (%)	50†	70	10
Volume of distribution (L/kg)	1.1	5.5–9.5	2
Clearance (ml/min/kg)	10–15	6–10	2–3
Half-life (hours)	1–8	9–12	11–13
Therapeutic serum concentration (mg/L)	1.5–5.5	0.8–2.0	3–10

*Renal excretion is pH dependent; greater excretion in acid urine.
†Concentration dependent; 30 per cent bound at 20 mg/L.

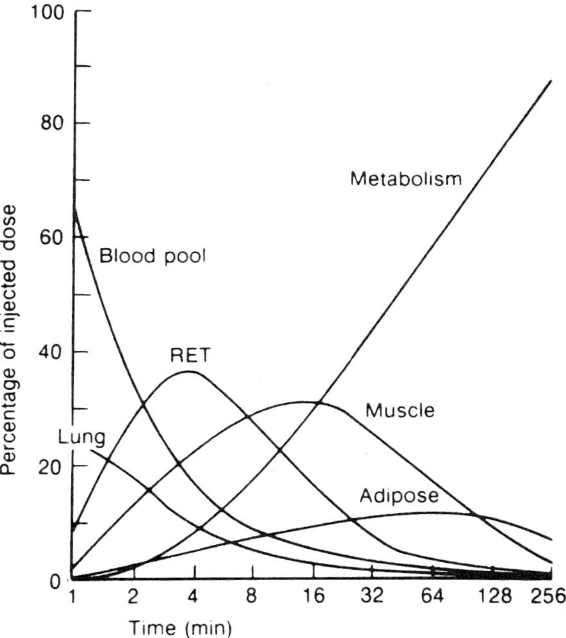

Figure 96–1. Computer simulation based on a perfusion model of the distribution of lidocaine to various human tissues after a 1-minute intravenous infusion (note log time scale). (RET, rapidly equilibrating tissues, such as brain and heart.) The initial rapid decline in blood concentration is due primarily to drug distribution to tissues. RET lidocaine concentration peaks at 4 minutes, and blood lidocaine concentration from this time onward parallels RET concentration. Distribution of lidocaine to other tissues is slower, and blood lidocaine concentration continues to decline rapidly for 20 to 30 minutes because of tissue uptake. The subsequent slower decline in blood lidocaine concentration is primarily due to metabolism. (From Benowitz N, Forsyth RP, Melmon KL, et al: Lidocaine disposition kinetics in monkey and man. I. Prediction by a perfusion model. Clin Pharmacol Ther *16*:87–98, 1974.)

thesia or after oral ingestion of it or other type IB antiarrhythmic drugs.

Lidocaine and tocainide are moderately lipophilic, with volumes of distribution of 1.1 to 2 times body weight, whereas mexiletine is extremely lipophilic and tissue bound, with a volume of distribution of 5.5 to 9.5 L/kg. This means that lidocaine and tocainide are potential candidates for accelerated drug removal by hemoperfusion or hemodialysis, whereas mexiletine is not.

Elimination

Lidocaine and mexiletine are extensively metabolized. Tocainide is eliminated by both hepatic metabolism and renal elimination. Lidocaine is de-ethylated to monoethylglycinexylidide (MEGX), which is subsequently hydrolyzed to glycine xylidide (GX). Both metabolites are active and are excreted in the urine to a greater extent than is lidocaine. The half-lives of MEGX and GX are 2 hours and 1 hour, respectively.[34, 35] These metabolites may contribute to the toxicity of lidocaine, particularly after oral ingestion of lidocaine or in patients with severe heart failure or renal failure receiving prolonged infusions.[36]

Mexiletine is hydroxylated whereas tocainide is conjugated, primarily by glucuronidation. The metabolism of tocainide is stereoselective. At steady state, the concentration of the S(−) isomer is fourfold greater than that of the more active R(+) isomer of tocainide. Variability in the R:S isomer ratio may explain the wide therapeutic range for total tocainide concentration. Neither mexiletine nor tocainide produces pharmacologically active metabolites.

As the drugs in this class are weak bases, renal excretion is pH dependent. Therefore, renal clearance is higher in acid and lower in alkaline urine.

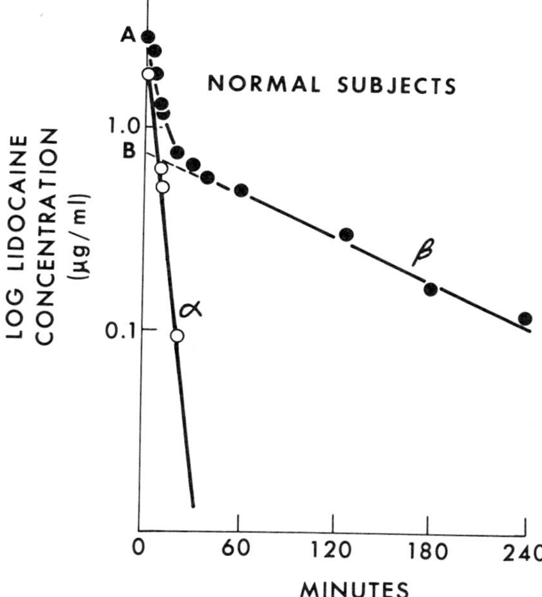

Figure 96–2. Lidocaine blood concentration–time curve after intravenous injection of 50 mg in a healthy volunteer can be described by a biexponential curve. The short and long phases are represented by α and β. (From Thomson PD, Rowland M, Melmon KL: The influence of heart failure, liver disease, and renal failure on the disposition of lidocaine in man. Am Heart J *82*:417–421, 1971.)

Lidocaine is eliminated with an average elimination half-life of 1.5 to 2 hours in healthy people (see Fig. 96–2); the half-life is longer in the presence of disease states, as described later. Toxicity from lidocaine may persist from as briefly as 1 minute (after bolus injection) to as long as several hours (after prolonged infusion or after injection for local anesthesia). In contrast, the half-lives of mexiletine or tocainide are long, averaging about 10 hours (longer in disease states). The long half-lives are due to extensive tissue distribution and low clearance for mexiletine and tocainide, respectively. In both cases, intoxication can be expected to be protracted, lasting for 24 hours or longer.

Effect of Disease States and Drug Interactions

Lidocaine is the prototypic drug displaying blood flow–limited metabolism. That is, the rate of metabolism is proportional to liver blood flow. In states of reduced liver blood flow, such as cardiac failure or shock or with administration of drugs such as beta-blockers, the rate of metabolism of lidocaine is slowed, with a corresponding prolongation of half-life.[37–39]

Since lidocaine and mexiletine are extensively metabolized by oxidative enzymes, their clearance is reduced in the presence of severe liver disease. The glucuronidation of tocainide is not affected by liver disease. Tocainide clearance, however, is significantly reduced in the presence of renal failure.

Elimination of all drugs in this class may be slowed during acute myocardial infarction, resulting in two- to threefold increases in half-life. In addition to reducing clearance, circulatory insufficiency states slow the movement of lidocaine from the blood to body tissues, resulting in a smaller initial volume of distribution. Immediately after a bolus injection of a particular dose, blood levels are twice as high in patients with cardiac failure as in healthy people.[39] In dogs administered lidocaine during cardiopulmonary resuscitation, lidocaine levels were severalfold higher than in dogs with normal circulatory function (Fig. 96–3).[40]

Drug interactions that affect the kinetics of lidocaine are primarily those that reduce cardiac output and liver blood flow. Thus beta-blockers and myocardial depressant drugs may reduce the clearance and prolong the half-life of lidocaine. Cimetidine has been reported to reduce the clearance of lidocaine, but the data on this interaction are conflicting.[41]

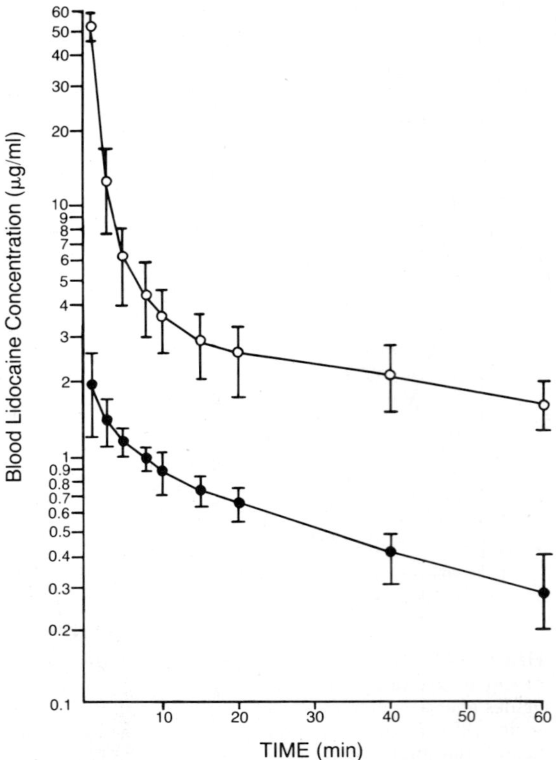

Figure 96–3. Mean right atrial blood lidocaine concentrations of five control (•—•) and three CPR (○—○) dogs after administration of 2 mg/kg of lidocaine via peripheral vein as a bolus dose. Initial concentrations of lidocaine in CPR dogs are approximately 10 times higher than those in control dogs because of a reduction in the volume of the central compartment. The decline in blood lidocaine concentration after 30 minutes in control animals is determined by the rate of lidocaine in metabolism, whereas the rate of decline of blood lidocaine concentration after 30 minutes in CPR animals is contributed to by both drug metabolism and distribution of drug to poorly perfused tissues. Thus, the slope of the blood lidocaine concentration curve after 30 minutes in CPR animals is not a true elimination half-life. (From Chow MSS, Ronfeld RA, Hamilton RA, et al: Effect of external cardiopulmonary resuscitation on lidocaine pharmacokinetics in dogs. J Pharmacol Exp Ther *224*:531–537, 1982.)

Mexiletine undergoes interactions with drugs that affect liver metabolism.[42] Thus metabolism is accelerated by phenobarbital, rifampin, and phenytoin and slowed by cimetidine, isoniazid, disulfiram, and some other drugs.

All drugs in this class potentially can interact with myocardial depressant drugs, such as beta-blockers, calcium channel blockers, or other antiarrhythmic drugs, to depress cardiac conduction or contractility additively in patients with pre-existing conduction defects or myocardial dysfunction.

LABORATORY TOXICOLOGY

Therapeutic blood concentration ranges are given in Table 96–2. Subjective effects of lidocaine may be noted within the therapeutic range, at concentrations of 3 to 5 μg/ml. Physical signs of toxicity are more likely seen at levels above 6 to 10 μg/ml. As described previously, toxicity may occur following rapid intravenous injection due to transiently high blood and brain concentrations, but blood levels measured a few minutes later may be therapeutic or lower. A few patients experience central nervous system toxicity with relatively low lidocaine levels. This toxicity may be due to accumulation of active metabolites.[36, 43]

Blood lidocaine concentrations in patients who die from lidocaine toxicity range from 6 to 33 μg/ml, with liver, heart, and brain tissue concentrations usually greater than 15 μg/ml.[2, 44] The absence of much MEGX in blood and tissues suggests an acute intoxication, whereas levels of MEGX that are 20 to 60 per cent those of lidocaine are expected following a prolonged infusion of lidocaine.[36, 45]

Patients receiving lidocaine during a cardiac arrest may have blood lidocaine concentrations well in the toxic range owing to impaired distribution out of the vascular space.[40, 46] Chow and associates measured blood lidocaine concentrations in patients during cardiopulmonary resuscitation and found great variability in both the maxiumum concentration and the time at which this concentration was achieved.[46] In seven patients who received a 100-mg bolus dose, the peak concentrations in blood ranged from 1.5 to 15.9 μg/ml, which occurred 2 to 13 minutes after administration. The variability is presumably due to differences in extent of organ perfusion, resulting in different initial volumes of distribution and to differing rates of drug delivery to the central circulation from the intravenous site of administration.

Tocainide levels of 385 and 74 μg/ml were measured postmortem after ingestions of 16 grams and an unknown dose, respectively.[12, 47]

MANAGEMENT OF OVERDOSE
(Table 96–3)

General management is similar to that described for other drug overdoses. Intravenous lidocaine should be discontinued immediately. Evaluation and monitoring of intoxicated patients should continue until absorption from the gastrointestinal tract or local anesthetic sites (lidocaine) is complete.

Central Nervous System Toxicity

Seizures should be treated with diazepam initially and then phenytoin and phenobarbital if necessary. Most lidocaine-induced seizures are brief in duration, but in massive poisoning status epilepticus may ensue. In status epilepticus refractory to anticonvulsive medications, barbiturate anesthesia should be considered.

Table 96–3. MANAGEMENT OF LIDOCAINE, MEXILETINE, AND TOCAINIDE OVERDOSE

General Management
- Oral ingestion: lavage and charcoal
- Seizures: diazepam, 5–10 mg IV; phenytoin, 15 mg/kg IV (rate ≤ 50 mg/min)

Impaired Myocardial Conduction
- Sodium bicarbonate: 50 mEq IV; repeat every 5–10 min to maintain artrial pH of 7.4–7.5

Arrhythmias
- Bradyarrhythmias
  - Isoproterenol
  - Cardiac pacemaker
- Ventricular tachycardia
  - Isoproterenol
  - Overdrive pacing
  - (Avoid other type Ib antiarrhythmic drugs)

Hypotension
- Normal saline: 200 ml every 10 min until 1000–2000 ml or evidence of pulmonary edema
- If still hypotensive, consider pulmonary arterial catheter
- If low systemic vascular resistance, dopamine or norepinephrine
- If low cardiac output, isoproterenol, dobutamine, epinephrine
- If intractable cardiogenic shock, intra-aortic balloon pump assistance or cardiopulmonary bypass

Accelerated Drug Removal
- Lidocaine: in massive poisonings with circulatory and/or liver failure consider hemoperfusion (possibly combined with cardiopulmonary bypass)
- Mexiletine: not useful
- Tocainide: consider hemoperfusion or hemodialysis, especially with renal insufficiency

Arrhythmias

Bradyarrhythmias producing hypotension may be temporarily managed by infusion of isoproterenol. However, insertion of a temporary pacemaker is the treatment of choice. Asystole due to a massive accidental overdose of lidocaine during coronary artery bypass graft surgery was treated successfully with combined atrial pacing and infusion of isoproterenol, allowing discontinuation of cardiopulmonary bypass.[48]

Hypotension

Hypotension may be due to decreased cardiac output, arrhythmias or myocardial depression, or decreased systemic vascular resistance. Hypotension should be treated with fluids and, if necessary, vasoconstrictor drugs such as norepinephrine or dopamine. Isoproterenol or other inotropic drugs may be useful in the presence of depressed myocardial contractility. Theoretically, hypertonic sodium bicarbonate should be of benefit in massive intoxications with prolongation of the QRS interval on the electrocardiogram (see Chapter 95 on quinidine). Extracorporeal circulatory assistance may provide short-term support for the patient, allowing time for lidocaine to be metabolized.[26, 48]

Accelerated Drug Removal

Charcoal in repeated doses has not been evaluated for treatment of intoxication of any of the drugs in this class. In theory, charcoal should be of some benefit for treatment of intoxication with tocainide, which has a relatively small volume of distribution and low intrinsic clearance and is not highly protein bound.

Acidification of the urine will increase the renal clearance of all drugs in this class; however, it is unlikely to be of clinical significance, except for tocainide, which is excreted to a considerable extent in the kidney and has a relatively low intrinsic clearance. In considering acidification therapy, the risks in convulsing patients of aggravating acidemia, with the associated aggravation of adverse renal effects due to myoglobinuria (if present), need to be weighed against the benefits of accelerated renal clearance.

Cardiopulmonary bypass as a means to maintain liver circulation and allow lidocaine to be metabolized has been evaluated in experimental animals and has been used to manage two patients who were accidentally overdosed by injection of a 20 per cent lidocaine solution.[26, 48] Because lidocaine has a moderate volume of distribution, hemoperfusion is potentially beneficial, particularly when metabolic clearance is reduced owing to circulatory collapse or severe liver disease. Hemodialysis is expected to be of less benefit because of the degree of protein binding.

Tocainide is significantly removed by hemodialysis[49] and similarly should be effectively removed by hemoperfusion. Since the intrinsic clearance of tocainide is low (200 ml/min, or less than in the presence of renal insufficiency), adding a hemoperfusion or hemodialysis clearance of 200 to 300 ml/min should substantially accelerate removal. However, because of the long half-life, these procedures need to be continued for at least several hours.

Mexiletine is rapidly metabolized, highly protein bound, and extensively distributed to tissues. Therefore, it is unlikely that any extracorporeal drug removal procedure will be of use in managing intoxications with this drug.

References

1. Kempen PM: Lethal/toxic injection of 20% lidocaine: A well-known complication of an unnecessary preparation? Anesthesiology *65*:564–565, 1986.
2. Peat MA, Deyman ME, Crouch DJ, Margot P, Finkle BS: Concentrations of lidocaine and monoethylglycylxylidide (MEGX) in lidocaine-associated deaths. J Forensic Sci *30*:1048–1057, 1985.
3. Pfeifer HJ, Greenblatt DJ, Koch-Weser J: Clinical use and toxicity of intravenous lidocaine. A report from the Boston Collaborative Drug Surveillance Program. Am Heart J *92*:168–173, 1976.
4. Davison R, Parker M, Atkinson AJ Jr: Excessive serum lidocaine levels during maintenance infusions: Mechanisms and prevention. Am Heart J *104*:203–207, 1982.
5. Alfano SN, Leicht MJ, Skiendzielewski JJ: Lidocaine toxicity following subcutaneous administration. Ann Emerg Med *13*:465–467, 1984.
6. Grimes DA, Cates W Jr: Deaths from paracervical anesthesia used for first trimester abortion. N Engl J Med *295*:1397–1399, 1976.
7. Hess GP, Walson PD: Seizures secondary to oral viscous lidocaine. Ann Emerg Med *17*:725–727, 1988.
8. Boston Collaborative Drug Surveillance Program: Drug-induced convulsions. Lancet 2:677, 1972.
9. Aldrete JA, Narang R, Sada T, Liem ST, Miller GP: Reverse carotid blood flow—a possible explanation for some reactions to local anesthetics. J Am Dent Assoc *94*:1142–1145, 1977.

10. Shira RB: Cephalic kinetics of intra-arterially injected lidocaine. Oral Surg *44*:167–172, 1977.
11. Yagiela JA: Intravascular lidocaine toxicity: Influence of epinephrine and route of administration. Anesth Progr 32:57–61, 1985.
12. Clarke CWF, El-Mahdi EO: Fatal oral tocainide overdosage. Br Med J *288*:760, 1984.
13. Kim WY, Pomerance JJ, Miller AA: Lidocaine intoxication in a newborn following local anesthesia for episiotomy. Pediatrics *64*:643–645, 1979.
14. Woods LA, Haggart J: Apneic and hypotensive effects of local anesthetic drugs in dogs and mice under general anesthesia. Anesthesiology *18*:831–840, 1957.
15. Englesson S, Paymaster NJ, Hill TR: Electrical seizure activity produced by xylocaine and Citanest. Acta Anaesthesiol Scand *16*:47–50, 1965.
16. Adriani J, Zepernick R, Hyde E: Influence of the status of the patient on systemic effects of local anesthetic agents. Anesth Analg *45*:87, 1966.
17. Campbell RWF: Mexiletine. N Engl J Med *316*:29–34, 1987.
18. Roden DM, Woosley RL: Tocainide. N Engl J Med *315*:41–45, 1986.
19. Jeresaty RM, Kahn AH, Landry AB: Sino-atrial arrest due to lidocaine in a patient receiving quinidine. Chest *61*:683–685, 1972.
20. Cheng TO, Wadhwa K: Sinus standstill following intravenous lidocaine administration. JAMA *223*: 790–792, 1973.
21. Lichstein E, Chadda KD, Gupta PK: Atrioventricular block with lidocaine therapy. Am J Cardiol *31*:277–281, 1973.
22. Klein HO, Jutrin I, Kaplinsky E: Cerebral and cardiac toxicity of a small dose of lignocaine. Br Heart J *37*:775–778, 1975.
23. Finkelstein F, Kreeft J: Massive lidocaine poisoning. N Engl J Med *301*:50, 1979.
24. Badui E, Garcia-Rubi D, Estanol B: Inadvertent massive lidocaine overdose causing temporary complete heart block in myocardial infarction. Am Heart J *102*:801–803, 1981.
25. Edgren B, Tilelli J, Gehrz R: Intravenous lidocaine overdosage in a child. Clin Toxicol *24*:51–58, 1986.
26. Freedman MD, Gal J, Freed CR: Extracorporeal pump assistance—novel treatment for acute lidocaine poisoning. Eur J Clin Pharmacol *22*:129–135, 1982.
27. Cocco G, Strozzi C, Chu D, Pansini R: Torsades de pointes as a manifestation of mexiletine toxicity. Am Heart J *100*:878–880, 1980.
28. Engler RL, Le Winter M: Tocainide-induced ventricular fibrillation. Am Heart J *101*:494–496, 1981.
29. Howard JJ, Mohsenifar Z, Simons SM: Adult respiratory distress syndrome following administration of lidocaine. Chest *81*:644–645, 1982.
30. O'Donohue WJ, Moss LM, Angelillo VA: Acute methemoglobinemia induced by topical benzocaine and lidocaine. Arch Intern Med *140*:1508–1509, 1980.
31. Benowitz NL, Meister W: Clinical pharmacokinetics of lignocaine. Clin Pharmacokinet *3*:177–201, 1978.
32. Greenblatt DJ, Benjamin DM, Willis CR, Harmatz JS, Zinny MA: Lidocaine plasma concentrations following administration of intraoral lidocaine solution. Arch Otolaryngol *111*:298–300, 1985.
33. Fruncillo RJ, Gibbons W, Bowman SM: CNS toxicity after ingestion of topical lidocaine. N Engl J Med *306*:426–427, 1982.
34. Strong JM, Mayfield DE, Atkinson AJ, Burris BC, Raymon F, Webster LT Jr: Pharmacological activity, metabolism, and pharmacokinetics of glycinexylidide. Clin Pharmacol Ther *17*:184–194, 1975.
35. Blumer J, Strong JM, Atkinson AJ: The convulsant potency of lidocaine and its *N*-dealkylated metabolites. J Pharmacol Exp Ther *186*:31–36, 1973.
36. Halkin H, Meffin P, Melmon KL, Rowland M: Influence of congestive heart failure on blood levels of lidocaine and its active monode-ethylated metabolite. Clin Pharmacol Ther *17*:669–676, 1975.
37. Svendsen TL, Tango M, Waldorff S, Steiness E, Trap-Jensen J: Effects of propranolol and pindolol on plasma lignocaine clearance in man. Br J Clin Pharmacol *13*:223S–226S, 1982.
38. Graham CF, Turner WM, Jones JK: Lidocaine–propranolol interactions. N Engl J Med *304*:1301, 1980.
39. Benowitz NL, Meister W: Pharmacokinetics in patients with cardiac failure. Clin Pharmacokinet *1*:389–405, 1976.
40. Chow MSS, Ronfeld RA, Hamilton RA, Helmink R, Fieldman A: Effect of external cardiopulmonary resuscitation on lidocaine pharmacokinetics in dogs. J Pharmacol Exp Ther *224*:531–537, 1982.
41. Jackson JE, Bentley JB, Glass SJ, Fukui T, Gandolfi AJ, Plachetka JR: Effects of histamine-2 receptor blockade on lidocaine kinetics. Clin Pharmacol Ther *37*:544–548, 1985.
42. Bigger T: The interaction of mexiletine with other cardiovascular drugs. Am Heart J *107*:1079–1085, 1984.
43. Strong JM, Parker M, Atkinson AJ: Identification of glycinexylidide in patients treated with intravenous lidocaine. Clin Pharmacol Ther *14*:67–72, 1973.
44. Poklis A, Mackell MA, Tucker EF: Tissue distribution of lidocaine after fatal accidental injection. J Forensic Sci *29*:1229–1236, 1984.
45. Collinsworth KA, Strong JM, Atkinson AJ Jr, Winkie RA, Perlroth F, Harrison DC: Pharmacokinetics and metabolism of lidocaine in patients with renal failure. Clin Pharmacol Ther *18*:59–64, 1975.
46. Chow MSS, Ronfeldt RA, Ruffet D, Fieldman A: Lidocaine pharmacokinetics during cardiac arrest and external cardiopulmonary resuscitation. Am Heart J *102*:799–801, 1981.
47. Barnfield C, Kemmenoe AV: A sudden death due to tocainide overdose. Hum Toxicol *5*:337–340, 1986.
48. Noble J, Kennedy DJ, Latimer RD, Hardy I, Bethune DW, Collis JM, Wallwork J: Massive lignocaine overdose during cardiopulmonary bypass. Successful treatment with cardiac pacing. Br J Anaesth *56*:1439–1441, 1984.
49. Wieger U, Hanrath P, Kuck KH, Pottage A, Graffner C, Augustin J, Runge M: Pharmacokinetics of tocainide in patients with renal dysfunction and during haemodialysis. Eur J Clin Pharmacol *24*:503–507, 1983.
50. Benowitz N, Forsyth RP, Melmon KL, Rowland M: Lidocaine disposition kinetics in monkey and man. 1. Prediction by a perfusion model. Clin Pharmacol Ther *16*:87–98, 1974.
51. Thomson PD, Rowland M, Melmon KL: The influence of heart failure, liver disease, and renal failure on the disposition of lidocaine in man. Am Heart J *82*:417–421, 1971.

CHAPTER 97

NEW CARDIAC ANTIARRHYTHMIC AGENTS

Paul R. Pentel, M.D.
David N. Dunbar, M.D.

The newer Class IC and Class III antiarrhythmic agents have proved to be useful drugs, but each has important toxic effects that can limit its use. Of greatest interest is their acute, potentially life-threatening cardiac toxicity. This may occur during therapeutic use or from drug overdose. As many as 5 to 15 per cent of patients using antiarrhythmic agents therapeutically will develop new or more frequent arrhythmias (proarrhythmic effect) rather than the intended therapeutic effect.[1] Some antiarrhythmic agents also can depress myocardial contractility and cardiac output. The effects of overdoses of these drugs are less well described but appear to be largely an exaggeration of the toxic effects observed with therapeutic doses.

The toxic effects of antiarrhythmic agents can generally be anticipated from an understanding of their electrophysiologic actions. Drugs within a given class tend to have similar therapeutic and toxic properties. This chapter provides a brief overview of the electrophysiologic basis of antiarrhythmic drug toxicity and considers several selected Class IC and III agents in more detail.

CARDIAC CELL ACTION POTENTIAL

The cardiac cell action potential is a series of voltage changes across the cell membrane (Fig. 97–1). In the resting state, an electrical potential exists across the cell membrane, with the interior negatively charged due to marked differences in ion concentrations across the cell membrane. This electrochemical gradient is maintained by the sodium pump, which transports sodium out of the cell in exchange for extracellular potassium. When the cardiac cell reaches a critical threshold voltage, sodium channels in the cell membrane open to allow positively charged sodium ions to enter the cell rapidly. The resulting rapid depolarization is represented by phase 0 of the action potential. Depolarization of the cardiac cell creates localized currents that cause adjacent cells to reach threshold voltage and depolarize. In this manner, depolarization is propagated through the specialized conducting tissues and myocardium. The rate of propagation, or conduction velocity, is directly related to the magnitude of the inward sodium current. Ventricular depolarization is represented on the electrocardiogram by the QRS complex. The duration of the QRS complex reflects the time required for ventricular depolarization and is inversely related to conduction velocity.

After a brief and limited repolarization (phase 1 of the action potential), the cardiac cell enters a "plateau" phase in which depolarization is maintained primarily by opening of the slow calcium channel (phase 2). During this period, there is little change in membrane potential, represented by the ST segment on the electrocardiogram. Repolarization occurs during phase 3 because of movement of potassium out of the cell, along with inactivation of the inward calcium and sodium currents. Myocardial repolarization is represented by the T wave on the electrocardiogram. The cardiac cell is refractory to stimuli until it is sufficiently repolarized during phase 3 to allow it to depolarize again.

Phase 4 of the action potential encompasses diastole, with maintenance of the resting membrane potential. In cells that demonstrate automaticity, the negative potential inside the cardiac cell gradually decreases until threshold voltage is reached and the cell depolarizes once again.

CLASSIFICATION AND ELECTROCARDIOGRAPHIC EFFECTS OF ANTIARRHYTHMIC DRUGS

(Fig. 97–2)

Class I. Class I drugs act principally by decreasing the fast inward sodium current in

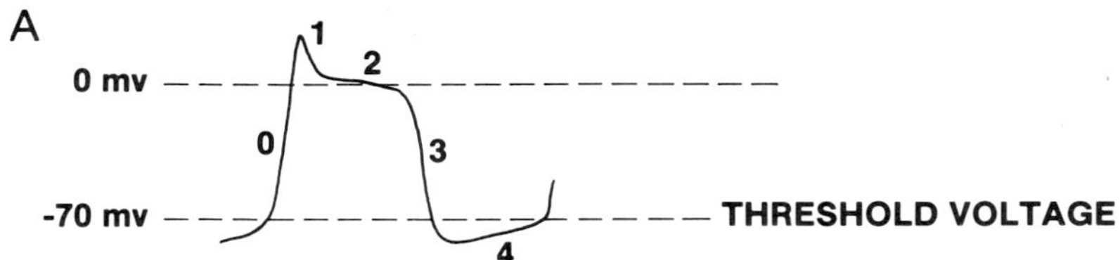

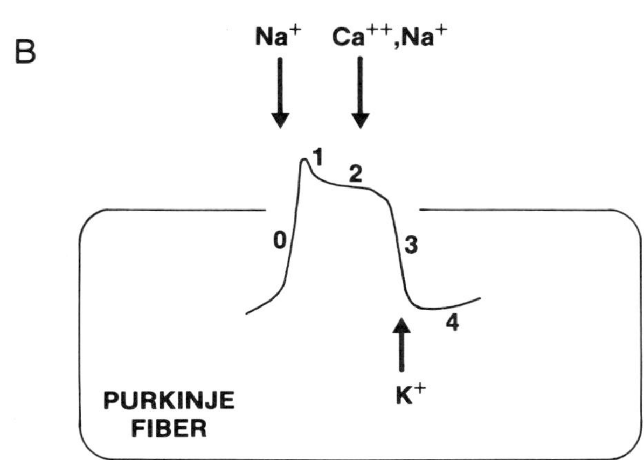

Figure 97–1. *A*, Normal Purkinje fiber action potential with phase 0 (depolarization), phase 1 (overshoot), phase 2 (plateau), phase 3 (repolarization), and phase 4 (spontaneous depolarization). *B*, Major ion currents in the normal Purkinje fiber action potential. Phase 0 is due to activation of the fast sodium channel and the resulting inward sodium current. The plateau phase is maintained by an inward current caused by calcium and sodium, and repolarization is due in part to an outward potassium current. (From Pentel PR, Benowitz NL: Tricyclic antidepressant poisoning. Med Toxicol *1*:101–121, 1986.)

a dose-dependent manner.[2] This action slows the rate of phase 0 depolarization (Vmax) and the rate of conduction of the cardiac impulse. Although all Class I drugs diminish Vmax, they differ markedly in the magnitude of this effect and the circumstances under which it occurs, and have been divided into three subclasses.[3]

Class IA drugs, which include quinidine, procainamide, and disopyramide (and perhaps imipramine and other tricyclic antidepressants) depress Vmax and slow conduction modestly at therapeutic doses. The QRS interval is normal or minimally prolonged with therapeutic dosing but is markedly prolonged with excessive doses. Type IA drugs also prolong action potential duration, resulting in an increase in the effective refractory period. Because action potential duration is a determinant of the electrocardiographic J-T interval (representing repolarization), Class IA drugs prolong the J-T interval.

Class IB drugs include lidocaine, tocainide, mexiletine, moricizine, and phenytoin. These drugs have little effect on Vmax of normal cardiac tissue, but slow Vmax markedly in abnormal (i.e., ischemic) tissue. Because Vmax in normal tissue is not affected, the electrocardiographic QRS interval is not changed, even with excessive or toxic doses of these drugs. Class IB drugs shorten action potential duration minimally and have no discernible effect on the J-T interval.

Class IC drugs include flecainide, encainide, propafenone, lorcainide, and indecainide. These drugs markedly depress Vmax, resulting in slowing of conduction. The QRS duration is prolonged, even at therapeutic doses. Class IC drugs have little effect on action potential duration and do not prolong the J-T interval. Prolongation of the QT interval is due to the QRS prolongation.

Class III. The primary action of Class III drugs is to prolong the action potential duration and effective refractory period. The electrocardiographic J-T interval is prolonged. Examples of Class III drugs include bretylium (limited to acute parenteral use) and amiodarone.

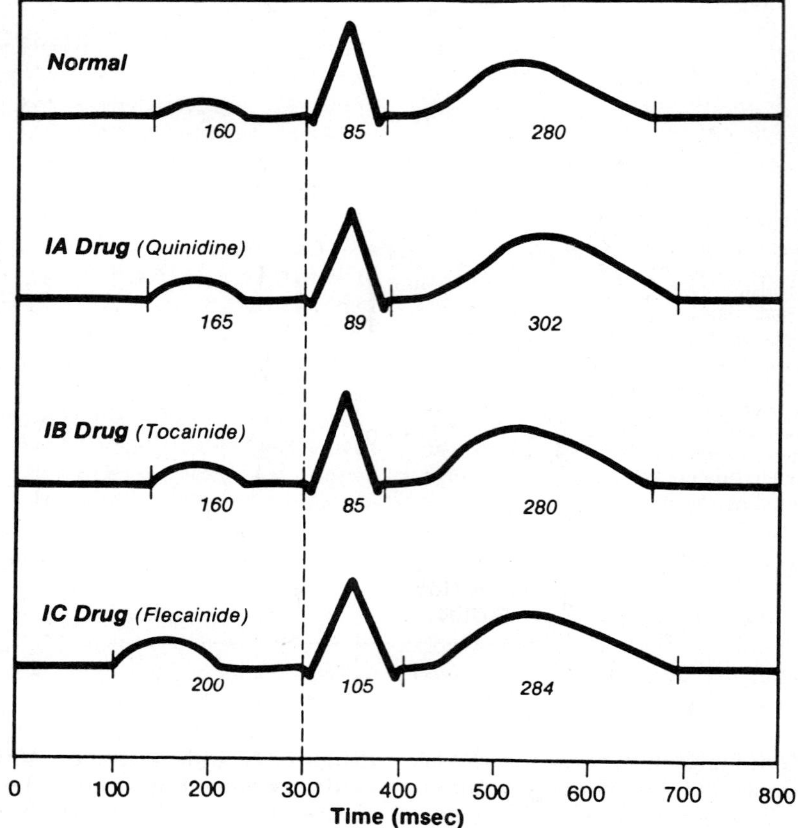

Figure 97–2. Graphic depiction of RR, QRS, and J-T intervals in normal patients (average intervals of 600 normal ECGs from patients receiving quinidine,[73] tocainide,[74] and flecainide.[73] Observed intervals have been adjusted to reflect a heart rate of 75 bpm. Class IA drugs prolong the J-T interval (measured from the end of the QRS complex to the end of the T wave) but affect QRS duration only minimally. Class IB drugs do not prolong either the QRS or J-T intervals. Class IC drugs prolong the QRS complex substantially but have little effect on the J-T interval. (Courtesy of Dr. Morrison Hodges.)

MECHANISM OF ANTIARRHYTHMIC DRUG TOXICITY

Impaired Automaticity. Automaticity is a normal property of certain cells in the specialized conduction system, such as the sinus node, parts of the atrium, and the His-Purkinje system. During phase 4, these cells spontaneously depolarize because of an inward sodium current[4, 5] until the threshold voltage is reached and an action potential results. The intrinsic rate of firing of these pacemaker cells is determined by the level of maximum diastolic potential (most negative potential to which the cell is repolarized), the rate of phase 4 depolarization, and the threshold potential. The pacemaker cells with the highest intrinsic rate are normally located in the sinus node. Subsidiary pacemakers at other sites have lower intrinsic rates and are normally inhibited by propagation of impulses originating in the sinus node.

Abnormal automaticity may develop in working atrial or ventricular myocardial cells that are partially depolarized by myocardial disease processes, such as ischemia.[6–8] Antiarrhythmic agents may act therapeutically by suppressing abnormal automaticity in ectopic foci. They can, however, cause arrhythmias by suppressing normal automaticity. All Class I drugs decrease the slope of phase 4 depolarization. Class IA and IC drugs further suppress automaticity by decreasing the maximum diastolic potential and increasing threshold voltage.[9] This increases the amount of phase 4 depolarization necessary to achieve threshold potential.

Both IA and IC drugs may markedly suppress sinus node function; IB drugs generally have little effect.[9] Clinically important sinus node suppression is generally limited to patients with pre-existing sinus node disease.[10] Drug-induced arrhythmias include sinus bradycardia, sinus pause, and sinus asystole. Significant sinus bradycardia or pauses may allow the emergence of subsidiary pacemakers in the form of ectopic atrial, junctional, or idioventricular escape rhythms. Slow heart rates also may predispose to the development of torsades de pointes (see later).

Conduction Block. Slowed conduction caused by Class I antiarrhythmic agents can lead to failure of the cardiac impulse to propagate. This is more common with Class IA and Class IC drugs, because of their greater effect on conduction, than with Class IB drugs. Sinus pauses may result from impaired conduction between the sinoatrial node and atrium, termed sinus node exit block. This drug effect is most common in patients with pre-existing sinus node disease. Class I drugs also may impair atrioventricular conduction, usually at the level of the His-Purkinje system. Electrophysiologic studies have shown the greatest HV prolongation with Class IC drugs, less HV prolongation with Class IA drugs, and little change in HV intervals with the IB drugs. Patients with pre-existing conduction system disease, such as bifascicular bundle branch block, are at increased risk of developing advanced or third-degree atrioventricular block during treatment with Class I drugs, particularly the IC drugs. These drugs are contraindicated in patients who have Mobitz II or advanced atrioventricular block without pacemaker support.

Drug-Induced Ventricular Arrhythmias. The spectrum of proarrhythmic effects of antiarrhythmic drugs includes the worsening of existing arrhythmias or the appearance of new arrhythmias. Aggravation of existing arrhythmias may include increasing the number of ventricular premature beats or couplets, increasing the frequency or duration of nonsustained ventricular tachycardia, or accelerating ventricular tachycardia. New and potentially lethal ventricular arrhythmias may develop, such as torsades de pointes, polymorphic ventricular tachycardia, ventricular fibrillation, or the conversion of nonsustained to sustained ventricular tachycardia. Proarrhythmic effects have been observed in 5 to 15 per cent of trials with antiarrhythmic drugs,[1] and all antiarrhythmic agents appear to have this potential. Risk factors associated with serious arrhythmias and death include the presence of structural heart disease, a history of sustained ventricular tachycardia, and rapid dosage escalation.[11, 12]

Re-entrant Tachycardias. Normally, cardiac impulses are conducted through the atria and ventricles until all excitable myocardium has been depolarized and only refractory tissue remains. Re-entry can occur if an area of slow conduction and block allows the cardiac impulse to persist for a sufficient time to re-excite areas that have been repolarized, and are no longer refractory. Most tachyarrhythmias are caused by re-entry mechanisms. Class I drugs may act therapeutically by altering the relationship between conduction and refractoriness in a re-entrant pathway, thus interrupting the re-entrant rhythm. However, they may also alter this relationship unfavorably (e.g., by slowing conduction more than refractoriness) and thereby provide a more suitable substrate for a re-entrant tachycardia. This may be one mechanism by which antiarrhythmic drugs cause ventricular tachycardia. This type of drug-induced rhythm is often quite difficult to terminate.

Polymorphous Ventricular Tachycardia and Torsades de Pointes. In addition to the usual (monomorphic) ventricular tachycardia in which all QRS complexes are similar, ventricular tachycardia may less commonly occur with a changing QRS morphology (polymorphous ventricular tachycardia). When the amplitude or polarity of QRS complexes twists about an isoelectric baseline in association with a prolonged QT interval, it is referred to as torsades de pointes.[13] The mechanism of these arrhythmias is unclear. Class IA and Class III antiarrhythmic drugs, which prolong repolarization, predispose to the development of torsades de pointes. Polymorphous ventricular tachycardia may occur with the use of IC agents, although monomorphic ventricular tachycardia is more common.

External Pacemaker Function. Class IA

and IC antiarrhythmic agents, especially in high doses, may interfere with external pacemaker function by increasing stimulation thresholds, resulting in loss of capture.[14, 15] The mechanism likely involves increasing refractoriness (IA drugs) and/or decreasing conduction velocity and membrane responsiveness (IA and IC drugs). IB drugs generally do not affect stimulation thresholds, although lidocaine has been observed to cause failure to capture in patients with myocardial disease.[16]

Myocardial Contractility. Depolarization of myocardial cells triggers contraction through the release of calcium from the sarcoplasmic reticulum. Drugs that slow depolarization, therefore, may also impair myocardial contractility. Significant decreases in cardiac output are uncommon with therapeutic doses of most antiarrhythmic agents, although flecainide can aggravate pre-existing congestive failure. Markedly impaired cardiac output, however, is common with overdoses of Class IA or IC drugs.

FLECAINIDE

Flecainide acetate is a fluorinated analogue of procainamide and the first Class IC drug released for clinical use in the United States.[17] The drug's most important action is blockade of the sodium channel, and therapeutic use is characterized by modest (10 to 30 per cent) prolongation of the QRS interval. Flecainide has a variable effect on action potential duration, decreasing it in Purkinje fibers and increasing it in ventricular muscle.[18] QT interval prolongation occurs with therapeutic use, owing to the prolonged QRS complex with little or no prolongation of repolarization (J-T interval).[19] Atrial and atrioventricular (AV) conduction are also impaired by flecainide, perhaps due to inhibition of the calcium channel. Lengthening of the PR interval occurs with therapeutic dosing, and AV block is a feature of flecainide toxicity. In contrast to quinidine and procainamide, flecainide has no anticholinergic or alpha-blocking activity.

Pharmacokinetics (Table 97–1). Flecainide is well absorbed orally, with little first-pass metabolism. Elimination is primarily by metabolism. Renal excretion is quite variable due to marked pH dependence. Drug excreted unchanged in urine ranges from 7.4 per cent in alkaline urine (pH, 7.5 to 8.3) to 44.7 per cent in acid urine (pH, 4.4 to 5.4), with corresponding elimination half-lives of 33 and 8 hours.[20] When urine pH is not controlled, renal excretion of unchanged drug in healthy subjects averages 25 per cent, with a half-life of 14 hours (range, 7 to 23 hours).[21] The elimination half-life is prolonged by congestive heart failure (range, 14 to 26 hours) or severe renal insufficiency.[21, 22] Several metabolites of flecainide are active but are present in serum in low concentrations and probably contribute little to therapeutic effect or toxicity. Important drug interactions include decreased flecainide clearance due to cimetidine or propranolol, and additive negative inotropic effect with propranolol.[23, 24]

Toxicity. Primary toxic effects of flecainide are arrhythmias, conduction delays, bradycardia, and impairment of cardiac output. Proarrhythmic events complicating therapeutic use are most likely to occur in patients with severe ventricular dysfunction or a history of sustained ventricular tachycardia, or in those who are taking more than 400 mg per day.[25] Deaths that occur during therapeutic dosing are often accompanied by excessive plasma flecainide concentrations (>1 μg/ml).[17, 26] Toxic effects are also more common in patients with more than 20 to 30 per cent prolongation of QRS or PR intervals.[19]

The most common arrhythmia complicating therapeutic dosing is monomorphic ventricular tachycardia.[17, 26, 27] The negative inotropic action of flecainide is generally modest, but it may cause or aggravate congestive heart failure in patients with impaired left ventricular function. The negative inotropic effect may contribute to hypotension caused by arrhythmias. For example, three cases of ventricular tachycardia are reported that were accompanied by hypotension despite modest ventricular rates of 100 to 150 beats/min. Flecainide also increases the threshold for electrical pacing of the ventricle.[28] This effect could hinder efforts to use a pacemaker to treat toxic rhythms due to flecainide.[26]

Few cases of acute flecainide overdose have been reported. Toxicity is generally similar to the adverse effects of therapeutic dosing, with QRS prolongation, AV block, bradycardia, ventricular tachycardia, and hypotension.[29] One patient on previous flecain-

Table 97–1. CLINICAL PHARMACOKINETICS OF CLASS IC AND CLASS III ANTIARRHYTHMIC AGENTS

DRUG	ACTIVE METABOLITES	VOLUME OF DISTRIBUTION (L/kg)	SYSTEMIC CLEARANCE (L/min)	% RENAL EXCRETION	ELIMINATION HALF-LIFE	PROTEIN BINDING (%)	THERAPEUTIC DOSE	THERAPEUTIC SERUM CONCENTRATION (ng/ml)
Class IC								
flecainide*		10	0.7	10–50*	14–19 hr	32–47	100–300 mg bid	200–1000
encainide†	ODE‡ MODE	3.8	1.8 (FM) 0.2 (SM)	low	1–3 hr (FM) 11–13 hr (SM)	70–80	25–75 mg qid	SM: encainide, 250–1400 FM: ODE, 100–300 MODE, 60–280
propafenone†	5-OH-propafenone	3.0	1.1	1	2–32 hr	97	up to 300 mg tid	Not established (range 64–1044)
lorcainide**	norlorcainide	6–17	1.0	3	8–13 hr		200–600 mg daily	lorcainide, 10–270 norlorcainide, 50–950
Class III								
amiodarone	? desmethyl-amiodarone	10–70	0.2–0.6	low	19–52 days	90	200–400 mg daily	500–3000

*Renal excretion markedly pH-dependent.
†Polymorphic metabolism with distinct population of slow metabolizers (SM) and fast metabolizers (FM).
‡ODE = *o*-Demethyl encainide, MODE = 3-methoxy ODE.
**Saturable first-pass metabolism.

ide therapy developed signs of toxicity from a single dose of 600 mg, but the relationship of toxicity to dose ingested or serum flecainide concentration is not well established.[30] A healthy patient who ingested a single dose of 2000 to 4000 mg of flecainide developed prolonged electrocardiographic intervals (PR = 0.24 sec, QRS = 0.12 sec) and mild drowsiness but no arrhythmias or hypotension despite a serum flecainide concentration of 3350 ng/ml 12 hours post-ingestion. This concentration is considerably higher than those associated with several fatalities occurring during therapeutic use of flecainide.[17] A comparable serum flecainide concentration proved fatal, however, in a patient who also ingested a large dose of propranolol.[31]

Treatment. There is no established specific therapy for flecainide toxicity. One potentially interesting approach that has been suggested is the use of therapies known to reverse tricyclic antidepressant toxicity. Like the Class IC antiarrhythmic agents, toxic doses of tricyclic antidepressant act on the fast sodium channel to slow phase 0 depolarization. Hypertonic solutions of alkali (sodium lactate or sodium bicarbonate) can partially reverse this slowing of phase 0 by increasing the extracellular pH and sodium concentrations. The rapid infusion of hypertonic sodium bicarbonate is effective in both animals and humans in reversing conduction delays, ventricular arrhythmias, and hypotension due to tricyclic antidepressant toxicity.[32] By analogy, Chouty et al treated three patients for flecainide toxicity with hypertonic sodium lactate (250 to 500 mEq over 30 to 60 min). Hypotension and QRS prolongation improved coincident with treatment.[29] Hypertonic sodium bicarbonate also has been used with apparent clinical benefit for a patient with encainide toxicity,[33] suggesting that further study of the use of hypertonic alkali for toxicity due to Class IC drugs is warranted.

The use of other Class IC or IA antiarrhythmic agents is contraindicated in the treatment of Class IC drug toxicity, because these agents may aggravate sodium channel blockade. Renal flecainide excretion can be enhanced by acidification of urine.[20] The expected benefit of this maneuver is limited, because urine pH is normally somewhat acidic, but some patients, especially those with a higher urine pH, might benefit from this therapy. Hemodialysis is not expected to enhance flecainide elimination appreciably because of the drug's high lipid solubility. Hemoperfusion might add modestly to flecainide clearance, but its use has not been reported.

ENCAINIDE

The electrophysiologic properties of encainide are similar to those of flecainide. Therapeutic use is associated with up to 45 per cent prolongation of the QRS and P-R intervals, and prolongation of the QT interval due to the prolonged QRS complex.[34, 35] The pharmacokinetics of encainide is complex, because both parent drug and the major metabolites *o*-demethylencainide (ODE) and 3-methoxy-ODE (MODE) are pharmacologically active. In addition, genetic polymorphism of encainide metabolism exists, resulting in populations of fast and slow metabolizers.[36] Therapeutic use of encainide is associated with a less negative inotropic effect than is flecainide.[37]

Pharmacokinetics (see Table 97–1). Metabolism of encainide is under genetic control, with distinct populations of fast and slow metabolizers.[38, 39] In fast metabolizers (90 per cent of patients), the half-life of ODE is much longer than that of encainide, and serum concentrations of ODE exceed those of encainide during chronic dosing. In addition, ODE is 5 to 50 times as potent as encainide. The therapeutic effect in fast metabolizers, therefore, is due primarily to ODE.[40, 41] Slow metabolizers do not achieve therapeutic concentrations of ODE but may accumulate encainide to levels that are sufficient to provide antiarrhythmic activity. Interpretation of drug levels, therefore, must take account of both encainide and ODE. Genetic control of encainide metabolism appears to be linked to the well-described genetic control of debrisoquin hydroxylation.[41, 42]

MODE is also active, but its contribution to therapeutic and toxic effects is less clear. Both ODE and MODE are eliminated in part by renal excretion and accumulate in patients with renal failure.

Toxicity. Minor but bothersome side effects are common with therapeutic use of encainide, including headache, dizziness, blurred vision, tremor, confusion, and nausea.[43] The most common serious side effect is ventricular tachycardia. Winkle and associates reported 11 patients who developed ventricular tachycardia that required cardioversion or CPR while receiving encainide.[44] All patients had a previous history of sustained ventricular tachyarrhythmias. This contrasts with quinidine-induced arrhythmias, which often occur without such a history. The encainide-induced arrhythmia usually occurred within several days of starting therapy or increasing the encainide dose. Ventricular tachycardia was most often monomorphic, but periods of polymorphic ventricular tachycardia were noted in half of these patients. Encainide-induced arrhythmias typically were sustained and difficult to treat with cardioversion or other standard therapies. Mean QRS prolongation prior to the onset of tachycardia was 33 per cent, and two patients had only 13 per cent and 14 per cent prolongation. Thus, excessive QRS prolongation may be a risk factor for development of ventricular tachycardia but is not always present. The hazard of attempting to treat encainide toxicity with other Class I antiarrhythmic agents was illustrated by one patient in this series who received 500 mg of procainamide because of several brief episodes of encainide-induced ventricular tachycardia. This resulted in multiple recurrences of sustained ventricular tachycardia and cardiac arrest over a period of 20 hours. The patient had previously received procainamide alone without adverse effect.

A case of acute encainide overdose (3 to 3.5 gm) has been reported in a previously healthy patient.[33] Presentation was characterized by marked QRS prolongation, hypotension, bradycardia, seizures, and coma. Seizures were controlled with diazepam. Administration of 100 mEq of hypertonic sodium bicarbonate (1 mEq/ml) was associated with modest improvement in blood pressure and heart rate. Several hours later, when the patient had a normal heart rate, blood pressure, and arterial blood gases but persistent marked QRS prolongation, hypertonic sodium bicarbonate was again administered. A brief improvement in QRS duration was noted (Fig. 97–3). This finding is of interest because hypertonic sodium bicarbonate has been shown partially to reverse the cardiac toxicity of tricyclic antidepressants, drugs

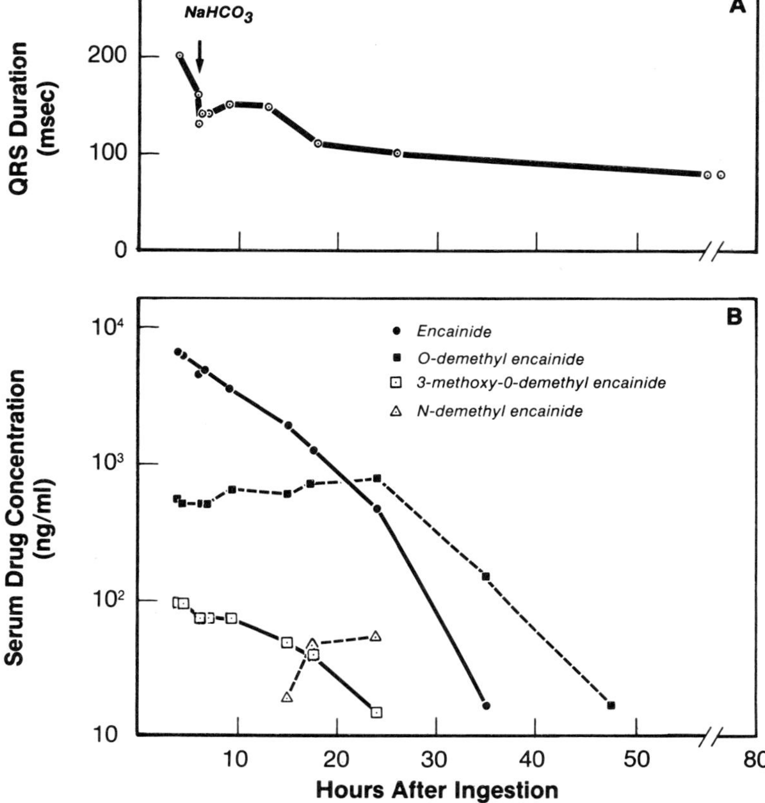

Figure 97–3. *A*, QRS duration after ingestion of encainide (estimated dose: 3.0 to 3.5 grams). Administration of 100 mEq of hypertonic sodium bicarbonate (arrow) increased the arterial pH (7.40 to 7.48) and serum sodium concentration (139 to 142 mEq/liter) and was followed by a transient decrease in QRS duration. *B*, Serum encainide and metabolite concentrations, demonstrating that the effect of hypertonic sodium bicarbonate was not mediated by changes in these concentrations. (From Pentel PR, Goldsmith SR, Salerno DM, et al: Effect of hypertonic sodium bicarbonate on encainide overdose. Am J Cardiol 57:878–880, 1986.)

that also act by inhibiting the sodium channel (see discussion of flecainide toxicity). Further study is needed to assess whether hypertonic sodium bicarbonate may be of benefit in treating the cardiac toxicity of encainide and, perhaps, other Class IC antiarrhythmic drugs.

Treatment. As with flecainide, there is no established therapy for encainide toxicity. The use of hypertonic sodium bicarbonate may be of benefit for QRS prolongation or arrhythmias. The use of other Class IA or Class IC antiarrhythmic agents to treat encainide-induced arrhythmias is clearly contraindicated, as they may aggravate conduction delays. The potential benefit of hemoperfusion is difficult to predict because of encainide's complicated pharmacokinetics. In fast metabolizers, encainide serum concentrations during chronic dosing contribute little to toxicity, but encainide concentrations following an acute overdose may be high enough to produce toxicity.[33] Encainide clearance in fast metabolizers, however, is quite rapid (1800 ml/min) and hemoperfusion (maximum possible clearance about 300 ml/min) would be expected to add little to this. The efficacy of hemoperfusion in removing the active metabolite ODE is unclear, because its volume of distribution and clearance are not known. For slow metabolizers, encainide clearance is low. Hemoperfusion might be of benefit, but this has not been reported. Hemodialysis is unlikely to be useful for either encainide or ODE because both are highly lipid soluble. The possibility of enhancing renal encainide or ODE excretion has not been studied.

PROPAFENONE

Propafenone is an investigational Class IC drug that has some structural resemblance to propranolol.[45] Like other Class IC drugs, it prolongs the PR and QRS intervals. In addition to its effect on the sodium channel, it has weak beta-blocking and calcium channel antagonist actions in vitro. It is unclear whether these additional actions contribute to its therapeutic or toxic effect. Propafenone has been used orally for suppression of chronic ventricular arrhythmias and intravenously to terminate supraventricular tachycardia.

Pharmacokinetics (see Table 97–1). Oral absorption is rapid and complete, but bioavailability is low and variable due to first-pass metabolism. This process appears to be saturable, so that plasma propafenone concentrations increase disproportionately as the dose is increased.[46] The principal metabolite, 5-OH-propafenone, may be more active than the parent compound. Populations of fast and slow metabolizers of propafenone have been identified.[47] This observation, along with dose-dependent first-pass elimination, may explain the wide range in reported propafenone half-lives (2 to 32 hours) and therapeutic serum propafenone concentrations (64 to 1044 ng/ml).[48] The activity of a second metabolite, *N*-depropylpropafenone, is not known.

Toxicity. Cardiovascular side effects of propafenone include ventricular arrhythmias, bundle branch block, bradycardia, and congestive heart failure.[49, 50] It is unclear whether these effects are related to serum propafenone or metabolite concentrations. Conduction delays and bradycardia are most likely to occur in patients with underlying conduction abnormalities, and congestive heart failure is most likely to develop in patients with underlying left ventricular dysfunction. Therapeutic efficacy of propafenone correlates with QRS and PR prolongation. By analogy with encainide and flecainide, excessive prolongation of these intervals may be useful in anticipating toxicity.

Acute propafenone overdose (133 mg/kg) has been reported in a 2 year old child.[51] Toxicity was generally similar to that reported for flecainide or encainide overdose: seizures, marked QRS prolongation, first-degree AV block, hypotension, and progressive bradycardia leading to cardiac arrest. Resuscitation using atropine, dopamine, and sodium bicarbonate was successful, but the contribution of each to the outcome is not clear.

Treatment. There is no established therapy for propafenone toxicity (see discussions of flecainide and encainide for general principles).

LORCAINIDE

Lorcainide is an investigational Class IC drug used intravenously or orally for suppression of chronic ventricular arrhythmias, slowing the ventricular response during atrial fibrillation and flutter, and terminating reciprocating tachycardias associated with the Wolff-Parkinson-White syndrome.[52] Electrophysiologic and clinical actions of lorcainide are generally similar to those of flecainide.[53] However, chronic oral dosing produces prolongation of atrial and ventricular refractoriness that is not observed after acute intravenous administration. This may be due to the presence of an active metabolite, norlorcainide, with oral dosing.[54]

Pharmacokinetics (see Table 97–1). Lorcainide undergoes saturable first-pass elimination with oral dosing. Bioavailability increases from less than 30 per cent with the first dose to nearly 100 per cent with chronic dosing.[55] As a result (and despite lorcainide's half-life of 8 hours), steady-state lorcainide concentrations in serum may not be achieved until 4 to 5 days after therapy is initiated or a dose is changed. The elimination half-life of norlorcainide is longer than that of the parent compound, and norlorcainide serum concentrations exceed those of lorcainide with chronic dosing. Norlorcainide appears to contribute to antiarrhythmic efficacy during chronic lorcainide administration.[56]

Toxicity. The most frequent adverse effect of therapeutic dosing is central nervous system toxicity: insomnia, vivid dreams, and occasionally tremor.[57] Ventricular arrhythmias also have been noted. There is little experience with lorcainide overdose, and no specific therapy for toxicity. Hemoperfusion would likely be of limited efficacy because of lorcainide's large volume of distribution.

AMIODARONE

Amiodarone is an iodinated compound initially developed as an antianginal agent because of its coronary and systemic vasodilating action. It is currently approved in the United States for the treatment of chronic ventricular arrhythmias, but it is also effective for some supraventricular arrhythmias.[58] Amiodarone is usually classified as a Class III antiarrhythmic agent because it prolongs repolarization of myocardial tissue.[59] It is now recognized that amiodarone also prolongs depolarization, an effect that may contribute to its antiarrhythmic action.[60, 61] Beta-antagonist activity and possible calcium channel blockade also have been described, but their clinical importance is unclear. Amiodarone slows the sinus rate and atrioventricular conduction. Common effects of therapeutic doses of amiodarone on the electrocardiogram include PR prolongation and repolarization changes, such as abnormal T waves and U waves, and QT prolongation. QRS prolongation is not observed.

Pharmacokinetics (see Table 97–1). Oral bioavailability of amiodarone is low (28 to 50 per cent) due to incomplete and erratic intestinal absorption.[62] First-pass metabolism is low. The metabolite desmethylamiodarone is electrophysiologically active in vitro, but its contribution to the clinical activity of amiodarone is not known. Enterohepatic recycling of amiodarone has been postulated, and amiodarone concentrations in bile 50 times those of serum have been reported.[63] The steady-state volume of distribution of amiodarone is quite large (10 to 70 L/kg), and disposition is complex owing to very extensive distribution of drug to some tissues; three- and four-compartment models have been used to describe the time course of serum concentrations. Elimination is almost entirely by metabolism. Because of the modest systemic clearance and the very large volume of distribution, the elimination half-life of amiodarone has been reported to be 19 to 52 days.[64] Steady-state concentrations, and therapeutic effect, may be delayed weeks to months after initiation of therapy. Loading doses can reduce this interval.[65] The slow onset and termination of therapeutic effect of this drug have made establishing a therapeutic serum concentration range difficult, but values of 0.5 to 3.0 μg/ml are commonly used.[58] No clear relationship has been established between serum concentrations and the cardiac toxicity of amiodarone.

Toxicity. Chronic noncardiac toxicity of amiodarone, particularly pneumonitis, may be life threatening[58] but will not be considered here. The most important acute complications of therapeutic use of amiodarone are ventricular arrhythmias and sinus bradycardia.[66–68] Because steady-state serum concentrations of amiodarone are achieved slowly with therapeutic dosing, the onset of toxicity is most often delayed for several weeks.[68] Toxicity may develop more rapidly with the use of loading doses. As anticipated with amiodarone's long elimination half-life, the duration of toxicity may be prolonged. Reports vary from resolution within 1 to 3 days[66, 67] to as long as 10 days.[68, 69a]

The proarrhythmic effect of amiodarone may be less common than with other antiarrhythmic agents, but both monomorphic and polymorphic ventricular tachycardia can occur. Monomorphic ventricular tachycardia is occasionally resistant to both antiarrhythmic therapy and cardioversion.[66, 67] Torsades de pointes is likely a consequence of amiodarone's effects on ventricular repolarization. The concurrent use of other antiarrhythmic drugs that prolong repolarization, such as quinidine, may increase the risk of developing this arrhythmia.[70] Sinus arrest has been reported in three patients. All had normal sinus node function prior to therapy but were taking digoxin concurrently. Progression of atrioventricular block has also been reported.[66] Amiodarone may impair cardiac output and aggravate congestive heart failure, but this is uncommon.

A single case of acute amiodarone overdose has been reported.[71] Ingestion of 8 gm produced no clinical toxicity, and no therapy was required. A small decrease in heart rate and an increase in the QT interval were noted within hours of the ingestion and persisted for 3 days. The peak amiodarone serum concentration was 1.1 μg/ml but decreased within hours to the usual therapeutic range. The rapid onset of cardiac effects in this patient illustrates that the usual delay in onset of therapeutic effect of amiodarone is due to the slow dosing rate rather than slow distribution of amiodarone to myocardium. Further support of this point is provided by the observation that intravenous amiodarone can produce conversion of atrial fibrillation in some patients within 5 to 10 minutes.[72]

Treatment. Experience in treating arrhythmias caused by amiodarone is limited. Torsades de pointes has been reported to respond to the usual measures for this arrhythmia: isoproterenol and pacing.[68] Monomorphic ventricular tachycardia may respond to Class Ib antiarrhythmic agents or propranolol.[67] The use of Class Ia drugs that prolong repolarization may increase the risk of producing polymorphic ventricular tachycardia.[70]

Because amiodarone is extensively protein bound, hemodialysis clearance is low. The use of hemoperfusion for acute amiodarone ingestion may possibly be of benefit if it is initiated before extensive tissue distribution has taken place, but this has not been reported. The use of repeated doses of oral activated charcoal to interrupt enterohepatic recycling also might be of benefit if used early, but this has not been studied.

References

1. Velebit V, Podrid P, Lown B, Cohen BH, Graboys TB: Aggravation and provocation of ventricular arrhythmias by antiarrhythmic drugs. Circulation *65*:886–894, 1982.
2. Vanghan Williams EM: Classification of antiarrhythmic drugs. *In* Sandoe E, Flenstod-Jensen E, Olesen K (eds): Cardiac Arrhythmias. Sodertalje, Sweden, Ad Astra, 1970, pp 449–473.
3. Harrison DC: Antiarrhythmic drug classification: New science and practical applications. Am J Cardiol *56*:185–187, 1985.
4. DiFrancesco D, Ojeda C: Properties of the current if in the sino-atrial node of the rabbit compared with those of current $1K_2$ in Purkinje fibers. J Physiol (Lond) *308*:353–367, 1980.
5. DiFrancesco D: A new interpretation of the pacemaker current in Purkinje fibers. J Physiol (Lond) *314*:359–376, 1981.
6. Friedman PL, Stewart JR, Wit AL: Spontaneous and induced cardiac arrhythmias in subendocardial Purkinje fibers surviving myocardial infarction in dogs. Circ Res *33*:612–626, 1973.
7. Hordof A, Edie R, Malin J, Hoffman BF, Rosen MR: Electrophysiologic properties and response to pharmacologic agents of fibers from diseased human atria. Circulation *54*:774–779, 1976.
8. Singer DH, Baumgarten CM, Ten Eck RE: Cellular electrophysiology of ventricular and other dysrhythmias: Studies on diseased and ischemic heart. Prog Cardiovasc Dis *24*:97–156, 1981.
9. Estes NAM III, Garan H, McGovern B, Ruskin JN, Class J: Antiarrhythmic agents; Classification, electrophysiologic considerations, and clinical effects. *In* Reiser HJ, Horowitz LN (eds): Mechanisms and Treatment of Cardiac Arrhythmias: Relevance of Basic Studies to Clinical Management. Baltimore, Urban Schwarzenberg, 1984, pp 183–199.
10. Bigger JT Jr, Reiffel JA: Sick sinus syndrome. Annu Rev Med *30*:91–118, 1979.
11. Morganroth J: Risk factors for the development of proarrhythmic events. Am J Cardiol *59*:327–376, 1987.
12. Morganroth J, Anderson J, Gentzkow G: Classification by type of ventricular arrhythmia predicts frequency of adverse cardiac events from flecainide. J Am Coll Cardiol *8*:607–615, 1986.
13. Smith WM, Gallagher JJ: "Les torsades de pointes." An unusual ventricular arrhythmia. Ann Intern Med *93*:578–584, 1980.
14. Gay RJ, Brown DF: Pacemaker failure due to procainamide toxicity. Am J Cardiol *34*:728, 1974.
15. Hellestrand KF, Burnett PF, Milne JR, et al: Effect of antiarrhythmic agent flecainide acetate on acute and chronic pacing thresholds. PACE *6*:892, 1983.
16. Moss AJ, Goldstein S: Clinical and pharmacologic factors associated with pacemaker latency and incomplete pacemaker capture. Br Heart J *31*:112, 1969.
17. Roden DM, Woosley RL: Drug therapy: Flecainide. N Engl J Med *315*:36–40, 1986.

18. Ikeda N, Sungh BN, Davis LD, Hauswirth O: Effect of flecainide on the electrophysiologic properties of isolated canine and rabbit myocardial fibers. J Am Coll Cardiol *5*:303–310, 1985.
19. Salerno DM, Granrud G, Sharkey P, et al: Pharmacodynamics and side effects of flecainide acetate. Clin Pharmacol Ther *40*:101–107, 1986.
20. Muhiddin KA, Johnston A, Turner P: The influence of urinary pH on flecainide excretion and its serum pharmacokinetics. Br J Clin Pharmacol *17*:447–451, 1984.
21. Conard GJ, Ober RE: Metabolism of flecainide. Am J Cardiol *53*:41B–51B, 1984.
22. Franciosa JA, Wilen M, Weeks CE, Tanenbaum R, Kram DC, Miller AM: Pharmacokinetics and hemodynamic effects of flecainide in patients with chronic low output heart failure. J Am Coll Cardiol *1*:699, 1983.
23. Tjandra Maga TB, Verbesse HR, Van Hecken A, Van Melle P, De Schepper PJ: Oral flecainide elimination kinetics: Effects of cimetidine (abs). Circulation *68*(Suppl3):111–416, 1983.
24. Lewis GP, Holtzman JL: Interaction of flecainide with digoxin and propranolol. Am J Cardiol *53*:52B–57B, 1984.
25. Morganroth J, Horowitz LN: Flecainide: Its proarrythmic effect and expected changes on the surface electrocardiogram. Am J Cardiol *53*:89B–94B, 1984.
26. Sellers TD, DiMarco JP: Sinusoidal ventricular tachycardia associated with flecainide acetate. Chest *85*:647–649, 1984.
27. Spirack C, Gottlieb S, Miura DS, Somberg JC: Flecainide toxicity. Am J Cardiol *53*:329–330, 1984.
28. Hellestrand KJ, Nathan AW, Bexton RS, Camm AJ: Electrophysiologic effects of flecainide acetate on sinus node function, anomalous atrioventricular connections, and pacemaker thresholds. Am J Cardiol *53*:30B–38B, 1984.
29. Chouty F, Funck-Brentano C, Landau JM, Lardoux H: Efficacite de fortes doses de lactate molaire par voie veineuse lors des intoxications au flecainide. Presse Med *16*:808–810, 1987.
30. Ward SR, personal communication, 1986.
31. Brown CR, Buchanan JF: Combined flecainide and propranolol overdose. Clin Toxicol Update *8*:9–12, 1986.
32. Pentel PR, Benowitz NL: Tricyclic antidepressant poisoning. Med Toxicol *1*:101–121, 1986.
33. Pentel PR, Goldsmith SR, Salerno DM, Nasraway SA, Plummer DW: Effect of hypertonic sodium bicarbonate on encainide overdose. Am J Cardiol *57*:878–880, 1986.
34. Roden DM, Reele SB, Higgins SB, et al: Total suppression of ventricular arrhythmias by encainide. N Engl J Med *302*:877–882, 1980.
35. Lynch JJ, Lucchesi BR: New antiarrhythmic agents: part II. The pharmacology and clinical use of encainide. Prac Cardiol *10*:109, 1984.
36. Woosley RL, Wood AJJ, Roden DM: Encainide. N Engl J Med *318*:1107–1115, 1988.
37. Sami MH, Derbekyan VA, Lisbona R: Hemodynamic effects of encainide in patients with ventricular arrhythmia and poor ventricular function. Am J Cardiol *52*:507–511, 1983.
38. Wang T, Roden DM, Wolfenden HT, Woosley RL, Wood AJJ, Wilkinson GR: Influence of genetic polymorphism on the metabolism and disposition of encainide in man. J Pharm Exp Ther *228*:605–611, 1984.
39. Roden DM, Duff HT, Altenbern D, Woosley RL: Antiarrhythmic activity of the *O*-demethyl metabolite of encainide. J Pharm Exp Ther *221*:552–557, 1982.
40. Carey EL, Duff HJ, Roden DM, Kirby Primm R, Wilkinson GR, et al: Encainide and its metabolites; Comparative effects in man on ventricular arrhythmia and cardiographic intervals. J Clin Invest *73*:539–547, 1984.
41. Kates RE, Harrison DC, Winkle RA: Metabolite cumulative during long-term oral encainide administration. Clin Pharmacol Ther *31*:427–432, 1982.
42. Woosley RL, Roden DM, Dai G, Wang T, Altenbern D, et al: Co-inheritance of the polymorphic metabolism of encainide and debrisoquin. Clin Pharmacol Ther *39*:282–287, 1986.
43. Berchtold-Kanz E, Schwart G, Hust M, Nitsche K, Just H: Increased incidence of side effects after encainide: A newly developed antiarrhythmic drug. Clin Cardiol *7*:493–497, 1984.
44. Winkle RA, Mason JW, Griffin JC, Ross D: Malignant ventricular tachyarrythmias associated with the use of encainide. Am Heart J *102*:857–864, 1981.
45. Salerno DM, Hodges M: New therapy focus: Propafenone. Cardiovasc Rev Rep *6*:924–931, 1985.
46. Connolly SJ, Kates RE, Lebsack CS, et al: Clinical pharmacology of propafenone. Circulation *68*:589–596, 1983.
47. Siddoway LA, McAllister CB, Want T, et al: Polymorphic oxidative metabolism of propafenone in man (abs). Circulation *68*(Suppl 3):64, 1983.
48. Siddoway LA, Roden DM, Woosley RL: Clinical pharmacology of propafenone: Pharmacokinetics, metabolism and concentration-response relations. Am J Cardiol *54*:9D–12D, 1984.
49. Hodges M, Salerno D, Granrud G: Double-blind and placebo-controlled evaluation of propafenone in suppressing ventricular ectopic activity. Am J Cardiol *5*:45D–50D, 1984.
50. Connolly SJ, Kates RE, Lebsack CS, et al: Clinical efficacy and electrophysiology of oral propafenone for ventricular tachycardia. Am J Cardiol *52*:1208–1213, 1983.
51. McHugh TP, Ferina DG: Propafenone ingestion. Ann Emerg Med *16*:437–440, 1987.
52. Pottage A: Clinical profiles of newer class 1 antiarrhythmic agents—tocainide, mexiletine, encainide, flecainide and lorcainide. Am J Cardiol *52*:24C–31C, 1983.
53. Meinertz T, Kasper W, Kersting F, Just H, Bechtold H, Jahnchen E: Lorcainide. II. Plasma concentration-effect relationship. Clin Pharm Ther *26*:196–204, 1979.
54. Echt DS, Mitchell LB, Kates RE, Winkle RA: Comparison of the electrophysiologic effects of intravenous and oral lorcainide in patients with recurrent ventricular tachycardia. Circulation *68*:392–399, 1983.
55. Jahnchen E, Bechtold H, Kasper W, Kersting F, Just H, Heykants J, Meinertz T: Lorcainide: Saturable presystemic elimination. Clin Pharmacol Ther *26*:187–195, 1979.
56. Mead RH, Keefe DL, Kates RE, Winkle RA: Chronic lorcainide therapy for symptomatic premature ventricular complexes: Efficacy, pharmacokinetics and evidence for norlorcainide antiarrhythmic effect. Am J Cardiol *55*:72–78, 1985.
57. Vlay SC, Mallis GI: Intravenous and oral lorcainide: Assessment of central nervous system toxicity and

antiarrhythmic efficacy. Am Heart J *111*:452–455, 1986.
58. Mason JW: Drug therapy: Amiodarone. N Engl J Med *316*:455–466, 1987.
59. Singh BN, Williams EMV: The effects of amiodarone, a new anti-anginal drug, on cardiac muscle. Br J Pharmacol *39*:657–667, 1970.
60. Mason JW, Hondeghen LM, Katzung BG: Amiodarone blocks inactivated cardiac sodium channels. Pflugers Arch *396*:79–81, 1983.
61. Idem: Block of inactivated sodium channels and of depolarization-induced automaticity in guinea pig papillary muscle by amiodarone. Circ Res *55*:277–285, 1984.
62. Holt DW, Tucker GT, Jackson PR, Storey GCA: Amiodarone pharmacokinetics. Am Heart J *106*:840–846, 1983.
63. Andreasen F, Agerbaek H, Bjerrgaard P, Gotzsche H: Pharmacokinetics of amiodarone after intravenous and oral administration. Eur J Clin Pharm *19*:293–299, 1981.
64. Latini R, Tognoni G, Kates RE: Clinical pharmacokinetics of amiodarone. Clin Pharmacokin *9*:136–156, 1984.
65. Hager JJ, Prystowsky EN, Zipes DP: Relationships between amiodarone dosage, drug concentrations, and adverse side effects. Am Heart J *106*:931–935, 1983.
66. McGovern B, Garan H, Kelly E, Ruskin J: Adverse reactions during treatment with amiodarone hydrochloride. Br Med J *287*:175–180, 1983.
67. Zipes DP, Prystowsky EN, Heger JJ: Amiodarone: Electrophysiologic actions, pharmacokinetics and clinical effects. JAAC *3*:1059–1071, 1984.
68. Sclarovsky S, Lewin RF, Kracoff O, Strasberg B, Arditti A, Agmon J: Amiodarone-induced polymorphous ventricular tachycardia. Am Heart J *105*:6, 1983.
69. Gallastegui JL, Bauman SL, Anderson JL, et al: Worsening of ventricular tachycardia by amiodarone. J Clin Pharmacol *28*:406–411, 1988.
69a. Fogoros RN, Anderson KP, Winkle RA, Swedlow CD, Mason JW: Amiodarone: Clinical efficacy and toxicity in 96 patients with recurrent, drug-refractory arrhythmias. Circulation *68*:88–94, 1983.
70. Tartini R, Steinbrunn W, Kappenberger L, Meyer UA: Dangerous interaction between amiodarone and quinidine. Lancet *1*:1327–1329, 1987.
71. Bonati M, D'Aranno V, Galletti F, Fortuati MT, Tognoni G: Acute overdose of amiodarone in a suicide attempt. J Toxicol Clin Toxicol *20*:181–186, 1983.
72. Holt P, Crick JCP, Davies DW, Curry P: Intravenous amiodarone in the acute termination of supraventricular arrhythmias. Int J Cardiol *8*:67–76, 1985.
73. Hodges M, Salerno D, Granrud G, et al: Flecainide vs. quinidine: Results of a multicenter trial. Am J Cardiol *53*:66B–71B, 1984.
74. Horowitz LN, Josephson ME, Farshidi A: Human electropharmacology of tocainide, a lidocaine congener. Am J Cardiol *42*:276–280, 1978.

CHAPTER 98
SYMPATHOMIMETICS

Michael T. Kelley, M.D.

A large proportion of the medications used in modern medicine accomplish their desired effects by altering autonomic nervous system functions. Cardiac output and vascular resistance are altered to control blood pressure. Bronchioles are dilated to control asthma. Nasal vessels are constricted to control the symptoms of the common cold. The autonomic nervous system is divided into parasympathetic and sympathetic divisions. This chapter focuses on the toxicology of drugs that stimulate the sympathetic division.

Drugs that stimulate the sympathetic division of the autonomic nervous system are called sympathomimetics. The sympathomimetics exert their effects by interacting with alpha- and beta-adrenergic receptors. The alpha adrenergic receptors are further subdivided into alpha$_1$- and alpha$_2$-receptors. Only a few times in this chapter are the subclassifications of the alpha-receptors considered, since stimulation of both receptor types usually has similar physiologic effects.

The beta adrenergic receptors are also subdivided into beta$_1$- and beta$_2$-receptors. Selective stimulation of the beta receptors produces differing physiologic effects. Table 98–1 lists the physiologic effects of stimulation of the alpha-, beta$_1$-, and beta$_2$-receptors.

Unless multiple drugs have been ingested, the diagnosis of an overdose of a sympathomimetic medication can often be made by

Table 98–1. SYMPATHOMIMETIC EFFECTS

Alpha-Stimulation	$Beta_1$-Stimulation
pupillary dilatation	increased heart rate
arterial vasoconstriction: skin, mucosal, skeletal, cerebral, pulmonary, visceral, renal, salivary	increased cardiac contraction
systemic venoconstriction	increased cardiac automaticity
decreased bowel motility	**$Beta_2$-Stimulation**
increased GI sphincter tone	skeletal muscle, pulmonary, visceral, and renal arterial dilatation
increased trigone and urinary bladder sphincter tone	relaxation of bronchial smooth muscle
pilomotor contraction	decreased GI motility
increased sweating in palms	relaxation of urinary bladder
decreased pancreatic secretions	increased glycogenolysis and gluconeogenesis
platelet aggregation	increased lipolysis
	increased pancreatic and glandular secretions
	hyperkalemia

recognizing patterns of specific physiologic responses. These have been termed "autonomic clinical syndromes."[1] By noting the effects on blood pressure, pulse, pupil size, skin and mucous membrane moisture, lung sounds, and bowel sounds, an overdose of a particular drug often can be classified into a particular syndrome. Proper treatment can then proceed in a logical manner. Table 98–2 summarizes the sympathetic clinical syndromes.

Sympathetic Syndromes

The alpha-adrenergic syndrome is caused by relatively pure alpha-agonists. The blood pressure is increased owing to constriction of the peripheral arteriolar beds. Reflex bradycardia often accompanies this rise in blood pressure. The pupils are dilated. The mucous membranes are dry due to decreased blood flow to the capillary beds, but sweating is frequently present. Bowel sounds are decreased because of decreased gut motility.

Some of the beta-adrenergic agents are selective therapeutically, but in overdose usually both $beta_1$- and $beta_2$-receptors are stimulated,[2] producing the beta-adrenergic syndrome. Heart rate is increased because of $beta_1$-receptor stimulation. $Beta_2$-stimulation causes vasodilation and hypotension. Gut motility may be decreased. The pupils are relatively unaffected by beta-stimulation.

A mixed alpha- and beta-adrenergic syndrome is seen with both agents, which increase central sympathetic output as well as those that stimulate both alpha- and beta-receptors. Blood pressure is increased because of vasoconstriction as well as $beta_1$-stimulation of the heart (positive inotropic effect). Because of the $beta_1$-stimulation, tachycardia is also seen (positive chronotropic effect). The combination of hypertension with tachycardia differentiates this syndrome from the pure alpha adrenergic syndrome, in which hypertension occurs with reflex bradycardia. The pupils are dilated in the mixed adrenergic syndrome. Mucous membranes are dry, but sweating is often present. Bowel sounds are diminished because of decreased gut motility.

SPECIFIC AGENTS

Phenylpropanolamine

Many of the sympathomimetics are available for over-the-counter as well as prescription use. It is intriguing that when used as a nasal decongestant, a 75-mg dose of phenylpropanolamine is a prescription medication (Entex-LA), but the same 75-mg dose can be purchased without a prescription in the form of an appetite suppressant (Dexitrim). Table 98–3 lists over-the-counter agents that contain phenylpropanolamine at the time of this writing. However, even though the trade names may remain the same, the ingredients often change. The patent is for the name,

Table 98–2. SUMMARY OF SYMPATHOMIMETIC SYNDROMES

	BP	PULSE	PUPIL SIZE	SWEATING	PERISTALSIS
Alpha-adrenergic	+ +	−/0	+ +	+	0/−
Beta-adrenergic	+/−	+ +	0	0	0
Mixed adrenergic	+ +	+ +	+ +	+ +	0/−

+, Increased; −, decreased; 0, variable or no effect.

(Modified from Olsen KR, Pentel, PR, Kelley MT: Physical assessment and differential diagnosis of the poisoned patient. Med Toxicol 2:52–81, 1987.)

Table 98–3. COMMERCIAL PREPARATIONS OF OTC PHENYLPROPANOLAMINE

	AMOUNT	TYPE
4-Way Cold Tablets	12.5 mg	comb, as, ch
Acutrim	75 mg	sing
Allerest Allergy Tablets	18.7 mg	comb, ch,
Allerest 12 Hour Caplets	75 mg	comb, ch
Allerest Sinus Pain Formula	18.7 mg	comb, ch, ac,
Allerest, Headache Strength	18.7 mg	comb, ch, ac
Allerest, Children's	12 mg	comb, ch
Allergy Relief Medicine	25 mg	comb, ch
Bayer Children's Cold Medicine	3.125 mg	comb, as
Bayer Children's Cough Medicine	9 mg/5 ml	comb, dx, al
Cheracol Plus	25 mg/15 ml	comb, ch, dx, al
Chexit	25 mg	comb, ph, py, dx, th, ac
Congesprin, Children	6.25 mg/5 ml	comb, ac, al
Contac	75 mg	comb, ch
Contac, Severe Cold	25 mg	comb, ch, ac, dx
Coricidin Demilets	6.25 mg	comb, ch, ac
Coricidin Max Strength	12.5 mg	comb, ch, ac
Coricidin 'D'	12.5 mg	comb, ch, ac
Demazin Nasal Decongestant	25 mg	comb, ch
Dexatrim Capsules	50 mg	sing
Dexatrim Maximum Strength	75 mg	sing
Dexatrim Max Str Pre-Meal	25 mg	sing
Dimetapp Tablets	25 mg	comb, br
Dimetapp Exentabs	75 mg	comb, br
Dimetapp Plus Caplets	12.5 mg	comb, ac, br
Dimetapp Elixir	12.5 mg/5 ml	comb, br, al
Naldecon DX, Children	9 mg/5 ml	comb, gu, dx, al
Naldecon EX, Pediatric	9 mg/1 ml	comb, gu, al
Naldecon DX, Pediatric	9 mg/1 ml	comb, gu, dx, al
Naldecon DX, Adult	18 mg/5 ml	comb, gu, dx
Naldecon CX, Adult	18 mg/5 ml	comb, gu, co
Naldecon EX, Children	9 mg/5 ml	comb, gu, al
Pyrroxate Capsules	25 mg	comb, ch, ac,
Robitussin-CF	12.5 mg/5 ml	comb, gu, dx, al
Sinarest Extra Strength	18.7 mg	comb, ac, ch
Sinarest Regular	18.7 mg	comb, ac, ch
Sine-Off Sinus Medication	12.5 mg	comb, as, ch
St. Joseph Cold Tablets	3.125 mg	comb, ac
Sucrets Cold Decongestant	25 mg	sing
Triaminic Chewables	6.25 mg	comb, ch
Triaminic Allergy Tablets	25 mg	comb, ch
Triaminic Cold Syrup	12.5 mg/5 ml	comb, ch
Triaminic Cold Tablets	12.5 mg	comb, ch
Triaminic Expectorant	12.5 mg/5 ml	comb, gu, al
Triaminic-12 Tablets	75 mg	comb, ch
Triaminic-DM Cough	12.5 mg/5 ml	comb, gu
Triaminic Tablets	25 mg	comb, ch, ac
Triaminicol Cold Syrup	12.5 mg/5 ml	comb, ch, dx
Triminicol Cold Tablets	12.5 mg	comb, ch, dx
Trind	12.5 mg/5 ml	comb, ch, al
Trind-DM	12.5 mg/5 ml	comb, ch, dm, al
Tussagesic Tablets	25 mg	comb, ph, py, dx, th, ac

ac = acetaminophen
al = alcohol
as = aspirin
br = brompheniramine
ch = chlorpheniramine
co = codeine
dx = dextromethorphan
gu = guaifenesin
ph = pheniramine
ps = pseudoephedrine
py = pyrilamine maleate
th = terpin hydrobromide
comb = combination
sing = single

not the drugs in the product. Therefore, the treating physician should contact the regional poison center for current product ingredients.

Phenylpropanolamine (PPA) is used clinically as a decongestant and an anorectic. On the street it may be sold illegally in "speed" look-alikes. The "speed" look-alikes often contain up to 50 mg of PPA, as well as ephedrine and caffeine. Some of the slang names for these drugs are "pink ladies," "black beauties," and "speckled pups."

Pharmacology

Phenylpropanolamine (D,L-norephedrine) is structurally similar to amphetamine and ephedrine.[3] PPA crosses the blood-brain barrier and therefore has central nervous system (CNS) activity.[3] Its CNS activity, however, is less than that of amphetamine. Unfortunately, the lower CNS activity often leads to overdose with PPA because the abuser does not experience the expected amphetamine high. Phenylpropanolamine is almost a pure alpha-agonist. It has some beta-agonist activity, but in overdose, the alpha-effects predominate.

In addition to direct stimulation of the alpha-receptors, PPA also causes the release of norepinephrine at the nerve terminals.[1–6] The half-life after a therapeutic dose is 3 to 4 hours. The major route of elimination (80 to 90 per cent) is via the kidney, and acidification of the urine can hasten elimination.

Phenylopropanolamine is a relatively safe drug when taken as directed. However, it has a low therapeutic index in that adverse symptoms can occur at doses two to three times normal.[7] The recommended daily dose is 75 to 150 mg.

Clinical Presentation

Hypertension is a common presenting problem seen in phenylpropanolamine overdose.[8–11] Hypertension is a result of increased cardiac output, increased peripheral vascular resistance, increased stroke volume, and increased ejection fraction.[10] Accompanying the increase in blood pressure is a decrease in heart rate.[10] Hypertensive crisis, manifested by severe headache and encephalopathy,[12] and intracerebral hemorrhage have been reported after PPA overdose.[8, 9]

Phenylpropanolamine overdose has caused cardiac arrhythmias.[8, 9, 11, 13] Bradycardia is the most common arrhythmia, but if PPA is combined with antihistamines or other sympathomimetics, tachycardia may occur.

Seizures have also been reported with PPA,[12] but there is some question whether the seizures were caused by PPA or by another ingredient in the combination drug. Anxiety, hallucinations, agitation, and psychotic behavior, often seen with amphetamine abuse, can occur with phenylpropanolamine overdose.[8, 9]

Muscle tremors, increased sweating, nausea and vomiting are also common presenting symptoms.

Treatment (Table 98–4)

Decontamination and removal of the drug are important steps in managing any drug overdose. However, in the treatment of a patient with severe hypertension, chest pain, or CNS changes, consideration should be given to lowering the blood pressure before inducing emesis or performing lavage, as both therapies may further increase intracranial pressure. Activated charcoal should be

Table 98–4. THERAPEUTIC DRUGS

	INDICATION	DOSE *(Adult)*	*(Child)*
phentolamine	hypertension	2.5–5 mg IV*	0.05–0.1 mg/kg*
	extravasation	5–10 mg in 10 ml saline locally	0.1–0.2 mg/kg locally
nitroprusside	hypertension	0.5–10 μg/kg/min†	0.5–10 μg/kg/min
propranolol	tachycardia	0.5–1.0 mg IV slow	10–20 μg/kg IV
labetalol	hypertension	20 mg IV q 10 min to max 30 mg	0.5 mg/kg IV 0.25 mg/kg q 2 hr
esmolol	tachycardia	50–200 μg/kg/min after 500 μg/kg/min bolus	unknown
diazepam	seizures	5–10 mg	0.1–0.3 mg/kg

*Dose can be repeated in 5 to 10 minutes to attain the desired effects.
†Titrate as needed.

administered as soon as possible to prevent further systemic absorption of the drug.

Hypertension should be treated on the basis of symptoms and not on absolute blood pressure. It is not uncommon for an adolescent with a PPA overdose to present with a blood pressure of 190/110. Although some elderly adults with long standing hypertension can tolerate that pressure, most adolescents have baseline pressures in the 100/60 range. Before treating the hypertension an intracerebral bleed has to be ruled out by a good physical examination. Lowering the blood pressure too much or too fast in the presence of an intracerebral bleed can increase brain destruction.

Initial therapy can begin with placing the patient in an upright position to maximize orthostatic effects. Phentolamine, a short acting alpha antagonist, will lower the blood pressure by direct alpha receptor blockade. In an overdose the duration of PPA toxicity may last longer than the duration of the effects of phentolamine. Therefore, frequent blood pressure monitoring is needed to determine the need for repeat doses of phentolamine. Sodium nitroprusside or other vasodilators also may be used to lower blood pressure rapidly.

Tachycardia is rare, but if it compromises cardiac function, propranolol or another beta-blocker can be used.[10] However, a beta-blocker should not be used without also administering an alpha-blocker. Blocking the beta-receptors in the periphery may cause unopposed alpha-vasoconstriction, leading to a further increase in blood pressure. Bradycardia should not be treated unless the patient is hypotensive. Bradycardia is normally a physiologic reflex to the hypertensive state. For the same reason treatment with an anticholinergic like atropine may also worsen hypertension.

Although acidification of the urine will enhance the clearance of phenylpropanolamine, this therapy is rarely warranted. PPA excretion is rapid and toxicity often lasts less than 6 hours. In PPA overdoses, increased muscular activity is often seen. The increased muscular activity or vasoconstriction or both that accompany PPA overdose may cause myoglobinemia. Acidification of the urine may cause precipitation of myoglobin in the kidney and acute renal failure. Furthermore, specific antagonists available to treat PPA toxicity avoid the risks of urine acidification and probably outweigh the benefits of this formerly recommended practice.

Should seizures occur, diazepam is an appropriate treatment, although barbiturates are also effective. The occurrence of seizures should increase the index of suspicion of a cerebral bleed. If computed tomography (CT) of the head cannot be performed, the blood pressure should be lowered slowly and carefully.

Pre-existing medical conditions that increase toxicity and complicate treatment include coronary artery disease, hypertension, arrhythmias, glaucoma, hyperthyroidism, prostatic hypertrophy, and concurrent beta-blocker therapy. Such patients require close observation, and symptoms should be treated accordingly.

Phenylephrine

Phenylephrine is used as a nasal decongestant and as a topical ophthalmic mydriatic in 2.5 and 10 per cent solutions. Phenylephrine is primarily an alpha-agonist, with very few beta-effects. Cardiovascular reactions have been reported after the use of topical phenylephrine in infants, in geriatric patients, and in patients with underlying cardiovascular disease or hypertension.[14, 15] Myocardial infarction[15] and subarachnoid hemorrhage secondary to hypertension[16] have been reported as adverse effects of topical phenylephrine.

The duration of action of phenylephrine is short, on the order of 30 to 60 minutes. However, in some cases toxicity can persist; if necessary, therapy should follow the guidelines for phenylpropanolamine.

Ephedrine and Pseudoephedrine

Ephedrine and its optical isomer pseudoephedrine are also common over-the-counter medications. Their major use is in oral preparations as nasal decongestants. Ephedrine also has $beta_2$-effects and can produce bronchodilation. It is combined with theophylline in some preparations because of this effect. Unfortunately, this combination has been shown to potentiate the toxic effects of theophylline without improving the therapeutic response.

Pharmacology

Both ephedrine and pseudoephedrine have alpha- and beta-adrenergic agonist effects. The pharmacologic effects of these drugs result from direct stimulation of the adrenergic receptors and the release of norepinephrine. The serum half-life of ephedrine depends on urine pH.[17] At a urine pH of 5.6, the half-life is 1.9 hours, whereas at a pH of 7.4, it is 21 hours.

Clinical Presentation

Typical findings in overdose are diaphoresis, hypertension, headache, ventricular ectopy, tachycardia, agitation, psychosis, and seizures.[8, 18] Intracerebral hemorrhage, presumably due to a direct cerebral vascular effect has also been reported.[19]

Treatment (See Table 98–4)

The majority of overdoses with these medications are mild, and no therapy except decontamination and activated charcoal is necessary. Acidification of the urine will enhance elimination of the drug, but the risk of this procedure probably exceeds any potential benefit.

Hypertension and tachycardia can be treated with the combined alpha- and beta-antagonist.[20] As with phenylpropanolamine, the use of a beta-blocker alone can lead to unopposed alpha-effects and worsening hypertension. Blood pressure should be monitored carefully. Combination therapy with phentolamine and a beta-blocker like propranolol also can be used.

Agitation and psychosis should be treated with reassurance and, if necessary, benzodiazepine. The antipsychotic agents should be avoided, as they can complicate the cardiovascular toxicity by producing anticholinergic effects.

Epinephrine

Epinephrine, a natural catecholamine, has many therapeutic uses. Asthma, anaphylaxis, cardiac arrest, hemostasis, nasal decongestion, and glaucoma are some examples of the variety of conditions treated with epinephrine preparations.

Pharmacology

Epinephrine is a potent stimulator of both alpha- and beta-adrenergic receptors. The duration of action for epinephrine is relatively short. It is metabolized in the blood by the catechol-*O*-methyl transferase (COMT) and monoamine oxidase (MAO) systems.

Clinical Presentation

Adverse effects and symptoms of overdose have been seen after conventional doses.[21] Most problems occur after the inadvertent intravenous administration of concentrations intended for subcutaneous delivery. In general, epinephrine should not be administered intravenously to anyone who has a normal blood pressure.

After administration of epinephrine, vasoconstriction of the vascular beds in the skin, mucosa, and kidney causes a rapid, dose-dependent rise in blood pressure. A large increase in blood pressure may lead to a reflex bradycardia. However, beta-agonist activity usually produces an increase in heart rate and force of contraction. The resulting rapid rise in blood pressure may produce headache, encephalopathy, and cerebral hemorrhage.

Myocardial infarction can occur secondary to the increased cardiac work and oxygen consumption. Infarction is not a result of coronary artery constriction. Epinephrine actually dilates coronary arteries.[22]

Epinephrine can also produce cardiac arrhythmias.[23] The arrhythmias probably result from a combination of factors. The increased oxygen demand creates an ischemic myocardial state. There is direct myocardial irritation due to stimulation of the beta-receptors. Further, epinephrine administration produces a hypokalemia secondary to stimulation of the $beta_2$-receptor.[24]

Diaphoresis and mydriasis also occur in overdose.

Treatment (See Table 98–4)

Because the duration of action for epinephrine is short (20 to 30 minutes), treatment may not be necessary. A combination of an alpha- and beta-blocker, such as labetalol or phentolamine plus propranolol, can be used. Nitrites or sodium nitroprusside also can be used for hypertension. Arrhythmias can be treated with a beta-blocker, but a beta-blocker should not be used alone because unopposed alpha-stimulation may worsen hypertension. If epinephrine has extravasated into the local subcutaneous tissues or has been injected inadvertently into a digit, phentolamine should be infused into the area to relieve vasoconstriction and prevent ischemia and necrosis.

Norepinephrine

Norepinephrine is a naturally occurring catecholamine neurotransmitter that has a limited clinical use except for the treatment of severe hypotension.

Norepinephrine stimulates alpha- and beta$_1$-receptors, but, when compared with epinephrine, it has very few beta$_2$-effects.

The pharmacologic effects of norepinephrine include hypertension with reflex bradycardia or tachycardia, depending on the dose. Adverse effects include headache, mydriasis, diaphoresis, and arrhythmias.

Treatment (See Table 98–4)

Because the duration is short, stopping a norepinephrine infusion is the major treatment modality. In the case of inadvertent administration or overdose, a combination of alpha- and beta-antagonists, as in the treatment for epinephrine, can be used.

Subcutaneous extravasation from an infiltrated intravenous line is a common complication of norepinephrine therapy. If extravasation occurs, prompt treatment with local infiltration of phentolamine can correct local ischemia and prevent tissue loss. However, if it is absorbed, phentolamine can block the therapeutic effect of norepinephrine.

Imidazolines

The imidazolines have alpha-adrenergic stimulation properties.[25] Clonidine, rilmenidine and guanabenz are alpha$_2$-agonists that act centrally to decrease the sympathetic output from the brain. As such, they are used to treat hypertension. Because they act as sympatholytic agents, they will not be discussed in this chapter. Clonidine was initially developed for use as a nasal decongestant. Other imidazolines are used clinically for their ability to produce local vasoconstriction when topically applied and are categorized as sympathomimetics.

Oxymetazoline, Xylometazoline, Tetrahydrozoline, Naphazoline

The imidazoline derivatives oxymetazoline, xylometazoline, tetrahydrozoline and naphazoline are common ingredients in topical ophthalmic and nasal decongestant products. Many formulations are available for over-the-counter purchase. Abuse and overuse of these produces is common. They are generally used as topical vasoconstrictors in the nose and eye, but systemic absorption and adverse effects can occur.

The clinical effects and consequently the adverse effects are mediated through stimulation of the alpha$_2$-receptors. As a group, the imidazolines are potent vasoconstrictors. However, like their antihypertensive cousins, they can have central effects. Psychosis and hallucinosis has occurred with chronic nasal use.[26] Central stimulation of alpha$_2$-receptors increases vagal tone and may cause bradycardia. Glazener and colleagues reported a case of a patient who was about to undergo a pacemaker placement because of syncope secondary to bradycardia and hypotension. Surgery was cancelled when it was noted that she frequently used an oxymetazoline-containing nasal spray. When the nasal spray was discontinued, the bradycardia resolved.[27] In children, oxymetazoline can cause sedation, seizure, agitation, insomnia, and hallucinations.[28]

Retinal artery occlusion has been reported after topical ophthalmic use. The occlusion was thought to be secondary to alpha-receptor–stimulated increase in platelet aggregation.[29] Constriction of uterine vessels and decreased perfusion led to uteroplacental insufficiency in a near term woman using nasal spray.[30]

These agents are sometimes used as fillers in illicit cocaine. Nine cases of intravenous injection of what was supposed to be cocaine but was actually 97 per cent naphazoline was reported by van Montfrans and associates.[31] After intravenous injection, diaphoresis, nausea, drowsiness, headache, syncope, and seizures occurred. In addition, a sinus bradycardia with normal blood pressure was present. One of the patients was treated with atropine because of bradycardia and ectopic beats. She subsequently had an abnormal rise in blood pressure and an intracerebral hemorrhage.

Treatment (See Table 98–4). Generally, all that is necessary is observation for mildly symptomatic cases. Intravenous phentolamine is effective treatment for the adverse alpha-effects of the drug. Seizures should be treated with diazepam.

Beta-Agonists

The beta-adrenergic receptor stimulators are primarily used clinically for the treatment of bronchospasm. Isoproterenol has the added therapeutic role of increasing heart rate in symptomatic bradycardia unresponsive to atropine.

Isoproterenol

Isoproterenol stimulates $beta_1$- and $beta_2$-receptors but has almost no alpha-agonistic effects. It has been used as a bronchodilator, but it is no longer the drug of choice since more selective $beta_2$-agonists are available.

Headache, flushing of skin, cardiac arrhythmias, and myocardial ischemia from increased oxygen demand are some of the major untoward effects of isoproterenol use. Peripheral vasodilation and hypotension can also occur secondary to the stimulation of $beta_2$-receptors.

Treatment (See Table 98–4)

Treatment of the adverse effects begins with stopping drug infusion. Blood pressure initially should be supported with fluids and position. Arrhythmias can be treated with a beta-blocker, and the nonselective antagonist propranolol is the most logical treatment. In asthmatic patients, in whom the blockage of the $beta_2$-receptor may not be advantageous, the short-acting, $beta_1$-selective antagonist esmolol may be indicated.

$Beta_2$-Agonists

The selective $beta_2$-agonists are used in the therapy of bronchospasm. They can be administered via inhalation, by mouth, or subcutaneously. Drug toxicity is reduced when they are administered via inhalation. The amount of drug in an entire albuterol inhaler canister is only slightly more than the 24-hour oral dose of the drug.[32]

Metaproterenol actually stimulates both $beta_1$- and $beta_2$-receptors. However, when inhaled, the $beta_1$-effects are minimized.

Terbutaline is also relatively selective in stimulating the $beta_2$-receptor. However, when given parenterally, it loses its selectivity. A reflex tachycardia can occur from $beta_2$-induced vasodilatation. Skeletal muscle tremors are also more frequent after oral or subcutaneous administration.

Albuterol has relatively selective $beta_2$-stimulation. A fine tremor, hypotension, and reflex tachycardia are side effects of albuterol.

These compounds are relatively nontoxic. A review of albuterol overdoses with up to 20 times the oral daily dose revealed no deaths.[33] In overdose tremor, hypotension and tachycardia can occur. Arrhythmias caused by the beta-stimulation of the heart or the $beta_2$-induced hypokalemia may also be seen.[34]

A case is reported of myocardial infarction that occurred after the intravenous infusion of albuterol.[35] The patient became hypotensive, and an ECG showed ST segment depression and multiple ventricular premature beats. Symptoms resolved in 30 minutes; however, significant cardiac enzymes elevation was noted.

A 7 year old girl had seizures from a dose of terbutaline that was three times normal.[36] She responded to treatment with diazepam.

Intravenous fluids are usually adequate for the treatment of hypotension caused by these drugs. Tachycardia, if compromising cardiac function, can be treated with propranolol or esmolol.

SUMMARY

Overdoses with the sympathomimetic preparations are not uncommon. Treatment requires a good understanding of autonomic physiology as well as autonomic pharmacology.

Many of the drugs listed in this chapter are used in combination with other drugs. These other drugs may have their own toxicity and symptomatology. For instance, antihistamines are commonly combined with the decongestants phenylpropanolamine, ephedrine, and pseudoephedrine. The antihistamines have anticholinergic effects and can alter the expected symptoms.

Decontamination is usually the appropriate initial therapy. However, lavage can cause vagal stimulation or increased intracranial pressure. In some cases, specific therapies are needed first.

In general, vital signs should be supported. However, abnormal vital signs do not always need to be treated. Treatment of bradycardia in the hypertensive patient may just make the symptoms worse.

Finally, the underlying medical conditions of the patient should be considered. Consultation with the local poison center and a toxicologist is often necessary for appropriate treatment.

References

1. Olsen KR, Pentel PR, Kelley MT: Physical assessment and differential diagnosis of the poisoned patient. Med Toxicol 2:52–81, 1987.
2. Benowitz NL, Goldschlager N: Cardiac disturbances in the toxicologic patient. *In* Haddad LM, Winchester JF (eds): Clinical Management of Poisoning and Drug Overdose. Philadelphia, WB Saunders, 1983, pp 65–98.
3. Bravo EL: Phenylpropanolamine and other over-the-counter vasoactive compounds. Hypertension *11* (Suppl II):II7–II10, 1988.
4. Nickerson M, Nomagochi G: Response to sympathomimetic amines after Dibenamine blockade. J Pharmacol Exp Ther *107*:284–299, 1953.
5. Greiner TH, Garb S: The influence of drugs on the irritability and automaticity of heart muscle. J Pharmacol Exp Ther *98*:215–233, 1950.
6. Trendelenberg U, de La Sierra BGA, Muskus R: Modification by reserpine of the response of the atrial pacemaker to sympathomimetic amines. J Pharmacol Exp Ther *141*:301–309, 1963.
7. Horowitz JD, Land WJ, Howes LG: Hypertensive response induced by phenylpropanolamine in anorectic and decongestant preparations. Lancet *1*:60–61, 1980.
8. Pentel P: Toxicity of over-the-counter stimulants. JAMA *252*:1898–1903, 1984.
9. Berstein E, Diskant BM: Phenylpropanolamine: A potentially hazardous drug. Ann Emerg Med *11*:311–315, 1982.
10. Pentel PR, Asinger RW, Benowitz NL: Propranolol antagonism of phenylpropanolamine-induced hypertension. Clin Pharmacol Ther *37*:488–494, 1985.
11. Pentel PR, Mikell FL, Zavoral JH: Myocardial injury after phenylpropanolamine ingestion. Br Heart J *47*:51–54, 1982.
12. Mueller SM, Solow EB: Seizures associated with a new combination "pick-me-up" pill. Ann Neurol *11*:322, 1982.
13. Mecklenburg RS, Benson EA, Benson JW, et al: Atrioventricular conduction block caused by phenylpropanolamine. JAMA *253*:2646–2647, 1985.
14. Fraunfelder FT, Meyer SM: Possible cardiovascular effects secondary to topical ophthalmic 2.5% phenylephrine. Am J Ophthalmol *99*:362, 1985.
15. Fraunfelder FT, Meyer SM: Possible adverse effects from topical ocular 10% phenylephrine. Am J Ophthalmol *85*:447–453, 1978.
16. Solosko D, Smith RB: Hypertension following ophthalmic 10% phenylephrine. Anesthesiology *36*:187–189, 1972.
17. Brater DC, Kaojarern S, Benet LZ, et al: Renal excretion of pseudoephedrine. Clin Pharmacol Ther *28*:690–694, 1980.
18. Hughes DTD, Empey DW, Land M: Effects of pseudoephedrine in man. J Clin Hosp Pharm *8*:315–321, 1983.
19. Loizou LA, Hamilton JG, Tsementzis SA: Intracranial hemorrhage in association with pseudoephedrine overdose. J Neuro Neurosurg Psychiatr *45*:471, 1982.
20. Mariani PJ: Pseudoephedrine-induced hypertensive emergency: Treatment with labetalol. Am J Emerg Med *4*:141–142, 1986.
21. Barach EM, Nowak RM, Lee TG, Tomlanovich MC: Epinephrine for treatment of anaphylactic shock. JAMA *251*:2118–2122, 1984.
22. Weiner N: Norepinephrine, epinephrine, and the sympathomimetic amines. *In* Gilman AG, Goodman LS, Rall TW, Murad F (eds): The Pharmacological Basis of Therapeutics. New York, Macmillan, 1985, pp 145–180.
23. Sullivan TJ: Cardiac disorders in penicillin-induced anaphylaxis: Association with intravenous epinephrine therapy. JAMA *248*:2161, 1982.
24. Brown MJ: Hypokalemia from $beta_2$-receptor stimulation by circulating epinephrine. Am J Cardiol *56*:3D–9D, 1985.
25. Timmermans PB, deJonge A, von Zwieten PA: Comparative quantitative studies on central and peripheral alpha-adrenoceptors. Chest *83*:354–357, 1983.
26. Eschobar J, Karno M: Chronic hallucinosis from nasal drops. JAMA *247*:1859–1860, 1982.
27. Glazener F, Blake K, Gradman M: Bradycardia, hypotension, and near-syncope associated with afrin (oxymetazoline) nasal spray. N Engl J Med *309*:731, 1983.
28. Soderman P, Sahlberg D, Wiholm BE: CNS reactions to nose drops in small children. Lancet 1:573, 1984.
29. Margargal LE, Sanborn GE, Donoso LA, Gonder JR: Branch retinal artery occlusion after excessive use of nasal spray. Ann Ophthalmol *17*:500–501, 1985.
30. Baxi LV, Gindoff PR, Pregenzer GJ, Parras MK: Fetal heart rate changes following maternal administration of a nasal decongestant. Am J Obstet Gynecol *153*:799–800, 1985.
31. van Montfrans GA, van Steenwijk RP, Vyth A, Borst C: Intravenous naphazoline intoxication. Acta Med Scand *209*:429–430, 1981.
32. Spangler DL: Review of side effects associated with beta agonists. Ann Allergy *62*:59–62, 1989.
33. Prior JG, Cochrane GM, Raper SM, Christine A, Volans GN: Self-poisoning with oral salbutamol. Br Med J *282*:1932, 1981.
34. Higgins RM, Cookson WO, Lane DJ, John SM, McCarthy GL, McCarthy ST: Cardiac arrhythmias caused by nebulized beta-agonist therapy. Lancet *2*:863–864, 1987.
35. Santo M, Sidi Y, Pinkhas Y: Acute myocardial infarction following intravenous salbutamol. S Afr Med J *58*:394, 1980.
36. Freidman R, Zitelli B, Jardine D, Fireman P: Seizures in a patient receiving terbutaline. Am J Dis Child *136*:1091–1092, 1982.

CHAPTER 99
ERGOT

Donald B. Kunkel, M.D.
David S. Jallo, R.Ph.

It is not precisely known when human beings first suffered the diverse, debilitating (and often fatal) effects of ergotism. Allusions to a "noxious pustule in the ear of grain" appeared in an Assyrian tablet, ca. 600 BC. Later pre-Christian writings seem to indicate that the ancients, at least on occasion, associated infested grain with illness and abortion. Not until the ninth century A.D. was the first Western reference to ergotism made. An epidemic of ergotism was described wherein "a great plague of swollen blisters consumed the people by a loathsome rot so that their limbs were loosened and fell off before death."[1] Convulsive ergotism and mixed convulsive/gangrenous presentations were recorded in the literature of the eleventh century, but it is not clear that earlier associations with "noxious pustules" in grain were appreciated in the Middle Ages. The opposite is probably true, as cures were achieved by pilgrimages to the shrine of St. Anthony, where an incidental change of diet literally "cured the patient." Thus the naming of the disease "holy fire" or St. Anthony's fire.

Epidemics of ergotism have continued into the twentieth century despite the recognition of a causal connection between the ingestion of "ergot of rye" and clinical disorders in 1676. Outbreaks were reported in Russia (1926), in Ireland (1929), in 1951 in France and India; and as late as 1977–1978 in Ethiopia. No human epidemics due to ingestion of contaminated grain have been reported recently, although future human exposure remains a concern and livestock poisoning is an ongoing reality.[2]

Ergotism continues as a subject of medical concern as a result of therapeutic applications of ergot compounds, especially the various natural and semisynthetic alkaloids. Historically, ergot was used as a medicinal by midwives in antiquity in China. As early as 1582, ergot was recognized as being able to promote uterine contractions. The use of ergot in obstetrics quickly spread in the United States following published reports in the early nineteenth century, but limitations on its safe use were quickly realized. In the nineteenth century, reports on the use of ergot in migraine headache appeared. The isolation of an active principle from ergot in 1906 (ergotoxine, actually a mixture of alkaloids), followed by the isolation of ergotamine in 1920, signaled the beginning of modern pharmaceutical applications of specific ergot alkaloids.

Botany

The term "ergot" is generally used to describe species of the fungal genus *Claviceps,* the sclerotia formed by the fungi (specifically *Claviceps purpurea*), and the wide range of unique alkaloids produced by the fungi following infestation of grain.

Three species of *Claviceps (C. purpurea, C. paspali,* and *C. cinerea)* have been known to parasitize the grains of various cultivated and wild grasses in the United States, with resultant animal disease.[3] On a historical basis, however, *Claviceps purpurea* infection of rye grain has been closely associated with human illness worldwide, and the sclerotium of this fungal species has become the source of many pharmacologically active principles.

Infection of grain takes place at the time of flowering of the grass. A parasitic spore of *Claviceps* germinates within the ovary of the grass and penetrating hyphae form a dense mass of tissue (mycelium), which supplants the ovary. This mass gradually hardens into a dark purplish resting body known as a sclerotium. The small club-shaped (hence the name *Claviceps*) sclerotium may superficially resemble the host grain and may be processed and consumed with the grain itself. Strict controls over maximal concentrations of sclerotia in grain exist today, greatly accounting for the reduced incidence of natural ergotism.

Sclerotia of *Claviceps purpurea* contain, in addition to certain pharmacologically active alkaloids to be discussed, alkaloids of unproved pharmacologic use. Also isolated, among other diverse chemicals, have been such compounds as tyramine, tyrosine, tryptophan, histamine, histidine, choline, acetylcholine, and ergosterol.[4]

Chemistry

The ergot alkaloids are derivatives of the tetracyclic compound 6-methylergoline. The ergoline aspect of the chemical structure, present in all ergot alkaloids, bears a structural relationship to the biogenic amines epinephrine, norepinephrine, dopamine, and serotonin. This similarity may account for the various receptor site activities of the ergot alkaloids.[5]

The ergot alkaloids that are of therapeutic interest belong to two main chemical categories: the amine alkaloids and the amino acid alkaloids, or ergopeptides (Table 94–1). Natural ergot alkaloids include ergonovine and ergotamine. Clinically important derivatives of the amine alkaloids include lysergic acid diethylamide (LSD), methylergonovine, and methysergide. Several useful derivatives of the ergopeptide group also have been synthesized. Hydrogenation of ergotamine yields dihydroergotamine. The hydrogenated derivatives of the ergotoxine group are dihydroergocornine, dihydroergocristine, and alpha- and beta-dihydroergokryptine, which are the active ingredients in Hydergine. The hydrogenated derivatives are generally less toxic than the natural alkaloids.

Lergotrile, lisuride, and methergoline are preparations that are related to the ergot alkaloids, yet differ in that they are not derivatives of lysergic acid. These drugs have been studied in the treatment of parkinsonism because of their strong dopaminergic actions.

Pharmacology

The pharmacologic activities of the ergot alkaloids and their semisynthetic derivatives are extremely varied and complex. They have been used therapeutically in obstetrics, endocrinology, migraine and other vascular headaches, venostasis, senile cerebral insufficiency, and in Parkinson's disease. "There simply is no such single entity as ergot from the pharmacologic, toxicologic, biologic, or clinical point of view."[6] This complexity of effects may be explained by the ability of the ergot alkaloids to interfere with more than one type of specific receptor site. The different ergot compounds may interact with tryptaminergic, dopaminergic and alpha-adrenergic receptors. In addition, the intrinsic activities of each alkaloid vary at the receptor site, resulting in a broad range of effects. Thinking simply of vasoconstriction and uterine contractions when considering the pharmacology of the ergot alkaloids does not accurately reflect the spectrum of pharmacologic activities of these drugs, which includes alpha-adrenergic receptor interference (both agonist and antagonist), pressor effects, uterotonic action, emetic activity, dopaminergic effects, serotonin receptor activity (agonist and antagonist), and hyper- or hypothermia. It is essential to have an understanding of the intrinsic activity and receptor specificity of each ergot alkaloid in order to accurately assess its clinical and toxicologic effects.

Ergotamine and Dihydroergotamine. The

Table 99–1. CLINICALLY SIGNIFICANT ERGOT ALKALOIDS AND THEIR DERIVATIVES

AMINE ALKALOIDS	ERGOPEPTIDES
ergonovine Ergonovine Maleate (Wyeth, Purepac) Ergotrate (Lilly)	ergotamine Bellergal (Dorsey) Cafergot (Sandoz) Ergostat (Parke-Davis) Ergomar (Fisons) Wigraine (Organon)
methylergonovine Methergine (Sandoz)	dihydroergotamine D.H.E. 45 (Sandoz)
methysergide Sansert (Sandoz)	dihydrogenated ergot alkaloids (ergoloid mesylates) Hydergine (Sandoz)
lysergic acid diethylamide (LSD)	bromocriptine Parlodel (Sandoz)
lisuride	
lergotrile	
methergoline	

Table 99–2. PHARMACOLOGIC ACTIVITY OF ERGOT ALKALOIDS

	ERGOTAMINE	DIHYDRO-ERGOTAMINE	METHYL-ERGONOVINE	BROMO-CRIPTINE	METHY-SERGIDE	DIHYDRO-ERGOTOXINE
Pressor activity	1000	120	<10	<10	30	30
Alpha-adrenergic blockade	50	350	<0.4	230	<0.4	1000
Emetic activity	1000	85	210	410	<1	540
Serotonin-blocking activity	10	40	250	3	1000	10
Uterotonic activity	500	Inhibition of Me-ergonovine	1000	Inhibition of Me-ergonovine	40	Inhibition of Me-ergonovine

Based on an arbitrary potency of 1000 for the most active compound. (Adapted from Berde B, Sturmer E: Ergot alkaloids and related compounds. *In* Berde B, Schild HO (eds): Handbook of Experimental Pharmacology. Vol 49. Berlin, Springer-Verlag, 1978, p 4.)

"classic" natural ergot alkaloid is ergotamine, which causes many of the symptoms found in St. Anthony's fire. Its hydrogenated derivative, dihydroergotamine, shares many of ergotamine's pharmacologic properties, differing mainly in its degree of activity (Table 94–2).

Ergotamine possesses the most potent vasoconstrictor activity of the ergot alkaloids, producing constriction of both veins and arteries. This vasoconstriction is probably due mainly to mediation by alpha-adrenergic receptors, tryptaminergic receptors, or both.[7, 8] These alkaloids also may inhibit receptor reuptake of norepinephrine at sympathetic nerve endings, which increases the vasoconstrictive action. Dihydroergotamine has comparatively less vasoconstrictive action than ergotamine; however, its constrictive ability may be appreciable, especially in capacitance vessels, which is the rationale behind using dihydroergotamine in orthostatic hypotension. Ergotamine and dihydroergotamine may cause bradycardia as a result of their effects of increasing vagal activity, possibly decreasing sympathetic tone, and causing direct myocardial depression.[9]

Ergotamine has a potent emetic effect through stimulation of the chemoreceptor trigger zone and may cause nausea and vomiting, which is a common finding upon acute overdose. Dihydroergotamine is 12 times less active in emetic potential than is ergotamine. Ergotamine has the most potent uterotonic effect of the amino acid alkaloids; however, it has only about half the activity of ergonovine. Dihydroergotamine has much less oxytocic effect than does ergotamine.

The amino acid alkaloids, including ergotamine and dihydroergotamine, are incompletely and irregularly absorbed. Peak blood levels are reached about 2 hours after oral administration. Caffeine slightly increases the water solubility of ergotamine, which increases its dissolution rate and rate of absorption. Caffeine is a common ingredient in combination products with ergotamine and can add its own toxic effects with overdoses of these combinations. Ergotamine and dihydroergotamine are both extensively metabolized in the liver, and reduction in liver function may lead to accumulation. Ergotamine may sequester in various tissues, which probably accounts for its long-lasting effects despite a short plasma half-life of about 2 hours.

Dihydroergotoxine Mesylate. The dihydroergotoxine mesylate salts have been used therapeutically for the treatment of selected symptoms in elderly patients, including mood depression, confusion, unsociability, and dizziness. In contrast to ergotamine, dihydroergotoxine has little or no vasoconstrictor activity. Indeed, it usually causes peripheral vasodilation, due primarily to central nervous system depression of vasomotor nerve activity and its potent alpha-adrenergic receptor blocking action. This usually results in a slight decrease in blood pressure and heart rate. Dihydroergotoxine has a fairly strong emetic potential, about half that of ergotamine. Dihydroergotoxine has no oxytocic activity but will actually block the effects of methylergonovine on the uterus, owing to its strong alpha-adrenergic blocking activity.

Bromocriptine. Bromocriptine is an ergopeptide derivative that possesses strong dopaminergic activity, making it useful in the treatment of parkinsonism and in the suppression of prolactin secretion. It does not have hormonal or estrogenic effects. Like other drugs with strong dopamine agonist activity, bromocriptine may cause hypotension. Bromocriptine has a moderate emetic effect, and nausea and vomiting can cause discontinuation of the drug in a small percentage of patients. Like dihydroergotoxine, bromocriptine has no uterotonic effects but will antagonize the oxytocic effects of methylergonovine. Bromocriptine is rapidly and completely absorbed, peak blood levels occurring within 2 to 3 hours after oral administration. Bromocriptine is extensively metabolized, with excretion of the metabolites mainly through the bile.

Lysergic Acid Diethylamide (LSD). In the amine alkaloid group, lysergic acid diethylamide (LSD) is well known for its extremely potent psychedelic effects. LSD is discussed in Chapter 42.

Ergonovine. Ergonovine presently has a major clinical use in assessment of coronary artery spasm during cardiac catheterization. It is a natural ergot that has very potent uterotonic actions. In smaller doses, ergonovine increases the frequency of amplitude of uterine contractions. Larger doses also elevate the basic tone, which makes ergonovine useful in decreasing blood loss from the postpartum uterus. The sensitivity of the uterus to ergot varies, but even the immature uterus may be stimulated. This uterine-stimulating activity seems to be mediated through stimulation of alpha-adrenergic receptors in the uterus, and may be blocked by alpha-blocking agents such as phenoxybenzamine.

Ergonovine has mild emetic properties, being about one fifth as potent as ergotamine. Its vasoconstrictor effects are less than those of ergotamine; however, ergonovine may cause an increase in blood pressure in oxytocic doses and should be used with caution. Outside the United States, ergonovine is recognized by its British name of ergometrine.

Methylergonovine shares many of the pharmacologic properties of its parent drug, ergonovine. Methylergonovine has a more powerful and prolonged effect on the uterus than does ergonovine. Methylergonovine causes less vasoconstriction and is less likely to precipitate hypertension than is ergonovine.

Methysergide. Methysergide is a very potent 5HT (serotonin)-antagonist, which makes it useful in the therapy of vascular headache. While methysergide is a competitive antagonist of serotonin peripherally, it may act as a serotonin agonist in the central nervous system, especially in the brain stem. The antiserotonin effects of methysergide include inhibition of serotonin-induced vasoconstriction and inflammation. This alkaloid also inhibits the release of histamine from mast cells.

Methysergide has very weak uterotonic and emetic actions. In addition, it has very weak vasoconstrictor ability. Unlike LSD, methysergide has comparatively little effect on the nervous system in usual doses, although central nervous system effects have been reported.

Toxicity

Ergotism is the term used to describe a patient who clinically presents with ergot toxicity. Historically, ergotism has been divided into "gangrenous" and "convulsive" forms. In epidemics, one form or the other seems to predominate, although mixed presentations in a single epidemic may occur. It is unclear whether variables in toxic contents of sclerotia, dose effects, or population susceptibilities are considerations.

With the advent of pharmacologic utilization of specific alkaloids, toxic syndromes have been clarified somewhat, although acute toxicity is poorly documented as compared with more commonly reported subacute or chronic peripheral vascular spasm.

Acute toxicity may be precipitated by attempts at abortion, may be associated with obstetric complications, or may occur with suicide attempts or childhood accidents. Pediatric-age exposures are especially worthy of note because of high mortality rates associated with perinatal accidents[10] and toddler ingestions.[11] Administration of ergot alkaloids to individuals with sepsis, hepatic damage, vascular disease, renal disease, or toxemia may cause acute effects, either as a result of underlying disease states or impaired ability to metabolize the drug.

Chronic toxicity is commonly the result of therapeutic misadventures involving ergotamine tartrate. Typically, the patient will experience increased headaches and will increase the frequency of dosing the drug. It is of interest that ergotamine itself may cause headache. Also, discontinuance of the drug may precipitate a withdrawal state with more severe headache, necessitating resumption of ergotamine at possibly higher levels by the patient. Frequently, the patient may be taking ergot alkaloids for tension headache, utilizing a rather continuous pattern of dosing, as opposed to the intermittent drug-dosing pattern of migraine. Smokers may be at increased risk of vascular injury occasioned by ergot use.

Clinical Presentation

Symptoms of *acute intoxication* include nausea, vomiting, diarrhea, severe thirst, tingling of the skin (formication), evidence of skin hypoperfusion, chest pain, bradycardia or tachycardia, hypotension or hypertension, confusion, convulsions, or coma. Fatal doses are difficult to determine; however, deaths following cardiac arrest have been reported after small doses of ergonovine during evaluations for variant angina pectoris.[12]

Vascular complications are usually evident in *chronic exposures*. Presentations are highly variable, based upon the vascular structures most affected. Most generally, the legs are involved, and this may be unilateral. A pulseless, cold, pale, or cyanotic extremity may be present, and the patient may complain of burning pain and numbness. Demarcated ischemia may be observed in advanced cases. Arteriography usually reveals marked diffuse spasm of major arteries, with poor visualization of the distal vasculature. Collateral vessels are usually prominent. Evidence of clot formation may be present but is not a usual finding. The upper extremities may be similarly involved. Unusual presentations have included acute myocardial infarction, sudden blindness, bilateral foot drop, ischemic bowel disease, and renal failure, all the result of vascular impairment. Alopecia and retroperitoneal/pleural fibrosis have been reported, the latter associated with methysergide administration. Residual sensory loss and/or paresthesias may persist following acute intoxication.

Ergot alkaloids have been reported to cause a wide variety of central nervous system effects, including nausea, vomiting, headache, fatigue, insomnia, restlessness, excitement, delirium, dementia, seizures, and respiratory depression. Hallucinogenic effects have, of course, been well documented for LSD (see Chapter 34) but have also been demonstrated for ergonovine, methylergonovine, methysergide, and bromocriptine.

Treatment

Acute ingestions of ergot-containing preparations would best be approached with vigorous gut decontamination efforts, especially in children, with emesis or gastric lavage followed by administration of activated charcoal and a cathartic. Supportive measures, including nitroglycerin administration for coronary vasospasm, may be necessary. Effective removal of ergot alkaloids by use of extracorporeal techniques (hemodialysis and hemoperfusion) is probably impossible because of minute blood levels and significant tissue distribution. It is conceivable that peripheral vasospasm may be severe enough to warrant consideration of the use of vasodilators and anticoagulants (to be discussed). Other drug components in formulations with the ergot alkaloids will warrant separate considerations in cases of acute ingestions.

In situations of *chronic* exposure with vasospasm, withdrawal of the drug will effect a reversal of toxicity in the great majority of cases. In situations of severe arterial vasospasm, various intra-arterial vasodilators have been used (with mixed results), including tolazoline, ethanol, niacin, and papaverine. Intravenous heparin and low molecular weight dextran have been recommended in order to minimize thrombosis caused by stasis and endothelial damage. Sympathetic blockade is controversial because of the direct action of ergot on smooth muscle receptors.[13]

More recently, intravenous nitroglycerin has been used with success for the treatment of ergotamine-induced vasospasm.[14] Intravenous or intra-arterial nitroprusside seems to be the present drug of choice for reversal of severe spasm, due to its direct action on smooth muscle and its rapid onset and cessation of action.[15] Prazosin has more recently been recommended because of its close similarity in pharmacologic action to nitroprusside.[16] It has the advantage of oral administration, thus making it suitable for use in cases of lesser severity, or conceivably, in cases in which inaccessible peripheral veins preclude intravenous therapy. Verapamil recently has been used to reduce coronary artery spasm previously provoked by ergonovine testing,[17] but no therapeutic application of verapamil in ergot alkaloid toxicity is noted as yet. Nifedipine has been used clinically in ergotamine tartrate–induced peripheral vascular spasm and may be recommended when aggressive treatment with nitroprusside is not indicated.[18]

Acute Bromocriptine Toxicity

Special note is made of a growing body of literature concerning the acute effects of bromocriptine in overdose amounts. Bromocriptine, through its structural relationship to dopamine, acts to stimulate dopamine receptors. Curiously, possibly via direct dopamine activity in large doses or by the activity of bromocriptine metabolites, both sympathomimetic signs (tachycardia, hypertension, hallucinations, paranoid behavior) and anticholinergic findings (mydriasis, flushed skin, tachycardia, fever, hallucinations, confusion, mania) may be noted in bromocriptine overdose.[19] Nausea, vomiting, dizziness, lethargy, pupillary dilatation, hypotension, and tachycardia seem to be common presenting signs.[20]

Recovery is usually rapid with adequate gut decontamination and supportive care, with particular attention to airway, hypo- and hypertensive crises and management of delirium. No human deaths have been reported as yet as a result of bromocriptine overdose, and the drug seems to have a relatively large margin of safety.[19]

References

1. Merhoff CG, Porter JM: Ergot intoxication. Ann Surg *180*:773, 1974.
2. Kingsbury JM: Poisonous Plants of the United States and Canada. Prentice-Hall, Englewood Cliffs, NJ, 1964, p 86.
3. Kingsbury JM: Poisonous Plants of the United States and Canada. Prentice-Hall, Englewood Cliffs, NJ, 1964, p 80.
4. Morton JF: Major Medicinal Plants. Charles C Thomas, Springfield, Ill., 1977, p 6.
5. Berde B, Sturmer E: Ergot alkaloids and related compounds. *In* Berde B, Schild HO (eds): Handbook of Experimental Pharmacology. Vol. 49. Springer-Verlag, Berlin, 1978.
6. Berde B: Pharmacology of Ergot Alkaloids in Clinical Use. Med J Aust Special Supplement, Nov. 4, 1978, p 3.
7. Berde B, Sturmer, E: Ergot alkaloids and related compounds. *In* Berde B, Schild HO (eds): Handbook of Experimental Pharmacology. Vol. 49. Springer-Verlag, Berlin, 1978.
8. Miller-Schweinitzer E, Weidmann H: Ergot alkaloids and related compounds. *In* Berde B, Schild HO (eds): Handbook of Experimental Pharmacology. Vol 49. Springer-Verlag, Berlin, 1978.
9. Autonomic drugs. *In* Reilly JR (ed): American Hospital Formulary Service. American Society of Hospital Pharmacists, Bethesda, Md, 1978.
10. Edwards WM: Accidental poisoning of newborn infants with ergotamine maleate. Clin Pediatr *10*:257, 1971.
11. Jones EM, Williams B: Two cases of ergotamine poisoning in infants. Br Med J *1*:466, 1966.
12. Buxton A, et al: Refractory ergonovine-induced coronary vasospasm: Importance of intracoronary nitroglycerin. Am J Cardiol *46*:329, 1980.
13. Henry LG: Ergotism. Arch Surg *110*:929, 1979.
14. Husum B, et al: Nitroglycerine infusion for ergotism. Lancet *2*:794, 1979.
15. Husted JW, et al: Intra-arterial nitroprusside treatment for ergotism. Am J Roentgenol *131*:1090, 1978.
16. Cobaugh DS: Prazosin treatment of ergotamine-induced peripheral ischemia. JAMA *244*:1360, 1980.
17. Waters DD, et al: Ergonovine testing to detect spontaneous remissions of variant angina during long-term treatment with calcium antagonist drugs. Am J Cardiol *47*:179, 1981.
18. Dagher FJ, et al: Severe unilateral ischemia of the lower extremity caused by ergotamine: Treatment with nifedipine. Surgery *97*:369, 1985.
19. Mack RB: Mairzy doats and dozy doats and a kiddle eat almost anything: Bromocriptine (Parlodel) overdose. NC Med J *49*:17, 1988.
20. Vermund SH, et al: Accidental bromocriptine ingestion in childhood. J Pediatr *105*:838, 1984.

CHAPTER 100
THEOPHYLLINE

Sally M. Ehlers, M.D.

Theophylline is commonly used in treating both acute and chronic illness. Its reputation for causing toxicity is great, as it has a very low therapeutic index. Many of the problems associated with its early use were due to a lack of knowledge of its elimination kinetics.

At one time, use of theophylline was discouraged because of the frequency and severity of toxicity. Erratic absorption from suppositories or intramuscular injection was partially responsible for these problems, but most difficulties resulted from lack of studies on the effect of age on theophylline clearance. Since 1972, when Jenne and associates noted marked individual differences in theophylline clearance,[1] the list of factors that alter elimination of the drug continues to lengthen.

Another difficulty in management of theophylline therapy was unsatisfactory laboratory determinations of theophylline concentrations in the blood. Now, with the use of high-pressure liquid chromatography and enzyme immunoassay, there are few potential interfering factors. Recent proliferation and use of slow-release formulations may be responsible for more complex management concerns with theophylline. Appreciation of individual variation in the handling of theophylline, in association with measurement of drug concentrations and individualizing doses, should result in appropriate management with the drug. Clinicians are often confronted by very ill patients who have inadvertently received too much theophylline, who have become toxic because of a change of their theophylline clearance, or who have ingested the medication in a suicide attempt. In such patients, toxicity may be severe and management difficult; death may occur.

PHARMACOKINETICS

A methylxanthine similar to caffeine (1,3,7-trimethylxanthine), theophylline (1,3-dimethylxanthine) is rapidly and efficiently absorbed from the gastrointestinal tract when taken orally. Peak blood levels occur within 2 hours of ingestion, with approximately 96 per cent of administered dose being absorbed from plain, uncoated theophylline tablets. Sustained-release preparations are widely used now, but there is marked variability in rates of absorption and elimination among products and among patients; diurnal variation also has been observed in some patients.[2–5] Peak concentrations with sustained-release formulas usually occur at 4 to 6 hours after ingestion.[6] In general, the presence of food or antacids will delay peak absorption but not the total percentage absorbed, although there is variation with slow-release formulations here, too. Because of the differences in the various slow-release preparations, they are not interchangeable for clinical use. Absorption of theophylline from rectal suppositories and from intramuscular injections is less predictable.

Only 8 to 10 per cent of theophylline is excreted unchanged in the urine. Most of the drug undergoes metabolism in the liver, mediated by cytochrome P-450 microsomal enzymes. Both linear and nonlinear kinetics occur with theophylline; nonlinearity is believed caused by saturability of hepatic metabolism.[7] Major metabolites include 1,3-di-methyluric acid, 3-methylxanthine, and 1-methyluric acid, all of which are excreted in the urine. The percentage of each tends to remain the same under most conditions, but some differences have been described with dietary manipulation,[8] in liver disease, and with different preparations. The most active metabolite is 3-methylxanthine, which possesses 30 to 70 per cent of the biologic activity of theophylline.

The metabolism of theophylline in the neonate is considerably different from that of other age groups. About one half is excreted unchanged in the urine, and one third is metabolized to caffeine.[9, 10] Metabolism is altered in advanced age as well, with a smaller percentage excreted unchanged and a greater percentage excreted as 1-methyluric acid.[11] One half to two thirds of theophylline is protein bound, though less binding is observed in neonates, elderly people,[11] cirrhotic patients, and those with increasing theophylline concentrations.[6]

Placental transfer of theophylline has been demonstrated, with similar serum theophylline concentrations in both neonate and the mother who is receiving theophylline for asthma.[12] Although alterations in volume of distribution and half-life have been seen in pregnancy, theophylline clearance is not changed significantly.[13] Theophylline is found in breast milk, though less than 1 per cent of the total amount of drug eliminated was recovered from the milk.[14] Thus, no dosage change is necessary in treatment of the nursing mother, but this potential source of theophylline to the nursing infant must be considered if theophylline is used in the infant's therapeutic regimen.

Although the volume of distribution of theophylline of 0.5 L/kg is the same in most groups of patients studied, clearance and half-life are quite variable. An appreciation of factors influencing theophylline elimination is necessary to prevent toxicity as well as to understand the cause and course of toxicity in some patients. The average clearance and half-life of theophylline in a healthy nonsmoking adult are 50 to 60 ml/kg/hr and 6 to 8 hours, respectively. The most readily identifiable influences on theophylline clearance are age (Table 100–1), smoking, liver disease, and drugs (Table 100–2), although the mechanisms are not fully understood. Several drugs also affect theophylline clearance, and this list grows steadily. Factors that affect theophylline clearance must be considered in arriving at maintenance drug regimens as well as in evaluating the patient with theophylline toxicity.

Wide fluctuations of theophylline clearance and half-life have been observed in the pediatric age group, from the premature infant to the adolescent. After adolescence and into the adult age groups, however, clearance and half-life tend to be relatively stable. In the premature infant, theophylline clearance is significantly less than in the full-term infant, averaging 18 to 24 ml/kg/hr, with a half-life of 24 to 30 hours (see Table 100–1). Clearance progressively increases and half-life progressively decreases from birth until the age of approximately 9 months, presumably as hepatic enzyme systems mature. Maximal clearance is achieved during the ages of 1 to 9 years. Clearance then decreases into adolescence and stabilizes in the mid-teens. Although there may be some decrease in clearance in patients over 60 years old, half-life is not significantly affected;[23–25] Antal and colleagues found that overall plasma clearance was reduced by 30 per cent when altered plasma protein binding was taken into consideration in those between 70 and 85 years of age.[11]

Decreased theophylline clearance in hepatic disease can be expected, since all but 8 to 10 per cent of the drug is metabolized by the liver (see Table 100–2). This decrease may be peculiar to certain disease states, however, and requires significant liver impairment before its effect is manifested. Mangione and associates describe decreased theophylline clearance in decompensated cirrhosis and acute hepatitis but not in cholestasis or compensated hepatic cirrhosis.[26] In cirrhosis, theophylline clearance has been shown to correlate inversely with serum bilirubin[26] and half-life inversely with serum albumin.[27, 28] Theophylline clearance may continue to

Table 100–1. AGE AND THEOPHYLLINE ELIMINATION

AGE	AVERAGE CLEARANCE (ml/kg/hr)	AVERAGE HALF-LIFE (hr)	REFERENCE NUMBER(S)
Infants			
Premature	18–24	24–30	10, 15, 16
10–20 wk	17–34	9–19	17
3 mo to 1 yr	64–89	4–5.5	18, 19
Children			
1–9 yr old	94–100	3–5	10, 20–22
10–18 yr old	77	—	22
Adults			
All	51–66	6–7	10, 22
Elderly	28–42	5.4–9.0 hr	23
(>60 years)	43	—	24
(70–85 years)	29	9.8	11

Table 100–2. FACTORS OTHER THAN AGE AND THEOPHYLLINE CLEARANCE

STUDIES SHOW NO OR INSIGNIFICANT EFFECT	DECREASE CLEARANCE/ INCREASE HALF-LIFE	INCREASE CLEARANCE/ DECREASE HALF-LIFE
Drugs		
Allopurinol (standard dose)	Allopurinol (high dose)	Barbiturates
Antacids	Antibiotics	Pentobarbital
Antibiotics	Erythromycin (5 d or more)	Phenobarbital
Amoxicillin	Quinolones	Secobarbital
Ampicillin	Enoxacin	Carbamazepine
Cefaclor	Ciprofloxacin	Isoniazid
Cephalexin	Troleandomycin	Isoproterenol (IV)
Cotrimoxazole	H_2-blocker	Rifampin
Doxycycline	Cimetidine (dose- and age-dependent)	Sulfinpyrazone
Josamycin	Propranolol	
Midacamycin		
Metronidazole		
Tetracycline		
β-Agonists (oral)		
Caffeine		
H_2-blockers		
Famotidine		
Rantidine		
Medroxyprogesterone acetate		
Metaclopramide		
Metoprolol		
Nicotine gum		
Steroids		
Diseases		
Renal failure	Hepatic cirrhosis	Cystic fibrosis
Fever	Acute hepatitis	Hyperthyroidism
Cholestasis	Congestive heart failure	
COPD without acute illness or cor pulmonale	Acute influenza	
	Pneumonia	
	Severe acute illness	
	Cor pulmonale	
	COPD with hypoxemia	
Miscellaneous		
Influenza vaccination (nonviable split virus)	Increased dose	Cigarette smoking
	High carbohydrate diet	Marijuana
Gender	Cessation of smoking	High protein diet
Pregnancy		

change for several weeks following the onset of acute hepatitis; during the acute phase of infection, theophylline toxicity is a risk because of prolonged half-life. Later, as liver function steadily improves, asthma exacerbations may occur because of progressive increase of theophylline clearance as it returns back to baseline.[29] Decreased clearance of theophylline in congestive heart failure has been attributed to hepatic congestion.[30] Cystic fibrosis and hyperthyroidism are the only diseases associated with an increased theophylline clearance.[31]

Cigarette smoking increases theophylline clearance, an effect that reverts to or toward normal after cessation of smoking.[30] Induction of hepatic microsomal enzyme systems by polycyclic hydrocarbons is thought to explain the decreased half-life of theophylline in smokers, rather than a nicotine effect. Lee and associates show no difference in theophylline clearance between chewers of nicotine gum and of placebo gum.[32] When those taking theophylline discontinue smoking, there is a decrease in theophylline clearance, increasing the likelihood of developing theophylline toxicity.

Other factors that alter theophylline clearance include exacerbation of chronic obstructive pulmonary disease in adults with hypoxemia or cor pulmonale, use of marijuana, dietary manipulation, and influenza A or B infection in children. Induction of interferon is believed responsible for inactivating the hepatic P-450 system. Although influenza vaccination with a trivalent split-virus reduced theophylline clearance, several other investigators have shown no significant change and lack of interferon production with other vaccines.[31]

Many drugs have been evaluated in terms of their effect on theophylline clearance, often prompted by reported cases of alteration of serum theophylline concentration in the patient. The H_2-blocker cimetidine decreases theophylline clearance, and it has resulted in significant theophylline toxicity in patients previously stabilized on that drug.[33–35] Single night-time dosing affects clearance less than several doses during the day.[36] Neither ranitidine nor famotidine has affected theophylline clearance in studies,[37, 38] but ranitidine has been implicated in causing symptomatic toxicity.[39, 40] Barbiturates will decrease half-life and increase clearance of theophylline, ranging from a 17 per cent increase in clearance with phenobarbital to a 340 per cent increase with secobarbital.[34] Two other antiepileptic agents, phenytoin and carbamazepine, also increase theophylline clearance.[33] Allopurinol has been shown to cause no change in theophylline clearance when given at a dose of 300 mg daily,[41] but it causes an increased theophylline half-life when given at a higher dose.[42] The calcium channel blockers nifedipine and verapamil have been implicated in cases of theophylline toxicity.[43–45] Caffeine ingestion and furosemide also may alter theophylline metabolism, although conflicting data exist.[1, 8, 24, 33] Several antibiotics have been studied (see Table 100–2); the quinolones enoxacin and ciprofloxacin also appear to affect theophylline clearance.[46–48]

The relationship of theophylline clearance to theophylline dosage remains unclear. In case reports of theophylline toxicity, there is a decrease of clearance in some instances and normal clearance in others. Vaucher and associates found first-order elimination in two infants with theophylline overdose (peak levels of 64 and 141 μg/ml).[49] The half-life was 9 hours in an adult, with a maximal drug serum concentration of 270 μg/ml.[50] For a 17 month old child, Kadlec and associates found a half-life of 12.6 hours as the serum theophylline concentration decreased from 100 to 34 μg/ml, and then of 5.4 hours as the level decreased further to 4.5 μg/ml.[20, 21] In a premature infant, theophylline clearance was only 12.7 ml/kg/hr, and the half-life was 24.7 hours.[51] Lawyer and colleagues[52, 53] and Fleetham and associates[54] observed a changing half-life in patients with theophylline toxicity. In studies of altering theophylline dosage for treating pulmonary disease, dose-dependence has been demonstrated[1, 55, 57] and is felt secondary to saturation of the hepatic metabolic pathway for only one of the metabolites (3-methylxanthine). Of course, in individuals ingesting theophylline, continued gastrointestinal absorption of the drug must be considered in assessment of serum drug concentrations and determination of half-life. Considerable evidence exists for some element of dose-dependence in theophylline elimination.

In patients with very high serum concentrations of drug, the half-life may be greater than normal for one or more of the reasons listed in Table 100–2. Half-life also may be above normal because of a greater amount of drug being administered, or there may be no change. Therefore, half-life must be determined in each patient to predict the course and to help determine factors contributing to the cause of toxicity.

THERAPEUTIC USES AND MECHANISMS OF ACTION

Three major indications for the use of theophylline in clinical medicine exist at present: *asthma, pulmonary edema,* and *apnea of prematurity.* Dilation of bronchial smooth muscle by theophylline was first described in the early 1920s, and theophylline has been used in treating asthma since the mid-1930s, but its mechanism of action is still unknown. Several mechanisms have been proposed for the smooth muscle relaxation in the bronchi observed in asthma, including inhibition of prostaglandins, phosphodiesterase inhibition, alteration of intracellular calcium and cyclic AMP, and antagonism of adenosine receptors mediating bronchoconstriction. None of these provides a satisfactory answer, however.

Theophylline causes a positive inotropic effect on the heart at therapeutic serum concentrations and a dose-dependent chronotropic effect.[13] Catecholamines are released and may be responsible for these effects. Peripheral vasodilation also occurs. Cardiac output is increased by a direct effect on the myocardium, hence theophylline's usefulness in pulmonary edema.

Since 1973, theophylline has been used in treating apnea of prematurity. Direct stimulation of respiratory and vasomotor centers of the brain causes an increased rate and depth of breathing and decreases the number of apneic attacks.[58, 59] Beneficial effects on lung maturation and weaning from ventilator support are being investigated.[9] Use of theophylline in premature infants has further extended understanding of the variability of theophylline clearance in relation to age.

Although theophylline is often prescribed for patients with chronic obstructive pulmonary disease, its role is controversial. It can increase the efficiency of diaphragmatic contractility and decrease the susceptibility of the diaphragm to fatigue; cardiac function and chronic obstructive pulmonary disease can improve with theophylline.[60, 61] Most studies indicate no objective positive effects of theophylline, though subjective improvement with the drug is noted. Recommendations are for further study of its effect and prudent use, if any, in patients with chronic lung disease.[62, 63]

PREPARATIONS

A variety of preparations containing theophylline and aminophylline are available in tablet, capsule, and liquid form. Preparations are of plain theophylline or theophylline plus other ingredients, including phenobarbital, guaifenesin, and/or ephedrine. The theophylline component in the shorter-acting preparations is 100 per cent available, and approximately 96 per cent is absorbed; peak action is 1 to 2 hours from ingestion. Several forms of sustained-release preparations are available and may have varying absorption and half-life. Because of the lack of uniformity of these products, it is important to avoid interchanging them; one should be alert to the possibility of either toxicity or underdosage if this is done. Of particular concern in terms of variable absorption is Theo-dur Sprinkles, which is markedly less absorbed when taken with food compared with Theo-24, which demonstrated markedly increased absorption with food to the point of toxic symptomatology.[64]

Although most sustained-release formulations will provide for steady state therapeutic levels in normal nonsmoking adults, there may be wide fluctuations in serum theophylline concentration in individuals who exhibit a very short half-life (Table 100–3). Children and smokers, who usually have more rapid elimination rates, require more frequent dosing than average.[65] Each individual will require adjustments of dosing according to elimination rate and absorption of the preparation used. Several regimens are suggested for use in dosing various types of individuals.[2, 31]

For individuals sensitive to the ethylenediamine in aminophylline, dyphylline (7-[2,3-dihydroxypropyl] theophylline) may be used. Because its metabolism and excretion are less dependent upon the liver, it may be useful in patients with severe hepatic dysfunction. In one study, 44 per cent of the dose given intravenously was recovered unchanged from the urine.[53]

The various forms of theophylline all have the same mechanism of action, differing in the amount available, peak blood concentra-

Table 100–3. SLOW-RELEASE THEOPHYLLINE PRODUCTS

Absorption (%)		
95–100	**85–94**	**Variable; Fasting /with Food**
Quibron—T/SR (Bristol)	Elixophyllin SR (Forest)	Constant-T (Geigy)
Respbid (Boehringer Ingelheim)	Theobid (Glaxo)	Slo-Bid Gyrocaps (Rorer)
Slo-Phylline* (Rorer)	Theovent (Schering)	Theo-24 (Searle & Co) 71/100
Slo-Phylline Gyrocaps* (Rorer)		Theo-Dur Sprinkle (Key) 91/94
Somophylline-CRT (Fisons)		Uniphyl* (Purdue Frederick)
Sustaire (Pfizer)		
Theoclear LA* (Central)		
Theo-Dur (Key)		
Theolair* (Riker)		
Theolair-SR (Riker)		
Theospan-SR* (Laser)		

*These drugs show great fluctuations of serum theophylline concentration outside the therapeutic range in patients who exhibit a short half-life.

tion, and duration of action. Caldwell and associates have shown that the metabolism of aminophylline and theophylline is not identical, however.[66]

TOXICITY

Serum theophylline concentration is most accurately determined by high-pressure liquid chromatography. Other methods used have included ultraviolet spectrophotometry and gas liquid chromatography; enzyme immunoassay is now accurate and readily available for clinical use. Salivary theophylline concentrations correlate well with blood levels but have been used primarily in experimental circumstances or in evaluation of infants and children. Cerebrospinal fluid theophylline concentrations have been found to correlate with serum concentrations, in most instances, but are not used clinically.[67]

Both clinical response and symptoms of toxicity correlate with serum concentrations of theophylline. When used in treating apnea of prematurity, serum concentrations of 4 to 12 μg/ml are considered therapeutic; therapeutic serum concentrations in asthma are 10 to 20 μg/ml, though some effect may be observed with levels as low as 5 μg/ml. For individual dosages, drug concentrations should be determined after 24 hours with constant infusion; for sustained-release formulation, it is best to measure serum concentration 4 hours after a dose, with the patient on a consistent regimen for 72 hours prior to the dose.[2]

The therapeutic index is low with theophylline, however. *Thirty per cent of patients with serum theophylline concentrations greater than 15 μg/ml had toxic reactions, and 78 per cent of patients with concentrations greater than 25 μg/ml had symptoms of toxicity.*[68] Whether the overdose is acute or chronic also affects the severity and types of symptoms that may be seen. With the widespread availability and use of slow-release theophylline products, very prolonged toxicity is possible. Several patients demonstrated a marked increase in serum theophylline concentration and worsening symptoms several hours after suicide attempts with sustained-release preparations.[69–71] Olson and associates found peak levels to occur 1 to 24 hours after ingestion, with a mean of 11 hours.[72]

Clinical Symptoms and Signs of Theophylline Toxicity

Theophylline toxicity should be suspected in patients with nausea, vomiting, tachyarrhythmias, agitation, or seizures. Symptoms of theophylline toxicity can involve several systems, and, although symptomatology relates to serum drug concentrations, there is no predictable step-wise relationship. The acuteness or chronicity of toxicity also determines severity of symptoms. "Acute" toxicity refers to an ingestion with suicidal intent, whereas "chronic" toxicity occurs in the patient receiving excessive intravenous theophylline or an excessive oral dosage for the individual's clearance rate. Gastrointestinal symptoms of nausea and vomiting are common with serum concentrations greater than 20 μg/ml. These symptoms are not necessarily present before more severe central nervous system or cardiovascular abnormalities occur, however. Of 18 patients receiving intravenous theophylline who showed signs and symptoms of theophylline toxicity (plasma theophylline concentration greater than 20 μg/ml), only 5 experienced nausea and vomiting; less than half of those with seizures or severe arrhythmias had preceding nausea and vomiting.[73] Nausea and vomiting occur by local effect on gastric mucosa and by a central effect as well. Foster and colleagues have shown that gastric acid secretion is increased with use of both oral and intravenous theophylline, even when serum drug concentrations are in the therapeutic range.[74] In cases of severe acute theophylline toxicity, gastrointestinal bleeding may occur.[20, 21, 49, 50, 75, 77] Diarrhea may be present, but with very high levels ileus may occur.[10]

Seizures may occur with serum theophylline concentrations as low as 25 μg/ml but are more common when the concentration is greater than 40 μg/ml in chronic or inadvertent toxicity and may be refractory.[10] An infant with a serum concentration as high as 330 μg/ml had only questionable seizure activity.[78] In acute overdose, seizures are unlikely unless the serum theophylline concentration is greater than 80 to 100 μg/ml.[6, 10, 72] Baker reported seizures in two acutely intoxicated children who had serum theophylline concentrations under 50 μg/ml.[79] Agitation, confusion, and lethargy also are often seen.

Tachyarrhythmias may also occur when the

serum theophylline concentration is greater than 20 μg/ml. A supraventricular origin is most common, but ventricular premature beats, tachycardia, and fibrillation may occur with severe toxicity; prior cardiac disease predisposes to arrhythmias, and ventricular tachycardia occurred in a 71 year old patient with a serum theophylline concentration of only 29 μg/ml who had inadvertent toxicity.[88] Cardiovascular collapse and respiratory arrest are rare unless the concentration is greater than 50 μg/ml in the chronic overdose or greater than 100 μg/ml in acute toxicity. Tachycardia is the most common sign in both acute and chronic toxicity.

The experimental ventricular fibrillation threshold was reduced by 30 to 40 per cent during the infusion of theophylline. It was reduced even further when respiratory failure from hypoventilation was present during the theophylline infusion.[81] Shortly after the completion of the infusion period the threshold rose to above the normal ventricular fibrillation threshold. Peak drug concentrations should correspond with the time of the lowest threshold, and the subsequent rising threshold should correlate with the falling drug concentration. For 60 per cent of patients in whom the precipitating event for cardiac arrest was thought to be drug related, injection of theophylline through a central venous catheter was implicated.[82] The arrhythmias that occur during infusion of theophylline, particularly bolus infusion, presumably may be related to this decrease of ventricular fibrillation threshold. Camarata and associates speculate that rapid infusion through the central venous route was related to such toxicity.[82] Multifocal atrial tachycardia in patients receiving theophylline was associated with a decreased survival compared with those not receiving theophylline,[83] and was observed even in some patients with therapeutic theophylline concentrations.[84]

Other significant clinical manifestations of theophylline toxicity include rhabdomyolysis,[85–88] increased CK-MB isoenzymes,[89] bezoar formation in the stomach,[90] psychosis,[91] and electrolyte abnormalities. Severe hypokalemia, hypophosphatemia, hypercalcemia, hyperglycemia, and metabolic acidosis are present in acute overdosage, believed related to elevated catecholamines and beta-adrenergic stimulation.[92–96] Rhabdomyolysis may occur following theophylline-induced seizures or because of profound hypokalemia.[87]

MORBIDITY AND MORTALITY

Although isolated case fatalities from theophylline toxicity continue to be reported, the mortality rate in large series of cases of serious theophylline toxicity is low (Table 100–4). Children in particular seem to survive very high serum theophylline concentrations and show less morbidity than adults. Elderly patients have both greater morbidity and mortality than younger adults and children, presumably due to pre-existent pulmonary disease, which may well be accompanied by cardiovascular impairment; they are therefore more likely to have a delayed elimination rate of the drug. Elderly patients are also more likely to be toxic because of a chronic or inadvertent overdose, and with chronic toxicity there is a lower threshold for seizures and arrhythmias. In both acute and chronic toxicity, death or permanent neurologic deficit is a result of either very prolonged seizure activity or severe cardiac arrhythmias with cardiovascular collapse.[104] Of the 12 deaths compiled from series in Table 100–4, 6 were caused by acute ingestion, with ages ranging from 11 months to 60 years, contrasting with a range of 61 to 84 years of age in those who died because of chronic overdose. Peak serum theophylline concentrations in the acute overdose deaths ranged from 138 to 228 μg/ml, but several individuals whose peak serum theophylline concentrations were in the 100 and 200 μg/ml range have survived acute overdose without sequelae. Wells and Ferlauto reported an infant who survived theophylline toxicity with a peak serum theophylline concentration of 330 μg/ml.[78] On the other hand, those dying because of chronic toxicity had peak serum theophylline concentrations of from 30 to 46 μg/ml, the usual range seen in patients with chronic toxicity. Serum theophylline concentrations greater than 90 μg/ml are unusual in patients with inadvertent overdose.

Other problems associated with theophylline use include eczematous dermatitis and urticaria as a result of hypersensitivity to the ethylenediamine component in aminophylline,[105, 106] and increase of left ventricular out-

Table 100–4. MORTALITY IN SERIOUS THEOPHYLLINE TOXICITY

INVESTIGATOR(S)	NO. OF PATIENTS/ EPISODES*	TYPE OF OVERDOSE	AGE RANGE (yr) *(Mean)*	PEAK OR ADMISSION THEOPHYLLINE CONCENTRATION, *mg/ml (Mean)*	DEATHS
Baker[79]	44* 21*	acute chronic	¼–16 (7.4)	<20–101.9	0
Bertino and Walker[97]	19/20*	chronic	(67)	19.4– 43.9 (31.6)	0
Frewin and Cooper[98]	8	chronic	70–85 (78)	28.8 to >40	2
Gaudrealt et al[99]	28	acute	3⅓–21 (15.5)	24 to >120 (89)	0
Greenberg et al[100]	2	acute	35, 52	80, 180	0
	8	chronic	48–77 (66)	30–79 (45)	0
Hall et al[92]	22	acute	15–69 (25.3)	40–228 (87.6)	2
Mountain and Neff[101]	21/22*	chronic	46–86 (63)	22.4–104.8 (42.8)	0
Olson et al[72]	15	chronic	½–75	24–70 (39)	1
Park et al[102]	6	acute	<1–44 (20)	71–150 (92)	1
	22	chronic	12–87 (51)	(37)	0
	8	iatrogenic	48–77 (64)	30–81 (48)	3
Woo et al[103]	26	acute	(31)	76–205	3

flow obstruction when it is used to treat pulmonary edema in idiopathic, hypertrophic, subaortic stenosis.[107]

TREATMENT

Treatment of theophylline toxicity is predominantly supportive and directed at symptoms. Obviously the drug should be discontinued and not reinstituted until serum concentrations are well within the therapeutic range or even at subtherapeutic levels for both symptomatic patients and asymptomatic patients. *Activated charcoal* adsorbs the drug well within the gastrointestinal tract and should follow gastric lavage in both symptomatic and asymptomatic patients with large oral ingestion. It is more effective in reducing peak concentration and absorption than ipecac.[108]

Activated charcoal and a cathartic such as magnesium citrate or sorbitol should be given orally or by nasogastric tube to those who have ingested slow-release formulations, in particular to enhance elimination from the gastrointestinal tract and to prevent the very prolonged absorption that can be seen with overdoses of these agents. Half-life was significantly reduced when oral activated charcoal doses were given every 1 to 6 hours[6, 109–112] or even as a continuous nasogastric infusion.[113] Generally, 0.5 to 1 gm/kg should be given every 2 to 4 hours as tolerated. Such treatment may be inhibited by vomiting, however. Gastrointestinal symptoms will usually resolve readily as the drug level decreases, though antiemetics and the H_2-blockers ranitidine or famotidine may be helpful in the interim.

Arrhythmias may be difficult to treat, but the beta-blocker *propranolol* may be most efficacious for this problem. Verapamil, lidocaine, procainamide, and digoxin are not always beneficial. Intravenous propranolol also has been effective in increasing blood pressure and in improving the metabolic abnormalities that often accompany theophylline toxicity (hypokalemia, hyperglycemia, hypophosphatemia, hypercalcemia, and metabolic acidosis).[93, 95, 114, 115] Response to a beta-blocker may be expected because of theophylline's effect on stimulating the release of catecholamines. *Correction of hypokalemia* is, of course, important in managing arrhythmias, and supplemental potassium may be required in some of these patients as well because of deficits from gastrointestinal losses. Close cardiac monitoring is advisable because catecholamine-induced intracellular potassium shifts may play a more significant role than actual potassium losses, and hyperkalemia could result as potassium shifts back out of cells.[116]

Seizures may be very difficult to control; *diazepam* is probably the most effective and phenytoin the least effective agent, though seizures may be refractory to both. Diazepam should be used as the drug of choice in any instance and barbiturates next. Seizures in children with theophylline toxicity may be more responsive to therapy than those in adults.[79, 99]

Because toxicity correlates well with serum theophylline concentrations, enhanced removal of drug would be expected to and does result in improvement in symptoms. Efforts to remove drug have been reported by several investigators. Use of oral activated charcoal has been called "gastrointestinal dialysis." Half-life was reduced from 24 hours to 2 hours,[112] 17.2 hours to 5.9 hours,[109] and 18.7 to 4.6 hours[110] using oral activated charcoal. Exchange transfusion in pediatric patients has not been effective in treating toxicity.[78, 117] Peritoneal dialysis gives a clearance of only 0.7 ml/kg/min at best[6] and is not beneficial in treating toxicity, though 25 per cent of administered theophylline was removed from rats with peritoneal dialysis.[117] Hemodialysis has been used in evaluating theophylline removal in uremic patients measuring a dialysis clearance of 32.8 ml/min[118] to 88 ml/min.[119] Krishna and colleagues showed a reduction in half-life from 14.8 hours before to 3.4 hours during hemodialysis in a patient with chronic toxicity;[120] half-life increased from 3.5 and 4.5 hours during hemodialysis to 25 and 7 hours after dialysis in two patients who ingested slow-release theophylline.[103]

Both *charcoal and resin hemoperfusion* have been used successfully in treating severe theophylline toxicity.[52, 54, 72, 75, 76, 100, 102, 103, 114, 121–123] Maximal clearances were 113 to 223 ml/min for charcoal and 225 ml/min for resin hemoperfusion. An estimated two thirds of the ingested dose of theophylline was removed by charcoal hemoperfusion in a 3 year old child.[75] When to institute hemoperfusion in treating theophylline overdose remains controversial.[10, 124, 125] Confusion as to its efficacy exists because of the absence of controlled studies in its application, use of the procedure so very late in a patient's course that irreversible damage may already have been done, and lack of recognition until recently of the differences in manifestations and outcome of toxicity depending on age and acuteness or chronicity of toxicity.

Most patients with theophylline toxicity can be treated satisfactorily with supportive measures. Those who do not respond may benefit by aggressive efforts to remove the drug by hemoperfusion. Resin hemoperfusion and charcoal hemoperfusion are both very effective, and even hemodialysis with a large surface area dialyzer and rapid blood flows can remove theophylline. Patients who are most likely to respond poorly to supportive care and symptomatic treatment alone and hence are most likely to benefit from hemoperfusion are (1) those with acute toxicity and a serum theophylline concentration greater than 80 to 100 μg/ml; (2) patients who have chronic toxicity, age greater than 60 years or less than 6 months, with a serum theophylline concentration greater than 40 μg/ml, or (3) those with liver disease, congestive heart failure, or other factors that significantly increase theophylline half-life.[6, 10, 72, 99, 104] Patients with status epilepticus, uncontrollable arrhythmias, and/or cardiovascular collapse should be treated with hemoperfusion, as their outlook with these conditions is very poor.

Because of prolonged absorption of slow-release preparations, it is necessary to follow serum theophylline concentrations in patients with theophylline toxicity, for the level at the time of admission may give a false sense of security. Peak theophylline concentrations have been documented as long as 12 to 17 hours after ingestion in acute overdose.[69, 71, 90] Remeasurement in 2 to 4 hours after admission or ingestion, or with any worsening of the patient's condition, will allow for adequate assessment of late toxicity.

References

1. Jenne JW, Wyze E, Rood FS, MacDonald FM: Pharmacokinetics of theophylline: Application to adjustment of the clinical dose of aminophylline. Clin Pharmacol Ther *13*:349, 1972.
2. Hendeles L, Massanari M, Weinberger M: Update on the pharmacodynamics and pharmacokinetics of theophylline. Chest *88*:103S–111S, 1985.
3. Karim A: Effects of food on the bioavailability of theophylline from controlled-release products in adults. J Allergy Clin Immunol *78*:695–703, 1986.
4. Szefler SJ: Theophylline and its fickle unpredictability of absorption. Ann Allergy *55*:580–583, 1985.
5. Pedersen S: Effects of food on the absorption of theophylline in children. J Allergy Clin Immunol *78*:704–709, 1986.
6. Gaudreault P, Guay J: Theophylline poisoning: Pharmacological considerations and clinical management. Med Toxicol *1*:169–191, 1986.
7. Lesko LJ: Dose-dependent kinetics of theophylline. J Allergy Clin Immunol *78*:723–727, 1986.
8. Monks TJ, Caldwell J, Smith RL: Influence of methylxanthine-containing foods on theophylline metabolism and kinetics. Clin Pharmacol Ther *26*:513, 1979.
9. Aranda JV, Chemtob S, Laudignon N, Sasyniuk BI: Pharmacologic effects of theophylline in the newborn. J Allergy Clin Immunol *78*:773–780, 1986.
10. Albert S: Aminophylline toxicity. Pediatr Clin North Am *34*:61–73, 1987.
11. Antal EJ, Kramer PA, Mercik SA, Chapron DJ, Lawson IR: Theophylline pharmacokinetics in advanced age. Br J Clin Pharmacol *12*:637–645, 1981.
12. Arwood LL, Dasta JR, Friedman C: Placental transfer of theophylline: Two case reports. Pediatrics *63*:844, 1979.
13. Bukowskyj M, Nakatsu K, Munt PW: Theophylline reassessed. Ann Intern Med *101*:63–73, 1984.
14. Stec GP, Greenberger P, Ruo TI, Henthorn T, Morita Y, Atkinson AJ, Patterson R: Kinetics of theophylline transfer to breast milk. Clin Pharmacol Ther *28*:404, 1980.
15. Brazier J-L, Renaud H, Ribon B, Salle BL: Plasma xanthine levels in low birth weight infants treated or not treated with theophylline. Arch Dis Child *54*:194, 1979.
16. Jones RAK, Baillie E: Dosage schedule for intravenous aminophylline in apnea of prematurity, based on pharmacokinetic studies. Arch Dis Child *54*:190, 1979.
17. Nassif EG, Weinberger MM, Shannon D, Guiang SF, Hendeles L, Jimenez D, Ekwo F: Theophylline disposition in infancy. J Pediatr *98*:158, 1981.
18. Rosen JP, Danish M, Ragni MC, Saccar CL, Yaffe SJ, Lecks HI: Theophylline pharmacokinetics in the young infant. Pediatrics *64*:248, 1979.
19. Simons FER, Simons KJ: Pharmacokinetics of theophylline in infancy. J Clin Pharmacol *18*:472, 1978.
20. Kadlec GJ, Ha LT, Jarboe CH, Richards D, Karibo JM: Theophylline half-life in infants and young children. Ann Allergy *40*:303, 1978.
21. Kadlec GJ, Jarboe CH, Pollard SJ, Sublett JL: Acute theophylline intoxication. Biphasic first order elimination kinetics in a child. Ann Allergy *41*:337, 1978.
22. Zaske DE, Miller KW, Strem EL, Austrian S, Johnson PB: Oral aminophylline therapy—increased dosage requirements in children. JAMA *237*:1453, 1977.
23. Nielsen-Kudsk F, Magnussen I, Jakobsen P: Pharmacokinetics of theophylline in ten elderly patients. Acta Pharmacol Toxicol *42*:226, 1978.
24. Jusko WJ, Gardner MJ, Mangione A, Schentag JJ, Koup JR, Vance JW: Factors affecting theophylline clearances: Age, tobacco, marijuana, cirrhosis, congestive heart failure, obesity, oral contraceptives, benzodiazepines, barbiturates, and ethanol. J Pharmaceut Sci *68*:1358, 1979.
25. Cusack B, Kelly JG, Lavan J, Noel J, O'Malley K: The effect of age and smoking on theophylline kinetics. Br J Clin Pharmacol *8*:384P, 1979.
26. Mangione A, Imhoff TE, Lee RV, Shum LY, Jusko WJ: Pharmacokinetics of theophylline in hepatic disease. Chest *73*:616, 1978.
27. Piafsky KM, Sitar DS, Ogilvie RI: Effect of phenobarbital on the disposition of intravenous theophylline. Clin Pharmacol Ther *22*:336, 1977.
28. Piafsky KM, Sitar DS, Rangno RE, Ogilvie RI: Theophylline disposition in patients with hepatic cirrhosis. N Engl J Med *296*:1495, 1977.
29. Feinstein RA, Miles MV: The effects of acute viral hepatitis on theophylline clearance. Clin Pediatr *24*:357–358, 1985.
30. Ogilvie RI: Clinical pharmacokinetics of theophylline. Clin Pharmacokin *3*:237, 1978.
31. Jenne JW: Effect of disease states on theophylline elimination. J Allergy Clin Immunol *78*:727–735, 1986.
32. Lee BL, Benowitz NL, Jacob P: Cigarette abstinence, nicotine gum, and theophylline disposition Ann Intern Med *106*:553–555, 1987.
33. Jonkman JHG, Upton RA: Pharmacokinetic drug interactions with theophylline. Clin Pharmacokin *9*:309–334, 1984.
34. Jonkman JHG: Therapeutic consequences of drug interactions with theophylline pharmacokinetics. J Allergy Clin Immunol *78*:736–742, 1986.
35. Freston JW: Safety perspectives on parenteral H_2-receptor antagonists. Am J Med *83*(Suppl 68):58–67, 1987.
36. Frank WO: Safety: Cimetidine and concomitant theophylline or warfarin-drug interactions and their implications. Clin Ther *8*(Suppl A):57–68, 1986.
37. Seggev JS, Barzilay M, Schey G: No evidence for interaction between ranitidine and theophylline. Arch Intern Med *147*:179–180, 1987.
38. Chremos AN, Lin JH, Yeh KC, Chiou R, Bayne WF, Lipschultz K, Williams RL: Famotidine (F) does not interfere with the disposition of theophylline (T) in man—comparison to cimetidine (C) (abs). Clin Pharmacol Ther *39*:187, 1986.
39. Fernandes E, Melewicz FM: Ranitidine and theophylline. Ann Intern Med *100*:459, 1984.
40. Gardner ME, Sikorski GW: Ranitidine and theophylline. Ann Intern Med *102*:559, 1985.
41. Vozeh S, Powell JR, Cupit GC, Riegelman S, Sheiner LB: Influence of allopurinol on theophylline disposition in adults. Clin Pharmacol Ther *27*:194, 1980.
42. Manfredi RL, Vesell ES: Inhibition of theophylline metabolism by long-term allopurinol administration. Clin Pharmacol Ther *29*:224, 1981.
43. Harrod CS: Theophylline toxicity and nifedipine. Ann Intern Med *106*:480, 1987.
44. Parrillo SJ, Venditto M: Elevated theophylline blood

levels from institution of nifedipine therapy. Ann Emerg Med *13*:216–217, 1984.
45. Burnakis TG, Seldon M, Czaplicki AD: Increased serum theophylline concentrations secondary to oral verapamil. Clin Pharm *2*:458–461, 1983.
46. Wijnands WJA, vanHerwaarden CLA, Vree TB: Enoxacin raises plasma theophylline concentrations. Lancet *2*:108–109, 1984.
47. Maesen FPV, Teengs JP, Baur C, Davies BI: Quinolones and raised plasma concentrations of theophylline. Lancet *2*:530, 1984.
48. Raoof S, Wollschlager C, Khan FA: Ciprofloxacin increases serum levels of theophylline. Am J Med *82*(Suppl 4A):115–118, 1987.
49. Vaucher Y, Lightner ES, Walson PD: Theophylline poisoning. J Pediatr *90*:827, 1977.
50. Adam RD, Robertson C, Jarvie DR, Stewart MJ, Proudfoot AT: Clinical and metabolic features of overdosage with Amesec. Scot Med J *24*:246, 1979.
51. Loughnan PM, McNamara JM: Paroxysmal supraventricular tachycardia during theophylline therapy in a premature infant. J Pediatr *92*:1016, 1978.
52. Lawyer CH, Aitchison J, Sutton J, Bennett W: Treatment of theophylline neurotoxicity with resin hemoperfusion. Ann Intern Med *88*:516, 1978.
53. Lawyer CH, Bardana EJ, Rodgers R, Gerber N: Utilization of intravenous dihydroxypropyl theophylline (dyphylline) in an aminophylline-sensitive patient, and its pharmacokinetic comparison with theophylline. J Allergy Clin Immunol *65*:353, 1980.
54. Fleetham JA, Ginsburg JC, Nakatsu K, Wigle RD, Munt PW: Resin hemoperfusion as treatment for theophylline-induced seizures. Chest *75*:741, 1979.
55. Lesko LJ: Dose-dependent elimination kinetics of theophylline. Clin Pharmacokin *4*:449, 1979.
56. Sarrazin E, Hendeles L, Weinberger M, Muir K, Riegelman S: Dose-dependent kinetics for theophylline: Observance among ambulatory asthmatic children. J Pediatr *97*:825, 1980.
57. Weinberger M, Ginchansky E: Dose-dependent kinetics of theophylline disposition in asthmatic children. J Pediatr *91*:820, 1977.
58. Dietrich J, Krauss AN, Reidenberg M, Dreyer DE, Auld PAM: Alterations in status in apneic pre-term infants receiving theophylline. Clin Pharmacol Ther *24*:474, 1978.
59. Kuzemko JA, Paala J: Apnoeic attacks in the newborn treated with aminophylline. Arch Dis Child *48*:404, 1973.
60. Aubier M: Effect of theophylline on diaphragmatic muscle function. Chest *92*:27S–31S, 1987.
61. Matthay RA: Favorable cardiovascular effects of theophylline in COPD. Chest *92*:22S–26S, 1987.
62. Rice KL, Leatherman JW, Duane PG, Snyder LS, Harmon KR, Abel J, Niewohner DG: Aminophylline for acute exacerbations of chronic obstructive pulmonary disease: A controlled trial. Ann Intern Med *107*:305–309, 1987.
63. Jenne JW: Theophylline as a bronchodilator in COPD and its combination with inhaled β-adrenergic drugs. Chest *92*:7S–14S, 1987.
64. Hendeles L, Weinberger M, Milavetz G, Hill M III, Vaughan L: Food-induced "dose-dumping" from a once-a-day theophylline product as a cause of theophylline toxicity. Chest *87*:758–765, 1985.
65. Hendeles L, Iafrate RP, Weinberger M: A clinical and pharmacokinetic basis for the selection and use of slow release theophylline products. Clin Pharmacokin *9*:95–135, 1984.
66. Caldwell J, Monks TJ, Smith RL: A comparison of the metabolism and pharmacokinetics of intravenously administered theophylline and aminophylline in man. Br J Pharmacol *63*:369P, 1978.
67. Auritt WA, McGeady SJ, Mansmann HC Jr: The relationship of cerebrospinal fluid and plasma theophylline concentrations in children and adolescents taking theophylline. J Allergy Clin Immunol *75*:731–735, 1985.
68. Jacobs MH, Senior RM, Kessler G: Clinical experience with theophylline—relationships between dosage, serum concentration, and toxicity. JAMA *235*:1983, 1976.
69. Corser BC, Youngs C, Baughman RP: Prolonged toxicity following massive ingestion of sustained-release theophylline preparation. Chest *88*:749–750, 1985.
70. Robertson NJ: Fatal overdose from a sustained-release theophylline preparation. Ann Emerg Med *14*:154–158, 1985.
71. Clayton D, Bochner F: Delayed toxicity with slow-release theophylline. Med J Aust *144*:386–387, 1986.
72. Olson KR, Benowitz NL, Woo OF, Pond SM: Theophylline overdose: Acute single ingestion versus chronic repeated overmedication. Am J Emerg Med *3*:386–394, 1985.
73. Hendeles L, Bighley L, Richardson RH, Hepler CD, Carmichael J: Frequent toxicity from IV aminophylline infusions in critically ill patients. Drug Intell Clin Pharm *11*:12, 1977.
74. Foster LJ, Trudeau WL, Goldman AL: Bronchodilator effects on gastric acid secretion. JAMA *241*:2613, 1979.
75. Chang TMS, Espinosa-Melendez E, Francoeur TE, Eade NR: Albumin-collodion activated charcoal hemoperfusion in the treatment of severe theophylline intoxication in a 3-year-old patient. Pediatrics *65*:811, 1980.
76. Ehlers SM, Zaske DE, Sawchuk RJ: Massive theophylline overdose—rapid elimination by charcoal hemoperfusion. JAMA *240*:474, 1978.
77. Gal P, Roop C, Robinson H, Erkan NV: Theophylline-induced seizures in accidently overdosed neonates. Pediatrics *65*:547, 1980.
78. Wells DH, Ferlauto JJ: Survival after massive aminophylline overdose in a premature infant. Pediatrics *64*:252, 1979.
79. Baker MD: Theophylline toxicity in children. J Pediatr *109*:538–542, 1986.
80. Siemons LJ, Parizel G: Prolonged runs of ventricular tachycardia as a complication of theophylline intoxication: Report of a case. Acta Cardiol *41*:457–464, 1986.
81. Horowitz LN, Spear JF, Moore EN, Rogers R: Effects of aminophylline on the threshold for initiating ventricular fibrillation during respiratory failure. Am J Cardiol *35*:376, 1975.
82. Camarata SJ, Weil MH, Hanashiro PK, Shubin H: Cardiac arrest in the critically ill. I. A study of predisposing causes in 132 patients. Circulation *44*:688, 1971.
83. Habibzadeh MA: Multifocal atrial tachycardia: A 66 month follow-up of 50 patients. Heart Lung *9*:328, 1980.
84. Levine JH, Michael JR, Guarnieri T: Multifocal atrial tachycardia: A toxic effect of theophylline. Lancet *1*:12–14, 1985.
85. MacDonald JB, Jones HM, Cowan RA: Rhabdo-

myolysis and acute renal failure after theophylline overdose. Lancet *1*:932–933, 1985.
86. Modi KB, Horn EH, Bryson SM: Theophylline poisoning and rhabdomyolysis. Lancet *2*:160–161, 1985.
87. Rumpf KW, Wagner H, Criee C-P, Schwarck H, Klein H, Kreuzer H, Scheler F: Rhabdomyolysis after theophylline overdose. Lancet *1*:1451–1452, 1985.
88. Wight JP, Laurence S, Holt S, Forrest ARW: Rhabdomyolysis with hyperkalaemia after aminophylline overdose. Med Sci Law *27*:103–105, 1987.
89. Ng RH, Roe C, Funt D, Statland BE: Increased activity of creatinine kinase isoenzyme MB in a theophylline-intoxicated patient. Clin Chem *31*:1741–1742, 1985.
90. Cereda J-M, Scott J, Quigley EMM: Endoscopic removal of pharmacobezoar of slow release theophylline. Br Med J *293*:1143, 1986.
91. Wasser WG, Bronheim HE, Richardson BK: Theophylline madness. Ann Intern Med *95*:191, 1981.
92. Hall KW, Dobson KE, Dalton JG, Ghignone MC, Penner SB: Metabolic abnormalities associated with intentional theophylline overdose. Ann Intern Med *101*:457–462, 1984.
93. Kearney TE, Manoguerra AS, Curtis GP, Ziegler MG: Theophylline toxicity and the beta-adrenergic system. Ann Intern Med *102*:766–769, 1985.
94. Sawyer WT, Caravati EM, Ellison MJ, Krueger KA: Hypokalemia, hyperglycemia and acidosis after intentional theophylline overdose. Am J Emerg Med *3*:408–411, 1985.
95. McPherson ML, Prince SR, Atamer ER, Maxwell DB, Ross-Clunis H, Eslep HL: Theophylline-induced hypercalcemia. Ann Intern Med *105*:52–54, 1986.
96. Niggli F, Fanconi S, Ghelfi D: Hypokalemia in theophylline intoxication. J Pediatr *111*:157, 1987.
97. Bertino JS Jr, Walker JW Jr: Reassessment of theophylline toxicity: Serum concentrations, clinical course, and treatment. Arch Intern Med *147*:757–760, 1987.
98. Frewin DB, Cooper DJ: Accidental coadministration of intravenous aminophylline and theophylline by mouth: A hazardous practice. Med J Aust *144*:481–482, 1986.
99. Guadreault P, Wason S, Lovejoy FH Jr: Acute pediatric theophylline overdose: A summary of 28 cases. J Pediatr *102*:474–476, 1983.
100. Greenberg A, Piraino BH, Kroboth PD, Weiss J: Severe theophylline toxicity: Role of conservative measures, antiarrhythmic agents and charcoal hemoperfusion. Am J Med *76*:854–860, 1984.
101. Mountain RD, Neff TA: Oral theophylline intoxication: A serious error of patient and physician understanding. Arch Intern Med *144*:724–727, 1984.
102. Park GD, Spector K, Roberts RJ, Goldberg MJ, Weismann D, Stillerman A, Flanigan MJ: Use of hemoperfusion for treatment of theophylline intoxication. Am J Med *74*:961–966, 1983.
103. Woo OF, Pond SM, Benowitz NL, Olson KR: Benefit of hemoperfusion in acute theophylline intoxication. Clin Toxicol *22*:411–424, 1984.
104. Goldberg MJ, Park GD, Berlinger WG: Treatment of theophylline intoxication. J Allergy Clin Immunol *78*:811–817, 1986.
105. Botet MG: Systemic eczematous contact dermatitis due to the ethylenediamine fraction of aminophylline. Bol Asoc Med Puerto Rico *72*:14, 1980.
106. Booth BH, Coleman WP, Mitchell DQ: Urticaria following intravenous aminophylline. Ann Allergy *43*:289, 1979.
107. Awan NA, Miller RR, DeMaria AN, Lee G, Mason DT: Effects of morphine and aminophylline on the severity of obstruction to left ventricular outflow in idiopathic hypertrophic subaortic stenosis: Potential adverse effects in treatment of pulmonary edema. Clin Cardiol *1*:16, 1978.
108. Neuvonen PJ, Vartiainen M, Tokola O: Comparison of activated charcoal and ipecac syrup in prevention of drug absorption. Eur J Clin Pharmacol *24*:557–562, 1983.
109. Gal P, Miller A, McCue JD: Oral activated charcoal to enhance theophylline elimination in acute overdose. JAMA *251*:3130–3131, 1984.
110. Sessler CN, Glauser FL, Cooper KR: Treatment of theophylline toxicity with oral activated charcoal. Chest *87*:325–329, 1985.
111. Amitai Y, Yeung AC, Moye J, Lovejoy FH Jr: Repetitive oral activated charcoal and control of emesis in severe theophylline toxicity. Ann Intern Med *105*:386–387, 1986.
112. Rygnestad T, Walstad RA, Dahl K: Self-poisoning with theophylline: The effect of repeated doses of oral charcoal on drug elimination. Acta Med Scand *219*:425–427, 1986.
113. Ohning BL, Reed MD, Blumer JL: Continuous nasogastric administration of activated charcoal for the treatment of theophylline intoxication. Pediatr Pharmacol *5*:241–245, 1986.
114. Biberstein MP, Ziegler MG, Ward DM: Use of β-blockade and hemoperfusion for acute theophylline poisoning. West J Med *141*:485–490, 1984.
115. Amin DN, Henry JA: Propranolol administration in theophylline overdose. Lancet *1*:520–521, 1985.
116. D'Angio R, Sabatelli F: Management considerations in treating metabolic abnormalities associated with theophylline overdose. Arch Intern Med *147*:1837–1838, 1987.
117. Emonds AJG, Driessen OMJ: Treatment of theophylline intoxication: A model study utilizing peritoneal dialysis. Clin Toxicol *13*:505, 1978.
118. Levy G, Gibson TP, Whitman W, Procknal J: Hemodialysis clearance of theophylline. JAMA *237*:1466, 1977.
119. Lee CS, Marbury TC, Perrin JH, Fuller TJ: Hemodialysis of theophylline in uremic patients. J Clin Pharmacol *19*:219, 1979.
120. Krishna GG, Zahrowski JJ, Nissenson AR: Hemodialysis for theophylline overdose. Dial Transplant *12*:40–42, 1983.
121. Russo ME: Management of theophylline intoxication with charcoal-column hemoperfusion. N Engl J Med *300*:24, 1979.
122. Kelly WJW, Parkin WG: Charcoal hemoperfusion treatment of severe theophylline toxicity. Aust NZ J Med *15*:75–77, 1985.
123. O'Regan S, Robitaille PO, Mongeau JG, Yazbeck J, Boisvert F: Charcoal hemoperfusion for drug and poison intoxication in pediatric patients. Dial Transplant *14*:609–611, 1985.
124. Garella S, Lorch JA: Hemoperfusion for acute intoxication. Clin Toxicol *17*:515–527, 1980.
125. Garella S: Hemoperfusion in treatment of theophylline intoxication. Am J Med *77*:A105, 1984.

Miscellaneous Agents

CHAPTER 101
NITRATES, NITRITES, AND OTHER SOURCES OF METHEMOGLOBINEMIA

J. Ward Donovan, M.D.

Nitrates and nitrites are potent smooth muscle relaxants that produce cardiovascular effects through coronary and peripheral vasodilation. Their toxic effects are most notably an ability to induce methemoglobinemia, a property shared with a long list of other chemicals and medicinals. The proliferation of inorganic nitrites in agriculture, and the widespread abuse of organic nitrites as aphrodisiacs, make these the most common sources of methemoglobinemia. Congenital causes of methemoglobinemia also exist, as well as conditions of increased sensitivity to methemoglobin formation.[1, 2]

History and Incidence

The vasodilatory effects of the alkyl nitrites were described in 1859, and in 1867 were first used to relieve angina pectoris.[3, 4] Amyl nitrite was marketed as a prescription drug in 1937, but this restriction was lifted in 1960, leading to early reports of abuse as an over-the-counter aphrodisiac.[3] The prescription requirements for amyl nitrite were reinstated in 1968, and nitroglycerin or other organic nitrates replaced it as the preferred angina treatment.[3, 4] Butyl and isobutyl nitrite have proliferated as abused inhalants since the early 1970s, accounting for 5 to 15 $\times$ 10^7 ml used each year in the United States.[5] Up to 9 per cent of high school students have used inhaled nitrites recreationally, with 0.5 to 1 per cent using them regularly.[3] Their abuse among homosexuals ranges from 30 to 80 per cent of this group, although this has decreased recently owing to fears of a relationship between their use and acquired immune deficiency syndrome.[3, 4]

The first report of methemoglobinemia from well water contamination with nitrogen fertilizers appeared in 1945.[6] These fertilizers contain nitrites and nitrates and are often applied in excess of 200 pounds per acre per year. This has resulted in 27 to 50 per cent of private wells in some regions exceeding EPA nitrate-nitrogen standards, and 9 to 20 per cent having dangerous levels.[6, 7] Added to this is our daily dietary intake of 75 to 100 mg of nitrates.

Despite the widespread exposure to these and other methemoglobin-inducing oxidant agents, treatment of methemoglobinemia with methylene blue was reported only 117 times by American poison centers in 1987–1988.[8] This most likely reflects frequent missed diagnoses or the lack of clinically significant symptoms in most cases.

PATHOPHYSIOLOGY

Physiologic Effects of Nitrates/Nitrites

Nitrates and nitrites produce relaxation of smooth muscles in coronary arteries and peripheral arteries and especially veins, meningeal vessels, uterus, gastrointestinal tract, bronchi, biliary system, and ureters.[5, 9] Venous pooling in the lower extremities leads to a decreased cardiac preload and output, compounding the hypotension and thus ischemia of vital organs. Compensatory increases in pulse rate and arteriolar constriction ameliorate these effects, but with arteriosclerotic or cardiac disease these reflexes are limited. Inhalation of the alkyl nitrites causes upper respiratory tract irritation and, in high concentrations, may cause reflex irritation of the medullary centers, resulting in temporary hypertension and bradycardia.[5]

Physiologic Methemoglobinemia

Methemoglobin is an abnormal hemoglobin in which the usual reduced ferrous (Fe^{++}) state of the heme iron molecule is oxidized to the ferric (Fe^{+++}) form.[10–12] Some oxyhemoglobin, in fact, also exists in the ferric state physiologically through an electron transfer from oxygen to form superoxo-ferriheme ($Fe^{+++}O_2$).[12] This reactive oxidizing O_2 is protected in the hydrophobic pocket of the heme molecule. The release of oxygen occurs after the electron shift reverses and iron is returned to the normal ferrous state of oxyhemoglobin.

In contrast, methemoglobin is formed from deoxygenated hemoglobin and differs from oxyhemoglobin in that the sixth coordination position of the iron atom is bound to either a water molecule or a hydroxyl group instead of oxygen.[2, 9] It is estimated that about 3 per cent of hemoglobin is autoxidized to methemoglobin daily during the oxygenation-deoxygenation process of oxygen transport.[12] In addition to oxygen, leukocytes, drugs, and chemicals are capable of oxidizing the heme iron. Methemoglobin is incapable of reversibly binding and transporting oxygen or carbon dioxide.[10] In addition, the presence of the oxidized iron on the heme molecule increases its oxygen affinity and thereby reduces oxygen release to the tissues. This leftward shift of the oxyhemoglobin dissociation curve intensifies tissue hypoxia and cyanosis.

Methemoglobin is normally present as less than 1 per cent of the total hemoglobin under physiologic conditions.[2, 11, 12] These levels are maintained as a balance between the daily oxidation of hemoglobin and two continuously operating reducing mechanisms: the reduction of oxidizing compounds, and the reduction of formed methemoglobin back to hemoglobin.[10, 11, 13] Reduced nicotine adenine dinucleotide phosphate (NADPH) from the pentose phosphate shunt reduces glutathione, which in the presence of the enzyme glutathione reductase combines with oxidants (Fig. 101–1, pathway B).[10, 14] Oxidants are also inactivated by the enzyme catalase, and directly by ascorbic acid, sulfhydryls, and glutathione. Oxidant reduction plays a minor role in controlling methemoglobin levels, as evidenced by the fact that individuals deficient in ascorbic acid, glutathione, and catalase are not methemoglobinemic.[2, 10]

Reduction of methemoglobin occurs via two enzymatic pathways in erythrocytes. The most active physiologically is the NADH-dependent methemoglobin reductase system, also called Diaphorase I, or cytochrome b_5 reductase (see Figure 101–1, pathway C).[2, 15] NADH combines with methemoglobin in the presence of the enzyme to form hemoglobin plus NAD, and this accounts for 95 per cent of methemoglobin reduction.[10] The second pathway is catalyzed by NADPH-dependent methemoglobin reductase (Diaphorase II, or NADPH-dehydrogenase), in which NADPH combines with MetHb in the presence of the cofactor methylene blue to yield ferrous hemoglobin plus NADP (Fig. 101–1, pathway D). This pathway is dependent on a functioning hexose monophosphate shunt, which requires in its first step glucose-6-phosphate dehydrogenase (G6PD). This system accounts for less than 5 per cent of methemoglobin reduction physiologically but is a reserve system that is accelerated at least tenfold in the presence of an exogenous electron carrier such as methylene blue or riboflavin.

Methemoglobinemia is defined as a methemoglobin concentration of greater than 1 per cent, and it occurs when the production of methemoglobin exceeds the erythrocyte's reducing capacity. This may be caused by a deficiency in the normal reducing pathways, an alteration in the structure of hemoglobin rendering it resistant to reduction, or an excess of oxidizing agents like nitrites.[2, 16] The first two conditions cause congenital methemoglobinemia, while the last is defined as causing acquired, or toxic, methemoglobinemia.

Congenital Methemoglobinemia

This rare disorder is usually related to a deficiency of NADH-dependent methemoglobin reductase, which is an autosomal recessive trait.[17] Those people homozygous for the trait must utilize the less effective NADPH methemoglobin reductase and nonenzymatic pathways to reduce methemoglo-

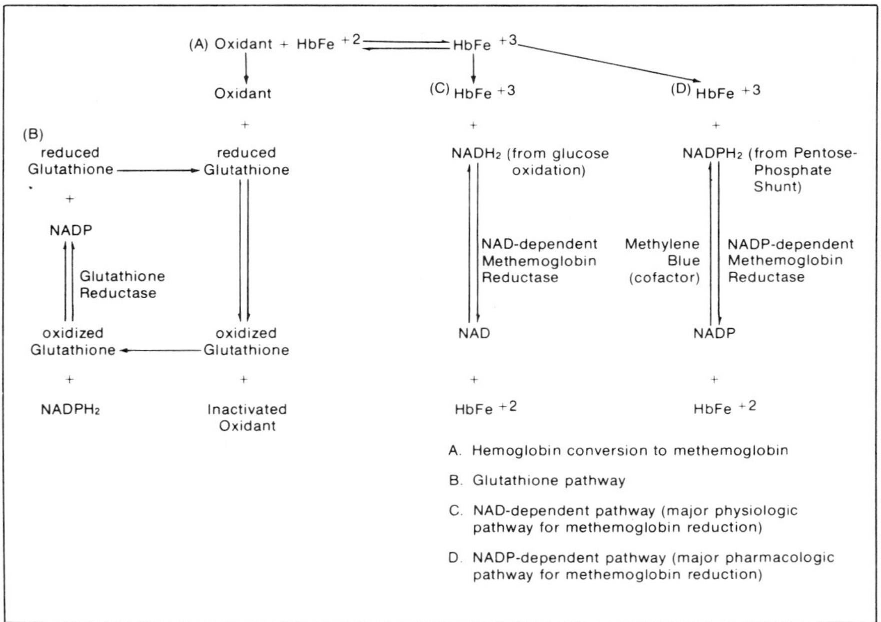

Figure 101–1. Hemoglobin ⇆ methemoglobin metabolic pathways. (From Schimelman MA, Soler JM, Muller HA: Methemoglobinemia: Nitrobenzene ingestion. J Am Coll Emerg Phys 7:406, 1978.)

bin, and chronically they have 10 to 50 per cent methemoglobin levels. Heterozygous individuals usually have normal methemoglobin concentrations, but they are particularly sensitive to oxidizing agents. The heterozygous state is reported to occur in 0.03 to 0.4 per cent of the population.[12] Some individuals with NADH methemoglobin reductase deficiency have an associated severe neurologic disorder with mental retardation owing to reductase deficiency not confined to erythrocytes. Individuals deficient in G6PD or in NADPH methemoglobin reductase do not exhibit congenital methemoglobinemia.

Hemoglobin M variants have amino acid substitutions near the heme-binding sites, causing very stable bonds between the amino acid and the heme iron.[2] These hemoglobins are readily oxidized and maintained in the ferric state and resist the normal reductive processes.[12, 18] Hemoglobin Ms are transmitted as codominant characteristics and only heterozygotes exist, since the homozygous state is incompatible with life. Those with this rare disease have methemoglobin levels of 25 to 30 per cent, and there is no effective therapy.[11, 18]

Acquired Methemoglobinemia: Sources

Agents that induce methemoglobin production at a rate faster than can be physiologically reduced include chemicals and drugs that are direct oxidants, and others that have oxidizing metabolites. Nitrites and nitrates are the greatest source of toxic methemoglobinemia and exist in organic and inorganic forms. They are found in fertilizers, anticorrosives, room odorizers, vegetables and meats, home remedies, inks, and dyes, and in pharmaceuticals to treat coronary disease, cystitis, diarrhea, vomiting, burns, and cyanide poisoning.[5, 10, 13, 14] Nitrites are much stronger oxidizing agents than nitrates, which must be converted by bacteria to nitrites.[19]

The inorganic nitrates include potassium, sodium, and calcium nitrates, also known as saltpeter.[20] Ingestion of these compounds is most commonly due to well water contaminated by nitrogenous fertilizers, animal organic waste, or seepage from septic tanks. The nitrate ion is formed from the oxidation of ammonia by soil or water microorganisms or both.[6, 7] Methemoglobin production depends upon conversion to nitrites by gastrointestinal microorganisms having nitrate reductase.[21] These include *Escherichia coli, Pseudomonas aeruginosa,* and *Aerobacter aerogenes* found in saliva and in the intestines.[22–24] The use of well water contaminated with 94 mg/L of nitrate nitrogen for home dialysis has caused severe methemoglobinemia.[23]

This was probably due to passive transport of nitrates into the bowel where conversion to nitrites occurred and was complicated by the patient's existing anemia. Another major natural source of nitrates is vegetables, which, through chemical reduction within the plants or from bacterial contamination during preparation, yield nitrites.[25] Carrots, cabbage, beets, celery, lettuce, and spinach contain the highest amounts of nitrates, greater than 1500 mg/kg.[7, 25] Bismuth subnitrate used as an antidiarrheal and ammonium nitrate used for diuresis also have caused toxicity.[23, 26] Silver nitrate has induced methemoglobinemia when used for the local treatment of burns and cystitis, and molten nitrate salts have caused fatal methemoglobinemia.[15, 24, 27]

Inorganic nitrites are also found in soil, water, and sewage because of reduction of nitrates or ammonia by microorganisms.[13] Overuse of nitrite salts as curing agents, preservatives, and color enhancers in meat, cheeses, and fish has caused methemoglobinemia.[13, 28, 29] Accidental exposures leading to isolated epidemics have occurred from confusing sodium nitrite for table salt. Contamination of foods with cooling fluid containing sodium nitrite as an anticorrosive has resulted in deaths.[13] Finally, sodium nitrite is used therapeutically to treat cyanide toxicity, inducing methemoglobin production and the formation of cyanmethemoglobin. Methemoglobin concentrations as high as 58 per cent have occurred even with proper dosing.[30]

The organic nitrates are used as coronary and peripheral vasodilators for the treatment of angina and heart failure. Formulations include the short-acting nitroglycerin and the long-acting preparations isosorbide dinitrate, pentaerythritol tetranitrate, and erythrityl tetranitrate. Methemoglobin may be produced after the metabolism of these agents to nitrites by reductive hydrolysis, catalyzed by glutathione organic nitrate reductase in the liver.[22] Usual doses of these agents do not induce significant methemoglobin elevations, but excessive use has led to clinical symptoms in the presence of anemia or cardiac disease.[22, 31, 32] Nitroglycerin is used in explosives manufacturing, and workers have been reported to suffer coronary vasospasm upon withdrawal from chronic exposure.[5, 33]

The organic nitrites amyl, butyl, and isobutyl nitrite are now widely abused by inhalation as aphrodisiacs to enhance penile erection and to relax the anal sphincter and smooth muscle of the rectum.[5, 34] They are also claimed to heighten sexual stimulation, prolong duration, and delay ejaculation, all possibly due to the sensation of the cerebral rush.[4, 35] They are sold in liquid form as room odorizers, or in small glass ampules known as "snappers" or "poppers." Amyl nitrite is also included in the Lilly Cyanide Kit to induce methemoglobinemia, but in the recommended doses the level induced is insignificant.[36] However, abuse by inhalation and particularly ingestion of the volatile nitrites can cause severe toxicity and death.[9, 35, 37] Ethyl nitrite is found in a folk remedy called sweet spirits of nitre and caused the death of a child following ingestion.[38]

Non-nitrate therapeutic agents reported to cause methemoglobinemia include sodium nitroprusside, metoclopramide, sulfamethoxazole, prilocaine, benzocaine, lidocaine, phenazopyridine, quinone antimalarials, and dapsone.[39–46] Chlorate salts used in toothpastes and throat soothants, and potassium permanganate in herbal preparations, are other "medicinals" causing methemoglobinemia by accidental or suicidal overdose.[47, 48] Toxic cases with these drugs are usually the result of accidental, suicidal, or iatrogenic overdose, or from use in those with deficient reduction systems. Rare cases result from recommended doses in normal adults.[18, 41, 43, 45, 49]

Aniline has been a common methemoglobin-inducer due to its ready absorption from dermal and ingested sources, such as inks, dyes, shoe polish, paints, varnishes, and gasoline additives.[21, 50–52] It is postulated that aniline must be metabolized to the oxidative intermediate phenylhydroxylamine to cause methemoglobinemia and then is cyclically oxidized and reduced, increasing the duration and severity of toxicity.

Smoke inhalation has been suggested to induce methemoglobinemia, presumably by inhalation of oxides of nitrogen from burning plastics.[53] Reported methemoglobinemia levels of 12 to 19 per cent, together with carbon monoxide impairment of oxygen transport and release, could cause significant clinical effects.

A list of modern methemoglobin-inducing agents and their common uses can be found in Table 101–1.

Table 101–1. METHEMOGLOBIN-INDUCING AGENTS

AGENT	USE/SOURCE	REFERENCE
Aniline	Inks, dyes, shoe polish, photo developers, varnish, paints, fuel additive	21, 50–52
Benzocaine	Topical anesthetic	18, 56
Betanaphthol disulfonate	R salt	19
Chlorate salts	Matchheads, toothpaste, throat soothants	47
Chloroquine	Antimalarial	11
Copper sulfate	Emetic, fungicide, astringent	59
Dapsone	Dermatologic, antimalarial	39, 54
Lidocaine	Local and IV anesthetic, antiarrhythmic	18, 49
Metoclopramide	Antiemetic	44, 46
Methylene blue	Medical dye, methemoglobin therapy	60
Monolinuron	Urea herbicide	58
Naphthalene	Mothballs, deodorizers	11
Nitrates		
Sodium, potassium, calcium nitrate	Contaminated water, fertilizers, food preservatives, vegetables	6, 19, 20, 21, 23, 25
Bismuth subnitrate	Antidiarrheal	23, 26
Ammonium nitrate	Diuretic, fertilizer	10, 23
Silver nitrate	Topical burn therapy	24
Isosorbide dinitrate/tetranitrates	Vasodilator	22, 55
Nitrites		
Amyl nitrite	Cyanide therapy, vasodilator, abused inhalant	5, 57
Butyl nitrite	Room odorizers, abused inhalant	5, 57
Isobutyl nitrite	Room odorizer, abused inhalant	5, 9, 35, 37
Sodium nitrite	Cyanide therapy, food preservative, anticorrosive	13, 15, 29, 30
Ethyl nitrite	Folk medicine	38
Nitrobenzene	Solvent, polishes	14
Nitrogen oxide	Fires, silage	53
Nitroglycerin	Vasodilator, explosives	31–33
Permanganate salts	Folk remedy	48
Phenacetin	Analgesic	11
Phenazopyridine	Urinary tract analgesic	42
Phenols	Disinfectants	61
Prilocaine	Local, caudal, epidural anesthesia	45
	Epidural anesthetic	10
Primaquine	Antimalarial	54
Sulfonamides	Antibacterial	43
Toluidine	Methemoglobin antidote, dye, artificial fingernails	30, 56

Infant Methemoglobinemia

Infants are particularly sensitive to methemoglobin inducers due to their transient deficiency in methemoglobin reductase, their low levels of erythrocyte NADH, and the greater susceptibility of hemoglobin F (fetal hemoglobin) to oxidation.[1, 21, 29, 46] NADH-dependent methemoglobin reductase activity in neonates is 60 per cent of adult levels, and hemoglobin F is 60 to 80 per cent of the circulating hemoglobin.[6, 21, 26] Near-adult levels of methemoglobin reductase and hemoglobin A are reached by 4 months of age.[21, 25] Another factor increasing infant risk is their greater nitrate intake from food and contaminated water relative to body weight and total hemoglobin. Additionally, a higher gastric pH in infants from limited acid secretion allows bacterial proliferation and thus increased conversion of dietary nitrates to nitrites. This may be exaggerated in infants with gastroenteritis, who can develop a syndrome of dehydration, acidosis, and methemoglobinemia.[1, 26] These risks have led to recommendations that, for infants, water for preparing formulas always contain less than 10 ppm of nitrate-nitrogen, that the therapeutic use of oxidants be limited, and that vegetables with high nitrate content not be included in infant diets.[21, 25, 62]

Hemolysis

Nitrates, nitrites, and other oxidizing agents can precipitate an intravascular hemolysis with formation of Heinz bodies, which are aggregates of denatured hemoglobin.[50, 51, 57] The resultant anemia compounds the hypoxic effects of methemoglobinemia. Implicated substances have included volatile nitrites, cresol, hydroxyquinone, chlorate salts, aniline, nitrobenzene, dapsone, phenazopyridine, toluidine, and methylene blue.[14, 47, 50, 51, 56, 57]

RANGE OF TOXICITY

Nitrates and Nitrites

Acute ingestion of 10 mg of sodium nitrite has caused flushing and headache because of the vasodilatory effects.[28] Administration of 600 mg to an adult for treatment of cyanide toxicity resulted in a methemoglobin level of 58 per cent.[30] The estimated lethal dose ranges from 2 to 6 grams in adults.[13] It is thought that doses of less than 10 mg/kg/day of nitrates and 0.8 mg/kg/day of nitrites will not cause methemoglobinemia in adults, but infants and those with reducing deficiencies may tolerate much less.[15–21] However, infants ingesting 1 to 15 mg/kg/day of nitrates in well water did not exhibit clinical methemoglobinemia, and the maximum methemoglobin level was 5.3 per cent.[21] The U.S. Public Health Service maximum recommended levels in drinking water are 45 ppm (mg/L) for nitrate (NO_3) or 10 ppm for nitrate-nitrogen (NO_3–N).[1, 21] An infant death was traced to formula prepared for 2 months with well water containing 150 ppm of NO_3–N.[62] Although 80 per cent of contaminated well water cases had concentrations greater than 100 ppm, NO_3–N levels as low as 10 to 20 ppm in water have led to mild methemoglobinemia.[21] Use of well water containing 94 ppm of NO_3–N for hemodialysis resulted in methemoglobinemia; maximum water levels of 2 ppm of NO_3 are recommended for this use.[21, 23]

Recreational inhalation of the volatile organic nitrites over a period of several hours has caused significant methemoglobinemia, and ingestion of 10 to 15 ml has caused severe symptoms and death.[9, 34, 35, 37] Workers exposed to ambient butyl nitrite concentrations of 25 to 155 ppm in a bottling plant developed average methemoglobin levels of 5 per cent but no clinical effects.[37] Inhalation of amyl nitrite from the Lilly Cyanide Kit for 5 minutes yielded maximum levels of only 2.2 per cent.[36]

Intravenous nitroglycerin has been reported to induce a methemoglobin level of over 12 per cent and contributed to death at infusion rates of 10 to 58 μg/kg/min for several hours.[31] An average of 77 mg/day of oral isosorbide dinitrate produced average methemoglobin levels of only 1.78 per cent and a maximum of 5.1 per cent. Forty mg of sublingual nitroglycerin with 60 mg of isosorbide dinitrate over 36 hours resulted in a level of 7 per cent.[22, 32]

Other Oxidants

Ingestion of 25 to 65 mg of aniline can cause methemoglobinemia, and as little as 1 gram has caused death.[51] Benzocaine doses greater than 15 to 25 mg/kg can induce clinically appreciated methemoglobinemia, and ingestion of 560 mg (40 mg/kg) elevated the methemoglobin concentration to 59 per cent.[63] The administration of 1 to 6 mg/kg of metoclopramide over 2 days to infants has resulted in methemoglobin levels of 20 to 23 per cent.[44, 46]

PHARMACOKINETICS

The nitrates and nitrites are ordinarily very rapidly absorbed, but the duration of metabolism, elimination, and effects depends upon multiple factors. Intravenous injection of sodium nitrite causes peak effects within 30 minutes.[30] The organic nitrates by inhalation show onset of cardiovascular effects within 10 seconds, peak at 30 to 60 seconds, and normalize by 90 seconds.[36, 37] They are hydrolyzed almost immediately to the nitrite ion and alcohol.

The required metabolism of nitrates to the methemoglobin-inducing nitrites would be expected to delay the onset of effects. Nitrates are metabolized in the liver by glutathione reductase to nitrites, which are eliminated by the kidneys.[31] Hepatic and renal dysfunction, therefore, may prolong the metabolism and excretion. Isosorbide dinitrate peaks at 1.5 hours and undergoes hepatic biotransformation.[55] This process becomes saturated with high chronic oral doses, and significant concentrations persist for 3 to 4 hours.

The elimination half-life of physiologic methemoglobin is 55 minutes by first-order kinetics, but this is prolonged in methemoglobin reductase–deficient patients to 126 minutes.[64] The elimination process appears to become saturated, because the spontaneous half-life at methemoglobin levels of 80 per cent is 15 to 20 hours.[42, 65]

CLINICAL EFFECTS

Acute

Nitrates and Nitrites

The effects of nitrates and nitrites depend upon the form, route, and dosage but in general involve the cardiovascular, metabolic, and neurologic effects of vasodilation and hypoxia. Inhalation of the volatile nitrates cause a fall in systolic blood pressure within 30 to 60 seconds, with maximum effect in 1 to 3 minutes.[5, 37] The diastolic pressure changes lag behind the systolic fall and recovery, so the pulse pressure is initially reduced and then increases. The pulse rate reflexively increases, and there may occur flushing in skin, pulsatile headache, euphoria, weakness, blurred vision, increased ocular pressure, confusion, lightheadedness, diaphoresis, and syncope.[3–5] Nausea and vomiting may occur with ingestion or inhalation. Pulmonary irritation and even respiratory failure may occur with the inhaled nitrites, and cardiovascular collapse can occur from marked vasodilation, decreased cardiac output, and vital organ anoxia. The volatile nitrites also have been reported to cause transient inversion of T waves and ST depression.[4, 57]

Methemoglobinemia

The initial manifestation of methemoglobinemia is darkened blood and a slate gray cyanosis, which in mild cases may appear only on the lips and mucous membranes. The blood and skin color is due to the spectral color characteristics of the abnormal pigment rather than being manifestations of hypoxia.[66] The patient may appear deeply cyanotic and yet be completely asymptomatic at lower concentrations. Total methemoglobin of 1.5 gm/dl, equivalent to 10 to 15 per cent of the circulating hemoglobin in a non-anemic individual, imparts a cyanosis equivalent to that seen when 5.0 gm/dl of hemoglobin is deoxygenated.[31, 48] The appearance of cyanosis also depends on the total hemoglobin, oxygen saturation, skin pigmentation, and ambient lighting.[12] The clinical effects are determined by the cardiopulmonary status and the total methemoglobin rather than just the methemoglobin percentage. Those methemoglobin-inducing agents that also cause a hemolytic anemia compound the effects. An anemic individual will be less tolerant of an increased methemoglobin level, which in effect reduces further the red cells available for oxygen transport.

In normal individuals, methemoglobin levels must be greater than 10 per cent to be clinically recognized, and only mild symptoms of headache, fatigue, and nausea occur at levels of 20 to 30 per cent.[23, 29, 37] Dyspnea on exertion, lethargy, and tachycardia may be noted at 30 to 45 per cent levels, and at

50 to 70 per cent, arrhythmias, coma, seizures, respiratory distress, and lactate acidosis develop. Levels greater than 70 per cent cause cardiovascular collapse and have a high degree of mortality if untreated. Deaths from nitrates/nitrites or other oxidants are relatively uncommon but have resulted from large suicidal ingestions, prolonged abuse of volatile nitrites, ingestion of contaminated food, herbal medication use, industrial accidents, and chronic ingestion of well water in infants.[9, 13, 15, 34, 38, 62]

Chronic Effects of Nitrates and Nitrites

Repetitive abuse of nitrite inhalants can cause crusting skin lesions and tracheobronchial irritation, with hemoptysis and dyspnea.[3, 4] Telangiectasia has resulted from chronic abuse of the organic nitrates, presumably due to prolonged vasodilation.[67] Industrial exposure by inhalation of organic nitrites has caused respiratory failure, left ventricular hypertrophy, and fatal myocardial infarctions upon withdrawal.[4, 5, 33, 68]

Mutagenic, Teratogenic, and Carcinogenic Effects

Inorganic and organic nitrites can react with amines and amides (amino acids, peptides, proteins) to form *N*-nitrosamines and nitrosamides, which are known to be carcinogenic, mutagenic, and teratogenic.[4, 68] Inorganic nitrates in food are also a source of *N*-nitroso compounds through their conversion to nitrites by salivary and gastric microorganisms.[69] *N*-Nitroso compounds have been found to cause gastric, bladder, esophageal and intestinal cancer in animals but have not been linked to human cancer.[3, 4, 68, 69] Studies of nitrate fertilizer workers showed no increase in cancer rates or death over cohorts despite the presence of significantly increased *N*-nitroso compounds.[69] Volatile nitrites also have immunosuppressive effects that can occur after only a few hours of exposure. This and the carcinogenic effect of nitrosamines have led to suggestions of a relationship between the abuse of nitrites by homosexuals with AIDS and the development both of opportunistic infections and Kaposi's sarcoma.[3]

A relationship between fetal malformations and maternal ingestion of high-nitrate drinking water has been suggested. However, studies in animals have not been able to identify nitrates as specific teratogens.[21] Very high nitrate concentrations in water ingested by breast-feeding mothers have been reported to cause methemoglobinemia in infants, but appreciable amounts of nitrate transfer in human milk ordinarily does not occur. Nitrites can cross the mammalian placenta, but there is no evidence of fetal effects, and the fetus was not affected in a case of nitrite-induced maternal methemoglobinemia.[21, 70]

DIAGNOSIS

The diagnosis of nitrate, nitrite, or other oxidizing agent toxicity is usually made by a history of exposure, the presence of hypotension, and a deep cyanosis of the skin and mucous membranes. Cardiac and pulmonary dysfunction cause cyanosis because of large amounts of circulating deoxyhemoglobin, but, unlike methemoglobinemia, they respond at least partially to high-flow oxygen. The cyanosis of methemoglobinemia is disproportionate to the symptoms in mild-to-moderate cases and has been described variously as a chocolate brown or slate gray color. An aid in the differential diagnosis is to expose or shake the blood in air, which will turn deoxyhemoglobin red but not affect methemoglobin. Comparing a drop of the dried blood on filter paper with normal blood may be of limited help in recognizing the chocolate appearance. In one study, all examiners perceived the blood to be dark at methemoglobin concentrations of 35 per cent, but only half described a chocolate color.[71] At methemoglobin concentrations of 12 to 14 per cent, only one half of examiners appreciate any color difference at all. The blood pH may alter the color change, since methemoglobin is reddish-brown in alkaline medium and brown in acidemia.[12]

Cyanide and carbon monoxide toxicity may cause respiratory depression and cyanosis, which will clear with pulmonary support and oxygen, in contrast to methemoglobin. Confusion between cyanide and nitrobenzene toxicity may occur because both can have a bitter almond odor.[14, 16] Victims of smoke inhalation can have a combination of carboxyhemoglobinemia, methemoglobinemia, and cyanide toxicity.[53]

Sulfhemoglobin is another abnormal pigmented molecule that is an ineffective oxygen carrier and produces a clinical picture similar to that of methemoglobinemia.[66] Unlike methemoglobin, sulfhemoglobin is neither naturally occurring nor reversible to reduced hemoglobin and remains until the erythrocyte is destroyed or removed by exchange transfusion. The patient with sulfhemoglobinemia appears even bluer than those with methemoglobinemia, owing to different spectral characteristics. Symptoms are milder, however, because sulfhemoglobin shifts the oxyhemoglobin dissociation curve to the right, enhancing oxygen release to tissues. The blood colors are similar, but methemoglobinemia can be differentiated from sulfhemoglobinemia by diluting the blood 1:100 in deionized water with a crystal of potassium cyanide. Methemoglobinemic, but not sulfhemoglobinemic, blood turns pink owing to the formation of cyanomethemoglobin.[10] The causes of sulfhemoglobin overlap with agents causing methemoglobin and include phenacetin, acetanilid, sulfonamides, dapsone, hydroxylamine, and hydrogen sulfide.[66]

LABORATORY STUDIES

With significant nitrate/nitrite toxicity and methemoglobinemia, arterial blood gases reveal a lactate metabolic acidosis from tissue ischemia and hypoxia. The PO_2 remains normal, but the measured (not calculated) oxygen saturation will be low. Transcutaneous pulse oximetry estimations of oxygen saturation will be lowered by methemoglobinemia.[41] Spuriously high pulse oximetry readings are possible with increasing concentrations, so it is advisable to measure oxygen saturation directly if methemoglobinemia is suspected. Methylene blue used for therapy will cause a spurious pulse oximeter desaturation despite clinical improvement.

Methemoglobin concentrations should be quantified by spectrophotometry and repeated serially because of prolonged methemoglobin induction by some agents. Concentrations will be falsely low if not measured immediately, through the action of endogenous methemoglobin reductase.[37, 72] Methemoglobin may be reported as a percentage of the total hemoglobin or as an absolute amount in gm/dl. To convert the latter to a percentage, simply divide the amount of methemoglobin by the total hemoglobin and multiply by 100.

If a co-oximeter is used, the presence of sulfhemoglobin may cause falsely elevated methemoglobin levels.[72] Sulfhemoglobinemia can be differentiated from methemoglobinemia by spectrophotometry when potassium cyanide is added to the sample. The characteristic methemoglobin absorption peak at 630 nm disappears because of cyanmethemoglobin formation, but the sulfhemoglobin band at 620 nm remains.[12] Because this technique does not differentiate sulfhemoglobin from certain abnormal hemoglobins, further spectrophotometric and isoelectric focusing methods are recommended.[66]

All patients with methemoglobinemia should have hemoglobin electrophoresis performed to check for dyshemoglobinemias. Evaluation also should include determination of methemoglobin reductase and G6PD activity.[2, 12] Urinalysis may show a brown-black color, and casts or protein may be found.[10, 11]

TREATMENT

General

The cyanotic patient initially should receive airway management, respiratory support, and high-flow oxygen therapy. If the level of consciousness is depressed, administer naloxone and 50 per cent dextrose. For ingestions, gastric decontamination is indicated if done within 2 to 4 hours after exposure. Activated charcoal will adsorb most methemoglobin inducers and also should be given. Because of the high dermal and pulmonary absorption of some oxidizing agents, remove contaminated clothing, flush the skin, and protect health care workers from exposure. Hypotension from nitrate/nitrite vasodilation or reduced cardiac output usually responds to intravenous fluids and the Trendelenburg position, but it may require vasopressors. Patients with symptomatic methemoglobinemia require intensive care monitoring until symptoms clear and the methemoglobin level is below 15 per cent.

Methylene Blue

Methylene blue is the antidote of choice for acquired (toxic) methemoglobinemia.[10, 11, 50, 51] It acts as an exogenous cofactor to greatly accelerate the NADPH-dependent methemoglobin reductase system (see Fig. 101–1, pathway D).[2, 10] This system requires the production of reduced NADPH by the pentose phosphate shunt, as well as the presence of the enzyme and cofactor.[12, 51] Methylene blue in its oxidized form is reduced to the colorless leukomethylene blue by accepting electrons from NADPH. Leukomethylene blue in turn acts as an electron donor to reduce methemoglobin to hemoglobin (Fig. 101–2). Leukomethylene blue is excreted in the urine and bile.[10, 50]

Treatment with methylene blue is indicated for acquired methemoglobinemia when the level is greater than 35 to 40 per cent and the patient has cardiorespiratory symptoms.[10, 12, 50] These guidelines do not apply to patients with pre-existing anemia or cardiovascular disease, who may warrant therapy with levels as low as 15 per cent, or about 2 to 3 gm/dl of methemoglobin.[23, 31] The initial dosage is 1 to 2 mg/kg, or 0.1 to 0.2 ml/kg of the 1 per cent solution given intravenously over 5 minutes.[50, 51] Response occurs within 1 hour and reduces the elimination half-life of severe methemoglobinemia to 45 to 90 minutes.[50, 65] Methemoglobin levels should be checked 1 hour after infusion, and a repeat dose may be warranted if levels remain high and the patient is still symptomatic.

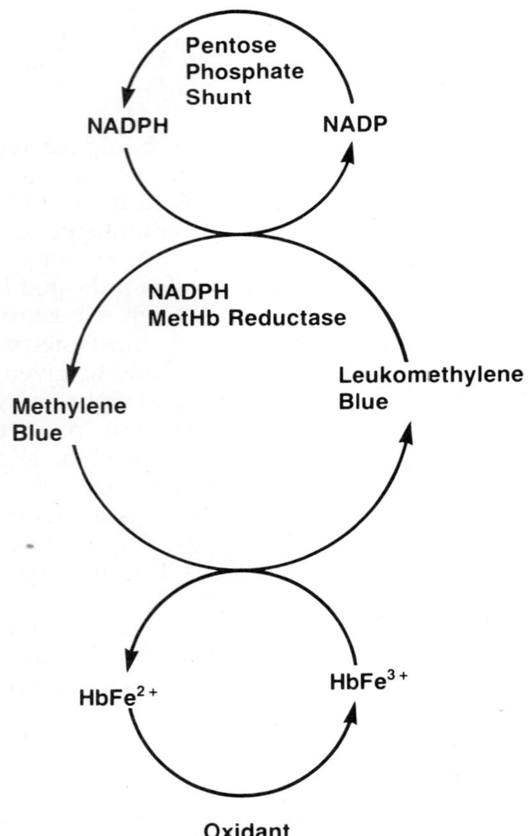

Figure 101–2. Reduction pathway of methemoglobin by methylene blue.

Failure to respond to methylene blue can result from errors in diagnosis, inborn metabolic deficiencies, or characteristics of the toxin. Sulfhemoglobinemia has no effective treatment, and its presence alone or in conjunction with methemoglobinemia will yield a partial or no response. A G6PD deficiency in the pentose phosphate shunt impairs NADPH production and thus the necessary conversion of methylene blue to leukomethylene blue. A deficiency of NADPH methemoglobin reductase likewise limits this conversion. Therefore, treatment failures should be tested for these abnormalities. G6PD activity may be falsely normal if the sample is obtained in the presence of hemolysis and should be repeated later.[51] Exposure to toxins such as aniline or dapsone, which have prolonged absorption and cyclic production of methemoglobin, may respond incompletely or even worsen with multiple doses of methylene blue.[50–52] Phenylhydroxylamine, a metabolite of aniline, also competitively blocks the uptake of methylene blue into erythrocytes and may further limit its efficacy.[52] Another oxidant, hydroxylamine, not only blocks the uptake of methylene blue but also inhibits the activity of methemoglobin reductase.

Hazards of Methylene Blue. Methylene blue in therapeutic doses causes a bluish discoloration of the urine and skin, creating a cyanotic appearance and confusing clinical assessment. Excretion in the urine can cause bladder irritation.[12] In higher doses, methylene blue itself is an oxidizing agent, and as little as 5 mg/kg has caused asymptomatic methemoglobinemia.[35, 60] Cumulative doses greater than 7 mg/kg have an increased risk of methemoglobin induction and can cause chest pain, nausea, vomiting, dizziness, hypertension, confusion, diaphoresis, tremor, dyspnea, and cyanosis.[50, 63] However, a total dose of 15 mg/kg produced no untoward effects in one reported case.[51]

Excess methylene blue can cause hemolysis, particularly in infants and in those with

G6PD deficiency.[9, 16, 50, 51] Administration of 2 to 4 mg/kg of methylene blue to neonates has induced a Heinz body hemolytic anemia.[73] Methylene blue is contraindicated in G6PD deficiency because of this risk and its ineffectiveness.

Hemolysis is also a particular risk when treating aniline toxicity with methylene blue, so additional doses should be given with caution. The hemolytic anemia may be delayed for 1 week, and methemoglobin formation may be prolonged in these patients.[51]

Methylene blue is hazardous in cases of methemoglobinemia caused by the use of sodium nitrite for cyanide toxicity, because of the release of cyanide, which may cause enhanced toxicity.[30]

Adjunctive Therapies of Methemoglobinemia

If therapy of acquired methemoglobinemia with methylene blue is contraindicated, ineffective, or unavailable, other modalities may have some effect. Ascorbic acid is often mentioned as an alternative therapy, but its reducing effect is probably too slow to have significant benefit.[10, 11] One case of 70 to 80 per cent methemoglobinemia and G6PD deficiency was reported to survive with oxygen and intravenous ascorbate treatment, but supportive care alone may be successful.[12] In addition to offering little advantage over normal endogenous pathways, ascorbic acid may acidify the urine and increase the risk of myoglobinuric renal failure.[51]

Exchange transfusion is indicated in severe cases if methylene blue fails, for it has the advantage of replacing methemoglobin, correcting hemolytic anemia, and removing the absorbed toxin.[13, 51, 52, 65] Exchange transfusions equal to less than the total blood volume and up to greater than twice the volume have been used.[14, 16, 65]

Hyperbaric oxygen may be helpful as a temporizing or additional measure and has been shown to reduce methemoglobin levels and mortality in mice.[16, 74] In addition to bypassing the oxygen transport dysfunctions of methemoglobin, hyperbaric oxygen may limit the oxidation of hemoglobin.[65, 74]

Therapy of Congenital Methemoglobinemia

Those with hereditary methemoglobinemia due to NADH–methemoglobin reductase deficiency tolerate levels of up to 40 per cent without serious effects but may have exertional dyspnea as well as cosmetically displeasing cyanosis.[10, 12] Ascorbic acid nonenzymatically reduces methemoglobin and is the preferred treatment for these cases, in a dosage of 200 to 1000 mg orally daily.[10, 75] Unfortunately, it can cause bladder and gastric irritation, increased oxalate excretion, and nephrolithiasis.[12, 75] An alternative is oral methylene blue in a dosage of 100 to 300 mg daily (3 to 5 mg/kg), but it discolors the urine and also can cause bladder and gastric irritation.[17]

Riboflavin has been reported to be effective in activating the NADPH reductase system, and it appears to be useful for the treatment of congenital methemoglobinemia.[17, 75] This therapy is particularly useful in those unable to tolerate methylene blue or ascorbate and may be the drug of choice because of its lack of untoward reactions. Oral doses of 20 to 120 mg per day in divided doses have been used.

There is no therapy for congenital methemoglobinemia caused by hemoglobin M or unstable hemoglobins, but fortunately these are usually benign conditions.[12]

References

1. Dagan R, Zaltzstein E, Gorodischer R: Methaemoglobinemia in young infants with diarrhea. Eur J Pediatr *147*:87–89, 1988.
2. Jaffe ER: Methemoglobin pathophysiology. *In* The Function of Red Blood Cells: Erythrocyte Pathobiology. New York, Liss Inc, 1981, pp 133–151.
3. Haverkos HW, Dougherty J: Health hazards of nitrite inhalants. Am J Med *84*:479–482, 1988.
4. Newell GR, Mansell PWA, Spitz MR, Reuben JM, Hersh EM: Volatile nitrites: Use and adverse effects related to the current epidemic of the acquired immune deficiency syndrome. Am J Med *78*:811–816, 1985.
5. Haley TJ: Review of the physiological effects of amyl, butyl and isobutyl nitrites. Clin Toxicol *16*:317–329, 1980.
6. Lukens JN: The legacy of well-water methemoglobinemia. JAMA *257*:2793–2795, 1987.
7. Johnson CA: Methemoglobinemia: Is it coming back to haunt us? Health Environ Digest *1*(12):3–4, 1988.
8. Litovitz TL, Schmitz BF, Matyunas N, Martin TG: 1987 Annual report of the American Association of Poison Control Centers national data collection system. Am J Emerg Med *6*:479–515, 1988.
9. Dixon DS, Reisch RF, Santinga PH: Fatal methemoglobinemia resulting from ingestion of isobutyl nitrite. J Forensic Sci *26*:587–593, 1981.
10. Curry S: Methemoglobinemia. Ann Emerg Med *11*:214–221, 1982.
11. Hall AH, Kulig KW, Rumack BH: Drug and chemi-

cal-induced methaemoglobinaemia: Clinical features and management. Med Toxicol *1*:253–260, 1986.
12. Mansouri A: Review: Methemoglobinemia. Am J Med Sci *289*:200–209, 1985.
13. Ten Brink WAG, Wiezer JHA, Luijpen AFMG, et al: Nitrate poisoning caused by food contaminated with cooling fluid. J Toxicol Clin Toxicol *19*:139–147, 1982.
14. Schimelman MA, Soler JM, Muller HA: Methemoglobinemia: Nitrobenzene ingestion. J Am Coll Emerg Phys *7*:406–408, 1978.
15. Harris JC, Rumack BH, Peterson RG, McGuire BM: Methemoglobinemia resulting from absorption of nitrates. JAMA *242*:2869–2871, 1979.
16. Harrison MR: Toxic methaemoglobinemia. Anaesthesia *32*:270–272, 1977.
17. Hirano M, Matsuki T, Tanishima K, et al: Congenital methaemoglobinemia due to NADH methaemoglobin reductase deficiency: Successful treatment with oral riboflavin. Br J Haematol *47*:353–359, 1981.
18. O'Donohue WJ, Moss LN, Angelillo VA: Acute methemoglobinemia induced by topical benzocaine and lidocaine. Arch Intern Med *140*:1508–1509, 1980.
19. Johnson PN, Sullivan FM, Lewander WJ: Methemoglobinemia following occupational exposure to sodium betanaphthol disulfonate (R salt). Vet Hum Toxicol *29*:460, 1987.
20. Patterson JW: Chemical composition for saltpeter. J Am Acad Dermatol *11*:309–310, 1984.
21. Fan AM, Willhite CC, Book SA: Evaluation of the nitrate drinking water standard with reference to infant methemoglobinemia and potential reproductive toxicity. Regul Toxicol Pharmacol *7*:135–148, 1987.
22. Arsura E, Lichstein E, Guadagnino V, et al: Methemoglobin levels produced by organic nitrates in patients with coronary artery disease. J Clin Pharmacol *24*:160–164, 1984.
23. Carlson DJ, Shapiro FL: Methemoglobinemia from well water nitrates: A complication of home dialysis. Ann Intern Med *73*:757–759, 1970.
24. Cushing AH, Smith S: Methemoglobinemia with silver nitrate therapy of a burn: Report of a case. J Pediatr *74*:613–615, 1969.
25. Keating JP, Lell ME, Strauss AW, Zarkowsky H, Smith GE: Infantile methemoglobinemia caused by carrot juice. N Engl J Med *288*:824–826, 1973.
26. Yano SS, Danish EH, Hsia YE: Transient methemoglobinemia with acidosis in infants. J Pediatr *100*:415–418, 1982.
27. Jerkins GR, Noe HN, Hill DE: An unusual complication of silver nitrate treatment of hemorrhagic cystitis: Case report. J Urol *136*:456–458, 1986.
28. Henderson WR, Raskin NH: Hot dog headache: Individual susceptibility to nitrite. Lancet *2*:1162–1163, 1972.
29. Walley T, Flanagan M: Nitrite-induced methemoglobinemia. Postgrad Med J *63*:643–644, 1987.
30. Van Heijst ANP, Douze JMC, Van Kesteren RG: Therapeutic problems in cyanide poisoning. Clin Toxicol *25*:383–398, 1987.
31. Bojar RM, Rastegar H, Payne DD, et al: Methemoglobinemia from intravenous nitroglycerin: A word of caution. Ann Thorac Surg *43*:332–334, 1987.
32. Marshall JB, Ecklund RE: Methemoglobinemia from overdose of nitroglycerin. JAMA *244*:330, 1980.
33. Przybojewski JZ, Heyns MH: Acute myocardial infarction due to coronary vasospasm secondary to industrial nitroglycerin withdrawal. S Afr Med J *64*:101–104, 1983.
34. O'Toole JB, Robbins GB, Dixon DS: Ingestion of isobutyl nitrite, a recreational chemical of abuse, causing fatal methemoglobinemia. J Forensic Sci *32*:1811–1812, 1987.
35. Shesser R, Mitchell J, Edelstein S: Methemoglobinemia from isobutyl nitrite preparations. Ann Emerg Med *10*:262–264, 1981.
36. Galdun JP, Weiss LD, Paris PM, Kaplan RM, Stewart RD: Methemoglobin levels following inhalation of amyl nitrite. Ann Emerg Med *16*:484–485, 1987.
37. Wason S, Detsky AS, Platt OS, Lovejoy FH: Isobutyl nitrite toxicity by ingestion. Ann Intern Med *92*:637–638, 1980.
38. Chilcote RR, Williams B, Wolff LJ, Baehner RL: Sudden death in an infant from methemoglobinemia after administration of sweet spirits of nitre. Pediatrics *59*:280–282, 1977.
39. Berlin G, Brodin B, Hilden JO, Martensson J: Acute dapsone intoxication: A case treated with continuous infusion of methylene blue, forced diuresis, and plasma exchange. Clin Toxicol *22*:537–548, 1984–1985.
40. Bower PJ, Peterson JN: Methemoglobinemia after sodium nitroprusside therapy. N Engl J Med *293*:865, 1980.
41. Eisenkraft JB: Pulse oximeter desaturation due to methaemoglobinemia. Anesthesiology *68*:279–282, 1988.
42. Chakraborty TK, Filshie RJA, Lee MR: Methaemoglobinemia produced by phenazopyridine (Pyridium) in a man with chronic obstructive airways disease. Scot Med J *32*:185–186, 1987.
43. Damergis JA, Stoker JM, Abadie JL: Methemoglobinemia after sulfamethoxazole and trimethoprim therapy. JAMA *249*:590–591, 1983.
44. Kearns GL, Fiser DH: Metoclopramide-induced methemoglobinemia. Pediatrics *82*:364–366, 1988.
45. Ludwig SC: Acute toxic methemoglobinemia following dental analgesia. Ann Emerg Med *10*:265–266, 1981.
46. Wilson CM, Bird SG, Bocash W, Yang LL, Merritt RJ: Methemoglobinemia following metoclopramide therapy in an infant. J Pediatr Gastroenterol Nutr *6*:640–642, 1987.
47. Klendshoj NC, Burke WJ, Anthone R, Anthone S: Chlorate poisoning. JAMA *180*:1133–1134, 1962.
48. Mahomedy MC, Mahomedy YH, Canham PAS, Downing JW, Jeal DE: Methaemoglobinemia following treatment dispensed by witch doctors. Anesthesia *30*:190–193, 1975.
49. Weiss LD, Generalovich T, Heller MB, et al: Methemoglobin levels following intravenous lidocaine administration. Ann Emerg Med *16*:323–325, 1987.
50. Harvey JW, Keitt AS: Studies of the efficacy and potential hazards of methylene blue therapy in aniline-induced methaemoglobinemia. Br J Haematol *54*:29–41, 1983.
51. Kearney TE, Manoguerra AS, Dunford JV: Chemically induced methemoglobinemia from aniline poisoning. West J Med *140*:282–286, 1984.
52. Mier RJ: Treatment of aniline poisoning with exchange transfusion. Clin Toxicol *26*:357–364, 1988.
53. Hoffman RS, Sauter D: Methemoglobinemia resulting from smoke inhalation. Vet Hum Toxicol *31*:168–170, 1989.
54. Jaeger A, Sauder P, Kopferschmitt J, Flesch F: Clinical features and management of poisoning due to antimalarial drugs. Med Toxicol *2*:242–273, 1987.
55. Shane SJ, Iazzetta JJ, Chisholm AW, Berka JF, Leung

D: Plasma concentrations of isosorbide dinitrate and its metabolites after chronic high oral dosage in man. Br J Clin Pharmacol *6*:37–41, 1978.

56. Potter JL, Krill CE, Neal D, Kofron WG: Methemoglobinemia due to ingestion of *N-N*-di-methyl-*p*-toluidine, a component used in the fabrication of artificial fingernails. Ann Emerg Med *17*:1098–1100, 1988.
57. Bogart L, Bonsignore J, Carvalho A: Massive hemolysis following inhalation of volatile nitrites. Am J Hematol *22*:327–329, 1986.
58. Proudfoot AT: Methaemoglobinemia due to monolinuron—not paraquat. Br Med J *2*:285, 1982.
59. Chugh KS, Singhal PC, Sharma BK: Methemoglobinemia in acute copper sulfate poisoning. Ann Intern Med *82*:226–227, 1975.
60. Whitwam JG, Taylor AR, White JM: Potential hazard of methylene blue. Anaesthesia *34*:181–182, 1979.
61. Chan TK, Mak LW, Ng RP: Methemoglobinemia, Heinz bodies, and acute massive intravascular hemolysis in Lysol poisoning. Blood *38*:739–744, 1971.
62. Johnson CJ, Bonrud PA, Dosch TL, et al: Fatal outcome of methemoglobinemia in an infant. JAMA *257*:2796–2797, 1987.
63. Potter JL, Hillman JV: Benzocaine-induced methemoglobinemia. J Am Coll Emerg Phys *8*:26–27, 1979.
64. Horne MK, Waterman MR, Simon LM, Garriott JL, Foerster EH: Methemoglobinemia from sniffing butyl nitrite. Ann Intern Med *91*:417–418, 1979.
65. Smith RP: Toxic responses of the blood. *In* Klaassen CD, Amdur MO, Doull J (eds): Casarett and Doull's Toxicology: The Basic Science of Poisons. New York, Macmillan, 1986, pp 223–244.
66. Park CM, Nagel RL: Sulfhemoglobinemia: Clinical and molecular aspects. N Engl J Med *310*:1579–1584, 1984.
67. Lycka B: Amyl and butyl nitrites and telangiectasia in homosexual men. Ann Intern Med *106*:476, 1987.
68. Tannenbaum SR: *N*-Nitroso compounds: A perspective in human exposure. Lancet *1*:629–631, 1983.
69. Forman D, Al-Dabbagh S, Knigh T, Doll R: Nitrate exposure and the carcinogenic process. Ann NY Acad Sci *534*:597–603, 1988.
70. Moore PJ, Braatvedt GD: Acquired methemoglobinemia in pregnancy. S Afr Med J *67*:23–24, 1985.
71. Henretig FM, Gribetz B, Kearney T, Lacouture P, Lovejoy FH: Interpretation of color change in blood with varying degree of methemoglobinemia. J Toxicol Clin Toxicol *26*:293–301, 1988.
72. Zwart A, Buursma A, Oeseburg B, Zijlstra WG: Determination of hemoglobin derivatives with the IL 282 co-oximeter as compared with a manual spectrophotometric five-wavelength method. Clin Chem *27*:1903–1907, 1981.
73. Kirsch IR, Cohen HJ: Heinz-body hemolytic anemia from the use of methylene blue in neonates. J Pediatr *96*:272–278, 1980.
74. Goldstein GM, Doull J: Treatment of nitrite-induced methemoglobinemia with hyperbaric oxygen. Proc Soc Exp Biol Med *138*:137–139, 1971.
75. Kaplan JC, Chirouze M: Therapy of recessive methaemoglobinemia by oral riboflavine. Lancet *2*: 1043–1044, 1978.

CHAPTER 102
THYROID

Paul W. Ladenson, M.D.
J. Douglas White, M.D.

Over 400 million thyroid hormone–containing tablets are prescribed each year in the United States to an estimated 4 per cent of the adult population.[1] In light of the ready availability of thyroid hormone supplements, it is somewhat surprising that only 2231 thyroid hormone ingestions (based on extrapolation from National Capital Poison Center statistics) were documented in the United States in 1986. This probably reflects the relative tolerance of most victims, especially children and otherwise healthy adults, to even relatively large overdoses of these preparations.

THYROID PHYSIOLOGY

Thyroid Hormone Synthesis and Circulating Forms

Iodine plays a central role in thyroid physiology, being a major constituent of thyroid hormones. Dietary iodine is reduced in the gastrointestinal tract to iodide, absorbed within an hour, and actively transported from blood into thyroid follicular cells. Iodide is then oxidized to a higher valence state capable of binding to tyrosyl residues in thyroglobulin. This organification of iodine,

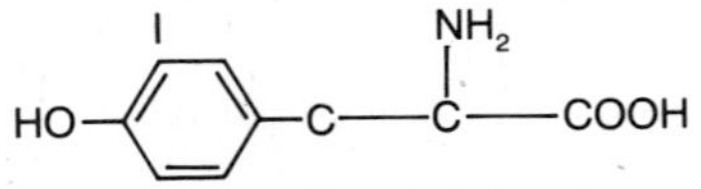

3-Monoiodotyrosine

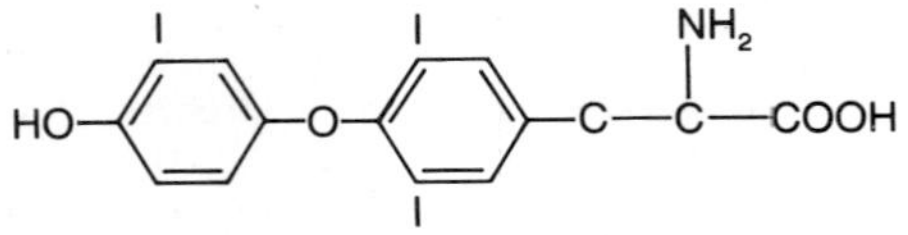

3′,3-5-Triiodothyronine (T_3)

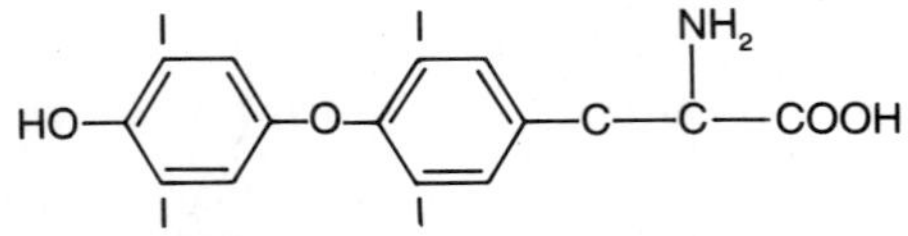

3,5,3′,5′-Tetraiodothyronine (thyroxine, T_4)

Figure 102–1. Iodothyronines.

catalyzed by thyroid peroxidase, results in the formation of hormonally inactive monoiodotyrosine (MIT) and diiodotyrosine (DIT). These precursors then undergo oxidative condensation, or coupling, to yield a variety of iodothyronines, including 3,3′,5,5′-tetraiodothyronine (thyroxine, T4) and 3,3′,5-triiodothyronine (T3) (Fig. 102–1). Thyroglobulin is then secreted into the follicular lumen, where it is stored as colloid, until it is reabsorbed by pinocytosis into follicular cells. Within lysosomal vesicles, T3 and T4 are hydrolyzed from thyroglobulin and released from the cell. Biologically inactive iodotyrosines and iodothyronines are stripped of iodine by an intrathyroidal deiodinase, with subsequent reutilization of the liberated iodine. All these steps in thyroid hormone biosynthesis are stimulated by thyrotropin (thyroid-stimulating hormone, TSH).

The thyroid gland normally secretes 80 to 90 μg of T4 and 8 μg of T3 daily. Most total daily T3 production, approximately 30 μg, actually results from extrathyroidal monodeiodination of T4, an enzymatically catalyzed process that occurs in all thyroid hormone–responsive tissues.[2] Circulating T4 is almost entirely bound (99.97 per cent) to plasma proteins, predominantly thyroxine-binding globulin (TBG, 70 per cent), but also thyroxine-binding prealbumin (TBPA, 15 per cent) and albumin (10 per cent). Plasma T3 is bound to a lesser extent (99.7 per cent). Target tissue responses are related principally, if not exclusively, to concentrations of the small free fractions of circulating thyroid hormones. In overdosages, the concentration of TBG is changed little, and the concentration of free hormone will increase directly or even disproportionately with the total serum hormone concentration. T3 is approximately three times as potent as T4. Indeed, T4 has been considered by some to be simply a plasma prohormone and T3 to be the biologically active thyroid hormone in target tissues.

Thyroid function is regulated by the hypothalamic-pituitary axis and by intrathyroidal mechanisms. Thyrotropic cells of the anterior pituitary secrete TSH, which stimulates both thyroid growth and hormone biosynthesis. TSH synthesis and secretion are, in turn, controlled by hypothalamic thyrotropin-releasing hormone (TRH). Production of both TRH and TSH is inhibited by thyroid hormone feedback on the hypothalamus and pituitary, respectively.

Thyroid Hormone Metabolism and Actions

The normal serum half-life for T4 is 7 days,[3] whereas the serum T3 half-life is approximately 1 day. T4 has a metabolic clearance rate of 0.8 to 1.4 L/day, a volume of distribution of 0.15 L/kg, and a fractional turnover rate of 10 to 14 per cent per day. The metabolic clearance of both T4 and T3 is altered by patient age and underlying thyroid status. The T4 half-life may be prolonged in elderly[4] and hypothyroid patients.[9] Conversely, the serum T4 half-life may be halved in children[6] and decreased in hyperthyroidism.[7] Although most observations on thyroid hormone metabolism in hyperthyroidism have been made in patients with Graves' disease, these have been corroborated by studies of factitious hyperthyroidism from ingested thyroid hormone preparations.[8] Little is actually known about the time required for these changes in T4 and T3 kinetics and metabolic clearance to occur.

The most important intermediate product of T4 metabolism is T3, which is present in significant amounts within 1 hour of intravenous T4 administration. The three main pathways of thyroid hormone degradation are (1) deiodination, (2) side-chain metabolism, and (3) conjugation with glucuronic acid and sulfate. The first pathway accounts for 80 per cent of T3 and T4 disposal. This process probably occurs in all tissues, but deiodinases are present in highest concentrations in liver, kidney, muscle, brain, and heart.[9] The iodothyronines are eventually totally deiodinated, but the diphenyl-ether link of the thyronine nucleus is left intact.[10] The alanine side-chain of T3 and T4 is also subject to attack by enzyme systems in the peripheral tissues, yielding pyruvic, lactic, and acetic acids. An additional pathway involving conjugation of the hydroxyl group and biliary excretion accounts for a substantial amount (20 per cent) of thyroid hormone degradation.[11]

In contrast to the similar disposal of T3 and T4 by deiodination and side-chain metabolism, conjugates of the iodothyronines are handled quite differently; sulfoconjugation is most important for T3, whereas T4 undergoes glucuronidation.[12] Absence of the conjugates in the stool suggests that hydrolysis occurs in the gut, probably by bacterial enzymes. Thyroid hormone released from conjugates in the gut is available for reabsorption, but the magnitude of their enterohepatic circulation in humans is unknown. Theoretically, the use of activated charcoal or cholestyramine to interrupt this enterohepatic circulation might be an adjunct to the management of thyroid hormone intoxication, but there are no clinical studies validating their use. A small amount of hormone is normally excreted by the kidney.

Intravenously administered T4 usually takes 6 to 8 hours to exert clinical effects, which may not peak until the following day. After massive oral overdoses of T4 administration, however, clinical effects have been observed as soon as 3 to 16 hours. Approximately a third of extrathyroidal hormone is stored in the liver, and circulating thyroid hormone slowly saturates other tissues to reach equilibrium in several days. T4 has a volume of distribution of 0.15 L/kg. Placental transfer of thyroid hormones from the maternal to fetal circulation is limited. Within hours, thyroid hormones stimulate intracellular mRNA and protein synthesis, increase mitochondrial oxidative phosphorylation, and enhance certain membrane transport functions in all tissues but brain, spleen, and testes. In addition to affecting many cellular metabolic processes, thyroid hormones are crucial for normal fetal neurologic development and childhood growth and have positive inotropic and chronotropic effects on myocardium.

Orally administered thyroid hormone preparations are readily absorbed from the gastrointestinal tract, predominantly from the stomach, within hours. T3 is 95 per cent absorbed, whereas T4 absorption is approximately 80 per cent.[13]

Laboratory Tests of Thyroid Function

Serum total T4 and T3 concentrations are readily determined by a number of specific, accurate, and widely available radioimmunoassay (RIA) techniques. Because serum protein binding of the thyroid hormones may be altered by nonthyroidal disease processes and drugs (Table 102–1), hyperthyroxinemia is not pathognomonic of hyperthyroidism. Furthermore, decreased serum protein binding of thyroid hormones can mask thyroid hormone excess. Therefore, it is important to define the levels of free thyroid hormones in blood.

Two techniques—direct free T4 RIA and the calculated free T4 index (FTI)—are commonly employed. The FTI is the calculated product of the serum total T4 concentration and the T3 resin uptake (T3RU), which is determined by adding a tracer amount of radiolabeled T3 to a serum sample and incubating until equilibrium is established between the labeled T3 and previously unoccupied protein binding sites. Then a resin capable of binding large quantities of small organic molecules, including the remaining unbound labeled T3, is added, allowed to equilibrate, and separated from the serum sample by centrifugation. Thus, the amount of labeled T3 associated with the resin varies inversely with the number of unoccupied binding sites on TBG. The calculated FTI is useful in distinguishing deranged TBG binding from states of true thyroid hormone excess or deficiency. The FTI generally corre-

Table 102–1. CLINICAL SITUATIONS ASSOCIATED WITH ALTERATIONS OF TBG CONCENTRATION

INCREASED TBG	DECREASED TBG
Oral contraceptives and other estrogens	Androgens
Acute intermittent porphyria	Chronic liver disease
Chronic active hepatitis	Active acromegaly
Acute hepatitis	Nephrosis
Pregnancy	

lates well with results of both the free T4 RIA and the more complex determination of free T4 level by equilibrium dialysis.[14] It must be remembered that the T3RU does not measure the patient's serum T3 level. Ingestions of thyroid hormone preparations that contain solely T3 or are composed of a major T3 component (see later) will not be accurately assessed without also determining a serum T3 concentration by RIA.

COMMERCIAL THYROID HORMONE PREPARATIONS

T4 is the thyroid hormone preparation of choice in most clinical circumstances and the most commonly prescribed agent. Both T4 and T3 are satisfactorily absorbed from the gastrointestinal tract. Levothyroxine (T4, Synthroid, Levothroid), desiccated thyroid extract, porcine thyroglobulin (Proloid), and synthetic T4 plus T3 combination agents (Liotrix, Thyrolar, Euthroid) generally have a slower onset and a longer duration of action than liothyronine (Cytomel), i.e., pure T3. The full target tissue effects of T4-containing preparations may not be seen for at least 1 week, whereas the maximal effect of T3 is generally apparent within 24 hours and maintained for 72 hours.

Thyroid hormone is used clinically as replacement therapy in treatment of primary and central hypothyroidism. In addition, thyroid hormone is used for suppression of some benign nontoxic nodular goiters, chronic autoimmune thyroiditis, and thyroid carcinoma. Other indiscriminate uses of thyroid hormones are unjustified and potentially dangerous. Thyroid preparations should not be used for dietary, somatic, menstrual, and fertility disorders not specifically related to thyroid disease. A list of the most common preparations and their comparative effects on metabolic rate is shown in Table 102–2.

Levothyroxine Sodium. The monosodium salt of the levoisomer of T4 synthetically prepared for commercial use is a hygroscopic, cream-colored, odorless, tasteless powder, slightly soluble in alcohol and water. The sodium salt is better absorbed from the gut than the free acid. It may be administered orally or intravenously when reconstituted with saline. T4 is also available as an aqueous preparation that may be given parenterally. Daily maintenance doses are usually between 75 and 200 μg but may range from 25 μg to 300 μg.

Table 102–2. THYROID PREPARATIONS

GENERIC	COMMON BRAND NAMES
Desiccated thyroid	Thyroid Strong, Thyrar, S-P-T, Thermoloid, Thyro-Teric, Thyrocrine, Tuloidin
Thyroglobulin	Proloid
Levothyroxine sodium (T_4, L-thyroxine)	Synthroid, Levothyroid, Noroxine, L-T-S, Levoid
Liothyronine Sodium (T_3)	Cytomel, Cytomine
Liotrix	Thyrolar, Euthyroid
Calorigenic Equivalence	
Thyroid USP	65 mg (1 grain)
Thyroglobulin	65 mg
Levothyroxine (T_4)	0.1 mg (100 μg)
Liothyronine (T_3)	25 μg
Liotrix (T_4 and T_3)	50 μg T_4 plus 12.5 μg T_3

Liothyronine Sodium. The sodium salt of the L-isomer of T3 differs from T4 only in the absence of an iodine atom at the 5′ position. It is prepared as a tan, crystalline powder, slightly soluble in water and alcohol. Available only as an oral preparation, the usual maintenance dose is 25 to 75 μg/day but may range from 5 to over 100 μg/day. When a patient is transferred from another thyroid preparation to sodium liothyronine, the initial thyroid preparation should be discontinued and therapy initiated with a low, daily dose of liothyronine because of its rapid onset of action.

Liotrix. This synthetic combination contains T4 and T3 in a 4:1 ratio by weight. Commercially available preparations alter the amount of each drug but preserve this ratio. The manufacturers claim calorigenic equivalence, but brands should not be interchanged without considering the possible differences in bioavailability and potency.

Thyroid USP. Thyroid USP is the desiccated form of thyroid gland obtained from hogs, cattle, and sheep. This yellow insoluble powder, containing both T4 and T3, has a characteristic odor (meatlike) and a saline taste. Usual maintenance doses are 60 to 180 mg/day.

Thyroglobulin. Thyroglobulin is an extract of hog thyroid gland containing T3 and T4. When the potency is standardized to meet USP requirements for iodine and animal bioassay, it has no clinical advantage over thyroid USP. Available in tablets or as a tan, poorly soluble powder, thyroglobulin is administered orally in usual maintenance doses of 60 to 180 mg/day.

THYROID HORMONE TOXICITY

Clinical Features

Thyroid hormone intoxication typically occurs in several settings: childhood ingestions, suicidal overdosages, and subacute or chronic iatrogenic or factitious thyrotoxicosis. Although massive overdoses are decidedly uncommon, mild overdoses can result from medication errors by physicians, pharmacists, nurses, or patients. Some patients may become iatrogenically thyrotoxic on thyroid hormone doses that were previously considered appropriate[15] or that become excessive as hormone metabolism declines with aging. Rarely, epidemics of thyrotoxicosis have followed the contamination of ground beef with thyroid tissue.[16]

Effects of thyroid hormone overdosage are observed primarily in the cardiovascular, gastrointestinal, and neurologic systems. Typical hemodynamic responses include tachycardia, increased force of myocardial contraction, palpitations, cutaneous vasodilation, and systolic hypertension. Hypotension, congestive heart failure, and cardiovascular collapse can occur if the cardiovascular system is stimulated beyond its reserve capacity. Typical associated tachyarrhythmias are sinus tachycardia, paroxysmal atrial tachycardia, atrial flutter, and fibrillation.[17] Electrocardiographic changes are common but nonspecific.[18] Gastrointestinal symptoms are most often diarrhea and vomiting, but acute abdominal pain and peptic ulceration have been reported.[19] Neurologically, patients may evidence excessive sympathetic nervous system activity, including anxiety, mydriasis, diaphoresis, and agitation. Rare central nervous system manifestations of thyroid hormone intoxication are acute psychosis,[20] seizures, and coma. Patients have been reported to develop periodic paralysis in subacute overdoses,[21] a phenomenon most often seen in Oriental males. Constitutional features of thyroid hormone intoxication may be fever and malaise. Glucose intolerance and hypercalcemia may be encountered, as well as slight elevations in liver function tests, BUN, and creatinine.

Euthyroid persons appear to have a wide range of tolerance to the effects of acute or chronic overdose. Patients without underlying heart disease generally tolerate intravenous T4 doses of 750 μg.[22] Some cardiologists contend that women tolerate thyroid excess less well than men,[23] and all authorities concur that an aged or debilitated cardiovascular system can be vulnerable to even modest overdoses.[21] On the other hand, enhanced kinetics and metabolism may allow children to tolerate overdoses of up to 45 grains (2.8 gm) of thyroid extract without symptoms or signs of poisoning.[24] Indeed, an overdose of 132 grains in a 3 year old child with only modest symptoms has been reported.[25] Nonetheless, a small enough child (15 months) taking a similar dose (5 grain/kg) can appear quite toxic, although complete clinical recovery may be expected within 12 to 18 hours and complete chemical resolution in less than a week.

The clinical course of a thyroid hormone overdose depends on the preparation involved. Ingestion of up to 1600 μg of T3 may be well tolerated[26] and rapidly eliminated from the vascular compartment. However, patients ingesting T4 may remain well until several days after the ingestion, when peripheral conversion of T4 is significant and the patient becomes thyrotoxic.[27]

Differential Diagnosis of Thyroid Hormone Intoxication

Clinical Findings. Patients in full-blown thyroid "crisis" or "storm" are rare. The absence of dramatic clinical manifestations or even a satisfactory history in some individuals makes the differential diagnosis of thyroid hormone intoxication challenging. A thorough inquiry should be made about the availability of thyroid preparations, e.g., a personal or family history of thyroid disease, previous neck surgery, or "weight problems" treated with "medications." T4 tablets come in standardized colors so that a specific description of the drugs ingested yields valuable dose information. Most cases of factitious hyperthyroidism occur in paramedical personnel[28] or in patients eager to lose weight.

Findings on physical examination may be

nonspecific, but attention should be focused on the cardiovascular system and possible signs of sympathetic nervous system hyperactivity. Systolic hypertension, tachycardia, a hyperdynamic point of maximal cardiac apical impulse, and systolic flow murmur may be observed; tremor, diaphoresis, and eyelid lag also may be present. Neurologic findings may include restlessness, delirium, and rarely psychosis or coma.

Occasionally, conditions posing a major physiologic stress may mimic thyroid overdose, e.g., infection, sepsis, hemorrhage, trauma, or profound pain. The clinical setting must be relied upon for recognition of these patients and those with heat stroke. The physician must always assess both the temperature of a patient in thyroid crisis and consider (at least clinically) the thyroid status of any hyperthermic patient.

It is important to distinguish between endogenous thyrotoxicosis and overdose. Primary hyperthyroidism is distinctly unusual before the age of 5 years.[24] The absence of ophthalmopathy and normal gland size also help inculpate thyroid ingestion.

Few compounds stimulate cellular metabolism to the same extent as thyroid hormone, and most of these other agents induce symptoms rapidly. A toxicologic analysis will exclude many of these substances (amphetamines, cocaine, tricyclic antidepressants, salicylates). Salicylates (aspirin, oil of wintergreen) share many of the same symptoms as thyroid excess; however, the acid-base, glucose, and coagulation abnormalities of salicylism are typical and may be ruled out rapidly with a urine ferric chloride test. Like salicylates, phenol derivatives (dinitrophenol, pentachlorophenol) uncouple oxidative phosphorylation and produce an increase in diaphoresis, oxygen consumption, body temperature, pulse rate, and respiratory rate. These are caustic agents, however, and ingestions are characterized by pronounced gastrointestinal and mucous membrane toxicity. Unlike the case in thyroid excess, anoxia, acidosis, and delayed renal and hepatic damage may be prominent.

Nicotine (tobacco, insecticides) in small doses may be ruled out in the absence of salivation and miosis. Anticholinergic overdose must be considered, but the absence of diaphoresis should help implicate this possibility. Cocaine and amphetamine ingestion may be easily confused with thyroid excess; however, abuse of these drugs may be recognized by their uniformly rapid onset. Although thyroid excess may be accompanied by mydriasis, hypertension, and psychosis, these findings are more frequent and pronounced with stimulant abuse.

Laboratory Testing. In the hours following ingestion, serum thyroid hormone levels may be markedly elevated in the absence of clinical thyrotoxicosis. Although serum thyroid hormone concentrations are clearly valuable to confirm the nature and approximate amount of ingested thyroid hormones, early results are of limited use in defining the prognosis for patients with an overdose[1] or in mandating the aggressiveness of therapy. Sudden death has been reported with only modest serum thyroid hormone elevations and during periods when levels are decreasing. Furthermore, accurate laboratory assessment of thyroid status may be obscured in patients who are critically ill for any reason.[29] Infectious, hepatic, and renal diseases, among others, can lower serum T4, and particularly serum T3, concentrations.

With significant sustained thyroid hormone excess, the serum TSH concentration is generally suppressed to the lower limit of detection in conventional assays, both basally and following exogenous TRH administration. With acute thyroid hormone ingestion, however, circulating TSH may remain temporarily detectable as pituitary thyrotropes respond to thyroid hormone excess and circulating TSH is metabolically cleared.

On occasion, it may be necessary to distinguish endogenous hyperthyroidism from thyrotoxicosis attributable to thyroid hormone ingestion. Thyroid scintigraphy is helpful in differentiating between these possibilities, since thyroidal uptake of ^{123}iodine or ^{99m}technetium will be suppressed by supraphysiologic doses of exogenous thyroid medication, whereas it is increased in the most common forms of hyperthyroidism (i.e., Graves' disease and toxic nodular goiter). The specificity of a diminished radionuclide uptake is limited, however, by the fact that certain less common forms of endogenous hyperthyroidism (e.g., subacute and lymphocytic thyroiditis) are also associated with low fractional thyroid tracer uptakes. The serum thyroglobulin is suppressed by excessive thyroid medication but is increased in virtually all types of endogenous thyrotoxicosis. As with serum TSH, the radionuclide thyroid uptake and serum thyroglobulin may be incompletely suppressed during the first hours after an acute ingestion.

TREATMENT OF THYROID HORMONE TOXICITY

Several factors should determine the aggressiveness with which a patient who has ingested thyroid hormone should be managed: the form of thyroid hormone (i.e., T4, T3 or both), estimated dose of medication, time since ingestion and—perhaps most important—the age and underlying cardiac status of the patient. As noted previously, healthy individuals, particularly children, may tolerate even relatively large overdoses well without serious consequences.[25, 30] On the other hand, life-threatening toxicity does occur, particularly in adults with underlying cardiac disease, and even in children.[31]

Special considerations apply to management of intoxication with each of the biologically active thyroid hormones. T3 ingestions tend to be more serious, with clinical manifestations appearing relatively soon after ingestion, whereas the more common T4 ingestions are generally milder, but maximal thyrotoxicosis may be delayed for days.

The initial clinical evaluation should include the most precise possible history regarding the form, dose, and time of thyroid hormone ingestion; current symptoms and signs of thyrotoxicosis; and any past history or signs of cardiac or other significant underlying disease. Unless there are specific contraindications, emesis should be induced, followed by administration of activated charcoal and a cathartic. Although serum T3 and T4 levels should be requested of the laboratory to confirm the type and general dosage of the ingestion, the limitations of serum thyroid function testing in assessing the severity and prognosis of thyroid hormone intoxication, particularly for T4, have been previously discussed.

Patients who have ingested more than 100 μg/kg of T4 or 30 μg/kg of T3, who have serum T4 concentrations greater than 50 μg/dl, who are severely symptomatic, or who have a history of significant underlying cardiopulmonary disease generally should be admitted to hospital. Supportive measures include correction of hyperpyrexia, maintenance of fluid and electrolyte balance, and monitoring cardiac rhythm and respiratory status. Acetaminophen should be used as an antipyretic since aspirin can increase the serum free T4 fraction. In T3 ingestion, hospital observation should continue until the patient is only mildly symptomatic and the serum T3 has fallen to less than 400 ng/dl. For T4 ingestion in adults, hospitalization generally should be continued for 4 days after the peak serum T4 concentration. A briefer period of hospital observation may be reasonable for children, whereas more prolonged inpatient care is often appropriate for individuals with known cardiac disease or other complications. In pure T3 ingestions, these criteria may be satisfied within 12 to 24 hours, whereas hospitalization for 1 to 2 weeks can be anticipated for some T4 ingestions in adults not treated with extracorporeal detoxification (see following). Asymptomatic or mildly symptomatic and otherwise healthy patients may be followed at home for approximately 1 week, particularly if T4 was the major thyroid hormone ingested.[27]

Propranolol is useful to ameliorate tachycardia, systolic hypertension, diaphoresis, and tremulousness accompanying hyperthyroidism. Oral propranolol, 10 to 80 mg every 6 hours, or intravenously, 0.1 to 3 mg every 4 hours, may be used in patients with no contraindication (e.g., pulmonary edema, bronchospasm, heart block) to beta-adrenergic blockade. Children should receive a lower oral dose, no more than 0.2 mg/min IV. The propranolol dose should be titrated to the patient's response; a heart rate less than 120 beats per minute is a reasonable goal. A completely normal heart rate is not easily restored; an attempt to achieve it may cause hypotension.

Cardiac glycosides may augment control of atrial fibrillation in patients but should be expected to be less effective in controlling heart rate than in euthyroid individuals. Although the metabolic clearance rate for digoxin is increased in hyperthyroidism, toxicity will still result if the dosage is titrated based on heart rate. Chlorpromazine has been suggested as a useful therapeutic adjunct as an adrenergic and cholinergic antagonist and antiemetic with sedative properties. However, it also may depress cardiac and ventilatory functions[25] and exacerbate hyperthermia.

No evidence supports the older concept of relative adrenal insufficiency in thyroid crisis. Nonetheless, glucocorticoids may be useful in diminishing T4 to T3 conversion. Propylthiouracil (PTU), iopanoic acid, other radiocontrast dyes, and amiodarone all share the ability to impair extrathyroidal T4 to T3 conversion but have no clearly demonstrated place in the usual management of thyroid hormone ingestions. Because the thionamides PTU and methimazole (Tapazole) do not block release or action of previously synthesized thyroid hormones, they have no other role in treating exogenous thyroid hormone intoxication.

Diuresis and hemodialysis are not useful in accelerating clearance of thyroid hormones because of their binding to plasma proteins too large to pass through glomerular capillary and dialysis membranes, respectively. Peritoneal dialysis, the first effective method for speeding thyroid hormone removal, reduces the T4 half-life to less than 24 hours.[32] Exchange transfusion[33] with donor blood effectively provides unsaturated serum proteins but has the disadvantages attendant to any blood transfusion.

These approaches have been supplanted by two newer techniques, plasmapheresis and charcoal hemoperfusion, which have proved valuable in severe cases of thyrotoxicosis. Plasmapheresis with reinfusion of cells is the less effective but safer technique.[34] Hemoperfusion with activated charcoal has emerged as the most effective approach to remove circulating thyroid hormone quickly. Charcoal hemoperfusion for 8 hours or less has produced dramatic clinical improvement and normalization of serum T3 and T4 levels within 36 hours.[35] Both protein-bound and free hormones are adsorbed, the hazards of transfusion are avoided, and the procedure can be accomplished quickly and safely in experienced hands. Charcoal or XAD-4 resin hemoperfusion may be appropriate in patients with severe existing or potential cardiac toxicity, or following failure of conventional supportive and beta-adrenergic antagonist therapy after 24 hours.

INTOXICATIONS WITH THYROID ANTAGONISTS

Agents used to treat hyperthyroidism work by (1) depriving the gland of iodine substrate (e.g., perchlorate or thiocyanate), (2) inhibiting hormone biosynthesis (e.g., thionamides) or release (e.g., iodide, lithium), (3) interfering with extrathyroidal T4 to T3 conversion (e.g., PTU, glucocorticoids, iopanoic acid, and other iodinated radiocontrast dyes), or (4) blocking the target tissue sympathomimetic actions of thyroid hormones (e.g., propranolol). The toxicity of iodine (Chapter 63), lithium (Chapter 35), and beta-adrenergic antagonists (Chapter 92) is discussed elsewhere.

The thionamide antithyroid drugs PTU and methimazole inhibit organification of iodide and especially the coupling of iodotyrosines to form hormonally active iodothyronines. Both are white, slightly soluble, and light-sensitive powders, which are readily absorbed from the gastrointestinal tract within an hour. The volume of distribution for PTU is approximately 0.3 L/kg and 80 per cent is protein bound; methimazole circulates unbound. The serum half-lives of PTU and methimazole are 1 to 2 hours and 4 to 6 hours, respectively. Intrathyroidal accumulation of drug occurs.[36] Both drugs, particularly methimazole, cross the placenta and appear in human milk.

The most common side effect of both thionamides, of course, is hypothyroidism. Hypersensitivity reactions (e.g., fever, urticaria, other rashes, and arthralgias) occur in approximately 5 per cent of patients but are not dose related and generally occur within the first 3 months of therapy. Idiosyncratic agranulocytosis is a rare occurrence (0.2 per cent), but a mild, dose-dependent leukopenia occurs in up to 10 per cent of patients. Other side effects may include gastrointestinal distress, hepatitis, arthritis, and rarely headache, drowsiness, vertigo, visual and hearing disturbances, ageusia, allergic vasculitis, aplastic anemia, and coagulopathy. Hepatic injury is generally mild but rarely may be life-threatening.[37]

In one reported case of PTU overdose, a 12 year old patient ingested between 5 and 13 grams.[38] Urinary levels of PTU were 90 mg/dl 17 hours after ingestion. Serum thyroid hormone levels declined for several days, with the expected greater reduction in T3 than T4. Although this massive PTU ingestion was well tolerated, ideal conditions for rapid clearance of PTU existed, since the patient had normal renal function. PTU overdose may prove more complicated in patients with previously impaired renal or liver function.

In the event of thionamide overdosage, liver and renal function tests and the leukocyte count should be monitored daily for at least 3 days. The transient antithyroid activity should not require treatment in previously euthyroid individuals. Milder allergic reactions simply can be observed or treated with antihistamines or glucocorticoids if severe. There is no experience with extracorporeal detoxification for PTU; in view of its serum protein-binding, only hemoperfusion techniques would seem promising.

References

1. Nystrom E, Lindstedt G, Lundberg PA: Minor signs of toxicity in a young woman despite massive thyroxine ingestion. Acta Med Scand *207*:135, 1980.
2. Braverman LE, Ingbar SK, Sterling K: Conversion of T_4 to T_3 in athyreotic subjects. J Clin Invest *49*:855, 1970.
3. Nicoloff JT, Dowling JT: Studies of peripheral thyroxine metabolism. J Clin Invest *47*:2000, 1968.
4. Rosenbaum RL, Barzel US: Levothyroxine replacement dose for primary hypothyroidism decreases with age. Ann Intern Med *96*:53–55, 1982.
5. Sterling K, Chodos RB: Radiothyroxine turnover studies in myxedema, thyrotoxicosis and hypermetabolism without endocrine disease. J Clin Invest *35*:806–813, 1956.
6. Haddad HM: Rates of I^{131}-labelled thyroxine metabolism in euthyroid children. J Clin Invest *39*:1590, 1960.
7. Sterling K, Chodos RB: Radiothyroxine turnover studies in myxedema, thyrotoxicosis and hypermetabolism without endocrine disease. J Clin Invest *35*:806, 1956.
8. Rose E, Sander TP, Webb WL: Occult factitial thyrotoxicosis. Ann Intern Med *71*:309, 1969.
9. Sprott WE, Maclagan NF: Metabolism of thyroid hormones. Biochem J *59*:288, 1955.
10. Lissitsky S, Bennett MT, Rouges M, Roch J: Sur la desiodation des iodotyrosine. Bull Soc Chim Biol (Paris) *41*:1329, 1959.
11. Pittman CS, Chambers JB: Carbon structure of thyroxine metabolites in urine. Endocrinology *84*:705, 1969.
12. Taurog A, Briggs FN, Chaikoff IL: I^{131} labelled L-thyroxine: Nature of excretion product in bile. J Biol Chem *194*:655, 1952.
13. Fish LH, Schwartz HL, Cavanaugh J, Steffes MW, Bantle JP, Oppenheimer JH: Replacement dose, metabolism, and bioavailability of levothyroxine in the treatment of hypothyroidism: Role of triiodothyronine in pituitary feedback. N Engl J Med *316*:764–770, 1987.
14. Anderson BG: Free thyroxine in serum in relation to thyroid function. JAMA *203*:135, 1968.
15. Bhasm S, Wallace W, Laurence JB, Lesch M: Sudden death associated with thyroid hormone. Am J Med 70:887, 1981.
16. Hedberg CW, Fishbein DB, Janssen RS, et al: An outbreak of thyrotoxicosis caused by the consumption of bovine thyroid gland in ground beef. N Engl J Med *316*:993–998, 1987.
17. Rogers HM: Cardiovascular manifestations of induced thyrotoxicosis. Ann Intern Med *26*:914, 1947.
18. Sandler G: Effect of thyrotoxicosis on the electrocardiogram. Br Heart J *21*:111, 1959.
19. Garbart AC: Simultaneous occurrence of active peptic ulcer and active hyperthyroidism. J Mount Sinai Hosp *17*:787, 1951.
20. Roberts JA: Correct use of thyroxine. Med J Aust 2:650, 1975.
21. Layzer RB, Goldfield E: Periodic paralysis caused by the abuse of thyroid hormone. Neurology *24*:949, 1974.
22. Ridgway EC, McCammon JS, Benotti J, Maloof F: Acute metabolic responses to large doses of intravenous L-thyroxine. Ann Intern Med *77*:549, 1972.
23. Likoff WB, Levine SA: Thyrotoxicosis as the sole cause of congestive heart failure. Am J Med Sci *206*:425, 1943.
24. Dahl IL: Thyroid crisis in a three year old. Acta Paediatr Scand *57*:55, 1968.
25. Funderburk SJ, Spaulding JS: Sodium levothyroxine intoxication in a child. Pediatrics *48*:295, 1970.
26. Dahlberg PA, Karlsson FA, Wide L: Triiodothyronine intoxication. Lancet 2:700, 1979.
27. Von Hofe SE, Young RL: Thyrotoxicosis after a single ingestion of levothyroxine. JAMA *237*:1361, 1977.
28. Gorman CA, Wahner HW, Tauxe WM: Metabolic malingerers. Am J Med *48*:708, 1970.
29. Wartofsky L, Burman KD: Alterations in thyroid function in patients with systemic illness: The "euthyroid sick syndrome." Endocrinol Rev *3*:164–216, 1982.
30. Jahr HM: Thyroid poisoning in children. Nebraska State Med J *21*:388, 1936.
31. Levy RP, Gilger WG: Acute thyroid poisoning. N Engl J Med *256*:459, 1957.
32. Herrman J, Schmidt HJ, Kruskemper HL: Thyroxine elimination by peritoneal dialysis in experimental thyrotoxicosis. Hormone Metab Res *5*:180, 1973.
33. Ashkar FS, Katims RB, Smoak WM, Gilson AJ: Thyroid storm treatment with blood exchange and plasmapheresis. JAMA *214*:1275, 1970.
34. Huekelon S, Kinderen PJ, Vingerhoed AC: Plasmapheresis in L-thyroxine intoxication. Vet Hum Toxicol *21*:7, 1979.
35. Seyffart G: Dialysis and Hemoperfusion in Poisonings. Fresenius Foundation, Bad Homburg, 1977.
36. Marchant B, Alexander WD, Lazarus JH, Lees J, Clark DH: Accumulation of ^{35}S antithyroid drugs by the thyroid gland. J Clin Endocrinol Metab *34*:847, 1972.

37. Weiss M, Hassin D, Bank H: Propylthiouracil-induced hepatic damage. Arch Intern Med *140*:1184, 1980.
38. Jackson GL, Flickinger FW, Wells LW: Massive overdosage of propylthiouracil. Ann Intern Med *91*:418, 1979.
39. Ladenson PW: Diseases of the thyroid gland. Clin Endocrinol Metab *14*:145–173, 1985.

CHAPTER 103
VITAMINS A AND D AND THEIR ANALOGUES

C. Patrick Mahoney, M.D.

Current prescribing practices and the metabolic characteristics of vitamins A and D account for their relative high rate of toxicity compared with other vitamins. Accidental poisonings and inappropriate prescribing of large doses of these vitamins continue to produce new cases of hypervitaminosis A and D. The main source of intoxication, however, arises from the pharmacologic use of vitamin A analogues (retinoic acid derivatives) for skin diseases and vitamin D_3 for disorders of calcium and phosphorus metabolism. At therapeutic levels, these agents have many side effects and are teratogenic when taken during pregnancy.

The licensure, in 1982, of the first retinoic acid analogue, isotretinoin, to treat severe acne illustrates the magnitude of the problem. By 1985, an estimated 160,000 women of childbearing age had taken isotretinoin, even though it is as teratogenic as thalidomide.[1] Many of the women exposed during pregnancy had spontaneous or therapeutic abortions, and more than 30 infants were born with the characteristic malformations of the fetal retinoic acid syndrome.[1]

Unlike water-soluble vitamins, vitamins A and D are stored in the body. Daily doses that do not cause symptoms initially can lead to progressive increase in body stores over several weeks or months, resulting in chronic intoxication. Individuals vary in their ability to metabolize vitamin D, and certain diseases, such as sarcoidosis and infantile hypercalcemia, appear to alter vitamin D metabolism so that intoxication occurs at low dosage.

VITAMIN A

Vitamin A is required in higher animals to maintain normal reproduction, vision, differentiation of epithelium, and mucus secretion. Only its role in the visual cycle is understood. Vitamin A aldehyde, or retinal, is the prosthetic group for the photosensitive pigment in rods and cones of the retina. Outside the visual cycle, vitamin A appears to play a role in insuring normal structure and function of biologic membranes.[2]

Pathophysiology of Intoxication

Vitamin A is absorbed and esterified within the epithelial cells of the small bowel, transported in chylomicrons via the lymphatic system to the blood stream, and deposited mainly in the liver. Vitamin A is mobilized from hepatic stores as the unesterified free alcohol retinol, which is bound to its specific carrier protein, retinol-binding protein. About 95 per cent of plasma vitamin A in the fasting state exists in the form of retinol bound to its carrier protein as an equimolar complex.[2, 3] Retinol-binding protein protects tissues from the surface-active properties of vitamin A.

In hypervitaminosis A, the capacity of retinol-binding protein is exceeded, and the surfeit of vitamin A begins to circulate as retinyl esters nonspecifically bound to plasma proteins. When delivered to peripheral tissues in this manner, the surface-active properties of vitamin A cause tissue damage by producing unstable cellular membranes.[3]

Only commercial vitamin preparations and liver contain sufficient vitamin A to produce acute or chronic toxicity. Excessive intake of carotene-containing foods does not produce toxicity, because the conversion of carotene to vitamin A is limited in the presence of large stores of vitamin A. Acute vitamin A intoxication has ensued after a single ingestion of liver from polar bears, seals, or sharks; chronic poisoning has occurred after daily intake of chicken or beef liver for several months.[4, 5]

A single dose of vitamin A in the range of 2 million international units (IU) in adults and 75,000 IU in infants causes acute intoxication. Daily vitamin A intake for several months of 18,000 IU in infants, 80,000 IU in prepubertal children, and 100,000 IU in adults results in chronic intoxication. In general, daily intake of 3000 IU/kg is sufficient to cause chronic intoxication.[6]

Clinical Signs of Intoxication

The cardinal manifestations of vitamin A intoxication are central nervous system symptoms, dermatitis, bone pain, liver disease, fatigue, and anorexia (see differential diagnosis in Table 103–1). Hypervitaminosis A causes increased intracranial pressure which, in turn, gives rise to headaches, vomiting, diplopia, visual field defects, papilledema, and, in infants, bulging fontanels. Cutaneous signs include red, desquamating skin, especially over the hands and feet; lip fissures; and hair loss. Bone tenderness, muscle stiffness, and edema of the lower extremities are frequently noted. Polydipsia and polyuria probably are due to bone reabsorption leading to hypercalcemia and calciuria. Hepatomegaly is common, and it is occasionally accompanied by pallor and a bleeding tendency. Excess vitamin A intake during pregnancy is teratogenic and produces fetal craniofacial and musculoskeletal malformations.[7, 8]

Table 103–1. DIFFERENTIAL DIAGNOSIS OF THE MANIFESTATIONS OF VITAMIN A INTOXICATION

Increased intracranial pressure
Benign increased intracranial pressure
CNS tumor
Intracranial hemorrhage
Hydrocephalus
Corticosteroid or tetracycline therapy
Addison disease or hypoparathyroidism
Papuloerythematous dermatitis
Eczematous dermatitis
Drug eruptions
Exanthematous diseases
Corticohyperostosis and hypercalcemia
Caffey disease
Hypervitaminosis D
Hepatomegaly and abnormal liver function test
Hepatitis
Obstructive liver disease
Genetic-metabolic disorders
Infiltrative-vascular diseases of liver

In cases of acute intoxication, signs of increased intracranial pressure develop within 8 to 12 hours, and cutaneous desquamation follows in a few days.[9] It usually takes a few months for symptoms to appear in chronic intoxication. Recovery should be expected in acute intoxication, but occasionally liver disease and skeletal deformities are permanent in chronic intoxication.

Radiographic Signs

Infants given excess vitamin A frequently show thin cranial bones and widened sutures. The long bones of toddlers may exhibit corticohyperostosis (Fig. 103–1) and an increased angle of metaphyseal flare ("pagoda" sign). Rarely, premature epiphyseal fusion leads to localized growth arrest and unequal leg lengths. Bone scans may demonstrate increased uptake in the long bone diaphysis even when conventional radiographs are normal.[10] Cerebrospinal fluid pressure is often increased, but computed tomography of the brain may show variable changes in the ventricular system, including normal, small, or large ventricles.[4]

Laboratory Findings

Serum calcium, alkaline phosphatase, bilirubin, prothrombin time, and erythrocyte sedimentation rate are often elevated. Mild anemia and hypoalbuminemia also have been reported. The normal total vitamin A concentration is 20 to 60 μg/dl. Total vitamin A concentrations above 100 μg/dl are usually associated with poisoning. However, levels that cause toxicity vary according to the concentration of retinol-binding protein. In cirrhosis, retinol-binding protein concentration is low, and vitamin A levels as low as 60 μg/dl can be compatible with intoxication. Retinol-binding levels are raised in renal disease, so that a vitamin A concentration of

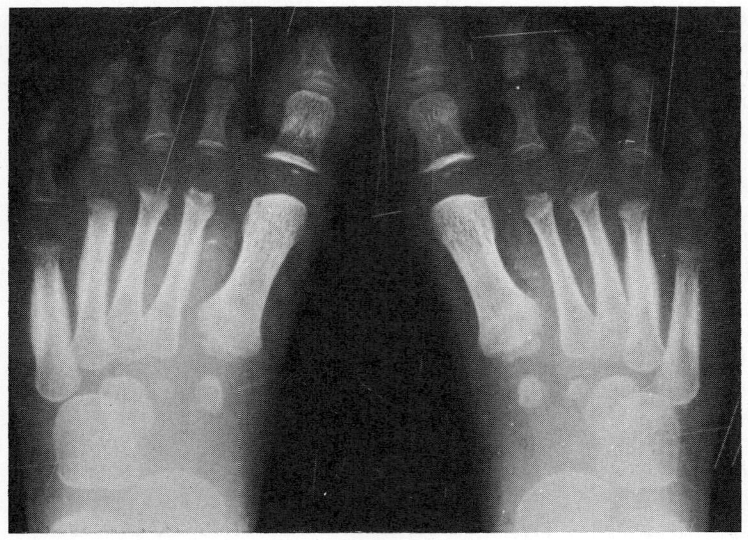

Figure 103–1. Metaphyseal flare and corticohyperostosis of vitamin A intoxication in a toddler.

100 μg/dl may not indicate overdose. Therefore, measurements of retinol-binding protein concentration are useful in these situations.[3]

Treatment

Ordinarily no therapy is necessary for vitamin A intoxication other than withdrawing the vitamin. Headaches, papilledema, and diplopia regress spontaneously within several weeks after vitamin A withdrawal. Therefore, repeated spinal taps to relieve increased intracranial pressure are rarely necessary. The management of hypercalcemia is discussed under the treatment of vitamin D toxicity. Abnormal liver function tests require follow-up, since liver damage may be permanent.

VITAMIN A DERIVATIVES (RETINOIDS)

The term *retinoids* refers to the naturally occurring forms of vitamin A and the over 1000 synthetic analogues of retinoic acid.[2] Retinoic acid analogues have lost vitamin A's actions on vision and reproduction, but they have retained its roles of regulating epithelial differentiation and mucus production. Retinoic acid analogues have been developed to treat acne and keratinization disorders. Isotretinoin (13-cis-retinoic acid) is very effective against recalcitrant nodulocystic acne.[11] The synthetic retinoids etretin and etretinate are being used to treat severe psoriasis and keratinization disorders.[12] Unfortunately, at the doses required to treat these disorders, retinoic acid analogues are now producing most of the adverse effects previously chronicled in vitamin A poisonings.

The early side effects are manifested within 2 weeks of therapy—often within 48 hours.[13] Nearly all patients experience a temporary flare-up of acne. The vast majority also show cheilitis, facial erythema, and xerosis of the face and scalp. Dry mucous membranes probably account for the common additional symptoms of nosebleeds and rectal and vaginal itching.

Side effects appearing 1 month or later in the course of therapy include musculoskeletal symptoms, fatigue, minor depression, insomnia, decreased libido, menstrual irregularities, visual complaints, and hair loss.[13] Musculoskeletal symptoms, such as stiff or aching joints and backache, are noted in about one third of patients. Vague symptoms of fatigue and malaise, which cannot always be explained by abnormal liver function tests, occur in 10 per cent to 25 per cent of patients.[13]

Laboratory tests frequently reveal the hepatic side effects of retinoic acid therapy. Abnormal liver function tests and elevated levels of triglycerides and cholesterol are found in 10 per cent to 20 per cent of patients.[13] The high serum concentrations of low and very low density lipoproteins suggest that the hyperlipidemia associated with retinoic acid therapy stems from enhanced hepatic synthesis of lipoproteins.[17]

Radiographic changes in the skeleton can be demonstrated in the majority of patients receiving isotretinoin for over a year, even though half the patients remain asymptomatic.[14] The spectrum of changes includes generalized diminished bone density, premature fusion of epiphyses, ossification of ligaments, and osteophyte formation, particularly of the cervical spine.[14, 15] Premature epiphyseal fusion can lead to unequal extremities in children.[16]

The risk of bearing a malformed infant when a pregnant women is exposed to isotretinoin in the first trimester is in the range of 20 per cent to 25 per cent.[1] A characteristic pattern of malformations has arisen, involving the head, heart, thymus, and brain. The malformations include central nervous system defects, retinal or optic nerve abnormalities, small or absent ears, micrognathia, cleft palate, thymic defects, and conotruncal heart defects or aortic arch abnormalities. Thymic hypoplasia leads to progressive attrition of circulating T lymphocytes, which, in turn, predisposes the infants to infection and contributes to their high mortality.[18] The pattern of malformation closely mimics the retinoid teratogenesis induced in experimental animals.[1, 19] The retinoic acid dysmorphic syndrome may stem from the deleterious effects of retinoic acid on the developing cephalic–neural crest cells in the embryo.[1]

Retinoids are not mutagenic, so that subsequent pregnancies appear to be safe once these compounds are fully excreted.[1] Isotretinoin and etretin are not retained in tissues; unfortunately, etretinate, like vitamin A, is probably stored in the liver. The half-lives of isotretinoin, etretin, and etretinate after chronic administration are 16 to 20 hours, 2 to 4 days, and 84 to 168 days, respectively.[20] Hence, although conception is probably safe within a few months after discontinuing isotretinoin or etretin, pregnancy should be avoided for several years after chronic use of etretinate.[1, 12, 20]

VITAMIN D AND DERIVATIVES

Metabolism

Dietary vitamin D*† is absorbed in the duodenum and jejunum and reaches the portal circulation via the intestinal lymphatics. Most circulating vitamin D is taken up by hepatic cells for further metabolism, but small amounts are stored in adipose tissue and muscle. Vitamin D released from storage sites is transported in the circulation bound to a specific carrier protein, transcalciferol.[21, 22]

Hepatic vitamin D is hydroxylated at the 25 position to form 25-OH-D, which rapidly leaves the liver to become the major form of vitamin D in circulation. Levels of circulating 25-OH-D reflect vitamin D intake and body pool size. Hepatic hydroxylation is not influenced by parathyroid function or calcium metabolism and is only weakly inhibited by 25-OH-D blood levels.

In the kidney, 25-OH-D is further hydroxylated at the 1 position to form $1,25(OH)_2D$, or calcitriol. Production of $1,25(OH)_2D$ is stimulated by elevated concentrations of parathormone and phosphate and inhibited by rising levels of calcium and calcitriol. Calcitriol is a potent stimulator of calcium absorption at physiologic levels and of bone reabsorption at supraphysiologic levels. In terms of potency, 1 μg of vitamin D and 0.01 μg of calcitriol are equivalent to 40 IU of antirachitic activity.

Pathophysiology of Intoxication

Toxic doses of vitamin D for children range from 10,000 IU/day for 4 months to 200,000 IU/day for 2 weeks, with most cases receiving from 25,000 to 60,000 IU/day for 1 to 4 months. Twenty per cent of normal adults receiving 100,000 IU/day for several weeks or months develop hypercalcemia. Doses in the range of 1000 to 3000 IU/kg should be considered dangerous.[5]

Hypervitaminosis D produces hypercalcemia, hypercalciuria, and decreased fecal fat. Hypercalcemia is derived mainly from intestinal calcium absorption and, to a lesser degree, from bone reabsorption and diminished glomerular filtration. The pathologic effects of hypercalcemia are compounded by the damaging action of excessive vitamin D on membranes. As a result, calcium is deposited in soft tissues, including the myocardium, arterial walls, basement membrane of renal tubules, and alveolar septa of lung. Massive doses of vitamin D (10,000 IU/kg) during pregnancy are teratogenic, producing arterial stenosis in rabbits and possibly in humans.[23]

---

*The term vitamin D without a subscript is nonspecific and refers to both vitamin D_2 (ergocalciferol) and vitamin D_3 (cholicalciferol).

†Cutaneous vitamin D biosynthesis will not be considered since it is not a source of intoxication.

Patients who are hypersensitive to vitamin D develop toxicity even from relatively low doses. Vitamin D intake of 1000 to 4000 IU/day may be toxic to infants with idiopathic hypercalcemia syndrome (Williams' syndrome) and at any age in patients with chronic granulomatous disease, especially sarcoidosis.[24] Recent studies suggest that elevated circulating 1,25$(OH)_2D_3$ is responsible for the abnormal calcium metabolism in sarcoidosis; hypercalcemia develops in about 30 per cent of these patients.[25]

Clinical Signs of Intoxication

Symptoms and signs generally appear 2 to 8 days after acute intoxication with massive doses of vitamin D. Conversely, it may take several weeks or months for sufficient vitamin D accumulation to produce symptoms during chronic intoxication. The manifestations are related to hypercalcemia and in the early stages include weakness, fatigue, headache, nausea, vomiting, and diarrhea (Table 103–2). Polyuria and polydipsia usually develop because hypercalcemia inhibits the action of antidiuretic hormone on the distal tubule. Prolonged hypercalcemia produces nephrocalcinosis and metastatic calcifications of the cardiovascular system, leading to hypertension, cardiac insufficiency, renal failure, azotemia, and anemia. In contrast to vitamin A intoxication, tissue damage and metastatic calcification from vitamin D can be fatal.

Table 103–2. DIFFERENTIAL DIAGNOSIS OF HYPERCALCEMIA DUE TO HYPERVITAMINOSIS D

Hyperparathyroidism, primary, or secondary to renal disease
Paget's disease of bone
Neoplasms: lung, bone, renal
Nonparathyroid endocrinopathies
Hyperthyroidism
Adrenal insufficiency
Pheochromocytoma
Acromegaly
Other pharmacologic agents
Milk-alkali syndrome
Thiazide diuretics
Vitamin A
Calcium or lithium
Hypersensitivity to vitamin A
Granulomatous disease, especially sarcoidosis
Idiopathic infantile hypercalcemia
Miscellaneous
Newborn physiologic hypercalcemia
Immobilization
Phosphate depletion in uremia patients
Hypophosphatasia

Laboratory and Radiographic Findings

Blood calcium is elevated above 11 mg/dl, providing a good, albeit nonspecific, screening test for vitamin D intoxication (see differential diagnosis in Table 103–2). The blood citrate concentration is high, and the alkaline phosphatase low. Hypercalciuria, mildly elevated levels of serum phosphorus and blood urea nitrogen, and hypochromic anemia are commonly found. It is unclear whether doses of calcitriol too low to cause hypercalcemia are harmful to renal function.[26]

Bone radiographs show increased periosteal thickening and intense mineralization of the provisional line of calcification. Rarefaction of diaphysis is also present if mineral reabsorption has been severe. Radiologic evidence of metastatic calcifications can be demonstrated in kidneys (usually first and most severe), blood vessels, lungs, adrenal glands, cerebral membranes, and muscles (Fig. 103–2).

Commercial methods for measuring vitamin D are available.[23] Both vitamin D and 25-OH-D are elevated in vitamin D intoxication, but only blood 1,25$(OH)_2D_3$ is high in calcitriol overdose. The normal range for both vitamin D and 25-OH-D_3 is 10 to 50 pg/ml; values of 200 to 500 are often found in vitamin D intoxication. The normal range for 1,25$(OH)_2D_3$ concentration is 10 to 20 pg/ml; concentrations of 50 to 80 are reported in calcitriol overdosage. Because of the short half-life, the concentration of 1,25$(OH)_2D_3$ depends on the time of the last dose.

Treatment

Therapy depends on the vitamin D preparation used and the severity of hypercalcemia. Blood calcium usually falls to normal levels within a few days after stopping calcitriol, whereas hypercalcemia may persist for several days or even months after discontinuing vitamin D because of body storage.[23, 27] Moderate hypercalcemia (below 14 mg/dl) persisting beyond a few days after stopping vitamin D therapy should be treated with a low-calcium diet and prednisone (1 mg/kg/day).[28] Prednisone decreases calcium absorption from the gut and decreases

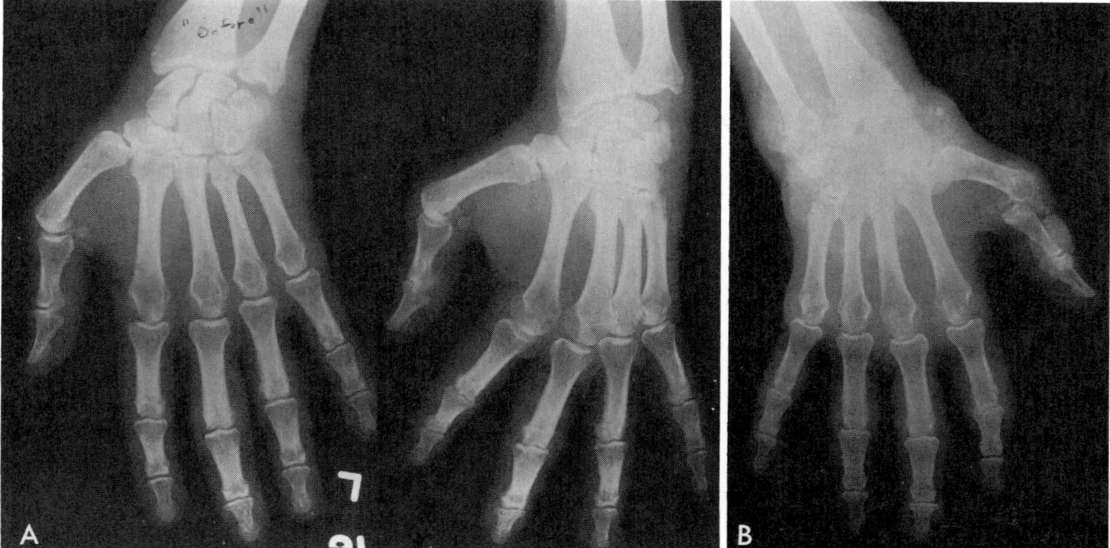

Figure 103–2. Periosteal thickening and intense mineralization of provisional line of calcification before (*A*, 1949) and after (*B*, 1954) vitamin D intoxication.

calcium mobilization from bone.[29] Prednisone also reduces 1,25$(OH)_2D_3$ levels to normal in sarcoidosis.[25] Persistent or severe hypercalcemia (above 14 mg/dl) can be treated additionally with hydration and calcitonin-salmon (4 to 8 IU/kg intramuscularly every 6 to 12 hours).[28, 30] Calcitonin acts by blocking bone reabsorption. Hydration (at least 100 to 200 ml/kg/day) and furosemide diuretics (0.5 to 1.0 mg/kg intravenously every 6 hours) will result in calciuresis and amelioration of hypercalcemia. The patient should be monitored for excessive urinary losses of sodium, potassium, phosphate, and magnesium. Peritoneal dialysis and hemodialysis can be utilized if large volumes of intravenous fluids are contraindicated in individuals with cardiac or renal insufficiency.[31] In cases of prolonged hypercalcemia due to massive vitamin D overdosage, treatment with inducers of hepatic microsomal enzyme synthesis (e.g., glutethimide) may be useful to enhance the rate of vitamin D degradation by the liver.[32]

References

1. Lammer EJ, Chen DT, Hoar RM, Agnish DN, et al: Retinoic acid embryopathy. N Engl J Med *313*:837, 1985.
2. Goodman DS: Vitamin A and retinoids in health and disease. N Engl J Med *310*:1023, 1984.
3. Smith RF, Goodman DS: Vitamin A transport in human vitamin A toxicity. N Engl J Med *294*:805, 1976.
4. Mahoney CP, Margolis MT, Knauss TA, Labbe RF: Chronic vitamin A intoxication in infants fed chicken liver. Pediatrics *65*:893, 1980.
5. Inkeles SB, Conor WE, Illingworth DR: Hepatic and dermatologic manifestations of chronic hypervitaminosis A in adults. Am J Med *80*:491, 1986.
6. Hayes KC, Hegsted DM: Toxicity of Vitamins in Toxicants Occurring Naturally in Food. 2nd ed. Washington, DC, National Academy of Science, 1973.
7. Fantel AG, Shepard TH, Newell-Morris LL, Moffett BC: Teratogenic effects of retinoic acid in pigtail monkeys *(Macaca nemestrina)*; General features. Teratology *15*:65, 1977.
8. Strange L, Carlstrom K, Erickson M: Hypervitaminosis A in early pregnancy and malformations of the central nervous system. Acta Obstet Gynecol Scand *57*:289, 1978.
9. Braun IG: Vitamin A excess, deficiency, metabolism, and misuse. Pediatr Clin North Am *9*:935, 1962.
10. Schaywitz B, Siegel NJ, Pearson HA: Megavitamins for minimal brain dysfunction: A potentially dangerous therapy. JAMA *238*:1749, 1977.
11. Peck GL, Olsen TG, Yoder FW, Strauss JS, et al: Prolonged remissions of cystic and conglobate acne with 13-cis-retinoic acid. N Engl J Med *300*:329, 1979.
12. Madhok R, Muller SA, Dicken CH: Treatment of psoriasis with etretin: A preliminary report. Mayo Clin Proc *62*:1084, 1987.
13. Bruno NP, Beacham BE, Burnett JW: Adverse effects of isotretinoin therapy. Cutis *33*:484, 1984.
14. Lawson JP, McGuire J: The spectrum of skeletal changes associated with long-term administration of 13-cis-retinoic acid. Skeletal Radiol *16*:91, 1987.
15. DiGiovana JJ, Helgott RK, Gerber LH, Peck GL: Extraspinal tendon and ligament calcification associated with long-term therapy with etretinate. N Engl J Med *315*:1177, 1986.

16. Prendiville J, Bingham EA, Burrows D: Premature epiphyseal closure—a complication of etretinate therapy in children. J Am Acad Dermatol *15*:1259, 1986.
17. Marsdsen J: Hyperlipidemia due to isotretinoin and etretinate: Possible mechanism and consequences. Br J Dermatol *114*:401, 1986.
18. Cohen M, Rubinstein A, Li JK, Mathenson G: Thymic hypoplasia associated with isotretinoin embryopathy. Am J Dis Child *141*:263, 1987.
19. Willhite CC, Hill RM, Irving DW: Isotretinoin-induced craniofacial malformations in humans and hamsters. J Craniofac Genet Dev Biol (Suppl 2):193, 1986.
20. Brazzell RK, Coburn WA: Pharmacokinetics of the retinoids isotretinoin and etretinate. J Am Acad Dermatol *6*:463, 1982.
21. Schnoes HK, DeLuca HF: Recent progress in vitamin D metabolism and the chemistry of vitamin D metabolites. Fed Proc *39*:2723, 1980.
22. Favus MJ: Vitamin D physiology: Some clinical aspects of the vitamin D endocrine system. Med Clin North Am *63*:1291, 1978.
23. Taussio HB: Possible injury to the cardiovascular system from vitamin D. Ann Intern Med *65*:1195, 1966.
24. Zaweda ET, Lee DB, Kleeman CR: Causes of hypercalcemia. Postgrad Med J *66*:91, 1979.
25. Chesney RW, Hamstra HA, DeLuca HF, et al: Elevated serum 1,25-dihydroxyvitamin D concentrations in the hypercalcemia of sarcoidosis: Correction by glucocorticoid therapy. J Pediatr *98*:919, 1981.
26. Massry SG, Goldstein DA: Is calcitriol (1,25[OH]$_2$D$_3$) harmful to renal function? JAMA *242*:1875, 1979.
27. Chan JCM, Hsu AC: Vitamin D and renal disease. Adv Pediatr *27*:117, 1980.
28. Inesi G: Emergency management of hypercalcemia. Drug Ther (Hosp) *3*:14, 1978.
29. Streck WF, Waterhouse C, Haddad JG: Glucocorticoid effects in vitamin D intoxication. Arch Intern Med *139*:974, 1979.
30. Bergquist E, Sjoberg HE, Hjern B, Hallberg D, Caustrom A: Calcitonin in the treatment of hypercalcemic crisis. Acta Med Scand *192*:385, 1972.
31. Cardella CJ, Birkin BC, Roscoe M, Rapoport A: Role of dialysis in the treatment of severe hypercalcemia: Report of two cases successfully treated with hemodialysis and review of literature. Clin Nephrol *12*:283, 1979.
32. Igbal SJ, Taylor WH: Treatment of vitamin D$_2$ poisoning by induction of hepatic enzymes. Br Med J *285*:541, 1982.

CHAPTER 104
BABY POWDER, BORATES, AND CAMPHOR

A. Baby Powder

Thomas O. Stair, M.D.

Baby powder is a hazard when aspirated into the tracheobronchial tree. A sibling may throw powder in the face of an infant, or during a diaper change a toddler may grab a canister with a loose top and, mistaking it for a bottle, raise it to its mouth, only to gasp and aspirate when the contents fall out. Swallowed baby powder tends to be poorly absorbed and is relatively nontoxic.[1]

Initial reports of baby powder aspiration tended to be single, fatal cases.[2, 3] Subsequently more survivors were reported because of both better case finding and improved respiratory support techniques.[4–9] Logs of poison centers now reveal many more mild cases, most with no symptoms and requiring follow-up but no treatment.[1, 10]

Early symptoms of baby powder aspiration include coughing, sneezing, dyspnea, and vomiting. Enough powder can produce acute airway obstruction. Even if initially asymptomatic, aspiration pneumonitis can soon proceed to wheezing, tachypnea, and respiratory distress. Secondary bronchopulmonary inflammation can produce respiratory failure in a few hours.[1]

Several reports describe this asymptomatic interval,[3, 6, 7] and one case has been reported only because of progressive inflammatory pulmonary talcosis noted 8 years after aspiration.[11] Thus, every possible aspiration of baby powder, no matter how innocuous appearing at first, should be followed up and parents informed of possible late sequelae.

Severe aspiration pneumonitis may require

endotracheal intubation, ventilatory support, and positive end expiratory pressure (PEEP). Corticosteroids may reduce late respiratory failure in a few cases,[4, 5, 8] but prophylactic antibiotics have shown no obvious benefit. Bronchial washing has been used successfully, but its value is limited by the insolubility of the powder.[7, 9]

There are many formulations of baby powder, but the major ingredient is usually talc, a commercially mined mineral of naturally variable composition, primarily composed of hydrated magnesium silicate. Talc from some sources has a higher content of asbestos, but no carcinogenic effect has been demonstrated from cosmetic-grade talcum powder.[12]

Talc particles in dusting powders average about 1 μm in diameter, which means they may be small enough to filter down to the alveolar level.[2] When chronically inhaled, talc can produce a pneumoconiosis; acutely it produces an intense inflammatory reaction.

Other common ingredients of baby powder include calcium and zinc salts, kaolin, phynyl mercury borate, petrolatum, and perfume. Cornstarch is a major ingredient in "talc-free" baby powder. All of these substances can, when inhaled, produce a similar aspiration pneumonitis.

There is no real need to put powder on babies. Baby powder's absorptive capacity is negligible compared with that of a diaper; its fragrance and friction-reducing effects are transient; it is less effective as a vehicle for medication than a cream or lotion; and parents are not often aware of the danger of aspirating baby powder.[10]

References

1. Mofenson HC, et al: Baby powder—a hazard. Pediatrics *68*:265, 1981.
2. Molnar JJ, Nathanson G, Edberg S: Fatal aspiration of talcum powder by a child: Report of a case. N Engl J Med *266*:36–37, 1962.
3. Jenkins MQ: Poisoning of the month: Dusting powder inhalation. J South Car Med Assoc *59*:62–63, 1963.
4. Hughes WT, Kalmer T: Massive talc aspiration: Successful treatment with dexamethasone. Am J Dis Child *111*:653–654, 1966.
5. Lund JS, Feldt-Rasmussen M: Accidental aspiration of talc: Report of a case in a two-year-old child. Acta Pediatr Scand *58*:295–296, 1969.
6. Gould SR, Bernardo ED: Respiratory distress after talc inhalation. Br J Dis Chest *66*:230–233, 1972.
7. Pfenninger J, D'Apuzzo V: Powder aspiration in children: Report of two cases. Arch Dis Child *52*:157–159, 1977.
8. Brouilette F, Weber ML: Massive aspiration of talcum powder by an infant. Can Med Assoc J *119*:354–355, 1978.
9. Motomatsu K, Adachi H, Uno T: Two infant deaths after inhaling baby powder. Chest *75*:448–450, 1979.
10. Moss MH: Dangers from talcum powder. Pediatrics *43*:1058, 1969.
11. Cruthirds TP, Cole FH, Paul RN: Pulmonary talcosis as a result of massive aspiration of baby powder. South Med J *70*:626–628, 1977.
12. Cosmetic talc powder (editorial). Lancet *1*:1348–1349, 1977.

B. Borates

N. John Stewart, M.D., FACEP
Terrance P. McHugh, M.D., FACEP

Borates are salts or esters of boric acid, H_3PO_3. Borax, also known as sodium borate or sodium tetraborate, is an alkaline salt having the chemical formula $Na_2B_4O_7 \cdot 10H_2O$ and has been used as a cleansing agent since ancient Greek and Roman times. Originally imported into the United States from China and Japan, by the mid 1800s large borax deposits were discovered in California's Death Valley, which continues to be the principal US domestic source.

In 1702, William Homberg formed boric acid by mixing borax with mineral acid. He introduced boric acid into medical usage as a sedative, antispasmodic, and analgesic known as sal sedativum Hombergi (Homberg's Sedative Salt).[1] Joseph Lister, in 1875, is credited with the first antiseptic application of boric acid, thus promoting its use in a multitude of products.[2] The first two deaths from boric acid solutions were reported in 1881; a boric acid solution was used to irrigate the pleural cavity in one victim and a lumbar abscess in a second.[2]

Sources

Boric acid has been used as a gastric, colonic, thoracic, wound, joint, and eye irrigant, usually as a 5 per cent solution. Boric compounds have also been used in baby powders, in topical ointments as buffering or antifungal agents, in mouthwashes and dentifrices, in eyewashes, and as a food preservative. In recent years, boric acid has gained popularity as an insecticide, deployed in a tablet or powder form that is 99 per cent pure. Because boric acid is not bactericidal and only weakly bacteriostatic, its therapeutic uses have been supplanted by newer, safer, and more effective compounds. Nevertheless, numerous preparations containing boric acid are still available (Table 104–1).

Pharmacology

Boric acid is a colorless, odorless, nonstaining compound available in granule, crystal, or powder form and in solution. Boric acid is rapidly absorbed through the gastrointestinal tract and across mucous membranes, serous cavities, and abraded or denuded skin; it is not well absorbed across healthy intact skin.[3, 4] Boric acid is distributed throughout the body but has an affinity for the liver, brain, and kidneys.[3, 5] Borate excretion occurs mainly through the kidneys; greater than 50 per cent of an oral dose is excreted unchanged by the kidneys within 24 hours and 90 per cent by 96 hours.[3, 4] The half-life of boric acid is reported to vary between 5 and 21 hours.[4, 6–8]

Neither the minimal symptomatic dose nor the median lethal dose (LD_{50}) for humans is known. Systemic poisonings have occurred in humans after ingestion of 0.2 gm/kg.[9] Although the LD_{50} in various animal species ranges from 0.8 to 6.4 gm/kg,[9] the adult human LD_{50} probably exceeds 30 gm (1 teaspoon of pure boric acid crystals contains approximately 3 to 5 gm of boric acid).

Boric acid is teratogenic in chick embryos; the resulting malformations resemble those caused by riboflavin deficiency, and supplemental administration of riboflavin reduces their incidence.[8, 10] In animal models, the supplemental administration of riboflavin caused a decreased incidence of boric acid toxicity.[11] In humans, an increase in the urinary excretion of riboflavin has been documented following boric acid ingestion.[10] Although supplemental riboflavin may prove a future therapeutic tool in cases of human boric acid poisoning, no studies to date have demonstrated such efficacy.[8, 10]

TABLE 104–1. EXAMPLES OF PRODUCTS CONTAINING BORATES

Medications
Wyanoid hemorrhoidal suppositories (Wyeth)
Borofax ointment (Burroughs-Wellcome)
Eye Preparations
Collyrium eye lotion (Wyeth)
Murine Plus eye drops (Abbott)
Clear Eyes eye drops (Abbott)
Contact lens solutions
Cleansing Products
20 Mule Team Borax
Boraxo Powdered Hand Soap
Uni-Wash skin cleanser (United)
Insecticides
Roach-Pruf roach powder
Harris Famous Roach Tablets
Industrial Products
Kodak photographic F5A hardener
Fireproofing of clothing

Toxicology

The principal toxic effects of borates involve the gastrointestinal tract, central nervous system, skin, liver, and kidneys; these effects may be delayed hours to days following exposure.[12] Infants are more susceptible to borate intoxication than adults and have a higher risk of death.[9]

Because reports in the literature vary widely, it is difficult to determine an exact minimum lethal dose (MLD). The MLD has been estimated to be between 3 and 5 gm for an infant and between 15 and 20 gm for an adult.[5, 10] Individual susceptibility varies widely. Schillinger and associates[3] reported a 44 year old female who ingested 14 gm of boric acid and, although she developed exfoliative dermatitis, renal failure, and elevated liver function tests, fully recovered after a 2-week hospital stay. However, Linden and colleagues[9] reported a 14 month old infant who ingested 20 gm without apparent symptoms and a 27 year old who ingested 297 gm and developed vomiting as the sole symptom.

In 1962, Valdes-Dapens and Arey[2] reviewed 175 cases of boric acid poisoning collected from the world literature; 86 of the cases were fatal. Fatal cases appeared to follow the use of boric acid as an irrigation solution within body cavities or as a powder applied to burned or denuded skin.[1, 2, 5] Most deaths occurred during the earlier years of the review, with the last adult death from a single acute ingestion having been reported in 1928.[4, 9]

Litovitz and coworkers[4] recently reported 792 cases of acute ingestions, including exposures up to 88.8 gm; no deaths were noted, and 88 per cent of the patients were totally asymptomatic. They concluded that, *in adults*, a single large dose of boric acid was essentially nontoxic. A 1986 report from the American Association of Poison Control Centers lists 2335 exposures to borates and boric acid, excluding topical medications and insecticides.[13] Of these cases, no deaths occurred.

A major tragedy of the past was the frequency of infant poisonings. A powdered form of boric acid applied to raw diaper areas has been implicated in a number of severe cases.[2, 14, 15] The accidental use of boric acid solutions in infant formulas has occurred frequently, even in hospital nurseries. Wong and associates[16] reported on 11 infants in a newborn nursery fed formula prepared with a 2.5 per cent boric acid solution; five of the infants died. Baker and Bogema[6] reported two siblings (24 days old and 14 months old) fed a solution of boric acid that originally had been prepared as an eye wash; both of these infants survived. Cases such as these prompted the American Academy of Pediatrics to recommend the elimination of boric acid from the newborn nurseries and pediatric wards of all hospitals.[17]

Chronic borate exposure can also lead to toxicity; repeated small doses are more dangerous than a single acute ingestion.[14] Chronic intoxication has been reported following the ingestion of 4 to 5 gm of boric acid daily over a 3- to 4-week period or the ingestion of 6 to 20 gm of borax daily for several months.[2, 3] Stein and colleagues[18] reported a case of toxic alopecia from repeated ingestion of mouthwash containing boric acid, and Tan[19] reported another case of a storekeeper who daily filled a dispenser with a washing powder containing borax. O'Sullivan and Taylor[20] reported seizures in seven infants that resolved following termination of use of a honey and borax mixture on their pacifiers.

Borax dust exposure can also act as an irritant. In a study of borax workers, Garabrant and associates[21] found that boric acid or borax dust particles act as an irritant to the eyes and repiratory tract. Small changes in the respiratory function of smokers, as measured by forced expiratory volume (FEV_1), have been reported following dust exposure.[22] The American Conference of Governmental Industrial Hygienists has proposed a threshold limit value of 10 mg/m^3 and a short-term exposure limit of 20 mg/m^3 for boron oxide.[21]

Clinical Presentation

Acute borate ingestion produces a clinical syndrome akin to acute gastroenteritis. Abdominal cramps, nausea, vomiting, and diarrhea are all typical complaints and may develop irrespective of the route of administration. Although not consistent findings, a blue-green discoloration and blood have often been noted in the feces or vomitus.[4, 6] The most striking clinical finding involves the skin and arises 1 to 3 days after ingestion. The skin becomes very erythematous—the "boiled lobster" appearance—and then progresses to general desquamation and exfoliation over the next 1 to 2 days.[6] This process can involve the mucous membranes as well as the skin. In infants, this rash resembles toxic epidermal necrolysis—scalded skin syndrome or Lyell's or Ritter's disease—and boric acid poisoning should be considered in its differential diagnosis.[6, 23] This rash can also be confused with cases of scarlet fever or Kawasaki's disease.[5] Neurologic manifestations of borate toxicity include confusion, headache, weakness, lethargy, coma, and seizures.[6] Although irritability is commonly seen in infants, central nervous system (CNS) depression is more common in adults. Oliguria and proteinuria may herald acute tubular necrosis, but renal symptoms are not common. Mild liver function abnormalities and jaundice also have been reported.[4]

Chronic borate exposure may produce any of the following signs or symptoms: alopecia, anemia, menstrual disorders, skin disorders, anorexia, weight loss, vomiting, chronic diarrhea, seizures, or death.[19, 20]

Laboratory Assessment

Most hospital laboratories are incapable of measuring either boric acid or boron levels in a timely fashion. However, this is not critical since the results do not correlate well with either the amount ingested or the resulting clinical state.[4, 9] Measured values are of interest in documenting exposure but should not dictate treatment.[9] The US Borax and Chemical Co. can provide assistance in analyzing serum for borates; they can be reached at their 24-hour telephone number (714–774–2673). They require that blood, in an unbreakable container, and a case report be sent via express overnight mail to US Borax Research, 412 Crescent Way, Anaheim, CA 92801; results should be available the next day (personal communication).

Small amounts of boric acid are normally present in the body as a result of dietary intake of fruits, vegetables, bread, and cereals; normal serum boric acid levels range from 1.4 to 2.5 μg/ml.[2] In infants, the average blood borate level was found to be 0.25 μg/ml with a range of 0.0 to 1.25 μg/ml.[24] In adult males the mean was 0.6 μg/ml. Symptoms of toxicity are usually associated with blood levels of 20 to 150 μg/ml.[6, 16, 20]

Some laboratories measure serum boron levels instead of boric acid levels. If boron levels are measured, the relationship between serum boric acid and serum boron is expressed by the following equation:[4, 9, 25]

$$\text{serum boric acid (mg/dl)} = \text{serum boron level (mg/dl)} \times 5.72$$

A simple bedside test was once widely used to detect boron.[16] The patient's urine was acidified and then applied to turmeric paper. A pink to brown color change indicated the presence of boron. However, because this test is capable of detecting even normal dietary boron, it is too sensitive and should no longer be used.[2]

Treatment

There is no antidote for boric acid poisoning, and good supportive care remains the mainstay of treatment. Following acute ingestions, gastric emptying should be induced with syrup of ipecac, 30 ml for an adult and 15 ml for a child, or by means of gastric lavage. Cathartics should be administered to speed bowel transit. Activated charcoal has been shown to be ineffective in absorbing boric acid and is not indicated in a pure borate ingestion; however, it should still be given in cases of multiple drug ingestion.[12] Intravenous fluid administration may become necessary, especially if severe dehydration or shock develops from prolonged vomiting or diarrhea. In select cases, laboratory measurement of electrolytes and liver or renal function tests should be considered. If skin desquamation occurs, local skin care is of paramount importance, and antibiotics should be given only if secondary bacterial infection develops. Following chronic exposures, immediate suspension of contact with boric acid or other compounds of boron is essential.

Exchange transfusions, peritoneal dialysis, and hemodialysis have all been shown to have varying degrees of success in lowering plasma boron levels.[4, 15, 16, 26] Exchange transfusion has many limitations and is generally no longer used.[16] Of the other two procedures, hemodialysis appears to be the most effective. It is interesting that some authors suggest dialysis following large ingestions even in asymptomatic patients, whereas others feel this is not necessary since most acute ingestions are so benign.[4, 9, 26] Baker and Bogema[6] recommend consideration of dialysis in the presence of severe clinical symptoms or when serum boric acid levels are in excess of 200 μg/ml. Hemodialysis is clearly indicated in patients with oliguric renal failure or those whose severe fluid or electrolyte abnormalities cannot be corrected by conventional therapy.

Litovitz and coworkers[4] have recommended the following treatment protocol for *acute* ingestions. If the patient weighs less than 30 kg, observation only is recommended for ingestions of less than 200 mg/kg, ipecac syrup for ingestions of between 200 and 400 mg/kg, and measurement of blood levels 2 to 3 hours post ingestion for ingestions of more than 400 mg/kg. If the patient weighs more than 30 kg, observation only is recommended for ingestions of less than 6 gm, ipecac syrup for ingestions of 6 to 12 gm, and measurement of blood levels for ingestions that exceed 12 gm. The blood tests are used to document ingestion, not to guide therapeutic decisions. Hemodialysis should be considered for greatly elevated blood levels or if serious symptoms develop. It should be noted that this protocol does not apply to newborns or patients suffering from chronic exposure to borates.

Summary

Boric acid has caused many toxic problems since its introduction into medical practice. Fortunately, since the medical community has realized the toxicity of borates and no longer uses them as irrigation solutions or in powders applied to open or raw skin, deaths have become exceedingly rare. With adults, single large ingestions are almost always nonfatal and aggressive therapy usually is not necessary. Infants, however, appear to be at a greater risk, and newborns fed formulas contaminated with borates have the highest risk of death. Every effort should be made to avoid their use in this age group. A potential new threat is the availability of 99 per cent pure boric acid in some insecticides.

References

1. Goldbloom RB, Goldbloom A: Boric acid poisoning: Report of four cases and a review of the world literature. J Pediatr *49*:631–643, 1959.
2. Valdes-Despena MA, Arey JB: Boric acid poisoning: three fatal cases with pancreatic inclusions and a review of the literature. J Pediatr *61*:531–546, 1962.
3. Schillinger BM, Berstein M, Goldberg LA, et al: Boric acid poisoning. J Am Acad Dermatol *7*:667–673, 1982.
4. Litovitz TL, Klein-Schwartz W, Odera GM, et al: Clinical manifestations of toxicity in a series of 784 boric acid ingestions. Am J Emerg Med *6*:209–213, 1988.
5. Siegel E, Wason S: Boric acid toxicity. Pediatr Clin North Am *33*:363–367, 1986.
6. Baker MD, Bogema SC: Ingestion of boric acid by infants. Am J Emerg Med *4*:358–361, 1986.
7. Schou JS, Jansen JA, Aggerbeck B: Human pharmacokinetics and safety of boric acid. Arch Toxicol *7*(Suppl):232–235, 1984.
8. Roe DA: Recollections of nutrition and the chemical environment. J Nutr *117*:416–420, 1987.
9. Linden CH, Hall AH, Kulig KW, et al: Acute ingestions of boric acid. J Toxicol Clin Toxicol *24*:269–279, 1986.
10. Pinto J, Huang VP, McConnell RJ, et al: Increased riboflavin excretion resulting from boric acid ingestion. J Lab Clin Med *92*:126–135, 1978.
11. Roe DA, McCormick DB, Lin RT: Effects of riboflavin on boric acid toxicity. J Pharm Sci *61*:1081–1085, 1972.
12. Odera GM, Klein-Schwartz W, Insley BM: In vitro study of boric acid and activated charcoal. Clin Toxicol *25*:13–19, 1987.
13. Litovitz TL, Martin TG, Schmitz BS: 1986 annual report of the American Association of Poison Control Centers National Data Collection System. Am J Emerg Med *5*:405–445, 1987.
14. Skipworth GB, Goldstein N, McBride WP: Boric acid intoxication from "medicated talcum powder." Arch Dermatol *95*:83–86, 1967.
15. Balih T, MacLeish H, Drummond KN: Acute boric acid poisoning: Report of an infant successfully treated by peritoneal dialysis. Can Med Assoc J *101*:166–168, 1969.
16. Wong LC, Heimbach MD, Truscott DR, et al: Boric acid poisoning: report of 11 cases. Can Med Assoc J *90*:1018–1023, 1964.
17. American Academy of Pediatrics, Subcommittee on Accidental Poisonings: Statement on hazards of boric acid. Pediatrics *26*:884, 1960.
18. Stein KM, Odom RB, Justice GR, et al: Toxic alopecia from ingestion of boric acid. Arch Dermatol *108*:95–97, 1973.
19. Tan TG: Occupational toxic alopecia due to borax. Acta Dermatol (Stockholm) *50*:55–58, 1970.
20. O'Sullivan K, Taylor M: Chronic boric acid poisoning in infants. Arch Dis Child *58*:737–749, 1983.
21. Garabrant DH, Bernstein L, Peters JM, et al: Respiratory and eye irritation from boron oxide and boric acid dust. J Occup Med *26*:584–586, 1984.
22. Garabrant DH, Bernstein L, Peters JM, et al: Respiratory effects of borax dust. Br J Ind Med *42*:831–837, 1985.
23. Rubenstein AD, Musher DM: Epidemic boric acid poisoning simulating staphylococcal toxic epidermal necrolysis of the newborn infant: Ritter's disease. Pediatr Pharmacol Ther *77*:884–887, 1970.
24. Fisher RS, Freimuth HC: Blood boron levels in human infants. J Invest Dermatol *30*:85–86, 1958.
25. Weir RJ, Fisher RS: Toxicologic studies on borax and boric acid. Toxicol Appl Pharmacol *23*:351–364, 1972.
26. Martin GI: Asymptomatic boric acid intoxication: Value of peritoneal dialysis. NY State J Med *71*:1842–1844, 1971.

C. Camphor

Robert C. Kopelman, M.D.

Camphor (2-camphanone) is a cyclic ketone of the hydroaromatic terpene group.[1] It was listed in the US Pharmacopeia as a topical rubefacient, antipruritic, and mild local anesthetic agent. Camphor is obtained naturally by steam distilling chips of the camphor tree or synthetically from pinene ($C_{10}H_{10}$), a hydrocarbon obtained from turpentine oil.[2]

Camphor's strong medicinal odor undoubtedly explains its continued use in more than 20 popular over-the-counter external analgesic rubs in the absence of acknowledged efficacy (Table 104–2).[3] Less appreciated is its toxicity. Camphor is rated very toxic, with a probable human lethal dose of 50 to 500 mg/kg.[4]

The AAPCC National Data Collection System in 1987 reported 4691 exposures to camphor, requiring 1499 patients to be treated in a health care facility.[5] The Committee on Drugs of the American Academy of Pediatrics has recommended removal of camphor from all products as it "has no established, therapeutic role in scientific medicine."[6] Over 21 fatalities have been recorded.

It is striking that all the fatalities have occurred either because a camphor-containing preparation was substituted in error for an intended efficacious drug or a child accidentally ingested a preparation intended for topical use. The most common substitutions have been camphor for castor oil, cod liver oil, and Castoria.[7] Camphorated oil contains 20 per cent camphor in cottonseed oil, and many over-the-counter preparations contain 5 to 10 per cent camphor. One teaspoon of camphorated oil is potentially lethal for an infant, and the quantities of the more dilute preparations necessary to cause significant morbidity or mortality are modest. Poisoning by topical application and inhalation are demonstrated by the case of a 7 year old child who developed seizures after crawling through spilled spirits-of-camphor and had recurrent seizures 1 year later after camphor vapor inhalation.[8]

Parenteral camphor was employed by Meduna in 1933 for the purpose of inducing seizures in the treatment of catatonic stupor.[9] He evaluated the dose response in animals necessary to produce seizures without pathologic changes in the brain. Hundreds of schizophrenic patients were probably treated with intramuscular camphor in oil prior to the development of pentylenetetrazol as a seizure-inducing agent. Insulin and electroconvulsive therapy (ECT) have replaced these toxic agents. Attempts to use camphor in the treatment of mental illness by induction of seizures dates to the late 18th century. At least one death associated with camphor ingestion for such treatment purposes has been reported.

TABLE 104–2. A PARTIAL LISTING OF OVER-THE-COUNTER PREPARATIONS CONTAINING CAMPHOR

	MANUFACTURER	% CAMPHOR
Camphorated oil	Various	20.00
Campho-Phenique	Glenbrook	10.80
Camphor spirits	Various	10.00
Soltice Hi-Therm Analgesic Balm	Chattem	7.00
Ben-Gay Children's Rub	Pfizer	6.00
Soltice Quick-Rub (Adult)	Chattem	5.10
Sayman Salve	Carson	5.00
Vicks Vaporub	Vick	4.81
Panalgesic	Polythress	4.00
Heet	Whitehall	4.00
Soltice Quick Rub (Children's)	Chattem	3.75
Sloan's Liniment	Standard	3.40
Guia-Camp	Dorsey	3.00
Soltice Hi-Therm Arthritic Lotion	Chattem	3.00
Lini-Balm Aerosol Foam	Arnar-Stone	2.00
Analbalm	Central	1.50
Sloan's Balm	Standard	0.50
Rhulicream	Lederle	0.30
Musterole	Plough	?
Penetro Quick Acting Rub	Plough	?
Va-Tro-Nol	Vick	?
Mother's Friend	SSS	?

All products are for external analgesic rub.

(Adapted from Phelan WJ III: Camphor poisoning: Over-the-counter dangers. Pediatrics 57:428, 1976. Copyright American Academy of Pediatrics 1976.)

Clinical Signs of Intoxication

The most important clinical signs of camphor intoxication are (1) nausea, vomiting, and burning epigastric pain; (2) changed mental status; (3) increased muscular irritability; and (4) grand mal seizures. The amount of ingested camphor absorbed increased by 80 per cent when mixed with a solvent.[10] Symptoms begin 5 to 90 minutes after ingestion and are often abrupt in onset. Vomiting is frequently the first sign, with the odor of camphor being readily apparent.[11] Because vomiting is so common, the actual absorbed dose is usually unknown.

Generalized grand mal seizures may occur without prior warning or after premonitory movement disorders or mental confusion or hallucinations. Seizures have been treated by standard antiepileptic agents, but recurrent seizures, resolving only after active measures for removal of camphor, have been reported in more severe cases. Barbiturates may be protective of permanent central nervous system damage and have therefore been recommended by some investigators.[12]

Benz reported a unique experience in 1919.[13] Twenty children, aged 4 to 10 years, were given 1 to 1.5 tablespoonfuls of camphorated oil instead of castor oil. All became ill, beginning 45 minutes after the ingestion. Most had seizures, and one child had recurrent seizures and coma lasting 20 hours but was reported well at 29 hours.

Complete recovery has been reported in all survivors, although careful follow-up is usually lacking. Several observations suggest that this statement must be guarded. Smith and Margolis reported pathologic changes in the brain of a 19 month old infant who expired 5 days after ingestion of 5 ml of camphorated oil.[12] The investigators report that "extensive degenerative changes selectively involving neurons and sparing glial and vascular structures . . . were most severe in Sommer's section of the hippocampus, where virtually every pyramidal cell was necrotic."

The investigators then evaluated the role of pentobarbital administered along with camphor intraperitoneally in mice. Convulsions were prevented in all mice and the brains were pathologically normal, as were pentobarbital-administered controls. Based on these observations, they recommended administration of barbiturates. No other anticonvulsants were investigated.

Jimenez and coworkers[14] reported a case of a 6 month old infant who was admitted with suspected Reye's syndrome based on hepatic injury associated with rapid neurologic deterioration following a respiratory infection. When liver histology was inconsistent with Reye's syndrome, a repeat history revealed that the mother had been administering a home remedy that was shown to contain 3 per cent camphor and 33 per cent alcohol. It had been given in small amounts for 5 months, with an estimated 300 mg/kg administered in the 3 days prior to admission. The infant developed brain death on the fifth hospital day. The pathologic findings in the brain were similar to those previously described in an infant by Smith and Margolis.[12]

In another report,[3] a 3 year old female had onset of seizures approximately 3 hours after ingestion of an estimated 0.7 gm of camphor. She was treated with conservative supportive measures and appeared well 21 hours after the ingestion. An electroencephalogram obtained 18 hours after the seizures revealed "excessive slow activity in the bianterior and bicentral regions without specific paroxysmal discharges." The electroencephalogram was unchanged at 15 days but normal at 90 days.

Management of Camphor Poisoning

Management of camphor intoxication is guided by awareness of the clinical spectrum and chemical nature of camphor. The possibility of camphor is suggested by the history or the odor of camphor on the breath or in the gastric contents or urine. The medicine bottle should be checked for contents, as castor oil and camphor in oil are frequently made by the same companies and sold in nearly identically labeled containers placed alphabetically adjacent on the pharmacy shelf. The possible abrupt development of seizures dictates the use of emergency transportation. The patient should not be left unattended. Activated charcoal and cathartics should be administered. Gastric lavage should be used in recent (less than 2 hours) ingestions. Unsupervised use of emetics is hazardous because of the risk of seizures. Oils may enhance the absorption of camphor and should not be administered.[7, 10]

Since the majority of ingestions are small and of low toxicity, one goal in management is assessment of risk. Two groups have developed guidelines for use in poison control centers. Geller and colleagues recommend home observation for ingestions of less than 10 mg/kg; activated charcoal and cathartics for ingestions of 10 to 30 mg/kg; and transport to an emergency medical facility for ingestions of more than 30 mg/kg.[15] Siegel and Wason use a higher threshold, with observation alone for up to 1000-mg ingestions; use of charcoal and cathartics for ingestions greater than 1000 mg; and admission only with symptoms or ingestions greater than 3000 mg.[16]

Active measures to remove camphor have been undertaken in five reported cases with recurrent seizures. Ginn and associates first employed hemodialysis with lipid dialysate and a Klung plate dialyzer.[17] Soybean oil was used because of the high lipid solubility of camphor. The patient was described as alert after 3 hours of dialysis. The procedure was stopped after 4.5 hours, and the patient made a complete recovery. Antman and colleagues also employed lipid dialysis, using soybean oil and a 1 m^2 coil dialyzer.[18] They reported cessation of seizures and clearing of the camphor odor on the patient's breath coincident with the appearance of the camphor odor in the soybean oil bath. These workers suggested that hemoperfusion with Amberlite XAD-4 resin might be effective.

Kopelman and colleagues reported treatment of a 37 year old man with recurrent seizures with combined lipid (Wesson oil) hemodialysis and Amberlite XAD-4 hemoperfusion.[19] The patient awoke after 2.5 hours of active removal and made an uneventful recovery. Measurement of plasma camphor levels revealed complete extraction by the Amberlite XAD-4 resin but only 60 per cent extraction when lipid hemodialysis alone was used.

Mascie-Taylor and colleagues reported on a patient treated with a Haemocol charcoal hemoperfusion cartridge and a 10 per cent Intralipid dialysate bath in series.[20] The patient had experienced two seizures prior to arrival in the emergency department and was obtunded on arrival without hyperreflexia. Plasma camphor concentrations revealed essentially complete clearance by the charcoal cartridge. The Intralipid dialysate was discontinued owing to suspected hemolysis, and its ability to adsorb camphor could not be measured.

Köppel and colleagues also used Amberlite XAD-4 resin hemoperfusion to treat a 54 year old female with recurrent seizures, coma, and respiratory depression.[10] They stated that the seizures ceased but "extracorporeal detoxification had no marked influence on the stage of coma." The patient recovered fully. Camphor was cleared by the resin with 89 to 95 per cent efficiency, but the total amount actively removed was only 35 mg.

The exact role of active removal of camphor is undetermined. Active seizures ceased during hemoperfusion in all cases and did not recur. However, it was not clear if the subsequent period of coma or recovery was altered. Because of a very large volume of distribution of camphor, only a small percentage of the total body load is removed with hemoperfusion despite effective clearance from plasma. The relative importance of plasma to total body camphor has not been defined.

Limited information exists on toxic plasma levels of camphor. Kelly and associates report the development of a simple gas chromatographic procedure with a detection limit of 0.1 μg/ml.[1] Using this methodology, the plasma camphor level in the case reported by Kopelman and colleagues was 1.7 μg/ml when the patient had seizures at the start of the therapy. The plasma camphor level fell to 0.4 μg/ml with clinical recovery and remained at that level during the subsequent 20 hours of observation. Mascie-Taylor and coworkers reported an initial camphor level of 3.1 μg/ml at the start of their hemoperfusion in the absence of active seizures or deep coma.[20] Köppel measured a camphor level of 5.5 μg/ml on admission to the intensive care unit (ICU) and 2.4 μg/ml at the start of hemoperfusion, when the patient had active seizures. It was 0.8 μg/ml at the end of the procedure when the seizures had resolved.[10]

Routine laboratory studies often have been reported to show a moderate transient leukocytosis. In addition, several reports mention modest abnormalities in liver function tests, with derangements primarily of a hepatocellular nature.

Camphor ingestion during pregnancy deserves special comment. There are four case reports of camphorated oil being taken in error for castor oil in an attempt to induce labor. In two,[21, 22] early labor did not follow, and subsequently normal infants are believed to have resulted. In the other cases, labor occurred at or near term. One infant died 30 minutes after birth,[23] and in the second case no neonatal problems were observed other than mild, transient increases in serum glutamic oxaloacetic transaminase (SGOT) and serum glutamic pyruvic transaminase (SGPT).[24] In both cases, the odor of camphor was present on the infants' breath and in the amniotic fluid. The infant who died had additional risk factors. Camphor was detectable in the maternal blood 15 minutes after the ingestion, but not in three further maternal blood samples prior to delivery. It was detectable in amniotic fluid at amniocentesis 20 hours after ingestion and at birth. It was also detectable in cord blood and infant brain, liver, and kidney. In the second case, delivery of a normal infant occurred 22 hours after ingestion. Camphor was reported "just detectable" in the infant's blood and in "large amounts" in a maternal sample obtained 24 hours after ingestion. In neither case were the camphor levels or the methodology described.

These observations confirm that camphor readily crosses the placenta and may be toxic to the neonate. Since camphor is detoxified in the liver,[25] a delay in delivery may be preferable to take advantage of the maternal glucuronidase system.

Summary

Camphor poisoning is an uncommon event, often caused by substitution of camphor for other compounds or ingestion of topical liniments. It is potentially fatal, with abrupt onset of vomiting and seizures from 5 to 90 minutes after ingestion. Most cases are successfully treated conservatively; however, fatalities have been reported with ingestions of more than 60 mg/kg. Thus, prompt transfer to a hospital where emesis, respiratory depression, and seizures can be managed is mandatory. Charcoal hemoperfusion or lipid dialysis may be considered in severe cases with recurrent seizure activity.

References

1. Kelly RC, Kopelman RC, Sunshine I: A simple gas chromatographic procedure for the determination of camphor in plasma. J Anal Toxicol *3*:76, 1979.
2. Reid F: Accidental camphor ingestion. J Am Coll Emerg Phys *8*:339, 1979.
3. Phelan WJ III: Camphor poisoning: Over-the-counter dangers. Pediatrics *57*:428, 1976.
4. Gleason MN, Gosselin RE, Hodge HC, Smith RP: Clinical Toxicology of Commercial Products. 3rd ed. Baltimore, Williams & Wilkins, 1969, p 56.
5. Litovitz TL, Schmitz BF, Matyunas N, Martin TG: 1987 Annual Report of the American Association of Poison Control Centers National Data Collection System. Am J Emerg Med *6*:479, 1988.
6. Committee on Drugs: American Academy of Pediatrics. Camphor: Who needs it? Pediatrics *62*:404, 1978.
7. Aronow R: Camphor poisoning. JAMA *235*:1260, 1976.
8. Skoglund RR, Ware LL, Schanberger JE: Prolonged seizures due to contact and inhalation exposure to camphor. Clin Pediatr *16*:901, 1977.
9. Fink M: Meduna and the origins of convulsive therapy. Am J Psychiatr *141*:1034, 1984.
10. Köppel C, Martens F, Schirop T, Ibe K: Hemoperfusion in acute camphor poisoning. Intensive Care Med *14*:431, 1988.
11. Craig JO: Poisoning by the volatile oils in childhood. Arch Dis Child *28*:475, 1953.
12. Smith AG, Margolis G: Camphor poisoning. Am J Pathol *39*:857, 1954.
13. Benz RW: Camphorated oil poisoning with no mortality. JAMA *72*:1217, 1919.
14. Jimenez JF, Brown AL, Arnold WC, Byrne WJ: Chronic camphor ingestion mimicking Reye's syndrome. Gastroenterology *84*:394, 1983.
15. Geller RJ, Spyker DA, Garrettson LK, Rogol AD: Camphor toxicity: Development of a triage strategy. Vet Hum Toxicol *26*(Suppl 2):8, 1984.
16. Siegel E, Wason S: Camphor toxicity. Pediatr Clin North Am *33*:375, 1986.
17. Ginn HE, Anderson KE, Mercier RK, Stevens TW, Matter BJ: Camphor intoxication treated by lipid dialysis. JAMA *203*:230, 1968.
18. Antman E, Jacob G, Volpe B, Finkel S, Savona M: Camphor overdosage: Therapeutic considerations. NY State J Med *78*:896, 1978.
19. Kopelman R, Miller S, Kelly R, Sunshine I: Camphor intoxication treated by resin hemoperfusion. JAMA *241*:727, 1979.
20. Mascie-Taylor BH, Widdop B, Davison AM: Camphor intoxication treated by charcoal haemoperfusion. Postgrad Med J *57*:725, 1981.
21. Blackmon WP, Curry HB: Camphor poisoning: Report of a case occurring during pregnancy. J Florida Med Assoc *18*:999, 1957.
22. Weiss J, Catalano P: Camphorated oil intoxication during pregnancy. Pediatrics *52*:713, 1973.
23. Riggs J, Hamilton R, Homel S, McCabe S: Camphorated oil intoxication in pregnancy. Obstet Gynecol *25*:255, 1965.
24. Jacobnizer H, Roybin H: Camphor poisoning. Arch Pediatr *79*:28, 1962.
25. Robertson JS, Hussain M: Metabolism of camphors and related compounds. Biochem J *113*:57, 1969.

CHAPTER 105
CYANOACRYLATE (SUPER GLUE)

Shawn Gazaleh, M.D., FACEP
Marilyn Rogers, M.D., FACEP

Cyanoacrylate (Super Glue, Magic Glue, Krazy Glue, Instant Glue, Miracle Glue) is manufactured by numerous companies and used for its adhesive properties. Its widespread use in industry and the home has led to an increasing number of accidents requiring emergency care.

Cyanoacrylate adhesives are monomers that almost instantaneously polymerize in the presence of a small amount of water or weak base to form a strong bond. It bonds human tissue, including skin and other epithelial tissue, in seconds. Surgery should *never* be used to separate accidentally bonded skin or other tissues.

In this chapter, the complications and treatment of accidental contact with cyanoacrylate will be discussed; however, it should be mentioned that the substance has been used successfully in the management of corneal perforations,[1, 2] retinal detachments,[3] non–suture closure of wounds,[4] bronchial artery occlusion for severe hemoptysis,[5] arteriovenous malformations,[6] medical splenectomy,[7] and female sterilization[8] and in the occlusion of carotid cavernous fistulas with preservation of carotid artery flow.[9]

Clinical Effects

Dermal. Cyanoacrylate bonds skin instantly. If this occurs, immerse the bonded surfaces in warm soapy water. Peel or roll the surfaces apart with the aid of a blunt edge such as a spoon handle or spatula. Do not try to pull the bonded surfaces apart with a direct opposing action.

If peeling is impractical or unsuccessful, soak the affected area in acetone for 3 to 5 minutes.

Physical attempts to remove residue are not necessary. Residue will come off by itself in a few days.

Contact dermatitis secondary to cyanoacrylate has been reported.[10–12]

On solidification, cyanoacrylates give off heat. In rare cases, a large drop will produce enough heat to cause a burn. If this occurs, the burn should be treated after the lump of cyanoacrylate is released from the tissue.

Oral. If the lips are accidentally bonded together, apply a stream of water to the lips and encourage maximum wetting and pressure from saliva from inside the mouth. Peel or roll the surfaces apart gently. Do not try to pull the lips apart with direct opposing action.

It is almost impossible to swallow cyanoacrylate. The adhesive polymerizes, solidifies, and adheres to the mouth and tongue, producing a grayish-white plaque that will disappear in 12 hours to 2 days. The process may be hastened by gentle abrasion with a toothbrush.

If a lump forms in the mouth, position the patient to prevent ingestion or aspiration when the lump detaches.

No cases of esophageal adhesion or toxicity of a generalized nature have been reported.

Ophthalmic. When cyanoacrylate adhesive comes into contact with the lid margins and lashes, adherence of the lids to each other will usually occur. If the eyelids are only partially closed, try to evaluate the eye for the presence of any foreign material. Do not try to pull the lids apart, but irrigate the eye thoroughly with warm water for about 15 minutes. Then try to gently remove some of the adhered material. A gauze patch should then be applied, and the eye will open spontaneously in 1 to 4 days.

Cyanoacrylate introduced onto the eye surface will adhere immediately, and there will be increased adherence to the conjunctiva and cornea with pressure of the eye (as would occur with tightly shutting the lids). The chemical causes the most severe reaction to the conjunctiva, with marked injection, chemosis, weeping, and double vision. Corneal irritation and abrasion are common. The eye should be irrigated with warm water. Acetone, a solvent for cyanocrylate, should not be used, as it burns and will dry the corneal epithelium. Generally, the glue will spontaneously dissociate from the surface of the eye within a matter of hours. The eye should then be treated with antibiotics, cycloplegics, and a patch, particularly if there is evidence of corneal abrasion.

Respiratory. Cyanoacrylate vapor causes chemical irritation to the respiratory tract. Asthma and rhinitis due to cyanoacrylate have been reported.[13, 14]

Management of the chemical bronchitis seen after acute inhalation includes removal from the environment, general supportive care, and oxygen and aminophylline if air hunger or bronchospasm is present. Since pneumonitis or other pulmonary complications may develop, such patients should be hospitalized. Antibiotics may be indicated if secondary infection develops.

References

1. Hirst LW, Stark WJ, Jensen AD: Tissue adhesives: New perspectives in corneal perforations. Ophthal Surg *10*:58, 1979.
2. Streit S, Ackerman J, Kanarek I: Cyanoacrylate. Ann Ophthalmol *13*:315, 1981.
3. Folk J, Dreyer RF: Cyanoacrylate adhesive in retinal detachment surgery. Am J Ophthalmol *101*:486, 1986.
4. Dalvi A, Faria M, Pinto A: Non-suture closure of wound using cyanoacrylate. J Postgrad Med *32*:97, 1986.
5. Grenier P, Cornud F, Lacombe P, Viau F, Nahum H: Bronchial artery occlusion for severe hemoptysis. AJR *140*:467, 1983.
6. Bank WO, Kerber CW, Cromwell LD: Treatment of intracerebral arteriovenous malformations with isobutyl 2-cyanoacrylate: Initial clinical experience. Radiology *139*:609, 1981.
7. Goldman ML, Philip PK, Sarrafizadeh MS, Sarfeh IJ, Salam AA, Galambos JT, Powers SR, Balint JA: Intra-arterial tissue adhesive for medical splenectomy in humans. Radiology *140*:341, 1981.
8. Neuwirth RS, Richart RM, Stevenson T, Bolduc LR, Zinser H, Baur H, Cohen J, Eldering G, Rivas GA, Nilsen PA: An outpatient approach to female sterilization with methylcyanoacrylate. Am J Obstet Gynecol *136*:951, 1980.
9. Kerber CW, Bank WO, Cromwell LD: Cyanoacrylate occlusion of carotid-cavernous fistula with preservation of carotid artery flow. Neurosurgery *4*:210, 1979.
10. Rycroft RJG: Contact dermatitis from acrylic compounds. Br J Dermatol *96*:685, 1977.
11. Calnan CD: Cyanoacrylate dermatitis. Contact Dermat *5*:165, 1979.
12. Shelley E, Shelley W: Chronic dermatitis simulating small plaque parapsoriasis due to cyanoacrylate adhesive used in fingernails. J Am Acad Dermatol *252*:2455, 1984.
13. Kopp S, McKay R, Moller D, Cassedy K, Brooks S: Asthma and rhinitis due to ethylcyanoacrylate instant glue. Ann Intern Med *102*:613, 1985.
14. Lozewicz S, Davison A, Hopkirk A, Burge P, Boldy D, Riordan J, McGivern D, Platts B, Davies D, Newman Taylor A: Occupational asthma due to methyl methacrylate and cyanoacrylates. Thorax *40*:836, 1985.

CHAPTER 106
COSMETICS AND TOILET ARTICLES

Clyde M. Burnett

Cosmetics of one form or another are part of practically every household. They have been associated with humankind for thousands of years and show no sign of diminished importance in everyday life. Our pharmacies, department stores, and supermarkets abound with cosmetic bottles, tubes, and packages of every description, and the shelves and drawers of American homes contain an amazing array of these products.

Cosmetics are subject to requirements of the US Food, Drug, and Cosmetic Act, enforced by The Food and Drug Administration (FDA). The Act defines cosmetics as:

"(1) articles intended to be rubbed, poured, sprinkled, or sprayed on, introduced into, or otherwise applied to the human body or any part thereof for cleansing, beautifying, promoting attractiveness, or altering the appearance, and

(2) articles intended for use as a component of

any such articles; except that such term shall not include soap."

It is interesting to note that cosmetics also may be classified as drugs if health claims are made in their labeling. Examples are a lipstick that the manufacturer claims will protect from the harmful effects of wind or sun, such as chapping, or a product sold as a suntan cream (cosmetic) but for which sunscreen claims are made (drug).

The colors used in cosmetics are those allowed by the FDA after careful safety screening. Only hair color preparations are permitted to contain dyes that are not otherwise on the FDA's approved lists, and then only if the hair dye label contains the statement "CAUTION—this preparation contains ingredients that may cause skin irritation in certain individuals, and a preliminary test according to accompanying directions should first be made. This product must not be used for dyeing the eyelashes or eyebrows; to do so may cause blindness" and the package provides the directions for performing a patch test 24 hours prior to application.

The fundamental requirement for cosmetics in The Act is that they not be poisonous or deleterious when used as directed in the package labeling. The Act also requires that cosmetics be clean and stored under sanitary conditions and that cosmetic containers do not cause the content to become injurious.

One very useful aid to physicians and others in identifying the ingredients in cosmetics is the cosmetic package labeling. Today, the names of ingredients in cosmetics are listed either on the immediate container label or on the cosmetic carton. The listing appears on cosmetic products sold at retail, and beginning in 1990 there will be a listing of ingredients on salon products. If the label or carton bearing the ingredient listing is available, it may greatly aid the doctor in selecting proper emergency treatment. The names of ingredients as used on cosmetic labels may not always be familiar. However, the Cosmetic, Toiletry, and Fragrance Association, Inc., at 1110 Vermont Ave., N.W., Washington, DC 20005, publishes the CTFA Cosmetic Ingredient Dictionary (third edition now available), which catalogues the ingredient names alphabetically and provides significant information about them: the chemical name, structure, other synonyms, references for further information, and so on. The Dictionary has been recognized by the FDA as the controlling compendium for cosmetic ingredient labeling.

Cosmetics are also subject to requirements of the Poison Prevention Packaging Act, which is basically designated to prevent accidental ingestion of toxic substances by requiring special packaging (i.e., caps or closures that are difficult if not impossible for young children to remove) and to the Fair Packaging and Labeling Act, which has as its purpose the prohibition of unfair and deceptive packaging and labeling.

NOTE: Information in this section that deals with suggested first aid measures is for emergency purposes. Unless seriously misused, it is not anticipated that cosmetics generally pose any significant threats to health.

The purpose of the rest of this chapter is to provide general information on the composition of the various kinds of cosmetic products and, for each category, brief information on emergency first aid measures in cases of accidental ingestion, eye irritation, skin irritation, and allergic hypersensitivity.

HAIR COLOR

Products intended to color hair are for the most part divided into three types: *permanent, semipermanent* and *temporary,* depending on their composition, manner of use, and the length of time the color resists wear-off and shampooing.

Permanent Hair Colors. The permanent hair colors, sometimes referred to as "oxidation" hair colors, depend on chemical interaction between an oxidizer and dye intermediates to produce coloring molecules that become fixed in the hair shaft. The oxidizing substance most used in modern permanent hair colors is an aqueous solution of hydrogen peroxide, usually containing 6 per cent H_2O_2. The other component, which is mixed equivolume with the peroxide just before application, is a mixture generally containing dye intermediates such as paraphenylenediamine, resorcinol, aminophenols, and substituted phenylenediamines in a base consisting of a water solution of soap, such as ammonium oleate, or synthetic detergent, along with other ingredients to affect such factors as wetting, spreadability, viscosity, penetration, and so on.

A typical oxidation or permanent type of hair color may include a broad selection of ingredients:

water	glycerine
ammonium hydroxide	propylene glycol
ammonium oleate	antioxidant
isopropanol	fragrance

dyes/intermediates such as paraphenylenediamine and its derivatives and resorcinol and aminophenols

Semipermanent Hair Colors. A "semipermanent" hair color is so called because its coloring effect lasts through a few (5 to 6) shampoos, the duration lying between permanent and temporary types. Semipermanent hair color does not rely on the use of hydrogen peroxide or other oxidizers for development of color. The coloring molecules are preformed and are deposited on the cuticle of the hair shaft. They are used essentially to cover gray hair and do not lighten the natural hair color pigment, as do the oxidation types.

A typical semipermanent type of hair color may include the following ingredients:

water	
coconut or other fatty acid	propylene glycol
cellulose ether	isopropanol
fatty acid amines	low concentrations of disperse dyes and aromatic nitroamine compounds
alkanolamines and esters	

Temporary Hair Colors. "Temporary" hair colors, so called because they last only through one shampoo, are less frequently used today. They contain dyes that are deposited only on the surface of the hair shaft, frequently resulting in undesirable rub-off. A typical temporary hair color might contain the following:

fatty acid alcohols
selected quaternary detergents
water
certified and textile dyes
preservatives

Emergency First Aid Measures

Ingestion. The oxidation or "permanent" types of hair colors are moderately toxic orally. However, because of the free ammonia present in most oxidation-type hair colors (ethanolamine may replace ammonia in some), it would seem improbable that a significant amount could be consumed accidentally without reflex vomiting. The acute oral toxicity of the oxidation hair color after being mixed with the developer (hydrogen peroxide solution) is less than that of the dye solution. (Six per cent hydrogen peroxide solution has very low toxicity.)

In case of ingestion, rinsing the mouth and administering milk will help alleviate oral and gastric irritation. In my experience, accidental ingestion of hair color has not caused significant health problems.

The semipermanent and temporary hair colors are significantly lower in acute oral toxicity, having rat LD_{50} values in the range of 10 to 15 gm/kg. Rinsing the mouth and administering milk is recommended if accidentally ingested.

Skin Irritation/Allergic Reactions. Hair dyes, particularly oxidation/permanent types, may elicit allergic response in hypersensitive people, although the occurrence is rare. Instructions accompanying retail packages of hair colors include directions for performing a patch test 24 hours prior to application and caution against using the product if adverse symptoms appear at the patch site. Observing this recommended procedure should prevent exposure of hypersensitive individuals. If allergic response does occur, conventional therapeutic measures for the management of topical hypersensitivity are indicated.

Eyes. Temporary irritation of the conjunctiva may occur, accompanied by burning and itching. The eyes should be washed immediately and thoroughly (several minutes) with lukewarm water. Soothing eye drops may be helpful. No lasting adverse effects are anticipated.

SHAMPOO

The number and diversity of types of shampoos marketed today are greater than ever before, due in no small part to the emphasis, particularly in the younger market, on more frequent shampooing. Essentially gone are the soap-based shampoos—now replaced almost entirely by synthetic detergent-based compositions.

Shampoo compositions vary from relatively simple to complex. They may range in form from watery liquids to thick gels or pastes. Variation in such factors as fragrance, color, opacity, conditioners, thickeners, and so on, make it clear that shampoos are complex mixtures. They are among the most popular cosmetic-toiletry items purchased and can be expected to be present in practically every household.

Due to the variability in the kinds of shampoos and the number of ingredients that may be used in the manufacture of any particular type, it is doubtful that a "typical" shampoo formulation can be projected. The following list contains a limited but representative selection of chemicals used in popular shampoos marketed today.

- nonionic and anionic surfactants (in some cases, amphoteric and cationic surfactants)
- preservatives
- sequestering agents
- certified colors
- fragrance
- water

Emergency First Aid Measures

Ingestion. There is little danger of any significant adverse systemic effect from ingestion unless rather large amounts are swallowed. The rat LD_{50} for these products is in the range of 5 to 15 ml or gm/kg body weight, making them only slightly toxic. Gastric irritation with nausea and vomiting may occur. Milk may be given to help soothe the gastric mucosa and dilute the shampoo. However, none of the ingredients is significantly hazardous.

Skin Irritation/Allergic Reaction. Excessive use may result in dryness of the scalp with consequent itching, but no injury to the skin should be expected. Allergic response, although rare, may be treated using conventional therapy for topical hypersensitivity.

Eyes. Irritation and stinging, such as that from getting soap in the eye, may result from accidentally getting shampoo in the eyes. Rinsing eyes with lukewarm water promptly and thoroughly should relieve the condition. If the eyes have been exposed for an undue time, mild temporary conjunctivitis can occur. Soothing eye drops may be helpful.

PEROXIDES

Hydrogen peroxide solution, or so-called "peroxide," is essential to bring about development of color when mixed with the permanent (oxidation)-type hair color products. It is also used in admixture with inorganic persulfates and ammoniacal soap solution for lightening or bleaching the hair, either for just that purpose or preparatory to toning the hair with high-fashion colors.

Almost all "peroxide" solutions for use on hair are 6 per cent hydrogen peroxide in purified deionized water plus a trace of inorganic stabilizer. A few may contain up to 12 per cent hydrogen peroxide. Rarely, one may encounter a solid peroxide for use with colors, such as urea peroxide, but these preparations have fallen into disfavor. The 6 per cent hydrogen peroxide solutions are commonly referred to in the trade as "20 volume," meaning that 1 milliliter of the solution releases 20 milliliters of oxygen.

Some liquid peroxide preparations may contain thickeners to improve viscosity in order to prevent running when in use on the hair. They may be colored with trace amounts of FDA-certified dyes.

Emergency First Aid Measures

Ingestion. Hydrogen peroxide solutions as used in the cosmetic industry are considered practically nontoxic. The rat LD_{50} of these products is generally 15 ml/kg or higher. If swallowed, the principal ingredient, hydrogen peroxide, decomposes in the stomach to form water and oxygen. Should some be ingested, no particular first aid measure is indicated.

Skin Irritation/Allergic Reaction. Allergies to hydrogen peroxide, to the best of our knowledge, are unknown. Moreover, the products are not known to be harmful to skin though they are capable of lightening the skin.

Eyes. Inadvertent splashing into the eyes of 6 per cent hydrogen peroxide may cause a stinging sensation. Rinsing thoroughly and promptly with lukewarm water should prevent any serious consequences. However, in case of eye contact with 30 or 40 volume hydrogen peroxide, the person should be advised to rinse the eyes thoroughly and present to an emergency room as soon as possible for evaluation and treatment.

HAIR LIGHTENER SYSTEMS

The color of hair may be lightened somewhat by use of hydrogen peroxide solution alone. However, this would be inefficient and slow. For achieving significant lightening, such as the palest stage necessary before use of toners, a more efficient system is required and is obtained by combining hydrogen peroxide with lotions and powders before application. The lotions provide ammonia, while the powders accelerate the lightening action by reason of their oxidizer components.

Lightener powders usually contain oxidizers such as ammonium, potassium, or sodium persulfate (singly or in combination), along with lesser amounts of silicates (anticaking), metasilicates (alkalizers), sodium lauryl sulfate (detergent), disodium EDTA (sequestrant), sodium or aluminum stearates (thickeners), and certified or other FDA-listed colors.

Lightener lotions are essentially ammoniacal soap solutions containing lesser amounts of other ingredients such as thickeners, emulsifiers, stabilizers, dispersants, and so on. The pH of these solutions generally ranges between 9.5 and 11.5.

Emergency First Aid Measures

Ingestion. *Lightener powders* are moderately toxic. Ingestion of a significant amount of the lightener powder would probably be difficult due to the disagreeable taste and gritty sensation in the mouth. Should ingestion occur, the mouth should be rinsed thoroughly and promptly with water. If a significant amount is swallowed, the clinician should be alert to possible electrolyte imbalance. Animal tests have shown these materials to be highly emetic.

Lightener lotions also are moderately toxic. If any should contact the mouth, rinsing with water promptly and thoroughly should follow. If any are ingested, milk may be given for its dilution and soothing properties.

Skin/Allergic Reactions. Directions for use of lightener powders and lotions stress that contact with the skin of the scalp or surrounding areas of the face, neck, and ears should be avoided. However, if contact should occur, the skin should be washed promptly with water or saline to avoid significant primary irritation, particularly in sensitive individuals.

Allergic response to these products is rare. Should it occur, generally accepted procedures for allergic hypersensitivity may be used.

Eyes. See the immediately preceding topic, "Peroxides."

HAIR WAVING PREPARATIONS

In brief, hair waving consists of softening the hair by use of chemicals to temporarily alter its molecular structure, shaping it in the curl or wave form desired, then re-hardening or stiffening it to its original state. This process is carried out in two steps, using first a "waving lotion," that remains on the hair for a time and is then rinsed out, and second, a "neutralizer" to interrupt the action of the waving lotion. Finally, the neutralizer is rinsed from the hair, which is then set and dried.

Waving lotions, which are applied to the hair before or after winding onto curler forms, are generally of two types: those containing thioglycolic acid salts, and those utilizing sodium or ammonium sulfites for the hair "softening" step.

Neutralizers are generally solutions of hydrogen peroxide or sodium bromate in mildly acidic solution.

Emergency First Aid Measures

Ingestion. *Sulfite-type waving lotions* have mildly alkaline bases (pH between 7 and 8.5) and are generally only slightly to moderately toxic. Milk may be helpful for dilution and soothing effects.

Thioglycolate-type waving lotions are moderately toxic. (A preparation containing 15 to 16 per cent ammonium thioglycolate was determined in our laboratories to have a rat LD_{50} of 4.7 ml/kg.) Because of their rather high alkalinity, ingestion of this type of lotion can cause irritation of the mouth and throat and may cause nausea, vomiting, and diarrhea. Rinse mouth with water and administer large amounts of milk.

Neutralizers of the *hydrogen peroxide* type pose no particular threat if ingested, the hydrogen peroxide being converted into oxygen and water. However, the *bromate types* are generally regarded as quite toxic. Provided the bromate concentration is sufficiently high, 1 or 2 teaspoonsful can produce serious poisoning in children. The human adult lethal dose of sodium bromate is estimated at 10 grams. Serious poisoning has been reported in young children (1.5 to 3 years of age) following ingestion of 1.5 to 3.0 grams of a 2 per cent solution. Emesis or gastric lavage or both may be indicated, using generally accepted procedures when bromate ingestion is recognized. Renal failure is the cause of death as the bromates are primarily nephrotoxic (see Chapter 9 for management).

Skin/Allergic Reactions. Waving lotions used other than as directed (such as in overly prolonged contact) or in hypersensitive individuals can cause skin irritation, including edema and erythema. Skin irritation may be reduced by rinsing thoroughly but gently with copious amounts of water.

Allergic hypersensitivity to waving lotions and/or neutralizers is extremely uncommon and not anticipated; should it occur, conventional measures for topical hypersensitivity are indicated.

Eyes. Waving lotions, due to their possibly high alkalinity (thioglycolate type), may be quite irritating to the eye, which should be immediately and thoroughly rinsed with lukewarm water. The same should be done for neutralizers in the eye. In the healthy eye, neither the waving lotion nor the neutralizer should cause any lasting effects if rinsing is prompt and thorough. Typical waving lotions (both sulfite and thioglycolate types) and neutralizers (both bromate and hydrogen peroxide types) tested in our laboratories for rabbit eye irritation showed only minimal conjunctival effects, which disappeared before the third day.

HAIR STRAIGHTENERS

Cosmetic products offered for straightening, relaxing, or uncurling the hair are based on the same scheme as are waving preparations—that is, to chemically soften or "relax" the hair, then fix it in the desired shape. Hair straightening requires somewhat stronger treatment of the hair than does waving, consequently greater concentrations of hair-softening chemicals are required, or the chemicals selected must be stronger. Sodium hydroxide in the range of 1 to 3 per cent is used for relaxing/straightening. Precise application techniques, and following directions exactly, are necessary to avoid burning or irritation of the skin or eyes and damage to hair. These preparations are highly alkaline (pH 13). Once the relaxer is thoroughly rinsed out, an acidic shampoo is used to neutralize lingering alkali. *Hair straighteners are considered the major toxic cosmetic.*

Emergency First Aid Measures

Ingestion. If accidental ingestion has occurred, the material should be washed from the mouth immediately using lukewarm water. Milk is indicated to neutralize and dilute the alkali. The mouth and esophagus should be carefully checked for possible caustic burns. Once in the stomach, the pH of the normal stomach contents should be sufficient to neutralize the material (see Chapter 65 for management of caustics).

Skin Irritation/Allergic Reaction/Eye Irritation. Hair straightening/relaxing preparations are severe irritants to the skin and eyes. If accidental contact with either occurs, the material should be washed away immediately with plenty of lukewarm water. No allergic reaction is anticipated.

HAIR SPRAYS

Hair sprays are among the most popular cosmetics and are used to hold the hair once it is combed into the desired style. Their effect is produced by the dried film formed on the hair when a solution of a resin in a suitable solvent is sprayed on the hair and allowed to dry. The solvent is usually ethyl alcohol and is usually present as the main ingredient, sometimes amounting to 95 per cent of the formula. Resins used vary from the now nearly defunct shellac to the more modern polymers such as methyl vinyl ether/maleic anhydride, acrylamide with acrylic acid or methacrylic acid as their esters, vinyl acetate with crotonic acid, methyl vinyl ether with maleic anhydride, and many others of lesser popularity.

Hair sprays are dispensed either from a hand-pumped container or from a self-pressurized container by means of a compressed gas (so-called "aerosol" type). Aerosol propellants currently popular include butane, isobutane, and propane, usually in mixtures. Since it became suspect that chlorofluorocarbons (fully halogenated chlorofluoroalkanes) interfere with the amount of ozone in the stratosphere, the FDA banned their use as propellants for aerosol cosmetics after April, 1979.

Emergency First Aid Measures

Ingestion. The high proportion of ethyl alcohol in hair sprays will cause typical effects such as dizziness or stupor, depending on the amount consumed. Since most hair sprays contain 90 per cent or more of alcohol by weight, alcohol intoxication should be looked for and guarded against.

Skin/Allergic Response. Hair sprays are not generally recognized as causes of allergic response but should such occur, the conventional therapeutic measures for allergic hypersensitivity should be followed by the physician.

Our experience has indicated no problems are associated with skin irritation following use of hair sprays.

Eyes. If the spray is unintentionally directed into the eye, a stinging sensation may occur. It should be flushed out thoroughly and promptly with lukewarm water, and, if discomfort or other symptoms persist, a physician should be consulted. Normal use of hair spray should cause no harmful effects on the eyes.

HAIR CONDITIONERS, CREAM RINSES, AND HAIR DRESSINGS

These products vary in their function and in composition but are generally practically innocuous. They serve to alter the character of the hair in order to hold it in place, or make it easier to comb, or cause less fly-away and frizziness and to add luster or sheen.

Conditioners. Conditioners are applied to the hair and either left on the hair or rinsed with water. The rinse-out conditioner typically may contain natural or synthetic fatty derivatives, higher fatty alcohols, quaternary ammonium compounds, specially selected proteins, preservatives, perfume, and water. The leave-in types of conditioners are similar but may also contain film-forming resins or polymers.

Hair Dressings. This group may include a number of different kinds of products, each having a different desired effect—brilliantines, pomades, alcohol-based lotions, cream emulsions, gels, and so on. Their composition is as diverse as their kind and form. Generally, mineral oil or petrolatum or both are major ingredients in the brilliantines and pomades, while the liquid forms may contain alcohol to improve spreadability and uniformity. The cream emulsions commonly employ magnesium, zinc, or aluminum stearates as emulsifiers for mineral oil, but other emulsifiers such as ethoxylated fatty alcohols and lanolin alcohols may be used.

Emergency First Aid Measures

Ingestion. None of the products in this category are toxic if ingested accidentally, although some gastric upset may occur. An exception is the case of a product containing a significant proportion of alcohol, in which case the classic symptoms of alcohol intoxication should be looked for and treated accordingly.

Skin/Allergic Reactions. None of these products are potential skin irritants nor do they contain the kinds of ingredients usually associated with possible allergic response. Should irritation appear, the conventional therapeutic measures for topical hypersensitivity should be followed.

Eyes. Normal use of these products as directed should not pose problems with eye irritancy. However, should eye exposure occur, flushing with lukewarm water for a few minutes should be sufficient to alleviate any possible discomfort. If symptoms persist, a physician should be consulted.

BUBBLE BATH

A typical bubble bath preparation may contain essentially anionic and nonionic detergents, with lesser amounts of emulsifiers, preservatives, sequestrants, fatty alcohol, certified colors, and fragrance. However, marketed formulations may vary widely in composition.

Emergency First Aid Measures

Ingestion. Some gastric upset with possible nausea and vomiting may occur if the undiluted bubble bath preparation is swallowed. Administration of milk or water would be advisable unless a large amount has been ingested, in which case gastric lavage may be indicated, with care to prevent foaming.

Skin Irritation/Allergic Response. At the recommended levels in the bath and under normal exposure conditions, no skin or mucosal irritation is expected. These products do not contain ingredients recognized as sensitizers. However, should allergic response occur, conventional therapeutic measures should be followed.

Eyes. Splashing a small amount of the bath water containing properly diluted bubble bath into the eye should produce no more than slight transient irritation. If the undiluted material contacts the eye, it should be rinsed immediately but gently with large volumes of lukewarm water for several minutes.

BATH OILS AND BATH SALTS

These preparations generally contain vegetable or mineral oil (bath oils), various surfactants/emulsifiers, fragrance, and preservatives. The "salts" are inorganic, e.g., sodium chloride.

Emergency First Aid Measures

Ingestion. These preparations are generally regarded as practically nontoxic, although some minor gastric disturbance could occur. If excess of bath salts is consumed, electrolyte imbalance should be guarded against.

Skin Irritation/Allergic Response. No problems of this type are anticipated. Should allergic sensitivity occur, though unlikely, it should be treated by conventional procedures.

Eyes. If any of these products get in the eyes, they should be flushed thoroughly but gently with lukewarm water. No serious eye problem is anticipated.

EYE MAKE-UP PRODUCTS

Eyebrow pencils, eyebrow colorants, liquid and cake or wax eyeliners and powder, and stick or cream eyeshadows all contain relatively innocuous ingredients. The colors chosen for them must be specified by the FDA as acceptable for use in the area of the eye.

Mascaras are essentially water, selected colors, waxes, thickeners, a film-forming material, and preservative. The "waterproof" type is based on mineral spirits in place of water.

Eye make-up removers may be of the "water" type which generally contain amphoteric surface-active agents in water along with color and preservative. The "oily" type contains mineral or vegetable oil, color, fragrance, and preservative.

Emergency First Aid Measures

Ingestion. The probability of any acute hazard from accidental ingestion of this group of products is extremely remote due to their small package sizes. As a group, they are generally recognized as practically nontoxic. However, fluids such as milk or water may be given liberally for dilution should ingestion occur.

Skin Irritation/Allergic Response. None anticipated, but should either occur, wash off thoroughly; allergy may be treated by conventional procedures but is highly unlikely.

COLOGNES, TOILET WATERS, BODY SPLASHES, PERFUMES

These products are essentially hydroalcoholic solutions with smaller amounts of fragrance (perfume oils). Certified colors and propylene glycol or similar "bodifiers" may be added. Alcohol levels may range from 50 to 95 per cent or more.

Emergency First Aid Measures

Ingestion. Because of the alcohol content, ingestion may cause dizziness or stupor, depending on amount ingested. Conventional therapy for alcohol ingestion may be indicated (see Chapter 26).

Skin Irritation/Allergic Response. None anticipated.

Eyes. May irritate eyes. Wash out with plenty of lukewarm water.

COSMETIC POWDERS (DUSTING, BODY, TALCUM, BABY)

A general formula for the body-type powders would include talc or starch or both as the major ingredient with lesser amounts of inorganic carbonates, zinc stearate, kaolin, fragrance, and, possibly, preservatives.

Emergency First Aid Measures

Ingestion. The powders described are generally recognized as practically nontoxic.

Eyes. They should be flushed gently using plenty of lukewarm water.

Inhalation. Inhalation of a massive amount may restrict breathing passages, causing severe respiratory distress. Clear airways and maintain respiration while providing symptomatic and supportive treatment (see Chapter 104).

FACIAL MAKE-UP COSMETICS

Blushers, foundations, make-up bases, and blemish covers of the liquid, cream, or stick variety contain waxes, oils, fats, and water, for the most part, with lesser amounts of fillers, humectants, thickeners, colors (certified and selected color additives), fragrance, and preservative. Powder blushers are mostly talc with kaolin, stearates, mineral or vegetable oil, fatty acid esters, magnesium carbonate, color, preservative, and fragrance.

Emergency First Aid Measures

These preparations are, as a group, practically nontoxic. No adverse symptoms would be anticipated. In case of topical hypersensitivity, conventional therapeutic measures would be indicated.

LEG AND BODY PAINTS

Alcohol and water are the chief ingredients, some containing up to 50 per cent alcohol. Lower amounts of emulsifiers, fillers, humectants, color additives, and preservatives are included.

Emergency First Aid Measures

Ingestion. These preparations may be moderately toxic due to the possibly higher alcohol content. Dizziness or stupor can occur depending on the amount of alcohol in the formula and the amount ingested. Conventional measures for alcohol intoxication may be indicated.

Skin Irritation/Allergic Response. None anticipated. In case of irritation, wash off with water and mild soap if necessary. Allergic response can be treated with conventional therapy.

Eyes. Flush with plenty of lukewarm water.

LIPSTICK

The familiar lipsticks are mainly composed of mineral or vegetable oils, waxes, and FDA-approved colors. They may also contain lanolin or lanolin derivatives, fragrance, preservative, antioxidant, and possibly a flavoring agent.

Emergency First Aid Measures

Lipsticks are virtually nontoxic with no symptoms expected or treatment indicated.

NAIL POLISH

Nail polishes, also called nail lacquer, nail gloss, and so on, are composed essentially of solvents such as xylene, toluene, acetone, ethyl acetate, ethanol or methanol, and plasticizer (butyl acetate, dibutyl phthalate, camphor) with nitrocellulose or other resin. In some cases, a pearlescent agent may be added (see Chapters 37 and 79 for further discussion).

Emergency First Aid Measures

Ingestion. Because of the small-sized packages marketed (usually 30 ml or less), the hazard is low. If ingested, nausea, vomiting, and possibly depression or even narcosis could occur, depending on the amount swallowed. If less than 20 ml has been swallowed, milk may be given liberally. If more, gastric lavage may be advisable, with symptomatic treatment and supportive measures. Depending on the chemical, further management may be indicated (refer to the appropriate chapter).

Skin Irritation/Allergic Response. None anticipated.

Eyes. Flush with plenty of lukewarm water.

NAIL POLISH REMOVERS

Solvents such as acetone and ethanol are the chief ingredients. Lanolin, oils, fatty alcohol, and fragrance also may be present (see Chapter 37 for further discussion of acetone).

Emergency First Aid Measures

Ingestion. Due to the solvents present, these preparations may be slightly to moderately toxic. Treatment is same as for ingestion of nail polish.

Skin Irritation/Allergic Response. None anticipated.

Eyes. May cause irritation on contact. Flush thoroughly but gently with a large volume of lukewarm water.

DENTIFRICES

Preparations for cleaning the teeth may be in powder, paste, gel, or liquid form. Formulas vary with form, the powder generally containing calcium phosphate, alumina, an abradant such as silica, calcium carbonate, flavor, and anionic surfactants. Paste and liquid forms usually contain silica or other abradant, humectants, gum binder, flavor, anionic surfactants, color, and water. Gel types generally contain silica or other abradant, humectants, anionic surfactant, flavor, and color. Any of the dentifrices also may contain fluoride to help prevent cavities.

Emergency First Aid Measures

Dentifrices are generally regarded as virtually nontoxic. If a significant amount has been swallowed, mild gastrointestinal irritation may occur. Freely administering milk may be helpful.

MOUTHWASHES AND BREATH FRESHENERS

These products may be packaged in ready-to-use form or as a concentrate for dilution with water. Generally they contain alcohol, water, flavor, sweetener, preservative, color and an astringent.

Emergency First Aid Measures

Ingestion. The ready-for-use type is practically nontoxic, whereas the concentrate, owing to its usually higher alcohol concentration, can cause alcohol intoxication symptoms, and gastrointestinal irritation may be present. Rinse mouth with water if concentrate has been ingested; treat for alcohol intoxication if symptoms so indicate.

Eyes. Either type may be irritating to the eyes on contact, the concentrate more so than the ready-for-use type. Flush the eyes immediately with a large volume of lukewarm water.

DENTURE CLEANSERS

The liquid nonbleaching type of cleansers (used with a brush) generally contain water, anionic and amphoteric surfactants, polishing agents, alcohol, chelating and buffering agents, flavor, fragrance, and color. The bleaching types (solids) usually contain potassium persulfate, sodium perborate, sodium carbonate, trisodium phosphate, and fragrance.

Emergency First Aid Measures

Ingestion. The liquid nonbleaching cleanser is practically nontoxic, but the bleaching type is slightly toxic and may be moderately irritating, causing a burning sensation in the mouth and throat with possible epigastric pain and vomiting. Flush mouth with water and administer milk freely. General supportive measures should be provided as needed.

Eyes. Flush immediately with a large volume of lukewarm water.

SOAP

Soaps are available in solid bar forms and as liquids, the essential difference being the amount of water. Both forms contain surfactants (anionic and nonionic), humectants, vegetable or mineral oils, fragrance, and colors. The bar soaps, in particular, may contain antibacterial agents.

Emergency First Aid Measures

Ingestion. Soaps are generally regarded as nontoxic. If a significant amount is swallowed, gastrointestinal irritation, nausea, and vomiting may occur. Milk may be given liberally for dilution.

Skin Irritation/Allergic Response. No significant irritation of the skin is expected. Prolonged exposure of the hands, for example, can cause dryness and minor irritation. Hypersensitive individuals should discontinue use and conventional measures for topical hypersensitivity should be undertaken.

Eyes. Soap in either form will cause smarting and irritation if it gets in the eyes. Flush thoroughly but gently with lukewarm water.

DEODORANTS AND ANTIPERSPIRANTS

Deodorants serve either to mask body odor or to help prevent bacterial decomposition of excreted perspiration. They generally contain, if in liquid form, alcohol, water, color, and a deodorizing agent (0 to 5 per cent by weight). Some liquid forms are propellant dispensed (''aerosols''). Waxes, soap, and humectants may be present in minor proportions in stick forms. Roll-on types and creams are similar in composition, with the addition of emulsifier and thickeners.

Antiperspirants have bases very similar to deodorants in their various forms but contain, in addition, an antiperspirant chemical such as aluminum hydroxychloride (also known as aluminum chloride hydroxide, aluminum chlorohydroxide, aluminum chlorohydrate), which, by its astringent action, serves to inhibit or reduce the flow of perspiration.

Emergency First Aid Measures

Ingestion. These preparations are generally considered practically nontoxic orally. The mouth should be flushed out, and milk may be given for its soothing and diluting effect.

Skin Irritation/Allergic Response. The products are nonirritating to most people, but, should an individual be sensitive, the preparation should be washed off thoroughly. A substitute brand may prove less irritating. Should true allergic hypersensitivity develop (rare), conventional therapeutic measures may be undertaken.

Eyes. Propellant-dispensed types may cause eye irritation. The eyes should be flushed carefully with lukewarm water for a few minutes. Soothing eye drops may be helpful.

Inhalation. Normal use has not been shown to be harmful. However, as is the case with possibly any household ''aerosol'' (propellant-dispensed) product, intentional misuse by breathing of captured vapors (such as from a plastic bag into which the product is dispensed) can be harmful or even fatal due to cardiac toxicity (see Chapter 85 for further discussion).

CREAMS AND LOTIONS (SKIN CARE)

Products for cleansing the skin are based essentially on an emulsion in water of various oils, fats, or waxes by use of surfactants/emulsifiers. Humectants, certified colors, fragrances, and preservatives are usually included. Creams or lotions intended for softening, moisturizing, and esthetic/cosmetic effects contain essentially water, wax, fat or oil, witch hazel, humectants, alcohol (usually 10 per cent or less ethyl alcohol), thickeners, color, fragrance, and preservatives.

Emergency First Aid Measures

Ingestion. These products are generally considered to be nontoxic orally. If large quantities are ingested, general gastrointestinal distress may occur. Milk or water given liberally should prove helpful.

Skin Irritation/Allergic Response. No irritation anticipated. Allergic response should be treated by conventional therapeutic measures, but these products do not contain recognized sensitizers.

Eyes. Flush thoroughly and gently with lukewarm water.

DEPILATORIES (HAIR REMOVERS)

Depilatories rely on the action of alkali and thioglycolic acid salts (usually ammonium, but calcium, strontium, or others may be used) to accomplish their purpose: to soften and partially dissolve hair so that it may be wiped away. The thioglycolate content may be as high as 10 per cent by weight while the alkali component (usually sodium or calcium hydroxide) may vary from 1 to 10 per cent by weight. The remaining ingredients are usually water, emulsifier, humectants, and waxes.

Emergency First Aid Measures

Ingestion. Depilatories are moderately toxic. Symptoms such as nausea, vomiting, and diarrhea may occur, depending on the amount ingested. Dilute with milk in large volume. Gastric lavage with water may be indicated if a large amount has been ingested (see Chapter 65 on caustics).

Skin Irritation/Allergic Response. Due to their alkalinity, these products can be irritating, particularly to mucous membranes. Should such occur, the affected tissues should be very thoroughly flushed with large volumes of lukewarm tap water to free the tissue of alkali.

Eyes. Depilatories are irritating to eyes on contact. Flush the eyes thoroughly but gently with lukewarm water for 15 to 30 minutes.

SKIN LIGHTENERS

Also known as "spot removers," these preparations today are based on hydroquinone for their action, usually at from 1 to 5 per cent by weight. The remainder of a typical formulation may consist of water, glyceryl stearate, glycerine, stearic acid, and fragrance.

Emergency First Aid Measures

Ingestion. Since typical skin lightener creams contain up to about 5 per cent hydroquinone, these products can be regarded as slightly to moderately toxic, depending on the amount ingested and the concentration of hydroquinone in the particular brand. Ingestion of toxic quantities could cause dyspnea, cyanosis, and convulsions. Gastrointestinal irritation may occur, as may possibly other symptoms typically associated with hydroquinone ingestion. If it is believed that a toxic quantity has been ingested, gastric lavage is indicated. Supportive therapy may be indicated.

Skin Irritation/Allergic Response. No irritation of skin or allergic response is expected with normal use of skin lighteners. Should irritation develop, wash off the preparation with mild soap and plenty of water. Conventional therapeutic measures for topical allergic hypersensitivity may be followed should allergic reaction develop.

Eyes. The typical skin lightener cream is not expected to cause other than temporary eye irritation. It should be immediately but gently flushed with large volumes of lukewarm water for several minutes to assure complete removal.

General References

Arena, JM: Poisoning—Toxicology, Symptoms, Treatments. 4th ed. Charles C Thomas, Springfield, Ill, 1979.

Clairol, Incorporated, Research and Development Division, Stamford, Conn: Unpublished data.

CTFA Cosmetic Ingredient Dictionary. 2nd ed. The Cosmetic, Toiletry, and Fragrance Association, Washington, DC, 1976.

Federal Food, Drug, and Cosmetic Act, current, as amended. Superintendent of Documents, US Government Printing Office, Washington, DC.

Gosselin RE, Hodge HD, Smith RP, Gleason MN: Clinical Toxicology of Commercial Products. 4th ed. Williams & Wilkins, Baltimore, 1976.

Kirk RE, Othmer DF (eds): Encyclopedia of Chemical Technology. 3rd ed. Vol 12. John Wiley & Sons, New York, 1980.

Weiss G (ed): Hazardous Chemicals Book. Noyes Data Corporation, Park Ridge, NJ, 1980.

CHAPTER 107
THE VOLATILE OILS

Timothy J. Rittenberry, M.D., FACEP
Richard Feldman, M.D., FACEP

The volatile oils are a group of complex mixtures of hydrocarbons derived from plant sources that share the characteristic of readily evaporating at room temperature. Also known as ethereal or essential oils, these compounds generally impart agreeable odors or pleasant tastes at extremely low concentrations when combined with other materials. Since antiquity such spice extracts have been valued as perfumes, flavorings, and medicaments, making them prominent and influential factors in the commercial intercourse of nations.[1] Today, their medical role is extremely limited; medical interest is almost entirely confined to the treatment of accidental ingestion of or topical exposure to these oils.

Recently renewed interest in herbal medicines and self-treatment as well as the ready availability of a number of concentrated volatile oils from health food stores, mail order establishments, and pharmacies has increased the likelihood of a toxic incident. As food additives, use of these oils is regulated by the Food and Drug Administration (FDA) (concentrations limited to less than 300 ppm), making toxicity through ingestion of flavored foodstuffs a trivial risk. However, as herbal or nondrug preparations there is no such regulation, and the threat of serious toxicity exists.[2, 3] The more common volatile oils include chenopodium, clove, cinnamon, pennyroyal, peppermint, lemon grass, eucalyptus, pine, sandalwood, and sassafras oils (Table 107–1).[4]

Chenopodium Oil

Chenopodium oil, also known as American wormseed oil, is a pale yellow liquid with an unpleasant odor and bitter taste distilled from the American wormseed or Jerusalem oak plant. The week is common in the southeastern United States. Once a standard part of the physician's armamentarium for the treatment of ascariasis and other intestinal parasitic infestations, chenopodium is now of largely historical interest, having been abandoned in favor of other less toxic anthelminthics. Its principal component is ascaridole, with lesser amounts of cymene, camphor, and limonene.[5] Oil of chenopodium is a strong local irritant, causing inflammation of mucous membranes.[6] Minor toxic reactions following ingestions include nausea, vomiting, abdominal pain, dizziness, headache, and paresthesias, whereas in fatal ingestions central nervous system (CNS) symptoms such as seizures, paralysis, or coma predominate.[7] Acute ingestions have also been associated with mydriasis, temporary impairment of vision, and postingestion optic atrophy.[8] Salant approximated the fatal

Table 107–1. THE VOLATILE OILS

OIL	PLANT SOURCE	PRINCIPAL COMPONENT	PLANT PART
chamomile	*Anthemis flores*	Tiglic oil	Flowers
chenopodium	*Chenopodium ambrosiodes* (American wormseed)	Ascaridole	Plant tops
cinnamon	*Cinnamomum loureirii* or *zeylanieum*	Cinnamaldehyde	Bark, leaves
clove	*Eugenia caryophyllus*	Eugenol	Flowerbuds
eucalyptus	*Eucalyptus dives* or *radiata*	Eucalyptol	Leaves
juniper	*Juniperus communis*	Pinene	Fruit
lemon grass		Citral	Leaves
pennyroyal	*Mentha pulegium* *Hedeoma pulegiodes*	Pulegone	Leaves
peppermint	*Mentha piperita*	Menthol	Leaves
sandalwood	*Santalum album*	Santalol	Leaves
sassafras	*Sassafras albidum*	Safrol	Root

oral dose of chenopodium in rabbits at 250 mg/kg, noting that lesser ingestions repeated after 1 or 2 days caused increased toxicity.[9] Autopsy findings in man give evidence for acute cerebral edema, enteritis, nephritis, and hepatitis as well as interstitial pulmonary edema.[5, 10]

Pennyroyal Oil

Pennyroyal oil or tea (made from the leaves of the immature *Mentha pulegium* or *Hedeoma pulegiodes* plant) has been used since the days of Rome as a stimulus for menses and as an abortifacient. Its actions are believed by herbalists to involve irritation of the uterus and bladder, triggering contractions.[11] Ingestions of as little as 3.5 ml in an adult have been associated with protracted emesis, abdominal pain, erythematous skin rash, delirium, and seizures.[12–15] Sullivan and associates reported one fatality from the ingestion of 1 oz of pennyroyal oil.[15] The patient, an 18 year old female who was attempting to abort a suspected pregnancy, presented with generalized rash and persistent emesis, which was positive for blood. Her steadily downward course over the next 7 days was significant for metabolic acidosis, disseminated intravascular coagulation (DIC), hepatocellular dysfunction with markedly elevated liver enzymes, pneumonia, and subsequent renal failure. Postmortem findings demonstrated congestion and consolidation of the lung parenchyma as well as massive centrilobular hepatic necrosis. Vallance[16] reported a similar case in which a 24 year old female presented with fever and generalized rash after ingesting an unknown amount of pennyroyal oil. Nausea, vomiting, abdominal pain, and diarrhea progressed to anuric renal failure, spontaneous abortion of an approximately 12-week pregnancy, hemolysis, and pneumonia over a 10-day course. Necropsy revealed renal tubular degeneration with pigmented casts consistent with acute hemolysis and "transfusion kidney," cerebral edema, and consolidated pulmonary parenchyma. Acute hepatic and pulmonary necrosis has been caused in mice at doses of 400 mg/kg, with the major constituent of pennyroyal oil, R-(+)-pulegone, being primarily responsible.[17] There is suggestive evidence that pulegone may cause tissue necrosis via a toxic intermediate in a fashion similar to acetaminophen.

Peppermint Oil

Peppermint oil has long been used medically as a carminative, augmenting relaxation of gastrointestinal smooth muscle both in vivo and in vitro. Doses of 0.2 ml have provided some improvement in symptoms of irritable bowel syndrome.[18] The toxicity of peppermint oil is generally considered to be minimal, yet its two major constituents (up to 90 per cent menthol and up to 30 per cent menthone) have been implicated in toxic reactions. Menthol is a ubiquitous constituent of over-the-counter medications, toothpastes, mouthwashes, shaving creams, and analgesic balms as well as foods and candies. It has been found to cause hypersensitivity reactions when used topically, causing hot flashes, dermatitis, and urticaria.[19] Menthol has also been implicated in the development of chemical pneumonitis in an infant after exposure to a medicated aerosol and jaundice in neonates with G6PD deficiency treated with menthol-containing powders.[20, 21] The menthone component of peppermint oil is considered a strong topical irritant. Parys reported a case of chemical burn secondary to peppermint oil exposure proceeding to frank skin necrosis, which he ascribed to the menthone component.[22] Oral exposure to peppermint oil has caused acute allergic reactions in the mouth with massive edema of oral and pharyngeal tissues.[23] Large ingestions of peppermint oil have resulted in the development of cataracts in rabbits, whereas topical exposure has caused temporary corneal clouding. Accidental rubbing of the eyes with menthol or peppermint oil in humans, however, has caused only a transient burning sensation.[8] The oral median lethal dose (LD_{50}) of menthol at 48 hours in rats was found to be approximately 2.5 gm/kg, consistently producing CNS symptoms of seizures, ataxia, limb paralysis, and respiratory depression.[24]

Eucalyptus Oil

Eucalyptus oil is a clear to pale yellow liquid with a distinctive aroma and pungent taste. Since first described by an Australian physician in 1790, it has been used as a traditional remedy for a variety of common ailments, particularly of the respiratory tract. It is among the most toxic of the volatile oils. The predominant constituent is 8-cineole, or eucalyptol, which constitutes up to 70 per cent of the oil. The safe oral adult dosage is quoted as 0.06 to 0.2 ml.[25]

A review of 31 fatalities due to eucalyptus ingestion from the British and Australian literature by Gurr notes that burning of the oral mucosa, abdominal pain, and vomiting are common early findings. Pulmonary involvement includes acute bronchospasm, bronchorrhea, tachypnea, and the development of chemical pneumonitis.[26] Dizziness, slurred speech, giddiness, ataxia, headache, and drowsiness are common neurologic symptoms. Serious ingestions may rapidly progress to coma with loss of deep tendon reflexes and respiratory depression.[26–28] Seizures have occurred in children but have not been common in adults.[29] Death in adults has followed ingestion of as little as 4 ml.[30] Convalescing patients may have the odor of eucalyptus on their breath for days, and work by Boyd and Pearson suggests that the respiratory excretion of eucalyptol may be responsible for pulmonary irritation.[31]

Clove Oil

Clove oil contains eugenol, a phenolic compound, in concentrations up to 92 per cent, with lesser amounts of caryophillin and vanillin. It is ubiquitous as a flavoring and fragrance added to candies, medications, toothpastes, and soaps. It is often applied to the gingiva as a traditional treatment for odontalgia. The principal compound, eugenol, is an effective disinfectant and a rapidly acting anodyne, making it useful in dentistry for root canal procedures as well as in the treatment of hyperemic and inflamed pulp.[32] Topical exposure to clove oil causes irritation to the skin and oral mucosa. Prolonged contact with eugenol in dental packs has caused inflammation and frank necrosis.[33, 34] As with many of the other volatile oils, clove oil is capable of eliciting allergic reactions when mucosal or skin surfaces have been previously sensitized. It has been responsible for cases of contact dermatitis and stomatitis.[35, 36] The initial stinging and irritation after topical exposure may progress to permanent local anesthesia and anhidrosis if contact is prolonged.[37] This is supported by Kozam, whose studies with eugenol on frog sciatic nerve indicate a direct, progressive, dose-related neurotoxic effect.[38] Clove oil splashed into the eye may cause acute pain, blepharospasm, lacrimation, and conjunctival edema, with loss of corneal epithelium.[39] When injected into the cornea, an acute inflammatory reaction with hypopyon of the anterior chamber results.[8]

Reported cases of clove oil ingestion in humans have been infrequent; subsequent toxicity can only be inferred from animal studies. Dogs given oral doses of 0.25 gm/kg of eugenol demonstrated vomiting, weakness, lethargy, and ataxia.[40] At 0.5 gm/kg, eugenol is capable of causing coma and death within 24 hours.[29] The LD_{50} of eugenol in rats has been determined to be 1.8 ml/kg (1.93 gm), with postmortem findings consistent with sudden cardiovascular collapse.

Clove cigarettes (40 per cent dried clove and 60 per cent tobacco) also cause toxicity; they are imported from Indonesia and are readily available throughout the United States. Nausea, vomiting, dyspnea, bronchospasm, pulmonary edema, hemoptysis, and epistaxis have been reported and may be due to the direct effects of eugenol or as a result of eugenol-induced anesthesia of the mucous membranes, allowing more vigorous inhalation of the tobacco constituent.[41, 42] When instilled directly into the trachea of rats, eugenol causes interstitial hemorrhage, acute emphysema, and acute pulmonary edema.[42] Moreover, the low LD_{50} of 11 mg/kg in these rats emphasizes the potential toxicity of clove oil if aspirated during ingestion or gastric removal.

Cinnamon Oil

Cinnamon oil is predominantly composed of cinnamic aldehyde (60 to 80 per cent) with lesser amounts of other volatile components, including eugenol. Most cases of toxicity have been related to hypersensitivity reactions or direct irritation when contacting skin or mucous membranes. In addition to allergic contact dermatitis and stomatitis, perioral leukoderma due to exposure to cinnamon-flavored toothpastes has been reported.[43, 44] Prolonged topical exposure has been noted to cause a chemical burn.[45] Cinnamon oil has been used by herbalists as a carminative and an antidiarrheal in adults in doses of 0.06 to 0.2 ml, whereas larger doses have been associated with gastrointestinal irritation. Cases involving severe toxicity or death from ingestion have not been published, yet similarities to other volatile oils, as well as limited experience in animal models, suggest that 5 to 10 ml taken orally may be capable of inducing seizures, respiratory depression, and altered mentation.[46, 47]

Lemon Grass Oil

The predominant constituent of lemon grass oil is citral, a diolefinic aldehyde, which may constitute up to 80 per cent of the oil. It is often used in fragrances, cosmetics, and flavorings as well as in disinfectants and pet repellants. As with several of the other volatile oils, it too may be a primary irritant or sensitizing agent, giving rise to contact dermatitis with topical exposure.[48, 49] In animal studies using rabbits and monkeys, vascular endothelial damage has been caused with single oral doses as small as 5 μg/kg.[50] Human beings seem less sensitive to citral. Two grams of orange peel contains approximately 50 μg of citral, yet such toxicity has not been reported in humans ingesting orange peel.

Sassafras Oil

Oil of sassafras was once used as a treatment for pediculosis capitus, as an abortifacient, and as a flavoring and fragrance. Containing 80 per cent safrol with small amounts of pinene and camphor, its use dropped dramatically in 1960 when the FDA prohibited its use in foods, citing evidence that safrol was a proven carcinogen in rats and mice. Today, its availability is limited to health food stores in the form of sassafras tea or small quantities of the oil. The acute toxicity profile of sassafras oil is similar to that of eucalyptus oil. Craig reviewed five cases of sassafras oil ingestion in young children, which rapidly caused vomiting, vertigo, aphasia, stupor, and shock. An adult male died after taking 1 teaspoon of the oil.[28] Chronic use of sassafras teas, with as much as 200 mg of safral available in one tea bag,[51, 52] may increase the risk for hepatocarcinoma.

TREATMENT

Clinical experience with volatile oil poisoning is extremely limited. Treatment is basically *symptomatic* and *supportive*. Owing to their common irritant and allergenic sensitizing qualities, skin and eye exposures should be handled with rapid removal and copious irrigation. Following eye exposure, a complete ophthalmologic examination with appropriate referral is necessary, especially with oil of cloves. Ingestions of seemingly small amounts of the oils should be aggressively treated with rapid gastric removal. Because of the danger of aspiration pneumonitis and the altered mental status often seen with the volatile oils, emesis with ipecac is potentially hazardous. Finally, ingestion of these oils must be considered hydrocarbon ingestions (eugenol has a viscosity similar to that of turpentine), and their likely aspiration with emesis or gastric lavage may cause pneumonitis.[53] Prudent care would dictate protection of the airway with endotracheal intubation whenever possible. Dialysis has been used in one case in which ethanol and eucalyptus oil were coingested with dubious improvement.[26] Presently, dialysis is only indicated in the presence of progressing renal failure. Although there is no clear evidence that any chemotherapeutic agent may act as an antidote in volatile oil ingestion, further investigation may be fruitful. Work to date suggests that the toxicity of lemon grass and pennyroyal oils may be mechanistically similar to the hepatotoxicity of acetaminophen.[15] Pretreating mice prior to pennyroyal challenge with diethylmaleate has been noted to decrease hepatic glutathione levels by 30 per cent with an associated increase in hepatic injury.[17] That the toxic effects of citral can be reversed in animals by administration of antioxidant sulfhydryl compounds such as cysteine supports this assumption.[50]

Acknowledgement

The authors would like to thank Ms. Rose Sturghill-Bradford for her assistance in preparing this chapter.

References

1. Gildemeister E: The Volatile Oils. Vols 1 and 2, 2nd ed. New York, John Wiley & Sons, 1913.
2. Lewin NA, Howland MA, Goldfrank LR, Flomenbaum NE: Herbal preparations. *In* Toxicologic Emergencies. 3rd ed. Norwalk, CT, Appleton-Century-Crofts, 1986, p 560.
3. Doull J (ed): Casarett and Doull's Toxicology, the Basic Science of Poisons. 2nd ed. New York, Macmillan, 1980, p 600.
4. Morton JF: Major Medicinal Plants. Springfield, IL, Charles C Thomas, 1977, pp 359–381.
5. Gayton WL: Poisoning due to oil of chenopodium. JAMA *132*:330, 1946.

6. Salant W, Nelson ER: The toxicity of oil of chenopodium. Am J Physiol *36*:440, 1915.
7. Birnberg TL, Steinberg CL: Case of oil of chenopodium poisoning: Treatment with forced perivascular (spinal) drainage. Arch Pediatr *56*:304, 1939.
8. Grant WM: Toxicology of the Eye, 3rd ed. Springfield, IL, Charles C Thomas, 1986, pp 199, 576.
9. Salant W: The pharmacology of the oil of chenopodium. JAMA *69*:2016, 1917.
10. Ingham SD, Courville CB: Diffuse cerebral changes in poisoning with oil of chenopodium. Bull Los Angeles Neurol Soc *1*:152, 1936.
11. Gunby P: Plant known for centuries still causes problems today. JAMA *241*(21):2246, 1979.
12. Early DF: Pennyroyal poisoning: A rare case of epilepsy. Lancet *2*:580, 1961.
13. Holland GW: A case of poisoning from pennyroyal. Virg Med Semimonthly *7*:319, 1902.
14. Kimball HW: Poisoning by pennyroyal. Atlant Med Wkly *9*:307, 1898.
15. Sullivan JB, Rumack BH, Thomas H, Peterson RG, Bryson P: Pennyroyal oil poisoning and hepatotoxicity. JAMA *242*(26):2873, 1979.
16. Vallance WB: Pennyroyal poisoning: A fatal case. Lancet *2*:850, 1955.
17. Gordon WB, Forte AJ, McMurtry RJ, Gal J, Nelson SD: Hepatotoxicity and pulmonary toxicity of pennyroyal oil and its constituent terpenes in the mouse. Toxicol Appl Pharmacol *65*:413, 1982.
18. Rees WDW: Treating irritable bowel syndrome with peppermint oil. Br Med J *2*:835, 1979.
19. Papa CM, Shelly WB: Menthol hypersensitivity. JAMA *189*(7):546, 1964.
20. Krueger RP: Chemical pneumonitis from medicated vapor aerosol spraying. Clin Pediatr *6*(8):465, 1967.
21. Olowe SA, Ransome-Kuti O: The risk of jaundice in glucose-6-phosphate dehydrogenase deficient babies exposed to menthol. Acta Pediatr Scand *69*:341, 1980.
22. Parys BT: Chemical burns resulting from contact with peppermint oil mar: A case report. Burns *9*:374, 1983.
23. Smith ILF: Acute allergic reaction following the use of toothpaste. Br Dent J *125*:304, 1968.
24. Eickholt TH, Box RH: Toxicities of peppermint and *Pycnanthemun albescens* oils, Fam. Labiateae. J Pharm Sci *547*:1071, 1965.
25. Martindale W: The Extra Pharmacopoeia. 27th ed. London, Pharmaceutical Press, 1977.
26. Gurr FW: Eucalyptus oil poisoning treated by dialysis and mannitol infusion. Aust Ann Med *4*:238, 1965.
27. Foggie WE: Eucalyptus oil poisoning. Br Med J *1*:359, 1911.
28. Craig JO: Poisoning by the volatile oils in childhood. Arch Dis Child *28*:475, 1953.
29. Patel S, Wiggins J: Eucalyptus oil poisoning. Arch Child Dis *55*:405, 1980.
30. MacPherson J: The toxicology of eucalyptus oil. Med J Aust *1*:313, 1925.
31. Boyd EM, Pearson GL: On the expectorant action of volatile oils. Am J Med Sci *211*:602, 1946.
32. Gurney B: Eugenol utility versus toxicity. Oral Hygiene *55*:74, 1965.
33. Waerhaug J, Loe H: Tissue reaction to gingivectomy pack. Surgery *10*:923, 1957.
34. Guglani LM, Allen F: Connective tissue reaction to implants and peridontal packs. J Peridontol *36*:279, 1965.
35. Sternberg L: Contact dermatitis: Cases caused by oil of cloves and by oil of camomile tea. J Allergy *8*:185, 1937.
36. Silvers SH: Stomatitis and dermatitis venanata with purpura resulting from oil of cloves and oil of cassia. Dent Items Interest *61*:649, 1939.
37. Isaacs G: Permanent local anaesthesia and anhidrosis after clove oil spillage. Lancet *1*:882, 1983.
38. Kozam G: The effect of eugenol on nerve transmission. Oral Surg *44*:799, 1977.
39. Libby GF: Ocular injury from oil of cloves. Ophthalmic Rec *21*:189, 1912.
40. Lauber FU, Hollander F: Toxicity of the mucigogue, eugenol, administered by stomach tube to dogs. Gastroenterology *15*:481, 1950.
41. Centers for Disease Control: Illnesses possibly associated with smoking clove cigarettes. MMWR *34*:297, 1985.
42. LaVoie EJ, Adams JD, Reinhardt J, Rivenson A, Hoffman D: Toxicity studies on clove cigarette smoke and constituents of clove. Determination of the LD_{50} of eugenol by intratracheal instillation in rats and hamsters. Arch Toxicol *59*:78, 1986.
43. Drake TE, Maibach HI: Allergic contact dermatitis and stomatitis caused by a cinnamic aldehyde–flavored toothpaste. Arch Dermatol *112*:202, 1976.
44. Mathias CGT, Maibach MI, Conant MA: Perioral leukoderma simulating vitiligo from use of a toothpaste containing cinnamic aldehyde. Arch Dermatol *116*:1172, 1980.
45. Sparks TS: Cinnamon oil burn. West J Med *142*:835, 1985.
46. Osal A: The Dispensatory of the United States of America. 25th ed. Philadelphia, JB Lippincott, 1955.
47. Rumack BH: Poisindex, Denver, Micromedex, Inc., 1989.
48. Rothenborg HW, Menne' T, Sjolin KE: Temperature dependent primary irritant dermatitis from lemon perfume. Contact Dermatitis *3*:37, 1977.
49. Mendelsohn HV: Lemon grass oil—a primary irritant and sensitizing agent. Arch Dermatol Syph *53*:94, 1946.
50. Leach EH, Lloyd JPF: Citral poisoning. Proc Nutr Soc *15*:15, 1956.
51. Segelman AB, Segelman FB, Karliner J, Sofia D: Sassafras and herb tea—potential health hazards. JAMA *236*:477, 1976.
52. Hagan EC, Jenner PM, Jones WI, Fitzhugh OG, Long EL, Brouwer JG, Webb WK: Toxic properties of compounds related to safrol. Toxicol Appl Pharmacol *7*:18, 1965.
53. Weast RC (ed): CRC Handbook of Chemistry and Physics. 68th ed. Boca Raton, FL, CRC Press, Inc, 1987.

CHAPTER 108
MISCELLANY

Lester M. Haddad, M.D., FACEP

The purpose of this chapter is to include information on a variety of subjects that the physician will either face or be queried about in practice from time to time.

It is not the purpose of this chapter to provide an exhaustive review of miscellaneous toxic chemicals and agents. Physicians who need information concerning a particular agent not listed in this text may call an approved, functional Poison Control Center. If the identity or toxicity of a particular agent still cannot be ascertained, the physician should utilize a general approach in treating the patient, as outlined in Chapter 1.

Aquarium Products

A common phone call to emergency departments and poison control centers concerns products used for home aquariums. Aquarium products include antimicrobials used to control algae, fungi, bacteria, and parasites; antichlorine products, such as sodium thiosulfate; pH indicators, such as bromothymol blue; and miscellaneous substances, including vitamins, aquarium salts, and copper sulfate.[1]

With the exception of copper sulfate, these products generally are of low toxicity, although some pH test kits do contain sodium hydroxide. Should one be consulted about any of these substances, the physician should inquire about the particular ingredient on the label in case the product contains any potentially toxic ingredients.

Birth Control Pills (Oral Contraceptives)

Pediatric ingestion of birth control pills is very common. They usually contain estrogen or progesterone or their derivatives, either in combination or in sequence. Oral contraceptives presently are not considered harmful in pediatric ingestion.

Calamine Lotion

Calamine lotion or cream is a 1 per cent solution of calamine and is often used either alone or with diphenhydramine for the relief of itching caused by poison ivy or oak and insect bites, and for soothing relief of mild sunburn. Calamine itself is a pink powder composed of roughly 99 per cent zinc oxide and 0.5 per cent ferric oxide. Ingestion of large quantities of either calamine lotion or Caladryl (calamine/diphenhydramine combination) has caused gastritis and vomiting. Supportive therapy may be indicated.

Cantharidin (Spanish Fly)

Spanish fly, or cantharides, is a powder derived from certain beetles belonging to the family Meloidae, which contain roughly 0.6 per cent of the active ingredient cantharidin.[1–4] Spanish fly has an intense irritant action on mucous membranes. An irritation of the urethra results in priapism, thereby giving Spanish fly an undeserved popular reputation as an aphrodisiac. In fact, Spanish fly, when ingested, is extremely toxic and often lethal. The adult lethal dose is usually considered to be 50 to 75 mg. Spanish fly ingestion causes intense burning of the throat, dysphagia, hematemesis, and mucosal sloughing of the upper gastrointestinal tract from mouth to pylorus. Following absorption, renal failure secondary to acute tubular necrosis, hematuria, and urgency of micturition occur, as does priapism, and usually death.

Management is strictly supportive. The management of the esophageal injury is similar to that for lye ingestion. Hemodialysis may be necessary in the event of renal failure.

Dimethyl Sulfoxide (DMSO)

DMSO is an excellent solvent and has found extensive use as both an industrial and military solvent. It has a distinct garlic-like odor. The Food and Drug Administration has approved the use of dimethyl sulfoxide solely for the symptomatic relief of patients with interstitial cystitis. Dimethyl sulfoxide is presently available as Rimso-50, in a 50 per cent aqueous solution; it is used via intravesical instillation by urinary catheter for the treatment of interstitial cystitis.

When injected, DMSO caused intravascular hemolysis with hemoglobinuria and subsequent renal failure; liver necrosis has also been observed.[5]

Douches

Vaginal douches are recommended for routine cleansing at the end of menstruation, after the use of contraceptive creams or jellies, or as a rinsing of the residue of prescribed vaginal medication. Douches come in disposable packages, liquid concentrates, or powder. They variously contain germicides, borates, detergents, ethanol, aromatics such as oil of eucalyptus or menthol, various coloring dyes, chemicals such as citric acid, lactic acid, sorbic acid, and sodium bicarbonate to affect vaginal pH, and other agents.

Because they are brightly colored and often accessible to exploring children in bathrooms, pediatric ingestion of douches is rather common. Generally, douches are of low toxicity, and therapy is supportive.

Fenfluramine (Pondimin)

Fenfluramine is a sympathomimetic amine, the pharmacologic activity of which differs from that of amphetamine in that it produces more central nervous system depression than stimulation. It is indicated in the management of infantile autism, and in Great Britain it has found use as an appetite suppressant.

Several reports of intentional overdose are noted in the literature. One fatal case involved a 17 year old girl who ingested 1600 mg of fenfluramine and presented within 3 hours of ingestion with agitation and sinus tachycardia. She subsequently developed seizures, cardiac arrhythmia, and cardiopulmonary arrest; she did not respond to resuscitative measures.[6]

In the event of ingestion of fenfluramine, aggressive gastric decontamination with instillation of activated charcoal and careful monitoring of clinical parameters with supportive therapy may be indicated (see Chapter 98 on sympathomimetic toxicity for further discussion).

Fertilizers

Fertilizers are plant foods that contain one or more of the three chemical elements necessary for plant growth: nitrogen, phosphorus, and potassium. Most commercial fertilizers bear a series of three numbers indicating the content of these three elements. For example, Vigoro 5–10–5 fertilizer indicates that the product contains 5 per cent by weight of elemental *nitrogen*, 10 per cent of *phosphorus* as phosphoric acid anhydride (P_2O_5), and *potassium* compounds equivalent to 5 per cent of potash. Nitrogen is usually supplied by an organic compound such as ammonium nitrate, sodium nitrates, or ammonium sulfate or ammonium phosphate. Phosphorus is usually present in the form of animal bone meal, superphosphate, or potassium phosphate. Potassium is usually provided in the form of potash.

Pediatric ingestion of fertilizers that contain *only* these three elements usually causes no symptoms other than vomiting or diarrhea. It is possible that the nitrate present in these compounds may produce methemoglobinemia, particularly in children under the age of 1 year. A few products presently on the market may also contain calcium cyanamides, borates, herbicides and insecticides, or other additives that in themselves may prove toxic. Other chemicals such as ammonia may be used as fertilizer.[3] Specific management for these additive or other chemicals may be indicated, as well as supportive therapy.

Hydrogen Peroxide

Hydrogen peroxide is commercially available as a 3 per cent solution. It is a popular home antiseptic. Pediatric ingestions are common but are generally of low toxicity, as hydrogen peroxide rapidly decomposes to water and oxygen in the gastrointestinal tract prior to absorption. Since 1 ml of 3 per cent hydrogen peroxide liberates 10 ml of oxygen,[7] ingestion of large quantities of hydrogen peroxide may cause gastric distention.

Oral ingestion of industrial strength hydrogen peroxide (30 to 40 per cent) has been associated with three fatalities.[8–10] Recently reported was a patient who suffered seizures, metabolic acidosis, diffuse hemorrhage and edema of the stomach, and respiratory arrest but survived with aggressive airway and ventilatory management and general supportive care.[11]

Hypoglycemic Agents

Both accidental and intentional overdoses of insulin and the oral hypoglycemic agents are seen in patients, particularly those undergoing treatment for diabetes mellitus, and the reader is referred to standard textbooks in emergency medicine[12] and internal medicine[13] for a thorough discussion of this subject. In addition, multiple agents have been implicated in producing hypoglycemia, the more common being ethanol, salicylates, and propranolol. As hypoglycemia is a common cause of coma in an emergency department, a brief discussion follows.

Insulin. Unintentional overdose or therapeutic use of insulin with inadequate food intake is the most common cause of hypoglycemia[12] presenting to an emergency department. Deliberate overdoses relating to the use of insulin generally involve the use of the long-acting insulins. Insulin has also been implicated in cases of attempted and successful homicides.

Oral Hypoglycemic Agents. Since the biguanide phenformin was removed from the American market in 1977 because of its association with lactic acidosis, the sulfonylureas are the only group of oral hypoglycemic agents presently prescribed for the treatment of adult-onset diabetes mellitus. The sulfonylureas presently in use in the United States include tolbutamide (Orinase), chlorpropamide (Diabinese), acetohexamide (Dymelor), tolazamide (Tolinase), and the "second-generation" sulfonylureas[14–16] glipizide (Glucutrol) and glyburide (Micronase, Diabeta). The sulfonylureas act by stimulation of pancreatic secretion of insulin. Individual variation exists among the different agents with respect to hepatic metabolism and renal clearance. Glyburide and glipizide are effective in smaller doses but otherwise differ little from the traditional sulfonylureas in their overall effect. Of these agents, chlorpropamide has the longest serum half-life (up to 38 hours) and consequently has the longest duration of action. Chlorpropamide is the drug most commonly reported in accidental and suicidal hypoglycemia to date.[17, 18] *Hypoglycemia is less common with the sulfonylureas than with insulin, but when it occurs it tends to be severe and prolonged.*

Following the diagnosis of hypoglycemia in the patient in coma or with altered mental status, the treatment is straightforward: administration of glucose to maintain normal serum glucose levels. The usual pitfalls of therapy include insufficient glucose quantities and premature cessation of therapy.[17] Maintenance intravenous therapy with 10 per cent glucose, with repeated boluses of intravenous 50 per cent glucose (or up to 25 per cent glucose in the pediatric age group[19]) may be indicated. Glucocorticoids or glucagon or both occasionally may be indicated.

Prolonged hospitalization may be necessary to insure that a patient remains euglycemic following apparent stabilization. Finally, patient education, and psychiatric intervention in the event of suicidal attempts, may be appropriate.

Licorice

Natural licorice is an extract of the root of *Glycyrrhiza glabra* and contains glycyrrhizinic acid, a compound with well-documented mineralocorticoid activity. The syndrome of pseudoprimary hyperaldosteronism is a known complication of chronic excessive licorice ingestion.[20] This syndrome is rarely reported in the United States, since commercial products usually contain artificial licorice flavoring. In areas of the world such as the Middle East where anise (which has a similar flavor but a different chemical structure) is used for flavoring, this syndrome is not observed. Patients demonstrate the classic features of exogenous mineralocorticoid excess: depressed serum renin and serum aldosterone levels, hypokalemia, hypertension, renal potassium wasting, sodium retention, and metabolic acidosis.[20] Treatment involves withdrawal of the offending agent and potassium supplementation, which usually suffices to correct the problem.

Methocarbamol (Robaxin)

Methocarbamol is commonly used for the relief of discomfort associated with acute, painful musculoskeletal conditions. Although thought to be a muscle relaxant, methocarbamol in fact possesses a central nervous system depressant effect. Commercially marketed as Robaxin, it is available in tablets and in injectable form for intramuscular and intravenous use.

Intravenous Robaxin often produces hypotension, which readily responds to placing the patient in the Trendelenburg position and administering intravenous fluids. An overdose of oral methocarbamol is occasionally seen, either alone or in combination with alcohol or other drugs, and is marked by coma, altered mental status, or other signs of central nervous system depression. Treatment is symptomatic and supportive.

"Pencil Lead"

The "lead" in pencils is not elemental lead at all but rather graphite, which is biologically inert. This is a common cause of emergency department visits, especially of children who have been stabbed accidentally by sitting on a pencil, or stabbed intentionally by a schoolmate. When informed that the pencil is in fact harmless, parents still insist often that the pencil point be removed for cosmetic reasons. Depending on multiple factors, I may or may not remove the pencil point, but I always try to please the patient and the family—if possible.

Phosphate Compounds

Sodium phosphate compounds are frequently used as osmotic laxatives. Fleet's enema and the oral preparation Phospho-Soda are common commercial preparations utilizing a combination of sodium biphosphate and sodium monophosphate. Hyperphosphatemia, hyperosmolar dehydration, hypocalcemia and tetany, metabolic acidosis, shock, and death have been reported[21–25] following the absorption of inorganic phosphates from enemas in both adults and children, especially those with Hirschsprung's disease, and in patients with chronic renal failure.

The administration of intravenous saline, and parenteral calcium in the event of hypocalcemic tetany, and use of general supportive measures may be indicated in the event of toxicity.

Podophyllum

Podophyllum resin is extracted from the dried rhizome of *Podophyllum peltatum* (mandrake or May apple). It contains numerous lignins and flavonols, including podophyllotoxin and alpha- and beta-peltatins. Podophyllum resin is a powerful cytotoxin, which arrests cell mitosis.

The usual treatment for venereal warts or condyloma acuminatum involves the use of topical podophyllum. Podophyllum is usually administered in a 20 per cent podophyllum solution in tincture of benzoin, which is applied locally to the venereal lesions. The patient is instructed to wash off the medication after a varying period of time.

A significant number of case reports[26–30] describe significant neurologic, hematologic, hepatic, and renal sequelae and death following the application of podophyllum. These are generally related to the generous use of podophyllum for multiple and widespread lesions.

Podophyllum is an extremely toxic agent that is a violent purgative and acts as a mitotic poison when applied locally. At the same time, it is medically useful, and podophyllum, 20 per cent in tincture of benzoin, is still in use for *isolated* venereal warts. Its use is contraindicated in pregnancy.

Thermometers

Physicians often receive frantic calls from parents because their child has broken off the end of a thermometer and swallowed the glass and mercury contents. Reassure the parent that the ingestion of the free metal from a broken thermometer is normally harmless, since mercury in the free state is not absorbed from the gastrointestinal tract (see Chapter 56, Mercury, for further discussion). As long as the child has not sustained lacerations, has no superficially imbedded glass in the oropharynx, and has no trouble breathing or swallowing, the ingested glass should not pose a problem, and observation is all that is usually indicated.

Outdoor thermometers usually contain less than 1 ml of xylene, toluene, alcohol, or other chemicals and thus generally do not pose a problem.

Acknowledgements

I wish to thank Donna Flake, librarian at Memorial Medical Center, Savannah, and Geri Charlesworth, R.N., at Beaufort Memorial Hospital, for their research efforts; Carol Young, Michelle DeLong, Jennie Williams, and Joyce Davidson for their secretarial help; my two daughters, Elizabeth Anne and Madeleine Haddad, for their assistance in proofreading; and my son Daniel Haddad for helping plan the new book cover.

References

1. Arena JM: Poisoning: Toxicology, Symptoms, Treatment. 4th ed. Springfield, IL, Charles C Thomas, 1979.

2. Gosselin RE, Hodge HC, Smith RP, Gleason MN: Clinical Toxicology of Commercial Products. 4th ed. Baltimore, Williams & Wilkins, 1976.
3. Rumack BH: POISINDEX. Denver, Micromedex, 1989.
4. Presto AJ, Muecke EC: A dose of Spanish fly. JAMA *214*:591, 1970.
5. Yellowlees P, Greenfield C, McIntyre N: Dimethyl sulfoxide–induced toxicity. Lancet *1*:1004, 1980.
6. Veltri JC, Temple AR: Fenfluramine poisoning. J Pediatr *87*:119, 1975.
7. Reynolds JEF: The Extra Pharmacopeia. 28th ed. London, Pharmaceutical Press, 1982, p 1232.
8. Jozwik T, Molenda R: A case of poisoning with hydrogen peroxide. Pol Tyg Lek *23*:1606, 1968.
9. Giusti GV: Fatal poisoning with hydrogen peroxide. Forensic Sci Int *2*:99, 1973.
10. Zecevic D, Gasparec Z: Death caused by hydrogen peroxide. Z Rechtsmed *84*:57, 1979.
11. Giberson TP, Kern JD, Pettigrew DW, Eaves CC, Haynes JF: Near-fatal hydrogen peroxide ingestion. Ann Emerg Med *18*:778, 1989.
12. Tintinalli JE, Rothstein RJ, Krome RL: Emergency Medicine—A Comprehensive Study Guide. New York, McGraw-Hill, 1985.
13. Braunwald E, Isselbacher KJ, Petersdorf RG, Wilson JD, Martin JB, Fauci AS: Harrison's Principles of Internal Medicine. 11th ed. New York, McGraw-Hill, 1987.
14. Lebovitz HE, Reaven GM: Proceedings of a Symposium: New perspectives in noninsulin-dependent diabetes mellitus and the role of glipizide in its treatment. Am J Med *75*:58, 1983.
15. Prendergast BD: Glyburide and glipizide—second-generation oral sulfonylurea hypoglycemic agents. Clin Pharmacol *31*:473, 1984.
16. Glyburide and glipizide. Med Let *26*:79, 1984.
17. Bobzien WF: Suicidal overdoses with hypoglycemic agents. J Am Coll Emerg Phys *8*:467, 1979.
18. Ludman B, Mason P, Joplin GF: Dangerous misuse of sulfonylureas. *293*:1287, 1986.
19. Chameides L (ed): Pediatric Advanced Life Support. Dallas, TX, American Heart Association, 1988.
20. Blachley JD, Knochel JP: Tobacco chewer's hypokalemia: Licorice revisited. N Engl J Med *302*:784, 1980.
21. Wason S, Tiller T: Severe hyperphosphatemia, hypocalcemia, acidosis, and shock in a 5-month-old child following the administration of an adult Fleet enema. Ann Emerg Med *18*:696, 1989.
22. Geffner ME, Opas LM: Phosphate poisoning complicating treatment of iron ingestion. Am J Dis Child *134*:509, 1980.
23. Oxnard SC, O'Bell J, Grupe WE: Severe tetany in an azotemic child related to a sodium phosphate enema. Pediatrics *53*:105, 1974.
24. Chesney RW, Haughton PB: Tetany following phosphate enemas in chronic renal disease. Am J Dis Child *127*:585, 1974.
25. Loughan P: Brain damage following a hypertonic phosphate enema. Am J Dis Child *131*:1032, 1977.
26. Ward JW, Clifford WS, Monaco AR, Bickerstaff HJ: Fatal poisoning following podophyllum treatment of condyloma acuminatum. South Med J *47*:1204, 1974.
27. Clark ANG, Parsonage MJ: A case of podophyllum poisoning with involvement of the central nervous system. Br Med J *2*:115, 1957.
28. Chamberlain MJ, Reynolds AL, Yeoman WB: Toxic effect of podophyllum application in pregnancy. Br J Med *3*:391, 1972.
29. Baluciani M, Zellers DD: Podophyllum resin poisoning with complete recovery. JAMA *189*:639, 1964.
30. Montaldi DH, Giambrone JR, Courey JP, Taefi P: Podophyllum poisoning associated with the treatment of condyloma acuminatum: A case report. Am J Obstet Gynecol *119*:1130, 1974.

APPENDIX

CHEMICAL CONVERSIONS OF TOXICOLOGIC LABORATORY VALUES

Thomas S. Herman, Ph.D.

THE INTERNATIONAL SYSTEM OF UNITS

Laboratory values today are expressed in the United States in traditional units—for example, mg/dl.

In 1960, the Eleventh General Conference on Weights and Measures (CGPM) established the International System of Units (SI, or Système Internationale)[1-4] as a practical system of units of measurement. The SI System is the laboratory standard in Europe, the Commonwealth countries, and others. An example of international units is moles/liter.

In the United States, the National Committee for Clinical Laboratory Standards (NCCLS) has recommended phasing in most SI units in reporting clinical laboratory data.[4] Many American medical and scientific journals require the reporting of both traditional and SI units. Thus, until the SI system is universally accepted, practitioners should be conversant with two measurement systems.

Several aids for the interconversion of traditional and SI units commonly encountered in toxicology are given here. The conversion aids are designed for traditional units reported as or converted to metric mass per volume and require the relative molecular or atomic mass (M_r) of the compound/element of interest. The M_r of many toxicologic compounds is listed in Table 2.

To Convert American (Traditional) Units to SI Units

1. Determine the factor from Table 1 by matching the desired SI unit column with the traditional unit row.
2. Determine the relative molecular or atomic mass (M_r) of the particular compound/element in Table 2.
3. SI unit = traditional unit ÷ (M_r × factor)
   Example: Convert 1.5 μg/L of digoxin to nmol/L:
   SI unit = 1.5 μg/L ÷ (781 × 10^{-3}) = 1.92 nmol/L

To Convert SI Units to Traditional Units

1. Determine the factor from Table 1 by matching the desired traditional unit row and SI unit column.
2. Determine the relative molecular or atomic mass (M_r) of the compound/element in Table 2.
3. Traditional unit = SI unit × (M_r × factor)
   Example: Convert 80 μmol/L of phenytoin to mg/dl:
   Traditional unit = 80 μmol/L × (252 × 10^{-4}) = 2 mg/dl

[1]Doumas BT: IFCC documents and interpretation of SI units—A solution looking for a problem. Clin Chem *25*:655, 1979.

[2]Lines JG: SI units: Another view. Clin Chem *25*:1331, 1979.

[3]Page CH, Vigouraux P (eds): The International System of Units (SI). NBS Special Publication 330, US Government Printing Office, Washington, DC, 1974.

[4]Quantities and Units: SI. NCCLS Proposed Position Paper: PCP-11. National Committee for Clinical Laboratory Standards, Villanova, PA, 1979.

Table 1 FACTORS FOR INTERCONVERSION OF SI UNITS AND TRADITIONAL UNITS

TRADITIONAL UNITS	SI UNITS nmol/L	μmol/L	mmol/L	mol/L
pg/ml	1	10^{3}	10^{6}	10^{9}
pg/dl	10^{2}	10^{5}	10^{8}	10^{11}
pg/L	10^{3}	10^{6}	10^{9}	10^{12}
ng/ml	10^{-3}	1	10^{3}	10^{6}
ng/dl	10^{-1}	10^{2}	10^{5}	10^{8}
ng/L	1	10^{3}	10^{6}	10^{9}
μg/ml	10^{-6}	10^{-3}	1	10^{3}
μg/dl	10^{-4}	10^{-1}	10^{2}	10^{5}
μg/L	10^{-3}	1	10^{3}	10^{6}
mg/ml	10^{-9}	10^{-6}	10^{-3}	1
mg/dl	10^{-7}	10^{-4}	10^{-1}	10^{2}
mg/L	10^{-6}	10^{-3}	1	10^{3}
g/ml	10^{-12}	10^{-9}	10^{-6}	10^{-3}
g/dl	10^{-10}	10^{-7}	10^{-4}	10^{-1}
g/L	10^{-9}	10^{-6}	10^{-3}	1

Table 2 THE RELATIVE MOLECULAR MASS (M_r) OF SELECTED PRODUCTS[1-6]

PRODUCT	TRADE NAME	M_r
acetaminophen	Tylenol	151.16
acetone		58.08
aluminum		26.98
amitriptyline	Elavil	277.41
ammonia		17.03
amphetamine	Benzedrine	135.21
amyl nitrate		117.15
aniline		93.12
arsenic		74.92
borate		58.83
bromide		79.90
butabarbital	Butisol	211.25
butalbital	Fiorinal	224.26
caffeine		194.19
carbamazepine	Tegretol	236.26
carbaryl	Sevin	201.22
carbon monoxide		28.01
carbromal	Carbrital	237.11
carisoprodol	Soma	260.33
chloral hydrate	Noctec	165.40
chloramphenicol		323.14
chlordiazepoxide	Librium	299.76
chlorpromazine	Thorazine	318.86
chlorpropamide	Diabinese	276.74
chlorazepate	Tranxene	313.72
cocaine		303.35
codeine		299.36
cyanide		26.03
desipramine	Norpramin	266.39
diazepam	Valium	284.75
diazinon		304.36
digitoxin		764.96
digoxin		780.95
diphenhydramine	Benadryl	255.37
disopyramide	Norpace	339.47
doxepin	Sinequan	279.39
ethanol		46.07
ethchlorvynol	Placidyl	144.60
ethinamate	Valmid	167.21
ethosuximide	Zarontin	141.17
ethylene glycol		62.07
fluoride		18.99
flurazepam	Dalmane	387.88
formaldehyde		30.03
glutethimide	Doriden	217.27
haloperidol	Haldol	375.87
halothane		197.38
heroin		369.42
hydrogen sulfide		34.08
hydromorphone	Dilaudid	285.33
imipramine	Tofranil	280.40
lidocaine	Xylocaine	234.33
lindane		290.83
lithium		6.94
LSD		323.44
meperidine	Demerol	247.35
meprobamate	Miltown	218.25
methadone	Dolophine	309.45
methanol		32.04
methaqualone	Quaalude	250.29
methocarbamol	Robaxin	241.25
methotrexate		454.44
methsuximide	Celontin	203.24
methyl bromide		94.95
methyprylon	Noludar	183.25
morphine		285.33
nicotine		162.23
nortriptyline	Aventyl	263.37
oxazepam	Serax	286.72
oxycodone	Percodan	315.38
parathion		291.27
PCP	Phencyclidine	243.38
phenobarbital		232.23
phenytoin	Dilantin	252.26
procainamide	Pronestyl	235.33
promethazine	Phenergan	284.42
propoxyphene	Darvon	339.49
propranolol	Inderal	259.34
protriptyline	Vivactil	263.38
salicylate		180.15
secobarbital	Seconal	238.29
theophylline		180.17
thioridazine	Mellaril	370.56
tobramycin	Nebcin	467.52
tolbutamide	Orinase	270.35
toluene		92.13
valproic acid	Depakene	144.21
warfarin	Coumadin	308.32
xylene		106.16
zinc		65.37

NOTE: The molecular mass (M_r) reflects the weight of the principal base, anhydrous compound *only.* Cations such as sodium or anions such as chloride are *not* included. For example, 308.32 is the M_r for warfarin; *not* for warfarin sodium.

[1] The United States Pharmacopeia. 20th rev. US Pharmacopeia Convention, Publishers, Rockville, Md, 1980.

[2] Osol A, Pratt R (eds): The United States Dispensatory. 27th ed. J.B. Lippincott Company, Philadelphia, 1973.

[3] Physicians' Desk Reference. 34th ed. Medical Economics Company, Oradell, NJ, 1980.

[4] The Merck Index. 9th ed. Merck and Company, Rahway, NJ, 1976.

[5] Baselt RC: Analytical Procedures for Therapeutic Drug Monitoring and Emergency Toxicology. Biomedical Publications, Davis, Cal, 1980.

[6] Baselt RC: Biological Monitoring Methods for Industrial Chemicals. Biomedical Publications, Davis, Cal, 1980.

THE METRIC SYSTEM

1 kilogram (kg) = 1000 grams (gm)
1 gram (gm) = 1000 milligrams (mg)
1 milligram (mg) = 1000 micrograms (mcg or μg)
1 microgram (μg or mcg) = 1000 nanograms (ng)

1 nanogram (ng) $= 0.001$ *or* 1×10^{-3} *or* $\frac{1}{1000}$ microgram

$= 0.000001$ *or* 1×10^{-6} *or* $\frac{1}{1,000,000}$ milligram

$= 0.000000001$ *or* 1×10^{-9} *or* $\frac{1}{1,000,000,000}$ gram

1 milliliter (ml) = 1 cc = 1 gram = 15 drops or minims
5 ml ≅ 1 teaspoon
15 ml ≅ 1 tablespoon
30 ml ≅ 1 ounce
100 ml = 1 deciliter (dl)
1000 ml = 1 liter (L) = 1 kilogram (kg)
1 mg % (milligram per cent) = 1 milligram per 100 ml = 1 mg/dl = 1000 mcg/dl or μg/dl = 1,000,000 ng/dl
1 nanogram/ml = 0.001 μg/ml

CALCULATION OF MILLIEQUIVALENTS

1 milliequivalent (mEq) =

$$\frac{\text{the relative atomic mass of a substance in grams}}{\text{valence} \times 1000}$$

Example: How many mEq of sodium are in a 3 gram sodium diet?

1. Determine the atomic mass from the periodic table of the elements. Na = 23
2. Thus, 1 mEq of Na $= \frac{23}{1 \times 1000} = 0.023$ g or 23 mg.
3. Thus, 1 mEq of Na = 23 mg of sodium.
4. Per 3 grams of sodium, there are $\frac{3000 \text{ mg}}{23 \text{ mg}} = 130.4$ mEq of sodium.

OTHER CONVERSIONS

1 grain = 60 mg (occasionally rounded off to 65 mg)
ppm = parts per million = mg/liter
ppb = parts per billion = μg(mcg)/liter

Percentage Expressions

As 0.1% ethanol = 100 mg/100 cc = 0.1 g/dl = 1 g/L = 100 mg/dl = 1 mg/ml
As 10% Mucomyst = 10 grams/100 cc = 10 g/dl = 100 g/L = 10000 mg/dl = 100 mg/ml

Example: Calculation of the Dose of Mucomyst for Acetaminophen Overdose

The initial dose of *N*-acetylcysteine (Mucomyst) for acetaminophen overdose is 140 mg/kg; subsequent doses are 70 mg/kg.

Suppose the patient weighs 132 pounds and your pharmacy has 10% Mucomyst. How much Mucomyst do you give your patient?

1. 1 kilogram = 2.2 pounds   132/2.2 = 60 kilograms
2. 10% Mucomyst means that there is 1 gram of Mucomyst in 10 ml of Mucomyst. The initial dose is 140 mg/kg. Thus the patient should receive 60 × 140 or 8400 mg or 8.4 grams of Mucomyst (*N*-acetylcysteine).

Answer: The patient should receive 84 ml of 10% Mucomyst or 42 ml of 20% Mucomyst.

THE PERIODIC TABLE OF THE ELEMENTS

Ru Ruthenium 44 101.07	
Ru	symbol
Ruthenium	element
44	atomic number
101.07	atomic weight†

Period \ Group	1	2							
1	**H** Hydrogen **1** 1.01								
2	**Li** Lithium **3** 6.94	**Be** Beryllium **4** 9.01							
3	**Na** Sodium **11** 23.00	**Mg** Magnesium **12** 24.31							
4	**K** Potassium **19** 39.10	**Ca** Calcium **20** 40.08	**Sc** Scandium **21** 44.96	**Ti** Titanium **22** 47.90	**V** Vanadium **23** 50.94	**Cr** Chromium **24** 52.00	**Mn** Manganese **25** 54.94	**Fe** Iron **26** 55.85	**Co** Cobalt **27** 58.93
5	**Rb** Rubidium **37** 85.47	**Sr** Strontium **38** 87.62	**Y** Yttrium **39** 88.91	**Zr** Zirconium **40** 91.22	**Nb** Niobium **41** 92.91	**Mo** Molybdenum **42** 95.94	**Tc*** Technetium **43** 98.91	**Ru** Ruthenium **44** 101.07	**Rh** Rhodium **45** 102.91
6	**Cs** Cesium **55** 132.91	**Ba** Barium **56** 137.34	**La** Lanthanum **57** 138.91	**Hf** Hafnium **72** 178.49	**Ta** Tantalum **73** 180.95	**W** Tungsten **74** 183.85	**Re** Rhenium **75** 186.2	**Os** Osmium **76** 190.2	**Ir** Iridium **77** 192.22
7	**Fr*** Francium **87** (223)	**Ra*** Radium **88** 226.02	**Ac*** Actinium **89** (227)	**Rf*** Rutherfordium **104** (260)	**Ha*** Hahnium **105** (262)				

Lanthanide series	**Ce** Cerium **58** 140.12	**Pr** Praeseodymium **59** 140.91	**Nd** Neodymium **60** 144.24	**Pm*** Promethium **61** (145)	**Sm** Samarium **62** 150.4
Actinide series	**Th*** Thorium **90** 232.04	**Pa*** Protactinium **91** 231.04	**U*** Uranium **92** 238.03	**Np*** Neptunium **93** 237.05	**Pu*** Plutonium **94** (244)

* All isotopes are radioactive.
( ) Indicates mass number of longest known half-life.
† All atomic weights have been rounded to .01.

THE PERIODIC TABLE OF THE ELEMENTS *(Continued)*

In each A group, the number of electrons (#e⁻)
in the outer shell of each element is the same.

In each period, the identifying number (*n*)
for the outer shell of each element is the same.

			3	4	5	6	7	8
								He Helium **2** 4.00
			B Boron **5** 10.81	**C** Carbon **6** 12.01	**N** Nitrogen **7** 14.01	**O** Oxygen **8** 16.00	**F** Fluorine **9** 19.00	**Ne** Neon **10** 20.18
			Al Aluminium **13** 26.98	**Si** Silicon **14** 28.09	**P** Phosphorus **15** 30.97	**S** Sulfur **16** 32.06	**Cl** Chlorine **17** 35.45	**Ar** Argon **18** 39.95
Ni Nickel **28** 58.71	**Cu** Copper **29** 63.55	**Zn** Zinc **30** 65.37	**Ga** Gallium **31** 69.72	**Ge** Germanium **32** 72.59	**As** Arsenic **33** 74.92	**Se** Selenium **34** 78.96	**Br** Bromine **35** 79.90	**Kr** Krypton **36** 83.8
Pd Palladium **46** 106.4	**Ag** Silver **47** 107.87	**Cd** Cadmium **48** 112.40	**In** Indium **49** 114.82	**Sn** Tin **50** 118.69	**Sb** Antimony **51** 121.75	**Te** Tellurium **52** 127.60	**I** Iodine **53** 126.90	**Xe** Xenon **54** 131.30
Pt Platinum **78** 195.09	**Au** Gold **79** 196.97	**Hg** Mercury **80** 200.59	**Tl** Thallium **81** 204.37	**Pb** Lead **82** 207.2	**Bi** Bismuth **83** 208.98	**Po*** Polonium **84** (210)	**At*** Astatine **85** (210)	**Rn*** Radon **86** (222)

Eu Europium **63** 151.96	**Gd** Gadolinium **64** 157.25	**Tb** Terbium **65** 158.93	**Dy** Dysprosium **66** 162.50	**Ho** Holmium **67** 164.93	**Er** Erbium **68** 167.26	**Tm** Thulium **69** 168.93	**Yb** Ytterbium **70** 173.04	**Lu** Lutetium **71** 174.97
Am* Americium **95** (243)	**Cm*** Curium **96** (247)	**Bk*** Berkelium **97** (247)	**Cf*** Californium **98** (251)	**Es*** Einsteinium **99** (254)	**Fm*** Fermium **100** (257)	**Md*** Mendelevium **101** (257)	**No*** Nobelium **102** (255)	**Lr*** Lawrencium **103** (256)

(From Berlow PB, Burton DJ, Routh JI: Introduction to the Chemistry of Life. Saunders College Publishing, Philadelphia, 1982.)

INDEX

Note: Page numbers in *italics* refer to figures; page numbers followed by t refer to tables.